Facial Plastic and Reconstructive Surgery

Third Edition

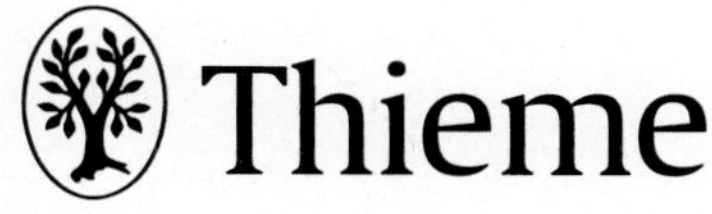

Facial Plastic and Reconstructive Surgery

Third Edition

Ira D. Papel, MD
Associate Professor of Otolaryngology–
Head and Neck Surgery
Division of Facial Plastic Surgery
Department of Otolaryngology–Head and Neck Surgery
The Johns Hopkins University School of Medicine
Facial Plastic Surgicenter
Baltimore, Maryland

John L. Frodel, MD
Director of Facial Plastic and Reconstructive Surgery
Department of Otolaryngology–Head and Neck Surgery
Geisinger Medical Center
Danville, Pennsylvania
Private Practice
Marietta, Georgia

G. Richard Holt, MD, MSE, MPH, MABE
Professor and Program Director
Department of Otolaryngology–Head and Neck Surgery
The University of Texas Health Science Center at San Antonio
San Antonio, Texas

Wayne F. Larrabee Jr., MD
Clinical Professor of Otolaryngology–Head and Neck Surgery
Department of Otolaryngology–Head and Neck Surgery
University of Washington
Seattle, Washington

Nathan E. Nachlas, MD
Private Practice
Boca Raton, Florida

Stephen S. Park, MD
Professor and Vice-Chair
Division Chair of Facial Plastic and Reconstructive Surgery
Department of Otolaryngology–
Head and Neck Surgery
The University of Virginia
Charlottesville, Virginia

Jonathan M. Sykes, MD
Professor of Otolaryngology–Head and Neck Surgery
Department of Otolaryngology–Head and Neck Surgery
University of California Davis Medical Center
Director, Facial Plastic and Reconstructive Surgery
Sacramento, California

Dean M. Toriumi, MD
Professor of Otolaryngology–
Head and Neck Surgery
Division of Facial Plastic and Reconstructive Surgery
Department of Otolaryngology
University of Illinois at Chicago
Chicago, Illinois

Thieme
New York · Stuttgart

Thieme Medical Publishers, Inc.
333 Seventh Ave.
New York, NY 10001

Consulting Medical Editor: Esther Gumpert
Managing Editor: J. Owen Zurhellen
Editorial Assistants: Judith Tomat and Jacquelyn DeSanti
Vice President, Production and Electronic Publishing: Anne T. Vinnicombe
Production Editor: Heidi Pongratz, Maryland Composition
Vice President, International Marketing and Sales: Cornelia Schulze
Chief Financial Officer: Peter van Woerden
President: Brian D. Scanlan
Compositor: Thomson Digital
Printer: Everbest Printing Co.
Cover image: Réunion des Musées Nationaux/Art Resource, NY

Library of Congress Cataloging-in-Publication Data

Facial plastic and reconstructive surgery / [edited by] Ira D. Papel. – 3rd ed.
p. ; cm.
Includes bibliographical references and index.
ISBN 978-1-58890-515-4
1. Face–Surgery. 2. Surgery, Plastic. I. Papel, Ira D.
[DNLM: 1. Face–surgery. 2. Cosmetic Techniques. 3. Esthetics. 4. Neck–surgery.
5. Reconstructive Surgical Procedures–methods. WE 705 F141 2008]
RD119.5.F33F32 2008
617.5'20592–dc22

2008025283

Important note: Medical knowledge is ever-changing. As new research and clinical experience broaden our knowledge, changes in treatment and drug therapy may be required. The authors and editors of the material herein have consulted sources believed to be reliable in their efforts to provide information that is complete and in accord with the standards accepted at the time of publication. However, in view of the possibility of human error by the authors, editors, or publisher of the work herein or changes in medical knowledge, neither the authors, editors, nor publisher, nor any other party who has been involved in the preparation of this work, warrants that the information contained herein is in every respect accurate or complete, and they are not responsible for any errors or omissions or for the results obtained from use of such information. Readers are encouraged to confirm the information contained herein with other sources. For example, readers are advised to check the product information sheet included in the package of each drug they plan to administer to be certain that the information contained in this publication is accurate and that changes have not been made in the recommended dose or in the contraindications for administration. This recommendation is of particular importance in connection with new or infrequently used drugs.

Printed in China

5 4 3 2 1

ISBN 978-1-58890-515-4

Contents

Foreword

I am pleased and flattered to have been asked to write this foreword for the new third edition of *Facial Plastic and Reconstructive Surgery* by my friend Ira D. Papel. I have had the pleasure of working with Ira for over a decade, following him as the AAFPRS President, ABFPRS Secretary, and ABFPRS Treasurer, and now working with him at the *Archives of Facial Plastic Surgery*. This book reflects his personality—thorough, focused, and a great resource. Our field had long needed a concise, yet comprehensive text. This is that text. The bestselling prior editions of this book have been our residents' favorite facial plastic and reconstructive resource. The AAFPRS Fellows have told me that this is the single best text that they use during their training and in preparation for the Fellowship Exam. It is well written and provides coverage of the breadth of facial plastic and reconstructive surgery with insights from experienced surgeons. Another book like it cannot be found.

Enjoy this book and, as you read it, also be pleased that all the royalties will be used to support the Foundation of the American Academy of Facial Plastic and Reconstructive Surgery.

Peter A. Hilger, MD
University of Minnesota

Preface

Facial plastic and reconstructive surgery is a dynamic specialty, offering surgeons a constant stream of clinical challenges. At an ever-increasing rate, technology and surgical innovations have provided an expanding choice of treatment options, often of unknown efficacy. This new third edition of *Facial Plastic and Reconstructive Surgery* provides updated information on the wide variety of facial plastic surgery procedures and treatments. The contributing authors have updated most chapters, and created new ones where needed, focused on both cosmetic and reconstructive problems. The book chapters continue to be constructed according to the successful formula of those in previous editions—they provide core information in the subject area, backed by appropriate basic science, clinical details, and references. Readers are then prepared to pursue more detailed research into clinical or surgical care.

New areas covered in this edition include anti-aging medicine, ambulatory surgery considerations, autologous fat augmentation, pediatric rhinoplasty, tissue engineering, and nonablative skin resurfacing techniques.

I would like to thank the contributing editors and authors for their continuous support of this project, whose first edition was published in 1992. As with past editions, all royalties generated by *Facial Plastic and Reconstructive Surgery*, third edition, will be donated to the Education and Research Foundation of the American Academy of Facial Plastic and Reconstructive Surgery, so that education in facial plastic surgery can be supported in perpetuity.

Acknowledgments

This project would not have been possible without the help and support of Thieme Publishers in New York. Special thanks to Esther Gumpert, Judith Tomat, and J. Owen Zurhellen IV at Thieme for ensuring that the third edition stayed on track throughout the editorial and production process. I thank Dr. Natarajan Balaji of Glasgow, Scotland, for his thorough review of this book's draft manuscript.

Contributors

Peter A. Adamson, MD, FRCSC, FACS
Professor of Otolaryngology–Head and Neck Surgery
Department of Otolaryngology–Head and Neck Surgery
Toronto General Hospital
Toronto, Ontario, Canada

Donald J. Annino Jr., DMD, MD
Assistant Professor of Otolaryngology–Head and Neck Surgery
Department of Otolaryngology–Head and Neck Surgery
Tufts University, New England Medical Center
Boston, Massachusetts

Babak Azizzadeh, MD, FACS
Assistant Clinical Professor of Surgery
Division of Head and Neck Surgery
David Geffen School of Medicine at UCLA
Los Angeles, California

Shan R. Baker, MD
Professor of Otolaryngology
Department of Otolaryngology
University of Michigan
Livonia, Michigan

Daniel G. Becker, MD
Clinical Associate Professor of Otolaryngology–Head and Neck Surgery
Department of Otolaryngology–Head and Neck Surgery
Universities of Pennsylvania and Virginia
Sewell, New Jersey

William H. Beeson, MD
Clinical Professor of Dermatology and Otolaryngology–Head and Neck Surgery
Departments of Dermatology and Otolaryngology–Head and Neck Surgery
Indiana University School of Medicine
Indianapolis, Indiana

Richard Bennett, MD
Clinical Professor of Medicine
Dermatology Division
University of California Los Angeles
Santa Monica, California

William J. Binder, MD, FACS
Assistant Clinical Professor of Facial Plastic and Reconstructive Surgery
Division of Head and Neck Surgery
David Geffen School of Medicine at UCLA
Attending Surgeon
Audrey-Kenis Skirball Center for Plastic and Reconstructive Surgery
Cedars-Sinai Medical Center
Los Angeles, California

Andrew Blitzer, MD, DDS
Professor of Clinical Otolaryngology
Department of Otolaryngology
Columbia University College of Physicians and Surgeons
New York, New York

Kofi D. O. Boahene, MD
Assistant Professor of Facial Plastic Surgery
Department of Otolaryngology–Head and Neck Surgery
The Johns Hopkins University School of Medicine
Baltimore, Maryland

Daniel Buchbinder, MD
Professor of Oral, Maxillo-Facial Surgery, and Otolaryngology
Chief, Division of Oral and Maxillo-Facial Surgery
Director, Oral, Maxillo-Facial Surgery Residency Training Program
Mt. Sinai School of Medicine
New York, New York

Alan J. C. Burke, MD
Private Practice
Medical Director, Ageless Remedies–
Medical Skincare and Apothecary
Richmond, Virginia

Brian B. Burkey, MD
Associate Professor of Otolaryngology
Department of Otolaryngology
Vanderbilt University Medical Center
Nashville, Tennessee

Patrick J. Byrne, MD
Associate Professor of Otolaryngology–
Head and Neck Surgery
Department of Otolaryngology–Head and Neck Surgery
Director of Facial Plastic and Reconstructive Surgery
The Johns Hopkins University School of Medicine
Baltimore, Maryland

Randolph B. Capone, MD, MS
Assistant Professor of Otolaryngology–
Head and Neck Surgery
Department of Otolaryngology–Head and Neck Surgery
The Johns Hopkins University School of Medicine
Director, The Baltimore Center for Facial Plastic Surgery
Co-Director, Greater Baltimore Cleft Lip and Palate Team
Baltimore, Maryland

Paul J. Carniol, MD, FACS
Clinical Associate Professor of Otolaryngology–
Head and Neck Surgery
Department of Otolaryngology–Head and Neck Surgery
University of Medicine and Dentistry of New Jersey
Newark, New Jersey

Benjamin S. Carson Sr., MD
Professor of Neurological Surgery
Director of Pediatric Neurosurgery
Department of Neurological Surgery
The Johns Hopkins University School of Medicine
Baltimore, Maryland

Richard D. Castellano, MD
Private Practice
Facial Plastic Surgery
Tampa, Florida

Donn R. Chatham, MD
Private Practice
Facial Plastic and Reconstructive Surgery
New Albany, Indiana

J. Madison Clark, MD
Private Practice
Alamance ENT and Facial Plastic Surgery
Burlington, North Carolina

John R. Coleman Jr., MD
Private Practice
Atlanta Center for Facial Plastic Surgery
Atlanta, Georgia

Ted A. Cook, MD, FACS
Professor of Otolaryngology–Head and Neck Surgery
Department of Otolaryngology–Head and Neck Surgery
Oregon Health and Science University
Portland, Oregon

Peter D. Costantino, MD
Associate Professor of Clinical Otolaryngology–
Head and Neck Surgery
Director of Cranial Base Surgery
Vice-Chairman, Department of Otolaryngology–
Head and Neck Surgery
St. Luke's-Roosevelt Medical Center
New York, New York

Roger L. Crumley, MD, MBA
Professor and Chairman of Otolaryngology–
Head and Neck Surgery
Department of Otolaryngology–Head and Neck Surgery
UCIrvine Medical Center
Orange, California

Robert J. DeFatta, MD, PhD
Clinical Professor of Surgery
Division of Otolaryngology
Department of Surgery
Albany Medical College
Albany, New York
Private Practice
Williams Center for Facial Plastic Surgery Specialists
Latham, New York

Timothy D. Doerr, MD, FACS
Associate Professor and Program Director
Department of Otolaryngology–Head and Neck Surgery
University of Rochester School of Medicine and Dentistry
Rochester, New York

Kristin K. Egan, MD
Chief Resident
Department of Otolaryngology
University of California San Francisco
San Francisco, California

Jami Eidem, MD
Resident Physician
Department of Anesthesiology
McGaw Medical Center
Chicago, Illinois

David W. Eisele, MD, FACS
Professor and Chairman of Otolaryngology–Head and Neck Surgery
Department of Otolaryngology–Head and Neck Surgery
University of California
San Francisco, California

George W. Facer, MD
Department of Otolaryngology
Mayo Clinic
Scottsdale, Arizona

Edmund Fisher, MD
Private Practice
Fisher Cosmetic Facial Surgery
Bakersfield, California

Mark V. Fletcher, MD
Director of Anesthesia
Department of Anesthesia
Meridian Plastic Surgery Center
Indianapolis, Indiana

Hossam M. T. Foda, MD
Private Practice
Facial Plastic Surgery Associates
Houston, Texas

Craig D. Friedman, MD, FACS
Visiting Surgeon
Department of Surgery/Otolaryngology
Yale New Haven Hospital
New Haven, Connecticut

Oren Friedman, MD
Assistant Professor of Otorhinolaryngology and Facial Plastic Surgery
Department of Otorhinolaryngology and Facial Plastic Surgery
Mayo Clinic
Rochester Methodist Hospital
Rochester, Minnesota

John L. Frodel, MD
Director of Facial Plastic and Reconstructive Surgery
Department of Otolaryngology–Head and Neck Surgery
Geisinger Medical Center
Danville, Pennsylvania
Private Practice
Marietta, Georgia

Jaime R. Garza, DDS, MD
Clinical Professor of Plastic Surgery
Clinical Professor of Otolaryngology–Head and Neck Surgery
University of Texas Health Science Center at San Antonio
San Antonio, Texas

Holger G. Gassner, MD
Staff Consultant
Department of Otorhinolaryngology
University of Regensburg
Regensburg, Germany

Eric M. Genden, MD, FACS
Professor and Chairman of Otolaryngology–Head and Neck Surgery
Department of Otolaryngology–Head and Neck Surgery
Director, Head and Neck Cancer Center
Mount Sinai Medical Center
New York, New York

Mark J. Glasgold, MD
Clinical Associate Professor of Surgery
Department of Surgery
Robert Wood Johnson University Hospital
University of Medicine and Dentistry of New Jersey
Piscataway, New Jersey

Robert A. Glasgold, MD
Clinical Assistant Professor of Surgery
Department of Surgery
Robert Wood Johnson University Hospital
University of Medicine and Dentistry of New Jersey
Piscataway, New Jersey

George S. Goding Jr., MD
Associate Professor of Otolaryngology–Head and Neck Surgery
Department of Otolaryngology–Head and Neck Surgery
University of Minnesota, Twin Cities
Attending Staff
Hennepin County Medical Center
University of Minnesota Hospitals and Clinics
Minneapolis, Minnesota

Daniel R. Gold, MD
Department of Otolaryngology
Tufts University
New England Medical Center
Boston, Massachusetts

H. Devon Graham III, MD, FACS
Clinical Assistant Professor of Otolaryngology–Head and Neck Surgery
Department of Otolaryngology–Head and Neck Surgery
Tulane University School of Medicine
Ochsner Health Systems
New Orleans, Louisiana

Steven D. Gray, MD†
Professor of Otolaryngology–Head and Neck Surgery
Department of Surgery
University of Utah School of Medicine
Salt Lake City, Utah

Michael Guarnieri, PhD
Emeritus Faculty, Senior Staff
Department of Neurological Surgery
The Johns Hopkins University School of Medicine
Baltimore, Maryland

Robert A. Guida, MD, PC
Private Practice
New York Plastic Surgery
New York, New York

Mark M. Hamilton, MD
Clinical Assistant Professor of Otolaryngology–Head and Neck Surgery
Department of Otolaryngology–Head and Neck Surgery
Indiana University School of Medicine
Indianapolis, Indiana

Matthew M. Hanasono, MD
Assistant Professor of Plastic Surgery
Department of Plastic Surgery, The University of Texas
MD Anderson Cancer Center
Houston, Texas

Christopher B. Harmon, MD
Clinical Instructor of Dermatology
Department of Dermatology
University of Alabama, Birmingham, Alabama

David A. Hecht, MD, PC
Private Practice
Facial Plastic Surgery
Scottsdale, Arizona

John D. Hendrix Jr., MD
Private Practice
Charlottesville, Virginia

†deceased

Peter A. Hilger, MD
Private Practice
Facial Plastic and Reconstructive Surgery Specialists
Edina, Minnesota

John F. Hoffmann, MD
Private Practice
Spokane Center for Facial Plastic Surgery
Spokane, Washington

G. Richard Holt, MD, MSE, MPH, MABE
Professor and Program Director
Department of Otolaryngology–Head and Neck Surgery
The University of Texas Health Science Center at San Antonio
San Antonio, Texas

David B. Hom, MD, FACS
Professor of Otolaryngology–Head and Neck Surgery
Department of Otolaryngology–Head and Neck Surgery
Director, Division of Facial Plastic and Reconstructive Surgery
University of Cincinnati College of Medicine
Cincinnati Children's Hospital Medical Center
Cincinnati, Ohio

Lisa E. Ishii, MD
Assistant Professor of Facial Plastic Surgery
Department of Otolaryngology–Head and Neck Surgery
The Johns Hopkins University School of Medicine
Baltimore, Maryland

Yong Ju Jang, MD
Associate Professor of Otolaryngology
Department of Otolaryngology
Asan Medical Center
University of Ulsan College of Medicine
Seoul, Korea

Albert Jen, MD
Clinical Assistant Professor of Otolaryngology
Department of Otolaryngology
Columbia University College of Physicians and Surgeons
New York, New York

Sara A. Kaltreider, MD
Private Practice
Oculoplastics and Orbital Consultants, PLC
Charlottesville, Virginia

Amir M. Karam, MD
Clinical Instructor of Otolaryngology–
Head and Neck Surgery
Division of Facial Plastic and Reconstructive Surgery
Department of Otolaryngology–
Head and Neck Surgery
University of California Irvine
Orange, California

Jan L. Kasperbauer, MD
Professor of Otolaryngology
Department of Otolaryngology
Mayo Clinic
Rochester, Minnesota

Robert M. Kellman, MD
Professor and Chair of Otolaryngology
and Communication Sciences
Departmenta of Otolaryngology
and Communication Sciences
SUNY Upstate Medical University
Syracuse, New York

Paul E. Kelly, MD
Private Practice
Facial Plastic Surgery Associates
Houston, Texas

Eugene B. Kern, MD, MS
Emeritus Endocott Professor in Medicine
Emeritus Professor in Rhinology and Facial Plastic Surgery
Department of Otolaryngology
Mayo Clinic
Rochester, Minnesota

David W. Kim, MD
Director, Division of Facial Plastic
and Reconstructive Surgery
Assistant Professor, Department of Otolaryngology–
Head and Neck Surgery
University of California San Francisco
San Francisco, California

R. James Koch, MD, MS
Private Practice
Lifestyle Lift
San Mateo, California

Mimi S. Kokoska, MD
Professor of Otolaryngology–Head and Neck Surgery
Department of Otolaryngology–Head and Neck Surgery
Indiana University School of Medicine
Indianapolis VA Medical Center
Indianapolis, Indiana

Theda C. Kontis, MD
Assistant Professor of Otolaryngology–
Head and Neck Surgery
Department of Otolaryngology–Head and Neck Surgery
The Johns Hopkins University School of Medicine
Baltimore, Maryland

Russell W. H. Kridel, MD, FACS
Clinical Professor of Otolaryngology–
Head and Neck Surgery
Division of Facial Plastic and Reconstructive Surgery
Department of Otolaryngology–Head and Neck Surgery
University of Texas
Houston, Texas

Keith A. LaFerriere, MD, FACS
Clinical Professor of Otolaryngology–
Head and Neck Surgery
Department of Otolaryngology–
Head and Neck Surgery
University of Missouri
Springfield, Missouri

Samuel M. Lam, MD
Private Practice
Luminaire Laser Center
Dallas, Texas

Wayne F. Larrabee Jr., MD, MPH
Clinical Professor Otolaryngology–Head and Neck Surgery
Department of Otolaryngology–Head and Neck Surgery
University of Washington
Seattle, Washington

Roger P. Levin, DDS
Private Practice
Levin Group, Inc.
Baltimore, Maryland

Timothy S. Lian, MD, FACS
Associate Professor of Otolaryngology–
Head and Neck Surgery
Department of of Otolaryngology–Head and Neck Surgery
Resident Program Director
Louisiana State University, Health Sciences Center
Shreveport, Louisiana

Jason A. Litner, MD, FRCSC
Private Practice
Profiles Beverly Hills
West Hollywood, California

Garrett B. Lyons Jr., DDS
Private Practice
Montchanin, Delaware

Corey S. Maas, MD, FACS
Private Practice
The Maas Clinic
San Francisco, California

Brian P. Maloney, MD, FACS
Private Practice
The Maloney Center for Facial Plastic Surgery
Atlanta, Georgia

Stephen H. Mandy, MD
Clinical Professor of Dermatology
Department of Dermatology
University of Miami
Miami Beach, Florida

Lawrence J. Marentette, MD, FACS
Professor of Otolaryngology and Neurosurgery
Division of Facial Plastic and Reconstructive Surgery
Director of Cranial Base Program
University of Michigan Medical Center
Ann Arbor, Michigan

Robert H. Mathog, MD
Professor and Chairman of Otolaryngology–Head and Neck Surgery
Department of Otolaryngology–Head and Neck Surgery
Wayne State University School of Medicine
Detroit, Michigan

John A. McCurdy Jr., MD, FACS
Private Practice
Honolulu, Hawaii

Scott A. McLean, MD, PhD
Senior Staff Surgeon
Department of Otolaryngology–Head and Neck Surgery
Henry Ford Medical Center
Detroit, Michigan

Tanya K. Meyer, MD
Assistant Professor of Otolaryngology–Head and Neck Surgery
Department of Otolaryngology–Head and Neck Surgery
University of Maryland
Baltimore, Maryland

Harry Mittelman, MD
Private Practice
Mittelman Plastic Surgery Center
Los Altos, California

Gary D. Monheit, MD
Private Practice
Total Skin and Beauty Dermatology Center
Birmingham, Alabama

Sam P. Most, MD
Associate Professor and Chief of Facial Plastic Surgery
Division of Facial Plastic Surgery
Department of Otolaryngology–Head and Neck Surgery
Stanford University School of Medicine
Stanford, California

Craig S. Murakami, MD, FACS
Clinical Associate Professor of Facial Plastic Surgery and Otolaryngology
Departments of Facial Plastic Surgery and Otolaryngology
Virginia Mason Medical Center
Seattle, Washington

Nathan E. Nachlas, MD
Private Practice
Boca Raton, Florida

Shervin Naderi, MD, FACS
Private Practice
Naderi Facial Plastic Surgery
Herndon, Virginia

Steven S. Orten, MD
Private Practice
Lifestyle Lift Dallas
Dallas, Texas

Ira D. Papel, MD
Associate Professor of Otolaryngology–Head and Neck Surgery
Division of Facial Plastic Surgery
Department of Otolaryngology–Head and Neck Surgery
The Johns Hopkins University School of Medicine
Facial Plastic Surgicenter
Baltimore, Maryland

Stephen S. Park, MD
Professor and Vice-Chair of Otolaryngology–Head and Neck Surgery
Division Chair of Facial Plastic and Reconstructive Surgery
Department of Otolaryngology–Head and Neck Surgery
The University of Virginia
Charlottesville, Virginia

Norman J. Pastorek, MD
Clinical Professor of Facial Plastic Surgery
Department of Otolaryngology
Weill Medical College of Cornell University
New York Presbyterian Hospital
New York, New York

Stephen W. Perkins, MD
Clinical Assistant Professor of Surgery
Department of Otolaryngology–
Head and Neck Surgery
Indiana University School of Medicine
Indianapolis, Indiana

Judy Pinborough-Zimmerman, MD
Adjunct Professor of Communication Disorders
Department of Communication Disorders
University of Utah
Program Manager, Child Development Clinic
Utah Department of Health
Salt Lake City, Utah

Vito C. Quatela, MD
Clinical Associate Professor Facial Plastic Surgery
Department of Otolaryngology
University of Rochester Medical Center
Rochester, New York

John S. Rhee, MD, MPH
Associate Professor of Otolaryngology
Department of Otolaryngology
Medical College of Wisconsin
Milwaukee, Wisconsin

Marion B. Ridley, MD
Professor of Otolaryngology–
Head and Neck Surgery
Department of Otolaryngology–
Head and Neck Surgery
University of South Florida
College of Medicine
Tampa, Florida

W. Russell Ries, MD
Associate Professor of Otolaryngology
Department of Otolaryngology
Vanderbilt University Medical Center
Nashville, Tennessee

Daniel E. Rousso, MD
Private Practice
Rousso Facial Plastic Surgery
Birmingham, Alabama

Robert O. Ruder, MD
Private Practice
Beverly Hills Cosmetic Surgery Center
Beverly Hills, California

Paul Sabini, MD
Private Practice
Panzer Dermatology and Cosmetic Surgery
Hockessin, Delaware

Cecelia E. Schmalbach, MD, MS
Assistant Professor of Otolaryngology–
Head and Neck Surgery
Department of Otolaryngology–
Head and Neck Surgery
Wilford Hall Medical Center
Lackland Air Force Base, Texas

David A. Sherris, MD
Professor and Chairman of Otolaryngology
Department of Otolaryngology
University of Buffalo
Buffalo, New York

William W. Shockley, MD
Professor and Vice-Chair of Otolaryngology–
Head and Neck Surgery
Department of Otolaryngology–
Head and Neck Surgery
University of North Carolina
Chapel Hill, North Carolina

Russell S. Shu, MD
Private Practice
Norwood, Massachusetts

Robert L. Simons, MD
Clinical Professor of Otolaryngology–
Head and Neck Surgery
Department of Otolaryngology–
Head and Neck Surgery
University of Miami
Miami, Florida

Craig L. Slingluff, MD
Professor of Surgery
Division Head, Division of Surgical Oncology
University of Virginia
Charlottesville, Virginia

Marshall E. Smith, MD
Associate Professor of Otolaryngology
Department of Otolaryngology
University of Utah
Salt Lake City, Utah

Christian L. Stallworth, MD
Chief Resident of Otolaryngology–Head and Neck Surgery
Department of Otolaryngology–Head and Neck Surgery
University of Texas Health Science Center
San Antonio, Texas

Robert B. Stanley Jr., MD, DDS
Professor of Otolaryngology–Head and Neck Surgery
Department of Otolaryngology–Head and Neck Surgery
University of Washington School of Medicine
Seattle, Washington

Dow Stough, MD
Private Practice
The Stough Clinic
Hot Springs, Arkansas

E. Bradley Strong, MD
Associate Professor of Otolaryngology
Department of Otolaryngology
University of California Davis Medical Center
Sacramento, California

Fred J. Stucker, MD
Professor and Chairman of Otolaryngology–
Head and Neck Surgery
Department of Otolaryngology–Head and Neck Surgery
Louisiana State University Health Sciences Center
Shreveport, Louisiana

Sandeep Sule, MD
Private Practice
Dallas, Texas

Jonathan M. Sykes, MD
Professor of Otolaryngology–Head and Neck Surgery
Department of Otolaryngology–Head and Neck Surgery
Director, Facial Plastic and Reconstructive Surgery
University of California Davis Medical Center
Sacramento, California

Edward Szachowicz III, MD
Private Practice
Edina, Minnesota

Monica Tadros, MD
Assistant Professor of Otolaryngology–
Head and Neck Surgery
Director of Facial Plastic Surgery Education
Columbia University College of Physicians and Surgeons
New York Presbyterian Hospital
Director of Facial Plastic Surgery Education
Roosevelt Hospital
Director of Aesthetic Facial Surgery
The Center for Facial Reconstruction and Restoration
New York, New York

M. Eugene Tardy Jr., MD
Private Practice
Oak Park, Illinois

J. Regan Thomas, MD
Lederer Professor and Chairman
Department of Otolaryngology–
Head and Neck Surgery
University of Illinois
Chicago, Illinois

Geoffrey W. Tobias, MD
Instructor of Otolaryngology
Department of Otolaryngology
Mount Sinai Hospital
Englewood, New Jersey

Whitney D. Tope, MD
Associate Physician
Advancements in Dermatology, PA
Edina, Minnesota

Dean M. Toriumi, MD
Professor of Otolaryngology–Head and Neck Surgery
Division of Facial Plastic and Reconstructive Surgery
Department of Otolaryngology
University of Illinois at Chicago
Chicago, Illinois

Behrooz A. Torkian, MD
Clinical Instructor of Otolaryngology–
Head and Neck Surgery
Division of Facial Plastic and Reconstructive Surgery
Department of Otolaryngology–
Head and Neck Surgery
University of California Irvine
Irvine, California

Gilbert J. Nolst Trenité, MD, PhD
Professor of Otolaryngology
Department of Ear, Nose, and Throat
University of Amsterdam
Amsterdam, The Netherlands

Rudy J. Triana Jr., MD
Private Practice
The Triana Institute
Manalapan Island, Florida

Steven M. VanHook, MD
Attending Physician
Department of Infectious Diseases
and Internal Medicine
St. Thomas Hospital, Nashville, Tennessee

Mark L. Urken, MD
Chief, Division of Head and Neck Surgical Oncology
Department of Otolaryngology
Director, Head and Neck Surgical Oncology
of Continuum Cancer Centers of New York
Co-Director, Institute for Head and Neck
and Thyroid Cancers
Beth Israel Medical Center
New York, New York

Craig Vander Kolk, MD
Professor of Plastic Surgery
Associate Director of Plastic Surgery
Department of Plastic and Reconstructive Surgery
The Johns Hopkins University School of Medicine
Mercy Medical Center, Baltimore, Maryland

Karin Vargervik, DDS
Larry L. Hillblom Professor in Craniofacial Anomalies
Director, Center for Craniofacial Anomalies
University of California San Francisco
San Francisco, California

Tom D. Wang, MD
Professor of Facial Plastic and Reconstructive Surgery
Department of Otolaryngology–Head and Neck Surgery
Oregon Health and Science University
Portland, Oregon

Jeffrey M. Whitworth, MD
Assistant Professor for Dermatology
New Jersey Medical School
Warren Dermatology Associates
Warren, New Jersey

Edwin F. Williams III, MD
Clinical Professor of Surgery
Department of Surgery
Albany Medical College
Private Practice
Director, Williams Center for Facial Plastic
Surgery Specialists
Latham, New York

Maria Wittkopf, MD
Resident of Otolaryngology–Head and Neck Surgery
Department of Otolaryngology–Head and Neck Surgery
Vanderbilt University School of Medicine
Nashville, Tennessee

Matthew Wolpoe, MD
Private Practice
Ear, Nose, and Throat Associates
Billings, Montana

Kenneth C. Y. Yu, MD
Staff, Otolaryngology–Head and Neck Surgery
Travis Air Force Base, California

I

Principles of Facial Plastic and Reconstructive Surgery

1 Anatomy and Physiology of the Skin

Richard Bennett

The skin is a complex tissue that is transected, manipulated, and rearranged during cosmetic and reconstructive surgery. Yet most surgeons view the skin as a simple barrier to be cut through rather than a complicated organ structure. This viewpoint has led to a paucity of cutaneous research within surgical programs and a general lack of understanding of basic cutaneous anatomy and physiology. This chapter focuses on the surgically relevant features of cutaneous anatomy and physiology. For more detailed descriptions of cutaneous anatomy and physiology, refer to several books listed in the references.[1–3]

Surface Characteristics of the Skin

If the skin is considered an organ, it is the heaviest organ, whereas the lung is the largest organ in terms of surface area. However, if the skin is considered a tissue, it is not the heaviest tissue. Goldsmith[4] states that the weight of skin is ~3.79 kg, which ranks it the fourth heaviest organ after fat, bone, and muscle.

The skin invests the body and is draped over the bony prominences. It is an important component of outward beauty. Because the skin is the initial structure seen by others, it takes on extreme importance. At the orifices, the skin changes texture, and its composition changes from dry to moist. In the very young, the skin is smooth and lacks surface growths and irregularities.

Modifications occur with aging; in childhood nevi appear, in middle age the skin starts to sag, and in old age wrinkles appear. With aging the skin may be marred by areas of hyperpigmentation, scars, areas of atrophy, and a variety of cutaneous lesions. These events are the result of physiological changes that occur over time, and many patients wish to reverse the effects rather than grow old gracefully.

The skin is not a uniform organ macroscopically, microscopically, physiologically, or when viewed in the fourth dimension, time. There are regional and temporal variations in the epidermal thickness, dermal thickness, elastic fiber content, presence and number of hair follicles, sebaceous glands, apocrine glands, and eccrine glands. Parts of the skin are hair bearing and others are not. The skin may be dry as on the trunk or arms, moist as in the groin or axillae, or oily as on the face. In addition, there are individual variations with regard to these cutaneous differences. For instance, some individuals have small pores and smooth skin on the cheeks (**Fig. 1.1A**),

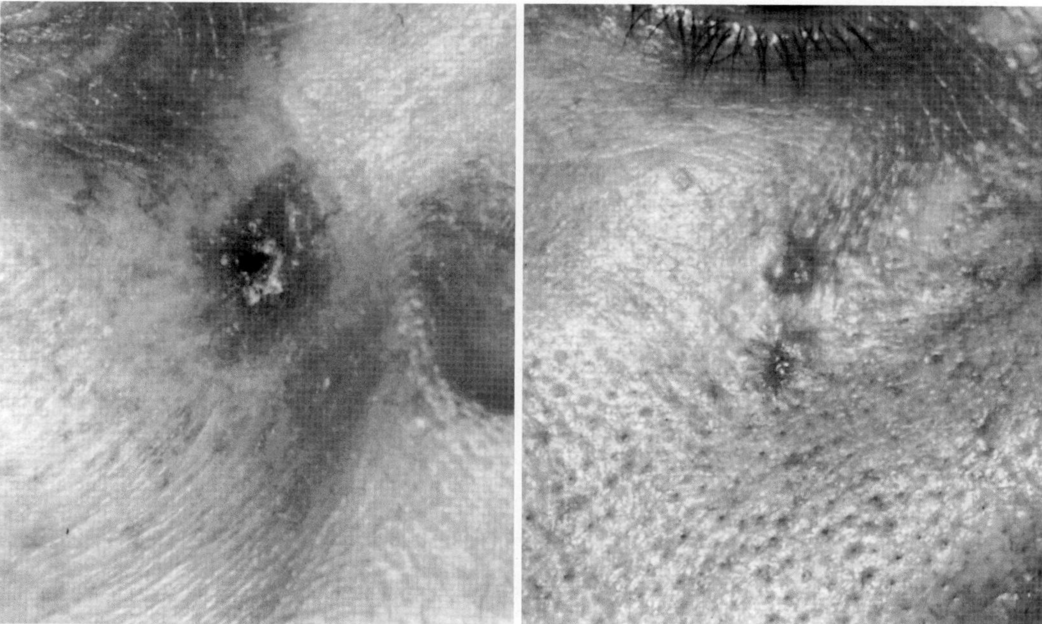

Fig. 1.1 (**A**) An individual with smooth cheek skin with small inconspicuous pores. (**B**) An individual with cheek skin with large patulous conspicuous pores.

Table 1.1 Cutaneous Lesions Directly or Indirectly Influencing Appearance of Future Cutaneous Scars

Hypertrophic scars	Hypertrophic scars
Keloids	Keloids
Dupuytren	Contracture
Hyperpigmentation	Hyperpigmentation
Lichen planus Psoriasis Discoid lupus erythematosus	Koebner phenomenon resulting in lichen planus or psoriasis or discoid lupus erythematosus in scars
Spread scars	Spread scars
Double jointedness	Telangiectasia around scars
Ruddy complexion	

whereas other individuals have patulous pores and oily skin on the face and are prone to acne (**Fig. 1.1B**). Some individuals with unusually dry skin are prone to xerosis and atopic dermatitis.

Before surgery is performed on the skin, the patient's skin should be assessed for clues that will influence the outcome of surgery (**Table 1.1**). For instance, hypertrophic scars, keloids, hyperpigmentation, and double joints should be noted. An important phenomenon to take into account is the Koebner phenomenon. This phenomenon is the predisposition of certain cutaneous diseases to localize in areas of scars regardless of how carefully the surgery is performed. Important common skin diseases that will localize in scars include psoriasis, lichen planus, and discoid lupus erythematosus (**Fig. 1.2**).

Aging skin is extremely important to the cosmetic surgeon. Aged skin has changes that are either endogenous or exogenous in origin. The endogenous changes include fine wrinkling, dermal atrophy, and a decrease in subdermal adipose tissue. This atrophy is particularly marked on the face and dorsum of the hands. In addition, there is a loss of elastic fibers and laxity of the skin. The exogenous changes occur largely because of chronic sun exposure and are characterized by coarse folds and a leathery appearance to the skin.

The term *photoaging* has been used to describe these changes.[5,6] The leathery appearance results from a buildup of elastotic material in the papillary portion of the dermis. Also, there is a homogenization of collagen fibers that become basophilic, and an accumulation of glycosaminoglycan and proteoglycan complexes within the dermis.[7] Recent interest has focused on topical creams, such as tretinoin (Retin-A, Janssen Pharmaceutica, Inc., Titusville, NJ), that help reverse some of the changes associated with aging.[7]

Anatomy of the Skin

The skin is divided into three layers—the epidermis, the dermis, and the superficial fascia (**Fig. 1.3**). As is true with the skin surface, each of these three layers has a different appearance in different areas of the body.

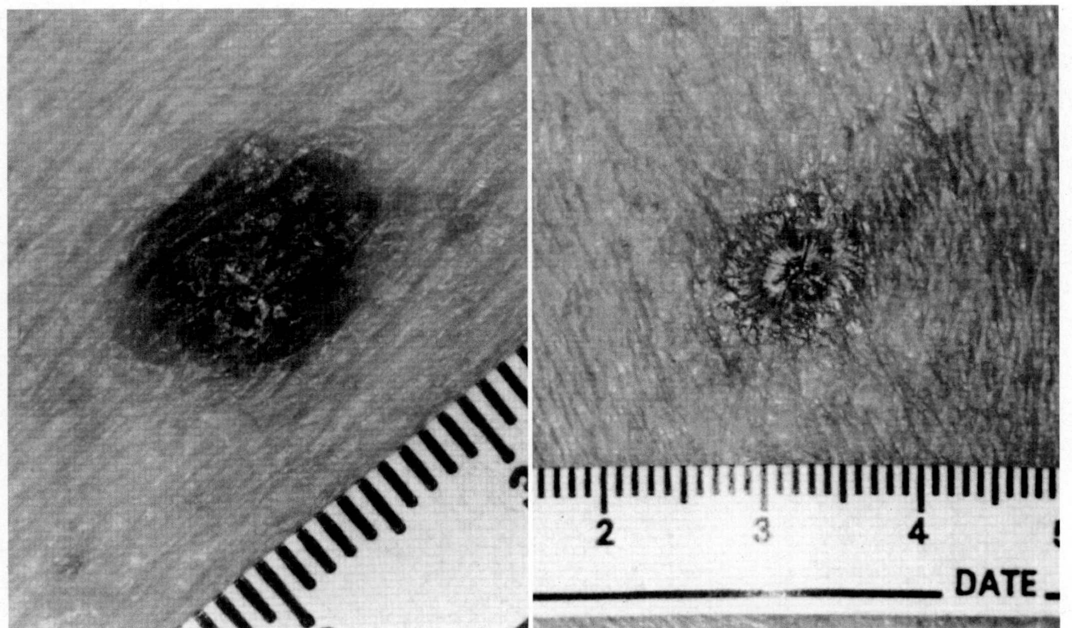

Fig. 1.2 Psoriasis localized to skin biopsy site. (**A**) Prebiopsy superficial melanoma. (**B**) Postbiopsy; note scaly area around biopsy. Patient had extensive psoriasis elsewhere.

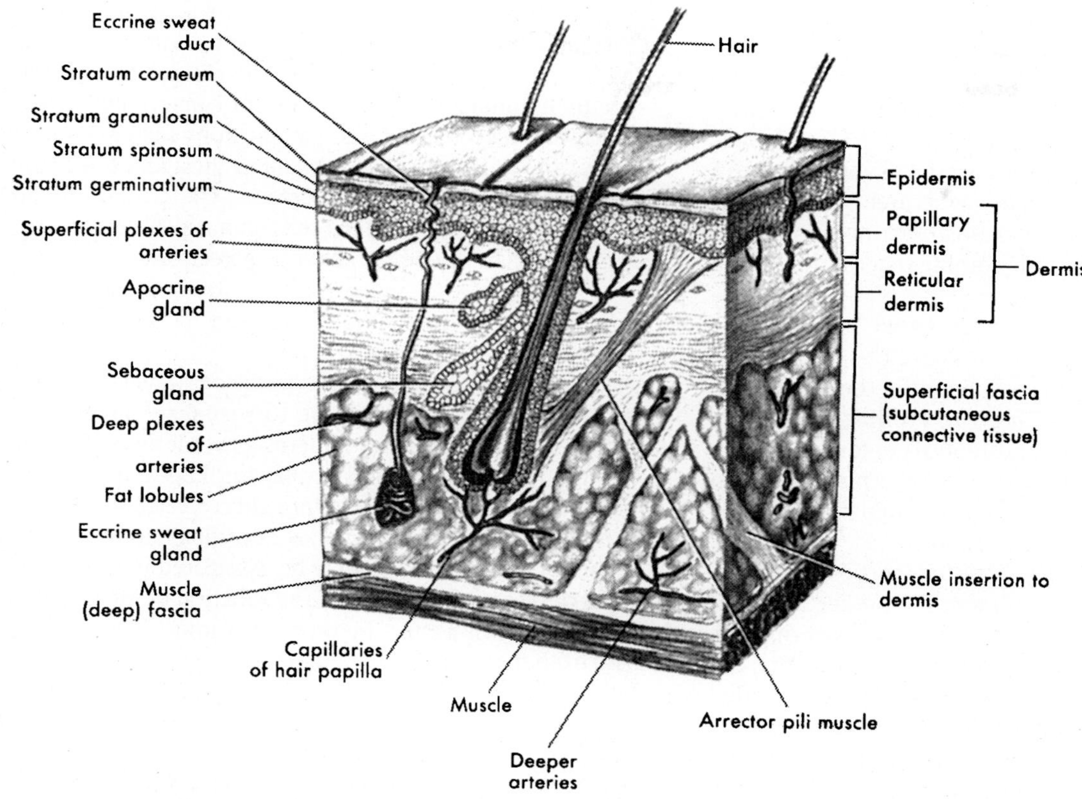

Fig. 1.3 The three layers of the skin: epidermis, dermis, and superficial fascia. (From Bennett RG. Fundamentals of Cutaneous Surgery. St Louis: CV Mosby; 1988. With permission.)

The Epidermis

The epidermis is the top layer of the skin. It contains four distinct cell types—keratinocytes, melanocytes, Langerhans cells, and Merkel cells. About 80% of the cells in the epidermis are keratinocytes. Keratinocytes are subclassified by their location within the epidermis and their degree of keratinization. The epidermis is divided into five layers. The basal cell layer, the stratum germinativum, is the bottom layer of the epidermis. It is composed of a single layer of cuboidal cells, the basal cells. Basal cells have a slightly basophilic cytoplasm and divide to give rise to the next layer above, the prickle cell layer. The basal cells rest on the basement membrane and are connected to each other through desmosomes and to the basement membrane by hemidesmosomes. Between some of the basal cells are melanocytes, the pigment-producing cells of the body. For every 10 basal cells there are approximately one or two melanocytes. However, this ratio varies in different areas of the body.

The next layer above the basal cell layer is the prickle cell layer, the stratum spinosum. This layer is usually three to four cells thick and is composed of polygonal cells with preformed keratin. This keratin gives these cells a definite cytoplasmic eosinophilia. Even under light microscopy, the desmosomal attachments between the prickle cells are evident.

The attachments appear as small spines emanating from the cells and give rise to the name *prickle cells*. The next layer above the prickle cell layer is the granular cell layer, the stratum granulosum. This layer is one to four cells thick; the cells contain coarse cytoplasmic granules that are deeply basophilic and represent preformed keratin granules, keratohyalin granules, that will coalesce to help form the next layer, the cornified layer, the stratum corneum. The stratum corneum is the outermost layer of the epidermis and is formed from the extremely flattened, anucleated keratinocytes and compacted keratin granules.[8] The cell borders and nuclei are lost as the keratin granules fuse, and this layer is often described as having a basket-weave pattern. The stratum corneum is usually several cell layers thick and may reach enormous proportions in the palms and soles.

On the palms and soles a fifth layer of epidermis is often identified, the stratum lucidum. This clear area appears between the stratum corneum and the stratum granulosum.

Cell Types

Keratinocytes

Of great importance in epidermal cells is keratin. Within the stratum corneum, 60% of its mass and 85% of its cellular proteins are made up of keratin filament. Keratin filaments are complex tubular structures formed first by three keratin polypeptide chains twisting together to form a coil, and then nine coils coming together to form a tubular structure.[9]

Keratin filaments become aggregated between the granular and cornified layers of the skin. This aggregation occurs because of a protein component of the keratohyalin granules known as profilaggrin. Profilaggrin undergoes dephosphorylation and proteolysis to form filaggrin. It is filaggrin that catalyzes the aggregation of keratin filaments. The complex of keratin filaments within the filaggrin matrix is known as macrofibril.

The cornified cells of the stratum corneum contain a cell envelope deep to the plasma membrane. The cell envelope is ~12 mm wide and acts as an impermeable barrier. The major precursor proteins found in the cell membrane are keratolinin and involucrin. When cornified cells pass through the outer half of the stratum corneum, the cell plasma membrane becomes discontinuous, and the cell envelope becomes the outermost barrier of the outermost cornified cells.

Certain keratin filaments are also known as tonofilaments and connect the desmosomes at the cell surface with the nuclear membrane of the cell. Keratin filaments thus provide a cytoskeleton to the cell and may also serve as a communication system between the cell surface and the nucleus.

Keratin filaments are intermediate filaments that are 10 mm in diameter and are used as a marker for the epithelial cells. There are 19 antigeneticly different keratins. Monoclonal antibodies to all 19 keratins have been developed and are used to identify the origin of neoplasms or specific dermatologic disorders.

Langerhans Cells

Within the epidermis are a few additional cells that are important. Langerhans cells are clear cells found mainly within the prickle cell layer. Under light microscopy these cells resemble melanocytes. These cells are difficult to see unless a special stain, the gold-chloride stain, or electron microscopy is used. With the gold-chloride stain, Langerhans cells appear dendritic. Langerhans cells contain cytoplasmic organelles, Birbeck granules, seen under electron microscopy. Langerhans cells have many features of monocytes and macrophages and are thought to migrate to the skin from the bone marrow. These cells are probably the mediators of immunologic responses within the skin.[10,11] The dendritic processes of the Langerhans cells efficiently capture and process antigens within the skin. The Langerhans cells then present the antigen to the skin-specific lymphocytes. The number of Langerhans cells is greatly enhanced during allergic reactions such as contact dermatitis. With aging or exposure to ultraviolet light the number of Langerhans cells decreases. Thiers et al[12] found a 15% decrease in Langerhans cells on buttock skin on subjects older than 65 compared with subjects under age 24.

Merkel Cells

Merkel cells are found in the basal cell layer and, like Langerhans cells, are difficult to visualize under light microscopy. Under electron microscopy, Merkel cells have membrane-bound granules similar to those found in neuroendocrine tissue cells. Therefore, this cell is probably part of the amine precursor uptake decarboxylation (APUD) system of the body[13] and may be associated with the terminal nerves within the skin. The function of Merkel cells is unknown. However, Merkel cell tumors occasionally arise from these cells.

Melanocytes

Melanocytes are found within the basal cell layer and are specialized to produce melanin pigment. Melanocytes may be variable in appearance but appear with routine hematoxylin-eosin (H&E)–stained sections as cuboidal cells with a clear cytoplasm and eccentrically placed, crescent-shaped nuclei. Under special stains, such as the Dopa stain, melanocytes appear as stellate cells. The melanin granules produced by these cells are donated to adjacent keratinocytes via their stellate projections. In blacks, these melanocytes are particularly active. In those with vitiligo, melanocytes are absent altogether. In those with albinism, the melanocytes are present but lack the enzyme tyrosinase so that tyrosine cannot be transformed into melanin. The ratio of melanocytes to basal cells varies with anatomical location but not with race. With aging, the melanocytic density decreases with each decade by 6 to 8%.[14] In addition, the melanocytic enzyme tyrosine declines in activity with age.[15] Therefore, the elderly do not tan as easily as when they were young. Melanocytes in older skin are also somewhat pleomorphic as are the keratinocytes.[1] Melanocytes in the elderly may show some nuclear atypia and variations in size, shape, and staining quality.

Dermal–Epidermal Junction

Basement Membrane

The area between the epidermis and the dermis is a well-defined area known as the basement membrane zone. On

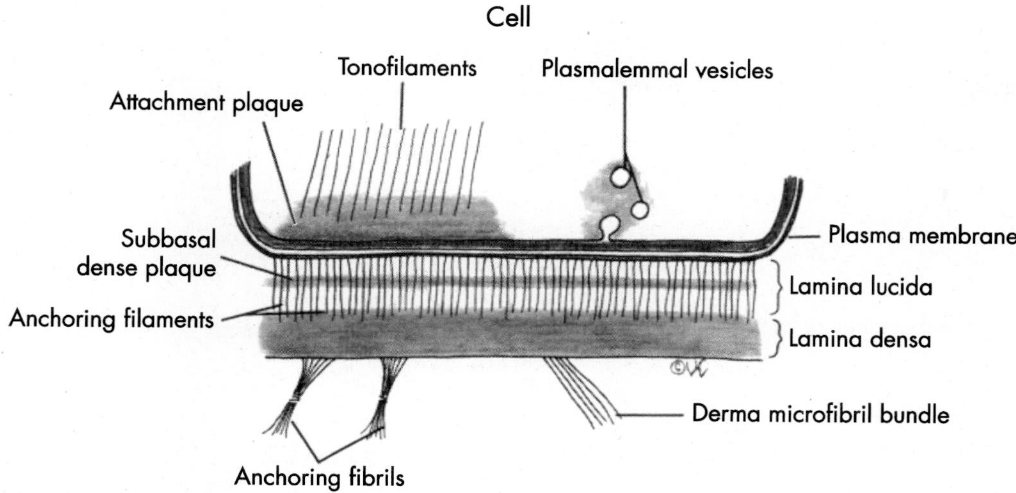

Fig. 1.4 Basement membrane anatomy.

H&E–stained sections this zone appears as a thin (i.e., 1 to 2 mm), poorly defined band of eosinophilic material. The basement membrane actually functions in the following three ways: it attaches the epidermis to the dermis, provides mechanical support to the epidermis, and provides a barrier to chemicals or cells. The basement membrane is actually a complex structure, consisting of several layers seen on electron microscopy[16] (**Fig. 1.4**). The hemidesmosome is within the basal cell plasma membrane and consists of tonofilaments from within the basal cell that condense and attach to an electron-dense thickening, identified as the attachment plaque. Plasmalemmal vesicles are part of the intracellular basal cell structure; these vesicles participate in endocytosis and exocytosis of low-molecular-weight solutes, soluble macromolecules, and small colloidal particles. The lamina lucida rests on top of the lamina densa. Within the lamina lucida are the subbasal dense plate and anchoring filaments. Attached to the undersurface of the lamina densa are anchoring dermal microfibril bundles and anchoring fibrils. Dermal microfibril bundles represent terminations of the dermal elastic system and contribute somewhat to the anchorage of the basement membrane. Anchoring fibrils are specialized collagen fibrils that consist of type VII collagen and have been described as wheat stack–shaped structures.[17] Their function is to anchor the epidermis and the epidermal–dermal junction to the dermis. Anchoring fibrils are absent in early scars and are less numerous in sun-exposed areas compared with sun-protected areas.[18] The basement membrane zone continues around hair follicles and sweat ducts.

Anchoring Fibrils

The anchoring fibrils in skin, like other types of collagen, are susceptible to degradation by collagenase. Collagenase may be stimulated by the cytokinin interleukin-1. Interleukin-1 in turn may be produced by keratinocytes that are stimulated by ultraviolet light.[19,20] Collagenase may also be inhibited by topically applied tretinoin, which may explain the improved stability of tretinoin-treated skin. Woodley et al[21] showed that topical tretinoin, when applied to the forearm, increased the anchoring fibril density. They speculated that this increased density was due to the drug's property of inhibiting collagenase. On electron microscopy, the number of anchoring fibrils appeared to increase with tretinoin applications.[22]

Rete Ridges

The contour of the bottom of the epidermis is irregular with numerous projections, the rete pegs. These projections help to anchor the epidermis into the dermis. When viewed in three dimensions, the rete pegs form a netlike pattern and are more properly referred to as rete ridges (**Fig. 1.5A**). The corresponding upward elevations of the dermis that interdigitate with the rete ridges are the dermal papillae. In scars the rete pegs are lost (**Fig. 1.5C**), and the epidermis has a smooth bottom. The lack of rete pegs in scar tissue is one reason why scar epidermis may shear off more easily than normal epidermis. With aging there is a decrease in the length of the dermal papillae and rete pegs and the dermal–epidermal junction appears flattened[23,24] (**Fig. 1.5B**). The relative decrease in interface allows dermal–epidermal separation to occur more readily in the elderly and probably leads to a propensity for torn skin after minor trauma. The decreased length of the dermal–epidermal junction also leads to a decrease in the quantity of available keratinized cells because of a decrease in the number of basal cells per unit area. This promotes dry skin.[24] The decline in surface area of the

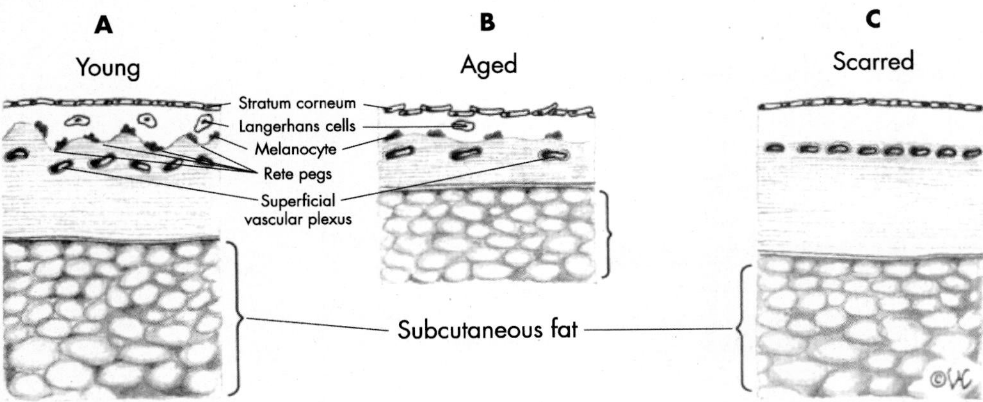

Fig. 1.5 The changes in the skin with time and scarring. (**A**) Young skin. (**B**) Aged skin. (**C**) Scarred skin.

dermal–epidermal interface also lessens communication and nutrient transfer between the dermis and epidermis.

Hair Shafts

Piercing the epidermis at intervals are hair shafts. Hair shafts are complex structures that arise within hair follicles. The hair follicle is composed of several cell layers. It is important to understand that the outer cell layer, the external root sheath, is really an extension of the surface epidermis. As such, some diseases in the epidermis tend to involve the outermost sheath of the hair follicle. For instance, Bowen disease carcinoma and lentigo maligna melanoma can be seen not only within interfollicular epidermis but also within the external root sheath of hair follicles. The fact that these skin cancers extend down hair follicles has certain implications regarding cure rates by various treatment methods. The remainder of the hair anatomy is discussed later in this chapter.

Effects of Aging

With aging the normal and neat epidermal architecture is lost. Epidermal cells vary in size, shape, and staining qualities.[25] There is some loss of polarity, and the orderly progression from basal cell layer to granular cell layer is not so pronounced. Cellular heterogenicity is seen. With aging the epidermis appears thinner under the microscope. It is believed that the thin epidermis in the elderly is actually a misconception; in the young the epidermis appears thicker because the dermis is more contractile.[26] The time progression from the basal cell layer to the stratum granulosum is ~2 weeks; from the lowest layer of the stratum corneum to the surface of the skin takes an additional 2 weeks. In the elderly the epidermal replacement is decreased by 30 to 50% and may account for slower wound healing.[27] Cellular proliferation within the epidermis may also be under control of various stimulatory substances that include nerve growth factor and epidermal growth factor (EGF). EGF is predominantly located in the basal cell layer with lesser amounts in the more differentiated cell layers.[28] With increasing degrees of differentiation, EGF binding decreases.[29] EGF has been found to be increased in transitional cell carcinoma of the bladder where it was associated with poor differentiation and invasion.[30]

The Dermis

The dermis is divided into two parts, the papillary dermis and the reticular dermis (see **Fig. 1.3**). The papillary dermis is relatively thin, is located just below the dermal–epidermal junction, and is composed of loose collagen, blood vessels, and fibrocytes. The reticular dermis is below the papillary dermis, is relatively thick, and makes up the rest of the dermis. The reticular dermis is composed of compact collagen with few fibrocytes. Cutting across the dermis are peripheral branches of the vascular and nervous systems and epidermal appendages (i.e., pilosebaceous, apocrine, and eccrine units). The papillary dermis surrounds the adnexal structures and is called the adventitial dermis.

Structural Components

The main structural components of the dermis are collagen, reticulin, and elastic fibers embedded in a matrix of glycoproteins. This matrix is referred to as the ground substance. The collagen is made up of collagen fibers that are synthesized by fibrocytes. The collagen bundles are easily seen on H&E–stained sections as eosinophilic fibers that are bundled together. Because the collagen bundles are oriented in various directions, normal dermal collagen is birefringent in polarized light. In scars the collagen is often not so randomly directed but is laid down instead in the direction of wound stress. When scar collagen is polarized, it is thus not birefringent.

Collagen

Collagen is continuously turning over in the skin. The rate of turnover depends on the rate of synthesis and the rate of degradation. The latter is controlled by collagenase that is located largely in the papillary dermis and synthesized by fibroblasts.[31–33] With aging skin, collagen synthesis decreases and the skin collagen content decreases.[34] Skin collagen decreases by 1% per year throughout adult life.[35] In addition, collagen fibers change their appearance. In infancy, collagen bundles are small and oriented parallel to the skin surface. In young adulthood, collagen bundles appear randomly arranged in the papillary dermis, but in the reticular dermis the collagen bundles are large, loosely interwoven, and tightly packed. In the elderly, collagen is more compact, perhaps because of the loss of ground substance that is normally found between individual collagen bundles. Collagen in the elderly is arranged in thick, coarse bundles or as loosely woven, straight fibers.[36] Some of the enzymes (i.e., galactosyltransferase and glucosyltransferase) that modify collagen within the cell are decreased with aging.[37]

Reticulin and Elastic Fibers

Reticulin fibers are also found in the dermis. These fibers are thin, small fibers that are probably early collagen fibers soon after extrusion from fibrocytes. Elastic fibers are wavy eosinophilic fibers that vary in length and width. Elastin is the functional protein component of the elastic fiber.[38] Surrounding the elastin is a microfibrillar component that can be seen on electron microscopy. Elastic fibers extend from the dermal–epidermal basement membrane into the reticular dermis, but only in the deeper portion of the dermis are they invested with elastin and thus can be seen under the microscope as elastic fibers.[39] In sun-damaged skin the elastic fibers are usually thick and abundant in the papillary dermis. These thickened elastic fibers are referred to as elastotic fibers. Their origin from elastic fibers is shown by the fact that they stain positively with an antielastin antibody (HB8) and disappear with elastase.[40] With age, elastic fibers in the reticular dermis increase in number and become thicker, more branched, and haphazardly arranged. There are areas of focal loss and focal proliferation of elastic fibers.[41] In the papillary dermis, however, elastic fibers disappear with age. There is a decrease in the diameter and number of elastic fibers and the fibers are often fragmented.[42] Thus, with aging, there is a lack of functional elastic fibers, and the skin becomes loose, pendulous, and devoid of recoil. Striae cutis distensae are linear flat or atrophic areas in skin that has been subjected to stress. Striae cutis distensae are probably the result of attenuation or rupture of elastic fibers.[43] Within the dermis are also microfibrillar fibers that can be seen on electron microscopy. These fibers appear as linear bundles containing many individual microfibrils. The microfibrils are very small and have an average diameter of 10 to 12 mm. One component of microfibrils, fibrillin, is a glycoprotein that was recentlycharacterized.[44] These fibers serve as a scaffolding for the deposition of elastin during elastogenesis. In 1990, Hollister et al[45] reported finding a deficiency of the microfibrillar–fiber system in the skin and cultured fibroblasts of patients with Marfan syndrome.

Fibrocytes

The main cell in the dermis is the fibrocyte. These cells are abundant in the papillary dermis but sparse in the reticular dermis. The fibrocyte may become modulated during wound healing to become an active collagen-producing cell with abundant endoplasmic reticulum. The fibrocyte may also become a contractile cell during wound contraction. The contractile fibrocyte has intracytoplasmic filaments that resemble actin on special stains. Therefore, the fibrocyte is a versatile cell, responding to wound injury and stress. Fibrocytes decrease with age, which perhaps accounts for slower healing in the elderly. Andrew et al[46] counted the number of dermal nuclei and found that the abdomen at 80 years of age had less than half the number of nuclei present at 1 year of age. Mast cells may also be found within the dermis, mostly around blood vessels in the papillary dermis. In scars, mast cells can be abundant. The ground substance is also made by fibrocytes and is composed of glycoproteins and glycosaminoglycans. The ground substance is fluid and can be displaced by pressure. For instance, sleeping with an arm on a sharp object may produce a depression in the skin resulting from displacement of the ground substance. However, within a few hours this displaced fluid returns to its normal position as the arm is used. Hypertrophic scars and keloids also contain considerable ground substance. Therefore pressure massage of hypertrophic scars will reduce their swelling resulting from a reduction of the ground substance.

The Superficial Fascia

Below the dermis but above the underlying muscle is the superficial fascia. Although this layer has been called the subcutis, the panniculus adiposus, or simply the subcutaneous fat layer. All of these terms are either poor or misleading, and the term *superficial fascia* is preferred. This structure is composed of both a fatty component (fat cells) and a fibrous component (the fibrous septae) (**Fig. 1.6**). In some areas of the body, such as the scalp, the fibrous component predominates, and it is therefore impossible to undermine the skin. On the trunk and extremities, the

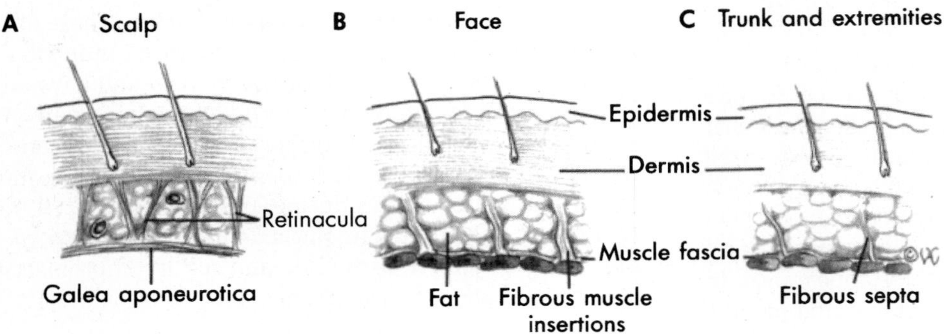

Fig. 1.6 The superficial fascia in certain anatomical areas. (**A**) The scalp. (**B**) The face. (**C**) The trunk and extremities.

fat component predominates, making undermining relatively easy. On the face, there is a mixture of fibrous septae and fat. Here the fibrous septae actually run from the underlying deep (muscle) fascia investing muscles to insert into the overlying dermis. On the lateral face the fibrous septae of the superficial fascia may become organized between the adjoining fibrous septae giving rise to a structure known as the superficial musculoaponeurotic system (SMAS). The thickness of the superficial fascia varies from one region of the body to another, from one gender to another, and from one individual to another. Because it contains abundant fat, this layer obviously reflects the nutritional status of the individual.

The Vascular Network

The blood vessels of the skin consist of a superficial network and a deep network (**Fig. 1.7**). The deep network, the deep plexus, lies in the superficial portion of the superficial fascia. From this deep network, small arteries pass vertically upward to the papillary dermis where they give rise to small arteries that interconnect to form a superficial arteriolar network, the superficial plexus. The superficial plexus gives rise to capillary loops that ascend into the dermal papillae and descend into the papillary dermis where they connect with venules that form the superficial venular network, the superficial venular plexus. The latter connects with veins in the superficial fascia. On the face the arteriolar portion of the capillary loops may be dilated, whereas on the extremities the venular side of the capillary loop may be distended. Because of the difference in the portion of the capillary loop dilated in these two areas, the response to sclerosing agents or laser is not the same. The telangiectatic vessels on the face are arteriolar, red, and respond well to lasers emitting wavelengths in the yellow portion of the electromagnetic spectrum but respond poorly to sclerosing agents. In contrast, the telangiectatic vessels on the legs are venular, bluish, and respond well to sclerosing agents but poorly to lasers. On the distal extremities there are shunts between the arterioles and venules in the superficial plexuses. These shunts are controlled by glomus cells that are innervated by adrenergic fibers. Glomus cells are polygonal in shape and group around vessels. The microscopic appearance of cutaneous vessels is similar to that of vessels elsewhere in the body. The vascular lumen is surrounded by endothelial cells that sit on a basement

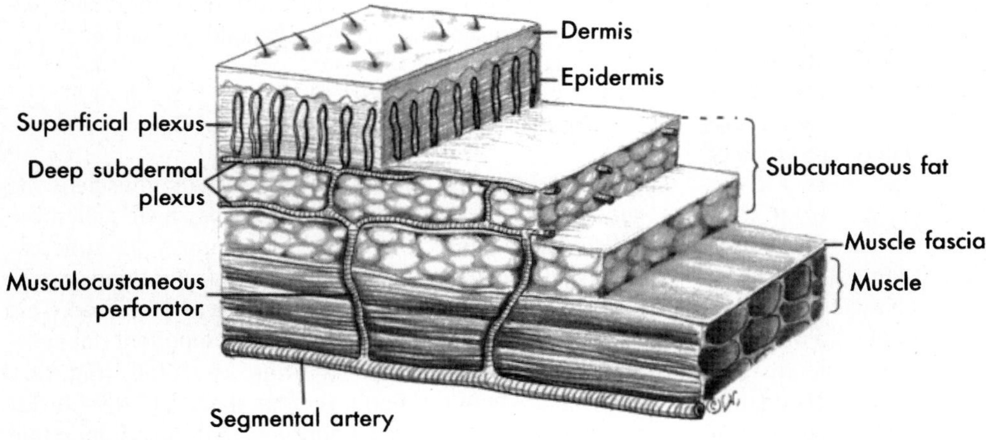

Fig. 1.7 The vascular network of the skin.

membrane, which is surrounded by smooth muscle cells, pericytes, and connective tissues. With aging the pericytes surrounding the vessels decrease in number and synthetic activity.[47] These changes parallel the thinning of vascular walls with aging and, along with the decrease in stromal support, explain the susceptibility of bruising in the elderly. Dermal blood vessels normally do not have a surrounding infiltrate. However, within photodamaged skin, a lymphohistiocytic perivenular infiltrate with numerous mast cells is present. Skin with this infiltrate has been labeled chronic heliodermatitis.[48] In the elderly, dermal blood vessels may be collapsed, disorganized, or absent.[24] The skin also contains lymphatics. The lymphatics begin in the superficial papillary dermis as blind-ended vessels that are lined by endothelial cells without a basal lamina. The more proximal portion of the lymphatic system within the superficial fascia contains thicker walls and valves.

Nerves

The nerves in the skin are distributed in a network that resembles the vascular network previously described. Cutaneous nerves are either sensory or autonomic. Nerves in the skin appear as nerves elsewhere in the peripheral nervous system. With routine H&E stains, the sensory nerves cannot be distinguished from the autonomic nerves. The sensory nerves are afferent nerves that carry the sensations of pain, itching, temperature, pressure, and proprioception. The sensory impulses begin in nonencapsulated receptors or encapsulated receptors. The nonencapsulated receptors include the end organs, which reside in the dermal papillae and wrap around the hair follicles, and the neural–Merkel cell complexes. The encapsulated receptors include the Meissner and Vater-Pacini corpuscles. The Meissner corpuscles that mediate the sensation of touch are located in the dermal papillae and appear as a string wound around a spindle. The Vater-Pacini corpuscles that mediate the sensation of pressure are located in the superficial fascia, most abundantly in the palms and soles, and appear as oval bodies with internal concentric lamellae. The efferent nerves in the skin are mainly autonomic and originate in the sympathetic system. These nerves innervate the glomus bodies, the smooth muscles of blood vessels, the smooth muscles, the arrector pili (i.e., smooth muscles connected to hair follicles), and the apocrine and eccrine glands. Innervation of these nerves thus causes the blood vessels to constrict, hair to stand, goose bumps to appear, and sweating to occur.

Pilosebaceous Unit

The pilosebaceous unit consists of the hair, hair follicle, sebaceous gland, sensory end organ, and arrector pili muscle. This unit makes hair and an oily, fatty emollient; it also has a sensory and motor function. In many areas of the skin, such as the scalp, the hair is dense and thick. This hair is referred to as the terminal hair. In other areas of the body, such as the temples, the hair is thin and almost imperceptible. This fine hair is vellus hair. In some areas of the body, such as the nose, the sebaceous portion of the pilosebaceous unit is enlarged and is the predominant part of the unit; in other areas, the hair portion of the pilosebaceous unit is prominent and the sebaceous portion minimal. Only on the palms, soles, and mucous membranes is the pilosebaceous unit absent.

Hair and Hair Follicle

The hair follicle, a structure from which a hair arises, is composed of three portions (**Fig. 1.8**). The topmost portion is the infundibulum, which extends from the surface of the skin to the level of the opening of the sebaceous gland duct into the follicle. When apocrine glands are also present, these may empty into the infundibulum. The isthmus connects the infundibulum with the area at which the arrector pili muscle inserts into the follicle. The inferior portion is the portion of the follicle below the insertion of the arrector pili muscle. Hair arises from the hair bulb, the lowest portion of the hair follicle. The hair bulb is a rounded structure that contains the hair matrix. The hair matrix consists of cells with vesicular nuclei and basophilic cytoplasm that give rise to the hair. Also found within the hair bulb are melanocytes that are incorporated into growing hairs. The hair bulb surrounds as a cap the papilla that contains specialized mesenchymal cells and is a dermal structure. The hair papilla influences the activity within the hair matrix from which the hair shaft and inner and outer root sheaths arise.

The hair shaft is formed by keratinization of the cells within the hair matrix. The mature hair shaft has a complicated structure with several distinct layers. The innermost portion is the medulla, which is absent in vellus hair but present in nonvellus hair. The next layer is a cortex and a hair cuticle, which consists of shingles of overlapping cells. Above the matrix more layers appear. The inner and the outer root sheaths are keratinized layers that form support for the growing hair. Surrounding the outer root sheath is the vitreous, an eosinophilic band that is continuous but thicker than the epidermal basement zone. The final two layers are the fibrous root sheath and the periadventitia dermis.

Hair growth occurs in cycles with anagen, catagen, and telogen stages. The anagen stage is the growth stage. During this stage the inferior portion of the hair elongates and forms a bulb that contains the matrix within which is the dermal papilla. The catagen stage is an involutional stage in which the inferior portion of the hair ascends to

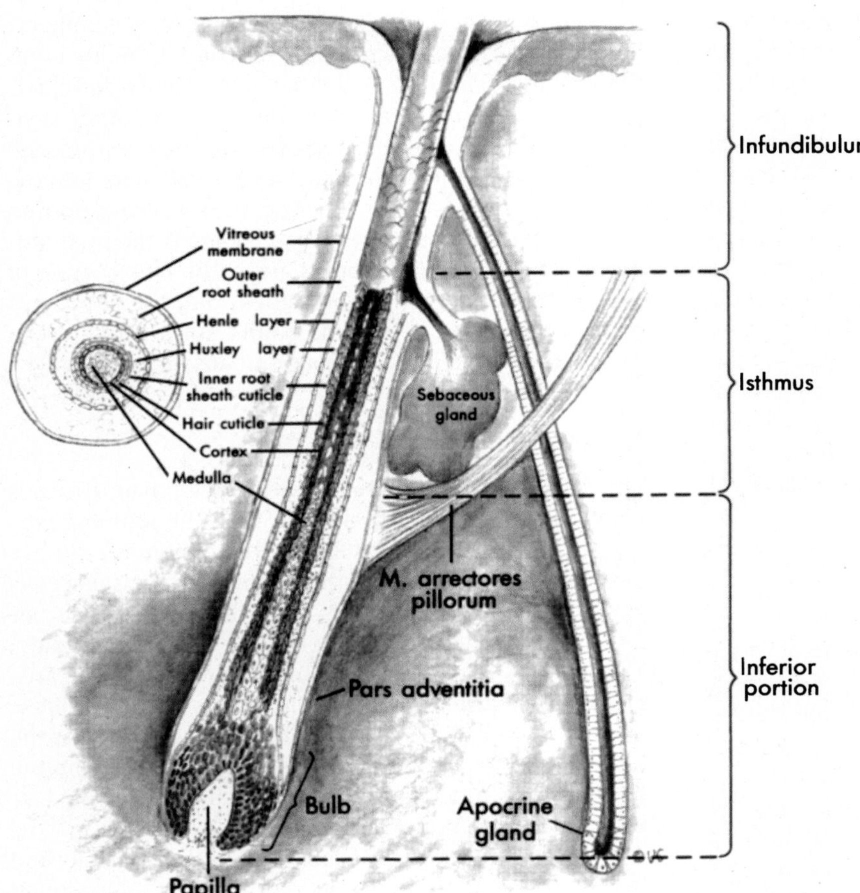

Fig. 1.8 Hair shaft and hair follicle.

the level of the attachment of the arrector pili muscle. In its path of retreat, a band of collagen can be distinguished. The telogen phase is the resting phase. During this stage, the inferior portion of the follicle is absent. With aging, the number, rate of growth, and diameter of hair shafts declines. Gray hair is also seen with advanced age and results from decreased amounts of pigment within hair shafts. On electron microscopy, gray hair contains melanocytes but with large vacuoles in their cytoplasms. The melanosomes are not fully melanized.[14]

Arrector Pili Muscles

Associated with hair follicles are the arrector pili muscles. These small muscles insert onto the hair follicles below the sebaceous gland duct and extend obliquely upward into the papillary dermis where they are anchored. Contraction of the arrector pili muscles is caused by sympathetic nerves and causes the hair to be pulled from an oblique position to a more vertical position. Clinically, this contraction results in slight elevations of the skin, known as cutis anserina or goose bumps.

Sensory Nerves

Also associated with hair follicles are the sensory nerves (the end organs) that ramify in a netlike fashion around the isthmus and inferior portions of the follicle. As the hairs are brushed, these sensory nerves are activated.

Sebaceous Gland

The sebaceous gland is associated with the hair follicle, and its duct empties into the hair follicle. In some areas of the body, the hair follicle is so small that the sebaceous glands appear to empty directly onto the skin. Sebaceous glands produce a fatty secretion, sebum, that provides emollients for the hair and skin. Sebum production peaks in late adolescence and is associated with acne. Thereafter, sebum production declines by ~23% per decade in men and 32% per decade in women.[49] This decrease is associated with a decreased androgen production. However, the decreased glandular production in the elderly does not parallel the sebaceous gland size, which actually increases with age.[50] A common lesion in middle-aged adults and the elderly is sebaceous hyperplasia. Sebaceous glands are present in most areas of the body except the palms and soles. There is a high density of sebaceous glands on the face, chest, and back. In some anatomical areas, sebaceous glands have special names (e.g., Fordyce spots on the lips, Tyson glands on the prepuce and labia minora, Montgomery tubercles on the areola, and meibomian glands on the eyelid). The sebaceous gland is unilobular or multilobular and empties into the hair follicle via a short duct. This duct is composed of squamous epithelium and ends in the infundibulum of the hair follicle. The cells on the periphery of the sebaceous gland are cuboidal with basophilic cytoplasm. These cells differentiate into larger lipid-filled cells whose borders disintegrate as the cells approach the sebaceous duct. The secretions of the sebaceous glands are holocrine and are under the influence of male and female sex hormones.

Eccrine Glands

The eccrine glands produce sweat. Eccrine glands are found everywhere on the skin surface except at the mucocutaneous junctions and the nail beds. Eccrine glands are particularly numerous on the palms, soles, and forehead. With aging the number and function of eccrine glands decrease. The eccrine unit is composed of the following three parts: a secretory gland, an intradermal duct, and an intraepidermal duct. The secretory gland is coiled and is situated in the deep dermis or subdermal fat. The lumen of the gland is surrounded by two types of secretory cells—clear cells that contain glycogen and dark cells that contain mucopolysaccharides. These secretory cells lie on a basal lamina that is surrounded by myoepithelial cells and periadnexal dermis. The gland itself is innervated by nonmyelinated cholinergic and adrenergenic fibers. The intradermal duct ascends through the dermis with a relatively straight course. The duct is lined by an eosinophilic cuticle produced by basophilic duct cells. Like the gland portion of the eccrine unit, the intradermal duct is surrounded by myoepithelial cells and periadnexal dermis. The intraepidermal duct spirals through the epidermis to the surface. The lumen of the intraepidermal duct is lined by cells that are keratinized.

Apocrine Glands

Apocrine glands produce a secretion that is odorless but when acted on by bacteria becomes odoriferous. Apocrine glands, unlike sweat glands, are found only in certain locations on the body. They are most numerous in the axillae and groin. In some areas of the body apocrine glands have special names (e.g., Moll glands on the eyelids, mammary glands on the breast, and ceruminous glands of the external auditory canal). The apocrine unit also consists of a secretory coil, an intradermal duct, and an intraepidermal duct. The secretory coil is located within the subdermal fat and has a large lumen. The secretory cells surrounding the lumen are cuboidal cells with eosinophilic cytoplasm. These cells show apical budding. The secretory cells rest on a basal lamina and are surrounded by elongated myoepithelial cells and periadnexal dermis. These glands are under both cholinergic and adrenergic stimulation. The intradermal portion of the duct ascends relatively straight and usually empties into the hair follicle above the sebaceous duct orifice. The duct may also open directly onto the skin surface. The intradermal portion of the duct has a double layer of basophilic cells resting on a basal lamina. The basal lamina is in turn surrounded by myoepithelial cells and periadnexal dermis.

Summary

The skin is a complex structure both anatomically and physiologically. Understanding this organ will enhance a surgeon's ability to predict its response to injury and to achieve the optimal cosmetic and functional result for the patient.

References

1. Hood AF, Kwan TH, Burnes DC, et al. Primer of Dermatology. Boston: Little, Brown; 1984
2. Murphy GF. Histology of the skin. In: Elder D, Elenitsas R, Jaworsky C, Johnson B, eds. Lever's Histopathology of the Skin. 8th ed. Philadelphia: JB Lippincott; 1997
3. Montagna W, Parakkal PF. The Structure and Function of the Skin. 3rd ed. New York: Academic; 1974
4. Goldsmith LA. My organ is bigger than your organ. Arch Dermatol 1990;126:301
5. Gilchrest BA. Physiologic and pathologic alterations in old skin. In: Platt D, ed. Geriatrics. 3rd ed. Berlin: Springer-Verlag; 1984
6. Gilchrest BA. Skin and photoaging: an overview. J Am Acad Dermatol 1989;21:610
7. Weiss JS, Ellis CN, Headington JT, et al. Topical tretinoin improves photoaged skin: a double-blind vehicle-controlled trial. JAMA 1988; 259:527
8. Fukugama K, Inone W, Suzuki H, et al. Keratinization. Int J Dermatol 1976;15:274
9. Muramatsu MS. Epidermal structural proteins. J Assoc Mil Dermatol 1990;16:28
10. Stingl G, Katz SI, Clement L, et al. Immunologic functions of Ia-bearing epidermal Langerhans cells. J Immunol 1978;121:2005
11. Streilein JW, Toews GB, Bergstresser PR. Langerhans cells: functional aspects revealed by in vivo grafting studies. J Invest Dermatol 1980;75:17
12. Thiers BH, Maize JC, Spicer SS, et al. The effect of aging and chronic sun exposure on human Langerhans cell populations. J Invest Dermatol 1984;82:223
13. Winkelmann RK. The Merkel cell system and a comparison between it and the neurosecretory or APUD cell system. J Invest Dermatol 1977;69:41

14. Gilchrest BA, Blog FB, Szabo G. Effects of aging and chronic sun exposure on melanocytes in human skin. J Invest Dermatol 1979; 73:141
15. Hu F. Aging of melanocytes. J Invest Dermatol 1979;73:70
16. Briggaman RA, Wheeler CE Jr. The epidermal-dermal junction. J Invest Dermatol 1975;66:71
17. Sakai LY, Keene DR, Morris NP, et al. Type VII collagen is a major structural component of anchoring fibrils. J Cell Biol 1986;103:1577
18. Tidman MJ, Eady RAJ. Ultrastructure morphometry of normal human dermal-epidermal junction: the influence of age, sex, and body region on lamina and nonlaminar components. J Invest Dermatol 1984;83:448
19. Hauser C, Saurat JH, Schmitt A, et al. Interleukin-1 is present in normal human epidermis. J Immunol 1986;136:3317
20. Postlethwaite AE, Lachman LB, Mainardi CL, et al. Interleukin-I stimulation of collagenase production by cultured fibroblasts. J Exp Med 1983;157:801
21. Woodley DT, Zelickson AS, Briggaman RA, et al. Treatment of photoaged skin with topical tretinoin increase epidermal–dermal anchoring fibrils. JAMA 1990;263:3057
22. Zelickson AS, Mottaz JH, Weiss JS, et al. Topical tretinoin in photoaging: an ultrastructural study. J Cutan Aging Cos Dermatol 1988;1:41
23. Grove GL, Duncan S, Kligman AM. Effect of aging on the blistering of human skin with ammonium hydroxide. Br J Dermatol 1982;107:393
24. Montagna W, Carlisle K. Structural changes in aging human skin. J Invest Dermatol 1979;73:47
25. Bhawan R. Histology of epidermal dysplasia. J Cutan Aging Cos Dermatol 1988;1:95
26. Evans R, Cowdry EV, Nielson PE. Aging of human skin. Anat Rec 1943; 86:545
27. Grove GL. Age-related differences in healing of superficial skin wounds in humans. Arch Dermatol Res 1982;272:381
28. Nanney LB, McKanna JA, Stoscheck CM, et al. Visualization of epidermal growth factor receptors in human epidermis. J Invest Dermatol 1984;82:165
29. O'Keefe EJ, Payne RE Jr. Modulation of the epidermal growth factor receptors of human keratinocytes by calcium ion. J Invest Dermatol 1983;81:231
30. Neal DE, Bennett MK, Hall RR, et al. Epidermal-growth factor receptors in human bladder cancer: comparison of invasive and superficial tumors. Lancet 1985;1:366
31. Eisen AZ. Human skin collagenase: relationship to pathogenesis of epidermolysis bullosa dytrophica. J Invest Dermatol 1969;52:449
32. Seltzer JL, Eisen AZ, Bauer EA, et al. Cleavage of type VII collagen by interstitial collagenase and type IV collagenase (gelatinase) derived from human skin. J Biol Chem 1989;264:3822
33. Stricklin GP, Bauer EA, Jeffrey JJ, et al. Human skin collagenase: isolation of precursor and active forms from both fibroblast and organ cultures. Biochemistry 1978;17:2331
34. Uitto J. Collagen biosynthesis in human skin: a review with emphasis on scleroderma. Ann Clin Res 1971;3:250
35. Shuster S, Black MM, McVitie E. The influence of age and sex on skin thickness, skin collagen, and density. Br J Dermatol 1975;93:639
36. Lavker RM, Zheng PS, Dong G. Aged skin: a study by light, transmission electron, and scanning electron microscopy. J Invest Dermatol 1987;88:44s
37. Anttinen H, Oikarinen A, Kivirikko KI. Age-related changes in human skin collagen galactosyltransferase and collagen glucosyltransferase activities. Clin Chim Acta 1977;76:95
38. Sandberg LB, Soskel NT, Leslie JG. Elastin structure, biosynthesis, and relation to disease states. N Engl J Med 1981;304:566
39. Cotta-Pereira G, Guetta RF, Bittencourt-Sampaio S. Oxytalan, elaunin, and elastic fibers in the human skin. J Invest Dermatol 1976;66:143
40. Bouissou H, Pieraggi MT, Julian M, et al. The elastic tissue of the skin: a comparison of spontaneous and actinic (solar) aging. Int J Dermatol 1988;27:327
41. Braverman IM, Fonferko E. Studies in cutaneous aging, I: The elastic fiber network. J Invest Dermatol 1982;78:434
42. Frances C, Robert L. Elastin and elastic fibers in normal and pathogenic skin. Int J Dermatol 1984;23:166
43. Pinkus H, Keech MK, Mehregan AH. Histopathology of striae distensae, with special reference to striae and wound healing in the Marfan syndrome. J Invest Dermatol 1966;46:238
44. Sakai LY, Keene DR, Enguall E. Fibrillin, a new 350-kD glycoprotein, is a component of extracellular microfibrils. J Cell Biol 1986; 103:2499
45. Hollister DW, Godfrey M, Sakai LY, et al. Immunohistologic abnormalities of the microfibrillar-fiber system in the Marfan syndrome. N Engl J Med 1990;323:152
46. Andrew W, Behnke RH, Sato T. Changes with advancing age in the cell population of human dermis. Gerontologia 1964–1965;10:1
47. Braverman IM, Fonferko E. Studies in cutaneous aging, II: The microvasculature. J Invest Dermatol 1982;78:444
48. Lavker RM, Kligman AM. Chronic heliodermatitis: a morphologic evaluation of chronic actinic dermal damage with emphasis on the role of mast cells. J Invest Dermatol 1988;90:325
49. Jacobsen E, Billings J, Frantz R, et al. Age-related changes in sebaceous wax ester secretion rates in men and women. J Invest Dermatol 1985; 85:483
50. Plewig G, Kligman AM. Proliferative activity of the sebaceous glands of the aged. J Invest Dermatol 1978;70:314

2 Wound Healing

Edmund Fisher and John L. Frodel Jr.

Cutaneous wound repair involves a complex yet coordinated series of biological events. Although complete understanding of all biochemical steps is probably unnecessary, it is essential for the facial plastic surgeon to know the basic stages of wound healing to achieve the best result. Virtually all wounds produce visible scars; even when the healing process is normal, functionally disabling scars may occur. Abnormal wound healing may involve hypertrophic scarring and keloid formation, which further compromise appearance and function. Accordingly, the surgeon must approach an acquired or iatrogenic wound carefully, considering the factors involved in wound repair. This chapter reviews basic cutaneous anatomy and the phases of wound healing and discusses factors affecting wound repair and scar formation.

History

Wound healing has been a concern throughout recorded history. The Edwin Smith Papyrus (1600 BC) represents the first documentation of wound care and healing.[1] War and the treatment of its casualties accounts for most of the information recorded in other ancient literature. Nearly 150 descriptions of wounds are included in Homer's account on the siege of Troy by the Greeks (*The Iliad*, 1000 BC). The use of so-called sovereign medicines was noted in the treatment of these wounds, along with a high mortality rate. By the time of Hippocrates (460 to 370 BC), established wound management included removal of foreign bodies, cleansing and drying of the wound, suturing (with crude techniques), and application of clean, dry dressings. Celsus (25 BC to AD 50) appears to be the first to discuss inflammation, but Galen (AD 130 to 200), in his treatment of Roman gladiators and soldiers, developed the doctrine of laudable pus (suppuration) as an important aspect of wound healing. Unfortunately, this notion was generally accepted until the fourteenth century when Henry de Mondeville (1260 to 1320) advised that wounds be cleaned and suppuration avoided. His doctrines were considered unacceptable by many but eventually prevailed. With the advent of gunpowder in the fourteenth century, a new type of wound was established. Cauterization with hot oil was the treatment of choice, with little reverence for cleanliness. Only when French surgeon Pare (1520 to 1590) found his oil supply exhausted and was forced to apply milder compounds (e.g., egg yolk, oil of roses, and turpentine) did this inhumane, ineffective treatment end.[1] Wound treatment has continued to evolve since the sixteenth century, although subsequent advances have been related primarily to the creation of optimal conditions for wound repair. Advances include debridement of necrotic tissues and foreign bodies, wound edge apposition, and use of aseptic technique (the Lister principle). Of comparable validity are the following tenets of Halsted that should be known and respected: gentle handling of tissue, aseptic technique, sharp anatomical dissection of tissue, careful hemostasis, obliteration of dead space, avoidance of tension, and reliance on rest.[2] Although the biological processes of wound healing have been more thoroughly described in this century, control over the healing process and thus the final outcome remains the goal.

Anatomical Considerations

Knowledge of the basic anatomical components of skin is essential to understanding wound healing.[3] Skin has two layers—the epidermis and the dermis—that contribute to wound healing (**Fig. 2.1**).

The epidermis is a protective, waterproof layer characterized by color, texture, and, unfortunately, scar tissue. The basal, or germinal, layer continually replicates, pushing dying keratin to the surface. Destruction of this superficial layer by an abrasion or burn allows tissue fluid weeping and exposes the wound to outside substances, such as bacteria or medications. Because the basal layers remain intact in such injuries, healing generally occurs without scarring. However, given that melanocytes are found in the epidermis, these injuries may result in discoloration. Because the epidermis contains no collagen fibers, wound strength is minimal. It does, however, have considerable growth potential, enabling rapid epithelial cell migration to seal fresh wounds within a few hours. The epidermis rests on the dermis in an irregular papillary surface interface (papillary ridges) that makes the two parts difficult to separate. Collagen, the most important component of this layer, is produced as a fibrous protein and, through extensive cross-linking, provides intrinsic strength to this layer. The process of laying down the collagen requires much more time than the rapid process of epithelial closure. The dermis also contains the blood supply to the skin and various epithelial-lined skin appendages, such as sweat and sebaceous glands.

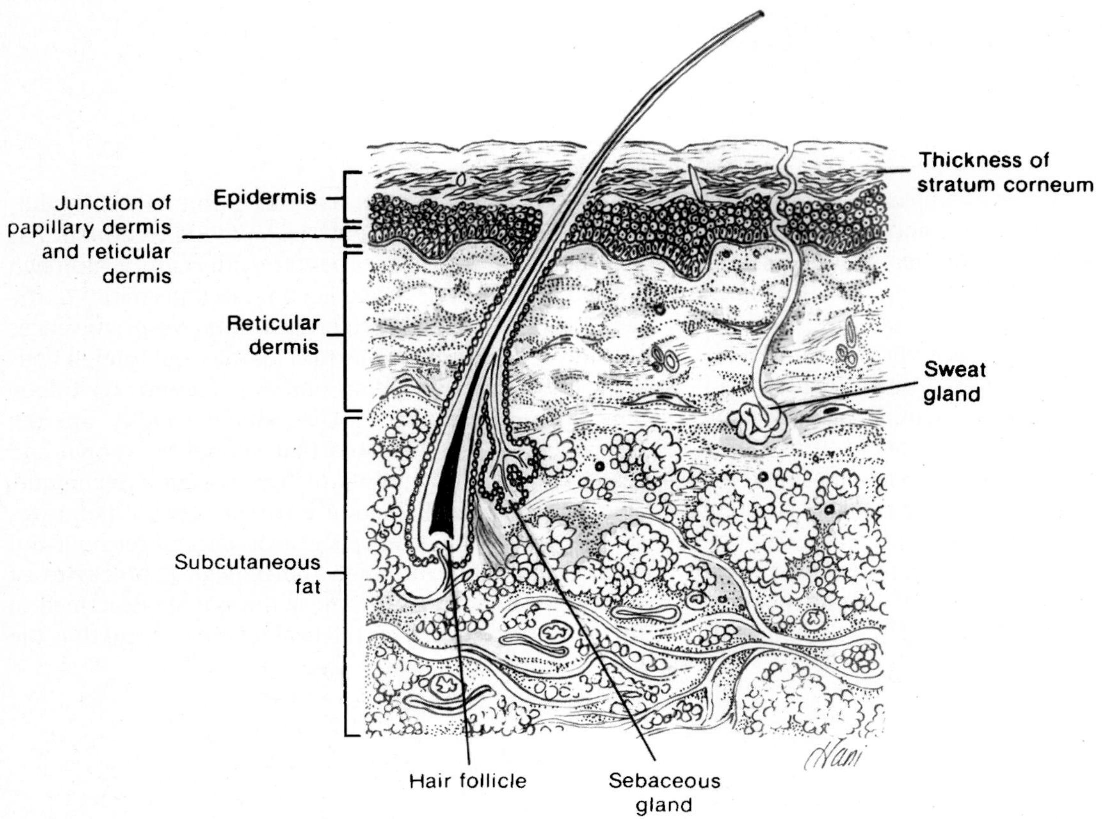

Fig. 2.1 Diagram of normal skin and appendages. (Modified from Koranda FC. Dermabrasion. In: Thomas JR, Holt GR, eds. Facial Scars: Incision, Revision, and Camouflage. St. Louis: CV Mosby; 1989. With permission.)

Sebaceous glands are epidermal-lined structures and the principal source of epithelial regeneration in dermal injuries.

Wound-Healing Phases

Wound healing is accomplished in multiple phases that occur over time (**Fig. 2.2**). Whether an injury is secondary to an abrasion, a burn, a contusion, or a laceration, an immediate vascular and inflammatory response occurs. Local vasoconstriction is the initial event and lasts 5 to 10 minutes. With endothelial cell injury, the coagulation cascade is activated, resulting in platelet adhesion and aggregation into clots or plugs. Activated platelets release a variety of biologically active substances, including prostaglandins and vasoactive materials (i.e., serotonin, histamine, proteases, thromboxane) that further affect vascular tone. Various chemotactic and proliferative factors are also released, including platelet-derived growth factor (PDGF), epidermal growth factor (EGF), insulin-like growth factor (IGF-1), transforming growth factor–β (TGF–β), and fibroblast growth factor (FGF), which activate their target epithelial, endothelial, and fibroblast cells.[3–5] **Table 2.1** lists cytokines involved in wound healing. After the initial vasoconstriction, active vasodilation takes place, probably secondary to histamine release from mast cells, and circulates serotonin. These factors, along with enzymes that affect norepinephrine and proteolytic enzymes that activate kallikrein, which in turn activates the kinins, significantly increase vascular permeability by allowing endothelial cell separation. Microvascular permeability changes increase for the first 48 to 72 hours, allowing the inflammatory phase to persist.[3] The cellular response in the inflammatory phase lags slightly behind the vascular changes. Fibronectin appears to be a major component of granulation tissue because it promotes the migration of neutrophils, monocytes, fibroblasts, and endothelial cells into the region. Cross-linking between the clot and fibronectin provides a temporary matrix by which epithelial cells and fibroblasts may proliferate in the wound.[5,6] Polymorphonuclear leukocytes (granulocytes) and monocytes appear shortly after injury. The granulocytes are stimulated by chemotactic factors and act primarily to remove bacteria and debris from the wound. These short-lived cells disappear rapidly in the

Table 2.1 Cytokines Involved in Wound Healing

Cytokine	Abbreviation	Source	Function
Human growth hormone	GH	Pituitary gland	Fibroblast proliferation; increases collagen content and tensile strength; anabolism; stimulates IGF-1
Epidermal growth factor	EGF	Platelets, bodily fluids (including epithelial cell and fibroblast saliva, urine, milk, and plasma)	Epithelial cell and fibroblast proliferation and migration; activates fibroblasts; angiogenic
Platelet-derived growth factor	PDGF	Platelets, macrophages, fibroblasts, endothelial cells, smooth muscle cells	Mitogenic for fibroblasts and smooth-muscle cells chemoattractant for neutrophils and macrophages; angiogenic
Fibroblast growth factor	FGF	Macrophages, brain, pituitary gland	Proliferation and migration of vascular endothelial cells; mitogenic and chemotactic for keratinocytes and fibroblasts
Transforming growth factors	TGF	Platelets, fibroblasts, neutrophils, macrophages, lymphocytes	Epithelial cell and fibroblast factors proliferation
Nerve growth factor	NGF	Schwann cell, muscle cells	Motor neurons, Schwann cells, muscle cells
Brain-derived neurotrophic factor	BDNF	Central nervous system, skeletal muscle, heart, lung	Support cranial and spinal factor motor neurons after axotomy
Ciliary neurotrophic factor	CNTF	Schwann cells	Promote survival and differentiation of neural and glial cells within the nervous system
Insulin-like growth factor–1	IGF-1	Fibroblasts, liver, plasma	Fibroblast proliferation, synthesis of proteoglycans and collagen
Tumor necrosis factor	TNF	Macrophages, mast cells, lymphocytes, other tissues and cells	Fibroblast proliferation
Interleukins	IL	Macrophages, lymphocytes, lymphocytes, other tissues and cells	Fibroblast proliferation, neutrophil chemotaxis
Interferons	IFN	Fibroblasts, lymphocytes	Inhibition of fibroblast proliferation and collagen synthesis
Keratinocyte growth factors	KGF	Fibroblasts	Epithelial cell proliferation

Source: Terris DJ. Dynamics of wound healing. In: Bailey BJ, ed. Head and Neck Surgery—Otolaryngology. Philadelphia: Lippincott-Raven; 1998. With permission.

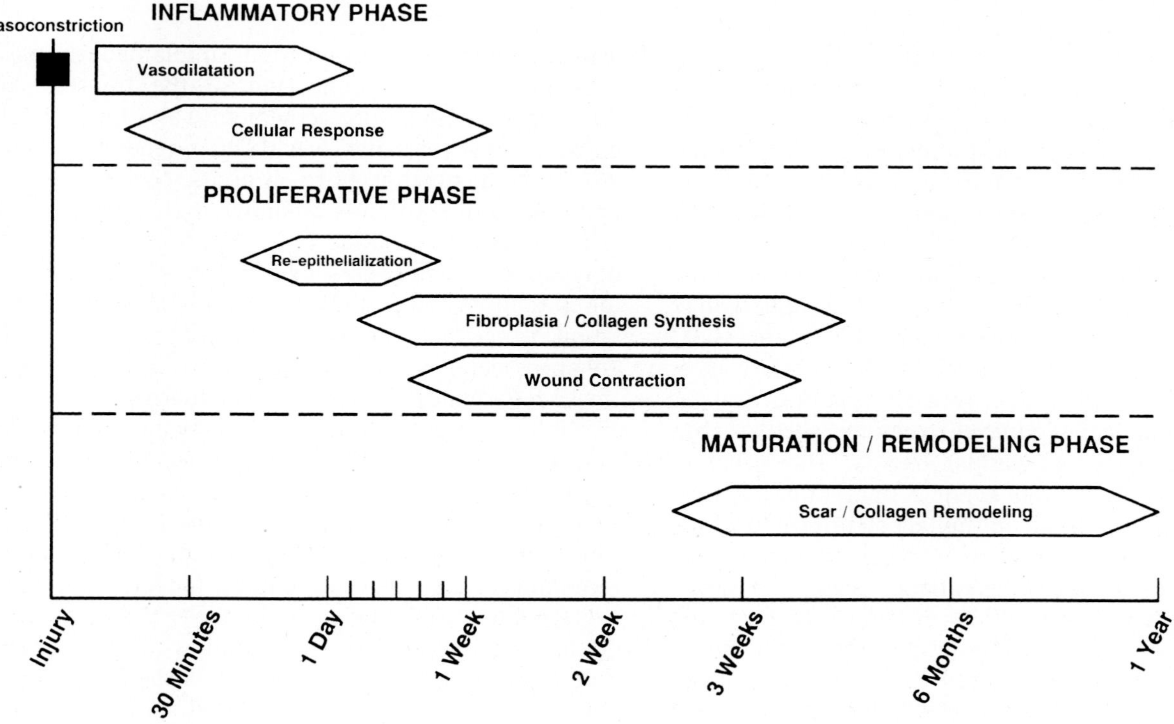

Fig. 2.2 Phases of wound healing.

noncontaminated wound. In the contaminated wound, however, granulocytes persist and prolong the inflammatory phase. This important extended inflammation may account for more severe end-stage scarring. Accordingly, it is important to progress from this stage as quickly as possible so that the wound may close and subsequent collagen deposit may begin.[3] In contrast, healing will proceed in the clean wound without the presence of granulocytes if there is normal macrophage, fibroblast, and endothelial cell function.[7] Perhaps the most important component of the cellular response of the inflammatory phase is the macrophage.[8] This becomes the predominant cell type by day 3 or 4.[3] Although phagocytosis and tissue debridement are an important function of macrophages, release of chemotactic and growth factors, including TGF–β, basic FGF, EGF, TGF–α, and PDGF, for endothelial cell and fibroblast proliferation may be the most significant functions.[9–11] In the context of poor macrophage function, granulation tissue formation, fibroplasia, and collagen production are impaired, as well as overall wound healing.[12] Lymphocytes produce TGF–β, interferons, interleukins, and tumor necrosis factor, which also interact with the macrophage during the inflammatory process, linking the immune response to wound repair.[13] The transition from inflammation to subsequent conditions illustrates the complexity and overlap of the concept of successive stages in wound healing. Interaction of the vascular and cellular responses prepares the wound for formation of granulation tissue, epithelial repair, and collagen deposition. In the first few days after injury, wound strength is minimal and relies primarily on fibrin clot and early epithelialization.[2,3] Only when inflammation subsides does collagen deposition begin, with subsequent increases in tensile wound strength. The next major aspect of wound healing is the proliferative phase, which includes epithelial regeneration, fibroplasia and collagen formation, wound contraction, and neovascularization. Epithelial regeneration plays a critical role in the wound repair process. With the completion of this process there is reestablishment of a barrier to protect underlying tissues from bacteria and foreign material. The process of reepithelialization begins within 24 hours of injury as a migration of epithelial cells from surrounding wound margins or from deeper adnexal structures, such as hair follicles or sebaceous glands, begins. The precise initiating stimulus for this event is uncertain, but the process begins with basal epithelial cell differentiation and separation from the underlying basement membrane and dermis.[3,9,14,15] This cell differentiation begins a complex process by which active mitosis of basal cells leads to migration across the wound (**Fig. 2.3**). The advancing front of epithelial cells continues until it comes into contact with similar epithelial cells. A contact inhibition of migration occurs, followed by further mitotic differentiation

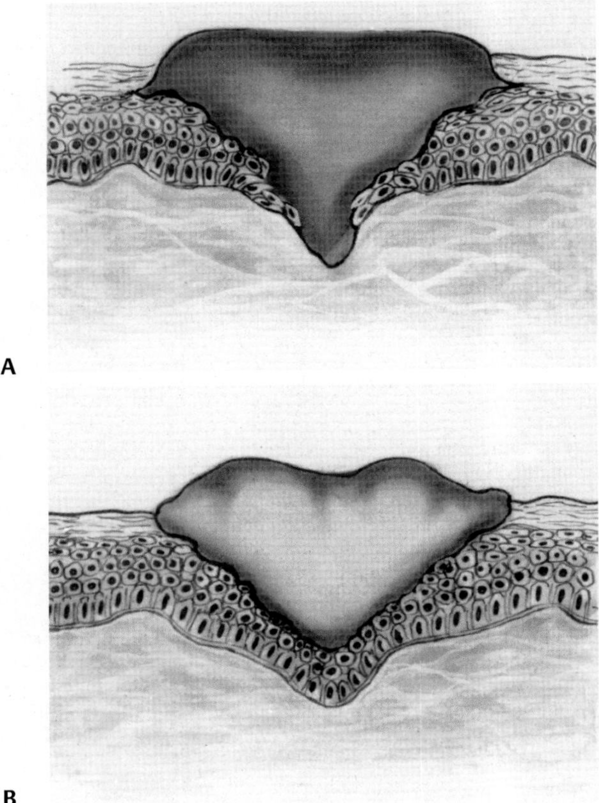

Fig. 2.3 (**A**) Differentiated and dividing basal epithelial cells migrating beneath dried clot. (**B**) Contact inhibition and further differentiation with epithelial stratification.

leading to epithelial stratification. Simultaneously, basal cells next to the wound and in the injured skin appendages begin mitotic activity, thus assisting in thickening the new epithelial layer.[14] This extended epithelial growth is maximal at 48 to 72 hours. The stimulus for epithelial proliferation is unknown, but it appears that EGF and its close relative TGF–α13 are involved. These polypeptides have been shown to function as mitogens for epithelium and stimulants for fibroplasia and granulation tissue.[9,16,17] Research also suggests that EGF enhances early wound healing, particularly in partial-thickness wounds.[18] Chalones, which are glycoproteins that inhibit epidermal replication, may also be involved in increasing epidermal proliferation in an open wound when they are temporarily lost until the epidermis regenerates.[19] In wounds closed primarily, epithelialization may be completed in 24 to 28 hours, but secondary intention wounds take considerably longer, especially if the wound is full thickness. In these cases, minimal epithelial migration usually continues for 3 to 5 days until a granulation bed has been established.[3] It has long been understood that a moist wound surface enhances normal wound healing. Conversely, wound desiccation

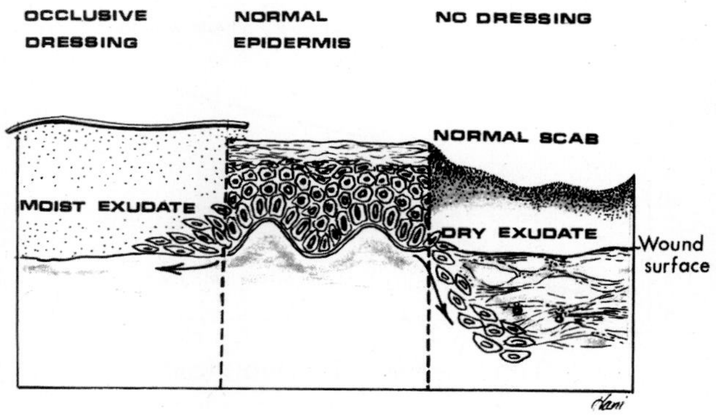

Fig. 2.4 Effects of moist occlusion on promoting more rapid epithelialization than when under dried clot. (Modified from Winter GD. Epidermal regeneration studied in the domestic pig. In: Maibach HI, Rovee DT, eds. Epidermal Wound Healing. Chicago: Year Book Medical Publishers; 1972. With permission.)

significantly impairs normal wound healing (**Fig. 2.4**).[20] When a crust or scab forms, the underlying dermis becomes desiccated and partially necrotic. Accordingly, the migrating epidermis takes a longer, less efficient route, thus delaying epithelialization. In occluded moist wounds, migration is direct and unimpeded, providing more rapid wound coverage.[5,21] As reepithelialization proceeds, granulation tissue forms beginning 3 to 4 days after injury. It consists of inflammatory cells, new blood vessels, and fibroblasts in a bed containing fibrin, glycoproteins, newly formed collagen, and glycosaminoglycans.[5] Granulation tissue persists until reepithelialization is completed. Fibroblasts appear in the wound as early as day 2 or 3 and play an important role in healing. Fibroblasts migrate and replicate in response to mediators (C5a, fibronectin, PDGF, FGF, and TGF–β).[22] Besides producing collagen, fibroblasts are important in the production of elastin, fibronectin, glycosaminoglycans, and collagenase, which is important in the later maturation and remodeling phase.[23] Fibroblasts, along with perivascular mesenchymal cells, differentiate into myofibroblasts, which are important for wound contraction.[5,24] Glycosaminoglycans are complex polysaccharides that are important to the early granulation tissue response. Hyaluronic acid initially predominates but is replaced by chondroitin 4-sulfate, dermatan sulfate, and other proteoglycans.[5] Together these make up the ground substance that is important for subsequent collagen formation.[14] Although collagen is present in the wound as early as day 3, the rate of synthesis increases dramatically by day 4. It is commonly believed that the fibroblastic aspect of the proliferative phase begins at this time.[25] Collagen molecules, or tropocollagen, are aggregated into filaments, which in turn are woven into fibrils via complex intermolecular bonding. Finally, the fibrils combine in a ropelike fashion to form the collagen fiber[14] (**Fig. 2.5**).

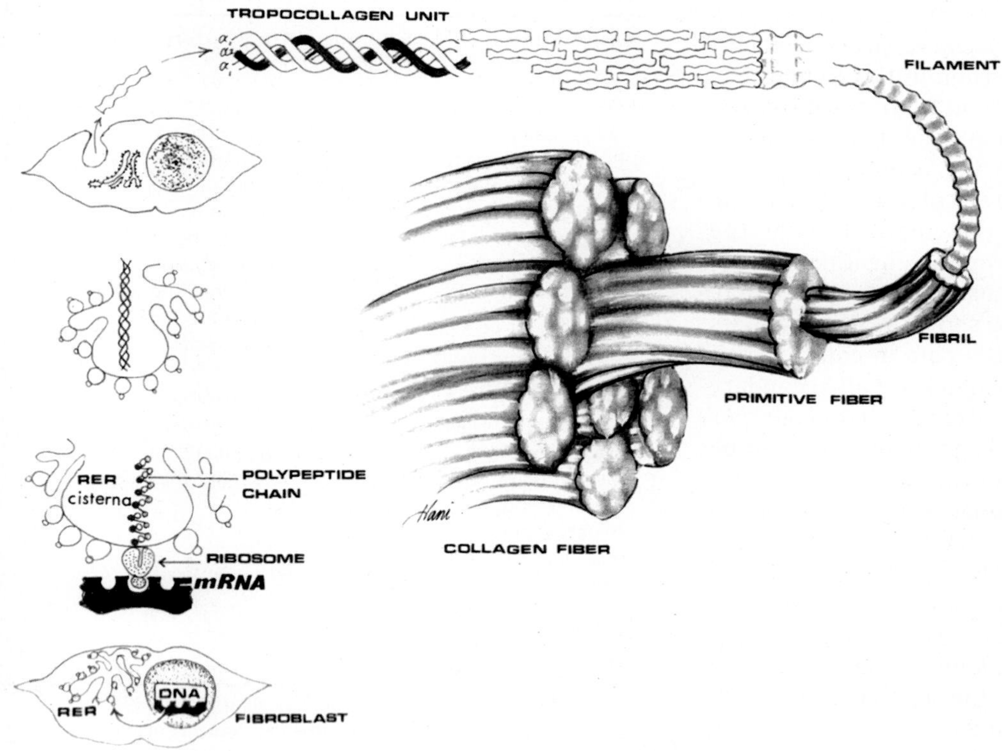

Fig. 2.5 Summary of collagen formation.

In the early period of fibroplasia, type III collagen predominates. As the scar matures, however, type I collagen is the major component of scar tissue.[9] Although wound tensile strength is minimal in the first few days, there is a gradual increase in strength corresponding to the amount of collagen in the wound. At the end of the inflammatory phase, ~5 to 7 days, the wound has only ~10% of its final tensile strength. Collagen synthesis and degradation reach a maximum ~3 weeks after injury.[3] A period of maturation follows, during which collagen formation subsides and fibroblasts decrease in the scar. Discussion of the proliferative phase is not complete without a discussion of wound contraction neovascularization. Because the wound must be essentially closed before other long-term healing phases will progress, an attempt to contract the wound is begun in full-thickness wounds. This contraction is centripetal, mediated by the myofibroblast, and maximal at 10 to 15 days. If a wound is left open for a long time, contraction may become severe, especially if significant inflammation is present.[3] In the presence of skin grafts, wound contraction is less severe but still a significant factor. Even with full-thickness skin grafts, 20% contraction will generally occur.[26] Neovascularization is obviously important to the healing wound. Early endothelial cell migration through the basement membrane is followed by angiogenesis, which is stimulated by macrophages, platelets, lymphocytes, and mast cells. These cells release numerous growth factors, including FGF, PDGF, TGF–α and β, and vascular endothelial growth factor. Low oxygen tension in the wound may stimulate an angiogenesis factor from macrophages, leading to the formation of new vascular channels.[27] As oxygenated blood reaches the wound, this factor decreases stimulation of neovascularization, leading to an eventual decrease in vascularization of the scar.[9] The final stage of wound healing is the maturation or remodeling phase. During this period, the scar becomes stronger and shows a decrease in its dimensions and erythema. It is pale in color, softer, and less protruding. These changes are all secondary to the remodeling and reorganization that occurs. As mentioned, type III collagen is gradually replaced by type I collagen. Water resorption around the scar allows further organization of the collagen fibers.[5] Although these fibers are initially in disarray, they gradually line up in a more parallel fashion, increasing tensile strength and improving appearance. Likewise, neovasculature regresses and the final scar is relatively avascular. Completion of the remodeling phase may take 12 to 18 months. At this time, the scar has ~70 to 80% of the tensile strength of unwounded normal skin (**Fig. 2.6**).

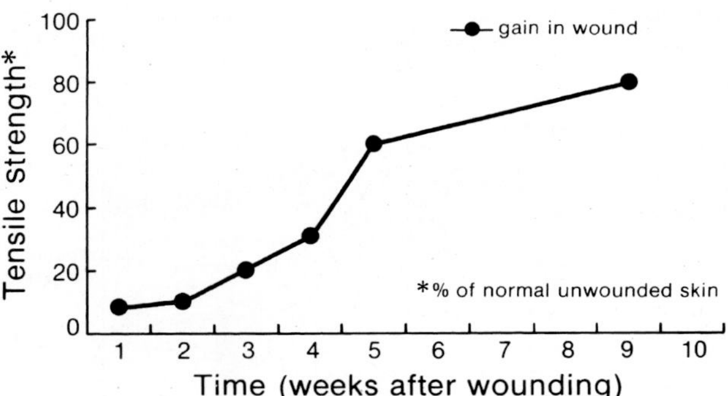

Fig. 2.6 Increase in wound tensile strength with time after injury. (Modified from Goslin JB. Wound healing for the dermatologic surgeon. J Dermatol Surg Oncol 1988;14(a):965. With permission.)

Clinical Considerations in Wound Healing

Although wound healing proceeds in a systematic fashion, local factors and systemic considerations may affect healing. Attempts have been made for hundreds of years to hasten the healing process, but no condition or substance has been shown unequivocally to achieve this goal. More importantly, certain local wound conditions and systemic deficiencies that impair optimal wound healing have been noted (**Table 2.2**).

Table 2.2 Factors That Impede Wound Healing

Disease States	Local Factors
Hereditary	Ischemia
Coagulation disorders	Infection
Ehlers–Danlos/Marfan syndrome	Tissue trauma
Prolidase deficiency	Retained foreign body
Werner syndrome	Desiccation
Vascular disorders	Medications
Congestive heart failure	Glucocorticoids
Atherosclerosis	Anticoagulants
Hypertension	Antineoplastic agents
Vasculitis	Colchicine
Venous stasis	Penicillamine
Lymphedema	Vitamin E
Metabolic	Salicylates (high dose)
Chronic renal failure	Nonsteroidals (high dose)
Diabetes mellitus	Zinc sulfate (high dose)
Malnutrition	Vitamin A (high dose)
Cushing syndrome	
Hyperthyroidism	
Immunologic deficiency states	
Others	
Chronic pulmonary disease	
Liver failure	
Malignancy	

Source: Terris DJ. Dynamics of wound healing. In: Bailey BJ, ed. Head and Neck Surgery—Otolaryngology. 2nd ed. Philadelphia: Lippincott-Raven Publishers, 1998. With permission.

Local Wound Healing Factors

Of absolute importance to normal wound healing is the local wound environment. Factors in this environment that may be affected by the clinician are reviewed in the following sections.

Wound Closure Techniques

Good surgical technique is essential for normal wound repair. Crushing skin edges with inappropriately large forceps, tying sutures too tightly, and cauterizing too excessively may result in local tissue inflammation, necrosis, and, potentially, infection. If improper suture material is used, similar events may occur. The surgeon must always take into account basic surgical principles as a major factor in the wound healing process.

Wound Desiccation

Adequate wound humidity is essential for proper healing. Studies suggest that epithelial cells migrate if there is adequate surface moisture.[20,28] Desiccated, crusted (i.e., scabbed) wounds heal much more slowly than those that are kept moist. As shown in **Fig. 2.4**, epithelial cells will select a pathway of migration at a proper moisture or humidity level deep to the crusted scab area in a desiccated wound. Not only is this often a longer route for epithelial closure, it is also one that requires increased energy expenditure by the cell. If the wound is kept moist, particularly with an occlusive dressing, migration proceeds more directly and efficiently.[5,28] Accordingly, numerous semiocclusive or occlusive dressings have been developed. Studies suggest that minimal atmospheric oxygen is directly absorbed through an open wound; thus, even totally occlusive dressings allow normal wound healing.[21,29] With either type of dressing, epithelialization is enhanced, thus decreasing epithelial closure time by up to 50%.[21,28,30,31] Occlusive dressings have the added advantage of promoting fibroblast, keratinocyte, and endothelial cell proliferation because of the fluid that collects under these impermeable membranes, which contains PDGF.[32–34] However, bacteria may have the opportunity to proliferate under such dressings. **Table 2.3** presents some of the commonly used biosynthetic occlusive or semiocclusive dressings.[9,21,35] Clinical evidence supports the use of such dressings after carbon

Table 2.3 Types of Newer Surgical Dressings

Name	Types of Composition	Transparent	Adherent	Absorbent	Gas Permeable	Fluid Permeable	Clinical Uses
Opsite	Polyurethane	Yes	Yes	No	Yes	No	Sutured wounds, cutaneous ulcers, skin graft sites, laser wounds
Tegaderm	Polyurethane	Yes	Yes	No	Yes	No	Same as for Opsite
Bioclusive	Polyurethane	Yes	Yes	No	Yes	No	Same as for Opsite
Ensure	Polyurethane	Yes	Yes	No	Yes	No	Same as for Opsite
Flexan	Two-layer polyurethane	No	Yes	Yes	Yes	No	Laser wounds
Revita-Derm	Three-layer polyurethane	No	Yes	Yes	Yes	No	Laser wounds
Vigilon	Polyurethane oxide/water	Partially	No	Yes	Yes	Yes	Dermabrasion, laser wounds
Second Skin	Polyurethane oxide/water	Partially	No	Yes	Yes	Yes	Dermabrasion, laser wounds, friction blisters
Duoderm	Hydrocolloid	No	Yes	Yes	No	No	Cutaneous ulcers, sutured wounds, dermabrasion, friction blisters
Comfeel Ulcus	Hydrocolloid	No	Yes	Yes	No	No	Same as for Duoderm
Biobrane	Silicone/nylon with collagen peptides	No	No	No	Yes	Yes	Thermal burns, dermabrasion
Silon-TSR	Silicone polymers	Yes	No	No	Yes	Yes	Laser wounds, dermabrasion
N-terface	Monofilament plastic	No	No	No	Yes	Yes	Skin grafts, dermabrasion, laser wounds

Source: Expanded and modified from Wheeland RG. The Miller surgical dressings and wound healing. Dermatol Clin North Am 1987;5(2):400.

dioxide (CO_2) laser skin resurfacing.[36,37] Topical medications are commonly utilized for abraded wounds and after wound closures. Eaglestein and Mertz noted the effect of various medications on the relative rate of healing.[38] For example, triamcinolone ointment hindered the relative rate of healing by 34% and petroleum jelly by 8%. On the other hand, polymyxin B sulfate (Neosporin ointment; Johnson & Johnson, Langhorn, PA) and silver sulfadiazine (Silvadene cream, King Pharmaceuticals, Inc., Bristol, TN) increased the healing rate by 28%.

Wound Tissue Ischemia

Local tissue ischemia caused by infection, hematoma, foreign bodies, anemia, or poor surgical technique may slow wound healing. Oxygen is consumed in higher quantities in a healing wound.[39] However, even under optimal wound healing conditions, tissue injury results in reduced oxygen when it is most needed. It should be noted that not all wound healing phases are affected by low oxygen tensions; chemotactic and growth factors, angiogenesis, and epithelial cell migration arepromoted by hypoxia.[9] However, for fibroblasts to proliferate and collagen synthesis to occur, a pO_2 of 30 to 40 mm Hg is necessary.[40] Oxygen supplementation, via hyperbaric oxygen administration, may improve the rate of epithelialization, but it appears not to have an impact on long-term wound healing results.[41]

Infection

Ischemic, contaminated states may lead to local bacterial wound infection. If this occurs, wound healing will be prolonged.[9] Bacteria delay normal healing phases by directly damaging cells of wound repair, by prolonging the inflammatory phase, and by competing for oxygen and nutrients within the wound.[9,42]

Systemic Wound-Healing Factors

Congenital Alterations

Genetic disorders affecting wound healing, rarely seen clinically, include Ehlers–Danlos syndrome, pseudoxanthoma elasticum, cutis laxa, osteogenesis imperfecta, progeria, and many others. Different types of the wound healing process causing pathological wound healing or defective collagen production result from congenital errors in metabolism.[42] Although diabetes mellitus may also be acquired, it is more commonly an inherited condition that affects wound healing in multiple ways. Microangiopathy diminishes oxygen delivery, whereas insulin deficiency is

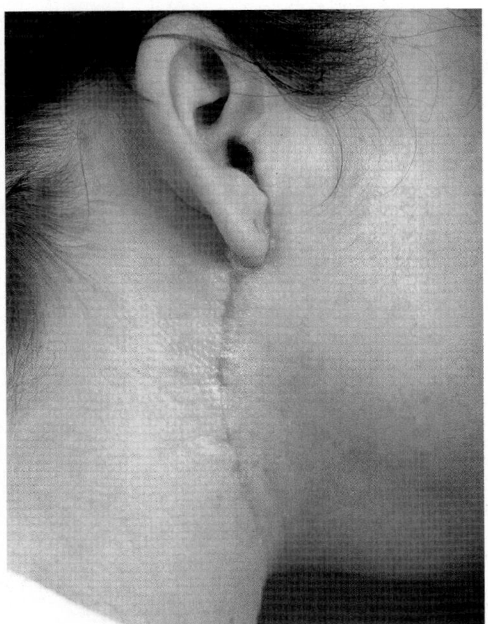

Fig. 2.7 Hypertrophic scar.

particularly significant in early wound healing phases when leukocyte function is defective. This combination of factors creates the potential for an increased incidence of wound infections.[39,42,43] Low insulin states also lead to defective collagen synthesis.[43] Early insulin therapy and supplemental vitamin A (25,000 units/day) appear to improve wound healing in patients with diabetes.[42,44] Hypertrophic scars and keloids represent genetic pathological "overhealing" states. The lesions are caused by excessive production and deposition of collagen and glycoprotein without equivalent degradation. Although a thorough discussion of hypertrophic scars and keloids is beyond the scope of this chapter, differences between the two are important for clinicians. Hypertrophic scars (**Fig. 2.7**) are elevated and remain within the original tissue injury site; they tend to regress with time. In contrast, keloids (**Fig. 2.8**) overgrow the boundaries of the original injury and invade the surrounding normal tissue.[42,45] Treatment of both hypertrophic scars and keloids is directed toward inhibiting collagen overproduction by a combination of intralesional corticosteroids and, occasionally, excision with postoperative pressure devices, silicon gel sheeting, interferon-α2b, or radiation.[46] However, recurrence is usually frequent, although one study reported only an 8% recurrence rate when surgery excision of keloids was combined with radiation or intralesional steroids and interferon-α2b.[47] Finally, TGF–β1 has been shown to induce keloid collagen growth. Future therapy may be aimed

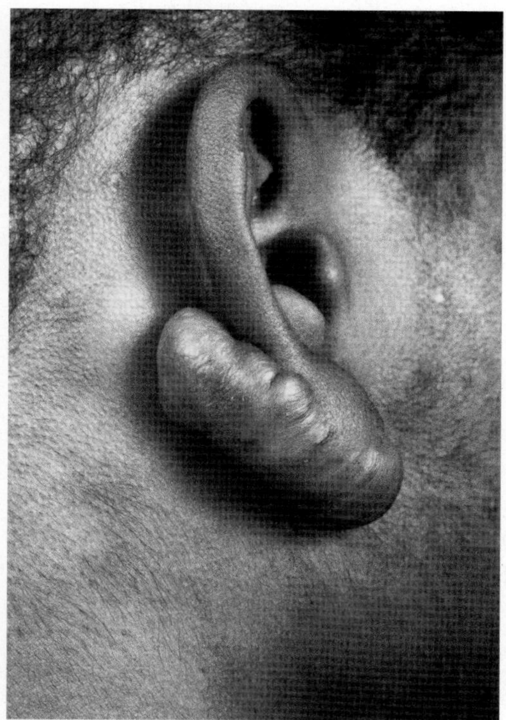

Fig. 2.8 Keloid.

at blocking the action of this growth factor in wounds prone to keloid formation.[22]

Acquired Alterations

Although no agent or process has been shown to improve wound healing unequivocally, certain deficiency and disease states are known to impair wound healing. Nutritional deficiencies rarely cause poor wound healing unless they are extremely severe, which may be the case in patients with cancer or alcoholism. Severe protein deficiency affects healing, and, in this circumstance, an effort to correct the nutritional state with administration of essential amino acids must be made to ensure normal wound healing.[9,25] Several vitamins play supportive substrate roles, and deficiencies may affect wound healing. Vitamin A deficiency inhibits epithelialization and wound closure, decreases collagen synthesis rates, and retards cross-linking of the collagen molecule.[3,5] As an important cofactor providing the hydroxylation of lysine and proline during collagen synthesis, vitamin C has long been known to be an important factor in wound healing. Because humans cannot synthesize vitamin C, bodily stores will only last 4 to 5 months before scurvy, with impaired wound healing, develops. Vitamin C is important in neutrophil function, serving as a reducing agent in superoxide radical formation. Thus deficiencies may increase wound infection and inhibit healing.[3,21] Because the production of clotting factors II, VII, IX, and X depend on cofactor vitamin K, prolonged bleeding and hematoma may occur in deficiency states; moreover, when the clot forms, it is similarly deficient in clotting factors and cannot develop a normal collagen matrix.[9,21,25] Vitamin E inhibits wound healing by decreasing collagen production and tensile strength but appears to have minimal impact on the healing process. Zinc and iron represent the most important trace elements involved in wound healing. Zinc is also an important component of enzymes in RNA and DNA synthesis and of collagenase.[5,21] Many diseases that are beyond the scope of this discussion also may impair wound healing. This group includes hereditary conditions, vascular diseases (e.g., congestive heart failure, atherosclerosis, venous stasis, lymphedema), metabolic disorders (e.g., chronic renal failure, diabetes, Cushing syndrome, hyperthyroidism), immune deficiency states, chronic liver disease, malignancies, and thrombocytopenic conditions.[5] Abnormal wound repair is commonly a result of poor nutrition or immunologic dysfunction in these medical conditions. Other aspects of wound healing are affected by the aging process. With age, healing proceeds more slowly, and thus there is decreased tensile strength.[21,48,49] Patients who have undergone radiation therapy are known to be at high risk for poor wound healing. Obliterative endarteritis may result in a wound with decreased collagen and poor tensile strength. In addition, other biochemical alterations at the molecular level probably play an important role.[25,50,51] Numerous systemic medications have an impact on wound healing, although only a few are clinically significant. Most important are the corticosteroids, which inhibit aspects of the inflammatory phase and eventually affect collagen synthesis and wound contraction.[52,53] Similarly, cellular defense mechanisms are affected, and the incidence of infection increases. Oral administration of vitamin A seems to reverse many of these adverse effects,[54] although routine administration of vitamins (e.g., vitamins C, A, E) or minerals (e.g., zinc) does not promote wound healing.[9] Various chemotherapeutic agents affect wound healing via their relationship to the inflammatory phase or by initiating collagen synthesis and wound contraction. Although early phases of wound repair may be inhibited by these agents, normal healing usually results.[55]

Future Considerations

Although a basic understanding of wound healing is evident in the literature, research in a variety of areas is needed, including the use of cutaneous growth factors and biological dressings. EGF along with polypeptides that stimulate RNA and DNA and protein synthesis have been shown to enhance the rate of healing of partial-thickness wounds.[18] Without question, further wound-enhancing modalities should be studied. Biological dressings and the use of cultured keratinocyte grafts merit watching in the future.[56] Large quantities of cultured autologous grafts can be grown and have been useful in the treatment of superficial wounds and as biological dressings.

Summary

The goal in management of cutaneous wounds is timely healing with an acceptable scar. Knowledge of the biology of tissue injury and repair is necessary to create optimal conditions for wound healing.

References

1. Howes PM. The latest wrinkles in wound healing. Am J Cosmet Surg 1985;2:42
2. Howes EL, Sooy JW, Harvey SC. The healing of wounds as determined by their tensile strength. JAMA 1929;92:42
3. Saski GH, Krizek TJ. Biology of tissue injury and repair. In: Giorgiade NG, et al, eds. Essentials of Plastic Maxillofacial and Reconstructive Surgery. Baltimore: Williams & Wilkins; 1967
4. Diegelmann RF. Cellular and biochemical aspects of normal and abnormal wound healing: an overview. J Urol 1997;157:298
5. Goslen JB. Wound healing for the dermatologic surgeon. J Dermatol Surg Oncol 1988;14:959
6. Grinnell F, Billingham RE, Burgess L. Distribution of fibronectin during wound healing in vivo. J Invest Dermatol 1981;76:181
7. Simpson DM, Ross R. The neutrophilic leukocyte in wound repair: a study with antineutrophil serum. J Clin Invest 1972;51:2009
8. Diegelmann RF, Cohen IK, Kaplan AM. The role of macrophages in wound repair: a review. Plast Reconstr Surg 1981;68:107
9. Goslen JB. Physiology of wound healing and scar formation. In: Thomas JR, Holt GR, eds. Facial Scars: Incision, Revision, and Camouflage. St Louis: CV Mosby; 1989
10. Kanzler MH, Gosulowsky DC, Swanson NA. Basic mechanisms in the healing cutaneous wound. J Dermatol Surg Oncol 1986;12:1156
11. Pierce GF. Macrophages: important physiologic and pathologic sources of polypeptide growth factors. Am J Respir Cell Mol Biol 1990;2:233
12. Leibovich SJ, Ross R. The role of the macrophage in wound repair: a study with hydrocortisone and antimacrophage serum. Am J Pathol 1975;78:71
13. Herndon DN, Nguyen TT, Gilpin DA. Growth factors: local and systemic. Arch Surg 1993;128:1227
14. Bryant WM. Wound healing. Clin Symp 1977;29:1
15. Peacock EE, Cohen IK. Wound healing. In: McCarthy JG, eds. Plastic Surgery. Vol 1. Philadelphia: WB Saunders; 1990
16. Burgess AW. Epidermal growth factor and transforming growth factor alpha. Br Med Bull 1989;45:401
17. King LE. What does epidermal growth factor do and how does it do it? J Invest Dermatol 1985;84:165
18. Brown GL, Curtsinger L, Brightwell JR. Enhancement of epidermal regeneration by biosynthetic epidermal growth factor. J Exp Med 1986;163:1319
19. Bullough WS, Lawrence EB. Mitotic control by internal secretion: the role of the chalone–adrenaline complex. Exp Cell Res 1964; 33:176
20. Winter GD. Effect of air drying and dressings on the surface of a wound. Nature 1963;197:91
21. Wheeland RG. The newer surgical dressings and wound healing. Dermatol Clin 1987;5:393
22. Hom DB. Wound healing in relation to scarring. Facial Plast Surg Clin North Am 1998;6:111
23. Van Winkle W. The fibroblast in wound healing. Surg Gynecol Obstet 1967;124:369
24. Stewart RJ, Duley JA, Dewdney J, et al. The wound fibroblast and macrophage, II: Their origin studied in a human after bone marrow transplantation. Br J Surg 1981;68:129
25. Rohrich RJ, Spicer TE. Wound healing/hypertrophic scars and keloids. Select Read Plast Surg 1986;4:1
26. Stegman SJ, Tromovich TA, Glogau RG. Grafts. In: Basics of Dermatologic Surgery. Chicago: Year Book Medical Publishers; 1982
27. Knighton DR, Hunt TK, Scheuenstuhl H, et al. Oxygen tension regulates the expression of angiogenesis factor by macrophages. Science 1983;221:1283
28. Hinman CD, Maibach H. Effect of air exposure and occlusion on experimental human skin wounds. Nature 1963;200:377
29. Varghese MC, Balin AK, Carter DM, et al. Local environment of chronic wounds under synthetic dressings. Arch Dermatol 1986;122:52
30. Goodson WH, Hunt TK. Wound healing in experimental diabetes mellitus: importance of early insulin therapy. Surg Forum 1978; 29:95
31. Winter GD. Formation of the scab and the rate of epithelialization of superficial wounds in the skin of the young domestic pig. Nature 1962;193:293
32. Alper JC, Tubbetts LL, Sarazen AA. The in vitro response to the fluid that accumulates under a vapor-permeable membrane. J Invest Dermatol 1985;84:513
33. Alvarez OM, Mertz PM, Eaglestein W. The effect of occlusive dressings on collagen synthesis and reepithelialization in superficial wounds. J Surg Res 1983;35:142
34. Katz MH, Alvarez AF, Kirsner RS, et al. Human wound fluid from acute wounds stimulates fibroblast and endothelial cell growth. J Am Acad Dermatol 1991;25:1054
35. Eaglstein WH. Effect of occlusive dressings on wound healing. Clin Dermatol 1984;2:107
36. Weinstein C, Ramirez OM, Pozner JN. Postoperative care following CO_2 laser resurfacing: avoiding pitfalls. Plast Reconstr Surg 1997;100:1855
37. Newman JP, Koch RJ, Goode RL. Closed dressings after laser skin resurfacing. Arch Otolaryngol Head Neck Surg 1998;124:751
38. Eaglstein WH, Mertz PM. "Inert" vehicles do affect wound healing. J Invest Dermatol 1980;74:90
39. Hunt TK. The physiology of wound healing. Ann Emerg Med 1988;17: 1265
40. Pai MP, Hunt TK. Effect of varying oxygen tensions on healing of open wounds. Surg Gynecol Obstet 1972;135:756
41. De Haan BB, Ellis H, Wilks M. The role of infection on wound healing. Surg Gynecol Obstet 1974;138:693
42. Carrico TJ, Mehrhof AI, Cohen IK. Normal and pathological wound healing. In: Giorgiade NG, et al, eds. Essentials of Plastic, Maxillofacial, and Reconstructive Surgery. Baltimore: Williams & Wilkins; 1987
43. Goodson WH, Hunt TK. Studies of wound healing in experimental diabetes mellitus. J Surg Res 1977;22:221
44. Seifter E, Rettura G, Padawer J, et al. Impaired wound healing in streptozotocin diabetes: prevention by supplemental vitamin A. Ann Surg 1981;194:42
45. Farrior RT, Stambaugh KI. Keloids and hyperplastic scars. In: Thomas JR, Holt GR, eds. Facial Scars: Incisions, Revision, and Camouflage. St Louis: CV Mosby; 1989
46. Terris DJ. Dynamics of wound healing. In: Bailey BJ, ed. Head and Neck Surgery: Otolaryngology. Philadelphia: Lippincott-Raven; 1998
47. Berman B, Bieley HC. Adjunct therapies to surgical management of keloids. Dermatol Surg 1996;22:126
48. Chvapil M, Koopman CF. Age and other factors regulating wound healing. Otolaryngol Clin North Am 1982;15:259

49. Goodson WH, Hunt TK. Wound healing and aging. J Invest Dermatol 1979;73:88
50. Reinisch JF, Puckett CL. Management of radiation wounds. Surg Clin North Am 1984;64:795
51. Rudolph R, Arganese T, Woodward M. The ultrastructure and etiology of chronic radiotherapy damage in human skin. Ann Plast Surg 1982;9:282
52. Pollack SV. Wound healing: a review, III: Nutritional factors affecting wound healing. J Dermatol Surg Oncol 1979;5:615
53. Reed BR, Clark RAF. Cutaneous tissue repair: practical implication of current knowledge. J Am Acad Dermatol 1985;13:919
54. Ehrlich HP, Tarver H, Hunt TK. The effects of vitamin A and glucocorticoids upon inflammation and collagen synthesis. Ann Surg 1973;177:222
55. Falcone RE, Nappi JF. Chemotherapy and wound healing. Surg Clin North Am 1984;64:779
56. Phillips TJ, Gilchrest BA. Cultured allogenic keratinocyte grafts in management of wound healing: prognostic factors. J Dermatol Surg Oncol 1989;15:1169

3 Soft Tissue Techniques

Ted A. Cook, Robert A. Guida, and Alan J. C. Burke

Expertise in facial plastic and reconstructive surgery requires knowledge and skills of basic soft tissue surgery. The face, with its excellent blood supply, variety of relaxed skin tension lines, and numerous anatomical boundary markers, offers great flexibility and challenge for rewarding cosmetic and reconstructive procedures. Superb results can be obtained if certain rudimentary principles are practiced. This chapter discusses equipment, techniques, and surgical principles that we consider necessary to achieve optimal results.

Best soft tissue technique requires a detailed understanding of our working substrate. Throughout the head and neck, the skin has widely different thicknesses (e.g., scalp vs eyelid), sebaceous content (alar vs cervical skin), vascularity, and other attributes, such as skin appendages like hair. Different areas require different handling. Care must be taken not to advance tissue from one anatomical unit to another because the quality of skin will often change, resulting in a disfiguring scar. The requirement for large or pedicled flaps and the need for tension applied to wound closure in turn requires an intimate knowledge of facial vascularity. Skin undermining and dissection should be done in the immediate subdermal layers to protect the dermal plexus of vessels in skin zones that receive watershed or random vascular supply. The random vascular supply refers to a blood supply from the musculocutaneous perforators that arborize in the subdermis. Axial flaps trace along the path of arterial vessels; therefore, they are more robust and can be more easily pedicled and transferred to areas of marginal vascular supply. Fortunately, the really excellent blood supply of the face provides for great resistance to infection and higher rates of wound healing in comparison with other tissues. At this juncture, it is important to note that smokers compromise their cutaneous circulation by causing prolonged vasoconstriction of the subdermal vascular plexus. Soft tissue viability following surgical manipulation can thus be seriously attenuated by smoking, affecting healing, scarring, and local flap viability.

Equipment

Soft Tissue Instrument Set

To obtain good soft tissue handling, proper instrumentation is mandatory. The basic soft tissue instrument set should include the 10 items listed and depicted in **Fig. 3.1**. Brown-Adson forceps are toothed to provide a firm grasp of deep soft tissue. For finer, less traumatic manipulation, as in skin closure, the delicate, single-toothed Bishop-Harman

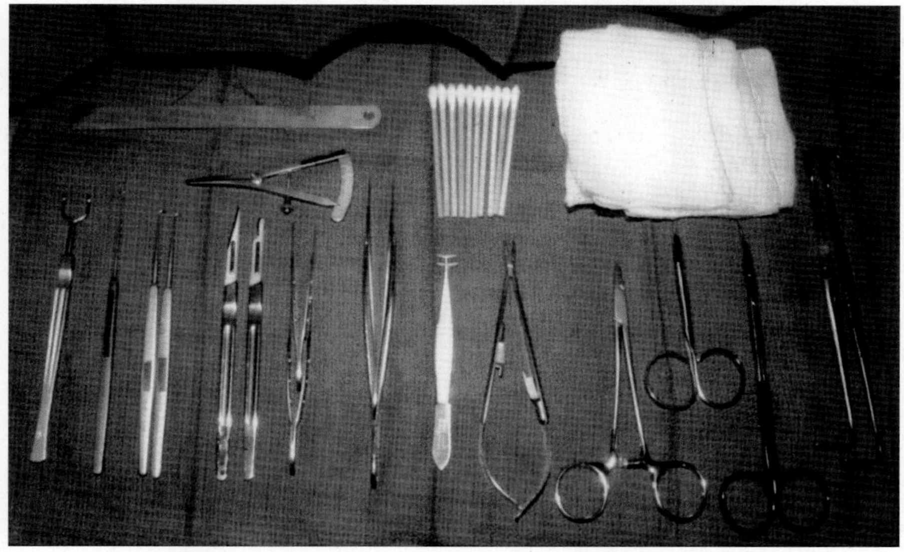

Fig. 3.1 Basic soft tissue instrument set: 1. Brown-Adson tissue forceps 2. Bishop-Harman tissue forceps 3. Single and double skin hooks 4. Webster needle holder 5. Castroviejo needle holder 6. Stevens tenotomy scissors 7. Castroviejo calipers 8. Small suture scissors 9. No. 15 knife blades 10. Moist sponges.

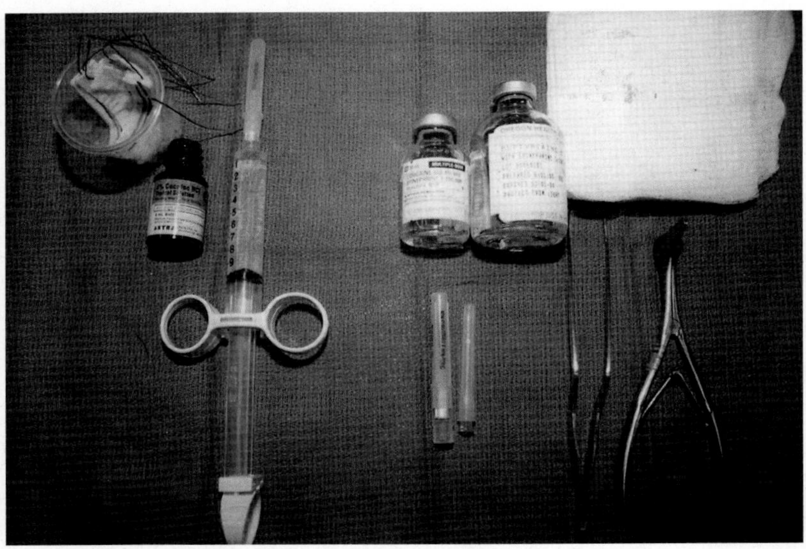

Fig. 3.2 Local anesthesia set.

forceps are used. Skin hooks inflict less tissue crushing than forceps and are essential for skin edge eversion and retraction needed in skin undermining or placement of subcuticular sutures. Two varieties of needle holders are used to effectively manage the smaller needles used for facial surgery. The Webster needle holder easily grasps smaller needles and is used for subcuticular or deep suturing of the head and neck. The delicate Castroviejo needle holder allows accurate placement of finer sutures for skin closure, nerve grafting, or other precise work. A variety of Stevens tenotomy scissors are used for undermining or cutting through soft tissues or skin. The tips are curved and blunted and should be used with the points directed upward when undermining and in the direction of the incision when cutting through skin. Smaller suture scissors are necessary to achieve more accurate cutting of the fine sutures used in facial work. Precision work and flap design frequently require measurement with Castroviejo calipers because of the easy maneuverability, 0 to 20 mm scale, and sharp tips that can be used for skin markings. Knife handles on the set include no. 3, no. 9, and the Beaver handle. The nos. 15 and 11 knife blades are the most frequently used in facial plastic surgery. The larger no. 10 blade is rarely required on facial skin. Finally, moist sponges are always used in soft tissue work on the face. A wet sponge causes less pulling and trauma to the soft tissue and blood vessels than a dry sponge.

Local Anesthesia Set

The majority of work done on the face can be accomplished with local anesthesia only (**Fig. 3.2**). The local set should consist of a 10 mL three-ringed syringe. The three-ringed holder offers control for injecting small amounts of anesthesia. A 30 gauge 1.5 in. needle minimizes the pain of injection. A sealed, packaged anesthetic agent, often 1% lidocaine with 1:100,000 epinephrine, is used in conjunction with sodium bicarbonate in a 9:1 mixture. Preservatives in the packaged anesthetic bottle lower the pH, causing increased pain on injection. This can be minimized by the buffering effect of the sodium bicarbonate. We most commonly use a 50:50 combination of 1% lidocaine, a short-acting amide, and 0.5% bupivacaine, a longer-acting amide, to provide longer-lasting local anesthesia. The addition of epinephrine reduces intraoperative bleeding by causing vasoconstriction and also prolongs anesthetic action by preventing leeching of anesthetic solution from the soft tissues (**Table 3.1**).

Photographic Equipment

A camera is an absolute necessity in the practice of facial plastic surgery. Not only is it helpful for insurance documentation and liability coverage, but it is most significant in maintaining good patient rapport. Important features include a 35 mm camera body, a macro lens with

Table 3.1 Lidocaine versus Bupivacaine: Onset, Dose, and Duration of Action

	Onset	Dose (mg/kg)	Duration (h)
Lidocaine	Rapid	3–5 5–7 with epinephrine	1–2
Bupivacaine	Delayed	3	2–4

a focal length of 105 mm that allows for portrait shots, an off-centered metered flash, and a sturdy carrying case capable of carrying extra miscellaneous equipment. Modern digital film technology now has an image fidelity that closely matches that of conventional 35 mm film. The latter is still regarded as the gold standard for image documentation, though the ease of use, image manipulation, and archiving are making digital photoprocessing a more popular option.

Excisions

Planning of Excisions and Incisions

Proper planning is necessary for achieving good results when excising lesions on the head and neck.[1] The face has several unique features that must be recognized before any surgical maneuvers can be planned. An abundance of anatomical boundary markers between aesthetic units can be found on the face (e.g., the sublabial crease, the nasolabial fold, and the preauricular crease) that are ideal for incision placement (**Figs. 3.3, 3.4, and 3.5**). The relaxed skin tension lines (RSTLs) and a lack of tension-loaded facial movements enable one to hide and minimize most facial incisions (**Figs. 3.6 and 3.7**). The RSTLs are equivalent to the lines observed originally by Langer when he excised circular punches of skin in cadavers and observed their resultant linear configuration. These RSTLs can be predicted based on the underlying facial musculature; they will always be perpendicular to the orientation of muscle fibers. The only exception is around the eye where the RSTLs parallel the musculus orbicularis oculi fibers, owing to the rigid scaffold provided by the tarsal plate. All incisions, especially in the face, must be made so that the long axis of the incision is in one of the RSTLs even if it curves or, in some instances, double curves. Incisions made in the RSTLs will close with minimal tension and without widening the scar; however, incisions made across the lines will close under significant tension and the scar will spread as it heals. Anatomical

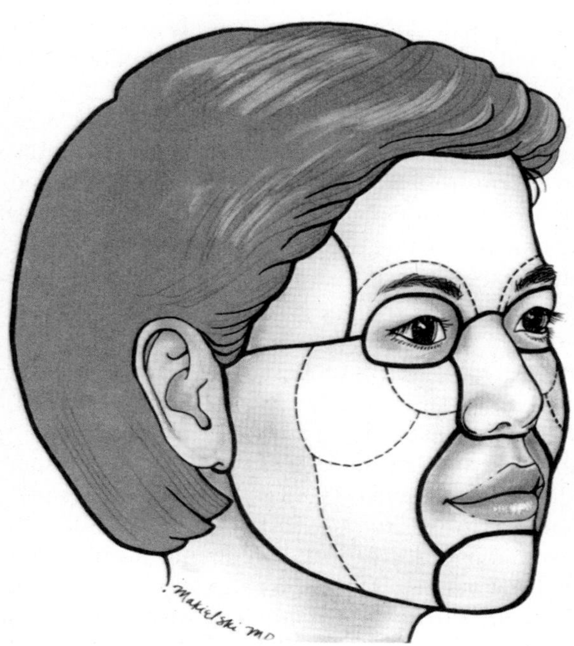

Fig. 3.3 Anatomical subunits of the face.

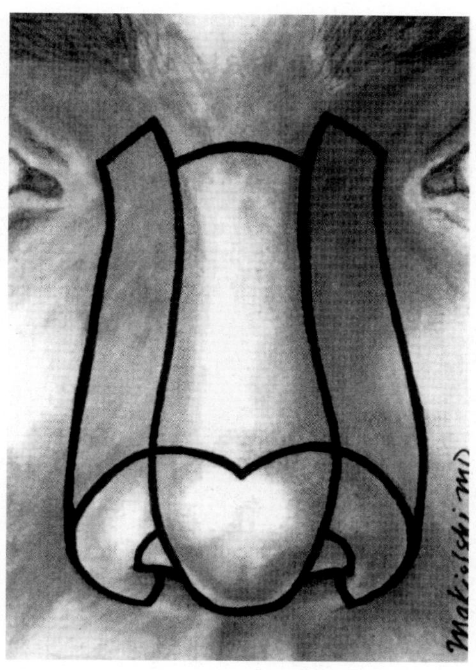

Fig. 3.4 Nasal subunits.

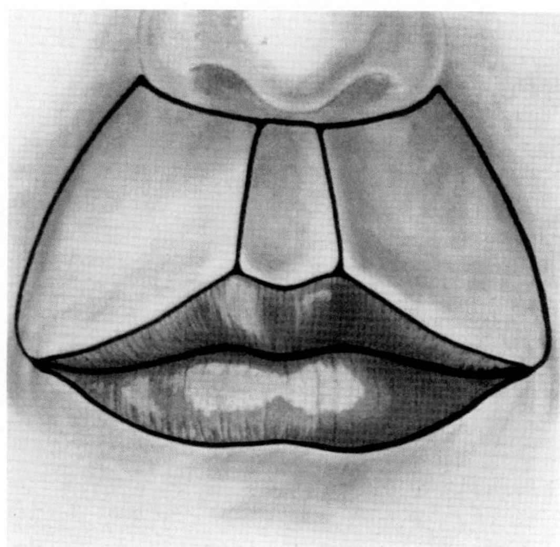

Fig. 3.5 Lip subunits.

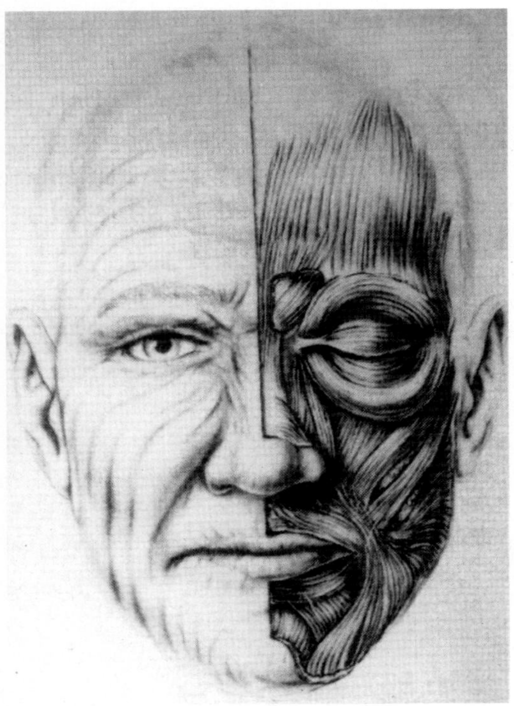

Fig. 3.6 Facial rhytids and relationship to underlying facial musculature. (From Larrabee WF, Makielski KH. Surgical Anatomy of the Face. New York: Raven Press; 1993. With permission.)

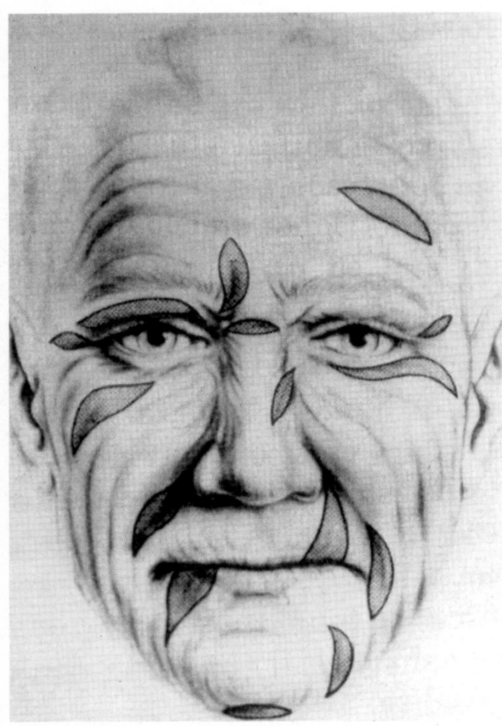

Fig. 3.7 Fusiform excisions along facial relaxed skin tension lines.

subunits distract visually from the perception of scars along the borders because of facial geometry, angulation, and shadowing. Many different access incisions can be hidden in orifices, such as endonasal or transconjunctival incisions. Utilizing anatomical structures as fencelike barriers works in select circumstances, such as placement of bilobe flaps around the ear or within the alar crease. The hairline or the hair itself provides excellent camouflage. Scars that are the result of endoscopic techniques are similarly camouflaged by the tunneling of access incisions to the site of interest.

Certain areas require exacting tissue handling and reconstitution. The mucocutaneous borders of the lip's vermilion and the eyelid's gray line are such examples. In these areas not only must the precise depth and alignment of the mucocutaneous junctions be restored but the exact structural integrity of the underlying supporting structures—the musculus orbicularis oris in the lip and the tarsal plate in the lid—must be meticulously reconstructed.

Often, structural or tension-bearing elements are required. The superficial musculoaponeurotic system (SMAS) layer provides an underlying supporting, tension-bearing trapeze in the subcutaneous layer of the skin. This can be utilized to place tension on structures and appose the epidermis in a tension free manner. Examples include the deep temporalis fascia or the canthal tendons, both of which can support great tension loads.

The simplest type of excision is a fusiform design commonly referred to as an ellipse. The fusiform excision involves wide undermining of all sides and bilateral advancement of tissue for closure. As mentioned previously, the fusiform must always be designed in an RSTL and with a length-to-width ratio of 2.5:1 to 3:1, thus helping to avoid the standing-cone or dog-ear deformity at the ends of the wound on closure (**Fig. 3.7**). The dog-ear or standing-cone deformity results from the rotation of skin around a pivot point. The excess skin and advancement collect in the shape of a cone. The formation of these dog ears can be predicted and prevented by the excision of excess tissue that permits the standing cone to lie flat. The Burow triangle is a simple example of this execution and should ideally be designed to parallel the excision lines in the RSTLs for best camouflage. To flatten a standing cone, an inferiorly based triangle is excised, akin to the door flap of a tepee.

Methods of altering the size of the fusiform excision can be usefully employed (**Fig. 3.8**). An M-plasty created at the ends of the fusiform will shorten the final length of the wound and decrease the volume of healthy skin excised.[2] However, the trade-off for shortening the overall incision length is to create an additional small incision on each side and a wound that is a bit more complex to close. The limbs of an M-plasty should be less than 30 degrees

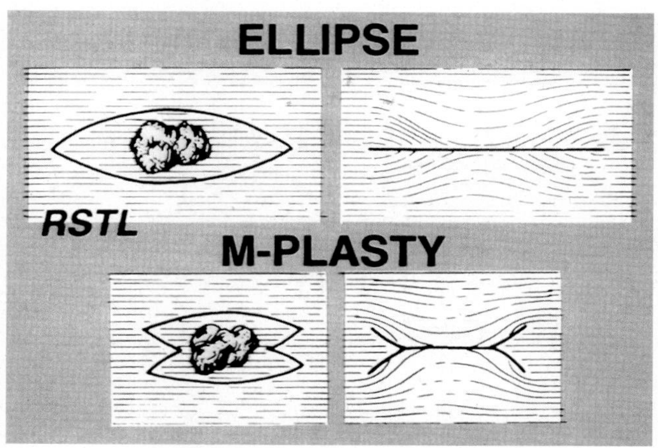

Fig. 3.8 Upper: Planning and creating a fusiform excision. Lower: M-plasty for a shorter scar. RSTL, relaxed skin tension line.

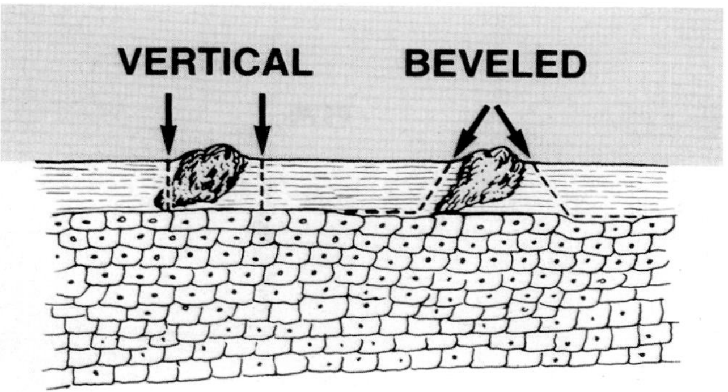

Fig. 3.9 Beveling outward from lesion when creating skin incision.

to help avoid the creation of standing-cone deformities. The closure is actually a V-to-Y maneuver that shortens the scar along its central axis. This technique is used when large defects may be closed as an ellipse and when avoiding extension of an ellipse across a normal anatomical border, such as the vermilion. Serial excisions at 2- to 3-month intervals will allow excision of larger defects with a final straight-line closure. Serial excisions are performed by excising and discarding scar tissue until a point is reached where the minimized scar can be excised from healthy tissue boundaries.

This technique has a similar background to tissue expansion where the dermis is stimulated to hypertrophy, increasing its surface area and thus affording larger flap expansion and the ability to excise a lesion in single or fewer stages. Tissue expanders have gained some popularity for large wound closures and in scalp excisions. Saline-filled expanders are sized and placed in subgaleal pockets to permit their fixation. Expansion takes place over the course of 3 to 6 weeks during which different regimens are used to inflate the expander with injected saline. Reexcision may be prevented in some areas, such as the scalp or forehead, by the use of tissue expanders at the sides of the defect before final closure.

Execution of Incisions

Most incisions in the facial region can be made with either a no. 15 or a no. 11 blade using a no. 9 knife handle. The no. 11 blade is most useful for straight cuts made perpendicular to the skin with a sawing-type motion (e.g., creating small cuts in a running W-plasty incision). The initial knife position is perpendicular to the skin edge, and the tip of the blade should be used to begin the incision. Then the handle of the knife should be arched downward so that the midportion of the incision is made with the belly of the blade. At the end of the incision, the handle should be arched upward again so that the end of the incision is made with the tip of the blade. The blade should always be perpendicular to the skin surface, and the incision should be made completely through skin and subcutaneous tissue for the entire length of the cut. When making an incision to excise a lesion, instead of creating the cut at right angles to the skin surface, bevel the incision outward (**Fig. 3.9**). This accomplishes the following: it aids in skin edge eversion, which is helpful in preventing depressed scars; it helps to create the plane for undermining; and it gives better assurance of completely excising around the lesion. A skin hook should then be placed into the starting end of the first-side incision, providing traction and stabilization for the second-side incision. Without this stabilization of the end of the wound it is difficult to make the second incision precise.

The final step in executing an excision before closure is undermining. This is performed in proportion to the amount of skin tension and to optimize suturing techniques. Undermining should be done in the immediate subdermal plane (**Fig. 3.10**). Around the central face, this plane avoids emerging motor nerves. The facial nerve branches pass deep to all of the mimetic musculature except those branches that emerge superficially to innervate the lateral fibers of the orbicularis oris, ~1 to 2 cm from the lateral commissure. Undermining should be used in virtually all surgical procedures in the skin of the head and neck and should be done completely around the incision, the ends as well as the sides, for a distance of ~2 cm from the wound edges. Studies have shown that undermining beyond 2 cm is probably counterproductive in removing tension from the wound edges.[3]

However, for advancement and rotation flaps, useful undermining should be performed 3 to 4 times the length of the arc of rotation, or size of the defect to be closed. The scalp requires special consideration. Despite extensive undermining in the scalp, little advancement can be

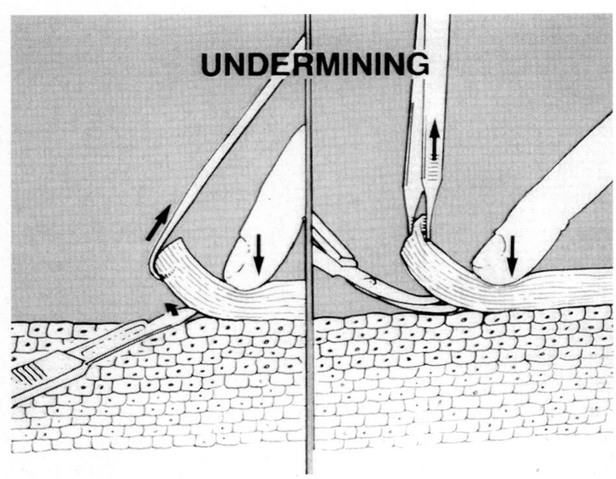

Fig. 3.10 (**A**) Undermining skin with skin hook and no. 15 blade versus (**B**) forceps and scissors.

achieved because of the tensile strength of the galea aponeurosis. This can be overcome by placing multiple galeotomies perpendicular to the line of scalp advancement to facilitate mobilization of scalp tissue. Although undermining has traditionally been performed with curved scissors and tissue forceps, the use of a skin hook and a no. 15 scalpel blade is more advantageous. The skin edge should be everted outward with the skin hook and middle finger, and the belly of the no. 15 blade beveled upward to scrape the undersurface of the skin to be undermined. This technique provides more effective skin eversion, less crushing of the skin edge tissue, and more accurate and less traumatic undermining. Undermining allows for movement of wound edges toward the center of a defect and decreases the tension on the wound edges. Also, with differential undermining one can move the center of the excision to a desirable spot. This principle is especially important when closing cheek defects arising from meiolabial flaps. The skin and soft tissue of the upper lip are not undermined to prevent upward distortion of this aesthetically important anatomical unit. The undermining is borne by the upper malar tissue, allowing its mobilization to the lip.

Closure of Excisions

By wound closure, we generally refer to the active process of primary-intention, suture-assisted healing. The goal of secondary-intention healing is not to appose the skin edges but to allow the wound to heal by the collection of granulation tissue from the base to the superficial layers of a wound over which epithelium migrates. Secondary intention healing is always an option, but rarely is it the best cosmetic option. The canthal areas of the eyes are particularly amenable to secondary-intention healing with

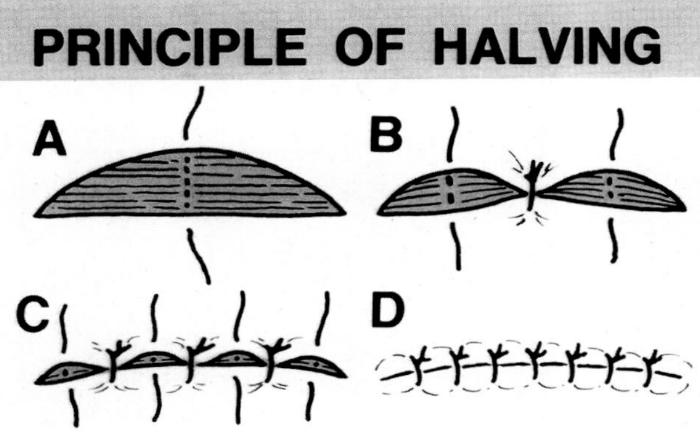

Fig. 3.11 Principle of halving.

a good cosmetic outcome. In these areas, the skin is thin, contoured in three dimensions, and subject to constant motion secondary to lid closure—all issues that might favor secondary-intention healing. Depending on the size and location of the defect, closure of an excision can be done primarily (e.g., in a fusiform defect), with a flap, or using a graft. Regardless of the technique chosen, the following three principles for achievement of better wound healing should be remembered: minimize trauma to the wound edges, place minimal tension on the wound edges, and provide eversion of the skin closure. When closing a defect, especially a fusiform excision, it is important to equalize the sides of the incision to avoid bunching at the ends of the wound. The best way to avoid this problem is to use the principle of halving (**Fig. 3.11**). This is done by placing the first suture in the center of the defect. The next suture should bisect the two remaining halves, and, by continuation of this halving, the wound will be closed with equal tension and eversion throughout, even if one side of the incision is initially longer than the other. Another technique to equalize the length of both sides of an excision is to remove a triangle of skin (Burow triangle) from the longer side of the wound (**Fig. 3.12**). Often, if

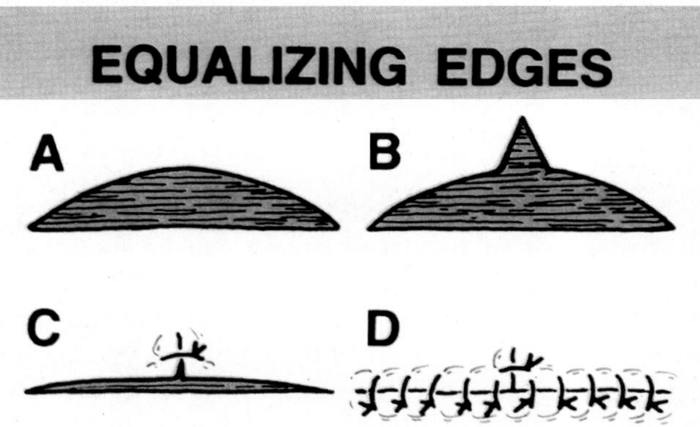

Fig. 3.12 Equalizing length of edges with a Burow triangle.

adequate undermining is performed, this step can be avoided.

There are several methods for closing a wound (**Fig. 3.13**). The standard simple suture should be inserted with the needle angled slightly outward to achieve slight eversion of the wound edge with the knot tied as far as possible from the wound edge (**Fig. 3.10A**). The simple suture provides little wound edge eversion and hardly any relief of wound edge tension; therefore, it is not the best approach to closure of facial skin. Vertical mattress suturing involves placing the small intracuticular portion of the suture first, holding up the wound edges with the suture, and causing eversion of the wound for placement of the wide portion of the suture (**Fig. 3.10B**). This suture provides both eversion and tension relief, and for this reason it can be useful in closing skin edges that will be under tension despite subcutaneous closure.

Tacking of wound corners can be accomplished either by placement of simple interrupted corner sutures or by use of the Gillies half-buried corner stitch. Here the corner tissue is tacked into place by a suture that begins in a transcutaneous position, passes through the dermal plane of the advancing tissue corner, and finishes with a

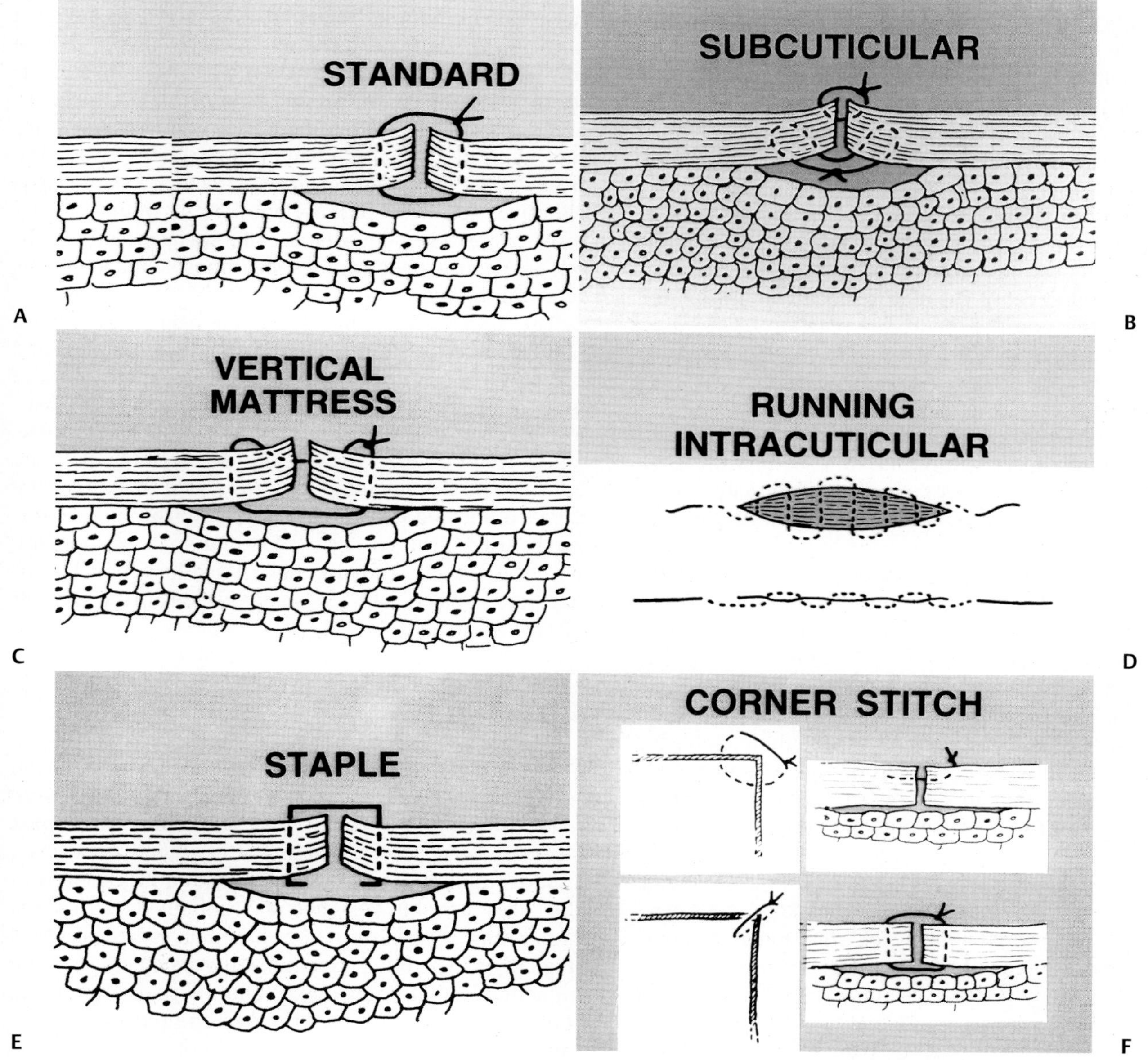

Fig. 3.13 Excision closure techniques. (**A**) Standard simple suture. (**B**) Subcuticular buried everting suture. (**C**) Vertical mattress suture. (**D**) Running intracuticular suture. (**E**) Stainless steel staple. (**F**) Corner stitch.

transcutaneous suture. This has the theoretical advantage of providing strength to a tissue closure without disrupting the skin. It often works best in narrow-based tissue remnants where passing a needle transcutaneously through the apex would otherwise be technically difficult and would result in unnecessary tissue trauma. The most useful suture technique for accomplishing both eversion of wound edges and relief of tension of the edges is the subcuticular buried everting technique (**Fig. 3.13B**). In placing the suture in the head and neck region, a small, one-half-curved, reverse cutting needle (such as the Ethicon P-2 needle, Ethicon, Inc., Somerville, NJ) is most helpful. The subcuticular suture is placed while everting the wound edge outward between a skin hook and the middle finger. The surgeon should reach back with the needle under the dermis and insert the suture 2 to 3 mm back from the wound edge, tying the knot in a buried fashion. The monofilament absorbable synthetic material polydioxinone (PDS) is preferred for the buried subcuticular suture because there is less chance of cutting the tissue in a cheese-wire fashion. The skin is then closed with fine monofilament or fast-absorbing gut to align the depth of the two sides of the wound. Stainless steel staples provide for wound eversion and ride above the level of the skin surface when in place. Because of this and the low tissue reaction from stainless steel there is very little incidence of skin marking from staples themselves. They are particularly useful for enclosing neck and scalp defects, providing full-thickness closure.

Simple interrupted sutures are most commonly used to reapproximate skin edges once the subcuticular layer has been placed. Because placement of such sutures can be time consuming, some clinicians prefer using simple running sutures or a running locking suture technique. The advantage of the running suture is that it is quicker to place and provides even tension throughout the length of the wound. However, if pulled too tightly, the running suture may compromise vascularity to the skin edge. The running intracuticular suture provides good closure of straight wounds, especially in children, but does not relieve tension from the wound edges. Although more time consuming and difficult to use, it can provide an excellent result once the technique is mastered.

When proper subcuticular closure of a facial wound has been done, there should be eversion of the skin edges, with the edges approximating each other under minimal tension. The skin can then be properly closed using a 6–0 fast-absorbing gut that has minimal tissue reaction and will dissolve spontaneously in 3 to 5 days. The repair is then reinforced with sterile strips to relieve wound edge tension further. For minimizing scar widening, wound taping for 4 to 6 weeks or more has been advocated (even though this can occur for up to 6 months) and is usually satisfactory in cosmetic-sensitive areas or in areas where the dynamic stretching of underlying musculature would otherwise put the wound under adverse tension (e.g., lip wounds).

Interest in the use of cyanoacrylate tissue adhesives for the closure of wounds, both traumatic and surgical, has grown rapidly.[4] Many authors feel that these adhesives will gain a significant role in wound care because of their ease of application, simplification of wound care, and good performance in comparison with that of traditional sutures. Their use has been limited by the histotoxicity of their degradation products, cyanoacetate and formaldehyde, though now products with lowered histotoxicity have been introduced. The use of cyanoacrylates has been particularly favorable in the emergency room due to ease of use, and with pediatric patients because of the ability to avoid the emotional and physical pain of needles. Some authors believe that there is no cosmetic difference between standard suture and cyanoacrylate closure. We believe that for selected wounds cyanoacrylate tissue adhesives hold great promise but that the wound characteristics are of key importance; superficial wounds without deep tissue penetration appear most suitable for this type of adhesive.

The final aspect of closing an excisional wound involves adequate dressing to provide protection and pressure to the site. This prevents collection of fluid or blood underneath the wound edges. The dressing usually involves antibiotic ointment, a nonadhesive gauze, and cotton or gauze sponge followed by tape. A tissue adhesive on the surrounding skin is used to prevent the tape from losing its firm attachment to the skin. Drains can be used if there is a risk of hematoma development, with the aim of removing these when less than 10 cm^3 has been collected in a 24-hour period in the face, or 30 cm^3 in the neck.

Local Flaps

The simplest local flap is the fusiform excision (discussed previously). As a general rule, one should favor the simplest repair and avoid more complex closures. Because the skin of the head and neck has a superb subdermal vasculature, almost all local flaps in this area can be designed as random-pattern flaps rather than axial-pattern flaps based on specific arteries (**Fig. 3.14**).[5] The flaps are almost always elevated in the immediate subdermal plane, and sharp undermining is necessary on all sides of the flap and receptor site in this same plane. The principles of soft tissue surgery previously mentioned should be strictly adhered to when one is executing these flaps.

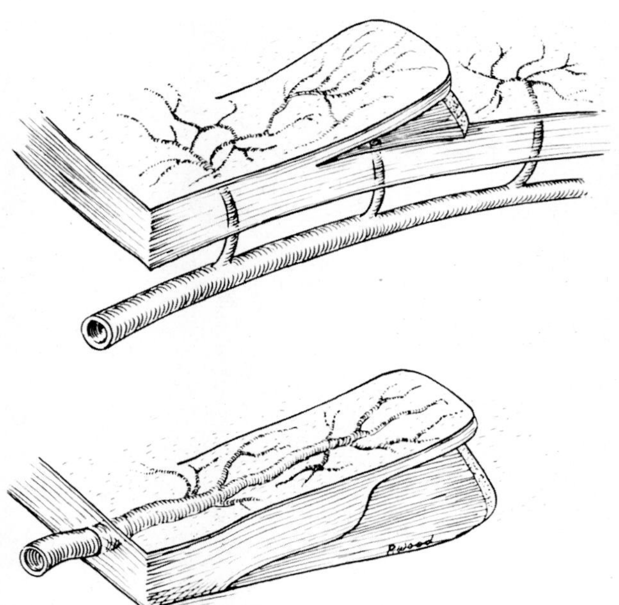

Fig. 3.14 Upper: random-pattern flap. Lower: axial-pattern flap.

Unilateral Advancement Flap

The classic, single-pedicled advancement flap moves entirely in one direction, advancing over the defect (**Fig. 3.15**). It has limited value in the head and neck because of its somewhat restricted flexibility. The forehead and lip, especially the upper lip, are the two areas where this flap may occasionally be useful. In the face, these flaps are rarely designed in a straight line but commonly follow the natural skin lines. The length-to-width ratio may be as high as 4:1 and seldom requires excision of Burow triangles for closure if adequate undermining is performed. For smaller defects, a variation of the single advancement flap is the V to Y flap. This design recedes the flap away from the defect and can be used to bulk up an area slightly widened and lengthen an axis of an area (**Fig. 3.16**).

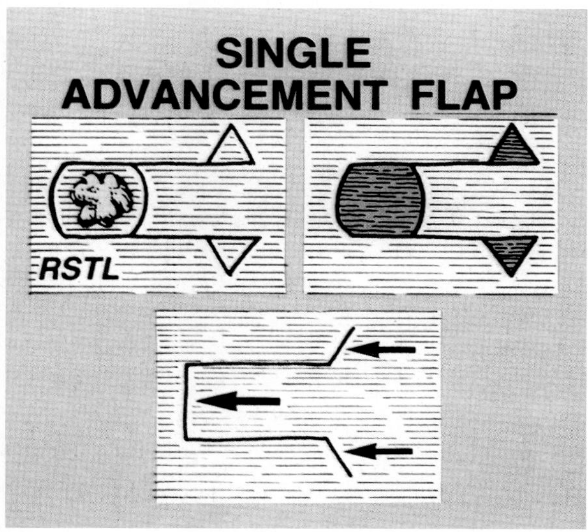

Fig. 3.15 Unilateral advancement flap. RSTL, relaxed skin tension line.

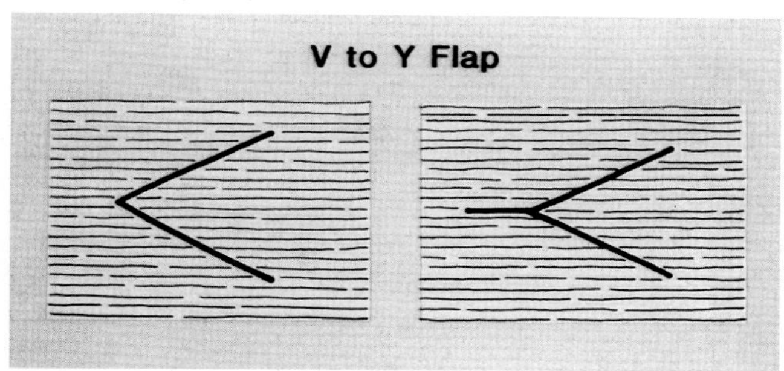

Fig. 3.16 V to Y advancement flap.

Bilateral Advancement Flap

The bilateral advancement flap is more flexible in terms of planning, although the same principles of design utilized for the single advancement flap also apply here. A flap is 4:1 advanced from both sides of a defect that is too large to be closed with a single advancement flap (**Fig. 3.17**). The two flaps need not be of equal length. The flap should be designed so that closure of the final line where the two flaps meet is placed in an optimal location, such as the philtrum of the upper lip. The bilateral advancement flap requires extensive undermining and long incision lines. With adequate undermining, closure without Burow triangles can be accomplished. Although limited in its use in the head and neck, it can close some forehead defects and, less often, dorsal nasal defects quite nicely.

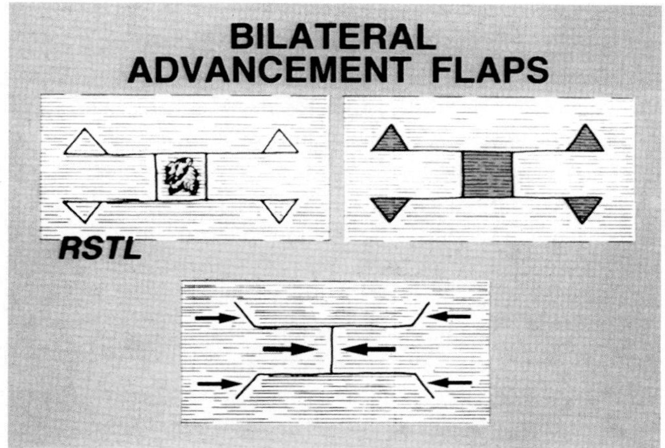

Fig. 3.17 Bilateral advancement flap. RSTL, relaxed skin tension line.

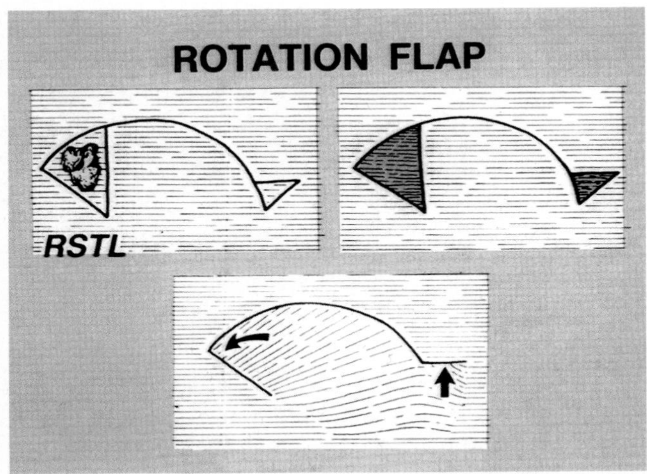

Fig. 3.18 Classic rotation flap. RSTL, relaxed skin tension line.

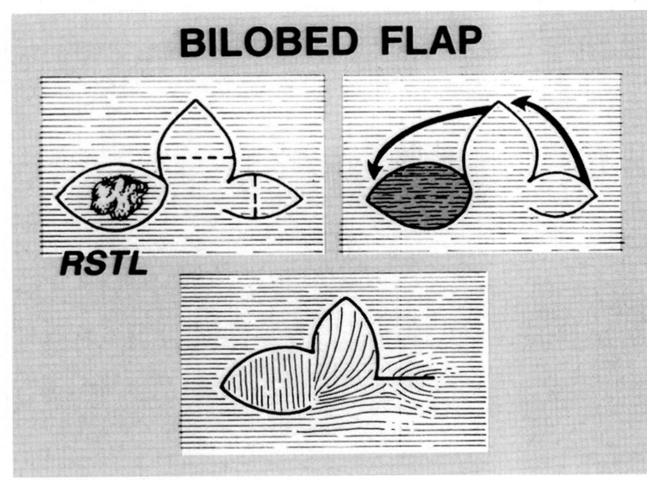

Fig. 3.19 Bilobed interposition flap. RSTL, relaxed skin tension line.

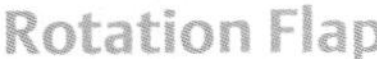

Rotation Flap

The classic rotation flap covers a triangular defect by rotating a semicircular flap around the pivotal point (**Fig. 3.18**). It is a versatile, broad-based flap capable of closing large defects in the head and neck. The length of the perimeter of the flap should be at least four times the width of the defect itself to allow easy closure with no donor site defect. The relaxing side incision should be placed in an RSTL or an anatomical borderline (i.e., nasolabial groove or preauricular crease). Rarely is there a need for an equalizing Burow triangle at the distal end of the flap if the surrounding tissue is undermined appropriately.

Interposition Flaps

Interposition flaps, sometimes called transposition flaps, are flaps that are raised from their donor site and rotated over adjacent tissue to be placed in the defect site.[6] This usually requires a combination of rotation and advancement of tissue. The interposition of flaps in such a manner provides great flexibility for closure of a variety of large and small defects in the head and neck. The bilobed flap is actually two transposition flaps. When a defect is too large to close primarily, a smaller flap is used to close the defect using a second, smaller flap to close the first donor site (**Fig. 3.19**). As a general rule, the first flap (A) should be slightly smaller than the original defect, and the second flap (B) should be half the diameter of the first. However, the combined length of both flaps must equal the length of the original defect. The flaps should be created as half-ellipses, with the direction of the final closure planned along the orientation of the RSTL. Flap A should be 90 degrees to the long axis of the original defect and flap B 180 degrees to that axis. Care must be taken so that the base of flap A, which becomes the common base of both flaps at final closure, is not made too narrow by extending the second side of flap B too far back for the defect. The rhombic (Limberg) interposition flap is a reliable alternative for closure of many smaller defects of the head and neck (**Fig. 3.20**).[7] This flap takes advantage of the elasticity of the skin adjacent to the defect by rotating and advancing that skin over the recipient site. The tension across the secondary defect is perpendicular to that of the original defect. After the flap is interposed into the defect, the secondary defect can be easily closed primarily. The flap can be designed from virtually any angle around a given defect so that the final closure can almost always be in the direction of the RSTL. All four sides of the basic defect and both legs of the flap must be of equal length.

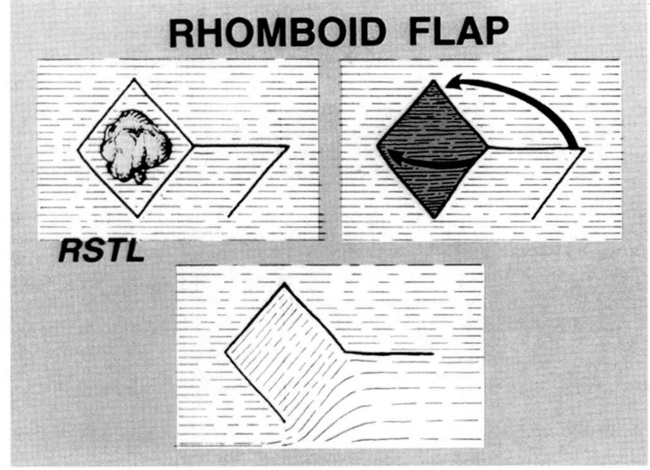

Fig. 3.20 Rhombic interposition flap. RSTL, relaxed skin tension line.

The outer edge of the flap must be parallel to the sides of the rhombic defect. The Webster 30-degree angle flap and the Duformental flap are other frequently used variations of the original flap design by Limberg.

Z-plasty

Z-plasty is an interposition technique whereby two equal and opposing flaps are raised and interposed around a shared axis. The best way to visualize the basic concept of this "double triangular flap" construction is to draw out a parallelogram with a short axis and a long axis. The result of interposing the flaps is to exchange the long axis with the short axis, borrowing tissue from one dimension and essentially donating it to the dimension at right angles. Thus the surgeon can lengthen a contracting scar (**Fig. 3.21**).[8] Z-plasty has the following three basic functions:

1. Rotate the long axis of a scar from an unfavorable to a favorable position
2. Lengthen a contracted scar line
3. Align anatomical lines that have been misaligned

By achieving the desired result when doing a Z-plasty, one accepts a new scar that is three times the length of the original. The amount of lengthening achieved by Z-plasty is related to the length of the central and lateral limbs, as well as the angle of the Z-plasty. In general, a 30-degree Z-plasty achieves a 25% increase in length of the axis to the central limb, a 45-degree Z-plasty achieves a 50% increase, and a 60-degree Z-plasty achieves a 75% increase (**Figs. 3.22 and 3.23**).[9] Our general rule is to use no Z-plasty with arms greater than 1 cm in the face or 1.5 cm in the neck. When a greater length gain is needed, the scar is broken up with two or more nonadjoining Z-plasties. Most often, we use a 60-degree angled Z-plasty, although we will work with angles from 45 degrees to 70 degrees, adjusting to the individual case.

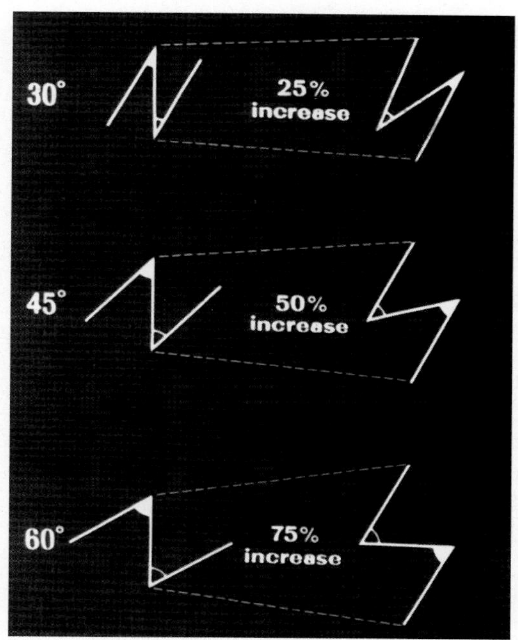

Fig. 3.22 Z-plasty angles.

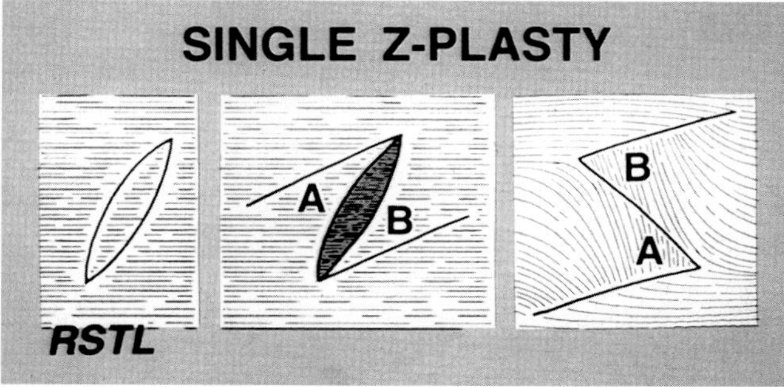

Fig. 3.21 Single Z-plasty. RSTL, relaxed skin tension line.

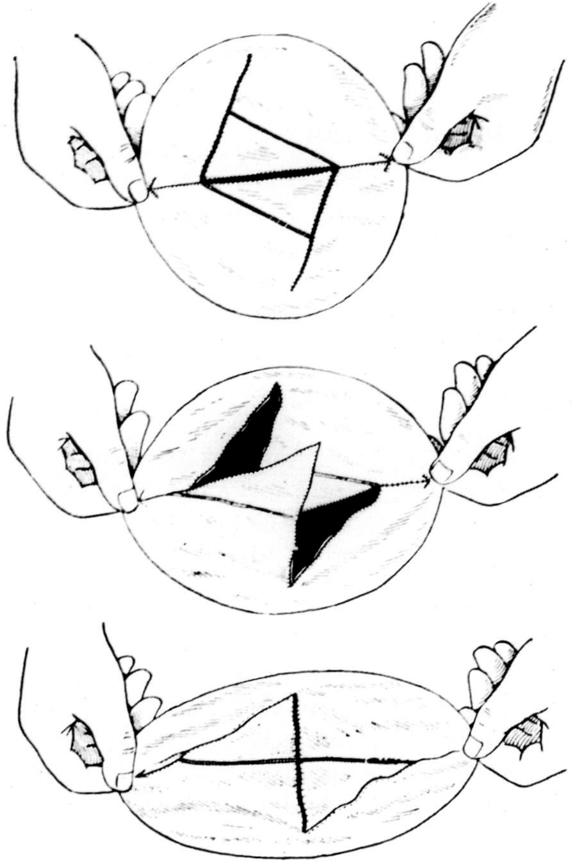

Fig. 3.23 Creation of a Z-plasty.

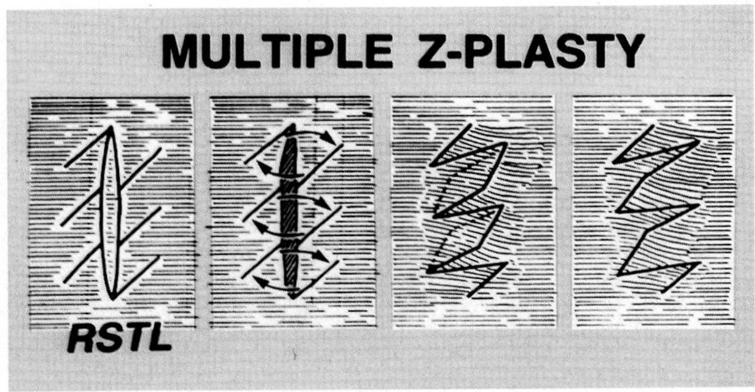

Fig. 3.24 Multiple Z-plasties. RSTL, relaxed skin tension line.

For longer scars, a multiple Z-plasty can be used (**Fig. 3.24**). All Z-plasties are planned, marked out with Castroviejo calipers, scratched out with the tip of an 18-gauge needle, and created with a no. 11 scalpel. Wide undermining is necessary at all sides for tension-free rotation of the interposing flaps. Closure depends on meticulous placement of interrupted subcuticular sutures of synthetic absorbable monofilament. Leveling of the sides of the wound edges is done with fine monofilament or fast-absorbing gut cutaneous sutures. The closure is then reinforced with sterile strips.

W-plasty and the Geometric Broken Line Closure

The running W-plasty and the geometric broken line (GBL) closure of Webster are two techniques that camouflage scars in the face that

1. Are not parallel to RSTL
2. Are not contracted
3. Do not cross anatomic boundaries
4. Are greater than 2 cm in length[10]

The objective is to excise the scar and close the defect to disguise a straight line (which is easy for the eye to follow) into a pattern (that is more difficult for the eye to follow). A GBL closure is the more effective of the two because of its random pattern; however, it is more complex in design and more of a challenge to execute properly. The W-plasty scar revision procedure was first described by Borges in 1959 (**Fig. 3.25**). It is important to realize that the running W-plasty is not a multiple Z-plasty and does not cause any increase in scar length. Scar revision of this type should be delayed as long as possible in persons younger than 21 years because delayed scar maturation will exaggerate the resultant defect. There are some general guidelines to aid in designing a W-plasty scar revision. The entire width of the original scar must be excised. No part of the pattern should cross into the scar. No leg of the scar

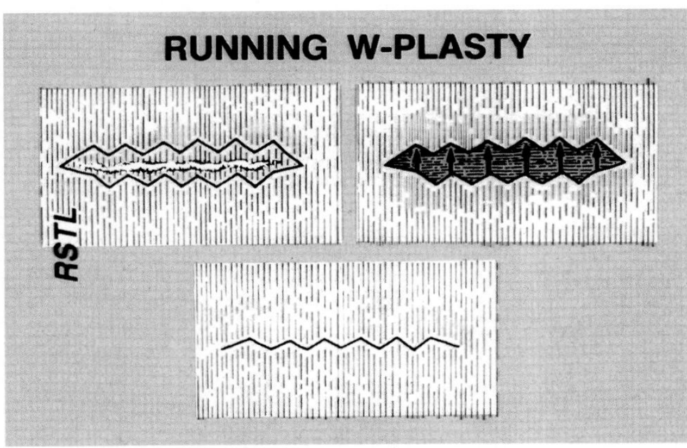

Fig. 3.25 Running W-plasty. RSTL, relaxed skin tension line.

should be greater than 6 mm in length, and the angles of the Ws should be ~60 degrees, with one set of legs in the direction of the RSTL. Avoid designing any flap that has an angle greater than 90 degrees and avoid designing a repair that disrupts a normal anatomical boundary line, such as the eyebrow or philtrum ridge. A GBL design should be predominantly squares and rectangles for optimal aesthetic appearance of the scar revision. Curved patterns have been found to be both difficult to create and ultimately more obvious to the eye. After one side is marked out, the mirror image on the other side is drawn. The design should be scratched in with the tip of an 18-gauge needle. A no. 11 blade should be used to make each cut toward the scar itself. The scar in the W-plasty should be excised as one piece. The techniques of skin-hook stabilization, wound edge handling, and wide, sharp undermining on all sides must be strictly adhered to. The sides are then brought together using interrupted, subcuticular, monofilament, or absorbable sutures at the tips of each point along one side only.

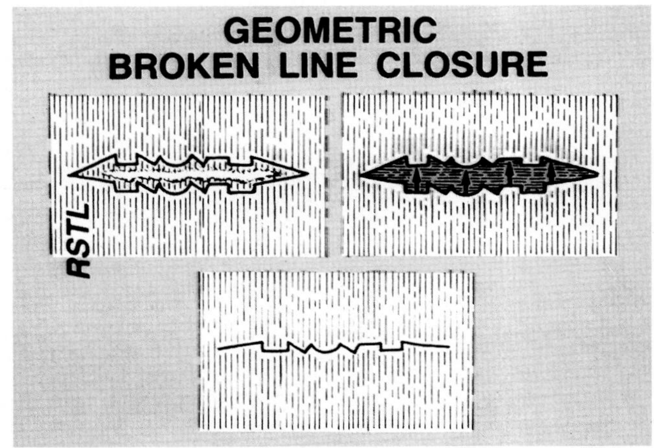

Fig. 3.26 Geometric broken line scar revision. RSTL, relaxed skin tension line.

Skin closure is accomplished with a running locked suture using 6–0 mild chromic catgut at each tip, up one side and then back down the other side. The wound is then reinforced with sterile strips. Although the design of the GBL closure is somewhat more complex, the same principles apply to its excision and closure (**Fig. 3.26**). Patients undergoing this type of scar camouflage must be warned that the wound will be somewhat erythematous for several months after surgery before turning pale. They should also plan for dermabrasion of the scar. The best time for this is at 8 to 10 weeks postoperatively, at the approximate end of the proliferative phase of wound healing and prior to complete wound contracture and scar fading. By blending raised edges with the surrounding skin or by lowering healthy skin to a recessed area, dermabrasion aids in resurfacing and blending scars into the surrounding skin. Of note is that dermabrasion is not good for raised, hypertrophic scars; rather, it is best for lowering the height of normal tissue to the level of the scar.

Summary

The basics of soft tissue surgery are not difficult to comprehend, yet their execution and daily practice require patience and discipline. By maintaining a working knowledge of these basic principles, a creative approach to facial soft tissue surgery, and good patient rapport, a surgeon can hope to achieve further improvement in surgical results.

References

1. Borges AF. Elective Incisions and Scar Revision. Boston: Little, Brown; 1973
2. Limberg AA. The Planning of Local Plastic Operations on the Body Surface: Theory and Practice. Lexington: Collamore Press; 1984
3. Cox KW, Larabee WF. A study of skin flap advancement as a function of undermining. Arch Otolaryngol 1982;108:151
4. Trott AT. Cyanoacrylate tissue adhesives: an advance in wound care. JAMA 1997;277:1559–1560
5. Tardy ME. Regional flaps: principles and applications. Otolaryngol Clin North Am 1972;5:551
6. Bernstein L. Transposed and interposed flaps in head and neck surgery. Otolaryngol Clin North Am 1972;5:531
7. Gunter JP. Rhombic flaps. Facial Plast Surg 1983;1:69
8. Borges AF. Historical review of Z-plastic techniques. Clin Plast Surg 1977;4:207
9. Gustafson J, Larabee WF, Borges AF. Experimental analysis of the adjunctive Z-plasty in the closure of fusiform defects. Arch Otolaryngol 1984;110:41
10. Webster RD, Davidson TM, Smith RC. Broken line scar revision. Clin Plast Surg 1977;4:263
11. Larrabee WF, Makielski KH. Surgical Anatomy of the face. New York: Raven Press; 1993

4 Skin Grafts and Local Flaps

Rudy J. Triana Jr., Craig S. Murakami, and Wayne F. Larrabee Jr.

In dealing with skin and soft tissue defects, the surgeon must have an in-depth knowledge of the anatomy and physiology of skin grafts and local flaps to ensure the success of the reconstructive effort. This knowledge provides the necessary insight to determine not only the wound requirements, such as skin only, skin and subcutaneous tissue, or a combination involving the underlying cartilage or bone, but also the limitations of the planned reconstructive graft or flap, such as contour, color, degree of vascularity, and presence of pilosebaceous units. With careful use of this information, a well-considered surgical plan can be developed. In many cases the preoperative planning is much more complicated than the procedure. This chapter provides a review of skin graft and local flap anatomy and physiology, with emphasis on the process of evaluation and aesthetic closure of skin and soft-tissue defects of the face.

Skin Grafts

A skin graft is an island of epidermis and dermis that has been surgically removed from a donor site; its blood supply is transferred and is dependent on the recipient site. Skin grafts can be categorized as split-thickness or full-thickness grafts.

Types of Skin Grafts

Split-Thickness Skin Grafts

Split-thickness skin grafts (STSGs), also known as Thiersch grafts, are usually harvested with a dermatome or razor blade. They consist of epidermis and a superficial segment of dermis (papillary dermis). Thin STSGs may measure 0.008 to 0.010 in. in thickness, whereas a thick (standard) STSG measures between 0.016 and 0.018 in. Epidermal and dermal thickness varies in different parts of the body, in different skin colors, and in different age groups, and it is generally thicker in males. The skin of an adult is 3.5 times thicker than the skin of a newborn. By age 5 years, the skin thickness approximates that of an adult.[1] Measurements of epidermal and dermal thickness taken from various age groups, sexes, and sites were found to vary from 0.017 to 0.15 in.[2] The skin of the eyelids is the thinnest, and the soles of the feet the thickest.

Though highly reliable, STSGs have limited usefulness in facial reconstruction because of their tendency to contract. The thinner the graft, the greater the degree of contraction, but also the higher the likelihood of graft survival. STSGs typically have a different texture as well as a lighter color and thickness than the neighboring tissue.[3] STSGs may be meshed to increase their surface area; however, this further thins the graft and may compromise the aesthetic result. STSGs in facial reconstruction have been used to repair large defects of the scalp, as well as defects associated with deeply invasive tumors or uncertain margins where close postoperative surveillance of the resection area is especially important (**Fig. 4.1**).[4,5]

Full-Thickness Skin Grafts

With full-thickness skin grafts (FTSGs), the entire thickness of the epidermis and dermis is harvested from the donor site and subsequently transplanted. The subcutaneous tissue may be trimmed from the graft to create the appropriate thickness. Hair follicles are preserved so that hair growth may be preserved. FTSGs do not contract and do not change in color or texture. These grafts are thicker than STSGs and are more slowly revascularized, with a higher graft failure rate. An adequate blood supply in the recipient site is required to ensure graft survival. FTSGs are much more resistant to sheering forces than STSGs. The donor sites for FTSGs include the pre- or postauricular skin, the supraclavicular skin, and, occasionally, the melolabial fold skin. The FTSG donor site contains no epithelial elements from which reepithelialization can take place; therefore, the donor site must be closed primarily or covered with an STSG. FTSGs are particularly useful for facial defects involving the nasal tip, lateral surface of the auricle, and eyelids (**Fig. 4.2**).

Dermal Grafts

Dermal grafts are harvested from the dermis after the overlying epidermis has been elevated. These grafts are very reliable, resistant to infection, and can be buried below the skin surface. When buried the epithelial elements atrophy and become inactive; however, a graft that is exposed or used as a resurfacing graft is capable of reepithelialization.[6] Dermal grafts have been used for intraoral coverage or for subcutaneous implantation to add bulk or contour. Currently, many facial plastic

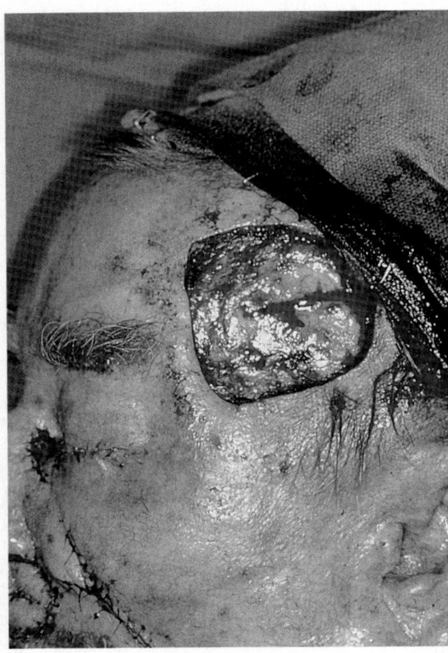
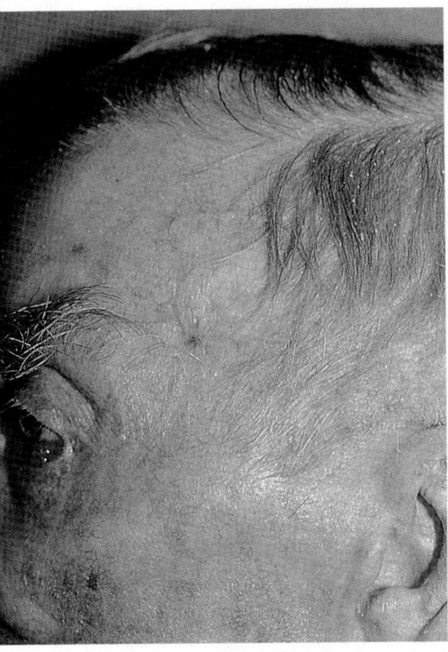

A,B

Fig. 4.1 Split-thickness skin graft. (**A**) Left temple defect 6 to 8 cm following resection of a deeply infiltrating squamous cell carcinoma of the skin. (**B**) The 4-month postoperative result using a split-thickness skin graft reconstruction.

surgeons have replaced the dermal graft with an acellular dermal graft (AlloDerm, LifeCell Corp., Branchburg, NJ) for adding bulk and contour to many facial defects.[7–9]

Vascularization of Skin Grafts

Both STSGs and FTSGs are a form of a free tissue transplant from a donor site to a recipient site where a new blood supply is acquired. The revascularization of skin grafts takes place in the following phases: imbibition, revascularization, and organization.

Serum Imbibition Phase

The initial phase of serum imbibition or plasmatic circulation lasts ~48 hours. Graft nutrition is dependent on plasma exudate from dilated capillaries in the host bed. Fibrinogen-free serum, not plasma, enters the graft to nourish it.[10] Erythrocytes penetrate the fibrin clot and are passively trapped. These trapped erythrocytes are suspended in the serum under the graft and are a source of edema of the graft. As revascularization occurs, new blood flow enters the graft, and plasmalike fluid is removed from the graft.[11]

Revascularization Phase

Vascular buds begin to grow into the supportive fibrin network during the first 48 hours. Revascularization occurs through both direct ingrowth of host blood vessels in the graft (neovascularization) and the formation of anastomoses between graft and host vessels (inosculation).[12–14] Although inosculation between graft and host vessels occurs, the primary mode of revascularization depends on the ingrowth of host vessels into the graft dermis.[15] Lymphatic circulation between the graft and the host bed is functional by the fourth or fifth postoperative day.

Organization Phase

The organization phase begins within 5 hours of transplantation. A fibrin clot forms an interface between the graft and the host bed. The fibrin clot also acts to adhere the graft to the host bed.[9] Leukocytes begin to infiltrate the deeper layers of the graft, and as revascularization proceeds they are removed and replaced by fibroblasts.[16] By the seventh or eighth postoperative day, fibroblast infiltration of the fibrin clot continues as a collagen matrix is being created. By the ninth day, the graft is firmly anchored by its new blood supply and fibroblast integration. Within 2 months, neural structures begin to regenerate and enter the graft through the base and the sides, following vacated neurilemmal cell sheaths.[17] Skin grafts rarely attain normal sensory innervation after healing is complete.[4]

Donor Sites

The surgeon must consider a variety of factors when choosing a donor site for an STSG. These factors include the characteristics of the donor skin (color, texture, thickness, and vascularity), the amount of skin needed, necessity of hair on the graft, convenience, and potential for deformity. Most donor sites in the head and neck have

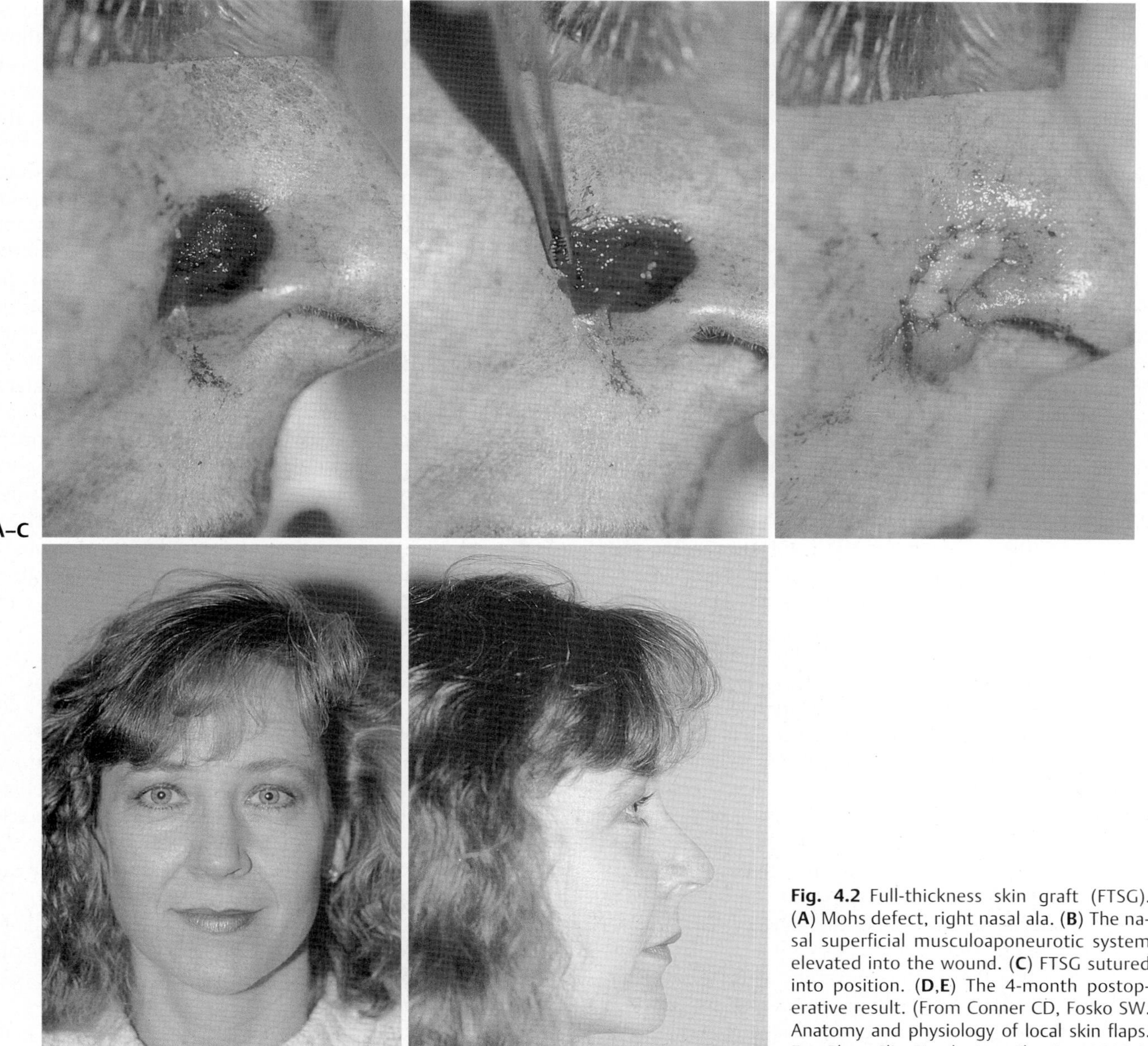

Fig. 4.2 Full-thickness skin graft (FTSG). (**A**) Mohs defect, right nasal ala. (**B**) The nasal superficial musculoaponeurotic system elevated into the wound. (**C**) FTSG sutured into position. (**D**,**E**) The 4-month postoperative result. (From Conner CD, Fosko SW. Anatomy and physiology of local skin flaps. Fac Plast Clin North Am, Elsevier, 1996;4: 447–454. With permission.)

a great vascular supply; however, several different donor sites are used to provide a range of skin color, texture, and thickness.

Good sites for harvesting skin grafts include pre- and postauricular skin, upper eyelid skin, melolabial skin, and skin from the surpraclavicular area and abdomen. The pre- and postauricular skin is thin, hairless, and has a good color and texture match for the face. FTSGs can be harvested from this region and used for defects of the nose and cheek. These donor sites usually allow for primary closure of the defect. FTSG of upper eyelid skin can be obtained from patients with excess upper eyelid skin. This graft is useful for covering defects of the opposite eyelid, concha, nasal vestibule, and external ear canal. Bilateral upper eyelid skin excisions should be performed to ensure symmetry. This donor site provides limited skin and requires primary closure of the donor site defect. Larger amounts of full-thickness skin may be obtained from either the supraclavicular or the abdominal skin. Full-thickness skin from the melolabial fold is useful for reconstructing cutaneous defects of the nose. The color, texture, and thickness of this skin make it suitable for restoring defects of the nasal tip. The melolabial donor site can be closed primarily, leaving an inconspicuous scar.

Composite (skin and cartilage) grafts can be harvested from segments of the external ear to reconstruct defects of the nasal rim or contralateral ear.[4,18]

The anterolateral thigh and abdomen provide larger areas for harvesting split-thickness and dermal grafts. Full-thickness grafts from these regions have a poor color and texture match with the face.

Surgical Technique

Instruments commonly used for harvesting skin grafts are a scalpel, or an electric or air-driven dermatome. Both the air-driven Brown (Padgett Corporation) or Zimmer dermatome (Zimmer, Inc., Warsaw, IN) and the Padgett electric dermatome (Integra, Plainsboro, NJ) are ideal instruments for obtaining a consistently uniform skin graft.

The donor site is prepped with a bactericidal solution and allowed to dry. A thin layer of mineral oil is applied to the donor site skin and to the blade of the dermatome. The Brown or the Padgett dermatome should be set between 0.010 and 0.018 in., depending on the thickness of the graft desired. The dermatome is placed at an approximately 45-degree angle to the donor skin and started prior to contact with the skin. Gentle traction is applied to the donor site skin as the dermatome is smoothly applied with even pressure. This technique ensures the harvest of a good graft. Bleeding from the dermal capillary bed will be noted in the donor site. Telfa soaked in a solution of epinephrine is applied to the donor site to provide hemostasis until the final dressing is applied. The donor site should be dressed with some type of semiocclusive dressing, such as OpSite (Smith & Nephew Healthcare, Hull, UK) or a piece of petrolatum gauze attached to the wound, followed by placement of a slight pressure dressing in the form of a Kerlix or Ace wrap. Reepithelialization of the donor site occurs over the following 2 to 3 weeks.

When obtaining a dermal graft, a strip of split-thickness skin (0.012 to 0.016 in.) is elevated as previously described but is left attached at one end. The dermatome-cutting tract should be narrowed so that a strip of dermis (0.012 to 0.014 in.) can be harvested and excised. The flap of split-thickness skin is placed over the defect and stapled or sutured into position.

Preparation of the host bed is important in ensuring the survival of the graft. This should include obtaining adequate hemostasis, debridement of necrotic tissue, and removal of infected tissue. Bone or cartilage that is not covered by periosteum or perichondrium does not provide a good vascular host bed for the graft and should be avoided.

The STSG can be passed through a graft mesh to provide greater surface area and allow for drainage of serous fluid from the reconstructed site. Unfortunately, meshing grafts creates a thinner graft, which is likely to contract and heal as shiny, thin, atrophic skin. If a graft of adequate size is obtained, a scalpel can be used to cut multiple small slits (5 to 6 mm) in the graft to allow serous fluid to drain from under the graft. The graft can be secured to the recipient site with staples or suture. The most important factor in ensuring the success of the STSG is graft immobilization and pressure over the site. This prevents the graft from migrating and thereby limits the shearing forces applied to the graft that act to disrupt any of the vascular connections that may have formed recently. Fibrin glue may be applied as both a hemostatic agent and an adhesive that helps bind the graft to the host bed.[4] A pressure dressing using cotton, fluffed gauze, or a sponge can be maintained in position using tie-over sutures. Sometimes a stent may be used to provide pressure on a graft, which is placed in the ear or hard palate. These dressings are usually removed within 7 to 10 days.

Skin grafts can be preserved by storage at low temperatures. Grafts can be wrapped in gauze soaked in Ringer's lactate or normal saline and stored in a sterile container at 4°C. The graft should never be totally immersed in saline because it will become macerated.[4] After 14 days of storage at 4°C, the respiratory activity of the skin graft is reduced by 50%.[17]

Skin Flaps

A skin flap is composed of skin and subcutaneous tissue that is transferred from one part of the body to another, with a connection to the body or vascular pedicle preserved for its blood supply. The relationship of the vascular pedicle to the flap may vary according to the orientation of the defect to the flap.[18] In some cases, the vascular pedicle can be transected and transferred to a distal site by microvascular anastomosis to another set of recipient (nourishing) vessels (microvascular free flap). Microvascular free tissue transfer may include fascia and skin, or a composite of skin, muscle, and bone.

Wounds or defects can be covered with either a skin graft or a skin flap. Although a skin graft should be considered first, there are many circumstances in which a flap is required. Skin flaps are frequently needed because either the recipient site is poorly vascularized and is unable to nourish a free skin graft or the transfer of a skin flap provides a better match of color and texture. When planning the reconstruction of a facial defect, the surgeon must consider the location of the defect, visibility of the site, and the patient's concern with the final aesthetic appearance. One unique situation involves resection of a tumor with a high chance of recurrence or where the surgical margins were uncertain. In these cases, it is advised to use a temporary STSG to allow close monitoring for tumor recurrence. If after an acceptable observation period there has been no tumor recurrence, reconstruction of the defect with the appropriate flap may be performed.[4]

Vascular Anatomy of the Skin

The anatomical variations in the blood supply of the skin must be understood before one embarks on using various local flaps in reconstruction. The skin is supplied by two principal vascular sources: musculocutaneous vessels and direct cutaneous vessels. Musculocutaneous vessels arise from segmental vessels; their anastomoses with axial vessels course below the muscles. From the muscle vasculature arise perforating musculocutaneous branches that enter the subcutaneous tissue.[19] The musculocutaneous vessels supply the majority of blood flow to the skin, especially in the trunk and extremities. After ascending to the deep reticular dermis, these vessels provide branches to two horizontally arrayed microvascular plexuses in the dermis. The deeper plexus, which is located at the dermal–subcutaneous junction, supplies the adnexal structures, the hair follicles, and the eccrine glands. Projections from this deep plexus anastomose with vessels in the superficial plexus located in the papillary dermis (**Fig. 4.3**).[20]

Segmental, anastomotic, and axial vessels also give rise to a limited number of direct cutaneous vessels that lie above the muscular fascia and are parallel to the skin. These arteries supplement the musculocutaneous arteries in providing additional nutritive and nonnutritive blood flow to the skin.[18] The direct cutaneous arteries have an associated subdermal vein in addition to paired venae comitantes. The direct cutaneous arteries send branches into the two dermal microcirculatory plexuses and account for the majority of the scalp and facial cutaneous vascular supply.

Flap Design

Random Flaps

Random flaps or random pattern flaps (local cutaneous flaps) are the most common type of flap employed in reconstruction of cutaneous defects of the head and neck. These flaps are created by dissecting the flap at the level of the subcutaneous fat. Their arterial supply comes from perforating musculocutaneous vessels at the flap base arising from segmental vessels that underlie muscle and subcutaneous tissue (**Fig. 4.4**). The blood flow to the free portion of the flap is supplied by the anastomoses between the deeper dermal–subcutaneous plexus and the more superficial papillary dermal plexus.[21,22] Random pattern flaps may be divided into two basic types: advancement flaps and rotation flaps (which can include transposition flaps).

The survival of random pattern flaps is unpredictable.[19] Milton[23] disproved the early teaching that a length to width ratio was required to ensure flap viability. Most flaps can be created with a length to width ratio of 3:1 and longer if the facial flap has an axial pattern vascular supply through direct cutaneous vessels (i.e., paramedian forehead flap).[18,24]

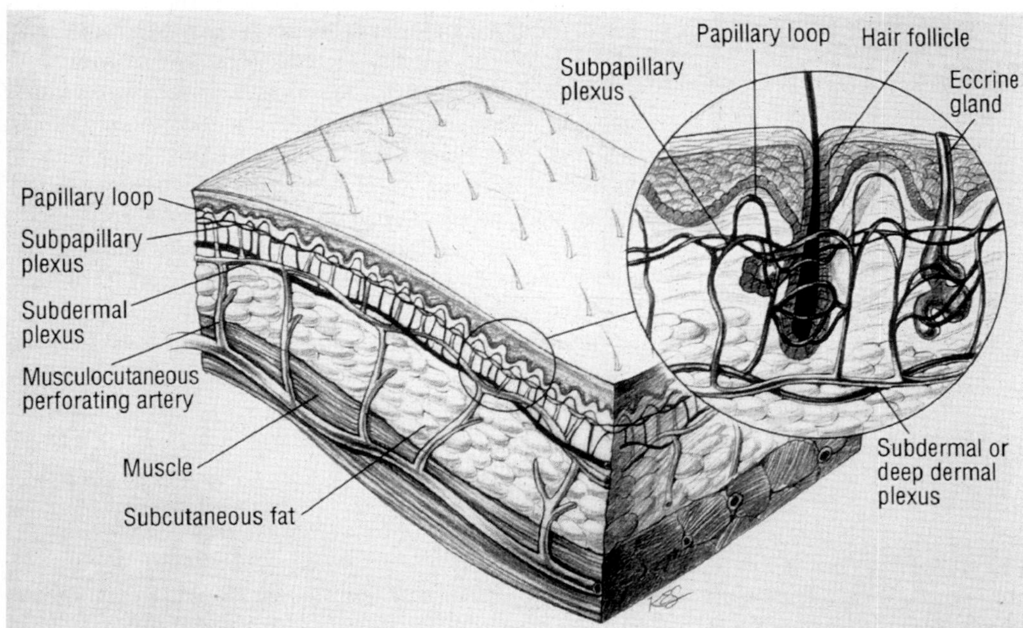

Fig. 4.3 Cutaneous vascular anatomy demonstrating the anastomoses between the subdermal and subpapillary plexuses. (From Conner CD, Fosko SW. Anatomy and physiology of local skin flaps. Fac Plast Clin North Am, Elsevier, 1996; 4:447–454. With permission.)

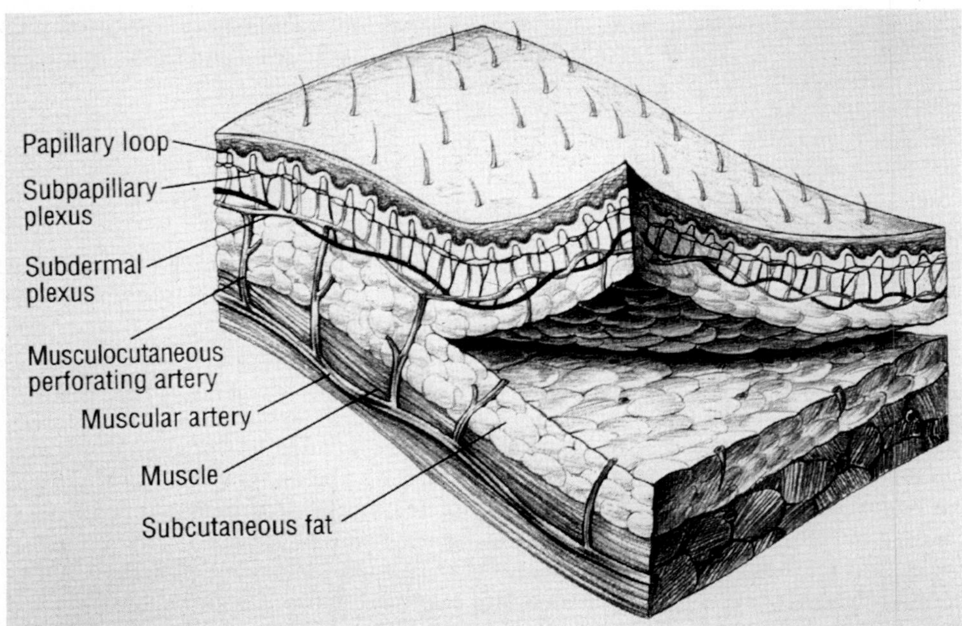

Fig. 4.4 Cross-section of a random pattern skin flap. The plane of dissection is in the subcutaneous fat. Musculocutaneous perforating arteries arising from underlying muscular arteries provide the blood supply to these flaps.

Axial Flaps

Axial flaps, or axial pattern flaps (arterial flaps), derive their blood supply from a direct cutaneous artery arising from a segmental, anastomotic, or axial artery.[25] Axial flaps can be of greater length to width ratios than random flaps. The distal free portion of the flap is a random flap by nature of its vascular supply. Hence, the dynamic vascular territory is larger than the anatomical territory. This supports the concept of the angiosome, which is the area of skin comprising the flap that is supplied by an axial vessel but may be extended by its communication with branches of an adjacent vessel.[26] Axial pattern flaps are supplied by an identifiable vessel: deltopectoral (internal mammary artery), forehead (supratrochlear artery), or scalp flap (superficial temporal artery). One advantage of the axial pattern flap is that a large area of skin coverage can be provided in a single procedure without the need for inclusion of the bulky underlying muscle. The base of the pedicle need only be wide enough to accompany the named vessel supplying the flap.

Free Flaps

Microvascular free tissue transfer or free flaps have evolved over the past decade through the technological advances in the field of microvascular surgery. These techniques allow the reconstructive surgeon to transfer free axial-pattern skin (fasciocutaneous), skin and muscle (musculocutaneous), or skin, muscle, and bone (osteomyocutaneous or osteocutaneous) flaps from a host donor site to a distant recipient site in a single-stage operation. The axial artery and vein that supply the flap are anastomosed under the microscope, with recipient vessels near the defect in the head and neck. Donor sites for skin (fasciocutaneous flaps) include the forearm (radial forearm free flap), lateral arm free flap, and lateral thigh free flap.[27–29] The parascapular, scapular, fibula, and iliac crest tissues are excellent donor sites where the defects include bone and surrounding soft tissue.[30–33] Rectus abdominis and latissimus dorsi are good donor sites where bulk is needed to reconstruct the defect.[34–36] These flaps are usually harvested as muscle with the overlying skin. Although free tissue transfer requires advanced surgical techniques, special equipment, and prolonged operative times, it provides the surgeon with an excellent alternative for reconstruction of complex head and neck defects.

The remaining portion of this chapter focuses on the use of various random pattern skin flaps for the reconstruction of facial defects.

Wound Closure

Surgical Planning

Most of the defects encountered by facial plastic surgeons may be repaired by primary closure or with local skin flaps. Selection of the appropriate method of closure of facial defects requires an understanding of the biomechanics of wound closure.

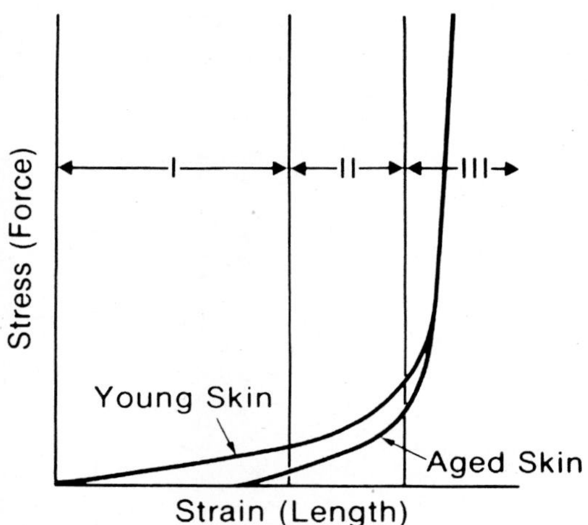

Fig. 4.5 Stress–strain curve for young and aged skin. (From Toriumi D, Larrabee WF. Skin grafts and flaps. In: Papel ID, Nachlas N, eds. Facial Plastic and Reconstructive Surgery. St. Louis: CV Mosby; 1992. With permission.)

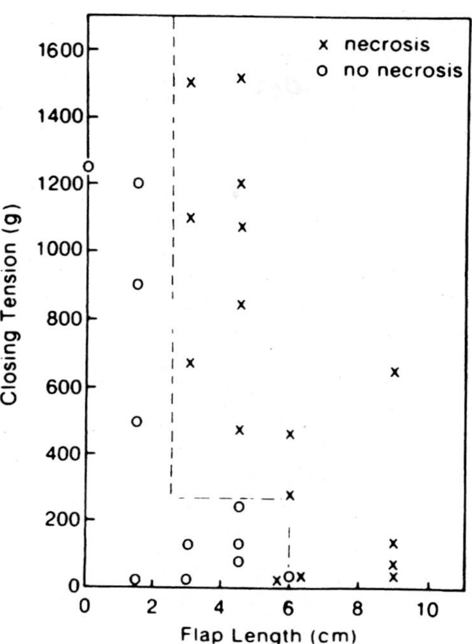

Fig. 4.6 Effect of closing tension on skin flap viability. (From Larrabee WF, Holloway GA, Sutton D. Wound tension and blood flow in skin flaps. Ann Otol Rhinol Laryngol 1984;93:112. With permission.)

Biomechanics of Wound Closure

Optimal wound closure requires an understanding of soft tissue mechanics and the principles of wound healing. The mechanical behavior of skin is primarily related to its collagen and elastin content.[36–38] Collagen types I and III provide the principal supporting framework of the extracellular matrix in the dermis. Elastic fibers in combination with collagen provide the elasticity or relative ease of deformation of the skin.[19] As skin is stretched, there is a period of easy deformation (section I) on the stress–strain curve that is controlled primarily by the fine elastin network (**Fig. 4.5**). In section II of the curve, randomly arranged collagen fibers begin to lengthen in the direction of the force, and deformation becomes more difficult. Lastly, in section III, all of the collagen fibers are oriented with the force, and little further deformation is possible. Clinically, when attempts to close a wound result in excessive tensions (section III of the stress–strain curve), little additional tissue can be advanced with more force, and other methods of closure (grafts or flaps) should be considered.[4,18]

Excessive tension in skin flaps can result in flap necrosis likely caused by reduced blood flow specifically in those flaps with borderline viability.[39] Larrabee et al[40] reported in their animal study using 2 cm wide random pattern skin flaps that any flap longer than 6 cm (length to width ratio being greater than 3:1) underwent necrosis regardless of tension (**Fig. 4.6**). Any flap less than 2 cm in length (less than 1:1 length to width ratio) was viable regardless of tension. Those flaps of intermediate length were most influenced by tension. Flaps closed under 250 g of tension or less tended to survive, whereas those closed under higher tensions underwent necrosis. This study reinforces the clinical impression that tension on flaps of borderline viability increases the incidence of necrosis.[4]

In another study, increasing tension was placed on a random pattern skin flap in piglets, and blood flow was measured at four sites along the flap with the Doppler laser. As shown in **Fig. 4.7**, there was decreased blood flow with increased tension, with the blood flow leveling off at ~250 g of tension. To summarize, tension does decrease blood flow in skin flaps; in flaps with excellent blood flow, tension may not be a critical factor, but with borderline viability it increases the incidence of necrosis.[4]

The forces in skin change over time.[38] Creep is the increase in strain (change in length to original length) seen when skin is placed under a constant stress (force or unit area). Stress relaxation refers to the decrease in stress when skin is held under tension at a constant strain. The surgeon who uses tissue expanders or the technique of serial excision of tissue routinely employs these time-dependent properties of skin.

The attachments of skin to subcutaneous tissue are mechanically critical because undermining the skin a moderate amount decreases wound-closing tensions and distributes skin deformation. Larrabee[39] studied the mechanical results of skin undermining in an animal model. A series of 2 × 6 cm fusiform defects were created, and undermining from the flap edge was performed

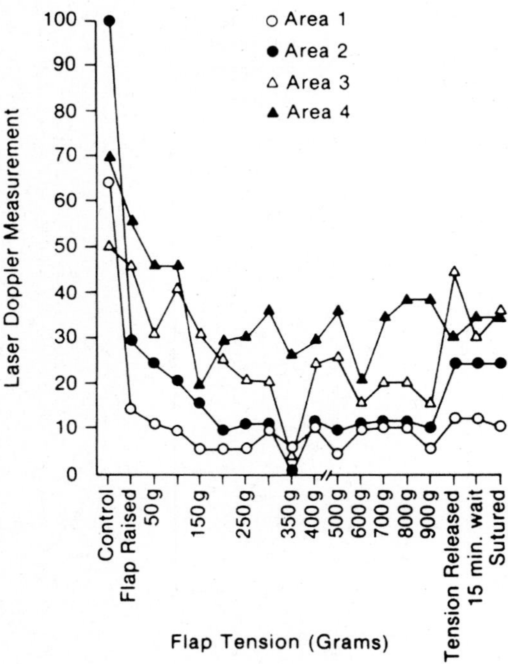

Fig. 4.7 Doppler laser measurement of blood flow in 3 to 6 cm skin flaps with increasing tension. Area 1 was at the end of the flap and area 3 at the base. Area 4 was in the region of the pedicle. (From Larrabee WF, Holloway GA, Sutton D. Wound tension and blood flow in skin flaps. Ann Otol Rhinol Laryngol 1984;93:112. With permission.)

in 2, 4, and 6 cm increments (**Fig. 4.8**). The flaps were advanced and a series of curves generated, showing the force required to advance the flap a given distance (**Fig. 4.9**). In each case, undermining of 2 to 4 cm caused the curve to shift to the right, thus denoting decreased tension on the flap for a given advancement. Undermining more extensively to 6 cm did not result in any significant change in forces and in some cases actually resulted in increased flap tension. In this model, moderate undermining was not helpful in decreasing flap tension but may have helped in tissue redraping.[4,18] Tissue redistribution can be controlled somewhat by altering the extent of undermining. Sometimes it is necessary to differentially undermine, meaning to limit undermining around a specific anatomical structure so as not to distort or deform (e.g., oral commissure, eyelids, brow, and nasal tip).

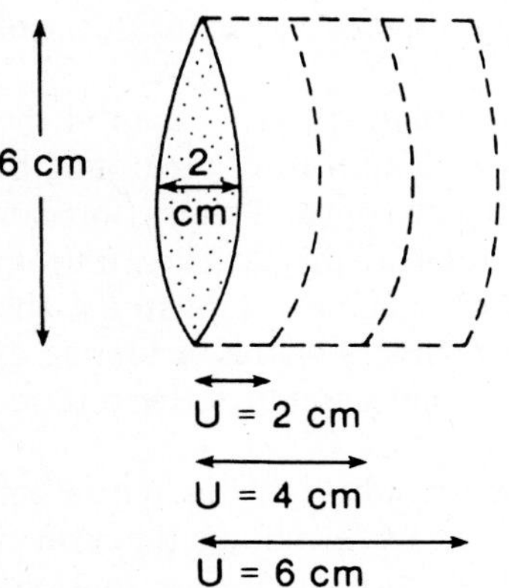

Fig. 4.8 Skin flaps undermined to 2, 4, and 6 cm. (From Toriumi D, Larrabee WF. Skin grafts and flaps. In: Papel ID, Nachlas N, eds. Facial Plastic and Reconstructive Surgery. St. Louis: CV Mosby; 1992:36. With permission.)

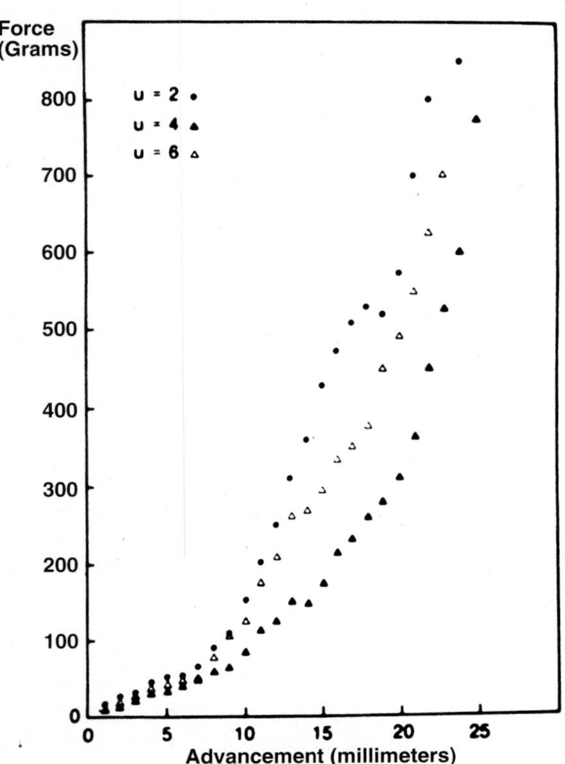

Fig. 4.9 Stress–strain curves with 2, 4, and 6 cm of undermining (U). (From Toriumi D, Larrabee WF. Skin grafts and flaps. In: Papel ID, Nachlas N, eds. Facial Plastic and Reconstructive Surgery. St. Louis: CV Mosby; 1992:36. With permission.)

Fusiform Repair

Most small facial lesions can be excised in a fusiform fashion and a simple closure performed with a good cosmetic result. The key to maximizing this technique is to place the lines of excision parallel to the relaxed skin tension lines (RSTLs) whenever possible (**Fig. 4.10**).[39] As a result, the maximal tension on the wound is parallel to the lines of maximal extensibility (LMEs). LMEs are usually perpendicular to the RSTLs and represent the direction in which closure can be performed with the least tension.[41] If the surgeon wishes to shorten the total length of the fusiform excision, an M-plasty can be used (**Fig. 4.11**). The M-plasty is especially useful when the

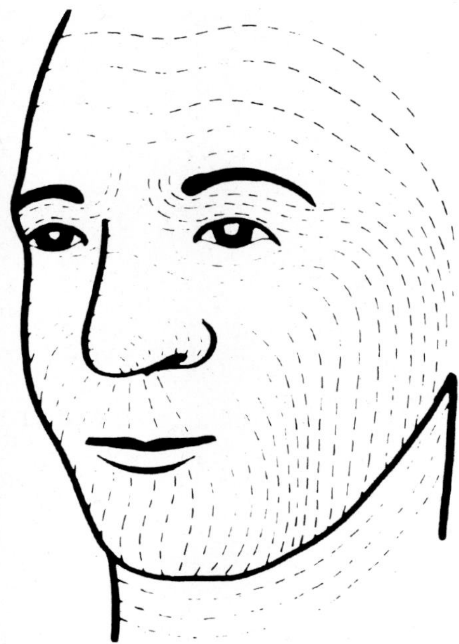

Fig. 4.10 Approximation of the relaxed skin tension lines (RSTLs) of the face. When excising a lesion on the face, the lines of excision should parallel the RSTL and parallel the lines of maximal extensibility.

standard fusiform excision would cross from one facial subunit to another or cross a normal facial groove (e.g., melolabial fold). A Gillies corner stitch should be used to close the corner of the M-plasty. This pulls the tips of the M-plasty toward the middle of the incision and prevents skin deformation at the end of the incision (i.e., dog-ear deformity).

Skin closure should be performed in multiple layers. An absorbable suture, such as Vicryl, Monocryl, polydiaxonone (PDS; Ethicon, Inc., Somerville, NJ), or Maxon (Davis and Geck), is placed in the subcutaneous tissue to evert and approximate the skin edges. Davidson[42] describes placing the subcutaneous sutures farther away from the skin edge to affect extreme wound-edge eversion and minimize tension on the healing incision.

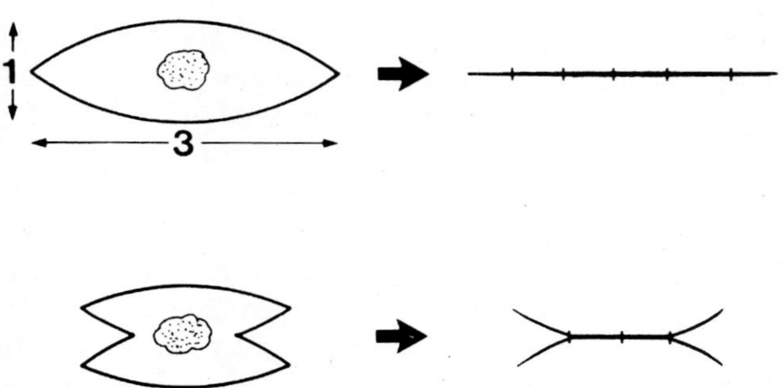

Fig. 4.11 M-plasty. A fusiform excision by inverting the end of the incision so that it creates a small M on either end. When these M-plasties are closed it is helpful to use a corner stitch to pull the tips of the M-plasty toward the middle of the incision.

Local Skin Flaps

The majority of facial defects that cannot be treated by primary closure can usually be closed with a local skin flap. The blood supply of these random pattern skin flaps is based on the subdermal plexus of vessels. Flaps are usually created with a flap length to width ratio of two to one (2:1). Some facial flaps have an axial pattern vascular supply through direct cutaneous vessels (e.g., forehead). These flaps tolerate much higher length to width ratios because the vascular supply is generally robust.[24]

All local facial flaps have rotational or advancement components, or both, in their movement from donor site to defect. Most flaps, including transposition flaps, have a component of both rotation and advancement, and the ratio of rotation to advancement can be tailored by flap design.[24] In the design of local skin flaps, many needs of the defect must be identified and analyzed. The depth and composition of the defect should be analyzed so that the reconstruction restores all layers of the defect. Regional differences in the thickness of the subcutaneous layer of facial skin must be appreciated when choosing the type of flap. For example, a skin-only defect of the eyelid is much thinner than a skin-only defect of the nasal tip.[43]

Advancement Flaps

The classically designed advancement flap has a length to width ratio of 2:1 and advances tissue a distance approximating the width of the flap (**Fig. 4.12**). These

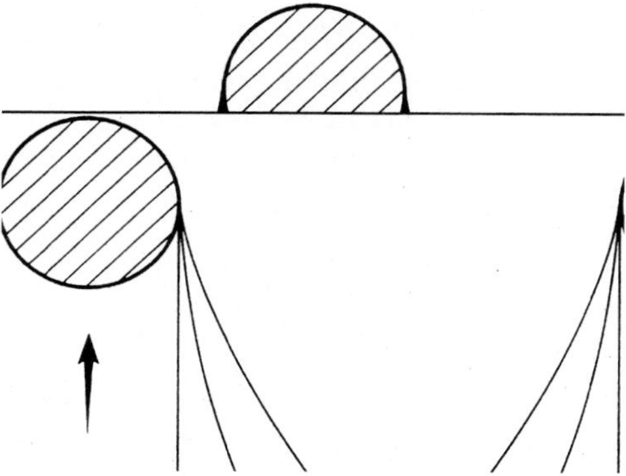

Fig. 4.12 Advancement flap design. Classically, these flaps have a length to width ratio of 2:1. Modifications can be made to follow the basic aesthetic units or the relaxed skin tension lines. Increasing the width of the flap does not necessarily increase the distal blood flow. (From Murakami CS, Nishioka GJ. Essential concepts in the design of local skin flaps. Fac Plast Surg Clin North Am, Elsevier, 1996;4: 455–468. With permission.)

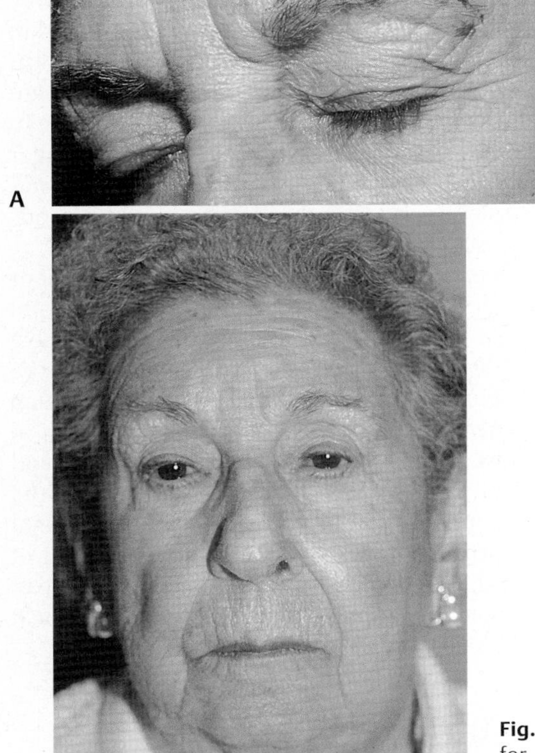

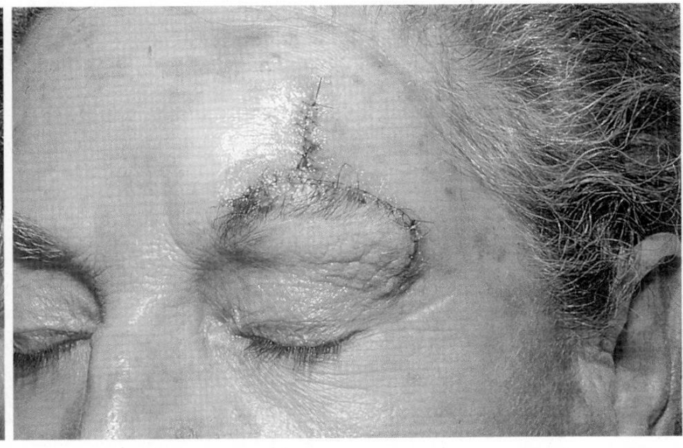

Fig. 4.13 Bilateral advancement flaps. (**A**) Proposed 2 cm defect for excision of a basal cell carcinoma (BCCA) of the eyebrow/forehead. (**B**) Bilateral advancement flap closure. (**C**) The 4-month postoperative result.

flaps are particularly useful for defects of the forehead. In the forehead, bilateral advancement flaps are designed with the horizontal components placed parallel to the RSTLs and adjacent to normal forehead creases (**Figs. 4.13 and 4.14**). Occasionally, Burow triangle excisions are needed but should not be performed until after the flap is advanced.

Rotation Flaps

All rotation flaps also have a component of advancement; therefore, many surgeons prefer the term *rotation–advancement flap*.[44] Lines of rotation tend to follow the natural contours of the face, such as face-lift flap and lower eyelid blepharoplasty flaps. The rotation–advancement flap is usually designed to move along an arc of less than 30 degrees. These flaps are easy to design and generally result in minimal tissue redundancy and wound-closing tension. Although tissue redraping may be improved by extending the rotation of the flap beyond 30 degrees, tension in the flap will increase and is found at the donor site, not along the longer length of the flap.[39] The amount of advancement of the rotation–advancement flap can be increased or decreased by alterations in flap design. The classic rotation flap is designed using a radius approximately two to three times the diameter of the defect and extending the length of the flap approximately four to five times the width of the defect, which creates an arc close to 90 degrees. The 90-degree arc flap will rotate 30 degrees to close the defect (**Fig. 4.15A**). Although usually unnecessary, the arc of the flap may be increased toward the maximum of 180 degrees.

Variations of the classic rotation flap can be created by increasing the radius of rotation (**Fig. 4.15B**). These changes

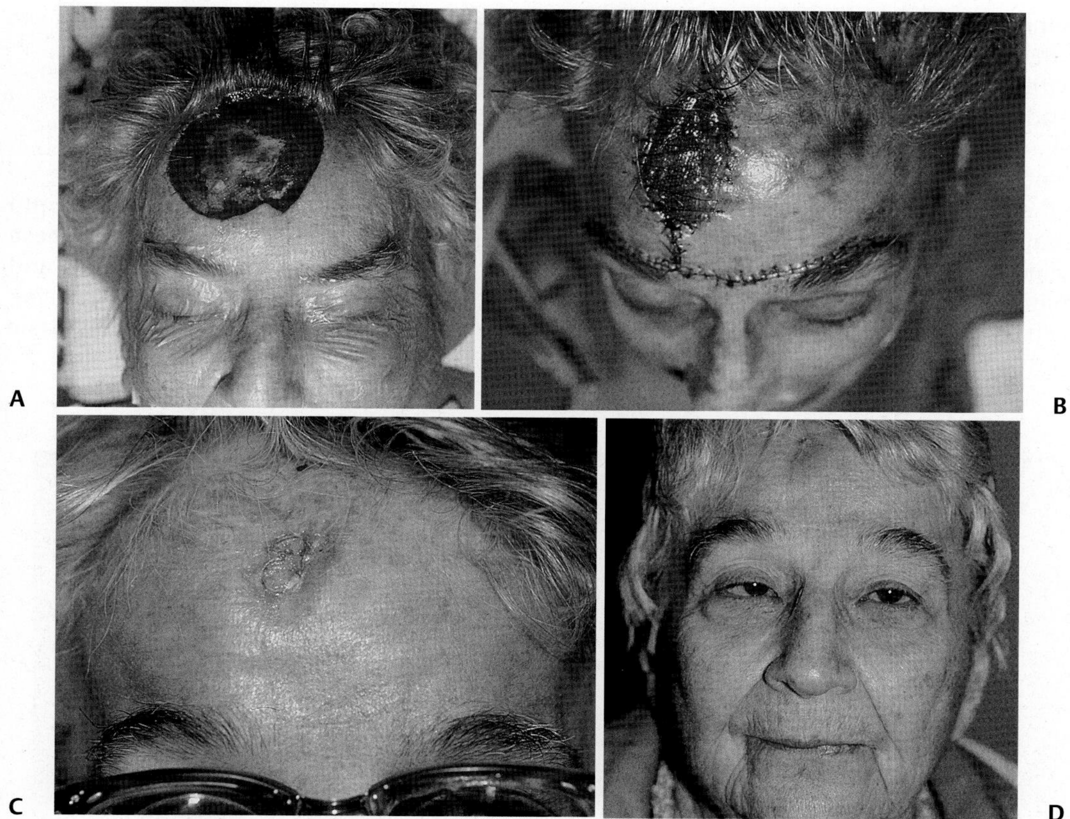

Fig. 4.14 Bilateral advancement flaps. (**A**) Large forehead Mohs defect approximately following excision of a basal cell carcinoma. (**B**) Bilateral advancement flaps used for partial closure. Central defect left open to heal by secondary intention. (**C**) The 1-month postoperative result, with significant healing noted. (**D**) The 3-month result with forehead completely healed.

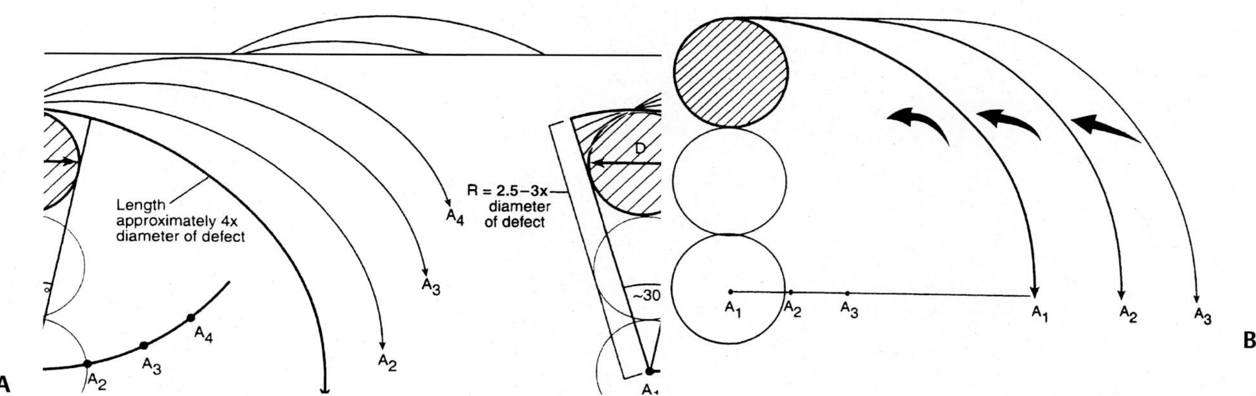

Fig. 4.15 Rotation–advancement flaps and modifications. (**A**) The basic rotation flap is drawn using a radius (R) that is 2.5 to 3 times the diameter (D) of the defect. The axis of rotation (A1–A4) can be moved along an arc to allow for greater rotation and less advancement. The base and the tip of the modified flaps become wider. (**B**) If the axis of rotation (A1–A3) is moved along a perpendicular line, the flap will have a greater advancement component and less rotation. (From Murakami CS, Nishioka GJ. Essential concepts in the design of local skin flaps. Fac Plast Surg Clin North Am, Elsevier,1996;4:455–468. With permission.)

alter the ratio of advancement and widen the width of the base and distal tip of the flap. The base of the flap is not fixed but advances with movement of the flap into the defect. The amount of advancement can be increased with a back-cut. Remember that this will advance the flap and decrease the amount of tension at its distal aspect, but narrows the width of the base of the flap and potentially results in vascular compromise if performed excessively.[24] Rotation–advancement flaps are useful for large cheek defects (**Fig. 4.16**). Any time there is a large triangular defect, such a flap should be considered. Two or three rotation–advancement flaps may be combined to close large circular defects. This is particularly useful for defects of the scalp.[45,46]

Transposition Flaps

Transposition flaps may be created and transposed into a defect with primary closure of the donor site. These flaps may be designed in many different shapes and sizes, making the choice of which flap to use for a given defect somewhat confusing.[24] There are three basic transposition flaps: rhomboid, bilobed, and Z-plasty.

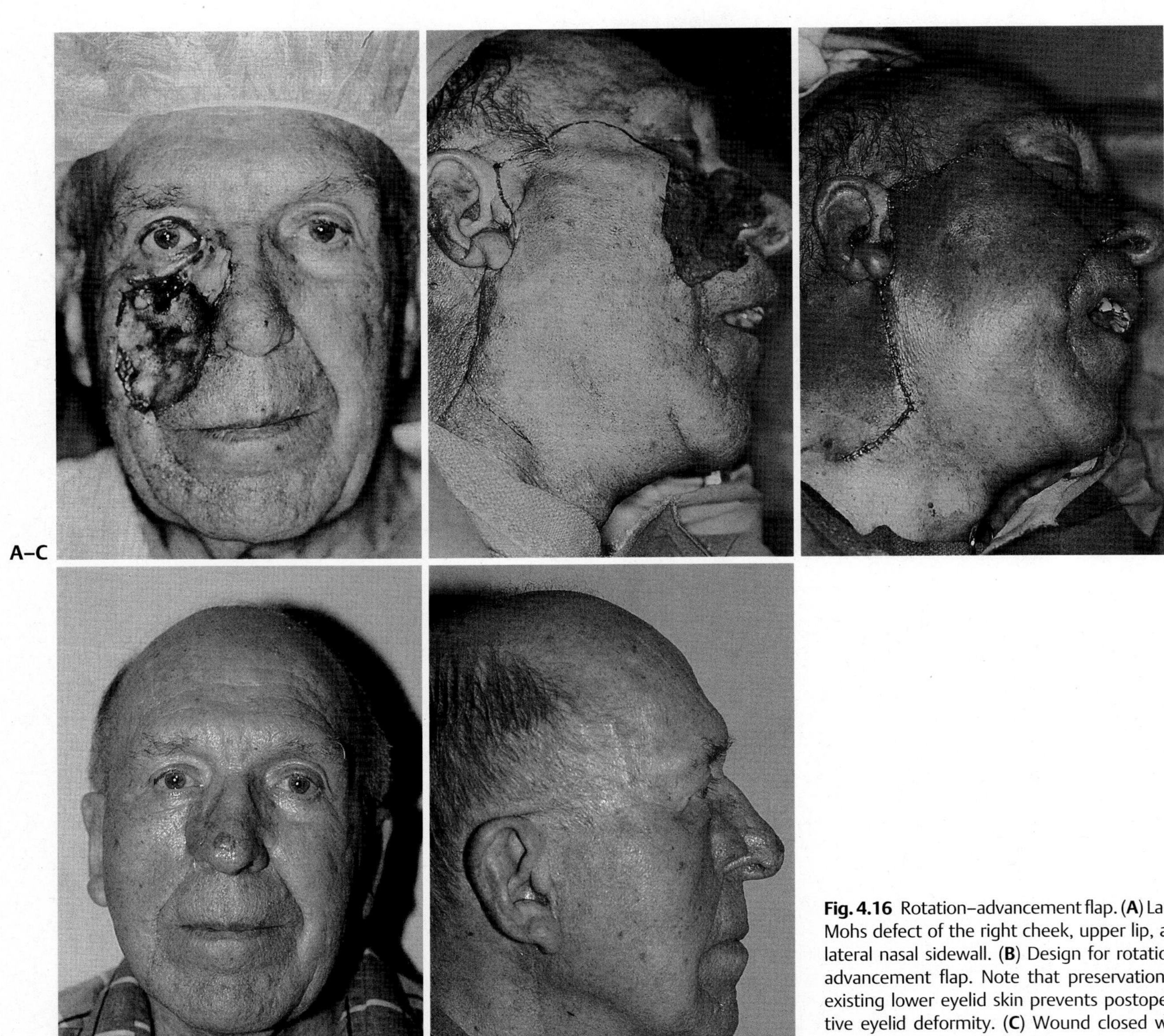

Fig. 4.16 Rotation–advancement flap. (**A**) Large Mohs defect of the right cheek, upper lip, and lateral nasal sidewall. (**B**) Design for rotation–advancement flap. Note that preservation of existing lower eyelid skin prevents postoperative eyelid deformity. (**C**) Wound closed with extension into the neck. (**D**) The 5-month postoperative result. (**E**) Lateral 5-month postoperative result.

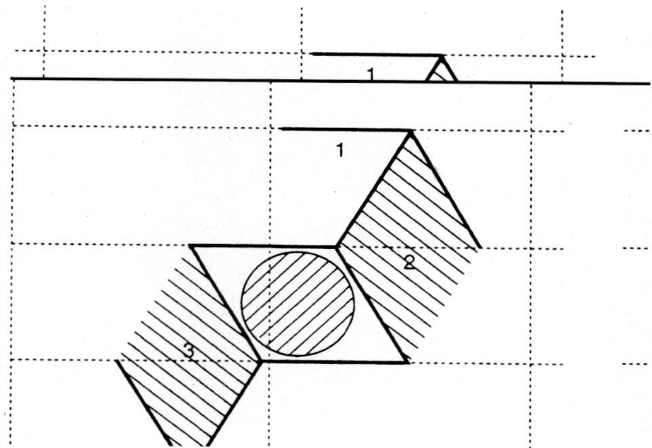

Fig. 4.17 Rhomboid flap. The basic 60-degree rhomboid or Limberg flap is designed using the relaxed skin tension lines (RSTLs) and the lines of maximal extensibility (LMEs). Four flaps can be created after the rhombus is placed around the defect. Only flaps 2 and 3 will have maximal wound closure in the LME. This design fails to take into account that defects are usually circular (not rhomboid), and the RSTLs and the LMEs are usually curvilinear. (From Murakami CS, Nishioka GJ. Essential concepts in the design of local skin flaps. Fac Plast Surg Clin North Am, Elsevier, 1996;4:455–468. With permission.)

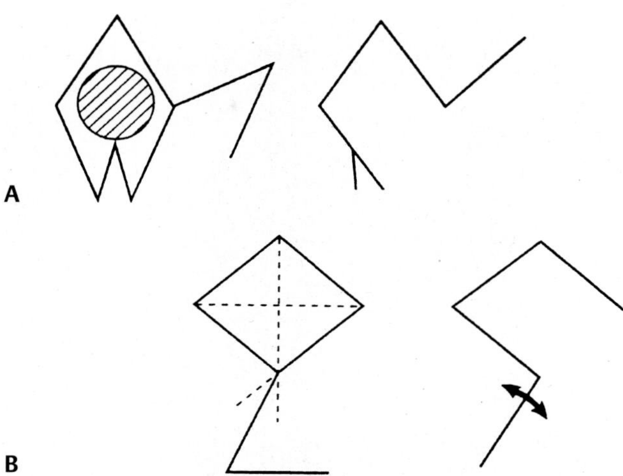

Fig. 4.18 Webster and Dufourmental flaps. (**A**) Webster's 30-degree flap. (**B**) Dufourmental flap. These modifications of the basic 60-degree rhomboid flap allow partial closure of the defect using secondary movement of surrounding tissue. The flaps also have smaller angles of rotation that result in smaller standing cones and redundancies. (From Murakami CS, Nishioka GJ. Essential concepts in the design of local skin flaps. Fac Plast Surg Clin North Am, Elsevier, 1996;4:455–468. With permission.)

Rhomboid Flap

The 60-degree rhomboid flap is a classic flap described by Limberg,[47] which consists of a rhomboid with two 60-degree angles and two 120-degree angles (**Fig. 4.17**). The greatest advantage of the rhomboid flap is its simple design, making it easy to position the flap so that maximum tension is positioned along an LME, with the borders of the flap lying in RSTLs.[48] A useful variation of the rhomboid design includes a 30-degree transposition flap that is transposed into a rhomboid defect that has been shortened with an M-plasty (**Fig. 4.18**).[49] Although somewhat more difficult to design, the 30-degree transposition flap is effective in decreasing the angle of rotation, thereby distributing the tension more evenly along the surface and minimizing dog-ear deformities. The Dufourmental flap is another modification of the rhomboid flap that may be applied to any rhombic defect, not just those of 60 or 120 degrees (**Fig. 4.18**).[50,51] It is useful for rhombic defects with an acute angle of 60 to 90 degrees, when the surgeon chooses not to excise additional skin to create a more acute angle.

The majority of the tension of a rhomboid flap is at the closure of the donor site.[48–51] Whenever possible, this line of tension at the donor site closure should be parallel to the LME. Double and triple rhomboids are very useful in the closure of large rectangular and circular defects. A standardized approach to rhomboid flap design allows selection of the optimal flap for a given defect.[40] The surgeon first draws two lines parallel to the LME and creates two rhomboids (**Fig. 4.17**). The four possible rhombic flaps for each figure are then drawn. Of these four flaps, one of the two flaps with a short diagonal parallel to the LME should be chosen.[50]

The rhomboid flap is particularly useful for defects in the cheek and temple area (**Fig. 4.19**). Although this flap is reliable, versatile, and easy to design, it does require forcing a facial defect into an arbitrary design. This may result in discarding normal tissue and making final scar placement more visible because of exact geometry.

Bilobed Flaps

The bilobed flap is another common transposition flap that consists of the mobilization of two flaps with a common base to cover the defect. The primary flap is the same size as or slightly smaller than the defect, and the secondary flap is slightly smaller than the primary flap (**Fig. 4.20**).[52] Early descriptions of the bilobed flap indicated that each flap rotated around an axis of 90 degrees, which often resulted in large redundancies of tissue and excess tension along margins of the flap.[53] Zitelli[54] redesigned the bilobed flap such that each flap rotates ~45 degrees. This reduces the amount of redundant tissue and the amount of tension at the flap margins. Sometimes the angles for these flaps are difficult to draw and calculate when the flaps are positioned over a convex or concave surface, such as the nasal dorsum.[24]

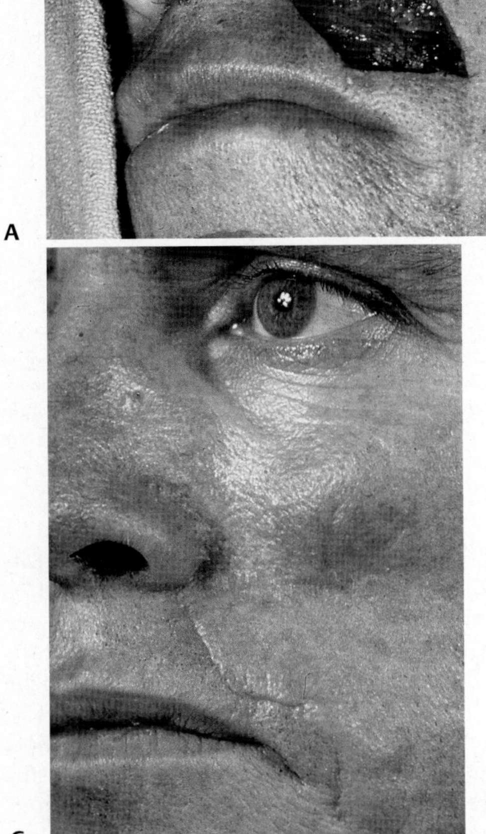

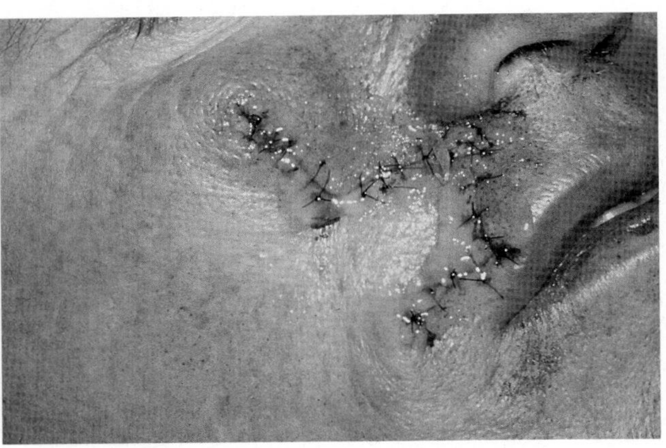

Fig. 4.19 Rhomboid flap. (**A**) Mohs defect of left upper lip. Wound modified to facilitate rhomboid design. (**B**) Wound closed. (**C**) The 1-month postoperative result.

The circular template technique makes it easy to design bilobed flaps that have primary and secondary flaps with appropriate sizes and angles of rotation.[55] The bilobed flap is commonly used for small defects (1 to 2 cm) of the dorsum and lateral side wall of the nose, or the lateral cheek (**Fig. 4.21**). The disadvantages of the bilobed flap are the length of the incisions, pin cushioning, and skin deformation.[4,18]

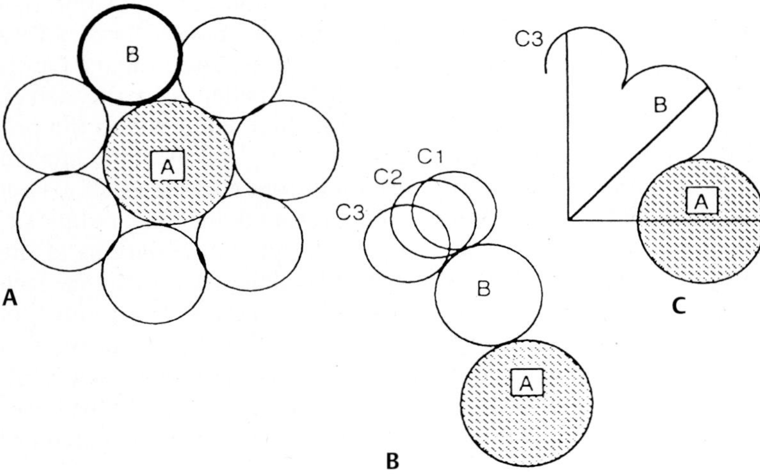

Fig. 4.20 Bilobed flap. (**A**) Template B is placed around defect A. (**B**) The C template is then drawn adjacent to circle B. The C position can be modified (C1–3) to control the rotation and advancement components. The C3 flap is at a 45-degree angle to the A–B axis. (**C**) If the C3 template is chosen and the bilobed flap is drawn around the B–C3 template, a bilobed flap similar to the Zitelli bilobed flap is created. (From Murakami CS, Nishioka GJ. Essential concepts in the design of local skin flaps. Fac Plast Surg Clin North Am, Elsevier, 1996;4:455–468. With permission.)

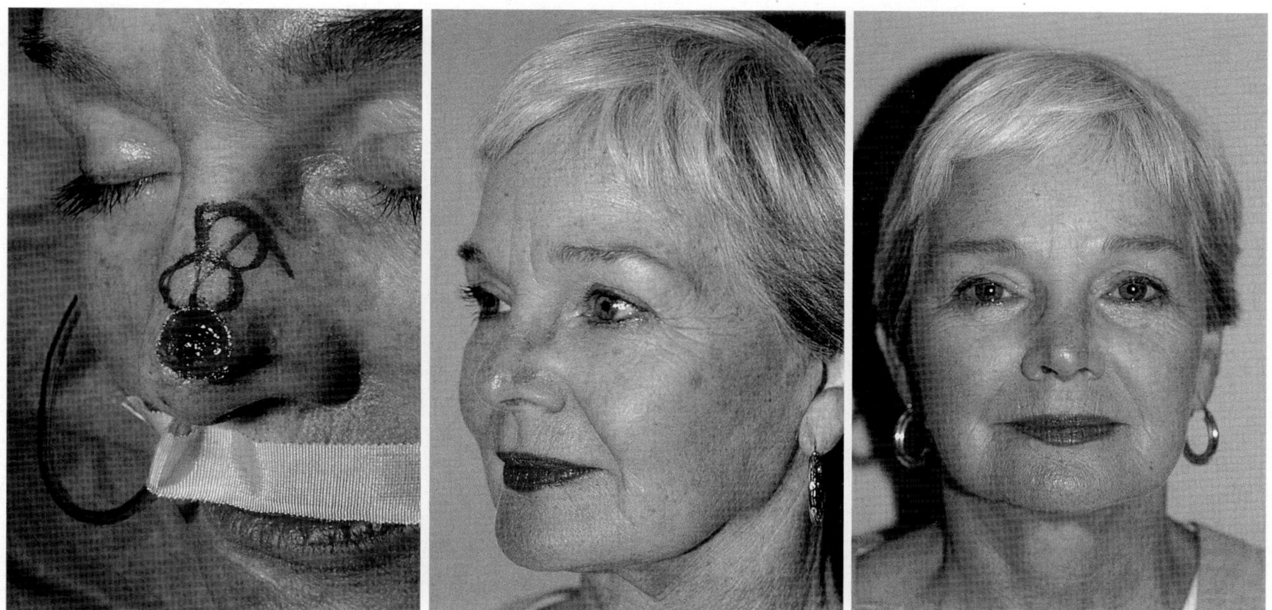

A–C

Fig. 4.21 Bilobed flap. (**A**) Mohs defect of the nasal tip. Bilobed flap designed. (**B**, **C**) The 3-month postoperative result.

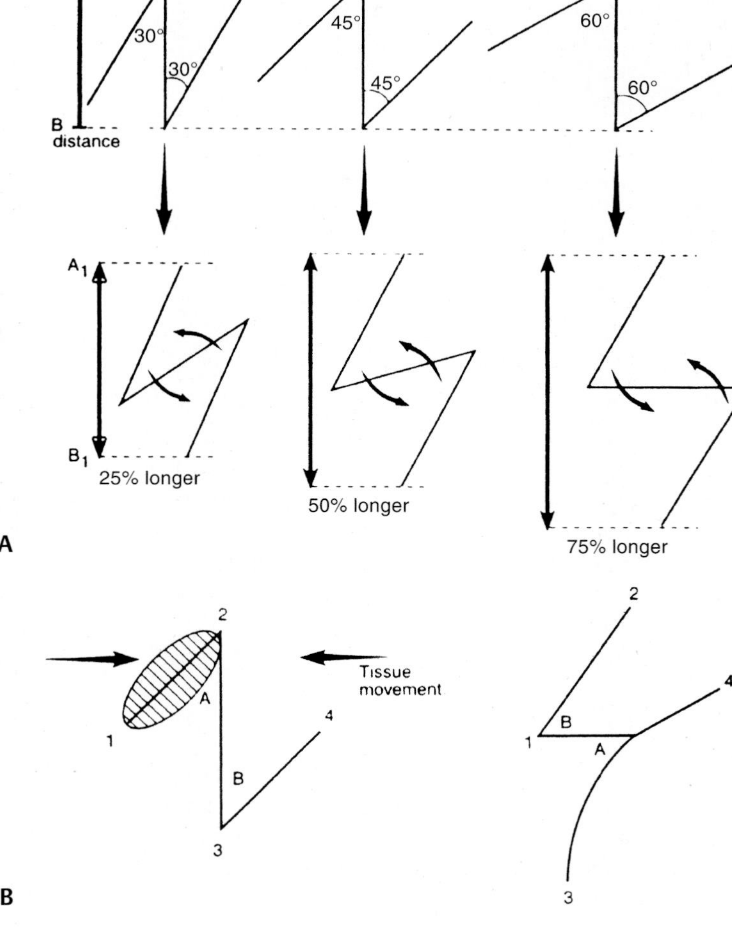

Fig. 4.22 Z-plasty flap. (**A**) The standard Z-plasty advances tissue from the lateral margins and expands the tissue along the 2–3 axis. A defect may be placed in any one of the three limbs of the Z-plasty. The A and B flaps must transpose across one another. The transposition of the A and B flaps occurs with all transposition flaps, although it may not be as obvious as in the Z-plasty flap. (**B**) A Z-plasty design used to close a defect placed along one of its three limbs. (From Murakami CS, Nishioka GJ. Essential concepts in the design of local skin flaps. Fac Plast Surg Clin North Am, Elsevier, 1996; 4:455–468. With permission.)

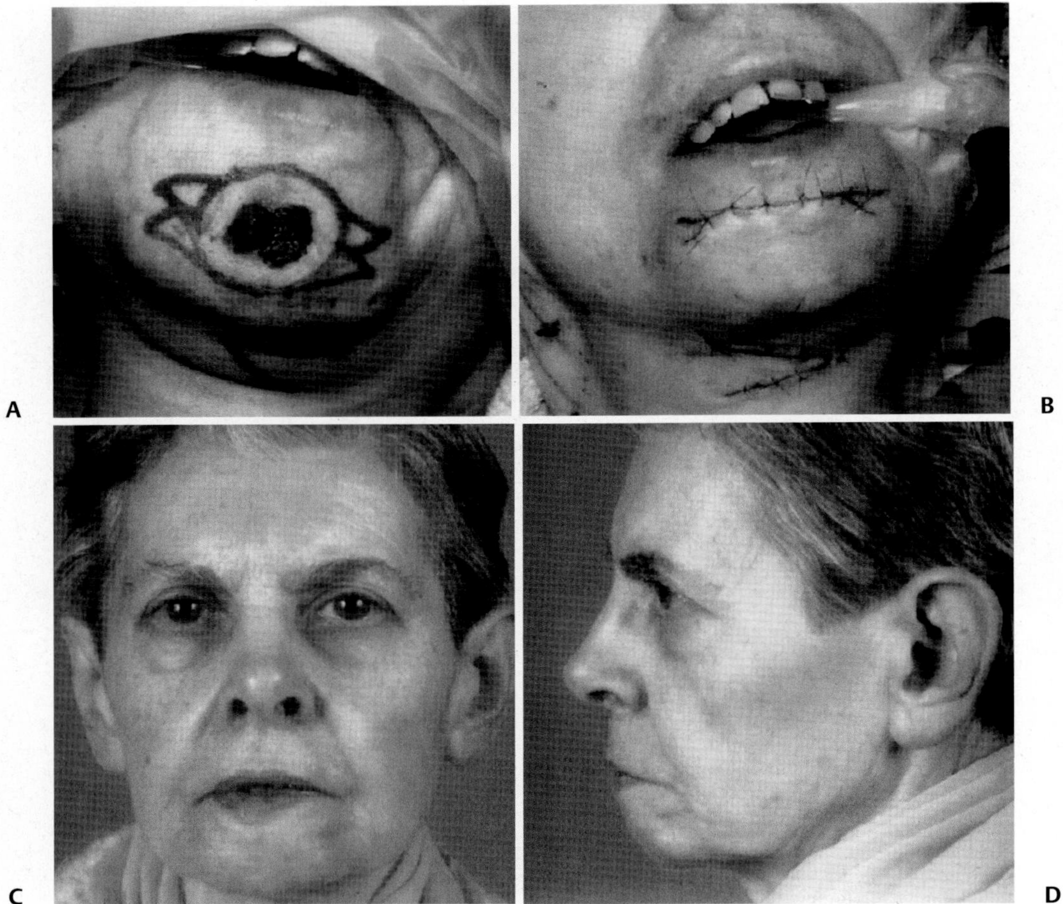

Fig. 4.23 Adjunctive Z-plasty. (**A**) Adjunctive Z-plasty designed to aid in fusiform closure of the large chin defect by borrowing tissue from the submental region. (**B**) Closure of both defects, with the Z-plasty hidden in the submental region. (**C, D**) The 6-month postoperative result. (From Toriumi D, Larrabee WF. Skin grafts and flaps. In: Papel ID, Nachlas N, eds. Facial Plastic and Reconstructive Surgery. St. Louis: CV Mosby; 1992:36. With permission.)

Z-Plasty

A Z-plasty is a double transposition of two flaps of equal size. Z-plasties are frequently used to revise scars by lengthening a contracted scar or changing the direction of scar so as to reorient it to favorable RSTLs or the basic aesthetic unit (BAU). The Z-plasty technique may be used to close a defect located on one of its three limbs (**Fig. 4.22**). Basically, two flaps of unequal size and unequal angles are transferred during closure of the defect. The concept is essentially the same in that there will be elongation in one dimension and contraction in the other with reorientation of the incisions. Lastly, Z-plasty may be helpful for closing wounds that cross the junction between BAUs or to avoid unnecessary traction on important anatomical structures, such as the eyelid, nose, and mouth (**Fig. 4.23**).

Subcutaneous Pedicle Flaps

Subcutaneous pedicle flaps are useful for moving a small amount of tissue a short distance. A triangle or kite-shaped area of skin is incised with its blood supply based on its subcutaneous pedicle.[56–58] It is then mobilized and advanced into the defect. The donor area is closed in a V to Y fashion (**Fig. 4.24**). The flap can also be designed for rotation or advancement into a nonadjacent defect.[4,18]

Summary

A comprehensive knowledge of the anatomy, physiology, biomechanics, and design of skin flaps must be achieved before embarking on the reconstruction of a soft tissue defect of the face. Each defect is unique, and the surgeon

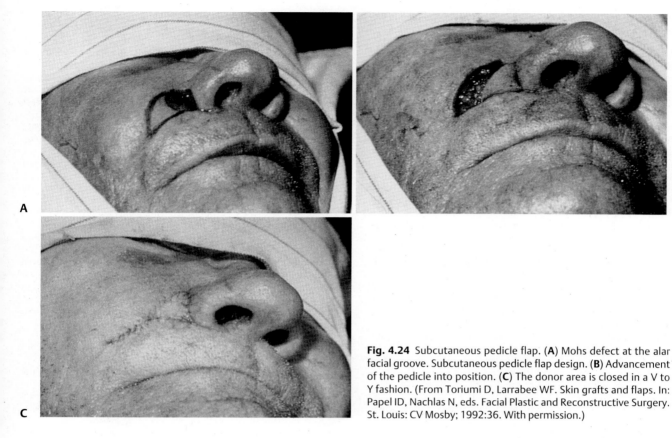

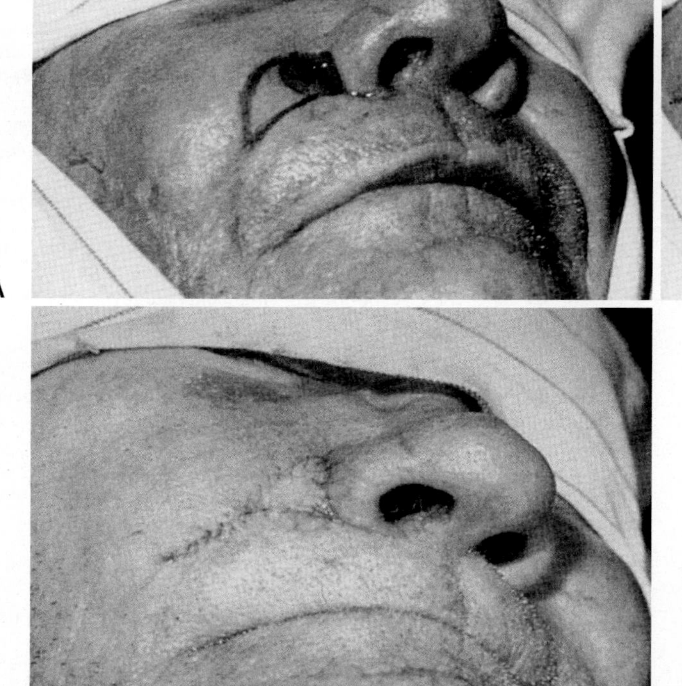
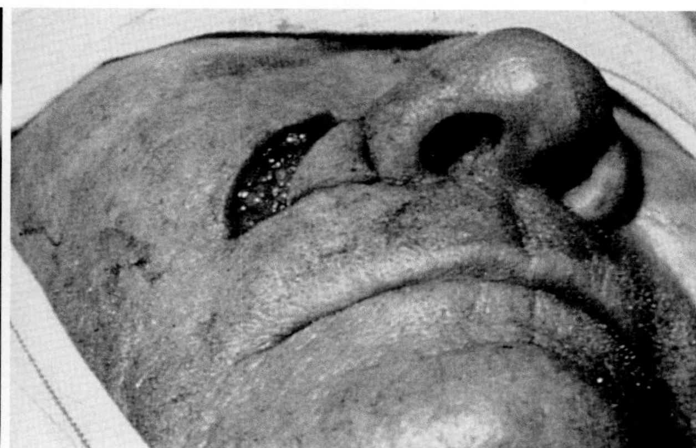

Fig. 4.24 Subcutaneous pedicle flap. (**A**) Mohs defect at the alar facial groove. Subcutaneous pedicle flap design. (**B**) Advancement of the pedicle into position. (**C**) The donor area is closed in a V to Y fashion. (From Toriumi D, Larrabee WF. Skin grafts and flaps. In: Papel ID, Nachlas N, eds. Facial Plastic and Reconstructive Surgery. St. Louis: CV Mosby; 1992:36. With permission.)

often relies on variations of the rotation, advancement, and transposition flaps to close defects based on their specific location, size, and donor tissue.[24] The better one understands these concepts, the better one is able to customize a local flap to suit the specific needs of the defect, avoid complications caused by miscalculations, and attain an aesthetically pleasing closure of the skin and soft tissue defect with minimal associated morbidity.

References

1. Kazanceva ND. Growth characteristics of skin thickness in children and its significance in free skin grafts. Acta Chir Plast 1969;11:71–78
2. Southwood WFW. The thickness of the skin. Plast Reconstr Surg 1955;15:423–428
3. Clevens RA, Baker SR. Defect analysis and options for reconstruction. Otolaryngol Clin North Am 1997;30:495–517
4. Toriumi DM, Larrabee WF. Skin grafts and flaps. In: Papel ID, Nachlas NE, eds. Facial Plastic and Reconstructive Surgery. St. Louis: Mosby-Year Book; 1992
5. Kaufman AJ. Adjacent-tissue skin grafts for reconstruction. Dermatol Surg 2004;30:1349–1353
6. Reed GF, Zafra E, Ghyselen AL, et al. Self-epithelialization of dermal grafts. Arch Otolaryngol 1968;87:518–521
7. Sclafani AP, Romo T. Alloplasts for nasal augmentation: clinical experience and scientific rationale. Facial Plast Surg Clin North Am 1999;7:43–54
8. Cox AJ, Wang TD. Skeletal implants in aesthetic facial surgery. Facial Plast Surg 1999;15:3–12
9. Jones F, Schhwartz B, Silverstein P. Use of a nonimmunogenic acellular dermal allograft for soft tissue augmentation. Aesthetic Surg Q 1996;16:196–201
10. Hynes W. The early circulation in skin grafts with a consideration of methods to encourage their survival. Br J Plast Surg 1954;6:257–262
11. Singer AJ, Clark RAF. Mechanisms of disease: cutaneous wound healing. N Engl J Med 1999;341:738–746
12. Converse JM, Smahel J, Ballantyne DL. Inosculation of vessels of skin graft and host bed: a fortuitous encounter. Br J Plast Surg 1975;28:274–280
13. Edgerton MT, Edgerton PJ. Vascularization of homografts. Transplant Bull 1955;2:98–102
14. Mir Y, Mir L. Biology of the skin graft: new aspects to consider in its revascularization. Plast Reconstr Surg 1951;8:378–384
15. Zitelli JA. Wound healing by secondary intention. J Am Acad Dermatol 1983;9:407–412
16. Kamrin BB. Analysis of the union between host and graft in the albino rat. Plast Reconstr Surg 1961;28:221–229
17. Fitzgerald MJT, Martin F, Paletta F. Innervation of skin grafts. Surg Gynecol Obstet 1967;124:808–814
18. Menick FJ. Facial reconstruction with local and distant tissue: the interface of aesthetic and reconstructive surgery. Plast Reconstr Surg 1998;102:1424–1433
19. Lawrence JC. Storage and skin metabolism. Br J Plast Surg 1972; 25:440–447
20. Connor DC, Fosko SW. Anatomy and physiology of local skin flaps. Facial Plast Surg Clin North Am 1996;4:447–454
21. Murujo AA. Terminal arteries of the skin. Acta Anat (Basel) 1961;58:289–295
22. Cormack GC, Lamberty BGH. The Arterial Anatomy of Skin Flaps. New York: Churchill Livingstone; 1986
23. Milton SH. Pedicle skin flap: the fallacy of the length-width ratio. Br J Surg 1970;57:502–508

24. Taylor GI, Minabe T. The angiosomes of mammals and other vertebrates. Plast Reconstr Surg 1992;89:181–215
25. Murakami CS, Nishioka GJ. Essential concepts in the design of local skin flaps. Facial Plast Surg Clin North Am 1996;4:455–468
26. McGregor IA, Morgan G. Axial and random pattern flaps. Br J Plast Surg 1973;26:202–213
27. Smith PJ. The vascular basis of axial pattern flaps. Br J Plast Surg 1973;26:150–157
28. Calhoun KH. Radial forearm free flap for head and neck reconstruction. Facial Plast Surg 1996;12:29–33
29. Clymer MA, Burkey BB. Other flaps for head and neck use: temporoparietal fascia free flap, lateral arm free flap, omental free flap. Facial Plast Surg 1996;12:81–89
30. Deschler DG, Hayden RE. Lateral thigh free flap. Facial Plast Surg 1996;12:75–79
31. Funk GF. Scapular and parascapular free flaps. Facial Plast Surg 1996;12:57–63
32. Chen ZW, Yan W. The study and clinical applications of the osteocutaneous flap of fibula. Microsurgery 1983;4:11–16
33. Urken M, Vickery C, Weinberg H. The internal oblique-iliac crest osteomyocutaneous free flap in oromandibular reconstruction. Arch Otolaryngol 1989;115:339–349
34. Taylor GI, Corlett RJ, Boyd JB. The versatile deep inferior epigastric (inferior rectus abdominis) flap. Br J Plast Surg 1984;37:330–350
35. Meland NB, Fisher J, Irons GB. Experience with 80 rectus abdominis free-tissue transfers. Plast Reconstr Surg 1989;83:481–487
36. Civantos FJ. Latissimus dorsi microvascular flap. Facial Plast Surg 1996;12:65–68
37. Daley CH, Odland GF. Age-related changes in the mechanical properties of human skin. J Invest Dermatol 1979;73:84–89
38. Gibson T, Stark H, Evans JH. Directional variations in the extensibility of human skin in vivo. J Biomech 1969;2:201–206
39. Larrabee WF. A finite element model of skin deformation. Laryngoscope 1986;96:399–405
40. Larrabee WF, Holloway GA, Sutton D. Wound tension and blood flow in skin flaps. Ann Otol Rhinol Laryngol 1984;93:112–115
41. Borges AF. Elective Incisions and Scar Revision. Boston: Little, Brown; 1973
42. Davidson TM. Subcutaneous suture placement. Laryngoscope 1985;97:501–505
43. Sykes JM, Murakami CS. Principles of local flaps in head and neck reconstruction. Oper Tech Otolaryngol Head Neck Surg 1993;4:2–10
44. Wexler DB, Gilbertson LG, Goel VK. Biomechanics of the rotation-advancement skin flap: experimental and theoretical studies. In: Barduch J, ed. Local Flaps and Free Skin Grafts in Head and Neck Reconstruction. St. Louis: Mosby–Year Book; 1992
45. Vecchione TR. Multiple pinwheel scalp flaps. In: Strauch B, Vasconez LO, Hall-Findlay EJ, eds. Grabb's Encyclopedia of Flaps–Head and Neck. Philadelphia: Lippincott-Raven; 1998
46. Orticochea M. New three-flap scalp reconstruction technique. Br J Plast Surg 1971;124:184–185
47. Limberg AA. The Planning of Local Plastic Operations on the Body Surface: Theory and Practice. Toronto: Cullamore Press; 1964
48. Larrabee WF, Tracy R, Sutton D. Rhomboid flap dynamics. Arch Otolaryngol 1981;107:755–757
49. Webster RC, Davidson TM, Smith RC. The 30-degree transposition flap. Laryngoscope 1978;88:85–88
50. Pletcher SD, Kim DW. Current concepts in cheek reconstruction. Facial Plast Surg Clin North Am 2005;13:267–281
51. Lister GD, Gibson T. Closure of rhomboid skin defects: the flaps of Limberg and Dufourmental. Br J Plast Surg 1972;25:440–445
52. Becker FF. Rhomboid flap in facial reconstruction: new concept of tension lines. Arch Otolaryngol 1979;105:569–573
53. Zimany A. A bilobed flap. Plast Reconstr Surg 1953;11:424–426
54. McGregor JC, Soutar DS. A critical assessment of the bilobed flap. Br J Plast Surg 1981;34:726–734
55. Zitelli JA. The bilobed flap for nasal reconstruction. Arch Dermatol 1989;125:957–959
56. Murakami CS, Odland PB. Bilobed flap variations. Oper Tech Otolaryngol Head Neck Surg 1993;4:76–79
57. Esser JF. Island flaps. N Y State J Med 1917;106:264–266
58. Baker SR. Regional flaps in facial reconstruction. Facial Plast Surg 1990;5:925–928

5 Scar Revision

Mimi S. Kokoska and J. Regan Thomas

The purpose of scar revision is to optimize scar camouflage. Although scar appearance can in many circumstances be improved, a scar cannot be completely removed. Patients should be informed as such. The ultimate appearance of a scar is dependent on many factors. The orientation of the scar, amount of tissue loss or injury, scar position on the face, age of the patient, patient's underlying health, genetic predisposition to abnormal scar formation, technique of wound closure, and presence of wound healing complication all contribute to the final scar result. Scar position, extent of tissue loss, patient age, genetic factors, and underlying health are for the most part beyond a surgeon's control. However, the surgeon can implement specific wound healing and scar formation principles in the surgical planning to effect an optimal outcome for the patient.

Understanding the mechanism of scar formation can be helpful in deciding on the method of scar revision. Blunt trauma, gunshot wounds, and burn scars tend to involve a larger surrounding area of injury than surgical incisional scars. Initially, it may be difficult to determine how much of the adjacent soft tissue is not viable, especially in wounds associated with thermal injury. Debridement during the initial stage of repair should be conservative to preserve as much viable tissue as possible. Scars resulting from these types of injuries may be less amenable to a satisfactory result or may require staged revisions.

There are some guidelines for optimizing initial scar formation, which in turn may facilitate later scar revision or even circumvent the need for a secondary procedure. All wounds should be as clean as possible, with removal of foreign bodies. Irrigation with sterile saline has been shown to decrease bacterial counts. Clearly devitalized tissue should be debrided with preservation of healthy tissue. The orientation of the scar should not necessarily be altered during the initial injury because scar irregularities may serve to help camouflage the scar, and neighboring tissues can be observed for viability and preserved for any required secondary procedures. During initial closure of traumatic injuries, soft tissues should be closed in multiple layers if the injury penetrates the subcutaneous tissues. Conservative undermining may be necessary to approximate wound edges without tension. Tension increases the risk for widened or hypertrophic scars. The wound surface should be kept moist with antibiotic ointment or an occlusive dressing.

Scar Analysis

The ideal scar is narrow, flat, and level with the surrounding skin. It has similar color match to the surrounding skin. The scar should be parallel or within the relaxed skin tension lines (RSTLs) (**Fig. 5.1**) and possibly in a junction between aesthetic subunits. The scar should not tent or bunch up the surrounding skin. Scar revision is indicated for scars that are hypertrophic, widened, depressed, perpendicular to RSTLs, webbed, trap-door, causing malalignment of a facial landmark (brows, vermilion), or interfering with facial function. Scars that are narrow, within the RSTLs, but hypertrophic may respond to intralesional triamcinolone injection alone (**Fig. 5.2**).

Timing of Scar Revision

All scars tend to improve spontaneously after a period of maturation of 1 year. However, the patient frequently wishes for earlier intervention, if warranted. The characteristics of a scar can help guide the timing of the scar revision. If a fresh scar is narrow, flat, situated within the RSTL, but erythematous, it may serve the patient better to reassess the scar after it matures because erythema usually dissipates. However, if the scar has significant unfavorable characteristics, such as malalignment, that will usually not improve with time, then earlier scar revision may be beneficial.

Minor revisions, such as dermabrasion, may be routinely performed ~8 weeks after the initial wound repair. Dermabrasion during this early period of wound healing may in theory benefit from the high fibroblast activity. At this time scars are usually still erythematous. Dermabrasion itself causes significant transient erythema. Therefore, early dermabrasion may decrease the total time that a patient has to endure an erythematous scar by overlapping the erythematous periods associated with early scar healing and dermabrasion.

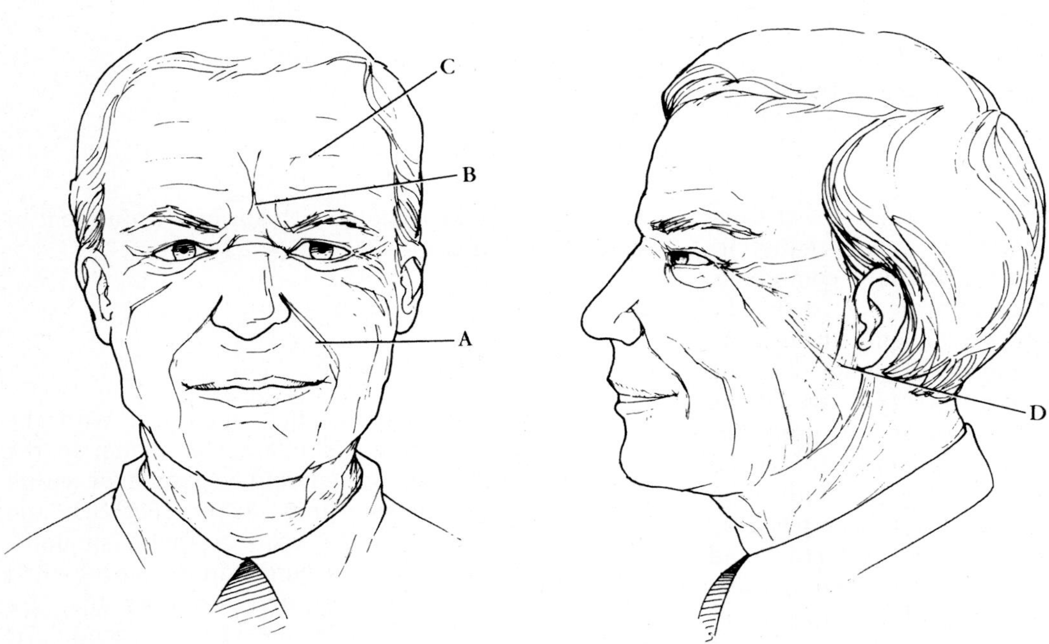

Fig. 5.1 Relaxed skin tension lines, which help guide the orientation of scar placement. Examples include the *A*, nasolabial creases; *B*, vertical glabellar furrows; *C*, horizontal forehead creases; and *D*, crow's feet. Junctions between aesthetic units can also be used to camouflage scars. For example, the adjacent wounds may be closed, with the scar placed in the melolabial fold.

Excisional Techniques

Scar Repositioning

Frequently scars can be repositioned to fall within RSTLs, borders between aesthetic units, or hair-bearing scalp. Scar repositioning requires the scar to be in proximity to the more hidden site. This concept can be applied to the facelift or postparotidectomy patient who has a noticeable preauricular scar. Often these scars can be repositioned close to the tragus, resulting in better camouflage (**Fig. 5.3**). Scars that cause malalignment of an aesthetic landmark can be excised and repositioned.

Simple Excision

Often scars that are malaligned or malpositioned can be improved by simple fusiform excision and redirection of the wound to a favorable position. Simple excisions can provide a finer scar with orientation into an RSTL or a junction of an aesthetic unit for scars that have healed under less than favorable conditions (**Fig. 5.4**). Fusiform excisions are ideal for small-diameter or short scars. If the ends of the planned fusiform excision approach another aesthetic unit or a facial landmark, an M-plasty can be performed to shorten the end of the ellipse. Fusiform excision angles should ideally be 30 to 60 degrees. Angles greater than 60 degrees result in a standing-cone deformity that requires either M-plasty or further extension of the wound to correct the tissue excess.

Serial Excisions

Serial partial excisions are utilized when the scar or skin lesion is too large to allow closure of the surrounding skin in a single stage. Some types of scars that may benefit from serial partial excisions include (1) large scars closed primarily with a skin graft and (2) burn scars. The initial incision is placed within the scar at one margin. The wound edges are undermined, a portion of the scar is excised after advancement, and the wound is closed. After 8 to 12 weeks during which the skin stretches, the procedure is repeated with the incision within the scar border.

In the last excision, the remaining scar is excised and normal skin margins in both sides of the wound are approximated. In this final closure, the skin margins can be approximated in a straight line, W-plasty, or broken-line closure. Skin has a great ability to stretch and accommodate wound closure. Serial excisions utilize

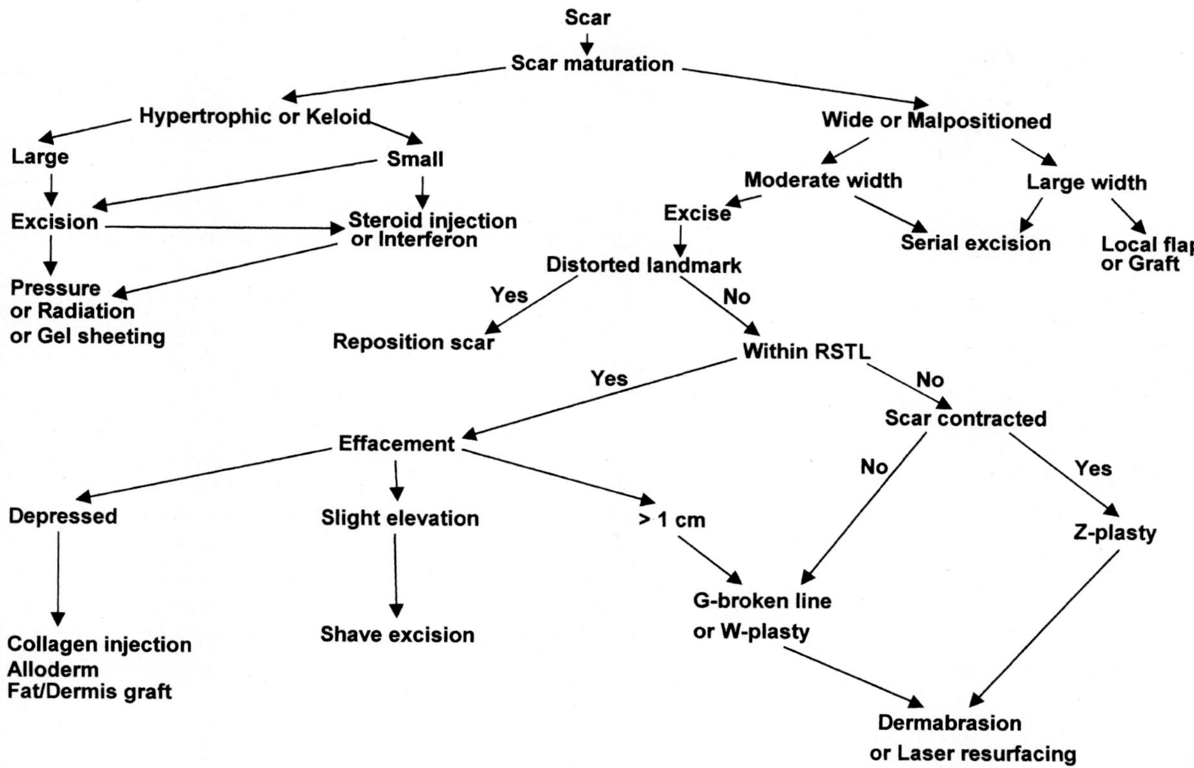

Fig. 5.2 This flow diagram demonstrates the preoperative analysis and treatment options for optimal scar revision. (Modified from Thomas JR. Facial scars. In: Thomas JR, Holt GR, eds. Facial Scars: Incision, Revision, and Camouflage. St. Louis: CV Mosby; 1989. With permission.)

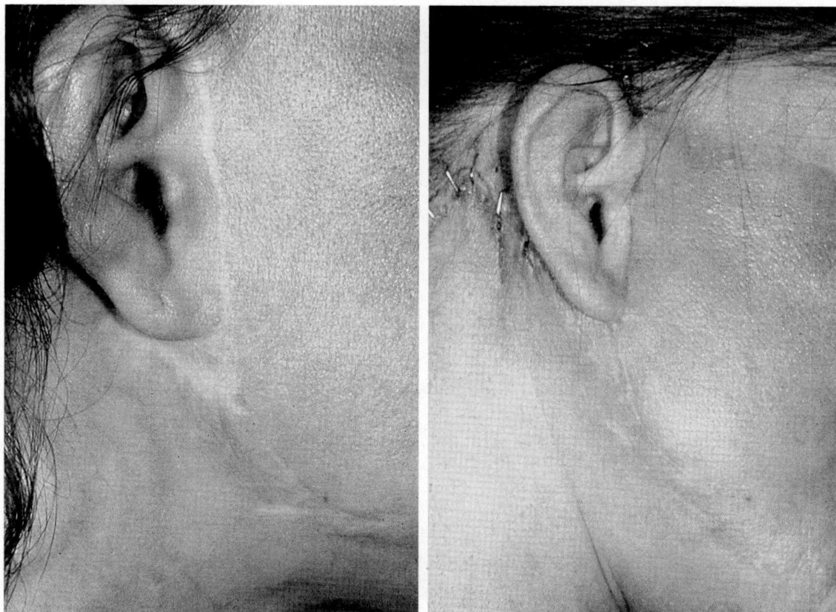

Fig. 5.3 (**A**) Patient with wide and malpositioned scar. (**B**) One week after scar repositioning.

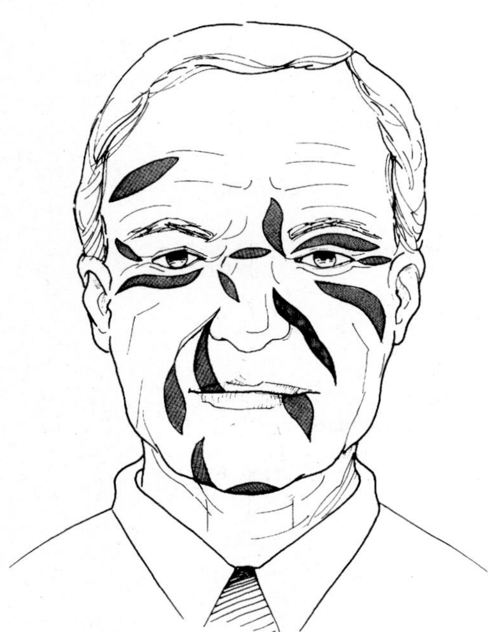

Fig. 5.4 Fusiform excisions are ideally situated in relaxed skin tension lines or aesthetic borders.

the extraordinary ability of the skin to stretch and slowly accommodate over time. Even large wounds that cover up to 50% of the forehead can be serially excised. In addition, serial excisions can be used to move scars to a site that provides better camouflage, such as junctions of aesthetic units, into hairlines and RSTLs.

Z-plasty

Z-plasty is a technique that provides irregularization of the scar while changing scar direction; it lengthens the scar and provides excision. It utilizes the transposition of triangular flaps around the scar that is the central member. The new orientation of the central member is perpendicular to the original scar. The classic Z-plasty has a central member and two peripheral members, which are equal in length, and two equal triangles (**Fig. 5.5**). The scar can be excised as the central member or multiple central members, as in multiple Z-plasties. After incision of the members, the triangular flaps are undermined. The triangular flaps are then transposed and sutured in place using multiple-layer closures. In theory, angles of 30 degrees will provide lengthening of 25%, whereas 45-degree angles will lengthen a wound by 50%, and 60-degree angles will yield a 75% lengthening. Therefore, the lengthening of the scar must be considered, especially when lengthening of the scar encroaches into another aesthetic unit or anatomical structure. For example, Z-plasty on a vertical forehead scar near the brow could cause distortion of the brow position after lengthening. The members should be less than 1 cm to assist in scar camouflage.

Unequal Z-plasty angles can be used to move tissue into an area of tissue deficiency. This is helpful in areas where scar contracture has caused retraction of an adjacent structure. The smaller-angle flap has greater rotational potential than the larger-angle flap. The smaller-angle flap is then used to provide additional tissue to the deficient area. Although it does not provide tissue lengthening in the direction of the original scar, it does provide additional tissue lengthening perpendicular to the original scar.

Multiple Z-plasties

Multiple Z-plasties are used to decrease the scar contracture associated with a wound by redirecting the tension along the entire scar (**Fig. 5.6**). This is accomplished without excessive member length, which would leave noticeable scars and limit the breakage of the scar line. Pin cushion or trap-door deformities are associated with circular or semicircular scars. There appears to be edematous tissue "trapped" by a surrounding area of wound contracture. Treatment options include intralesional steroid injections, application of pressure, and scar revision. The thickened flap can be undermined and

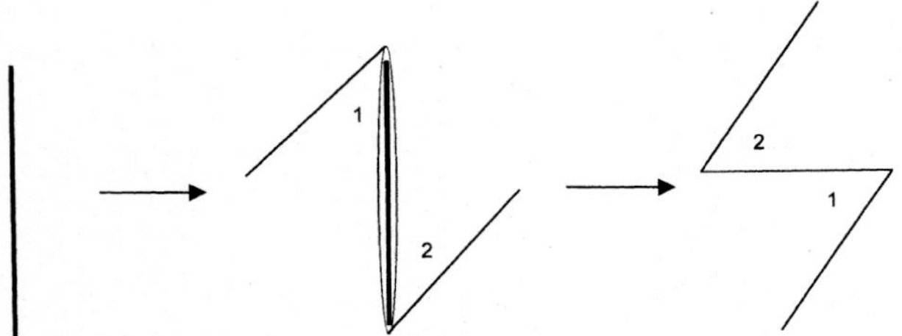

Fig. 5.5 Single Z-plasty. Two equal triangular flaps are transposed. Note that the original scar member has been excised and the scar length has increased.

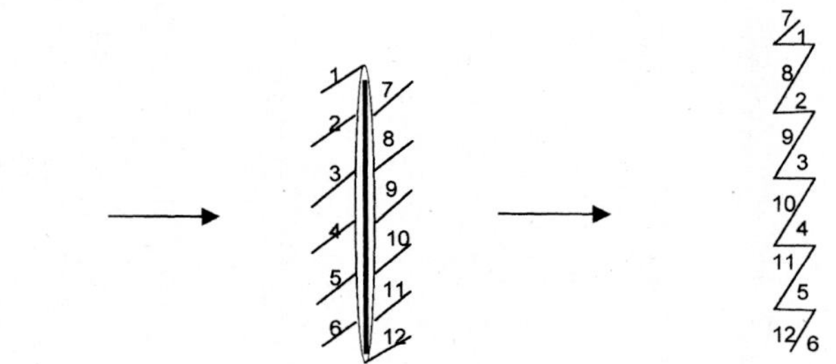

Fig. 5.6 Multiple Z-plasty. Placement of several small Zs along the wound allowing transposition of several small triangular flaps. Benefits from multiple Z-plasty include scar irregularization and distribution of wound tension into several vectors. Elongation of the wound is inevitable and must be anticipated.

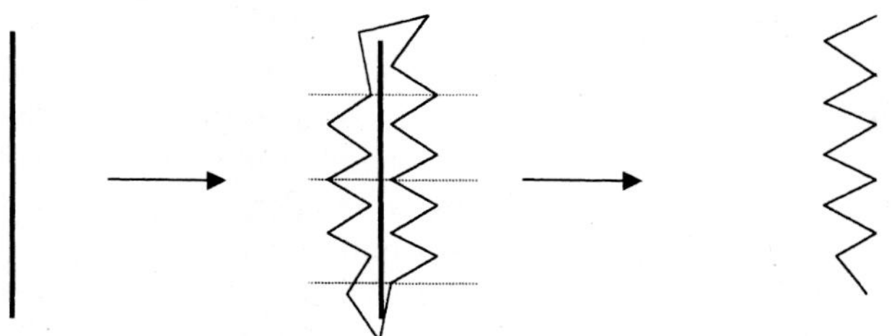

Fig. 5.7 W-plasty. Running triangular flaps are interposed resulting in a regular irregular scar. A single long scar can be reoriented into small scars that are situated within the relaxed skin tension lines.

debulked; then multiple Z-plasties can be used to redirect and lengthen the contracted scar. A web scar, which occurs frequently around the medial canthal region, can also be treated effectively with this technique.

W-plasty

W-plasty is utilized to irregularize and reorient a scar or wound that may lie perpendicular to the RSTL. It is performed by excising successive small triangular skin units from the perimeter of the scar or wound. The triangular flaps are advanced into its opposing triangular defects and the wound is closed (**Fig. 5.7**). In contrast to Z-plasty, there is no significant wound lengthening. Not only are the limbs of the W-plasty flaps in general shorter than the Z-plasty limbs, but there is no transposition of the W-plasty flaps. For long scars, W-plasty is less ideal than the geometric broken line closure (GBLC) technique. The regular irregular repeating units of the W-plasty wound are more readily identified by the eye than the asymmetric irregular units of the GBLC wound.

Geometric Broken Line Closure

The GBLC technique is a more complicated irregularization technique than the Z-plasty or W-plasty. It provides an irregular scar that is less detectable to the eye. It is ideal for lengthy scars that traverse an aesthetic unit, such as the cheek (**Fig. 5.8**).

A series of randomly alternating triangle, rectangle, trapezoid, semicircle, and square patterns are cut on one side of the wound, and its mirror image is cut on the other side of the wound (**Fig. 5.9**). The opposing sides are closed after removal of the cutout and intervening scar segment. The flap limbs should be less than 6 mm to facilitate scar camouflage because longer limbs tend to be followed by the eye.

Dermabrasion and Laser Skin Resurfacing

Either dermabrasion or laser skin resurfacing can be used to remove the superficial skin layers (epidermis and part of the papillary dermis). The wound is reepithelialized by

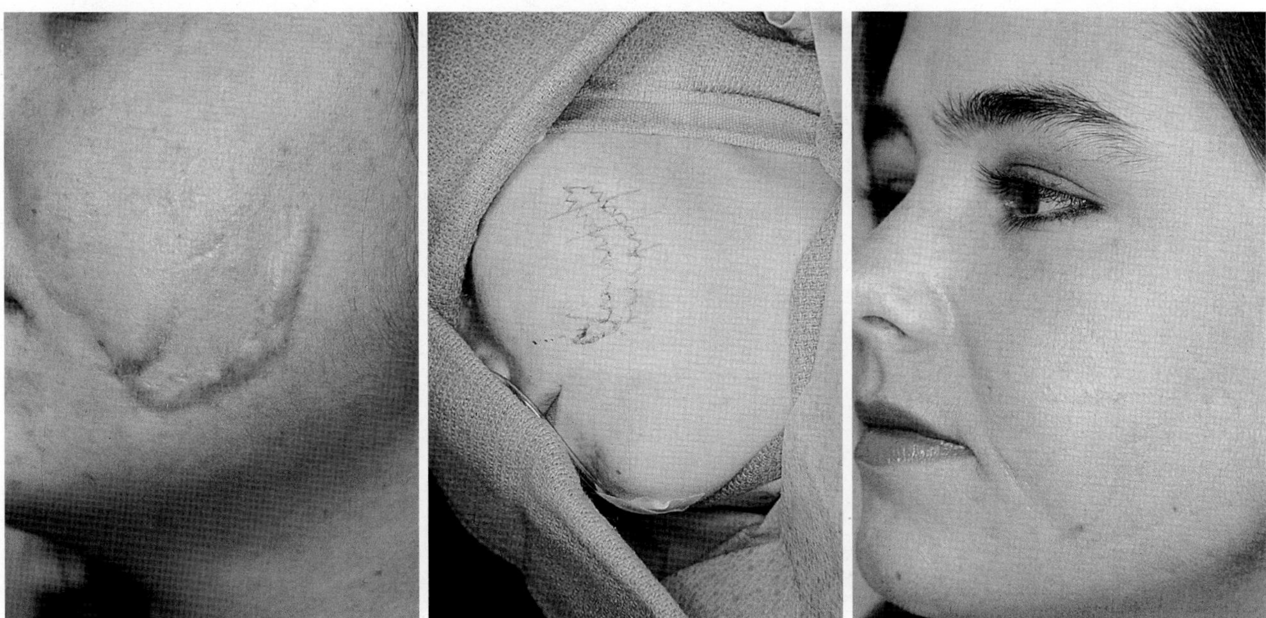

A–C

Fig. 5.8 (**A**) Preoperative hypertrophic and lengthy cheek scar. (**B**) Intraoperative geometric broken line closure. (**C**) One year after geometric broken line closure followed by secondary dermabrasion.

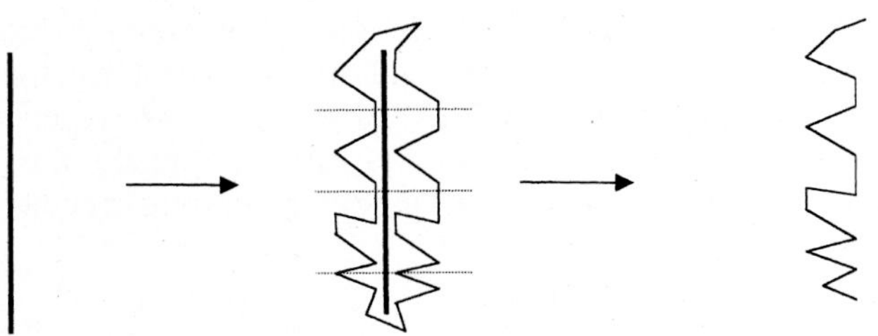

Fig. 5.9 Geometric broken line closure. Randomly alternating patterns result in an irregular scar with components oriented in the relaxed skin tension line.

surrounding epithelium and underlying adnexal structures.

These techniques can be used to level a scar, change the texture of a scar, and further blend the scar with the surrounding skin, thus improving the scar camouflage (**Fig. 5.10**). Dermabrasion can be performed with a diamond fraise or wire brush attached to a motorized hand piece. A local anesthetic is applied and the skin cleaned prior to dermabrasion. The skin is stretched and the fraise applied to the scar and surrounding skin. The fraise should be rotating in a clockwise fashion and applied perpendicular and oblique to the axis of the scar. Sponges should be kept away from the rotating fraise to avoid accidental snaring of the sponge into the dermabrader. The scar and surrounding skin are stretched taut to provide an even and firm surface for dermabrasion. Skin refrigerants are no longer used in most practices since freon was outlawed. Deep dermabrasion into the reticular dermis should be avoided to prevent further scarring. Dermabrasion is also valuable as a secondary stage of scar revision after Z-plasty, W-plasty, or GBLC. It can be performed 8 weeks after scar revision to further improve the scar camouflage.

Laser skin resurfacing is usually performed with a carbon dioxide or erbium laser. There may be theoretical advantages to laser skin resurfacing over dermabrasion for scar camouflage. It has been suggested that the laser offers increased collagen reorganization and therefore improved scar camouflage. However, the thermal damage associated with laser resurfacing may make the depth of penetration less predictable. Recent advances in laser scanner technology have provided more consistent skin resurfacing results. In addition, certain scanner patterns can selectively ablate the tissue around depressed areas, resulting in a more level plane.

Patient selection is important with either dermabrasion or laser skin resurfacing. Fair-skinned patients are less likely to develop noticeable pigmentary changes and

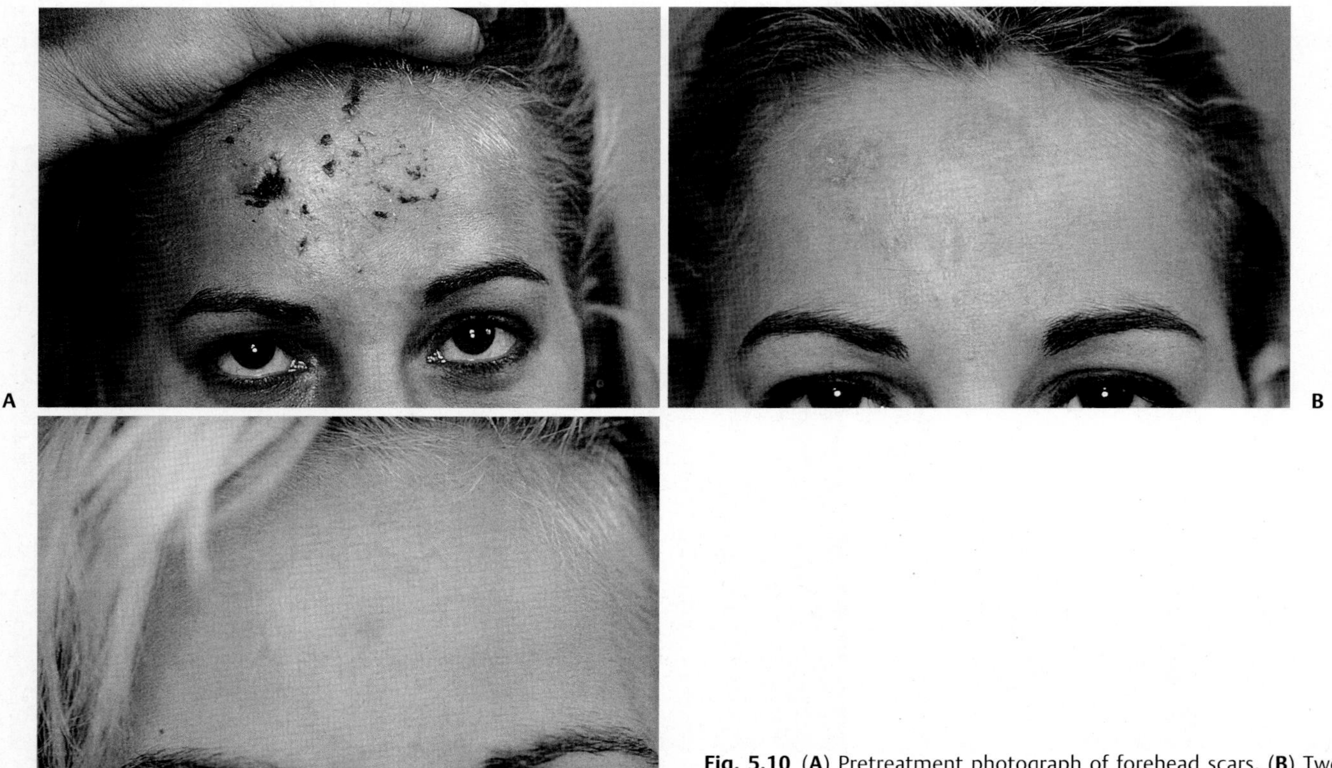

Fig. 5.10 (**A**) Pretreatment photograph of forehead scars. (**B**) Two weeks after dermabrasion. (**C**) One year postoperative result from dermabrasion alone.

hypertrophic or keloid scarring. Patients who are having perioral resurfacing are prophylaxed with antiviral medication against the herpes simplex virus. All candidates should be counseled on the risk of pigmentary changes, infection, scarring, and the possible need for multiple treatments.

Postoperative Care

After excisional scar revision or dermabrasion, an antibiotic ointment is applied to the suture line or wound for ~1 week. A dressing may be applied or the ointment may serve as a semiocclusive dressing. The sutures are usually removed at 1 week unless the patient has compromised wound healing. If any signs of hypertrophic or keloid scarring develop in the following weeks, triamcinolone acetonide (Kenalog, Bristol-Myers Squibb, New York, NY) 10 mg/mL is injected into the dermal portion of the scar. In addition to Kenalog, mechanical pressure (digital, earring clips) or Silastic gel sheeting (Dow Corning Corporation, Midland, MI) may be used to discourage further growth of the scar.

Suggested Readings

Borges AF. Improvement of antitension lines scar by the "W-plastic" operation. Br J Plast Surg 1959;12:29

Thomas JR, Holt GR, eds. Facial Scars: Incision, Revision, and Camouflage. St. Louis: CV Mosby; 1989

Webster RC, Smith RC. Scar revision and camouflage. Otolaryngol Clin North Am 1982;15:55

6 Synthetic Implants

Kofi D. O. Boahene

Synthetic implants include both natural and synthesized materials fabricated into devices to treat, augment, or replace defective organs or tissues in humans. The use of synthetic implants in medicine and dentistry can be traced 2000 years back to the Romans, Chinese, and Aztecs. However, it is only with the development of synthetic polymer systems in the past 2 decades that synthetic implants have gained a wider use in contemporary medicine. The use of synthetic implants in plastic and reconstruction surgery has greatly increased the options available for replacing or augmenting deficient tissue resulting from trauma, infection, cancer, and congenital anomalies. Recent advances in the fields of material science, tissue engineering, and nanotechnology have allowed the synthesis of biomaterials that mimic native tissue more closely, facilitating replacement, augmentation, and sometimes targeted delivery of drugs and growth factors. This chapter focuses on the evolving application of synthetic biomaterials in plastic and reconstructive surgery of the head and neck.

Evolution of Synthetic Implants

The turn of the century marked the increased use of synthetic materials in reconstructive surgery. The earliest materials selected for implants were made from readily available materials. Until a good understanding of the immune system developed, most of these "off-the shelf" implant materials proved to be either pathogenic or toxic. Since then, there have been significant changes in implant technology and application. Three generations of implants have evolved. First-generation synthetic implants were designed from materials with physical properties that matched those of the deficient tissue. The goal of these first implants was tissue replacement with materials that elicited little or no immunologic response from the host (i.e., bioinert). The majority of these first-generation implants were made from pure metals and their alloys. The first metal alloy developed specifically for human use was "vanadium steel" in the early 1900s. This material was used for bone plates in mandibular reconstruction. Material-related problems that resulted in premature loss of implant function, as evidenced by mechanical failure, corrosion, and poor biocompatibility, became quickly apparent. Material selection and biocompatibility remain the critical issues in today's synthetic implants. Currently, pure metals and alloys of iron, chromium, and titanium are the most commonly used metallic implants.

With the advancement in material technology, a second generation of implants evolved that shifted the emphasis from bioinert devices to bioactive implants. Bioactive implants include nonresorbable and resorbable polymers that promote implant–tissue interaction and integration. By the mid-1980s, bioactive implants, including bioactive glass, ceramic-glass composite implants, and synthetic hydroxyapatite, were commonly used in head and neck reconstruction. However, problems from stress shielding and particulate wear limited their widespread acceptance. With the development of biodegradable synthetic implants, some of the problems encountered with the earlier bioactive implants were solved. Biodegradable plates made from polyglycolic acid polymers gained popularity in craniofacial surgery, especially in children. Because they degraded over time, the issue of stress shielding was resolved. Nonetheless, one persistent limitation of second-generation implants was their inability to adapt to changing physiological demands such as weight-bearing forces and growth. Currently, intense research in tissue engineering is spurring the development of a third generation of synthetic implants that adapt more physiologically to the molecular environment of the surrounding tissue. These third-generation implants include different forms of synthetic absorbable scaffolds designed to allow seeding with embryonic or mesenchymal stem cells that are able to generate new bone, chondroid, or soft tissue matrix, totally replacing the implant over time. With the use of nanotechnology, biologically active proteins are being fused to these synthetic scaffolds to enhance tissue integration, regeneration, wound healing, and implant biocompatibility.

Selection of Implant Material

The selection of a biomaterial for a specific application must be based on several criteria. These include the biocompatibility of the implant, physicochemical properties and durability of the material, the desired function of the prosthesis, the nature of the physiological environment at the organ/tissue level, and adverse effects in case of failure. The most important factor in selecting a material for a synthetic implant is its biocompatibility.

Biocompatibility of Synthetic Implants

The biocompatibility of a synthetic implant refers to the ability of the implant to perform its intended function, with the desired degree of incorporation in the host, without eliciting any undesirable local or systemic effects. The biocompatibility requirements of synthetic implants is regulated by the International Organization for Standardization (ISO), which outlines guidelines for required testing for new implants.[1] Required testing includes evaluation for acute and chronic toxicity, carcinogenicity, genotoxicity, immunotoxicity, corrosion, neurotoxicity, and sensitization. Testing strategies that comply with the ISO 10993–1 are acceptable in Europe and Asia. In 1995, the Food and Drug Administration (FDA) adopted the ISO guidelines, although in some areas FDA's testing requirements exceed those of the ISO. There are many factors that influence the biocompatibility of an implant, such as implant size, shape, material composition and surface characteristics; host reaction to the physical characteristics of the implant material; the tissue site of implantation; and the surgical technique of placement.[2] The surface characteristics of an implant are pivotal to its biocompatibility.[3] Within seconds of implant insertion, a biolayer consisting of water, proteins, and other biomolecules from the physiological liquid is formed on the surface of the implant. Further interaction between the implant and the native tissue is mediated through this biolayer. Several methods have been used to modify the surface of synthetic implants to enhance their biocompatibility. One approach exploits the immobilization of bioactive molecules (cell adhesion peptides, albumin, fibrinogen, heparin, glycosaminoglycans) onto the implant surface by adsorption, covalent coupling, and tethering via an intermediate linker molecule. Once modified, the bulk of the implant interacts with the surrounding tissue through these bioactive molecules thereby enhancing their compatibility. Beyond the biocompatibility of an implant, the host tissue characteristics are important in ensuring long-term success of the implant. Important tissue characteristic include vascularity, proximity to contaminated cavities, mobility of surrounding tissue, cyclic loading, and stress and adequacy of soft tissue coverage.

Preventing Infection and Implant Failure

Intraoperative handling of the implant is important in minimizing synthetic implant failure. Extensive handling or exposure of the implant before insertion should be avoided. Once it is removed from its sterile package, the implant should be handled only by clean instruments with minimal contact with the contaminated gloved hand. Implant contact with the surrounding skin or oral cavity should be minimized to decrease bacterial inoculation. Under normal circumstances, 100,000 bacteria are necessary to cause clinically significant infection; however, in the presence of synthetic material, this number is significantly reduced.[4] Antibiotic prophylaxis is prudent but should not replace the use of sterile technique. The rationale for antibiotic coverage is to prevent or eliminate any bacterial inoculation that may have occurred on the implant surface. No large clinical trials have been conducted to confirm the efficacy of this approach. Additional antibiotic coverage is often sought by washing or soaking the implant before intraoperative insertion. This practice may be more valuable with implants with hydrophilic rather than hydrophobic surfaces. Whether this antibiotic impregnation actually lowers the postoperative infection rate is unknown. Some implant surfaces favor the development and maintenance of biofilm that is resistant to antibiotic treatment.[5–8] Such implants ultimately require removal when infected. Surface characteristics thought to promote biofilm adherence include chemical composition of the material (e.g., *Staphylococcus epidermidis* often causes polymer implant infection, *Staphylococcus aureus* is usually found in metal implant infections), surface roughness (irregular surfaces typically promote bacterial adhesion), surface configuration (bacteria colonize porous material surfaces preferentially), and surface hydrophobicity (hydrophilic materials are more resistant to bacterial adhesion than hydrophobic materials).[5–8]

Selected Implants and Implant Materials

Metals

Despite the great numbers of metals and alloys known to man, remarkably few possess the minimum properties for uses as implant materials. The relatively corrosive environment combined with the poor tolerance of the body to even minute concentrations of most metallic corrosion products eliminates from discussion most metallic materials. The main considerations in selecting metals and alloys for biomedical applications are biocompatibility, appropriate mechanical properties, corrosion resistance, and reasonable cost.

Gold

Gold is chemically inert and evokes minimal tissue reaction. It has poor mechanical properties in its purest form and usually functions best as an alloy when some structural integrity is needed, such as in dental implants. However, when used as a weight in upper eyelid reanimation procedures, the 24-carat, highly polished weight provides less reactivity, greater malleability, and greater success than simple tarsorraphy.[9,10]

Platinum

Platinum has long been recognized for excellent biocompatibility and is the preferred implant material for gold-sensitive patients undergoing eyelid-loading surgery for lagophthalmos.[11] Platinum is a lustrous, silvery-white, malleable, and ductile metal. Compared with gold, platinum eyelid implants are denser, allowing for lower profile implants that are less noticeable.[11]

Stainless Steel

Medical grade stainless steel used in biomaterial implants contain iron-chromium-nickel alloys and has good corrosion resistance. At least 17% composition of chromium should be present for steel to be called stainless steel. The addition of chromium generates a protective surface chromium oxide that improves corrosion resistance. Nickel was added to the alloy to harden it. The 316L alloy is used medically and represents the lowest carbon content (to prevent carbide formation), the highest nickel content (for hardening and strength), and adequate chromium (for anticorrosion).

Titanium

The superior strength to weight ratio of titanium compared with stainless steel and its outstanding corrosion resistance properties has made it the metal of choice in several implants. Light, strong, and totally biocompatible, titanium is one of few materials that naturally match the requirements for implantation in the human body. Additionally, the capacity for osseointegration makes titanium an attractive choice for bone replacement implants. The lower modulus of titanium alloys compared with steel is a positive factor in reducing bone resorption. Titanium is neither magnetic nor paramagnetic. Patients with these implants may safely undergo magnetic resonance imaging without concern about dislodgment of the graft or interference with the study. The use of customized titanium implants has seen a widespread indication for facial reconstruction following excision of orofacial tumors, in cases of severe maxillofacial trauma, and for congenital facial anomalies. Using rapid prototyping methodologies such as stereoscopic lithography or three-dimensional printing, customized titanium implants pretested for form and fit can be produced using computer-controlled milling before surgical implantation.[12] This cuts out guesswork, minimizes operative time, and improves aesthetic outcomes. In dental restoration surgery, osseointegrated titanium roots have greatly revolutionized dental rehabilitation in postcancer patients. Osseointegrated titanium screws also form the basis of more stable fixation of prosthetic devices used for nasal, auricular, and cheek reconstruction and as well as bone-anchored hearing aids.

Polymers

Silicon

Silicon is a polymer consisting of alternating elements of silicon and oxygen with organic side groups. It is the only form of noncarbon-chain polymer in clinical use today. One form of medical grade silicon is composed of dimethylsiloxane monomers, which contain a methyl side group. Linear chains of polymethylsiloxane with lower molecular weight and viscosity form liquid silicon, which is injectable. With an intermediate degree of cross-linking and viscosity, silicon gel is obtained. When the viscosity is extremely high (centistokes = 10,000) a solid state elastomer composed of a highly cross-linked gel filled with silica particles is formed. Silastic (Dow Corning, Midland, MI) is an example of high-viscosity cross-linked methylsiloxane polymer, forged from silica powder to modify its mechanical properties.

Injectable medical grade silicon was first introduced by Dow Corning (Midland, MI) in 1960. By 1990, over 100,000 patients had received silicon gel injections in the face, making it one of the most widely applied filler materials. The gel has desirable plasticity and is widely nontoxic and nonimmunogenic. Medical grade liquid silicone has been associated with numerous clinical abuses. Most abuses are related to an excessive number of injections and to the use of impure silicone. Adverse reactions presenting as inflammatory nodules, or "siliconoma," have been reported up to several years following injection.[13] Migration along the reticuloendothelial system into regional lymph nodes, liver, and spleen has been reported. The origin of these reactions is not well understood; they have been difficult to treat and often result in disfiguring defects. However, when applied in limited quantities (0.1 mL per area) using the microdroplet technique with a 30 gauge needle, the silicone appears to be stabilized by a fibrous capsule. Interval of injection should not be less than 4 weeks. In 1991, the FDA banned the use of injectable silicon in the United States, but it is still used in a limited fashion elsewhere.

A hybrid suspension of polyvinylpyrridone and silicone (Bioplastique, Uroplasty BV, Geleen, the Netherlands) was introduced in 1991. It consists of particles of polymerized silicon, 100 to 600 μm in size, surrounded by a resorbable carrier gel (polyvinylpyrridone). The gel surrounding the silicone is engulfed within a week and replaced by collagen within 6 weeks. The silicone particles, which are too large to be phagocytized, remain in the tissue and elicit a local foreign body reaction, ending in fibrosis, which contributes to the filling effect. As with medical grade silicone, successful use of Bioplastique depends on injection technique. Placement below the dermis is crucial for obtaining a lasting result. More superficial placement may result in extrusion. Persistent induration and swelling have been described, often requiring excision because antibiotics and

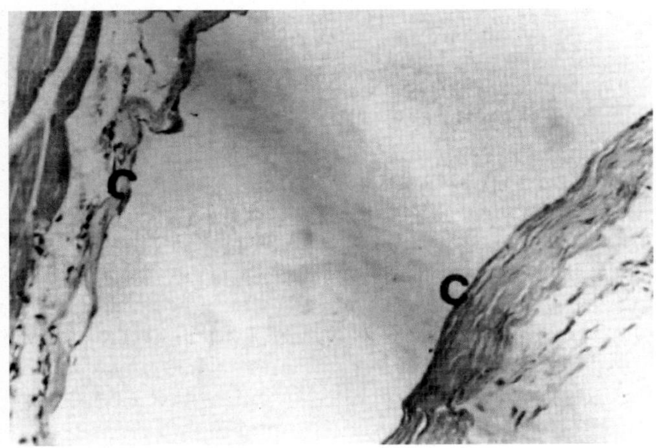

Figure 6.1 Thin fibrous capsule (C) showing scant number of mononuclear, chronic inflammatory cells. The cleft was left by the Silastic (Dow Corning, Midland, MI), which was dislodged during processing. (Courtesy of Jeanne S. Adams, MD.)

steroid injections have yielded a mixed and inconsistent response. Some authors have reported a curative response to the immune modulator imiquimod.[14]

The solid silicon elastomer, Silastic (Dow Corning), has been extensively used in head and neck reconstruction. Silastic blocks are easy to carve. It has been used in thyroplasties, cheek and chin implants, and nasal surgery. Histological studies of implants by several authors reveal that Silastic becomes enveloped by a thin organized capsule with a mild, chronic inflammatory reaction devoid of histiocytes and giant cells (**Fig. 6.1**). Because it is highly hydrophobic, there is no bonding between Silastic and its capsule, it is more prone to being dislodged. Silastic is more apt to be extruded when placed in a pocket with thin overlying coverage, and it gives the most persistent seromas. This is corroborated by the high extrusion rate of Silastic in nasal and auricular applications.[15]

Polymethylmethacrylate

Polymethylmethacrylate (PMMA), an acrylic polymer of high molecular weight, was one of the first polymers used as a biomaterial. Polymerization of the methylmethacrylate monomers yields a polymer of high strength and rigidity. Because of its biocompatibility, reliability, relative ease of manipulation, and low toxicity, PMMA has been used extensively in craniofacial reconstruction. PMMA is packaged as two components: liquid and powder. The liquid contains the PMMA monomer, stabilizer, and activator. The powder contains the polymer, a radiopaque substance and polymerization initiators. When added together and mixed, polymerization occurs. At first the cement is a relatively low viscosity glistening paste. The viscosity of the preparation steadily increases and the surface becomes dull. The rapid final phase of polymerization is associated with an exothermic reaction that can cause tissue injury. The material then becomes a solid resin. One distinct advantage is that it can be molded in situ. The ability to mold the implant in the tissues and remove it during the exothermic phase of polymerization enables one to obtain an accurate implant in size and shape without causing thermal damage. In cranioplasty, PMMA can be reinforced with a mesh for moderate-sized defects. For very large defects, computed tomographic (CT) scan–guided porous custom implants can be fabricated to facilitate a more accurate reconstruction. The best indication for use of PMMA in head and neck reconstruction is in patients with good-quality soft tissue, without previous infection, and with no connection to the sinuses. It is important to ensure immobilization of this material by onlay rigid fixation with screws because it can become loose with time.[16]

Polyethylene

Polyethylenes are polymers consisting of a large number of repeating monomeric units of ethylenes linked together to form highly branched macromolecules. Porous polyethylene implants are synthetic polymers that are biologically inert and nonbiodegradable in the body. MEDPOR (Porex Surgical, Inc., Newnan, GA) is a brand of high-density polyethylene (HDPE) solid implants that have been used since 1985 in facial augmentation for reconstructive or cosmetic purposes. Its porosity allows for soft tissue and vascular ingrowth, which helps to keep the implant in place. Mesh forms of HDPE include Prolene (Ethicon, Inc., Somerville, NJ) and Marlex. Porous high-density polyethylenes (HDPEs) (MEDPOR) with pore size 100 to 150 µm, encourages osseous tissue ingrowth with mature bony ingrowth into the surface pores at 1 year (**Fig. 6.2**). Histological analysis in an

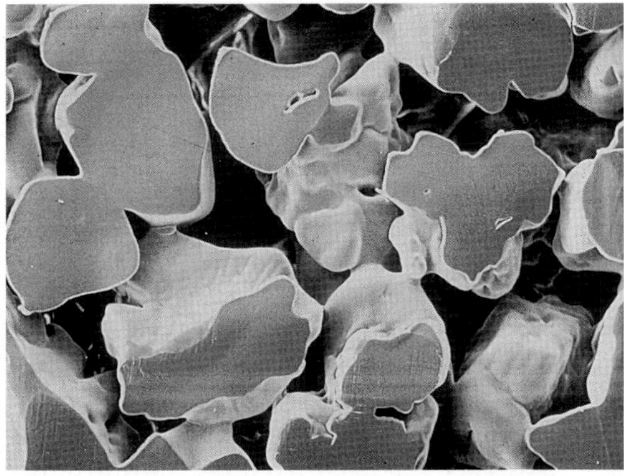

Fig. 6.2 Electron microscopic view of porous high-density polyethylene reveals architecture that allows ingrowth of fibrovascular tissue.

HDPE specimen revealed mature fibrous connective tissue ingrowth into pores with minimal foreign-body reaction.

Cenzi et al showed that the site of implantation (i.e., nose, maxilla, and ear) and diagnosis at admission (i.e., syndromic patients previously operated) is related to a higher risk of implant failure.[17] Recently, a porous polyethylene implant made from ultra-high molecular weight polyethylene (UHMWPE) (SynPOR, Synthes, Inc., West Chester, PA) or a combination of UHMWPE and titanium has become available for use in anatomical reconstruction of the craniofacial skeleton. With a pore size of 150 to 250 μm, it allows tissue ingrowth instead of encapsulation (**Fig. 6.3**).

Polyether Ether Ketone

Polyether ether ketone (PEEK) is a high-performance biomaterial that belongs to the polyaryletherketone family. The PEEKs have repeating monomers of two ether and ketone groups. PEEK is one of the highest-rated thermoplastic materials in terms of heat resistance, chemical and hydrolysis resistance, resistance to the effects of ionizing radiation, high strength, and extensive biocompatibility. Implants based on the PEEK polymer have been developed in the last decade as an alternative to conventional metallic devices. PEEK has found extensive use as an alternative to titanium in expandable vertebral replacement cages in spine surgery. PEEK devices may provide several advantages over the use of conventional materials, including the lack of metal allergies, radiolucency, low artifact on magnetic resonance imaging scans, and the possibility to tailor mechanical properties. In head and neck reconstruction, it has been used as customized healing caps for dental implants and as prefabricated implants for craniomaxillofacial defects (**Fig. 6.4**).

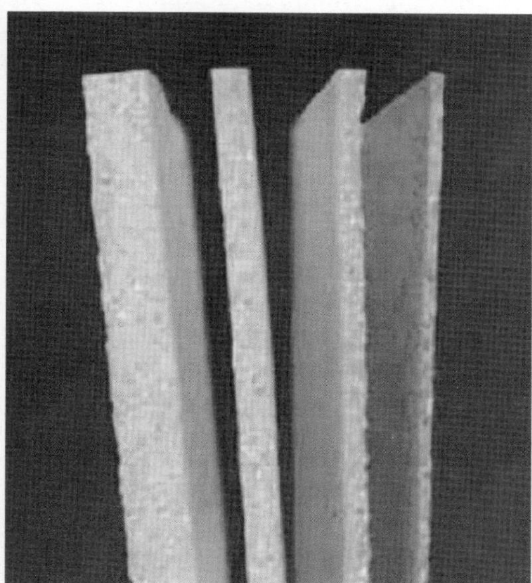

Fig. 6.3 Ultra-high-molecular-weight polyethylene (UHMWPE) (SynPOR, Synthes, Inc., West Chester, PA) implant for orbital floor repair.

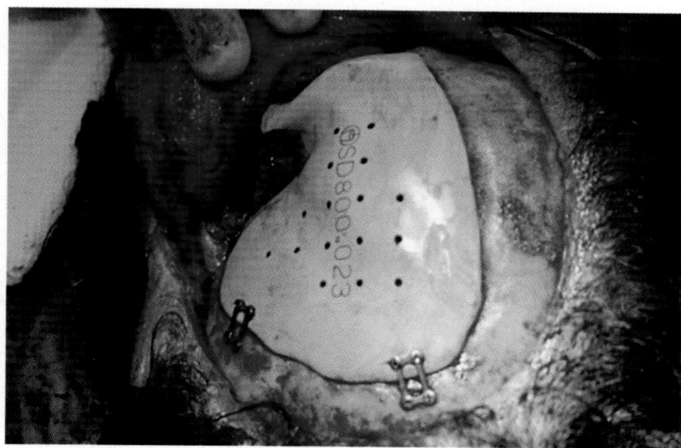

Fig. 6.4 Prefabricated polyether ether ketone implant in cranioplasty.

Expanded Polytetrafluoroethylene

Expanded polytetrafluoroethylene (Gore-Tex, W. L. Gore and Associates, Newark, DE) was first introduced as a vascular graft and subsequently for hernia repair before it became popular for facial augmentation. It is composed of nodules of solid polytetrafluoroethylene interconnected by thin, flexible polytetrafluoroethylene fibrils. Fibrillar length determines the interspacing of the molecules and hence actual pore size and accessibility of tissue ingrowth. A pore size ranging from 5 to 30 μm allows for adequate tissue ingrowth combined with ease of removal when necessary (**Fig. 6.5**). Current applications of ePTFE include lip enhancement; facial contouring; malar, nasal, and chin augmentation; filling soft tissue defects; and facial reanimation.[18] Complications associated with ePTFE include infection, extrusion, migration, shrinkage, and scarring.[19] To circumvent its shortcomings, various

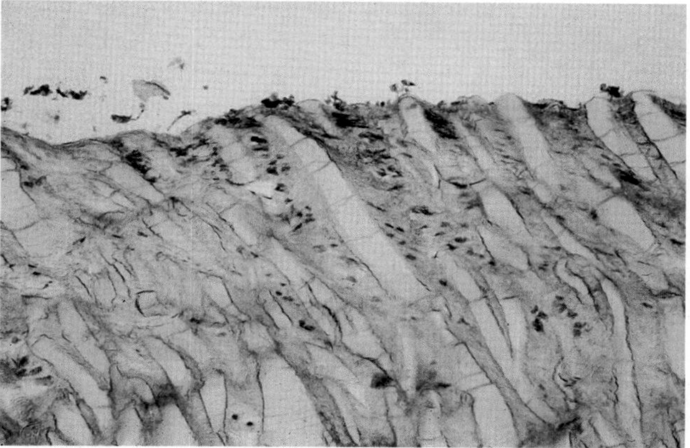

Fig. 6.5 Expanded polytetrafluoroethylene shows ingrowth of host tissue and minimal inflammatory response (N&E).

modifications of ePTFE continue to be developed. SoftForm (Collagen Corporation, Palo Alto, CA), a tube-shaped form of ePTFE, was developed for lip augmentation and treatment of deep facial furrows such as the nasolabial folds. Advanta (Atrium Medical Corporation, Hudson, NH) ePTFE is dual-porosity architecture consisting of a soft, open porosity central core of 100 µm integrated with a smooth, medium porosity outer layer of 40 µm. Advanta's dual-porosity structure provides a softer, less palpable facial implant.[20]

Biodegradable Implants

Bioabsorbable fixation devices are increasingly being used in craniomaxillofacial surgery. Implants are available for stabilization of fractures, osteotomies, bone grafts, and fusions. Because these implants are completely absorbed, the need for a removal operation is overcome, and long-term interference with the growing skeleton is avoided. The risk of implant-associated stress shielding, peri-implant osteoporosis, and infections is reduced. With resorbable implant, the initial acute inflammatory response is the same as for permanent synthetic implants. In contrast, the long-term problems of biocompatibility and the need for appropriate tissue–implant surface interaction is resolved as a result of the controlled chemical breakdown of the implant and its replacement with regenerating tissue. Widely used biodegradable materials include polyglycolic acid (PGA), poly-L-lactic acid (PLLA), poly-DL-lactic acid (PDLLA), PGA/trimethylenecarbonate copolymers (PGA/TMC), poly-p-dioxanone (PDS), and poly-β-hydroxybutyric acid (PBHBA). Biodegradable materials need to be hydrolytically labile and sturdy, at least for a period of time. Ultra-high-strength implants are manufactured from such polymers using self-reinforcing techniques. Biodegradable implants decompose into H_2O and CO_2 by nonspecific hydrolysis. During the first phase of degradation, water penetrates the biodegradable device, hydrolyzing long polymer chains into increasingly shorter fragments. In the second phase, the fragments are degraded into natural monomeric acids found in the body, such as lactic acid. These acids enter the Kreb (citric acid) cycle and are metabolized into CO_2 and water, which are then exhaled and excreted. The degradation rate and mechanical properties depend on the molecular weight, the surface quality, the composition of the polymers, crystallinity, manufacturing parameters, motion, shape, size, and site of the implant. Polymers with a high degree of L-lactides degrade more slowly (months to years) than mixtures of D and L isoforms (months). Some PLLA implants have been documented to take more than 5 years to absorb.[21] Implants made of PLLA occasionally have to be removed, conferring little advantage over metal. Polyglycolides degrade faster than polylactides. Homopolymer PGA implants therefore degrade very quickly, losing virtually all strength within 1 month and all mass within 6 to 12 months.[22] The newer generation of degradable implants is created from a blend of several polymers. These implants derive their physical properties from the varying proportions of the composite monomers: L lactide (provides strength to implants), D lactide (disrupts crystallinity), and trimethylene carbonate (TMC) (provides enhanced malleability and toughness). Due to the blending process, the overall degradation of these composite implants does not have the extreme degradation peaks sometimes seen in products made from one type of polymer. The likelihood of degradation-related inflammatory reactions is therefore usually lower than fast-degrading homopolymers. Biomechanical testing has shown blended implants to be of sufficient strength to be used in high-load mandibular areas and provide sufficient mechanical stability for primary healing. In a prospective clinical trial using self-reinforced poly-L/D-lactide plates and screws in 89 mandibular fracture, the authors demonstrated fracture stability after a mean follow-up of 24.4 months with only transient complication.[23]

Injectable Implants

Soft tissue augmentation using various injectable fillers has gained in popularity as more patients seek aesthetic improvement through minimally invasive approaches. The recent surge in available injectable implants has expanded the indications for injectable fillers as well as the number of practitioners offering them. Desirable product features include nonanimal origin, biocompatibility, biodegradability, a low risk of allergic reaction, durable but not permanent filling effect, ease of use, and minimal side effects, such as bruising, irritation, infection, migration, or tissue reactions.[24] The cosmetic effect of injectable facial fillers must address not only line filling but also the restoration of facial contours. A good understanding of the properties of common fillers is the first step in selecting the appropriate material for the intended result (**Table 6.1**).

Injectable Poly-L-Lactic Acid

Injectable PLLA (Sculptra, Dermik, Berwyn, PA) is a resorbable soft tissue augmentation filler of nonanimal origin containing microparticles of PLLA measuring an average of 40 to 63 µm in diameter. This particle size ensures that the particles are large enough to avoid phagocytosis by dermal macrophages or passage through the capillary walls but small enough to be easily injected intradermally or subdermally by needles as fine as 26 gauge. The microparticles are suspended in a sodium carboxymethylcellulose gel. PLLA is supplied as a lyophilized product that requires reconstitution with sterile

Table 6.1 Comparison of Injectable Fillers

Injectable Filler	Depth of Injection	Mode of Augmentation	Duration of Effect
New-Fill/Sculptra (Dermik, Berwyn, PA)	Deep dermis/ SubQ junction	Initial augmentation replaced by collagen and connective tissue reaction	1–2 years
Restylane (Medicis Aesthetics Holdings, Inc., Scottsdale, AZ)	Mid-dermis	Direct volume augmentation	6–8 months
Restylane Fine Lines, Touch (Medicis)	Upper dermis	Direct volume augmentation	3–6 months
Restylane Perlane (Medicis)	Deep dermis	Direct volume augmentation	9–18 months
Restylane SubQ (Medicis)	SubQ	Direct volume augmentation	Years
Artecoll/Artefill (Artes Medical, Inc., San Diego, CA)	Deep dermis	Encapsulation of PMMA sphere by collagen	Years
	Deep dermal/ subQ junction	Direct volume augmentation, collagen matrix	12–18 months
Radiesse (BioForm, Inc., Franksville, WI)	Upper dermis	Direct volume augmentation	2–5 months
CosmoDerm and Zyderm I and II (INAMED Aesthetics, Santa Barbara, CA)	Mid- to deep dermis	Direct volume augmentation	3–5 months
CosmoPlast and Zyplast (INAMED Aesthetics) Silicone	Deep dermis	Encapsulation	Years

Abbreviations: PMMA, polymethylmethacrylate.

water into a hydrocolloid suspension. Because the PLLA is of synthetic, nonanimal origin, allergy testing is not required before clinical use. After implantation, PLLA microparticles in the injection site gradually degrade and are replaced by a connective tissue response, which may augment the initial volume change. As a result, gradual approach to volume correction is recommended. The volume correction obtained following PLLA injection is reported to last from 18 to 24 months. Valantin and colleagues reported on the safety and efficacy of injectable PLLA in severely lipoatrophic patients with human immunodeficiency virus (HIV).[25] In contrast, others have noted many cases of granulomas and delayed inflammatory reactions and therefore recommend alternative fillers, especially in immunocompromised patients[26,27]

Hyaluronic Acid

Hyaluronic acid is a polysaccharide consisting of *N*-acetylglucosamine and glucuronic acid—a key structural component of all mammalian connective tissue. It is found in the extracellular space, and it functions as a space-filling, structure-stabilizing, and cell protective molecule. It is uniquely malleable and has superb biocompatibility. Cross-linked hyaluronic acid matrices are extremely viscoelastic and highly hydrophilic. Restylane and Perlane (Medicis, Inc., Scottsdale, AZ) are non-animal-stabilized hyaluronic acid (NASHA) gels that have been approved for soft tissue augmentation. Restylane is produced by cultured *Streptococcus* using NASHA technology. They appear to provide durable and aesthetic soft tissue augmentation and are useful adjuncts in facial cosmetic procedures. They rarely cause allergic reaction and generally do not require pretesting. Restylane was approved for nasolabial fold augmentation by the FDA in 2003. Hylaform Plus (Genzyme Corp., Cambridge, MA) is a naturally occurring cross-linked hyaluronic acid obtained from chicken combs. Hylaform was approved for aesthetic use by the FDA in April 2004. Results following injection of hyaluronic acid typically last from 3 to 6 months, depending on the type of cross-linked hyaluronic acid used and the area injected. For example, mobile areas, such as the lips and lower nasolabial folds, have a shorter duration than less mobile areas, such as the cheeks and zygoma. The temporary nature of hyaluronic acid—an advantage in itself—is both the primary advantage and disadvantage for patients seeking a longer-lasting effect. For patients new to facial rejuvenation procedures, guarantee of eventual dissipation can be reassuring. Intramuscular or subperiosteal injections are not recommended because much of the filler will be absorbed. Likewise, injections into dynamic areas associated with a great amount of movement, such as around the mouth, may lead to less satisfactory results because the motion will encourage absorption. Injection-related adverse effects—bruising, erythema, pruritis, discoloration—are common and should be described pretreatment to patients as expected sequelae. Delayed skin reactions, including granulomas, have been reported postinjection.[28] Granulomas often respond to injected corticosteroids, topical antihistamines, and digital pressure or manipulation.[28]

Injectable Hydroxyapatite

Radiesse (BioForm, Inc., Franksville, WI) is injectable filler composed of calcium hydroxyapatite (CaHA) microspheres suspended in an aqueous gel carrier. Because calcium molecules are visible on x-ray, it is radiopaque and has been used as a radiographic tissue marker. Radiesse FN contains microspheres ranging in size from 25 to 125 μm and can be injected through a 30 gauge needle, with occasional lumen occlusion, and freely through a 27 gauge needle. The carrier gel contains glycerin, sodium carboxymethylcellulose, and water, all commonly used carrier vehicles for intramuscular injections. Radiesse FN is cleared by the FDA for injection laryngoplasty and correction of craniofacial defects. Once injected the carrier vehicle gradually absorbs, degrades, and undergoes macrophage phagocytosis over a period of 6 to 8 weeks.[29] Concurrently a local fibroblastic response occurs resulting in fibrous encapsulation of the CaHA particles. When placed under the periosteum the matrix of CaHA spheres will be exposed to active osteoblasts, which may result in active bone formation. In clinical studies, bone formation in soft tissues has not been noted.[30] For this reason caution should be used when working near periosteum or bone. Radiesse FN is a thick, white, cohesive material best suited for subdermal or deep dermal placement. The material will feel firm for up to 2 to 3 months. There is a gradual softening during this period. Subdermal nodules are sometimes palpable but rarely visible and soften over a few months. Visible or palpable nodules can be treated with a small intralesional injection of Kenalog (40 mg/mL). Visible intradermal punctate (milia-like) nodules are best expressed at the time of implantation using a small needle or no. 11 blade to open the pocket and squeeze out the material. Left for more than a few days the CaHA spheres will become adherent to surrounding soft tissues and are difficult to remove. Radiesse FN has demonstrated good early results in the treatment of deeper folds, furrows, and creases, including the nasolabial folds (NLFs), frown lines, the labiomandibular grooves (LMGs), deeper glabelar furrows resistant to botulinum toxin injections, prejowl sulcus, and generalized facial volume augmentation.[31]

Polymethylmethacrylate

Artecoll (Artefill, Artes Medical, SanDiego, CA) is a suspension of PMMA microspheres in 3.5% bovine collagen solution. Artecoll is a nonbiodegradable filler that is expected to last at least 5 years. It has been used to correct atrophy of the malar fat pad as well as acne scars. After injections, the collagen solution eventually dissipates. The nonbiodegradable PMMA microspheres become engulfed by a fibrous reaction that is partially responsible for the long-term volume change. Hence, incremental correction over two to four injection sessions usually produces a smoother and more natural result. Because of the collagen content, allergy testing is required prior to injection. Undesirable outcomes are common when Artecoll is injected in areas of thin skin (e.g., lower eyelid or neck) or with improper placement intradermally instead of the upper subdermis. Delayed development of granulomatous reactions can lead to beading, ridging, and nodule formation that may require surgical removal.[26]

Future of Synthetic Implants in Plastic and Reconstructive Surgery

The increasingly intimate combination of engineering and biology has seen the transition from the use of bioinert synthetic implants to bioactive implants that offer the prospect of sophisticated tissue replacement or augmentation. Although the versatility of polymer-based implants in reconstructive surgery is well recognized, their lack of physiological adaptability remains a major limitation. The emergence of nanophase materials and nanotechnology holds a lot of promise in the development of a new generation of synthetic implants that are more physiologically adaptable.[32] Nanophase materials are defined as materials with constituent dimension less than 100 nm in at least one direction. To date, nanophase ceramics, metals, polymers, and composites have been developed and are being used in tissue engineering. Nanophase materials may be optimal synthetic implants not only because of their ability to simulate dimensions of proteins that make up tissues but also because of their higher reactivity for interactions of proteins that control cell adhesion and, thus, the ability to regenerate tissues. Another area of rapid advancement in the use of synthetic implants in plastic and reconstructive surgery is the use of tissue engineering approaches that combine degradable porous scaffolds with biological cells to promote tissue regeneration. Combined with advances in computational topology design of scaffolds, designer scaffolds are being tailored to individual clinical needs to create designer material/biofactor hybrids.

References

1. International Organization for Standardization (ISO) 10993 standards www.iso.org
2. Williams DF. Implantable prostheses. Phys Med Biol 1980;25:611–636
3. Baier RE, Meenaghan MA, Hartman LC, Wirth IE, Flynn HE, Meyer AE. Implant surface characteristics and tissue interaction. I. Oral Implantol 1988;13:594–606
4. Peterson PK, Fleer A. Foreign Body-Related Infections. Amsterdam: Excerpta Medica; 1987
5. Merritt K, Shafer JW, Brown SA. Implant site infection rates with porous and dense materials. J Biomed Mater Res 1979;13:101–108
6. Hogt AH, Dankert J, de Vries JA, Feijen J. Adhesion of coagulase-negative staphylococci to biomaterials. J Gen Microbiol 1983;129:1959
7. An YH, Friedman RJ. Concise review of mechanisms of bacterial adhesion to biomaterial surfaces. J Biomed Mater Res 1998;43:338

8. An YH, Friedman RJ, Draughn RA, Smith E, Qi C, John JF. Staphylococci adhesion to orthopedic biomaterials. Trans Soc Biomater 1993; 16:148
9. Sela M, Taicher S. Restoration of movement to the upper eyelid in facial palsy by an individual gold implant prosthesis. J Prosthet Dent 1984;52:88
10. Sobol SM, Alward PD. Early gold weight lid implant for rehabilitation of faulty eyelid closure with facial paralysis: an alternative to tarsorraphy. Head Neck Surg 1990;3/4:149
11. Bair RL, Harris GJ, Lyon DB, Komorowski RA. Noninfectious inflammatory response to gold weight eyelid implants. Ophthal Plast Reconstr Surg 1995;11:209–214
12. Eufinger H, Wehmoller M. Individual prefabricated titanium implants in reconstructive craniofacial surgery: clinical and technical aspects of the first 22 cases. Plast Reconstr Surg 1998;102:300–308
13. Ficarra G, Mosqueda-Taylor A, Carlos R. Silicon granuloma of facial tissues: a report of seven cases. Oral Surg Med Oral Pathol 2002;94: 65–73
14. Syed TA. A review of the applications of imiquimod: a novel immune response modifier. Expert Opin Pharmacother 2001;2:877–882
15. Davis PKB, Jones SM. The complications of Silastic implants: experience with 137 consecutive cases. Br J Plast Surg 1971;24:405
16. Smith AW, Jackson IT, Yousefi J. The use of screw fixation of methylmethacrylate to reconstruct large craniofacial contour defects. Eur J Plast Surg 1999;22:17–21
17. Cenzi R. Farina A, Zuccarino L, Carinci F. Clinical outcome of 285 Medpor grafts used for craniofacial reconstruction. J Craniofac Surg 2005;16:526–530
18. Panossian A, Garner WL. Polytetrafluoroethylene facial implants: 15 years later. Plast Reconstr Surg 2004;113:347–349
19. Brody HJ. Complications of expanded polytetrafluoroethylene (e-PTFE) facial implant. Dermatol Surg 2001;27:792–794
20. Yaremchuk MJ. Facial skeletal reconstruction using porous polyethylene implants. Plast Reconstr Surg 2003;111:1818–1827
21. Bergsma JE, de Bruijn WC, Rozema FR, Bos RR, Boering G. Late degradation tissue response to poly(L-lactide) bone plates and screws. Biomaterials 1995;16:25–31
22. Andriano KP, Pohjonen T, Tormala P. Processing and characterization of absorbable polylactide polymers for use in surgical implants. J Appl Biomater 1994;5:133–140
23. Yerit KC, Hainich S, Turhani D, et al. Stability of biodegradable implants in treatment of mandibular fractures. Plast Reconstr Surg 2005; 115:1863–1870
24. Klein AW. Skin filling: collagen and other injectables of the skin. Dermatol Clin 2001;19:491–508 ix.
25. Valantin MA, Aubron-Olivier C, Ghosn J, et al. Polylactic acid implants (New-Fill)(R) to correct facial lipoatrophy in HIV-infected patients: results of the open-label study VEGA. AIDS 2003;17:2471–2477
26. Saylan Z. Facial fillers and their complications. Aesthetic Surg J 2003; 23:221–224
27. Corbiget-Escalier F, Petrella T, Janin-Magnificat C, et al. Episodes d'angio-oèdemes de la face avec nodules de granulomes a corps étrangers deux ans après des injections d'un produit de comblement des rides: probable responsibilité du New-Fill. Nouv Dermatol 2003; 22:136–138
28. Lowe NJ, Maxwell CA, Lowe P, et al. Hyaluronic acid skin fillers: adverse reactions and skin testing. J Am Acad Dermatol 2001;45:930–933
29. Legeros RZ. Biodegradation and bioresorption of calcium phosphate ceramics. Clin Mater 1993;14:65–88
30. Hubbard W. Bioform Implants: Tissue Infiltration. Franksville, WI: Bioform Inc.; 2003
31. Flaharty P. Radiance. Facial Plast Surg 2004;20:165–169
32. Stylios GK, Giannoudis PV, Wan T. Applications of nanotechnologies in medical practice. Injury 2005;36(Suppl 4):S6–S13

7 Biological Tissue Implants

Fred J. Stucker and Timothy S. Lian

The adage "everything old is new again" rings particularly true in the use of biological implants in facial plastic and reconstructive surgery. As early as 1670, Van Meekren employed canine calvarial bone grafts to reconstruct a Russian soldier's skull defect.[1] Since then, an array of biological materials have been used in reconstructive surgery. Cartilage, dermis, fat, muscle, tendons, fascia, and even sclera have been used for a variety of facial plastic reconstructive purposes. These grafts have been derived from the patient (autologous), cadavers, other humans (homologous), and animals (allograft or xenograft). Surgeons often seek synthetic materials that are accepted by the host in lieu of biological implants. Although varying degrees of success have been achieved, many suffer from extrusion or other untoward reactions. These experiences prompt a bias toward autologous tissue and, to a lesser degree, homologous materials. This chapter outlines the advantages and disadvantages of a variety of biological materials, commonly used both as implants (nonbiological) and grafts (viable). These materials include cartilage, bone, dermis, dermal fat, and free fat.

Cartilage

Cartilage possesses several characteristics that satisfy the criteria for an ideal graft. It is easily carved and usually maintains it structural integrity. It is readily harvested from the patient or procured from donor banks and is easily preserved. Surprisingly, although autologous cartilage grafts were first used experimentally by Bert in the 1860s, they were not applied to humans until Koenig used them in 1896 by fashioning a rib for soft tissue augmentation.[2,3]

Classification and Early Controversy

Traditionally, cartilage is characterized according to its location, its function, and the type of fiber present. Thus the terms used in classification are *fibrous, articular*, and *elastic hyaline*.[4] However, Gibson points out that, for practical purposes, these categories are of little value because all cartilage contains the precursors to all of the other types, and when transplanted, metaplasia does not occur.[5] Therefore, transplanted cartilage from rib, septum, larynx, and all other sites maintains its respective structure, and each type should be considered individually.

The following three components are present in all cartilage: the chondrocyte, the matrix, and water. The matrix is secreted by the chondrocyte; it is composed of a collagen unique to cartilage and a proteoglycan matrix whose molecular structure permits large amounts of water to be covalently bonded. It is this water layer that allows nutrients to diffuse to the metabolically active chondrocytes. This is critical because cartilage is completely avascular. The matrix also serves to immunologically protect the chondrocyte, which is the more antigenic component of cartilage. Elves has conclusively shown a major histocompatibility group of antigens on this cell.[6] This explains the different findings among investigators. Those who use diced or carved cartilage implants exposed the chondrocytes, thus initiating an immunologic response. Clinically, this would also explain why several surgeons found a variable amount of absorption in homologous cartilage grafts.

There are a variety of methods used to preserve nonviable cartilage, including storage in thimerosal, boiling, freezing, formalin fixation, and megavolt radiation. Cartilage for implantation has been harvested from humans, cattle, pigs, and other animals. The main advantage of nonautologous cartilage is the unlimited supply and the fact that nonviable cartilage does not warp and is supposedly easier to carve than viable cartilage. Most report significant long-term absorption when using preserved cartilage.[7] Notably, the Soviet surgeon, Mikhelson, reported only three cases of absorption in more than 1800 cases using preserved cartilage.[8] His method of preservation consisted of maintaining the harvested human cartilage at a temperature below 6°C and implanting it within 3 months. Subsequent studies have noted that these cooled grafts are most likely still viable at the time of transplant.[9] A report by Schuller et al showed a mere 1.4% absorption rate in irradiated cartilage.[10]

In 1999, Kridel and Konior reported a low level of graft warping with irradiated homograft costal cartilage, which is consistent with other reports.[11] In 1998, Adams et al performed a controlled study that compared the in vitro warping characteristics of irradiated and nonirradiated homograft costal cartilage.[12] Their results demonstrated no significant difference. They also found that the warping continued over time for at least 4 weeks.

Donald and Cole in a 1981 survey of facial plastic surgeons indicated that most surgeons preferred autologous cartilage because of significantly less long-term absorption compared with all types of preserved cartilage except irradiated cartilage.[13] A subsequent animal study by Donald appears to contradict the claim of irradiated cartilage's longevity.[14] His 3-year follow-ups indicate that none of the implanted irradiated cartilages survived. In addition to the questionable absorption of homologous cartilage, many physicians and patients are concerned with the potential for transmission of pathogenic viruses. Although no case has been reported of a viral disease stemming from transplanted preserved cartilage and it is extremely unlikely that these viruses could survive the various devitalizing techniques, this concern of an anxious public is not likely to diminish. With these considerations, autologous fresh cartilage harvested from the nasal septum, auricular concha, or rib is used by most surgeons for a variety of procedures.

Common Uses of Cartilage Grafts

The most ubiquitous uses of cartilage grafts have been in cosmetic and reconstructive nasal surgery and ear reconstruction. Because rhinoplasty is the most commonly performed aesthetic operation, it is not surprising that it is also the most common application of cartilage grafts. The following specific problems that can be addressed by a cartilage graft were summarized by Ortiz-Monasterio et al: (1) retracted columella and nasal sine, (2) acute nasolabial angle, (3) vertically long upper lip, (4) insufficient anterior projection of the nose, (5) bulbous fatty nasal tip, (6) low bridge of dorsal defect, and (7) depressed piriform area.[15] Other nasal uses include effacing or deepening the nasofrontal angle, closing septal perforations, and correcting the nasal valve. There are also numerous uses in African Americans and Asians, as well as in patients with congenitally deformed noses, especially those with cleft lip and palate. The majority of grafts used in rhinoplasty are used for ether columellar support or tip augmentation. Dorsal augmentation is also a common use, but we prefer to restrict its application to replacement of structural support or to augmentation of no more than 3 to 4 mm. There are numerous techniques for harvesting and placement of such grafts. The rhinoplastic surgeon routinely harvests the autologous cartilage grafts from the septum. Less commonly, they are obtained from the concha and infrequently from the rib. Principles of utilization include care when handling and carving these grafts and insertion into an adequate but snug pocket. Absolute hemostasis is mandatory. Fixation is usually not necessary unless there is motion or if migration is possible. Migration results when the undermined area is larger than the graft. In these cases, fixation by suture is advocated. Conchal cartilage has been successfully employed in the nasal valve area to provide structural support for collapse of the cartilaginous valve (**Fig. 7.1**). Rib cartilage is used in auricular reconstruction for microtia and anotia. Use of the seventh and eighth rib, popularized by Tanzer and modified by Brent, is currently considered the gold standard in reconstruction of the auricle.[16,17] Orbital reconstruction and tarsal plate defects are also areas where cartilage grafts are used in facial plastic surgery.

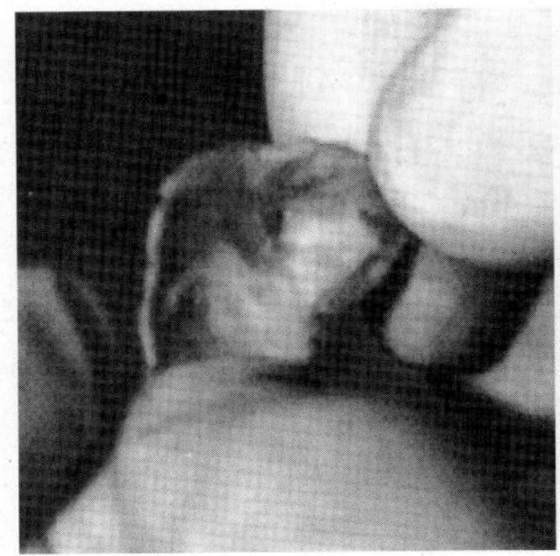

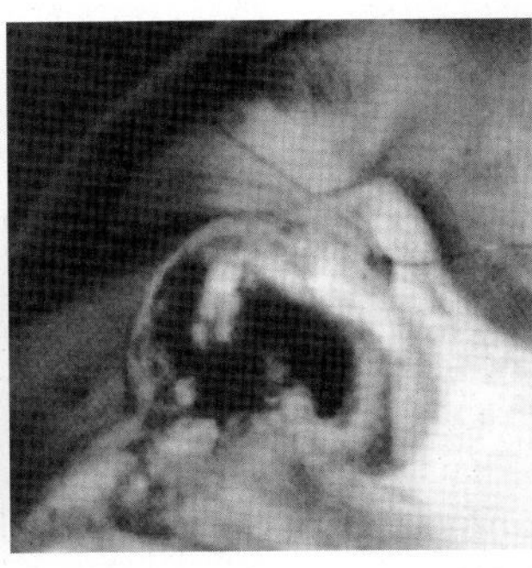

A B

Fig. 7.1 (**A**) Conchal cartilage graft fashioned for placement. (**B**) Percutaneous placement of mattress suture for fixation of cartilage graft and obliteration of dead space.

In conclusion, because of its ubiquity of donor sites, high degree of malleability, long-term viability, and resistance to resorption, autologous cartilage is a favored method used by many reconstructive facial plastic surgeons.

Bone

Classification, Type, and Structure

Bone, like cartilage, should be considered as a viable dynamic tissue. It is composed of cells (osteocytes) that occupy cavities (lacuna) in a dense matrix of condensed collagen and amorphous ground substance (calcium hydroxyapatite). Bone tissue is classified by its origin. Chondral bone is formed by epiphyseal cartilage slowly transforming into bone, and mesenchymal bone (membranous) is formed by the replacement of a preexisting membrane of mesenchyme.

All bone contains two types of tissue. Cortical tissue is the outer-component layer that is penetrated by small vascular canals (Volkmann canals). It is covered by a two-layer periosteum, an external layer of fibrocytes, and an internal layer of endothelial-like cells. Cancellous tissue is the other type of bone tissue. It forms a trabeculated framework, surrounding the marrow, traversed by haversian canals, and populated by osteoblasts.

The type and structure of bone is important when this tissue is used as a graft. Until recently, bone grafts were handled cavalierly, the same way a cabinet maker would handle wood. Historically, Ollier, a contemporary of Claude Bernard, was the first to demonstrate the importance of periosteum in new bone growth.[18] In 1914, Phemister was the first to note that split-graft survival rates were better than intact-bone survival rates when autotransplanted.[19] Robertson and Baron confirmed the superior osteogenic potential of cancellous bone and introduced the custom of drilling holes into grafts to expose cancellous bone and packing cancellous chips around the transplanted grafts.[20]

The steps involved in the assimilation of transplanted bone grafts were delineated in 1960. The first step is vascularization of the graft from the host vessels alone the graft's haversian system. Demineralization of the graft takes ~6 months, followed by a healing period of ~16 months. The bone graft is slowly recalcified and resumes the original donor osteon structure during the healing period. In addition, it had been found that membranous bone (i.e., calvarial) is revascularized twice as fast as endochondral bone. Experimental studies confirmed 90% maintenance of membranous bone compared with ~50% of endochondral bone.[21] Like cartilage, bone was once thought to be immunologically protected. In fact, this is not so, but the majority of antigenic sites are in the marrow and attached to soluble proteins. These can be reduced by a number of preservation techniques, thus allowing the use of homografts and xenografts. These preserved grafts should really be called implants because their nature requires nonviability, and they function as a scaffold. Even with good autolysis, osteogenesis will not occur in cancellous bone unless the host bed is well vascularized, adequately immobilized, and in apposition to viable host bone.

Primary Uses of Bone Grafts

The primary uses of bones grafts by the facial plastic and reconstructive surgeon have been for mandibular reconstruction, repair of traumatic midfacial defects, orthognathic surgery, and craniofacial surgery. More recently, particularly in terms of calvarial grafts, cosmetic and rhinoplastic applications have increased. Historically, the inner table iliac crest, the tibia, and rib grafts are common donor sites. More recently, calvarial bone grafts have been used because of harvesting ease and significantly less donor morbidity when compared with more traditional sources.

Grafts can be both free and vascularized. Vascularized bone grafts may be pedicled (e.g., pectoralis major with rib, temporalis with outer table calvarium, or trapezius with scapular spine) or be a free microvascularized graft (e.g., iliac crest osteomyocutaneous graft).

In addition to mandibular reconstruction, we regularly use bone grafts in areas of posttraumatic deficits where soft tissue grafts are not appropriate. This includes the orbit, forehead, zygoma, and total and partial nasal reconstruction where all or significant bony support is lost (**Fig. 7.2**). Craniofacial surgeons regularly use bone grafts to correct cranial and orbital synostoses, as in Treacher-Collins syndrome. We frequently fix grafts to neighboring solid bones using minicompression plates or lag screws (**Fig. 7.3**). External appliances or intermaxillary fixation is not necessary when plating is used. In total nasal reconstruction the bone graft can be doweled into the frontal bone and sinus and the flap draped over the newly constructed periosteal covered bony framework (**Fig. 7.4**).

Fat

Dermis and Dermal Fat

Soft tissue deficits and asymmetry are reconstructive deformities often seen by the facial plastic surgeon. When these defects are subcutaneous in nature, pliable autologous soft tissue is desirable for augmentation. Before 1914, surgeons utilized buried skin grafts for augmentation. These were complicated by the presence of epithelial cyst formation and chronic inflammation and infection. In 1914, Lexer was the first to use dermis to augment facial contours.[22] In addition, dermal fat grafts have been used in a variety of procedures, including tendon repair, hernia repair, mandibular ankylosis, closure of dural defects, great-vessel protection, and intraoral and oral pharyngeal cavity reconstruction. Dermal fat grafts were originally used in breast reconstruction and have since been applied to a variety of soft tissue deficit repairs, including hemifacial atrophy, gunshot trauma, and radical parotidectomy.

In 1959, Peer demonstrated that dermal fat grafts had significantly less resorption than free-fat grafts.[23] In spite of this, up to 80% were resorbed. Longacre used dermal fat flaps pedicled with a local blood supply for breast reconstruction, and Neumann used them for hemifacial atrophy reconstruction.[24,25] They postulated that the pedicled blood supply would allow for even less resorption. More recently, transfer of dermal fat flaps with microvascular reanastomosis has been performed.[26] We have also described the use of island pedicled flaps, particularly in relatively small areas of deficiency such as the inferior orbital sulcus.[27] The early concerns of many surgeons centered on epidermoid cyst formation.

The classis technique of obtaining free dermal and dermal fat grafts has been well described. Essentially, a split-thickness skin graft (0.14 to 0.16 in.) is lifted with a dermatome. The graft should be harvested in an area of relatively thick but hairless skin (i.e., buttock or thigh). If a dermal graft is also desired, a second pass is performed

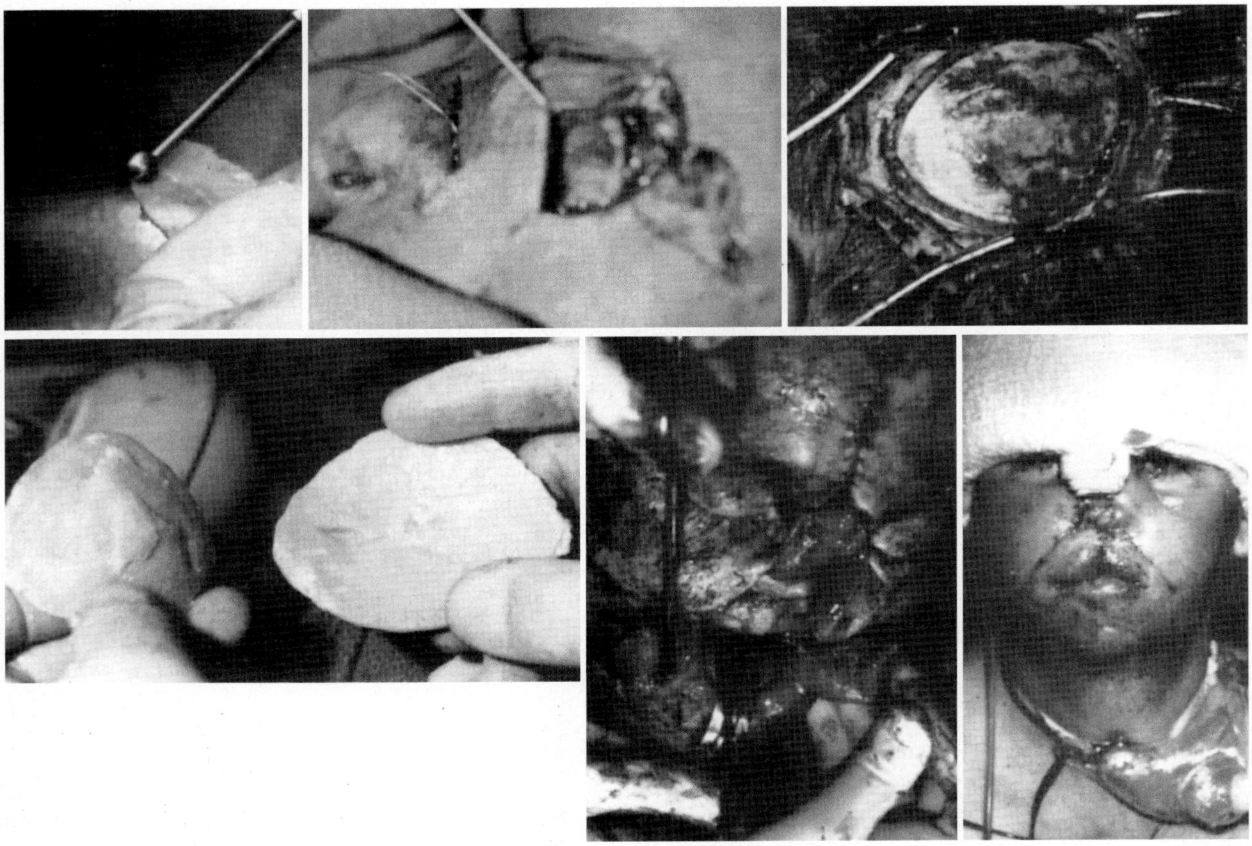

Fig. 7.2 (**A**) Shaping iliac bone graft with a drill. (**B**) Iliac bone graft to augment infraorbital deficit. (**C**) Periphery of calvarial bone graft drilled. (**D**) Inner and outer tables separated. One closes the skull defect, and the other serves as the graft. (**E**) Calvarial bone graft used for premaxillary replacement. (**F**) Calvarium replacing and stabilizing loss of entire midline bony structures.

with the dermatome at approximately the same thickness. A dermal fat graft is harvested using the knife, taking care to keep the fat attached to the dermis. It is important not to traumatize this tissue. Deepithelialization of skin may also be performed using the CO_2 laser. This technique is especially helpful when island or pedicled flaps are used. The handheld CO_2 laser is set at 10 W power using the 1 mm spot size. The area to be deepithelialized is systematically lasered by using the hand piece held far enough away to slightly defocus the beam. When the circumscribed area has been covered with the laser, it is wiped or debrided of the vaporized epidermal cell layers with a wet sponge. Often two or three passes with the laser are necessary to adequately deepithelialize the tissue. This is detected by a

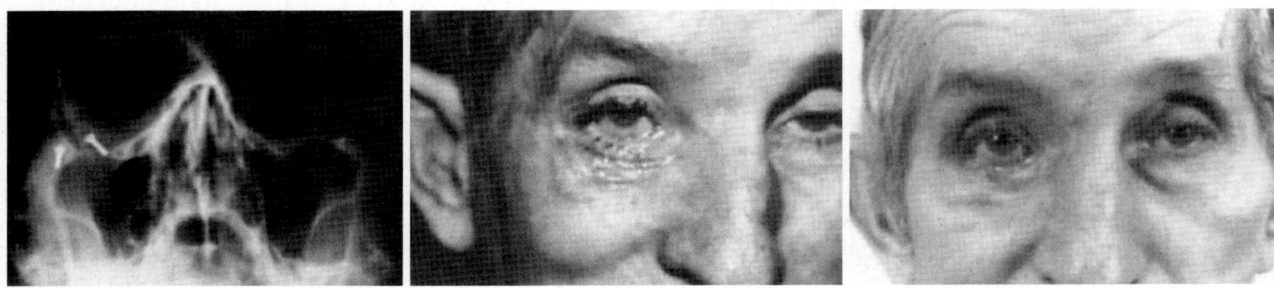

Fig. 7.3 (**A**) One-year postoperative x-ray demonstrating fixation of infraorbital bone graft with lag screws. (**B**) Postoperative view of infraorbital rim reconstructed with bone graft and covered with perichondrial cutaneous graft. (**C**) Six months after graft has been placed.

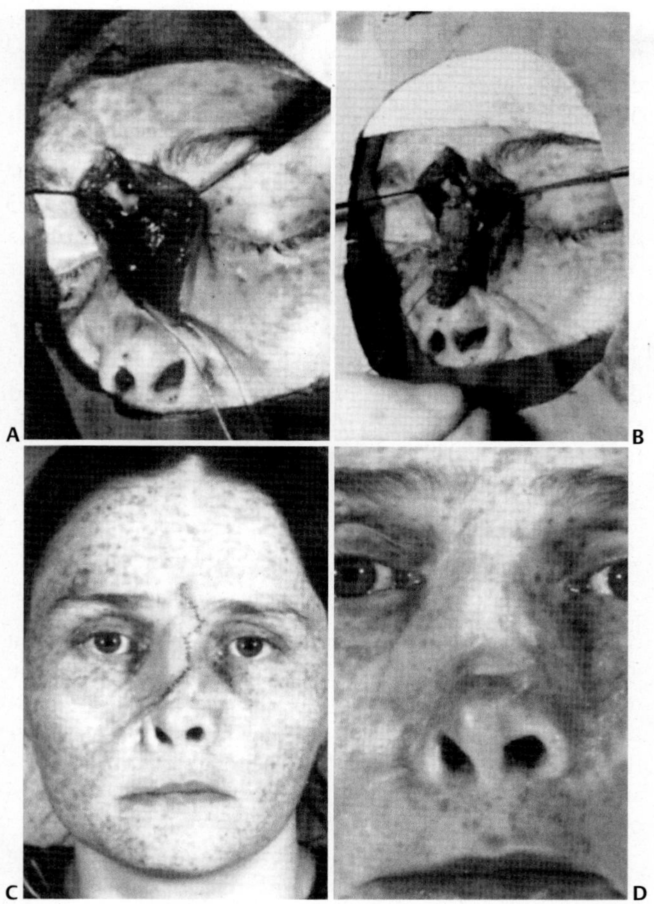

Fig. 7.4 (A) Hole drilled in frontal sinus as recipient for dowel end of bone graft. (B) Periosteal covered iliac bone graft with dowel fitted into hole. (C) Five days after surgery. (D) Two years after surgery.

notable white color and tissue contracture (**Fig. 7.5**). Care must be taken not to go deeper with the laser because this could potentially lead to permanent scarring. We have laser-deepithelialized many grafts and flaps, including pedicled fat grafts, and have found this technique to be reliable and expeditious, with limited long-term resorption.

Free Autologous Fat

Autologous fat transplantation has been performed for more than a century in the correction of facial defects. It was popularized in Europe by Czerny and Lexer in the 1890s.[28,29] It gained early and widespread acceptance in the early twentieth century. However, many surgeons are disappointed by the inordinate and relentless rate of resorption, reported to be from 30 to 100%.[30] Because of the increased reliability of dermal fat and the advent of collagen and synthetic silicone, free-fat augmentation was a neglected technique until recently. Despite Peer's elegant study in the 1930s, this demonstrated that transplanted fat does indeed survive indigenously and with its own blood supply. The popularity and interest in the free-fat grafts has recently resurfaced. In 1984, Illouz described the use of fat extracted from liposuction surgery and transplanted via injection to correct skin defects.[31] This provided the surgeon with an abundant supply of viable adipose tissue that could be used to augment soft-tissue deformities. Many others have since used this technique with success, incorporating several refinements. One refinement involves centrifuging to separate fat from serum and blood, thus reducing the inflammation and hopefully decreasing the

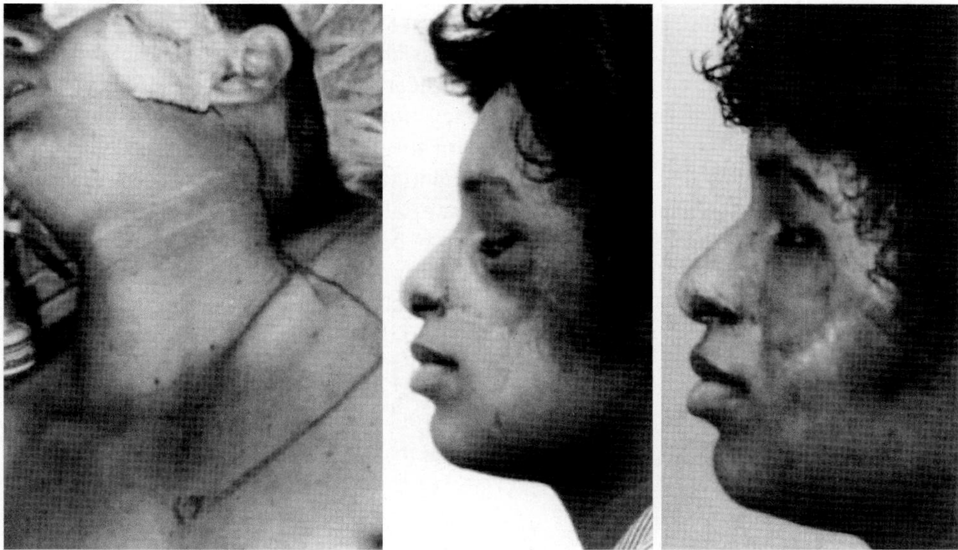

Fig. 7.5 (A) Laser deepithelialized split-thickness skin graft, allowing its burial beneath a rotating flap. (B) Preoperative photograph. (C) Postoperative placement of dermal graft from back to malar region.

amount of resorption.[32] Exposing the fat cells to an insulin-rich solution also reduces resorption because insulin is an antilipolytic agent.[33,34] This works in vitro but has not proved successful clinically. Another approach used only type I (i.e., genetic fat) cells. These cells have a high concentration of antilipolytic receptors (αI) and are therefore less likely to be resorbed. Anatomically, they are found in the abdominal and trochanteric regions. Conversely, adipose tissue in the face, arms, and upper torso has a high concentration of lipolytic (βII) receptors and is therefore a poor harvest site for fat transplantation.[35]

Acellular Dermal Grafts

Alloderm (Lifecell Corp., Woodlands, TX) was designed as a dermal replacement. Production of this dermal replacement entails removal of the entire epidermis and all of the dermal cells from cadaveric skin. The acellular dermis is then freeze-dried without damaging the extracellular matrix proteins. Immunohistochemical staining confirms the absence of antigens that induce rejection. This graft has been shown to integrate with the surrounding tissue both histologically and immunologically.[36]

The advantage of this material is that, because the body recognizes it as an "autograft," it becomes remodeled in the body and avoids donor site morbidity associated with harvest of autogenous tissue. As these types of grafts have become more popular, the concern over transmission of viral diseases has been raised. The cadaveric skin used in these grafts has been screened in accordance with the U.S. Food and Drug Administration's protocol on human tissue. The tissue banks used follow the appropriate protocol for donor blood testing and social screening. In addition, the process removes all cellular components, and the graft is treated with an antiviral agent that has been proved to inactivate concentrated human immunodeficiency virus. There have been no reported cases of viral transmission in any patient so far.[37]

This material has been used in the treatment of cutaneous burns. Cosmetic and reconstructive applications include nasal dorsal augmentation, lip augmentation, facial soft tissue filling, scar revision, and nasal septal perforation repair.[37,38]

Platelet Gels

Platelet gels or platelet rich plasma (PRP) has received increased attention recently secondary to reported advantages of its hemostatic and adhesive and, perhaps more interesting, its wound healing properties. PRP is a collection of blood products that contain a high concentration of platelets. In addition to concentrated platelets, there are also concentrated growth factors that play a role in wound healing. Growth factors include platelet-derived growth factor and transforming growth factor β.[39,40] It is postulated that with such concentrated growth factors in the surgical wound bed, postoperative healing is enhanced with resulting clinical manifestations of decreased edema, ecchymosis, erythema, and pain.[41,42] Autologous PRP is obtained by collecting a volume of the patient's blood, usually 40 to 60 mL, and separating out the platelets with use of a commercially available variable speed centrifuge. Blood is collected prior to making any incisions to avoid platelet activation. The PRP is applied topically to the wound bed using a double-barreled syringe in conjunction with topical thrombin, which is used to activate the platelets.

Future of Biological Tissue Implants

New cell culture techniques have made possible the in vitro creation of cartilage. The methodology involves the use of single cells rather than whole tissue for transplantation. In the liver, hepatocytes are used to support liver function. The possibility of cartilage transplantation in a similar manner may develop with increasing knowledge of chondrocyte differentiation.

Chondrocytes have been isolated from human tissue (i.e., septum) and have been transferred to a biodegradable scaffold (i.e., polyglycolic acid) in vitro. After 1 week, these were transferred to subcutaneous tissue of nude mice. Histological analyses after up to 24 weeks revealed growth of both type I and II collagen as well as vascular ingrowth. This method may become ideal for cartilage replacement in large defects.[43]

Autologous dermis and collagen implants may also be used in injectable form. Patients undergoing cosmetic surgery may now have their excised skin sent to a tissue bank for future use. When the need arises this tissue may be used in the form of injectable autologous collagen implant material (Dermalogen, Collagenesis, Inc., Beverly, MA). This may be used for soft tissue augmentation in the nasolabial fold, perioral rhytids, and vermilion augmentation. Future clinical studies will determine if the use of human autologous collagen injection results in a sustained clinical improvement due to decreased collagen degradation when compared with bovine collagen.

Summary

Repair of facial defects has long been a goal of the facial plastic surgeon. Many biological and synthetic materials have been used. No perfect material has been found for all types of defects. Because of this, it behooves the surgeon to be familiar with several reconstructive methods and techniques. We regularly use a variety of biological and synthetic materials successfully. Nevertheless, we and many others continue to search for more suitable materials.

References

1. Van Meekren J. Observation Medicochisurgicae. Amsterdam: Henrici and T. Bloom; 1670
2. Bert P. Sur la greffe animale. CR Acad Sci 1865;51:587
3. Koenig F. Zur Deckung von Defecten in der Vorderen Tracheal Wand. Berl Klin Wehnschr 1896;51:1129
4. Chaplan AI. Cartilage. Sci Am 1984;251:84
5. Gibson T. Transplantation of cartilage. In: Converse JM, ed. Plastic and Reconstructive Surgery. Vol 1. Philadelphia: WB Saunders; 1977
6. Elves MW. A study of the transplant antigens on chondrocytes from articular cartilage. J Bone Joint Surg Br 1974;56:178–185
7. Welling DB, Maves MD, Schuller DE, et al. Irradiated homologous cartilage grafts: long-term results. Arch Otolaryngol Head Neck Surg 1988;114:291–295
8. Mikhelson NM. Homogenous cartilage in maxillofacial surgery. Acta Chir Plast 1962;4:3
9. Curran RC, Gibson T. Absorption of autologous cartilage grafts in man. Br J Plast Surg 1956;9:177
10. Schuller DC, Bardach J, Krausse C. Irradiated homologous costal cartilage for facial contour restauration. Arch Otolaryngol 1977;103:12
11. Kridel RWH, Konior RJ. Irradiated cartilage grafts in the nose: a preliminary report. Arch Otolaryngol Head Neck Surg 1993;119:124–139
12. Adams WP Jr, Rohrich RJ, Gunter JP, et al. The rate of warping in irradiated and nonirradiated homograft rib cartilage: a controlled comparison and clinical implications. Plast Reconstr Surg 1999;103:265–270
13. Donald PJ, Col A. Cartilage implantation in head and neck surgery: report of a national survey. Otolaryngol Head Neck Surg 1982;90:85–89
14. Donald PJ. Cartilage grafting in facial reconstruction with special consideration of irradiated grafts. Laryngoscope 1986;96:786–807
15. Ortiz-Monasterio F, Olmedo AB, Oscoy LO. The use of cartilage grafts in primary aesthetic rhinoplasty. Plast Reconstr Surg 1981; 67:597–605
16. Brent B. Ear reconstruction with an expansive framework of autologous rib cartilage. Plast Reconstr Surg 1974;53:619–628
17. Tanzer RC. Total reconstruction of the auricle: the solution of a planned treatment. Plast Reconstr Surg 1971;47:523–533
18. Ollier L. Traite experimetale et clinique de la regeneration des os et de la prediction artificelle du tissue osseux. Paris: P Masson et Fils; 1976
19. Phemister DB. The fate of transplanted bone and regeneration of its various constituents. Surg Gynecol Obstet 1914;19:303
20. Robertson IM, Baron JN. A method of treatment of chronic infective osteitis. J Bone Joint Surg Am 1946;28:19
21. Craft PD, Sargent LA. Membranous bone bleeding and techniques in cellular bone grafting. Clin Plast Surg 1989;16:11–19
22. Lexer E. Free transplantation. Ann Surg 1914:60:166
23. Peer LA. Transplantation of Tissues. Vol 2. Baltimore: Williams & Wilkins; 1959
24. Longacre JJ. Use of local pedicle flaps for reconstruction of breast after subtotal or total mastectomy. Plast Reconstr Surg 1953;11:380
25. Neumann CG. The use of large buried pedicle flaps of dermis and fat, clinical and pathological evaluation in progressive hemiatrophy. Plast Reconstr Surg 1953;11:315
26. Baker DC, Shaw WW, Conley J. Microvascular free dermis-fat flaps for reconstruction after ablative head and neck surgery. Arch Otolaryngol 1980;106:449–453
27. Shockley WW, Stucker FJ. Dermal grafts and flaps in facial augmentation. Facial Plast Surg 1986;3:77
28. Czerny M. Reconstruction of the breast with a lipoma. Chir Kongr Besh 1895;2:216
29. Lexer E. Free Fat Grafting, IV Congress de Societe Internationale Chirurgie. New York: 1914
30. Peer LA. Loss of weight and volume in human fat grafts. Plast Reconstr Surg 1980;5:217
31. Illouz YG. L'aucnir de la neritralisation de la gresse après liposuccion. Rev Chir Esthet Lang Franc 1984;9:36
32. Asken S. Autologous fat transplantation micro and macro techniques. Am J Cosmet Surg 1978;4:111
33. Olafsky JM, Chang H. Insulin binding to adipocytes: evidence for functionally distinct receptors. Diabetes 1978;27:940
34. Pederson O, Hjøllund E, Beck-Nielsen H, et al. Insulin receptor binding and receptor-mediated insulin degradation in human adipocytes. Diabetologia 1981;20:636
35. Johnson GW. Body contouring by macro injection of autogenous fat. Presented at the First World Congress of the American Academy of Cosmetic Surgery, New Orleans, October 1986
36. Achauer BM, VanderKam VM, Celikoz B, Jacobson DG. Augmentation of facial soft tissue defects with alloderm dermal graft. Ann Plast Surg 1998;41:503–507
37. Tobin HA, Karas NK. Lip augmentation using an alloderm graft. J Oral Maxillofac Surg 1998;56:722–727
38. Kridel RWH, Foda H, Lunde KC. Septal perforation repair with acellular human dermal allograft. Arch Otolaryngol Head Neck Surg 1998;124: 73–78
39. Pierce GF, Mustoe TA, Altrock BW, Deuel TF, Thomason A. Rode of platelet-derived growth factor in wound healing. J Cell Biochem 1991;45:319–326
40. Pierce GF, Mustoe TA, Lingelbach J. Platelet-derived growth factor and transforming growth factor-beta enhance tissue repair activities by unique mechanisms. J Cell Biol 1989;109:429–440
41. Man D, Plosker H, Winland-Brown JE. The use of autologous platelet-rich plasma (platelet gel) and autologous platelet-poor plasma (fibrin glue) in cosmetic surgery. Plast Reconstr Surg 2001; 107:229–237
42. Whitman DH, Berry RL, Green DM. Platelet gel: an autologous alternative to fibrin glue with applications in oral maxillofacial surgery. J Oral Maxillofac Surg 1997;55:1294–1299
43. Rotter N, Aigner J, Naumann A, et al. Cartilage reconstruction in head and neck surgery: comparison of resorbable polymer scaffolds for tissue engineering of human septal cartilage. J Biomed Mater Res 1998;42:347

8 Tissue Engineering

G. Richard Holt and Jami Eidem

Over the past decade, great progress has been made in identifying the requisite major elements that will be required to produce new tissues, and how those elements will be three-dimensionally arranged and supported by enhancing chemical factors. The majority of the effort has been focused on producing new epithelial surfaces, complete with a vascular capillary network, structured engineering of cartilage, and enhanced regeneration of membraneous bone. All three of these tissues have tremendous clinical application in reconstruction of the face, head, and neck.

Initial success in tissue engineering came about through the culture and coalescing of epithelial cells, primarily on artificial strata, for the purpose of onlay skin grafting in patients with extensive burns and other tissue losses. This technology is well under way clinically and supports a small industry in producing autologous epithelial cells for transplant.

Following the success of this capability, the next challenge has been to fabricate a three-dimensional scaffolding system that would support the superficial epithelial stratum, as well as to provide a biocompatible network that could be inculcated into the fibrovascular bed of the defect. Encouraging results using biological polymers and dermal supporting cells have given impetus to the next step, the development of vascular capillary networks that integrate with both the overlying epidermal–dermal construct and the sublayered vascular buds of the host defect tissues.

Finally, exciting developments in producing chondrogenic tissue and regenerated bone tissue, primarily utilizing growth factors and mesenchymal stem cells in various combinations, gives promise to the future ability of the facial plastic and reconstructive surgeon to provide new tissues for those patients whose defects are too great for immediate implantation from the human body's great storehouse of "spare parts." Cartilage lacks an intrinsic capacity to repair itself, so tissue engineering may be utilized to facilitate extracellular matrix production and remodeling. Conversely, bone has regenerative capacity, and the current efforts in bone tissue engineering focus on implantation of biomaterials and factors that augment and stimulate the natural repair process in circumstances that normally will not heal primarily.

Cells for Tissue Engineering

Currently known as "skin equivalents," cultured cells to reconstitute the natural composite of epithelium are required to interact with each other as well as their substrata in the appropriate manner. Cell to cell adhesions in the epidermal basal layer, contact with the proteinaceous basement membrane, proper dermal–epidermal junctions, dermal matrix formation, and responsivity to chemical stimuli, all make up the very complex structure of living skin.[1] Of prime importance is the proper choice of cells to provide the appropriate differentiation and contact interactions that are required for proper function. Fully differentiated autologous cells are a reliable cell source without an immune response; however, their proliferative capacity is limited and long-term in vitro culturing can reduce their functional capabilities.

Because epithelium is a complex, layered network of cells that, of necessity, must interact with each other and the underlying dermal support structure to manifest its unique biomechanical properties, some research is under way to enhance the performance of this engineered skin. Gene-modified skin, using recombinant retrovirus encoding fibroblast growth factor-7, has been shown to modify diploid human keratinocytes genetically.[2] This modification transferred highly active antimicrobial properties against both gram-negative and gram-positive bacteria. This is a very important trait for engineered skin to possess because normal skin coexists with multiple skin bacteria that do not become pathological unless immunologic conditions dramatically change.

Embryonic stem cells have great potential, but many ethical issues, as well as regulatory issues, continue to reduce their practicality. Alternative sources of stem cell populations include bone marrow, muscle, and fat. Mesenchymal stem cells (MSCs) from adult bone marrow are nonhematopoietic stem cells. They are likely recruited from bone marrow for the intrinsic repair of injured tissues. They are easily isolated and expanded in culture, while maintaining the ability to differentiate into chondrogenic, osteogenic, and adipogenic lineages. It is conceivable that these MSCs might be capable of differentiating into neural cells as well. Therefore, they are considered by many scientists and ethicists to be an ethical alternative to embryonic stem cells.

Embryonic stem cells (ESCs) were harvested from human blastocysts and fetal tissues in the latter part of the twentieth century. Most stem cell populations being utilized for research purposes are descendants of the first ESCs. They exhibit ceaseless proliferation in vitro, along with the ability to differentiate into any cell type in the human body. Murine ESCs have been directed toward the chondrogenic and osteogenic lineages with limited success.

Autologous chondrocytes (ACs) represent the only cell-based cartilage repair product available in the United States at this time. When chondrocytes are removed from their native tissue environment and expanded in a monolayer culture, they experience a discouraging loss of chondrocytic phenotype, manifested by loss of spherical cell morphology, and production of type I collagen, instead of type II collagen for the matrix. However, the phenotype can be "rescued" by transferring the cells to a three-dimensional culture system, adding specific growth factors, and reducing oxygen tension.

With respect to the head and neck, auricular and septal cartilage are different from articular cartilage in many ways—they are covered by perichondrium, the biomechanical forces stored within the cartilage are unique and yet to be fully understood, the "gel" matrix flows within the substance of the cartilage when deformed, and there are "balanced" electrical charges on the sides of the cartilage itself. Slow application of force will allow the cartilage to bend and then reform to the original shape. The sudden application of force can overcome the "gel flow" and "balanced electrical forces" sufficiently to cause a deformation that remains altered after the force is removed—that is, the cartilage assumes a new shape with new biomechanical forces acting on it.

An exciting new field of study involves the "co-culturing" of cells, with the creation of enhanced capacity and phenotypic capabilities not seen with the single cell monolayer. Culturing multiple cell types together provides an opportunity for cells to have regulatory and synergistic effects. It may be that stem cell differentiation requires more complex "cues" than just adding a few growth factors. These cues may be provided by culturing multipotent cells with differentiated cells. Thus adult stem cells may demonstrate a "plasticity" in the sense that molecules from one cell could "reprogram" the gene expression of the other cell partner in a fused cell. Several examples have demonstrated this interaction.

When chondrocytes are co-cultured with MSCs in the absence of other stimulating factors, the MSCs have been found to undergo osteogenic differentiation. Expression of osteogenic markers is not as strong when MSCs are cultured with osteoblasts. In endochondral bone formation, a cascade of signs occurring between chondrocytes and osteoprogenitor cells ultimately leads to bone formation via a cartilage intermediate form.

When compared with bone formation from osteoblasts alone in a scaffold, a mixture of osteoblasts and chondrocytes in the same scaffold will exhibit accelerated bone tissue formation. Mixed cell implants are thought to reorganize themselves from a homogeneous distribution to specific bone and cartilage tissue regions. Intercellular interactions that exist between the chondrocytes and osteoblasts may lead to enhanced matrix production and tissue organization.

Scaffolds in Tissue Engineering

A scaffold provides cells with a three-dimensional structure upon which to adhere, proliferate, and produce matrix. It can function as a delivery vehicle for cells or can perform a tissue induction role such that, when implanted, cells from host tissue are encouraged to migrate into it and form functional tissue. Composite scaffolds and scaffolds with controlled architectures can influence the development and proper special orientation of the new tissues. For instance, nasal septal cartilage has an axial alignment of chondrocytes at the margins of the structure, but a cross-axial (horizontal) orientation in the center. This arrangement, coupled with the special gel matrix and specific electrical charges within the tissue, is such a unique and specialized combination that it has been quite difficult to reproduce. It is likely that the critical factor in the engineering of septal cartilage tissue would be the structure and function of the artificial scaffold.

A good scaffold must be porous to allow for effective transport of nutrients and waste products from the tissue, as well as being biocompatible with the host tissue in which it is implanted. The scaffold should eventually degrade as new tissue matrix is produced; the degradation products must be of low to no toxicity to the tissues. It must also have the correct physical and biomechanical properties for the given tissue application—very different for bone and cartilage, as well as skin.

For the most part, artificial skin has been a combination of cultured keratinocytes and fibroblasts isolated from skin biopsy of an uninvolved region of the body. Researchers continue to seek the best scaffolding for the transfer of these bicellular composites, which will result in a high rate of regeneration. One such simple scaffolding is human plasma. Human fibroblasts can be embedded in the three-dimensional matrix of the clotted plasma, with subsequent seeding of the cultured keratinocytes on that composite surface. This matrix combination has been tested successfully in immunocompromised mice and in human burn patients, with excellent success in growth of the confluence and long-term graft viability.[3]

Of particular interest in the head and neck region is the ability to reconstruct the oral cavity with a mucosal surface that will enhance the postsurgical/postradiation therapy functioning for the patient. Most reconstructive techniques utilize free or pedicled musculocutaneous flaps, or musculo-osseous flaps, which subsequently undergo some reepithelialization. It has been demonstrated that autogenous, preconfluent oral keratinocytes cultured in vitro can be successfully transferred to a muscle surface intraorally and create a mucosal surface similar to the natural state.[4] The grafting technique is performed in a single stage. Long-term studies on the mucosal surface's ability to regenerate and maintain integrity through the process of deglutition remain to be performed.

Most of the current scaffolds for bone formation contain inorganic compounds to enhance osteoconductivity—such as hydroxyapatite or calcium-phosphate cements. So-called designer scaffolds are usually composed of natural polymers that offer good cytocompatibility and bioactivity; synthetic polymers enable precise control of the physical–chemical properties of the tissue to be formed. The designer scaffolds range in biomaterials from natural (collagen and glycosaminoglycans) to synthetic (polylactic and polyglycolic acid or copolymer of these two).

A new type of designer scaffold is the injectable gel network. Injectable scaffolds can be used to fill irregularly shaped defects and can incorporate therapeutic agents or cells by simple mixing. Hydrogels are composed of highly cross-linked hydrophilic polymer chains to yield a highly swollen gel structure. Natural hydrogels such as fibrin (a natural peptide associated with wound repair) or synthetic hydrogels such as polyethylene oxide are both capable of soft tissue filling. Hydrogels are typically weaker than solid scaffolds unless added cells are encapsulated early on within a firmer nutritional "cocoon." Hydrogels can support chondrocyte survival and cartilage matrix synthesis—at least initially until new matrix is secreted—as they reproduce the gel matrix around the chondrocyte to maintain its spherical morphology. Hydrogels mixed with cell surface adhesion peptides can improve osteoblast adhesion and matrix synthesis within the three-dimensional polymer network.

Composite scaffolds use multiple lamellae to support layers of multiple cell types and to more closely approximate microanatomical structures. Cartilage–cartilage interfaces do not integrate well because of their non-adhesive matrix. However, bone integrates well with grafted bone tissue. To better integrate engineered cartilage tissue with host cartilage tissue, an osteochondral composite tissue implant allows the bony region to "anchor" the cartilage implant to a host structure (i.e., tissue-engineered implant to the nasal bones). Additionally, the cartilage and bone regions of an osteochondral composite scaffold may provide different physical and mechanical properties to an engineered implant that could be advantageous in regions where the two coexist, such as the nasal dorsum. It appears feasible to fabricate a three-dimensional composite scaffold using microstereolithography where the layers of the scaffold are laid down successively by the computer-generated design. Thus a certain architecture can be designed that matches the requirements of the host tissue.

Future modifications of the hydrogel scaffold might be to attach covalently certain adhesive particles (glycosaminoglycans) to serve as the cell–host interface; to increase the cross-linking density of the scaffold to survive injection into scar tissues, and through blending with soluble osteoinductive materials achieve a composite that will have bone formation capabilities in a bone conductive medium. It may also be possible to add a construct of chondrocytes and mesenchymal stem cells to facilitate maintenance of the chondrocytic phenotype. MSCs appear to differentiate and produce a mineralized matrix, perhaps through the exchange of regulating factors. This construct also appears to enhance collagen production. The scaffold can also be the transport medium for encapsulated, growth-factor loaded, biodegradable microspheres that can be differentially placed in different layers according to their site of action. Likewise, spatial orientation of different cell types within the multilayered scaffold can stimulate the true properties of mature cartilage or bone. One of the hardest properties of the hard tissues to reproduce will be matching the "imbedded" inherent biomechanical stresses and strains in the newly engineered tissue; perhaps through electrochemical or mechanical modulation it might be possible to achieve a successful reproduction of these unique but vital mechanical properties of skin, cartilage, and bone.

Angiogenesis of Engineered Tissue

The successful process of host tissue accepting autogenous grafted tissue (i.e., split-thickness or full-thickness skin graft) involves early imbibition and inosculation. Following these somewhat passive processes, it is commonly held that the subdermal vascular network, under the direction of angiogenic factors secreted by the hypoxic cycle, begins a budding process that eventually links with the "ghost" channels of the grafted dermal elements. The subdermal vascular plexus is eventually reestablished, and the normal nutritional supply of the skin elements is under way. Several novel techniques and strategies have been developed to add a vascularity to the composite tissue engineered system.

Interestingly, in one study, small vessel human dermal microvascular endothelial cells did not penetrate the artificial dermal scaffolding under the influence of angiogenic growth factors (vascular endothelial growth factor and basic fibroblast growth factor). However, two factors were identified that significantly enhanced endothelial cell penetration into the dermis—hypoxia and the site of endothelial cell transplantation.[5] It appeared that endothelial cells entered the dermis more readily when implanted into the papillary elements than when introduced into the reticular elements. Because the proper spacial arrangement of cells within the dermal matrix (and in proximity to the basement membrane) appears to be of high importance, the papillary dermis may be a site of "easy transit" between the collagen matrix and the basement membrane.

Another project has proposed that inosculation is a very important process in a successful vascularization of tissue-generated skin in a wound. After placing human endothelialized reconstructed skin in a collagen scaffolding, capillary-like structures were seen as early as 4 days after transplantation. The authors postulated that the early vascularization was likely the result of inosculation of the capillary-like network of the skin composite with the host tissue's capillaries, rather than direct neovascularization, which is a time-consuming process.[6]

In a slightly different model, it has been shown that autologous fibroblasts and endothelial cells implanted on a highly biodegradable three-dimensional scaffold of hyaluronic acid–derived polymer can be subsequently populated with autologous keratinocytes. The scaffold/supporting cell element composite is first allowed to equilibrate, then the epidermal skin cells are added. This complete dermal–epidermal substitute has been shown to be nourished by a microcapillary network within 21 days, formed from endothelial cells in a ringlike structure in the interstitial spaces that closely resembled an early vascular plexus.[7] An additional advancement in providing vascularity to the engineered tissue has come from using a polymer chamber, into which the engineered tissue and a small vascular pedicle are placed. The subcutaneous chamber allowed for a "flow through" vascular model which was most effective in developing angiogenesis in the extracellular matrix scaffold, with evidence that native cells could migrate into the scaffold and survive.[8]

Engineering Hard Tissues for Head and Neck Reconstruction

For most reconstructive requirements in the head and neck region, autologous cartilage from the auricle, nasal septum, or costal rib is sufficient. However, in some patients, there is insufficient cartilage in the ear or nose (having been resected previously), or donor rib harvesting is contraindicated (previous cardiopulmonary resuscitation or thoracic surgery). For application to grafting the laryngotracheal complex, or the ear or nose, tissue-engineered cartilage is a potential tool.

In one study using swine, auricular cartilage was harvested and processed, and cells were successfully cultured, with subsequent suspension in a biodegradable polymer.[9] This construct was then injected into the subdermal area of the animal. After 8 weeks, the construct was harvested and found to be solid enough to carve and possessing a neoperichondrial capsule. This structure was then implanted into the anterior laryngotracheal complex to simulate a reconstruction for stenosis. Bronchoscopy of the animals showed airway patency. After 3 months, the engineered cartilage grafts were incorporated into the substance of the cricoid cartilage, and the interior of the graft (luminal) possessed a mucosal lining.

Mesenchymal stem cells alone (harvested from bone marrow, processed liposuction waste, or patellar fat pad) have been shown to differentiate into progenitor cells of both bone and cartilage. However, there are likely multiple chemical factors in vivo that can drive these stem cells toward an osseous or a chondral matrix. One exogenous chemical, dexamethasone, can initiate the differentiation process, as can the morphogenic bone proteins. Other factors added to the matrix of mesenchymal stem cells can increase cartilage oligomeric matrix protein and collagen type II. Recently, dermal fibroblasts have been studied for their developmental potential when cultured on the cartilage matrix proteoglycan, aggrecan.[10] Pretreatment with insulin-like growth factor 1 induced the fibroblasts to differentiate in culture on aggrecan. After only 24 hours in culture, early aggregates that resembled condensate of mesenchymal stem cells were identified. These cells then were seen to express collagen type II messenger RNA. Because adult human fibroblasts are far easier to obtain than mesenchymal stem cells, this research is promising.

Vascularized pedicle or free flaps incorporating a bone component have been generally successful in head and neck reconstruction. However, any technique that will enhance the performance of bone allografts or even free autografts is worth investigating. Recently, a study has indicated that the transplantation of a tissue-engineered periosteum provided progenitor cells that markedly increased osteogenesis, primarily through differentiation and proliferation of these donor progenitor cells.[11] Such studies may provide clinical assistance in the form of autologously prepared periosteum when the reconstruction bone graft does not possess this important source of driver osteogenesis cells.

Summary

Head and neck reconstruction often requires multiple tissue replacement—skin, muscle, bone, and cartilage. In some cases, for medical or tissue loss reasons, it is not possible to utilize large autografts from the patient. Laboratory-engineered tissue has been on a refinement path for over 10 years now, with some definite clinical applications in production. New horizons for tissue engineering include the induction of cells to produce a nonnative tissue, fabrication of new "designer" scaffolds that allow for more precise reproduction of the natural state of the dermis and matrix, and the application of a wide variety of chemical factors that can enhance or stimulate formation of the precise tissue required (i.e., perichondrium or periosteum). The future for this technology is exciting, and advancements are likely to provide the facial plastic and reconstructive surgeon with a wider range of options than ever before.

References

1. Black AF, Bouez C, Perrier E, Schlotmann K, Chapuis F, Damour O. Optimization and characterization of an engineered human skin equivalent. Tissue Eng 2005;11:723–733
2. Erdag G, Medalie DA, Rakhorst H, Krueger GG, Morgan JR. FGF-7 expression enhances the performance of bioengineered skin. Mol Ther 2004;10:76–85
3. Llames SG, Del Rio M, Larcher F, et al. Human plasma as a dermal scaffold for the generation of a completely autologous bioengineered skin. Transplantation 2004;77:350–355
4. Schultze-Mosgau S, Lee B-K, Ries J, Amann K, Wiltfang J. In vitro cultured autologous preconfluent oral keratinocytes for experimental prefabrication of oral mucosa. Int J Oral Maxillofac Surg 2004;33:476–485
5. Sahota PS, Burn JL, Brown NJ, MacNeil S. Approaches to improve angiogenesis in tissue-engineered skin. Wound Repair Regen 2004;12:635–642
6. Tremblay P-L, Hudon V, Berthod F, Germain L, Auger FA. Inosculation of tissue-engineered capillaries with the host's vasculature in a reconstructed skin transplanted on mice. Am J Transplant 2005;5:1002–1010
7. Tonello C, Vindigni V, Zavan B, et al. In vitro reconstruction of an endothelialized skin substitute provided with a microcapillary network using biopolymer scaffolds. FASEB J 2005;19:1546–1548
8. Cronin KJ, Messina A, Knight KR, et al. New murine model of spontaneous autologous tissue engineering, combining an arteriovenous pedicle with matrix materials. Plast Reconstr Surg 2004;113:260–269
9. Kamil SH, Eavey RD, Vacanti MP, Vacanti CA, Hartnick CJ. Tissue-engineered cartilage as a graft source for laryngotracheal reconstruction—a pig model. Arch Otolaryngol Head Neck Surg 2004;130:1048–1051
10. French MM, Rose S, Canseco J, Athanasiou KA. Chondrogenic differentiation of adult dermal fibroblasts. Ann Biomed Eng 2004;32:50–56
11. Zhang X, Xie C, Lin ASP, et al. Periosteal progenitor cell fate in segmental cortical bone graft transplantations: implications for functional tissue engineering. J Bone Miner Res 2005;20:2124–2137

9 Tissue Adhesives

Kristin K. Egan, David W. Kim, and Dean M. Toriumi

Since the introduction of the first fibrin sealant in the 1940s, the use of surgical tissue adhesives has expanded significantly. For surgeons, the advantages have been clear: increased strength to tissue coaptation, reduced operative time, and fewer complications. Patients benefit from better tissue immobilization and decreased trauma, which translates into enhanced healing and cosmesis. As the science and technology of these materials advance, so too have the potential applications in surgery. These tools are especially valuable in surgery of the face, where a rich vascular supply underlies the most cosmetically sensitive part of the body. With the increasing trend toward minimally invasive strategies in facial plastic surgery, the use of tissue adhesives provides numerous benefits (**Table 9.1**).

Characteristics and Uses of Tissue Adhesives

Tissue adhesives have undergone significant advances in the last 5 years. Fibrin tissue adhesives were first described in 1944 and primarily used for skin grafts. A commercial fibrin sealant was first produced in 1978 from human plasma and is a two-component system. It has proven effective in hemostasis, sealing of tissues, and wound healing. Subsequently, their use expanded into Mohs reconstruction and rhytidectomy. Cyanoacrylates were first synthesized in 1949 but not used in surgical areas for 10 years. They were first developed for the rapid closure and repair of lacerations and provoked severe foreign body reactions. They were chemically engineered to decrease the host reaction, and their use has expanded into surgery as an alternative to traditional suture closure.

The ideal adhesive should possess five cardinal characteristics.[1] First, the material must be safe for use in the patient population with respect to allergic response, tissue fibrosis, and the possibility of disease transmission. Second, the adhesive must be able to eliminate potential spaces to decrease tissue swelling and seroma formation. Third, the material should be easy to use. This includes the work required for preparation of the material as well as ease of handling by the surgeon on the operating field. Fourth, the material should be cost effective. And finally, the clinical benefit of the material should justify its cost and use. The regulations set forth by the Food and Drug Administration (FDA) and the approval by this committee should be acknowledged, especially when off-label use is contemplated.

Numerous tissue adhesives are now available for surgical use. The two main applications are for tissue sealing/gluing and tissue hemostasis, but many adhesives possess both sealing and hemostatic qualities. Because of these properties, these agents are well suited to enhance the outcomes of wound closure during surgery. In particular, adhesives reduce tissue trauma and therefore enhance healing from surgical incisions. They minimize suturing needed to close a wound, and thereby reduce or circumvent violation of the skin. The ability of tissue adhesives to seal off vessels and lymphatics decreases surgical complications. Finally, these adhesives have the potential to carry medications and growth factors, which may further enhance the wound healing process and result in better scar cosmesis. Two main types of tissue adhesives are used in surgery: fibrin-based adhesives and cyanoacrylates. Each is discussed in the next sections.

Table 9.1 Common Tissue Adhesives

Name	Type	Main Application	Comments	Possible Applications in FPRS
TISSEEL (Baxter, Deerfield, IL)	Fibrin	Hemostatic/glue	Deep tissue use	Facelift, cutaneous reconstruction, brow and forehead lift, rhinoplasty
Platelet rich plasma	Fibrin	Hemostatic	Deep tissue use	Facelift, cutaneous reconstruction, brow and forehead lift, rhinoplasty
Dermabond (Ethicon, Inc., Somerville, NJ)	Cyanoacrylate	Glue	Superficial tissue use	Most cutaneous closure
BioGlue (CryoLife, Inc., Kennesaw, GA)	Bovine serum albumin and glutaraldehyde	Glue	Vascular use Deep tissue use	Brow and forehead lift

Abbreviations: FPRS, facial plastic and reconstructive surgery.

Fibrin Tissue Adhesives

Fibrin sealant was the first major tissue adhesive to be approved by the FDA and therefore has the longest history of safe and effective use in the United States. It consists of two major components: fibrinogen and thrombin, which in the presence of small amounts of factor XIII and calcium react to form polymerized fibrin, the final form of this biological tissue adhesive. The commercially available product is derived from pooled human plasma from screened human donors. It contains bovine aprotinin as a stabilizer and antifibrinolytic agent, which acts to reduce its biological degradation. Calcium acts as a catalyst in the reaction between the included fibrinogen and thrombin. Presently, heat pasteurization and ultrafiltration are utilized in the prevention of disease transmission.[2]

The strength of a fibrin tissue adhesive is determined by the fibrinogen concentration present in the mixture. The bonding strength of the adhesive is directly proportional to increasing concentrations of fibrinogen. The concentration of thrombin present in the mixture determines the rate at which the fibrin clot polymerizes. The specific use dictated by the surgeon should determine which concentration of thrombin is used. Rapid polymerization is typically used when the fibrin tissue adhesive is meant to act predominantly as a hemostatic agent. If the surgeon needs time to manipulate tissues (e.g., to position a skin flap), then a slower-polymerizing adhesive mixture is preferred.

The material must be refrigerated and requires approximately 20 minutes of preparation and should be used within 4 hours for maximal effectiveness. Fibrin tissue sealant can be delivered into the wound through various devices. A dual-syringe device allows its delivery through a needle-tipped applicator to specific suture lines (**Fig. 9.1**). A gas-driven spray device can apply small droplets of highly mixed material across broad surface areas, which rapidly polymerizes to a firm material (**Fig. 9.1**). Endoscopic delivery systems are also available (**Fig. 9.1**). The polymerization of the fibrinogen and thrombin are maximized by thorough mixing of the components. A spray delivery method results in a highly effective mixing and allows the surgeon to deliver less volume of the adhesive to the surgical field. Studies have shown that a thin layer of fibrin tissue adhesive results in the greatest degree of component mixing and ultimately the strongest adhesive.[3] This also allows the surgeon to use less volume of adhesive with a highly effective result (**Fig. 9.1**). A thick layer of fibrin adhesive may act as a barrier to healing and slow revascularization.

Clinical Uses

Fibrin tissue adhesives can significantly reduce the development of postoperative swelling and ecchymosis. In any procedure in which a large tissue flap must be elevated, such as facelifts and brow and forehead lifts, these adhesives are ideally suited to promote fixation and reduce bleeding.

In endoscopic brow lifting, fibrin adhesives have the added benefit of aiding in suspension of the flap. Typically, a malleable applicator tip is used to deliver the material for precise fixation of the brows. About 2 mL of the homologous fibrin tissue adhesive is applied along the orbital rim and in the midline surrounding the lysed corrugator and procerus musculature.[4] The flap is manually positioned and held in place while the adhesive polymerizes. In the lateral compartments, the adhesive may be used as an additional form of fixation to the fixation sutures. In this method, the lateral fixation sutures may be placed but are not tied until the adhesive has polymerized with the flap manually positioned at the desired level. Pressure applied to the glabellar region for 5 to 10 minutes after application will help the adhesive to polymerize and decrease postoperative bruising and edema (**Fig. 9.2**).

The use of fibrin tissue adhesive in facelift surgery can assist in skin flap positioning. In this case, a lower concentration of thrombin should be utilized with a spray applicator. The use of a spray applicator for the skin flaps ensures a thin application, which minimizes the barrier to wound healing and revascularization. The fixation sutures are again placed but not tied until the fibrin spray is applied and has polymerized. Pressure on the flap after the fixation sutures and fibrin spray have been placed helps to ensure that an effective bond between the fibrin clot and the tissues has been created. Reconstructive skin flaps after Mohs excision also provides an excellent opportunity to use fibrin tissue adhesive. The skin flaps are trimmed and positioned with fixation sutures placed and the fibrin is sprayed in a thin layer. The fixation sutures are tied and pressure is applied. The use of fibrin tissue adhesives may allow for the elimination of drains in these operations[4] (**Fig. 9.3**).

Platelet-Rich Plasma: A Fibrin-Based Adhesive

This tissue adhesive consists of a gel with a high concentration of platelets and a native concentration of fibrinogen harvested by centrifugal separation of autologous whole blood. This mixture is then combined with bovine thrombin, which creates a gel-like consistency. It can be made from ~70 mL of a patient's own whole blood and is especially attractive for those patients concerned about the use of homologous fibrin tissue adhesive.

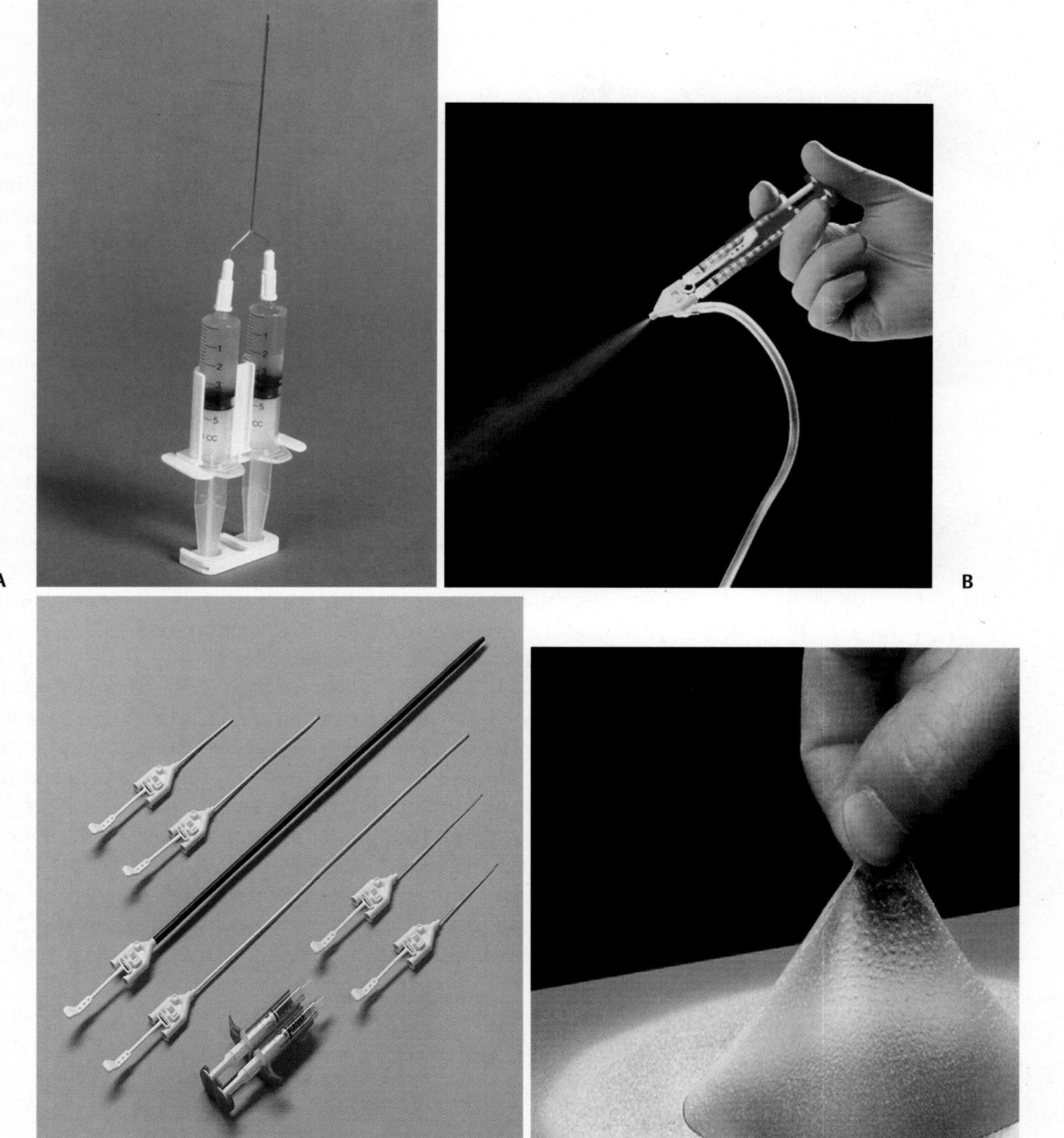

Fig. 9.1 **(A)** Dual syringe device for precise fibrin sealant delivery. **(B)** Gas driven spray device for broad delivery of fibrin sealant. **(C)** Endoscopic delivery system. **(D)** Even a thin layer of fibrin sealant can form a strong bond. (Photos courtesy of Baxter Medical.)

However, the concentration of fibrinogen in platelet-rich plasma is much lower than that in homologous fibrin tissue adhesive, resulting in a less effective adhesive. Platelet-rich plasma has a lower tensile strength and less hemostatic effect. Current literature has suggested that it may have a greater use in the immunocompromised patient population. It has the theoretical ability to improve healing in wounds that are chronic, nonhealing, or previously irradiated.

Clinical Uses

The uses of platelet-rich plasma overlap with those of fibrin tissue adhesive due to the similarity of their components. The endoscopic brow lift and facelift procedures can both be performed with the use of platelet-rich plasma in patients concerned about the transmission of infectious diseases. However, there are discussions of a risk of coagulopathy in patients who develop antibodies

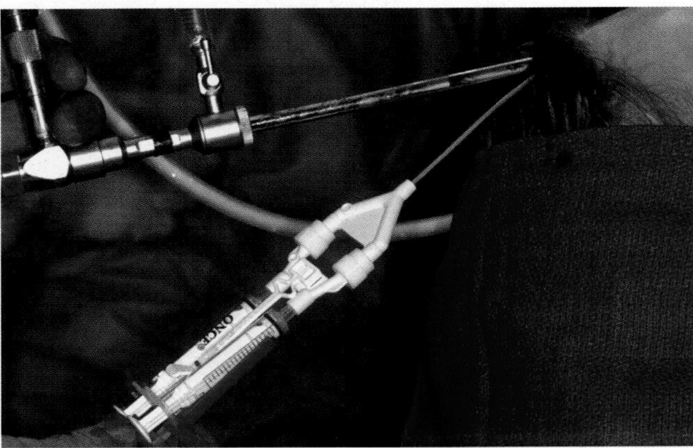

Fig. 9.2 Dual syringe system used for delivery of fibrin sealant during endoscopic brow-lift surgery.

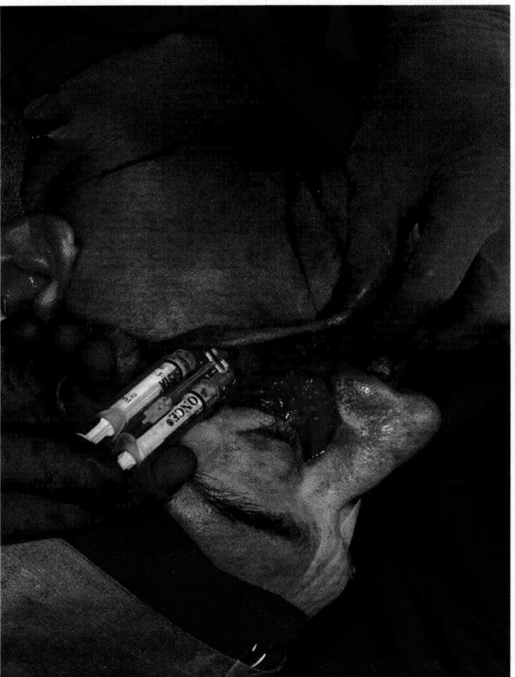

Fig. 9.3 Fibrin sealant used for flap fixation in cutaneous reconstruction following Mohs surgery for skin cancer.

to factor V contaminants in the bovine thrombin, especially if the patient has had previous uses of this adhesive.[5] The delivery method in the use of this adhesive is also important. Spray applicators are again better able to deliver a thin layer and provide better mixing.

Cyanoacrylate Tissue Adhesives

Butyl-cyanoacrylate derivatives were the first tissue adhesives to be used for the closure of skin. The material gained popularity because it provided a more rapid, less invasive method of wound closure. The early cyanoacrylate adhesives were short-chained derivatives with relatively rapid breakdown. This led to more rapid slough of the material, placing wounds at risk of early dehiscence. In addition, it was evident that the breakdown products of cyanoacrylate, formaldehyde, and cyanoacetate could create a histotoxic reaction if they infiltrated beneath the skin surface. The material was therefore modified to reduce these problems. Octyl-cyanoacrylates were subsequently developed. This derivative has a longer side chain and therefore forms a more flexible and stronger bond. The three-dimensional breaking strength of 2-octyl cyanoacrylate is four times that of butyl-2-cyanoacrylate.[6] The FDA approved derivative is 2-octyl cyanoacrylate or Dermabond (Ethicon, Inc., Somerville, NJ). This adhesive polymerizes in the presence of moisture and forms a bond much stronger than those possible with fibrin tissue adhesives. The longer chain on the cyanoacrylate derivative that octyl-2-cyanoacylate possesses allows a slower rate of degradation and theoretically a lower rate of tissue inflammatory response secondary to toxic by-products below the epidermal level.[7] The applicator for octyl-2-cyanoacrylate contains an initiator in the tip that accelerates the process of polymerization. Octyl-2-cyanoacrylate also contains a plasticizer in its formulation that allows conformation to the site of application and freedom of movement even in areas of maximum tension. However, the use of octyl-2-cyanoacrylate over joints and mobile surfaces has not been carefully studied (**Fig. 9.4**).

Toriumi and associates compared wound closure at 5 to 7 days and at 90 days using the modified Hollander wound evaluation scale between those wounds closed

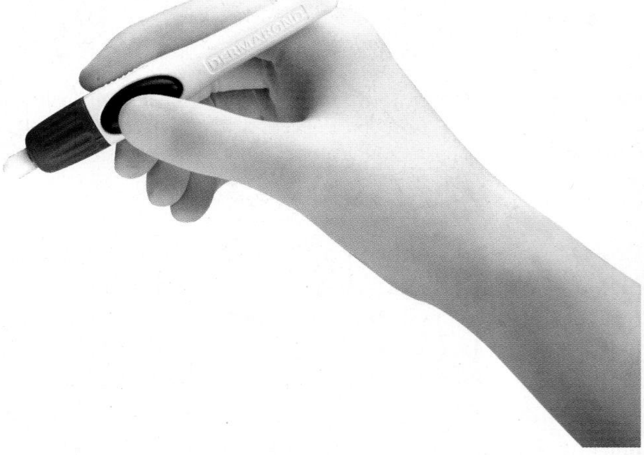

Fig. 9.4 Dermabond "hand-pen" (Ethicon, Inc., Somerville, NJ) allows precise application of octyl-2-cyanoacrylate. (Photo courtesy of Ethicon.)

with traditional suture materials and those using octyl-2-cyanoacrylate. The results showed essentially equivalent outcomes for sutures and octyl-2-cyanoacrylate across all time periods.[8] The costs associated with octyl-2-cyanoacrylate are much higher than traditional suturing material, but those costs must be weighed against the decreased number of postoperative visits for suture removal and the decreased risk of secondary tissue infection and inflammation requiring further treatment.

Clinical Uses

Cyanoacrylate tissue adhesives are designed solely for superficial skin closure. Because these adhesives circumvent the need for skin sutures, they are particularly advantageous for traumatic injuries, particularly in children, and in the closure of long incisions, which would otherwise be very time consuming. The cyanoacrylate adhesives have been used successfully for wound closure in most facial incisions, including facelift incisions, blepharoplasty incisions, closure of facial defects, and scar revisions (**Fig. 9.5**).

Reliance on a surface adhesive for skin closure places an increased emphasis on the importance of the orientation of the subcutaneous sutures. Traditionally, surface sutures are placed in a manner to create eversion of the skin edges to counteract forces of inward scar contracture and thus maximize cosmetic appearance. With adhesive skin closure, the deeper subcutaneous sutures must bear the responsibility of the creation of wound edge eversion. If the adhesive is used to close the skin without proper suture closure of the deeper layers, the skin edges may become inverted secondary to scar contracture in the postoperative period. The elimination of subcutaneous dead space and the eversion of skin edges may be achieved with proper placement of the deep layer of subcutaneous sutures. In addition, the use of fine forceps to position the skin edges in an everted orientation and the placement of the surface adhesive in small volumes precisely along the incision line can further increase eversion.

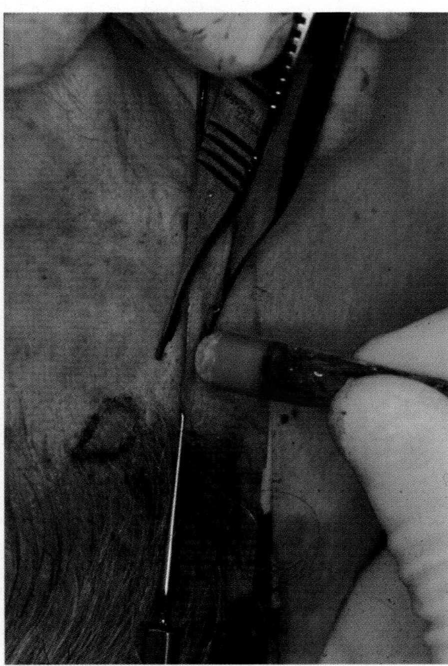

Fig. 9.5 Deep subcutaneous closure of the wound with traditional suture technique must be completed prior to application of octyl-2-cyanoacrylate for superficial skin closure. The skin edges should be placed into light eversion with fine instruments such as forceps while the adhesive is applied.

The operative time required for wound closure procedure can also be effectively decreased through the use of octyl-2-cyanoacylate. Complex scar revisions, such as Z-plasties, geometric broken line closures, or W-plasties can require a large time investment on the part of the surgeon to place numerous sutures. Octyl-2-cyanoacylate can be applied quickly and with a time limit of two to three minutes between layered applications can substantially decrease operative time and result in cosmetically acceptable results **(Fig. 9.6)**.

The application of multiple layers is advised to achieve a strong, uniform bond. Because application of this material creates a dose-related exothermic reaction, placement of more numerous thin layers will result in less discomfort than placement of fewer thick layers. It is advisable to wait 2 to 3 minutes between applications of the octyl-2-cyanoacrylate to allow previous layers to fully polymerize. It is critical to apply the adhesive only onto and above the skin surface with no penetration into the deeper tissue to prevent tissue toxicity.

Some have advocated the use of interspersing 6–0 fast-absorbing catgut vertical mattress sutures to further evert the skin edges prior to placement of the octyl-2-cyanoacrylate. These sutures will peel off with the surface adhesive naturally over time. This technique may be useful in those areas in which precise cutaneous apposition is most critical, such as the preauricular portion of the facelift incision.

In use around the eye, the patient should be positioned in a manner so that any excessive adhesive will tend to drip away from the eye. The use of small aliquots and multiple thin layers will also prevent eye exposure. If octyl-2-cyanoacrylate does contact the eye during the procedure, antibiotic ophthalmic ointment should be applied immediately. The octyl-2-cyanoacrylate will peel off over time without damage to the cornea. A fine applicator tip and a more viscous formulation that enhances control and site-specific application of the product are now available for periorbital use. The heat produced with application is slightly higher in this more viscous form,

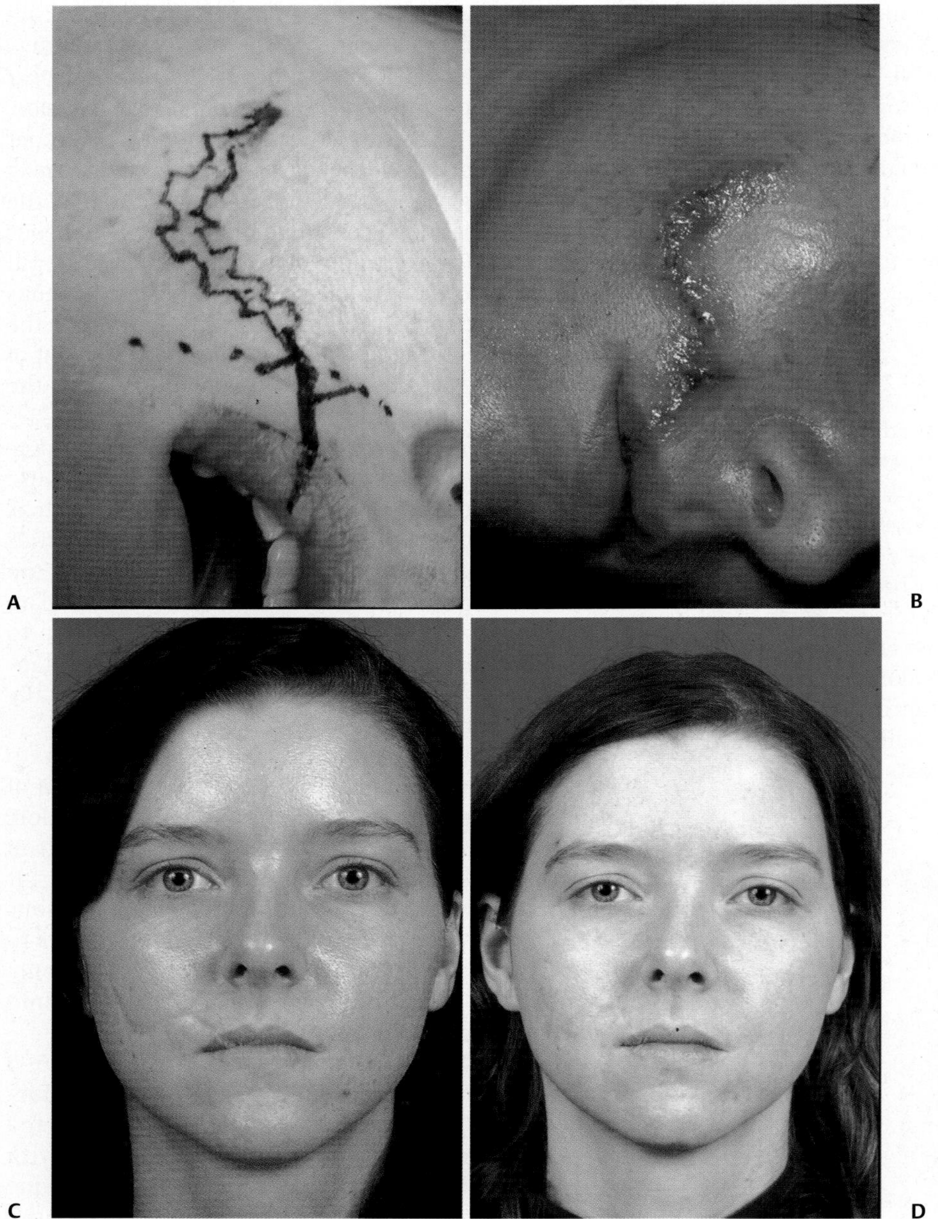

Fig. 9.6 **(A)** Geometric broken line closure design for depressed, wide scar. **(B)** Scar has been excised, deep subcutaneous layer closed with absorbable sutures, and skin layer has been closed with octyl-2-cyanoacrylate. **(C)** Preoperative photo. **(D)** Twelve-month postoperative photo.

further necessitating the application of thin layers. For use near the hairline, the application of petroleum ointment will minimize the adherence of the polymer to the hair follicles.

The use of octyl-2-cyanoacrylate is especially advantageous in pediatric patients in whom the process of suture placement and removal can be painful and difficult. Proper wound eversion with subcutaneous sutures becomes important in these patient populations. In large defects, a 5–0 Prolene running intradermal suture (Ethicon, Inc., Somerville, NJ) can be used temporarily to approximate the skin edges and removed after the octyl-2-cyanoacrylate has polymerized.[4]

BioGlue

BioGlue (CryoLife, Inc., Kennesaw, GA), which is composed of purified bovine serum albumin and glutaraldehyde, is a tissue adhesive primarily in use for vascular anastomoses.

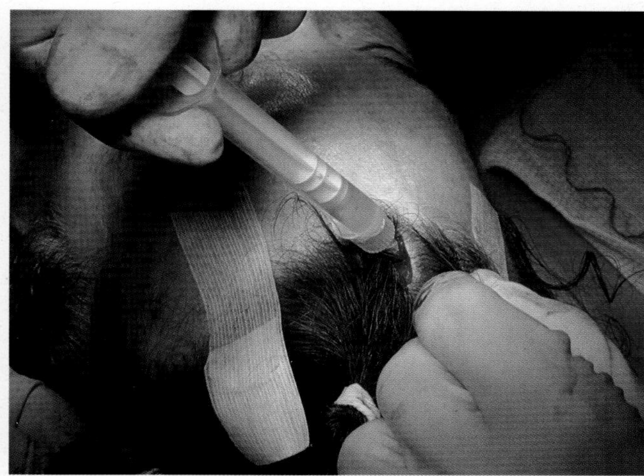

Fig. 9.7 Example of BioGlue (CryoLife, Inc., Kennesaw, GA) placement for fixation during endoscopic brow lift. (Photos courtesy of Dr. Corey Maas).

The delivery device is designed to mix the solution upon dispension and cross-linking can begin. It has been FDA approved for use as an adjunct in open repair of large vessels such as the aorta and femoral and carotid arteries. Recently, this material has been used with success as an adhesive for fixation of forehead flaps in endoscopic brow lifting (**Fig. 9.7**).

Summary

The use of tissue adhesives in the setting of facial plastic surgery can provide many benefits for both the surgeon and the patient. The fixation of tissue and adequate hemostasis can be achieved with the use of fibrin tissue adhesives, which can lead to decreased edema and ecchymosis. For the cosmetic surgery patient, this can translate to an earlier return to full activities. The use of octyl-2-cyanoacrylate while limited to superficial skin closure can result in a shorter operative time and eliminate the need for painful postoperative suture removal in both cosmetic and pediatric patients. The varied applications of these tissue adhesives are not mutually exclusive in the same patient. Frequently, fibrin tissue adhesives are used for deeper wound approximation and skin flaps while the superficial skin incisions can be successfully closed using octyl-2-cyanoacrylate.

The trend in facial plastic surgery is toward minimally invasive and outpatient procedures with less morbidity and a faster recovery. Tissue adhesives are a natural component of this equation, lending themselves easily to endoscopic procedures and reducing the postoperative sequelae. Tissue sealants enhance the results of minimally invasive surgery by reducing the rate of complications such as hematoma, seroma, bruising, and swelling. They may also facilitate the elimination of postoperative drains from many procedures. Fibrin tissue adhesives are applied under the skin but over the soft tissues, and a spray applicator can facilitate their application. The applicator ensures that less glue is wasted, and the fine mist delivers the glue evenly to avoid clumping, which may impede healing and neovascularization. Octyl-2-cyanoacrylate serves to glue wound margins in a shorter time period than is possible with traditional suturing techniques. The cost-effectiveness of this material is apparent in the shorter operative times required for long wounds. It also avoids the necessity for postoperative suture removal, which is important in both the cosmetic and pediatric populations.

The contemporary surgeon must be aware of new developments on the surgical horizon to cater to patient requests for rapid and less painful recovery and also to maximize the cost-effectiveness of the operation. The use of tissue adhesives can have a positive impact for both the surgeon and the patient and it is imperative that their use be contemplated in appropriate surgical situations.

References

1. Spotnitz WD. History of tissue adhesives. In: Sierra D, Saltz R, eds. Surgical Adhesives and Sealants, Current Technology and Applications. Lancaster, PA: Technomic Publishing; 1996:3–8
2. Radosevich M, Goubran HA, Burnouf T. Fibrin sealant: scientific rationale, production methods, properties, and current clinical use. Vox Sang 1997;72:133–143
3. O'Grady KM, Agrawal A, Bhattacharyya TK, Shah A, Toriumi DM. An evaluation of fibrin tissue adhesive concentration and application thickness on skin graft survival. Laryngoscope 2000;110:1931–1935
4. Toriumi DM, O'Grady KM. Use of surgical tissue adhesives in facial plastic surgery. In: Saltz, R, Toriumi DM, eds. Tissue Glues in Cosmetic Surgery. St. Louis, MO: Quality Medical Publishing; 2004:88–109
5. Nichols W. Adverse antibody-mediated reactions to topical bovine thrombin and fibrin glue. Symposium on Fibrin Sealant: Characteristics and Clinical Use. Bethesda, Uniformed Services University of the Health Sciences; 1994:5–10
6. Perry LC. An Evaluation of Acute Incisional Strength with Traumaseal Surgical Tissue Adhesive Wound Closure. Leonia, NJ: Dimensional Analysis Systems; 1995
7. Leonard F, Kulkarni RK, Brandes G, et al. Synthesis and degradation of poly (alkyl alpha-cyanoacrylates). J Appl Polym Sci 1966;10:259
8. Toriumi DM, O'Grady K, Desai D, Bagal A. Use of octyl-2-cyanoacrylate for skin closure in facial plastic surgery. Plast Reconstr Surg 1998; 102:2209–2219

10 Lasers in Facial Plastic Surgery

W. Russell Ries and Maria Wittkopf

Around the turn of the century, Einstein, in a publication titled "The Quantum Theory of Radiation," theorized the processes that must take place for a laser to radiate energy.[1] The first laser was built in 1960 by Maiman.[2] Since then, there has been an explosion of laser technology development leading to a great diversity of lasers that encompasses the entire electromagnetic spectrum. Increasingly, lasers are being coupled to other technologies, including imaging systems, robotics, and computers, to improve delivery of the laser to its target. Through the marriage of the fields of physics and bioengineering, medical lasers have become an important part of the armamentarium of surgeons in the treatment of disease. Initially, these lasers were cumbersome to work with, and their use required surgeons who had been specially trained in the physics of lasers. In the past 15 years, medical laser design has evolved toward ease of use, and many surgeons are taught the fundamentals of laser physics during residency or through continuing medical education programs.

This chapter discusses laser biophysics, laser–tissue interactions, lasers currently used in facial plastic and reconstructive surgery, general laser safety precautions, and future considerations in the field of cutaneous laser surgery.

Laser Biophysics

Lasers emit light energy that travels in a waveform, which is also true with any ordinary light (**Fig. 10.1**). The wavelength is the distance between two successive peaks of a wave. The amplitude is the height of the peak and is related to the intensity of the light. Frequency, or the period of the light wave, is the amount of time required for one full wave cycle. To understand how a laser functions, it is important to review quantum mechanics. The term *laser* is an acronym that stands for *l*ight *a*mplification by *s*timulated *e*mission of *r*adiation. If a photon, a unit of light energy, strikes an atom, it will raise one of its electrons to a higher energy level. The atom in this excited state is unstable and will re-emit a photon as the electron drops to its original lower energy level. This is a process known as spontaneous emission (**Fig. 10.2A**). If an atom is in a high-energy state and is struck by another photon, it will emit two photons that have the same wavelength, direction, and phase when the electrons revert to lower energy levels. This process is known as stimulated emission of radiation and is the underlying principle of laser physics (**Fig. 10.2B**).

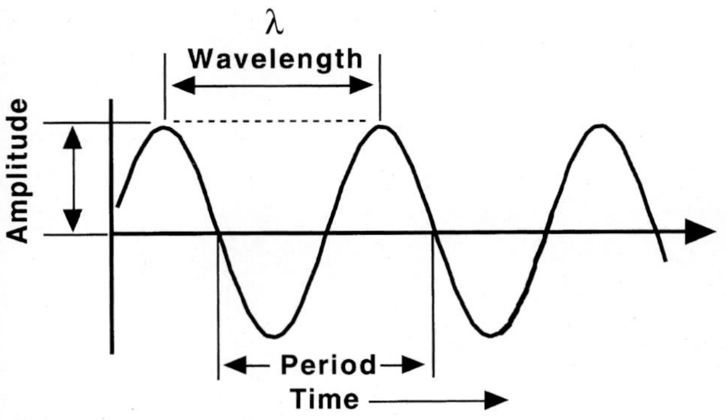

Fig. 10.1 Wave properties of light.

Regardless of type, all lasers contain four main components: an excitation mechanism or power source, a laser medium, an optical cavity or resonator, and a delivery system (**Fig. 10.3**). Most clinical lasers used in facial plastic surgery use an electrical excitation mechanism. Some lasers (e.g., flashlamp-excited dye laser) use light as an excitation mechanism. Others may use high-energy radio frequency waves, and still others may use chemical reactions to provide the energy for excitation. The excitation mechanism pumps energy into the resonating chamber that contains a laser medium, which may be a solid, liquid, gas, or semiconductive material. The energy dumped into the resonating chamber elevates electrons of the laser medium atoms to a higher energy state. When half the atoms in the resonating chamber have reached this highly excited state, a population inversion has occurred. Spontaneous emission occurs with photons radiating in all directions, with some striking atoms in an already excited state, leading to stimulated emission of paired photons. Amplification of stimulated emission takes place as the photons that travel along the axis between the mirrors are preferentially reflected back and forth between the mirrors. This leads to further stimulation as these photons strike other excited atoms. One mirror is 100% reflective and the other is partially transmissive, allowing radiant energy to escape from the resonating chamber. This energy is transmitted to the intended tissues by a delivery system. Most lasers have a fiberoptic delivery system. A notable exception is the carbon dioxide (CO_2) laser, which has mirrors in an articulated arm system. Waveguides for use with the CO_2 laser are available, but they limit the spot size and power output.

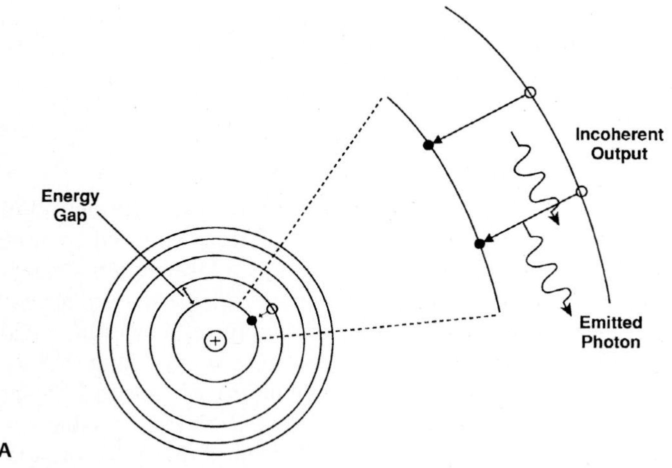

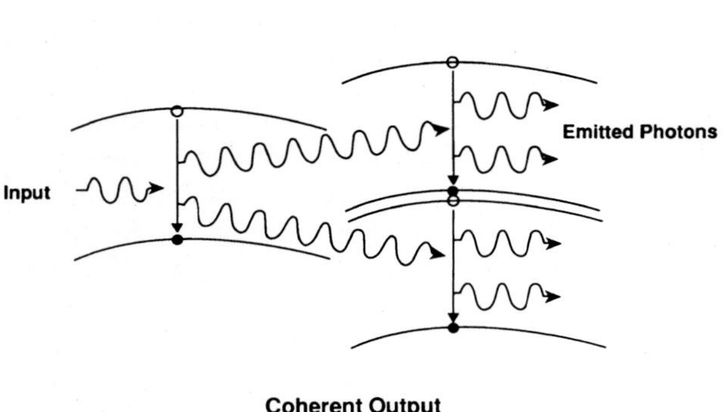

Fig. 10.2 **(A)** Spontaneous emission. **(B)** Stimulated emission.

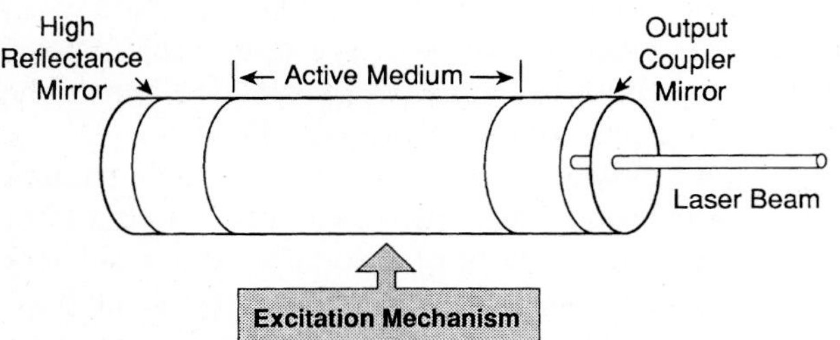

Fig. 10.3 Laser components.

Laser light, when compared with ordinary light, is more organized and intense in its qualities. Because the lasing medium is one kind of molecule or atom, the photons emitted by the stimulated emission are of one wavelength, thus creating the quality of monochromaticity. Ordinary light diverges widely when emitted from a source. Laser light is collimated; thus it diverges little as it travels, giving laser energy its persistent intensity over long distances. Not only do photons of laser light move in the same direction, but they are also in the same temporal and spatial phase. This is called coherence. These properties of monochromaticity, collimation, and coherence differentiate laser light energy from the disorganized energy of ordinary light (**Fig. 10.4**).

Laser–Tissue Interaction

There is a spectrum of effects that a laser can have on biological tissue, from modulation of biological function to vaporization (**Fig. 10.5**). Most of the laser–tissue interactions currently clinically available use the thermal effects of lasers to coagulate or vaporize. In the future, lasers may be used in a nonthermal capacity as probes to control cellular function without cytotoxic side effects.

The effect that a particular laser has on a specific tissue depends on the following three factors: tissue absorption, laser wavelength, and laser energy density.

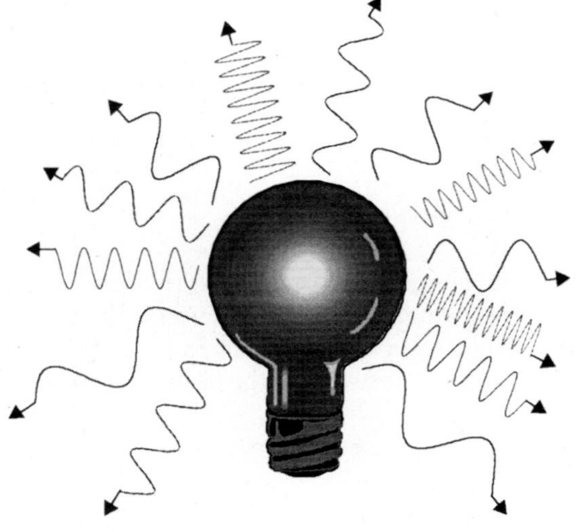

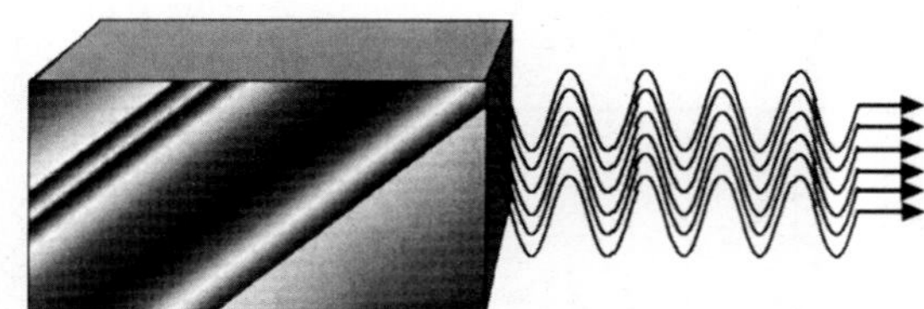

Fig. 10.4 **(A)** Ordinary light. **(B)** Characteristics of laser light: collimated, monochromatic, coherent.

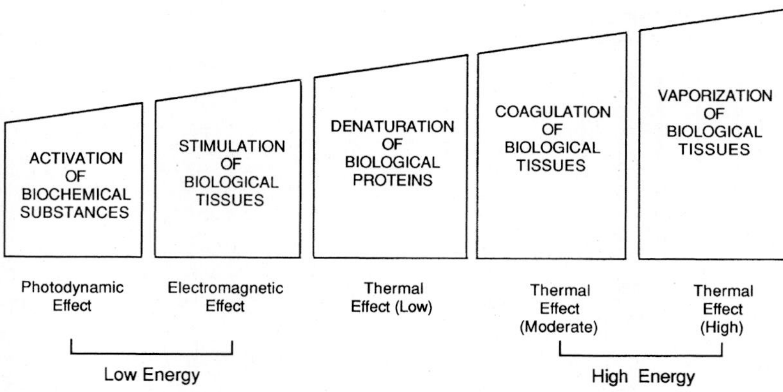

Fig. 10.5 Spectrum of biological laser effects.

As a laser beam impacts tissue, its energy may be absorbed, reflected, transmitted, or scattered (**Fig. 10.6**). In any particular laser–tissue interaction, all four processes occur in varying degrees, with absorption being the most important. The extent of absorption depends on the chromophore content of a tissue. Chromophores are substances that absorb a particular wavelength efficiently. For example, CO_2 laser energy is absorbed by soft tissues of the body. This is due to the CO_2 laser wavelength being well absorbed by water molecules, which make up 80% of soft tissues. In contrast, the CO_2 laser is minimally absorbed by bone. This is due to the low water content of osseous tissue. Initially, as a tissue absorbs laser energy, its molecules begin to vibrate. Absorption of additional energy causes protein denaturation, coagulation, and, finally, vaporization.

When tissue reflects laser energy, the tissue is unaffected because energy is deflected at the surface. Similarly, if laser energy is transmitted through overlying tissues to a deeper layer, the intervening tissue is unaffected. If a laser beam is scattered within tissue, the energy is not absorbed at the surface but is dispersed in deeper layers in a random fashion.

The third factor affecting laser–tissue interaction is energy density. Energy density is equal to the power density of the incident beam multiplied by the time for which the tissue is exposed. Power density is the power expressed in watts divided by the cross-sectional area of the laser beam (spot size).

$$\text{Energy density} = \text{power density} \times \text{time}$$

$$\text{Power density} = \frac{\text{Power (W)}}{\text{Cross-sectional area of laser beam (spot size)}}$$

In a laser–tissue interaction, with all other factors held constant, varying the spot size or the time of exposure can alter the tissue effects. As the spot size of a laser beam decreases, the amount of power reaching a particular volume of tissue increases. Conversely, as the spot size increases, the energy density of a laser beam decreases. To change the spot size, the delivery system can be focused, prefocused, or defocused on the tissue. With both, the prefocused and defocused beams, the spot size is larger than the focused beam, leading to less power density.

Another method of varying tissue effects is pulsing of laser energy. All pulsed modes of irradiation alternate periods of power on with periods of power off (**Fig. 10.7**). Because energy is not reaching tissue during the off periods, heat is allowed to dissipate during those intervals. If the off periods are longer than the thermal relaxation time of the targeted tissue, there is less chance of damaging the surrounding tissue by heat conduction. The thermal relaxation time is the amount of time required for an object to dissipate one half of its heat. The ratio of the on interval to the on-plus-off interval is termed duty cycle.

$$\text{Duty cycle} = \frac{\text{on}}{\text{on} + \text{off}}$$

There are a variety of pulsed modes available. Energy can be pulsed by setting the time that the laser is on (e.g., 0.1 s). The energy can be shuttered, in which case the continuous wave is blocked for specified intervals by a mechanical shutter.[3] In a superpulse mode the energy is not simply blocked but is stored within the power supply of the laser during the off interval and then released during the on interval. Thus

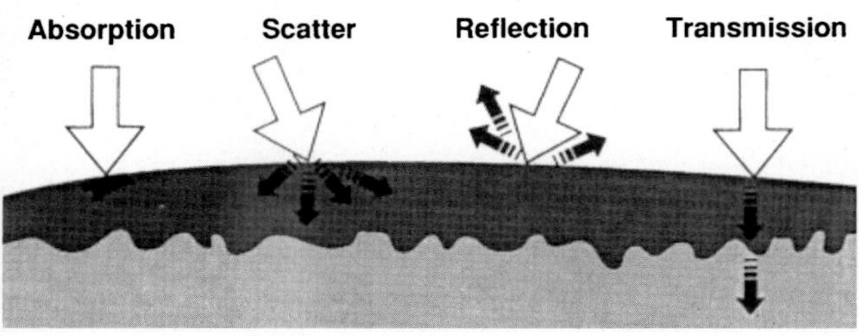

Fig. 10.6 Possible interactions of laser at tissue surface.

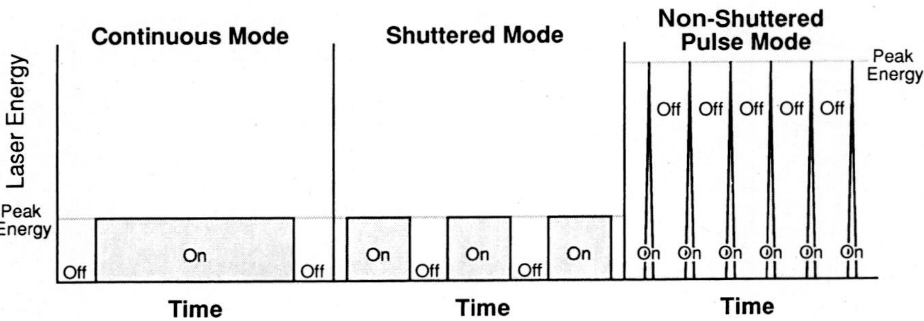

Fig. 10.7 Continuous versus pulsed mode.

the peak energy of the superpulse mode greatly exceeds that of the continuous or shuttered modes.

In a Q-switched laser, the energy is also stored during the off time, but it is stored in the laser medium. This is accomplished by a shutter mechanism in the resonating chamber between the two mirrors. The shutter in the closed position prevents lasing but allows energy to be stored on either side of the shutter. When the shutter is in the open position, the mirrors interact, causing the emission of a highly energized laser beam. The peak energy of a Q-switched laser is extremely high with a short duty cycle. A mode-locked laser is similar to a Q-switched laser in that a shutter exists between the two mirrors of the resonating chamber. The mode-locked laser opens and closes its shutter in synchrony with the time required for light to reflect between the two mirrors.

Laser Characteristics

Electrically Excited Lasers

Carbon Dioxide Laser

The CO_2 laser is the most commonly used laser in otolaryngology—head and neck surgery. Its wavelength is 10,600 nm, an invisible wavelength that is in the far-infrared (far-IR) range of electromagnetic radiation (**Fig. 10.8**). A helium-neon laser aiming beam is necessary to allow the surgeon to visualize the intended area of impact. The laser medium is CO_2 gas. The CO_2 laser wavelength is well absorbed by water molecules in tissue. Its effects are superficial because of high absorption and minimal scatter. Currently, it can be delivered only through mirrors and specialized lenses placed in an articulated arm. The articulated arm may be attached to a microscope to allow for microscopic vision and precision. The energy may also be delivered through a focusing handpiece attached to the articulated arm.

Neodymium:Yttrium-Aluminum-Garnet Laser

The neodymium:yttrium-aluminum-garnet (Nd:YAG) laser's wavelength is 1064 nm, in the near-IR spectral region. This is not visible to the human eye and requires a helium-neon aiming beam. The laser medium is neodymium:yttrium-aluminum-garnet. Most tissues in the body do not absorb this wavelength well. However, pigmented tissue absorbs it better than nonpigmented tissue. It is transmitted through the superficial layers of most tissues and is scattered into the deeper layers.

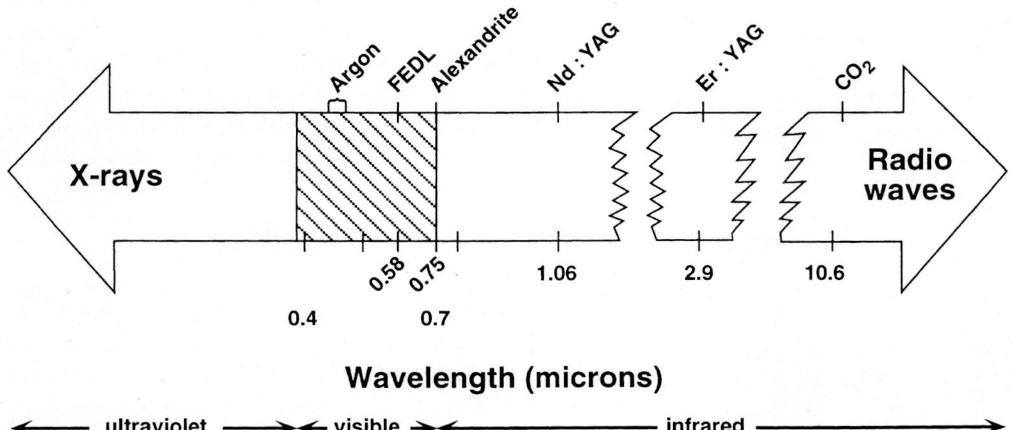

Fig. 10.8 Electromagnetic spectrum. Er:YAG, erbium:yttrium-aluminum-garnet; FEDL, flashlamp-excited dye laser; Nd:YAG, neodymium:yttrium-aluminum-garnet.

Compared with the CO_2 laser, the scatter of the Nd:YAG is considerably greater. Therefore, the depth of penetration is greater, and the Nd:YAG is well suited for coagulating deeper vessels. Experimentally, the depth of maximum coagulation is ~3 mm (coagulation temperature 60°C).[4,5] Apfelberg et al[6] report good results in treatment of perioral deep capillary and cavernous lesions with the Nd:YAG laser. Others report successful laser photocoagulation of hemangiomas, lymphangiomas, and arteriovenous malformations.[7-9] The increased depth of penetration and nonselective destruction, however, also predispose a patient to increased postoperative scarring. Clinically, this is minimized by conservative power settings, a pointillistic approach to the lesion, and avoidance of treatment in areas of thin skin. The use of the Nd:YAG in port-wine stains has been virtually replaced by the yellow-wavelength lasers. However, it is useful as an adjuvant laser in cases of nodular port-wine stains.[10]

In both fibroblast cultures and normal skin in vivo the Nd:YAG laser has been shown to suppress collagen production.[4] This suggests an advantage of this laser in the treatment of hypertrophic scars and keloids.[4] Clinically, however, the recurrence rate in keloid excision is high unless vigorous local steroid treatment is used adjunctively.[5]

Contact-Tip Nd:YAG Laser

The use of the Nd:YAG laser in the contact mode drastically alters the physics and absorption properties of the laser. The contact tip consists of a sapphire or quartz tip that attaches to the end of the laser fiber. The contact tip is directly applied to tissue and functions as a thermal scalpel to cut and coagulate simultaneously. A wide range of soft tissue surgery using the contact-tip laser has been reported. Its applications are closer to those of an electrocautery unit than to the noncontact mode of the Nd:YAG. In essence, the surgeon is no longer using the original laser wavelength to cut tissue, but rather to heat the tip. Therefore, the principles of laser–tissue interaction do not apply. The response time of the contact-tip laser is not immediate like the free fiber, and therefore there is a lag time for heating up and for cooling down. With experience, however, this laser is useful for raising cutaneous and muscular flaps.

Potassium Titanyl Phosphate Laser

The potassium titanyl phosphate (KTP) laser is an Nd:YAG laser whose frequency is doubled (wavelength halved) by passing the laser energy through the KTP crystal. This results in a green light (wavelength 532 nm) that corresponds to an absorption peak of hemoglobin. Its tissue penetration and scattering effects are intermediate between the CO_2 and the Nd:YAG lasers. The laser energy is delivered by a fiber. In the noncontact mode the laser vaporizes and coagulates. In the semicontact mode the tip of the fiber barely touches the tissue as it becomes a cutting instrument. The higher the energy setting used, the more the laser behaves like a hot knife, analogous to the CO_2 laser. Lower energy settings are used primarily to coagulate.

Argon Laser

The argon laser is a visible wavelength laser that has a range from 488 to 514 nm. Because of the makeup of the resonating chamber and the molecular structure of the lasing medium, a band of wavelengths is produced by this type of laser. A particular model may contain a filter that limits the output to a single wavelength. Similarly to the KTP laser, argon-laser energy is well absorbed by hemoglobin, and its scattering effect is intermediate between the CO_2 and the Nd:YAG lasers. The delivery system for the argon laser is a fiberoptic carrier. Because of the high absorption in hemoglobin, vascular lesions of the skin absorb argon laser energy.

Continuous Yellow Dye Laser

The continuous-wave, yellow dye laser is a visible wavelength laser that produces yellow light at 577 nm, which is well absorbed by hemoglobin. Like the flashlamp-excited dye laser discussed later, it is tunable by changing the dye within the activation chamber of the laser. An argon laser excites the dye. The delivery system for this laser is also a fiberoptic cable that may be focused to variable spot sizes. The laser light may be pulsed by mechanical shutters, or a Hexascanner handpiece can be used at the end of the fiberoptic system. The Hexascanner places the pulses of laser energy in a random pattern within a hexagonal outline. Because of its absorptive properties, the continuous-wave yellow dye laser is ideally suited for treating benign vascular lesions of the face.

Copper Vapor Laser

The copper vapor laser is a visible-wavelength laser that produces two separate wavelengths: a pulsed green wavelength at 511 nm and a pulsed yellow light at 578 nm. The laser medium is copper that is excited (vaporized) electrically. A fiberoptic system delivers the energy to a handpiece that has variable spot sizes ranging from 150 to 1,000 μm. The exposure time is variable from 0.075 seconds to continuous operation. The time between pulses is also variable from 0.1 to 0.8 seconds. The yellow light of the copper vapor laser is used in treating benign vascular lesions of the face. The green wavelength may be used to treat pigmented lesions such as freckles, nevi, and keratoses.

Diode Laser

Diodes using superconducting materials have been directly coupled to fiberoptic delivery devices resulting in laser light emission of varying wavelengths (depending on the characteristics of the materials used). The characteristic of diode lasers is their efficiency, as well as the portability of some. Diode lasers can convert incoming electrical power to light at efficiencies of 50%. This efficiency, resulting in less heat production and power input, allows compact diode lasers to be constructed without large cooling systems. The emitted light is delivered fiberoptically.

Flashlamp Excited Lasers

Flashlamp-Excited Dye Laser

The flashlamp-excited dye laser (FEDL) was the first medical laser designed specifically to treat benign, vascular cutaneous lesions. It is a visible-light laser with a wavelength of 585 nm. This wavelength closely coincides with the third absorption peak of oxyhemoglobin (577 nm), and therefore the laser energy from the FEDL is preferentially absorbed by hemoglobin. In the 577 to 595 nm range there is also less absorption by competing chromophores, such as melanin, and less scatter of the laser energy in the dermis and epidermis.

The laser medium is a rhodamine dye that is excited optically by a flashlamp, and the delivery system is a fiberoptic carrier. The handpiece of the FEDL has an interchangeable lens system that allows the use of 3, 5, 7, or 10 mm spot size. The laser is pulsed at 450 µs. This pulse width was chosen based on the thermal relaxation time of ectatic vessels found within benign vascular cutaneous lesions. However, more recent advancements in the area of the pulsed dye lasers have explored lengthening the wavelength to 600 nm for deeper tissue penetration and treatment of resistant port-wine stains. This has required the increase of the pulse duration to 1.5 msec to achieve the higher fluences required with the longer wavelengths.[11–13]

Although initially designed specifically for the treatment of vascular cutaneous lesions, the FEDL has proven useful in the treatment of scars, resulting not only in reduction of erythema within the scar but also leading to improvements in scar texture and decrease in scar height.[14]

In addition, hypertrophic scars treated with this laser have a lower rate of recurrence than those treated with the erbium:YAG (Er:YAG) and CO_2 lasers.[15]

Erbium Laser

The Er:YAG laser takes advantage of the 3000 nm band of the water absorption spectrum. Its wavelength, 2940 nm, corresponds to this peak and results in strong tissue water absorption (about 12 times that of the CO_2 laser). This laser, which is in the near-IR spectrum, is invisible and must be used with a visible aiming beam. The laser is a flashlamp-pumped laser, macropulsed with pulse width ranges from 200 to 300 µs, which themselves are composed of trains of micropulses. These lasers are used with a handpiece attached to an articulated arm. Scanners can also be incorporated into the system, allowing for more rapid and even removal of tissue.

Ruby Laser

The ruby laser is a flashlamp-pumped laser emitting light at 694 nm. This laser, located in the red region of the spectrum, is visible. It can be Q-switched to achieve short pulse widths and deep tissue penetration (greater than 1 mm). The long pulse ruby laser is used to deliver preferential heating to hair follicles for hair removal. This laser is transmitted using mirrors and an articulated arm system. It is not well absorbed by water but is strongly absorbed by melanin. Various pigments used in tattoos also absorb the 694 nm beam.

Alexandrite Laser

The alexandrite laser, a solid-state laser that can be flashlamp-pumped, has a wavelength of 755 nm. This wavelength, although in the red region of the spectrum, is not visible and thus requires an aiming beam. It is absorbed by blue and black tattoo pigments as well as by melanin but not by hemoglobin. It is a relatively compact laser and can be delivered with a flexible-light guide. This laser achieves relatively deep penetration, making it a useful tool in hair and tattoo removal. Seven and 12 mm spot sizes are available.

Filtered Flashlamp Intense Pulsed Light

Although not a laser, intense pulsed light (IPL) is currently being used to treat a variety of skin conditions, including telangiectasias and skin discolorations, as well as for hair removal and for combating the effects of photoaging. It is an intense, noncoherent, pulsed spectrum. The system utilizes crystal filters to emit light with wavelengths of 590 to 1200 nm. The pulse widths and fluences, also adjustable, do satisfy the criteria for selective photothermolysis. Based on the patient's skin type, the settings can be customized to select the wavelengths, number of pulses, duration of pulses, delay between pulses, and power delivered to best match the relative depth, size, and absorption characteristics of the intended target, and avoid causing damage to the areas that need to be preserved, thus allowing for a wide range of patients to benefit from this therapy. IPL intervention has been more useful for prevention of the effects of photoaging, and therapy often requires maintenance treatments.

Laser Applications

Vascular Lesions

The vascular lesions of the face and neck differ in cause and natural history. They do, however, share important characteristics that allow them to be selectively treated by lasers. The lasers useful in this area can inflict damage on the abnormal vessels while sparing surrounding tissue. The specific lesions discussed here include port-wine stains, telangiectasias, and hemangiomas.

Port-Wine Stains

Port-wine stains, which are more correctly termed congenital capillary vascular malformations, are benign vascular lesions that commonly involve the face and neck. Approximately 5% of port-wine stains are associated with Sturge-Weber syndrome and Klippel-Trenaunay syndrome.[16] Unlike hemangiomas, port-wine stains are usually apparent at birth. They usually appear as flat, pink-to-red lesions. As the patient ages, they often become darker in color and develop a thickness and nodularity of their surface. Hemangiomas, on the other hand, often undergo spontaneous involution. Histologically, port-wine stains are composed of large ectatic vessels located in the reticular dermis. Hemangiomas have endothelial hyperplasia in the ectatic vessels. This distinguishes them histologically from port-wine stains.[17]

Laser Selection

Some surgeons have used the CO_2 laser to treat port-wine stains.[18–20] However, to eradicate the vessels within the dermis, the overlying epidermis and a portion of the dermis must be vaporized with the CO_2 laser, and this can lead to scarring and hypopigmentation.[21] The argon laser has been used extensively for the treatment of port-wine stains because its blue-green light in the 488 to 514 nm range is absorbed by oxyhemoglobin.[22,23] A variety of treatment techniques using the argon laser have been described, but regardless of technique, hypertrophic scarring has been a complication.[24–26] Differing degrees of success in treating port-wine stains with the KTP laser[27] and the Nd:YAG laser[8] have been reported. In a study of 107 patients of Chinese descent treated with pulsed dye laser (PDL) or Nd:YAG, Ho et al reported that these patients required an average of 6.1 treatments for maximal lesional resolution.[28] Another study of 22 Chinese patients found that the Nd:YAG laser was only partially effective and requiring higher fluences for optimal results.[29]

The yellow-wavelength lasers (FEDL, copper vapor laser, continuous dye laser) have provided a breakthrough in the treatment of port-wine stains. In addition, the recently developed nonlaser IPL systems were found to be a highly effective and safe treatment for port-wine stains by one study.[30] These lasers function based on the principle of selective photothermolysis that was described by Anderson and Parrish.[31,32] This process is the selective heating of the ectatic vessel within a cutaneous lesion by preferential light absorption and heat production. To achieve ablation of a port-wine stain, the ectatic vessel must be heated to a temperature high enough to damage the endothelial lining. The yellow-wavelength lasers accomplish this by heating the blood within the vessel; the heat is conducted to the vessel wall. Simply coagulating the blood within the vessel without damaging the vessel wall allows recannulation to occur. Localizing the heat to the target vessel and sparing the surrounding tissue is attained by using the proper wavelength and by taking into account the thermal relaxation time of the tissues being treated. The wavelength of the yellow lasers is in the 577 to 585 nm range. The 577 nm wavelength precisely matches the third absorption peak of oxyhemoglobin. In comparison with other laser wavelengths such as the KTP or argon, there is a decrease in absorption by the competing chromophore melanin and less scatter in the dermis and epidermis[33] (**Fig. 10.9**). Tan et al[34] showed that the FEDL at 585 nm

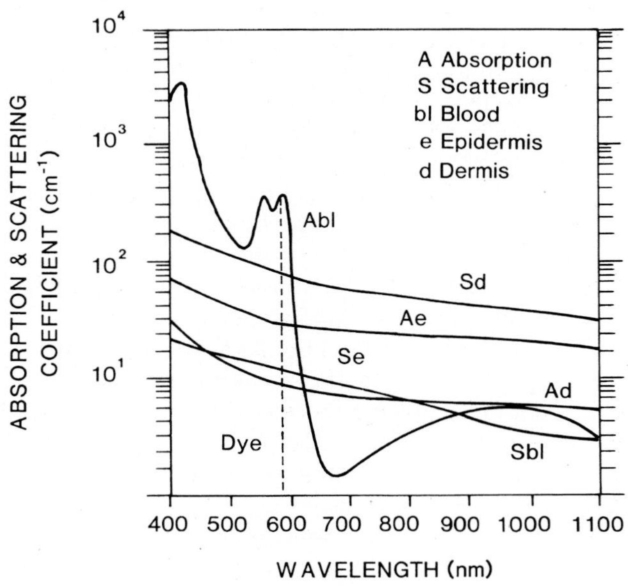

Fig. 10.9 Hemoglobin absorption curve.

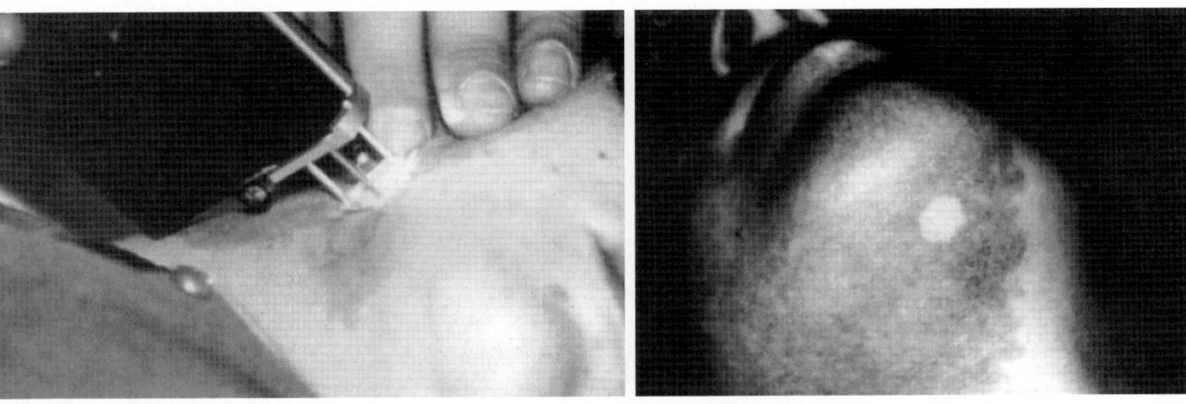

Fig. 10.10 **(A)** Application of yellow dye laser energy using Hexascanner. **(B)** Hexagonal pattern of clearing after using the Hexascanner.

causes deeper penetration of laser energy with no loss of vascular selectivity. With deeper penetration, there is faster clearing of the lesion.

The yellow-wavelength lasers use different mechanisms to obtain adequate thermal relaxation times for the ectatic vessels within port-wine stains. The FEDL has a set pulse width of 450 μs; this was calculated on the average diameter of vessels within port-wine stains. The copper vapor laser allows for variability in setting the pulse width and the time between pulses. The continuous-wave yellow dye laser may be used with a Hexascanner, a device that mechanically varies the position of laser pulses placed within a hexagonal pattern. By placing pulses in nonadjacent areas, the previously treated tissue has time to cool (**Fig. 10.10**).[35] In theory, longer wavelengths would minimize the number of treatments needed for complete resolution of vascular lesions as dermal scattering decreases allowing for greater penetration. A new generation of pulsed dye lasers with wavelengths between 585 nm and 600 nm has been introduced and shown to be clinically effective in the treatment of port-wine stains and telangiectasia.[11,36] However, the absorption of oxyhemoglobin decreases significantly at wavelengths longer than 585 nm, requiring an increase in the fluence. Increasing the energy targeted at the lesion increases the incidence of thermal damage to the surrounding normal skin. Thus skin cooling techniques such as cryogen spray cooling were developed. Cooling allows skin to be treated with more than twice the laser energy used in clinical settings without inducing thermal injury to the epidermis.[37–39] Furthermore, the effect of the cryogen cooling spray on the laser–tissue interaction were shown to be negligible.[40] Other methods of cooling, such as using a sapphire thermal surface conductor has shown beneficial in decreasing the transient temperature and related post-treatment purpura seen with the FEDL.[41]

Treatment

When the FEDL is used to treat facial port-wine stains, the first step is to determine the correct laser energy to be used for that particular patient. This is done by performing a purpuric threshold determination on normal skin of the volar aspect of the patient's forearm. Beginning at 2.0 J/cm^2 and increasing by 0.5 J/cm^2, successive pulses of laser energy are applied until the entire area of the spot is purple. The energy level at which this purpuric lesion appears is the patient's threshold level. This value is then multiplied by 1.5 or 2 times to obtain the energy density to be used for a test area. The test area is then performed by placing 10 to 20 slightly overlapping spots in a representative area of the patient's lesion. The test area is assessed at 6 weeks after treatment, at which time adjustments in the energy density are made depending on the patient's response. Any crusting or blistering is an indication that the energy density should be decreased. An irregular pattern of clearance is an indication that the energy density should be increased. After the correct energy density is determined, the lesion is treated in aesthetic units. Patients with darker skin may require increases in energy density. Lesions involving the eyelids, upper lip, mucosa, and neck often require less energy. An area may be retreated every 6 weeks. The number of treatments necessary to clear a facial port-wine stain varies according to the size, color, and location of the lesion (**Fig. 10.11**). An average of 6.5 laser treatments per lesional area was reported by Tan in a series of 35 children with port-wine stains.[42]

When using the copper vapor laser to treat port-wine stains, a test area is also performed. The 100 μm spot size is used and the power setting is varied, depending on the age of the patient and type of port-wine stain being treated. Application of the laser energy is done with the

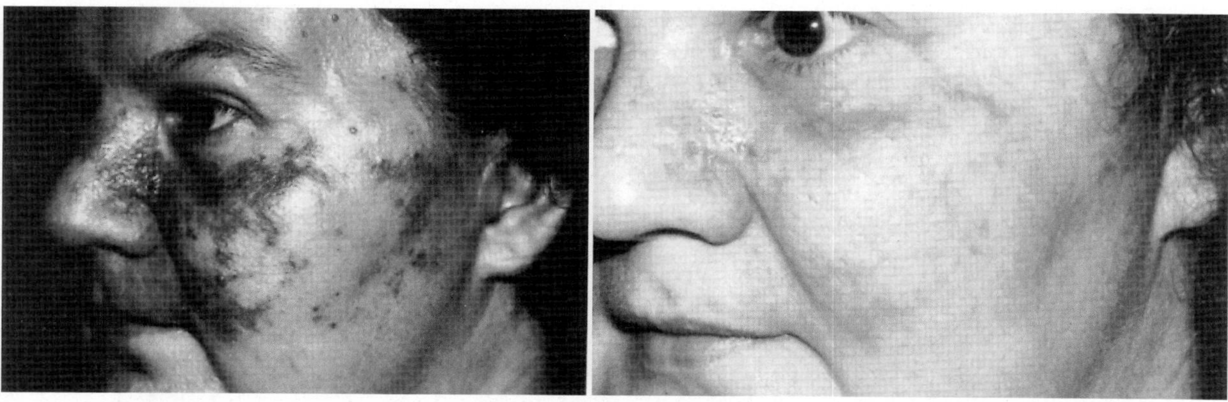

Fig. 10.11 (A) Pretreatment view of left facial port-wine stain. **(B)** Appearance after treatment using the flashlamp-excited dye laser (eight treatments).

surgeon using 6 × magnifying loupes. For lesions in which individual vessels are clearly identified under magnification, the clinical end point is where the vessel disappears. The handpiece must be moved at the correct speed, which depends on the power setting. For lesions in which no distinct vessels are identified, the area to be treated is painted by moving the laser rapidly from one area to another. The power setting determines the speed at which the laser must be moved.

The test spot is evaluated at 6 weeks and modifications in the power setting are made depending on the clearing of the test area. Treatment is begun using the correct power setting. Areas of 2 cm^2 are outlined, and the lesion within the defined area is treated.

The technique using the continuous-wave dye laser is similar to that used with the copper vapor laser. If a Hexascanner is used, then nonadjacent areas of the lesion are treated with the hexagonal pattern and the intervening areas are treated on return visits. If the Hexascanner is not available, then the lesion may be treated with a beading technique, vessel blanching with magnification, or laser painting. The beading technique is performed by placing successive pulses of laser energy in a pattern of nonoverlapping circles to cover the desired treatment area.[17,20]

The vessel blanching technique is often termed the Australian method and is similar to that described for the copper vapor laser. The individual vessels are treated under 6 × magnification.

With the paintbrush technique, laser energy is applied to the lesion until blanching is noted. This technique is often useful with thick nodular port-wine stains or for touch-ups of intervening areas where no individual vessels are readily identified. The laser must be moved rapidly over the lesion to avoid damage to the dermis and epidermis that may result in scarring or pigmentation changes.

Telangiectasias

Telangiectasias of the face are small ectatic vessels within the dermis. They occur in a variety of types, including linear, arborizing, reticular, punctate, and spider. Spider telangiectasias are often called spider nevi or spider angioma. These are acquired vascular marks that commonly appear on the face of young children. A study by Anderson[44] found spider telangiectasias in 47.5% of 1380 healthy school children. Lesions of similar appearance have been noted during pregnancy. They most frequently appear in the second trimester and enlarge until delivery. The spider telangiectasias of pregnancy are similar to the lesions found in patients with liver disease. Estrogen is thought to play a role in their formation.[45]

Telangiectatic lesions have also been noted after nasal surgery (e.g., the red nose of rhinoplasty). Other patients seem to have a hereditary predisposition to developing facial telangiectasias, and these lesions are classified as essential hereditary facial telangiectasias.

Laser Selection and Treatment

The copper vapor laser and continuous-wave yellow dye laser may be used to treat facial telangiectasias, and the treatment techniques are similar. Using a spot size that is adequate to obliterate the dilated vessel (0.1 to 0.2 mm), the vessels are traced until the dilated vessel disappears. The smallest spot size and lowest power should be used to minimize damage to the surrounding normal tissue and reduce the incidence of posttreatment scarring (**Fig. 10.12**). Spider telangiectasias require a slightly different technique; the radial vessels are first obliterated from the periphery toward the center and then the larger central vessel is treated.

When using the FEDL to treat facial telangiectasias, the 3 mm spot size is used to treat individual vessels

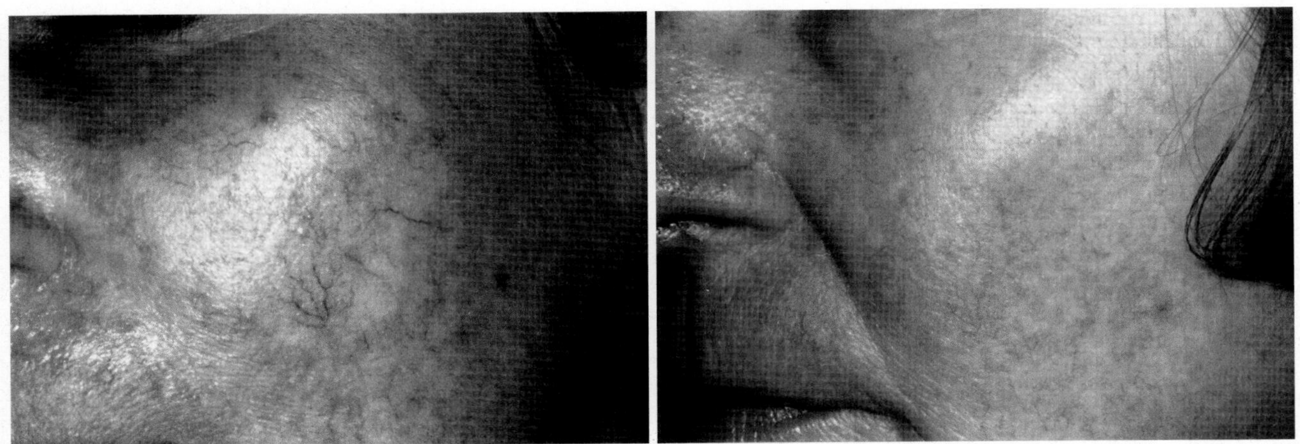

Fig. 10.12 (A) Telangiectasias of the face, pretreatment. **(B)** Appearance after single treatment with the potassium titanyl phosphate laser.

and the 5 mm spot size is used for treating vessels that have associated erythema. The laser spots are placed in a contiguous or slightly overlapping pattern over the vessel. As with the other yellow lasers, when treating the spider lesions, the radial vessels are treated first from the periphery toward the center, then the central vessel is treated. The energy densities used for treating telangiectasia are usually lower than those for treating port-wine stains and are often in the range of 5.5 to 6.0 J/cm^2. Retreatment with yellow dye lasers can usually be performed safely 6 to 8 weeks after the previous treatment.

The 532 nm long-pulse diode laser has been used successfully in the treatment of telangiectasia. Wavelength A 10 to 50 msec pulse duration is used, which is close to the thermal relaxation of the blood vessels targeted. This allows for the gradual heating of the vessel, therefore preventing vessel rupture and the related posttreatment erythema, commonly observed with the pulsed dye lasers.[11]

Hereditary Hemorrhagic Telangiectasia

Hereditary hemorrhagic telangiectasia (HHT), or Osler-Weber-Rendu syndrome, is an inherited autosomal dominant disease manifested by multiple telangiectatic lesions that appear on the skin and mucosal membranes.[46] Epistaxis, caused by bleeding from the nasal lesions, is the most common presenting symptom. Bleeding from lesions of the lips, gingiva, tongue, buccal mucosa, or hard palate may also occur. Histologically, ectatic vessels with incomplete surrounding muscular layers are observed.[47]

Patients with severe epistaxis have been treated successfully using septal dermatoplasty.[48] However, recurrent telangiectasias may appear at the edges of the graft or in some cases in the graft itself. Estrogen therapy has been advocated for the treatment of HHT. It is thought to be effective by reducing squamous metaplasia of the nasal mucosa and thereby reducing the incidence of bleeding.[49]

Laser Selection

The CO_2 laser,[50] argon laser,[51] Nd:YAG laser,[52] and KTP laser[53] have been used to photocoagulate the nasal and oral telangiectasias found in HHT. The CO_2 laser is not ideal for the treatment of telangiectasias because its effects are superficial and vaporization of the overlying mucous membrane covering the lesion may cause bleeding. In addition, fiber-directed lasers (Nd:YAG, KTP, and argon) have the advantage of accessibility to posterior sites and lateral nasal wall sites. The argon and KTP lasers with preferential oxyhemoglobin absorption offer the theoretic advantage of vascular selectivity. In addition, dedicated nasal instruments available with the KTP laser facilitate its usage in the constricted nasal cavity. Although the Nd:YAG laser is not preferentially absorbed by oxyhemoglobin, its deeper penetration makes it extremely effective in coagulating these lesions (**Fig. 10.13AB**).

Treatment

Whichever fiber laser is chosen, the free fiber is held above the mucosal surface and the individual vessels are treated in a rosette fashion by first encircling the central portion of the lesion with pulses of laser energy and then coagulating the central lesion (**Fig. 10.14**). For the Nd:YAG laser, power settings usually range from 10 to 25 W and the exposure time used is 0.5 seconds. With the KTP laser, the power is set to 6 W, exposure time

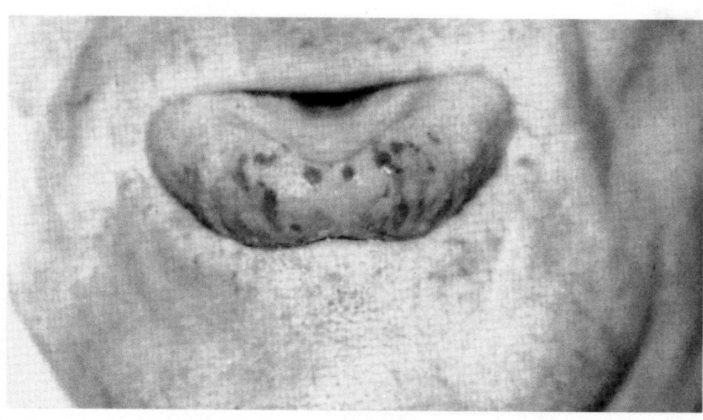
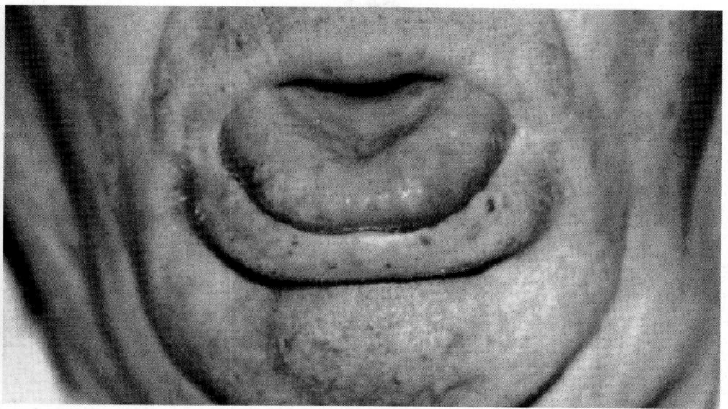

Fig. 10.13 **(A)** Lingual telangiectasia, pretreatment. **(B)** Appearance 2 weeks after treatment using the neodymium: yttrium-aluminum-garnet laser.

is 0.5 seconds, and the beam is used in a slightly defocused mode. The laser energy should be applied perpendicular to the mucosal surface. This obviously becomes more difficult as lesions deeper in the nasal cavity are treated.

Hemangiomas

The treatment of capillary or cavernous hemangiomas has been reported with CO_2, Nd:YAG, argon, and KTP lasers.[6,9,27,54] The vascular specificity of the KTP and argon lasers enhances the selectivity of the photocoagulation.[20] Nevertheless, the Nd:YAG laser is useful in nodular lesions when a greater depth of coagulation is desired (**Fig. 10.14**).[9] The maximum tissue penetration is ~1 cm, which limits external treatment of large lesions. In these cases, even large hemangiomas can be treated with intralesional application of the Nd:YAG laser utilizing the bare fiber inserted through a puncture site (**Fig. 10.15**).[55] Rosenfeld et al[8] reported on Nd:YAG laser treatment of 37 capillary and cavernous hemangiomas, with improvement in 29 cases. Only two cases of scarring were reported. Similar success rates were reported by Apfelberg et al.[6]

KTP and argon lasers offer the advantage of selectivity and decreased depth of penetration compared with the Nd:YAG laser. The potential to minimize risks of scarring exists with either laser. Excision of large hemangiomas of the nasal cavity and paranasal sinuses is facilitated by the KTP or contact-tip Nd:YAG lasers that complement traditional surgical approaches.

Pigmented Lesions

Cutaneous pigmented lesions include benign pigmented lesions and exogenous pigment (tattoos). Benign pigmented lesions include lentigines, freckles, café au lait spots, congenital nevi, and melasma. Exogenous tattoos can occur as a result of professional tattooing

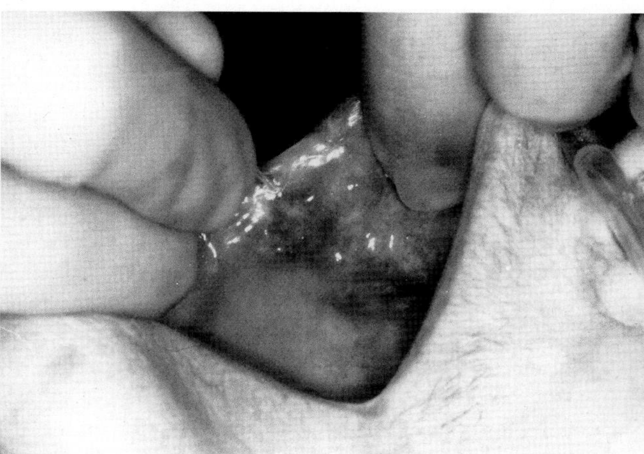
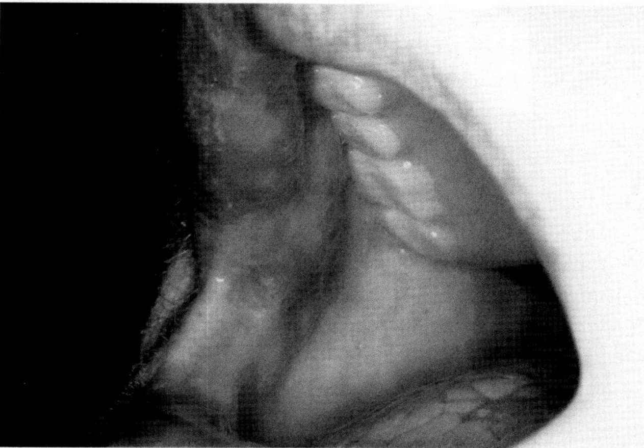

Fig. 10.14 **(A)** Pretreatment view of a right buccal hemangioma. **(B)** Posttreatment appearance after use of the noncontact neodymium:yttrium-aluminum-garnet laser.

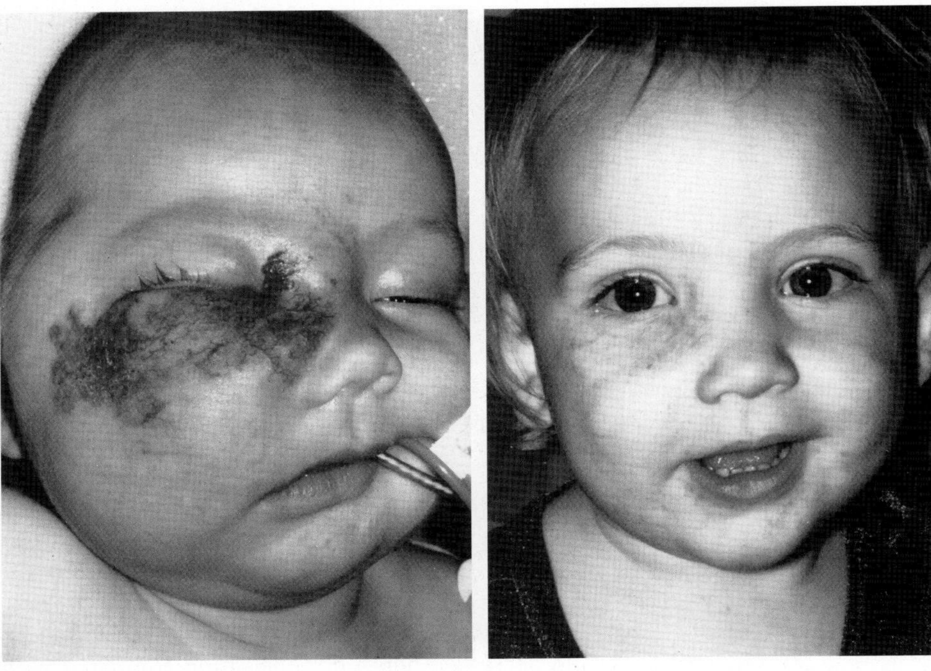

Fig. 10.15 (A) Right periorbital hemangioma in a 2-month-old. **(B)** Clinical response to intralesional neodymium: yttrium-aluminum-garnet laser. This lesion was also treated with intralesional corticosteroids and the flashlamp excited dye laser (three treatments). (Courtesy Archives of Otolaryngology, Head and Neck Surgery.)

or accidental tattooing as in an explosion or puncture injury. Both selective and nonselective lasers have been used to remove pigmented lesions. For example, nonselective vaporization of the lentigines and freckles has been accomplished with the CO_2 and erbium lasers. The principle of selective photothermolysis has guided the development of several lasers that reliably remove pigment without damaging surrounding tissue. The mechanism of pigment destruction is not completely understood, but it is probably a combination of photoacoustic damage to the cell by rapid heating and expansion of melanosomes, breakup of pigment, and systemic rephagocytosis and clearing.

Laser Selection

Lasers that target pigment include the pulsed dye laser (510 nm), copper vapor (511 nm), frequency doubled Q-switched Nd:YAG (532 nm), KTP (532 nm), Q-switched and long-pulsed ruby (694 nm), Q-switched and long-pulsed alexandrite (755 nm), and the Q-switched Nd: YAG (1064 nm).

The pulsed dye laser, with characteristic short wavelength and shallow tissue penetration, is excellent in clearing epidermal pigmented lesions such as lentigines, freckles, and café au lait spots, but less ideal for dermal pigment removal such as tattoos. However, it can effectively remove brightly colored pigments such as red, purple, and orange.[56] The shallow depth also leads to treatment of melanosomes but not melanocytes, which may partially explain recurrence rates in café au lait spots, Becker nevi, and melasma.[57]

The ruby laser (694 nm) is minimally absorbed by hemoglobin, preferentially absorbed by melanin, and has deeper tissue penetration, making it more effective in the dermis than the pulsed dye laser. The Q-switched ruby laser is highly effective for the removal of amateur tattoos, moderately effective for the removal of black professional tattoos, and less effective for the removal of brightly colored professional tattoos. Amateur tattoos respond more favorably in fewer treatments than professional tattoos do.[58] Green tattoos respond variably,[59] whereas red tattoos are most problematic.[60] One study, which compared the three lasers, found the Q-switched ruby laser to be most efficacious in removing blue-black tattoos, the Q-switched alexandrite laser was best for blue and green tattoos, and the frequency doubled Q-switched Nd:YAG was useful for red tattoos.[61]

The Q-switched alexandrite laser is also useful in treating pigmented lesions. As with the ruby laser, a longer wavelength (755 nm) allows for deeper penetration. Lentigines, freckles, and café au lait spots can be removed with the alexandrite laser. It is best at removing green tattoos, but less effective at removing blue-black or brightly colored tattoos. Long-pulsed ruby and alexandrite lasers have also been shown effective in treating laser-resistant congenital nevi.[62] The Q-switched Nd:YAG's usefulness can be expanded by placing a doubling crystal in the laser beam's path resulting in a laser that can be operated at 532 nm or 1064 nm, giving the clinician greater flexibility. The 532 nm wavelength is well absorbed by melanin and hemoglobin, making it useful in the treatment of both vascular and pigmented lesions. For the treatment of lentigines in dark-skinned patients a study of 34 patients showed that the long-pulsed 532 nm Nd:YAG laser was more effective than the Q-switched Nd:YAG laser.[63] Epidermal lesions such as keratoses and lentigines can be lightened considerably. Pigment in the deep dermis can be removed using the 1064 nm Q-switched Nd:YAG laser. The Q-switched Nd:YAG laser clears most amateur blue black tattoos.[64]

More recently, the KTP laser has been used for treating solar lentigines and other dyschromias associated with photoaging, although darker skin types are more difficult to treat and have a higher side effect profile.[65]

Treatment

In general, superficial lentigines and freckles can often be treated in one treatment. Congenital nevi, dermal tattoos, melasma, and café au lait spots generally require multiple treatments and still may recur in some cases. Q-switched lasers are often used without a local anesthetic or with a topical application like lidocaine/prilocaine cream. In the case of tattoos with multiple pigments, more than one laser may be needed. Higher fluences may be required to affect some congenital nevi and tattoo pigments. Treatments with the pulsed dye laser are initiated at 2 to 3 J/cm^2 using a 5 mm spot. The frequency-doubled Q-switched Nd:YAG should be initiated using fluences of 2 to 2.5 J/cm^2 in 2 mm spots at 5 to 10 Hz. Higher fluences are needed for the red lasers, including the ruby and alexandrite. The ruby laser uses fluences 5 to 6 J/cm^2 through an articulated arm to a 6.5 mm spot. Five to 10 J/cm^2 can be used for tattoos. Tattoo removal usually requires five to 10 treatments. The alexandrite laser should be begun with fluences of 6 to 8 J/cm^2. Finally, the Q-switched Nd:YAG is operated at fluences of 3 to 12 J/cm^2.

Hair Removal

Consumers spend over $500 million annually for products to remove unwanted body hair. Laser-assisted hair removal is a new and effective means for removing unwanted body hair. Although none of the currently approved lasers can boast permanent hair removal, laser-assisted hair removal is less painful than electrosurgical hair removal and provides longer-lasting results than the more traditional means of hair removal, including shaving, waxing, plucking, electrolysis, and use of depilatories. Removing hair from any body area, including the face, groin, extremities, and axilla is now safely done with appropriate laser systems and settings. The principle underlying hair removal is selective photothermolysis. As previously mentioned, this involves the selective absorption of light energy by the hair follicles with suitable pulse energies and pulse durations that are equal to or less than the thermal relaxation time of targeted follicles in the skin. In laser-assisted hair removal, the target chromophore is the pigment melanin. Lasers with wavelengths between 690 and 1100 nm are in the approximate range. This includes red-light lasers (694 nm ruby), infrared (755 nm alexandrite, 800 nm diode, 1064 nm Nd:YAG), and filtered flashlamp intense pulsed light producing a spectrum of 590 to 1200 nm. Pulse duration is also an important parameter in laser-assisted hair removal in that the pulse width must approximate the thermal relaxation time to provide sufficient heating to the target follicles. Ideally, this is done without causing damage to the surrounding epidermis (which also contains melanin). Cooling systems are utilized in hair removal lasers systems to decrease collateral thermal damage.

Laser Selection

The long-pulsed ruby and alexandrite, the diode, and the Nd:YAG (used in conjunction with a carbon suspension) are the primary lasers used for hair removal today. The long-pulsed ruby laser emits light at 694 nm, which is strongly absorbed by melanin, and has sufficient tissue penetration to reach the depth of the hair follicles. Several studies have confirmed the efficacy and safety of using long-pulsed ruby-based systems for the temporary removal of hair and long-term hair reduction.[64,66–68] The long-pulsed alexandrite laser (755 nm) is also strongly absorbed by melanin. It also achieves selective heating of the hair follicles and adequate tissue penetration, resulting in effective hair reduction,[69] although a high incidence of nonpermanent posttreatment pigmentary changes has been reported.[70] The diode lasers, emitting light in the 800 nm range, are also available. In addition, the filtered flashlamp IPL, using a noncoherent spectrum of light is also useful for hair removal and has somewhat adjustable features for treating different skin types and tones. The soft light system, utilizing an exogenous chromophore (a topical carbon suspension) and the Nd:YAG laser, has also been shown to effectively provide temporary and long-term hair reduction.

Treatment

In general, the previously mentioned lasers all produce light in the visible and near-IR spectrum utilizing the selective absorption of melanin for the destruction of the hair follicle. As also mentioned, the pulse duration should be less than or equal to the thermal relaxation time, which has been calculated to be ~10 to 100 msec. For hair removal, treating at the maximum tolerated fluences results in better long-term results. However, as with any treatment utilizing the laser, initial parameters should be conservative and increase once it is demonstrated that they will be well tolerated by the patient. Dark-haired, light-skinned people have the best results with laser-assisted hair removal. Darker skin tones are at higher risk for hypopigmentation at fluences required to remove hair. In general, patients with darker skin types are more safely treated with the longer wavelength lasers, such as the alexandrite and the Nd:YAG lasers.[71] More recently, a new laser technique of skin cooling in combination with longer-pulse widths has optimized the efficacy of laser-assisted hair removal and minimized the side effect profile in darker skin type patients.[72,73]

The biggest hurdle to long-term results, however, has to do with the biology of hair growth itself. Hairs in the growth or anagen phase are sensitive to laser irradiation because they are associated with melanocytes during this active phase (**Fig. 10.16**). Hairs in the catagen and telogen phases are much less affected. Hairs in these latter stages of the hair growth cycle lose much of their melanin, which is the target of the currently used laser systems. In addition, portions of the hair follicle are resorbed altogether.[74] The amount of hair in any given phase varies among patients and anatomical sites. Multiple sessions are therefore required to treat all of the hairs in any given region.

The long-pulse ruby lasers are generally started at fluences of 10 to 20 J/cm^2 or lower if the laser system does not have an incorporated cooling mechanism in the handpiece or cooling gel. The alexandrite lasers are similar in setting. The filtered flashlamp IPL uses a software system to determine initial settings based on the patient's skin type and produces fluences of 30 to 65 J/cm^2. The soft light system uses the Nd:YAG laser at lower fluences to propel the carbon into the hair follicles followed by another pass at higher fluences (2 to 3 J/cm^2) for hair removal. The diode laser produces fluences of 5 to 40 J/cm^2 over a 9 × 9 mm area. A cooled sapphire lens is incorporated into the handpiece to provide for additional epidermal protection. Most patients require more than one treatment for permanent hair reduction, although temporary hair removal can easily be accomplished in one treatment. Typically, two to five treatments are necessary for permanent hair reduction depending on the laser selected.

Rhinophyma

Rhinophyma is a disease of the nose and skin of the midface that occurs almost exclusively in men.[75] It usually begins in midlife or later and is characterized by hyperplasia of the sebaceous glands and connective tissue.[76]

Henning and von Gemert[77] reported the use of the argon laser for the treatment of rhinophyma; however, most laser surgeons use the CO_2 laser[78,79] because it offers distinct advantages. The ability to precisely excise and ablate the rhinophymatous tissue allows the surgeon to sculpt the nose. Intraoperative bleeding is kept to a minimum because of the hemostatic properties of the CO_2 laser. Postoperative pain is minimal and wound care usually requires only antibiotic ointment. Most laser surgeons use the CO_2 laser in a range of 5 to 10 W and in the continuous mode. Large nodules of rhinophymatous tissues arc excised; then the laser is defocused to ablate the remaining portion of the lesion in the paintbrush fashion. This may require several applications of energy to reach the appropriate depth of tissue ablation. The carbonaceous debris and char is removed between each application of laser energy (**Fig. 10.17**).

Skin Resurfacing and Rejuvenation

Laser resurfacing offers potential advantages of improved control and reproducibility in comparison to traditional methods of chemical peeling and dermabrasion. The principle involved, selective photothermolysis, utilizes the

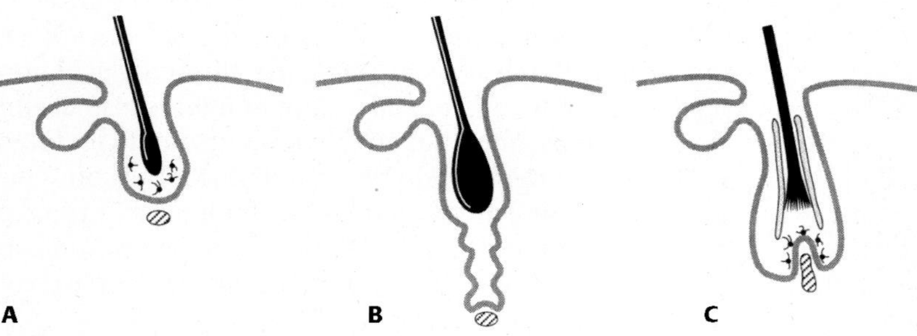

Fig. 10.16 **(A)** Phases of hair growth: the growth phase or anagen, **(B)** the transitional phase (catagen), and **(C)** a resting stage (telogen).

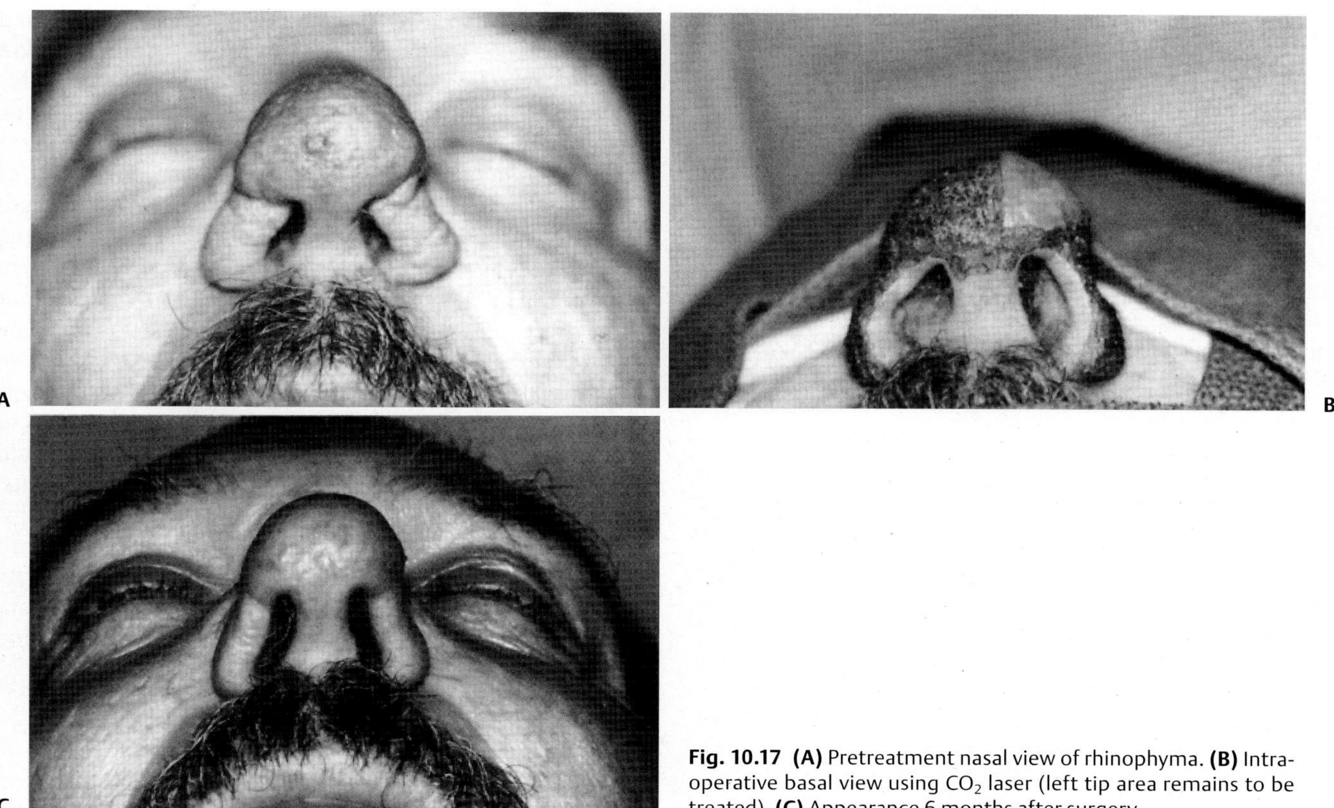

Fig. 10.17 (A) Pretreatment nasal view of rhinophyma. **(B)** Intraoperative basal view using CO_2 laser (left tip area remains to be treated). **(C)** Appearance 6 months after surgery.

chromophore water as a target to vaporize thin layers of tissue with minimal heat diffusion. As described previously, the target must be exposed to the laser light for a period less than or equal to its thermal relaxation time. Thus resurfacing lasers must be capable of delivering sufficient fluence during this brief time to achieve vaporization during a single laser pulse. For skin, this is ~5 J/cm^2 delivered in less than 1 msec.

Patients who may benefit from laser resurfacing include those with rhytids (**Fig. 10.18**), photoaging (including actinic keratosis, actinic chelitis, and dyschromias), and scarring resulting from trauma, iatrogenic causes, or acne. Small areas or the entire face can be treated in one setting. The laser is also useful in procedures that require deepithelialization of a flap or a portion of a flap. A few of the specific clinical entities are mentioned in the following sections.

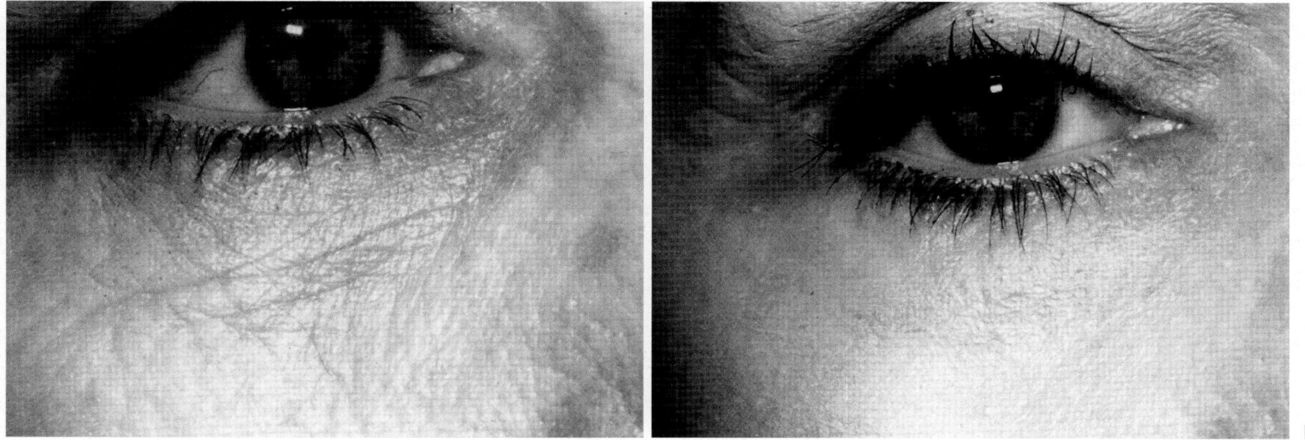

Fig. 10.18 (A) Pretreatment view of periorbital rhytids. **(B)** Posttreatment after resurfacing with the CO_2 laser.

Laser Selection

CO_2 and erbium lasers are the primary ones used in resurfacing. Both lasers utilize tissue water as the ablative target and have been engineered to achieve fluences for tissue vaporization. Although laser–tissue interaction is similar, two types of technologies have been developed for resurfacing. The first are high-energy, short-pulsed systems capable of producing single pulses of 600 msec duration with fluences 5 to 7 J/cm^2 for the CO_2 laser. Thermal damage, which occurs when heat is conducted to surrounding tissue, is directly proportional to the length of time energy is applied to the tissue. High-energy, short-pulsed systems allow ablation of thin layers while minimizing thermal damage. A computer pattern generator, used in conjunction, produces patterns up to 19 mm in diameter. The individual patterns are composed of a series of collimated beams that are overlapping by varying degrees to maximize uniformity. The second type of technology that has proved useful in resurfacing is scanning. Scanning technology utilizes a continuous laser beam with a microprocessor-controlled scanner that rapidly moves the focused beam across the tissue. The pattern of movement is designed to ensure that dwell time on any point is less than the thermal relaxation time (simulating a pulse). Fluences of 5 to15 J/cm^2 for the CO_2 laser are delivered with this system. Scanning diameters may be varied from 3 to 16 mm. Both the CO_2 laser and the erbium laser are useful in resurfacing. The differences between the two primarily lie in the biophysics of each. The CO_2 laser, in contrast to the erbium laser, has an additional thermal effect in the base of the treated wound. This thermal effect gives the CO_2 laser its characteristic ability to coagulate and to induce collagen remodeling in the dermis.[80] The erbium laser, with its much higher absorption coefficient, rapidly ablates tissue with very little thermal effect (a rim of 20 to 50 μm). Histologically, this translates into less tissue shrinkage[81] and more rapid reepithelialization.[82] Wound healing after erbium laser resurfacing is similar to that after such cold techniques as dermabrasion. The depth of tissue injury corresponds closely to the depth of ablation because thermal damage is extremely limited. This allows for quicker healing and for less postoperative erythema.

The CO_2 laser has also been used successfully in laser-assisted blepharoplasty. The scalpel-like cutting and effective coagulation properties of the continuous-wave mode, in combination with the ablative skin resurfacing properties of the pulsed laser mode, make it an ideal tool for this type of procedure.[83]

A recent trend toward using nonablative laser technologies for rejuvenating facial skin has evolved from the desire to minimize patient recovery time and possible complications.[84] The idea behind this approach is the use of lasers that lead to improvement in skin turgor and appearance while preserving the most superficial skin layers. Nonablative lasers used in the treatment of rhytids include IPL, pulsed dye lasers, and the Nd:YAG lasers. Lasers emitting shorter wavelength light work better in combating the vascular and pigmentation effects of photoaging, whereas longer wavelength lasers are more effective against wrinkles.[85] In animal models, both the pulsed dye laser and the Nd:YAG laser have been shown to work by inducing dermal collagen remodeling without affecting the epidermis.[86,87] The IPL systems work by targeting hemoglobin, melanin, and water to improve pigmentation and turgor.[85] Nonablative laser technology has proven safe and beneficial in the rejuvenation of patients with darker skin types. Because these systems do not affect the melanin-rich epidermis in these patients, posttreatment hyperemia, hypopigmentation, and postinflammatory hyperpigmentation, commonly seen with ablative laser technologies, are minimized.[73,89] The benefits of the nonablative approach to facial rejuvenation are under ongoing investigation, thus far showing promising results.[85,89,90]

Treatment

Preoperative planning is critical to the appropriate treatment of resurfacing patients. Skin tones and textures, thickness of the areas to be resurfaced, areas previously resurfaced with the laser or skin treatments, and a history of sun exposure, isotretinoin (e.g., Accutane, Hoffmann-La Roche, Inc., Nutley, NJ) usage, and exposure to radiation are all important. Perioperative care, including skin preparation, herpes prophylaxis, and the appropriate use of local anesthesia are also important to achieve optimal cosmetic results. Local anesthesia then is used with a weak epinephrine solution (1:200,000) so that severe vasoconstriction will not obliterate the color indicators of depth. The surgeon should be familiar with the ablation characteristics of the laser system used. A pink color indicates removal of the epidermis, a uniform gray appearance signals the papillary dermis, and a chamois yellow appearance heralds the reticular dermis. These important end points may be altered in patients who were previously treated, in patients taking isotretinoin, or in those with a history of radiation exposure.

Complete superficial laser ablation of anatomical units is performed. Several passes are usually needed, depending on the degree of photodamage and the laser used. In general, the erbium laser requires more passes than the CO_2 laser because its tissue effects depend almost completely on the depth of ablation and not the thermal effect. Residual tissue is then removed completely with a very moist saline sponge between passes. Fluences typically range from 5 to 10 J/cm². The erbium and CO_2 lasers can be used in a complementary fashion as well. For example, the epidermis can be removed with the CO_2 laser, and the erbium laser can be used to sculpt scars in finer detail. This technique combines the heating properties of the CO_2 laser with the ablation characteristics of the erbium laser.[91] Most recently, a combination laser has been developed that can deliver simultaneous erbium pulses and continuous-wave CO_2 beams.[92]

These same principles of tissue ablation can also be applied to the removal of specific photodamage lesions that have the potential for malignant transformation. Actinic cheilitis and keratoses are examples of precancerous dermatosis that occurs in patients with a history of chronic sun exposure.[93,94] Actinic cheilitis, appearing as superficial milky or silver-gray lesions of the lower lip, is often atrophic, and focal areas of scaling or crusting can be found. Because of the superficial nature of this lesion and its high water content, vaporization of the lesion using the CO_2 laser is an excellent treatment option. Continuous lasers have been used to ablate and excise these lesions including those used in laser vermilionectomy.[95] Newer technologies, such as the development of the high-energy, short-pulsed CO_2 laser coupled with the computer pattern generator, and the scanning continuous laser, have led to better results and improved healing rates.[91] Complete reepithelialization of the lip should occur in less than 4 weeks.

For the nonablative facial rejuvenation using the pulsed dye laser at wavelength of 585 to 595 nm, studies showing efficacy used fluences of 2.4 to 6.5 J/cm² and spot size of 5 to 10 mm with 350 μs pulses.[96–98] The Q-switched Nd:YAG laser has been shown to be effective for facial rejuvenation at fluences of 5.5 to 7 J/cm² and a spot size of 3 mm.[85] With respect to IPL, various settings have been tested and shown to be effective. Cutoff filters of 550 nm, 560 nm, and 640 nm have been used with fluances of 30 to 45 J/cm² and spot sizes of 8 to 45 mm.[89,90] The optimal settings for these lasers in facial rejuvenation are still under investigation.

Cutaneous Malignancies

Laser Excision

Basal and squamous cell carcinomas may be excised using the CO_2 laser as a light scalpel. The CO_2 laser offers some distinct advantages in performing excision surgery of facial cutaneous lesions.[79] One advantage is homeostasis. The CO_2 laser can seal blood vessels up to 0.5 mm in diameter when used in the focused mode. In the defocused mode, it can seal even larger vessels. Another advantage of the CO_2 laser is in flap elevation or undermining. Since the instrument does not contact the skin, there is theoretically less tissue trauma and edema. By using the CO_2 laser for excisional surgery, nerve endings are sealed; this reduces postoperative pain. A frozen section evaluation of the margins of resection has not been difficult when the CO_2 laser is used (**Fig. 10.19**).[99]

Photodynamic Therapy

Photodynamic therapy (PDT) is currently an experimental treatment modality that combines the use of light-sensitive drugs and lasers to destroy nonmelanoma skin malignancies. Photosensitizing drugs are administered intravenously and are taken up by all cells of the body but are preferentially

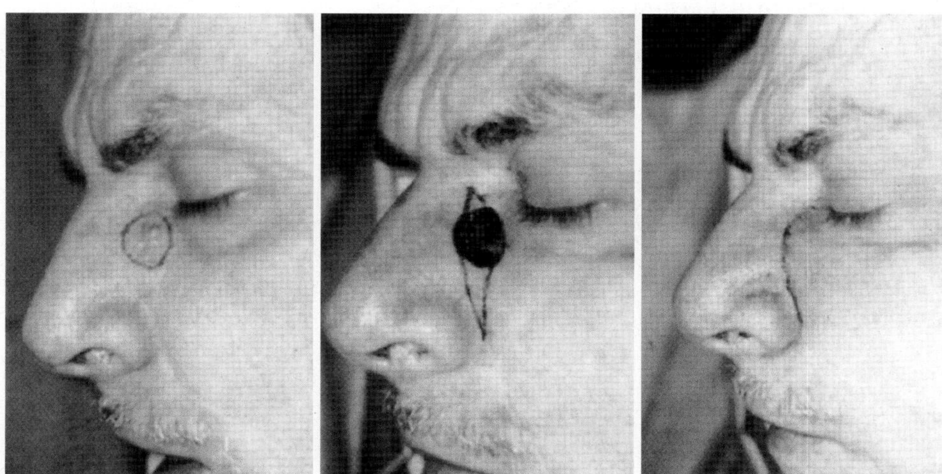

Fig. 10.19 **(A)** Left nasal basal cell carcinoma outlined for CO_2 laser excision. **(B)** Completion of laser excision and outline of areas to be excised with laser before closure. **(C)** Immediate postoperative appearance after closure of defect.

concentrated in tissues of the endothelial system and in tissues with rapid turnover, such as skin and neoplasms. Approximately 48 to 72 hours after administration of the drugs, they are activated by a laser light. The laser energy then drives an oxidative phototoxic reaction that results in cell death. Several photosensitizing drugs are being investigated for their potential in treating cutaneous and noncutaneous malignancies in the head and neck. Most of the work done in PDT so far has involved the use of hematoporphyrin derivative (HPD) and its commercially available preparation, Photofrin (Wyeth-Ayerst Lederle, Inc., Madison, NJ). More than 20 compounds are currently under evaluation.

Many studies have been published to date establishing the efficacy of PDT in treating patients with cutaneous malignancies of the head and neck. The most dramatic effects have been on localized basal and squamous cell tumors without extensive invasion. Many new drug delivery models and drug–laser combinations hold promise for treatment of many malignancies in a targeted way.

Safety Considerations

Any chapter on laser surgery would be incomplete if it did not address the issue of safety. Lasers are potentially hazardous instruments. Eye damage, skin damage, and endotracheal tube ignition are some of the problems that may occur during laser surgery. An understanding of how they occur and how to avoid them is essential. Ocular damage can result from corneal or retinal burns. Wavelengths ranging from 400 to 1400 nm that are in the visible and near-IR range of electromagnetic radiation cause retinal damage. This occurs because laser energy is focused on the retina to a small spot size by the cornea and lens of the eye. Laser wavelengths of less than 400 nm (ultraviolet), or greater than 1400 nm (far-IR) produce corneal injury. If the injury is of a recurrent or chronic nature, cataracts may develop.[100]

The eyes of the patient, surgeon, and operating room personnel must all be protected during surgery. If operating near a patient's eyes, corneal protectors should be used. If the surgery proposed is not in close proximity to the eyes, then eye pads with overlying reflective material, such as aluminum foil, can be applied to the eyes. With the CO_2 laser, wet eye pads are applied to the closed eyelids and taped in place. For the surgeon and operating room personnel, eyeglass protection of an appropriate tint, recommended by the laser manufacturer, should be worn. When laser surgery is being performed in the operating room, signs should be posted on all entrances to prevent personnel from entering without eye protection.

Inadvertent laser irradiation of unintended skin areas, due to direct or reflected beams, is a problem that is particularly important to the facial plastic surgeon. This can be prevented by placing the laser on standby or turning it off when it is not in use. It is also important to cover as much of the patient's skin as possible with wet towels, with the obvious exception of the area to be treated. In many instances during facial plastic procedures, the patient's skin is marked with a pen to delineate areas of intended surgery. It is important to realize that these marks may change the absorption of a particular wavelength and alter the intended tissue effect.

Laser irradiation may be used close to an endotracheal tube, particularly when treating perioral or intraoral lesions. If a laser beam strikes an unprotected, nonlaser-resistant endotracheal tube, a fire can easily occur. The surgeon is responsible for ensuring that a laser-resistant tube is used. The ventilating gas mixture should contain the least amount of oxygen possible combined with helium. Helium decreases the combustibility of the upper airway gas mixture during anesthesia.[101]

It is imperative that every hospital performing laser surgery has a laser safety committee. This committee establishes guidelines and protocols for performing laser surgery and setting the basic minimum requirements for a surgeon to acquire laser surgery privileges. The committee is also responsible for ensuring that the surgeon, anesthesiologist, and operating room personnel are all up to date on the latest safety precautions as they relate to the different wavelength lasers. Hands-on laser surgery courses attended by otolaryngologist/head and neck surgeons have decreased the incidence of laser complications. Similar courses should be required for all surgeons that plan to use lasers in their practice.

Future of Lasers in Facial Plastic Surgery

The use of lasers in facial plastic surgery is well established and even the treatment of choice for certain lesions and applications. Laser technology, utilizing the principle of selective photothermolysis, allows the surgeon to choose a tool for a very specific purpose. Further improvements in laser–tissue interaction by optimizing laser wavelength, pulse parameters, and energy delivery will certainly lead to new lasers with unique applications. Improvements in these parameters will also lessen the deleterious effects of lasers, including hypopigmentation and scarring.

Existing laser systems are also getting smaller and less expensive, increasing their use and usefulness. Further developments in materials manipulation will lead to more versatile lasers. Recently, portable diode lasers have emerged, increasing their versatility. It is hoped that making the technology more widely available will lead to further innovations by physicians who previously did not have access to certain types of lasers.

The coupling of laser technology with computers, robotics, and imaging systems will probably be the area of greatest progress in the near future. The precise and efficient control of the laser utilizing these technologies will not only maximize results but will also reduce morbidity. Delivery systems that increase the speed, uniformity, and versatility of laser application not only support the development of new uses but also make the current applications more tolerable. As a result, many patients who previously had few options for treatment will have laser therapies available to them.

Finally, new drugs useful in photodynamic therapy will be developed. Targeting tumors with agents that interact with laser light in a lethal way has revolutionary potential. Molecular markers unique to certain tumor cells could be targeted with antibody-delivered chemicals with specific absorption characteristics. When exposed to a particular wavelength of laser light, a lethal blow could be delivered to tumor cells with minimal damage to surrounding normal tissue. With proper delivery, the same technologies can be extended to the treatment of benign lesions as well. Many exciting improvements in clinical practice are to be expected for the facial plastic surgeon who stays abreast of the advances in this field.

References

1. Einstein A. Zur Auanten Theorie der Strahlung. Phys Zeit 1917;18:121
2. Maiman TH. Stimulated optical radiation in ruby. Nature 1960;187:493
3. Johnson JR. Introduction to Laser Biophysics. Orlando, FL: Photon Publishing Division of Photon Dynamics LTD; 1988:11
4. Brackett KA, Sankar MY, Joffe S. Effects of Nd:YAG laser photoradiation on intra-abdominal tissues: a histological study of tissue damage versus power density applied. Lasers Surg Med 1986;6:123
5. Marchesini R, Andreola S, Emanuelli H, et al. Temperature rise in biological tissue during Nd:YAG laser irradiation. Lasers Surg Med 1985;5:75
6. Apfelberg DB, Smith T, Lash H, et al. Preliminary report on use of the neodymium:YAG laser in plastic surgery. Lasers Surg Med 1987;7:189
7. Dixon JA, Davis RK, Gilbertson J. Laser photocoagulation of vascular malformations of the tongue. Laryngoscope 1986;96:537
8. Rosenfeld H, Sherman R. Treatment of cutaneous and deep vascular lesions with the Nd:YAG laser. Lasers Surg Med 1986;6:20
9. Rosenreid H, Wellisz T, Reinisch JF, et al. The treatment of cutaneous vascular lesions with the Nd:YAG laser. Ann Plast Surg 1988;3:223
10. Dixon JA, Gilbertson J. Argon and neodymium:YAG laser therapy of dark nodular port-wine stains in older patients. Lasers Surg Med 1986;6:5
11. Travelute Ammirati C, Carniol P, Hruza G. Laser treatment of facial vascular lesions. Facial Plast Surg 2001;17(3):193–201
12. Bernstein E. Treatment of a resistant port wine stain with the 1.5 millisecond pulse duration, tunable, pulsed dye laser. Dermatol Surg 2000;26:1007–1009
13. Kelly K, Nanda V, Nelson J. Treatment of port-wine stain birthmarks using the 1.5-msec pulsed dye laser at high fluences in conjunction with cryogen spray cooling. Dermatol Surg 2002;28(4):309–313
14. Chang CWD, Ries WR. Nonoperative techniques for scar management and revision. Facial Plast Surg 2001;17(4):283–288
15. Bradley D, Park S. Scar revision via resurfacing. Facial Plast Surg 2001;17(4):253–262
16. Jacobs HA, Walton RG. The incidence of birthmarks in the neonate. Pediatrics 1976;58:218
17. Enzinger FM, Weiss SW. Soft tissue tumors. In: Benign Tumors and Tumor-like Lesions of Blood Vessels. St. Louis: CV Mosby; 1983
18. Buecker JW, Ratz JL, Richfield D. Histology of port-wine stain treated with carbon dioxide laser. J Am Acad Dermatol 1984;10:94
19. Patseavouras LL. Expanded applications of carbon dioxide laser in facial plastic surgery. Fac Plast Surg 1990;6:151
20. Ratz J, Balin P, Levin H. CO_2 laser treatment of port-wine stains: a preliminary report. J Dermatol Surg Oncol 1982;8:1039
21. Bailin PL. Treatment of port-wine stain with the CO_2 laser: early results. In: Amdt KA, Noe JM, Rosen S eds. Cutaneous Laser Therapy: Principles and Methods. New York: John Wiley and Sons; 1983
22. Noe JM, Barsky SH, Geer DE. Port-wine stains and the response to argon laser therapy: successful treatment and predictive role of color, age, and biopsy. Plast Reconstr Surg 1980;65:130
23. Silver L. Argon laser photocoagulation of port-wine stain hemangiomas. Lasers Surg Med 1986;6:24
24. Apfelberg DB, Flores JT, Maser MR, et al. Analysis of complications of argon laser treatment for port-wine hemangiomas with reference to striped technique. Lasers Surg Med 1983;2:357
25. Cosman B. Experience in the argon laser therapy of portwine stain. Plast Reconstr Surg 1980;65:119
26. Dixon J. Huether S, Rotering R. Hypertrophic scarring in argon laser treatment of port-wine stains. Plast Reconst Surg 1984;73:771
27. Apfelberg DB, Bailin P, Rosenberg H. Preliminary investigation of KTP>532 laser light in the treatment of hemangiomas and tatoos. Lasers Surg Med 1986;6:38
28. Ho WS, Chan H, Ying S, et al. Laser treatment of congenital facial port-wine stains: long-term efficacy and complication in Chinese patients. Lasers Surg Med 2002;30:44–47
29. Chan H, Chan E, Kono T, et al. The use of variable width frequency doubled Nd;YAG 532 nm laser in the treatment of port-wine stains in Chinese patients. Dermatol Surg 2000;26(7):657–661
30. Angermeier MC.Treatment of facial vascular lesions with intense pulsed light. J Cutan Laser Ther 1999;1:95–100
31. Anderson RR, Parrish JA. Microvasculature can be selectively damaged using dye lasers: a basic theory and experimental evidence in human skin. Lasers Surg Med 1983;1:263
32. Anderson RR, Parrish JA. Selective photothermolysis: precise microsurgery by selective absorption of pulsed radiation. Science 1983;22:524
33. Von Gemert MJC, Welch AJ, Amin AP. Isthereanoptimal lasertreatment forport-winestains? LasersSurg Med 1986;6:76
34. Tan OT, Murray S, Surban AK. Action spectrum of vascular specific injury using pulsed irradiation. J Invest Dermatol 1989;92:868
35. Mordon SR, Rotteleur G, Buys B, et al. Comparative study of the “point-by-point technique” and the “scanning technique” for laser treatment of port-wine stain. Lasers Surg Med 1989;9:398
36. Dover J, Arndt K: New approaches to the treatment of vascular lesions. Lasers Surg Med 2000;26:158-163
37. Dai T, Pikkula B, Tunnell J, et al.: Thermal response to human skin epidermis to 596-nm laser irradiation at high incident dosages and long pulse duration in conjunction with cryogen spray cooling: and ex-vivo study. Lasers Surg Med 2003;33:16-24
38. Geronemus R, Quintana A, Lou W, et al.: High-fluence modified pulsed dye laser photocoagulation with dynamic cooling of port-wine stains in infancy. Arch Dermatol 2000;136:942-943
39. Chang CJ, Nelson J.Cryogen spray cooling and higher fluence pulsed dye laser treatment improve port-wine stain clearance while minimizing epidermal damage. Dermatol Surg 1999;25:767–772
40. Edris A, Choi B, Aguilar G, et al. Measurements of laser light attenuation following cryogen spray cooling spurt termination. Lasers Surg Med 2003;32:143–147
41. Ries WR, Speyer M, Reinisch L. Effects of thermal conducting media in the skin surface during laser irradiation. Laryngoscope 2000;110: 575–584
42. Tan OT, Sherwood K, Gilchrest BA. Treatment of children with port-wine stains using the flashlamp-pulsed tunable dye laser. N Engl J Med 1989;320:416
43. Scheibner A, Applebaum J, Wheeland RG. Treatment of port-wine hemangiomas in children. Lasers Surg Med Suppl 1989;1:42
44. Anderson MR. Spider nevi: their incidence in healthy school children. Arch Dis Child 1963;38:286

45. Barter RH, Letterman GS, Schurter M. Hemangiomas in pregnancy. Am J Obstet Gynecol 1963;87:625
46. Ries WR. Flashlamp-excited dye laser: treatment of vascular cutaneous lesions. Fac Plast Surg 1989;6:167
47. Osier W. On a familial form of recurring epistaxis, associates with multiple telangiectasias of the skin and mucous membranes. Bull Johns Hopkins Hosp 1901;12:333
48. Janeke V. Ultrastructure of hereditary telangiectasia. Arch Otolaryngol Head Neck Surg 1970;91:262
49. Saunders WH. Septal dermatoplasty for control of nose bleeds caused by hereditary hemorrhagic telangiectasia or septal perforations. Trans Am Acad Ophthalmol Otolaryngol 1960;64:5
50. Harrison DF. Use of estrogen in treatment of familial hemorrhagic telangiectasia. Laryngoscope 1982;92:314
51. Ben-Bassat M, Kaplan I, Levy R. Treatment of hereditary hemorrhagic telangiectasia of the nasal mucosa with the CO2laser. Br J Plast Surg 1978;31:157
52. Parkin JL, Dixon JA. Laser photocoagulation in hereditary hemorrhagic telangiectasia. Otolaryngol Head Neck Surg 1981;89:204
53. Levine HL. Lasers and endoscopic rhinologic surgery. Otolaryngol Clin North Am 1989;22:739
54. Hobby LW. Further evaluation of the potential of the argon laser in the treatment of strawberry hemangiomas. Plast Reconstr Surg 1983;71:481
55. Clymer MA, Fortune DS, Reinisch L. Interstitial Nd:YAG photocoagulation for vascular malformations and hemangiomas in childhood. Arch Otolaryngol Head Neck Surg 1999;125:431–436
56. Fitzpatrick RE, Goldman MP, Ruiz-Esparza J. Laser treatment of benign pigmented lesions using a 300 nanosecond pulse and 510 nm wavelength. J Dermatol Surg Oncol 1993;19:341–346
57. Alster TS. Complete elimination of large café-au-lait birthmarks by the 510nm pulsed dye laser. Plast Reconstr Surg 1995;96:1660–1664
58. Wheeland RG. Q-switched ruby laser treatment of tattoos. Lasers Surg Med 1991;11(Suppl 3):64
59. Goyal S, Arndt KA, Stern RS, et al. Laser treatment of tattoos: a prospective, paired, comparison study of Q-switched Nd:YAG, frequency doubled Q-switched Nd:YAG, and Q-switched ruby lasers. J Am Acad Dermatol 1997;36:122–125
60. Levine V, Geronemus RG. Tattoo removal with the Qswitched ruby laser and the Nd:YAG laser: a comparative study. Cutis 1995;55:291–296
61. Zelickson BD, Mehregan D, Zarrin A, et al. Clinical, histological, and ultrastructural evaluation of tattoos treated with three laser systems. Lasers Surg Med 1994;15:364–372
62. Veda S, Imayama S. Normal-mode ruby for congenital nevi. Arch Dermatol 1992;133:355
63. Chan H, Fung W, Ying S, Kono T. An in vivo trial comparing the use of different types of 532 nm Nd;YAG lasers in the treatment of facial lentigines in Oriental patients. Dermatol Surg 2000;26(8):843–849
64. Kilmer SL, Anderson RR. Clinical use of the Q-switched ruby and the Q-switched Nd:YAG (1064nm and 532nm) lasers for the treatment of tattoos. J Dermatol Surg Oncol 1993;19:330–338
65. Bassichis B, Swamy B, Dayan S. Use of the KTP laser in the treatment of rosacea and solar lentigines Facial Plast Surg 2004;20:77–83
66. Grossman MC, Dierickx CC, Farninelli WA, et al. Longpulsed ruby laser hair removal: comparison between 2 pulse widths (0.3 and 2 msec). Lasers Surg Med 1997; (supplement 9):36
67. Elman P, Noren A, Waldman M, et al. Non-invasive hair removal with the dual mode ruby laser. Austr J Dermatol 1997;38(suppl2):52
68. Allison K, Kiernan M, Waters R, et al. Evaluation of the ruby 694 chromos for hair removal in various skin sites. Lasers Med Sci 2003;18:165–170
69. Finkel B, Eliezri YD, Waldman A, et al. Pulsed alexandrite laser technology for non-invasive hair removal. J Clin Laser Med Surg 1997;15:225–229
70. Weisberg N, Greenbaum S. Pigmentary changes after alexandrite laser hair removal. Dermatol Surg 2003;29:415–419
71. Hamilton M, Dayan S, Carniol P. Laser hair removal update. Facial Plast Surg 2001;17(3):219–222
72. Nahm W, Tsoukas M, Falanga V, et al.: Preliminary study of fine changes in the duration of dynamic cooling during 755-nm laser hair removal on pain and epidermal damage in paritents with skin types III-V. Lasers Surg Med 2002;31:247–251
73. Nottingham LK, Ries WR: Update on lasers in facial plastic surgery. Curr Opin Otolaryngol Head Neck Surg 2004;12:323–326
74. Pashayan AG, Gravenstein JS. Helium retards endotracheal tube fires for carbon dioxide lasers. Anesthesiology 1985;62:274
75. Ries WR, Duncavage JA, Ossoff RH. Carbon dioxide laser treatment of actinic chelitis. Mayo Clin Proc 1988; 63:294
76. Marks R,Wilkinson DS.Rosacea and perioral dermatitis. In: Rook A, Wilkinson DS, Ebling FJG, eds. Textbook of Dermatology. Vol 2. Ed 3. Oxford: Blackwell Scientific; 1979
77. Henning JPH, von Gemcrt MJC. Rhinophyma treated by argon lasers. Lasers Surg Med 1983;2:211
78. Shapshay SM, Strong MS, Anastas GW, et al. Removal of rhinophyma with carbon dioxide laser: a preliminary report. Arch Otolaryngol 1980;106:257
79. Bohigian RK, Shapsay SM, Hybels RL. Management of rhinophyma with carbon dioxide laser: lahey clinic experience. Lasers Surg Med 1988;8:397
80. Ross E, Naseef G, Skrobal M, et al. In vivo dermal collagen shrinkage and remodeling following CO2 laser resurfacing. Lasers Surg Med 1996;18:38
81. Jaffe BH, Walsh JT Jr. Water flux from partial-thickness skin wounds: comparative study of the effects of Er:YAG and Ho:YAG lasers. Lasers Surg Med 1996;18(1):1–9
82. Khatri K, Ross E, Grevelink J, et al. Comparison of erbium:YAG and CO2 lasers in skin resurfacing. Lasers Surg Med Suppl 1997;9:37
83. Munker R. Laser blepharoplasty and periorbital laser skin resurfacing. Facial Plast Surg 2001;17(3):209–217
84. Hirsch R, Dayan S. Nonablative resurfacing. Facial Plast Surg 2004; 20(1):57–61
85. Sadick N. Update on nonablative light therapy for rejuvenation: a review. Lasers Surg Med 2003,32:120–128
86. Dahiya R, Lam S, Williams E III. A systematic histological analysis of nonablative laser therapy in a porcine model using the pulsed dye laser. Arch Facial Plast Surg 2003;5:218–223
87. Dayan S, Damrose J, Bhattacharayyya T, et al. Histological evaluation following 1,064-nm Nd;YAG laser resurfacing. Lasers Surg Med 2003; 33:126–131
88. Negishi K, Tezuka Y, Kushikata N, et al. Photorejuvenation for Asian skin by intense pulsed light. Dermatol Surg 2001;27:627–632
89. Bitter PH. Noninvasive rejuvenation of photo damaged skin using serial, full face intense pulsed light treatments. Dermatol Surg 2000;26:835–883
90. Goldberg DJ, Cutler KB. Nonablative treatment of rhytids with intense pulsed light. Lasers Surg Med 2000;26:196–200
91. Alster T, Apfelberg D, eds. Cosmetic Laser Surgery: A Practitioner's Guide. 2nd Ed. New York: Wiley-Liss; 1999
92. Koch R. Office-based procedures in facial plastic surgery. Otolaryngol Clin North Am 2002;35:119–133
93. Nicolau SG, Balus L. Chronic actinic chelitis and cancer of the lower lip. Br J Dermatol 1964;76:278
94. Shapshay SM, Oliver P. Treatment of hereditary hemorrhagic telangiectasia by Nd:YAG laser photocoagulation. Laryngoscope 1984;94:1554
95. Dufresne RG, Garrett AB, Bailin PL, et al. Carbon dioxide laser treatment of chronic actinic cheilitis. J Am Acad Dermatol 1988;19:876
96. Bjerring P, Clement M, Hickendorff L, Egevist H, Kiernan M. Selective non-ablative wrinkle reduction by laser. J Cutan Laser Ther 2000;29:15
97. Restan E, Boves L, Iyer S, Fitzpatrick R. A double-blind side-by-side comparison of low fluences long-pulse dye laser for coolant treatment of wrinkling of the cheeks. Cosmet Laser Ther 2001;3:129–136
98. Zelickson B, Kilmer S, Bernstein E. Pulsed dye laser therapy for sun-damaged skin. Lasers Surg Med 1999;25:229–236
99. Mehregan AH. Actinic keratosis and actinic squamous cell carcinoma: a comparative study of 800 cases observed in 1968 and 1988. Cutan Aging Cosmet Dermatol 1988;2:151
100. Bmmmitte DW, Mang TS, Cooper M, et al. Use of photodynamic therapy for the treatment of extensive basal cell carcinomas. Fac Plast Surg 1989;6:185
101. American national standard for the safe use of lasers in healthcare facilities. The Laser Institute of America; September 1988.

11 Aesthetic Facial Proportions

Marion B. Ridley and Steven M. VanHook

During every recorded age of history, and undoubtedly even earlier, humankind has sought to define and measure beauty and thereby be enabled to create it. Indeed, it has been stated that the prime requisites of a civilization are intellectual energy, freedom of the mind, and a sense of beauty.[1] *Aesthetic* is derived from the Greek word *aisthesis*, which means having a sense or love of that which is beautiful. Individuals have unique perspectives on aesthetics that are related to their personalities and environmental milieux.[2] Thus no two people would likely describe their concept of beauty in exactly the same way. Although a universal canon of beauty cannot be established because of differences in time, culture, ethnicity, and age, there are found proportion and harmony among the parts of certain faces, which confer on the whole a timeless beauty.[3]

Defining an ideal beauty has been an elusive, unattainable goal of every civilization. In interpreting the definition of ideal beauty from civilizations past, we are limited in the resources available. Often we are left to interpret the most popular artistic creations of the time and assume that this is how society felt beauty should be portrayed. At other times, we are able to read the historical record and writings about the subject from the people of those eras. The people of ancient Greece attempted to describe beauty through the perfection of the mind and body in an ordered universe. Their civilization focused on art, literature, and politics, while also prizing the value of beauty in society. There were rewards for those of society with beauty, and often people were referred to with names that described specific aspects of their beauty.[4] Attempts were made to define beauty through mathematical equations and geometric formulas (i.e., laws by which much of nature seemed to abide).[5] The Athenian philosopher Plato stated that "the qualities of measure and proportion invariably constitute beauty and excellence." He wrote that there are three wishes of every man: to be healthy, to be rich by honest means, and to be beautiful. Although Plato started defining beauty in terms of mathematics, he also realized that beyond physical proportions, beauty was also the result of good taste and balance.

History of Beauty in Art

Several other Greek figures played important roles in helping to define ideal beauty. Polyclitus developed a canon of proportions in the fifth century BC that he felt produced a figure with a flawless body. He experimented with proportions taken from nature and from those proportions created figures appearing more aesthetically pleasing to onlookers. Even more influential in the development of an ideal beauty was the Greek sculptor Praxiteles. His work in the fourth century BC led to a depiction of ideal beauty that held for the next 100 years.[4] He sculpted the figure of Aphrodite, the goddess of love, in what is considered the first completely nude image of the goddess created. In his interpretation he crafted a female figure that appeared much more gentle than previous sculptures, in which females seemed more like males with breasts attached to their chests.[6] His Aphrodite showed human expression, and this figure, modeled after a well-known woman of his society, was to be imitated and revered for many years.

In the first century BC the Roman architect Marcus Vitruvius Pollio wrote that the proportions of humans should be used when creating sacred buildings. He reasoned who the human body is a model of perfect proportions; thus architecture would benefit if buildings were modeled on nature. He described the proportions of humans who he felt created the most ideal figure. He also attempted the task of trying to contain the human figure within a circle and square by having the figure with arms and legs extended (later to be referred to as the Vitruvian man). Although his work was not appreciated in his time, he provided a great influence for several of the Italian Renaissance painters.

The late fourteenth century through the middle of the sixteenth century in western Europe was referred to as the Renaissance period. During this time there was a renewed interest in ancient Greece, and the ideals of classic beauty reappeared. Women were starting to receive formal education and were attaining some increased degree of independence. People were also regarding female intelligence as compatible with beauty.[4] This increased reverence for women was also met with new advances in artistic techniques. Masaccio (1401–1428) developed the artistic technique of perspective, allowing the creation of figures that appeared more realistic and human.[6] Artists during this time found that copying beauty was no longer the goal; they wanted to *perfect* beauty. Female faces would often be created with the combination of various features from different models.[4]

Leonardo da Vinci (1452–1519) devised a new version of the Vitruvian man and developed an obsession with the infinity of geometric transformation as exhibited by his

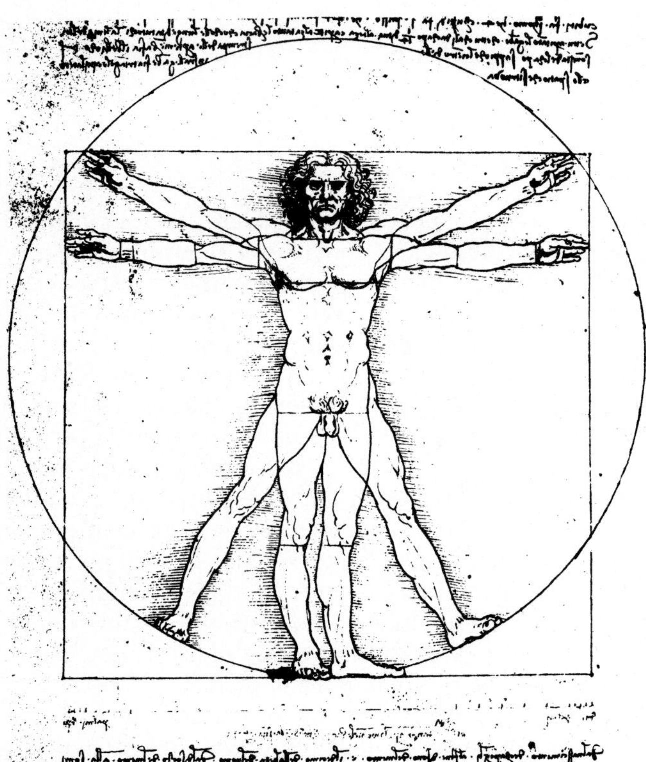

Fig. 11.1 Leonardo da Vinci's proportions of the ideal human body. (Courtesy Historical Pictures Service, Chicago.)

attempt to square the circle (**Fig. 11.1**). The image he created, recognizable to most people, was far more aesthetic in appearance than the original created by Vitruvius.[7] This figure uses the golden proportion (discussed later) prominently, as do many of da Vinci's other works.

Another artist who was inspired by the Vitruvian notion of perfect proportions was the German painter and printmaker Albrecht Dürer (1471–1528). He tested the human proportions devised by Vitruvius that would create the perfect body. By applying these principles, he created drawings of the female figure as described by Vitruvius. Unfortunately, the image that resulted was a round-bellied, drooping-breasted, large-hipped woman with gigantic feet. Without becoming discouraged, Dürer continued in his pursuit to define beauty by writing four books on human proportions. The Italian monk Agnolo Firenzuolo (1493–1543), also interested in defining ideal beauty, wrote a catalog of desirable female traits. Basically analyzing every feature of the female body, Firenzuolo described the size, shape, and proportions of what he considered the ideal woman.[4]

Perhaps the artist most renowned for defining the Renaissance ideal of beauty was the Florentine painter Sandro Botticelli (1445–1510). In his art he was able to combine the social preferences of his time with the classic ideals of antiquity. His images of women show classical bodies, but they also have the Renaissance style of high foreheads and high coloring.[4] The women appear voluptuous but not cumbersome. In his most famous work, *The Birth of Venus* (c. 1480), the image of Venus appears to be floating, despite having her feet touching the shell beneath her.[6] Her face is long and angular rather than oval, as had been common. Although ideals change from generation to generation, this image of the female figure exhibits many of the traits still deemed ideal.

After the Renaissance period, the ideal of beauty changed to the long-fingered, long-necked, graceful female figures of the Mannerist period. Artists of this time tried to convey an unearthly beauty by greatly extending and distorting the natural proportions.[4] After this period, which lasted 75 years, the Baroque period, a Counterreformation response of the Catholic Church to Protestantism, inspired many splendorous works of art. Peter Paul Rubens (1577–1640) was one of the great artists of this period. His figures, recognized throughout the world, depict females as robust, round, pink nudes that were cheerful and playful in appearance. For a brief period of time Rubens's nudes were seen as the ideal beauty of women, perhaps due to the energy portrayed by the subjects rather than the appearance of the figures themselves.[6]

From the middle of the eighteenth century until early in the nineteenth century, the definition of beauty switched back and forth between the classical images of the Greeks to the Romantic images of the time. In the nineteenth century, doll-like females began to emerge as the epitome of beauty. These women, with pale, rounded faces, portrayed purity in addition to beauty. No longer did the ideal female possess certain physical traits, but the role of fashion in the determination of beauty came to the forefront.

The twentieth century has seen the concept of beauty change with each successive decade. The advent of motion pictures and later television facilitated the widespread dissemination of images of models and actresses who represented the beauty of their generation. The ideal beauty at the turn of the century was personified by "the Gibson girl," and later in the 1920s by the "flapper." The "pin-up girl" of the 1940s gave way to the "new look" of the 1950s. The "flower child" of the 1960s made the natural look, with long, flowing hair, no makeup, and simple clothing, popular. The 1970s brought excess in hair styles, makeup, and clothing, followed by an emphasis on a healthy, fit appearance at the end of the century. Undoubtedly, the look of beauty will continue to change at an even more rapid pace in the twenty-first century.

To perceive beauty is an emotional experience. The regard for beauty is perhaps one of the most precious of human qualities, and in its most basic form is intuitive or instinctive.[8] Recognizing and appreciating beauty in different forms and analyzing proportion and harmony can be learned. Even though tastes, fashions, and standards of beauty change from age to age, there appear to be certain facial proportions and relationships that provide a basis for diagnosis and planning in facial surgery.

Considerations in Facial Analysis

To form a basis for analysis of the facial components, several general considerations should be taken into account. These factors help shape our concept of beauty and therefore should be noted first. Performing a generalized analysis of the whole before considering the individual parts will create some general impressions on which a more detailed analysis can be constructed.

Age

Consideration of the patient's age is of primary importance in facial analysis. The effect of the aging process is often the main factor involved in the patient's desire for surgery. Although senescence of the facial structures is a normal physiological process, there may be a discrepancy between chronological age and perceived age because of an acceleration of these processes. Many patients desire to have their perceived age rolled back to have a facial appearance more appropriate for their actual physical or mental state.

Infants and children have a large amount of subcutaneous fat in their faces. Combined with highly elastic skin and a facial skeleton that is not yet fully developed, this imbues them with a round-faced, cherubic appearance. Growth of the facial skeleton during puberty and adolescence results in the characteristic curves and angles of the adult face.

The effects of senescence on the face have been described by Gonzales-Ulloa and Flores (**Fig. 11.2**).[9] The effects of aging begin to appear at about age 30. Skin laxity is first noted when the upper eyelids begin to overhang the palpebral lines. The inferior palpebral sulci and nasolabial folds become noticeable.

At about age 40 the forehead wrinkles and glabellar furrows begin to appear. Laxity of eyelid skin develops into noticeable excess, and crow's feet begin to appear at the lateral canthi. Sagging of the mandibular line also becomes detectable.

By 50 years of age the forehead and glabellar wrinkles have become permanent and may unite to form continuous lines. Upper-lid sagging may reach the level of the lashes. The outer canthi begin to tilt downward, and the nasal tip begins to droop. Fine wrinkles develop around the mouth and along the neck. Sagging of the cheek skin indicates early loss of subcutaneous facial fat.

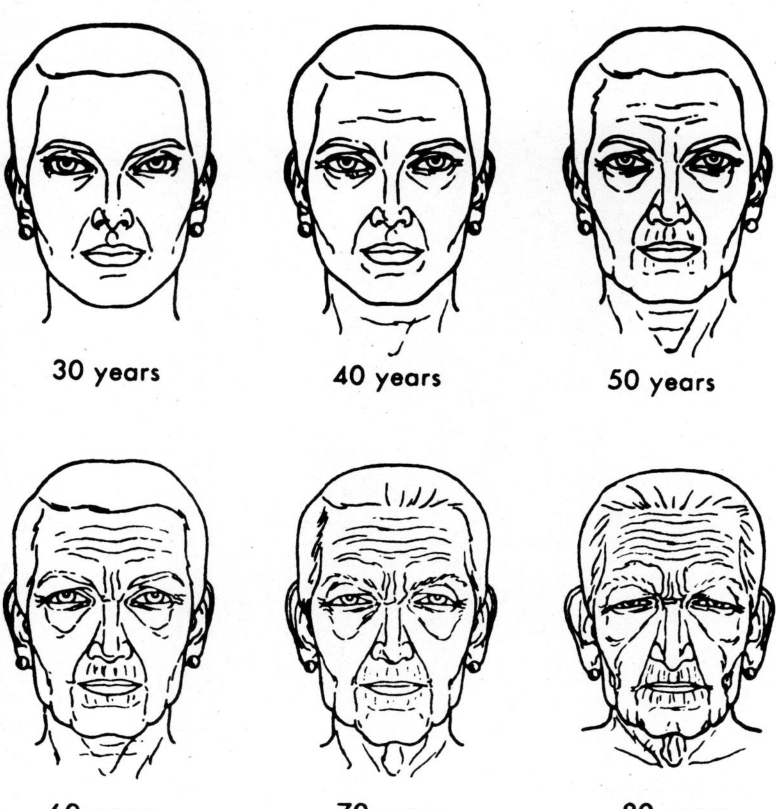

Fig. 11.2 Progressive effects of senescence upon the face. (From Gonzales-Ulloa M, Flores ES. Senility of the face: basic study to understand its causes and effects. Plast Reconst Surg 1965;36:240. With permission.)

At age 60 all skin wrinkles deepen and begin to coalesce. There is a perceived diminution in the size of the eyes resulting from progressive encroachment of the surrounding lid skin. Skin thickness begins to decrease, and the loss of subcutaneous adipose tissue accelerates, producing noticeable deficits in the temporal, orbital, and buccal areas.

By age 70 the nasal tip has descended even further, and the excess skin of the lower eyelids may have developed baglike deformities. Continued loss of subcutaneous fat makes the malar complexes appear quite prominent and the orbits more hollow.

At 80 years of age minute wrinkles coalesce about the face to produce the typical appearance of advanced senescence. Loss of skin thickness, absence of subcutaneous fat, and diminution in the size of the cranial vault combine to make the facial skeleton more conspicuous than at any other time in life.

Sex

Sex differences in facial appearance are the result of hormonal and cultural influences. In general, men tend to have stronger, more angular facial features. Women tend to have rounder, more curved lines defining the face. The gonial angle of the mandible is more defined and prominent in men. The chin is more prominent. Consequently, a receding chin in a man may cause him to be perceived as weak and ineffective. The forehead and zygomatic bones are more apparent in men. The eyebrows are thicker, straighter, and positioned at the supraorbital rim in men. Women's brows are usually thinner, more arched, and positioned above the level of the supraorbital rim. Facial skin is usually thicker and more textured in men.

Numerous differences are noticeable regarding the ideal noses of men and women. Men usually have larger, broader noses with a dorsum that is straight to slightly convex. Women tend toward smaller noses with a slightly concave dorsum. Their nasolabial angle is preferably obtuse, whereas most men prefer a nasolabial angle of no more than 90 degrees. Overall nasal contour is strongly associated with sex identity. Individuals may wish to masculinize or feminize their facial features to better harmonize with their self-image (**Fig. 11.3**).[10]

Body Habitus

Just as the parts of the face cannot be evaluated independently, the face cannot be analyzed without regard for the body on which it rests. Different faces are right for different body types. In general, the overall body type is reflected in the face. Tall, slender individuals will usually have longer, thinner faces, whereas short, stout people tend to have rounder faces with less height and more width. Obviously, this type of body and face will tolerate a shorter, broader nose. However, a long, narrow nose would appear out of place on a short, stocky build. Overall, the individual aesthetic units of the face must be in proportion

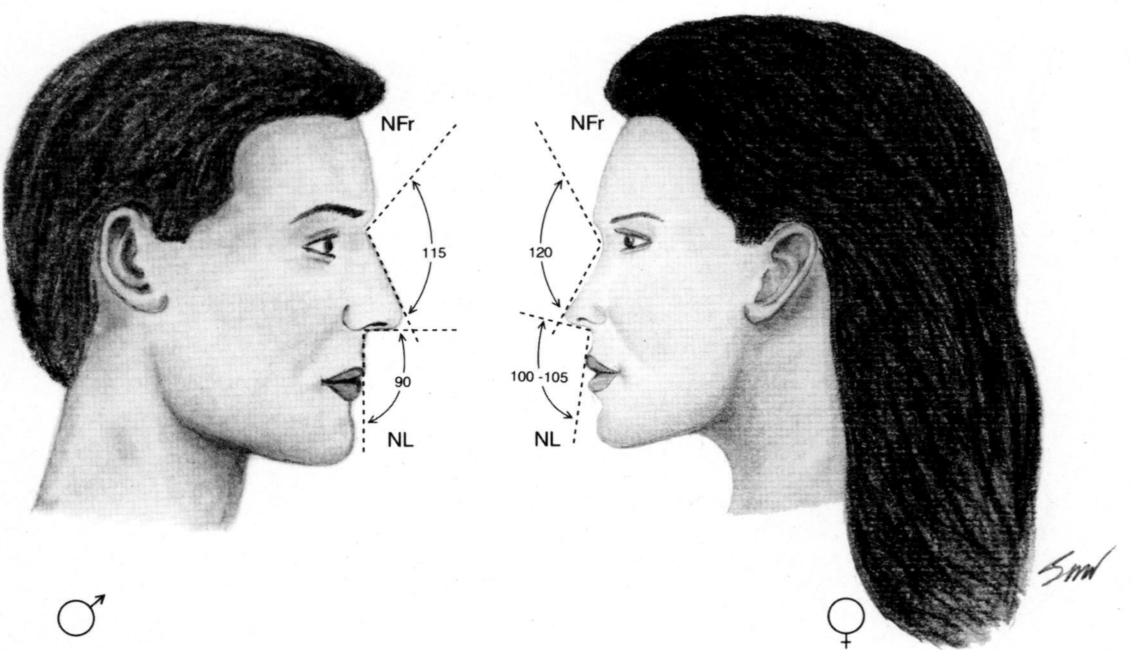

Fig. 11.3 Differences between male and female ideals for the nasofrontal and nasolabial angles. NFr, nasofrontal angle; NL, nasolabial angle.

with the rest of the face and, likewise, the face with the rest of the body.

Ethnicity

Aesthetic value is strongly associated with ethnic, cultural, and social background. Facial structure and body habitus are primarily genetically dependent. Skin type, scarring, and the ability to camouflage facial incisions may vary widely among various ethnic groups. Many patients wish to retain certain ethnic and cultural features that are important to their self-image. Most of the widely accepted standards of facial harmony are drawn from the art and culture of Western civilization,[11] but it is ill-advised to assume that all patients want westernization of non-Caucasian features. There is increasing interest in defining the standards of beauty for those of African and Asian descent.[12–15] Many of the facial proportions are constant throughout a wide range of ethnicities; however, significant differences do exist.[16] Increasingly heterogeneous ethnic and racial backgrounds in each successive generation will undoubtedly result in the continued evolution of our concept of beauty.

Personality

Assessing personality traits is part of the general impression gained during the facial evaluation. These characteristics usually cannot be inferred from static photographs. While awake the face is in a perpetual state of movement and dynamic change. This facial movement allows expression of the spectrum of human emotion. Relative movement among the various components of the face provides an endless array of expressions through which a wealth of nonverbal information is communicated. A certain proportion or harmony among the parts gives the face a personality that is perceived to be a reflection of the individual's personality. Surgery should neither distort nor deceive in this regard. An extrovert with a bubbly personality fits well with upturned facial lines and features, whereas a more somber, serious person would most likely be unhappy with such an incongruous appearance.

Hair

Hair can be styled to manipulate the space around the face. Hairstyles can camouflage less attractive aspects of the face and draw attention to the more pleasing features. Although the forehead is the most difficult aspect of the face to alter surgically, it is easily camouflaged by the hair. Protruding ears and preauricular and postauricular scars can likewise be minimized by judicious use of hairstyling.

Facial Proportions

For facial harmony to exist there must be some degree of relative proportion of the various parts through which an overall balance is achieved. No individual component of the face exists or functions in isolation from the other integral parts. Any change in one part of the face will have a real or perceived effect on the other facial parts and on the whole.

The most basic facial proportions are those that are learned by beginning art students drawing the face. The ancient Greeks taught that the ideal human stature must equal eight times the height of the head.[17] The length of the neck is approximately one-half the length of the head. This distance is measured from the suprasternal notch to the chin and from the chin to the vertex of the skull.

Relative proportions of the hand to the face play an important role for the portrait artist in establishing facial proportions.[1] The length of the hand is three fourths the length of the head or the length of the face as measured from the chin to the hairline. The width of the hand is one half the width of the face. Placed transversely, the hand will cover one fourth the length of the head or one third the length of the face. Leonardo da Vinci described the relationship of the forehead, nose, and chin on the lateral view as lying along an arc produced by a radius based at the external auditory canal.[17]

The Golden Proportion

A mathematic phenomenon that was recognized at least as early as the fifth century BC by the Greeks and probably much earlier by the Egyptians is referred to as the golden ratio or proportion. This ratio is described by a line consisting of two unequal segments such that the ratio of the shorter segment to the longer segment is the same as the ratio of the longer segment to the whole line. The numerical value of this ratio is 1.61803 and is represented by the Greek letter phi (Φ).

Numerous mathematic phenomena surround this proportion. The ratio of 1.0:1.618 is equal to the ratio of 0.618:1.0. It has the unique property of being the only number that, when reduced by 1, is its own reciprocal. If 0.618 is added to 1.618, the sum is 2.236, which is the square root of 5.8.

The Egyptian rectangle was 8 parts long and 5 parts wide. The ratio of 8:5 is 1.6. Ancient Greek temples and statues are replete with examples of the golden proportion. The

Hellenist Greeks found numerous proportions between the parts of the human body that corresponded to the golden proportion.[18] The golden proportion figures prominently in the paintings of Leonardo da Vinci and has even been called Leonardo's square, despite its origins in antiquity. This ratio has an intrinsic harmony or beauty, can be found throughout nature, and is particularly appealing to the human eye. Frequent examples of the golden proportion are also seen in the human face, including the ratio of the length to the width of the head and the ratio of the upper face (trichion to nasion) to the midface (nasion to nasal tip).

Symmetry

Facial symmetry is assessed by bisecting the face through the midsagittal plane and comparing the halves. Although minor asymmetries will be noted in almost everyone, the midline points of the forehead, nose, lips, and chin should lie on this axis. Facial width is then divided into fifths and evaluated for balance among the parts (**Fig. 11.4**). The width of one eye should equal one fifth of the facial width or the intercanthal distance. Lines dropped from the outer canthi should approximate the width of the neck.[19] The lateralmost fifths of the face on frontal view extend from the lateral canthus to lateralmost point of the helical rim.

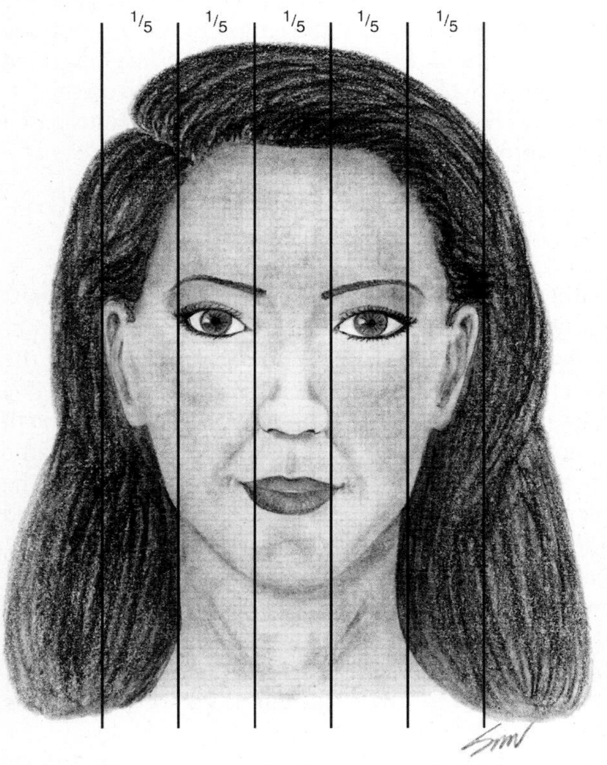

Fig. 11.4 The width of the face is divided into five equal parts; each part is equal to the width of one eye.

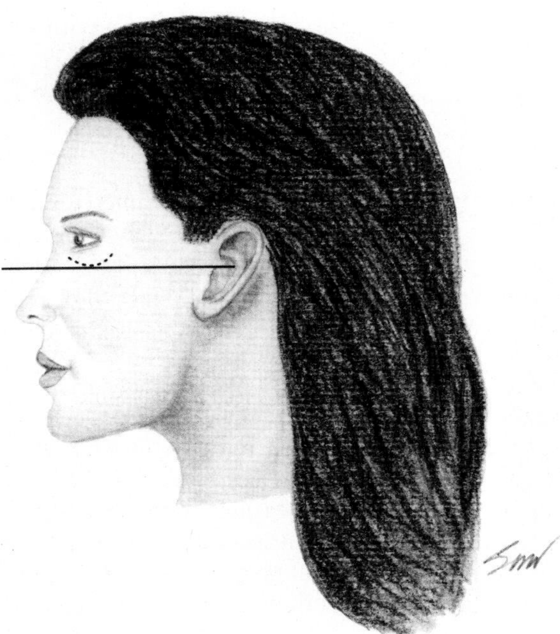

Fig. 11.5 The Frankfort horizontal may be approximated on lateral photographs by constructing a line from the superior margin of the tragus to the junction between the lower eyelid and the cheek skin.

Reference Points

The Frankfort horizontal is the standard reference for patient positioning in photographs and cephalometric radiographs. A line drawn from the superior aspect of the external auditory canal to the inferior aspect of the infraorbital rim is placed parallel to the plane of the floor to achieve this standardized position. Obviously, these points are more easily determined on lateral skull radiographs than photographs. When determining this position for patient photographs the hair must be pulled back sufficiently to reveal the tragus. The superior edge of the tragus approximates the superior aspect of the external auditory canal. The point of transition between the skin of the lower eyelid and the skin of the cheek is usually discernible and approximates the level of the infraorbital rim (**Fig. 11.5**).

For measurements of the face to provide meaningful information for communication with colleagues or for accurate records, standard reference points must be used. These have been standardized for use in facial surgery by Powell and Humphreys.[20]

Aesthetic Assessment

The initial assessment of the face is to determine facial height. This is measured in the midline from the hairline (trichion, Tr) to the lowest contour point of the chin (menton, Me). In those with a receding hairline, the

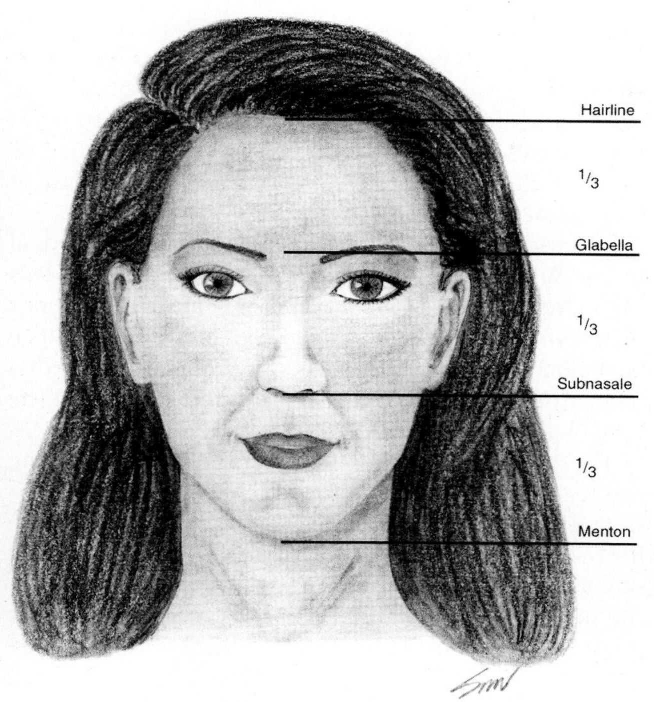

Fig. 11.6 The length of the face is divided into three equal divisions at the levels shown.

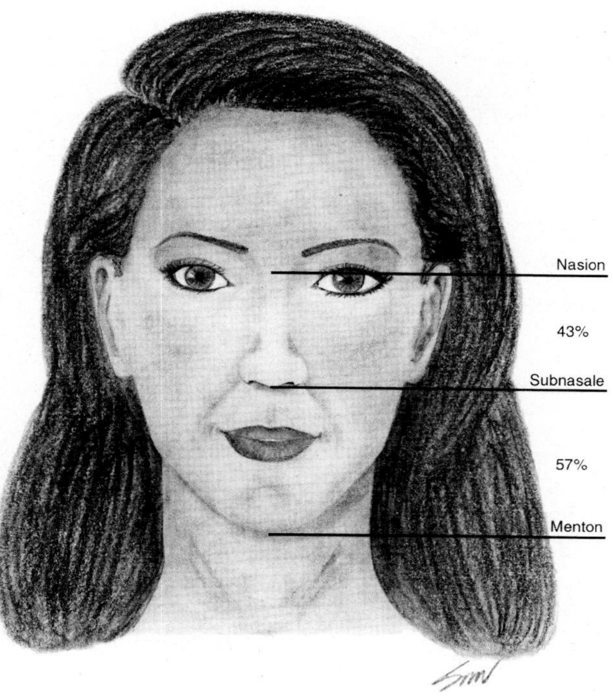

Fig. 11.7 The lower face is divided into a ratio as shown, 43:57.

trichion (Tr) may be determined by the uppermost point of action of the frontalis muscle. The face can then be divided into thirds at the most prominent point of the forehead (glabella, G) and the point at which the nasal columella merges with the upper cutaneous lip (subnasale, Sn). The upper, middle, and lower portions of the face should be equal using this method (**Fig. 11.6**).

A second method for assessing facial height takes into account only the middle and lower portions of the face. The initial measurement is taken from the deepest depression at the root of the nose (nasion, N) to the menton (Me). Midfacial height (N–Sn) should be 43% of the total, and lower facial height (Sn–Me) should be 57% of the total length (**Fig. 11.7**). The following are advantages of this method over the first: (1) the nasion (N) is a more reproducible landmark than the glabella (G) and (2) imbalance of the upper third of the face (forehead) is not easily amenable to surgical intervention.

The face is then subdivided into the following five major aesthetic units for further analysis: forehead, eyes, nose, lips, and chin. In addition, the ears and neck should be considered separately and as they relate to the face as a whole.

Forehead

The forehead comprises the entire upper one third of the face. It forms a stable mass that is not readily modified. The aesthetically pleasing forehead produces a gentle convexity on profile with its most anterior point just above the nasion (N) at the level of the supraorbital ridge. Other possible forehead shapes include protruding, flat, and sloping.

The nasofrontal angle (NFr) is formed at the transition between the nose and forehead, where the nasal dorsum merges with the glabella (G). The angle is determined by a tangent passing through the glabella (G) and the nasion (N), and another tangent along the nasal dorsum. This angle should ideally be 115 to 135 degrees (**Fig. 11.8**).

The eyebrows separate the upper and middle portions of the face and frame the eyes. The medial edge of the eyebrow lies on a perpendicular that passes through the lateralmost portion of the ala nasi and ~1.0 cm above the medial canthus of the eye. The brow should begin medially with a slight clublike configuration and gradually taper toward its lateral end. In women the brow should rest just above the level of the supraorbital rim. An arch is desirable in women, with its highest point at the level of the lateral limbus. The brow should end laterally at an oblique line that begins at the ala nasi and passes tangentially along the lateral aspect of the lower lid. The medial and lateral ends of the brow should lie on the same horizontal plane. In men the brow may form less of an arch and lie slightly lower at the level of the supraorbital rim (**Fig. 11.9**).[21]

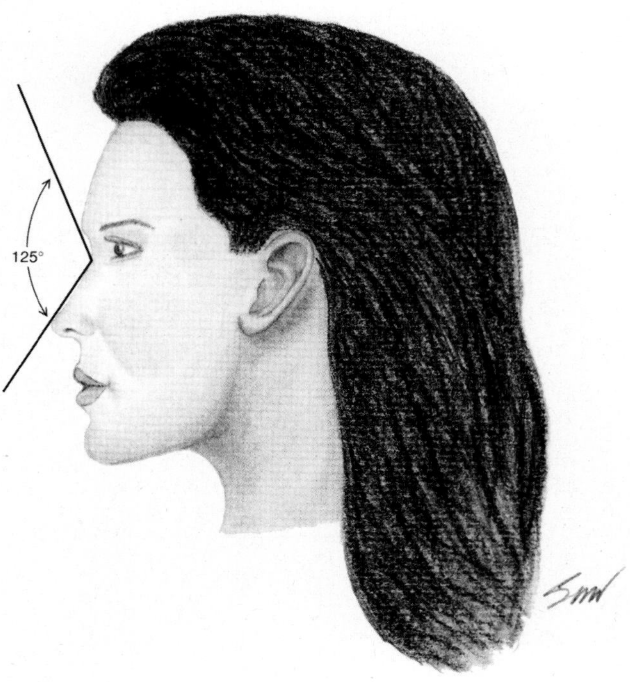

Fig. 11.8 The nasofrontal angle.

Eyes

The eyes are perhaps the most expressive part of the face and have been referred to as the window of the soul. Nowhere else in the body are asymmetries more noticeable than in the eyes. The effects of aging become apparent in the eyes sooner than in the other parts of the face. With increasing laxity of the skin of the eyelids, the eyes may project a tired, humorless expression that may be quite out of line with actual physical and mental state of the patient.

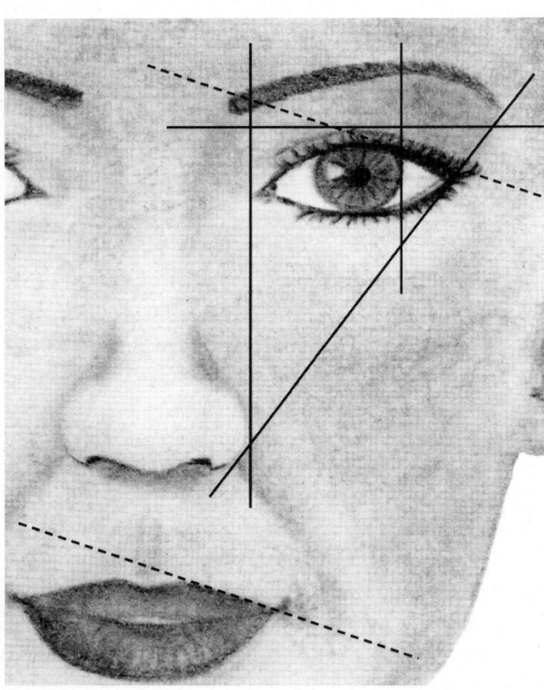

Fig. 11.9 Relationships of the eyebrow, eyelids, limbus, nasal ala, and upper lip.

The width of the eye from canthus to canthus is equal to one fifth the width of a well-proportioned face. This same measurement should approximate the distance between the medial canthi (see **Fig. 11.4**). The distance between the midpoints of the pupils should equal the distance from the nasion (N) to the vermilion border of the upper lip (labrale superius, LS).

The supraorbital rim lies slightly anterior to the infraorbital rim when the head is in the neutral position. The lateral canthus is attached posterior to the level of attachment of the medial canthus. The lateral canthi may lie on the same horizontal plane with the medial canthi or slightly above. The superiormost point along the arch formed by the free margin of the upper lid is at the level of a vertical passing through the medial limbus. The lateral portion of the free margin of the upper eyelid should parallel a tangent passing along the lateral vermilion border of the upper lip (**Fig. 11.9**).

The inferiormost point of the curve of the lower lid margin is along a vertical passing through the lateral limbus. If the lateral one third of the lower lid does not form a line rising steadily toward the lateral canthus, a subtle defect referred to as lateral scleral show may be present (**Fig. 11.10**). This may result from excessive excision of lower-eyelid skin during blepharoplasty.

The distance from the lash line to the lid crease in the upper lid varies from 7 to 15 mm and is related to body weight, skin thickness, and ethnicity. The upper eyelid normally covers a small portion of the iris but does not touch the pupil. The lower lid is within 1 to 2 mm of the iris on neutral gaze.[19]

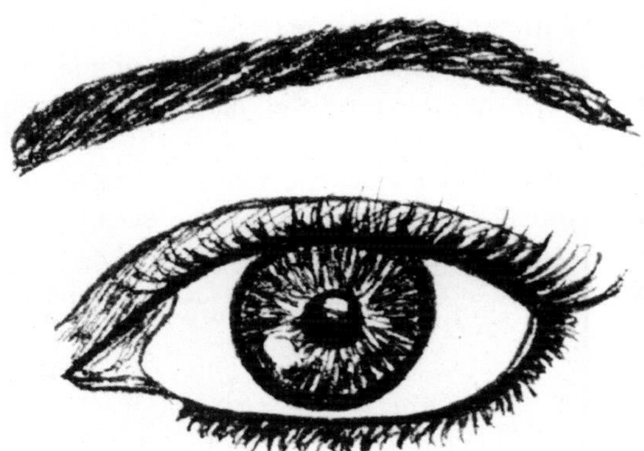

Fig. 11.10 Lateral scleral show.

Nose

The nose is the central focus of facial appearance by virtue of its position in the midline of the central third of the face. The tremendous significance of its form and function is reflected in the earliest writings of the Judeo-Christian tradition: "God formed man and breathed into his nostrils the breath of life."[22] Slight changes in the structure of the nose can sometimes produce dramatic improvements in facial harmony and the perception of the surrounding aesthetic units. The ideal nose should appear natural and in harmony with its surrounding features and not draw attention to itself.[23]

The nose is the central aesthetic unit of the face. It can be further subdivided into aesthetic or topographic subunits. These include the dorsum, sides, tip, alae, and soft triangles.[24] The borders of these subunits allow for camouflage of scars resulting from reconstruction of nasal surface defects (**Fig. 11.11**). When incisions lie along the margins of these natural anatomical subunits, the eye is less apt to recognize the scar. Excising additional nasal skin to make the defect fit an aesthetic subunit before reconstruction will ultimately produce a less noticeable incision.

The issue of nasal measurement is made quite complex by the plethora of methods available in the literature and the lack of standardization. The various methods have been reviewed by Powell and Humphreys[20] and are summarized here.

Angle Measurements

The nasofrontal angle (NFr) has been described previously (see **Fig. 11.8**), but a second angle measurement is necessary to define the proportions of the aesthetic nose. The nasofacial angle (NFa) is the incline of the dorsum of the nose in relation to the plane of the face (**Fig. 11.12**). On the lateral profile a line is drawn from the glabella (G) to the most anterior point of the chin (pogonion, Pg). The nasofacial angle (NFa) is defined when this line is intersected by the line of the dorsum of the nose. The dorsal line should intersect the nasion (N) and the tip (T) and should be drawn through any dorsal hump that exists.

The third angle measurement in the evaluation of the nose is the nasolabial angle (NL) (see **Fig. 11.3**). Lines are constructed between the upper mucocutaneous border of

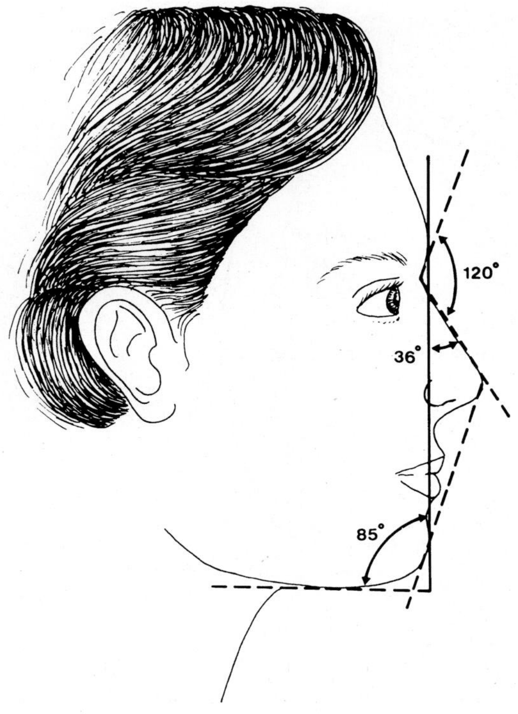

Fig. 11.12 The nasofacial angle.

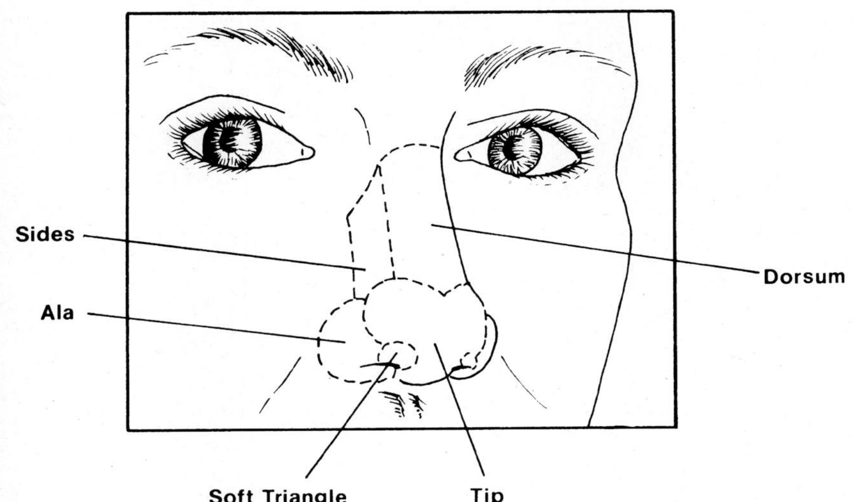

Fig. 11.11 Aesthetic or topographic subunits of the nose. (From Burget GC. Aesthetic restoration of the nose. Clin Plast Surg 1985;12:463. With permission.)

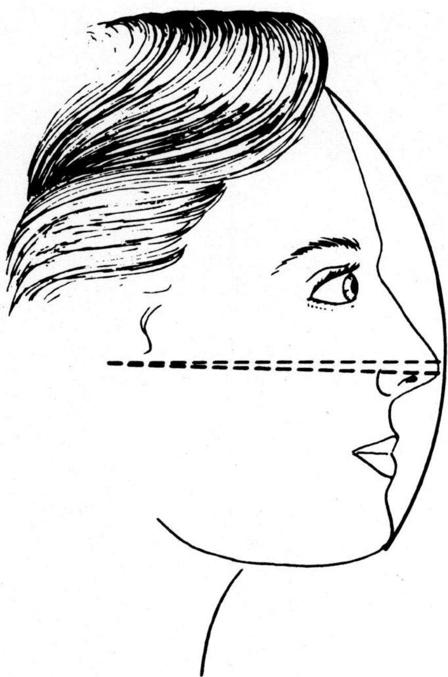

Fig. 11.13 Nasal tip rotation occurs along an arc based at the external auditory canal.

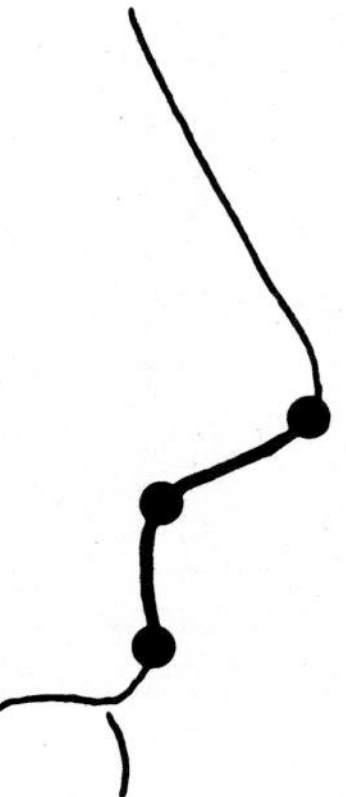

Fig. 11.14 Relationship of nasal tip projection to the length of the upper lip.

the lip (LS) and the subnasale (Sn), and between the subnasale (Sn) and the most anterior point on the columella of the nose (Cm). This angle defines the relationship between the nose and the upper lip. It is susceptible to abnormalities of the facial skeleton and dentition. This angle should measure 90 to 95 degrees in men and 95 to 105 degrees in women. Shorter individuals tolerate a more obtuse angle, whereas taller people require a nasolabial angle at the low end of the range for their gender.

Projection

It is necessary to differentiate between nasal projection and rotation. These two quantities are closely related perceptually. Cephalic movement of the lower lateral cartilages combined with lowering of the nasal dorsum can give the illusion of increased tip projection, even though actual projection has not changed. Tip rotation generally occurs along an arc produced by a radius based at the external auditory canal (**Fig. 11.13**).

Simons[25] prefers to measure tip projection in relation to the length of the upper lip. The upper lip is measured from the vermilion border (LS) to its junction with the nasal columella (Sn). The length of the nasal tip (T) is measured from the subnasale (Sn) to the anteriormost point of the nose. The ratio of these measurements should be as shown in (**Fig. 11.14**). Accurate measurement of these distances is difficult because of the complex topography of these structures, even when done on lateral photographs.

The method also assumes that the length of the upper lip is normal. Given the variability of upper lip lengths and the difficulties encountered in changing this measurement surgically, this method does not address all circumstances related to the measurement of tip projection.

Goode[20] uses a vertical line drawn from the nasion (N) to the alar groove and constructs a perpendicular line to the nasal tip (T) to evaluate tip projection. The ratio of the length of the perpendicular line to the nasal length as measured from the nasion to the tip (N–T) should be 0.55 to 0.60. This will maintain a nasofacial angle (NFa) of 36 to 40 degrees (**Fig. 11.15**).

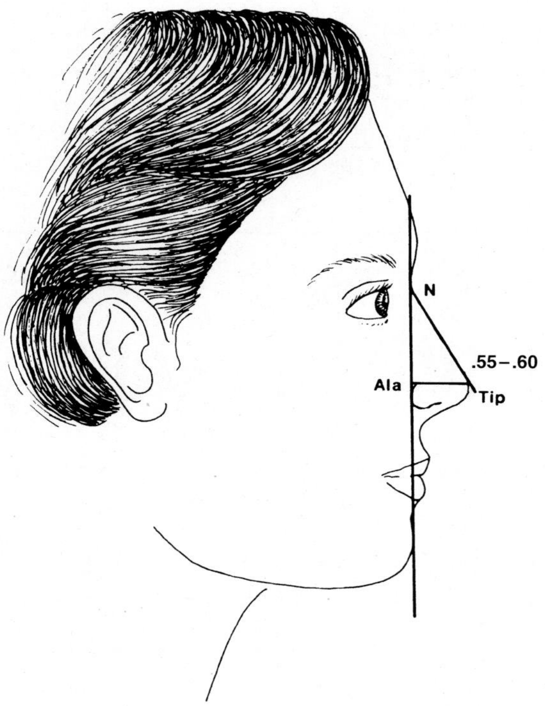

Fig. 11.15 The Goode method of measuring nasal tip projection.

Length

Nasal length has already been discussed in relation to facial proportions (i.e., glabella to subnasale is one third of the height, and nasion to subnasale is 43% of the distance from the nasion to the menton). However, these methods do not take the nasal tip (T) into consideration. Any subjective assessment of nasal length demonstrates the importance of the distance between the nasion (N) and the nasal tip (T). This measurement corresponds more precisely with the subjective impression of nasal length than do measurements taken to the subnasale (Sn).

Width

Nasal width is proportional to the width of one eye at the nasal base. If the distance between the medial canthi is proportionate (i.e., one eye-width), verticals drawn from the medial canthi should pass along the lateral alae (see **Fig. 11.4**).

Another method for determining proportional nasal width is to measure the nasal length from nasion (N) to tip (T) and calculate a desired nasal width as 70% of this number.

Basal View

The tip represents about one third of the total height of the base on basal view of the nose. The nares account for about two thirds of this distance. When viewed from its basal aspect, the nares are ovoid and obliquely slanted toward the tip. The anterior end of the naris is narrow, whereas the posterior end is wider and rounder. On frontal view the nares are barely visible with the head in a neutral position. Close inspection will reveal the facets of the nasal tip that are a reflection of the underlying soft tissue triangle of the rim. When viewed in profile, the columella is seen 2 to 3 mm below the level of the alae (**Fig. 11.16**).

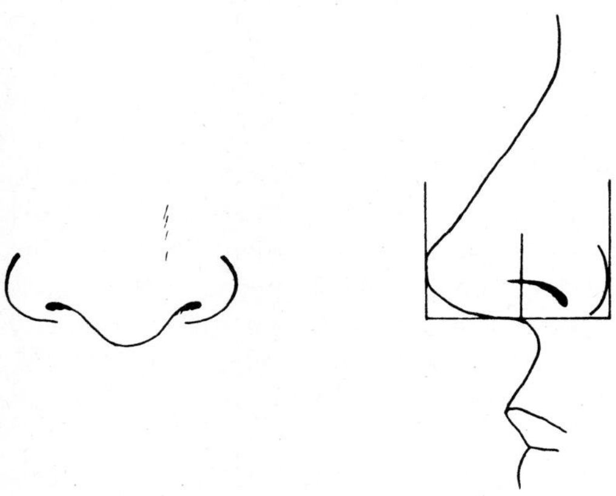

Fig. 11.16 The nasal tip. (**A**) Frontal view. (**B**) Lateral view showing tip-to-ala ratio.

Lateral View

On lateral view the ala-to-tip lobule ratio should be about equal. Tip lobular excess is more pleasing aesthetically than alar excess.[26] The nasal tip (T) in profile has a double break produced by the tip-defining point of the lobule anteriorly and the junction of the lobule with the columella inferiorly. Just above the tip there should exist a slight depression in the line of the nasal profile known as the supratip break. A more pronounced supratip break is acceptable in women than in men. A straighter nasal dorsum is desirable in men.

Lips

The lips are a dynamic and expressive aesthetic unit of the face. Fullness of the lips and strong definition of the philtrum are associated with youth. A thin vermilion, loss of lip highlights, and flatness are associated with aging.

The posture of the lips, designated as procumbent or recumbent, greatly depends on the underlying dental support. On frontal view the oral commissures are on a line vertical with the medial limbus. The lips are contained within the boundaries of the lower one third of facial height. The upper lip is measured from the subnasale (Sn) to the lowermost point on the vermilion of the upper lip. The lower lip is measured from the uppermost point on its vermilion to the menton (Me). The length of the lower lip should be about twice the length of the upper lip, using these points for measurement.

Horizontal lip position can be determined by constructing a line between the subnasale (Sn) and the soft tissue pogonion (Pg). The distance along a perpendicular from this line to the most anterior point of each lip defines its horizontal position (**Fig. 11.17**). The upper lip should rest 3.5 mm anterior to this line and the lower lip 2.2 mm.[27]

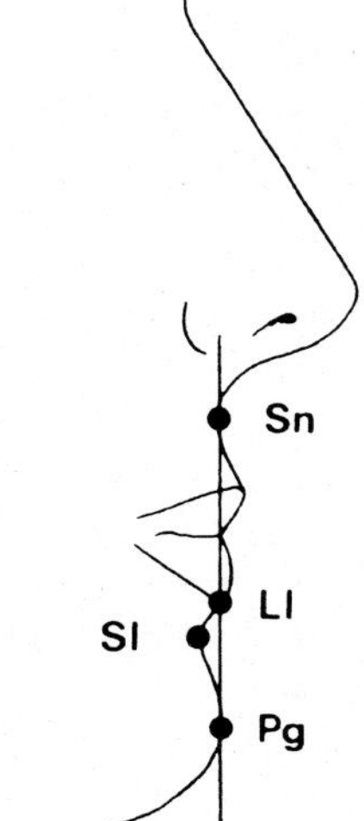

Fig. 11.17 The horizontal position of the lips and the mentolabial sulcus relative to a line drawn from the subnasale to the pogonion. Sn, subnasale; Pg, pogonion.

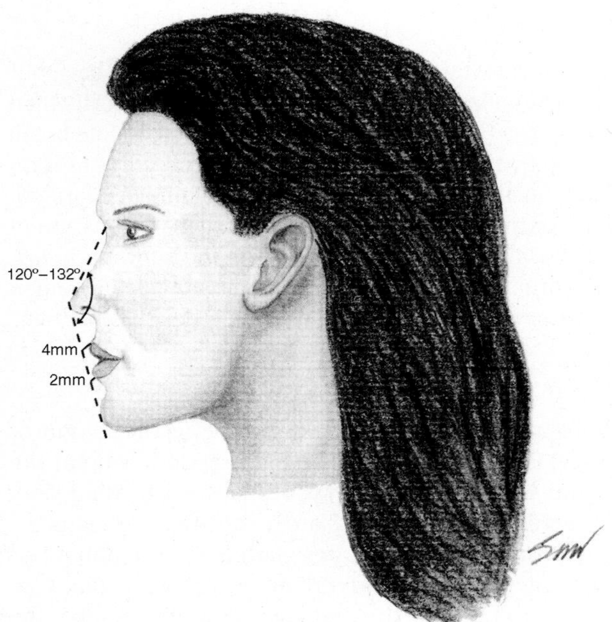

Fig. 11.18 The nasomental angle is formed by the intersection of the line of the nasal dorsum and the nasomental line. The upper lip should fall 4 mm posterior to this line and the lower lip 2 mm behind it.

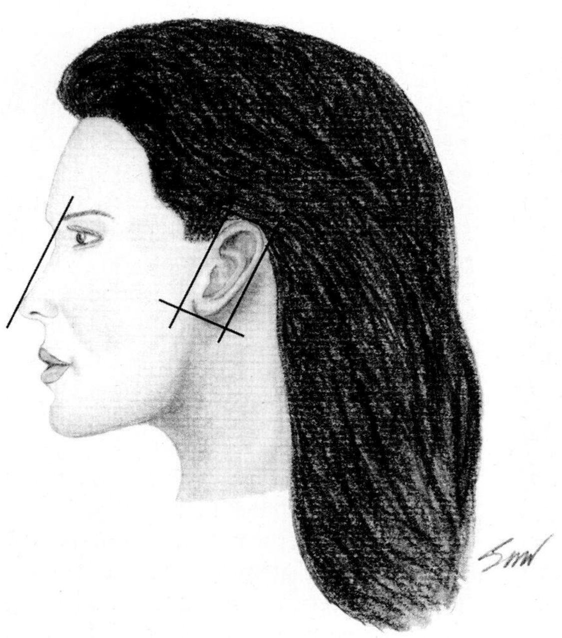

Fig. 11.19 The long axis of the ear is parallel to the line of the nasal dorsum. Ear width should be 55 to 60% of its length.

A second method of assessing horizontal lip position is to construct a line between the nasal tip (T) and the pogonion (Pg) termed the nasomental line (**Fig. 11.18**). The lips should lie posterior to this line. The lower lip ideally falls 2 mm posterior to this line and upper lip 4 mm behind it. This concept was described by Ricketts as the E-line and has been incorporated into the aesthetic triangle by Powell and Humphreys.[20]

Chin

The chin is the aesthetic unit that confers strength to the face. The anterior limit is at a vertical dropped from the brow. For the chin to have pleasing form it must be well defined from both frontal and lateral views without appearing knoblike.[19] There should be a definite, but gentle, mentolabial sulcus separating the cutaneous lower lip from the chin.

The chin is included in measurement of the lower portion of the face (Sn to Me), as well as being part of the length of the lower lip (to Me). The lower lip and chin compose two thirds of the lower portion of the face.

When measured from a line drawn between the vermilion border of the lower lip (labrale inferius, LI) to the pogonion (Pg), the deepest point of the mentolabial sulcus (Si) should lie ~4 mm behind this line (**Fig. 11.17**).

Ears

An additional facial feature to be considered is the ear. This flaplike, cartilaginous appendage has multiple convolutions and is attached to the scalp approximately one ear length posterior to the lateral brow. The superior aspect of the ear is at the level of the brow, and its inferior aspect is at the level of the ala nasi.

The width of the ear is 55 to 60% of its length. The line of the posterior aspect of the auricle roughly parallels the dorsal plane of the nose.[28] The long axis of the ear is posteriorly rotated ~15 degrees from the vertical plane (**Fig. 11.19**). The auricle produces an angle of ~20 degrees with the mastoid posteriorly. The superior portion of the helix should rest at ~15 to 20 mm from the squamous portion of the temporal bone.

Neck

Although the neck is not usually considered one of the major aesthetic units of the face, its shape, especially in the upper portion, can have a marked impact on the appearance of the chin and lower portion of the face. A low-lying hyoid bone, excessive submental fat, or laxity of the platysma can cause the neck–chin contour to be obtuse and create the perception of a chin deformity that does not exist.

Powell and Humphreys[20] have defined the mentocervical angle (MC), which relates the line of the neck to that of the entire face. The angle is produced by constructing

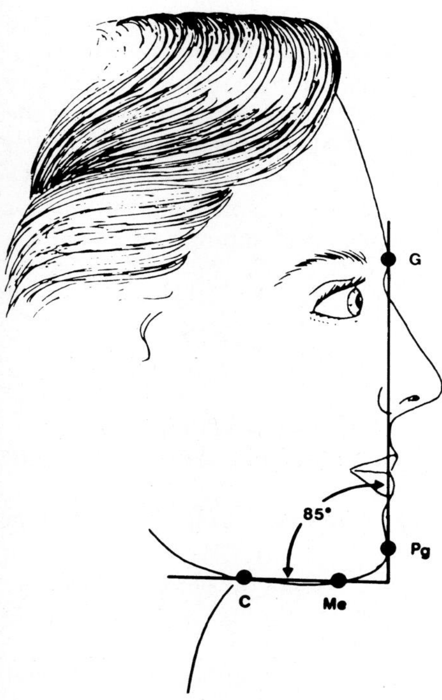

Fig. 11.20 The mentocervical angle. Relative degree of upper, middle, and lower facial protrusion or retrusion. This method does not take into account the angle of the neck or the projection of the nose in the facial analysis. C, cervical point; G, glabella; Me, menton; Pg, pogonion.

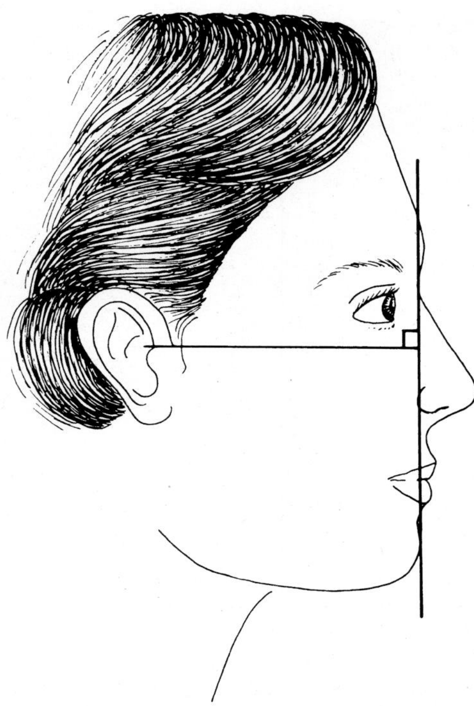

Fig. 11.21 The zero meridian of Gonzales-Ulloa.

the facial plane from the glabella (G) to the pogonion (Pg), and intersecting a line drawn from the menton (Me) to the innermost point between the submental area and the neck (the cervical point, C). This angle should ideally be between 80 degrees and 95 degrees (**Fig. 11.20**).

Aesthetic Analysis of the Face

Gonzales-Ulloa[29,30] based his method of facial profileplasty on the relationship of the facial structures to the facial plane, which he termed the zero meridian (**Fig. 11.21**). In the ideal facial profile, the facial plane lies 85 to 92 degrees relative to the Frankfort horizontal when constructed through the nasion (N). On the forehead, the glabella (G) lies just anterior to the plane and then slopes gently posteriorly. The alar crease is posterior to the plane. In the lower face the anteriormost point of the chin should lie within the plane. Using this concept a plane constructed approximately perpendicular to the Frankfort horizontal through the nasion (N) will indicate the relative degree of upper, middle, and lower facial protrusion or retrusion. This method does not take into account the angle of the neck or the projection of the nose in the facial analysis.

The aesthetic triangle was described by Powell and Humphreys in 1984.[20] This method of facial analysis allows for consideration of all of the major aesthetic masses of the face and illustrates their interdependence. Angles that have been considered separately can now be assessed simultaneously to evaluate facial harmony. It is first necessary to define one additional angle that has not yet been considered. The nasomental angle is formed by the intersection of the dorsal line of the nose and the nasomental line (**Fig. 11.18**).

The analysis begins at the forehead, which is relatively stable and the least amenable to surgical alteration. The facial plane is constructed between the glabella (G) and the pogonion (Pg). The facial plane determined by this method should intersect the Frankfort horizontal plane at an angle of 80 to 95 degrees. The glabella (G) is used as the reference point on the forehead rather than the nasion (N) (as used by Gonzales-Ulloa) because the position of the nasion (N) can be changed relatively easily by deepening the nasofrontal angle (NFr).

The nasofrontal angle (NFr) is then drawn as described previously. This angle should ideally be between 115 degrees and 135 degrees. The nasofacial angle (NFa) can now be measured from these lines as well. This angle should lie in the range of 30 to 40 degrees (**Fig. 11.22**).

The nasomental line is then constructed between the pogonion (Pg) and nasal tip (T). This creates the most important angle of the aesthetic triangle, the nasomental angle. The ideal range for this angle is 120 to 132 degrees. The upper line of this angle, the dorsal line of the nose, is primarily dependent on nasal projection. The lower line,

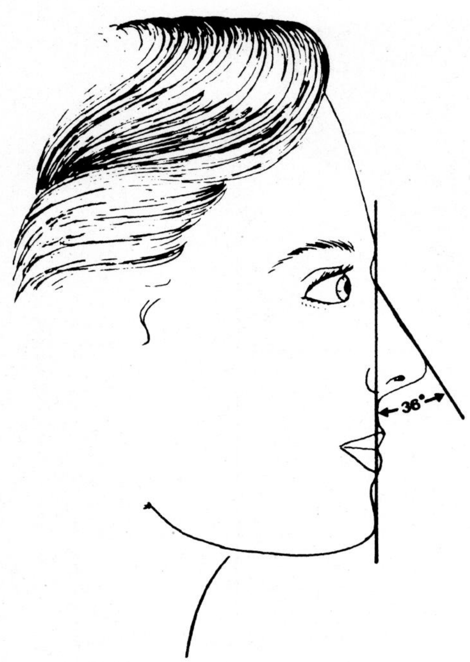

Fig. 11.22 Facial analysis using the aesthetic triangle of Powell and Humphreys. Components include the following: (1) the facial plane, (2) the nasofrontal angle (NFr), (3) the nasomental angle, and (4) the mentocervical angle (MC).

the nasomental line, is readily modified by the position of the chin. The nasomental line also allows horizontal position of the lips to be assessed. The upper lip should lie ~4 mm behind this line and the lower lip ~2 mm behind it (**Fig. 11.18**).

Finally, the mentocervical angle (MC) is measured. This angle evaluates the neck line and its relationship to the lower face. It is determined by constructing a line between the cervical point (C) and the lowermost point on the chin (Me) to intersect the facial plane. This angle should measure between 80 and 95 degrees (**Fig. 11.20**).

The aesthetic triangle is therefore affected by the nasofrontal angle (NFr) or depth of the nasion (N), the degree of nasal projection, and the position of the chin. Its appropriateness can be confirmed by the range of normal values for the primary, or nasomental, angle and by the relationship of its upper and lower lines to the facial plane; that is, the nasofacial angle (NFa) and to the horizontal position of the lips (i.e., 4 mm to the upper lip and 2 mm to the lower lip).

Summary

Numerous methods have been presented for assessment of the individual aesthetic units of the face and for the determination of their relative proportions in evaluating the face as a whole. Other factors, such as age, ethnicity, body habitus, and personality, must also be taken into account in the aesthetic assessment of the face. Although no precise algorithm for the determination of facial beauty exists, preoperative facial measurements assist in the determination of which facial features need to change to produce harmony with the face as a whole. Postoperative determination of the same measurements allows for assessment of the adequacy and appropriateness of the change.

Glossary

alar groove junction of the ala nasi with the cheek
cervical point (C) innermost point between the submental area and the neck
columella point (Cm) anteriormost soft tissue point on the nasal columella
dorsal line line passing through the nasion (N) and the nasal tip (T); should be drawn through any dorsal hump that exists
facial plane coronal plane passing through the face at the glabella (G) and pogonion (Pg)
Frankfort horizontal line drawn from the superior aspect of the bony external auditory canal to the inferiormost aspect of the infraorbital rim on a lateral radiograph; approximated on photograph by a line from the superior tragus to lower eyelid–cheek skin junction
glabella (G) most prominent point of the forehead on profile; usually at the level of the supraorbital rim
gonion most inferior, posterior, and lateral point on the external angle of the mandible
labrale inferius (LI) vermilion border of the lower lip
labrale superius (LS) vermilion border of the upper lip
mentocervical angle (MC) angle of a line drawn from the menton (Me) to the cervical point (C) relative to the facial plane
menton (Me) lowest contour point of the chin
nasion (N) point of deepest depression at the root of the nose
nasofacial angle (NFa) incline of the dorsum of the nose in relation to the facial plane
nasofrontal angle (NFr) angle defined by a tangent passing from the nasion (N) through the glabella (G) and the dorsal line of the nose
nasolabial angle (NL) angle between the line of the nasal columella (Sn–Cm) and the line of the upper lip (Sn–LS)
nasomental angle intersection of the dorsal line of the nose and a line from the pogonion (Pg) to the nasal tip (T)
nasomental line a line connecting the pogonion (Pg) and the nasal tip (T)
pogonion (Pg) anteriormost point of the chin

stomion inferius (stmi) uppermost point on the vermilion of the lower lip
stomion superius (stms) lowermost point on the vermilion of the upper lip
subnasale (Sn) point at which the nasal columella merges with the upper cutaneous lip
tip, nasal (T) anterior-most point on nasal profile
trichion (Tr) anterior hairline at the midline; may be determined in those with a receding hairline as the superiormost point of action of the frontalis muscle.

Acknowledgments

Illustrations by Steven M. VanHook, MD, and Renée Clements, BAA.

References

1. Patterson CN, Powell DG. Facial analysis in patient evaluation for physiologic and cosmetic surgery. Laryngoscope 1974;84:1004–1019
2. Fordham SD. Art for head and neck surgeons. In: Ward PH, Berman WE, eds. Plastic and Reconstructive Surgery of the Head and Neck: Proceedings of the Fourth International Symposium. St. Louis: CV Mosby; 1984
3. Gonzalez-Ulloa M. A quantum method for the appreciation of the morphology of the face. Plast Reconstr Surg 1964;34:241–246
4. Romm S. The Changing Face of Beauty. St. Louis: Mosby–Year Book; 1992
5. Tolleth H. Concepts for the plastic surgeon from art and sculpture. Clin Plast Surg 1987;14:585–598
6. Janson H. History of Art. 4th ed. New York: Harry N. Abrams; 1991
7. Whiting R. Leonardo: A Portrait of the Renaissance Man. New York: Knickerbocker; 1998
8. Ricketts RM. Divine proportion in facial esthetics. Clin Plast Surg 1982;9:401–422
9. Gonzalez-Ulloa M, Flores ES. Senility of the face: basic study to understand its causes and effects. Plast Reconstr Surg 1965;36:239–246
10. Davidson TM, Murakami WT. Rhinoplasty Planning: Aesthetic Concepts, Dynamics, and Facial Construction. 2nd ed. Washington, DC: American Academy of Otolaryngology–Head and Neck Surgery Foundation; 1986
11. Farkas LG, Hreczko TA, Kolar JC, Munro IR. Vertical and horizontal proportions of the face in young adult North American Caucasians: revision of neoclassical canons. Plast Reconstr Surg 1985;75:328–338
12. Jeffries JM III, DiBernardo B, Rauscher GE. Computer analysis of the African American face. Ann Plast Surg 1995;34:318–321
13. Abdelkader M, Leong S, White PS. Aesthetic proportions of the nasal aperture in 3 different racial groups of men. Arch Facial Plast Surg 2005;7:111–113
14. Choe KS, Sclafani AP, Litner JA, Yu GP, Romo T III. The Korean American woman's face: anthropometric measurements and quantitative analysis of facial aesthetics. Arch Facial Plast Surg 2004;6:244–252
15. Sim RS, Smith JD, Chan AS. Comparison of the aesthetic facial proportions of southern Chinese and white women. Arch Facial Plast Surg 2000;2:113–120
16. Rhee SC, Kang SR, Park HS. Balanced angular profile analysis. Plast Reconstr Surg 2004;114:535–544
17. Beeson WH. Facial analysis. In: Beeson WH, McCollough EG, eds. Aesthetic Surgery of the Aging Face. St. Louis: Mosby; 1986
18. Seghers MJ, Longacre JJ, deStefano GA. The golden proportion and beauty. Plast Reconstr Surg 1964;34:382–386
19. Tolleth H. Concepts for the plastic surgeon from art and sculpture. Clin Plast Surg 1987;14:585–597
20. Powell N, Humphreys B. Proportions of the Aesthetic Face. New York: Thieme-Stratton; 1984
21. Rafaty FM, Brennan G. Current concepts of browpexy. Arch Otolaryngol 1983;109:152–154
22. Bible, Genesis 2:7. King James Version
23. Tardy ME, Becker OJ. Surgical correction of facial deformities. In: Ballenger JJ, ed. Diseases of the Nose, Throat, and Ear. Philadelphia: Lea & Febiger; 1977
24. Burget GC. Aesthetic restoration of the nose. Clin Plast Surg 1985;12:463–480
25. Simons RL. Nasal tip projection, ptosis, and supratip thickening. Ear Nose Throat J 1982;61:452–455
26. Bernstein L. Aesthetics in rhinoplasty. Otolaryngol Clin North Am 1975;8:705–715
27. Burstone CJ. Lip posture and its significance in treatment planning. Am J Orthod 1967;53:262–284
28. Krugman ME. Photoanalysis of the rhinoplasty patient. Ear Nose Throat J 1981;60:328–330
29. Gonzalez-Ulloa M. Quantitative principles in cosmetic surgery of the face (profileplasty). Plast Reconstr Surg Transplant Bull 1962;29:186–198
30. González-Ulloa M, Stevens E. The role of chin correction in profileplasty. Plast Reconstr Surg 1968;41:477–486

12 Computer Imaging for Facial Plastic Surgery

Ira D. Papel

Computer imaging in clinical practice has changed enormously since its introduction in the 1980s. Enhanced technologies in computer hardware and software, combined with extensive public information about facial surgery, have increased the popularity and availability of imaging systems in surgeons' offices. Imaging systems have been used for diverse purposes such as resident and fellow education,[1] patient–surgeon communication,[2] detailed facial analysis,[3] archiving of patient images, and marketing of surgical practices.[4] There are many practical, ethical, and legal issues that have been raised by the advent of computer imaging. In this chapter we will try to address the highlights of this interesting tool in facial plastic surgery.

Historical Background

The earliest forms of patient imaging involved freehand sketches of anticipated surgical results by surgeons. Photographic techniques were not practical or affordable until the second half of the nineteenth century. As emulsion photography became more available, alterations of these images were used to communicate changes to the patient. Patient images in profile against dark backgrounds could be used to demonstrate reduction rhinoplasty or rhytidectomy procedures. In the twentieth century it became possible to print photographs on paper, and this made the foregoing techniques more practical. Drawing on the back of photographic prints could be used to envision profile changes against a background light. Instant photography provided another tool for swiftly demonstrating patient characteristics and could be drawn upon to suggest changes.

Another method of demonstrating changes is to project 35 mm slides onto a white drawing tablet. This allows freehand alteration of the projected image to demonstrate potential surgical changes. When computer imaging became available the relative ease and speed of the computer overshadowed all of these time-tested methods. Although the early computer graphic programs were cumbersome and required practice, the newer systems are much more user-friendly. The common element in any imaging system is that surgeons must have a clear idea of what they would like their patients to see and understand. This requires that the surgeon have a well-developed sense of facial analysis and aesthetics, and the ability to express this with the computer tools available.

System Requirements

Modern imaging systems may be purchased from various vendors with a variety of features. The core of each system involves an image capture device, such as a digital video or still camera. Digital cameras are now commercially available with up to 14 megapixels per image. A camera with a 6 to 8 megapixel capacity will serve very well for most imaging techniques. The image is then downloaded into a computer and archived for current or future use. Each imaging system utilizes special software developed for patient image modification. Graphics boards, digital drawing tablet, large hard drive, backup tape system, monitor, and lighting system are essential. The computer should include at least 1 gigabyte of RAM, a 100 gigabyte hard drive, and a central processing unit of at least 3.0 MHz speed to cope with the large memory and speed demands of graphic imaging. The equipment should be situated so that patient and surgeon may sit near the monitor and discuss proposed surgical techniques and anticipated changes. Many offices combine the lighting used for traditional photography and computer imaging in one multimedia room. A printer may be used to make hard copies of computer images if desired.

Many commercial systems are available for purchase in a wide range of prices. Those systems with purely digital image capture systems and sophisticated hardware can run as high as $30,000. Basic systems can cost a fraction of this. It is possible to assemble reasonable hardware and purchase software to reproduce these graphic systems for a much lower cost. This requires the ability to integrate computer software and hardware into a working unit.

The patient background should be a consistent color and shade to facilitate a fair comparison of images. A light blue background seems to be aesthetically pleasing and provides good contrast with natural skin tones.[5] Lighting should be provided that eliminates shadows but does not flatten out the details of the face and skin. Indirect modeling lights with umbrellas and diffusers

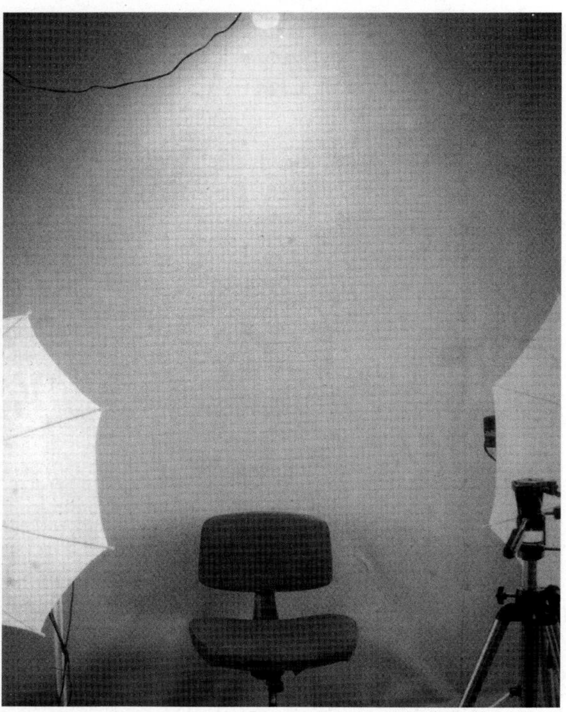

Fig. 12.1 Demonstration of lighting system used for computer imaging.

from at least two directions will provide excellent images (**Fig. 12.1**).

Images are captured in the same patient positions as with conventional photography. Soft tissue reference points, such as the tragus, angle of mandible, and anterior hairline, should be visible to enhance analysis potential. It is recommended that all images be stored on the hard disk prior to initiating graphic changes. These will prevent loss of images if there is a computer failure. Each system should have an external backup, such as a tape drive or off-site facility, to download files at the end of each day.

In 1998 it was estimated that 8 to 10% of cosmetic surgery practices were utilizing computer imaging in some capacity. This number was expected to grow to 40% by 2001.[6]

Analysis and Applications

Computer imaging provides an opportunity to assess patient characteristics in a quantitative fashion. These analytical data can be used in conjunction with aesthetic judgment to plan potential facial surgery. Imaging also gives the patient a chance to assess the surgeon's goals, thus creating a very important communication device that was lacking before sophisticated imaging systems were available. The surgeon may also assess whether the patient has realistic ideas of what facial surgery can attain. Based on this interaction either patient or surgeon may decide that surgery is not indicated due to patient–surgeon incompatibility. This is beneficial for surgeon and patient alike.

In planning facial surgery the relationship to quantitative facial ideals may be considered. With the imaging systems it is fairly easy to generate data based on quantitative facial measurements as defined by several authors to assist in facial analysis.[7–10] These techniques have been used for instruction in facial analysis for resident surgeons and fellows. The most common key points for facial analysis, definitions, and aesthetic norms are listed in the glossary and **Tables 12.1 and 12.2**.

Table 12.1 Definition of Measurements

Frankfort and vertical planes	Intercept of tragion to infraorbital rim with glabela to pogonion line
Nasofrontal angle	Intercept of glabela to nasion line with nasion to tip line
Nasofacial angle	Intercept of glabela to pogonion line with nasion to tip line
Nasomental angle	Intercept of nasion to tip line with tip to pogonion line
Mentocervical angle	Intercept of glabela to pogonion line with menton to cervical point line
Nasal height	Nasion to subnasale
Lower facial height	Subnasale to menton
Legan facial convexity angle	Intercept of glabela to subnasion line with subnasion to pogonion line
Nasolabial angle	Intercept of columella point to subnasale line with subnasale to labrale superioris line
Columellar show	Midnares to subnasion
Goode nasal projection ratio	Alar point to tip divided by nasion-to-tip distances; alar point defined by intercept of nasion-to-ala line with perpendicular line to tip
Alar lobule ratio	Tip to posterior lobule divided by posterior lobule to ala
Mentolabial sulcus	Distance from labrale inferioris to pogonion line to mentolabial sulcus

Table 12.2 Aesthetic Norms for Facial Analysis

Profile Analysis	
Frankfort and vertical planes	80–95 degrees
Aesthetic triangle	
Nasofrontal angle	115–130 degrees
Nasofacial angle	30–40 degrees
Nasomental angle	120–132 degrees
Mentocervical angle	80–95 degrees
Anterior facial height	
Nasal height ratio	47%
Lower facial height ratio	53%
Legan facial convexity angle	8–16 degrees
Nasolabial angle	90–120 degrees
Columellar show	3–5 mm
Goode nasal projection ratio	0.55–0.60
Alar lobule ratio	1:1
Vertical lip ratio	1:2
Mentolabial sulcus	4 mm
Frontal Analysis	
Facial height	
Nasal height ratio	47%
Lower facial height ratio	53%
Nasal width	Equal to intercanthal distance
Intercanthal distance	25.5–37.5 female; 26.5–38.7 male

Rhinoplasty and Mentoplasty

As an example of quantitative analysis using the computer imaging system, consider the case of a 30-year-old man with a history of trauma resulting in septal and nasal deformity. The preoperative computer analysis is shown in **Fig. 12.2**. The measurement indicates that the nasal tip projection is adequate, and the Legan angle of 20 degrees indicates poor chin projection. All other parameters were within normal range. A computer-generated revision is shown and compared with the preoperative image in **Fig. 12.3**. The patient elected to undergo septorhinoplasty and mentoplasty. The postoperative profile is compared with the computer-generated image in **Fig. 12.4**. The postoperative analysis is shown in **Fig. 12.5**, with all measurements now in the normal range. It is also important to use aesthetic sense to judge if the results are pleasing to the eye as well as statistically correct.

Rhytidectomy

A 50-year-old woman is shown on the left in her preoperative appearance before rhytidectomy surgery (**Fig. 12.6**). The center image is the computer-generated anticipated result and the right the actual 1-year surgical result. Note that the jawline, neck, and midface can be addressed with computer imaging.

Augmentation Rhinoplasty

Figure 12.7 demonstrates a patient with previous rhinoplasty leaving an overresected dorsum and overprojected tip. The left image is the preoperative appearance; the center is the computer-generated changes, and the right

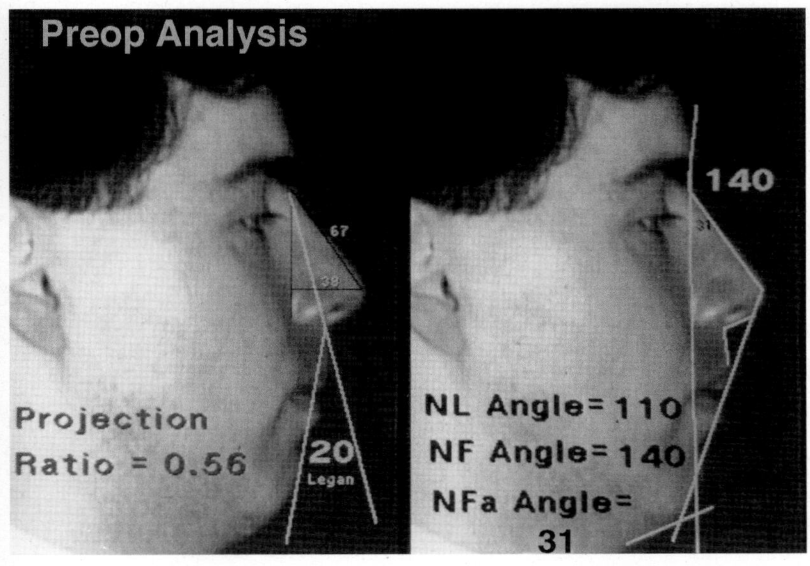

Fig. 12.2 Preoperative analysis of patient with nasal and chin deformities.

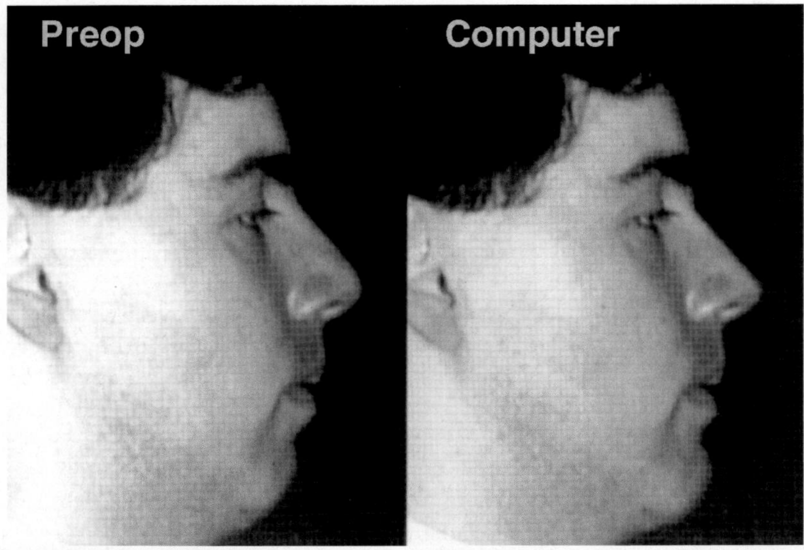

Fig. 12.3 Computer-generated changes are compared with the preoperative images.

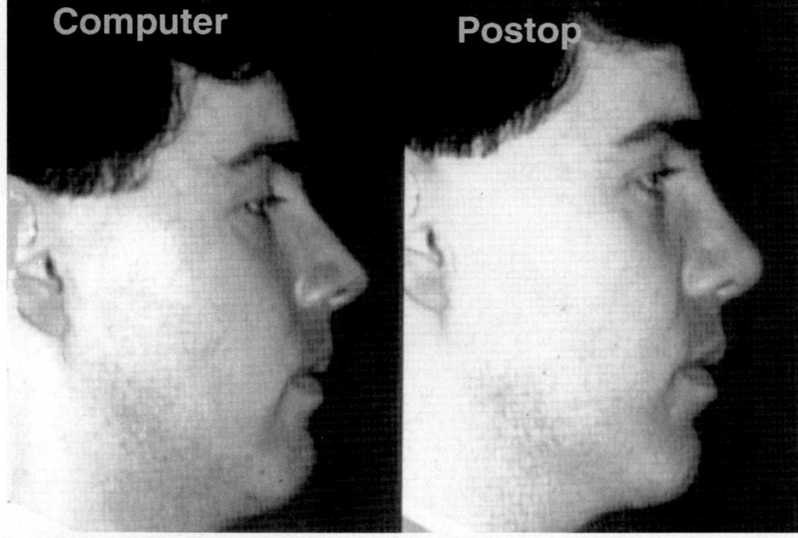

Fig. 12.4 The computer image generated before surgery is compared with the actual postoperative image.

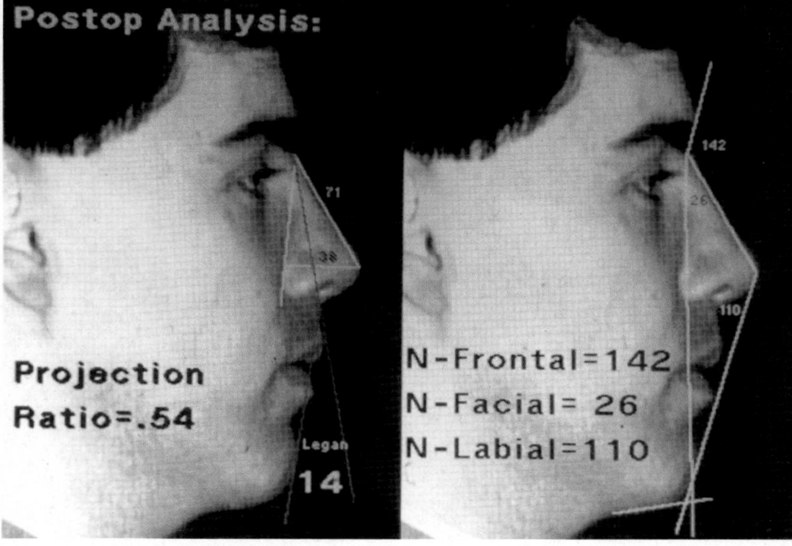

Fig. 12.5 Postoperative analysis showing better relationship to aesthetic ideals.

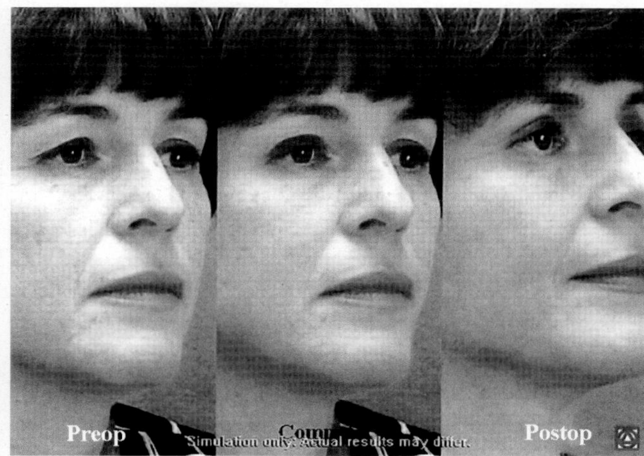

Fig. 12.6 (**A**) A 50-year-old woman prior to rhytidectomy. (**B**) The computer-generated changes. (**C**) The actual postoperative image.

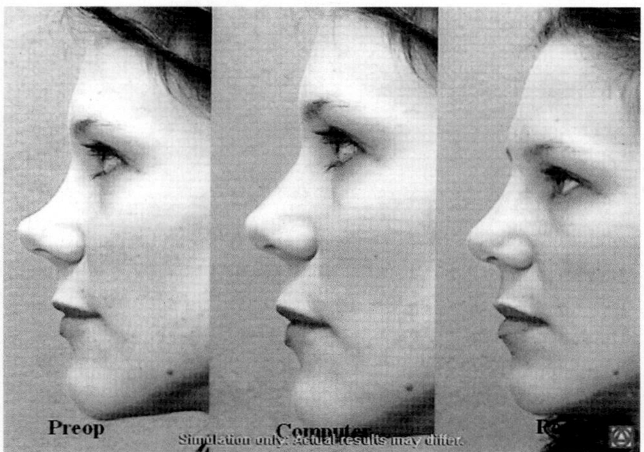

Fig. 12.7 This patient had a previous rhinoplasty with a residual overprojected tip and shallow dorsum. (**A**) Preoperative image. (**B**) Computer-generated image. (**C**) Actual postoperative image.

the actual postoperative profile. This is an example of the actual postoperative profile not being exactly like the computer projection. It is not unusual for the patient to prefer the actual surgical result to the computer prediction.

Reduction Rhinoplasty

Figure 12.8 demonstrates a 16-year-old girl desiring rhinoplasty. Analysis determined overprojection of the tip and shallow nasofrontal angle. The center image demonstrates computer-generated alterations. The right image shows the actual surgical result.

Blepharoplasty

Figure 12.9 shows the computer imaging for a 45-year-old blepharoplasty patient. The left image shows a preoperative

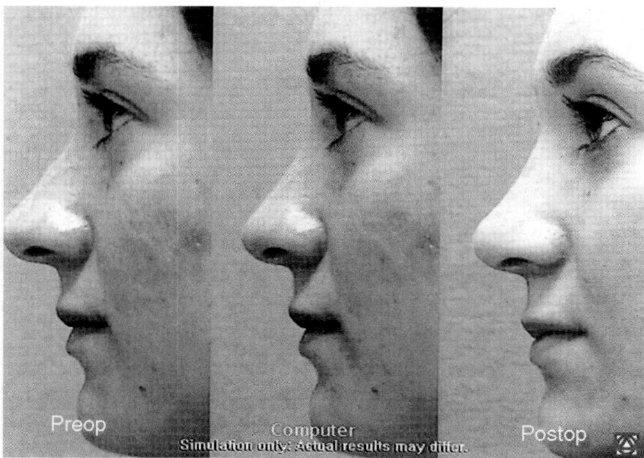

Fig. 12.8 A 16-year-old girl with overprojected tip and shallow radix. (**A**) The preoperative image. (**B**) Computer image. (**C**) Postoperative appearance.

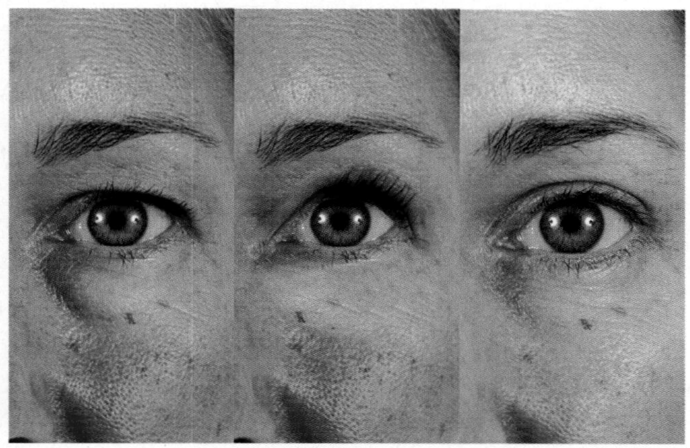

Fig. 12.9 A 45-year-old woman presented for blepharoplasty. (**A**) The preoperative photo. (**B**) Computer-generated image. (**C**) Postoperative photo.

close-up, the middle image a computer generation, and the right image is the postoperative appearance.

Advantages of Computer Imaging

Computer imaging has several obvious and enviable advantages in a plastic surgery practice. Imaging has great appeal among prospective patients and has become an expected part of a consultation in some cities. The computer imager can also be used to market the surgeon's practice with its "value-added" implications to potential patients.

The imaging system has tremendous potential for facial analysis and surgical planning. Surgeons in teaching situations can utilize this, as can residents and fellows independently to help develop better understanding of facial aesthetics. Imaging is also very useful for communication of anticipated surgical results to patients. Newer systems with high-quality digital cameras can also provide photographic archiving systems with excellent image quality. Although not as sharp as fine-grain 35 mm photography, digital imaging is improving rapidly and will match film emulsions in time. The cost factor of the imaging system then becomes more attractive when film purchase and processing in a busy surgical practice are eliminated.

Disadvantages of Computer Imaging

The major problems with computer imaging arise when a surgeon is overly optimistic about postoperative changes during the imaging session. Imaging must be approached with an honest and conservative attitude. There should be a direct and open discussion about the fact that computer imaging is not equivalent to surgery and should never be taken as a guarantee of a surgical result. The relative risks and benefits of demonstrating to patients projected surgical results have generated discussion related to medicolegal matters.[11] Chavez et al argue that a well-documented and honestly projected imaging session may actually reduce the risk of malpractice suits by better informing both the patient and the surgeon of the other's outcome concepts.[6] Some surgeons require that patients read and sign a consent form prior to any imaging session. As in any consultation, overly optimistic predictions and modifications will probably lead to patient dissatisfaction.

Additional disadvantages include the expense and time necessary to include computer imaging in a consultation. The hardware can occupy significant space but can be included in a photography room utilized by many surgeons. The time required for recording the images, generating modifications, and consulting with the patient about the images may add 30 minutes to a cosmetic consultation. The surgeon who personally performs all of these functions will experience a significant increase in time spent. Some surgeons employ their office staff to record and modify the images, followed by surgeon review and modification as needed.[12] This method does save some time at the initial consultation but requires a second visit and additional surgeon time.

In spite of the time and resource commitments, most surgeons who use computer imaging in their practices feel that the increased patient education, decreased anxiety, and easy demonstration of ancillary procedures make the investment worthwhile.

Ethical Issues

All surgeons who practice facial surgery are taught to be conservative in predicting surgical results. Computer imaging, especially in a young surgical practice, creates temptations for the surgeon to portray unrealistic results. The surgeon and staff must resist this pattern and honestly communicate realistic outcomes. Although imaging can be used to market a practice in a tasteful and honest manner, care must be taken to stay within realistic limits in predicting surgical outcomes. To stray beyond this limit will create dissatisfied patients and possible legal complications.

One more issue raised by digital and computer imaging is the problem with truthful presentation at medical meetings. The advent of computer-generated lecture presentations with all-digital visuals creates the potential for altered images presented as postoperative results. This possibility may call into question conclusions about surgical techniques. Some imaging programs have built-in icons, which identify altered images, but this is not universal and may be deactivated by a sophisticated computer user.

Summary

Computer imaging is a valuable tool in facial plastic and reconstructive surgery. Through computer graphic technology the surgeon can project realistic-looking postoperative predictions to share with patients and fellow surgeons. The ability to measure and evaluate facial features is invaluable for surgical planning and outcome analysis. Discussions about legal and ethical issues will continue, guided by a growing practical experience.

Glossary

cervical point Junction of tangents to neck and submental areas
columellar point Most anterior point of columella
glabella Most prominent portion of forehead in midsagittal plane
gnathion Intercept of subnasale to pogonion line with cervical point to menton line
mentolabial sulcus Most posterior point between lower lip and chin
menton Lowest point on contour of chin soft tissue
nasion Most posterior point at root of nose in midsagittal plane
pogonion Most anterior point of chin soft tissue
rhinion Junction of bony and cartilaginous dorsum
subnasale Junction of columella and upper lip
supratip Point cephalic to dome
tip Most anterior projection of nose
tragion Most anterior portion of supratragal notch
trichion Hairline at midsagittal plane

References

1. Papel ID, Park RI. Computer imaging for instruction in facial plastic surgery in a residency program. Arch Otolaryngol Head Neck Surg 1988;114:1454–1460
2. Koch RJ, Chavez A, Dagum P, Newman JP. Advantages and disadvantages of computer imaging in cosmetic surgery. Dermatol Surg 1998;24:195–198
3. Papel ID. Quantitative facial aesthetic evaluation with computer imaging. Facial Plast Surg 1990;7:35–44
4. Berman M. Marketability of computer imaging. Facial Plast Surg 1990;7:59–61
5. Tardy ME, Brown M. Principles of Photography in Facial Plastic Surgery. New York: Thieme; 1992
6. Chavez AE, Dagum P, Koch J, Newman JP. Legal issues of computer imaging in plastic surgery: a primer. Plast Reconstr Surg 1997;100:1601–1608
7. Gonzales-Ulloa M. Quantitative principles in cosmetic surgery of the face (profileplasty). Plast Reconstr Surg 1961;29:186
8. Crumley RL, Lancer M. Quantitative analysis of nasal tip projection. Laryngoscope 1988;98:202
9. Goode R. The five major aesthetic masses of the face. In: Powel N, Humphries B, eds. Proportions of the Aesthetic Face. New York: Thieme-Stratton; 1988
10. Legan H, Burstone C. Soft tissue cephalometric analysis for orthognathic surgery. J Oral Surg 1980;38:744
11. Gorney M. Preoperative computerized video imaging [letter]. Plast Reconstr Surg 1986;78:286
12. Schoenrock LD. Five-year facial plastic experience with computer imaging. Facial Plast Surg 1990;7:18–25

13 Photography in Facial Plastic Surgery

Theda C. Kontis

Photographic documentation of patients is an integral component of cosmetic and reconstructive surgery. Consistent standard photographic technique allows critical analysis of aesthetic features of the patient before and after surgery. Occasionally, preoperative review of photographs will demonstrate an irregularity or an asymmetry that was not recognized during the patient encounter. A frequently quoted dictum is that demonstration of these irregularities to the patient preoperatively is considered "counseling," whereas postoperative explanations are viewed by the patient as an "excuse" for a less than perfect result.

Preoperative photographs are essential for all plastic and reconstructive procedures. Insurance companies frequently use photographs for preauthorization purposes. Patients may "forget" how they looked before surgery, and some request to see their preoperative photos. Photographs are an important part of the patient record for medicolegal documentation. The surgeon can also refine and adjust technique from review of surgical successes and failures. Preoperative and postoperative photographs may also be used for marketing and patient education seminars.

Equipment

For the past 50 years, the gold standard for photodocumentation has been the single-lens reflex (SLR) 35 mm camera (**Fig. 13.1A**). Image standardization can be achieved with the SLR camera because the image seen in the view finder is identical to the photographic image generated.

Advancements in digital photography in the past 5 years have made 35 mm photography obsolete. By now, most surgeons have converted to a strictly digital format (**Fig. 13.1B**). For historical purposes, the essentials of 35 mm photography are discussed here. Techniques of patient positioning, lens choice, and lighting are similar to those used with digital format photography.

35 mm Photography

Camera

Although a high-quality 35 mm camera body provides excellent imaging, the body need not be the top-of-the-line

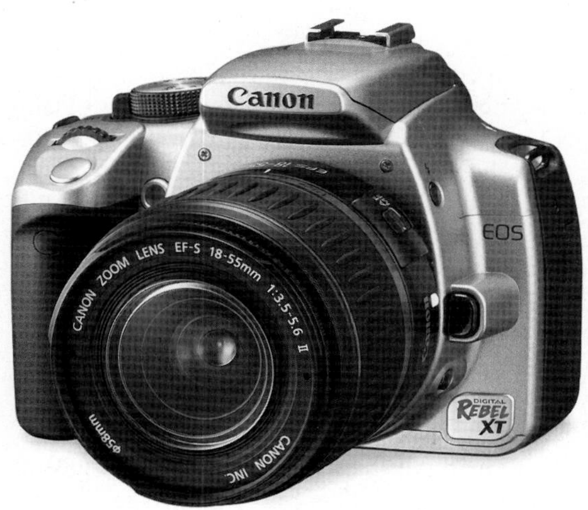

Fig. 13.1 The digital camera has replaced the 35 mm camera for surgical photodocumentation. (Photographs courtesy of Nikon, Inc., Melville, NY, and Canon, U.S.A., Inc., Lake Success, NY.)

model with extravagant features. Medical portrait photography does not require the ability to perform special effects, so the simpler cameras often suffice. A motor drive for film advancement allows for a smooth and rapid photographic session with the patient and may permit automatic exposure bracketing (see later). One disadvantage of the motor drive is the tendency to snap photos without allowing enough charge recycle time for the flash units. A good rule of thumb is to wait 2 seconds after the camera flash ready light is illuminated before taking the next picture.

A "databack" accessory prints the date or other important data on the photograph. This feature is standard in a few cameras or can be added to many 35 mm camera bodies. This can aid in patient identification and can be used to time the postoperative photographic sequence. A log book of patient photographs updated by a compulsive photographer can substitute for a databack.

Lens

The most important piece of photographic equipment (and often the most costly) is the camera lens. A 90 mm or 105 mm "macro" lens is recommended for portrait photography. The macro telephoto lens minimizes facial distortion by allowing a 1:1 representation onto the film.

An ultraviolet or skylight filter can be attached to the lens to protect it from dust, fingerprints, and scratches. Close-up filters can be purchased and provide an inexpensive way to obtain magnified views. However, magnifying filters are not required if a macro lens is used.

Aperture Setting (F-Stop)

The lens f-number determines the brightness of the image by adjusting the amount of light that enters the lens. The f-number series is equivalent to 1.4, 2, 2.8, 4, 5.6, 8, 11, 16, 22, 32. Changing to the next larger number decreases the image brightness by half. Lowering the f-stop to the previous number doubles the brightness of the photo. The larger the aperture (smaller f-number) the greater the maximum shooting distance, but the lower the depth of field (image sharpness). The larger the aperture, the shorter the flash recycling time.

In portrait photography, one must select the appropriate f-stop that maximizes image depth of field and shooting distance while keeping the image bright. Tardy[1] suggests determining the correct f-stop for a given studio setup by photographing a subject holding tongue depressors marked with the aperture setting used, analyzing the photos, then selecting the best image and using the f-stop labeled. One will find that this f-stop setting will generally work for most photography in the office studio, except on darker-skinned patients. The f-stop should be lowered one half to one f-stop when photographing these patients to open the lens aperture and brighten the image.

Because the surgeon cannot instantly view the photographs taken, it is often a safeguard to obtain photographs at different f-stop settings by using exposure "bracketing." This camera feature allows the photographer to select three to five different f-stops at one time, generally one half to one f-stop above and below the recommended f-stop setting. With one depression of the shutter release button, three to five images are taken with a range of selected aperture settings. Exposure bracketing can be performed manually with any camera.

Lighting

A studio setup is the most desirable method for obtaining standardized portraits. Most studios use background lighting and soft umbrella lighting (**Fig. 13.2**). A slave-triggered light can be installed on the ceiling behind the patient to prevent shadows behind the subject and to increase depth of field (**Fig. 13.3**). This key light or "kicker" flashes when the primary flash is triggered.

Two umbrella flashes, one placed on each side of the patient, allow soft lighting for portrait photography.

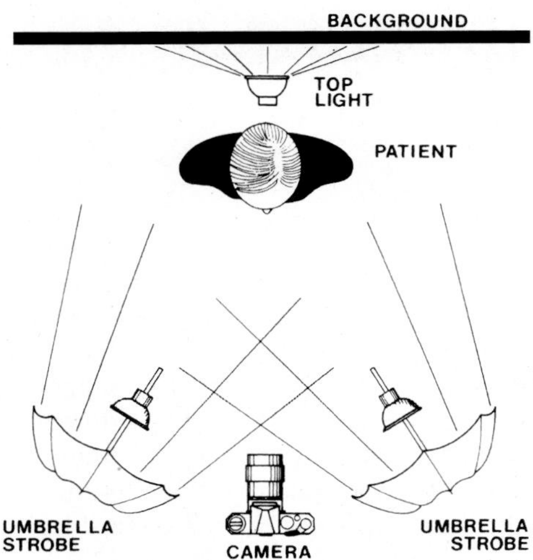

Fig. 13.2 Suggested placement of patient, lights, and camera for in-office studio.

Umbrellas are available in two types: the "reflector" type with an opaque inner lining of white, gold, or silver, and the "shoot-through" umbrella, which is made of a translucent material. The reflectors bounce the flash light off of the umbrella onto the patient. The shoot-through umbrellas (**Fig. 13.4**) let the flash light through the umbrella. For small studios with low ceilings, shoot-through types are preferred because they allow the flash unit to be positioned close to the subject. The umbrella flash units should be positioned at the same level and equidistant from the camera. A cable from one of the umbrella flashes is attached to the camera body accessory shoe.

Electronic flash units that attach to the camera body are required when patients are being photographed outside the studio setting. Because of the variability in flash units, it is recommended that trial photographs be taken

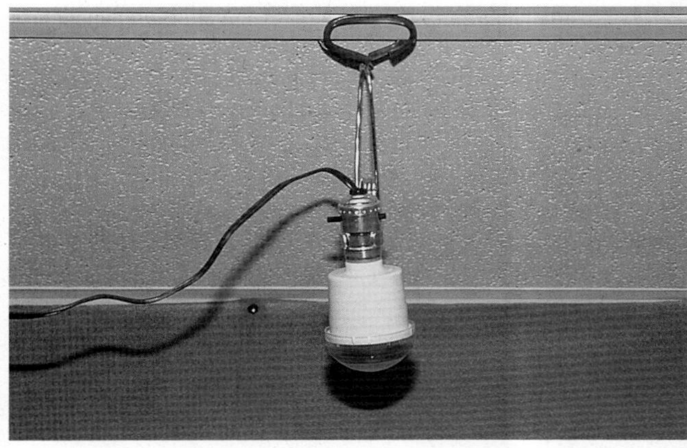

Fig. 13.3 A slave flash unit is mounted on the ceiling behind the patient. This flash is triggered by the camera flash unit or umbrella flash, and it eliminates background shadows.

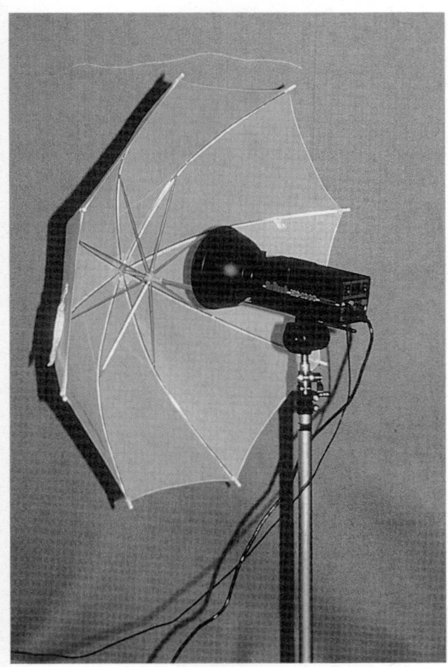

Fig. 13.4 "Shoot-through" umbrella light produces soft lighting of the subject.

using different f-stop settings to determine the optimal flash parameters. A "ring" flash is not used for portrait photography. These flash units provide shadowless lighting, which is optimal for photography of body cavities; however, the harshness of this lighting makes it unsuitable for portrait photography.

Background

The ideal color of the background in portrait photography is light blue or green. These colors do not overwhelm the subject, are appealing to the eye, and allow for a greater depth of field. A dark background appears to envelop the subject and diminishes the image's three-dimensional quality (**Fig. 13.5**). The background should be a single solid color, without folds or creases in the material. The background should be flat, not shiny, to avoid having light reflected back at the camera. Background materials include felt, window shades, or a papered or painted wall with a flat finish.

Film

Until recently, the 35 mm slide transparency has been the most common format for cosmetic surgery photodocumentation. There were two general types of Kodak slide film: Kodachrome and Ektachrome (Eastman Kodak, Rochester, New York); however, Kodak has discontinued Kodachrome film. Fuji (Elmsford, New York) also makes a film similar to Ektachrome (Fujichrome). Ektachrome and Fujichrome can be developed quickly using the widely available E-6 process. Ektachrome slides have a sharp image but must be stored in a cool, dark environment to limit image degradation and color fading.

Kodachrome film has a more stable emulsion. Kodachrome 25 and 64 are used for portrait photography because they produce photographs with excellent image quality and resolution. Kodachrome film is processed at fewer laboratories than Ektachrome. The film is usually mailed to processing centers with turnaround time of up to 10 days.

Film speed (ISO number) refers to the film sensitivity to light: the higher the number, the greater the sensitivity. A film speed of ISO 200 is twice as "fast" or "sensitive" as ISO 100. Films with lower ISO numbers (25 and 64) are used for portrait photography to reduce image grain. The studio setting, with adequate artificial light, allows for the use of lower-speed film. The fine grain

A 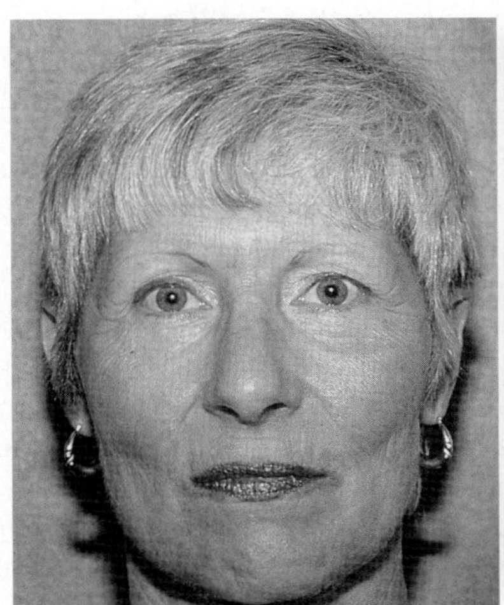

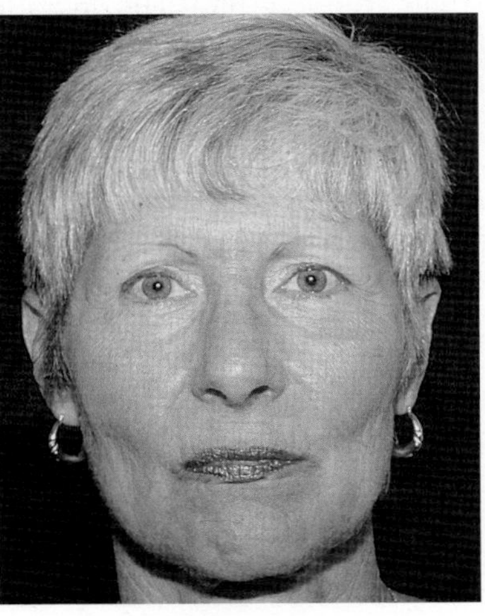 B

Fig. 13.5 The same patient is photographed using (**A**) light blue and (**B**) black backgrounds. A light blue background allows the patient to appear more three-dimensional and is aesthetically pleasing when printed in either color or black and white.

of the lower-speed films allows preservation of image sharpness for print enlargement or projection onto a screen during a presentation.

Portrait Photography

Consent

Consent for photodocumentation should be obtained from patients prior to the photographic session. These photographs may be used to demonstrate surgical results to other patients and physicians. At the time of consent, one may also obtain permission for use in publications, advertising, or transmission on the Internet. Patient confidentiality must be maintained, of course.

Standardization

Standardization of pre- and postoperative photographic views is of paramount importance in facial plastic surgery because it facilitates image comparison. Identical views should be obtained for each type of surgery performed. Photography can be standardized by photographing the patient in the same studio, with the same equipment, using the same focal length distance from the patient, and using a set of standardized views (**Table 13.1**). The major photographic goals are consistency and reproducibility. These goals can be met by having a simple protocol that is always followed (**Figs. 13.6 and 13.7**).

The patient is seated on a stool that can swivel and roll. The patient's feet should touch the floor. Preferably, the stool should have a short back to help the patient assume a straight posture. The patient is asked to "swivel" in the chair or "roll" the chair to obtain optimal positioning. One method of standardization of photographs uses permanent markers fixed on the walls of the studio. The patient is asked to swivel in the chair and look at each marker. This standardizes the position of the eyes and head for reproducible results. Patient positioning is the most difficult skill to master and is a common cause of unsatisfactory photographs.

A tripod reduces motion artifact and helps standardize patient images. A wall-mounted camera, with the camera mounted in the vertical position and perpendicular to the facial plane, can also be useful. Most physicians prefer to hold the camera, orienting it vertically or horizontally as needed. Motion artifact is minimal due to the short duration of the electronic flash.

Accurate and reproducible photographic techniques can be augmented by using a focusing screen with a grid pattern. This is a plate inserted into the body of the 35 mm camera with lines for orientation of the subject. Focusing screens can be used in many of the more expensive SLR camera models. The grid is viewed through the viewfinder but is not printed onto the photograph. Multiple grids have been designed to assist in portrait photography.[2,3] A horizontal line aids in positioning the frontal and base views by preventing head tilt. It also helps with the lateral view by lining up the Frankfort plane (an imaginary line from the top of the tragus to the inferior orbital rim, parallel to the orbital floor). Vertical lines assist in correctly "framing" the image on the screen. The experienced photographer can achieve accurate and symmetric photographs without using a grid. The photographer can "imagine" the vertical and horizontal lines for proper patient positioning. In the base view, the tip of the nose would be seen between the brows (**Fig. 13.6G,H**). Surgeons often disagree about patient positioning for the oblique view. Some photographers line up the tip of the nose with the edge of the opposite cheek,[4] whereas others feel that this extensive rotation results in a "five-sixths" view rather than a "three-fourths" view. Lesser rotation, by aligning the medial canthus with the oral commissure, may better demonstrate the relationship of the nose to the opposite cheek[2] (**Fig. 13.8**).

Table 13.1 Recommended Standardized Photographic Views for Specific Procedures.

Procedure	Views
Rhinoplasty	Frontal
	Base
	R/L lateral
	R/L oblique
Blepharoplasty	Frontal (full face)
	Frontal (close-up eyes)
	Eyes open
	Eyes closed
	Upward gaze
	R/L lateral
Rhytidectomy	Frontal
	R/L lateral
	R/L oblique
Otoplasty	Frontal
	Posterior
	R/L lateral
	R/L lateral close-up

Abbreviations: R, right; L, left.

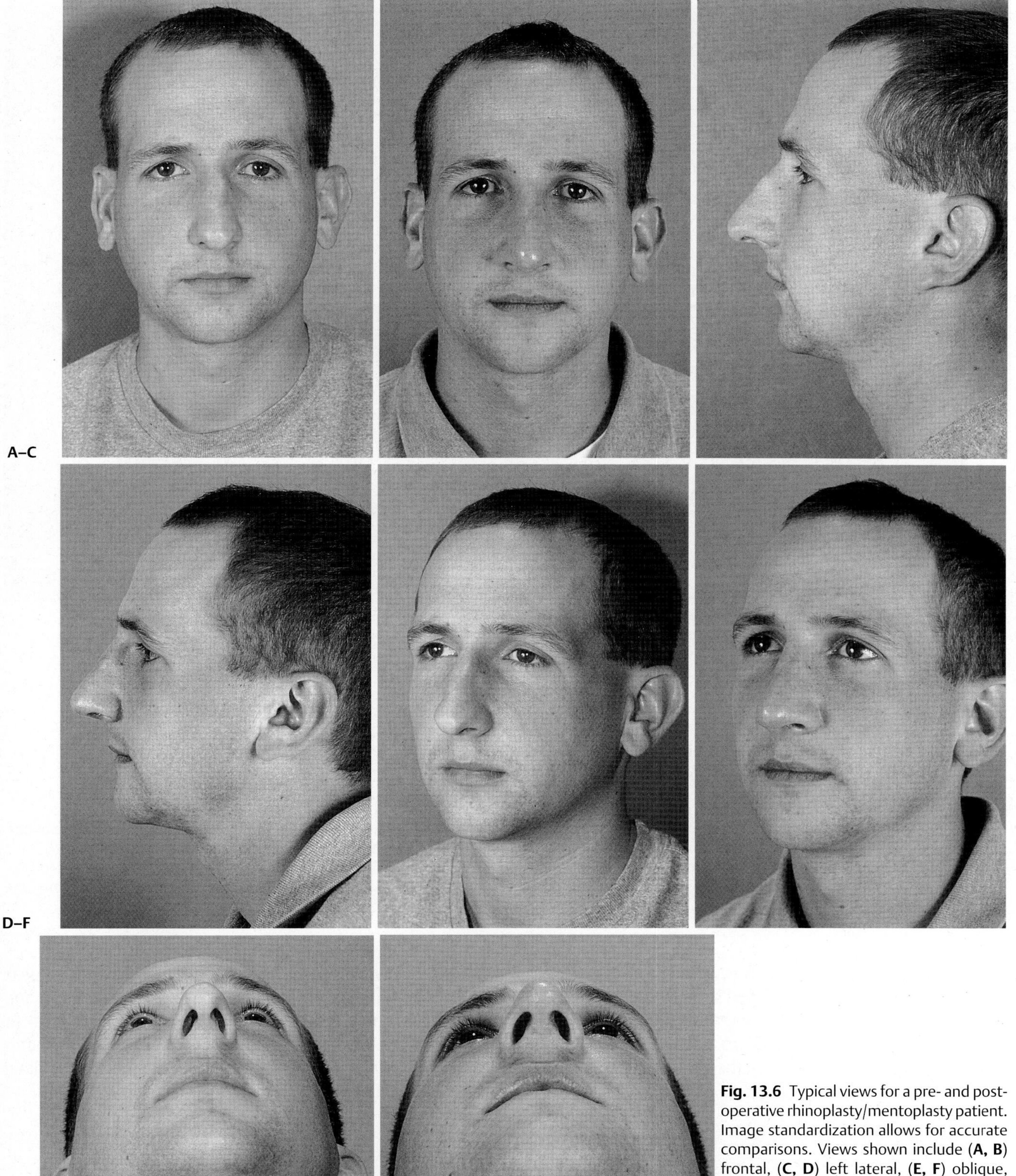

Fig. 13.6 Typical views for a pre- and post-operative rhinoplasty/mentoplasty patient. Image standardization allows for accurate comparisons. Views shown include (**A, B**) frontal, (**C, D**) left lateral, (**E, F**) oblique, and (**G, H**) base views.

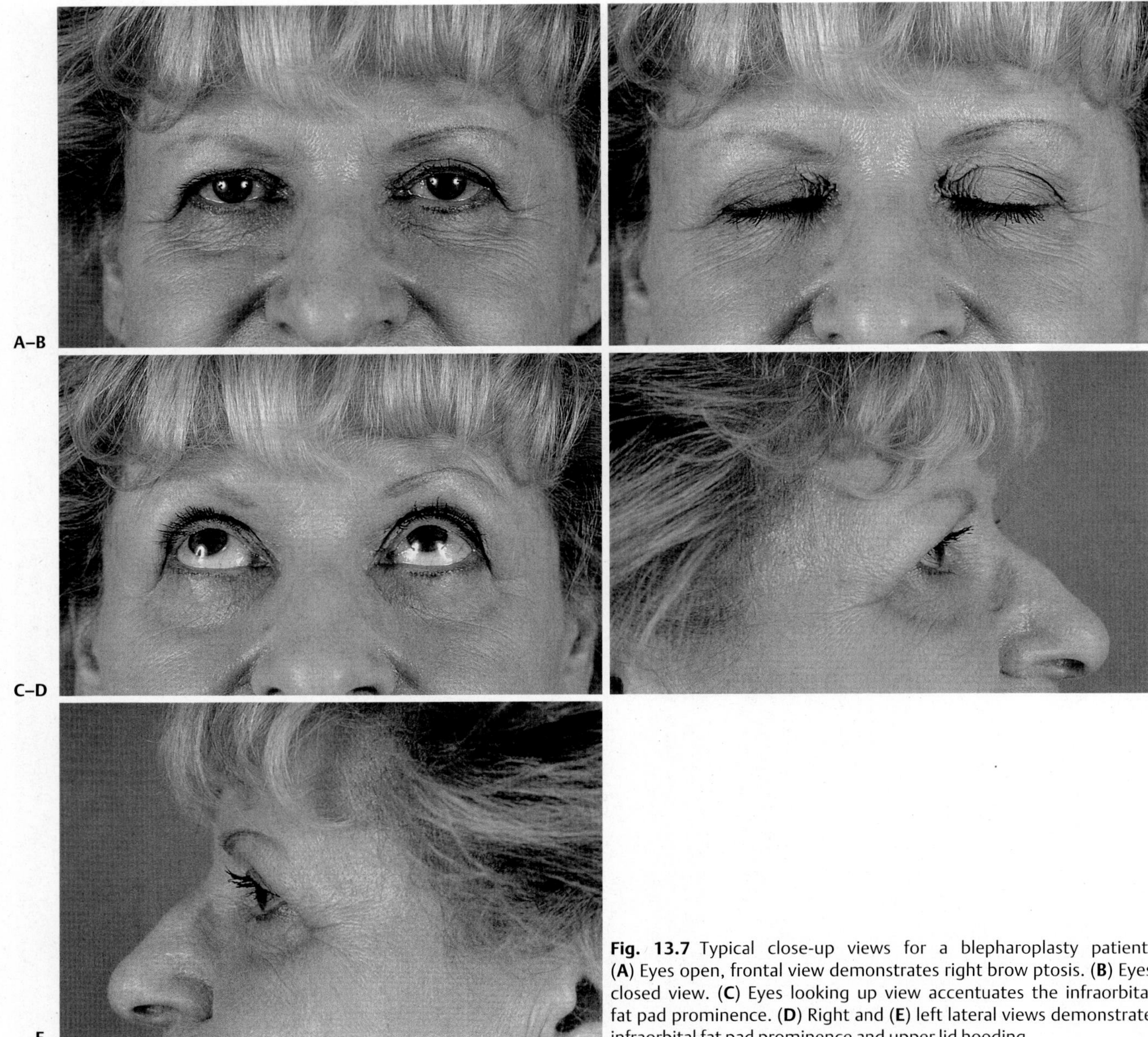

Fig. 13.7 Typical close-up views for a blepharoplasty patient. (**A**) Eyes open, frontal view demonstrates right brow ptosis. (**B**) Eyes closed view. (**C**) Eyes looking up view accentuates the infraorbital fat pad prominence. (**D**) Right and (**E**) left lateral views demonstrate infraorbital fat pad prominence and upper lid hooding.

Relevant anatomical details must be well visualized. Hair may need to be tied back or pinned back with bobby pins or hair clips, and glasses should be removed. Photographs of otoplasty and microtia patients are assisted by the use of a headband to pull hair away from the ears (**Fig. 13.9**).

Digital Photography

Because of the rapid improvement in technology, digital photography has become the standard for surgical photodocumentation. There are many advantages of digital photography. The photographs can be viewed in near real time, allowing the images to be saved or discarded, and retaken at the same sitting. The images are stored on a disk or other removable medium that can be loaded into a computer and saved indefinitely. Film purchasing and processing, along with issues of emulsion stability, are no longer relevant.

Camera

Digital photography, first developed in the 1970s, involves image capture onto a charged coupler device (CCD). This

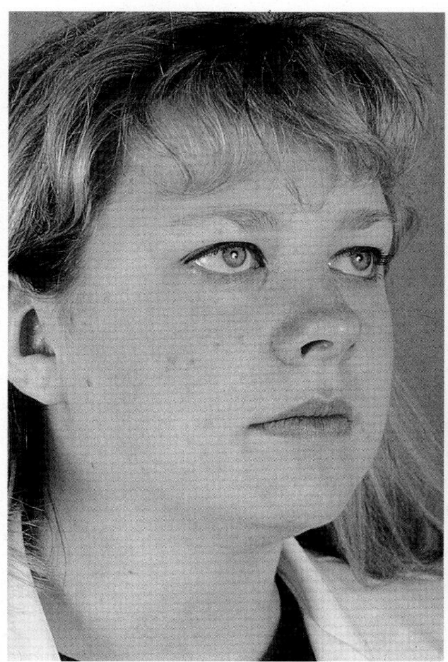

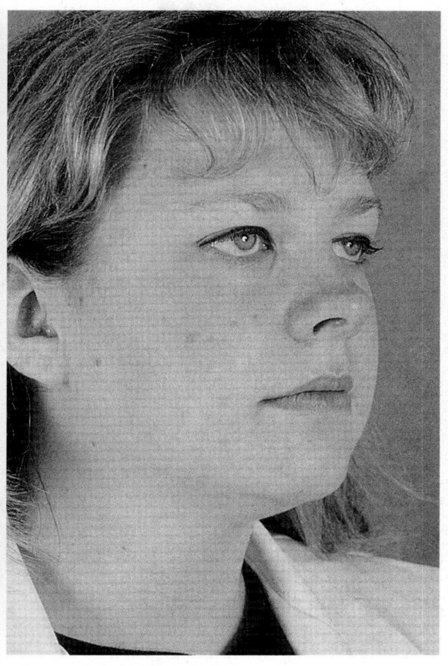

A B

Fig. 13.8 (**A**) The three-quarter oblique view places the medial canthus in line vertically with the lateral oral commissure. (**B**) The "five-sixths" oblique view aligns the tip of the nose with the edge of the cheek.

image is formatted by a digital signal processor into a digital code that is translatable by computer. The data are then stored on a memory device, temporarily within the camera, and usually downloaded onto a computer.

All of the major camera manufacturers (Nikon, Canon, Olympus, Sony) market digital cameras. The qualities of a digital camera in which one should be interested include the resolution, lens quality, zoom capabilities, and price. Currently, most digital cameras suitable for portrait photography are priced at around $1000. Although digital cameras are becoming less expensive, they can become superseded by improved technology in as little as 6 months.

Resolution is one of the most important characteristics of a digital camera. Digital photographic resolution has not yet approached the fine resolution of 35 mm photography. There are more than 35 million pixels (points of light with uniform color) in a 35 mm photograph, but only ~8 million with a digital photograph. However, a resolution of 1.5 million pixels is sufficient for medical photography.[5] In general, more than

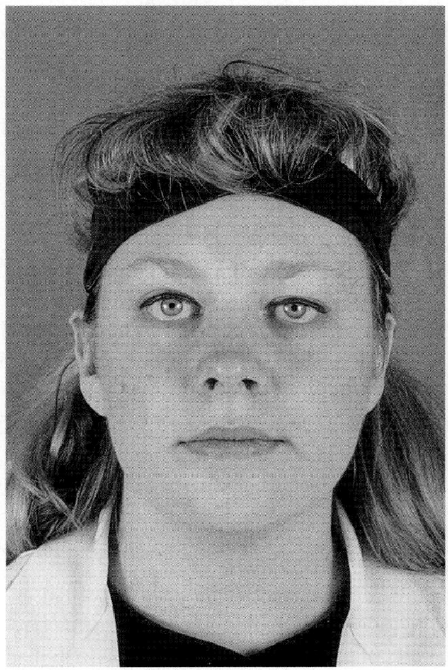

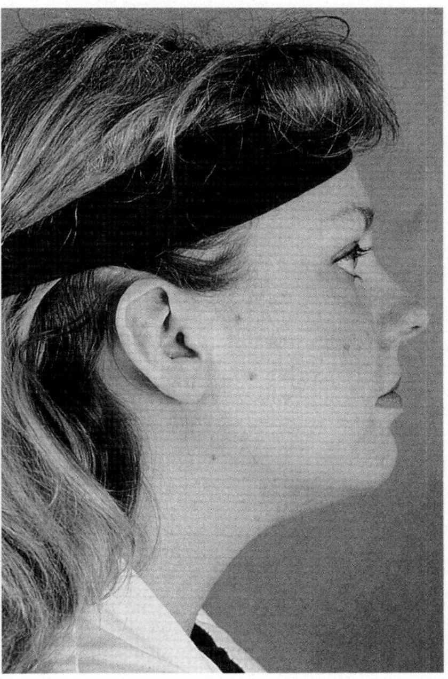

A B

Fig. 13.9 A headband can be used to pull hair away from the patient's ears when photographing otoplasty or microtia patients.

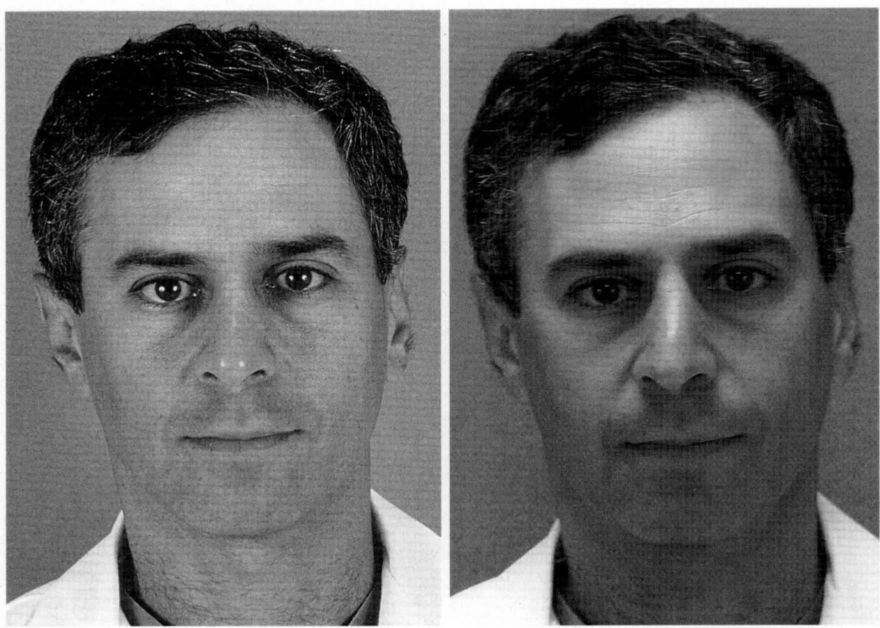

Fig. 13.10 Comparison of 35 mm (**A**) and digital (**B**) photos of the same studio setting. (Equipment used: Nikon 6006 35 mm camera with Kodachrome 64 film; Olympus D-620 digital camera, super high resolution.)

1.4 million pixels is required for a photograph to be acceptable. Higher resolution digital photography requires longer time for image loading and transfer and more memory for image storage. In general, images should be stored with a resolution of less than 3 million pixels for the greatest ease of manipulation and storage.

As in 35 mm photography, the lens system is also important in digital photography. The lens should be made of optical glass and have macro capabilities for close-up photography. Focusing is generally automatic with the lower quality digital cameras. The more sophisticated digital cameras possess capabilities for manual focusing, exposure settings, and flash settings. Some digital cameras accept interchangeable lenses. Some of the newer digital cameras allow a grid pattern to be superimposed during shooting and playback.

Digital cameras consume considerable amounts of battery power for image capture, viewing, and flash photography. For office photography, it is suggested that the camera have rechargeable batteries using the latest battery technology.

Lighting

An acceptable digital photograph can be taken with ambient natural lighting. One or two umbrella flashes and a slave light for background illumination are probably still required in the studio setting. If a photograph is not ideal, software packages can be used to eliminate shadows and manipulate shading after the photograph has been taken.

Image Storage

The number of images that can be stored in the camera itself can range from one to several hundred, depending on the size of the memory card. The higher the image quality, the fewer the number of photographs that can be stored on a card. Digital cameras currently use 128 megabyte (MB) to 4 gigabyte (GB) removable media cards (occasionally referred to as digital film and e-film). Most digital cameras do not come with a memory card, and this additional purchase is currently about $50. Removable media cards currently available include Memory Sticks, CompactFlash, SD (Secure Digital), and XD. Media cards that can store even larger numbers of images are becoming available as technology improves.

Hard drive storage of digital photographs on the personal computer requires adequate free disk space, usually at least 5 MB per photograph. The images can be compressed into a JPEG (Joint Photographic Experts Group) file, which allows 1 to 2000 images to be stored on 1 GB of hard drive space. File compression makes the files smaller and easier to manipulate, but may cause some degradation of the digital file. The images can also be stored onto a writable compact disc (CD), digital video disc (DVD), or microdrive.

Software

Digital cameras generally come with cables and software necessary for downloading images onto the personal computer. The software used is as important as, if not more important than, the selection of the digital camera. Digital file formats include JPEG, TIFF, and BMP. It is essential that the software used be compatible with these formats. Software packages are available, such as Adobe PhotoShop and Adobe PhotoDeluxe (Adobe Systems, Inc., Seattle, WA), which allow manipulation of the images once downloaded. Once digitized, there are numerous possibilities for image manipulation: shadows can be eliminated, photographs can be rotated, text can be added, photographs can be merged or added to the Web, and so forth (**Fig. 13.10**). The photos can also be placed into a slide format, such as PowerPoint (Microsoft, Redmond, WA), for presentations.

Printers

A printer is required for conversion of a digital image to a photograph. Ink Jet printers can print 4 × 6 photos for a cost of ~25 cents per print. A dye sublimation printer offers the best quality, and photograph production costs on average ~30 cents per photo. The cost of these printers is only about $100.

Making the Transition to Digital Photography

The conversion to digital photography requires the purchase of expensive equipment (camera, lens, storage media, printer, and photographic paper); however, the cost decreases dramatically after start-up because film purchasing and developing fees are not generated.[6]

It is a fallacy that surgeons converting from 35 mm slides to digital photography need to scan their entire collection of 35 mm slides into digital format. Actually, only classic, nonreproducible photos, or those with outstanding postoperative results need to be converted.[7] Slides can be converted to digital format by the use of a slide scanner or by a professional photography store.

35 mm versus Digital Photography: Advantages and Disadvantages

Digital photography has replaced the 35 mm camera as the medium of choice for patient documentation, and the personal computer has replaced the slide projector for image display for presentations. Gone are the days of trying to keep two slide projectors in exact sequence at presentations, and damaged slides that fail to "drop."

The advantages of the 35 mm camera include its familiarity and ease of use. Disadvantages of traditional photography include the expense of film purchasing and developing, and the delay in film processing. The images are not viewed immediately, so mistakes in patient positioning, lighting, and aperture setting are not seen until the slide has been developed and the patient has left the office. Virtually all surgeons have at one time or another operated on a patient only to find that the preoperative photographs "didn't turn out." (More often than not, the postoperative result is superb!)

The storage space required for slides is enormous. Slides can be stored in cabinets, boxes, notebooks, and so forth. The slides must be correctly labeled and cataloged accordingly so that they can be found with ease. Slides can be damaged, lost, or misfiled. Pertinent information about the subject of the image must be transcribed onto a slide or the date printed onto the slide using a databack accessory. Digital photographs have all the important information stored with the image, and the date or other information can easily be added or removed from the image. Hundreds of photographs can be stored on disks, obviating the need for notebooks full of 35 mm slides. Journals now accept digital photos for publication. National meetings have converted exclusively to electronic format. Of course, backup of digital photographs is crucial. Theoretically, one computer glitch can potentially destroy one's entire photograph collection. Backup of images should be performed frequently, preferably onto a medium that will not soon become obsolete.

Digital photography is more expensive than 35 mm photography to initiate but much less expensive to maintain. The image capture, storage, and retrieval are instantaneous. The photograph, once taken, is viewed immediately and can be deleted and retaken if necessary. The date and time information is stored as part of the file. There is no need for film purchase and developing, and no delay in image production. Motor drives are unnecessary because there is no film to advance. However, there is a learning curve with the use of digital photography and its software.

Image stability is superior with digital photography. Slide emulsions can degrade, but a digital photograph is stored as computer data. Despite compression, digital images will theoretically remain unaltered indefinitely.

Acknowledgment

The author thanks Matthew Cooper of Cooper's Camera Mart (Baltimore, MD) for his assistance with the technical aspects of this chapter.

References

1. Tardy ME. Principles of Photography in Facial Plastic Surgery. New York: Thieme; 1992
2. Ellenbogen R, Jankauskas S, Collini FJ. Achieving standardized photographs in aesthetic surgery. Plast Reconstr Surg 1990; 86:955–961

3. DiBernardo BE, Adams RL, Krause J, et al. Photographic standards in plastic surgery. Plast Reconstr Surg 1998;102:559–568
4. Zarem HA. Standards of photography. Plast Reconstr Surg 1984;74:137
5. Galdino GM, Vogel JE, VanderKolk CA. Standardizing digital photography: it's not all in the eye of the beholder. Plast Reconstr Surg 2001;108:1334–1344
6. Niamutu J. Image is everything: pearls and pitfalls of digital photography and Powerpoint presentations for the cosmetic surgeon. Dermatol Surg 2004;30:81–91
7. Hollenbeak CS, Kokoska M, Stack BC. Cost considerations of converting to digital photography. Arch Facial Plast Surg 2000;2:122–123

14 Ethics in Facial Plastic Surgery

Donn R. Chatham

Beginning in the early 2003 television season, with the emergence of numerous reality shows, several programs featured people undergoing cosmetic surgery. Some were based on extreme transformation of unattractive people in an attempt to make them attractive. Multiple procedures were sometimes performed at one time, and the physical transformation could be dramatic. Other themes included "beauty pageants" featuring surgically enhanced women. Other programs asked the question: who wants a face like a famous celebrity? Still others featured the personal and sometimes life-in-the-fast-lane stories of cosmetic doctors in Beverly Hills and Miami.

In the words of one program, these lucky people will have a "'Cinderella experience'—a real life fairy tale, changing not only looks . . . but lives and destinies." One writer called this a modern rite of passage, with surgical excision and death of the inadequate "old" and rebirth of the "new." Following surgery, a more attractive, sophisticated, and engaging personality emerges. As a result, spiritual and personal achievement are fulfilled. Sometimes, thousands of people would apply in the hope of being one of the chosen few, to receive a total surgical transformation and be featured on international television.

Some plastic surgeons enthusiastically embraced the opportunity to transform ordinary people to prettier and younger-looking ones. This sometimes led to local and national marketing efforts and garnered publicity for the surgical/cosmetic team as well as the television network. What emerged was a hybrid entity, sort of a "surgetainment" experience. It provided some ordinary people a chance to look more aesthetic while the world watched, gave cosmetic surgeons and others a chance to showcase their skills, and made fascinating programming.

This has not occurred without some controversy within the medical community. Some lay voices have voiced concern as well.

The British Columbia College of Physicians and Surgeons in 2004 issued a warning to its members that participating in an Extreme Makeover (E.M.) program could lead to ethical and legal problems: "where there is a high level of hype and emotion . . . may compromise the normal doctor relationship."

Speaking before the American Medical Association (AMA) council of ethical and judicial affairs, AMA member and American Academy of Facial Plastic and Reconstructive Surgery past president Russell Kridel, MD, called these shows "the Jerry Springers of medicine" and spoke of the importance of communicating with one's patients and ensuring that their expectations are realistic.

David David, MD, of the International Society of Craniofacial Surgeons in 2004 said in part that "E.M. uses vulnerable people for the entertainment of others . . . and trivializes surgery that is often complex and never certain . . . [and that] well-being is also determined by emotional . . . and spiritual states."

It also redefines what is "normal." As a result, "people whose features are not abnormal now fear becoming outcasts."

Rod Rorich, MD, of the American Society of Plastic Surgeons, in a 2004 press release cautioned its members by saying "do not be lulled into doing 12 procedures at once . . . don't substitute good surgical judgment just for good patient relations." He also cautioned the public, "Some patients on these shows have unrealistic and, frankly, unhealthy expectations about what plastic surgery can do for them."

However, in general, there has been little focus on the psychological, emotional, and ethical nature of these sorts of shows. Whether the producers and others participating in these events care to address it or not, some questions beg to be answered.

On the positive side, do these programs raise awareness and help create a more informed population and thereby produce a more positive effect on society? Do they find needy people who could never afford the procedures that really benefit them, then benevolently provide the new faces and bodies, forever improving their lives, and possibly the lives of those around them?

But other questions linger.

1. Is it OK to take ordinary people and, before millions of television viewers, dissect their appearance and then tell them if they want to be attractive, then they need redesigning?
2. Is it OK to tell these people that if they are ever to look attractive, they need lots and lots of different procedures?
3. Do these shows promote the idea that if a woman does not have pearly white teeth, D-cup levitating breasts, a small waist, and high brows, then she is not desirable?
4. Is the message sent that if one has self-esteem issues, then the solution is to have them surgically removed?

5. Do these shows portray cosmetic surgeons as amoral technicians guided only by their personal aesthetic preferences and the desires of their patients?
6. How much surgery performed at one time is "too much"? When all procedures are elective, general anesthesia is being utilized, and patients are immobilized for hours at a time, is it really in their best interests to have eight or 10 procedures performed one after the other?
7. Are patients portrayed as autonomous decision-makers, who really do know exactly what they want, impervious to others, and therefore the role of the surgeon is to simply fulfill their wishes?
8. Do these shows demonstrate to the viewer the seriousness of surgery, including the potential risks and complications, as well as the prolonged recovery required and discomfort experienced by these patients?
9. What is the impact on the families of these patients, especially when they are sequestered in another city for weeks at a time?
10. What are the effects on spouses and other significant people when one partner is now "attractive" and perhaps the other one is still "not that attractive"?
11. Are surgeons pressured to perform more surgeries than they would normally be comfortable with because there is a show to produce, and cameras and crew are looking over their shoulders the whole time? Is there room for honest curtailment when judgment would suggest it?
12. Does the message to the public become "in order to be truly happy with oneself it is necessary to look attractive and the standards will be those determined by Western culture and cosmetic surgeons"?
13. Would the public be more truthfully served if the shows also devoted some time on the complications of surgery?
14. Would the actual life-transforming results be more credible if these shows returned to interview these patients at a future date, once they and others adjusted more fully to the "transformed person"?

These are just some of the questions one could ask as the new breed of "television-entertainment-surgery-life transformation" has emerged. No doubt future programs will evolve in even new directions. And to ask ethical questions is not to condemn or negatively judge the people involved in this arena. Simply put, if the definition of ethics is "doing the right thing," then is it not important to answer some of these questions?

No doubt the majority of the surgeons, and other cosmetic caregivers, are talented, earnest, and competent professionals and keep the interests and welfare of their patients number one on the list of values. And most patients are no doubt wishing for a positive and life-enhancing transformation following their surgery. It is hoped that this is what they get.

But the questions remain. And there are sometimes no easy pat answers. Surgery is still an art and requires wisdom and discernment when decisions are made to put a patient under the knife, especially when the surgery is not necessary to sustain life. When medical judgment, cosmetic surgery, entertainment, and vulnerable patients are all in the mix, then wisdom and keen judgment are vital.

The First Ethics Tragedy

The Greek poet Pindar (474 BC) writes about the mythical physician Asklepios, who had an illustrious career in mending and healing:

"Those who came to him with flesh devouring sores, with limbs gored by gray bronze or crushed stones, all those with bodies broken, sun struck or frost bitten, he freed of their misery, each from his ailment, and led them forth—some to the lull of soft spells, others by potions, still others with bandages steeped in medications culled from quarters, and others he set right through surgery." [11:47–53]

But this comes to a tragic end:

"Even wisdom feels the lure of gain: gold glittered in his hand and he was hired to retrieve from death a man whose life was already forfeit; Zeus hurled flashing lightning and drove the breath, smoking from the breasts of savior and saved alike." [54–60]

Perhaps this fable highlights the first case of medical ethics. A competent physician was induced by greed to perform a forbidden medical service. He violated divine law and paid the penalty. Medical ethics, then and now, is about the physician's attitude and dealings with the price of saving and healing life.[1]

What Is Ethics

> Ethics is a subject that those colleagues beneath you need to be concerned with. Anon.

Although *ethics* is a word we hear often, we have a hard time defining it. It has been said that a man who is good in his heart is an ethical member of any group in society, whereas one who is bad in his heart is an unethical member. Ethics implies a state of goodness verging on saintliness to which we might aspire but which we are unable to achieve.[2] Random House defines ethics as "moral principles, philosophy of values dealing with the rightness or wrongness of certain actions and to the goodness and badness of the motives and ends of such actions." The fellowship pledge of the American College of Surgeons in part goes: "I pledge to pursue the practice of surgery with honesty, and to place the welfare and rights of my patient above all else."

Perhaps ethics is a personal expression of what one believes is right and one's capacity to give meaning to that belief. It is often associated with honesty and truthfulness. When one thinks about an ethical person, such as an ethical physician, one inherently believes that person will deal with patients in an honest and truthful manner and not put his or her own needs first. In a simplistic way, ethics can be thought of as doing what is right.

Historically, ethical codes have evolved from the time of Hippocrates, through Roman influences, into the writings of Thomas Percival in the eighteenth century, which in turn had an influence on the Code of Ethics of the AMA. (The original AMA ethics writings began as a set of admonitions to ensure peaceful relations between physicians!)

How do ethics relate to the facial plastic surgeon? Why is the existence of ethics important to all physicians? Who should decide what is ethical behavior and what is not? Ultimately, the most important ethical behavior involves the moral bond to which the physician commits in trying to help the patient. One of the goals of this chapter will be to better acquaint facial plastic surgeons with ethical concepts and guides.

Simple Ethical Questions Raised by Plastic Surgery

Several ethical questions come to mind when one is thinking about facial plastic surgery, both cosmetic and reconstructive:

- Is cosmetic surgery inherently ethical or not?
- Is reconstructive surgery more ethical?
- Who should be performing cosmetic and reconstructive surgery?
- What is the difference between a revolutionary new procedure and experimental surgery?
- Who should be primarily making decisions about another person's health?
- How should information about plastic surgery be communicated to the public?
- What is ethical advertising?
- What is ethical behavior with regard to one's peers?
- What is ethical behavior when one is running a business?
- What is ethical behavior with regard to one's patients?

This last, how the physician behaves with regard to the patient because the patient comes to the physician asking for help, is most important. In asking for help the patient presumes that ethical care will be delivered.

Surgeons generally have avoided issues of ethics, believing that if they work hard, study perennially, and do their best technically, all will be well, even though life's experiences teach us that such a notion is naive. But no longer can we just "do the best job that we can" and then move on, as we once did. What we have failed to do in the past, attorneys, insurers, governments, and hospitals now frequently do with ill-informed glee. For example, if we know that certain operations are unnecessary but perform them anyway, how can we protest when outside forces intervene?[3]

A Modern Fable about a Plastic Surgeon and a Patient

Once upon a time, Jane made an appointment with a plastic surgeon. She had never felt very comfortable with her appearance; now she wondered if plastic surgery could help make her happier and add to the quality of her life. After all, she had been reading the paper and seeing ads on TV that talked of the "miracles of cosmetic surgery." The results showed beautiful people—real patients who were smiling, looked great, and seemed very self-assured.

Jane had chosen Dr I. M. ZeBest because he had a very nice ad that extolled his many credentials. He claimed experience and competency in many procedures, and she liked his ability to provide "no-scar surgery." In addition, she had heard that she should only see a doctor who is "board-certified" and Dr. ZeBest was that.

On the day of her consultation, Jane found Dr. ZeBest's office to be palatial, with ornate furnishings. She was asked to complete some paperwork and told that payment was expected that day before the consultation. One of the questions asked was, "Have you ever had any cosmetic surgery in the past and were you happy with the results?" She had had a dermabrasion procedure several years earlier, with modest results and no real problems.

After a 2-hour wait she was escorted into the private office of Dr. ZeBest. When she met Dr. ZeBest, he introduced himself as the "premier plastic surgeon in this part of the country" and asked her what she needed to change. "Nothing drastic, Dr. ZeBest," were her words as she began to describe her feelings about her face. She wanted some subtle improvements. Dr. ZeBest interrupted Jane after a minute or so, telling her that she needed lots of work on her face if she wanted to be really attractive and thus happy. He suggested she have several procedures done. Dr. ZeBest asked her if she was satisfied with the work done by the previous surgeon. He looked at her scars, whistled as he shook his head and muttered, "um, um, umm."

One of the procedures Dr. ZeBest suggested was relatively new, but he had just returned from a seminar the previous week where he had heard about the technique. He felt that he knew just about enough to perform it. Certainly, after he had performed it a few times he would pick up the nuances, and some patient had to be first, after all. Jane asked about possible risks and complications. Dr. ZeBest told her not to worry, he "did not allow complications with his patients." He saw no need to worry Jane by revealing details about the three liability settlements that had been judged against him. Jane told him that she'd had some sort of "hepatitis thing once" but she believes she is over it now.

When it was time to discuss fees, Jane realized she did not have enough money to afford all of the procedures Dr. ZeBest recommended. He advised her to take out a short-term loan and told her that his staff would help her apply through a financing company with which he worked. Jane obtained the loan but later told Dr. ZeBest's receptionist that she had to sell some family jewelry to come up with the final amount.

Before Jane left Dr. ZeBest's office, his assistant told her about a "special personalized skin care regimen" to be started prior to surgery. "Dr. ZeBest wants all his patients on this and it is crucial you maintain this for the rest of your life." We have skin products that have been "developed especially for our patients, and can be purchased only through our office." Thirty minutes later, Jane left with a sack of several jars and bottles of skin rejuvenation lotions and creams and was $245 poorer.

Surgery was scheduled. Jane arranged with some difficulty to be off work for 10 days, and prepared herself. The day before her surgery, one of Dr. ZeBest's friends called him. "I. M., I have a tee time tomorrow at Augusta National for the two of us. Fly down with me in the morning and we will be back by nightfall." Being an avid golfer and Masters fan, Dr. ZeBest wanted to go, but doing so would involve postponing Jane's surgery, creating an inconvenience for her.

"What the heck," he reasoned, "patients change their plans all the time." So he decided to go. He asked his receptionist to call Jane to inform her about the "emergency surgery" he had to perform the next day. Because of her job commitments, it would be another 6 months before Jane could get back on the surgery schedule. She trusted Dr. ZeBest and didn't want to interview another surgeon, so she rescheduled despite losing some vacation time. The morning of surgery she wanted to speak with him one last time preoperatively, as he had promised. But the nurses gave her so much Versed she could barely keep her eyes open and she couldn't think of what she had wanted to say.

Dr. ZeBest was a bit tired that day. The previous day had been exhausting, and he had stayed out late having dinner and drinks at a friend's birthday celebration. This morning his headache was relieved with a Tylenol #3. "I can operate better when I'm tired than most other surgeons can on their best days," he boasted to himself. The surgery seemed to go well, except for a little extra bleeding. "All bleeding stops eventually," he chuckled to his assistant. He noticed a dark nevus on the back of the patient's shoulder that bothered him, even though Jane had never mentioned it, and he excised it for her and discarded it.

In the recovery room, the nurses paged the doctor to tell him that Jane's blood pressure was a bit high, ~200/150. He told them to either find the anesthesiologist or call one of the internists because hypertension was not his thing. Later Jane was discharged.

Jane called the office on postoperative day (POD) no. 4, a bit worried about some redness and swelling of one side of her face. She asked to speak with Dr. ZeBest, and the nurse told her he was seeing patients all day and could not be interrupted. She told Jane to put heat on the swelling and see them at her 1-week visit.

On POD no. 7 in the office, Dr. ZeBest said to Jane: "Darling, you look beautiful!" Jane thought she looked as if she had been hit by a train and she was depressed. There was an ugly dark blue swelling in her cheek, and one side of her mouth seemed not to move as well as it had. "Don't worry, dear, everything will heal perfectly," Dr. ZeBest said with a smile as he backed out of the door. She wanted to ask Dr. ZeBest several questions, but in 40 seconds he was gone, leaving his nurse to remove Jane's sutures. Jane asked when she was to see Dr. ZeBest again, and his nurse replied, "I will be the main person you will see, but we can make an appointment in about 6 months for the doctor to see you." At that moment, Jane did not feel very good about herself, or very beautiful.

Is Cosmetic Surgery Inherently Ethical or Not?

> The creed of the cosmetic surgeon: if you're happy, I'm happy.— J. Goin and M. K. Goin[4]
>
> It is just as important to make patients happy as it is to make them well.— Sir Wm. Osler[5]
>
> The only contraindication to repeat plastic surgery is poverty of funds or tissue.— David Hyman[6]

Plastic surgery generates a great deal of interest and analysis on the part of the public, the medical community, and the payers of health care. Especially significant is the distinction between reconstructive ("to restore") surgery and cosmetic ("to enhance") surgery. The ethics of cosmetic surgery creates interesting viewpoints. Is cosmetic surgery inherently ethical? Is it possible that some procedures themselves are unethical or perhaps are sometimes performed for unethical reasons?

Psychological studies of beauty suggest that more attractive people are thought to be more "sensitive, kind, interesting, strong . . . sociable . . . exciting" and to "experience happier and more fulfilling lives than less attractive people."[7]

For example, let's take the subject of aging. What is the morality of treating the affliction of aging? Is aging an actual disease, and must it be treated as such? Is it ethical to classify aging, which most people would consider a normal process, as an abnormality to be treated? Is there a message that we as practitioners of cosmetic surgery are sending to society to the effect that looking older is undesirable and must be addressed? Or has society already decided this for us, and are we merely responding to a need? If our society valued aging and the people who age the most, then wrinkles would be considered worthy of praise.[8]

Let us also examine the goal of cosmetic surgery. Traditionally the goal of medicine has been health, and this remains the goal for most of medicine, both Eastern and Western. But the ideal outcome of many cosmetic procedures has become not health but happiness with the surgical result. Is it ethical to replace "health" with "happiness with the result"? So now the measure of a surgical outcome is not whether the patient is healthier but whether he or she likes what was done. For example, if a patient requests we make an ornamental scar on one cheek, we know that this does not promote physical health. Would we hesitate to perform such a surgery? Yet the creation of a scar as a by-product of a cosmetic procedure (say, tightening of a sagging face) is a routine event.

What if a patient were to request removal of an organ because the person believes this would improve his or her self-esteem? Most surgeons would probably not agree. However, we routinely remove sections of skin from the face and lids (portions of the largest organ) solely in the hope that the new appearance will help the patient to feel better.[9]

If one decides that surgery performed solely for beautification is unethical, then other questions arise. Are cosmetic dental procedures ethical? Do procedures designed to simply whiten teeth or to position shiny veneers over existing teeth violate this prohibition against beautification? No one would argue that haircuts are in themselves unethical. Is the application of skin tattoos unethical? And what about application of ultraviolet radiation to skin for the purpose of darkening it? After all, one can make the case that this is inherently unhealthy, promoting a myriad of health problems.

On the other hand, is the application of nonionizing radiation to skin (i.e., laser "skin resurfacing") more ethical than the services of tanning centers? After all, a second-degree burn is intentionally created for the skin to take on a "more desirable" texture and color.

Today's medical model has the surgeon as a cafeteria worker, displaying the various therapies to patients and allowing them to choose on the basis of risk, price, benefit, or whatever else the patient considers to be important.[9]

And what of the question, Is reconstructive surgery more ethical than cosmetic surgery? One could argue that it may be. Or one could argue that surgery that ends up being mutilative (some head and neck cancer extirpations) perhaps is not as ethical as it could be. What of nasal surgery? Is reduction of a nasal fracture (reconstructive) more ethical than a pure rhinoplasty (cosmetic)? What about septorhinoplasty? Just what is unethical surgery and who is responsible for defining it?

Physician Qualifications: Who Should Be Performing Plastic Surgery?

> Cur'd yesterday of my disease I died last night of my physician.— Matthew Prior

Much has been made of the qualifications surgeons must hold before being allowed to call themselves "plastic surgeons" and perform procedures defined as "plastic surgery procedures." Who should the practitioners be? Should they all come from the ranks of a certain specialty, board, or society? Does the completion of a certain training program or board certification confer to a surgeon special qualities and qualifications that can only be obtained in this manner? Certainly a patient seeking plastic surgery should expect the surgeon to be well trained in the performance of that procedure and capable of handling any complications that might arise.

Some surgeons disparage the training, education, or skills of other surgeons. Is this ethical? On the other hand, if a surgeon knows that another physician is not trained to perform certain procedures and has seen serious complications arising from that physician's past surgeries, is there a moral obligation to warn the patient against surgery? Then there are those surgeons who masquerade as the knight in armor riding the white steed, whose mission in life is to save society from the surgeons who have invaded the others' turf. Some of these champions have been guilty of defending their own financial coffers while demonstrating little altruistic concern.

Today's plastic surgeon stands on the shoulders of giants who emerged from general surgery, orthopedics, otolaryngology, ophthalmology, maxillofacial surgery, and dermatology—so he or she should grumble least of all about territorial disputes.

Another issue is the development and use of new surgical procedures and devices. As no surgeon is born with the innate knowledge of how to perform a surgical procedure, all must be learned. Some are more complicated than others. Once in practice, the surgeon may learn of a new procedure while attending a medical conference or perusing a journal. When is it ethical to introduce a new and perhaps partially unproved procedure on one's patients? And is there anything wrong with that surgeon promoting her- or himself as the "first surgeon in this area" to become trained in this implicitly improved procedure?

Also along the lines of training and proficiency, is it possible for every surgeon to become an "expert" in every procedure related to his or her specialty? The standard of care does not say that any procedure must be perfect or the outcome guaranteed. But society does expect a certain baseline of competency from its physicians, including surgeons. The moral issue here is the competence of the surgeon.

Another question we must ask is, Should physicians be performing procedures in their own office or office surgical suite if they cannot gain privileges to perform the same procedure in an accredited surgical facility or hospital, which is subject to strict peer review? Should prospective patients be told that their surgeon does not have credentials to perform certain procedures in an outside licensed medical center? One could also argue that due to the imperfect system of credentialing, which is subject to local politics and sometimes the personal agendas of competing surgeons, it may be impossible in some institutions for a given physician to ever obtain credentialing by that body. Or one could argue that a lack of peer credentialing exposes the patient to excessive risk.

But who can disagree that the foremost goal of our profession should be the issue of competency. Don't all patients deserve a competent physician, and certainly a competent facial plastic surgeon? It would seem that rules, regulations, admonitions, and efforts that point in the direction of enhanced competency would be worthwhile goals.

It has been stated that "most surgeons have a defect, congenital or acquired, of exaggerating the number of operations they do and of underestimating the failures. Some may call this lying; the more forgiving might say that it is evidence of rampant optimism."[10]

So our final prayer may become, "God, please provide me with a surgeon who knows what he or she is doing."

Health Care Decision Making: Who Should Do It?

> From the poetry of Lord Byron they drew a system of ethics, compounded of misanthropy and voluptuousness.
> — Lord Macaulay

At first glance, this may appear to be a simple question. But in today's world, there are many players vying for center stage when surgery is contemplated.

First, of course, there is the *patient*. We assume the patient is competent to make an "informed decision." But is the patient always properly informed? Can we assume that the patient has heard all the pros and cons about the proposed surgery, even if the surgeon tried his or her best to delineate them? Are patients always of sound mind and judgment to make this sort of decision? Who should decide if they are or aren't? Isn't the advice of a physician implicitly coercive because the surgeon is the "powerful one" and the patient in the lesser position of seeking advice? Or, if a patient adheres to a set of aesthetic beliefs different from those of the surgeon, how does one reconcile the difference?

Then there is the *surgeon*. Is the judgment of the surgeon always sound? Can it be influenced from time to time by extraneous forces, sometimes without the surgeon's conscious understanding? If the surgeon is having a particularly good day or not-so-good day, does his or her own mood play an important role? Does the promise of money sometimes seduce the surgeon into scheduling an inappropriate surgery? And who decides if the surgeon has sufficient skill to perform a certain procedure, especially if it is a relatively new procedure?

Then there are other players. If a *third-party health insurer* is involved, should they decide if a procedure is medically necessary or should the surgeon? Should the surgeon withhold information or exaggerate symptoms if it helps the patient achieve precertification? Or, if the surgeon knows that a plan he or she participates in will likely pay for a surgery but at a greatly reduced rate, then should he or she file for insurance in the first place?

Let's presume that certain materials or medical devices are to be used in the surgery. Does the existence of a business relationship between the surgeon and the company that manufactures the devices matter? If the surgeon financially profits from use of this material, does this interfere with impartial judgment?

What if a material or drug is approved by the Food and Drug Administration (FDA) for use in a certain anatomical site but the patient requests use in an entirely different site? What if the patient requests volumes that greatly exceed the usual amount? Should the patient be the one to decide if a certain implant should be used or not? Is the patient capable of deciding? What if the patient has a potentially communicable disease? What if the patient has some form of viral hepatitis history? What if he or she is positive for human immunodeficiency virus (HIV)? Should cosmetic surgery still be done? What if a patient desires surgery but the surgeon refuses to operate because of HIV history? Should the surgeon have the right to refuse the patient? Does this violate constitutional rights of the patient? Conversely, does an HIV-positive surgeon have an obligation to inform the patient prior to surgery?[10]

It is clear that medical decision making can be very complex. And when the directions become unclear, what shall serve as the "ethical compass" that sets us back on the correct course?

Caveat Emptor: What Is Ethical Advertising?

> Some forms of advertising are economical with the truth.[11]

Once upon a time, physicians did not engage in advertising, at least in the sense of paid use of the media to exhort their virtues and skills. It was assumed that medicine was a profession above those of trades people and that a surgeon who was "able, affable, available, and affordable" would have patients knocking on his door.

Yet a student of medicine can find examples of early advertising. The hawking of potions and elixirs was common. Consider the following example by a nineteenth century "medical salesman" taken from the *Saturday Evening Post* on September 13, 1760:

> A prolifick elixir, the cure of barrenness in women, of imbecility in men, by promoting the cheerful curricule of the blood and juices, raising all the fluids from their languid state, to one more florid and sparkeling, increasing the animal spirits, restoring the juvenile bloom, and evidently replenishing the crispy fibers of the whole habit with a generous warmth and balmy moisture . . . and even seems to keep back the effects of old age itself.

It is interesting to compare the previous example with a more recent ad from a plastic surgeon:

> Lines and wrinkles smoothed away naturally. Being unhappy with lines and wrinkles that are making you look older than you feel is a problem you don't have to live with any more. We have also developed an exclusive skin care treatment program which, in addition to our long established collagen replacement therapy service, represents the most important advance in skin care by any cosmetic surgery group.[11]

In recent times, there has been rapid growth of physician advertising. This was preceded in many parts of the United States by advertising produced by other medical groups, including hospitals, health insurers, and other health-related organizations; dentists; chiropractors; and others. Advertising by attorneys can be viewed as a separate phenomenon. (One could write another treatise on "truthful advertising by the legal profession.") So many physicians and surgeons have joined the ranks of advertisers and marketers of their skills.

The question begs to be asked: Is advertising itself inherently ethical? Is it unethical? Shouldn't advertising be truthful and helpful? Just what is ethical advertising and who should decide?

For instance, does plastic surgery advertising target a more vulnerable population? Is it moral to create a desire for procedures (unnecessary markets) that carry morbidity and risk, especially when presented to susceptible patients with lower self-esteem? In advertising cosmetic procedures, how can the self-esteem of a prospective patient be enhanced by a procedure that carries the message that he or she is basically unacceptable? For example, by promoting younger faces, do we not promote the "cult of youth"? Are we creating an unnecessary market for our surplus surgical skills? Although we know the importance of having realistic expectations, are we not advertising "perfection" in the quest for the perfect face?

When it comes to the advertising world, who should monitor and decipher boundary disputes between competing specialties? Should advertising be regulated and subject to certain government statutes, or should the "free market" decide who should say what about themselves? Should there be limits on what advertising should say or not say? Should paid testimonials from patients be permitted? Should there be a limit on use of terms like *exclusive, specially trained, first to be certified*, and other pronouncements of special competency? Should words like *advanced* and *superior* be allowed to be used without proof of validity?

Do consumers and society as a whole benefit from increased advertising? Do plastic surgeons contribute to the betterment of their communities by print ads promising a new face or by infomercials describing the benefits of certain procedures? For that matter, does knowledge of the newest version of the "Ronco Vegematic" help us or does it really matter?

After all, shouldn't society have access to all kinds of information? We cannot ban certain types of services and allow promotion of others, can we? But how do we know when we are actually seeing accurate and truthful information?

Professional Conduct: Our Behavior with Patients, Peers, and the Public

With Patients

> Ethics are the only guarantee we have in doing what we think is best in helping our patients—in the end this must prevail.
> Postoperatively each surgeon must ask himself, What did the operation accomplish?— John Conley, MD[12]
> God has given you one face and you make yourselves another.— Shakespeare[13]

What is the primary duty of the physician in the doctor–patient relationship? Ultimately, how we treat our patients defines the state of our ethical development. Ideally, we listen to learn about the patient's needs, we try to communicate about possible treatment options, we help patients to become adequately informed, we use our skills to try to achieve the best possible surgical results, we guide our patients through the healing process, and we try to be there for them afterward, as they enjoy (we hope) their improved faces and spirits.

But things aren't always ideal.

Is it ethical to spend 20 minutes with a prospective patient and then decide to perform procedures that carry potential health risks and cost thousands of dollars? In the initial consultation, sometimes the surgeon does not develop a rapport with the patient. Is it best to choose not to pursue the doctor–patient relationship at this point? As the consultation develops, isn't the doctor's advice somewhat coercive? Is it not weighted by the lure of increased income made possible by offering more and more procedures? How does a surgeon communicate enthusiasm to the patient about a procedure without appearing to be "selling" the patient something that may not be wanted or needed?

Sometimes the patient's expectations are not met. Does this constitute treatment failure? Sometimes the surgeon may feel no compassion for the patient. Should compassion be faked? Or is that dishonest? If there really exists no human empathy for the patient, how should this be handled? What if the surgeon just does not like the patient at all? Does this mean that the patient–doctor relationship should be terminated? If so, what is the best ethical (not to mention medicolegal) way to terminate the relationship?

And what constitutes unethical surgery? When is surgery "experimental" and when is it "breakthrough" surgery? What is the difference between performing "research" on your patients and offering them the "latest advances" in plastic surgery? Is it ethical to try a new procedure on a patient after just hearing about it at a meeting? What of new devices or materials that have not been investigated in terms of their long-term consequences to the patient? Is it ethical for the surgeon to use a drug or material (e.g., collagen) in a patient for a non-FDA-approved use or at an anatomical site for which it was not intended?

Remember that the surgeon is running a business, and the patient is the consumer who requests goods or services in exchange for money. The success of the transaction, like all business transactions, is whether the customer is happy with the services. Correct? Or is there more to it than a mere business comparison? Does not the physician have a greater moral responsibility than the typical business person?

For example, if a typical business with a product or service to sell is approached by a consumer who has a lot of money, the business owner is interested in making a business transaction. Let's suppose the consumer offers a lot more money for some special deal or more services. For example, at the end of a routine consultation, the patient says: "I want all six procedures we discussed, I want surgery tomorrow, and I will double the quoted fee in exchange for your additional trouble, doctor." In most businesses, it would be considered smart to find a way to satisfy the customer and make the financial exchange. But what about our situation? Can one separate business from ethics?

There are many other questions one must answer in terms of how to deal ethically with patients who walk into the surgeon's office.

With Peers

> A good name is more desirable than great riches; to be esteemed is better than silver or gold.— Proverbs 22:1

The early codes of professional conduct dealt primarily not with proper care of patients but with rules of conduct between physicians. For example, turf battles are not new, and physicians have traditionally had trouble in dealing with each other. Certainly when well-educated, ambitious individuals with large egos find themselves competing with others of like mind, conflicts and disagreements ensue.

In the realm of ethical behavior, how should physicians best deal with members of their own profession who violate the most commonly agreed on ethical principles? There exist state and national licensing boards, hospital committees, and ethics panels that can, and sometimes do, investigate questionable behavior. But in day-to-day living, how does one physician deal with another physician who appears to be transgressing beyond certain boundaries? How does one deal with an incompetent surgeon? If a surgeon sees evidence of poor work on a patient, is it ever ethical to openly criticize the offending surgeon?

On another matter, is it ethical for the specialist plastic surgeon to not inform or confer with the primary care physician about a mutual patient? What if the primary care physician recommends that a patient not undergo an elective surgery? Is it ethical for the plastic surgeon to suggest a second opinion or even to disregard the advice and proceed with the surgery?

And what of a new procedure that has been "invented" by a surgeon? If it helps people, should it be made available to all interested surgeons? Or is it ethical to "patent the procedure" so that no one else will steal it? Or should the inventor surgeon just market it to others if they agree to pay some money for the right to learn the technique?

Finally, is it ethical for a surgeon who has a financial relationship with a company to encourage use of that company's products to other surgeons?

If plastic surgeons were asked, "How do you wish your medical colleagues to remember you?" what would be the likely answer?

With the Business Community—the Surgeon as Businessperson

> Physicians of the utmost fame were called at once, but when they came they answered, as they took their fees, there is not a cure for this disease.— Hilaire Belloc

A successful surgeon must become a successful businessperson or the surgery services will not be available for long. Can this be done in an ethical manner, or is "successful business" incompatible with "good ethical standards"? How does the surgeon balance being a responsible businessperson and a compassionate caregiver? In today's world, we have situations where physicians who are members of a health maintenance organization must make medical decisions for their patients that may sometimes affect the final reimbursement rates for the physicians in that group. By denying certain tests and treatments, their financial reward increases. The question is obvious: Do the financial interests of the organization outweigh the health interests of the patient?

Additional questions we must answer in today's climate are as follows: Is the sale of such products as skin care potions, nutritional supplements, and vitamins for profit in one's office ethical? Is the patient not being somewhat coerced to buy what the doctor recommends?

Is it acceptable for a surgeon with a financial relationship with a company to support use of that company's products by other surgeons? Is it okay to accept gifts from companies? Is it ethical for the plastic surgeon to align with lay "beauty businesses" and salons to sign up patients, exchanging reduced costs for exclusive referral of potential patients? Is it ethical to raffle a cosmetic surgery procedure at a fund-raising benefit event?

The necessity of coexisting with other businesses is a reality. How best to relate to such businesses is the question.

New Biotechnology, Materials, and Procedures: Breakthroughs or Experiments?

> New procedures and devices are good if the patient is benefited and the new ideas are significant, practical, and successful. But the patient is harmed if the procedure is based on premature presentation, inaccurate information, unrealistic hopes, and unprepared surgeons.[3]

Although "plastic" is rarely used in plastic surgery procedures, there is never a dearth of other alloplastic or homograft materials available for implantation in patients. We know that medical devices and preformed implants sometimes vary not only between countries but between training institutions. There exists a large cache of "legal" cosmetic and reconstructive materials that may find their way into human bodies on any given day. Who should be responsible for ensuring that these implants and materials are safe for human consumption? Should the FDA assume ultimate responsibility? Should it be the manufacturer or supplier of the device? Should it rest with the surgeon recommending the surgery? Or should it rest with the patients themselves?

For those who think it might not matter, please consider recent history and the ongoing morass featuring the silicone breast implants. In 1992 the FDA and its General and Plastic Surgery Devices Panel concluded that, after years of use, not a single entity involved in the use of silicone-filled breast implants could meet the statutory requirements for safety and effectiveness.[14] After years of retrospective clinical studies, emotional rhetoric, and ongoing legal battles featuring unhappy patients accompanied by hungry plaintiff jackals, and as we view the billion dollar spoils, we pause to assess the emotional, legal, and financial costs. The question begs to be asked, was this an abrogation of responsibility on the part of surgeons to not insist on answers from the companies that develop and sell such devices?[15]

Congress long ago decided that caveat emptor is not an acceptable standard for medical devices used in this country. A review of the literature (refer to the history of pacemakers and spine appliances) will reveal that plastic surgery is not alone in its confusion.

And what of new procedures? Sometimes there is a fine line between a revolutionary new procedure and experimental surgery. How does one judge the competency of surgeons to perform the "latest procedure"? We can test automobile drivers and airline pilots, along with others trusted with performing in the public realm. Can we test a surgeon's skill out of the operating theater before it is applied to a living face? Can patients have any real assurances of the competency of the person to whom they entrust their face?

Medical Missions: Have Scalpel, Will Travel

> So when you give to the needy, do not announce it with trumpets.— Matthew 6:1

It is not uncommon for surgeons to volunteer their services in locations far from the communities in which they practice. Apart from the career medical missionary, there seem to be numerous venues where plastic surgeons can serve as short-term, intermediate-term, and even very short term itinerant surgeons. Most of the volunteer work being performed in domestic and foreign communities is likely altruistic and provides a very positive service for those patients who are the beneficiaries. So what possible ethics problems might arise?

Well-meaning surgeons from developed countries visit less endowed countries briefly to operate on indigenous patients who do not have access to certain types of elective surgery. The motivation can be mixed: to improve the quality of life is noble, but to improve one's skills by practicing on others is something else (e.g., in an "overdoctored country" they might not have the chance to perform a cleft lip repair). To gain experience at the expense of a disadvantaged community implies that the patients are of lesser worth than those living in the doctor's own country.[16]

Relatively few are helped unless the visiting surgeon is also there to instruct local surgeons in the techniques. This also emphasizes the shortcomings of the host country.[4] After the trip is complete, the physician has the opportunity to parlay it into a public relations experience. One might ask, Who becomes the beneficiary of this latest media exposure? Is the resultant media attention "just news," produced for the benefit of the local community. Or is it savvy marketing, which positions the surgeon as the latest Dr. Albert Schweitzer? I know several generous and committed physicians who tirelessly tend to the needs of impoverished patients in very difficult conditions overseas. I have seen surgeons who participate in regular foreign medical missions state in newsletters to their patients that they don't really enjoy traveling every year to those exotic lands to render their skills; rather, they do it out of a sense of "calling" as a self-sacrifice.

But do motivations really matter if a good deed is offered to a person who otherwise might not have benefited? Is this colonial paternalism or a mission of mercy?

Teaching and Training: Practicing Medicine

> Doctor, will you be the one actually performing my surgery?
> — A modern patient

Because no physician is born with medical wisdom or possesses innate surgical technique, all doctors must learn and be trained. All physicians, including surgeons, learn by their experiences in treating live patients. Sometimes the practice of medicine is actually that—practice. How do we balance the rights of the novice surgeon to learn and of society to replenish its surgical force against the rights of the patient who seeks care in a "teaching institution"? What rights does the patient in a teaching and training institution have? For example, if the senior surgeon is "supervising" the case, does this mean that the senior member is helping guide the novice's hand, carefully positioned in the operating suite? Or is he or she "present" but in another operating room, or the lounge, or via cell phone from the golf course? If a patient agrees to a trainee doing the surgery under the supervision of the senior physician, then what role has the senior physician agreed to take? What if the patient is a member of the surgeon's given the patient's immediate family? Should the care given the patient be different from the care given another?

We encounter other questions as well. Is it ethical for a resident surgeon to perform a procedure requiring thoughtful judgment and technical dexterity while extremely fatigued, often secondary to a long on-call stint?

Summary

As we endeavor to excel in facial plastic and reconstructive surgery, we realize that it is fairly easy to teach surgical techniques and to acquire new information. What is more difficult is to teach judgment and to develop advanced skills in ethical decision making. Although many surgeons developed a sense of ethics as they grew from childhood to mature adult, and from novice surgeon to accomplished master surgeon, unfortunately not all have done so. We need to improve on the process whereby we screen candidates who apply for facial plastic surgery residencies and fellowships, as well as continue to emphasize the importance of ethical behavior in our practices. Let us not forget, too, that there are many as yet undescribed ethical dilemmas to come.

We have asked many questions but find it difficult to provide all of the answers. Nevertheless, it is important that the questions be stated. We will end with a few words of wisdom by others:

> Professionals without ethics are merely technicians who know how to perform work but who have no capacity to say why their work has any larger meaning.[17] What we need is to construct and maintain a way of life of which we are not ashamed and which we shall not, on reflection, regret or despise, and which we respect.[18]
>
> As a stream cannot rise above its source, so a code cannot change a low-grade man into a high-grade doctor, but it can help a good man be a better man, and a more enlightened doctor. It can quicken and inform a conscience, but not create one.[19]
>
> In the final analysis, honesty in all matters is the keystone to our ethical arch. We must follow our instincts, offering to those in our care only the operations we would wish for our own wife or daughter or mother, advising with the truthfulness and kindness that we would hope our own loved ones would encounter.[3]
>
> The most ethical position is that which helps the patient and family most, under the advice and counsel of the physician.[20]

References

1. Jonsen AR. The fall of Asklepios: medicine, morality, and money. Plast Reconstr Surg 1988;82:147–150
2. Ward CM. Defining medical ethics. Br J Plast Surg 1993;46:647–651
3. Lister BD. Ethics in surgical practice. Plast Reconstr Surg 1996;97:185–193
4. Goin J, Goin MK. Changing the Body: Psychological Effects of Plastic Surgery. Baltimore: Williams & Wilkins; 1981
5. Tardy ME Jr. Ethics and integrity in facial plastic surgery: imperatives for the 21st century. Facial Plast Surg 1995;11:111–115
6. Hyman DA. Aesthetics and ethics: the implications of cosmetic surgery. Perspect Biol Med 1990;33:190–202
7. Berscheid S, Gangestad S. The social and psychological implications of facial physical attractiveness. Clin Plast Surg 1982;9:289
8. Ringel EW. The morality of cosmetic surgery of aging. Arch Dermatol 1998;134:427–431
9. Hyman DA. Cosmetic surgery implications. Perspect Biol Med 1990;33:190–202
10. Goldwyn RM. Reporting or hiding a complication. Plast Reconstr Surg 1983;71:843–848
11. Ward C. Advertising and boundary disputes. Br J Plast Surg 1994;47: 381–385
12. Conley J. The meaning of life-threatening disease in the area of the head and neck. Acta Otolaryngol 1985;99:201–204
13. Shakespeare W. Hamlet. Act 3, Scene 1.
14. Kessler DA, Merkatz RB, Schapiro R. A call for higher standards for breast implants [editorial]. JAMA 1993;270:2607–2608
15. Ward CM. Surgical research, experiments, and innovation. Br J Plast Surg 1994;47:90–94
16. Ward CM. Teaching, training, and traveling. Br J Plast Surg 1994;47: 280–284
17. Churchill LR. Reviving a distinctive medical ethic. Hastings Cent Rep 1989;19:28–34
18. Hampshire S. Mortality and Conflict. Cambridge: Harvard University Press; 1983:168
19. World Medical Association. Code of Medical Ethics. London: World Medical Association; 1949
20. Conley J. Ethics in otolaryngology. Acta Otolaryngol 1981;91: 369–374

15 Ambulatory Surgery

William H. Beeson

Ambulatory surgery is on the rise for several reasons. The dramatic increase is due in part to improved anesthesia, improved surgical techniques, the increased desire to contain medical costs, and the realization that postoperative infections might well be decreased in the ambulatory versus hospital setting. Improved anesthesia has resulted in significantly less postoperative nausea and vomiting. This enables patients to return home for convalescence much earlier than with prior anesthetic techniques. Pharmacological advances have resulted in much improved analgesia during recovery.

Improved surgical techniques have resulted in a reduction of intraoperative time. In addition, advances have lessened the degree of tissue trauma, thereby facilitating recovery and reducing postoperative ecchymosis and pain. Improved hemostatic techniques have decreased the need for postoperative transfusions. The list goes on and on.

In 1979, less than 10% of all surgeries were done as outpatient procedures. By 1995, more than 50% were outpatient procedures. Currently, in the United States, more operations are done as outpatient (65%) than as inpatients (35%). It is estimated that 15 to 20% of all outpatient operations are done as office-based surgeries. This appears to be especially true with cosmetic procedures. ("Guidelines for Care of Office Surgical Facilities," American Academy of Dermatology, part 1, 1992, part 2, 1995).

General Considerations

Advantages and Disadvantages

There are many pros and cons for performing ambulatory surgery in a freestanding ambulatory surgery center. Some legal authorities feel that there is yet to be a standard of care for procedures performed in such a setting. Traditionally, the community standards required that one should perform surgery and render care equal to hospital standards, regardless of the location where such care was rendered. However, today there are those who believe that with more and more surgeries being done in an office surgical setting or in a freestanding ambulatory surgical facility a new standard may be evolving. In fact, some feel that this special standard for ambulatory surgical patients may actually be a higher standard. Some legal authorities believe that standards for such care regarding preoperative and postoperative instructions, postoperative monitoring, and follow-up care might actually be higher than that rendered in an inpatient setting. These opinions further emphasize the importance of establishing a thorough and effective risk-management program in any type of ambulatory surgical setting.

Surgical Procedure

Whether you are performing surgery in an office facility or in a freestanding ambulatory surgery center that you develop, you will have to establish protocols and operating procedures that are very similar to those utilized in the hospital setting. These protocols and operating procedures have to be designed to maximize the patient's safety. A primary tenet is close observation of the patient in the immediate postoperative period. This would dictate that vital signs be appropriately monitored and that recovery be provided in an area that affords the patients both privacy and convenience while making emergency resuscitative equipment and skilled personnel readily available, should such be necessary.

Many authorities believe that it is critical that patient education be maximized when surgery is performed in either an office surgical or a freestanding ambulatory surgical setting. Normally, in a hospital setting the floor nurse would be responsible for reviewing postoperative instructions with the patient and the family prior to discharge. However, when surgery is performed on an outpatient basis the responsibility rests with the physician and the physician's staff to provide these important instructions. Obviously, patients cannot care for themselves immediately following surgery. For this reason, it is critical that a responsible adult, who is cognizant of the postoperative instructions, stays with the patient. Such a person must be able to deal effectively with the normal postoperative sequelae that a floor nurse would ordinarily be responsible for in the hospital inpatient setting. Dressing changes, postoperative nausea and vomiting, and minor discomfort are all associated with surgical procedures and must be dealt with by the patient's caretaker. It is critical that instructions and additional medical support be readily available for the patient, should such be needed. The protocols must address all of these potential issues.

It is important that the physician and staff be readily available to answer questions and deal with emergency situations. It is critical that adequate backup systems be employed so that in an event such as paging batteries going dead, it does not preclude the patient or the patient's caretaker from obtaining a quick medical response to their questions.

Documentation has always been of medical-legal importance. It is extremely critical in the outpatient setting. Oftentimes the physician who has operated in the hospital setting takes for granted the degree of documentation that is required. But the physician and office staff are themselves responsible for the documentation when surgery is performed either in the office surgical setting or in the freestanding ambulatory surgical center. Inpatients have their vital signs, symptoms, and conditions frequently documented on the patient's record by the attending nurse. On an outpatient basis, a telephone call that the patient is having some nausea or has decreased oral intake of fluids will be important at a later time. It is extremely important that such information obtained from telephone calls be recorded in the patient's chart in a timely manner to facilitate and preserve the continuity of care. Protocols must be established to ensure this. Physicians performing surgery on an ambulatory basis must have a system to insure such phone calls and patient contacts can be recorded appropriately in the patient's medical record.

Quality of Care

Quality of care has always been of primary importance to physicians. With today's health care market being so competitive and with the health care market moving more toward the consumer-driven health care system, this takes on even more importance because consumers are looking for the best value for their health care dollar.

Quality of care is of paramount importance to both physicians and patients. It is important to address the issue of quality of care factually, whether the care is rendered as an inpatient or an outpatient in either a hospital, office surgical, or freestanding surgical center.

The Orkand study is often regarded as the best structured, best implemented, and most authoritative study assessment with quality of care in the ambulatory surgery. The study showed that the quality of care in ambulatory surgical units was no less than that obtained by hospital inpatients. In 1974, the Department of Health, Education, and Welfare awarded the Orkand Corporation of Silver Springs, Maryland, a 3-year contract to study cost, quality, and the effect on the American health care delivery system of surgery performed in a variety of settings. The study involved 900 patients in seven facilities in Phoenix, Arizona. Care was assessed in the following four settings:

1. Traditional hospital inpatients
2. Traditional hospital outpatients
3. Hospital ambulatory surgical centers
4. Surgical care rendered in freestanding centers

The findings related that independent freestanding units cost ~42.5 to 61.4% less than care rendered in an inpatient setting. Independent freestanding units cost ~14.3 to 44.9% less than similar care rendered in the hospital ambulatory units. Most important, however, it was the fact that the overall quality of care rendered in freestanding units was noted to be at least as good as care rendered in the other three settings. Understandably, such an extensive and expensive study as the Orkand project has not been repeated. However, it serves to subjectively justify and quantitate the quality of care that can be safely rendered in the office or freestanding ambulatory surgical arena.

Many physicians believe that quality of care actually increases when surgery is performed in the office surgical unit or the freestanding ambulatory surgical center because there is increased supervision in such arenas. The physician is constantly available to monitor all stages of the patient's care, including the preoperative sedation, postoperative recovery, and, frequently, the discharge. This is not the case in the hospital setting. The physician is also readily available to handle any complications that arise during the patient's treatment as well as to supervise the care that is being delivered. In the office surgical unit, the physician is able to supervise all employees directly and there is a direct accountability that should help to increase the quality of care delivered.

An important aspect is the fact that there is increased specialization when surgery is performed in the office surgical unit or in the freestanding surgical center versus the hospital setting. Essentially, this is the "focused factory" concept. The physician staff and those that are functioning at the surgical center are familiar with the routine being performed and have specialized equipment and the expertise necessary to carry out the patient's treatment efficiently and effectively. In the hospital setting, it is common to have operating room nurses who are not familiar with the procedure being performed or scheduling conflicts resulting in equipment being unavailable.

Many surgeons find that there is a significant reduction in wasted resources as compared with surgery being performed in the hospital setting. When employees are directly accountable for resources and supplies and when these are under the scrutiny of the physician and the supervisory staff, waste dramatically decreases.

Many believe that the office-based surgical unit and the freestanding ambulatory surgery center are more cost-effective and perhaps provide better quality of care than surgery performed in the hospital setting. However, the physician assumes increased responsibility when surgery is undertaken outside the hospital setting. Risks can increase dramatically if the surgeon does not prudently execute those responsibilities. Surgery in the ambulatory surgical setting requires a change in philosophy and a change in standard operating procedures. Today, it is important for physicians to deliver the care in the most cost-effective surrounding, with no sacrifice in the quality of care rendered.

Accreditation and Certification

One of the first legal problems faced by surgeons desiring to open an office surgical unit or a freestanding surgical center is the possible requirement for a certificate of need or state licensure. Certificate of need and licensure laws vary from state to state. It is important to check with the state board of health or other health care regulatory agencies regarding these issues. Oftentimes, a consultation with a legal counsel specializing in health care is also advisable.

In many states, an ambulatory surgical center must be licensed by the state, whereas in other states accreditation by a nationally recognized entity suffices. In many states, a physician's office exemption exists. However, there has been a trend in recent years for states to require office surgical units to be licensed by the state or accredited by a nationally recognized entity. With the increased number of surgical cases being performed in the ambulatory surgical setting, regulatory bodies are developing rules and regulations that provide more stringent oversight of outpatient surgery.

There are two levels of certification or accreditation for office surgical or freestanding surgery centers. The first level is accreditation by nationally recognized accrediting organizations such as the Accreditation Association for Ambulatory Health Care (AAAHC) or the Joint Commission on Accreditation of Healthcare Organizations (JCAHO). These are examples of organizations that are nonprofit and nongovernmental and provide independent review and accreditation for ambulatory surgical and office surgical facilities. These organizations have developed standards to regulate and govern ambulatory facilities. These organizations also have a survey process, which provides on-site review to evaluate employees of the organization and the care being provided. These entities emphasize procedures and protocols that ensure a high quality of care in the surveyed facilities.

A second level of accreditation or certification is state licensure or Medicare certification. In some areas, a certificate of need may be required to obtain Medicare certification or state licensure. The cost associated with obtaining this "second level" of certification can be extremely significant. There are increased administrative costs in applying for such certification and there may be considerable paperwork that must be completed. Assistance from a paid consultant is often required to complete the various forms and applications, which are necessary for state licensure and Medicare certification. In addition, there are strict physical plan requirements that may be extremely expensive. Many physicians have found that the structural cost for a facility to meet state licensure or Medicare requirements may be twice the cost as compared with an office surgical facility that could be approved by AAAHC or JCAHO. It is advisable to contact your state health care planning agency or board of health regarding specific physical plans, requirements, and regulations for freestanding surgical centers and office surgical facilities in your state. In addition, assistance from an architect experienced in building medical facilities may be advantageous.

There are numerous reasons why an organization would want to obtain certification or accreditation, even if it is not a state requirement. A great deal of satisfaction is obtained from knowing that an outside organization has placed its "stamp of approval" on your organization and your operations. The service industry has long recognized the promotional value that can be obtained from such recognition. It attests that the organization has established and continues to meet specific standards in the important areas of quality care and patient safety.

Some specialty societies require that their members provide care within an organization where there is peer review and quality assurance. This often means that they need to practice within a facility that is certified or accredited to maintain membership within the specialty society.

In an ever-increasing litigious climate, there may well be an advantage to having certification, should an untold event occur in your office surgical or freestanding ambulatory surgical center. Some legal authorities feel that the certification would help to establish that you have met or exceed the local community standards for quality of care in such a facility.

Reimbursement may be a consideration. Most third-party carriers will reimburse for surgery performed in a licensed freestanding ambulatory surgical center. Medicare will reimburse for procedures performed that they certify. However, in some cases, office surgical units may qualify for a facility fee or supply charge if the facility is certified or accredited by specific organizations. Although this activity is not uniform among carriers, it is an important consideration and it should be investigated on an individual basis.

The following are nationally recognized not-for-profit ambulatory surgery accrediting organizations:

Accreditation Association for Ambulatory Health Care, Inc., 3201 Old Glenview Road, Suite 300, Wilmette, IL 60091

American Association for Accreditation of Ambulatory Surgical Facilities, Inc., 1102 Allanson Road, Mundelein, IL 60060

The Joint Commission on Accreditation of Healthcare Organizations, One Renaissance Boulevard, Oakbrook Terrace, IL 60181

American Osteopathic Association, 142 East Ontario Street, Chicago, IL 60611

Guidelines for Development of Ambulatory Surgical Facilities

It is important to have basic policies and procedures, which help to guide the performance of surgery in the office surgical or freestanding ambulatory surgical center. These policies, procedures, and common protocols typically fall into three areas: administration, quality of care, and clinical. These protocols and guidelines are recommended to help ensure that high-quality care is delivered in a safe atmosphere that recognizes basic patient rights.

Administration

Administrative areas deal with the governance of the facility and ensuring basic patient rights. When developing policies and procedures regarding governance, it is important the facilities have policies that describe the organizational structure, including lines of authority, responsibility, and accountability. In most cases, there would be a governing body that has the ultimate responsibility. Frequently a "medical director" is identified as a chief supervisory person. Job descriptions for each position and a supervisory structure are important to ensure that quality health care is provided in a safe environment. An important aspect is to ensure the facility and personnel are adequate and appropriate for the type of procedures performed. It is advisable that policies and procedures which govern the orderly conduct of the facility be in writing. It is also critical that they be in keeping with state and federal laws and regulations pertaining to ambulatory surgical facilities. It is also important to realize that local laws and codes can vary among locales and must be observed. Policies and procedures must be reviewed by the governing body on an annual basis to ensure that they are timely and in compliance with applicable local state and federal regulations, as well as those of accrediting organizations (if the facility is accredited).

In recent years, federal regulations have called attention to the importance of privacy and confidentiality of patients and their health care records. It is important that patients be treated with respect, consideration, and dignity. Patients have the right to be informed concerning their diagnosis, evaluation, treatment options, and prognosis. The patient should also have the opportunity to participate in decisions involving their health care. It is important that the facilities have guidelines and protocols that address these important issues, including the ability for patients to request their personal medical records. Facilities must comply with all state and federal statutes and regulations regarding patient rights, the medical record, and patient confidentiality.

Quality of Care

Ambulatory surgery organizations must develop a system that assesses the quality of care delivered and strive to provide an environment for continuous quality improvement. In addition, regulations in many states require adherence to specific patient safety guidelines and timely reporting of certain "medical errors." The ambulatory surgical facility needs to have written guidelines and protocols as well as policies that address all of these issues. Personnel issues, credentialing, patient evaluation guidelines, informed consent, medical records, discharge criteria, emergency protocols, transfer agreements, and peer review are some of the critical areas that fall under "quality of care."

Hospitals have very strict and well-established procedures for privileging and credentialing of health care practitioners. It is critical that the ambulatory surgical facility adopt policies and guidelines that ensure appropriate licensure or certification and appropriate training and skills by health care practitioners to deliver the services provided by the facility. It is important that personnel assisting in providing health care services also be appropriately trained, qualified, and supervised and that there be sufficient numbers of health care personnel to provide proper care. Policies and procedures need to delineate the functional responsibilities of staff. They also need to include well-defined methods that will be employed to provide oversight of health care practitioners and personnel within the facility. An important consideration regarding qualifications and training is that at least one person with training in advanced resuscitated techniques such as advanced cardiac life support should be immediately available until all patients are discharged. In many states, this is a legal requirement and a necessary inclusion in facility protocols.

Credentialing and privileging are critical to the quality of care being delivered in the ambulatory surgical facility. Credentialing is a three-phase process that assesses and validates the qualifications of an individual to provide services. It is important that the facility have well-defined policies and procedures for objective credentialing of health care professionals who work in the facility. It is also important for the facility to establish that health care professionals have the specialized professional background that they claim and that the various positions require. The organization is asked to establish minimal training, experience, and other requirements for health care personnel working at the facility. There should be a review process that assesses and validates an individual's qualifications, including education, training, experience, certification, licensure, and other levels of competence. Some licensure and accreditation standards may dictate specific requirements in this area, such as validation of medical education, validation of current state licensure, proof of medical liability coverage, search of the National Practitioner Databank, and so forth.

Privileging is also a three-phase process. The goal of privileging is to determine the specific procedures that the health care personnel may perform at the facility. Initially the organization determines the clinical procedures and treatments that can be offered in the facility. The organization then needs to determine policies and protocols that determine the qualifications relating to training and experience required to authorize health care professionals to obtain each privilege. In addition, a process of peer review and continuous oversight should be instituted to ensure quality of care and to guide any recredentialing or reprivileging process within the facility.

Peer review is an important part of the quality assurance program for ambulatory surgical facilities. An appropriate peer review program would consist of two or more physicians who have no financial interest in the facility and have knowledge and expertise relative to the scope of practice for the facility.

The organization must develop policies and guidelines dealing with patient evaluation. Such policies would dictate a current patient history and assessment by the surgeon on the day of the procedure. Protocols would also outline what preoperative evaluation could consist of, such as patient history, physical exam, proper diagnostic tests, plan for anesthesia care, and rules and regulations regarding informed consent for the facility. Policies and protocols regarding intraoperative evaluation should be developed and include continuous clinical observation and vigilant anesthesia monitoring. The American Society of Anesthesiology has developed many excellent policies regarding preoperative evaluation, intraoperative monitoring, and monitoring in the postanesthesia care unit.

If the facility elects to provide services to infants and children, great care should be given to development of patient evaluation and monitoring of care guidelines specific to this patient population.

It is important to point out that the patient evaluation process makes a responsible determination as to the medical appropriateness for the patient to undergo treatment in the ambulatory surgical setting. This would be based upon responsible evaluation of the patient's condition, specific morbidities that complicate the operative and anesthesia management, the patient compliance, specific intrinsic risk involved with the procedure, and the ability of the facility to provide the equipment and staff necessary to provide the services being contemplated.

The facility should have established protocols regarding informed consent regarding the anesthesia planned and the surgery to be performed.

It is important that informed consent be in writing and be obtained from patients prior to the procedure. The policies of the organization need to dictate that informed consent be utilized to address the anesthesia planned and the surgical services to be performed and that consent will be obtained after discussion of the risks, benefits, and alternatives. Also, informed consent must be documented in the medical record. Even though individual surgeons may have a consent form specifically for their private practice, it is important that the facility establish written policy that a specific informed consent be obtained on behalf of the facility, whether it be an office surgical or freestanding ambulatory surgical center.

It is critical that medical records be legible, complete, comprehensive, and accurate. The entity needs to establish policies and procedures that outline what the medical record includes. The record should include a recent history, physical exam, pertinent progress notes, operative reports, laboratory reports, and x-rays, as well as communications from other medical personnel. Records should highlight allergies and untold drug reactions and list the specific medications and their dosages that patients are on preoperatively to provide for continuity of medical care. Written policies need to be established regarding retention of active records, retirement of inactive records, timely entry of data in the records, and release of information. It is important to note that various state and federal rules and regulations relate to many aspects of the medical record and more specifically to release of patient information. It is critical that the organization's policies and procedures comply with state and federal rules and regulations regarding medical records.

Discharging patients is the responsibility of either or both the surgeon and the individual responsible for anesthesia care and should occur only when patients have met specific physician-defined criteria. These criteria should be established by the organization and placed in writing. In addition, written instructions and emergency contact cell phone numbers should be provided to the patient and documented in the medical record. It is also important that the facility establish written policies that the patient should be released to a responsible adult who has received instruction with regard to the patient's care. Many state regulatory and accrediting organizations require that the facility contact the patient by telephone following discharge to ensure their status and understanding of discharge instructions and to ensure continuity of care. The facility needs to be sure that its policies and procedures are in compliance with local and federal regulations specific to the area.

Emergency and Transfer Protocols

Although rare, emergencies can occur in the ambulatory surgical setting, and written policies and procedures need to be in place to ensure that necessary personnel, equipment, and procedures are available to handle medical and other emergencies that may arise. At a minimum, there should be written protocols for handling emergency situations, which include not only medical emergencies but also internal and external disasters, including but not limited to hurricanes, tornadoes, and fires. All policies and protocols should be established to ensure that all personnel are appropriately trained in emergency protocols and that adequate equipment is available for appropriate cardiopulmonary resuscitation. In addition, written protocols need to be in place to provide for a timely and safe transfer of patients to prespecified facilities when extended emergency services are needed. Protocols should include written transfer agreements with a nearby hospital or that all physicians performing surgery have admitting privileges at the facility.

Clinical Care

The facility needs to establish policies, procedures, and protocols dealing with the delivery of clinical services within the facility. These protocols need to ensure that qualified health care professionals function in an environment that ensures patient safety. Policies and protocols need to address anesthesia, surgical services, and any ancillary services provided in the facility, and they should address the physical plant and equipment utilized in that facility.

Facility protocols need to address the level of anesthesia to be used at the facility and that which would be appropriate for the patient, the surgical procedure, the clinical setting, the education and training of personnel, and the equipment that is available at the facility. The American Society of Anesthesiologists has established excellent guidelines for development of preoperative evaluation, intraoperative monitoring, and postsurgical recovery policies for postanesthesia care units. Policies need to address the specific needs of patients while ensuring rapid recovery to normal function with maximum efforts to control postoperative pain, nausea, and other side effects. Policies need to be established to ensure that individuals administering anesthesia are licensed, qualified, and working within their scope of practice. Nonphysicians who administer anesthesia should work under the supervision of an anesthesiologist or the operating physician unless state law permits otherwise. It is also important to establish policies that provide for individuals with current training in advanced resuscitative techniques, such as advanced cardiac life support, to be continually present at the facility until patients are discharged.

Continuous clinical observation and vigilance are the basis for safe anesthesia care. Physiological monitoring of patients should be appropriate for the type of anesthesia and individual needs of the patient. Protocols regarding such monitoring should be written and a part of the overall anesthesia plan. At a minimum, provisions should be made for reliable sources of oxygen, suction, resuscitation equipment, and emergency drugs. In locations where anesthesia is administered, there should be appropriate anesthesia apparatus and equipment to allow monitoring of patients. All equipment should be maintained, tested, and inspected according to manufacturer specifications. Backup power sufficient to ensure patient protection in the event of an emergency should be available. Written protocols and policies should ensure this.

When anesthesia services are provided to infants and children, special policies and procedures need to be in place to ensure that the specialized equipment, medications, and resuscitative capabilities appropriate for children are provided.

The organization needs to establish policies ensuring that surgical procedures are performed only by appropriate health care practitioners who are licensed in the state in which they are practicing. Procedures need to be undertaken to ensure that health care professionals are practicing within their own scope of practice, training, and expertise and within the capabilities of the facility. Procedures should be of a duration and complexity that would permit the patient to cover and be discharged from the facility in less than 24 hours or within the maximum time allowed by state law, if applicable. Policies should be established to address handling of patients who have preexisting medical or other conditions that may be a particular risk for complications and to exclude patients whose procedures would be more appropriately performed at another facility, such as a hospital inpatient setting.

If laser surgery is performed, written policies and procedures should be established including but not limited to laser safety, education, and training. The policies should ensure that the facility adheres to ANSI Z136.2 Laser Safety and Healthcare Facility Guidelines. Evidence of safety inspections and preventive maintenance for equipment should be current and available. Policies need to be established to provide a safe environment for laser surgery.

Facilities and Equipment

Before establishing an office surgical unit or a freestanding surgical center, it is advisable to check with local health care authorities and the state board of health for appropriate guidelines. National accrediting organizations such as AAAHC offer additional information. The Centers for Disease Control and Prevention, the Office of Architecture and Engineering Healthcare Facilities Service of the US Public Health Service, and the National Fire Protection Association can also provide information pertinent to constructing your facility.

Centers for Disease Control and Prevention, 1600 Clifton Road, NE, Atlanta, GA 30333
Office of Architecture and Engineering Healthcare Facilities Services, US Public Health Service, 5600 Fishers Lane, Room 9–45, Rockville, MD 20852
National Fire Protection Association, 600 Battery March Park, Quincy, MA 02269

Surgical facilities have a variety of forms and designs. Some are extremely sophisticated and closely resemble hospital surgical suites. Others serve as combination office, examination, and surgical procedure rooms. Whatever design one chooses, it is important that a great deal of thought be put into establishing a surgical facility that will provide for the patient's safety and quality of care and be representative of national standards and compliant with applicable local state and federal regulations.

Sizes of surgical suites may vary. Many feel that a room of 20 × 20 feet is the best size because it allows the physician and surgical personnel easy movement within the room during the surgical procedure. Additional equipment such as lasers or liposuction units can easily be added without restricting the functional movement within the room. In some locales room size is regulated by local and state statutes.

It is important to take into consideration location of doors and hallways. There must be adequate space to quickly evacuate the patient on a stretcher in case of an emergency. A 4-foot doorway is ideal. Materials used in construction of an office surgical or ambulatory surgical facility should be easily cleaned and sanitized. Perforated, dropped ceilings allow for dust to collect and are not easily cleaned. However, smooth, vinyl-covered dropped ceilings such as the type used in food preparation areas can easily be cleaned and sanitized. Solid ceilings composed of dry wall or plaster are somewhat more expensive but provide a more durable ceiling.

Various types of wall coverings can be used. However, the finish must be washable and must meet certain standards for flame spread and smoke production. Some states and municipalities have regulations for interior finishes of surgical suites. The state department of health and local building code authority should be contacted early in the planning and design stage to identify requirements. When in doubt, references should be made to appropriate National Fire Protection Association (NFPA) codes.

Although installation costs for ceramic tile are higher than those for painted or vinyl-covered walls, many feel that the tile is better able to withstand frequent cleaning and maintains a more attractive finish. Tiling, however, will crack or chip if struck by a heavy object. Cracked or chipped tile must be removed properly because the exposed interior could generate dust and harbor microorganisms.

Lighting should provide sufficient illumination so that even the most delicate procedures can be performed. Light standards for surgical suites have been recommended by the health care committee of the Illuminating Engineering Society (IES). This committee suggests that general illumination should have the potential to provide 200-foot candles throughout the operating room. The minimum light delivered to the surgical field should be 2500-foot candles when the surgical field is 42 inches from the lamp cover and the light covers an area 78 in.^{2} or larger.

White light is a combination of colors and actually contains a variety of source colors. If the temperature rises, the color will change from red to yellow, then to white or even bluish white. Temperature is expressed in degrees Kelvin for reference purposes. Studies have shown that most surgeons prefer light at ~5000 K. This approximates the color of noon sunlight.

Emergency Lighting, Electrical Circuitry, and Emergency Power

Electrical circuitry in a surgical facility is extremely important. The more complex the electrical equipment being utilized in the operating room is, the greater the possibility of a complication related to its use. Macroshock is the most common complication. It can result from electrical current entering the body through the intact skin due to inadequate grounding or insulation defects that cause a surgeon or patient to act as a pathway to the ground. Microshock, on the other hand, occurs if the current is applied directly to the heart, bypassing skin impedance. Thus smaller voltages may be lethal because they can cause cardiac fibrillation.

In some geographic areas, electrical circuitry of an office surgical facility is closely regulated by state codes. In some areas, office surgical facilities must be on a separate circuit from the rest of the building or office. Other areas have no restrictions. It is advisable to contact an electrical engineer to produce an electrical floor plan for the facility and to insure that you are in compliance with local building codes.

The potential loss of power and the ability to conclude a procedure or conduct emergency resuscitation in the event of power loss must be considered. Electrical generators are available that will supply power to an entire office or surgical area during the power failure. Gasoline and diesel generators tend to require more maintenance.

Natural gas generators appear to be more reliable and require far less maintenance. In an office facility, the physician may not wish to incur the considerable expense of a generator. If not required by accreditation or local code, an electric inverter is an excellent alternative. An electrical inverter converts DC to AC and provides an alternative 60-cycle 117 V. The inverter also monitors line voltage, so that when there is a change, it instantaneously activates.

It is imperative that surgery be performed in a clean and appropriate environment. Ventilation of the operating suite is important for both the comfort and the well-being of the patient as well as the surgical staff. Extremes in temperature, toxic accumulation of anesthetic gases, and significant concentrations of airborne bacteria do not constitute a desirable operative room environment. Just how important ventilation is and exactly what constitutes "good" ventilation are points widely debated.

Most states have precise guidelines for ambulatory surgery center operating room ventilation systems. These guidelines usually state that air entering the operating room must be filtered by a mechanical filter with at least 95% efficiency rating on particle sizes of 1 to 5 μm. A prefilter is required to be upstream of air-conditioning equipment and must have a 25% efficiency rating. Air in the operating room should be exchanged at least 25 times per hour, and five of those exchanges should be fresh air. In addition, a positive pressure atmosphere should exist in the operating room.

Most accrediting organizations have recognized that the type of ventilation appropriate for a surgical environment can vary significantly and can be achieved in a variety of ways. The guidelines for Accreditation of Ambulatory Healthcare Facilities state that appropriate ventilation must be provided. Appropriate ventilation is defined as each operating room being designed and equipped in such a way as to ensure the physical safety of all persons in the operating room during surgery. A safe environment for treating surgical patients must include safeguards to protect the patient from cross-infection, and environmental controls must be implemented to ensure a safe, sanitary environment.

The type of environment you plan to create must take into account the rules and regulations existing in your state and city, as well as the type of surgical procedures you plan to perform. If you do not wish to have a sophisticated ventilation filtration mechanism, the services of a mechanical engineer with experience in design of medical facilities should be obtained. Specific units can be designed for your office that will provide not only maximal filtration but also exact climate and humidity control.

Monitoring equipment should be available in the operating and recovery room areas to monitor pulse, blood pressure, electrocardiac activity, and pulse oximetry. Data should be recorded either by attending personnel or by automatic recording devices.

It is imperative that appropriate medications be available to treat acute emergency medical conditions, such as cardiopulmonary arrest, anaphylactic reactions, and seizures related to anesthetic reactions. It is advisable that your drug cart contain all the medications recommended by the American Heart Association for treating acute cardiopulmonary disorders. In addition to medications, the crash cart should contain equipment for administering emergency intravenous fluids and medications and instrumentation for establishing an emergency airway. Commercial crash carts are available in portable suitcase-type kits, which are especially useful in office surgical facilities.

Medical gases and suction are a part of the surgical facility environment. Oxygen, nitrous oxide, nitrogen, and compressed air are the usual gases to be considered for an ambulatory surgical suite. Suction should also be considered because the construction goes hand in hand with placement of medical gases.

A variety of sterilization equipment can be utilized for ambulatory surgical facilities. Office surgical facilities may desire steam-powered autoclaves or gas sterilizers, which can fit on counters. These units are too small and require several cycles to sterilize all the equipment needed for large surgical cases. Larger steam sterilizers are utilized in larger freestanding ambulatory surgical centers. It is important that sterilization units have appropriate ventilating systems and meet Occupational Safety and Health Administration requirements. Whatever type of sterilization unit is selected, it is essential that the equipment be checked periodically to ensure proper functioning. Culture sterilization checks should be performed at least monthly and tests documented. Protocols need to be established regarding proper use, maintenance, and documentation of sterilization for the ambulatory surgical facility.

Space dedicated to recovery can be conservative, depending on the anticipated case load. Individual cubicles may be used to provide privacy. In other instances, large spaces separated by pull drapes may be utilized. An important principle to adhere to is that you must have adequately trained personnel in the immediate vicinity of the recovering patient until he or she is fully awake and alert. Nurse call systems can be installed in "stepdown" recovery areas so that the patient may be in the temporary care of a family member who in turn can summon staff when needed. However, in the immediate postanesthesia period, close monitoring by center staff is imperative. Proper monitoring equipment must be readily available as well as proper resuscitation equipment. When patients reach the appropriate postanesthesia stage, they can be transferred to a stepdown recovery area where family members may assist in the final stages of the recovery prior to discharge. It is important to have established protocols dealing with patient monitoring as well as discharge criteria following surgery. The American Society of Anesthesiology Guidelines can be extremely helpful in establishing your specific policies and procedures.

Summary

The two critical issues in developing an ambulatory surgical facility are quality of care and accountability. In establishing a facility, you need to be sure that you meet the community standards and that you are able to deal competitively with the problems and challenges to safety and credibility. This is accomplished by developing policies and procedures that address key administrative and quality of care issues. Your challenge is to establish a process that adheres to national standards, provides peer evaluation, and provides quality care in a cost-effective, patient-friendly environment.

Directory of Organizations Providing Services or Guidelines to Ambulatory Surgical Facilities

Accreditation Association of Ambulatory Healthcare, Inc., 3201 Old Glenview Road, Suite 300, Wilmette, IL 60091

American Association for Accreditation of Ambulatory Surgery Facilities, Inc., 1202 Allanson Road, Mundelein, IL 60060

American Association of Nurse Anesthetists, 220 South Prospect Avenue, Park Ridge, IL 60068

American College of Surgeons, 633 North Saint Clair Street, Chicago, IL 60611–3211

American Medical Association, 515 North State Street, Chicago, IL 60610

American Society of Anesthesiology, 520 North West Highway, Park Ridge, IL 60068–2573

Federated Ambulatory Surgery Association, 700 North Fairfax Street, Suite 306, Alexandria, VA 22314

Federation of State Medical Boards, 400 Fuller Wiser Road, Suite 300, Euless, TX 76039

Institute for Medical Quality, 221 Main Street, Suite 210, San Francisco, CA 94105–1906

Joint Commission on Accreditation of Healthcare Organizations (JCAHO), One Renaissance Boulevard, Oakbrook Terrace, IL 60181

Suggested Readings

Accreditation AAAHC. Handbook for Ambulatory Healthcare. Skokie, IL: Accreditation Association for Ambulatory Health Care; 2005

American Academy of Dermatology. Guidelines for Care of Office Surgical Facilities. Part 1, 1992, part 2, 1995. Schaumburg, IL: American Academy of Dermatology; 1992, 1995

American Association for Accreditation of Ambulatory Surgical Facilities. Standards and Checklist for Accreditation of Ambulatory Surgical Facilities. Gurnee, IL: American Association for Accreditation of Ambulatory Surgical Facilities; 2005

American Association of Nurse Anesthetists. Standards for Office-Based Anesthesia Practice. Park Ridge, IL: American Association of Nurse Anesthetists; 2001

American College of Surgeons, Board of Governors Committee on Ambulatory Surgical Care. Guidelines for Optimal Ambulatory Surgical Care and Office-Based Surgery. 3rd ed., May. Chicago, IL: American College of Surgeons; 2000

American Medical Association. Patient Safety and Office-Based Surgical Facilities and Standards of Care. Board of Trustees Report 13-A-01. Chicago, IL: American Medical Association, Annual Meeting, July 2001

American Osteopathic Association, AOA Board of Trustees. Draft: Policy Statement: Office-Based Surgery, October 2001. Chicago, IL: American Osteopathic Association; 2001

American Society of Anesthesiologists. Guidelines for Office-Based Anesthesia. October 1999. Park Ridge, IL: American Society of Anesthesiologists; 1999

Beeson WH, Tobin HA. Developing a Practice in Ambulatory Surgery. New York: Thieme; 1993

Committee on Quality Assurance and Office-Based Surgery. Clinical Guidelines for Office-Based Surgery. New York State Public Health Council, New York State Department of Health, December 2000

Hall MJ, Lawrence L. Ambulatory Surgery in the United States. U.S. Department of Health and Human Services, Centers for Disease Control and Prevention, National Center for Health Statistics; Advanced Data, # 300, August 12, 1998

Healthcare Financing Administration. Survey Procedures and Interpretive Guidelines for Ambulatory Surgical Services. State Operations Manual, appendix L, section # 416.2, 416.40–416.49

Institute for Medical Quality. Accreditation Standards for Ambulatory Facilities. San Francisco: Institute for Medical Quality; 2000

Joint American Academy of Dermatology/American Society of Dermatologic Surgery Liaison Committee. Current issues and dermatologic office-based surgery. J Am Acad Dermatol 2000;42:847

Joint Commission (on Accreditation of Health Care Organizations). Accreditation Manual for Office-Based Surgery Practices. Oakbrook Terrace, IL: Joint Commission; 2005

Office-Based Anesthesia Considerations for Anesthesiologists and Setting Up and Monitoring a Safe Office Anesthesia Environment. Park Ridge, IL: American Society of Anesthesiologists; 2000

Pellman TG. Office-based surgery and public safety: what are state medical boards doing to protect the patient? Journal of Medical Licensure and Discipline 2001;87:47–51

Sutton JH. Office-based surgery regulation: improving patient's safety and quality care. Bull Am Coll Surg 2001;86:8–12

Wasmer AL. Office-based surgery: the doctor is in, and more boards are watching. Journal of Medical Licensure and Discipline 2001;87:99–103

II

Aesthetic Facial Surgery

16 Aesthetic Facial Analysis

R. James Koch and Matthew M. Hanasono

Facial aesthetic surgery requires the surgeon to have a clear vision of the final outcome prior to any intervention. Therefore, the preoperative analysis of the face is as critical to the end result as careful surgical technique and thoughtful postoperative care. Facial surgery requires a deep familiarity with the "normal" face. Comprehensive assessment of the facial plastic surgery patient also depends on knowledge of the aesthetic ideal as it is influenced by age, sex, and body type, as well as cultural and contemporary trends in facial aesthetics. When the goal is to restore a youthful appearance, the surgeon also needs to understand the facial changes associated with aging.

Equipped with an appreciation for what makes a face attractive, the surgeon must then identify problem areas and determine priorities for surgery. In the preoperative facial analysis, thickness and texture of the skin and subcutaneous tissues, bony structure, and wrinkle patterns caused by the mimetic actions of the facial musculature must be considered. Changes caused by aging must be both assessed and anticipated. The preoperative analysis is unique to each patient, and solutions to problems must be fitted to specific needs.

Key concepts in facial aesthetics include balance, proportion, symmetry, and harmony. It is the combination of facial features in balance and proportion rather than any one specific characteristic that we equate with facial beauty. It should be remembered during facial evaluation that exceptions to the rules of facial proportion are sometimes encountered in beautiful faces that demonstrate unique and pleasing disproportion. Asymmetries should be pointed out to the patient prior to any intervention so that the patient understands that they were not caused by the surgery. The patient should be advised that some asymmetries cannot be surgically corrected. Harmony is achieved when the features of the face are congruent with each other and the rest of the body habitus. The challenge to the surgeon is to modify the facial appearance, sometimes in major ways, while effectively hiding incisions, and to alter the patient's features without creating an "operated on" appearance.

Facial Beauty

Historical Perspectives

Since ancient Egyptian times, the ideals of aesthetic facial surgery has been portrayed in art (**Fig. 16.1**). Modern facial analysis, however, began in Greece. Greek artists and philosophers analyzed the perceptions of beauty and established standards for ideal facial proportions and harmony (**Fig. 16.2**). Strongly influenced by the Greeks, artists and anatomists of the Renaissance period continued the study of aesthetic proportions (**Fig. 16.3**). Leonardo da Vinci's work is well known for its portrayal of ideal facial proportions. His study of facial anatomy included the concept that facial balance exists when the face can be divided into equal thirds from the frontal hairline to the nasal root, the nasal root to the nasal base, and the nasal base to the bottom of the chin.

Modern Concepts

Whereas some concepts of facial beauty endure across time and culture, others vary. In our culture, television, magazines, and motion pictures appear to have the greatest

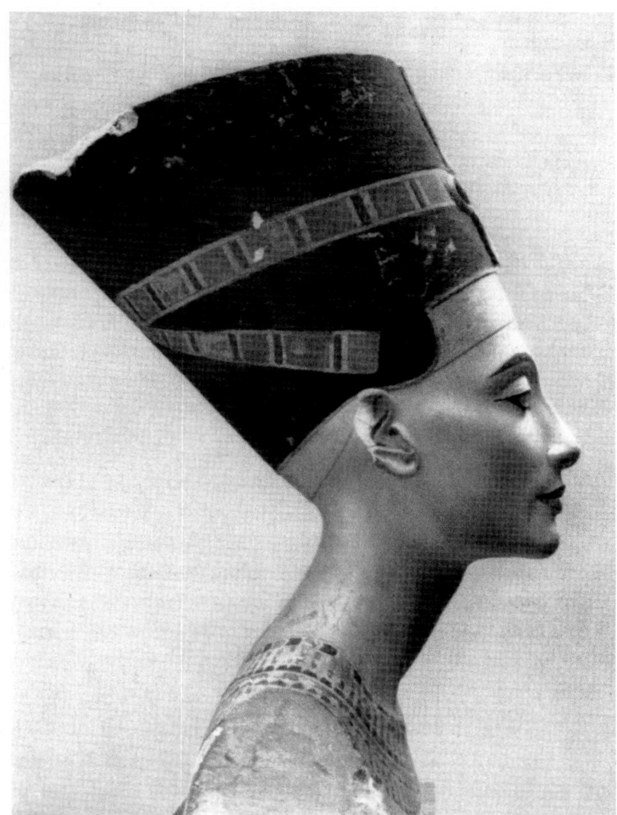

Fig. 16.1 The head of Queen Nefertiti, ca. 1365 BC. (Courtesy of the Berlin State Museum, Berlin, Germany.)

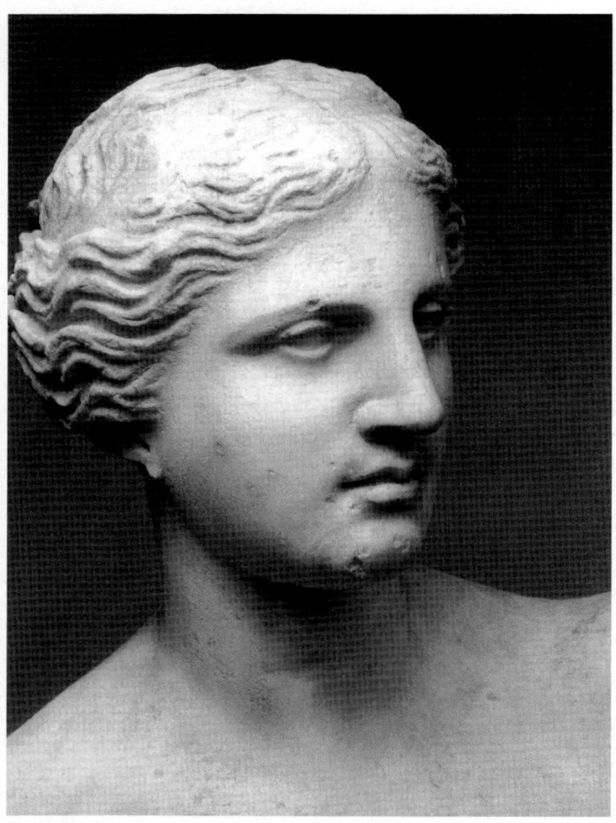

Fig. 16.2 *Venus De Milo*, Ca. 100 BC. (Courtesy of the Louvre, Paris, France.)

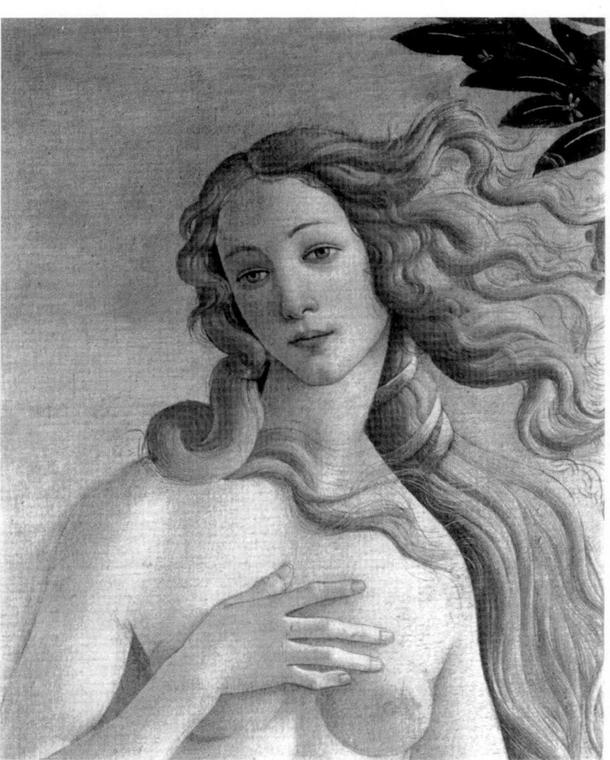

Fig. 16.3 The *Birth of Venus*, Botticelli, ca. 1480. (Courtesy of the Uffizi Gallery, Florence, Italy.)

impact on our perception of beauty. Temporal differences in the aesthetic ideal can be appreciated by observing popular media from recent decades.

Various sociological studies suggest at least some cultural differences in aesthetic tastes. Martin[1] conducted one such study in 1964. In that study, photographs of black female magazine models were ranked with respect to facial features considered to be most black and least Caucasian, to those felt to be least black and most Caucasian. These models were then ranked in terms of beauty by 50 college-age white American males, 50 college-age black African American males, and 50 college-age black Nigerian males. The beauty rankings of American whites and African American blacks both showed a positive correlation with models displaying more Caucasian, less black features. The beauty rankings of Nigerian blacks correlated with more black, less Caucasian features. Martin's study suggests that there is, or was at that time, a single cultural standard of beauty in American society, despite its multiracial composition, different from that of an African society that is predominantly based on the black facial model. Other studies show high interrater reliabilities in cross-cultural beauty, suggesting that some features are perceived as attractive regardless of the racial and cultural background of the viewer.

Recent research has sought to define facial beauty in terms that are more objective. It has sought to define preferences that appear to be biologically predetermined and cross-cultural. Langlois et al[2] showed that infants, whose inclinations presumably do not reflect culture-specific standards of beauty, prefer to look at adult faces that were perceived as more attractive. In a later study with adults, Langlois and Roggman[3] showed that a computer-generated face that was a composite of many faces was favored over any singular face of actual male and female subjects. This study suggests that "average" features (those that deviate least from the norm in terms of size, shape, location, and proportion) are the paragon of facial beauty.

More recently, Perrett et al[4] found that subjects preferred a computer-generated composite of attractive female faces to a composite of average female faces. Male subjects preferred a caricature in which the differences between the attractive composite and the average composite were increased by 50%. This preference was observed in British subjects judging British faces, Japanese subjects viewing Japanese faces, and British subjects viewing Japanese faces. British and Japanese women preferred an "attractive" male composite to an "average" male composite as well, but had no preference for a caricature over an attractive composite. Qualities found to be more attractive in female faces included large eyes, high cheekbones, narrow jaw, and smaller vertical third of the face.

Whether beauty is preprogrammed or exists only in the eye of the beholder, the most important goal for the facial plastic surgeon is to create a result that portrays beauty and contributes to a positive self-image in the mind of the patient. Certainly, one can accept that a face that is beautiful beyond a certain level is likely to be universally accepted as beautiful, transcending racial, cultural, and temporal preferences. In addition, in the present world with well-developed communications, frequent travel, and globalized media, beauty does not exist in a culture- or race-specific vacuum.

Aesthetic Facial Analysis

History and Physical Examination

A complete and systematic medical history and physical is as important in facial plastic surgery as any other surgical discipline. History taking should include information about medical problems, prior surgeries, medications, and allergies as well as smoking, illicit drug use, and drinking habits. As hematoma is among the most common complications of facial aesthetic surgery, risk factors for postoperative bleeding, such as hypertension and use of nonsteroidal anti-inflammatory drugs, should be elicited. Smoking history is pertinent to concerns for skin slough and flap necrosis.

Questions regarding dryness or irritation of the eyes should be posed to patients undergoing surgery in the periorbital region. Vision in each eye is assessed, and tests for adequate tear production are performed if the history is suggestive of decreased lacrimation.

Patients with rare skin disorders may present to the facial surgeon with premature aging or skin laxity. These conditions include Ehlers-Danlos syndrome, progeria, Werner's syndrome, cutis laxa, and pseudoxanthoma elasticum. The underlying pathological process must be taken into account in determining whether such patients are candidates for aesthetic surgery. Ehlers-Danlos is a genetic disease of connective tissue associated with thin, hyperextensible skin, hypermobile joints, and subcutaneous hemorrhages. Rhytidectomy is contraindicated due to high risk of postsurgical bleeding and poor wound healing. Plastic surgery is contraindicated in progeria, a disorder characterized by growth retardation, craniofacial disproportion, baldness, prominent ears, pinched nose, micrognathia, and shortened life span. Due to associated microangiopathy, cosmetic surgery is also contraindicated in Werner's syndrome, or adult progeria, a condition that also presents with scleroderma-like skin changes, including baldness, aged facies, pigmentation defects, short stature, muscle atrophy, osteoporosis, premature atherosclerosis, and diabetes. Cutis laxa, in which there is a degeneration of dermal elastic fibers, is associated with chronic obstructive pulmonary disease, cor pulmonale, hernias, as well as urologic and intestinal diverticula. Facial rejuvenation is generally safe in these patients as long as their overall health status is satisfactory. Finally, pseudoxanthoma elasticum is a degenerative disorder of elastic fibers resulting in premature skin laxity for which facial rejuvenation surgery is beneficial.

Preoperative Photography

Preoperatively, the surgeon should photograph the patient in standard views specific to each operative procedure. These photographs should include, at the minimum, a frontal view, left and right lateral views, and left and right oblique views, as well as close-up views of the regions to be addressed surgically. The photographs should be taken with the head in the Frankfort horizontal position. In the Frankfort horizontal, the supratragal notch is level with the infraorbital rim. Photographs assist in preoperative planning and intraoperative decision making, and postoperatively as a way of assessing results. They assist preoperatively in discussion with the patient as well as postoperatively during the counseling of patients who may not remember their exact preoperative appearance. Photographs are also necessary for medicolegal documentation. The reader is referred to Chapter 13, Photography in Facial Plastic Surgery.

Computers in Facial Analysis

There is no doubt that the use of preoperative computer imaging is an excellent tool to increase communication with patients. It allows the surgeon to visualize what the patient desires as a final result. The patient can articulate any desired modifications. It allows the surgeon and patient to compare their own aesthetic interpretations.

For procedures such as profile changes in rhinoplasty, it allows patients to view themselves from a different perspective, one that they normally do not see. Many times their self-image is not congruent with what others see. Also, the computer imager shows how different manipulations can yield very different results. This is important with procedures such as rhinoplasty where subtle or dramatic changes can be achieved by single maneuvers. It also shows the illusionary or secondary effects of a singular change. For example, apparent nasal tip rotation can be increased by removing a dorsal hump or augmenting the premaxilla. Such secondary effects can be visualized on the imager and are valuable in the planning of that procedure. The reader is referred to Chapter 12, Computer Imaging for Facial Plastic Surgery.

Skin Type

Due to the key role of skin in the facial appearance, evaluation of the skin deserves special mention. The texture, thickness, elasticity, and degree of sun damage to the skin of various facial regions should be evaluated by inspection and palpation. A gentle touch during this stage of the examination communicates to the patient the surgeon's technical delicacy. Skin lesions, scars, rhytids, and pigmentation should be noted and pointed out to the patient.

Fine, light skin with minimal subcutaneous tissue will tend to show even minor subcutaneous soft and bony tissue irregularities. Facial implants in such skin may prove problematic or unacceptable. Even minor abnormalities in contour require careful attention during surgery. On the opposite end of the spectrum, thick, oily skin tends to heal with scars that are more obvious. It also may conceal underlying structural changes. Somewhere between these two skin types lies the ideal skin for facial aesthetic surgery. Men tend to have thicker skin in the region of the beard, with an increased blood supply due to a richer subdermal plexus.

Textural imperfections, such as deep acne and chicken pox scars, may subtract from the desired result. Ice-pick acne scars penetrate through the dermal layer and fixate in the subcutaneous tissues, thus tethering the skin surface. Correction with injectable fillers or punch excision of depressed scars and sequential laser resurfacing/dermabrasion may be required (**Fig. 16.4**). Rhytidectomy frees scars from their underlying tethering and allows rotation and elevation of facial skin to an improved position.

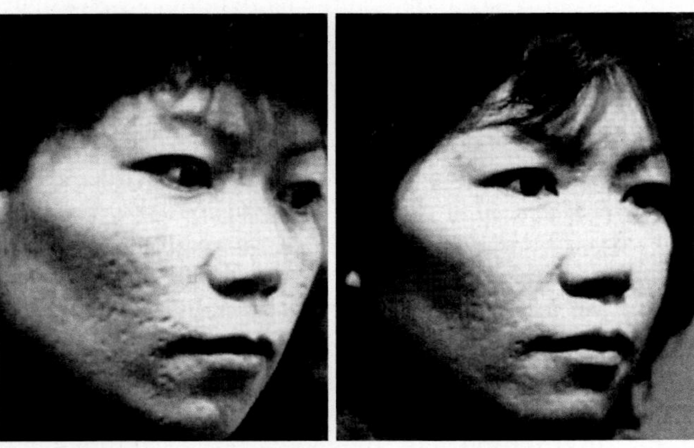

Fig. 16.4 Dermabrasion for chicken pox scarring. (Courtesy of Dr. John R. Hilger.)

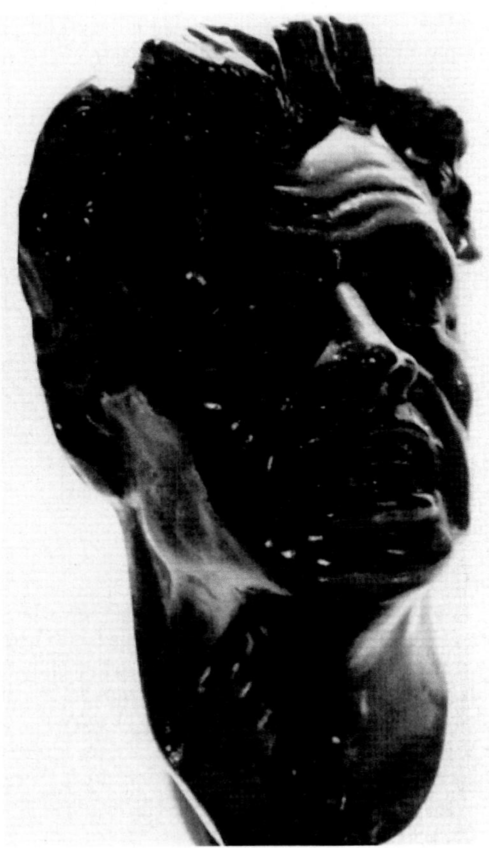

Fig. 16.5 Mimetic activation of facial musculature. (Courtesy of the Montreal General Hospital, Montreal, Canada.)

Skin aging is variable and depends on multiple intrinsic and extrinsic factors. Genetics, sun exposure, smoking history, radiation exposure, and amount of use of the facial mimetic musculature all play major roles in the development of facial rhytids. It is important to differentiate dynamic facial lines from true wrinkles. Dynamic furrows are caused by the repeated pull on the skin of underlying facial mimetic muscles and require that the underlying muscle(s) be addressed (**Fig. 16.5**). They are differentiated from wrinkles (sagging skin), which are caused by age-related laxity of the skin. Aging is also associated with a progressive decrease in the elasticity and thickness of the skin.

With age, the development of benign, malignant, and premalignant skin lesions may occur. It is important to biopsy any suspicious lesions. Keratoses, epitheliomata, and other hyperpigmented lesions may appear on the face. Environmental damage from both ultraviolet radiation and trauma may take a toll on facial skin. Actinic damage and regions of pigmentary change may occur. The presence of facial hypertrophic scars and keloids should be noted, as they may be a relative contraindication to certain types of surgery.

Table 16.1 Fitzpatrick's Sun-Reactive Skin Types

Skin type	Skin color	Tanning response
I	White	Always burns, never tans
II	White	Usually burns, tans with difficulty
III	White	Sometimes mild burn, tan average
IV	Brown	Rarely burns, tans with ease
V	Dark brown	Very rarely burns, tans very easily
VI	Black	No burn, tans very easily

When planning skin resurfacing, it is important to ascertain the patient's sun reactive skin type (Fitzpatrick) (**Table 16.1**). Those with type IV or type V skin (such as persons of Asian or Hispanic descent, respectively) or in anticipation of a hyperpigmentation problem are pretreated with hydroquinone topically.

Hair

Men tend to have recession of the frontal forehead hairline, with loss and thinning of hair, much earlier in life than women. The position of the hairline, temporal recession, and density of hair follicles should be taken into account when planning surgical incisions. For example, one may consider a coronal lift with a low forehead and Norwood classification type I hair pattern, a midforehead lift with androgenic baldness or thin, light hair, and a pretrichial lift with a high forehead and Norwood type I or II hair pattern.[5] When performing the pretrichial lift, a trichophytic incisional technique should always be used. An endoscopic browlift can be performed with most hair patterns, yet incision modifications may be necessary.

Facial Aesthetic Units

When all of the general considerations have been taken into account, a regional evaluation of the face is conducted. A practical method of doing this is by proceeding with a systematic evaluation of the individual facial aesthetic units. These units consist of the forehead and brow, the periorbital region, the cheeks, nose, the perioral region and chin, and the neck. However, one must remember to appreciate how the features of the various units interact with each other to produce a balanced or unbalanced appearance.

Forehead

Perhaps no other facial region has so many varied surgical approaches as the aging brow and forehead. A knowledge of the anatomy and aesthetics of the upper third of the face is necessary to select and perform the proper rejuvenation procedure. The layers of the forehead are in continuity with those of the scalp. The mnemonic SCALP describes the five layers of the forehead: S (skin), C (subcutaneous tissue), A (galea aponeurotica), L (loose areolar tissue), and P (pericranium). The skin (S) is adherent to the subcutaneous tissue (C). The galea aponeurotica (A) surrounds the entire skull. The galea divides to surround the frontalis and occipitalis muscles. Below the superior temporal line, the galea becomes the temporoparietal fascia. The loose areolar tissue (L) (subgaleal plane) is between the galea aponeurotica and the pericranium (P). This is an avascular layer that allows sliding of the other layers over the pericranium. The pericranium is a thick layer of connective tissue (periosteum) that is adherent to the outer table of the calvaria. At the temporal fusion line of the skull (where the superior and inferior temporal lines meet) the periosteum becomes confluent with the temporalis fascia. The periosteum also becomes continuous with the periorbita at the level of the supraorbital rims.

The movements of the forehead and eyebrows are due to four muscles: frontalis, procerus, corrugator supercilii, and orbital portion of the orbicularis oculi muscles. The paired frontalis muscles have a distinct midline separation. The frontalis originates from galea aponeurotica and inferiorly interdigitates with the procerus muscle, corrugator muscle, and the orbicularis oculi muscle. The frontalis muscle has no bony attachments. It is connected to the occipitalis muscle through its galeal attachments, and these two muscles act together to move the scalp. The function of the frontalis is eyebrow elevation. Transverse forehead creases result from chronic frontalis contraction. Loss of frontalis innervation results in brow ptosis on the affected side.

The paired corrugator supercilii muscles originate from the frontal bone near the superomedial orbital rim and pass through the frontalis and orbicularis muscles before inserting into the mideyebrow dermis. They pull the eyebrows medially and downward, and overuse (frowning) causes glabelar vertical furrows. The procerus is a pyramidal muscle that originates from the surface of the upper lateral cartilages and nasal bones, and inserts into the skin in the glabelar region. Contraction causes the medial aspect of the brows to descend and produces horizontal lines over the root of the nose. The orbicularis oculi muscle surrounds each orbit and extends into the eyelids. It originates from the periosteum of the medial orbital margin and inserts into the eyebrow dermis. It is divided into orbital, palpebral (preseptal and pretarsal), and lacrimal portions. The medial superior fibers of the orbicularis depress the medial brow. These fibers are called the depressor supercilii muscle. The corrugator, procerus, and orbicularis oculi muscles act together to close the eyes, are antagonistic to the movement of the frontalis, and their overuse creates horizontal and vertical glabelar lines.

The classically described brow position in a female has the following criteria[6]: (1) the brow begins medially at a vertical line drawn perpendicular through the alar base; (2) the brow terminates laterally at an oblique line drawn through the lateral canthus of the eye and the alar base; (3) the medial and lateral ends of the eyebrow lie at approximately the same horizontal level; (4) the medial end of the eyebrow is club shaped, and this gradually tapers down laterally; and (5) the apex of the brow lies on a vertical line drawn directly through the lateral limbus of the eye. Some feel that the apex or highest portion of the brow should ideally be in a more lateral position; that is, the apex set along a vertical line through the lateral canthus, as opposed to the lateral limbus.[7]

For males some of the classical criteria apply, including the apex lying on a vertical line through the lateral limbus, yet the entire complex is minimally arching and positioned at or just above the supraorbital rim. Overzealous lateral elevation, producing a high or arched brow, can feminize the male brow. Overzealous medial elevation produces a "surprised" look. Compared with the male, the female forehead is smoother and more rounded with a less developed supraorbital ridge and a less acute nasofrontal angle.

The two main age-related changes of the upper third of the face are brow ptosis and hyperdynamic facial lines. Brow ptosis is primarily a result of gravity and loss of elastic tissue support from collagen changes in the dermis. It can give a crowded or angry appearance to the eye and brow complex. The brow should be examined for any asymmetry accompanying bilateral ptosis. Also, any underlying etiologic factors (such as temporal branch paralysis) should be sought in unilateral ptosis. What at first appears to be excess upper eyelid skin (dermatochalasis) may in fact be ptotic forehead skin. Clinically, this most dramatically presents as "lateral hooding" over the upper eyelids. This may be severe enough to result in a superiolateral visual field defect, producing a functional indication for brow surgery. Attempts to excise the hooded skin via a blepharoplasty alone will only pull the lateral brow inferiorly, thereby worsening the brow ptosis.

In addition to brow ptosis, the aging brow and forehead may display hyperdynamic facial lines. These furrows are caused by the repeated pull on the skin of underlying facial mimetic muscles. Chronic contraction of the frontalis muscle in an upward effort leads to transverse forehead creases: the frontalis essentially performs its own nonsurgical browlift. Repeated frowning overutilizes the procerus and corrugator supercilii muscles. This, respectively, causes the development of horizontal creases at the root of the nose, and vertical interbrow furrows.

The need for ancillary procedures, such as blepharoplasty for upper eyelid dermatochalasis, should be recognized, as this will yield a potential camouflage incision site for the brow component. The height of the forehead should also be evaluated because some approaches will not only accomplish the lift but will secondarily improve (raise or lower) forehead vertical height. In general, whereas all forehead procedures elevate the brow as well as the forehead, browlifting procedures vary in their effects (if any) on the forehead.

Periorbital Region

The periorbital region includes the upper and lower eyelids, the medial and lateral canthal regions, and the globe. Again, the size, shape, position, and symmetry of the individual components should be assessed. The assessment should take into account the features of the remainder of the face. The intercanthal distance should be approximately equal to the width of one eye. In the Caucasian patient, the intercanthal distance should also be equal to the interalar width of the nasal base. In the Asian and African American patient, this rule does not necessarily apply due to typically greater interalar widths.

The primary muscle in this region is the orbicularis oculi. This muscle is innervated by the temporal and zygomatic branches of the facial nerve. The orbital portion of this muscle encircles the orbits and contracts as a sphincter to cause blinking. This portion of the muscle has lateral attachments to the anterior temporal and malar skin. This creates fine lines and wrinkling, known as crow's feet, as the face ages.

The eyelids often show the earliest signs of aging. The problems are mainly due to skin laxity (dermatochalasis), pseudoherniation of the orbital fat through the orbital septum, and orbicularis muscle hypertrophy. For the upper eyelids, dermatochalasis, followed by prominent fat pads, is the most common problem. The traditional skin–muscle upper eyelid blepharoplasty with fat removal addresses these problems well.

For the lower eyelids, problems with skin, fat, and muscle are often seen alone or in combination. Isolated lower eyelid pseudoherniated fat is commonly seen in younger patients and is managed by transconjunctival blepharoplasty. Mild dermatochalasis can be concurrently addressed by skin pinch excision, chemical peel, or laser resurfacing. Many younger patients also have isolated orbicularis muscle hypertrophy, usually secondary to frequent squinting or smiling. This is frequently observed in people who smile for a living, such as newscasters and politicians. This may appear as a firm roll along the margin of the lower eyelid and requires muscle excision or debulking.

Malar bags must be differentiated from festoons. Malar bags are edematous, sagging regions bordering onto the cheek aesthetic unit that accumulate fat or fluid with age. They sometimes require direct excision. Festoons, on the other hand, typically contain muscle and skin invaginations. They may be addressed via extended lower eyelid blepharoplasty.

Other periorbital problems, such as lid ptosis, enophthalmos, proptosis, exophthalmos, lower lid laxity or malposition, and lateral hooding, should be assessed. As noted previously, lateral hooding develops because of the descent of the brow as well as presence of redundant eyelid skin. The snap test, in which the lower lid is grasped between thumb and forefinger and pulled away from the globe, is routinely used to assess lower lid laxity. An abnormal result is delayed return to the globe surface or return only after blinking. Lower lid scleral show or ectropion (eversion of the eyelid margin) is also noted. Approximately 10% of the normal population have scleral show unrelated to aging. Enophthalmos may suggest prior orbital trauma and may require orbital reconstruction. Exophthalmos may suggest Graves' orbitopathy and requires endocrine evaluation. Globe malposition or extraocular muscle dysfunction requires ophthalmology consultation and orbital imaging studies.

Ptosis, entropion (inversion of the eyelid margin), ectropion, and excessive lower lid laxity can be corrected at the time of blepharoplasty. Hyperdynamic lines, such as crow's feet, cannot be eliminated except through alteration of the facial musculature. This may be achieved by paralysis or destruction of the facial nerve branches that supply the muscles. A practical method is chemical muscle paralysis with botulinum toxin.

Cheek

The cheeks form an aesthetic unit that extends from the preauricular crease laterally, to the nasolabial fold medially, as well as the zygomatic arch and inferior orbital rim superiorly, and to the inferior border of the mandible inferiorly. The most noticeable landmark on the cheek is the malar eminence. The malar eminence is composed of the zygomatic and maxillary bones. A prominent malar eminence is a sign of youth and beauty. The malar eminence lends form, strength, and shape to the facial appearance. Malar hypoplasia may be due to deficiency of the anterior face of the maxilla or, laterally, due to deficiency of the zygomatic prominence.

The muscles of the cheek can be divided into three layers. The deepest layer consists of the buccinator, which arises from the deep fascia of the facial area and blends with the orbicularis oris at the oral commissure. The next layer consists of the caninus, which originates at the canine fossa, and the quadratus labii superioris, which has three divisions that originate from the upper lip area. Both the caninus and quadratus labii superioris insert on the orbicularis oris. Finally, the zygomaticus and risorius interdigitate at the lateral commissure. All of these muscles originate from a bony landmark on the maxilla or the pterygomandibular raphe. They terminate in either the superficial fascia of the perioral skin or the deep musculature of the upper lip. They are innervated by the zygomatic and buccal branches of the facial nerve. These muscles cause an upward and lateral movement of the middle third of the face associated with expressions of happiness. The buccal fat pad is a consistent component of the masticatory space. Interestingly, it does not vary with the overall degree of adiposity of the individual. It is composed of a main body and three main extensions: temporal, buccal, and pterygoid. Significant jowling may be due in part to ptotic buccal fat. Clinically, ptotic buccal fat may present as inferior cheek volume or as a jowl with fullness in the midportion of the mandibular body.

The buccal fat pad is located through an intraoral incision above the third maxillary molar. The two surgically vulnerable structures are the parotid duct and the buccal branch of the facial nerve. It is therefore prudent not to chase buccal fat but to remove only that which buoyantly protrudes.

Deepening of the nasolabial crease and accentuation of the nasolabial fold, the portion of cheek lateral and adjacent to the crease consisting of the malar fat pad and overlying skin, are changes associated with aging. The nasolabial crease is perhaps the most noticeable crease on the face. It is a result of direct attachments of the mimetic muscles to the skin or forces of motion transmitted by the superficial musculoaponeurotic system (SMAS) to the skin by vertical fibrous septa. With age, there is atrophy of fat in the middle and upper face as well as deposition in the submental area. Development of submalar concavity associated with aging results in a hollow-cheeked look.

The malar eminence may be augmented with implants, which can be placed with an intraoral approach. Rhytidectomy with the appropriate vector of force in combination with malar augmentation may assist in diminishing the prominence of the nasolabial fold. The nasolabial crease may be directly addressed with implant augmentation or extended rhytidectomy. Complete eradication of this crease is not possible; neither is it probably desirable as it is an important facial landmark dividing the cheek aesthetic unit from the nasolabial unit. In extreme cases, direct excision of the nasolabial fold may be performed. Rhytidectomy may also improve the definition of the inferior mandibular border and can reposition the buccal fat pad.

Nose

The nose is the most noticeable of the facial aesthetic units owing to its central position in the coronal plane and its prominence in the sagittal plane. Minor asymmetry and variations are more conspicuous here than in other facial regions. Proportions of the nose should be in harmony with the rest of the face and the body habitus. A long, thin nose on a short, stocky person with a wide face appears out of place, as would a short, wide nose on a tall, thin person with a long face.

The muscles of the nasal pyramid are rudimentary in nature and have little influence on the static or dynamic appearance of the nose. Exceptions are the dilator muscles of the nostril and the depressor septi nasali, which extends from the upper lip to the floor of the nose and the nasal septum.

The nose is typically described in terms of its length, width, projection, and rotation. Numerous angles and measurements have been used to describe the nose and its relationship to the face.[8] In general, the dorsum follows a smooth curve downward from the medial aspect of the brows to the supratip region. A slight hump at the bony–cartilaginous junction is acceptable in either sex but is probably better tolerated in the male. The tip should show a double break, and 2 to 4 mm of columellar show is ideal. In the Caucasian, the base of the nose approximates an equilateral triangle. Wider interalar distances are normal in Asian and African American patients. Shorter people may be able to tolerate greater tip rotation than taller people.

With time, the cartilaginous skeleton of the nasal tip weakens causing broadening, tip ptosis, lengthening, and, potentially, airway obstruction. The nostrils may widen, and the columellar–labial angle may become sharper and more retruded. Thickening of the nasal skin may also occur, as in rosacea, for example.

A prominent nose associated with a hypoplastic mandible is aesthetically disagreeable and can usually be much improved when reduction rhinoplasty is combined with augmentation mentoplasty (**Fig. 16.6**). Conversely, nasal reduction should be conservative in patients with a prominent mandible and chin to preserve balance and facial harmony, and to prevent aggravation of a prognathic appearance, especially when viewed in profile.

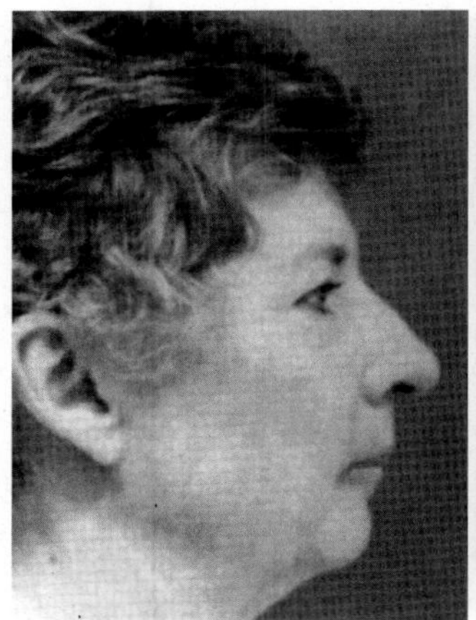
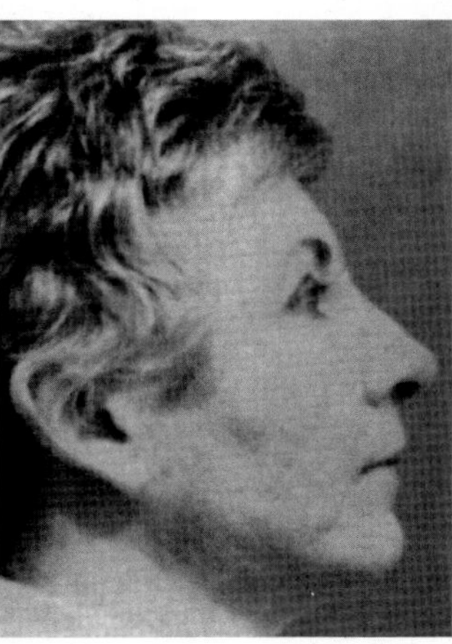

Fig. 16.6 Augmentation mentoplasty with reduction rhinoplasty. (Courtesy of Dr. John R. Hilger.)

Perioral Region and Chin

The perioral region includes the region of the face from the subnasal and nasolabial folds to the menton, the lower border of the soft tissue contour of the chin. The contour of the chin is determined by the shape and position of the mandible, as well as overlying soft tissues in the case of chin ptosis. Next to the nose, the chin is the most common site of abnormality in the profile view.

Muscles responsible for the mimetic actions around the mouth include the quadratus labii inferioris, mentalis, and triangularis muscles, which lie in a plane deep to the platysma. This group of muscles blends with the orbicularis oris in the lower lip. Nerve supply to this group of muscles comes from the marginal mandibular branch of the facial nerve. This muscle group serves to contract and depress the lower lip. All of the muscles of this group insert on the bony inferior rim of the mandible.

Microgenia literally means "small chin." In a patient with normal occlusion (Angle's class I: mesiobuccal cusp of the first maxillary molar aligns with the mesiobuccal groove of the first mandibular molar), microgenia is diagnosed by dropping a vertical line from the vermilion border of the lower lip to the chin. If this line falls anterior to the soft tissue pogonion, then the patient has microgenia. Specific preoperative analysis should focus on the lateral view, with the surgical goal being to extend the mentum to the vertical lip line. Slight overcorrection in men is acceptable, whereas undercorrection in women may be appropriate.

Overall facial balance on profile is best assessed by also considering the nasal dorsum projection. Many times the computer imager is helpful in illustrating the possible positive contribution of chin augmentation to the results of a rhinoplasty. The primary surgical choices for correction of microgenia are implant augmentation and genioplasty. The most commonly used alloplastic mandibular implants are Silastic (Dow Corning, Midland, MI).

Mandibular hypoplasia is an acquired condition secondary to varying degrees of bony resorption of the mandible. Adequate retained dentition can help combat overall loss of mandible size, especially that of alveolar height. With aging there is also specific progressive soft tissue atrophy and bone reduction in the region between the chin and jowl. The resulting groove has been termed the *prejowl sulcus*. This is of significance because although a well-performed facelift can improve the jowl area, it will leave this conspicuous groove behind.

Assessment of the patient with mandibular hypoplasia is similar to that of the microgenia patient, with attention to the presence of normal occlusion. One must not confuse mandibular hypoplasia with retrognathia. The latter condition demonstrates Angle's class II occlusion and benefits most from a bony advancement technique, such as sagittal split osteotomy.

The surgical approach to mandibular hypoplasia is the same as that described for microgenia. The main difference is in the type of Silastic implant used. An extended implant is selected if there is significant mandibular body hypoplasia. The implant design can also secondarily correct microgenia, if indicated. Certain patients lack mandibular definition in the region of the angle (usually congenitally), and may benefit from augmentation.

As with mandibular hypoplasia, dentition plays a major role in determining the shape of the lower face. Orthodontic correction can restore normal lip relationships in addition to restoring normal occlusal relationships of the teeth. Changes in dentition, specifically due to bone resorption in the edentulous mandible, may alter the proportions of the middle and lower thirds of the face. Absorption of alveolar bone, collapse of the vertical distance between the mandible and maxilla, and significant soft tissue disturbances may occur. These changes can only be partially compensated for by prosthetic dentition.

With aging, there is lengthening of the upper lip, thinning of the red lip portions, and midface retrusion. Perioral rhytids, which are vertical and extend from the vermilion borders of the upper and lower lips, also develop. Another phenomenon is the appearance and deepening of "marionette" lines, which are the bilateral inferior extensions of the nasolabial crease that resemble the vertical lines on the lower face of a ventriloquist's dummy. The chin as well as the malar eminences may become relatively underprojected as a result of redistribution of the overlying skin and subcutaneous tissues. The middle and lower facial skeleton also show a decrease in height with age.

Most procedures directed at lip alteration are for augmentation or reduction. Currently, full lips are favored. The upper lip should be fuller and project slightly anterior to the lower lip in profile. Lip augmentation has been performed with several various materials, including autogenous dermis or fat, homograft or xenograft collagen, and expanded polytetrafluoroethylene.

Neck

Restoration of cervicomental definition is an important component of rejuvenation surgery. The neck in youth has a well-defined mandibular line that casts a submandibular shadow. The skin of the submental triangle is flat and tight. The platysma muscle is smooth and has strong tone. In addition, the muscular attachments of the hyoid bone create a cervicomental angle of 90 degrees or less. These factors give the neck a youthful contour and appearance.

The unattractive neck may be the result of hereditary or acquired anatomical factors. Hereditary factors include a low-positioned hyoid–thyroid complex and accumulation of cervical fat both superficial and deep to the platysma. With aging, there are expected acquired changes in the lower face and neck. These include submandibular gland prolapse, platysmal banding, and skin redundancy. Microgenia, mandibular hypoplasia, jowling, chin ptosis, and prejowl sulci, all discussed previously, also have a great impact on the appearance of the neck.

Patients should be routinely assessed for the previously mentioned conditions. A standardized preoperative approach to the lower face and neck regions will ensure that the appropriate technique(s) is used.[9] Assessment for surgical rejuvenation of the neck follows a systematic approach: (1) assessment of skeletal framework adequacy, (2) need for management of the SMAS–platysma muscle complex, (3) need for fat contouring, and (4) need for skin tightening.

The hyoid bone is ideally positioned at the level of the fourth cervical vertebra. Patients with an anatomically low hyoid have an obtuse cervicomental angle, and this limits the surgical efforts. For cervical fat, the primary surgical approach is liposculpture using a suction cannula or direct lipectomy. The surgical correction of platysmal bands entails limited anterior horizontal myotomy with excision of the raised hypertrophic muscular edges. The newly defined anterior borders of the platysma are then reapproximated with sutures. Platysmal sling tightening will also help correct submandibular gland prolapse.

The preferred method to eliminate redundant neck skin is by superior lateral flap advancement during facelift. This bidirectional pull tightens the skin component of the sling. If persistent redundancy remains in the anterior neck, then a submental incision with local skin excision is necessary. Overzealous skin excision must be avoided as this produces standing cones at the lateral aspects of the closed incision. Excessive skin excision can also produce an acute cervical line that obliterates a youthful cervicomental contour. Certain patients with cervical fat and youthful, elastic skin with minimal redundancy may require only liposuction of the fat. This type of skin is not lax and still retains its memory. These patients do not require local skin excision, as the neck skin will draw superiorly and hug the submental contour.

Ears

Some patients with prominent ears can benefit from aesthetic surgery. The top of the auricular helix should be at the level of the lateral eyebrow. The inferior attachment of the ear lobe should be at the level of the alar–facial junction. The ear is posteriorly inclined on the lateral view, with its vertical axis offset slightly from the horizontal. This is important to remember during rhytidectomy to prevent creating a pulled-forward look that discloses surgical intervention. The width-to-length ratio of the ear is about 0.6:1. The ears should protrude from the posterior scalp ~20 to 25 degrees, and the midear should be no more than 2 cm from the head.

With age, there is an increase in lobe size. There is also increased prominence due to an increase in the conchoscaphoid angle, and there may be partial loss of the antihelical fold. An increased conchoscaphoid angle and loss of the antihelical fold can emphasize prominent ears. Changes to the ear lobe may also result from prolonged earring use.

Facial Analysis and the East Asian Patient

Facial aesthetic surgery specific to the Asian patient usually focuses on changing two aspects of the Asian face. This includes surgery to modify the upper eyelid to create a supratarsal fold, so-called double-eyelid surgery, and rhinoplasty with augmentation of the nasal dorsum.

The typical East Asian periorbital region differs from that of the Caucasian in several ways. The first is the presence of a persistent epicanthal fold. The epicanthal fold is present in all normal fetuses between the third and sixth fetal month but usually disappears in Caucasians by birth or by adolescence at the latest. Asians usually retain at least some trace of the epicanthal fold after maturity. Prominent epicanthal folds can be addressed with medial epicanthopexy. Another difference is that, unlike the Caucasian eye, the East Asian eye is not deep-set. Surgical management is not commonly pursued for this feature.

The third prominent feature is the presence of the so-called double eyelid in Caucasians that is lacking or less well developed in most Asians. The double eyelid in the Caucasian eye is attributed to a fold in the skin of the upper eyelid that is present when the eye is open, that is, the supratarsal fold, which is nearly parallel to the lid margin. Anatomically, this corresponds to the distal fibers of the levator aponeurosis, which run through the orbicularis oculi muscle above the tarsal plate to insert on the eyelid dermis near the ciliary margin. In the typical Asian eyelid, the levator aponeurosis terminates at the septum orbitale, with few or no fibers penetrating the orbicularis oculi and attaching to the dermal layer of the eyelids. As there are no connections between the levator and the dermis, the preseptal fat deep to the orbicularis oculi is able to drift anteriorly, which may further obscure the landmarks of the upper eyelid. In addition, the East Asian tarsal plate tends to be shorter (4 mm versus 10 mm in the Caucasian eyelid).

Several anatomical studies document the presence of a double eyelid in at least 50% of the Japanese population, so it is a misunderstanding that double eyelids are a uniquely Caucasian feature. Often this crease is prominent only in the central to lateral portion of the lid. The double eyelid is more common and better defined in Asian females than males. It is not uncommon for the double eyelid to be asymmetric, with one eyelid possessing a more prominent fold than the other.

The typical East Asian nose differs from the Caucasian nose in that it is smaller and somewhat differently shaped. The dorsum is wider and rounder. The Caucasian depression at the nasal root followed by a dorsal hump are features rarely seen in the East Asian nose. In comparison with the Caucasian nose, the tip is broad and drooping. In the East Asian nose, the ala are flared, and sometimes overhanging with a thicker nostril wall. Likewise, the nasal aperture is horizontally ovoid rather than vertically ellipsoid.

The nasal dorsum is the most common anatomical site for placement of alloplastic facial implants in Asian countries. A more defined nasal dorsum is considered to be aesthetically desirable in many Asian societies. The goal of the surgery is not necessarily to create an ideal Caucasian nose but to create a more well-proportioned nose that is in harmony with the patient's other facial features.

Facial Analysis and the African American Patient

The African American patient is often seen in consultation by the facial plastic surgeon for several somewhat specific issues and procedures, including rhinoplasty, central face rhytidectomy, cheiloplasty for enlarged lips, and scarring problems. The anatomical features of the nose and aging face are distinct from those of Caucasians. Again, the goal is not necessarily to create ideal Caucasian features but to create balanced features in harmony with the rest of the face and the body habitus.

Common complaints regarding the typical African American nose include a wide nasal dorsum that lacks anterior height, flared alae with a wide interalar distance, and poor tip projection and definition. Thick skin, abundant subcutaneous fat, and wide, flat crura all result in poor tip projection. These problems are addressed with dorsal augmentation, alar base resection, interalar reduction, and tip defatting, respectively.

The aging-related changes to the facial hard and soft tissues in African Americans are different from those in Caucasians. Male pattern baldness is common. Preauricular skin excess is uncommon, as is fine wrinkling, including periorbital crow's feet. Skin laxity is most common in the central face, along the nasolabial folds and submental area. Skin and fat along the infraorbital rim droop with age and contribute to nasolabial fold fullness, exaggerating malar hypoplasia. Facelift procedures may help but do not directly address the problems in the central face. Excision of the nasolabial folds and submental lipectomy may be performed, usually with good results for central face and submental skin and subcutaneous tissue redundancy.

Lip size is a concern among many African American patients. Central upper and lower lip heights of greater than 1 cm each are not uncommon. Visible pink vermilion on otherwise brown lips is felt by many to be undesirable. Optimally, the lower lip central height should be 50 to 75% greater than the upper lip central height. Dental assessment is part of the appropriate workup prior to offering cheiloplasty for reduction of lip size.

Excessive scarring, with the formation of hypertrophic and keloid scars, is seen with increased frequency in African American patients. Aberrant wound healing is most common on the chest, arms, and ears. Hypertrophic and keloid scars are rarely found on the eyelids, the nasolabial folds, the internal and external nose, the lips, and the submental area. Location of the incision, suture material, and surgical technique all play a role in prevention of hypertrophic and keloid scars.

Summary

Facial analysis is a critical element in successful facial aesthetic surgery. The surgeon must have a good grasp of contemporary facial ideal proportions, which must be put into perspective with the rest of the face and body habitus. Thorough anesthetic facial analysis allows the surgeon to select the appropriate procedures, and approaches to those procedures, for a specific patient. Baseline evaluation consists of a standard comprehensive history and physical, preoperative photography, appraisal of overall facial symmetry and balance, and systematic evaluation of the facial aesthetic units. Computer analysis is effective in conveying realistic expectations of surgical results to the patient and allows the surgeon and patient to compare their own aesthetic interpretations. Attention is paid to the quality of the skin, underlying bony landmarks, and contraction patterns of the facial musculature. Asian and African American patients may present specific concerns or areas they wish to address.

Acknowledgment

The authors thank Steve Ronson for his assistance in preparing this manuscript.

References

1. Martin JG. Racial ethnocentricism and judgement of beauty. J Soc Psychol 1964;63:59–63
2. Langlois JH, Roggman LA, Casey RJ, et al. Infant preferences for attractive faces. Dev Psychol 1987;23:363–369
3. Langlois JH, Roggman LA. Attractive faces are only average. Psychol Sci 1990;1:115–121
4. Perrett DI, May KA, Yoshikawa S. Facial shapes and judgement of female attractiveness. Nature 1994;368:239–242
5. Koch RJ, Troell R, Goode RL. Contemporary management of the aging brow and forehead. Laryngoscope 1997;107:710–715
6. Ellenbogen R. Transcoronal eyebrow lift with concomitant upper blepharoplasty. Plast Reconstr Surg 1983;71:490–499
7. Cook TA, Brownrigg PJ, Wang TD, et al. The versatile midforehead browlift. Arch Otolaryngol Head Neck Surg 1989;115:163–168
8. Powell N, Humphries B. Proportions of the Aesthetic Face. New York: Thieme-Stratton; 1984
9. Brennan HG, Koch RJ. Management of the aging neck. Facial Plast Surg 1996;12(3):241–255

17 Anesthesia in Facial Plastic Surgery

Mark V. Fletcher

Anesthesia for facial plastic surgery covers a gamut of techniques from local anesthesia without sedation to general anesthesia. The first sections of this chapter deal with the drugs we have at our disposal to perform anesthesia. The next section deals with deep-sedation anesthesia, also known as monitored anesthesia care, or "The Big MAC." The final sections deal with how anesthesia influences blood loss, monitoring standards, and a discussion of anesthetic costs.

Drugs Used as Anesthetics

Local Anesthetics

The first naturally derived local anesthetic was cocaine, isolated from the coca leaf in 1860. The first reported surgical procedure performed using local anesthesia was in 1884 when Koller reported using topical cocaine to facilitate ophthalmic surgery. The first synthetic local anesthetic, procaine, was synthesized in 1904. Lidocaine, the prototypical amide local anesthetic, was first synthesized in 1943.

All local anesthetics inhibit the inward flow of sodium ions that initiates a neural action potential. By progressively attenuating this inward current, they dampen and then totally eliminate neural conduction.

There are two classes of local anesthetics, esters and amides. The distinction is important for two reasons. First, an allergic response to amide local anesthetics is virtually unknown, whereas it is possible with the ester group. Second, all amide local anesthetics are metabolized in the liver, whereas all ester local anesthetics except cocaine are metabolized by pseudocholinesterase, a plasma enzyme.

Cocaine is unique among the local anesthetics in that it is the only ester local anesthetic partially metabolized in the liver and it is the only local anesthetic with vasoconstrictive properties. Both its psychoactive properties and its vasoconstrictive effect are due to blockade of norepinephrine reuptake. Thus, the combination of exogenous epinephrine and cocaine when administered nasally can result in significant tachycardia and hypertension in some patients. Pretreatment with a β-blocker can be beneficial.

Toxicity of local anesthetics is related to the peak plasma levels of the local anesthetic in the blood. The peak will be influenced by the following factors: quantity of drug injected, site of injection, presence or absence of a vasoconstrictor, and duration of administration.

Clearly, the more drug administered the higher the peak plasma concentration will be. In fact, there is a linear relationship between administered dose and plasma level.

The site of injection has tremendous impact on plasma concentrations. Obviously, injection into the vascular system itself results in a rapid rise in plasma level. Most toxic reactions to local anesthetics result from accidental intravascular injection. The differences between sites of injection are determined by their respective blood flows. The greater the vascularity, the sooner the peak is achieved and the higher the resulting concentration. The face has some of the highest cutaneous blood flow in the body. In particular, the nose and the mucous membranes of the mouth yield particularly rapid absorption.

Clinicians often add a vasoconstrictor, such as epinephrine, to a local anesthetic in an attempt to slow the rate of absorption of that anesthetic. This allows a higher total dose of local anesthetic without violating the safe plasma level. A second benefit of vasoconstrictor use is reduction in bleeding during surgery. When using epinephrine for vasoconstriction in facial surgery, the same quantity of drug should be used whether a local anesthetic is the primary anesthetic or a general anesthetic is used. The addition of local anesthesia with a vasoconstrictor to general anesthesia simplifies blood pressure management and ensures even and maximal vasoconstriction.

Maximal doses for local anesthetics are quoted as milligram per kilogram and are given as with and without epinephrine. Clinicians should consider both where the drug is injected and the time interval over which the drug is given. The toxic limit for a local anesthetic will be one quantity if the drug is given all at once and something quite different if the administration is stretched out over several hours. The redose intervals given in **Table 17.1** specify how often the maximal dose may be repeated.

Cocaine has poorly established maximal dosage limits. Cousins and Bridenbaugh give a limit of 150 mg in a typical adult,[1] whereas Goodman and Gilman are more liberal with 200 mg.[2] Many references do not publish a limit.

Table 17.1 Dosage Limits for Local Anesthetics (mg/kg)

Anesthetic	Plain	With Epinephrine	Redose Interval (min)
Lidocaine	4.5	7	90
Bupivacaine	2.5	3.2	180
Etidocaine	6	8	120–180

Source: Data from 1999 Physicians Desk Reference.

Ropivicaine is a newly introduced, long-acting, local anesthetic that is comparable to bupivacaine in duration and has a similar toxic limit of 3 mg/kg without epinephrine. In contrast, ropivicaine has a greater margin of safety for cardiotoxicity.

The two organ systems that manifest local anesthetic toxicity are the central nervous system (CNS) and the cardiovascular system. Fortunately, most patients express CNS toxicity with minimal to no cardiovascular toxicity. The earliest signs are a mild sedation, which then can progress to agitation, focal tics, and, finally, grand mal seizures. Patients will often report tinnitus, perioral numbness, and a metallic taste in the mouth.

Management of the early signs of CNS toxicity involves intravenous administration of a drug that will raise the seizure threshold. Benzodiazepines, such as midazolam and diazepam, or barbiturates, such as thiopental and methohexital, will suffice. Care must be taken not to sedate the patient to the point of airway compromise and hypoxia.

If the patient is seizing, the primary focus is on airway and oxygenation to prevent cerebral hypoxia. Termination of the seizure can then be accomplished as previously stated. Oxygen is indicated until the patient demonstrates normal blood oxygen saturation on room air.

Local anesthetics can also target the cardiovascular system, causing dysrhythmias, heart block, and reduced contractility. Fortunately, with most local anesthetics cardiovascular toxicity occurs at plasma levels twice those necessary to produce seizures. The one exception to this is bupivacaine, whereby cardiac and CNS toxicities occur at similar blood levels. Bupivacaine toxicity should be greatly respected as several fatalities have occurred. When treating cardiovascular toxicity with bupivacaine, prolonged resuscitation may be required as the drug binds tightly to the myocardium.

Epinephrine toxicity is also possible, manifesting as dysrhythmias, tachycardia, as well as increased contractility and blood pressure. Awake patients will often complain about rapid and forceful heartbeat, palpitations, and a sense of extreme anxiety. A common story from patients who have experienced this is that they are allergic to epinephrine or local anesthetics and that they "almost died" when they received them. More often than not this experience occurred in a dental chair with either rapid tissue absorption or accidental intravenous administration.

The most specific therapy for epinephrine toxicity is β-blockade. Sedatives may also help resolve the anxiety. Doses of less than 7 μg/kg of epinephrine are unlikely to cause dysrhythmias.[3,4]

Sedative Hypnotic Drugs

Simply stated, the ideal sedative hypnotic drug for outpatient facial cosmetic surgery would be inexpensive, free from side effects, and equally effective in short and long surgical cases. The commonly used hypnotic drugs for outpatient facial plastic surgery include propofol, thiopental, methohexital, and etomidate. Ketamine is also used, but much less frequently due to its unique properties. All of these drugs are capable of rapidly inducing complete unconsciousness in less than 1 minute. All of these drugs are used to induce general anesthesia, and some are used for sedation. They differ in cost, side effects, and pharmacokinetics.

Propofol

Propofol infusion has revolutionized the administration of outpatient, deep-sedation anesthesia. Propofol is very poorly soluble in water and is solubilized in a milky white suspension of soybean oil, glycerol, and egg lecithin. The suspension is responsible for the pain on injection noted with propofol, particularly when injected into a more distal, smaller caliber vein. The pain can be avoided or greatly diminished by immediately preceding the propofol with 20 to 30 mg of intravenous lidocaine and slowing the administration of propofol to 10 mg/second. There is a less than 1% risk of thrombophlebitis despite the potential for pain on injection, and both subcutaneous extravasation and accidental arterial injection are generally without sequelae.

Some practitioners have been concerned about the use of propofol in patients who report an allergy to eggs. Egg allergy develops to albumin, a component of the egg white. Egg lecithin used in the lipid suspension is a component of the yolk. For this reason, allergy to eggs is not a contraindication to the administration of propofol.

Propofol is a powerful sedative hypnotic with a rapid onset of action. Serious clinical effects include apnea, airway obstruction, loss of airway reflexes, and hypotension. When administered with other drugs, such as narcotics and benzodiazepines, cardiac output can be significantly reduced. Practitioners using this drug should be experienced in its use and be expert at airway management and resuscitation.

Propofol when used as an infusion has two distinct advantages for outpatient facial plastic surgery. First, it is rapidly and reliably titratable to a variety of anesthetic depths. Second, it is cleared rapidly from the patient's circulation. The clearance of propofol occurs by two mechanisms. The drug is conjugated by the liver and excreted by the kidney as inactive metabolites, and the drug is redistributed to more poorly perfused parts of the body. In the short term, these two mechanisms share the burden equally, but as infusion times lengthen, the plateau plasma concentration seen during recovery increases as redistribution sites are filled[5] (**Fig. 17.1**).

Propofol has other advantages, such as a reduced incidence of nausea and vomiting compared with thiopental.

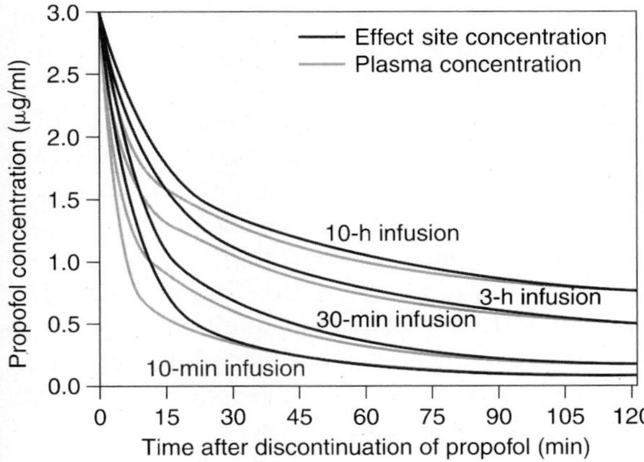

Fig. 17.1 Predicted plasma and effect site concentrations of propofol after various infusion times (10 minute to 10 hour). (From Kazama, T, Ikeda K, Morita K, Sanjo Y. Awakening propofol concentration with and without blood–effect site equilibrium after short-term and long-term administration of propofol and fentanyl anesthesia. Anesthesiology, Lippincott Williams & Wilkins, 1998;88:928–934. Reprinted by permission.)

It also usually induces a euphoric state, which gives the patient a sense of well-being and affection for the surgical team.

Thiopental

Thiopental was the first ultrashort-acting sedative hypnotic brought into clinical practice. It is a thiobarbiturate whose activity is terminated not by metabolism but by redistribution to more poorly perfused tissues. Even after single doses of thiopental, there is a residual serum level that persists for hours. This makes the drug inappropriate for continuous infusion. Its only clinical use in outpatient surgery is as a single dose to induce general anesthesia. Thiopental has two advantages in clinical practice: its long clinical history and its low cost. Where cost is not the limiting factor, propofol offers several advantages in the outpatient setting.

Methohexital

Methohexital is an oxybarbiturate with a pharmacological profile similar to that of thiopental. Its chief advantage is a shorter terminal elimination half-life. Patients will awaken somewhat more quickly with methohexital and will notice less of a hangover after 30 to 60 minutes. Patients managed with a methohexital infusion will develop a residual sedation secondary to accumulation in the redistribution sites, but this is less noticeable than with thiopental.

Etomidate

Etomidate is an imidazole derivative that is used as an ultrashort-acting sedative hypnotic for the induction of general anesthesia. Etomidate causes little or no depression of the patient's cardiovascular system and is often used to induce anesthesia in the sickest patients. Ideally, there would be little need for etomidate in a facial plastic surgery practice.

Initially, there was enthusiasm for using etomidate in a continuous infusion as a sedative for intensive-care patients. This ended when it was discovered that etomidate suppresses the pituitary adrenal axis.[6,7] Transient suppression is noted after even a single dose of etomidate.

Like propofol, etomidate is insoluble in water and is therefore solubilized in propylene glycol. Pain on injection is prominent with etomidate unless a small quantity of lidocaine is injected immediately before the drug is given.

Ketamine

Ketamine is a unique anesthetic that is fast-acting but not classified as a sedative-hypnotic. It functions as a dissociative anesthetic such that patients do not react to stimuli in an expected fashion. For example, painful stimuli may elicit a vocal response but not a withdrawal reflex. A portion of the drug effect is due to stimulation of narcotic receptors.[8] Ketamine is in the same drug classification as phencyclidine, better known as PCP or angel dust.

Ketamine is also unique among other sedative drugs in that it causes an increase in CNS sympathetic outflow, resulting in tachycardia and mild increases in blood pressure. This effect is blocked by prior administration of benzodiazepines or barbiturates. Its use in adults is limited by dysphoric reactions. These dysphoric episodes can also be prevented by a benzodiazepine effect that outlasts the ketamine effect. Children do not seem to be troubled with the dysphoric effects, thus making the drug very useful for short pediatric sedation cases, particularly as the drug is very effective when given intramuscularly. There is a tendency to excessive salivation, which can be treated with a low dose of an anticholinergic, such as glycopyrrolate or atropine.

The drug is a potent anesthetic and should only be used in the presence of oxygen, suction, and the ability to manage the airway should upper airway obstruction occur. The proper dose is 0.5 to 1 mg/kg intravenously or 3 to 5 mg/kg intramuscularly.

Narcotics

Sedative-hypnotics work well only in the absence of painful stimulation. The patient will continue to move in response to pain despite deep hypnosis. The solution is to include a narcotic in the sedation regimen.

Narcotics are poor sedatives when given alone. They are powerful analgesics and respiratory depressants, but poor amnestics and only mild sedatives. When the combination of narcotic and sedative-hypnotic drugs is given, profound synergism results. The patient will sleep, be amnestic, and have little to no response to moderately painful stimuli, such as local infiltration or tissue manipulation. The analgesic properties of narcotics make them the critical component of a successful deep-sedation regimen.

There are many different narcotics from which to choose. Cost and pharmacokinetics are the most important factors in choosing a narcotic. In general, it is cost-effective and efficient to choose a narcotic whose duration of action is similar to the length of the surgery. Long-acting narcotics, such as hydromorphone, for short, less painful surgical procedures is ill advised, particularly in the elderly patient. On the other hand, using a short-acting narcotic such as fentanyl for a 4-hour case will require multiple redosing. This has two effects. First, the cost rises in proportion to the number of redoses and second, the drug accumulates in the body, filling up the redistribution sites, converting the drug from a short-acting one (dependent on redistribution) to a long-acting one (dependent on hepatic elimination).

Longer-acting narcotics include morphine, meperidine, and hydromorphone. There is probably little difference in efficacy and side effects when equipotent doses are given. Recently, attention has been paid to normeperidine, a metabolite of meperidine, which tends to accumulate and can predispose to seizures.[9] This is of no consequence in the limited doses that patients undergoing facial plastic surgery would receive.

Antiemetics

Postoperative nausea and vomiting (PONV) is one of the top patient complaints with all anesthetics. Often PONV occurs later in the day or evening of surgery and disturbs both the patient and the on-call surgeon. When it occurs in the immediate postoperative period it can delay or prevent discharge from the postanesthesia care unit (PACU). At the minimum, this may increase overtime payroll, and at worst it may necessitate transfer of the patient from an outpatient facility to an inpatient one.

In keeping with the axiom "less is more," the less that is done to a patient the less likely he or she is to experience PONV. A patient who receives only local anesthetic with minimal or no sedation is very unlikely to suffer any ill effects.

Modern sedatives, such as propofol, and inhaled anesthetics, such as desflurane and sevoflurane, have less potential to cause PONV than older drugs with longer elimination times. In addition, we have new antiemetics—ondansetron and dolasetron—which have been shown to inhibit nausea without the problems of sedation or extrapyramidal side effects. The major drawback to the newer antiemetics is cost.

Traditional antiemetics, such as chlorpromazine, promethazine, and droperidol, are inexpensive and effective, but they are sedating and have the potential to cause muscular rigidity, akathisia, and torticollis as the most common extrapyramidal side effects.

As a routine, we administer promethazine 50 mg and metoclopramide 10 mg orally to all adult patients before administering general anesthesia or sedation anesthetics. As ondansetron is now available as a generic, most patients with intravenous access receive a dose.

Inhalational Anesthetics

Inhalational anesthetics have come a long way from the days of diethyl ether, methoxyflurane, and even halothane. As newer agents have been developed, there has been a constant effort to reduce side effects and toxicity. The ideal volatile agent would certainly have one property—speed. It would exhibit both rapid induction and emergence. Speed is quantified in volatile anesthetics by measuring the blood gas solubility coefficient. The lower the coefficient, the faster the onset and offset of the drug.

Halothane with a blood gas solubility coefficient of 2.54 was a great improvement over methoxyflurane and diethyl ether with a coefficient of 13 and 11, respectively. Isoflurane (coefficient = 1.46) was even better, but sevoflurane (coefficient = 0.69) and desflurane (coefficient = 0.42) have rivaled nitrous oxide (coefficient = 0.46). These properties are illustrated in **Figs. 17.2 and 17.3.**[10]

The first graph demonstrates the impact of blood gas solubility on anesthesia induction times. The more rapid the rate of rise of the alveolar concentration, the more rapid the induction. This information is critical to the anesthesiologist but less so to the surgeon.

The graph illustrating the recovery times is of greatest importance when considering outpatient surgery. Considering the logarithmic scale, desflurane and sevoflurane enjoy a 1.6-fold faster recovery than isoflurane. In this study, the duration of anesthesia was 30 minutes. With longer anesthesia times, the recovery difference becomes even more dramatic. At 1 hour postoperatively, both desflurane and sevoflurane levels are ~2% of full anesthetic levels. At 2 hours into recovery, levels have fallen to 1%. In comparison with propofol infusion, only infusions of 1 hour or less can match this recovery profile. The longer the infusion of propofol, the longer the recovery. Recovery from agents such as desflurane and sevoflurane are essentially independent of duration of anesthesia. Short recovery times reduce personnel costs by reducing overtime and perhaps decreasing the number of staff needed in the postanesthetic care unit. PONV are also reduced.

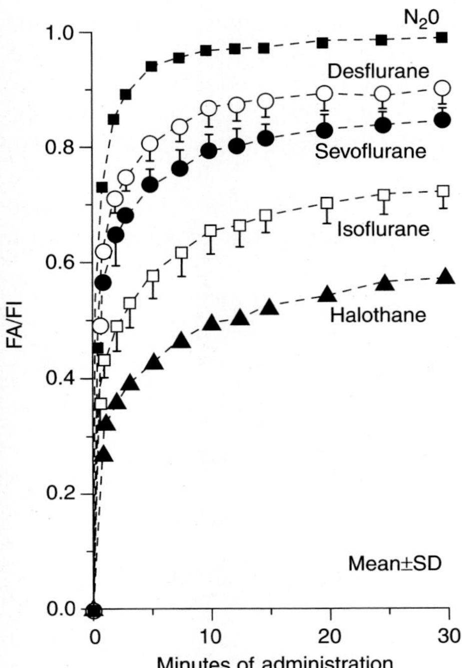

Fig. 17.2 The pharmacokinetics of sevoflurane and isoflurane during their administration are defined as the ratio of end-tidal anesthetic concentration to inspired anesthetic concentration. (From Yasuda N, Lockhart S, Eger EI II, et al. Comparison of kinetics of sevoflurane and isoflurane in humans. Anesthesia Analg, Lippincott Williams & Wilkins, 1991;72(3):316–324. Reprinted by permission.)

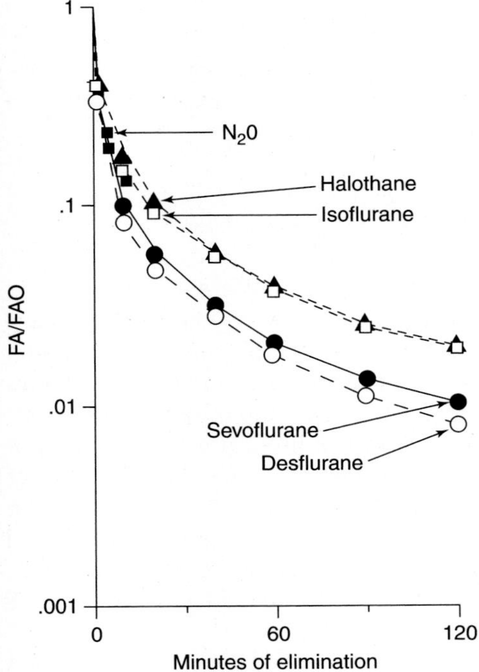

Fig. 17.3 Elimination of each anesthetic is defined as the ratio of end-tidal anesthetic concentration to that immediately before the beginning of elimination. (From Yasuda N, Lockhart S, Eger EI II, et al. Comparison of kinetics of sevoflurane and isoflurane in humans. Anesthesia Analg, Lippincott Williams & Wilkins, 1991;72(3):316–324. Reprinted by permission.)

Anesthesia Techniques

Before the successful public demonstration of ether anesthesia on October 16, 1846, sedation and a speedy surgery were the only comforts surgeons could offer their patients. Deep sedation was provided by one of two regimens: a near-toxic dose of alcohol or a near-toxic dose of opium. The outcomes were unpredictable and often unpleasant for both surgeon and patient. Today we are fortunate to have a variety of anesthetic regimens. For the purpose of this chapter these have been separated into four categories:

1. Minimal sedation
2. Moderate sedation/analgesia (also called conscious sedation)
3. Deep sedation/analgesia
4. General anesthesia

Any physician with appropriate training and facilities can administer the first two. The last two require specialty training in anesthesia. All may be supplemented with the use of local anesthetics to alleviate pain. The line between sedation and analgesia and deep sedation is a critical one. As published by the American Society of Anesthesiologists (ASA), moderate sedation/analgesia is defined as “a drug-induced depression of consciousness during which patients respond purposefully to verbal commands, either alone or accompanied by light tactile stimulation. No interventions are required to maintain a patent airway, and spontaneous ventilation is adequate.” In contrast, deep sedation/analgesia is defined as “a drug-induced depression of consciousness during which patients cannot be easily aroused but respond purposefully following repeated or painful stimulation. The ability to independently maintain ventilatory function may be impaired. Patients may require assistance in maintaining a patent airway, and spontaneous ventilation may be inadequate.”[11] The key difference is the patient’s response to verbal command and his or her ability to maintain a patent airway without assistance.

Practice guidelines for sedation and analgesia by non-anesthesiologists have been published by the ASA.[12] These include standards for preoperative assessment, intraoperative care, and postoperative management. A discussion of relevant standards is included in the section on monitoring.

The Big MAC

Monitored anesthesia care (MAC), the newest name for what used to be called local standby, comes in many different forms. In the simplest sense, there is a continuum of sedation from minimal to a level that approaches that of a light general anesthetic. Minimal sedation is used when the patient is critically ill and the primary role of the anesthesiologist is as a vigilant monitor of vital signs and an expert in resuscitation.

At the other end of the spectrum lies The Big MAC. The patient is profoundly sedated to the level of unconsciousness and is unresponsive to moderately painful stimuli. To many facial plastic surgeons, this is the Holy Grail of sedation anesthesia. The use of deep sedation is in many ways more difficult and nerve wracking than use of a garden variety general anesthetic would be. Not every anesthesiologist is comfortable with this technique. A good working relationship between the plastic surgeon and the anesthesiologist should be cultivated. Deep-sedation anesthesia is viewed with skepticism by many anesthesia training programs where there is a strong emphasis on airway control with an endotracheal tube or laryngeal mask airway. They refer to it as an uncontrolled general anesthetic or "unconscious sedation." When deep sedation is utilized without a controlled airway, most anesthesiologists become anxious. With experience, they can develop a repertoire of techniques as well as a level of personal comfort.

There are certain elements of a successful Big MAC. These are narcotics, airway management, and supplemental oxygen.

All deep-sedation anesthesia involves the use of sedatives, often benzodiazepines such as diazepam or midazolam. Anesthesiologists add such drugs as propofol or thiopental. Sedating an operative patient without the addition of narcotics will be unsatisfactory when the patient experiences a painful stimulus. The patient will be amnestic but will grimace or move purposefully during painful events, such as local anesthetic infiltration, nasal osteotomy, and so on. If a sufficiently high dose of sedative alone is given to prevent reaction or movement, the patient will be apneic and will almost certainly lose his or her airway and become hypoxic, in spite of supplemental oxygen.

If proper doses of narcotics are used, the dose of sedative drug can be greatly decreased, reducing the duration of any apneic period and motion in response to stimulation. Airway management and supplemental oxygen are still critical to the successful deep-sedation anesthetic. It is a rare patient who can be sedated to a level of unresponsiveness and still not require airway support. In short-duration anesthetics, neck extension and anterior jaw displacement may be all that is required. For longer cases and when the head and neck must be abandoned as part of the surgical field, nasal airways, oral airways, or laryngeal mask airways may be used. Nasal oxygen is often quite successful, and oxygen can often be jetted down the airway to preserve oxygenation.

At the Meridian Plastic Surgery Center, where the author practices, the anesthesiologists have been quite successful using a short nasopharyngeal airway as an oral airway. If the length is adequate to reach around the tongue to the glottic area without stimulating the glottis itself, this is ideal. The soft nasal airway is far better tolerated by the patient than a more rigid plastic oral airway and has the advantage of allowing jetted oxygen to be administered to the airway.

What follows are typical dosages for doing monitored anesthesia care during facelift or rhinoplasty on a typical adult patient:

Preoperatively

- Promethazine 50 mg orally
- Metoclopramide 10 mg orally
- Midazolam 1 to 2 mg intravenously for sedation

Preinduction

- Oxygen supplementation by nasal cannula

At induction

- Hydromorphone 1 mg intravenously
- Propofol 60 to 150 mg intravenously
- Airway support during local anesthetic administration, usually leading to insertion of nasal or oral airway with oxygen jetted at distal tip of airway.

Maintenance

- Propofol infusion at 50 to 150 μg/kg per minute.
- Patient may require one or two additional doses of hydromorphone of 0.25 to 0.5 mg.

Anesthesia and Blood Loss

Some surgeons have a strong preference for sedation over general anesthesia because they believe that general anesthetics are vasodilators that will increase blood loss. Multiple studies confirm that volatile anesthetics are indeed vasodilators, particularly of skeletal muscle.[13] There is no evidence in the literature to support that these agents will counteract the vasoconstricting effect of subcutaneous epinephrine on blood vessels. Although different patients appear to undergo vasoconstriction to a greater or lesser extent in response to injected epinephrine, this is not related to the choice of sedation or general anesthesia.

Blood loss is profoundly affected by systemic blood pressure. A sudden elevation in pressure is clearly reflected in increased bleeding at the surgical site. This is particularly noticeable where large cutaneous flaps are elevated or in nasal surgery. The best therapy is to address the cause of the hypertension. Appropriate measures to reduce blood pressure include deepening of the sedation or general anesthesia, extension of the local anesthetic to cover surgical areas incompletely anesthetized, or administration of vasoactive drugs.

Management of Hypertension

The use of subcutaneous epinephrine is critical in many facial plastic surgical procedures where direct control of all bleeding vessels is not practical or possible. Avoidance of hypertension is equally critical in the control of blood loss and the prevention of hematoma formation. Hypertension results from both intrinsic and extrinsic factors. The pain and stress of surgery can cause hypertension in a normotensive patient. The use of local anesthetics, narcotics, and sedatives will usually control this response. Many facial plastic surgical patients are elderly and suffer from intrinsic hypertension. It is critical that the medical condition of the patient be optimized and his or her antihypertensive regimen be maintained throughout the surgery and into the postoperative period. Additional antihypertensive drugs may be required to maintain tight control of blood pressure.

Tachycardia is very stressful for patients with coronary artery disease. It increases myocardial oxygen demand while decreasing myocardial oxygen supply.[14] It is good practice to avoid increases in heart rate that can occur with epinephrine injection or with a painful stimulus. β-Blockers are very effective in treating tachycardia secondary to increased adrenergic stimulation. For this reason, they are the first-line drugs for treatment of hypertension, unless the patient is already bradycardic. The most common β-blocker in our use is labetalol. Intravenous doses of 5 to 20 mg in an average adult are usually effective.

There is a ceiling effect with β-blockers seen when increased drug causes no reduction in pulse rate or blood pressure. This typically occurs at doses of labetalol greater than 0.5 mg/kg. Vasodilators such as hydralazine or calcium channel blockers such as verapamil or diltiazem are effective second-line drugs. Hydralazine causes a reflex tachycardia when given alone but less so after administration of a β-blocker. The usual intravenous dose for hydralazine is 5 to 10 mg. The onset time of hydralazine is delayed and it is necessary to wait 15 minutes to assess the effect of an intravenous dose. The author uses verapamil as a third-line drug in cases of resistant hypertension. The dose is 2.5 to 5 mg for the average adult.

Some practitioners have advocated the use of clonidine to control perioperative blood pressure. Clonidine is not available for injection but must be given either orally or transcutaneously as a patch. The onset time for the antihypertensive effect is slow, and the final effect is unpredictable. Patients who are started on oral clonidine for primary hypertension must be cautioned regarding postural hypotension. In the dynamic situation of surgery, it makes no sense to rely on a drug with a delayed onset and unpredictable effect when highly titratable drugs with rapid onset and predictable effect are available.

Hemodynamic control to limit bleeding not only is important intraoperatively but must continue into the postoperative period to prevent hematoma and decrease swelling. It may be necessary to initiate a 2-day course of β-blocker therapy with or without a vasodilator. The author's preference is to use atenolol 100 mg once or twice daily depending on previous response to intravenous β-blocker. In resistant cases, it may be necessary to add nifedipine 30 mg once daily.

The use of long-acting sedatives to control postoperative hypertension is not recommended. Only rarely will sedatives normalize the blood pressure in an otherwise hypertensive patient, and in situations where there may be bleeding into the airway they can be a recipe for disaster.

Where appropriate, the use of local anesthetics to reduce pain will often simplify postoperative management.

Monitoring

Intraoperative and postoperative standards for monitoring have been published by the ASA.[15] Following are the two published standards for intraoperative management.

Standard I

Qualified anesthesia personnel shall be present in the room throughout the conduct of all general anesthetics, regional anesthetics, and monitored anesthesia care.

The purpose of the first standard is to ensure the presence of competent personnel at all times during the administration of any deep sedation/analgesia or general anesthesia. This caregiver serves both to monitor the patient and to provide needed anesthesia care.

Standard II

During all anesthetics, the patient's oxygenation, ventilation, circulation, and temperature shall be continually evaluated.

An important distinction is made between "continually evaluated" and "continuously evaluated." Continual is defined as "repeated regularly and frequently in steady rapid succession," whereas continuous means "prolonged without any interruption at any time." This standard applies to all anesthetics and in its broadest interpretation might even apply to a patient receiving only local anesthesia.

To assess oxygenation, use of a pulse oximeter is required unless prohibited by surgical or anatomical factors. The use of skin color to assure adequate oxygenation is vastly inferior as cyanosis does not become apparent until more than 5 g/dL of desaturated hemoglobin is present.

Ventilation can be assessed in the sedated patient by feeling for exhaled gases, observing chest expansion, and watching for signs of obstruction, such as retractions, "rocking boat" respirations, and snoring sounds. Some practitioners advocate the use of end-tidal carbon dioxide monitoring in sedated patients, but it is virtually impossible to obtain a quantitative sample.

Circulation is assessed by continuous electrocardiography and intermittent blood pressure monitoring. ASA standards call for blood pressure determinations at least every 5 minutes.

Temperature monitoring must be available for all patients and utilized whenever clinically significant changes in body temperature are intended, anticipated, or suspected. The use of convective warming blankets is the most effective way to maintain body temperature in a cold operating room. Warm fluids should be used whenever large volumes of intravenous, irrigation, or tumescent fluid are used.

Whenever general anesthesia is employed, additional monitors must be used.[15] Inspired oxygen concentration as well as ventilatory volume and pressure are standard on all modern anesthesia machines. End-tidal carbon dioxide monitoring is now the standard, and agent analysis is an evolving standard.

The Bispectral Index (BIS) is a processed electroencephalographic monitor (Aspect Medical Systems, Newton, MA) that yields a number between 0 and 100 correlating with a patient's ability to recall events. An index of less than 60 virtually ensures total lack of recall, whereas an index greater than 70 puts the patient at progressively greater risk of recall. The monitor uses a proprietary electrode, which is applied to one side of the forehead just above the eyebrow. This position severely limits application of the BIS in facial plastic surgery. The company claims that BIS allows a reduction in anesthetic drug cost as well as a speedier discharge from recovery. The ultimate cost/benefit ratio has not been established.

The ASA standards for postoperative care can be summarized as follows. All patients who have received an anesthetic need to be monitored for an appropriate time in a PACU. Changeover from the caregiver in the operating room to the caregiver in the PACU is given at the time of transfer. Initial postanesthesia monitoring should include all of the same monitoring as was used in the operating room. Monitors can be withdrawn as the patient emerges from the effects of anesthesia. A physician is responsible for the discharge of the patient from the PACU.

Anesthetic Costs

Working at a privately owned surgery center has influenced the author's appreciation of costs. Because facility fees paid by cosmetic patients fund anesthesia drugs and materials as well as nursing costs, any reduction in anesthesia materials cost or personnel costs will have a direct effect on the bottom line. When costs of differing drugs and anesthetic techniques are borne by third-party payers or facilities such as hospitals, the anesthetic of choice is simply whatever the surgeon and anesthesiologist prefer. When drug costs are taken out of the fee paid to a facility owned by the surgeon, cheaper may well be better. Anesthesia costs can make or break the profitability of facility fees in a highly competitive environment.

Figure 17.4 shows hourly propofol costs for differing dosages. The patient is assumed to weigh 70 kg. The dosage range displayed covers the usual range required for a deep-sedation anesthetic (Big MAC). Costs will vary depending on the weight of the patient. This analysis ignores the costs of adjuvant drugs, such as narcotics and oxygen, as well as equipment, such as that for airway ventilation.

For comparative purposes, **Fig. 17.5** shows the relationship between fresh gas flows and hourly anesthetic costs for desflurane, sevoflurane, and isoflurane. Again, this analysis ignores the cost of equipment and supplies as well as adjuvant drugs. You will note that there are no data for sevoflurane at fresh gas flow rates less than 2 L/min. This is in keeping with Food and Drug Administration recommendations of a minimum flow rate of at least 2 L/min to avoid patient exposure to toxic breakdown products of sevoflurane.

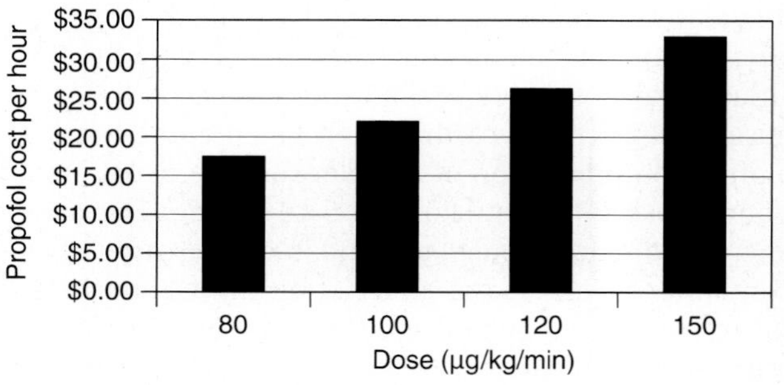

Fig. 17.4 The hourly cost of propofol at typical clinical infusion rates. The analysis is based on a 70-kg patient. (Data from the Meridian Plastic Surgery Center, Indianapolis, IN. Reprinted by permission.)

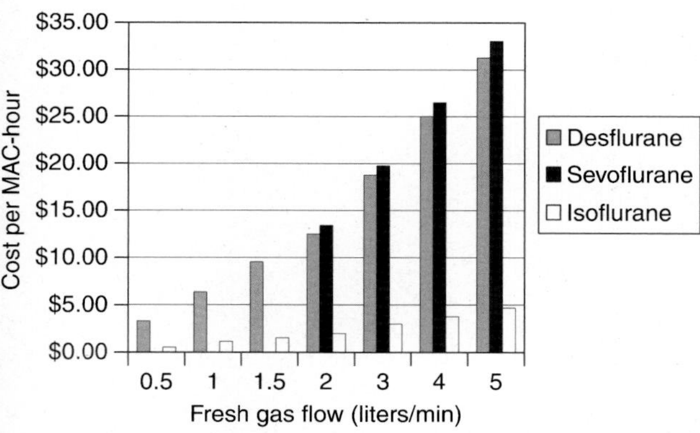

Fig. 17.5 Cost per MAC-hour for the major inhaled agents at different fresh gas flow rates. Costs for sevoflurane are not quoted below 2 L/min flow (see text). (Data from the Meridian Plastic Surgery Center, Indianapolis, IN. Reprinted by permission.)

Higher fresh gas flow rates are used at the onset of administration of a general anesthetic to compensate for the substantial uptake of agent early on. As time passes, flow rates can easily be reduced to below 2 L/min for desflurane and on long procedures can go as low as 500 mL/min. Profound cost savings can be realized with isoflurane at low flows if one is willing to accept a delay in emergence due to the higher blood gas solubility coefficient.

The obvious conclusion is that substantial cost savings can be realized over longer surgical procedures when general inhalation anesthesia is chosen over intravenous anesthesia with propofol. This is the same conclusion drawn by Alhashemi et al in their article on cost-effectiveness of inhalational, balanced, and total intravenous anesthesia.[16] On shorter procedures, the cost difference is not substantial and is therefore not a factor in choice of an anesthetic.

References

1. Cousins MJ, Bridenbaugh PO. Neural Blockade in Clinical Anesthesia and Management of Pain. 2nd ed. Philadelphia: JB Lippincott; 1988:113
2. Goodman LS, Gilman A. The Pharmacological Basis of Therapeutics. 5th ed. New York: Macmillan; 1970:393
3. Navarro R, Weiskopf RB, Moore MA, et al. Humans anesthetized with sevoflurane or isoflurane have similar arrhythmic response to epinephrine. Anesthesiology 1994;80:545–549
4. Moore MA, Weiskopf RB, Eger EI II, et al. Arrhythmogenic doses of epinephrine are similar during desflurane or isoflurane anesthesia in humans. Anesthesiology 1993;79:943–947
5. Kazama T, Ikeda K, Morita K, Sanjo Y. Awakening propofol concentration with and without blood-effect site equilibrium after short-term and long-term administration of propofol and fentanyl anesthesia. Anesthesiology 1998;88:928–934
6. Wagner RL, White PF, Kan PB, et al. Inhibition of adrenal steroidogenesis by the anesthetic etomidate. N Engl J Med 1984;310:1415–1421
7. Fragen RJ, Shanks CA, Molteni A, et al. Effects of etomidate on hormonal responses to surgical stress. Anesthesiology 1984;61:652–656
8. Hurstveit O, Maurset A, Oye I. Interaction of the chiral forms of ketamine with opioid, phencyclidine, and muscarinic receptors. Pharmacol Toxicol 1995;77:355–359
9. Stone PA, Macintyre PE, Jarvis DA. Norpethidine toxicity and patient controlled analgesia. Br J Anaesth 1993;71:738–740
10. Yasuda N, Lockhart S, Eger EI II, et al. Comparison of kinetics of sevoflurane and isoflurane in humans. Anesth Analg 1991;72(3):316–324
11. Continuum of Depth of Sedation. Definition of general anesthesia and levels of sedation/analgesia. American Society of Anesthesiologists Practice Guideline. Approved by the House of Delegates on October 13, 1999
12. Practice guidelines for sedation and analgesia by nonanesthesiologists. Anesthesiology 1996;84:459–471
13. Stevens WC, Cromwell TH, Halsey MJ, et al. The cardiovascular effects of a new inhalation anesthetic, Forane, in human volunteers at constant arterial carbon dioxide tension. Anesthesiology 1971;35:8–16
14. Loeb HS, Saudye A, Croke RP, et al. Effects of pharmacologically induced hypertension on myocardial ischemia and coronary hemodynamics in patients with fixed coronary obstruction. Circulation 1978;57:41–46
15. Standards for Basic Anesthetic Monitoring. American Society of Anesthesiologists Practice Standard. Approved by House of Delegates October 21, 1986, and last amended on October 21, 1998
16. Alhashemi JA, Miller DR, O'Brien HV, Hull KA. Cost-effectiveness of inhalational, balanced, and total intravenous anaesthesia for ambulatory knee surgery. Can J Anaesth 1997;44(2):118–125

18 Youthful Aging

Edward Szachowicz III

A whole new way of looking at the process of aging began with a curious question causing an incredible paradigm shift, "What if, for a moment, we scientists looked upon the process of aging not as an immutable process, but as a disease process that could be 'treated'?" This question arises at a critical time in our world history with the convergence of three major events: the simultaneous aging of a large demographic of postwar baby boomers who are presented with their parents' aging issues as well as their own, a worldwide commitment by scientists to decipher the human genetic code, and the growth of integrative medicine within the traditional academic medical centers.

In 2011, the baby boomer generation will begin to turn 65.

Looking at aging as a disease process should not be judgmental, in that youth is good and old is diseased; but instead, we should use the same diagnostic acumen as knowledgeable physicians to sift and sort information for our patients in regards to their medications, supplements, diet, and lifestyle that can help them live longer and better. As your individual practice embraces a youthful aging approach, your staff and patients will resonate with a healthy attitude, and your patients will be better surgical candidates, and will look and feel better from the inside out.

Youthful or healthy aging is not the same as anti-aging. Physicians cannot mislead patients to think that science has discovered the fountain of youth. The miracle is that what we can do to help our bodies is relatively simple, and early intervention can prevent or minimize chronic disease states such as type II diabetes, arthritis, osteoporosis, and cardiovascular disease that occur with more frequency as we age. Genetic science has demonstrated that although a person may possess an inherited genetic tendency, hormonal, diet, and lifestyle choices can determine whether the gene is actually expressed. The goal of youthful aging is to maintain the fidelity of transferring biological information between one's 60 trillion cells for as long as possible, so that wellness can be maintained into late in life.

Specifically, for surgeons devoted to rejuvenation procedures, it is desirable to help patients to not only appear younger, but also to have a physiological age 15 to 20 years less than their chronological age. A useful concept of youthful aging is the desire not to necessarily extend one's life span, but to proactively extend one's health span, that is, the time of health with limited morbidity. As physicians and teachers in facial plastic surgery, we can bring the message of youthful aging to our patients "for this inside as well as outside."

Theories of Aging

A useful theory about aging is based on reproduction. As a species, humans have evolved over thousands of years with intense pressure on both genders to survive to reproduce. In human males, testosterone enables the development of increased bone and muscle mass and libido, and mating for reproduction peaks in the twenties and then gradually declines with age. For women, the reproductive phase is longer, lasting into the late thirties, until the hormonal levels become variable until menopause. Then, one can theorize that beyond the time when the individual has passed on his or her genes and the offspring have begin to care for themselves, the "goal" of survival of the species is accomplished, and nature has little concern how the individual then ages.

After the peak in youthful sexual reproduction capacity (by the early 30s), we see the beginning of the onset of chronic diseases, that is, cardiovascular heart disease, loss of bone density, and the rise of genetic mutations (cancer). In a harsher environment, the more aged individual would not survive, whereas in more protected societies, an extended life span is possible. Two concepts can be derived from this theory: one being that an extended life span is demonstratively possible for a human in an enriched environment, and second, that a goal of hormonal replacement may be to maintain for as long as possible the neuroendocrine levels that a human has in the early 30s, before the onset of chronic diseases.

The theories of aging all coexist, each with a thoughtful contribution based on genetic, empiric, and nutritional science. Expect more information to evolve, especially as the human genome becomes more elucidated.

Free Radical Theory

This theory is based on the energetics of cellular survival. During the processes of routine cellular metabolism (converting the nutrients we eat into cellular energy) free radical are produced in all our mitochondria. A free radical is a molecule with an unpaired electron in its outermost ring, and has the capacity to damage other molecules, especially, the vulnerable DNA of the mitochondria. The mitochondrial DNA has a limited ability to repair itself (unlike our nuclear DNA) and over time, the free radical damage can begin to significantly interfere with the energy production within each individual cell. Antioxidants

(CoQ10, superoxide dismutase, glutathione, etc.) are produced within our cells to bind the free radicals. However, our body of 60 trillion cells also needs the external antioxidants derived from fruits and vegetables, which can include a panoply of phytonutrients, including vitamins C and E, and many that have not even been identified. As we encounter daily stressors (exercise, caffeine, daily life stress, prescription medications) the need for these antioxidants becomes more critical, and diet and supplements have been shown to significantly increase the circulating levels of important antioxidants.

Rapidly growing children also desperately need antioxidants, nutrient-rich food, and supplements. Organic food sources usually are more nutrient-rich, containing fewer chemicals, antibiotics, and hormones. Supplements containing vitamins, antioxidants, and phytonutrients should be considered in all individuals.

This theory also gives support to one of the few proven longevity programs in laboratory science, calorie restriction. By consuming at least 30% fewer calories, albeit while maintaining a diet with a balance of proteins, healthy fats, and proper nutrients, life span in animals can significantly and reproducibly be extended. Calorie restriction may be triggering genes to slow metabolism and increase body defenses to postpone reproduction until less stressful times. The result being that fewer calories produce fewer free radicals causing less mitochondrial damage and as well as other gene activation leading to an extended life span.

Neuroendocrine Theory

Hormones are important chemical messengers for our body, and the majority of these hormones, especially sex and growth hormones, decline as we age. Significantly, two hormones, cortisol and insulin, actually increase with age and can only be reduced by diet and lifestyle changes. The rapid senescence seen in salmon after their spawn has been linked to a dramatic and sustained release in cortisol, causing their flesh to deteriorate, their bones to decalcify, and their lenses to opacify all within weeks. Insulin's role in the body appears to be widespread and complex, and disturbances in insulin production or the response to it may not only play a role in obesity, but also in degenerative changes in aging and possibly cancer.

Controversy exists about the theory that questions whether hormone levels that are considered "normal" for an age-adjusted population in health and disease are normal for each individual's own specific biology and/or chronological age, and further whether these adjusted "normal" levels are desirable or optimal. One promise of the neuroendocrine theory of aging is replacement of each individual's hormones that have declined levels with balanced natural or bioidentical hormones to an ideal hormonal level present in people in their 30s, the age before the onset of chronic diseases. This would include at least the consideration of DHEA (dehydroepiandrosterone), testosterone, estrogens and progesterone, thyroid, and growth hormone.

All this is not without risk. Sex hormones and growth hormone may increase the risk of disease, including cancer, when used in a replacement regimen.

Telomere Theory

Telomeres are specialized proteins on the ends of our nuclear DNA. Each time a cell divides it loses a telomere protein, and Leonard Hayflick demonstrated that each cell type has a limited amount of times it can divide, which is predetermined by the number of telomere sequences. Germ cells, for example, spermatogonia cells in the male, contain a telomerase enzyme that rebuilds the telomere after cellular division. But somatic cells do not express this telomerase. It appears that this "Hayflick" limit is not reached during our lifetimes, but it may be important in the control of the replication of cancer cells.

Inflammation Theory

Inflammation is a common reactive pathway for every cell and organ in the body. Barry Sears and N. Perricone have popularized this theory of aging that states that certain foods and lifestyle choices are proinflammatory, whereas an antiinflammatory strategy will minimized cellular stress and thereby slow the process of aging. The most recent studies in Alzheimer research show that inflammation may play a key role in how our brain ages. Cortisol, an endogenous stress hormone, and insulin are major proinflammatory agents. The inflammation theory enlivens the pharmaceutical power of food; how each time we eat we have a renewed chance to decease the inflammation within our cells.

The glycation theory of cellular aging can be seen as belonging to part of the inflammation process. Eating carbohydrates that cause a rapid increase in blood glucose levels (high glycemic index foods) allows the excess glucose to coat the cellular proteins, including essential enzymes and cell membranes. This cross-linking of proteins with glucose, glycation, dramatically decreases the effectiveness of the all cellular energetics and thus accelerates aging.

Evaluation of Biomarkers of Biological Age and Chronic Diseases

- Albumin, g/dL (3.5–5)
- Cortisol AM, μg/dL (8–16)
- DHEA-sulfate, μg/dL (350–500)
- IGF (insulin-like growth factor)-1 ng/mL (250–320)

- Testosterone (free and total)
  - *Men*: free testosterone, pg/mL (130–190)
    total testosterone, ng/dL (700–900)
  - *Women*: free testesterone, pg/mL (7–10)
    total testosterone, ng/dL (50–70)
- Estradiol (in men and women)
  - *Female*: Follicular, pg/mL (39–189)
    Midcycle, pg/mL (94–508)
    Luteal, pg/mL (48–309)
    Postmenopausal, pg/mL (80–100)
- Thyroid (free T3, T4, and TSH [thyroid-stimulating hormone])
  - TSH, mIU/mL (0.4–5.5)
  - Free T3, pg/mL (2.3–4.2)
  - Free T4, ng/dL (0.8–1.8)
- Serum lipids
  - Cholesterol, mg/dL (140–180)
  - Triglycerides, mg/dL (40–100)
  - HDL (high-density lipoprotein) cholesterol, mg/dL (50–110)
  - LDL (low-density lipoprotein) cholesterol, mg/dL (8–110)
- Fasting insulin, µU/mL (1–5)
- Hemoglobin A1C % (3.5–5.1)
- *Women only*: LH (Luteinizing hormone)
  - Follicular, mIU/mL (1.9–12.5)
  - Midcycle, mIU/mL (8.7–76.3)
  - Luteal, mIU/mL (0.5–16.9)
  - Postmenopausal, mIU/mL (20–40)
- *Women only*: FSH (Follicle stimulating hormone)
  - Follicular, mIU/mL (2.5–10.2)
  - Midcycle, mIU/mL (1.6–18.8)
  - Luteal, mIU/mL (1.5–9.1)
  - Postmenopausal, mIU/mL (30–50)
- C-reactive protein. Indirect measure of inflammation in the arteries; if elevated, increases the risk of stroke and heart attack
- Homocysteine µmol/L (0–9). High homocysteine levels are associated with greater risk for cardiovascular disease, even if the lipid profile is normal.
- Lipoprotein(a) (<60). A unique lipid that appears to play a regulatory role in atherothrombosis; a serious risk factor if elevated
- *Women only*: Progesterone
  - Follicular, ng/mL (0.2–1.4)
  - Luteal, ng/mL (3.3–26)
  - Midluteal, ng/mL (4.4–28)
  - Postmenopausal, ng/mL (1–3)
- *Men only*: PSA (prostatic specific antigen), ng/mL (0–4)
- Body composition. Percentage of lean muscle mass by body weight. There are many ways to directly or indirectly calculate this figure, but the same tool should be used for comparison values. Ideal values for women would be <22% body fat; men <16%.
- Respiratory FEV_1. Usually a direct measurement
- VO_2 max (mL/kg/min). Can be directly measured, or more commonly can be estimated by exercise tolerance. Poor: 18–28; Fair/Average: 29–35; Good/High: 36–43; Excellent 44–60.
- Bone density. Often done as a DEXA (dual energy x-ray absorptiometry) scan, which can give you a body composition ratio in addition to bone density. Scoring is based on the sex and age of the individual, and testing is often measured at two sites in the skeleton (spine and hip).
- *Optional*: Rapid computerized tomographic (CT) heart scan. Somewhat controversial, but a rapid CT of the heart may image calcium deposits that are currently existing adjacent to or within the coronary vessels. The scoring is based on a percentile of people in a patient's age range. Another option to evaluate the present state of cardiac disease may be CT digital angiography, which may provide a baseline image for those with current or strong history of coronary vessel disease.

Human Growth Hormone (HGH)

HGH or somatotropin is produced in the pituitary to regulate metabolism, growth, and maturation. HGH is released in pulses throughout the day, and it is taken up by the liver where it stimulates the production of IGF-1, which is the active form causing a generalized systemic effect. As true with most other hormones, HGH levels decrease with age, so after the age of 30 levels begin to decline at a rate of ~14% per decade (**Table 18.1**).

In 1992, a 6-month study of HGH supplementation in 21 men demonstrated a significant increase in lean body mass (8.8%) and bone density (1.6%) and a decease in adipose tissue (14.4%) compared with untreated controls (Rudman et al). The decline in growth hormone in

Table 18.1 Specific Biomarkers for Reducing Disease and Morbidity Risk

HgbA1C <5.0%
Coronary risk ratio (total cholesterol/HDL) <3.5
Triglycerides/HDL <2
HDL >50
LDL <100
Triglycerides <100
Fasting insulin <5
Morning cortisol <18
Homocysteine <9
C-reactice protein <1
Body fat percentage women <25%; Men <20%

the elderly, called somatopause, seemed to be reversed with few patients experiencing side effects: dose-related edema, muscle and joint pain, carpal tunnel syndrome, hypertension, and hyperglycemia. Dr. Rudman's study, in part, gave rise to the new field of medicine devoted to the reversal of aging as he concluded, "The effects of 6 months of human growth hormone on lean mass and adipose-tissue mass were equivalent on magnitude to the changes incurred during 10 to 20 years of aging."

In the decade of study since, HGH may be an expensive, long-term therapy to maintain lean body mass, bone density, and exercise capacity for patients, and the effects may be most demonstrable in men. The main risk may be that HGH may encourage the growth of neoplastic tissue that is already present, although this risk is not high enough to become significant within the population thus far treated.

If the decision for HGH supplementation is made, generally the range of treatment dosing is 4 to 7 IU/week in a daily subcutaneous injection. Only HGH manufactured with recombinant DNA technology should be given.

As HGH causes increased efficiency of retrotubular absorption of sodium and water from the kidneys, edema is a frequent side effect when HGH is given in higher doses, but is usually transient and is treated with a reduction in dose. Synovial inflammation causing arthralgias (joint pain) and carpal tunnel syndrome may require stopping the therapy until symptoms resolve and then restarting the supplementation at one half the levels for 1 to 2 months before increasing the dose. Transient hyperglycemia needs to be monitored with fasting glucose and hemoglobin A1C levels, and diabetes is a relative contraindication. Serum monitoring of IGF-1 levels should be done to keep levels from rising too high: the optimal level in men is 290 to 350 μg/mL and in women 260 to 290 μg/mL. Serum levels of IGF-1 may not rise in all patients and may be variable depending on stress and exercise. The effects of a increase in lean body mass, bone density, and exercise tolerance, which are the most significant outcome measures, may not be seen unless the HGH supplementation is combined with a program of regular cardiovascular and weight training and a diet balanced for protein, good fats, and low-glycemic index carbohydrates. Outcomes measures such as body composition (percentage of body fat and lean muscle mass), bone density, and exercise endurance (VO_2 max) should be monitored at intervals to document progress.

Female Menopause

Menopause is a process over time wherein the sex hormone levels secreted by the ovaries—estrogens, progesterone, and testosterone—become erratic and then may drop dramatically. This is a time in which the outward signs of aging in women become manifest and often is the physiological cause for many patients seeking facial rejuvenation.

Estrogen Replacement

Estrogen replacement relieves the symptoms of menopause and seems to confer protective effects from cardiovascular disease and osteoporosis, but it possibly can increase breast and endometrial cancer as well. Estrogen replacement is not recommended if there is presence of liver disease, endometriosis, uterine fibromas, or gall bladder disease.

Some women request hormone replacement for the improvement on cognitive function and its positive effects in the incidence of Alzheimer disease.

Most of the scientific studies used Premarin, derived from pregnant horse urine, for estrogen replacement, and only now are studies being started using the human bioidentical form of estradiol. The metabolic consequence of foreign steroids in the human body may be substantially different in side effects than that of native sex steroids.

Generally, women with strong personal or family history of breast or endometrial cancer, with a past history or existing cardiovascular disease, or with a history of any clotting abnormality, stroke, or transient ischemic events should be cautioned to proceed with care and understanding of the risk of hormone replacement therapy. Genetic breast cancer patients should consider a Braca gene test. A breast cancer prevention diet would be high in antioxidants, coenzyme Q10, whole soy foods, and omega-3 fatty acids and would limit tobacco, alcohol, and weight gain.

If a female hormone replacement program is decided upon, then estrogens, progesterone, testosterone, and DHEA should all be considered as a program. A serum FSH level of greater than 50 mIU/mL and an estradiol less than 50 pg/mL confirms the failure of the ovaries to produce adequate sex hormones. Levels of DHEA-S, thyroid functions tests (TSH, free T3/T4), and testosterone should be done along with general chemistries including lipids.

Estrogen replacement is typical done with biestrogen (Bi-Est), a combination of estriol (E_3) 50 to 80% and estradiol (E_2) 20 to 50%. Although estriol is a weak estrogen, it is one of the estrogens that have some anticancer effects in breast tissue in mice, so it is included in Bi-Est.

Oral ingestion of estrogens results in the first-pass phenomenon, wherein the hormones are first taken to the portal (liver) circulation and are converted to metabolites, which are responsible for vasomotor symptoms and the formation of antiestrogens. A transdermal route with gels and creams, vaginal capsules and creams, or subcutaneous pellets all are well tolerated with consistent blood levels. The five most common side effects of replacement estrogen therapy include menstrual bleeding from excess estrogen (although spotting may occur for the first 3 months), breast tenderness, fluid retention from too much estrogen not balanced with progesterone, transient breakouts/ blemishes of the skin, and mood changes. A serum level of estradiol between 50 and 100 pg/mL is the target for the steady state of replacement.

Progesterone

Unopposed estrogens are associated with endometrial hyperplasia and carcinoma, so postmenopausal women with an intact uterus should be considered for progesterone replacement. Progesterone is a major precursor to other hormones, is as important for bone health as estrogens, and protects against fibrocystic beast disease and some breast cancers.

Natural progesterone derived form soybeans or Mexican yam roots do not have the side-effect profile of synthetic progesterones (Provera). There is poor oral absorption of progesterone, and also it is susceptible to rapid first-pass metabolism by the liver when taken orally. Therefore, a sublingual, oral lozenge or tansdermal preparations are recommended. After menopause, progesterone can be given cyclically (10–14 days each cycle) or continuously. Continuous therapy is suggested to lower LDL cholesterol, or in preventing osteoporosis. Serum blood levels in a premenopausal woman range from 4 to 25 ng/mL; target replacement levels in the postmenopausal female range from 10 to 20 ng/mL.

Andropause: Male "Menopause"

Men have an absolute and relative decrease in free testosterone as they age. Andropause is the name given to the decline of testosterone, the primary sex hormone for men, and 54 is mean age for these symptoms: reduction in libido, difficulty in initiating and maintaining an erection, fatigue, depression, and irritability. Testosterone production begins with the secretion of gonadotrophin-releasing hormone from the hypothalamus signaling the pituitary to produce LH, which finally stimulates the Leydig cells in the testes to produce testosterone. The testes in some men will eventually lose their ability to produce testosterone, regardless of the amount of LH stimulation; this is similar to what happens in the ovary during menopause for women.

Metabolically, testosterone is a hormone secreted by the ovaries, adrenal glands, and testes that results in widespread increase in cellular bioenergetics causing anabolic effects such as an increase in muscle mass, strength, exercise tolerance, and a decrease in body fat, serum cholesterol, and osteoporosis. Testosterone causes increased libido and sexual performance, improves mood and memory, improves glucose metabolism, cardiovascular dynamics, including blood pressure regulation, metabolic rate, and aerobic metabolism.

A concurrent hormone imbalance occurs in aging men as there is not only an absolute decrease in amount of free testosterone and but also the available testosterone may be increasingly converted to estrogen, most occurring in the intraabdominal or visceral fat. This fat contains an aromatase enzyme that effectively metabolizes testosterone and its precursors hormones into potent estrogens, which are powerful competitors of testosterone.

High serum levels of estrogen in men are implicated as a cause of prostatic cancer, and they can further lower free testosterone by primarily interfering with the stimulation of the pituitary to produce more LH, and secondarily by causing an increase in the body's production of sex hormone binding globulin (SHBG). This globulin binds free testosterone in the blood and makes more testosterone unavailable to cell receptor sites.

Treating Andropause

Eat less high-fat foods, and adopt a lifestyle to encourage normal weight. Phytonutrients from cruciferous vegetables such as broccoli and cauliflower promote excretion of excess estrogen by the liver. Review all prescription medications for their effects on liver function. Acetaminophen is not tolerated well and should be taken only as needed.

Excess body fat, especially visceral fat, turns on more aromatase production, which then rapidly converts testosterone to estrogen. Zinc (30–90 mg/day) is a natural aromatase enzyme inhibitor, or special aromatase inhibitor drugs, such as Arimidex (anastrozole), may be of value to aging men who have excess estrogen.

Heavy alcohol intake damages liver function; a healthy liver eliminates surplus estrogen and SHBG.

For optimal levels, free testosterone should be at the high-normal reference range; never should the testosterone be above the normal range as this can reverse all the beneficial effects of testosterone and cause serious health hazards.

Estradiol should be in the mid to lower normal range.

If the serum LH is low, human chorionic gonadotropin (HCG) can be given by subcutaneous injection two times per week. HCG functions similarly to LH and can restart the production of testosterone by the Leydig cells in the testes. But many practitioners believe that direct testosterone replacement therapy is safer and more effective. The goal with any testosterone replacement program is to elevate the levels of free testosterone to the upper one third of the reference range, but not to increase estradiol levels beyond 30. Testosterone replacement can be done with a patch, cream, subcutaneous pellets, or injection.

Blood tests are necessary every 30 to 45 days for the first 6 months during this therapy.

Contraindications to testosterone therapy include prostate cancer or elevated levels of PSA, for which one must rule out occult prostate cancer.

All men who begin on testosterone replacement therapy should be cautioned to be compliant with therapy and monitoring blood levels, as some men rapidly convert testosterone to estradiol ae treated as levels of estradiol approach 40 pg/mL.

DHEA is a steroid hormone produced mainly in the adrenal cortex, and it is a precursor of both male and female sex hormones. Natural production peaks during youthful sexual reproductive capacity (20s–30s) and then declines steadily. DHEA is thought of as an anabolic balance to the more catabolic adrenal hormone, cortisol. DHEA has been shown to decrease the accumulation of body fat, especially visceral (intraabdominal fat), which is associated with increased risk of cardiovascular disease and with metabolic syndrome and its associated insulin insensitivity. Studies have shown other cardiovascular benefits with the lowering of the "bad" LDL cholesterol, such as decreased rates of heart attacks and stroke. There are reported benefits to the immune system, mood and memory, and a role in supporting bone density. As a precursor to sex hormones, DHEA has been shown to increase libido in men and women and improve erectile dysfunction in men. DHEA appears to be quite safe, although one must caution women that some masculinizing features, especially acne, hair loss, and facial hair growth, may occur as the DHEA is naturally converted to testosterone in women. DHEA is not recommended for patients who have had breast or prostate cancer as there is an increase in sex hormone levels with supplementation.

This hormone is widely available as a supplement in the United States; consequently many patients may already be taking DHEA routinely. DHEA-S ("S" stands for sulfate) is a byproduct of DHEA, and plasma levels of DHEA-S are easier to measure and provide a rough estimate of DHEA levels. Oral supplementation ranges from 10 to 5 mg/day for women under age 50, 25 mg/day for women greater than age 50 or postmenopausal, to 50 mg/day for men. Optimal serum levels of DHEA-S for men range from 500 to 600 ug/mL and for women 250 to 300 μg/mL, adjusting downward for any masculunizing changes. DHEA supplementation to optimum levels is best done gradually, over a 1-year period.

Thyroid Hormone

Most physicians are aware of the importance of thyroid hormone in homeostasis and metabolism, especially carbohydrates and fats. The thyroid gland produces thyroxine (T4), a precursor to triiodothyronine (T3), the active form of the hormone. Low circulating levels of the protein-bound thyroid hormones are detected by the hypothalamus, which communicates with the pituitary gland to release TSH, which causes the release of thyroid hormones; 80% is held as the precursor T4, and 20% is the active form of the hormone, T3. T4 is converted into T3 by an enzyme, 5′-iodinase reductase, whose efficiency can be affected by levels of zinc, selenium, heavy metals, stress, and calorie reduction.

Clinical hypothyroidism is classically diagnosed as myxedema, with symptoms of fatigue, weight gain, depression, dry hair and skin, high cholesterol, and lower basal body temperature.

Interest of late has been the study of a "subclinical" hypothyroidism, that is, the condition that represents a slow decline in the amount of thyroid hormone produced as the gland shrinks in size over time, decreased efficiency in the conversion of T4 to the active T3 form, and the suggestion that even the active T3 hormone may be less effective on the membrane receptors on target cells as one ages or with exposure to heavy metals.

Serum measurement of TSH, free T4, and free T3 is recommended. TSH is not sufficient as a measure for TSH can be normal in the face of decreased conversion of the T4 to the active T3. Additionally, free T3 is necessary to monitor treatment, as the enzymatic conversion of T4 to the normal active T3 can also be shifted to create RT3 (reverse triiodothyronine), especially in a stress pattern.

Low T3 Syndrome

The range for "normal" free T3 levels are broad (230–420 pg/dL), and patients will describe a different energy level and quality of life when they function with a level of free T3 in the range of 3.3 versus 2.3. There will also be measurable differences as in lower cholesterol, body fat, depression, and improvement in the skin, hair, and nails. Patients whose serum levels are supplemented to elevate the free T3 into the middle range of "normal," will often have the energy to resume a more active lifestyle, and they report that they can eat normal portions of food without the concurrent weight gain. Many will report increased clarity of mental function and not feeling cold all the time.

Supplementation is controversial and is also being studied. Armour thyroid (an animal-derived compound of T3/T4) or newly compounded synthetic T3 drugs are recommended, and pure glandular preparations sold in health food stores are not recommended. Armour thyroid does not have as high a peak level when taken, and it should be supplemented slowly, usually starting at one-half grain, and increasing by one-quarter grain/month until desired levels are achieved. Synthetic T3 can be taken in smaller doses twice daily. Angina, hypertension, and history of supraventricular tachycardia are relative contraindications. Sweating, palpitations, and tremors are signs of supplementing too quickly in sensitive patients. Laboratory monitoring is suggested every 6 weeks until a steady state is achieved. Supplementation to restore free T3 serum levels to midrange should not suppress TSH levels to zero, only supply more active T3 hormone to the body.

Youthful Aging Strategies for Facial Plastic Surgery Patients

The space youthful aging has in your practice is very individual, but its purpose should start with patient education. The information available in magazines, media, and the Internet are tantalizing and confusing to the patient; the physician's true role is the teacher. The best way to bring youthful aging practices into the office is for the physician to educate him/herself and demonstrate to the staff and clients a healthy lifestyle, that is, assorted teas instead of coffee, healthy snacks at events, a leader who is smoke free and of normal weight.

Next, introduce healthy ways to prepare for surgery, adding supplements and nutritionals as adjuncts to healing, and encouraging healthy eating habits. Add lectures and seminars about demystifying the deluge of information about lifestyle and aging. Start gradually, with a more balanced lifestyle with dedicated space for sleep, exercise, and work. Get on track with understanding how everyone's body is aging, in appearance as well in terms of bone density and blood lipids. Get interested in what supplements your patients are taking and why, using their interests as a guide. The next layer would be proper nutritional supplements including bioavailable vitamins and minerals, and then add attention to areas of concern. This process will earmark your practice as one that recognizes the connection of inside health reflecting outside health. Some supplements that are worth considering in most patients over age 40 are:

- Omega-3 fish oils:
  - EPA (eicosapentaenoic acid), 1600 mg
  - DHA (docosahexaenoic acid), 800 mg
- Coenzyme Q10 ≤60 mg/day
- Calcium/boron/magnesium compounds
- Probiotics (mixture of beneficial bacteria for the gut)
- Indole-3-carbinol, 200–400 mg/day
- Multivitamin supplements that contain:
  - Vitamin E, 80–160 mg of the whole complex including mixed natural tocopherols, α tocopherol, and tocotrienols
  - Vitamin D, 400–1000 IU/day
  - Selenium, 200 μg/day
  - Mixture of carotenoids, including betacarotene, lutein, and lycopene
  - Vitamin C, 500–1000 mg/day
  - Vitamins A and B
  - Glucosamine/chondroitin sulfate
- For brain health
  - Alpha-lipoic acid, 100–400 mg/day
  - ALCAR (acetyl-L carnitine), 1000 mg day
  - Folate, 400–1600 μg/day

Many multivitamins preparations are formulated to meet basic nutrient needs. This list contains additional supplements that are not often contained in just a simple multivitamin. These nutrients/supplements are best taken in divided doses as their half-lives are shorter than a once per day regiment would allow. Men do not need to take iron as an additional supplement unless they donate blood very regularly.

As you begin your personal program and your energy improves, your exercise tolerance grows, and your body composition changes, you will notice that your biological age is slowly compared with your chronological age. Your success will spread to your family, staff, and patients. Soon your interviews will be just as much about lifestyle as facial plastic surgery.

Practice models have included having the primary surgeon and a nurse as the managers of the youthful aging program with development at courses or meetings to even having an association with medical physician partners to promote your youthful aging program. Personal trainers and nutritionists round out the offerings so that soon your patients can benefit from a team approach. Stress management and meditation soothe the mind and spirit.

Hold workshops on low glycemic index foods, anti-inflammatory diets, food choices that include abundant phytonutrients, and help patients respect food as the most potent daily medicine they partake. Food will become nutrition again, not a diet.

All this expands into "wellness" whose time is arrived. Wellness is not the next challenge, but today's invitation.

Incorporating Youthful Aging Strategies for Patients in Your Practice

To achieve a well-rounded rejuvenation, more than just facial plastic surgery is needed. A survey of your patient base may strangely reveal that many of your patients do not take supplements, have no consistent exercise regimen, don't understand nutrition, are overweight, and cannot manage stress. The dilemma is that as a surgeon, it is difficult to give complete surgical care and practice youthful aging medicine. Strategic partnerships with other medical specialists, such as those in integrative medicine and sports medicine, endocrinologists, obstetricians/gynecologists, chiropractors, nutritionists, instructors in yoga, meditation, and other forms of stress reduction. These other health and wellness professionals will educate you, your staff, and your patients about all aspects of youthful aging.

Education is the primary practice enhancement, through seminars, nutrition programs, Web site information, and advice on supplements and skin care.

One can begin a library for health topics, starting with your own readings and then reading the popular lay books for the public. The library also will become a resource for your patients as you expand your practice to include this broader range of rejuvenation.

A goal could be to expand your preoperative assessment to include the biomarkers of aging including laboratory tests, vitamin and antioxidant testing, pre- and postoperative nutritional care, and postoperative preventative/youthful aging management. An expectation for your surgery practice would be a healthier patient, who with proper nutritionals, heals well from the wounding and oxidative stress of surgery. After your successful surgery, the patient then can continue on a path of better health, nutrition, exercise, and stress management.

Summary

We cannot prevent the aging process, but hopefully we can mollify the chronic morbidities and increase our healthful life span. We as facial plastic surgeons see people who are willing to invest in themselves, and we can increase our integrity if we expand our focus to the message of youthful aging.

The inflammation theory of aging is gaining in science, and the antiinflammatory diet and lifestyle may help a large segment of our patients. The complexity of the human organism requires high-quality and specific supplements and nutrients each day to perform optimally, to repair and heal itself, and to be immunologically competent.

Healthy aging information is constantly changing and requires a dedicated interest to investigate new discoveries. Each of us should first enter into our own conscientious healthy aging program, learn as much along the way, and our patients will follow. Wellness centers are opening throughout the country as people seek the mind-body connection and now adopt a more proactive approach to all health issues.

Suggested Readings

Brand-Miller J, Wolever, T, Colagiuri S, Foster-Powell K, Leeds A. The New Glucose Revolution. 3rd ed. New York:Marlow & Co.; 2003

Cherniske, SA. The DHEA Breakthrough. New York: Ballantine Books; 1998

Khalsa DS, Stauth C. Brain Longevity. New York: Warner Books; 1997

Sinatra ST, Sinatra J, Lieberman RJ. Heart Sense for Women. Your Plan for Natural Prevention and Treatment. New York: Plume by the Penguin Group; 2001

Weil A. Healthy Aging. A Lifelong Guide to Your Physical and Spiritual Well-Being. New York: Knopf Group; 2005

Growth Hormone

Burman P, Johansson AG, Siegbahn A, et al. Growth hormone (GH)-deficient men are more responsive to GH replacement therapy than women. J Clin Endocrinol Metab 1997;82(2):550–555

Gibney J, Wallace JD, Spinks T, et al. The effects of 10 years of recombinant human growth hormone (GH) in adult GH-deficient patients. J Clin Endocrinol Metab 1999;84(8):2596–2602

Rudman D, Feller AG, Nagraj HS, et al. Effects of human growth hormone in men over 60 years old. N Engl J Med 1990;323(1):1–6

Vance ML, Mauras N. Growth hormone therapy in adults and children. N Engl J Med 1999;341(16):1206–1216

Testosterone

Friedrich MJ. Can male hormones really help women? JAMA 2000; 283(20):2643–2644

Hajjar RR, Kaiser FE, Morley JE. Outcomes of long-term testosterone replacement in older hypogonodal males: a retrospective analysis. J Clin Endocrinol Metab 1997;82(11):3793–3796

Tan R, Bransgrove L. Andropause: is there a place for hormone replacement therapy? Clin Geriatrics 1997;5(10):127–130

Winters SJ. Current status of testosterone replacement therapy in men. Arch Fam Med 1999;8:257–263

Female Hormonal Replacement

Hargrove J. Osteen K. An alternative method of hormone replacement therapy using the natural sex steroids. Infertil Reprod Med Clin 1995; 6(4):653–674

DHEA

Barrett-Connor E, Khaw KT, Yen SS. A prospective study of dehydroepiandrosterone sulfate, mortality, and cardiovascular disease. N Engl J Med 1986;315(24):1519–1524

19 Rhytidectomy

Stephen W. Perkins and Shervin Naderi

History

German and French surgeons are credited with pioneering facelift surgery. In 1906, Lexer is thought to have performed surgery to treat wrinkles, but it was Hollander in 1912 who was the first to report a case.[1] Other European physicians, including Joseph (1921) and Passot (1919), developed their own techniques for treatment of the aging face. However, these founding fathers were often guarded when it came to sharing their wisdom, and teaching was rare.

Following The Great War, the practice of reconstructive plastic surgery blossomed. Along with the explosion of new ideas and techniques came the inevitable increased interest in cosmetic surgery. Although still shrouded in secrecy, even the most prominent physicians of the time recognized its existence and demand. Many of these well-respected leaders were rumored to perform cosmetic surgery in their own private clinics or offices. Gilles in 1935 stated, "The operations for removal of eyelid wrinkles, cheek folds, and fat in the neck are justifiable if the patients are chosen with honest discrimination."[1]

Following World War II, with the advent of newer medications and improved anesthesia methods, elective surgery became more of a reality. In addition, a progressive affluent society expressed interest in equating appearance with a youthful outlook on life. However, the occult field of cosmetic surgery, surrounded by shameful secrecy, jealousy, and greed, had not allowed for the fostering of ideas and advancement that was common to the other surgical specialties of the time. Therefore, the results achieved by facelift surgery were marginal and not long lasting. Sam Fomon, a pioneer in facial cosmetic surgery and a founding father of what was to become the American Academy of Facial Plastic and Reconstructive Surgery (AAFPRS), was instrumental in teaching cosmetic surgery to all those interested. He recognized the limits of facelift surgery when he stated, "The average duration of the beneficial effects, even with the best technical skill, cannot be expected to exceed three or four years."[1]

At the time, facelift surgery techniques consisted of a limited subcutaneous dissection and skin elevation resulting in a tightening of the preauricular skin and, often, an obvious "operated look." Unfortunately, these methods did not change significantly until the 1970s. The social renaissance of the 1960s and 1970s brought a new openness and acceptance regarding cosmetic surgery. This fueled scientific advances and dialogue, leading to better surgical techniques and outcomes.

The first major contribution in a half-century was provided by Skoog, who touted the benefits of dissecting in a subfascial plane.[2] This allowed for a significant improvement in the lower third of the face. The validity of this new fascial plane was solidified by Mitz and Peyronnie's landmark article in 1976, defining this fascia as the superficial musculoaponeurotic system (SMAS).[3] To achieve a more natural look, numerous modifications have since been made in the sub-SMAS rhytidectomy including plication and imbrication techniques.

Early sub-SMAS dissections mostly provided for an improved jaw line. However, surgeons have attempted to concentrate efforts on improving the midface and nasolabial fold region. Hamra, the pioneer of the deep plane and composite rhytidectomy, continues to present the beneficial effects that can be achieved in the middle third of the face.[4,5] Others have concurred with the improved results possible with deep plane rhytidectomy.[6,7] Still, there are those designing different methods to achieve facial balance, including venturing into a subperiosteal plane.[8–10] And there are even those who are revisiting the subcutaneous dissection, considering it the method of choice in select situations.

The variety of anatomically sound rhytidectomy techniques offers the surgeon options in challenging the effects of aging. However, in addition to recent advances in surgical techniques, there is a new emphasis on recognizing the importance of patient individuality. Each surgical technique has its place. The key for the prudent surgeon is to appropriately evaluate each patient, both physically and emotionally, and then to utilize the correct treatment for the proper diagnosis.

Preoperative Evaluation and Preparation

Patients seeking aging face improvement, or in this case rhytidectomy, are treated in a standardized fashion along with all other cosmetic surgery patients in our respective practices. This includes having pleasant, knowledgable, and courteous receptionists and office staff and proper scheduling times to prevent undue waiting by the patient. Concise and well-organized literature is made available to the patients. On the day of the initial visit, photographs are taken by the photographer and used for preoperative photodocumentation as well as video imaging. This is becoming more and more prevalent and a key part of a coherent, realistic dialogue between the surgeon and patient. Standard preoperative photographic views for facelift surgery include the full-face frontal view, as well as full-face left and right oblique views, and left and right lateral views. One may choose a close-up perioral photograph, as well as a close-up showing more detail of the submental neck tissues. A close-up view of each auricle, with hair pulled behind the ears, earrings removed, and all photographs taken in a Frankfort horizontal line, is imperative. These photographs are best taken using a single lens reflex (SLR) camera with a macro 105 mm lens with appropriate lighting and background.

The initial consultation is done in a private setting to establish rapport as well as convey the surgeon's undivided attention to understand the patient's motivations and desires. It is imperative to understand if the patient's main concern is truly correctable by a standard facial rhytidectomy procedure. Often, the main concern may be true rhytids of the superficial surface of the face, which would be more appropriately treated by means other than a facelift procedure. If deep nasolabial folds are the primary problem and the patient is less concerned about jowling or submental skin and fat ptosis, a rhytidectomy may not be the appropriate procedure. A full consultation including medical and surgical history, inquiry about current and past-recent medications and drug allergies, in addition to an appropriate physical exam, is performed.

During this interaction it is the surgeon's responsibility to determine, with the patient's assistance, what the patient's true motivation for the surgery is. Being in the middle of a life-changing situation, such as divorce, is not in itself a contraindication for proceeding with facelift surgery. However, patients who expect the cosmetic surgical procedure or procedures to solve their situational dilemma may not be proper candidates for the procedure. Patients who truly believe they are doing this for their self-esteem and not for anyone else's benefit are more likely to have a successful psychological benefit. Patients must be realistic about what can and cannot be achieved by surgery, and it is incumbent on the surgeon to impart this information during the consultation. Video imaging greatly helps with this dialogue.

It is important to evaluate the patient's family history to determine the likely speed at which the loss of elasticity of the tissues and the overall aging process is occurring. One must determine lifestyle and social habits, taking into account issues such as solar exposure and smoking, which accelerate aging.

Our patients complete a detailed history questionnaire. Identifying whether or not the patient has had previous cosmetic surgery or any other surgery is important, including what the experience was, as well as whether or not there were difficulties with particular medications or anesthetic techniques. Preparing the patient for an appropriate positive mental experience is crucial. If the patient is terrified of anesthesia or the idea of surgery, it is imperative for the surgeon to find a way to get past this issue and ease the patient's mind to focus on the positive aspects of what can be achieved by surgery.

Certainly, it is important to take a complete medical history to ascertain which, if any, medical conditions exist that would preclude facelift surgery. Cardiovascular disease in itself is not a contraindication to surgery, but a complete clearance by a cardiologist is imperative prior to scheduling surgery. Certainly, an unstable cardiac history precludes any kind of anesthetic or surgical intervention. Liver and renal functions are important in determining the patient's sensitivity to anesthetics and ability to metabolize and excrete medications or agents.

There are a few diseases that would preclude facelift surgery. The history of advanced autoimmune diseases relating to the skin of the face may be a contraindication for facial surgery. Scleroderma and systemic lupus erythematosus are not contraindications to surgery unless the disease is manifesting in the face itself. Some of the other autoimmune diseases may be looked at with suspicion, particularly depending on the type of medication the patient is taking to suppress the autoimmune response. These medicines may suppress the patient's immune response or inhibit the healing process. Diabetes mellitus in itself is not a contraindication to surgery, nor is taking chronic steroids, particularly in the lower doses. Sjögren syndrome may be a relative contraindication, depending on the involvement of the parotid glands and stasis of salivary flow. The autoimmune diseases that relate to perivasculitis are of most concern due to the possible compromise to the vascularitiy of the skin.

A history of full-course radiation treatment to the preauricular regions or infraauricular neck would preclude surgical intervention. The long-term chronic vascular compromise to the skin's microvasculature will make skin flap elevation too risky. Use of isotretinoin (Accutane), though unusual in the facelift age group population, is only a relative contraindication to surgical intervention. There is very little evidence of delayed healing of incisions specifically due to isotretinoin treatment. Medications that would preclude the surgeon from using epinephrine in a local anesthetic or true allergy to any of the local anesthetic classes of medication would contraindicate the performance of facelift surgery given the importance of proper hemostasis.

Obesity in itself is not a contraindication to facelift surgery if you and the patient take into consideration that the results of the procedure may be less than satisfactory. Certainly, a patient who is overweight and plans dramatic weight loss in the ensuing 3 to 6 months should be counseled to lose the weight prior to having the facelift surgery. Generally, a loss or gain of 10 to 15 pounds postoperatively will not affect the overall results of the procedure. However, any patient who is in the midst of dieting that may diminish their vitamin and nutritional intake should be advised against surgery. Not only should one be healthy at the time of surgery, but a proper diet is critical for proper healing as well as for electrolyte balance during the surgery. There are some significantly overweight patients who should be advised against facelift surgery due to the inherent limitations of the procedure, even if a large amount of suction-assisted lipectomy is included. The facelift itself is not a weight reduction procedure, and thinning the midfacial tissues is inappropriate and fraught with complications. As a best-case scenario, overweight patients with heavy jowls and necks often require a revision or "tuck-up" procedures more frequently than less heavy neck patients.

During the physical examination, the surgeon should be able to advise the patient as to what outcome can be expected from the rhytidectomy. A physical examination is absolutely necessary before the surgeon can show the patient on the computer imaging system what his or her likely neck line and jaw line result will be. A good candidate for facelift surgery is a patient who has moderate thickness to the skin with minimal sun damage, and who has retained some hereditary elasticity to the skin, particularly appropriate for the chronological age. Those patients with premature loss of elasticity to their skin, despite it being smooth and nonphotodamaged, may have a less than satisfactory duration of improvement.

Thick-skinned and overweight patients should not expect too much from the results of the rhytidectomy procedure. Not only is the initial result limited, but the length of time for which soft tissues remain firm and in an upward positioned vector may be shorter than average due to the increased weight of the tissues and gravity.

The visible presence of loss of elasticity in the jowl tissues, as well as laxity in the skin, platysma, and fat of the submental and submandibular regions, is a prima fasciae reason to entertain the idea of a facelift as an appropriate procedure for the patient. Certainly, benefits have to be of a significant degree to warrant the surgical intervention required, given the potential risks involved. There do exist patients who have a minor degree of ptosis of soft tissues or presence of signs that a facelift can correct but who should be counseled either to consider other procedures or to return at a later date when the signs of aging have progressed and the procedure may be more indicated. Today's patient population may be slightly more anxious than they should be regarding when to begin the facelift process. It is incumbent on the surgeon not to be too eager to recommend, and on the patient not to be too eager to undergo, this procedure for marginal benefits. There are a variety of other procedures to be considered for these patients such as cheek lifts or submentoplasty.

Patients who are good candidates for facelift surgery may have a forward chin and strong bony structures such as particularly prominent cheek bones. Patients with heavy cheeks and jowls and minimum malar prominences may be disappointed in the outcome of soft-tissue lifting alone. Malar augmentation may enhance the overall angulation of the face. In addition, midfacial hypoplasia or loss of midfacial subcutaneous soft tissue due to hereditary and aging processes often necessitates submalar augmentation to achieve an appropriate rejuvenative result combined with a facelift procedure. The alternatives to these two augmentation procedures may involve a different approach to facelifting, such as midfacial lift or composite facelift. Equally, patients with class II malocclusion, hypoplasia of the mentum, or microgenia may be poor candidates for an improved neck line result. Orthognathic consultation or, at the minimum, alloplastic augmentation of the mentum at the time of the facelift is indicated to truly achieve a satisfactory aesthetic result. This is one of the values of preoperative video imaging whereby the patient can observe the results achieved by lifting soft tissues alone versus that combined with enhancing the bony architecture.

It is important for the surgeon to evaluate the cervical mental angle with respect to the underlying muscular tissues and position of the hyoid bone. Many patients are poor candidates for an improved neck angle due to a low-positioned hyoid, and this needs to be carefully shown to them, both through a mirror examination and on the video imaging monitor. The surgeon must not overcorrect the neck angle on the computer image with respect to the true angle of the underlying tissues of the patient's neck so as not to convey a false or unrealistic impression as to what the facelift result will be. This may determine whether or not the patient is satisfied postoperatively with the surgeon's work. Repositioning of the hyoid itself or sculpting of the digastric musculature has been described but is not recommended in the routine or standard neck portion of the rhytidectomy procedure. One must understand what can be accomplished with sculpting lipectomy and platysmaplasty, which can be remarkable at times but have inherent limitations. Overaggressive work in the submental area is fraught with complications.

Prior to leaving the consultation room, the surgeon must answer all of the patient's questions including a discussion of the entire procedure, its alternatives, risks, and limitations. It is also important for the patient to be fully aware of the location of each incision and resultant scar, however well placed and camouflaged it may be ultimately. The risks of anesthesia should be covered in terms of the choices and alternatives in a general sense. It is appropriate, however, that the risks of any particular anesthetic type be covered by the administering physician.

Following this the patient and surgeon view the morphed images on a video monitor and further issues may be pointed out and questions answered. At this point the patient has an opportunity to view other patients' operative results if they desire to see that the patients appear natural.

Anatomical Considerations and the Type of Facelift Performed

The fundamental decision as to what type of facelift will be required for an individual patient is primarily based on the preexisting condition of the patient as outlined and observed in the physical examination portion of the consultation. Not every patient requires the same degree of surgical aggressiveness to achieve a satisfactory result. Although the senior author has in the past described three types of facelift procedures, based on the general categories of surgical intervention required to achieve a satisfactory surgical result, recently we have modified the submental portion of the procedure in our practice (**Tables 19.1 and 19.2**).

The fundamental concept of rhytidectomy is based on certain anatomical relationships of the tissues. The elasticity and condition of the overlying skin, including its degree of photodamage and rhytid formation, is important. The relationship with the underlying subcutaneous tissue, including the vector of descent as a result of gravity, true ptosis, or abnormal accumulation and distribution of fat must be noted. Facial musculature is enveloped by continuous fascia that extends to the preparotid region. This fascia, which is contiguous with the platysma muscle of the neck, is the SMAS, first described as a dynamic contractile and fibromuscular web by Mitz and Peyronnie.[3] The fascia deep to this is the superficial layer of the deep cervical fascia that envelopes and covers the sternocleidomastoid muscle, as well as the parotid tissues and parotidomassoteric fascia. SMAS is also superficial to the superficial layer of the deep temporal fascia as well as to the periosteum of the forehead. The SMAS is contiguous with the galea of the scalp. In the neck anteriorly, the platysma muscle may or may not be interdigitated to form a connected sling depending on age. Often, there is a laxity and dehiscence of the anterior borders of the platysma muscle, creating banding in the neck.

Table 19.1 Ideal Candidates for Facelifting

Good skin tone with minimal photoaging and few wrinkles
Strong facial bony structures
Strong foreward chin
Prominent cheek bones
Fuller midface
Shallow cheek–lip grooves
Sharp cervicomental sulcus
Nonsmoker

Table 19.2 Poor Candidates for Facelifting

A low hyoid producing an obtuse cervicomental angle
Have receded or weak chins
Have low-slung submandibular glands
Deep oral commissure cheek–chin grooves
Deep nasolabial grooves and prominent cheek mounds or folds

It is the very nature and the existence of this SMAS layer that allows for a deeper plane of facelifting surgery than was performed in the original rhytidectomy procedures of the past. Only skin was lifted, elevated, excised, and resutured in a more cephalic and posterior position. Skin, due to its inherent creep phenomenon and rebound stretch characteristics, often does not hold for any length of time. Therefore, the effects of the facelift surgery were brief when this was the only layer approached. To achieve longer lasting results, tighter pulls were necessary resulting in a "stretched, operated" look as well as hypertrophic scars due to the tension. Unfortunately the skin-only rhytidectomy is still the method of choice for some surgeons.

Skin, particularly in the middle and more central portion of the face, is directly connected to the SMAS layer by firm dermal fibrous filaments. Often accompanying these dermal filaments is some penetrating vasculature from the deeper vascular systems to the superficial dermal plexus. It is easily demonstrable that lifting and pulling the SMAS layer with its integral attachment to the platysma muscle and midfacial muscles lifts and repositions the skin in the same fashion without undue tension on the skin edges (**Fig. 19.1**). A superior and posterior vector of pull of this fascia repositions the facial tissues in a more youthful position. The visible effect of gravity on these anatomical tissues is directly countered and improved by the facelifting procedures.

It is equally important to understand the anatomical relationships of the neurosensory and neuromotor branches supplying the face and neck. The fifth cranial nerve supplies sensation to the majority of cutaneous surfaces of the face, head, and neck. Facelifting surgery requires elevation of a certain amount of preauricular

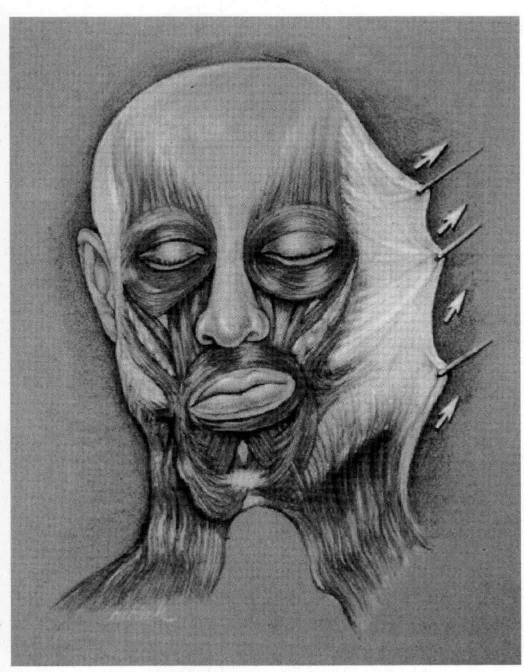

Fig. 19.1 Superficial musculoaponeurotic system (SMAS) connected with platysma and facial musculature.

and postauricular skin, interrupting the immediate innervation of this portion of the face. Typically, unless any major branch of the greater auricular nerve is interrupted, sensation returns to the skin in a relatively short time. The patient can expect return of sensation in the first 6 to 8 weeks, but occasionally 6 months to a year may be required for full return. In rare cases, the patient may report a decreased overall sensation to the skin than was there preoperatively, even beyond a year.

Sympathetic and parasympathetic reinnnervation of the skin proceeds more rapidly in the postoperative period. Although the most common major nerve branch injured in facelifting surgery is the greater auricular nerve as it crosses over the sternocleidomastoid, even this rarely causes permanent loss of sensation of the auricle or the preauricular skin. As one is dissecting skin and its dermal attachments away from the superficial layer of the sternocleidomastoid muscular fascia, if one interrupts this fascia, direct injury to this very large and visible nerve branch may occur. When recognized at the time of surgery, direct suture reanastomosis is indicated and return of nerve function within a year or two is expected.

Motor branches to the facial mimetic musculature are potentially in danger during facelift surgery. Branches of the facial nerve become very superficial as they extend beyond the parotid masseteric fascia. The marginal mandibular branch is at some risk as it crosses the mandibular margin, deep both to the platysma muscle and to the superficial layer of the deep cervical fascia. Techniques requiring elevation underneath the SMAS layer into the midface endanger branches to the orbicularis, zygomatic, and buccinator muscles, although innervation to these muscles is to the undersurface of the muscles, and deep plane technique at this point would be superficial to those muscles. Direct visualization of the nerve is part of this procedure and will be discussed further in this chapter.

The branch of the facial nerve most commonly injured in facelift surgery, with or without temporal lifting, is the frontal branch. This branch becomes very superficial at the level of the zygomatic arch and extends just beneath the subcutaneous tissues underlying the thin SMAS layer of the temporal region prior to its innervation of the deeper surface of the frontalis muscle. As it traverses this area, ~1.5 to 2 cm preauricular and halfway between the lateral orbital rim and the temporal tuft of hair, it is at greatest risk. It is imperative that the surgeon understand the anatomical relationships of the layers of the face and temporal region to prevent injury to the nerve. One can elevate the skin all the way to the lateral canthal region, the preauricular area overlying the zygomatic arch, up to the orbicularis muscle, as long as dissection is in the immediate subcutaneous layer. In addition, the surgeon can dissect freely under the frontalis fascia beneath the galeal layer superficial to the periosteum and the overlying superficial fascia of the temporalis muscle without injury to the frontal branch of the facial nerve, which is external to this avascular layer. However, at the level of the zygomatic arch, one needs to make the transition to beneath the periosteum or immediate transection of the facial nerve will occur as one follows the same plane overlying the zygomatic arch. Injury to the nerve in this area may or may not result in reinnervation of the frontalis muscle.

Surgical Technique

Incision planning and marking of the appropriate locations for the incisions for the facelift procedure is crucial to the long-term outcome. Changes in hairline or scars that are placed in visible locations may cause the patient to be totally dissatisfied with an otherwise good facelift. The natural look of the patient's hairline, the freedom with which hair styling can be done, and the invisibility of the scar lines separates the good facelifting surgeon from the one sought by patients as the best in the community. The facelift surgeon who pays attention to the details of incision placement and planning is often the one extolled and recommended by hairdressers and other cosmeticians who see the results from this aspect of the facelift.

There are three critical points that must be taken into consideration in planning the facelift incisions:

1. *How to manage and maintain the preauricular tuft of hair, including the sideburn.* Each patient is different in terms of the location of the lower portion of the sideburn and the width at which it extends anteriorly from the insertion of the helical curvature. If the preauricular sideburn hairline is 1 or 2 cm below the insertion of the superior portion of the helical insertion, it may be appropriate to design an incision that curves up into the temporal hair and allows some posterior superior lifting of the hairline. The curved hairline incision, rather than a straight vertical incision, is required to interrupt the forces of contracture, maintain a minimally wide scar, and avoid alopecia (**Fig. 19.2**). As long as the hairline is not lifted higher than the insertion of the superior helical insertion, the patient will have no cosmetic disturbance of this area. If the sideburn is at the helical insertion preoperatively, an inferior sideburn incision is required; this will usually be associated with a separate temporal incision if a lift is required in this region. At no time should the incision be carried anteriorly around the sideburn tuft and along the pretemporal hairline. All scars in this area will be visible and cannot be camouflaged by the fine, severely sloped hair as it exits the skin naturally in a posterior direction.
2. *Preauricularly, the incision must at least follow the apparent curvatures of the auricle itself.* There is a strong preference by the patient population for an incision hidden behind the posterior edge of the tragus so that the incision appears "inside the ear." No preauricular incision will be seen, as it otherwise follows the normal curvature of the helical insertion and goes behind the tragus ~1 to 2 mm, then exits at the junction of the earlobe with the face. As an alternative to this, for patients with hearing aids or very deep pretragal depressions and tall tragi, a curved incision extending into the incisura and then out around the curve in the helix may be acceptable. However, loss of pigmentation in the scar, no matter how thin, will leave a visible line forever and may necessitate a hairstyle modification in the future. In men care must be taken not to transplant hair bearing skin unto the tragus or lobule.
3. *Postauricularly, the incision must be directed up onto the posterior aspect of the auricle above the sulcus so that when the ear settles posteriorly and the scar heals with some contracture of the skin, the scar falls into the postauricular sulcus and not on the postauricular skin.* The incision should make a gentle curve across the junction of the auricle, with the postauricular skin not crossing the non–hair-bearing skin at the level of where the auricle meets the hairline. In most cases, the incision should be gently sloped back into the postauricular hair. When advancing the postauricular skin posteriorly and superiorly, the posterior hairline can then be approximated with no step-off or other deformity. However, when a patient has a significant amount of neck skin that must be repositioned posteriorly, it is often imperative that the incision be designed to run along the postauricular hairline before being swung posteriorly into the hair. In that way a large amount of skin can be moved posteriorly and superiorly without stepping off the postauricular hairline. At no time should the incision be left visible at the base of the hairline toward the anterior neck.

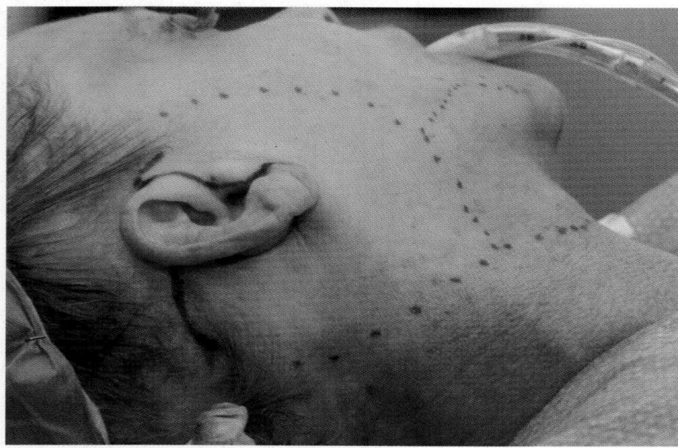

Fig. 19.2 Typical facelift incision for patient with a low sideburn tuft of hair.

In addition, a 2 to 3 cm incision is required in the submental area, just anterior to the preexisting deep submental crease, to facilitate the procedure that is required in the anterior neck. Prior to infiltration of anesthetic, a dotted line is often used to determine the area to be anesthetized and the area that will be subsequently undermined. Some surgeons prefer to mark the area of the zygomatic arch, McGregor's patch, and the angle of the mandible. Further outlining of the jowl and any platysma banding may be of benefit in highlighting areas that need correction during the operation.

One variation in the male facelift patient and the woman who has a fair amount of hirsute preauricular skin is an incision that is gently curved in the preauricular area in what is often a preexisting preauricular crease. This incision should not be entirely straight; rather, it should be a distance away from the incisura and in front of the tragus. One must leave a non–hair-bearing portion of skin when moving the bearded skin or hair-bearing

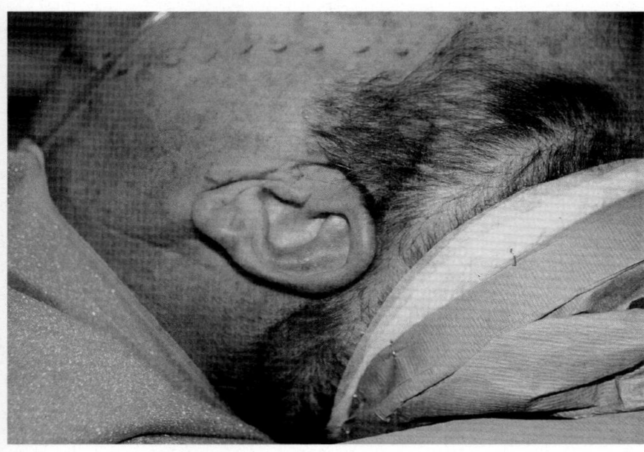

Fig. 19.3 Typical incision for a male with beard, preserving non–hair-bearing preauricular skin.

skin posteriorly and superiorly (**Fig. 19.3**). (It is a very important part of the consultation for you to outline exactly where you plan to make the incisions and note this in the chart, graphically as well as in written form.)

Anesthesia for facelift surgery requires an appropriate amount of local anesthetic infiltration combined with epinephrine to control cutaneous bleeding with a comfortable, sedated patient. Although many surgeons prefer inhalation anesthetics for a complete general anesthetic, this is not usually required. What is required is a patient who is intravenously sedated and fully monitored for continuous cardiac parameters, blood pressure, and oxygen saturation. A person is designated to monitor the patient, and this person can be an anesthesiologist, a certified nurse anesthetist, or a registered nurse under the direction of the operating surgeon. Having a patient who is well assured preoperatively is critical to the success of a conscious-sedation anesthesia. The patient who is comforted knowing that he or she will not experience pain, discomfort, or otherwise be mistreated during the operation will be mentally prepared for the appropriate effects of the sedation medicine administered. It is generally a good idea to provide the patient some oral medication for relaxation prior to administering intravenous sedation. Current medications confer a significant amount of amnestic effect, as well as proper sedation and analgesia. Any anesthetic administered should have some prolonged effect so that the patient remains comfortable for several hours in the immediate postoperative period. Infiltration of the incision lines is best accomplished with xylocaine 1% with 1:50,000 epinephrine. This provides not only good anesthesia but the maximum hemostasis for vasoconstriction that is possible. Infiltration of the areas to be undermined should be done with 0.5% xylocaine with 1:100,000 epinephrine. Some hemostasis is still required. Total volume of xylocaine must be carefully monitored. At no time should more than 500 mg of xylocaine with epinephrine be infiltrated at one time or within a 1- to 2-hour period. Overdosage of xylocaine with resultant toxicity can be a result of injudicious volume infiltration of this local anesthetic. It may be advisable to complete infiltration and surgery on one side of the face before proceeding to the other side. This sequential infiltration, as long as performed 10 to 15 minutes prior to the incision on that side, is safe and effective.

The patient must then be prepared for the surgical operation by having small bundles of hair twisted and secured away from the incision lines and operative field. This may require taping of these bundles prior to prepping. After the patient is prepped and draped with a head drape in the usual sterile manner, the operation may commence. No shaving of hair is required. Preoperative antibiotic prophylaxis is given to all patients, using a first-generation cephalosporin 1 day preoperatively and continuing for 4 days postoperatively.

Treatment of the Submentum, Jowl, and Neck

Initial treatment of the neck involves correction of the jowl, submandibular, and submental lipoptosis. In type I facelifts, there is generally little or no independent indication for intervention in the neck. However, since the previous edition of this chapter, we have been performing our standard platysmaplasty on nearly all patients to achieve a "sling" in the cervicomental area, which can then be used for posterior tightening of the skin–SMAS–platysma. In the majority of patients, some degree of liposuction is required.

In the rare situation where only debulking and reduction of this lipoptosis is required, a 1 cm incision is made in the submental crease to admit a liposuction cannula. If one has determined by examination that no platysma redundancy is present and there is some elasticity to the remaining skin, liposuction is performed as the only neck procedure. The initial 1 cm dissection is performed just beneath the skin in the middle of the fat layer or subcutaneous tissues. Small (1 mm) tunnels are started and then completed with a 2 or 3 mm liposuction cannula. No suction is applied initially, creating the tunnels all the way from the submental area across the mandibular margin into the jowl region, to the anterior border of the sternocleidomastoid and down and across the cervical mental angle to the area of the thyroid cartilage. This is done in a fanlike fashion from one jowl across the neck to the opposite jowl. A circular liposuction cannula with three openings on one side is used to perform this

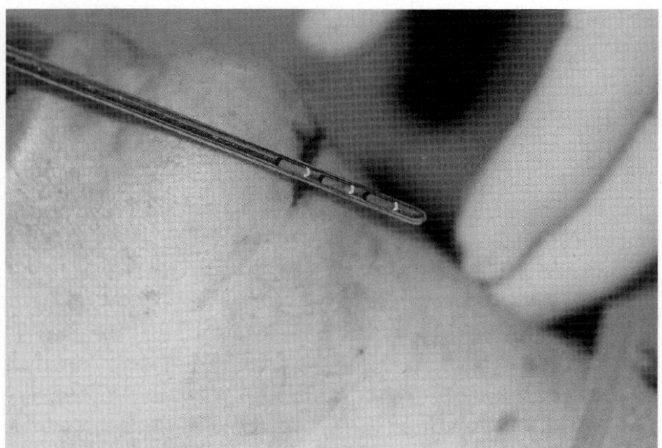

Fig. 19.4 A 3 mm three-opening liposuction cannula.

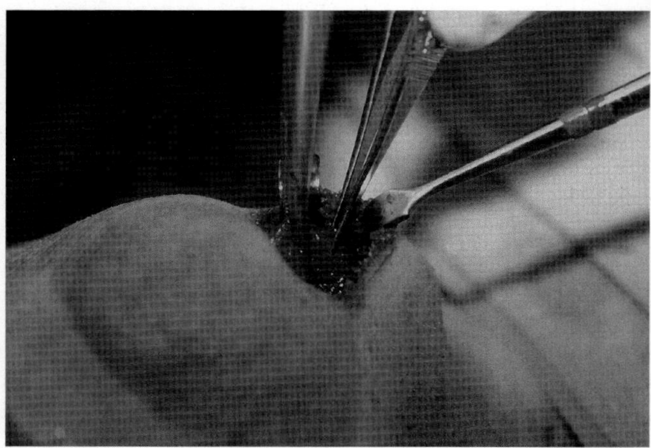

Fig. 19.5 Use of Kelly clamp to tighten anterior platysma and anterior submental fat for incremental excision.

liposuction maneuver (**Fig. 19.4**). Very careful and judicious liposuction in the jowl areas is performed so as to hold the tissues away from the mandibular margin and not create blunt trauma to the marginal mandibular nerve. Minimal liposuction is performed in an even fashion to prevent the creation of any furrows, tunnels, or dimpling. This can happen very easily in the jowl areas, so that care is taken to underdo this maneuver in this region. Depending on the amount of liposuction required in the submental and submandibular neck, a larger liposuction cannula may be required. A 4 mm or sometimes a 6 mm flat cannula with one opening on the inferior surface of the cannula is required to obtain adequate removal and contouring. Bimanual palpation is required to determine the symmetry and equality of the removal of the fat. Leaving a thin layer of subcutaneous fat is required to give supple skin contour. Caution should be excercised in terms of not being overly aggressive in performing liposuction across the cervical mental angle, as this has the potential for creating dermal injury and subdermal scarring, with late development of banding. Aggressive liposuction in the submental area may contribute to a cobra deformity as well.

In type II facelifts, as well as type III facelifts involving a tremendous amount of fat and some platysma ptosis and a significant collections of fat, laxity of skin, and platysma sagging, further work is required. This requires extension of the incision to at least 2.5 to 3 cm. Direct subcutaneous elevation is then performed after the liposuction to elevate the skin away from the platysma muscle. This is performed in a wide fashion, usually extending to the anterior border of the sternocleidomastoid and past the cervical mental angle. This then allows the surgeon to directly view the remaining lipoptosis beneath the platysma muscle and view the redundancy and laxity of the anterior platysma bands. Their dehiscence is readily visible.

The laxity and redundancy of these tissues is determined. Using a grasping Griffith's forceps and a long curved Kelly clamp, the tissues are tightened in the midline. Their redundancy is progressively excised, with care taken to maintain adequate hemostasis with bipolar cautery. Suturing the anterior transected borders of the platysma together into a midline corset is done. The excess fat and muscle are removed all the way down past the cervical mental angle (**Figs. 19.5 and 19.6**). Several mattressing sutures using 3–0 Vicryl (polyglycolic acid) (Ethicon, Inc., Somerville, NJ) are placed. In most men and in women with heavier necks 3.0 Tevdek permanent sutures (Teleflex Medical, Mansfield, MA) are added. After a firm muscular corset is created and a sharper

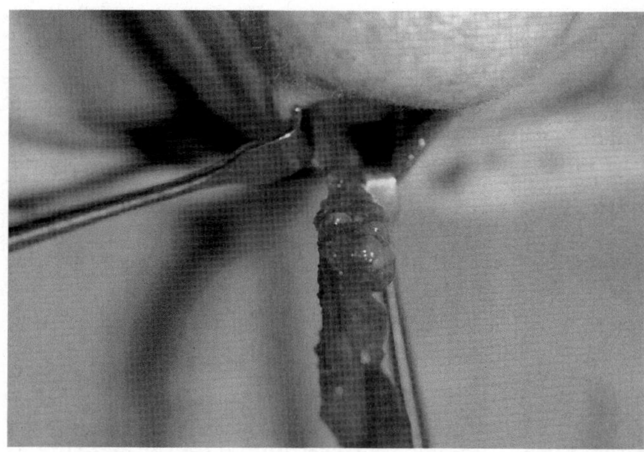

Fig. 19.6 Sequential removal of redundant submental muscle and fat past cervicomental angle.

cervical mental angle achieved, the remainder of the facelift skin undermining will be accomplished from the posterior position. Redundancy of skin in the submental area will be determined at the end of the operation following tightening of the bilateral pre- and postauricular skin in a superior posterior direction.

Skin Elevation and Undermining

The extent of undermining depends on the amount of redundancy of skin in the neck and to some degree on the facial tissues. With the use of SMAS lifting, the degree of undermining from older classic rhytidectomies is much less. A large degree of undermining increases the risk of vascular compromise as well as the development of small seromas, hematomas, and irregularities. However, when a large degree of skin and platysma redundancy is present in the neck, it is often necessary to separate the skin from the underlying platysma muscle to redrape each in a sequential fashion and achieve maximal improvement. Generally, lifting the SMAS and the deep facial tissues is as effective and much safer than separating the skin all the way out to the melolabial crease where the buccal branch of the facial nerve is at risk. Although some surgeons still prefer this older technique, today this large amount of undermining has not been shown to be more effective than the SMAS techniques in improving the jowl or deep melolabial fold.

Undermining of the skin begins in the postauricular area and can be done with a beveled facelift scissors in an advance-spreading technique (**Fig. 19.7**). Direct knife elevation is an alternative. It is important to begin deep to the level of the hair follicles in this region so as to not injure the hair follicles and create permanent alopecia. However, when the dissection is continued anterior to the postauricular hairline, it should be quite superficial in the immediate subcutaneous layer. This subcutaneous layer is minimal in the postauricular region and the skin very closely adherent to the overlying fascia of the sternocleidomastoid muscle. Care must be taken to separate this layer meticulously until the dissection is anterior to the sternocleidomastoid. Injury to the greater auricular nerve, as mentioned previously, is a real risk due to the lack of a thicker subcutaneous layer and adherent dermal attachments in this region. Elevation is then continued in the subcutaneous plane superficial to the platysma muscle and anteriorly as far as the amount of neck surgery dictates (**Fig. 19.8**). When this undermining is completed, it meets the undermining that was done previously in the submental area. Although the undermining may extend slightly above the mandibular margin, it is generally confined to the neck region.

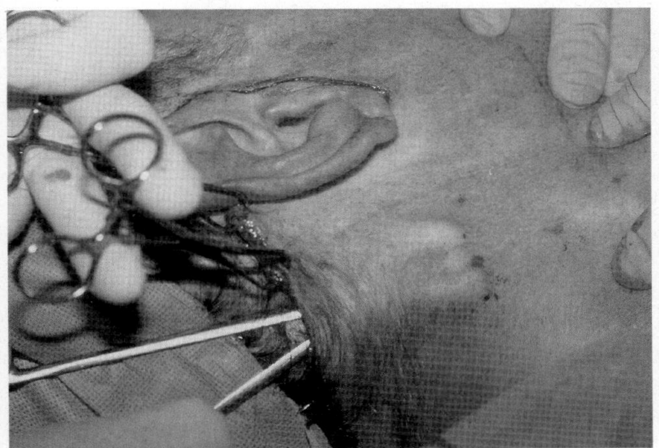

Fig. 19.7 Undermining with beveled facelift scissors with advance-and-spread technique.

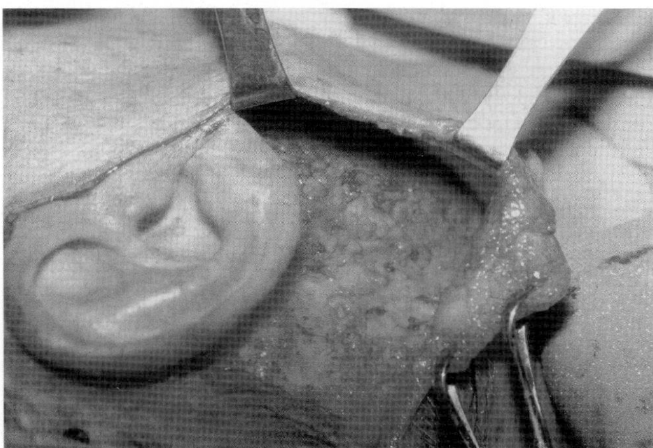

Fig. 19.8 Postauricular and neck flap elevated within subcutaneous fat layer over the sternocleidomastoid muscle.

Temporal Lift Technique

After the undermining of the neck has been achieved, undermining begins in the temporal area. Temporal lifting is required to achieve smoothing of the lateral canthal–temporal skin and lateral brow. Incisions are made down through the scalp tissues through the superficial galea and the superficial layer of the temporalis fascia is identified. Undermining can be performed in this layer all the way down to the lateral brow and the superior edge of the zygomatic arch. Elevation of the temporal unit is not required in all facelifts and is usually not required in type I facelifts. It is usually required when there is laxity of tissues in the lateral brow and lateral orbital region that must be redraped so as not to create bunching when the cheek tissues are brought up superiorly. The temporal lift may or may not be connected with other means of lifting the brow–forehead complex. Elevation is then begun in

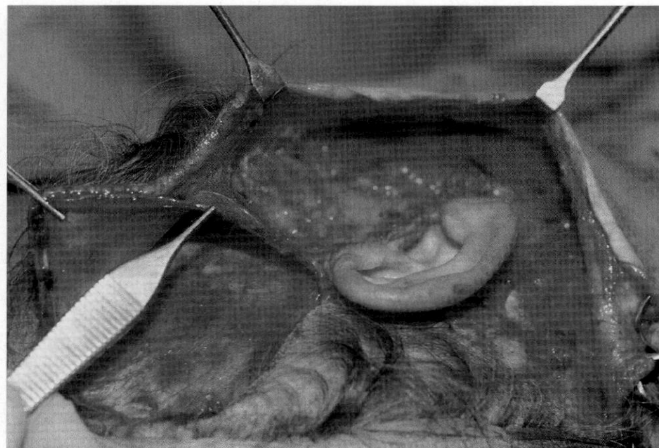

Fig. 19.9 Maintain a noninterrupted bridge of tissue in the temporal region to avoid injury to the frontal branch of the facial nerve.

the preauricular area at the level of the temporal tuft in the immediate subcutaneous layer. This is a layer distinctly different than that for the temporal elevation, and a noninterrupted bridge of SMAS and neurovascular bundles should be left intact that extends superiorly toward the frontalis muscle. By maintaining this bridge of tissue, one will not injure the frontal branch of the facial nerve which courses within this layer (**Fig. 19.9**). Undermining can then proceed to the malar area, extending in the preauricular region anywhere from 4 to 6 cm depending on the elasticity of the skin. This undermining is continued in the intraadipose layer, separating the subcutaneous dermal fat, leaving it with the skin flap, separate from the underlying fat overlying the SMAS. This preauricular space is connected to the same layer of elevation overlying the platysma muscle in the neck. Meticulous hemostasis is then assured under direct vision using bipolar cautery and a lighted retractor.

Depending on the nature of the facelift, one must determine the degree of intervention and manipulation of the SMAS layer. Even type I facelifts may require imbrication or deep plane maneuvers, depending on the need for elevation of the midfacial tissues. If only a small amount of jowl repositioning and posterior repositioning of the platysma muscle is required, some surgeons may prefer a plication of the SMAS (**Fig. 19.10**). However, one must remove the adipose tissue that is still on top of the parotid fascia in a semilunar fashion in the preauricular area so as to pull the SMAS over on itself while suturing. Otherwise, there will be no fibrous adherence of the SMAS and the lift may fail when the sutures give way. Some surgeons prefer a permanent suture for this plication or folding of the SMAS due to the fact that it needs to be maintained in this position over time.

Generally, facelifts do require some undermining of the SMAS layer and platysma so that it can advance superiorly and posteriorly (**Fig. 19.11**). The degree of this undermining will be dictated by the need for lifting of the jowl, platysma muscle, and midfacial tissues. This constitutes imbrication of the SMAS, whereby the SMAS is lifted, advanced, trimmed, and sutured end to end. This can be done with a long-term, but nonpermanent, suture.

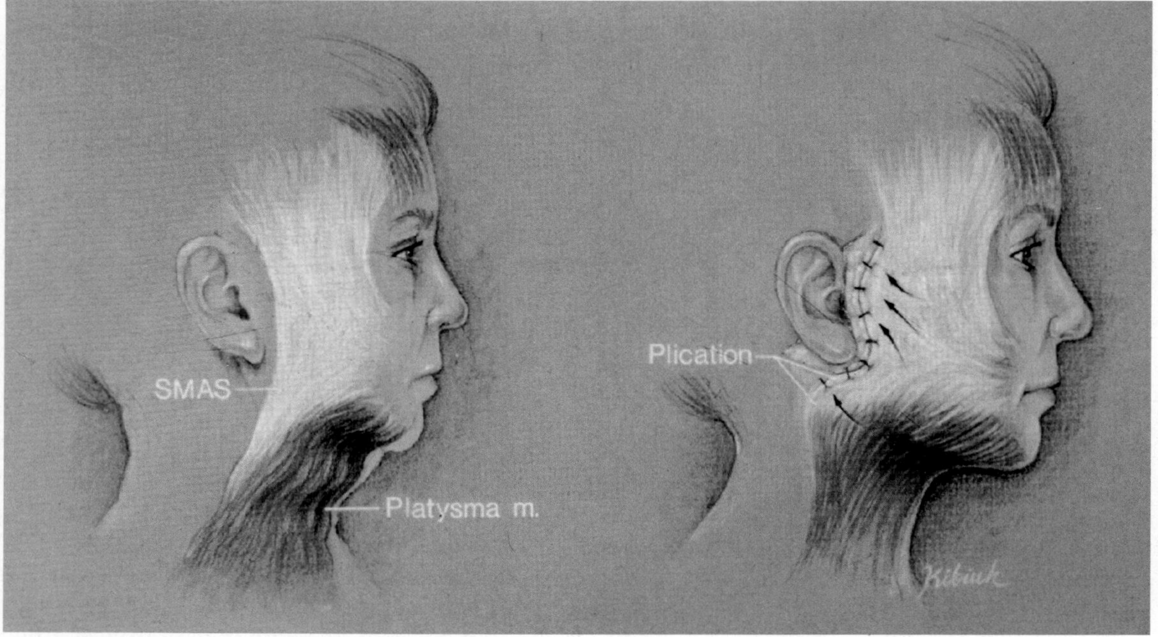

Fig. 19.10 Plication of the SMAS and platysma with posterior suspension.

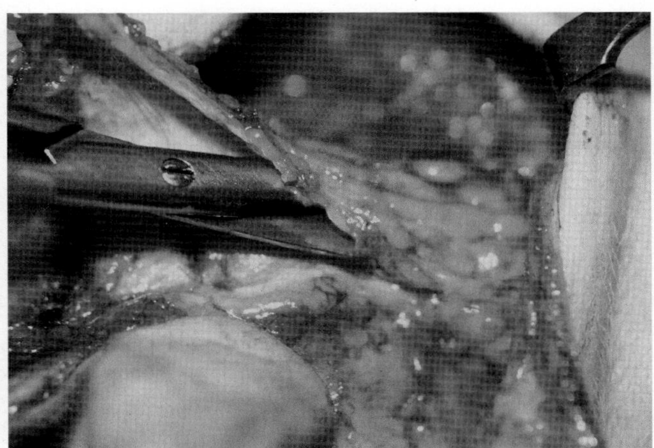

Fig. 19.11 Metzenbaum scissors elevation of the preauricular SMAS.

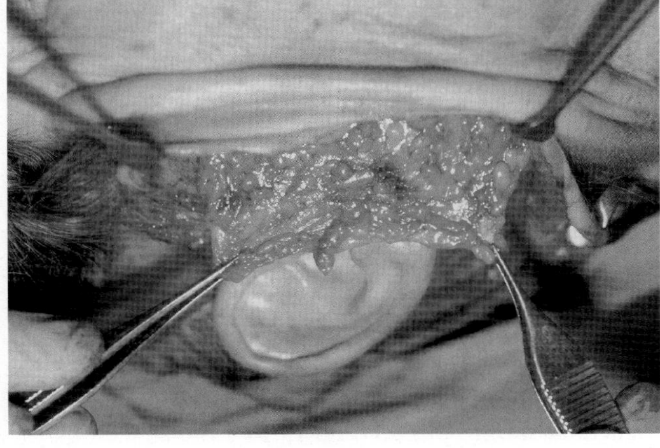

Fig. 19.12 Advancement of the undermined SMAS prior to imbrication.

Here again, permanent sutures may be added in men as well as women with heavy tissues. Imbrication after SMAS elevation creates scar between planes of tissue that result in longer-lasting surgical benefits.

For those patients requiring midfacial lift of the subcutaneous soft tissues, as a minimum, a modification of the deep plane facelift is performed. This requires elevation of the SMAS layer at the level of the zygomatic arch over the malar eminence and superficial to the zygomaticus muscle. Complete deep plane facelift techniques necessitate undermining the SMAS layer all the way anterior to the anterior border of the masseter muscle and connecting this to the elevation of the neck tissues superficial to the platysma muscle. Transition must be made, however, in the midcheek to the superficial layer overlying the zygomatic muscle or injury will occur to the nerve to this muscle, or the buccinator.

When the appropriate elevation of the midfacial tissues has been accomplished with the corresponding SMAS and platysma, this layer is advanced in an appropriate posterior superior direction (**Fig. 19.12**). Direct vision allows one to see the movement of the melolabial tissues, as well as the jowl, back and upward into a more youthful position. A slip of this SMAS fascia is brought up to the firm preauricular tissues as a sling suspension. Similarly, the SMAS is divided at the level of the earlobe and an inferior slip of SMAS/platysma is sutured with a 0-Vicryl suture as a supporting sling to the mastoid periosteum (**Figs. 19.13 and 19.14**). This provides crisp, sharp delineation of the cervical mental angle. Redundancies of platysma and SMAS are trimmed and a few sutures placed to the posterior postauricular fascial tissues. Anteriorly, the SMAS is trimmed, the excess is discarded, and the SMAS is sutured end to end with a long-lasting, temporary monofilament suture, such as 3–0 PDS (polydiaxonone).

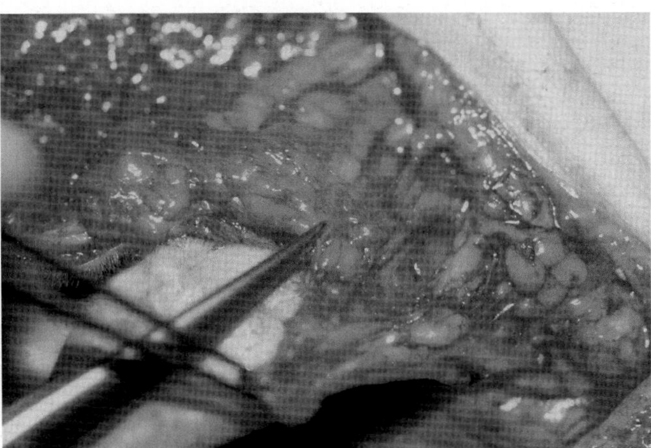

Fig. 19.13 Splitting the SMAS–platysma flap at the ear lobe for suspension of sling of platysma.

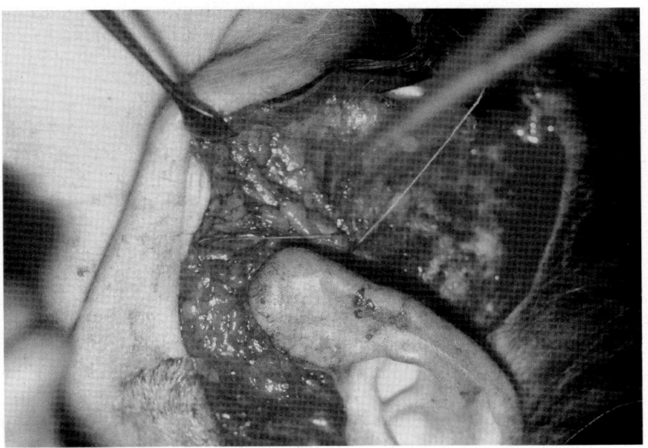

Fig. 19.14 Suspension of posterior slip of platysma–SMAS with 0-Vicryl suture to the mastoid periosteum.

Skin Flap Advancement

After adequate deep fascial lift has been completed for the long-term foundation of the facelift, the skin flap can be repositioned and modified as necessary. One can see, with minimum tension, the redundancy of skin that is draped over the ear in a posterior superior vector. The preauricular skin is moved mostly posteriorly and slightly superiorly, taking care not to let the sideburn tuft of hair be pulled too high. The neck skin is lifted in the postauricular area in a posterior but mostly superior fashion so as to not create a large step-off deformity of the postauricular hairline. When the skin has been secured in the high pre- and postauricular regions, incremental cuts are made and staples placed (**Fig. 19.15**). The skin along the postauricular occipital hair is incised in a beveled fashion, and surgical staples are used to approximate these scalp tissues. The skin in the non–hair-bearing postauricular areas is sutured in a running interlocking fashion with a 5–0 plain gut-type suture. As there is no tension, only one deep suture using 5–0 Dexon is placed in the post auricular area just superior to the lobule to allow a better seal for the suction drain. The earlobe is positioned with a deep 5–0 Dexon suture (Covidien, Mansfield, MA) and the skin trimmed so that the earlobe is tucked in a superior position. It is often important to exaggerate the upward lift to the earlobe so that when the tissues heal and drift inferiorly, the earlobe is not pulled down. It is critical to make the skin cut at the level of the lobule in a forward-horizontal fashion and avoid an inferior vector of cut to prevent an inferiorly distracted earlobe, which looks like a satyr's ear and is an obvious postoperative facelift deformity (devil's ear). The preauricular tissues are trimmed appropriately according to the planned preoperative incision. A tragal flap is left significantly redundant, so that when it is closed there is absolutely no tension in the flap. When this heals, it will contract and look extremely close to a normal tragus and not be pulled anteriorly due to overly tightened scar contracture from injudicious trimming of the flap. The preauricular skin is closed with a running interlocking 5–0 plain gut suture. No more than one or two deep 5–0 Dexon sutures are needed in this due to the lack of tension on the skin flaps. The temporal incision is closed, as was the occipital scalp, with interrupted surgical staples. Prior to complete closure, a flat, 7 mm or 4 mm, closed-suction drain is placed with an exit wound hidden in the postoccipital hair (**Fig. 19.16**). The drain is brought just to the level of the anterior angle of the mandible. The submental skin is then trimmed if there is excess, in a semilunar fashion with care taken not to create "dog ears" laterally or skin redundancies. "Chasing" of standing cone deformities in this area is not advised. This incision is closed using 5–0 running, locking plain gut suture in women and 5–0 nylon in men. Several deep Dexon sutures may be placed depending on tension.

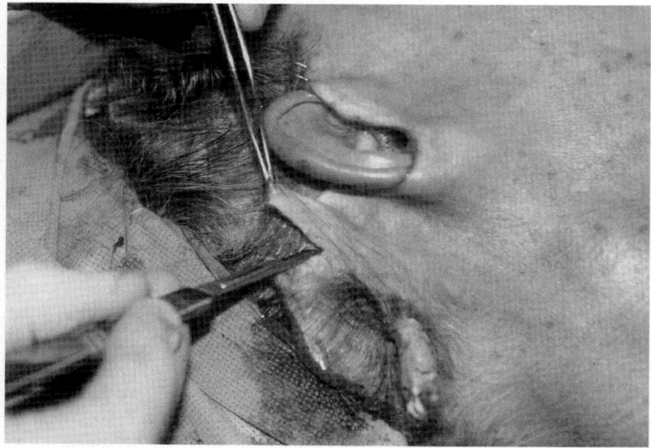

Fig. 19.15 Posterior draping of the skin flap requires alignment of the occipital hairline.

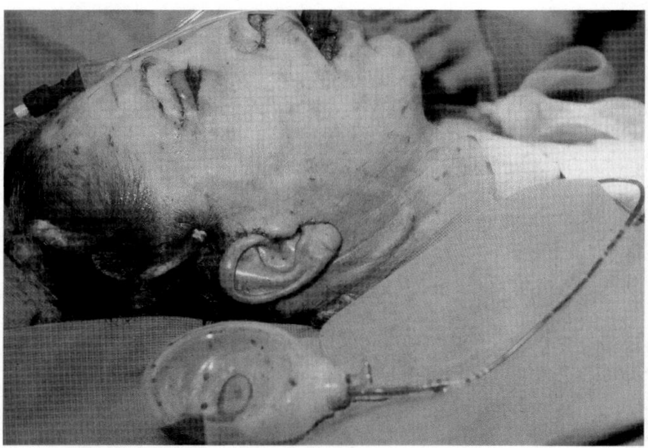

Fig. 19.16 A closed suction drain is used to prevent serohematomas.

Prior to placement of the dressing in the operating room, the patient's hair twirls are removed, the hair is washed, and any blood is rinsed at this time. An antibiotic ointment is applied to a nonadherent dressing that is placed in the pre- and postauricular areas. A few 4 × 4 sterile gauzes are placed over the undermined areas, and under the chin and over the top of the head. This is followed by a loose circumferential dressing including ABD pads followed by Kerlix (Covidien), and finally held in place with a minimally constrictive elastic-type chin strap. Care is taken not to apply excess pressure to the undermined skin flaps (**Fig. 19.17**).

The patient is discharged from the operating room to the recovery area. After adequate recovery has taken place, the patient is escorted to the car and driven home.

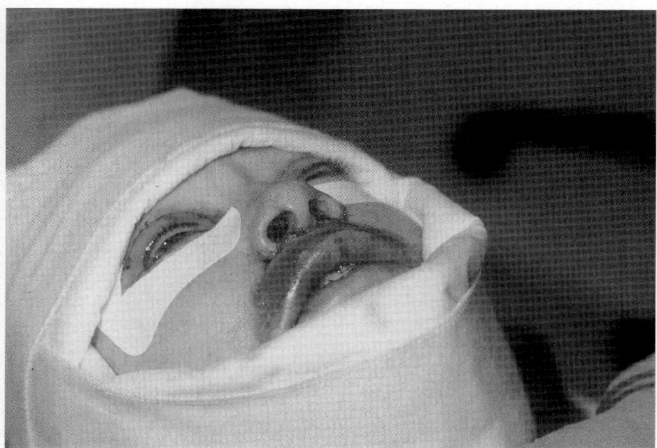

Fig. 19.17 Postoperative facelift dressing for mild compression.

Although not necessary, some patients make arrangements to stay overnight. The patient needs to be ambulatory with assistance before discharge and must have someone in attendance through the entire night. It is important to maintain phone contact with the patient that evening. The patient is required to stay within a 15- or 20-minute drive from the operative facility in the event that immediate postoperative care is required. The patient is requested to return the following morning, 12 to 18 hours postoperatively. At that time, the dressing is removed, the drains are generally removed, and facial nerve function and skin flaps are evaluated. The patient's hair is washed again as a courtesy and a light chin strap is applied for an additional 24 hours. The patient is asked to shower once a day for a week and to keep the wounds clean and moist with peroxide and antibiotic ointment. One week postoperatively, the patient returns for staple and suture removal.

The only permanent sutures placed were twp interrupted 5–0 nylon sutures at the apex of each ear lobule, which are removed around postoperative day 10 at which time the patient is reexamined and given the opportunity to meet with a makeup artist. The patient is instructed regarding appropriate makeup coverage for any residual ecchymoses and is given a full skin-care lesson. The makeup artist introduces appropriate moisturizers, cosmetics, and sun screens, and informs the patient about future appropriate skin-care practices to maintain the facelift results. It is imperative to see the patient at 1 month, 3 months, 6 months, and 1 year postoperatively to follow the results (**Figs. 19.18 to 19.25**). In the second to fourth week, the patient often requires emotional support, as adjustment is still being made to the new appearance, and reassimilating to work or social activities. Many of the postoperative sensations being experienced, as well as minor healing variabilities that the patient was told would occur, have been forgotten and reassurance is needed that everything is progressing as expected. Continuous reaffirmation of postoperative instructions and expectations is critical to the happiness of these elective cosmetic surgical patients. Your office should be a place

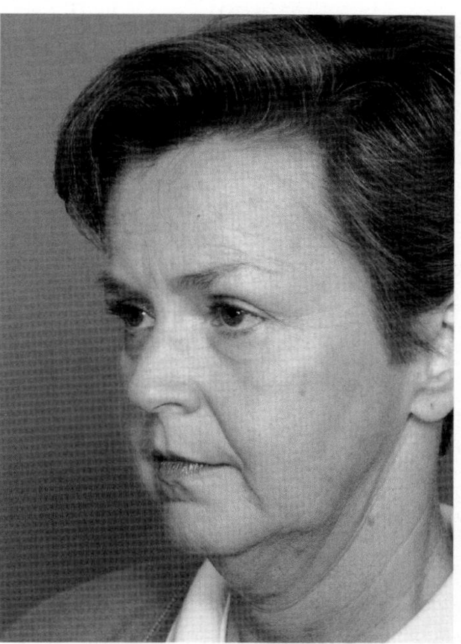

Fig. 19.18 Preoperative facelift, oblique view.

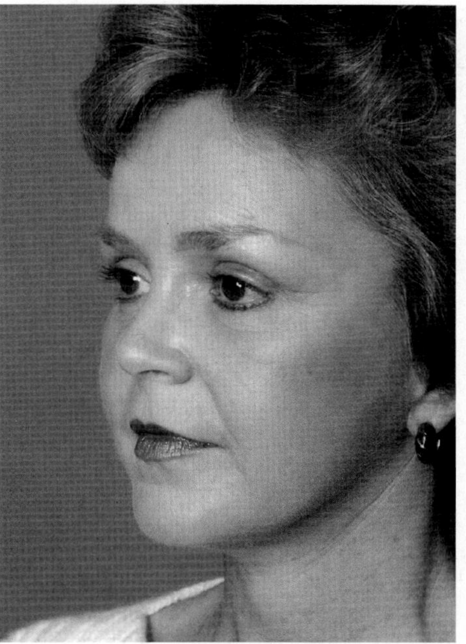

Fig. 19.19 Six months postoperative facelift, oblique view.

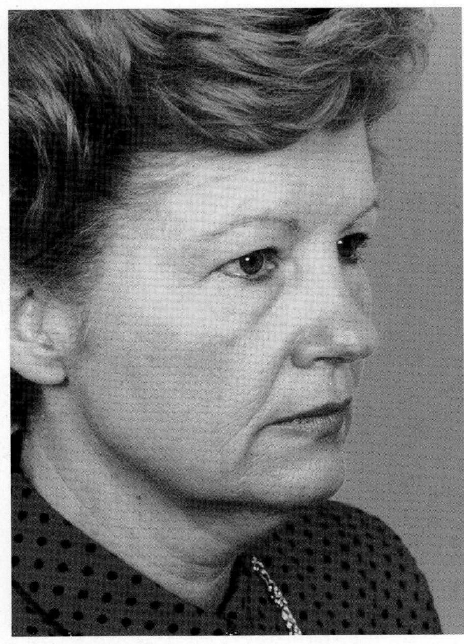

Fig. 19.20 Preoperative facelift, oblique view.

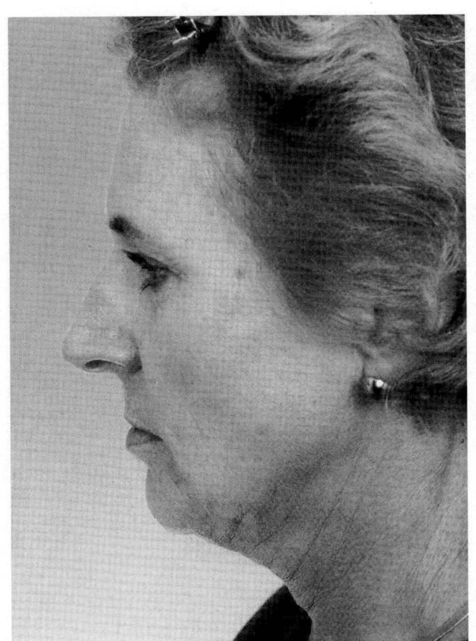

Fig. 19.22 Preoperative facelift, lateral view.

they feel comfortable calling, as well as returning to, in this immediate postoperative time. Patients must feel that you are there for them, to answer questions and reassure them. This is critical to their long-term satisfaction. For longer-term follow-up, it is important that you intervene if there is any tendency toward hypertrophic healing in the postauricular areas. Intralesional steroids may occasionally be required to settle down a slightly thickening postauricular scar. In addition, at the 4- to 6-week postoperative period, if the patient is going to experience some

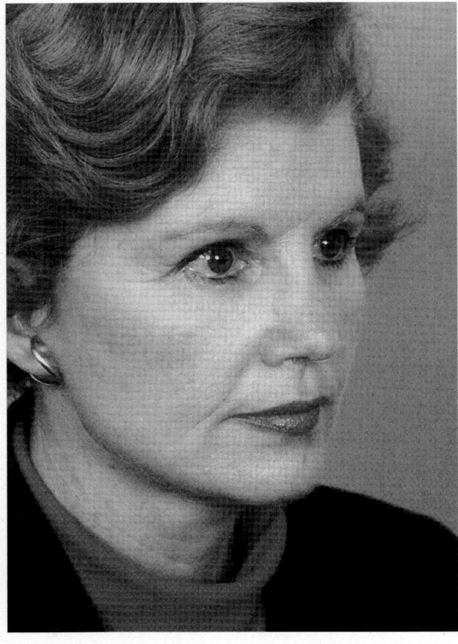

Fig. 19.21 Two years postoperative facelift, oblique view.

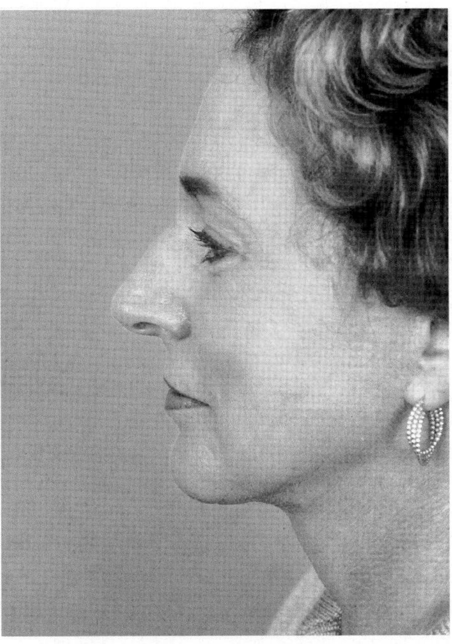

Fig. 19.23 Eighteen months postoperative facelift, lateral view.

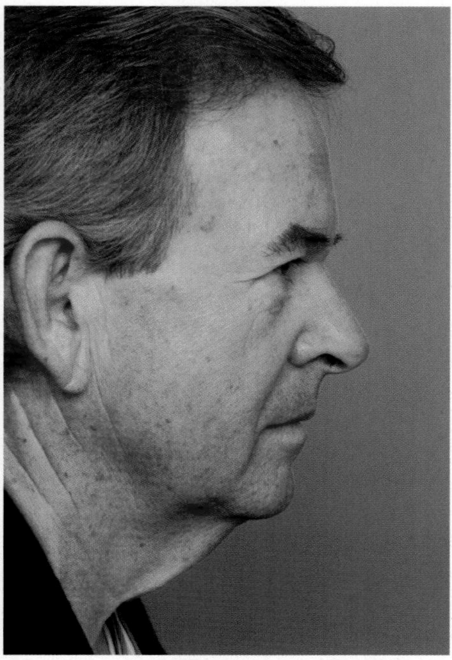

Fig. 19.24 Preoperative male facelift, lateral view.

temporary surgical alopecia in the hair-bearing areas, he or she needs complete reassurance that these hair follicles will regenerate hair shafts and that within 4 to 6 months all of the hair will grow back. The patient further needs reassurance throughout the first 3 to 6 months that hypersensitivities and neuresthesias are completely normal and part of the healing process.

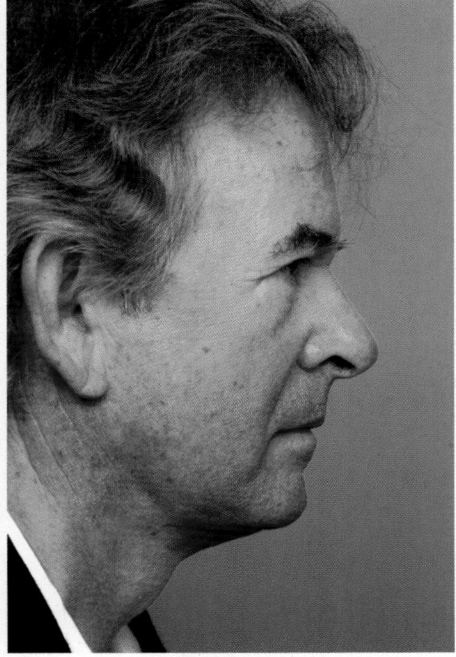

Fig. 19.25 Ten months postoperative male facelift, lateral view.

Tuck-ups and Secondary Rhytidectomy

As you follow your patients in the 6-month to 1-year postoperative period, it is inevitable that they will experience a certain degree of rebound relaxation in the superficial tissues of the face and neck. This is despite excellent efforts on your part to give them a long-term tightened jaw line and neck line. This is very much a function of their inherent hereditary loss of elasticity, which occasionally requires a small procedure to improve the overall results. Submental tuck-up procedures to take care of small residual submental bands or fullness may be required in 5 to 10% of patients, depending on their preoperative condition and skin elasticity. This should be offered to them as part of the overall facelift experience. It has nothing to do with your overall technique. More rarely, the jowl, due to its fullness and presurgical condition, will revert enough to require a cheek tuck-up. This is the area most likely to disappoint patients in terms of overall results. Whatever area needs to be addressed must be to achieve the long-term results and satisfaction they had expected.

However, despite all good efforts in the first year, there are patients whose facelift results do not last as long as they desire. This is often related to the age of the patient, the condition of the facial skin, and heredity. Patients must understand that a secondary facelift is never required; that they will continue to age and look normal, but will always look better than if they had never had the facelift. They will always look younger than their chronological age. A repeat facelift can indeed be done in the future but is not usually necessary for 5 to 8 years postoperatively. Techniques similar to those used in the original facelift may be required, depending on the advancement of the aging process in all layers of tissue involved. Care must be taken in SMAS elevation in that branches of the facial nerve may be more proximally encountered than in a virgin face.

Complications

Hematoma

The most common complication following rhytidectomy is hematoma formation, occurring in 2 to 15% of patients.[11,12] Major hematoma requiring reoperation and exploration usually presents within the first 12 hours postoperatively (**Figs. 19.26 and 19.27**). Hematoma formation is heralded by pain and increasing facial edema. Interestingly, there is no correlation between the volume of intraoperative blood loss and hematoma occurrence. Conversely, hypertension

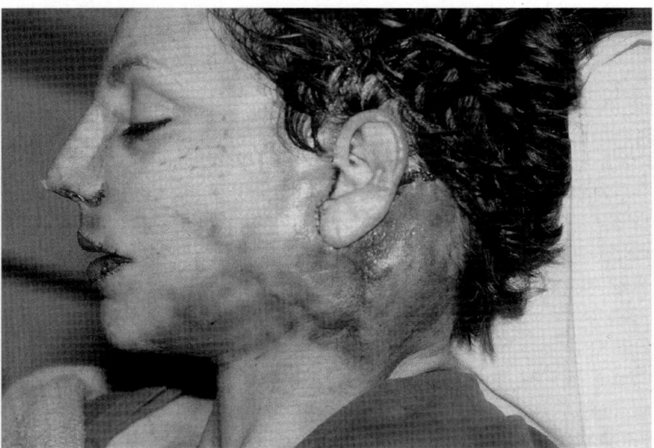

Fig. 19.26 Acute hematoma, 1 hour postfacelift.

predisposes to hematoma formation, increasing its incidence 2.6 times.[13] The importance of blood pressure control cannot be overstated; it must be closely monitored both intraoperatively and throughout the postoperative period. Particular attention should be paid to assuring a smooth emergence from anesthesia and avoidance of postoperative nausea, vomiting, and anxiety. Other predisposing factors associated with hematoma formation include ingestion of aspirin-containing products, nonsteroidal antiinflammatory drugs, high doses of vitamin E, some herbal medications, male sex, and the dominantly inherited Ehlers-Danlos syndrome.[14] A detailed list of aspirin-containing medications should be distributed because many of these products are not obvious. All of these products should be stopped at least 2 weeks preoperatively and remain so for at least 1 week postoperatively.

Certainly, management of patients taking anticoagulants needs to be performed in conjunction with the prescribing physician. We routinely screen all patients for prothrombin time, partial thromboplastin time, and platelet counts, referring those for further workup whose abnormal values are noted twice. Special precautions should be afforded to male patients as consensus among most facial plastic surgeons is that they are more susceptible to hematoma occurrence. Although not proven, it is felt to be secondary to an increased blood supply to the skin and beard follicles or possibly undiagnosed hypertension.

Delay in treatment may lead to skin flap necrosis, especially in those with a malignant rapidly expanding hematoma. In addition, the fluid accumulation may become an ideal culture medium, increasing the chances of infection. Often at the time of evacuation it is difficult to identify a single vessel at fault; rather, the norm is a diffuse oozing. Treatment should consist of clot evacuation, irrigation, exploration, and cautery of suspicious bleeding vessels. Suction drains and pressure dressing should be reapplied. These acute hematomas often necessitate opening of all or major portions of the incisions for visualization.

Minor hematomas are commonly encountered and probably account for the large range of hematoma percentages reported. Minor hematomas are usually identified in the first week postoperatively and consist of small pockets of fluid, usually in the postauricular area. Once liquified, these fluid collections can be evacuated by 18 gauge needle aspiration under sterile conditions. If not yet liquified a small opening in the incision line may be necessary to remove the clot using a Yankaur suction, and a Penrose drain is placed. These patients are refitted with a pressure dressing, and an extended course of antibiotics is prescribed. Undetected hematomas lead to fibrosis, skin puckering, and discoloration, which can take months to resolve (**Fig. 19.28**). If such a course is encountered, serial steroid injection of triamcinolone acetonide (Kenalog) 10 mg/mL or 40 mg/mL may be helpful.

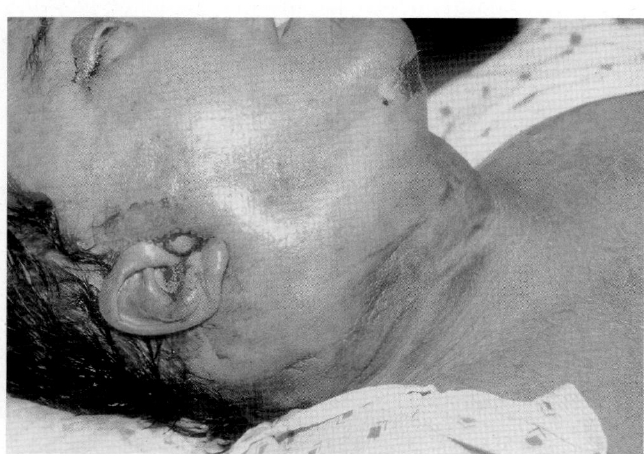

Fig. 19.27 Acute expanding hematoma, 3 hours postfacelift.

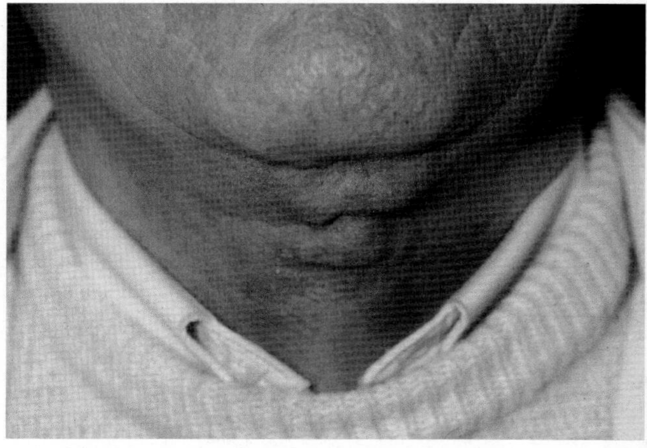

Fig. 19.28 Fibrosis and skin irregularities 2 months postoperative hematoma and seroma in submental neck.

Flap Necrosis

Skin flap necrosis occurs when blood supply to the distal ends of the random skin flap is compromised. Predisposing conditions include poor flap design, extended subcutaneous flap elevation, injury to the subdermal plexus, extensive closing tension, certain systemic medical conditions, large hematomas, and smoking. The postauricular area followed by the preauricular area are at greatest risk to necrosis. Deep plane and SMAS rhytidectomy benefit from decreased risk of necrosis by allowing for a more robust vascular flap and reduced closing tensions. The toxic effects of nicotine and smoking have long been identified as the most preventable cause jeopardizing blood supply in random skin flaps. The risk for flap necrosis is increased 12.6 times in smokers.[15] It is imperative that patients abstain from smoking for at least 2 weeks before and after surgery. Systemic diseases, such as diabetes mellitus, peripheral vascular disease, and multiple connective tissue disorders, may predispose patients to vascular compromise and warrant strong consideration preoperatively (**Fig. 19.29**).

Flap necrosis is preceded by venous congestion and flap discoloration. Frequent massaging of the area and an extended antibiotic course is instituted. Necrosis is usually accompanied by eschar formation. The compromised area should be treated conservatively with daily peroxide cleaning, limited debridement, and topical antibiotic ointment placement. Fortunately, most affected areas will heal nicely by secondary intention, but frequent postoperative visits and patient reassurance are necessary.

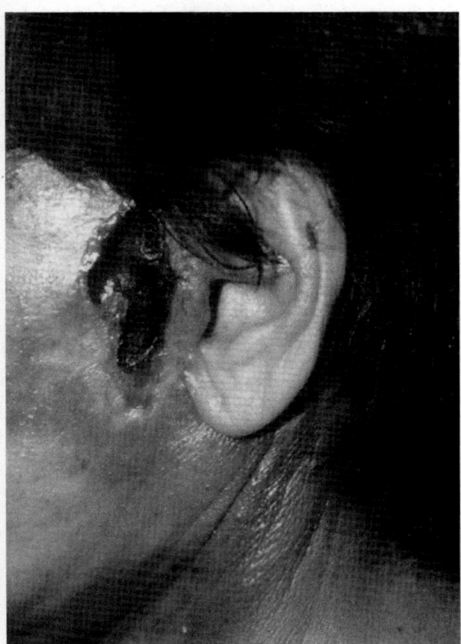

Fig. 19.29 Partial facelift flap necrosis in a patient taking immunosuppressive drug for severe arthritis.

Nerve Damage

A cervical sensory branch, the great auricular nerve, is the most commonly injured nerve in facelift surgery, occurring in 1 to 7% of patients.[16] Failure to repair the injury will lead to regional hypoesthesias and possibly painful neuroma formation.

Motor branch injury fortunately is much less common, occurring in 0.53 to 2.6% of facelift patients.[11,17] The two most commonly injured nerves are the temporal branch and the marginal mandibular branch of the facial nerve. The more commonly injured of the two branches depends on the method of surgery performed and the report cited. However, both of these injuries can lead to devastating outcomes for the patient and the physician. Rather than the single branch that is often depicted in textbooks, the temporal branch of the facial nerve consists of multiple rami. Anatomical studies have identified the rami crossing the middle portion of the inferior arch. Dissection in the immediate preauricular 10 mm of the arch and the distal 19 mm of the arch is safe. Unfortunately, injury to the facial nerve is usually not recognized at the time of surgery, but if it is, an attempt should be made for direct anastomosis. Microscopic assistance may be helpful. If immediate postoperative facial paralysis or paresis occurs, do not panic. Initially, allow at least a 4- to 8-hour time period for the effects of local anesthesia to dissipate. In the unfortunate event that a motor branch injury has occurred, surgical exploration and an attempt at anastomosis of these small distal branches is not practical. However, be reassured; clinical evidence has shown that a majority of these injuries (85%) will resolve with time.[6] The high incidence of recovery may be because injury was due to a temporary neuropraxia from local insult. Others theorize that, in the case of temporal nerve, multiple branches may allow for reinnervation even in the case of neurotemesis.[18] However, if recovery is not evident by at least 1 year, reconstructive options must be considered, including browlift, contralateral frontal branch neurolysis, and eyelid reanimation procedures.

Subplatysmal dissection places the marginal mandibular branch of the facial nerve at risk. Staying in the immediate subplatysmal plane and dissecting using a blunt scissors with the tines in a vertical motion will protect the nerve from injury. The nerve, which initially runs posterior and inferior to the mandible, enters a superficial plane over the mandible 2 cm lateral to the modiolus.[17] Dissection in the subcutaneous plane in this area is without benefit and fraught with disaster. Zygomaticus and buccal branch nerves surface at the anterior end of the parotid gland and

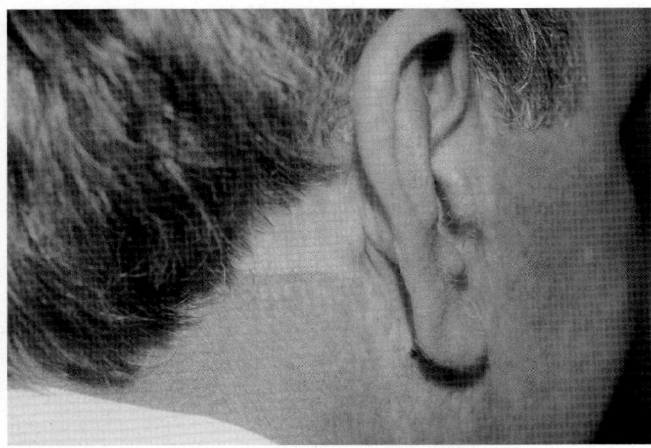

Fig. 19.30 Postauricular hypertrophic scar with widening due to excess tension on closure.

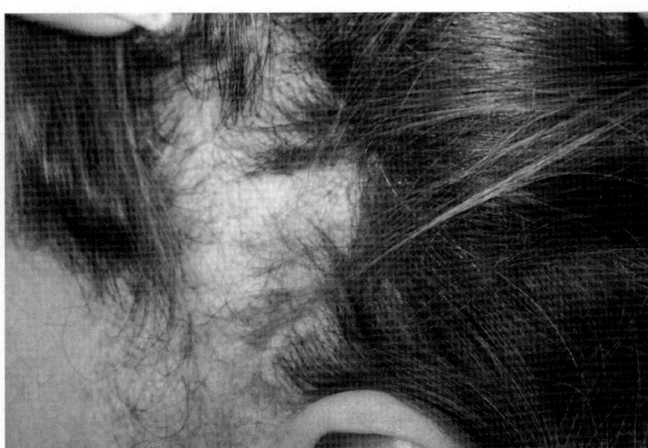

Fig. 19.31 Temporal alopecia secondary to excess tension and damage to hair follicles.

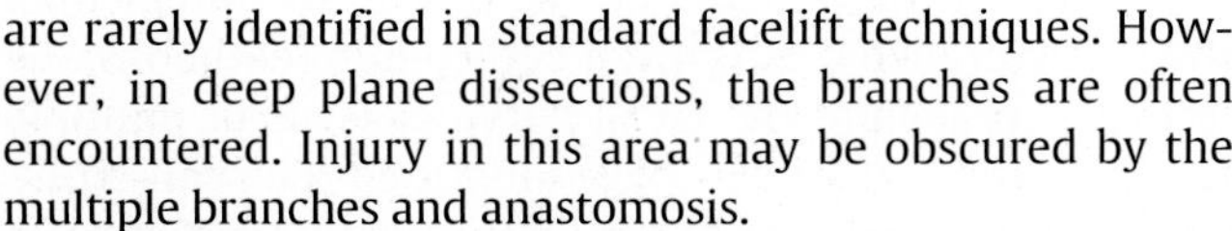

are rarely identified in standard facelift techniques. However, in deep plane dissections, the branches are often encountered. Injury in this area may be obscured by the multiple branches and anastomosis.

Bell's palsy recurrence has been reported following facelift surgery, and patients with a history of Bell's should be counseled to the possibility.[19] Total facial paralysis should be referred to the appropriate colleague for consultation. Electrical nerve testing may be of prognostic benefit in these patients, as well as in those with isolated motor branch injuries.

Hypertrophic Scarring

Hypertrophic scarring can occur if excessive tension is placed on flap closure and is most commonly associated with the isolated subcutaneous flap dissection (**Fig. 19.30**). Hypertrophic scarring can appear as early as 2 weeks postoperatively and usually occurs within the first 12 weeks. Interval intralesional injections with steroids can be helpful. Excision and primary closure of the hypertrophic scarring should be delayed for at least 6 months.

Incision Line Irregularities

Poor planning of incision lines may lead to loss of temporal tufts of hair, alopecia, excessive dog-ear formation, and hairline stair-stepping pattern. The temporal tuft of hair can be recreated with micrograft placement or through creative local flap designs. Hair loss is usually secondary to follicular shock (telogen effluvim), and reassurance can be given. However, if follicles were transected or tension on closure is excessive, hair loss may be permanent (**Fig. 19.31**). After a waiting period of 3 to 6 months, if there has been no hair recovery, alopecia areas may be excised and closed primarily. Micrografting can also help to camouflage the area.

Failure to advance and rotate the postauricular flap can lead to a stair stepping of the hairline. Fortunately, for most patients this area is easily hidden. However, if it is a problem for those interested in wearing their hair back, flap revision may be necessary.

Infection

Infection is rare in rhytidectomy patients. Mild cases of cellulitis will respond well to an extended antibiotic course covering the common variants of *Staphylococcus* and *Streptococcus*. These patients generally heal without sequelae. In the rare event of abscess formation, incision, drainage, and wound culturing are necessary (**Fig. 19.32**). Intravenous antibiotic administration should be considered.

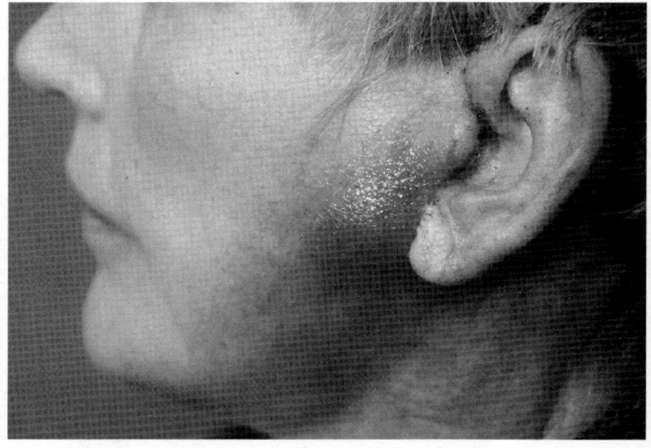

Fig. 19.32 Postoperative abscess and infection 1 week postfacelift.

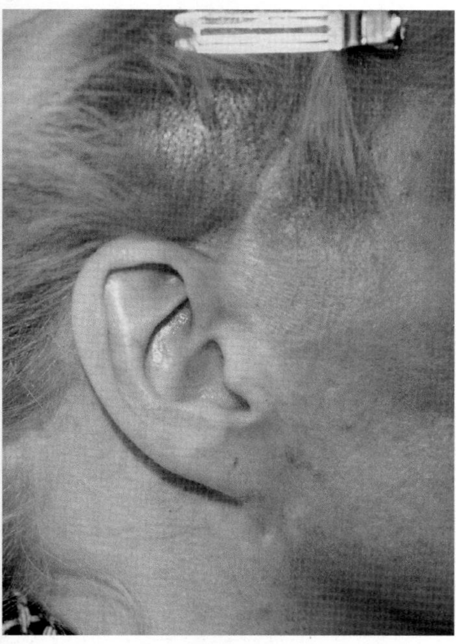

Fig. 19.33 Satyr's ear (devil's ear) with poor scar placement.

Earlobe Deformity

Satyr's ear (devil's ear) can occur if the earlobe is not tucked up properly. During the healing period, the earlobe is drawn inferiorly (**Fig. 19.33**). Poor placement of the earlobe can lead to the tell-tale signs of facelift surgery. Repair of the unnatural earlobe can be deceptively difficult. Classically, the best method to create the inferior lobe sulcus has been by V-Y plasty, delayed for at least 6 months after surgery. However most patients are not willing to accept a scar along the inferior portion of the lobule and a better method of repair is scar excision with tissue undermining and resuturing in an appropriate fashion allowing tension-free closure and tucking the lobule superiorly.

Submental Deformities

Cobra deformity is usually the result of overaggressive subdigastric/subplatysmal liectomy in addition to inadequate plastysma plication. Lateral standing cone deformities in the submental incision are often to do improper incision placement, direction, and shape. Attempts should be made to correct these; however, excessive chasing of these dog ears is not advisable.

Parotid Injury

Parotid parenchyma injury leading to sialocele or fistula formation is exceedingly rare. Intraoperative injury should be oversewn with available SMAS. Postoperative fluid accumulation may be treated with needle aspiration and pressure dressing. Persistent fluid accumulation may require a drainage procedure.

Sequelae of telangiectasias, hypertrichosis, and temporary hypoesthesias over the elevated flap tend to improve with time. However, persistent vascular lesions and problematical excessive hair can be effectively ameliorated with appropriate laser treatments.

References

1. Fomon S. The Surgery of Injury and Plastic Repair. Baltimore: Williams & Wilkins; 1939:1344
2. Skoog T. Plastic surgery: the aging face. In: Skoog, TG. Plastic Surgery: New Methods and Refinements. Philadelphia: WB Saunders; 1974: 300–330
3. Mitz V, Peyronnie M. The superficial musculoaponeurotic system (SMAS) in the parotid and cheek area. Plast Reconstr Surg 1976;58:80
4. Hamra ST. The deep plane rhytidectomy. Plast Reconstr Surg 1990; 86:53
5. Hamra S. Composite rhytidectomy. Plast Reconstr Surg 1992;90(1):1–13
6. Kamer FM. One hundred consecutive deep plane face lifts. Arch Otol Head Neck Surg 1996;122:17–22
7. Godin MS, Johnson CM. Deep plane/composite rhytidectomy. Facial Plast Surg 1996;12(3):231–239
8. Ramirez OM. The subperiosteal rhytidectomy: the third-generation facelift. Ann Plast Surg 1992;28:218–232
9. Psillakis JF, Rumley TO, Camargos A. Subperiosteal approach as an improved concept for correction of the aging face. Plast Reconstr Surg 1988;82:383–392
10. Baker SR. Triplane rhytidectomy. Combining the best of all worlds. Arch Otolaryngol Head Neck Surg 1997;123:1167–1172
11. Rees A. Complications of rhytidectomy. Clin Plast Surg 1978;5(1): 109–119
12. Lawson N. Male facelift. Arch Otolaryngol Head Neck Surg 1993;119: 539
13. Strath R, Raju D, Hipps C. The study of hematomas in 500 conservative facelifts. Plast Reconstr Surg 1983;52:694–698
14. Muenker R. Problems and variation in cervicofacial rhytidectomy. Facial Plast Surg 1992;8(1):33–51
15. Adamson P, Moran ML. Complications of cervicofacial rhytidectomy. Facial Plast Surg Clin North Am 1993;112:257–270
16. McKinney P, Katrana DJ. Prevention of injury to the great auricular nerve during rhytidectomy. Plast Reconstr Surg 1977;59:525–529
17. Liebman EP, Webster RC, Gaul JR, Griffin T. The marginal mandibular nerve in rhytidectomy and liposuction surgery. Arch Otolaryngol Head Neck Surg 1988;114:179–181
18. Gosain A, Sewall S, Yousif NJ. The temporal branch of the facial nerve: how reliably can we predict its path? Plast Reconstr Surg 1997;99(5):1224–1236
19. Castañares S. Facial nerve paralyses coincident with, or subsequent to, rhytidectomy. Plast Reconstr Surg 1974;54(6):637–643

20 Endoscopic Approach to the Brow and Midface

H. Devon Graham III, Vito C. Quatela, and Paul Sabini

Rarely does an individual's face age in an asymmetrical manner, yet for a long time surgery of the aging face was synonymous with a rhytidectomy and blepharoplasties. Often the upper and midface were inadequately addressed. Eventually surgeons began to focus attention on the contribution of brow position and often included a browlift as part of their treatment. The final piece of the puzzle emerged with the advent of endoscopic facial plastic surgery, first introduced in 1992 by Core et al[1] and by Liang and Narayanan.[2] The endoscope and its accompanying surgical instruments provide us with access to both the brow and the midface. It is now possible to treat an aging face without neglecting any component. In this chapter we will focus on the use of the endoscope in forehead and midfacial surgery. For clarification, an endoscopic forehead lift describes a procedure in which the dissection and suspension do not extend below the zygoma. When the dissection is carried below the zygomatic arch to the pyriform aperture and to the upper alveolar ridge, we refer to the suspension as a midface lift.

Smaller incisions, decreased risk of alopecia, and equivalent results to traditional browlifts are among the benefits of endoscopic forehead lifting. Dissection of the midface is an extension of this procedure and provides us with a means of repositioning the malar fat pad. Another advantage is the lack of hair-bearing skin excision, which serves to maintain the existing hairline. A relative disadvantage is the need for specialized equipment and an initial learning curve.

Forehead and Midfacial Anatomy

Surgeons often contrast surgical anatomy with anatomy to distinguish the unique perspective of the operative field from the gross anatomy laboratory. Endoscopic anatomy is an additional perspective that the facial plastic surgeon must master. Through the endoscope, familiar structures are viewed in an unfamiliar manner; therefore, a thorough grasp of the anatomy and the fascial planes is indispensable.

Scalp and Forehead Musculature

The scalp consists of the skin, subcutaneous tissue, aponeurosis or galea, loose areolar tissue, and periosteum. The galea is a tendinous inelastic sheet that connects the frontalis muscle to the occipitalis muscle. The galea merges laterally with the temporoparietal fascia, which is continuous with the superficial musculoaponeurotic system (SMAS) in the lower face. The frontalis muscle originates from the galea and inserts in the forehead skin. This muscle is the primary elevator of the brow, and its nerve supply is the frontal branch of the facial nerve. During the subperiosteal endoscopic forehead lift, the frontalis muscle is not visualized unless there is inadvertent tearing in the perisoteum. The depressor muscles of the brow include the paired corrugator supercilii, the orbicularis oculi, and the procerus muscle. The corrugator supercilii muscles are responsible for the vertical rhytides of the glabella. The procerus muscle, originating from the nasal bones, produces the transverse rhytides in the glabella.

Fascia

During an endoscopic forehead/midface lift, the dissection crosses several fascial planes. Endoscopic forehead lift occurs in both a supraperiosteal (laterally over the temporalis muscle) and a subperiosteal plane (in the forehead). Although midface lift has been described in a supraperiosteal plane,[3] we prefer a subperiosteal dissection. To safely approach the brow and the midface, it is necessary to have a thorough understanding of these different fascial planes.

The fascial planes are described in the order in which they are encountered during the procedure. The superficial temporal fascia, also known as the temporoparietal fascia (TPF), is located immediately beneath the skin and subcutaneous fat of the temporal area. The temporal artery and vein course superiorly within this fascial layer. Medially, over the forehead, the TPF merges with the galea. The TPF is continuous with the SMAS in the lower face. Beneath the TPF is the deep temporal fascia or true temporalis fascia. Dissection in the temporal region occurs on top of this fascia and therefore below the TPF. The deep temporal fascia splits at the level of the supraorbital ridge to become the intermediate temporal fascia and the deep temporal fascia with the intermediate fat pad in between (**Fig. 20.1**). The intermediate temporal fascia attaches to the superior edge of the zygomatic arch laterally

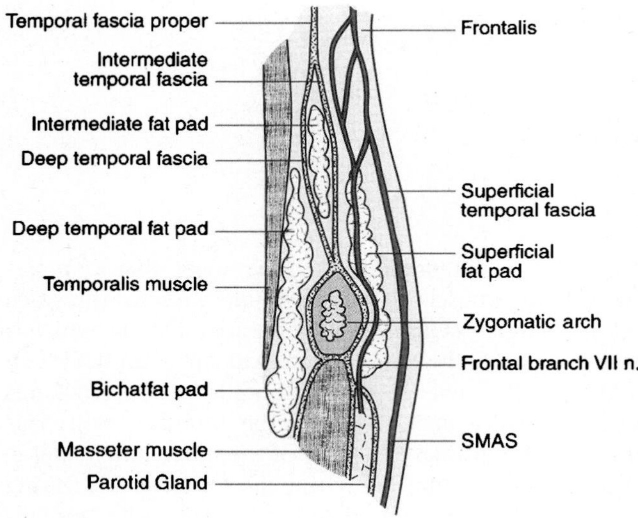

Fig. 20.1 A coronal slice at the level of the midzygomatic arch reveals the relationship of the fascial planes, facial nerve, and intermediate and deep temporal fat pads.

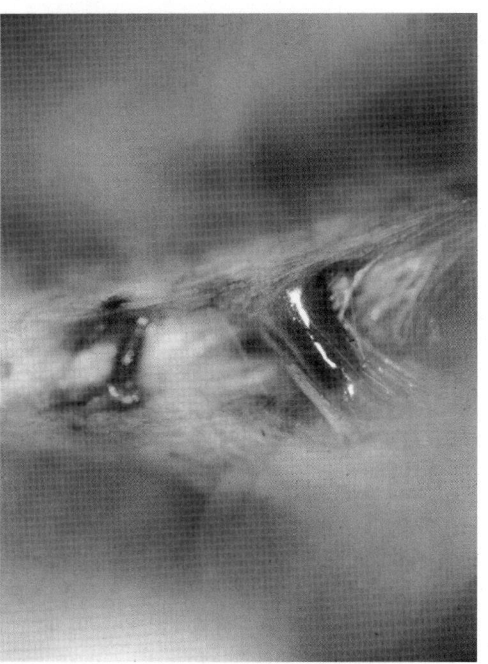

Fig. 20.2 During the temporal dissection, multiple vessels are encountered "bridging" the space between the temporoparietal fascia above and the deep temporalis fascia below. Often a substantially larger vessel (sentinel, vein on the right) is encountered adjacent to the superior edge of the lateral orbital rim. These veins indicate the precise location of a frontal branch of the facial nerve in the temporoparietal fascia above.

and the deep temporal fascia attaches medially. Deep to the deep temporal fascia is the deep temporal fat pad. Violation of the fascial covering of the deep temporal fat pad can result in atrophy of the fat and the appearance of temporal wasting.

Sensory and Motor Nerves in the Forehead

The facial nerve supplies all of the muscles of facial expression, including the corrugator and procerus. Sensation is provided by the trigeminal nerve. The supratrochlear and supraorbital branches emerge from the skull deep to the eyebrow. They are visualized and should be preserved when corrugator resection is performed. These nerves typically exit from the supraorbital notch or foramen; however, in up to 10% of cases one or both of these nerves may arise from a true foramen 1 to 2 cm superior to the orbital rim. In the latter situation, the nerves are at risk for transection if a blind non–endoscopic-assisted dissection is performed.[3]

The temporal branch of the facial nerve crosses the zygomatic arch halfway between the lateral canthus and the root of the auricular helix within the TPF. Sabini et al uncovered a more accurate means of identifying the precise location of the frontal branch of the facial nerve during endoscopic forehead surgery. A series of bridging vessels, including one larger sentinel vein, are encountered between the deep temporal fascia and the TPF during the dissection in the temporal region. These bridging vessels were shown to point to the frontal branch of the nerve as it coursed through the TPF[4] (**Fig. 20.2**).

Midfacial Anatomy

The malar prominence descends inferomedially with aging to deepen the nasolabial crease and expose the lateral orbital rim. It is composed of a subcutaneous malar fat pad with underlying orbicularis oculi muscle. Deep to this is the suborbicularis orbital fat (SOOF), which is intimately associated with the periosteum of the infraorbital rim and maxilla and the insertions of the zygomaticus major and minor muscles. Motor nerve supply to the muscles of the midface comes from the zygomatic and buccal branches of the facial nerve traveling along the deep surface of the muscles. Sensory innervation of the midface comes from the second division of the trigeminal nerve, the infraorbital nerve, which exits the infraorbital foramen, and the zygomaticotemporal branch of the trigeminal nerve that exits through the body of the zygoma.[5] The zygomaticotemporal nerve supplies the lateral temple region of the scalp and is encountered in a midfacial dissection, although it is rarely visualized. Transection of this branch, while not desirable, does not seem to adversely affect recovery of sensation in the lateral brow.

Aesthetics of the Orbital Complex

The surgeon should evaluate the orbital complex with consideration to all structures of the upper face. Consideration should be given to the brow position, glabella infrowning, amount of periorbital fat shifting that has occurred, and displacement of periorbital structures such as brow fat, lateral canthus, SOOF, and malar eminence.

The classic brow has its medial origin along a vertical line drawn through the nasal alar–facial junction. The lateral extent is along a line drawn from the nasal alar–facial junction through the lateral canthus. Both the medial and lateral brow should be at the same horizontal position. Generally, in women, the brow should arc delicately above the orbital rim, whereas in men it should be more horizontal. The male brow should rest on the superior orbital rim and the female brow extends well above this, with its highest point not at the lateral limbus, as often described, but at the lateral canthus (**Fig. 20.3**).[6] The more medial elevation tends to create an unnatural, surprised look. The glabella should not reveal infrowning at rest. The infraorbital fat should be slightly superficial to a plane tangential to the orbital rim. The inferior and lateral orbital rim should be padded with malar fat and SOOF. When the midfacial structures are ptotic and the orbital rim is exposed, the juxtaposition of prolapsed orbital fat and the fallen SOOF creates a double contour (**Fig. 20.4A**). Attempts to erase this double contour with lower-lid blepharoplasty and excessive fat removal result in a sunken, hollowed appearance. Other treatment options, including sub-orbicularis implantation and redistribution of orbital fat, camouflage the double contour; however, unlike

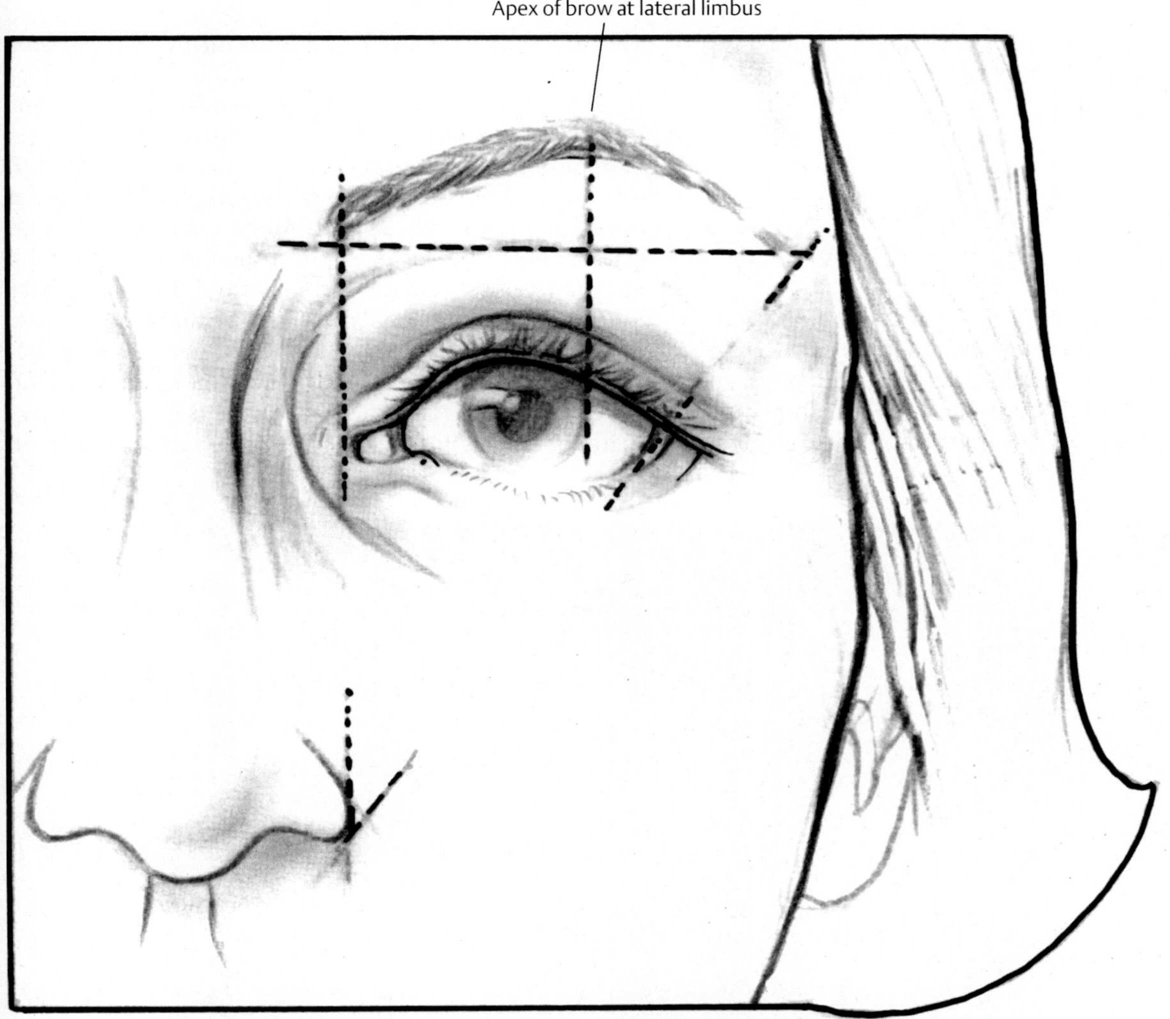

Fig. 20.3 Ideal brow position with the apex of the brow above the lateral limbus.

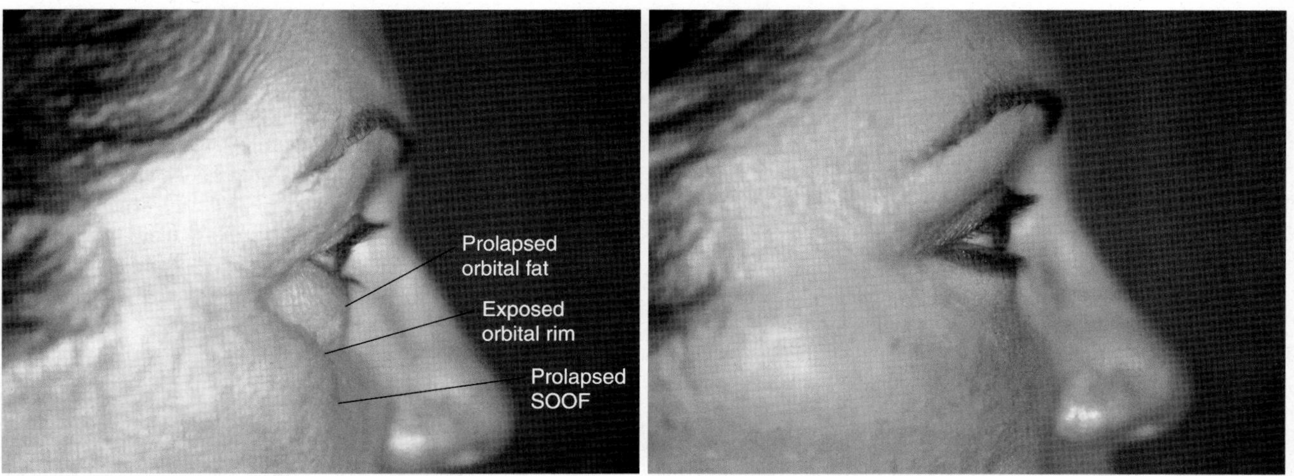

Fig. 20.4 (**A**) Juxtaposition of prolapsed orbital fat against the orbital rim creates a double contour. The lower half of the double contour is created with prolapse of the suborbicularis orbital fat, thereby exposing the orbital rim. (**B**) Postoperative midface lift shows correction of the double-contour deformity.

the midface lift, they do not have the advantage of restoring the fallen SOOF to its earlier youthful position (**Fig. 20.4B**).

Preoperative Assessment for Endoscopic Brow and Midface Lift

As with any facial plastic surgery procedure, patient selection is critical. Patient evaluation should begin with a thorough and complete history and physical examination. In the history, we typically elicit complaints about droopy eyelids and the appearance of weariness. The angry countenance of glabellar infrowning is also a frequent concern of the patient. Botulinum toxin injections are very effective for this; however, the endoscopic approach with partial resection of the corrugator supercilii and procerus muscles yields a more lasting result. Physical examination of the periorbital area may reveal brow ptosis, a ptotic SOOF, a ptotic malar fat pad, and scleral show. The latter is often seen in a patient who has had an overaggressive lower lid blepharoplasty with subsequent scleral show. The midface suspension reduces the downward pull on the lower lid and effectively raises the lower lid position and reduces scleral show (**Fig. 20.5**). A midface suspension can also improve mandibular jowling. If this were the patient's isolated

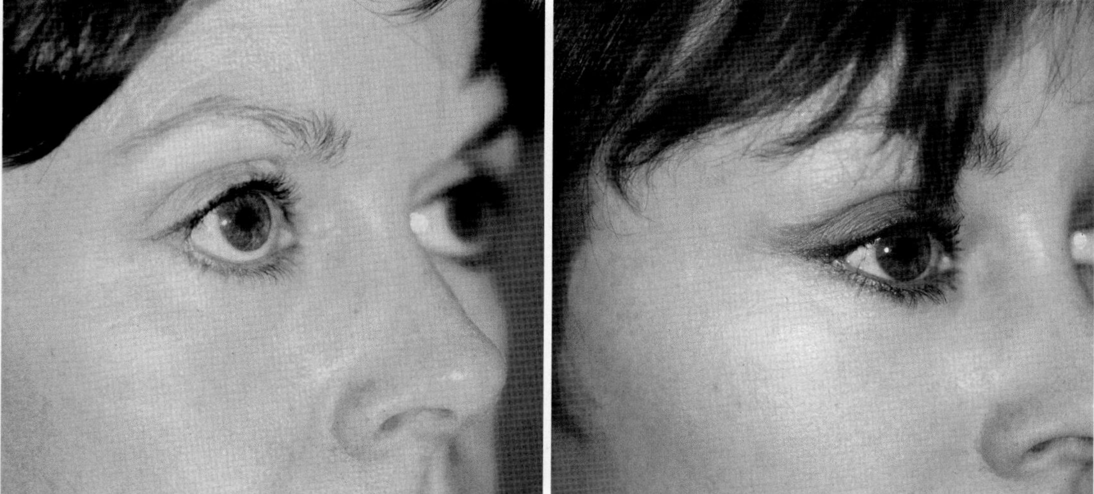

Fig. 20.5 Improvement of scleral show following a midface lift. (**A**) Preoperative. (**B**) Postoperative.

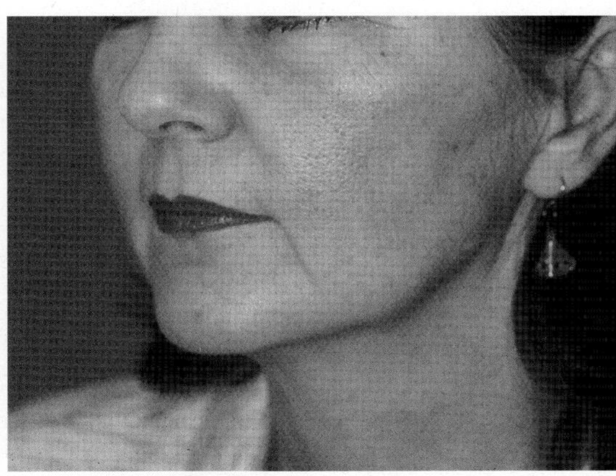
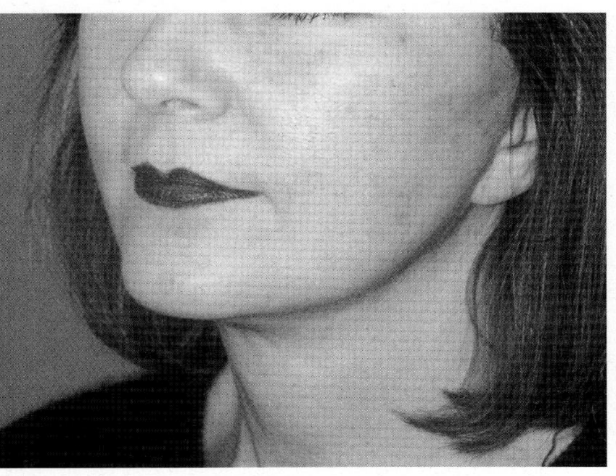

A B

Fig. 20.6 Moderate improvement in the mandibular jowl is a consequence of the midface lift. (**A**) Preoperative. (**B**) Postoperative.

complaint, we would not propose a midface lift in lieu of a rhytidectomy; nevertheless, we have observed dramatic improvement in mandibular jowling following the procedure (**Fig. 20.6**).

The ideal candidate is in good mental and physical health without systemic disease existing in an uncontrolled state. Preoperative screening for diseases and conditions that could adversely affect the patient's surgical experience is standard. Patient education is a powerful and effective tool for reducing anxiety and establishing realistic postoperative goals and should begin at the initial consultation. A patient who is a candidate for a midface lift deserves special mention. This procedure induces a more protracted period of postoperative edema (4 to 6 weeks) secondary to the subperiosteal dissection. These patients will require more intensive pre- and postoperative counseling to guide them through the normal healing of this deeper dissection.

Evaluation of the Brow

Matching patient deformity to surgical technique is tantamount to good results. Achieving the desired result makes for both a happy patient and a happy surgeon. Thus selecting an appropriate candidate for brow and forehead lifting requires careful evaluation of the aging upper face because one size most assuredly does not fit all. Not all patients are candidates for the endoscopic technique. Patients with a high hairline and a rounded frontal bone present a significant surgical challenge as it relates to the endoscopic technique. The endoscopes utilized are rigid and thus have limited angle of sight. A more appropriate approach for these patients would be a pretricheal or trichophytic technique, which would preserve the frontal hairline and actually offer the option of lowering it slightly.

When examining a patient for aging upper face, the patient should be in front of a mirror so that the surgeon and patient may together make observations and develop a plan. When evaluating the forehead and eyes, the patient should face forward with the head level, utilizing the Frankfort horizontal plane. The patient closes his or her eyes and relaxes the forehead for a full 15 to 20 seconds. Next the patient opens the eyes just enough to look straightforward without raising the brows. In this manner, the level of the brows can be evaluated in repose without the effects of exaggerated muscle contraction. The shape and position of the brows as they relate to the underlying orbit are then evaluated and compared with the classic brow. Usually in cases involving the aging upper face, the brow fat pad, which is designed to lie on and cushion the orbital rim, is ptotic, lying to various degrees on the upper eyelid. This is seen in the majority of these patients while in true repose and indicates the need for brow repositioning. A mistake that is often made is to overlook the brow position and simply address this as upper lid dermatochalasis. By performing an upper lid blepharoplasty without repositioning and fixating the brows, the natural spaces between the lateral canthus and lid crease as well as the lid crease and brow are shortened, sometimes markedly, leaving an abnormal appearance. It is important to diagnose brow ptosis if present because blepharoplasty performed without initial repositioning and stabilizing of the brow can exacerbate the problem and result in additional lowering of the brow. The upper third of the face should always be evaluated as a whole and not as individual components. Falling into this trap can lead to poor results and create problems that are virtually uncorrectable. A helpful guideline is to maintain a distance of ~1.5 cm between the eyebrow and the upper eyelid skin crease.[7]

Evaluation of the Midface

In the mid- to late thirties the aging process results in a descent of the midface. The malar prominence shifts inferomedially, resulting in exposure of the lateral orbital rim and a deepening of the nasolabial and alar groove. The SOOF descends revealing the inferior orbital rim and orbital fat, causing a double contour (**Fig. 20.4**). The endoscopic midface suspension effectively repositions these tissues and counters this aging process. This procedure reduces jowling and partially effaces the nasolabial groove. However, there is no benefit to the neck contour.

Surgical Technique for Endoscopic Brow and Midface Lift

Forehead and Brow

The forehead/browlift is the most common application for the endoscopic technique because of the excellent optic cavity created between the frontal bone and the soft tissues of the region. This surgery is designed to minimize the length of incisions thus preventing some of the common sequelae of the open approach such as scar alopecia and persistent forehead/scalp numbness as well as decreasing postoperative discomfort and recovery time.

Upon selection of an appropriate candidate for endoscopic brow and forehead lifting, a useful adjunct, though not a necessity is injection of botulinum toxin A to the central brow and glabella depressor muscles 2 weeks before the surgical procedure. This allows not only an excellent aesthetic improvement but also redraping and reattachment of the elevated periosteum unencumbered by depressor muscle action pulling the brows downward. Alternatively, in patients with strong and thick corrugator supercilli muscles these can be partially resected during the procedure. Care should be taken here, however, for overresection of the musculature of the glabellar region can lead to abnormal widening of the medial brows.

The procedure begins in the holding area prior to administration of anesthetic. The patient is examined in the sitting position and the brow position is assessed. The amount of medial brow elevation desired is measured. Despite its name, an endoscopic browlift does not always result in brow elevation. The procedure may be useful in a patient for whom glabellar infrowning is treated and brow position is kept neutral. The planned vectors of pull are determined and marked on the patient's forehead and temporal area. In women the vectors are typically more superior and lateral, whereas in men the emphasis is on a slightly more lateral than superior vector (**Fig. 20.7**). These markings are performed with the patient in the upright position, allowing gravity its full effect. If concomitant blepharoplasty is to be performed, the lower limb of the blepharoplasty incision corresponding to the existing lid crease is marked at this time. Additional preoperative marking includes the supraorbital notch bilaterally, glabellar infrowning lines, and the frontal branch of the facial nerve (**Fig. 20.8**).

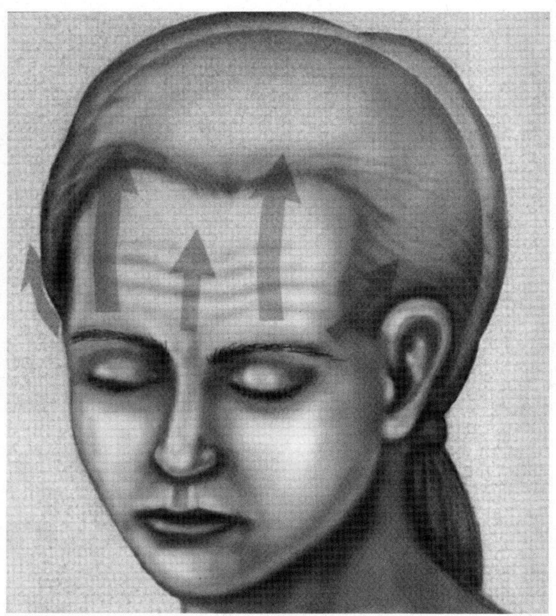

Fig. 20.7 Planned vectors of pull.

The patient is then brought to the operating suite where the equipment is arranged for proper visualization and function (**Fig. 20.9**). Intravenous analgesics are administered, followed by infiltrative local anesthesia using nerve and field blocks. After 15 or 20 minutes has been allowed for localization and vasoconstriction, two or three 1 to 1.5 cm incisions are made in a vertical fashion ~1.5 to 2.0 cm posterior to the anterior hairline in the midline and in the paramedian areas corresponding to the desired vectors of pull (**Fig. 20.10**). The vectors of pull, the need for central fixation, and the method of fixation all determine whether two or three incisions are used in this area. The incisions are made with a no. 15 blade through all layers down to the skull. The periosteum is then elevated carefully in the region of the incision utilizing a caudal elevator, with care taken not to fray or damage the periosteum. Complete continuity of the periosteum around this incision is necessary, as this will be vitally important when the time comes for fixation. Elevation then proceeds blindly utilizing endoscopic dissectors in the subperiosteal plane to a level ~1.5 cm above the orbital rims inferiorly, to the temporal lines laterally, and 3 to 4 cm posteriorly.

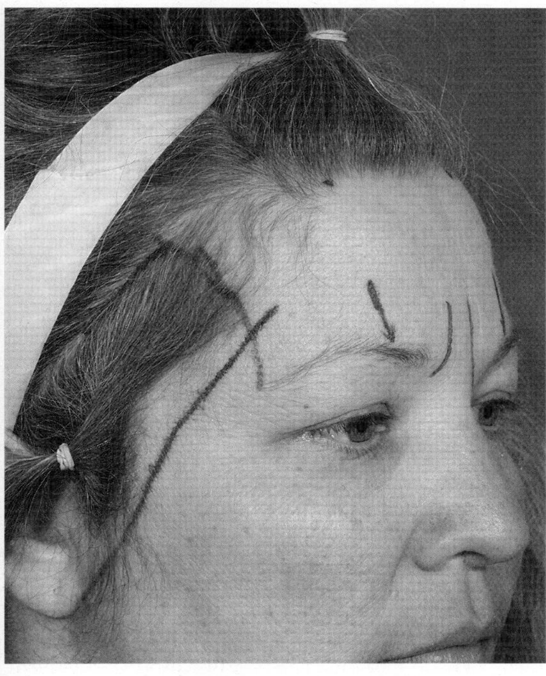

Fig. 20.8 Preoperative markings highlight the topographic course of the frontal branch of the facial nerve, the incisions, the location of the supraorbital notch, and the surface rhytides secondary to the action of the corrugator supercilii.

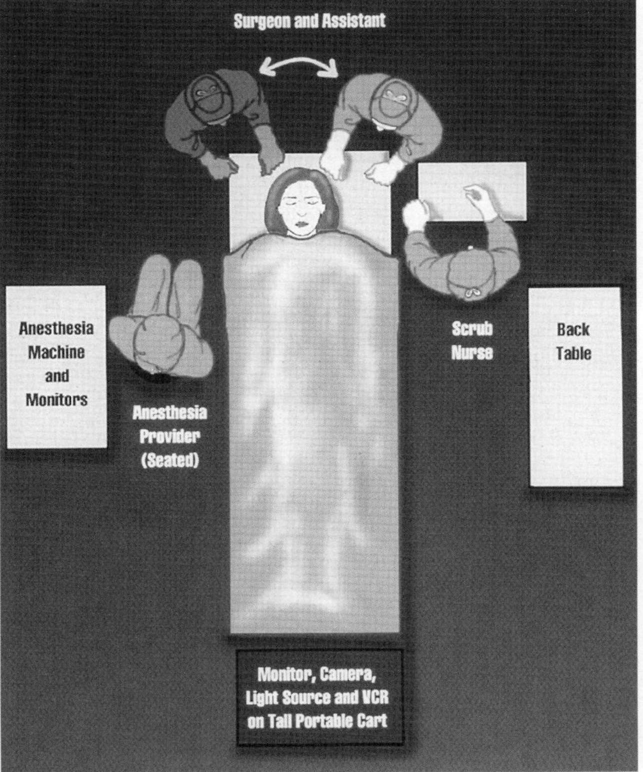

Fig. 20.9 Arrangement of operating room equipment and personnel during endoscopic brow- and facelifting.

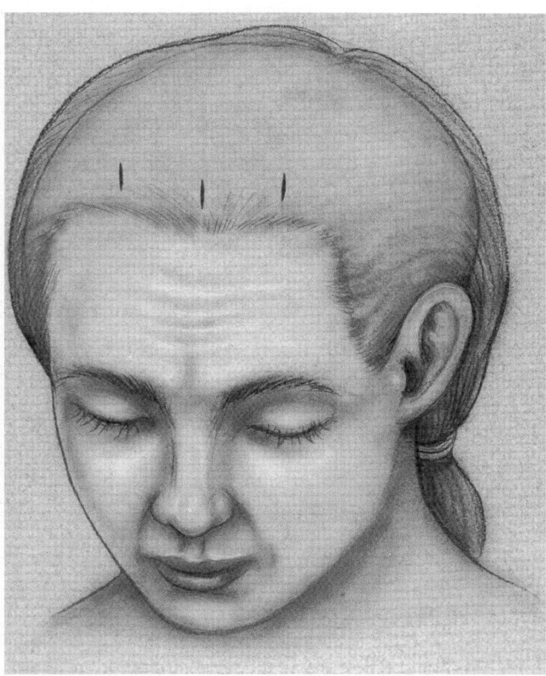

Fig. 20.10 Central pocket incisions.

At this point the 30-degree endoscope with sheath is introduced and the dissection proceeds inferiorly under direct vision. The visualized optic cavity should be almost bloodless, with excellent contrast between the underlying bone and overlying periosteum (**Fig. 20.11**).

Attention is directed to the area of the supraorbital neurovascular bundles. Care must be taken when dissecting toward this area as 10% of patients will have their neurovascular bundle exit through a true foramen as opposed to a supraorbital notch (**Fig. 20.12**). If corrugator and procerus resections are performed, the neurovascular

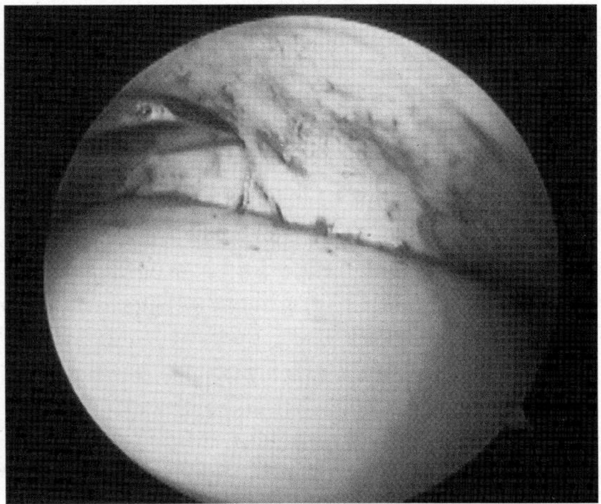

Fig. 20.11 Central optic cavity.

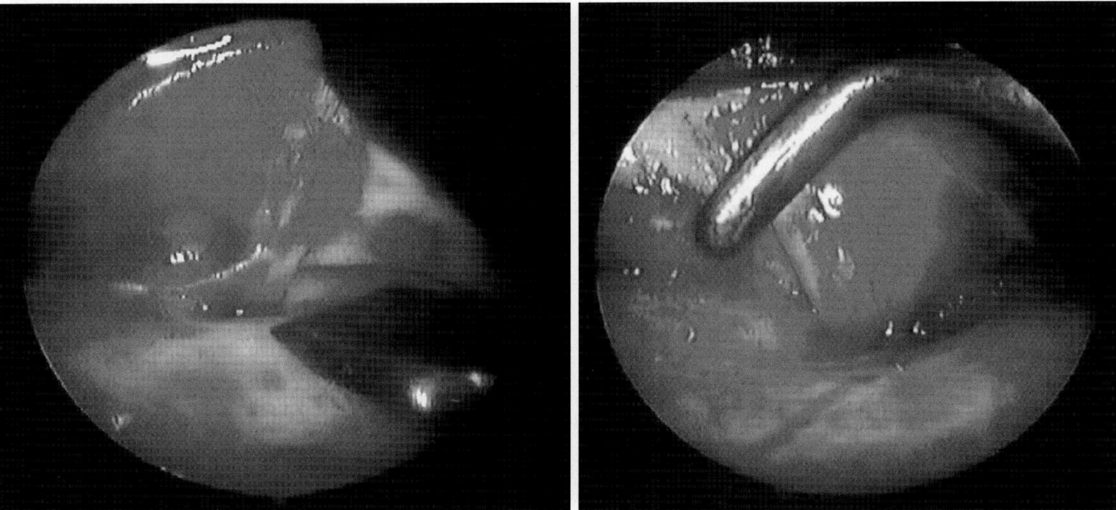

Fig. 20.12 (**A**) Supraorbital neurovascular bundle exiting skull through a true foramen. (**B**) Supraorbital neurovascular bundle exiting skull through the supraorbital notch.

bundle can be delineated with blunt dissection parallel to the fibers using a small dissector. A temporary transcutaneous stitch may be placed in the medial brow and lifted by an assistant to help open the pocket of dissection or the medial brow may be grasped between the thumb and index finger of the nondominant hand. If called for, the corrugator supercilii and procerus muscles are resected or simply divided. Cauterization is rarely needed for hemostasis. Orbicularis oculi myotomies may be performed by making multiple radial incisions in the muscle deep to the brow with a Colorado tip cautery, with caution to avoid the frontal branch of the facial nerve. We have performed unilateral orbicularis myotomies on the depressed brow to allow for increased single-brow elevation in patients with asymmetrical brows. Once the neurovascular bundles have been located, dissection is continued medially and laterally to these continuing inferiorly over the orbital rim releasing the periosteum at the arcus marginalis (**Fig. 20.13**). A gentle prying maneuver causes the periosteum to separate, revealing the overlying brow fat pad or retroorbicularis oculus fat (ROOF) (**Fig. 20.14**). It is critical that this periosteal separation be performed at the arcus marginalis, which lies below the level of the eyebrows. Only by a complete release at this level can the periosteum be elevated and resuspended as a bipedicled flap (**Fig. 20.14B**). In patients with very heavy brows and thick corrugator musculature, the muscle may be divided and a portion removed if warranted. After work is completed in the central pocket, attention is turned to elevation of the temporal pockets bilaterally. These will then be connected to the central optic cavity for completion of the elevation. The temporal pocket lies over the temporalis muscle and is bordered by the cephalic edge of the zygomatic arch inferiorly, the orbital rim anteriorly, and the temporal line superiorly.

Temporal pocket access is obtained through a 1.5 to 2 cm incision within the hairline of the temporal tuft corresponding to the superior and lateral vector of pull desired for the brow. If a midface lift is planned in addition, this incision is extended to ~3 to 4 cm. The incision is made through the skin, subcutaneous tissues, and TPF. The incisions should be beveled according to the direction of hair growth to preserve the follicular units and minimize alopecia (**Fig. 20.15**). The dissection proceeds inferiorly in the plane deep to the TPF and above the deep temporal fascia covering the temporalis muscle. This dissection is performed carefully using a

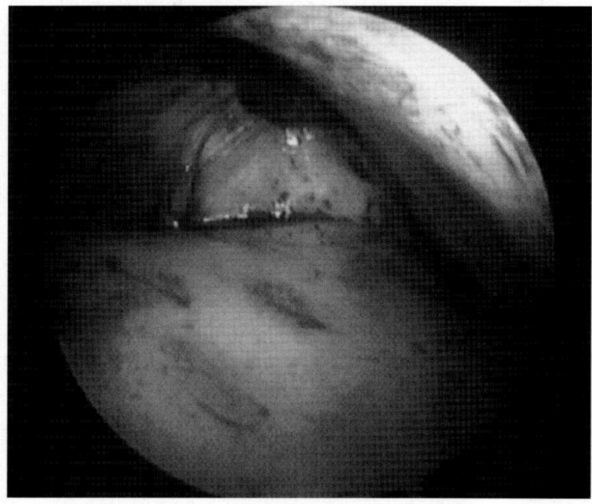

Fig. 20.13 The periosteum is released at the arcus marginalis.

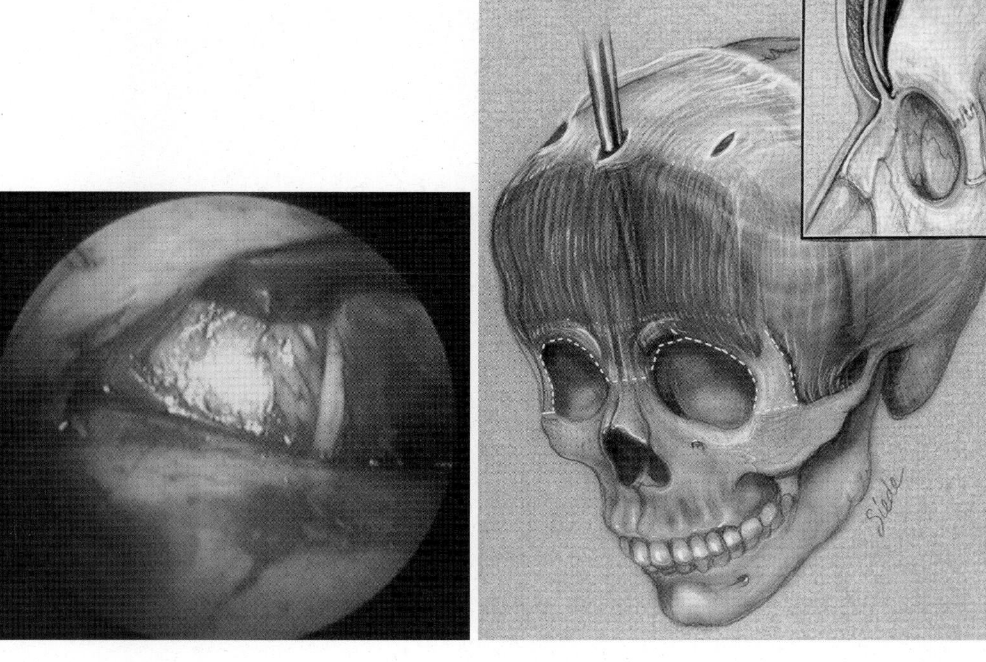

Fig. 20.14 (**A**) Release at the arcus marginalis reveals the retroorbicularis oculus fat (ROOF). (**B**) Complete release of the periosteum at the arcus marginalis bilaterally is essential.

blunt endoscopic dissector under direct visualization using the 0-degree endoscope.

In a standard brow and forehead lift, the inferior dissection is complete at a level just superior to the zygomatic arch approximating a horizontal line from the lateral canthus. A consistent landmark is the zygomaticotemporal vessel know here as the sentinel vein. The temporal pocket is then joined to the central pocket under direct visualization by sharp and blunt dissection of the temporal line attachments consisting of periosteum, galea, and temporal fascias (**Fig. 20.16**). The dissection to join the temporal and central pockets should proceed in a lateral to medial direction to maintain the proper plane. Once the two pockets have been joined under direct visualization superiorly, the dissection proceeds inferiorly using the beveled edge of the endoscopic elevator to elevate the temporal attachments. This is carried inferiorly to the area of the lateral orbital rim where dense connected tissue attachments to the bone are encountered. This conjoined tendon is sharply elevated in the subperiosteal plane using an endoscopic dissector, scissors, or endoscopic knife (**Fig. 20.17**). Once this dissection has been completed, the contralateral side is performed in the same manner. With this completed, the entire forehead–brow complex will be quite mobile and can be slid superiorly and inferiorly over the underlying bone.

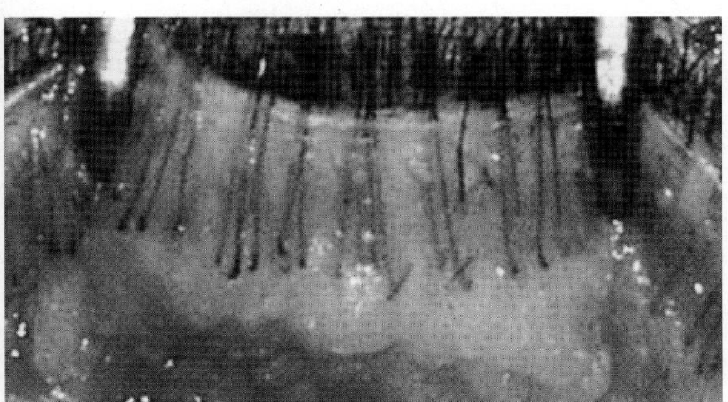

Fig. 20.15 A cut beveled in the direction of hair growth preserves the maximal number of follicular units and prevents traumatic alopecia.

After the entire elevation has been completed, the TPF is suspended through the temporal incision to the deep temporal fascia utilizing a heavy absorbable suture such as a 3–0 PDS (polydiaxonone). Maximal support in this area should be obtained, as this region cannot be overcorrected. After this has been completed bilaterally, suspension in the central region is begun. There are multiple approaches to fixation of the forehead, including permanent microscrews left under the scalp, cortical tunnels to fix the galeal pericranium with Prolene suture (Ethicon, Inc., Somerville, NJ), and external tied over foam dressing.[5] The method of

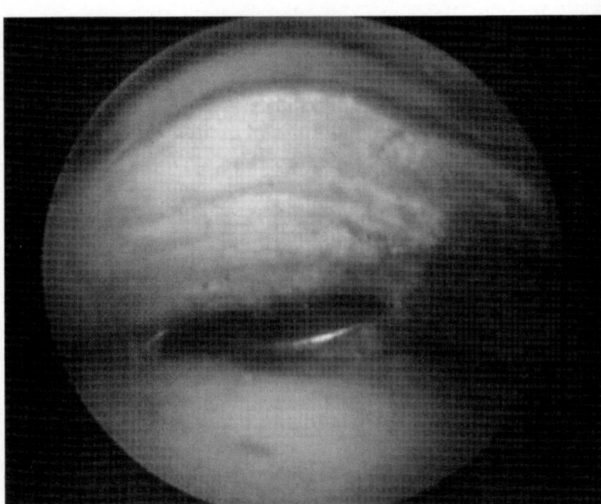

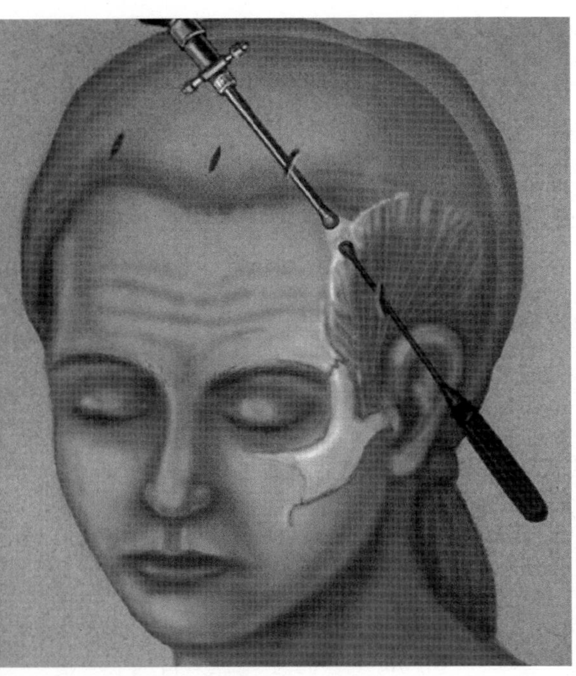

Fig. 20.16 Temporal pocket is joined to the central pocket from lateral to medial under direct visualization.

fixation reflects the surgeon's preference and should be based on patient comfort, surgical ease, and cost. One of the authors (HDG) preferred method depends on the length of the patient's forehead as well as hairline position. For the low to average hairline with short to average forehead length, the Endotine system (Coapt Systems, Inc., Palo Alto, CA) is the method of choice. For a patient with a slightly high hairline and/or a longer rounded forehead the method of choice is monocryl sutures tied around Bionx (Linvatec Biomaterials, Tampere, Finland) absorbable screws. In any case, complete surgical release of the entire forehead–brow complex is more significant than the method of suspension. Recent laboratory studies show that the elevated periosteum is completely reattached within a week and has achieved preoperative tensile strength within 12 days, indicating that long-term suspension may not be necessary.[8,9] In any event, final adjustments to brow height are made and suspension fixation is secured after the patient is brought to an upright sitting position, again allowing gravity its full effect. Incisions are then closed with skin staples. Computer analyses of long-term results have been gratifying and indicate that this technique will stand the test of time.

Fig. 20.17 The conjoined tendon often must be sharply dissected.

Endoscopic Midface Lift

The endoscopic forehead approach with midface suspension can be performed with or without elevation of the brows. In the majority of patients, the lower eyelid must be addressed during performance of an endoscopic forehead–midface lift, either with a lower lid skin pinch or periorbital laser resurfacing. This is because suspension of the midface elevates the cheek, frequently resulting in a bunching of skin under the eye. If lower lid fat removal is required, this is performed through a transconjunctival approach prior to placing the midface suspension stitches;

otherwise the lower lid will be too tightly approximated to the globe to allow access.

Attention is first directed to the lateral incision. This incision is made with care to bevel the incision so as not to transect the hair follicles. The incision is carried down to a level just superficial to the temporalis fascia proper. A set of endoscopic instruments is necessary for this dissection. A double hook is used to elevate the skin, whereas a no. 4 Ramirez or flat dissector is used to create a plane of dissection just superficial to the temporalis fascia proper. This plane can be elevated blindly to the superior aspect of the ear and posteriorly where it will become a subperiosteal dissection after leaving the temporalis muscle. A lighted Aufricht retractor provides better optical visualization. The dissection then continues inferiorly along the temporal line to the superior orbital rim as this subperiosteal plane is safe from the frontal branch of the facial nerve. The same dissector is then used to continue the plane of elevation over the temporalis fascia proper anteriorly using a gentle sweeping motion, keeping the temporal line as a landmark. Care must be taken here not to go too deep into the infratemporal fat, which can cause trauma and temporal wasting. Superficial dissection can traumatize the frontal nerve.

Multiple penetrating vessels will be encountered during the dissection (**Fig. 20.2**). They indicate the location of the frontal branch of the facial nerve. Dissect completely around the vessels and then, with traction, bipolar the deep aspect of the vessel so as to not cause thermal conduction trauma to the nerve that is superficial. This dissection is continued down to the superior orbital rim, and the periosteum is elevated off of the lateral aspect of the superior orbital rim. A bimanual elevation with one hand over the upper lid is performed to release the arcus marginalis. Attention is then directed to dissection to the zygomatic arch. The temporalis fascia proper splits at approximately the level of the supraorbital ridge to form an intermediate fascia and a deep temporal fascia with the intermediate temporal fat pad in between. Some surgeons prefer to continue the dissection in the middle of the intermediate fat pad, but our preference is to stay just superficial to the deep temporal fascia and elevate the intermediate temporal fat pad (**Fig. 20.18**). This plane can be more easily defined approaching the posterior one third of the zygomatic arch with moderate downward pressure on the flat dissector as the temporal fascia is thicker and stronger posteriorly. This plane of dissection is continued down to the superior edge of the zygomatic arch along its entirety. A lateral cuff of tissue of ~1 cm is preserved at the lateral canthus, depending on the amount of mobility desired in this region. The periosteum is incised at the superior aspect of the zygomatic arch with the dissector or a scalpel. A down-curved dissector is used to elevate the periosteum over the arch and release some of the masseteric aponeurosis attachments to the inferior aspect of the zygomatic arch. The dissection is then continued subperiosteally over the maxilla in a blind fashion. A finger is kept on the infraorbital foramen to protect the nerve as subperiosteal elevation is performed inferior to the nerve. An additional finger is placed over the inferior globe as dissection is performed along the infraorbital rim just superior to the infraorbital nerve (**Fig. 20.19**). Dissection is carried all the way to the nasal bones and piriform aperture. Bimanual elevation of the

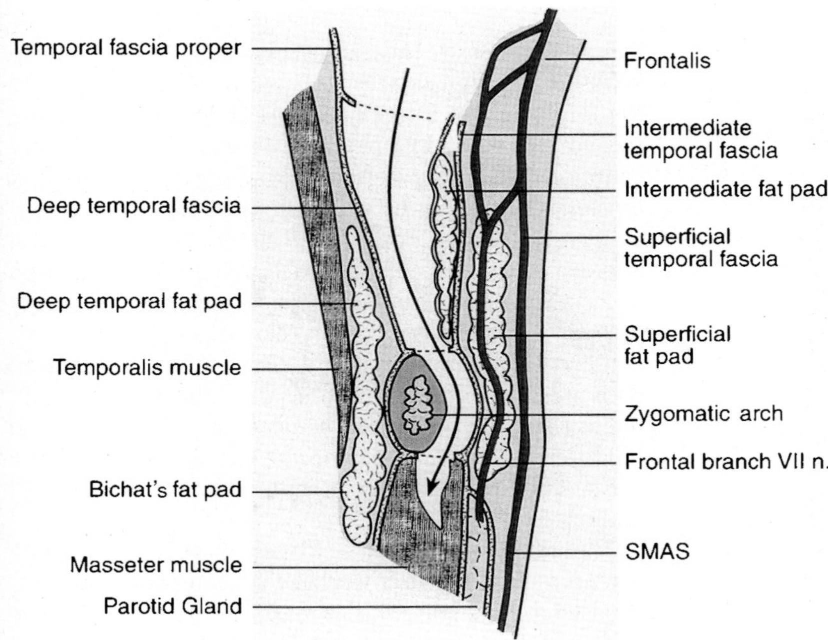

Fig. 20.18 The approach to the midface hugs the deep temporal fascia and elevates the intermediate temporal fat pad. This provides maximal protection to the frontal branch of the facial nerve. Violation of the intermediate fat pad impedes visualization; however, it does not seem to contribute to temporal wasting.

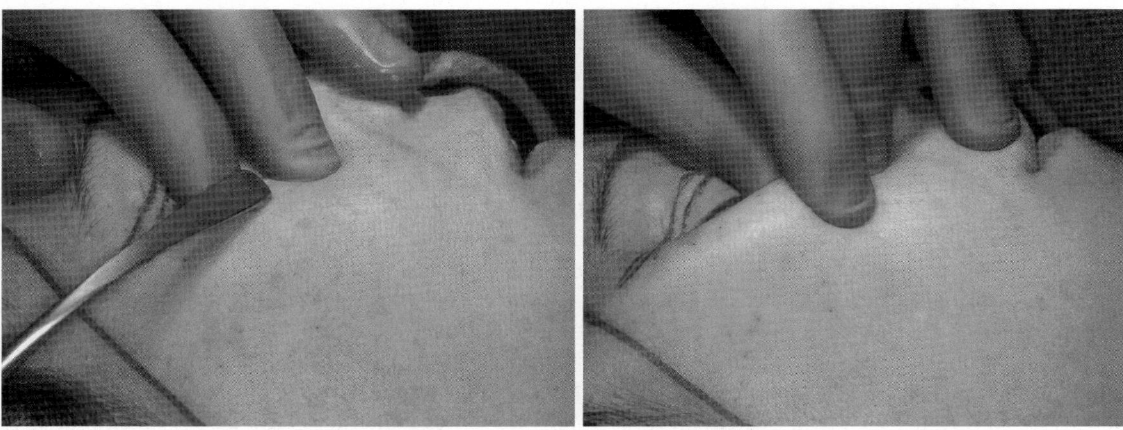

Fig. 20.19 The path of the midface dissection hugs the infraorbital rim. Placing a finger at the superior edge of the rim protects the globe.

cheek with the retractor further helps to release the periosteum, which is then tethered on the infraorbital nerve. A gauze is then placed in this cavity for hemostasis, and the identical procedure is performed on the other side.

The midface/SOOF is suspended with a large absorbable stitch placed through the periosteum just lateral to the zygomaticotemporal foramen and back to the temporalis fascia proper. Care is taken not to overcorrect with this suture. A second stitch is then placed proximal to the frontal nerve and back to the deep temporalis fascia. The excess skin in the temporal region is then smoothed out by placing three stitches in the superficial temporal fascia of the anterior skin edge and tacking it to the temporalis fascia proper posterosuperiorly. The skin is then closed with vertical mattress sutures to prevent a step-off deformity. Initially the skin will be puckered at this incision, but this will flatten relatively quickly and no skin excision is required.

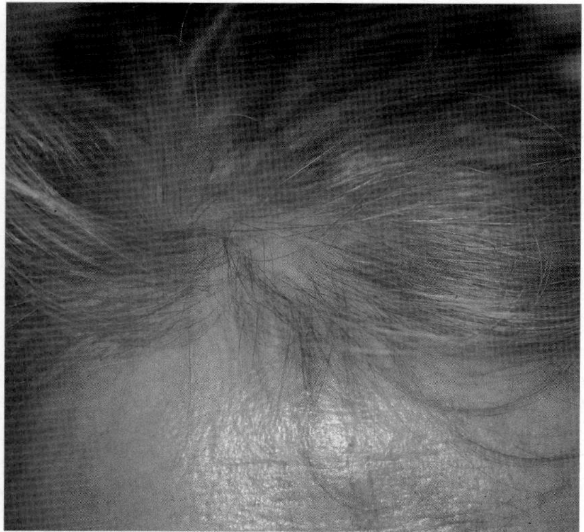

Fig. 20.20 Incisional alopecia can result in a generalized thinning. Typically this improves in 3 to 6 months.

A single small suction drain is placed at the level of the brows and exits laterally in the scalp. This is removed on postoperative day 1. Paper tape is placed on the forehead to minimize edema followed by a facelift pressure dressing, which is removed on postoperative day 1. Subperiosteal midface dissection induces more facial edema, and patients have to be prepared for this as well as a mild temporary distortion in the lateral canthal area. Patients are told that they will be presentable with makeup in 2 to 3 weeks but that edema and distortion do not completely resolve for 6 weeks.

Complications

Some numbness is invariably present following a forehead lift but typically resolves within 2 to 6 months in the forehead and 9 to 12 months at the crown. During recovery of sensation, paresthesia and itching are very common. There can be alopecia along the incisions if tension is placed during suspension, but hair growth generally returns in ~3 months (**Fig. 20.20**). Transient frontal nerve palsy has occurred and is felt to be a function of either thermal trauma secondary to electrocautery or overzealous temporal pocket elevation. An abnormal brow position may occur, which is initially treated with massage. If this does not achieve the desired result, releasing of the tissue may be necessary. Hematomas in the forehead or scalp may occur; however, the use of a closed-suction drain and/or compression dressings will minimize this.

The midface lift has a longer recovery and more potential pitfalls than a forehead lift. An expectation (as opposed to a complication) is masticatory tenderness. The release of the masseter combined with the suturing in the

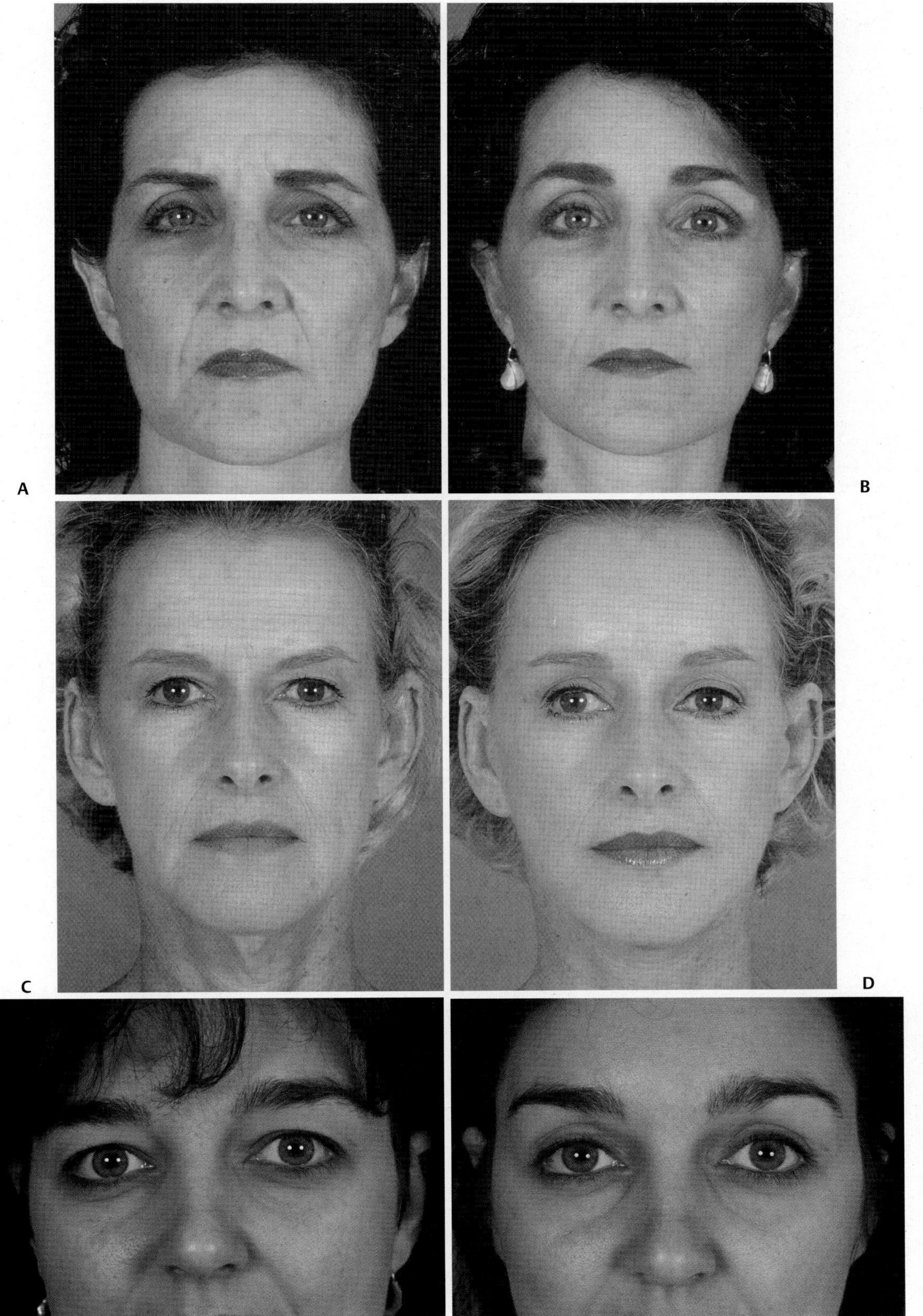

Fig. 20.21 Pre- and postoperative view (**A,B**) of a patient following endoforehead/midface lift. (**C,D**) Pre- and 1-year postoperative view of a patient following endoforehead lift along with facelift. (**E,F**) Pre- and 1-year postoperative view of a patient following endoforehead lift and upper blepharoplasty.

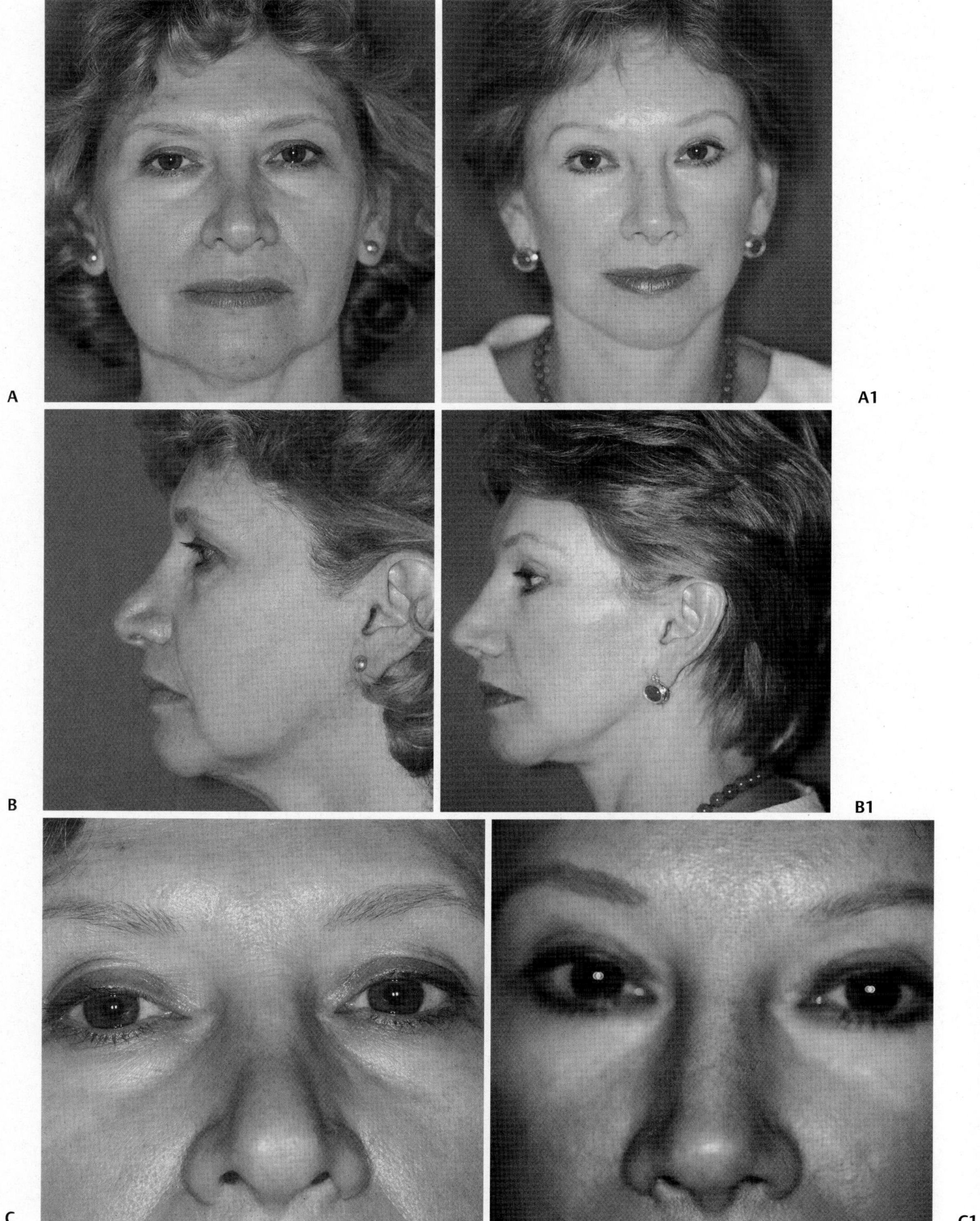

Fig. 20.22 Pre- and 1-year postoperative views of a patient following a forehead/midface lift. Close-up lateral views (**D**) highlight the double contour and its correction. The patient also underwent a rhytidectomy and rhinoplasty. The rhytidectomy and midface lift complement one another in their ability to improve the nasolabial and melolabial folds (**A–C**).

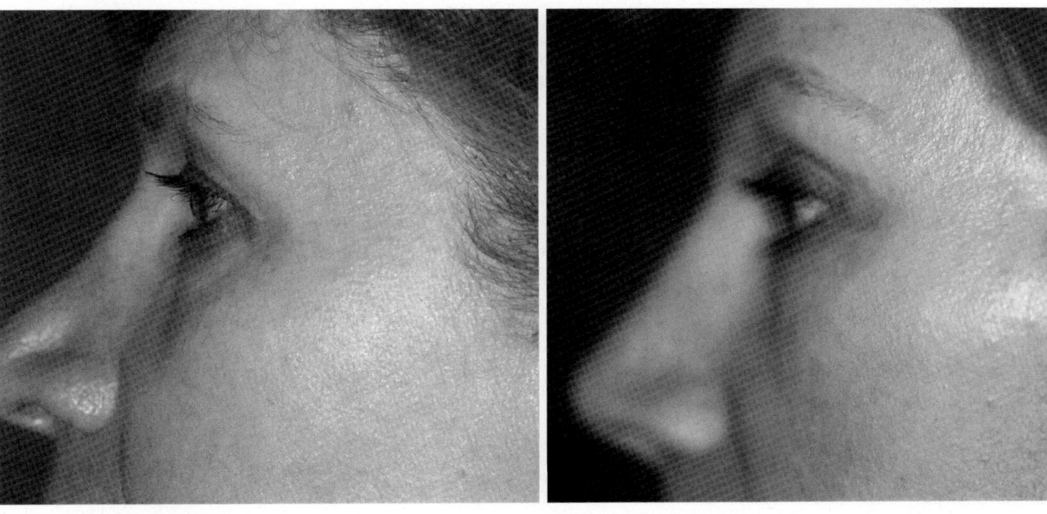

Fig. 20.22 (*Continued*)

temporalis muscle can trigger muscle spasm and simulate temporomandibular joint syndrome. This typically resolves within the first week. The patients are usually presentable at 3 weeks, but it is usually ~6 to 8 weeks before edema has resolved. Periorbital edema and chemosis may linger beyond 6 weeks postoperatively. Photosensitivity as well as dry-eye syndrome may occur in this context. As the edema resolves, orbicularis function returns to normal and the lower lid resumes its apposition to the globe. Asymmetry of eye shape is always present initially but usually resolves as patient massage coupled with the strong circular action of the orbicularis oculi muscle brings the lids back toward their baseline. Revision prior to 6 months is not recommended.

Summary

The endoscope and its accompanying equipment have provided facial plastic surgeons the opportunity to treat the aging brow and midface with smaller incisions and decreased risk of alopecia. The results are as reliable and impressive as those of more traditional techniques (**Figs. 20.21 and 20.22**). The more prolonged edema associated with the midfacial dissection does make the recovery longer, however, correction of the infraorbital complex at this time seems to justify the intervention.

References

1. Vasconez LO, Gore GB, Gamboa-Bobadilla M, et al. Endoscopic techniques in coronal brow lifting. Plast Reconstr Surg 1994;94:788–793
2. Liang M, Narayanan K. Endoscopic ablation of the frontalis and corrugator muscles: a clinical study. Plast Surg Forurm 1992;15:54
3. Isse NG. Endoscopic facial rejuvenation. Clin Plast Surg 1997;24(2):213–231
4. Sabini P, Wayne I, Quatela VC. Anatomic guides to precisely localize the frontal branch of the facial nerve. Presented at the Spring Meeting of the American Academy of Facial Plastic and Reconstructive Surgery; May 2000; Orlando, Florida
5. Ramirez OM. Endofacelift: subperiosteal approach. In: Ramirez OM, Daniel RK, eds. Endoscopic plastic surgery. New York: Springer-Verlag; 1996:109–126
6. Cook TA, Brownrigg PJ, Wang TD, Quatela VC. The versatile midforehead browlift. Arch Otolaryngol Head Neck Surg 1989;115:163–168
7. Connell BF, Lambros VS, Neurohr GH. The forehead lift: techniques to avoid complications and produce optimal results. Aesthetic Plast Surg 1989;13:217–237
8. Brodner DC, Crawford Downs J, Graham HD III. Periosteal readhesion after browlift in New Zealand white rabbits. Arch Facial Plast Surg 2002;4(4):248–251
9. Kim JC, Crawford Downs J, Azuola ME, Devon Graham H III. Time scale for periosteal readhesion after brow lift. Laryngoscope 2004;114(1):50–55

21 Surgical Approaches to the Midface Complex

Keith A. LaFerriere and Richard D. Castellano

Correction of the aging midface is now becoming an integral component of comprehensive facial rejuvenation. This central feature has largely been ignored through most of the history of facial plastic surgery. However, over the past 15 years midfacial rejuvenation has evolved as a versatile and indispensable adjunct to the field of facial plastic surgery. This chapter will define midface anatomy and the aging changes of the midface, review the history of midface procedures, and describe the common approaches currently utilized for rejuvenation.

Anatomy

Knowledge of the layers of midface and structures contained within is essential to understanding the aging changes and their correction. The boundaries of the midface include the inferior orbital rim and nasojugal groove superiorly, the melolabial fold inferomedially, and the zygoma laterally. The layers of the midface in the superior aspect differ from the layers within the inferior aspect. Starting from the "floor" to the "roof" of the superior midface, the layers include the bone, periosteum, preperiosteal fat, suborbicularis oculi fat (SOOF) pad, orbicularis oculi and facial muscles (levator labii superioris alaque nasi, levator anguli oris), subcutaneous fat, and skin. In the lower midface the layers include the bone, periosteum, facial musculature (zygomaticus major and minor), malar fat pad, subcutaneous fat, and skin (**Fig. 21.1**).

The layers of the midface attenuate and fuse inferomedially to form the melolabial or nasolabial crease. The malar fat pad is located between the inferior border of the orbicularis and the melolabial fold. This malar fat has been found to be anatomically indistinguishable from the subcutaneous fat of the infraorbital cheek skin. Sasaki and Cohen[1] performed cadaver studies that indicated the greatest average depth of the malar fat pad was ~6 mm, whereas the thickness at the melolabial fold was 2.2 mm. There are no demonstrable connections between the malar fat pad and the underlying superficial musculoaponeurotic system (SMAS) in this area.

In addition to these layers, three fascial connections are present that serve to attach the dermal roof to the bony floor. This includes the lateral orbital thickening, which is broadly based band over the frontal process of the zygoma, the orbicularis retaining ligament, which separates the prezygomatic space from the preseptal space of the lower eyelid, and the zygomatic-cutaneous ligaments, which originate from the inferior aspect of the zygoma (**Fig. 21.2**). For purposes of review, the prezygomatic space is bounded by these three ligaments, and the preseptal space is the tissue plane between the orbital septum and the orbicularis oculi.[2] The lateral orbital thickening and the orbicularis retaining ligament condense with one another, and serve as a durable anchor that tethers the midfacial structures from a superolateral position. Penetrating through the periosteum and preperiosteal fat, the second division of the trigeminal nerve ramifies into the cutaneous sensory branches of the midface.

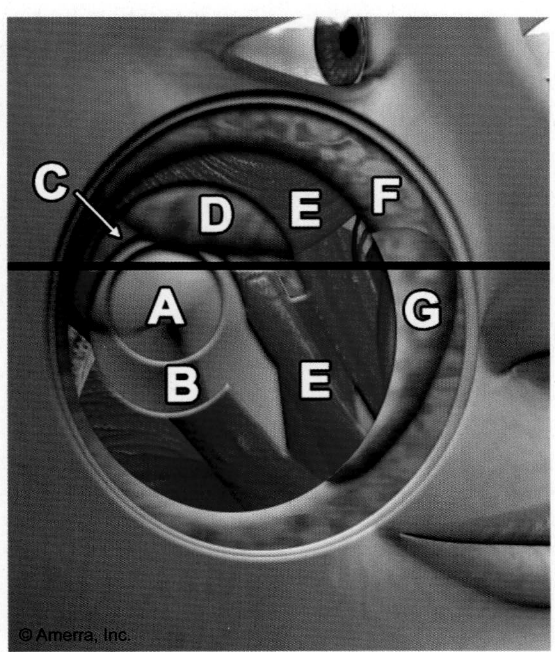

Fig. 21.1 Layers of the midface. In the upper midface, one can appreciate (from deep to superficial) the bone (A), periosteum (B), preperiosteal fat (C), suborbicularis oculi fat pad or SOOF (D), facial musculature (E: orbicularis oculi, levator labii superioris alaque nasi, and levator anguli oris), subcutaneous fat (F), and skin. In the lower midface the layers include the bone (A), periosteum (B), facial musculature (E: zygomaticus major and minor, levator labii superioris alaque nasi, and levator anguli oris), malar fat pad (G) and subcutaneous fat (F), and skin.

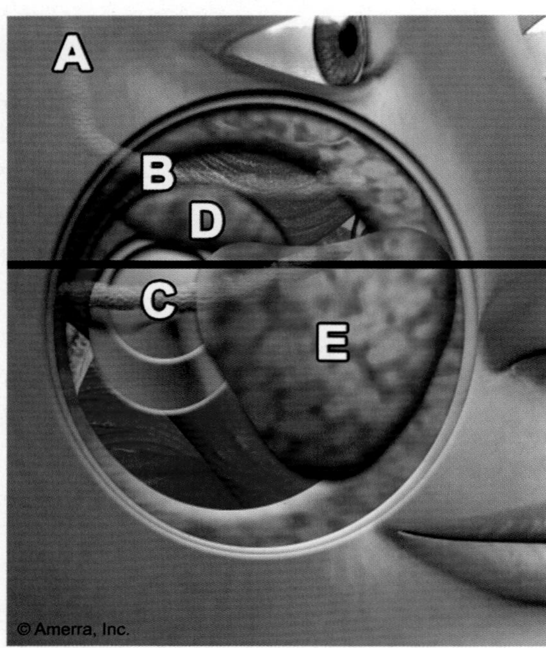

Fig. 21.2 Anatomical position of the facial ligaments and fat pads. Lateral orbital thickening (A), orbicularis retaining ligament (B), zygomatic-cutaneous ligaments (C), SOOF (D), and the malar fat pad (E).

Sensory innervation of the midface is supplied by the second division of the trigeminal (infraorbital nerve) along with the zygomaticofacial and zygomaticotemporal nerves. Sacrifice of the infraorbital nerve should be avoided as it is usually accompanied by permanent dysesthesia of the midface. Preservation of the zygomaticofacial and zygomaticotemporal nerves is also preferable, though the resultant sensory deficit tends to be temporary.

Aging Changes

Specifically, there are seven anatomical changes that signify midface aging: exposure of the nasojugal groove, paucity of soft tissue over the inferior orbital rim, presence of a double convexity of the lower eyelid/cheek complex, loss of malar fullness, increased distance from the lower eyelid to the malar fat pad, an inferomedial descent of the malar fat pad resulting in a deepening of the nasolabial fold, and a lateral infraorbital crescentic hollow. Often this is accompanied by a pseudoherniation of the orbital fat, which will accentuate the lower eyelid/cheek double convexity and prominence of the orbital rim (**Figs. 21.3 and 21.4**).

This compromise of the anatomical integrity is attributable to a combination of factors, including solar damage, thinning of the dermis, redistribution or atrophy of fat, and gravitational forces. The result is inferomedial

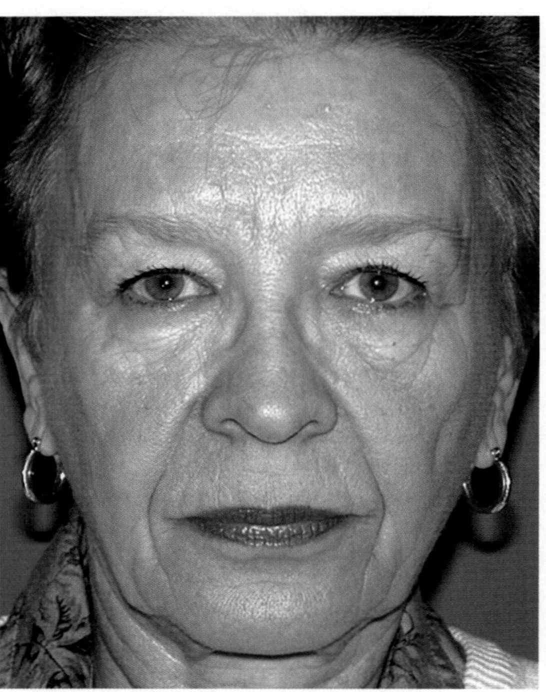

Fig. 21.3 Analysis of midface aging. One can see increased distance from the infraorbital rim to the ptotic cheek, paucity of soft tissue over the infraorbital rim, pseudoherniation of orbital fat, loss of malar fullness, cheek ptosis with deepening of the melolabial fold, and lateral infraorbital crescentic hollow.

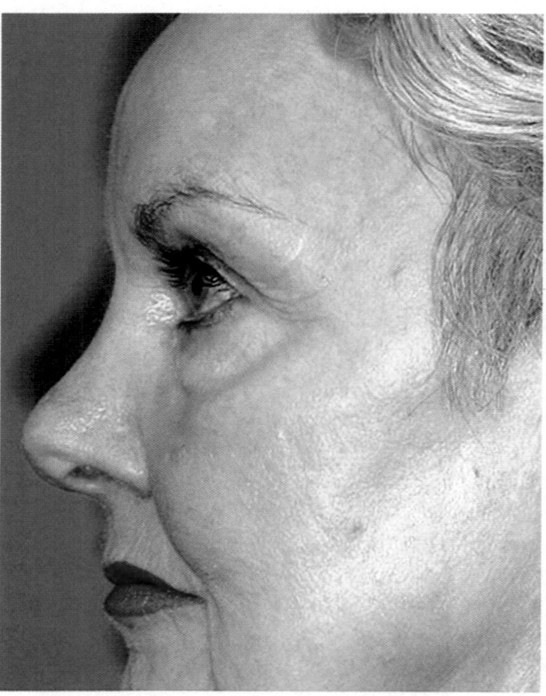

Fig. 21.4 Notice the double convexity caused by pseudoherniation of the infraorbital fat, and that of the malar fat pad, separated by the soft tissue paucity at the orbital rim.

descent of the midface structures, tethered superolaterally by the lateral orbital thickening and the orbicularis retaining ligament. This movement occurs against the melolabial fold, deepening the crease and augmenting the prominence with redundant tissue. Superiorly, the malar fat migration contributes to the crescent-shaped hollow below the lower edge of the orbicularis oculi muscle, deepens the nasojugal groove, and makes the infrazygomatic cheek concavity more prominent.[3] The anatomy of midface ptosis has also been well described by Lucarelli et al.[4] They demonstrated that attenuation of the orbitomalar, zygomatic, and masseteric cutaneous ligaments occur, but that midface ptosis results mainly from the inferior migration of skin and attached malar fat pad with relative sparing of the deeper tissues.

Patients less commonly present with malar bags; however, this chapter will not cover that topic in great depth. Malar bags represent excessive edema of the skin, manifesting as a bullae over the malar prominence, whereas malar festoons are the result of redundant orbicularis muscle below the orbital rim. Direct excision remains the primary treatment for bothersome malar bags, replacing this tissue redundancy with a thin scar. Laser resurfacing has also been used to address malar bags with mixed results, and extended blepharoplasty via a skin/muscle approach has been noted to provide some correction for both bags and festoons.

To adequately assess the midface, standard frontal, oblique, and lateral photographs of the face are essential. A bird's-eye view (i.e., a view from the top of the patient's head, aligning the chin and nasal tip) is often helpful as a comparison of midface position for preoperative and postoperative views. On frontal views, the distance from the lower eyelid margin to the beginning of the soft tissues of the youthful midface is comparable with the distance from the eyelid to the infraorbital rim. This distance increases with age and the surrounding structures descend, contributing to the double convexity of midface aging (**Figs. 21.3 and 21.4**). Additionally, when this double convexity is prominent, one should make note as to whether the lateral view shows the orbital rim to be posterior, anterior, or on the same plane of the cornea. If the plane of the orbital rim is posterior to the anterior plane of the cornea, the patient is said to have a negative vector, indicating that orbital fat repositioning is an excellent option for lower eyelid and midface restoration (**Fig. 21.5**). When a negative vector is present, these patients are often at risk for scleral show, which may be exacerbated by orbital fat removal. Ideally, the infraorbital region manifests a smooth convexity that masks the underlying infraorbital rim and nasojugal groove.[5] Fullness of the malar eminence is desirable as it will accentuate the eyes, and this feature is commonly emphasized in the application of makeup. As darkness gives the appearance of recession and light gives the appearance of coming forward, the application of a makeup that is darker than skin color underneath the malar eminence gives the illusion of an elevated cheek.

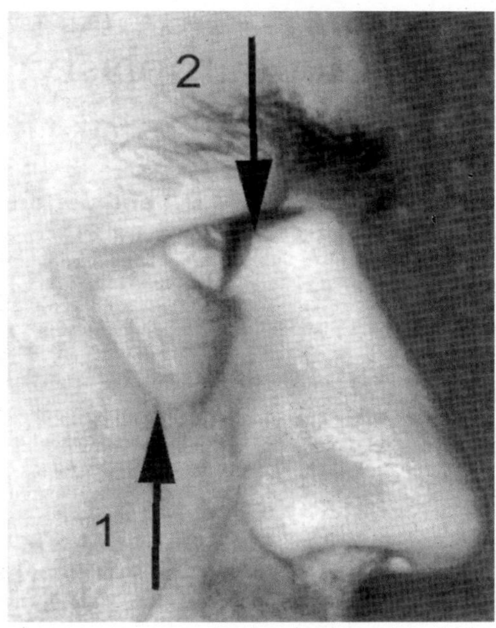

Fig. 21.5 A negative vector exists when the infraorbital rim (1) lies posterior to the anterior plane of the cornea (2). (From LaFerriere KA, Kilpatrick JK. Transblepharoplasty: subperiosteal approach to rejuvenation of the aging midface. Fac Plas Surg 2003 19(2):158. Reprinted by permission.)

History

Midface rejuvenation has evolved significantly over the past few decades. Paul Tessier[6] described the subperiosteal dissection of the midface in the late 1970s, paving the way for others to explore their respective techniques for similar rejuvenation of the midface. Hamra[7] went on to describe the composite rhytidectomy, which added a midface component to the rejuvenation by elevating the orbicularis oculi with the SMAS flap and superomedially fixating the muscle to the orbital rim. In the mid 1990s, Hamra further elaborated on periorbital fat preservation and arcus marginalis repositioning.[8] Ramirez then extended his endoscopic forehead lift to the midface, later suspending the SOOF, malar periosteum, and the buccal fat pad of Bichat.[9] Owsley and Zweifler[10] also described an extended rhytidectomy to address midface subperiosteally, and in 1998 McCord[11] et al discussed the transblepharoplasty subperiosteal midface lift (TBML) for tear trough and melolabial fold correction. This entailed a subperiosteal dissection of the midface, release of the periosteum, and suspension of the midface to the periosteum of the lateral orbital rim. A canthoplasty or canthopexy was utilized to support the lower lid. Gunter[12] later performed a similar procedure, however, without the lower lid canthoplasty or canthopexy except in cases of significant eyelid laxity. Goldberg[13] followed by elaborating on lower blepharoplasty fat repositioning that may be used in conjunction with midface lifting.

Preoperative Assessment

When evaluating patients preoperatively, it is important to verify whether the patient is a good candidate for midface repositioning, or whether additional or alternative procedures may be indicated. A patient with weak malar projection may benefit from a malar implant, or excessively hollow cheeks may be improved with submalar implants. Occasionally, soft tissue fillers may be used to temporarily address inadequacies of the cheek or midface; however, large volumes are usually required to achieve this transient effect. Fat transplantation is also a consideration for loss of volume. Patients in their 30s or 40s may be good candidates for melolabial plication if they are interested in less downtime. Of course, patients who undergo a subperiosteal midface lift must be counseled that swelling may persist for 3 to 6 weeks, and the eyes may appear to look East Asian until the edema resolves. For patients who are interested in total midface rejuvenation, it is appropriate to rank the procedures in order of most to least effective for the patient's anatomy and interests. This will allow patients to consider their options when deciding on multiple rejuvenative procedures, such as blepharoplasty, forehead lift, facelift, and resurfacing. As with all cosmetic procedures, a complete history and physical examination is necessary, along with a standard preoperative interview that explores patient motivations, psychological fitness, and emotional stability.

Surgical Techniques

The most commonly used approaches to the midface include the transtemporal subperiosteal midface lift (TTML), the transblepharoplasty subperiosteal (TBML), the transblepharoplasty SOOF lift, melolabial plication, and direct excision of the nasolabial folds. Choice of procedure depends on a variety of factors, including preferred outcome, tolerance for downtime, training bias, and concomitant procedures. The TTML may be easier to perform with an endoscopic forehead lift as they share dissection planes and temporal incisions. Similarly, the transblepharoplasty approaches are more easily done with concomitant blepharoplasty. **Table 21.1** briefly compares the merits of each approach.

Transtemporal Subperiosteal Midface Lift

The TTML is often performed in conjunction with an endoscopic forehead lift, and it can be achieved via an open or endoscopic approach. The subperiosteal layer is commonly utilized for the endoscopic forehead lift, and this plane is easily extended inferiorly to address midface ptosis. Please refer to the Chapter 20 for details on the forehead/brow lift procedure.

Temporal approaches to the midface traverse deep to the superficial temporal fascia. This fascial layer is the superior-most extension of the SMAS layer, and it is continuous with the galea across the forehead. The superficial temporal fascia is the most superficial of the temporal fascial layers, and it contains the frontal branch of the facial nerve and the temporal artery and vein. The relationship of the neurovascular structures within the superficial temporal fascia is analogous to that of the facial nerve and mimetic musculature found within the SMAS inferiorly. Pitanguy's line is used as a landmark for the frontal branch, delineating a line that runs from the lobule to the lateral canthus. As this line crosses the zygoma, at roughly the midpoint from the helical root

Table 21.1 Description of Midface Surgical Approaches

Approach	Vector of Pull	Shares Dissection	Downtime	Advantages	Disadvantages
Transtemporal (TTML)	Superolateral or superior	Endoforehead lift	3–6 weeks	Avoids eyelid	Downtime, potential for Asian-appearing eyes, widening of intermalar distance
Transbleph subperiosteal (TBML)	Superior	Blepharoplasty	3–6 weeks	Direct vector	Downtime, potential for eyelid malposition
Transbleph SOOF	Superior	Blepharoplasty	5–10 days	Direct vector	Less durable suspension of the midface structures
Melolabial plication	Superolateral	N/A	3–7 days	Quick, minimum downtime	Possible asymmetry, long-term results inconclusive
Nasolabial fold excision	Inferolateral	N/A	3–7 days	Direct nasolabial reduction	Scar in nasolabial fold

to the lateral canthus, this approximates the location of the frontal branch of the facial nerve.[14] Dissection in the temporal region is safest when deep to the superficial temporal fascia, as this will protect the facial nerve. In this plane one encounters bridging veins lateral to the lateral orbital rim that run from superficial to deep, traversing the temporal fascial planes. This vein, also known as the sentinel vein, is an important landmark that heralds the proximity of the frontal branch within 1 cm, and it should be preserved to avoid arborization of facial venous networks. When necessary, this vein is cauterized only along the deep aspect only to avoid thermal injury to the overlying nerve.[15]

The plane of dissection in the TTML is below the superficial temporal fascia and on top of the true fascia of the temporalis muscle. At the level of the supraorbital rim, the true temporalis fascia splits into superficial and deep layers, separated by the intermediate fat pad. This is distinct from the deeper fat pad of Bichat, which overlies the temporalis muscle and is deep to the temporalis fascia just described. The fat pad of Bichat is significant as violation of this plane may lead to atrophy of the fat with resultant temporal wasting. At the level of the zygomatic arch, the superficial layer of the temporalis fascia attaches to the superolateral surface of the zygomatic arch and the deeper layer attaches to the superomedial aspect of the zygomatic arch. Additional protection of the frontal branch of the facial nerve can be provided by incising the superficial layer of the temporalis fascia ~1 to 2 cm above the zygomatic arch and proceeding in the plane of the intermediate fat pad down to the zygomatic arch, and staying directly on the bone when dissecting over the arch. Gosain et al[16] confirmed with cadaveric studies that the frontal branch of the facial nerve ramifies as an average of three additional branches across the zygomatic arch, with all specimens possessing a distinct anterior and posterior trunk. These anatomical relationships confirm the need to remain beneath the superficial layer of the temporalis fascia when exposing the zygomatic arch, and this maneuver is best undertaken from anterior to the nerve, progressing posteriorly.[17]

When planning the TTML as an isolated procedure, a 3 to 5 cm temporal incision is made parallel to and behind the hairline (**Fig. 21.6**). Dissection proceeds down through the superficial temporal fascia to the level of the temporalis fascia, noted by its glistening white appearance. This plane is bluntly extended inferomedially, beyond the conjoined tendon, to the subperiosteal layer

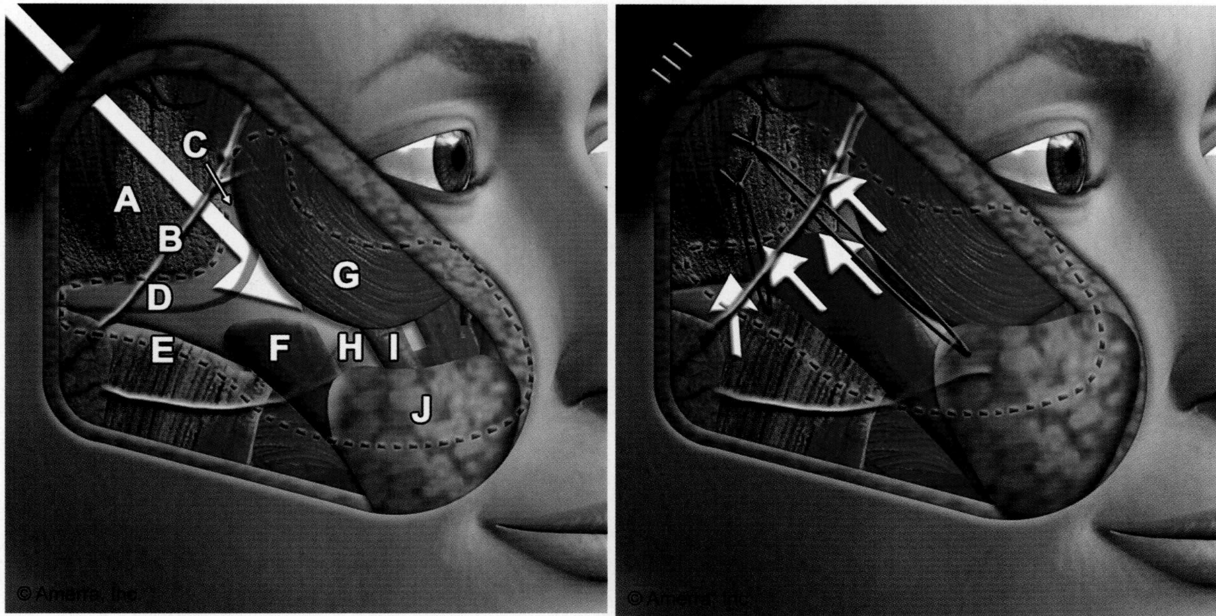

Fig. 21.6 (**A**) Transtemporal subperiosteal midfacel lift (TTML). The surgical approach illustrated is above the true temporalis fascia (A) and beneath the superficial temporal fascia containing the frontal branch of the facial nerve (B). The arrow represents the direction and plane of dissection in the subperiosteal pocket. The dotted line represents the extent of subperiosteal elevation, extending under the insertion of the masseter (E). Lateral orbital rim (C), zygomatic arch (D), zygomaticus major (F), orbicularis oculi (G), periosteum (H), zygomaticus minor (I), malar fat pad (J). (**B**) The tissues are repositioned in a superolateral vector and sutured to the temporalis fascia. Alternatively, if the dissection is carried posteriorly along the extent of the zygomatic arch, 1 to 2 cm under the fascia of the masseter muscle, a more direct, vertical vector of pull can be obtained. Note the repositioning of the zygomaticus major insertion.

at the frontal process of the zygoma. As mentioned previously, care is taken to avoid disruption of the sentinel vein, as this runs close to the frontal branch of the facial nerve and disruption of this vein can result in postoperative prominence of the cutaneous veins of the temporal region. Adequate release of the conjoined tendon is critical to avoid postoperative bunching after suspension of the midface. The arcus marginalis is also released, with care to preserve a 1 cm cuff of tissue around the lateral canthal periosteal attachment. Failure to preserve this periosteal cuff can lead to lateral canthal distortion. Periosteal elevation continues over the body of the zygoma to release the origin of the zygomatic major and minor muscles and over the anterior face of the maxilla, avoiding injury to the infraorbital nerve. The zygomaticofacial nerve exits the zygoma below the lateral aspect of the infraorbital rim, and this should be preserved (although disruption of this nerve does not result in long-term sensory deficits). As the dissection carries posteriorly along the zygomatic arch, care is taken to stay directly on the bone as the frontal branch of the facial nerve exists in the fascial plane just above the periosteum. Quatela et al[17] describe elevating the periosteum at the superior edge of the zygomatic arch to within 1 cm of the external auditory canal, though such a wide dissection is not universal. Depending on the desired mobility, the

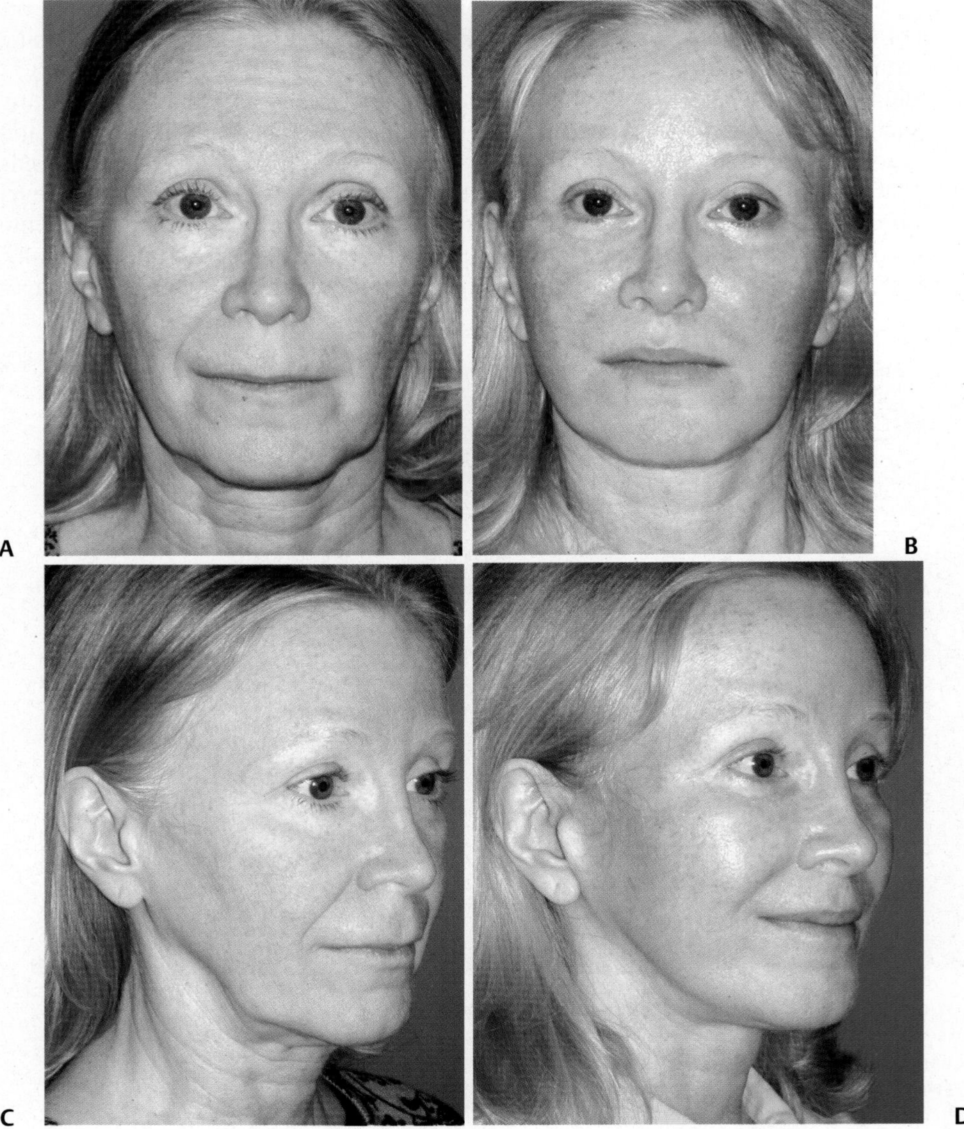

Fig. 21.7 One year results in a 59-year-old woman who had a transtemporal, subperiosteal midface lift with endoscopic brow lift, lower face lift, upper and lower blepharoplasty, and subnasal lip lift; preoperative (**A,C,E**) and postoperative (**B,D,F**).

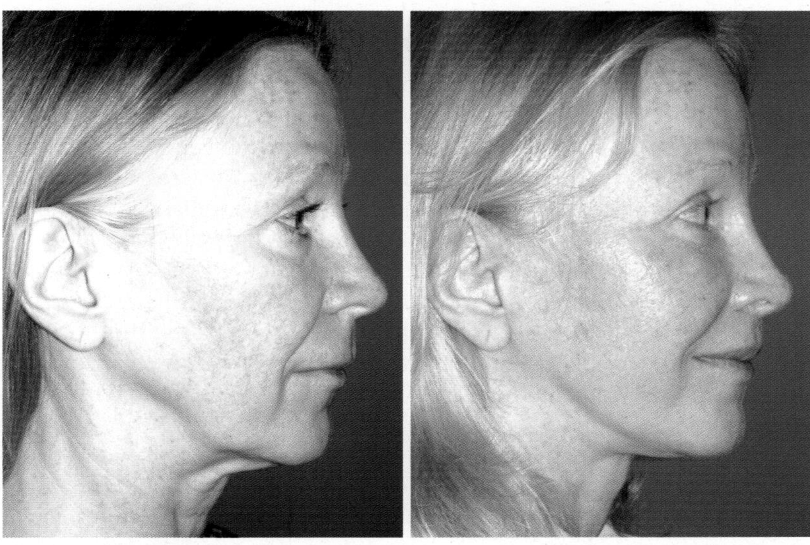

Fig. 21.7 (*Continued*)

dissection can proceed a few centimeters over the origins of the masseter muscle, giving added correction of the lower face as well. It has been found that when the subperiosteal elevation is carried laterally over the entire extent of the zygoma, the direction of pull can be almost vertical.[18]

Once the midface is adequately mobilized, it may be suspended either by suturing the malar fat pad, the periosteum, or both to the temporalis fascia in a superolateral vector.[14,19] As mentioned above, if the dissection has proceeded over the entire extent of the zygomatic arch and down under the masseteric fascia for a few centimeters, the pull can be more vertical. It has also been described to suspend the periosteum to the arcus marginalis,[9] though one should take caution to avoid excessive lower eyelid tension and ectropion. Skin incisions are closed with either sutures or staples. When this procedure is combined with an endoscopic forehead lift, the dissection is in a continuous plane from the forehead to the midface.

Advantages of the TTML include the ease of concomitant forehead lift and avoidance of blepharoplasty incisions that may result in eyelid malposition. The superolateral vector is reasonably effective in suspending the aging midface structures (**Fig. 21.7**). Disadvantages are risk of injury to the frontal branch of the facial nerve, lateral canthal distortion resulting in an Asian appearance, widening of the intermalar distance with repositioning of the origins of the zygomaticus major and minor muscles to a more superior position, and significant postoperative edema that necessitates a long recovery time. Facial nerve injury is usually avoided when in the appropriate plane of dissection over the zygomatic arch, and most neuropraxias are temporary. Lateral canthal distortions also resolve with time, and are best prevented with limited release of the arcus marginalis and periosteum in the immediate vicinity of the lateral canthus. Elevation and repositioning of the origins of the zygomatic major and minor muscles adds fullness to the area lateral to the orbits and can increase the appearance of the intermalar distance.

Transblepharoplasty Subperiosteal Midface Lift

This transcutaneous technique utilizes a subciliary incision and a standard skin–muscle flap, extending laterally in a natural skin crease ~1.5 to 2 cm beyond the orbital rim. The skin-muscle flap is elevated anterior to the orbital septum (**Fig. 21.8**). Excess skin and muscle is excised at this time, as would be done in a routine blepharoplasty. The temptation to remove more skin and muscle after the midface has been elevated will present itself and should be avoided due to the risk of eyelid malposition. A traction suture is placed in the pretarsal orbicularis at the midpoint of the lower lid and secured to the surgical drapes superiorly, placing the orbital septum under tension and protecting the cornea.

The dissection proceeds in the preseptal plane down to the level of the orbital rim, and it is best accomplished with two cotton-tipped applicators, using a pushing motion with one and countertraction with the other. The orbital rim is exposed to within 5 mm of the medial canthus and out to the lateral canthus. The periosteum is incised on the anterior surface of the orbital rim throughout its entire exposure, with a lateral extension over the orbital rim at the level of the lateral canthus. Care is taken to avoid the inferior oblique muscle that originates from the periosteum just inside the orbital rim. The periosteum is elevated over the anterior face of the maxilla medially over the ascending process down to the pyriform aperture to the level of the nasal ala. Laterally, the periosteum is elevated over the zygoma as far as the extent of the skin incision. The infraorbital nerve is always preserved, as is the zygomaticofacial nerve inferolaterally when possible. The periosteum is sharply incised medially, inferiorly, and laterally at the farthest extent of the dissection. Care is taken to gain a complete release of the periosteum and is accomplished by taking an elevator and releasing every periosteal band that is encountered.

Following complete periosteal release, the entire midface can be easily elevated into a more youthful position superiorly. If significant orbital fat pseudoherniation is present, it can be conservatively excised in the usual fashion or can be repositioned over the orbital rim and sutured to the undersurface of the midface at a point inferior enough so that it will be positioned over the orbital rim at the completion of the midface elevation. Elevation of the malar soft tissue alone is sufficient to eliminate mild evidence of fat pseudoherniation, and when this is the case, no fat is excised or repositioned. If lower lid laxity is present, the lid is supported by any of a variety of techniques available for canthoplasty or canthopexy. The authors' preference is a modification of the lateral retinacular suspension technique described by Jelks et al,[20] although canthopexy is used in mild cases of lid laxity. If normal lid position and tension are present preoperatively, there is no need for additional lid support with this midface technique, as the eyelid is very adequately supported by the midface elevation.

A cuff of periosteum is then elevated superiorly on the lateral orbital rim from the previous periosteal incision at the level of the lateral canthus. This creates a very sturdy attachment for the midface elevation and is the only point of suture fixation necessary to hold the midface structures in place until the periosteum has reattached in the elevated, more youthful position. The midface structures are then elevated superiorly in the desired position and the periosteum on the undersurface of the flap is sutured to the periosteal cuff of the lateral orbital rim with three 4–0 long-acting resorbable sutures (**Fig. 21.8**). At this point, there appears to be an excess of lower eyelid skin, and any temptation to resect more skin should be absolutely avoided. This appearance of skin excess will resolve in the postoperative period. Laterally, considerable bunching of tissues will be present and a conservative amount of skin can be excised in this area to avoid a dog-ear deformity. This can also be improved if a temporal or forehead/browlift accompanies this procedure. Regardless, there will be persistent fullness lateral to the eyelid that will settle out in time over the postoperative course.

Advantages of the TBML include a direct superior vector of midface elevation, a common preseptal plane of dissection with lower lid blepharoplasty, and less risk for lateral canthal distortion. The superior vector allows for

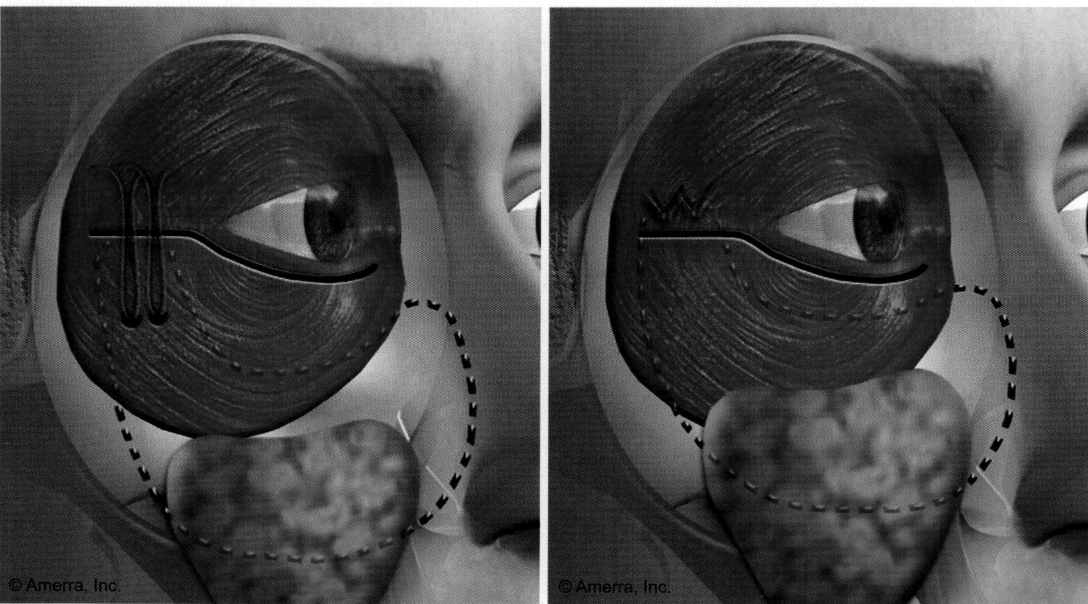

Fig. 21.8 (**A**) Extent of subperiosteal undermining in the transblepharoplasty midface lift (TBML). The bold line represents the transcutaneous approach, and the dotted line illustrates the periosteal release and incision. Suture placement is shown near the lateral orbital rim. (**B**) The repositioned midface is sutured to the periosteal cuff at the lateral orbital rim in a direct vertical vector.

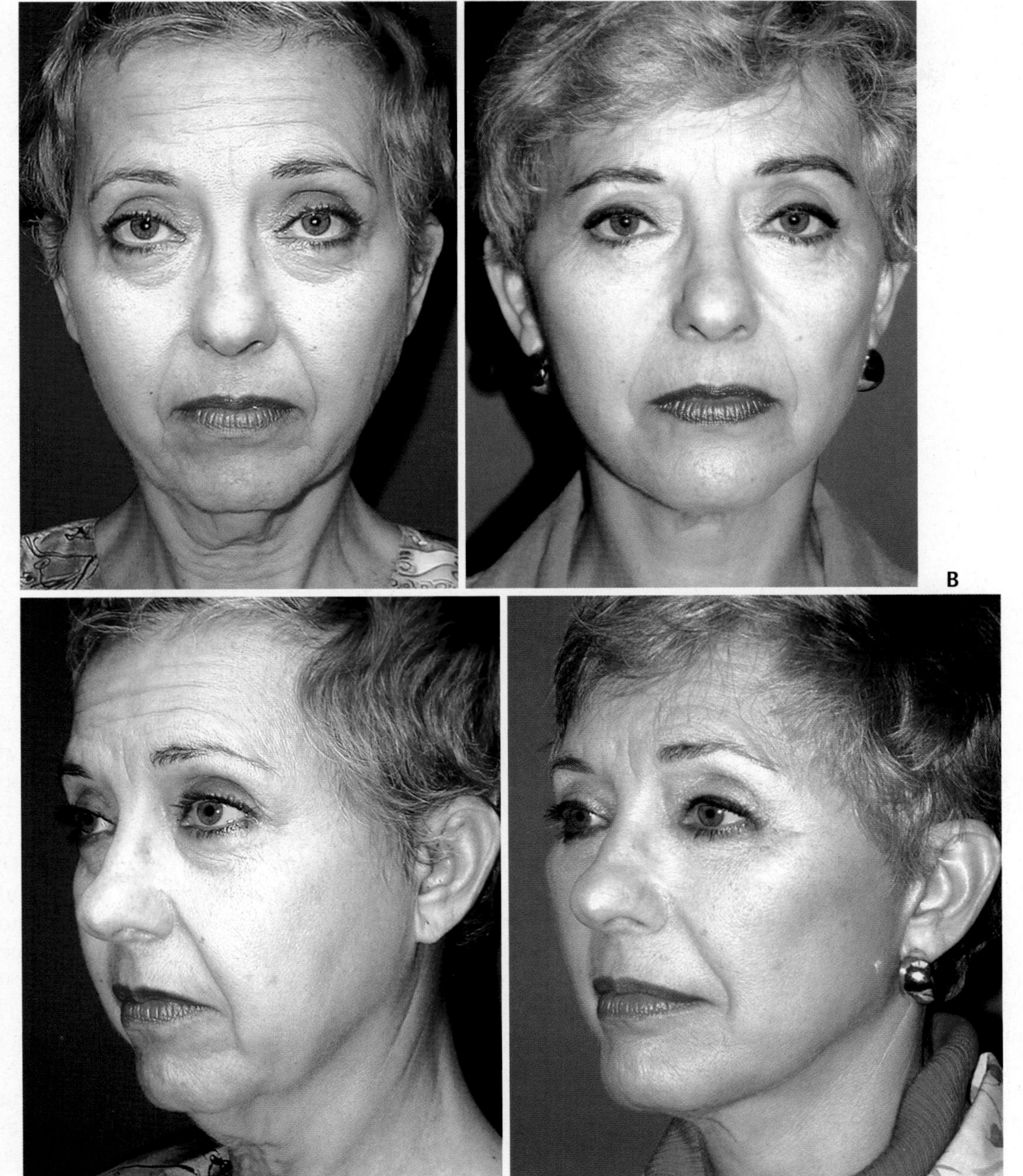

Fig. 21.9 One-year results in a 57-year-old woman who had a transorbital, subperiosteal midface lift with fat repositioning, lower cheek and neck lift, and chin augmentation. (**A,C,E**) Preoperative; (**B,D,F**) postoperative. (From LaFerriere KA, Kilpatrick JK. Transblepharoplasty: subperiosteal approach to rejuvenation of the aging midface. Fac Plas Surg 2003 19(2):157–170. Reprinted by permission.)

correction of the increased distance from the lower eyelid margin to the ptotic malar fat pad that is frequently seen with aging. The transblepharoplasty dissection allows for correction of fat pseudoherniation of orbital fat and skin excess if present (**Fig. 21.9**). Disadvantages are prolonged 3 to 6 weeks of recovery and possible eyelid malposition such as lateral rounding and scleral show. Edema may tend to be worse when midface procedures are combined with a browlift or lower facelift. However, eyelid malposition risk can be significantly reduced when the orbicularis is securely suspended to the periosteum of the lateral orbital rim just prior to skin closure. The authors' experience

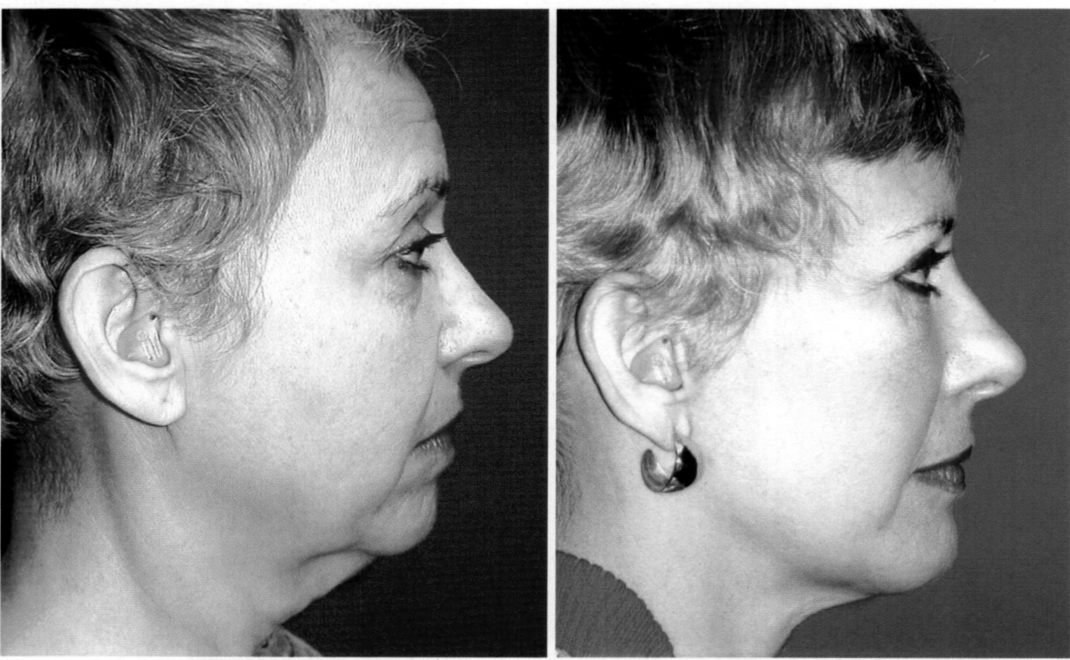

Fig. 21.9 *(Continued)*

using the techniques described has been remarkably free of such problems, largely due to the conservative resection of lower eyelid skin and attention to correction of lower eyelid laxity when present. Xerophthalmia is temporary, and of course it is screened for preoperatively in all patients. The lateral extent of the blepharoplasty incision will rarely require scar revision. Lateral periorbital skin excess is frequently seen in the early postoperative course, but this resolves spontaneously over time. Hester has added a technical modification to reduce this excess by extending the upper and lower blepharoplasty incisions and maximizing the amount of skin excision that is aided by wide undermining.[21] Apparent increase in lateral brow hooding has been present in patients with existing brow ptosis who did not undergo a simultaneous browlift. This is most likely a manifestation of tissue bunching from the elevated midface.

Transblepharoplasty SOOF lift

The approach can be via either a tranconjunctival incision or a skin/muscle flap, depending on the amount of excess skin and orbicularis festooning present. If excess skin and orbicularis are present, they are excised as in a routine blepharoplasty. As with the TBML, if excess skin appears to be present after the midface is lifted, the temptation to remove more skin is to be absolutely avoided, as postoperative eyelid malposition may occur.

The dissection proceeds anterior to the orbital septum down to the orbital rim as is described above with the TBML (**Fig. 21.10**). Fat pseudoherniation can be treated with excision when excessive or preservation of the medial and middle fat pads and cauterization of the orbital septum when pseudoherniation is mild. This cauterization will result in tightening of the septum, which will contour and minimize the pseudoherniation. Pseudoherniation of the temporal fat pad is routinely addressed by removal, as this is where persistent bulging of periorbital fat is frequently noted postoperatively. The inferior orbital rim is identified medial to lateral along its entire extent. An incision is made on the anterior face of the orbital rim down to but not through the periosteum. The dissection plane is on top of the periosteum and under the SOOF for several centimeters over the anterior face of the maxilla and the medial zygoma. This is best performed by a combination of sharp and blunt dissection with cotton swabs. The midface is then suspended in a superior direction by suturing the SOOF to the periosteum of the orbital rim at the arcus marginalis. Care is taken to get solid bites of the SOOF and the orbital rim periosteum with 4–0 long-acting absorbable sutures in multiple places along the orbital rim. Again, further removal of apparent excess skin is to be avoided at this time. The incisions are closed in the usual fashion.

Advantages of the transblepharoplasty SOOF lift are similar to the TBML, including a superior vector of midface elevation, a common preseptal plane of

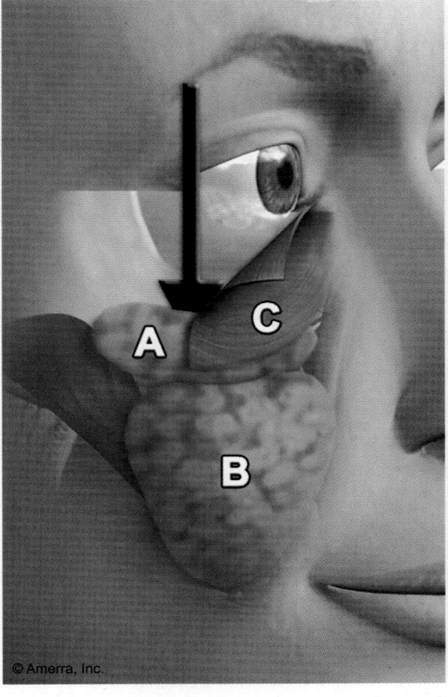

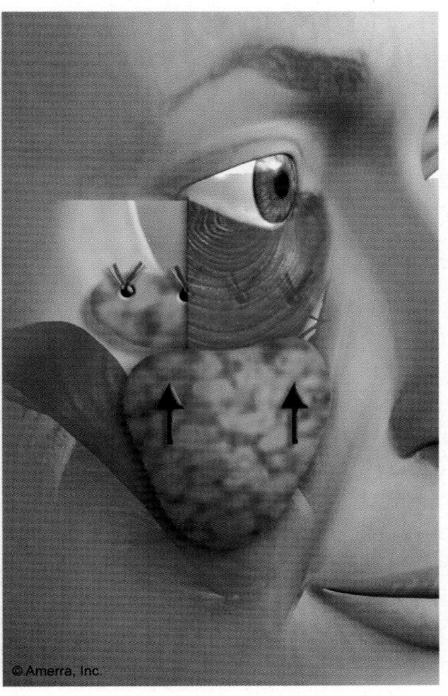

Fig. 21.10 (**A**) Transblepharoplasty SOOF lift. This represents a transconjunctival approach, and the arrow shows the preseptal plane of dissection. SOOF (A), malar fat pad (B), and orbicularis oculi (C). (**B**) As the SOOF is suspended to the periosteum of the inferior orbital rim, the malar fat pad is pulled superiorly to effect a change in the midface.

dissection with lower lid blepharoplasty, and less risk for lateral canthal distortion (**Fig. 21.11**). Disadvantages are a less substantial fixation of the SOOF to the periosteum (i.e., as opposed to suturing periosteum to periosteum). Again, eyelid malposition risk can be significantly reduced when the orbicularis is securely suspended to the periosteum of the lateral orbital rim, or when a transconjunctival approach is used.[22]

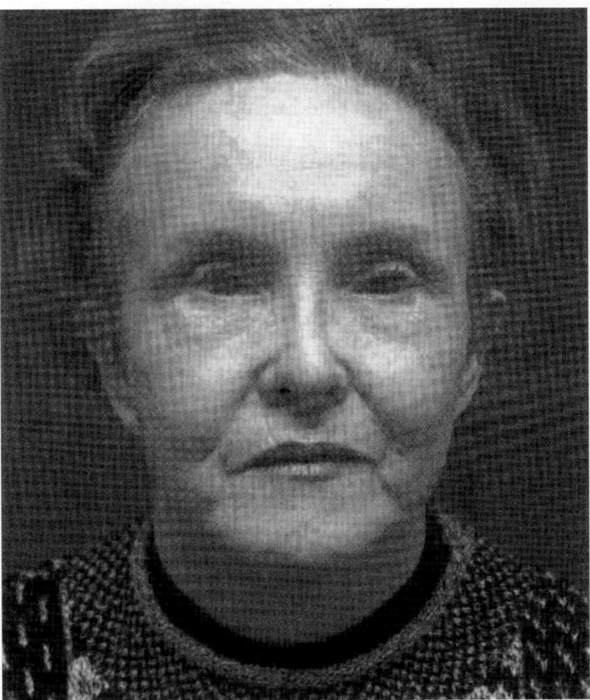

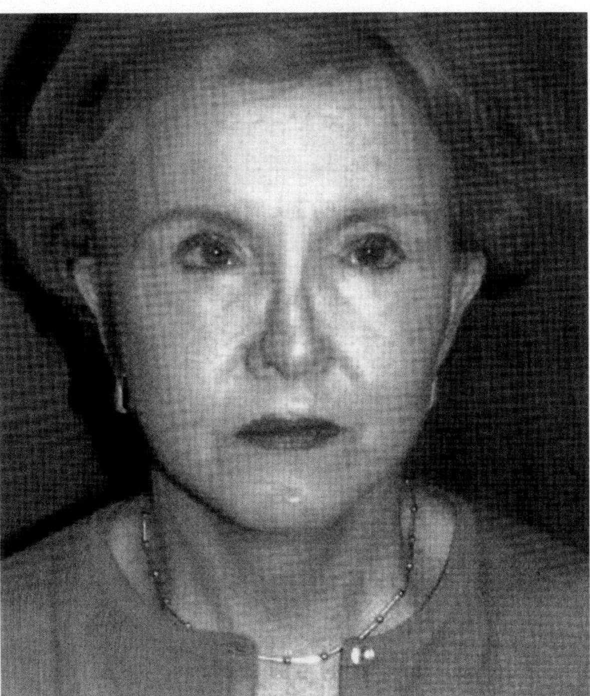

Fig. 21.11 SOOF lift, before and after. (From Freeman MS. Rejuvenation of the midface. Fac Plas Surg 2003;19(2): 233. Reprinted by permission.)

Melolabial Plication

Isolated melolabial plication will be most appropriate for patients in their 30s to late 40s whose main complaint is malar fat pad descent and deepening of the nasolabial fold. It is also useful in the older patient as an open procedure with a standard lower rhytidectomy. This procedure brings fullness to the midface through suture plication of the malar fat pad in a superolateral vector.

The cutaneous markings are performed, starting 1 cm lateral to the alar–facial groove, and 1 cm superolateral from the melolabial fold. A second mark is made 1 cm inferior to the first and parallel to the melolabial fold. The path of the suspension sutures is perpendicular to the melolabial fold and a second set of marks 1 cm and 2 cm away from the lateral orbital rim are made as a guide. A temporal incision is outlined posterior to the hairline and centered on the path from the melolabial and lateral orbital rim markings.

The sutures are prepared as demonstrated in the diagram (**Fig. 21.12**). The braided nature of the polygalactic acid suture allows for a sawing motion through the dermal remnants that would impede the seating of the e-PTFE (expanded polytetraflouroethylene; Gore-Tex, W. L. Gore & Associates, Inc., Flagstaff, AZ) pledget and thereby avoid dimpling of the skin.

The temporal incision is carried through the superficial temporal fascia to the superficial layer of the true temporalis fascia and the dissection proceeds on this plane to the previously marked areas adjacent to the lateral orbital rim. Full-thickness stab incisions are then made along relaxed skin tension lines at the marks adjacent to the melolabial folds. One of the Keith needles with the attached e-PTFE and polygalactic acid sutures threaded is inserted through the upper stab incision and carried down to the maxilla, retracted slightly, and directed superolaterally through the malar fat pad toward the medial mark at the lateral orbital rim, surfacing between the orbicularis oculi muscle and skin. Care is taken to make sure that the needle has not engaged the dermis to avoid dimpling in the skin but is superficial to the orbicularis oculi muscle. An Aufrecht retractor is inserted in the temporal incision to retrieve the Keith needle lateral to the orbital rim. The Keith needle is then advanced through the temporal incision. The retractor is deep to and protects the frontal branch of the facial nerve, which lies in the superficial temporal fascia. The ends of the two sutures are secured

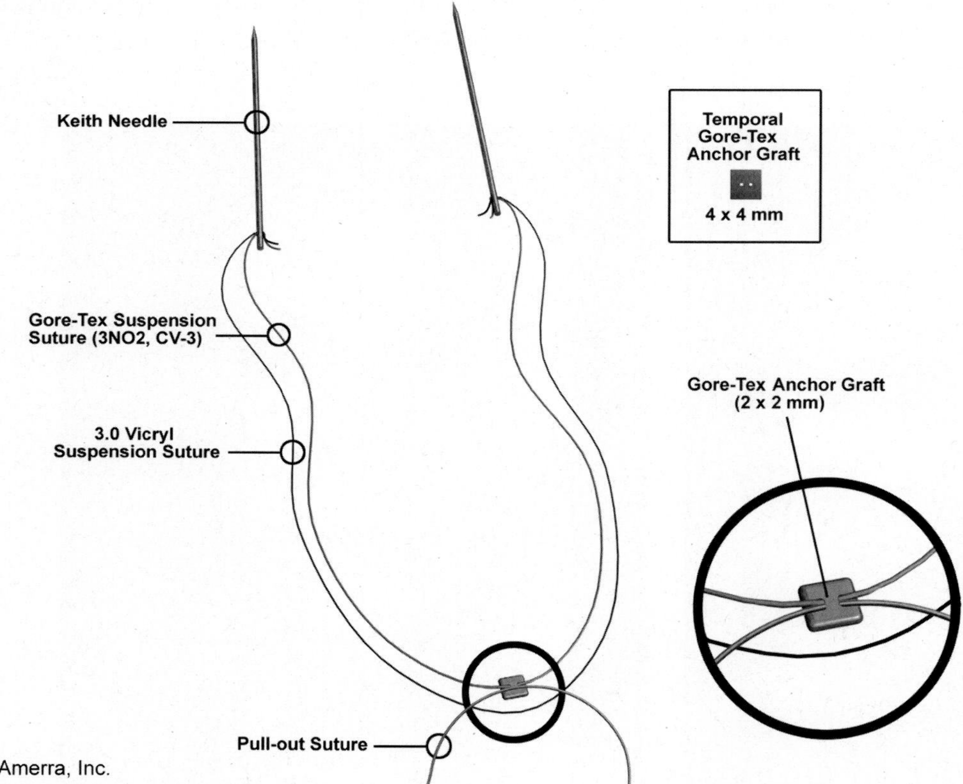

Fig. 21.12 Suture arrangement for melolabial plication. (Adapted from Sasaki, GH, Cohen AT. Meloplication of the malar fat pads by percutaneous cable-suture technique for midface rejuvenation: outcome study. Plast Reconstr Surg 2002;110:635–654.)

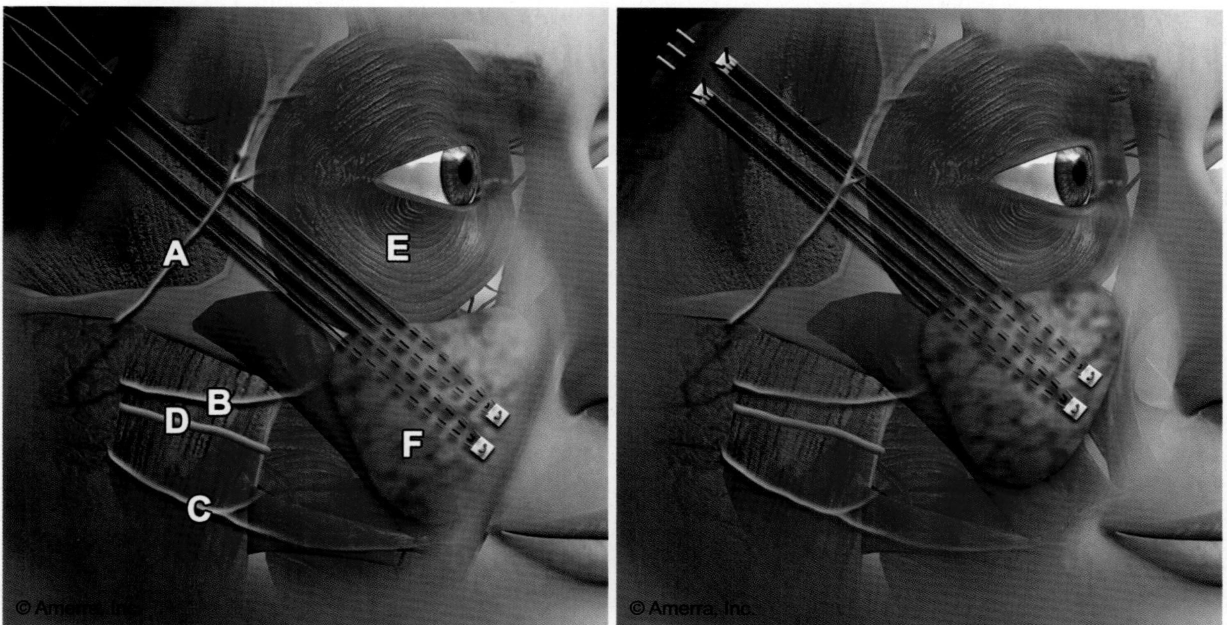

Fig. 21.13 (**A**) Melolabial plication (before). The suture apparatus is inserted 1 cm from the nasolabial fold, 1 cm apart from one another. Notice the path of the suture is through the malar fat pad, over the orbicularis, and under the frontal branch of the facial nerve (A), which lies within the superficial temporal fascia. Zygomatic branch of facial nerve (B), buccal branch of facial nerve (**C**), parotid duct (D), orbicularlis oculi (E), malar fat pad (F). (**B**) After suspension.

with a hemostat. The path of the suture is superior to the parotid duct, through the malar fat pad, above the orbicularis oculi muscle, and deep to the frontal branch of the facial nerve (**Fig. 21.13**).

In an identical fashion, the remaining Keith needle with the other end of the suture complex is passed through the same stab incision and delivered along the same path through the temporal incision. The e-PTFE patch on the e-PTFE suture is withheld from entering the stab incision by a guide suture through the e-PTFE pledget placed previously. From the temporal incision, the polygalactic acid suture is pulled through the stab incision and used to gently "saw" through the dermal attachments to prevent dimpling of the skin when the e-PTFE suture with the e-PTFE patch is seated. Excessive sawing of the polygalactic acid suture will penetrate through the entire malar fat pad, and should be avoided. Abrupt releases of the dermis or visualizing the effacement of the skin dimple are simple endpoints. The e-PTFE suture with the e-PTFE patch is pulled through the stab incision and seated to allow for plication of the malar fat pad. If dimpling of the skin is noted with the e-PTFE patch seated, it can be withdrawn back through the stab incision and further sawing of the polygalactic suture can be performed to release any remaining dermal attachments. The polygalactic suture is withdrawn when no dimpling of the skin is noted as the e-PTFE patch is seated.

This maneuver is repeated through the inferior stab incision adjacent to the melolabial fold and the second plication suture is seated. The superficial layer of the deep temporalis fascia is used to anchor both e-PTFE sutures at the level of the temporal incision with a French eye needle. Each suture is then tied over an additional 4×4 mm patch of 2 mm e-PTFE after suitable elevation of the malar fat pad is achieved. This e-PTFE patch is helpful in both securing the e-PTFE suture and in locating the suture at a subsequent time if additional suspension or modification is later desired. Malar fat pad elevation averages 3 mm, but may be more or less depending how much movement is desired. The result is a plication of the malar fat pad, not a repositioning of the entire skin and fat complex, thereby avoiding bunching of skin in the lateral orbital area. Temporal incisions are closed with surgical staples, and the opposite site is treated in identical fashion.[1,23,24]

Advantages of melolabial plication include minimal dissection and minimal recovery downtime. Additionally, the procedure can be reversed or adjusted as needed. Patient satisfaction is quite high in the authors' experience, but the long-term results are objectively inconclusive. Sasaki did show that of 137 patients undergoing this procedure, 82% maintained favorable results at 3 years.[1] The changes are often subtle and at times defy photographic documentation, but direct observation reveals a subtle youthfulness in the malar area (**Figs. 21.13 and 21.14**).

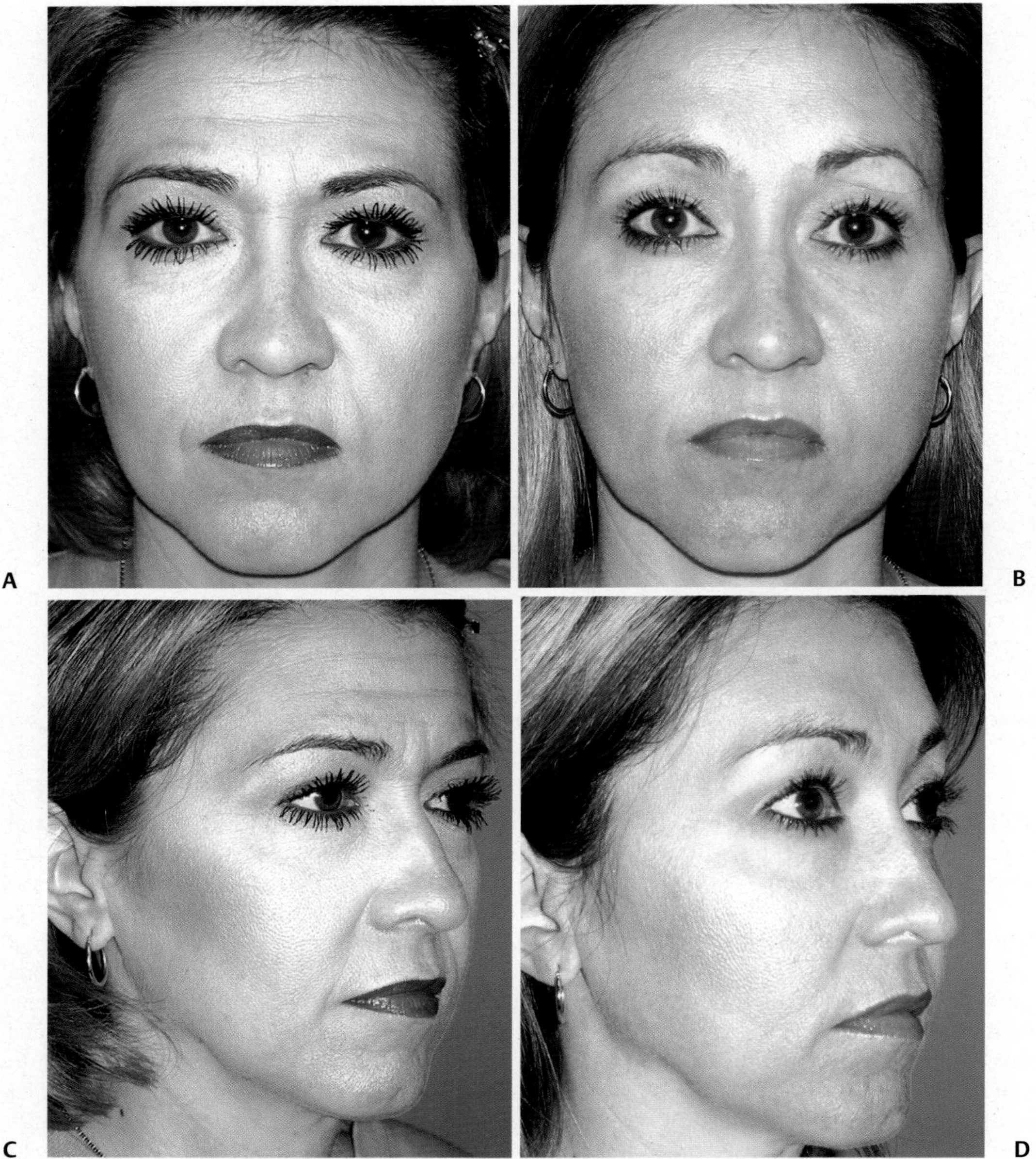

Fig. 21.14 Melolabial plication, preoperatively (**A,C**) and 18 months postoperatively (**B,D**). Notice the subtle change in light reflex that is significantly higher on the postoperative views. This is accompanied by a softening of the nasolabial mound. This patient also underwent an endoscopic forehead lift and browlift, along with a transconjunctival blepharoplasty with fat repositioning.

The main disadvantage is the potential for cheek asymmetry; however, this usually resolves in 1 to 2 months.

Direct Excision

When all other modalities are unsuccessful in correcting deep melolabial folds, direct excision is still a viable option. The incision is placed directly in the melolabial fold and the excess skin and fat are removed as desired from the cheek to diminish the appearance of a deep fold. Results are immediate, and complications rates are low; however, the patient must be willing to accept a scar within the nasolabial crease.[25,26]

Additional Options

In addition to surgical procedures, fillers and implants are also an option for the nasolabial crease. Alternatively, one may use liposuction for a prominent nasolabial fold, though this is uncommon and must be done very conservatively with a small liposuction cannula to avoid contour irregularities. Midfacial slings have also been fashioned with e-PTFE; however, this has only been reported by one author and merits further investigation.[27]

Midface suspension has also been achieved utilizing the Endotine (Coapt Systems, Inc., Palo Alto, CA) device. The path of the suspension is essentially the same as that of the meloplication described above, but the midface is approached transorally in the subperiosteal plane. The Endotine device is an absorbable device that has a long, flat strap with a head full of short suspension tines at one end. The malar repositioning is achieved by embedding the tines underneath the periosteum and soft tissues of the cheek adjacent to the melolabial fold. The other end of the strap is suture fixated to the superficial layer of the temporalis fascia giving the desired lift. Long-term results of this technique have not been published.

Polypropylene suture has also been utilized to lift the midface via opposing barbs that embed into the malar tissues. This is marketed under the trade name Aptos Suture (Surgical Specialties Corp., Reading, PA). Lycka et al described a series of 350 patients, noting a great deal of satisfaction though follow-up was limited to 2 years.[28] Silva-Siwady et al confirm the utility of this technique for minor, nonsurgical cosmetic improvements, though the authors do present a case report of a patient with one suture extruding 28 days after 10 were placed. This was easily removed and treated.[29]

Summary

Correction of midface aging is an evolving process that has achieved variable results, as is attested to by the fact that there are so many approaches that have been developed and there is no universally accepted technique. Initial outcomes for the various techniques appear quite promising, though published long-term results beyond 2 years postoperatively are scarce. Hamra has noted that midface ptosis tends to return 1 or 2 years after a deep plane facelift.[30] TTML has also been successfully performed; however, published long-term follow-up beyond 1 year is not yet available.[19] Hester notes persistent midface elevation in his TBML patients 3 and 4 years postoperatively, though these are isolated cases, and data are not provided for groups of patients.[21]

The TTML does achieve a favorable superolateral vector of tissue correction; however, effective midface lifting is limited in improving the soft tissue paucity at the medial half of the orbital rim. In addition, the temporal approach often still requires a lower blepharoplasty to fully address midface aging changes (i.e., lower blepharoplasty). Furthermore, the temporal approach relocates the origin of the zygomaticus major and minor muscles superolaterally, displacing them to a level that is not anatomical, creating a potential for fullness over the zygoma or a wider face on frontal view.

As noted by Hester et al,[21] complications of the TBML may range from lateral orbital skin excess, lateral canthal deformity, and lower lid malposition. Of their series of 757 patients, 19% underwent revision. Williams[31] reported on a variation of the TBML using an endoscope on 13 patients. Two of these patients required minor revisions to remove Prolene sutures (Ethicon, Inc., Somerville, NJ) suspending the periosteum at the lateral canthus, prompting the use of polydiaxonone (PDS) in subsequent patients, and follow-up was not discussed longer than 3 months. Gunter[12] presented 60 TBML patients, without routine canthoplasty or canthopexy, and a mean follow-up of 5 months, noting only four lower eyelid complications, two of which resolved without surgical intervention.

The TBML has the advantage of a purely vertical vector of midface elevation. The most striking improvement of the TBML is the return of the youthful distance between the lower eyelid and the soft tissue of the cheek. Melolabial and perioral improvement are also evident, though long-term improvement may be questionable. Several authors[12,32] have advocated performing a canthoplasty or canthopexy in all patients undergoing a TBML. The authors of this chapter reserve lateral canthal–tightening procedures only for those demonstrating lower lid laxity. Lower eyelid malposition and canthal asymmetries were encountered postoperatively in some patients in these earlier studies but have not occurred in our experience. Scleral show or ectropion may be attributed to excessive skin excision. To avoid this, one should excise redundant lower lid skin and muscle before midface suspension is performed. Considering the mechanics and vertical vector of TBML, less tension is placed on the lower eyelid postoperatively. In the absence of lower lid laxity, there should be no reason to expect lower eyelid malposition.

The transblepharoplasty SOOF lift is another valuable technique that takes advantage of this direct superior vector of midface correction. However, the fixation may not be as sturdy as the TTML or the TBML, and there are no long-term published results.

Melolabial plication offers a minimally invasive technique for midface correction, but again, it does not have data beyond 3 years to show long-term efficacy. Direct excision of the melolabial fold maximizes simplicity at the cost of a well-hidden facial scar, though this fails to correct the other aging changes of the midface.

Over the years, multiple approaches have been developed in an attempt to correct midface aging, and there is still no technique that is universally accepted. This can be considered as a testament to the degree of difficulty involved in midface rejuvenation. The surgeon is encouraged to maintain a variety of midface techniques in his or her armamentarium to maximize and individualize treatment of the aging midface.

References

1. Sasaki GH, Cohen AT. Meloplication of the malar fat pads by percutaneous cable-suture technique for midface rejuvenation: outcome study. Plast Reconstr Surg 2002;110:635–654
2. Mendelson BC, Muzaffar AR, Adams WP. Surgical anatomy of the midcheek and malar mounds. Plast Reconstr Surg 2002;110(3):885–896
3. LaFerriere KA, Castellano RD. Modern Blepharoplasty. Plastic Surgery Products. 2004.
4. Lucarelli MJ, Khwarq SI, Lemke BN, et al. The anatomy of midfacial ptosis. Ophthal Plast Reconstr Surg 2000;16(1):7–22
5. LaFerriere KA, Kilpatrick JK. Transblepharoplasty: subperiosteal approach to rejuvenation of the aging midface. Facial Plast Surg 2003;19(2):157–170
6. Tessier P. Lifting facial sous-perioste. Ann Chir Plast Esthet 1989;34:193
7. Hamra ST. The deep-plane rhytidectomy. Plast Reconstr Surg 1990;86(1):53–61
8. Hamra ST. Arcus marginalis release and orbital fat preservation in midface rejuvenation [see comment]. Plast Reconstr Surg 1995;96(2):354–362
9. Ramirez OM, Pozner JN. Subperiosteal minimally invasive laser endoscopic rhytidectomy: the SMILE facelift. Aesthetic Plast Surg 1996;20:463–470
10. Owsley JQ, Zweifler M. Midface lift of the malar fat pad: technical advances. Plast Reconstr Surg 2002;110(2):674–685
11. McCord CD Jr, Codner MA, Hester TR. Redraping the inferior orbicularis arc. Plast Reconstr Surg 1998;102(7):2471–2479
12. Gunter JP, Hackney FL. A simplified transblepharoplasty subperiosteal cheek lift. Plast Reconstr Surg 1999;103(7):2029–2035
13. Goldberg RA. Transconjunctival orbital fat repositioning: transposition of orbital fat pedicles into a subperiosteal pocket. Plast Reconstr Surg 2000;105(2):743–748
14. Quatela VC, Jacono AA. The extended centrolateral endoscopic midface lift. Facial Plast Surg 2003;19(2):199–205
15. Sabini P, Wayne I, Quatela VC. Anatomical guides to precisely localize the frontal branch of the facial nerve. Arch Facial Plast Surg 2003;5(2):150–152
16. Gosain AK, Sewall SR, Yousif NJ. The temporal branch of the facial nerve: how reliably can we predict its path? Plast Reconstr Surg 1997;99(5):1224–1233
17. Quatela VC, Choe KS. Endobrow-midface lift. Facial Plast Surg 2004;20(3):199–206
18. Quatela VC. Personal communication 2005.
19. Williams EF III, Vargas H, Dahiya R, Hove CR, Rodgers BJ, Lam SM. Midfacial rejuvenation via a minimal-incision browlift approach. Arch Facial Plast Surg 2003;5:470–478
20. Jelks GW, Glat PM, Jelks EB, Longaker MT. The inferior retinacular lateral canthoplasty: a new technique. Plast Reconstr Surg 1997;100(5):1262–1270
21. Hester TR, Codner MA, McCord MD, Nahai F, Giannopoulos A. Evolution of technique of the direct transblepharoplasty approach for the correction of lower lid and midfacial aging: maximizing results and minimizing complications in a 5-year experience. Plast Reconstr Surg 2000;105(1):393–406
22. Freeman MS. Rejuvenation of the midface. Facial Plast Surg 2003;18(2):223–236
23. LaFerriere KA, Castellano RD. Experience with percutaneous suspension of the malar fat pad for midface rejuvenation. Facial Plast Surg Clin North Am 2005;13(3):393–399
24. Keller GS, Namazie A, Blackwell K, Rawnsley J, Khan S. Elevation of the malar fat pad with a percutaneous technique. Arch Facial Plast Surg 2002;4:20–25
25. Rudkin G, Miller TA. Aging nasolabial fold and treatment by direct excision. Plast Reconstr Surg 1999;104(5):1502–1505
26. Sen C, Cek DI, Reis M. Direct skin excision fat reshaping and repositioning for correction of prominent nasolabial fold. Aesthetic Plast Surg 2004;28(5):307–311
27. Yousif NJ, Matloub MD and H, Summers AN. The midface sling: a new technique to rejuvenate the midface. Plast Reconstr Surg 2002;110(6):1541–1553
28. Lycka B, Bazan C, Poletti E, Treen B. The emerging technique of the antiptosis subdermal suspension thread. Dermatol Surg 2004;30(1):41–44
29. Silva-Siwady JG, Díaz-Garza C, Ocampo-Candiani J. A case of Aptos thread migration and partial expulsion. Dermatol Surg 2005;31(3):356–358
30. Hamra ST. A study of the long-term effect of malar fat repositioning in facelift surgery: short-term success but long-term failure. Plast Reconstr Surg 2001;110(3):940–951
31. Williams JV. Transblepharoplasty endoscopic subperiosteal midface lift. Plast Reconstr Surg 2002;110(7):1769–1775
32. Malcolm PD. A Simplified transblepharoplasty subperiosteal cheek lift [discussion]. Plast Reconstr Surg 1999;103(7):2040–2041

22 Upper Eyelid Blepharoplasty

Norman J. Pastorek

Successful upper lid blepharoplasty begins with the surgeon's artistic understanding of the relationship of the upper lid, eyebrow, forehead, and bony orbital rim and a general appreciation of the current concept of the beautiful American face. The latter can be seen on the cover of many magazines. Today's beautiful face is determined by the beauty editors who choose them, the photographers who record them, the advertising executives who hire them, and the product clients who endorse them. The beautiful eyelid is a fairly static concept. Although it is fashionable, it is not a rapidly changing fashion. Today's look is the result of a process that has been slowly evolving over the past 30 years. Today's female eyelid–brow appearance includes a relatively full brow positioned at the orbital rim, centrally or just slightly above the orbital rim, and laterally above the orbital rim. The upper lid crease is usually less than 10 mm above the lid margin. The sulcus below the orbital rim should not actually define the bony margin. The lateral lid is free of hooding or skin draping over the lateral orbital rim. The overall appearance of the eyelid is one of a healthy, assertive youth. Absent is the high, thin, arched brow placed entirely above the bony orbital rim; the high, dramatic lid crease; and the deeply sculpted lid sulcus. The gaunt, fragile, aloof appearance became a liability in the late 1980s and will continue to be so in the 2000s. New York's mannequin manufacturers have redesigned the standard beautiful American female image to incorporate the slightly heavier, healthier, fuller, and more assertive look. Some latitude is allowed for individual faces and individual tastes. For example, the young face with particularly heavy, ruddy skin, relatively low brows, and a weak chin–neck complex often looks much better with elevation of the brow–forehead unit to a relatively high level. Evaluation of the prospective blepharoplasty patient involves obtaining motivational and medical history, evaluation of the lid–brow complex, discussion of the proposed surgery, discussion of the preoperative and postoperative course and possible associated complications, and photographic documentation.

Preoperative Evaluation

Motivation for Surgery

The ideal candidate for upper lid blepharoplasty has had a relatively long-term desire for reversal of the progressive deterioration of the lid appearance. The patient is in an employment or social situation that warrants facial attractiveness and is realistic about the possible outcome. There should be no expectations of external-world changes as a result of the surgery (e.g., regaining a lost romance or obtaining an elusive job). The patient's questions, answers, forethought, and general dress and manner should appear correct and "feel right" to the interviewing facial plastic surgeon. Interestingly, almost all patients coming for blepharoplasty are good candidates. The psychological and motivational problems seen in rhinoplasty and facelift patients are much less common in blepharoplasty patients.

Medical History

Obviously, any general medical problem that contraindicates elective surgery also contraindicates upper lid blepharoplasty. Particular attention must be given to any condition that may be aggravated by the use of local anesthetic with epinephrine. Many of the newer psychological agents interact with the sympathomimetic amines and must be discontinued before surgery. Homeopathic medications are becoming a common part of many Americans' daily nutritional supplements. Many of these herbal preparations interact with medications used at surgery. St. John's wort, yohimbe, and licorice root can have a monoamine oxidase inhibitory effect. Gingko biloba, used for short-term memory loss, is a powerful anticoagulant. It is best to have a patient report all medications, including alternative medications.

Any condition that produces fluid retention, including the myxedema of hypothyroidism, must be considered in depth before surgery. Allergic dermatitis conditions, especially of the face and lid skin, should be controlled before blepharoplasty to avoid poor scarring or delayed wound healing.

Ophthalmic medical history is critically important. Use of eyeglasses, contact lenses, or eye medications must be documented. Any indication of dry eye syndrome (e.g., burning, tearing, use of artificial tears, waking at night with stinging pain in the eye, or sensitivity to windy conditions) merits a complete evaluation. Personally, the author will not perform upper lid blepharoplasty on any patient who presents with any degree of dry eye syndrome. Even minimal upper lid blepharoplasty can result in upper lid closure failure, exposing the corneal tissues and aggravating the dry eye syndrome with potentially severe complications. Judicious lower lid blepharoplasty can be performed in the presence of dry eye syndrome with much less worry about serious consequences. Unmasking or worsening the dry eye syndrome in an upper lid blepharoplasty patient creates one of the unrelenting postoperative problems in facial plastic surgery. It totally overwhelms even a perfect aesthetic surgical outcome.

A vision history should always be obtained. A nearvision (reading) acuity examination can easily be incorporated into the questionnaire the patient is given to fill out in the waiting area before consultation.

The history of previous upper lid blepharoplasty, even if done many years ago, is important. The possibility of lagophthalmos is always present in these patients, and the indication for conservative secondary surgery is imperative. These patients can present with an impressive amount of apparent upper lid skin redundancy. However, when the eyes are closed the amount of upper lid skin redundancy that can be removed without causing lagophthalmos is usually minimal.

Evaluation of the Brow–Lid Complex

Brow Evaluation

The assessment begins with simple observation while the patient is talking and listening. Eyebrow position during animation and during repose is noted. The patient with low-position eyebrows often elevates them when speaking, producing deep, horizontal forehead creases. In the female patient the lateral and central brow should ideally be above the superior orbital rim. If the lateral and central brow is at or below the orbital rim, a browlift procedure should be considered. An upper lid blepharoplasty performed on a patient with brows below the orbital will invariably pull the brows into a lower position. Of particular interest is a patient with unilateral brow ptosis. This patient invariably sees the problem as a unilateral excess upper lid skin and sees the surgery required as removal of more skin from one eyelid than from the other. This is understandable because patients with unilateral brow ptosis in repose observe this as their natural appearance in a mirror and in a lifetime of family photographs. These patients are quick to see that the problem is not the eyelid but the ptotic eyebrow and are amenable to a concomitant unilateral browlift. The patient with unilateral brow elevation present only with facial animation is also common. No attempt should be made to elevate the lower nonanimation eyebrow in these patients because this will only create an asymmetry in facial repose. After observation, the position of the eyebrow in relationship to the orbital rim is determined by palpation.

Lid Evaluation

The upper eyelid is examined. It should be kept in mind that in the simplest terms the aesthetic goals of upper lid blepharoplasty can be achieved by excision of redundant skin, removal of some part of the musculus orbicularis oculi when necessary, and resection of the pseudoherniated fat. The relative presence of medial fat and central fat is noted. The presence of a palpable lacrimal gland and lateral upper lid gland is also noted. The position of the eyelid crease at the superior tarsal margin is determined. The skin type is especially important in upper lid blepharoplasty. The patient with thin skin is usually an older individual requiring conservative resection of fat in the central compartment to avoid a retracted, hollow look postoperatively. Conservative muscle resection will also be required. In these patients, the eyelid appearance should be returned to one that was present at least a decade earlier. This can be demonstrated by using the wooden portion of a cotton-tipped applicator to roll the redundant skin toward the orbital rim while the patient is observing in the mirror. The patient with very heavy lateral orbital rims may be a candidate for removal of fat from beneath the orbitalis muscle in the region of the lateral brow. This procedure can be done in conjunction with upper lid blepharoplasty.

Special Considerations

The patient with heavy skin, and especially the younger patient with thick skin, has usually never had a discernible upper eyelid crease. Surgical creation of a sculpted eyelid requires excision of considerable fat and the musculus orbicularis oculi, and possibly a lateral extension of the lid skin excision. It is particularly important to show these patients how they will look postoperatively because they have never seen themselves with an eyelid sulcus. These patients often will say, “I've never had eyelids, not even when I was very young.” The patient with thick, heavy skin, especially in the outer third of the lid, may have some tendency toward scarring for several weeks after surgery. This should also be discussed with the patient. Also, when an upper lid blepharoplasty incision must cross the lateral orbital rim onto the facial skin (i.e., when there is considerable lateral hooding), the facial skin portion of the scar will take longer to mature.

The symmetry of the palpebral fissures is noted. The upper lid should cross the limbus just above the pupil in a bilateral symmetric position. A 2 to 3 mm noncorrectable, unilateral ptosis of the upper eyelid will often not be noted by the patient before surgery. Understandably, it is overlooked among the redundant skin and fat herniation. When blepharoplasty has eliminated all of the lid problems, the palpebral fissures asymmetry will be unmasked.

If the surgeon fails to identify this condition and carefully show it to the patient before surgery, it will become a point of contention between the doctor and the patient after surgery. It will be the first thing that friends notice. Any postoperative explanation, even with pictorial evidence, becomes an excuse. If this palpebral fissure asymmetry is noted before surgery, the patient will think of the surgeon as a careful and astute observer.

Notation is made of any associated skin lesion (e.g., xanthoma, syringoma, trichoepithelioma, hypertrophic sebaceous glands, skin pigmentation, enlarged veins, and telangiectasias). Whether these lesions will be removed at the time of surgery, at a later secondary procedure, or not at all must be discussed.

Preoperative Preparation

Decision to perform upper lid blepharoplasty is based on favorable results of psychological, general medical, and ophthalmologic examinations. It is vital that the patient's expectations are in balance with what is possible surgically. The patient should be prepared for the procedure with an in-depth discussion of preoperative recommendations, the surgical procedure itself, the usual postoperative course, and the possible complications.

Preoperative recommendations include asking the patient to avoid aspirin, vitamin E, ibuprofen, and other nonsteroidal antiinflammatory medications for 2 weeks before surgery. All of these medications are known anticoagulants. Use of any of these medications before surgery carries a possibility of intraoperative bleeding and almost certain postoperative moderate to severe ecchymosis. Alcohol ingestion in the immediate preoperative period can cause swelling, and the anticoagulative benefit of daily wine consumption is a detriment before surgery.

The patient should be aware of any physical activities, exercise programs, or travel plans that would adversely affect the immediate postoperative result. It is best to assume that the patient is totally ignorant of these matters at the time of the initial consultation.

Financial arrangements should be clearly understood by the patient so there is no confusion before the operation. Photographs of the patient are obtained either in the office or by a photographer. The standard views include full-face frontal, close-up frontal (eyes open, eyes up, and eyes closed), close-up oblique, and close-up lateral.

Surgical Technique

Most frequently, upper lid blepharoplasty can be done as an outpatient procedure under local anesthesia with minimal preoperative and intraoperative medication of choice.

Planning Incisions

The procedure begins with marking of the lids. To minimize "bleeding" of the skin marking and maximize the permanence of a fine-line drawing on the lid skin, the lids must be totally clean of natural skin oil. All makeup is removed the night before by the patient. The lids are degreased with alcohol or acetone before marking.

The initial lid marking is at the natural lid crease, which can almost always be seen clearly with a bright light and adequate magnification. This lid crease is at the upper margin of the underlying superior tarsal plate. If the natural lid crease is at 8 mm or more above the lid margin, it is always best to use this natural landmark. The lid crease is usually at the same level bilaterally. If there is a 1 mm discrepancy between lids, then adjustments in the lid crease marking are made so that both are 8 to 10 mm above the lid margin. The medial end of the incision is carried far enough nasally to include all of the fine creped skin but never beyond the nasal orbital depression to the nasal skin. Carrying the incision too far nasally causes almost irreversible webbing. Laterally the lid crease line is carried in the natural crease of the sulcus between the orbital rim and the eyelid. At this point, the line breaks laterally or slightly upward (**Fig. 22.1**). With the patient in a supine position, the real amount of the upper lid skin redundancy can only be determined after the brow is physically pushed downward. In the supine position the mobility and weight of the scalp and forehead pull the brow above the orbital rim. This is not the true, natural position of the brow. The upper lid skin redundancy is transiently

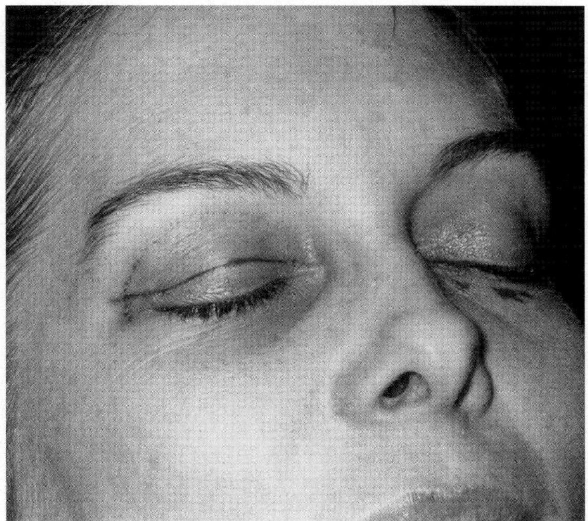

Fig. 22.1 The natural lid crease is used as the guide for the lower lid marking. It is marked on both eyes so that symmetry is achieved. The mark should naturally lie at 8 to 10 mm above the lid margin. If the mark is lower or higher than these limits, the scar may become obvious. In this patient the line has been extended laterally to encompass the lateral hooding. The dotted line shows the orbital rim.

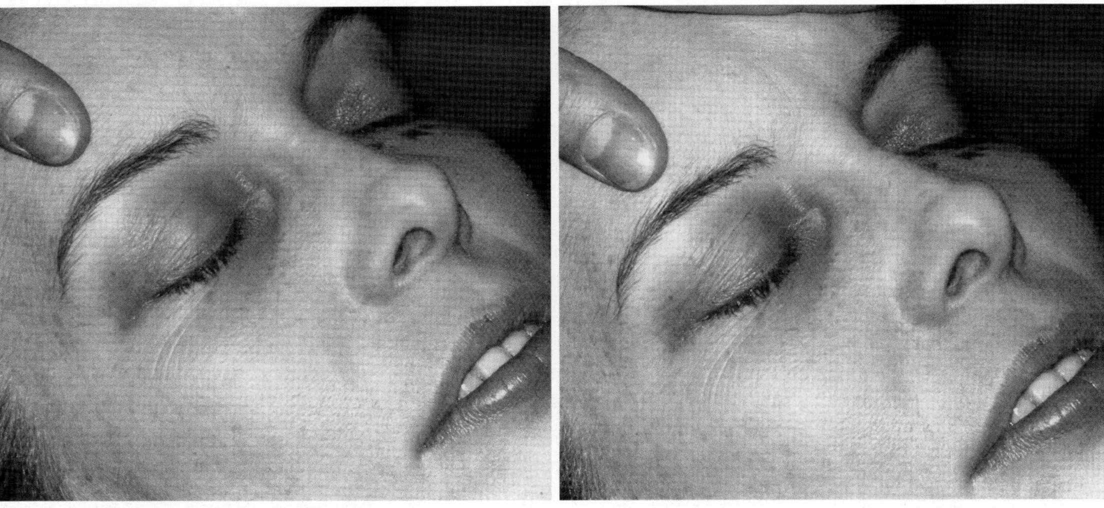

Fig. 22.2 (**A**) With the patient in the supine position, the brow position becomes elevated by the weight of the scalp. This elevates the lid skin and diminishes the amount of upper lid skin redundancy. The brow must be repositioned for lid marking. (**B**) With gentle pressure, the brow relocated downward. This is the position the brow would naturally assume if the patient were upright.

lessened. To plan the upper lid blepharoplasty correctly the brow must be gently pushed down toward the orbital rim into a position noted when the patient was seated or standing (**Fig. 22.2A,B**). The upper lid skin is then gently grasped with forceps. One blade of the forceps is at the previously marked lid crease. The other blade grasps just enough redundant skin to smooth the lid but not to move the lid margin upward. In other words, if the skin between the forceps blades were to be removed, surgical elevation of the lid margin and lagophthalmos should not occur (**Fig. 22.3**).

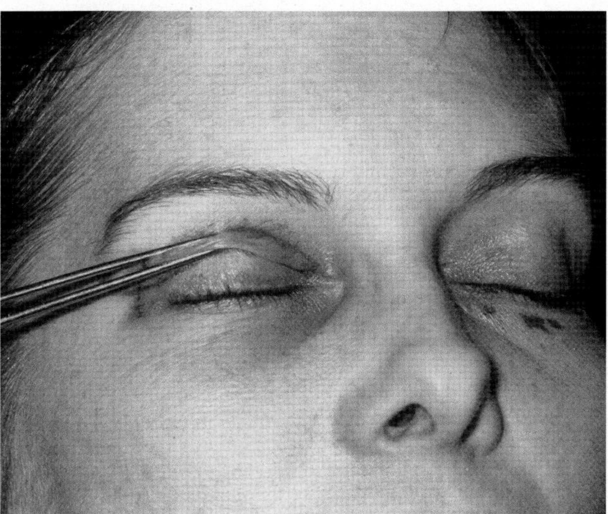

Fig. 22.3 The skin is grasped with a forceps so that all excess skin is incorporated. The lower blade of the forceps is on the mark indicating the natural lid crease. The lid should not open with this maneuver. Removal of enough skin to allow opening of the lid could cause lagophthalmos.

This marking technique is used at several points across the lid. As these points are connected a line is created that parallels the lid crease line. Medially and laterally the lines join at a 30-degree angle. The medial skin redundancy should always be slightly underestimated in patients with a large amount of medial fat. The defect created by the excision of a large amount of fat medially may cause a dead space to occur subcutaneously. If slightly less skin is excised medially the repaired medial end of the lid falls inward rather than tenting over the area of removed fat. If tenting of the medial lid skin occurs, dense scarring is almost a certainty in this region.

The lateral extent of the planned skin excision is determined by the amount of lateral hooding. If no hooding is present in a younger patient, the lateral excision ends just beyond the lateral canthus. If the lateral hooding is extensive, the excision may be carried 1 cm or more beyond the orbital rim laterally. The direction of the resultant scar should always lie between the lateral canthus and the lateral eyebrow (**Fig. 22.4**). In this position the incision can be camouflaged by eyeshadow makeup in the female patient (**Fig. 22.5**). The area demarcated by the surgical pen marking should be a gentle sinuous shape (**Fig. 22.6**).

Anesthesia

Once the marking is complete, local anesthesia can be infiltrated. Xylocaine 2% with epinephrine buffered 1:100,000 with sodium bicarbonate 8.4% is recommended. The ratio is 10 mL xylocaine to 1 mL bicarbonate. Approximately 1 mL is infiltrated into the upper lid subcutaneous space with a 1 in. or 25 to 27 gauge needle. To gain the maximal effect

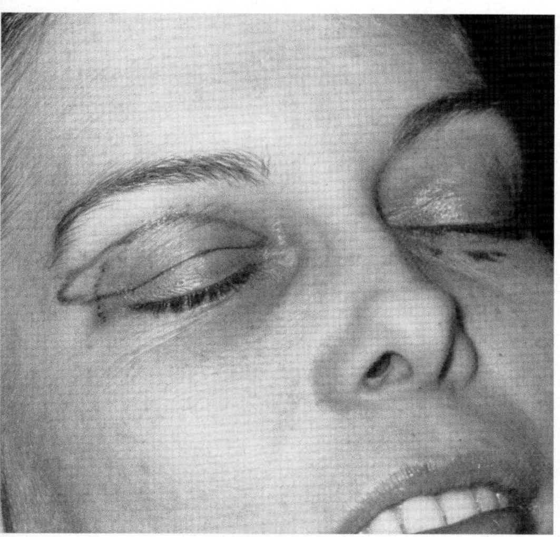

Fig. 22.4 With the patient's eyes closed, the amount of skin to be removed can be seen as a gentle sinuous shape extending beyond the lateral orbital margin.

from the epinephrine, at least 10 minutes must elapse before an excision is made.

Initial Incision and Muscle Excision

The initial incision is made by stretching the lid skin marking into a straight line and incising the lid crease marking with a no. 12 blade of choice (**Fig. 22.7**). A no. 67 Beaver blade is preferred because it is sharp and small. The upper limb of the incision is made, and the skin is removed with a forceps and curved Stevens scissors. At this point a decision is made about the underlying musculus orbicularis oculi. Some muscle is removed in almost all cases. Usually thin-skinned, older patients require less muscle excision, whereas younger and especially heavy-skinned patients require more muscle excision to gain a good aesthetic effect.

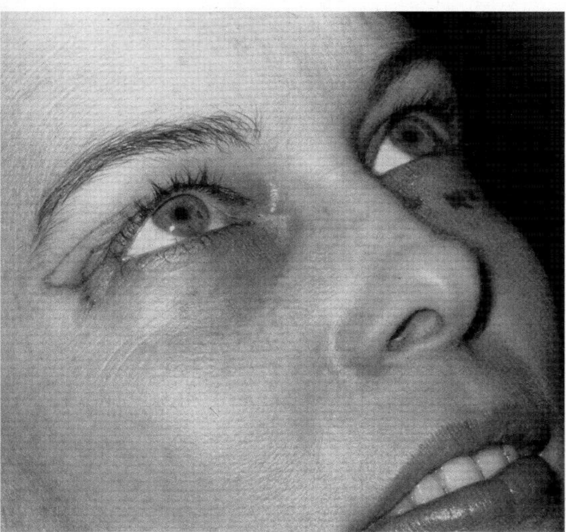

Fig. 22.5 With the patient's eyes open, the considerable amount of skin lateral to the palpebral fissure can be seen. The lateral excision will eliminate the lateral hooding.

The muscle excision is made along the path of the skin excision. The width of the skin excision is as wide or as narrow as necessary. The depth of the excision is to the orbital septum (**Fig. 22.8**).

Fat Removal

If there is an abundance of fat, it is probably wise to remove the central compartment before removal of the medial fat compartment. The central compartment can be opened by incising the orbital septum in one place or by opening along its entire length. A small fat pseudoherniation can be removed with one clamping. Larger amounts may require dividing the central compartment into two or more sections. The medial fat compartment is teased into the wound and excised. Although classically there is no lateral fat compartment in the upper lid, fat can be present external to the lacrimal gland in an apparent lateral compartment (**Fig. 22.9**). All fat is injected with a small amount of local anesthesia before clamping. The subcutaneously injected local anesthesia will not ordinarily penetrate the orbital septum. If additional anesthetic agent is not used, the patient will feel pain from the fat clamping. The fat is clamped with a small, narrow hemostat. It is then excised, leaving a small cuff of tissue available for cauterization. It is important not to actively pull fat from the orbit into the wound for removal. Only fat that comes into the wound easily should be removed. This is especially important in the area of the medial aspect of the central compartment. Removal of too much fat here can lead to a retraction of the lid and a pronounced overhang of the orbital rim. The resulting appearance can be that of aging and must be avoided.

The medial fat compartment may be elusive. It is important to analyze its significance preoperatively so that it is removed at surgery. At times, because of the patient's position, the medial fat falls back into a seemingly insignificant position. If it was seen to be a problem before surgery, then the medial fat pocket must be sought and removed. To underestimate the amount of redundant medial fat is the most common aesthetic error in upper lid blepharoplasty. The fat medially is whiter than yellow and also denser than the central compartment fat. Medial fat position is somewhat variable compared with all of the fat compartments in the upper and lower lids. The central and medial fat compartments are separated by the musculus obliquus superior oculi. In contrast with the musculus obliquus

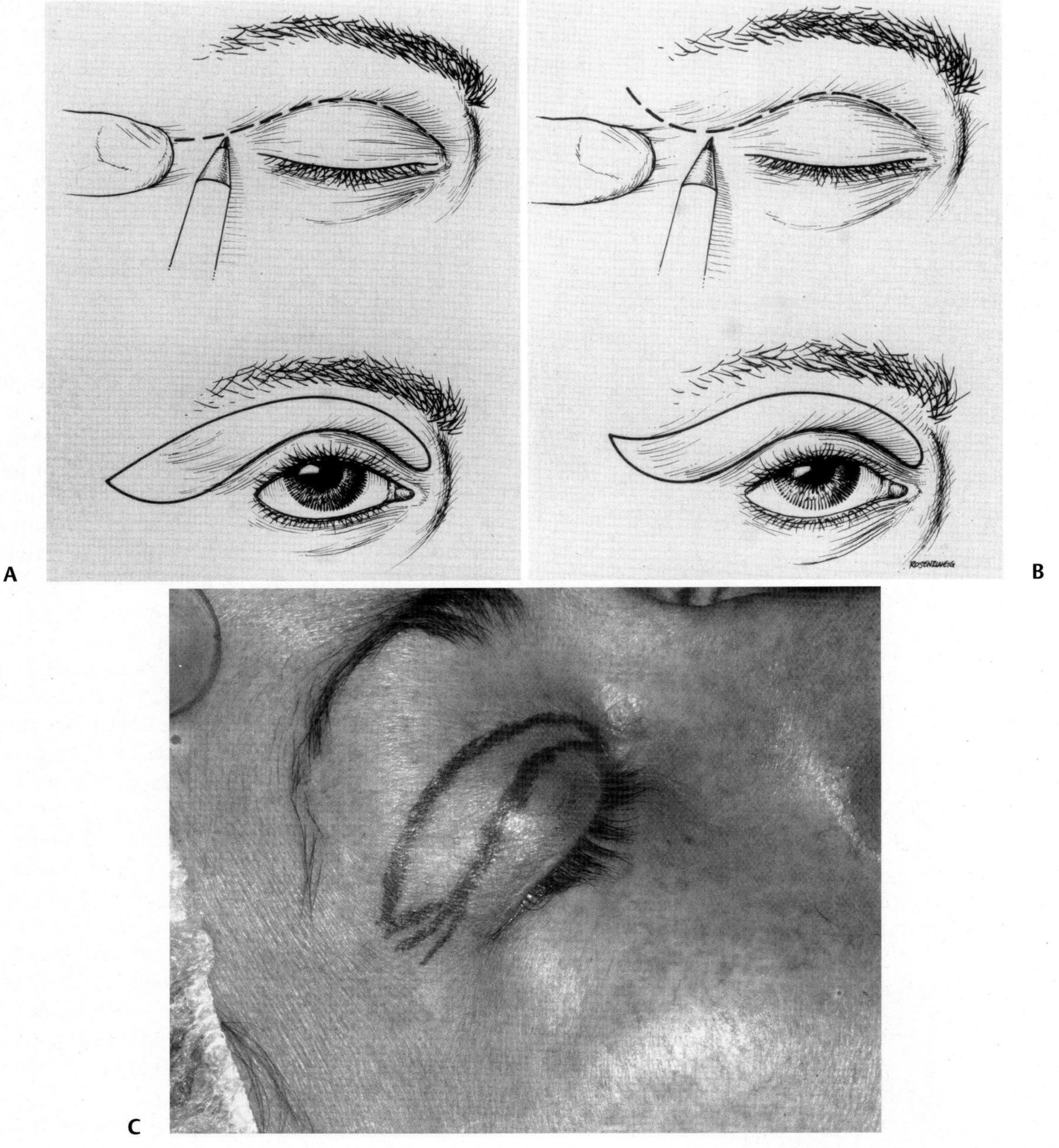

Fig. 22.6 (**A**) The classic skin excision follows the general line of the natural lid crease. The lateral extent of the incision tends to fall below the lateral hooding just beyond the orbital rim. The cleanness of the upper lid following excision of redundant skin may exaggerate the lateral hooding. (**B**) There are several advantages to moving the lateral extent of the incision upward at the lateralorbital rim. The resulting scar lies between the lateral brow and the lateral canthus. In this position the healing wound can be camouflaged by eyeshadow makeup in the first few days following blepharoplasty. Moving the lateral extent upward also avoids a permanent scar directly ina lateral crow's foot. The most significant advantage, however, is that the superior limb of the wound is stabilized by the firm subcutaneous tethering in this area. The idea for this modification came about when it was noted that the temporal skin cannot be drawn downward to close a defect in this area. (**C**) The surgical pen marking in this patient shows the various choices possible for skin incision in the lateral aspect of upper lid blepharoplasty. The most inferior position is the classic one placing the incision in a lateral rhytid. The midlevel mark would be used in a patient with minimal hooding. The superior mark (to be used in this patient) shows the best position for eliminating lateral hooding.

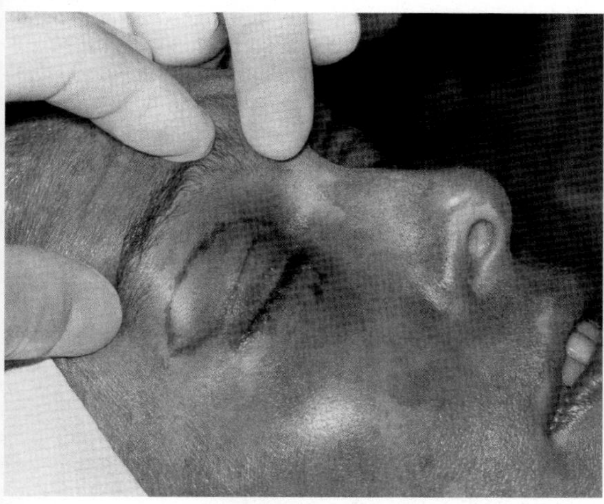

Fig. 22.7 The skin is stretched tightly in preparation for skin incision. The surgical mark should be made with the finest line possible. Natural skin oil on the lid surface may cause the surgical pen mark to widen. A thick mark can lead to excessive skin excision. It is always best to remove skin oil prior to marking.

inferior oculi, this muscle in the lower lid is rarely observed. Still its presence should always be sought before applying a hemostat to the fat.

If during the preoperative evaluation a lateral orbital rim fat pad has been noted to be a part of the aesthetic problem, it can be removed at this time. The upper outer limb of the incision is retracted. Blunt dissection beneath the orbicularis muscle exposes the lateral orbital rim fat pad. Scissors sculpting removes the fat. There are several small vessels in the fat. Hemostasis must be absolute and complete.

It is possible to remove fat from the medial compartment via a transconjunctival approach. The upper lid is everted with a lid retractor. Digital pressure is placed on the medial fat compartment. The fat will be seen as a bulge beneath the conjunctiva. The levator aponeurosis does not lie between the conjunctiva and the subseptal fat as it does in the central compartment. The conjunctiva is injected just as it is in the lower lid transconjunctival approach. The conjunctiva is opened sharply

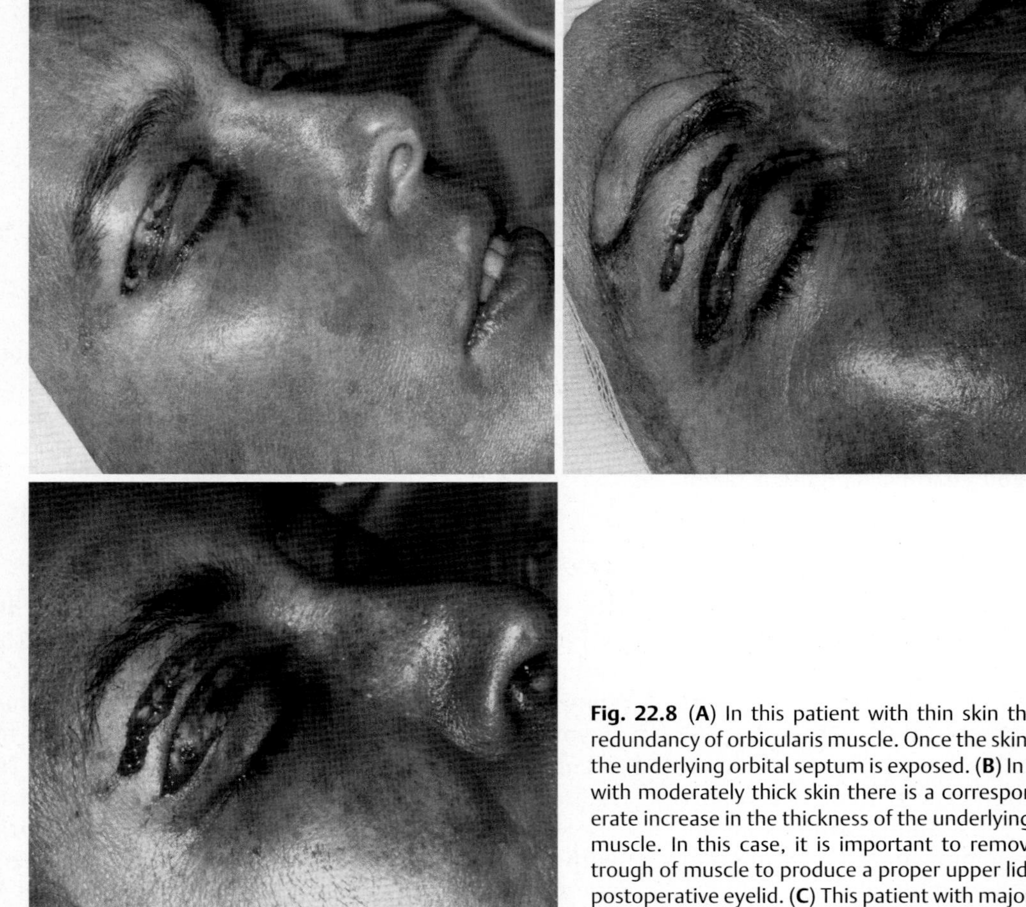

Fig. 22.8 (**A**) In this patient with thin skin there was no redundancy of orbicularis muscle. Once the skin is removed the underlying orbital septum is exposed. (**B**) In this patient with moderately thick skin there is a corresponding moderate increase in the thickness of the underlying orbicularis muscle. In this case, it is important to remove a central trough of muscle to produce a proper upper lid cleft in the postoperative eyelid. (**C**) This patient with major orbicularis muscle hypertrophy required a significant excision of muscle to allow definition of the upper lid cleft. If the muscle is not removed, the lid will continue to appear full.

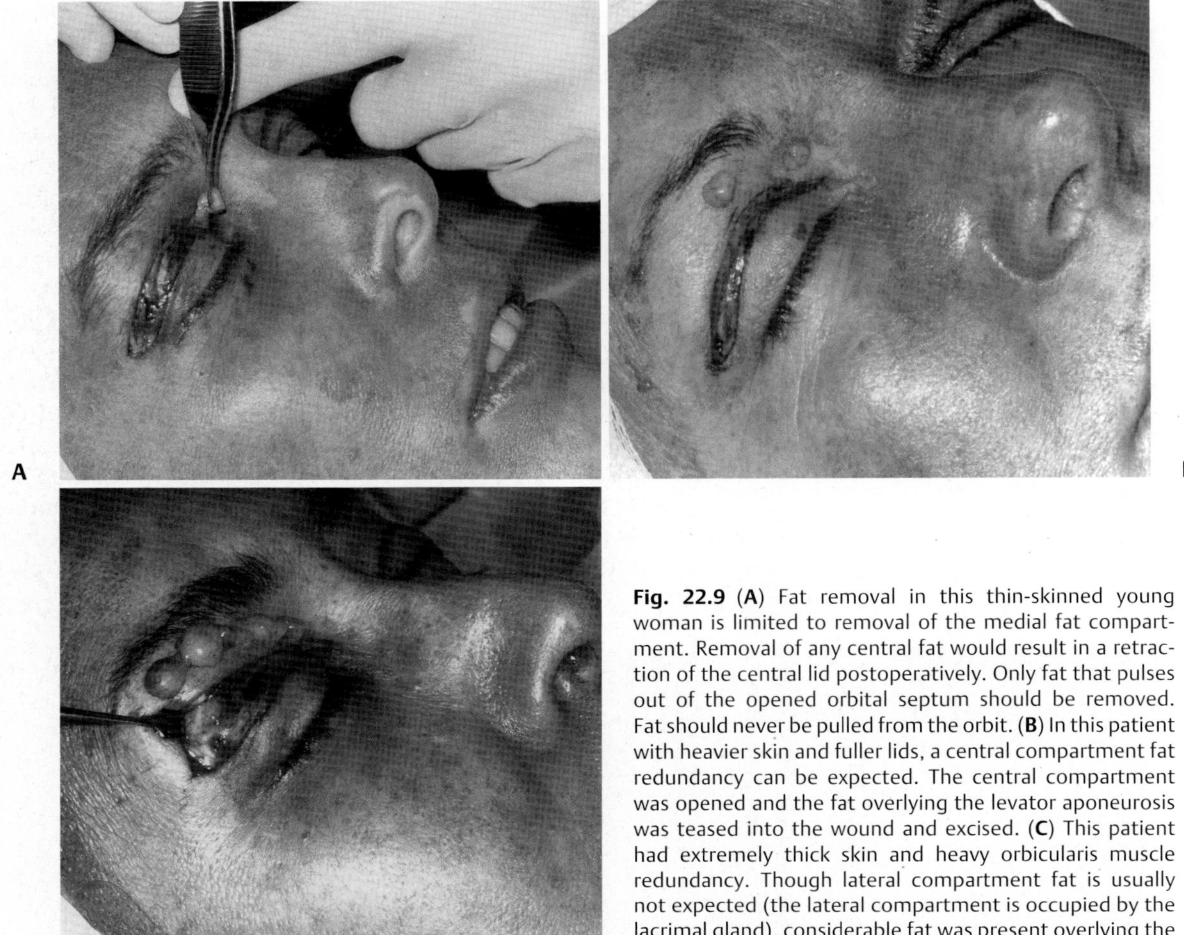

Fig. 22.9 (**A**) Fat removal in this thin-skinned young woman is limited to removal of the medial fat compartment. Removal of any central fat would result in a retraction of the central lid postoperatively. Only fat that pulses out of the opened orbital septum should be removed. Fat should never be pulled from the orbit. (**B**) In this patient with heavier skin and fuller lids, a central compartment fat redundancy can be expected. The central compartment was opened and the fat overlying the levator aponeurosis was teased into the wound and excised. (**C**) This patient had extremely thick skin and heavy orbicularis muscle redundancy. Though lateral compartment fat is usually not expected (the lateral compartment is occupied by the lacrimal gland), considerable fat was present overlying the lacrimal gland in this compartment.

and the fat is extracted, clamped, and excised. No suturing is necessary. This approach may be worth considering when the only problem is medial fat psuedoherniation. It may also be considered when medial fat is found to persist following upper lid blepharoplasty. Care is taken to avoid the superior oblique muscle.

Cauterization

A hot-tipped cautery is preferred; however, bipolar cautery may also be used. Unipolar electrocautery applied directly to the hemostat can cause the patient pain, especially under local anesthesia with light premedication. Apparently there is transfer of electrical impulses deep into the orbit. The patient will report pain "in the back of the eye." Animal studies at the University of Oregon have demonstrated transmission of heat up to a distance of 1 cm internal to the application of unipolar cautery to clamped fat. Thermal transmission was negligible to minimal with hot-tipped and bipolar cautery.

Hemostasis must be meticulous before wound closure. It is important not to be too aggressive with the cautery in the subcutaneous tissue at the incision margin because thermal injury here can interfere with the fine postoperative scar.

Wound Closure

The use of Prolene 6–0 suture (Ethicon, Inc., Somerville, NJ) for wound closure of the eyelids is preferred. This suture almost never leaves suture marks even if for some unpredictable reason the sutures remain in place beyond the usual 3- to 4-day ideal time. Also, the occurrence of suture tunnels or suture milia is rare. The lateral aspect of the wound where tension is the greatest is closed first (**Fig. 22.10A**). This area is repaired with several individual simple sutures. After the lateral one fourth of the wound is closed, the remainder of the wound is repaired with a running subcuticular 6–0 Prolene suture beginning medially. It is unnecessary to knot the Prolene at the entrance and exit of the skin

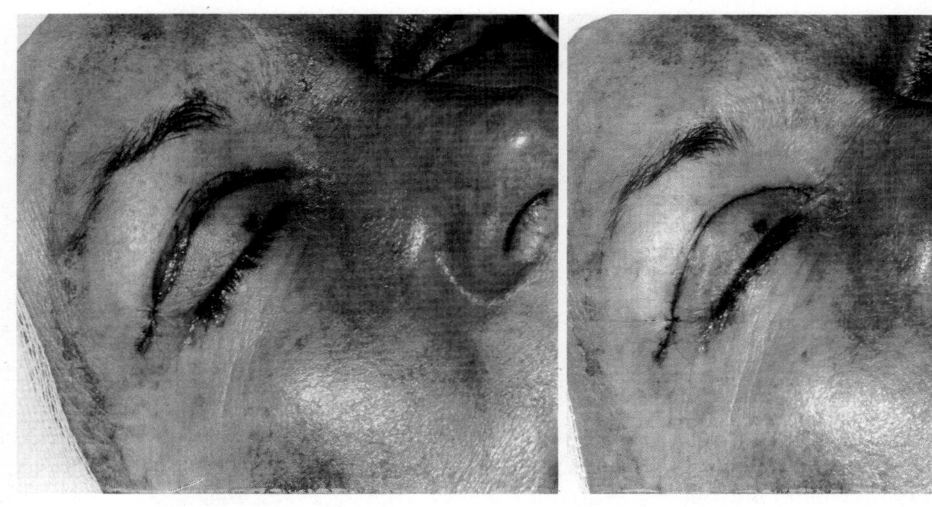

Fig. 22.10 (**A**) The lateral wound angle is closed first with individual 6–0 polypropylene sutures. The most tension is present in this area of transition between the eyelid skin and facial skin. It is most important that the angle be closed without any irregularity. (**B**) Following repair of the lateral aspect of the wound, the remainder of the wound is closed with a subcuticular running 6–0 polypropylene suture beginning at the medial angle of the wound. The suture repair can be supplemented with one-eighth inch. surgical tape over the wound and/or surgical glue to give further support.

(**Fig. 22.10B**). The ends of the subcuticular suture are taped to the forehead. When any suspicion of wound tension exists, the entire wound can be taped with inch-long surgical strips.

At the end of the procedure attention is directed to the medial aspect of the lid. Any remaining skin crepe can be excised as small triangles above and below the medial incision. These excisions can be opposite one another or staggered. The base of the triangle lies at the incision. Care is taken not to cut the subcutaneous suture during skin excision. These triangular defects can be taped closed with one-eighth inch surgical squares. Occasionally, a single 6–0 Prolene suture can be used to close the triangular defect. Most times the skin edges lie in approximation without any need to secure the wound. This final maneuver flattens the medial aspect of the lid. If any wound separation is noted at the conclusion of the surgery, an additional simple suture can be used at that area of tension.

Upper Lid Blepharoplasty in Men

Upper lid blepharoplasty surgery in women differs substantially from the procedure in men. In male patients, the surgeon must be extremely conservative. Extension of the lateral excision beyond the lateral canthal boundary, in general, should not be done in males. If the incision is carried beyond the lateral orbital rim, the immediate scar produced cannot be covered with makeup. The surgeon should always assume that the male patient would not wear cosmetics of any kind. The long-term scar, though very slight, may remain objectionable for years.

The surgical goal for the lid sulcus differs markedly in women and men. A deep superior lid sulcus is contraindicated in the male. It is not only feminizing but also radically changes the masculine appearance. It is not the usual male look. A man in today's society usually looks best with some upper lid skin redundancy, some skin crepe, and a lid crease just a few millimeters above the lid margin.

Postoperative Care

The patient is asked to remain quiet for the remainder of the day of surgery, preferably in a two-pillow supine position. Ice-cold compresses are used continuously during the waking hours and an ophthalmic ointment is used over the incision line several times a day. Pain is minimal and is relieved with acetaminophen or acetaminophen with codeine. The patient should not watch television or read for the next 24 hours. Individuals who are accustomed to a regular physical workout also must avoid physical exercise. Men especially must be counseled regarding what is expected in the postoperative behavior. The surgeon or staff must be available and approachable concerning any questions the patient or the patient's family or caretaker might have.

When Prolene is used to close the wound, the sutures are removed on the fourth postoperative day. The use of the other suture materials requires different schedules for suture removal. Silk sutures used in the eyelid should be removed within 24 hours to avoid suture tunnels or

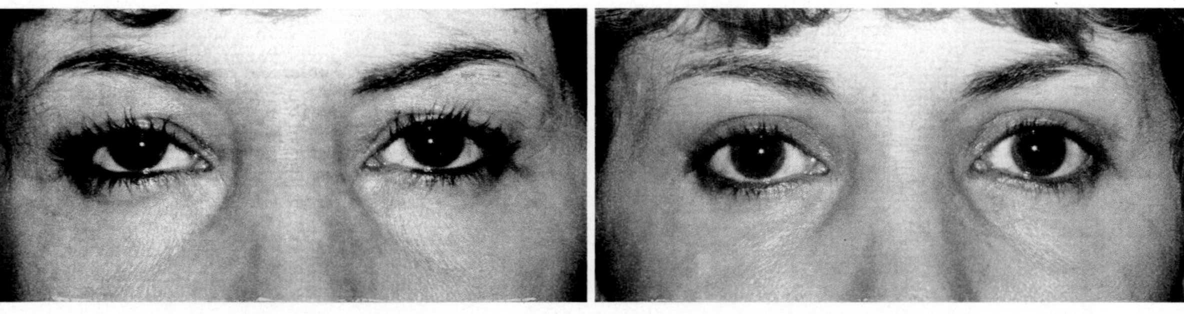

Fig. 22.11 (A) Preoperative frontal view of a 38-year-old woman with moderate upper lid blepharochalasis. (B) Postoperative view at 6 months.

track marks. Nylon also can leave marks if left in beyond 3 days. It is rare to find any suture reaction with Prolene. At the time of suture removal, the lateral wound must be closely observed for any minute wound-edge overlap or wound separation. Either condition warrants a "roughing up" of the wound edges and replacement of the sutures for 24 to 48 hours. The lateral eyelid wound, because it continues in many cases onto the facial skin beyond the limit of the orbital rim, has a tendency to become obvious. This is because of the difference in thickness of the eyelid skin and the facial skin beyond the orbital rim. The lateral wound will not show if great attention is given to it postoperatively. In any case, even if the wound looks perfect at the 4-day suture removal, inch-long surgical tape strips or surgical glue should be used to support this area for an additional 24 to 48 hours. The patient may apply cosmetics to the upper eyelid incision on the sixth postoperative day. Mild physical activity may begin at 10 days, progressing to full physical activity at 4 weeks. The patient should avoid direct, unprotected sun exposure for 6 weeks (**Figs. 22.11–22.14**).

Complications

Erythema along the incision, a sensation of tightness or minor tearing, numbness and edema of the lids, and obviousness of the lateral half of the surgical wound are all natural and transient events following upper lid blepharoplasty.

Hematoma

Hematoma is rare after upper lid blepharoplasty. The occurrence of unilateral swelling and discoloration immediately

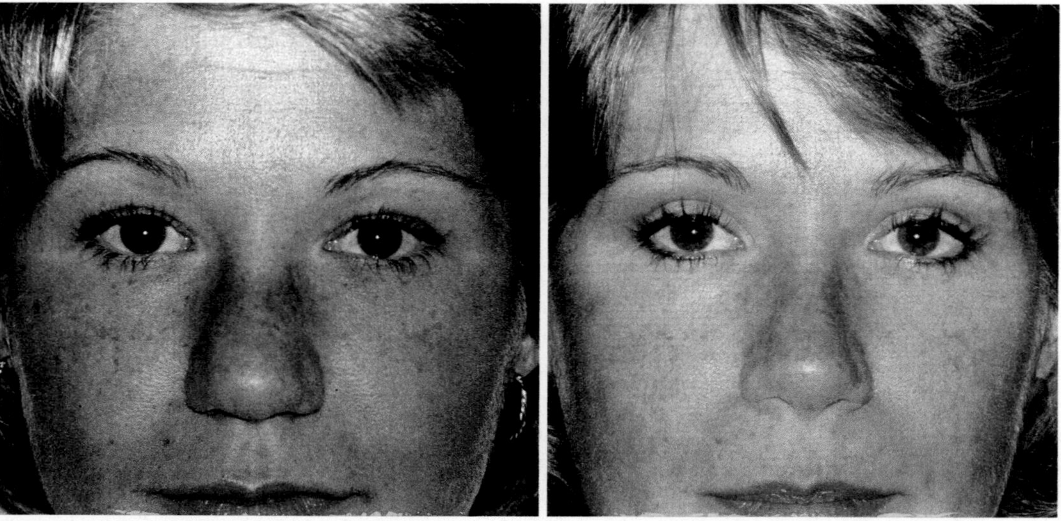

Fig. 22.12 (A) Preoperative view of a 32-year-old woman with long-term blepharochalasis. The fleshy appearance of the lids has been present since childhood. It is not unusual for these patients to also have a fleshy nasal appearance. Often the combination of rhinoplasty and blepharoplasty is synergistic. (B) Postoperative appearance 6 months following upper lid blepharoplasty and rhinoplasty.

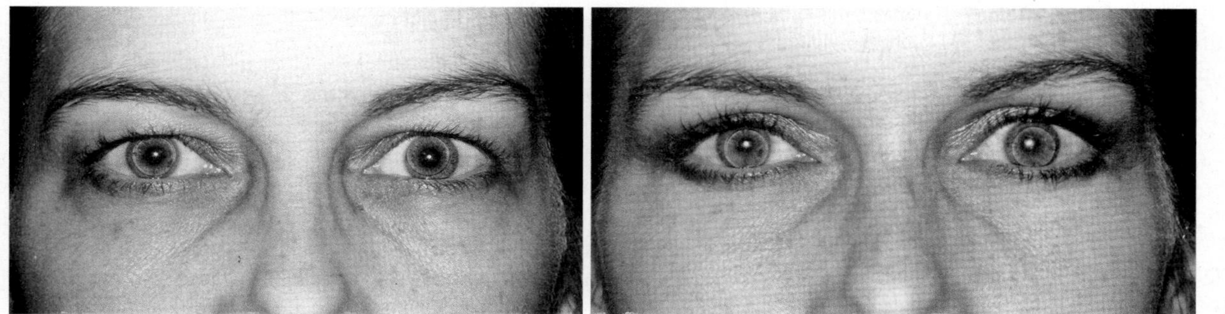

Fig. 22.13 (**A**) Preoperative frontal appearance of a 32-year-old woman with upper lid blepharochalasis. There is a slight asymmetry of the brows, which is common. This degree of asymmetry usually does not have to be addressed. Most patients are unaware of the condition. (**B**) Postoperative frontal view of the patient at 6 months following upper lid blepharoplasty.

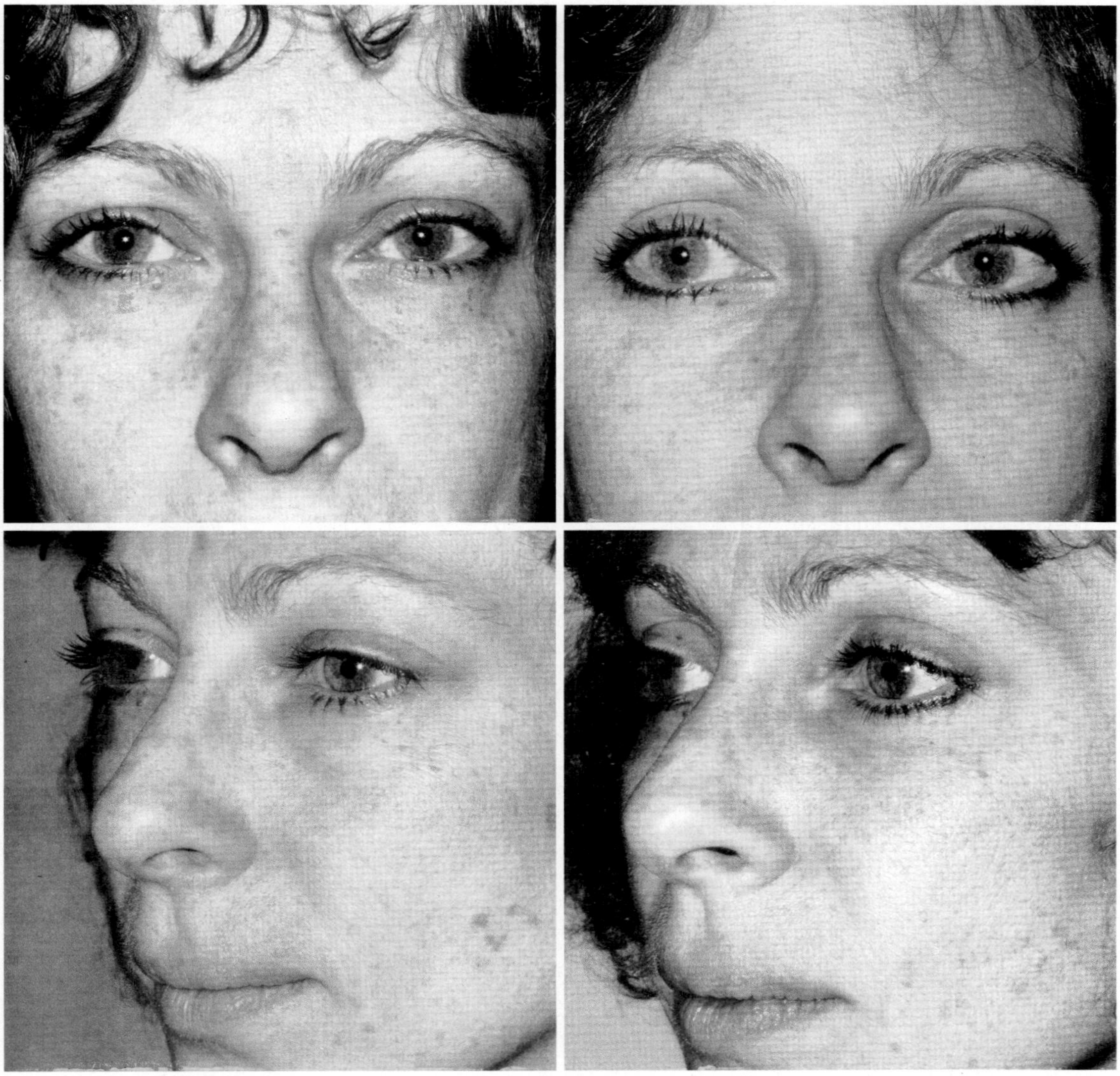

Fig. 22.14 (**A**) Preoperative frontal view of a 33-year-old woman with moderate upper and lower lid blepharochalasis. She has distinct medial fat compartments. (**B**) Postoperative frontal view of the patient 1 year after four-lid blepharoplasty. (**C**) Preoperative oblique view of the patient. (**D**) Postoperative oblique view of the patient at 1 year.

postoperatively should raise the suspicion of hematoma. The wound must be reopened. The bleeding vessel is cauterized and the wound is resutured.

Subconjunctival Ecchymosis

Subconjunctival ecchymosis is an unusual problem. Its cause is rarely obvious. Although it is usually frightening to the patient, it is only a cosmetic problem. The patient should be assured that within time the whiteness of the eye will return. The red discoloration persists for 3 weeks or more.

Chemosis

Chemosis (edema of the conjunctiva) is unusual in upper lid blepharoplasty. It can persist for 6 weeks after the procedure. Blephamide ophthalmic drops will shorten its course in most cases.

Lagophthalmos

Lagophthalmos is present for a short period postoperatively in many cases. It is most likely the cause of transient tearing and burning reported by some patients. The use of ophthalmic ointment initially and then daily use of synthetic tear drops and ointment quells the symptoms during the healing period. Persistent lagophthalmos can lead to dry eye syndrome. Surgical interference with the upper lid visor function of corneal protection mechanism is a serious problem that is most likely to occur when upper lid blepharoplasty is performed simultaneously with a forehead lift or during secondary upper lid blepharoplasty. It is difficult to estimate the amount of redundant upper lid at the time of forehead lift. It is never a mistake to postpone upper lid blepharoplasty until a few months following the forehead lift. Most of the acute problems resolve with time, but constant use of artificial tears, night taping of the lids, and ophthalmic consultation are often necessary.

Poor Scars

Obvious scars in the lateral upper lid wound may occur when wound separation at suture removal is not recognized or when sun exposure occurs to pigment the wound. In either case, a later secondary excision and repair procedure may be necessary. Poor medial scars are always due to excessive skin excision or unanticipated removal of large amounts of fat that leads to a wound closure tented over a dead space. These scars are best treated with minute injections of triamcinolone (Kenalog, 10 mg/mL).

Loss of Vision

Most reported cases of vision loss follow hematoma formation after lower lid or upper and lower lid blepharoplasty. Hypertension, old age, anticoagulant mediation, and metabolic diseases are also usually present. Vision loss secondary to bleeding in the upper lid blepharoplasty is distinctly rare. In all cases of hematoma, rapid decompression of the progressing retrobulbar hematoma is essential.

Suggested Readings

Burke AJ, Wang T. Should formal ophthalmologic evaluation be a preoperative requirement prior to blepharoplasty? Arch Otolaryngol Head Neck Surg 2001;127:719–722

Campbell JP, Lisman RD. Complications of blepharoplasty. Facial Plast Surg 2000;8:303

Kamer FM, Mingrone MD. Experiences with transconjunctival upper blepharoplasty. Arch Facial Plast Surg 2000;2:213–216

Mahe E, Harfaoui-Chanaaoui T, Banal A, Chappay C. Tran quoc chi. Different technical approaches for blepharoplasty in eyelid rejuvenation surgery. Arch Otorhinolaryngol 1989;246:353–356

McKinney P, Byun M. The value of tear film breakup and Schirmer's test in preoperative blepharoplasty evaluation. Plast Reconstr Surg 1999;104:566

Millay DJ. Upper lid blepharoplasty. Facial Plast Surg 1994;10:18–26

Siegel RJ. Essential anatomy of contemporary upper lid blepharoplasty. Clin Plast Surg 1993;20:209–212

Stambaugh KI. Upper lid blepharoplasty. Skin vs. pinch. Laryngoscope 1991;101:1233–1237

Wolfort FG, Vaughan TE, Wolfort SF, Nevaree DR. Retrobulbar hematoma and blepharoplasty. Plast Reconstr Surg 1999;104:2154–2162

23 Lower Eyelid Blepharoplasty

Roger L. Crumley, Behrooz A. Torkian, and Amir M. Karam

Lower eyelid blepharoplasty is an operation which is commonly performed to rejuvenate the lower eyelid region. It is considered a technically challenging operation with a myriad of technical variations and paradigms. The technical challenge of this procedure is due to the fact that a very fine line exists between an enhanced aesthetic outcome and significant functional and aesthetic complications. An intimate and thorough understanding of the anatomy, coupled with an understanding of the natural history of lower eyelid aging, is required to achieve a successful surgical outcome.

Periorbital Aging

The youthful lower eyelid should have a smooth gentle convexity and blend into the upper cheek mound. With age, weakening of the orbital septum results in variable degrees of bulging of the orbital fat. This coupled with descent of the malar fat pad, sagging of the orbicularis oculi muscle, lengthens the lid-cheek junction and reveals the bony outline of the inferior orbital rim. These factors combined results in a double-convexity contour deformity. The orbital fat is the superior convexity, directly below this is the relative concavity defined by arcus marginalis along the skeletonized inferior orbital rim, and the second concavity is defined by the cheek mound. This finding is a tell tale sign of aging of the central face. Tear-trough deformity or nasojugal fold is described by a depression at the transition of the medial aspect of the lower eyelid and upper cheek. The resultant deformity causes the periorbital region to have fatigued and aged appearance. This is a finding is caused by a deficiency of tissue, not excess. Therefore, removing skin, muscle, or fat from the lower eyelid will worsen this deformity. The etiology is caused by a descent of the cheek (malar mound) with age and/ or a deficient or hypoplastic infraorbital rim and maxilla.

The Female Eye

Periorbital skin should be smooth and free of rhytids or redundant folds. The glabella should be smooth, without vertical or horizontal deep rhytids. The junction of the lower eyelid and cheek should be smooth without obvious or severe convexities or concavities. The palpebral aperture should ideally have an almond shape. This is shape is desired in essentially all ethnicities. The canthal tilt is determined by drawing a horizontal line extending laterally from the medial canthus followed by a second line that extends from the medial canthus through the lateral canthus.[1] The distance measured in millimeters or degrees defines the canthal tilt. A positive value represents an upward tilt, which is thought be one of the most important features of the aesthetic eye. In women, the average canthal tilt equals + 4 degrees or 4.1 mm.[2]

The Male Eye

The goals for eyelid surgery are different for male patient. The surgeon must avoid maneuvers which will feminize the eye. In the male patient, slight fullness and redundancy of the tissue result in a more masculine outcome. The esthetics lower eyelid are similar to and parallel those of the female patient. The lower lid should be tight against the globe with no evidence of scleral show. There should be a slight incline of the canthal tilt ~ 2.1mm (+ 3 degrees).[3] More of an incline will give a more feminine appearance.

Anatomical Considerations

In no other area of facial aesthetic surgery is such a fragile balance struck between form and function as that in eyelid modification. Owing to the delicate nature of eyelid structural composition and the vital role the eyelids serve in protecting the visual system, iatrogenic alterations in eyelid anatomy must be made with care, precision, and thoughtful consideration of existing soft tissue structures. A brief anatomical review is necessary to highlight some of these salient points.

With the eyes in primary position, the lower lid should be well apposed to the globe, with its lid margin roughly tangent to the inferior limbus and the orientation of its respective palpebral fissure slanted slightly obliquely upward from medial to lateral (occidental norm). An inferior palpebral sulcus (lower eyelid crease) is usually identified ~5 to 6 mm from the ciliary margin and roughly delineates the inferior edge of the tarsal plate and the transition zone from pretarsal to preseptal orbicularis oculi[4] (**Fig. 23.1**).

Lamellae

The eyelids have been considered as being composed of two lamellae: (1) an outer lamella, composed of skin and the orbicularis oculi muscle; and (2) an inner lamella, which includes tarsus and conjunctiva. The skin of the lower

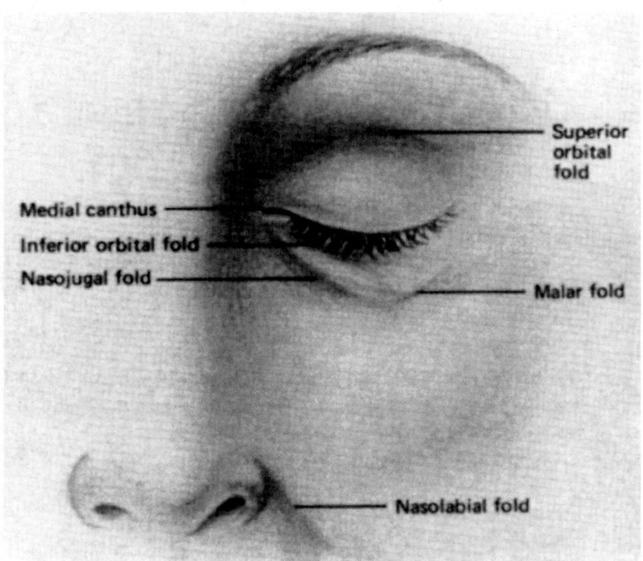

Fig. 23.1 Topographic anatomy of the eyelid, demonstrating natural folds. (From Kohn R. Textbook of Ophthalmic Plastic and Reconstructive Surgery. Philadelphia: Lea & Febiger; 1988. Reprinted by permission.)

eyelid, which measures less than 1 mm in thickness,[5] retains a smooth delicate texture until it extends beyond the lateral orbital rim, where it gradually becomes thicker and coarser. The eyelid skin, which is essentially devoid of a subcutaneous fat layer, is interconnected to the underlying musculus orbicularis oculi by fine connective tissue attachments in the skin's pretarsal and preseptal zones.

Musculature

The orbicularis oculi muscle can be divided into a darker and thicker orbital portion (voluntary) and a thinner and lighter palpebral portion (voluntary and involuntary). The palpebral portion can be further subdivided into preseptal and pretarsal components (**Fig. 23.2**). The larger superficial heads of the pretarsal orbicularis unite to form the medial canthal tendon, which inserts onto the anterior lacrimal crest, whereas the deep heads unite to insert at the posterior lacrimal crest. Laterally, the fibers condense and become firmly attached at the orbital tubercle of Whitnall, becoming the lateral canthal tendon.[6] Although the preseptal orbicularis has fixed attachments with the medial and lateral canthal tendons, the orbital portion does not and instead inserts subcutaneously in the lateral orbital region (contributing to crow's feet), overlies some of the elevator muscles of the upper lip and ala, and possesses attachments to the infraorbital bony margin.

Immediately beneath the submuscular fascia, extending along the posterior surface of the preseptal orbicularis, lies the orbital septum. Delineating the boundary between anterior eyelid (outer lamella) and intraorbital contents, it originates at the arcus marginalis along the orbital rim (continuous with orbital periosteum), and after fusing with the capsulopalpebral fascia posteriorly ~5 mm below the lower tarsal edge, it forms a single fascial layer that inserts near the tarsal base.

The capsulopalpebral head of the inferior rectus is a dense, fibrous, connective tissue expansion, which by virtue of its ultimate attachments to the tarsal plate allows for lower lid retraction during downward gaze. During its forward extension, it encompasses the musculus obliquus inferior, and after reuniting anteriorly, it contributes to the formation of Lockwood's suspensory ligament (inferior transverse ligament, at which point it is termed the ***capsulopalpebral fascia***, CPF).[7] Although the majority of its fibers terminate near the inferior tarsal border, some extend through orbital fat contributing to compartmentalization, some penetrate the preseptal orbicularis to insert subcutaneously about the lower

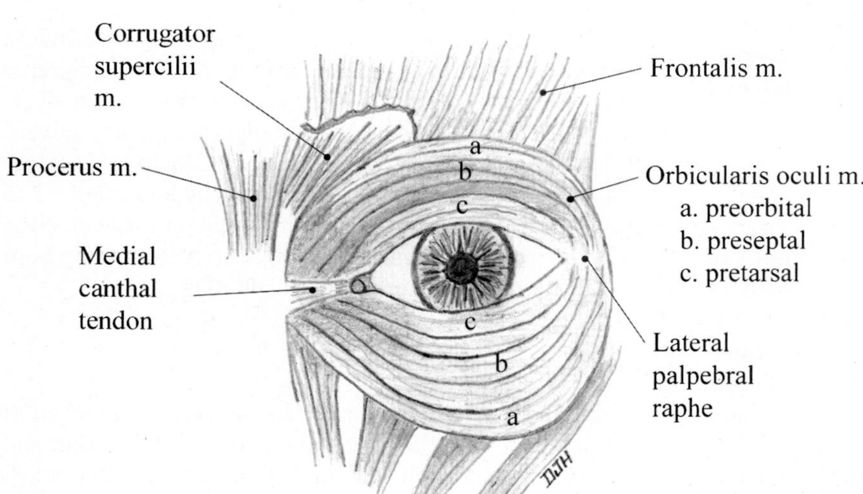

Fig. 23.2 Major divisions of the m. orbicularis oculi into pretarsal, preseptal, and orbital components.

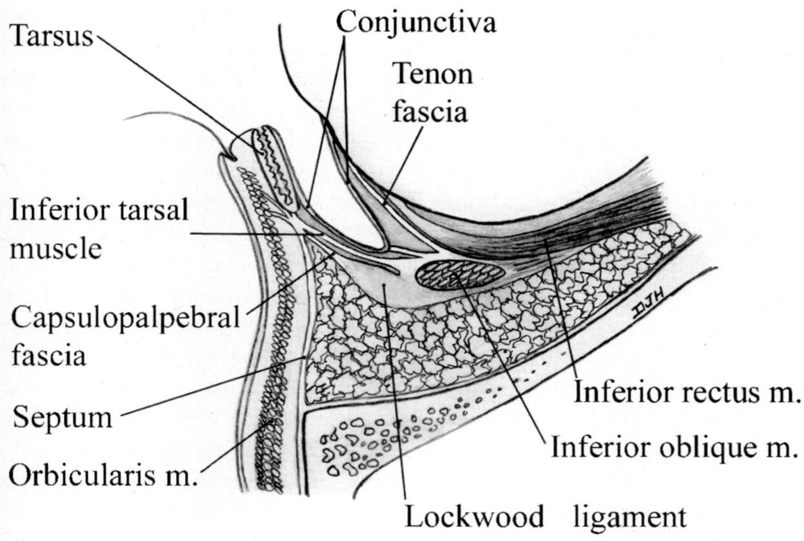

Fig. 23.3 Cross-sectional diagram of the lower eyelid demonstrating connective tissue expansion of inferior rectus into its terminal insertions.

eyelid crease, and others extend from the inferior fornix superiorly to contribute to Tenon's capsule (**Fig. 23.3**).

Orbital Fat

Contained behind the orbital septum and within the orbital cavity, the orbital fat has been classically segmented into discrete pockets (lateral, central, and medial), although interconnections truly exist.[8] The lateral fat pad is smaller and more superiorly situated, and the larger nasal pad is divided by the inferior oblique muscle into a larger central fat compartment and an intermediate medial compartment. (During surgery, care must be taken to avoid injury to the inferior oblique.) The medial pad has characteristic differences from its other counterparts, including a lighter color, a more fibrous and compact lobular pattern, and a frequent association with a sizable blood vessel near its medial aspect. The orbital fat can be considered an adynamic structure because its volume is not related to body habitus, and once removed it is not thought to regenerate.

Infraorbital and Midface Anatomy

The infaorbital area consists of skin, subcutaneous soft tissues, and fat overlying the bony orbital rim, arcus marginalis, and malar eminence. Two distinct fat pads in this area have been identified—the malar fat pad, and the suborbicularis occuli fat (SOOF) pad. The SOOF is defined as a collection of fat deep to the orbital portion of the orbilularis occuli muscle, overlying the inferior arcus marginalis. The malar fat pad is inferior to the orbicularis occuli muscle. These tissues mask the visibility of the inferior orbital rim in the youthful face. Inferior and medial descent of the malar fat and SOOF result in the aging infraorbital area characterized by volume reduction and exposure of the inferior orbital rim. Descent of these tissues coupled with pseudoherniation results in the tear trough or naso-jugal deformity.[9]

Innervation

Sensory innervation to the lower lid derives mainly from the infraorbital nerve with minor contributions from the infratrochlear and zygomaticofacial nerve branches. The blood supply is obtained from the angular, infraorbital, and transverse facial arteries. Situated 2 mm below the ciliary margin, between the orbicularis oculi and the tarsus, is the marginal arcade, which should be avoided if a subciliary incision is used. The motor innervation of the orbicularis is derived from the zygomatic and buccal divisions of the facial nerve.

Terminology

A number of descriptive terms are used pervasively in the literature of eyelid analysis and should be understood by those involved in surgical management of this area.

Blepharochalasis is a commonly misused term. It is an uncommon disorder of the upper eyelids, of unknown cause, which affects mainly young and middle-aged females. Blepharochalasis is characterized by recurrent attacks of painless unilateral or bilateral lid edema, causing a loss of skin elasticity and atrophic changes.

Dermatochalasis is an acquired condition of increased, abnormal laxity of the eyelid skin interrelated with genetic predisposition, natural aging phenomenon, and environmental influences. It is frequently associated with prolapsed orbital fat.

Steatoblepharon is a condition of true herniation or pseudoherniation of orbital fat behind a weakened orbital septum, causing areas of discrete or diffuse fullness in the eyelids. This condition and dermatochalasis are the two most common reasons why a patient presents to discuss eyelid surgery.

Festoons are single or multiple folds of orbicularis oculi in the lower lid that drape over onto themselves, creating an external, hammock-like bag. Depending on location, this bag may be preseptal, orbital, or jugal (cheek). It may contain fat.

Malar bags are areas of soft tissue fullness on the lateral edge of the infraorbital ridge and zygomatic prominence just superior to the palpebromalar sulcus. They are believed to be a result of recurrent dependent tissue edema and secondary fibrosis.

Preoperative Evaluation

A systematic and thorough preoperative assessment of blepharoplasty candidates is essential to minimize potential postoperative complications. Thus, patient analysis is directed to understanding the patient's desire and expectation, the etiology of the problem at hand, and development of the optimal treatment plan for the patient's unique needs.

Photography

High quality and standardized preoperative photographs are an essential component of all facial plastic surgery. They are required to document the preoperative condition, compare with postoperative outcomes, and evaluate the anatomy. Good lighting without the use of flash is ideal, as flash photography often washes out the fine details, such as rhytids, and the three dimensional features in this region. The standard views should include full face and close up AP with the patient in repose and during upward gaze; full face and close up bilateral oblique; full face and close up bilateral profile. The close up photographs should include the eyebrows superiorly and down to the level of the nasal ala inferiorly.

Risk Factors for Postoperative Dry Eye Syndrome

Realizing that the protective physiological functions of blinking and eyelid closure are temporarily impaired following blepharoplasty, an appropriate ocular history should elicit information that might put the patient at greater risk for postoperative dry eye syndrome. Excessive tearing, a burning or gritty sensation, ocular discomfort, foreign bodies, mucus production, eyelid crusting, and a frequent need to blink are all symptoms suggestive of borderline or inadequate tear production. A possible atopic cause has to be ruled out.

Certain systemic diseases, particularly the collagen vascular diseases (i.e., systemic lupus erythematosus, scleroderma, periarteritis nodosa), Sjögren syndrome, Wegener granulomatosis, ocular pemphigoid, and Stevens–Johnson syndrome, can interfere with the glandular lubricating function and should be identified.[10,11] The infiltrative ophthalmopathy of Graves disease can result in vertical eyelid retraction and inadequate corneal protection after surgery and should be managed with medical treatment preoperatively and surgical conservatism during surgery. Thyroid hypofunction associated with a myxedematous state may mimic the baggy eyelids of dermatochalasis and should be ruled out. Incomplete recovery of a previous facial nerve insult may interfere with eyelid closure and predispose a patient to dry eye syndrome.

Risk Factors for Postoperative Blindness

Postoperative blindness, the most catastrophic complication of blepharoplasty, is associated with retrobulbar hemorrhage.[12,13] Factors that influence bleeding tendencies should therefore be identified and controlled before surgery.[14] Ingestion of aspirin, nonsteroidal antiinflammatory drugs (NSAIDS), antiarthritics, cortisone preparations, and vitamin E should be withheld for at least 14 days before surgery because of qualitative effects on platelet function. Over-the-counter medications should be discontinued as well because gingko biloba, for example, has been implicated in excessive bleeding. Similarly, St. John's wort is known to have hypertensive effects through a monoamine oxidase inhibitor mechanism. Warfarin compounds, if medically feasible, should be withheld to normalize the prothrombin time and may be reinstituted 48 to 72 hours after surgery.

Any history of abnormal or easy bruising, prolonged clotting time, or family members with bleeding dyscrasia should be noted with appropriate coagulation profiles. Hypertensive patients should be medically stabilized at least 2 weeks before surgery to ensure a nonfluctuating normotensive state. Women have a greater bleeding tendency during their menstrual period than at other cycle times, and this should be considered in planning surgery. Other important factors include drinking and smoking history, as the former (in large amounts) may influence platelet function, and the latter has been associated with delayed wound healing and diminished flap viability. Finally, any patient with a documented or suspected history of glaucoma must be evaluated and managed by an ophthalmologist to normalize intraocular pressures and guard against a potential acute closed-angle attack prior to any eyelid surgery. Some facial plastic surgeons recommend a routine ophthalmologic exam for all of their patients preoperatively.

Ocular Assessment

Examination of the eyes should begin with an overall inspection. The eyelid should be assessed for symmetry (by noting palpebral fissure height and length), position of the lower eyelid margin with respect to the inferior limbus, scleral show, and the presence of ectropion/entropion or exophthalmos/enophthalmos. Scars or skin lesions should be noted because it may be possible to include these in the resection. Areas of skin discoloration or abnormal pigmentation should also be noted.

Other baseline features of the periorbital area should be pointed out to the patient, particularly in lieu of the inability of blepharoplasty to correct them.[15] The fine wrinkling and "crepe paper" appearance of the eyelid skin is not amenable to correction by blepharoplasty alone. Areas of abnormal pigmentation or discoloration (e.g., from venous stasis) will not be changed if outside the area of surgery and in fact may be more noticeable after surgery (because of light-refractile changes associated with conversion of a convex surface to a concave or flattened one). One of the greatest sources of dissatisfaction after lower blepharoplasty is the persistence of malar bags. The patient should realize that the upward tension necessary to attenuate such a soft tissue prominence would not be tolerated by the supporting structures of the lower lid and could lead to ectropion. Finally, lateral smile lines (crow's feet), despite the amount of lateral extension and undermining, are also not amenable to correction by standard blepharoplasty technique. All of these factors need to be discussed with the patient.

As a minimum, baseline ocular assessment should document visual acuity (i.e., best corrected vision if glasses or contact lenses are worn), extraocular movements, gross visual fields by confrontation, corneal reflexes, the presence of Bell's phenomenon and lagophthalmos. If there is any question of dry eye syndrome, the patient should be evaluated with Schirmer testing (to quantitate tear output) and tear film break-up times (to assess stability of precorneal tear film).[16] Patients who demonstrate abnormalities in either or both of these tests or who have past or anatomical evidence that would predispose them to dry eye complications should be thoroughly evaluated by an ophthalmologist preoperatively.

Assessment of Fat Pockets

Evaluation of the adnexal structures should include assessment of the fat pockets. Palpation of the infraorbital rim is an essential component of this examination. A surgeon must recognize that a prominent rim limits the amount of orbital fat that can be removed without creating disparities in confluence between the lower eyelid and the anterior cheek. What appears to be an appropriate fat resection may contribute to a sunken-eye appearance if the patient has a very prominent rim. Assessment of the fat pockets may be facilitated by directing the patient's gaze in certain directions; a superior gaze accentuates the medial and central pockets, whereas looking upward and to the contralateral side accentuates the lateral pocket. Further confirmation of fatty prominence may be obtained by gentle retropulsion of the globe with the eyelid closed and observation of the outward movements of the respective fat pads.

Assessment of Lid-Supporting Structures

Because the most common cause of lower lid ectropion after blepharoplasty is failure to recognize a lax lower lid before surgery, it is essential to properly assess the lid-supporting structures. Two simple clinical tests aid in this evaluation. A lid distraction test (snap test)[17] is performed by gently grasping the midportion of the lower eyelid between the thumb and index fingers and outwardly displacing the eyelid from the globe (**Fig. 23.4**). Movement of the lid margin greater than 10 mm indicates an abnormally lax supporting lid structure and suggests the need for a lid-shortening procedure. The lid retraction test[15] is used to assess lid tone as well as medial and lateral canthal tendon stability (**Fig. 23.5**). By using the index finger to inferiorly displace the lower lid toward the orbital rim, observations are made in terms of punctal or lateral canthal malposition (movement of puncta greater than 3 mm from the medial canthus indicates an abnormally lax canthal tendon and suggests the need for tendoplication). Releasing the eyelid, the pattern and rate of return of the lid to resting position should be observed. A slow return, or one that requires multiple blinks, indicates poor lid tone and eyelid support. Again, a conservative skin–muscle resection and lower lid–shortening procedure would be warranted.

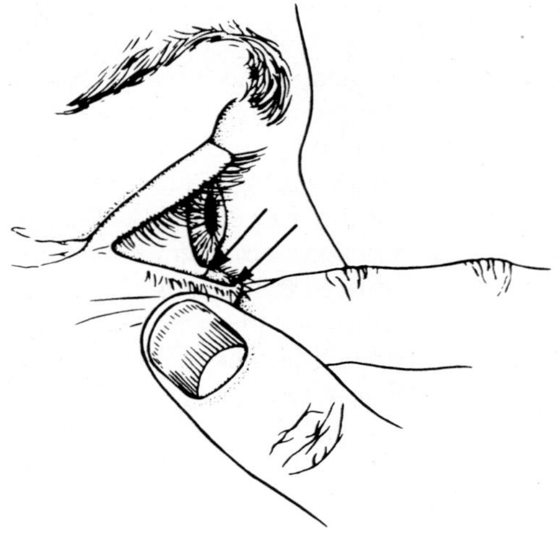

Fig. 23.4 Lid distraction test used to assess laxity of tarsoligamentous sling. (From Tenzel RR. Complications of blepharoplasty: orbital hematoma, ectropion, and scleral show. Clin Plast Surg, Elsevier, 1981;8:799.)

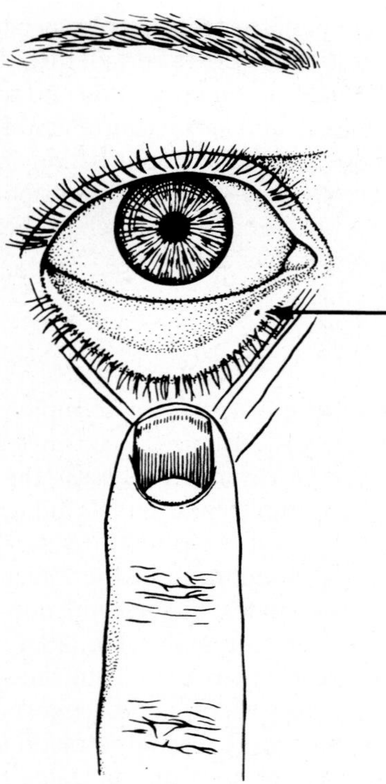

Fig. 23.5 Lid retraction test used to assess lower eyelid tone and stability of medial and lateral canthal tendon attachments. (From Tenzel RR. Complications of blepharoplasty: orbital hematoma, ectropion, and scleral show. Clin Plast Surg, Elsevier, 1981;8:800.)

Assessment of Tear Trough or Nasojugal Deformity

The tear trough deformity is frequently one of the first signs of aging in the central face. Often initially noticed in the early thirties, this deformity is defined as a loss of volume in the skin and soft tissues of the infraorbital area resulting in a depression in the medial lower eyelid-cheek junction extending obliquely from the medial canthus. It may also be associated with volume loss in the lateral aspect of the inferior orbital rim compounding the "tired" or "worn out" appearance of which affected patients complain. The tear trough deformity is important to recognize as is not generally addressed by standard lower eyelid procedures. Anatomically, the thinning of this area caused by descent of the infraorbital soft tissues exposes the infraorbital rim. This deformity may be accentuated by pseudoherniation of lower eyelid fat. The restoration of volume over the inferior orbital rim has been shown to improve the results of lower eyelid rejuvenation in affected patients.

Surgical Technique

Three basic surgical approaches have been described in lower lid blepharoplasty: (1) transconjunctival, (2) skin–muscle flap, and (3) skin flap.

Transconjunctival Approach

The transconjunctival approach to lower eyelid blepharoplasty was first described in 1924 by Bourquet.[18] Although it is not a new procedure, over the past 10 years there has been a surge of interest and a growth of proponents for this approach. The transconjunctival lower lid blepharoplasty respects the integrity of the orbicularis oculi, an active support structure of the lower eyelid. This minimizes the incidence of ectropion. Also, an external scar can be avoided.

Proper patient selection for the transconjunctival approach is required. Ideal candidates include older patients with pseudoherniation of orbital fat and a limited amount of skin excess, young patients with familial hereditary pseudoherniation of orbital fat and no excess skin, all revision blepharoplasty patients, patients who do not want an external scar, patients with a history of keloids, and dark-skinned individuals who have a small possibility of hypopigmentation of the external scar.[19,20] Because several authors have reported a significant reduction in short- and long-term complications with the transconjunctival approach to lower eyelid blepharoplasty compared with the skin–muscle method, the indications for the technique have been gradually expanding.[19,21] The presence of excess lower lid skin does not preclude use of the transconjunctival approach. In the senior author's practice, the most commonly performed lower lid procedure consists of transconjunctival fat excision, pinch excision of skin, and 35% trichloroacetic acid (TCA) peeling (described later).[19,22–24] The skin excision is needed to recontour the lower eyelid once the fat has been removed. There frequently is less excess than one initially estimates before the fat excision is performed.[21,25]

Preparation

While sitting upright, the patient is asked to look upward. This helps to refresh the surgeon's memory as to which fat pads are the most prominent, and these are marked. The patient is then placed supine. Two drops of ophthalmic tetracaine hydrochloride 0.5% are then instilled into each inferior fornix. Prior to the local injections, our patients typically receive some intravenous sedation composed of midazolam (Versed) and meperidine hydrochloride (Demerol). Ten milligrams of intravenous dexamethasone (Decadron) is also given to help minimize postoperative edema. A local anesthetic mixture, consisting of equal parts of 0.25% bupivacaine (Marcaine) and 1% lidocaine (Xylocaine) with 1:100,000 epinephrine to which is added a 1:10 dilution of sodium bicarbonate, is then injected into the lower lid conjunctiva using a 30 gauge needle. Experience has demonstrated that this mixture affords prolonged analgesic effect while minimizing the sting of initial infiltration through alkalinization of the local agent. The needle is advanced through the

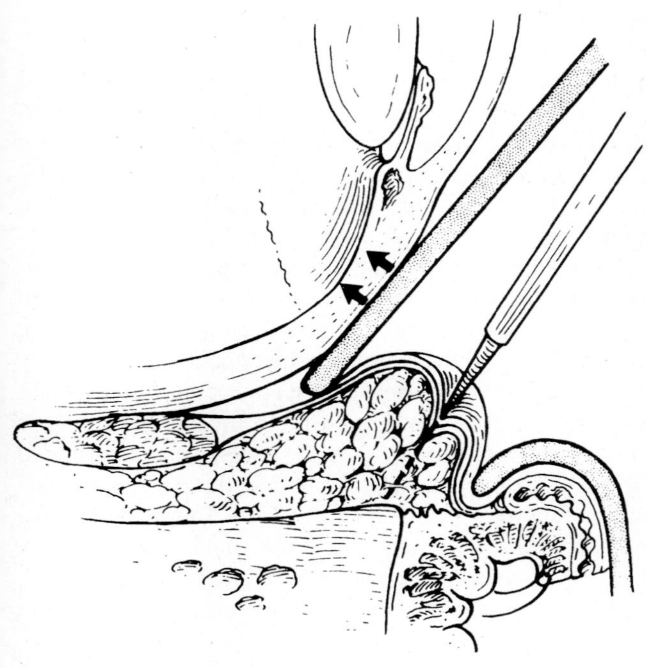

Fig. 23.6 Transconjunctival approach to lower eyelid fat pockets. Simultaneous eversion of the lower eyelid and ballottement of the globe produces a bulge of orbital fat that helps to guide the dissection. (From Baylis HI, Long JA, Groth MJ. Transconjunctival lower eyelid blepharoplasty: technique and complications. Ophthalmology, Elsevier, 1989;96:1027.)

conjunctiva until the bony orbital rim is palpated. The local is slowly injected as the needle is withdrawn. This is performed medially, centrally, and laterally. Several surgeons also like to inject transcutaneously, although we have found that this is usually not necessary and may lead to unnecessary bruising.

Incision

After waiting a full 10 minutes for vasoconstriction to occur, the lower lid is gently retracted by an assistant using two small, double-pronged skin hooks (**Figs. 23.6 and 23.7**). The upper lid is placed over the globe to protect it. Either a guarded needle-tip bovie on a low setting or a no. 15 blade is used (others prefer a laser) to make the transconjunctival incision 2 mm below the inferior edge of the inferior tarsal plate. This inferior tarsal edge appears gray through the conjunctiva. The medial aspect of the incision is in line with the inferior punctum. The incision is carried just 4 to 5 mm shy of the lateral canthus.

Immediately after the transconjunctival incision is made, a single 5–0 nylon suture is placed in the conjunctiva closest to the fornix and used to retract the posterior lamella over the entire cornea (**Fig. 23.8**). A small hemostat snapped onto the patient's headwrap is used to hold the sutures under tension. The conjunctiva acts as a natural corneal protector and the superior retraction allows for easier plane dissection. The two skin hooks are then carefully removed and a Desmarres retractor is now used to evert the free edge of the lower lid (**Fig. 23.9**).

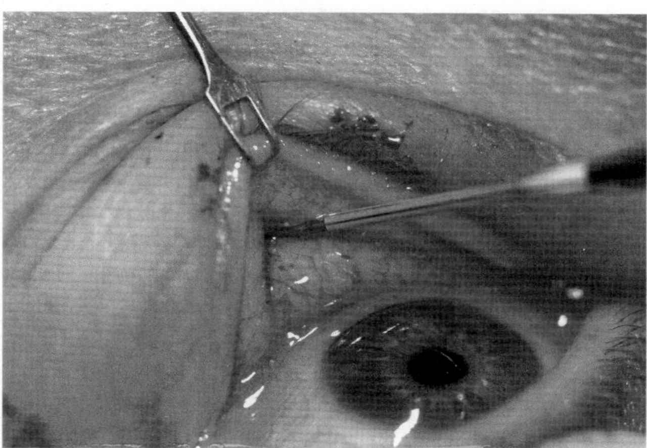

Fig. 23.7 The needle-tip bovie is poised to initiate the incision. (A corneal protector, or upper lid skin, is used for protection when the actual incision is made.)

The distance of the transconjunctival incision from the inferior edge of the inferior tarsal plate determines whether one will approach the orbital fat preseptally or postseptally.[20] We usually utilize the preseptal approach; therefore, our incisions are always ~2 mm below the tarsus. The preseptal plane is an avascular plane between the orbicularis oculi and the orbital septum.[26] Because the orbital septum is still intact while the preseptal plane is being developed, orbital fat does not bulge into one's view. The visualization obtained is closely similar to the orientation one is used to having when performing a skin–muscle

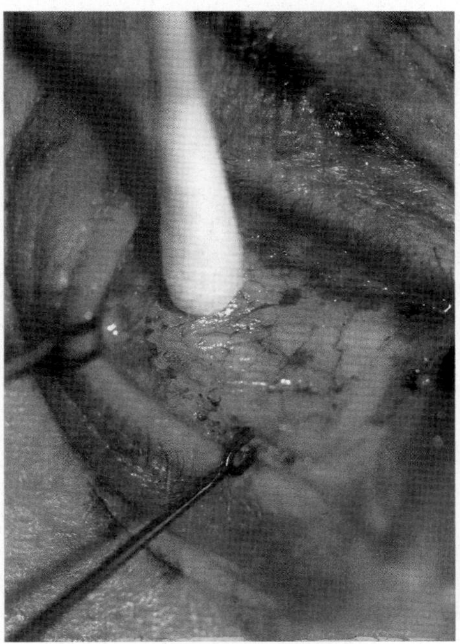

Fig. 23.8 Retraction suture in place; cotton-tipped applicator spreads incision site.

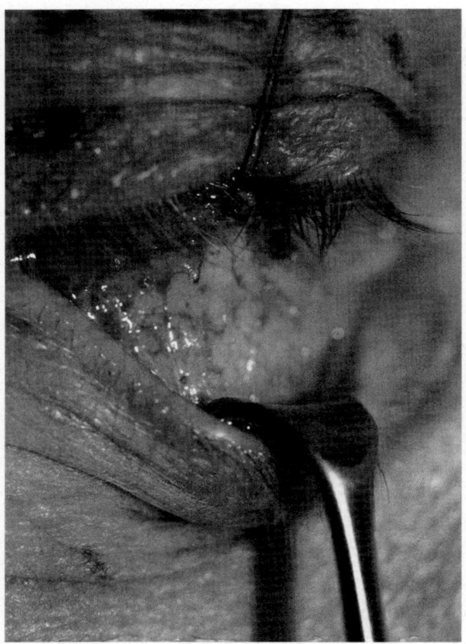

Fig. 23.9 Desmarres retractor exposes orbital septum.

flap blepharoplasty. The orbital septum will still have to be opened to access the orbital fat below (**Fig. 23.10**).

Others prefer the postseptal approach to the orbital fat.[23] To directly access the fat pads the conjunctiva is incised ~4 mm below the inferior border of the inferior tarsal plate and directly toward the anterior edge of the inferior orbital rim. The big advantage of this method is that the orbital septum is kept completely intact. Proponents for this technique state that the intact orbital septum adds to the support of the lower eyelid. One disadvantage is that the orbital fat immediately bulges into one's view. Care must be taken not to incise close to the conjunctival cul-de-sac to avoid the risk of synechiae.[20] Also, the view from the direct approach is one to which most facial plastic surgeons are less accustomed.

After the 5–0 suture retraction and Desmarres retractor are in place, the preseptal plane is developed with a combination of blunt dissection with a cotton swab and sharp dissection with scissors. It is mandatory to maintain a dry surgical field. Therefore, a bipolar cautery, "hot loop," or monopolar cautery is used to cauterize any bleeders.

The medial, central, and lateral fat pads are each individually identified through the septum with the help of some gentle digital pressure on the conjunctiva covering the globe. The orbital septum is then opened with scissors. Using forceps and a cotton-tipped applicator, the excess fat is carefully teased above the orbital rim and septum. Care must be taken to remove only the excessive and herniated fat because the eyes may take on a hollowed-out appearance following excessive fat excision. The ultimate goal is to achieve a lower eyelid contour that forms a smooth, gentle concave transition between it and cheek skin.

A 30 gauge needle is then used to inject a small amount of local anesthetic into the excess fat (**Fig. 23.11**). The bipolar cautery is used to cauterize across the fat stalk. When one is sure the entire stalk has been cauterized, scissors are used to cut across the cauterized area. Others, notably Cook, reduce fat volume with electrocautery, minimizing surgical excision. Many surgeons feel that the lateral fat pocket should be explored initially because its volume contribution becomes more difficult to assess after removal of its adjacent and interconnected central fat pad.[15,27] After excess fat has been removed from each compartment, the field is examined to make sure there is no bleeding. Although CO_2 laser fat excision has been advocated based on the advantages of hemostatic efficiency, precision, and reduced tissue trauma, the increased costs, requirements for highly trained personnel, and additional laser precautions have led us and others to abandon laser incisions for lower lid surgery.[28,29]

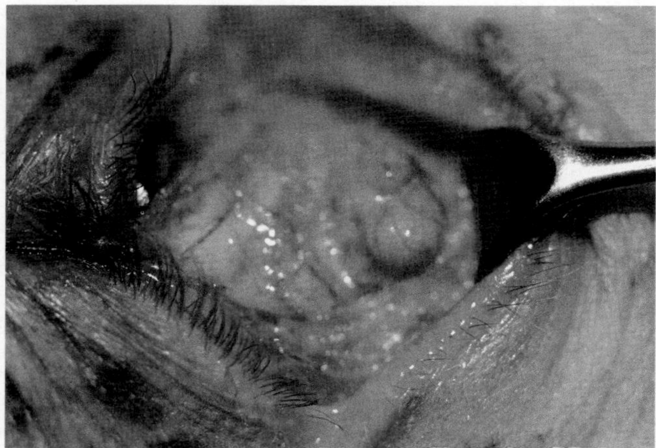

Fig. 23.10 Fat appearing through orbital septum.

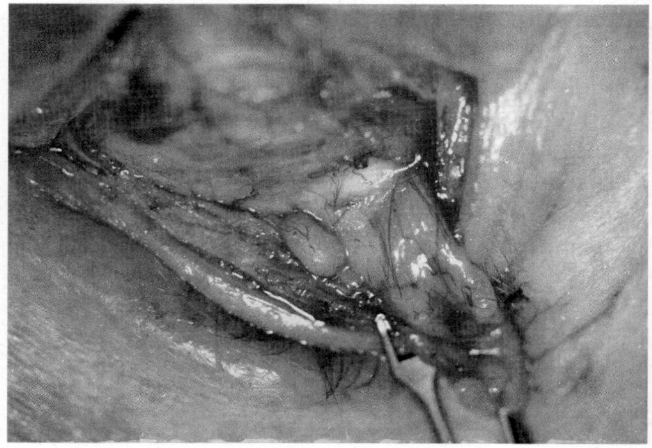

Fig. 23.11 Fat of medial compartment, partially excised.

The Desmarres retractor should be removed periodically and the lower eyelid redraped over the fat that remains in place to facilitate examination of the contour of the eyelid. The fat that is removed is retained on a gauze on the surgical field in order from lateral to medial, allowing for comparison with the fat removed from the opposite side. For example, if preoperatively the surgeon felt that the right lateral fat pad was much larger than all others, then intraoperatively that compartment would have the most fat removed.

The medial and central fat compartments are separated by the inferior oblique muscle. This muscle must be clearly identified prior to the excision of excess fat from these compartments to prevent muscle injury. The medial fat pad is whiter than the central and lateral fat pads. This helps in its identification. The lateral compartment is usually isolated from the central one by a fascial band off the inferior oblique muscle. This fascial band can be cut safely.

After each successive fat compartment is treated, the entire field must again be examined for bleeding. After all of the bleeding has been cauterized with the bipolar, the Desmarres and the retraction sutures are removed. The lower lid is gently elevated upward and outward and then allowed to snap back into its proper position. This allows for proper realignment of the edges of the transconjunctival incision. No suture is required, although some surgeons feel more comfortable closing the incision with one, buried 6–0 fast-absorbing gut stitch. Both eyes should then be irrigated with sodium chloride (ophthalmic balanced salt solution).

In an older patient with skin excess, a lower lid skin pinch or chemical peel may now be performed. Using fixation forceps or Brown–Adson forceps, a 2 to 3 mm raised fold of redundant skin is raised just below the ciliary margin (**Fig. 23.12**). The skin fold is excised with sharp scissors, with care taken not to cut the lower eyelashes (**Fig. 23.13**). The edges of the skin pinch are then brought together with interrupted 6–0 fast-absorbing gut stitches. Several authors have closed this incision with cyanoacrylate (Histoacryl) or fibrin glue.[19,30]

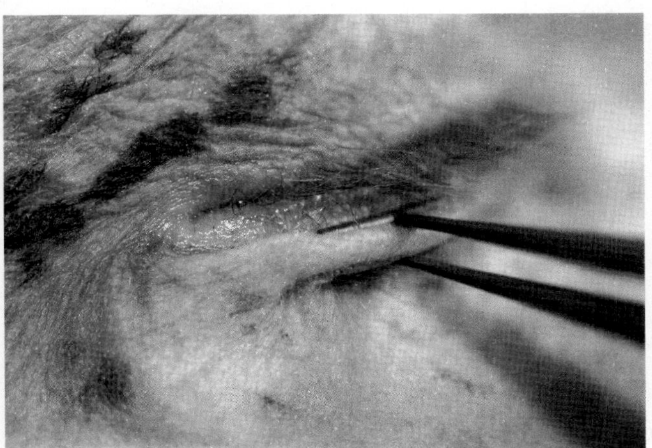

Fig. 23.12 Fixation forceps used to create ridge or mound for pinch excision.

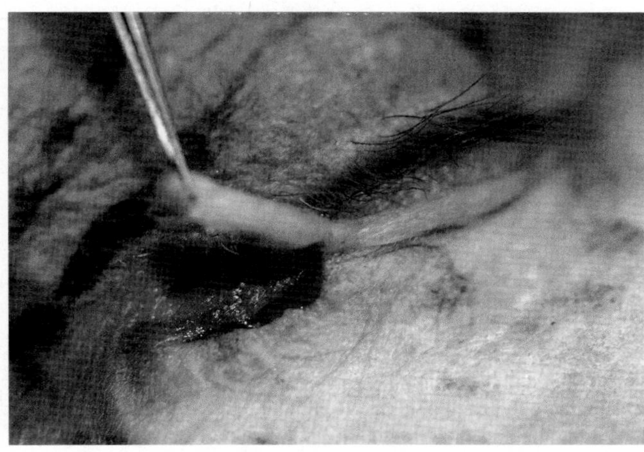

Fig. 23.13 Pinch excision progression.

Patients with crepey or fine lower eyelid rhytids are then treated with a 25 to 35% TCA peel. The TCA is applied immediately below the skin pinch incision. A typical "frost" is generated (**Fig. 23.14**). Phenol is not used for lower lids in our hands because the erythema and inflammation phase is much longer than the TCA peel.

Postoperative Care

Immediately after surgery, the patient is kept quiet with head elevated at least 45 degrees. Cold compresses are placed on both eyes and changed every 20 minutes. The patient is observed closely for at least an hour for any signs of bleeding complications. The patient is given strict instructions to limit physical activity for the next week. The patient who is diligent about the cold compresses

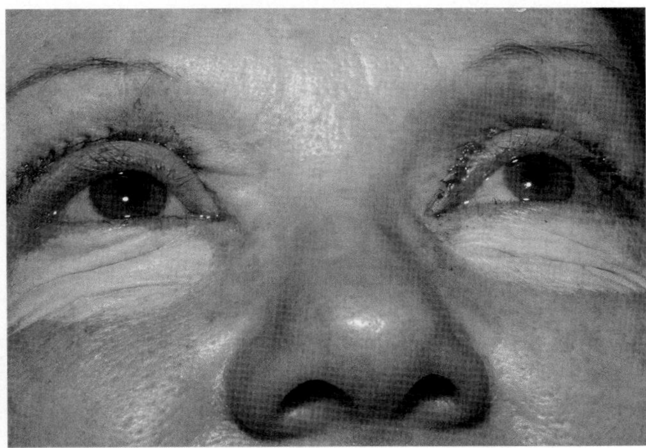

Fig. 23.14 Thirty percent trichloroacetic acid (TCA) lower lid peel frost. (Different patient in whom no pinch excision was done.) When the pinch technique is used, the TCA must not be applied any closer than 1 mm below the suture line.

and head elevation during the first 48 hours will experience substantially less swelling. Some physicians place their patients on sulfacetamide ophthalmic drops during the first 5 postoperative days to help prevent an infection while the transconjunctival incision is healing.

Skin–Muscle Flap Approach

The skin–muscle flap approach was perhaps the most commonly used method in the 1970s and early 1980s. In patients with a large amount of excess skin and orbicularis oculi as well as fat pseudoherniation, this is an excellent procedure. The advantages of this approach are related to the safety and facility of dissecting in the relatively avascular submuscular plane and the ability to remove redundant lower eyelid skin. One must realize that even with the skin–muscle flap one is limited by how much skin can safely be removed without risking scleral show and even an ectropion. Persistent rhytids often remain despite attempts to safely resect redundant eyelid skin.

Preparation

Preparation for this method is similar to that for the transconjunctival approach, except that tetracaine drops are not necessary. A subciliary incision is planned 2 to 3 mm beneath the eyelid margin and is marked with a marking pen or methylene blue with the patient in the sitting position. Any prominent fat pads are also marked. The importance of marking the patient in the upright position before injection relates to the changes in soft tissue relationships that occur as a result of dependency and infiltration. The medial extent of the incision is marked 1 mm lateral to the inferior punctum to avoid potential damage to the inferior canaliculus, whereas the subciliary extension is carried to a point ~8 to 10 mm lateral to the lateral canthus (to minimize potential for rounding of the canthal angle and lateral scleral show). At this point, the lateral-most portion of the incision achieves a more horizontal orientation and is planned to lie within a crow's-foot crease line. Care should be exercised in planning the lateral extension of this incision to allow at least 5 mm, and preferably 10 mm, between it and the lateral extension of the upper blepharoplasty incision to obviate prolonged lymphedema.

Our patients typically receive intravenous sedation composed of midazolam and meperidine hydrochloride after the preoperative marking has been accomplished and intravenous dexamethasone is in. Before surgical prepping and sterile draping, the incision line (beginning laterally) and entire lower lid down to the infraorbital rim are infiltrated (superficial to orbital septum) with our anesthetic mixture previously described.

Incision

The incision, which is begun medially with a no. 15 scalpel blade, is only through skin to the level of the lateral canthus, but through skin and musculus orbicularis oculi lateral to this point. Using a blunt-tipped, straight-dissection scissors, the incision is undermined in a submuscular plane from lateral to medial and is then cut sharply by orientation of the blades in a caudal direction (optimizing the integrity of the pretarsal muscle sling). A Frost-type retention suture, using 5–0 nylon, is then placed through the tissue edge above the incision to aid in counterretraction. Using blunt dissection (with scissors and cotton-tipped applicators), a skin–muscle flap is developed down to, but not below, the infraorbital rim to avoid disruption of important lymphatic channels.[31] Any bleeding points up to this point should be meticulously controlled with the handheld cautery or bipolar cautery, with conservatism exercised in the superior margin of the incision to avert potential thermal trauma to the eyelash follicles (Robinson L, Crumley RL, unpublished data 1990).

Fat Removal

If preoperative assessment suggests the need for fat-pad management, selective openings are made through the orbital septum over the areas of pseudoherniation and are guided by gentle digital pressure of the closed eyelid against the globe. Although alternatives aimed at electrocauterizing a weakened orbital septum exist[32] that may obviate violation of this important barrier, we are comfortable with the long-term results and predictability of our technique of direct fat-pocket management.

After opening the septum (usually 5 to 6 mm above the orbital rim), the fat lobules are gently teased above the orbital rim and septum using forceps and a cotton-tipped applicator. The fat resection technique is very much as described in the transconjunctival technique and is not repeated.

Access to the medial compartment may be limited in part by the medial aspect of the subciliary incision. This incision should not be extended; instead, the fat should be gently teased into the incision, taking care to avoid the inferior oblique muscle. The medial fat pad is distinguished from the central pad by its lighter color.

Closure

In preparation for skin excision and closure the patient is asked to open the jaw widely and gaze in a superior direction. This maneuver creates a maximal voluntary separation of the wound edges and assists the surgeon in performing accurate resection of the skin–muscle flap. With the patient maintaining this position, the inferior flap is redraped over the subciliary incision in a superotemporal direction. At the level of the lateral canthus, the extent of skin muscle overlap is marked and incised vertically. A tacking stitch of 5–0 fast absorbing gut is then placed to maintain the position of the flap. Using straight scissors, the areas of overlap are conservatively resected (medial and lateral to the retention suture) so that edge-to-edge apposition can be maintained without the need for reinforcement. It is important to bevel the blades caudally to allow for a 1 to 2 mm strip resection of orbicularis oculi on the lower flap edge to avoid a prominent ridge at the time of closure. Some surgeons refrigerate the resected skin (viable for at least 48 hours) in sterile saline in case replacement tissue graft is needed after an overzealous resection eventuating in ectropion. It is far better to prevent such complications by performing a conservative resection.

After fat removal from the second eyelid, simple interrupted 6–0 fast-absorbing gut sutures are placed to close the incision on the initial eyelid. Attention can then be redirected back to redraping, trimming, and suturing the second eyelid. Finally, inch-long sterile strips are placed to aid in temporal support, and a light application of antibiotic ointment is applied to the sutured incision after irrigating the eyes with sodium chloride (balanced salt solution).

Postoperative Care

Postoperative care after the skin–muscle approach is essentially identical to the aftercare used in the transconjunctival approach. Bacitracin ophthalmic ointment is given to the patient for the subciliary incision. Iced saline compresses, head elevation, and limited activity are stressed to all patients.

Skin Flap Approach

The skin flap approach is perhaps the oldest and the least frequently used. This method allows independent resection and redraping of lower eyelid skin and underlying orbicularis oculi and is effective in repositioning and redraping excessively wrinkled, redundant, or deeply creased skin.[29] In cases involving hypertrophy or festooning of the orbicularis oculi, direct access is provided for management, which allows for a greater and safer resection than would otherwise be tolerated if the flap were raised as a conjoined musculocutaneous unit. Disadvantages of this approach include a more tedious dissection that is associated with greater skin trauma (manifested by increased bleeding and eyelid induration), an increased risk of vertical eyelid retraction, and a higher demand placed on preoperative assessment of the fat pockets because of obscured subseptal observation by the overlying orbicularis oculi.[33,34]

The initial incision through skin is made only through the lateral extension of the subciliary marking to facilitate undermining. With an assistant maintaining downward traction on the lower eyelid skin (by placing a hand near the orbital rim), the lateral skin edge is grasped and pulled superiorly while sharp-scissors dissection carefully undermines the skin flap to a point just below the orbital rim. With the undermining accomplished, the subciliary incision is completed with the scissors. All bleeding points are precisely cauterized.

If the problem is skin redundancy or excessive wrinkling only, the skin flap is simply redraped in the manner described for skin–muscle flap. If access to the orbital fat compartments is required, these are approached by incising the orbicularis oculi ~3 to 4 mm inferior to the initial skin incision or via the transconjunctival approach. However, when orbicularis hypertrophy or festooning is present, optimal management is achieved by development of independent skin and muscle flaps. In this case, the muscle is incised (beveling caudally) across the extent of the incision, beginning ~2 mm below the skin incision to preserve the pretarsal muscle sling. Undermining of the muscle flap is carried to just below the most dependent muscle roll (with festooning) or to a point that will allow effacement of a prominent muscle bulge (with hypertrophy) after muscle resection. After fat-pad management, the muscle flap is reinforced by suturing of its lateral end to orbital periosteum with 5–0 Vicryl (Ethicon, Inc., Somerville, NJ) and reapproximation of its pretarsal muscle edges with a few interrupted 5–0 chromic sutures. Again, skin closure follows the pattern previously described.

Restoration of Infraorbital Volume

Restoration of volume in the infraorbital area must be addressed in the appropriate candidate. Several approaches have been described including, the use of injectable fillers, fat transfer, midface elevation, orbital fat repositioning, and SOOF elevation. Orbital fat repositioning and SOOF elevation may be preformed in conjunction with lower eyelid blepharoplasty without the need for additional incisions or approaches.

Injectable Fillers

Recent trends in nonsurgical treatment of facial aging have resulted in the creative application of the widely available injectable fillers in the periorbital area. Specifically, the use of non-animal, stabilized, hyaluronic acid (NASHA) fillers have enabled the treatment of early signs of aging in the infraorbital complex. Although the potentially longer-lasting calcium hydroxylapitite fillers have been used in the periorbital area, the authors feel that the particulate consistency of these materials expose the patient to unnecessary risks of retinal embolization when used in the immediate periorbital area.

Filling of the tear trough deformity and related lateral infraorbital hollows can be preformed in the office setting with topical and/or local anesthesia. If local anesthesia is to be employed, a block of the infraorbital and infratrochlear nerves is suggested. The zygomaticofacial nerve may also be blocked if treatment is to be extended into the lateral infraorbital hollow. Following nerve blocks a small amount of local anesthesia containing 1:100,000 or weaker of epinephrine can be injected directly into the treatment areas for vasoconstriction. Alternatively, ice packs may be applied before and after injection to decrease bruising.

Injections are preformed in slow, stepwise fashion, with the needle directed superiorly from a point approximately one centimeter inferior to the inferior orbital rim at the level of the medial limbus.[36]

The material should only be injected during retraction of the needle to prevent vessel embolization. Layered injections are suggested, beginning along the infraorbital rim, over the periosteum, and following with gentle layered "feathering" of the injectable material in multiple layers deep to the orbicularis muscle. Injection superficial to the orbicularis muscle can also be preformed, but it is suggested to attempt this only after mastery of the deeper injection technique. Gentle massage should be preformed after every few injections to disperse small isolated collections of material that may become palpable or visible as edema subsides. Risks specific to this treatment include bruising, palpable subcutaneous bumps, fluid collection in the injected area, and very remote risk of retinal embolus.

Orbital Fat Repositioning

Orbital fat repositioning has also been referred to as fat preservation blepharoplasty. This procedure employs the fat of the medial and middle inferior orbital compartments to restore volume over the inferior orbital rim, and efface the tear trough deformity and associated lateral infraorbital hollows. This can be approached through any lower eyelid approach that addresses the post-septal fat compartments. In the increasingly popular transconjunctival approach, the fat of the medial and middle fat compartments are dissected through a septal incision, and left attached as a pedicled flap transposed over the orbital rim and beneath the depression of the tear trough deformity. Fixation can be preformed using transcutaneous permanent sutures which are removed in 3–5 days, or absorbable sutures securing the fat to the periosteum of the infraorbital rim. This procedure may also be preformed in conjunction with the skin-muscle flap technique for lower blepharoplasty. In patients with excessive amounts of fat pseudoherniation, a small amount of fat may also be removed according to the techniques detailed above.

Sub-Orbicularis Occuli Fat Lift

SOOF lifting techniques may also be preformed via traditional transconjunctival and skin-muscle flap approaches. The SOOF is exposed by inferior dissection along the deep surface of the orbicularis occuli muscle, and over the periosteum of the inferior orbital rim. This dissection is carried to the inferior aspect of the nasojugal deformity. The SOOF is then encountered inferior to the nasojugal deformity, elevated and secured to the periosteum of the inferior orbital rim with absorbable mattress sutures.[37] Bleeding in this area is controlled with judicious bipolar cautery to prevent infraorbital nerve injury.

Structural Fat Grafting of the Infraorbital Region

Autologous fat grafting of the inferior periorbital region is used to restore volume loss along the skeletonized inferior bony rim, nasojugal region, and upper cheek in order to create a smooth soft tissue contour from the lower eyelids to the cheek. Specifically, by filling the concavities (orbital rim, nasojugal fold) the double convexity deformity is transformed into a single convexity which is present in youthful eyelids/upper cheek region. The fat is typically harvested from the abdomen or thighs using a low pressure liposuction technique. Then the fat is prepared by separating the serum and blood using a centrifuge. Once purified adipose tissue is isolated, it is injected using a microcanula along the orbital rim, nasogugal fold, and upper cheeks using a microinjection technique. The most common complication of this technique in this region is contour irregularities and palpable nodules. Due to the thin skin and bony nature of the periorbital region, successful treatment requires experience. When successfully performed the results are extremely pleasing and is synergistic when coupled with a conservative transconjunctival lower eyelid blepharoplasty.[38]

Complications

Complications after blepharoplasty are usually the result of overzealous skin or fat resection, lack of hemostasis, or an inadequate preoperative assessment.[39,40] Less commonly, an individual's physiological response to wound repair may lead to undesirable sequelae despite execution of the proper technique. The goal in minimizing complications consequent to blepharoplasty must therefore focus on prevention by identifying and managing known risk factors.

Ectropion

One of the most common complications after lower lid blepharoplasty is eyelid malposition, which may range in presentation from a mild scleral show or rounding of the lateral canthal angle, to a frank ectropion with actual eyelid eversion. In most cases resulting in permanent ectropion, a failure to address excessive lower lid laxity is the etiologic culprit. Other causes include excessive skin or skin–muscle excisions, inferior contracture along the plane of the lower lid retractors and orbital septum (greater in skin flap technique), inflammation of the fat pockets, and, rarely, destabilization of the lower lid retractors (a potential yet uncommon complication of the transconjunctival approach). Temporary ectropion has been associated with lid loading from reactionary edema or hematoma and muscle hypotonicity.

A conservative approach to management may include the following: (1) a short course of perioperative steroids with cold compresses and head elevation to manage edema; (2) warm and cool compresses alternated to hasten resolution of minor established hematomas and improve circulatory status; (3) repeated squinting exercises to improve muscle tonus; (4) gentle massage in an upward direction; and (5) supportive taping of the lower lid (upward and outward) to assist in corneal protection and tear collection.

When skin excisions are recognized to be excessive within the first 48 hours, the banked eyelid skin should be used as a replacement graft. If recognition is delayed, conservative measures to protect the eye should be used to allow the scar to mature and a full-thickness graft (preferably upper eyelid skin or, alternatively, postauricular skin, or foreskin in males) used to replace the deficit. In many cases, a lid-shortening procedure is combined with the tissue grafting and is the mainstay of treatment when an atonic lid is present. Management of persistent indurations, resulting from hematoma formation or inflammatory responses of the fat pockets, generally involves direct depot injections of corticosteroid.

Hematomas

Collections of blood beneath the skin surface can usually be minimized before surgery by optimizing coagulation profiles and normotensive status during surgery through delicate tissue handling and meticulous hemostasis and after surgery through head elevation, cold compressing, a controlled level of activity, and appropriate analgesic support. Should a hematoma develop, its extent and time of presentation will guide management.

Small, superficial hematomas are relatively common and are typically self-limiting. If organization occurs with the development of an indurated mass and resolution is slow or nonprogressive, conservative steroid injections may be used to hasten the healing process. Moderate or large hematomas recognized after several days are best managed by allowing the clot to liquify (7 to 10 days) and then evacuating the hematoma through large-bore needle aspiration or by creating a small stab wound over it with a no. 11 blade. Hematomas that are large and present early, that are expanding, or that represent symptomatic retrobulbar extension (decrease in visual acuity, proptosis, ocular pain, ophthalmoplegia, progressive chemosis) demand immediate exploration and hemostatic control. In the case of the latter, urgent ophthalmologic consultation and orbital decompression are the mainstays of treatment.

Blindness

Blindness, though rare, is the most feared potential complication of blepharoplasty. It occurs with an incidence of ~0.04%,[41] typically presents itself within the first 24 hours after surgery, and is associated with orbital fat removal and the development of a retrobulbar hematoma (medial fat pocket most commonly involved). Commonly implicated causes of retrobulbar hemorrhage include the following: (1) excessive traction on orbital fat resulting in disruption of small arterioles or venules in the posterior orbit; (2) retraction of an open vessel beneath the septum after fat release; (3) failure to recognize an open vessel because of vasospasm or epinephrine effect; (4) direct vessel trauma resulting from injections done blindly beneath the orbital septum; and (5) rebleeding after closure resulting from any maneuver or event that leads to an increased ophthalmic arteriovenous pressure head.

Early recognition of a developing orbital hematoma can be facilitated by delaying intraoperative closure (first side), avoiding occlusive-pressure eye dressings, and extending the postoperative observational period. Although many methods of management have been described to manage threatened vision resulting from elevated intraocular pressures (reopening the wound, lateral canthotomy, steroids, diuretics, anterior chamber paracentesis), the most effective definitive treatment is immediate orbital decompression, which is usually accomplished through medial wall and orbital floor resections.[12,42] Certainly, ophthalmologic consultation is advisable.

Epiphora

Assuming dry eye syndrome was ruled out before surgery or managed appropriately intraoperatively (conservative and staged resections), a dysfunctional lacrimal collecting system rather than a high glandular output state is typically responsible for postoperative epiphora (although reflex hypersection may be a contributing factor because of coexistent lagophthalmos or vertical retraction of the lower lid). This response is common in the early postoperative period and is usually self-limited. Causes include the following: (1) punctal eversion and canalicular distortion secondary to wound retraction and edema; (2) impairment of the lacrimal pump resulting from atony, edema, hematoma, or partial resection of the orbicularis oculi sling; and (3) a temporary ectropion resulting from lid loading. Outflow obstructions, secondary to a lacerated inferior canaliculus, are preventable by keeping the lower lid incision lateral to the punctum. Should laceration injury occur, primary repair over a Silastic stent (Crawford tube; Dow Corning, Midland, MI) is recommended. Persistent punctal eversion can be managed by cauterization or diamond excision of the conjunctival surface below the canaliculus.

Suture Line Complications

Milia or inclusion cysts are common lesions seen along the incisional line resulting from trapped epithelial debris beneath a healed skin surface or possibly from the occlusion of a glandular duct. They are typically associated with simple or running cuticular stitches. Their formation is minimized by subcuticular closure. If they develop, definitive therapy is aimed at uncapping the cyst (no. 11 blade or epilation needle) and teasing out the sac. Granulomas may develop as nodular thickenings within or beneath the suture line and are typically treated by steroid injections if small and by direct excision if large. Suture tunnels develop as a result of prolonged suture retention and epithelial surface migration along the suture tract. Preventive treatment includes early suture removal (3 to 5 days), and definitive treatment involves unroofing the tunnel. Suture marks are also related to prolonged suture retention and their formation can usually be avoided by using a rapidly absorbing suture (fast-absorbing gut or mild chromic), by removing a monofilament suture early, or by employing a subcuticular closure.

Wound Healing Complications

Although rare, hypertrophic or prominent lower eyelid scars may develop because of improper placement of the lower lid incision. If extended too far medially in the epicanthal region, bow-string or web formation may occur (conditions usually amenable to correction by Z-plasty technique). A lateral canthal extension (which normally overlies a bony prominence) that is oriented too obliquely downward or is closed under excessive tension predisposes an incision to hypertrophic scarring, and during healing the vertical contraction vectors act on the lateral lid to favor scleral show or eversion. If the lower lid incision is oriented too far superiorly or too close to the lateral aspect of the upper lid incision, the forces of contraction (now favoring a downward pull) provide conditions that predispose the patient to lateral canthal hooding. Again, proper treatment should be aimed at reorienting the direction of contracting vectors.

Wound dehiscence may develop as a result of closure under excessive tension, early removal of sutures, extension of an infectious process (unusual), or hematoma (more commonly). Skin separation is seen most often in the lateral aspect of the incision with the skin–muscle and skin techniques, and treatment is directed to supportive taping or resuturing. If tension is too great for conservative management, then a lid suspension technique and lateral grafting should be considered. Skin slough may develop as a result of devascularization of the skin segment. It is almost exclusively seen in the skin-only technique and typically occurs in the lateral portion of the lower eyelid after wide undermining and subsequent hematoma formation. Treatment consists of local wound care, evacuation of any hematomas, establishment of a line of demarcation, and early skin replacement to obviate scar contracture of the lower lid.

Skin Discoloration

Areas of skin undermining are frequently evident as hyperpigmentation in the early recovery period secondary to bleeding beneath the skin surface with subsequent hemosiderin formation. This process is usually self-limiting and often takes longer to resolve in darkly pigmented individuals. It is imperative during the healing process, and particularly in this patient population, to avoid direct sunlight because this may lead to permanent pigment changes. Refractory cases (after 6 to 8 weeks) may be considered for camouflage, periorbital peeling, or depigmentation therapy (e.g., hydroxyquinone, kojic acid). Telangiectasias may develop after skin undermining, particularly in areas beneath or near the incision, and most commonly occur in patients with preexisting telangiectasias. Treatment options may include chemical peeling or dye laser ablation.

Ocular Injury

Corneal abrasions or ulcerations may result from inadvertent rubbing of the corneal surface with a gauze sponge or cotton applicator, instrument or suture mishandling, or desiccation developing as a result of lagophthalmos, ectropion, or preexistent dry eye syndrome. Symptoms suggestive of corneal injury, which include pain, eye irritation, and blurred vision, should be confirmed by fluorescein staining and slitlamp examination by an ophthalmologist. Therapy for mechanical injury typically involves use of an antibiotic ophthalmic drop with lid closure until epithelialization is complete (usually 24 to 48 hours). Treatment for dry eye syndrome includes the addition of ocular lubricants, such as Liquitears and Lacri-lube.

Extraocular muscle imbalance, manifested by gaze diplopia, may be seen and is often transitory, presumably reflecting resolution of an edematous process. However, permanent muscle injury may result from blind clamping, deep penetration of the fat pockets during sectioning of the pedicle, thermal injury resulting from electrocauterization, suture incorporation during closure, or ischemic contracture of the Volkman type. Patients with evidence of refractory and incomplete recovery of muscle function should be referred to an ophthalmologist for evaluation and definitive treatment.

Contour Irregularities

Contour irregularities are generally caused by technical omissions. Overzealous fat resection, particularly in a patient with a prominent infraorbital rim, results in a lower lid concavity and contributes to a sunken-eye appearance. Failure to remove enough fat (common in lateral pocket) leads to surface irregularities and persistent bulges. A ridge that persists beneath the incision line is usually the result of inadequate resection of a strip of orbicularis oculi before redraping. Areas of induration or lumpiness below the suture line usually can be attributed to unresolved or organized hematoma, tissue reaction or fibrosis secondary to electrocauterization or thermal injury, or soft tissue response to fat necrosis. Treatment in each case is directed at the specific cause. Persistent fat bulges are managed by resection, whereas areas of lid depression can be managed by sliding fat-pad grafts, free-fat or dermal fat grafts,[43] or orbicularis oculi flap repositioning. Some patients with such bulges or prominences respond to direct injections of triamcinoline (40 mg/cm^3). In selected cases, infraorbital rim reductions distract noticeability from a hollow-eye appearance and may be used as an adjunctive technique. Unresolved hematomas and areas of heightened inflammatory response may be managed with conservative injections of steroids.

References

1. Volpe CR, Ramirez OM. The beautiful eye. Facial Plast Surg Clin N Am 2005;13:493–504
2. Bashour M, Geist C. Is medial canthal tilt a powerful cue for facial attractiveness? Ophthal Plast Reconstr Surg 2007;23(1):52–56
3. Bartlett SP, Wornom I 3rd, Whitaker LA. Evaluation of facial skeletal aesthetics and surgical planning. Clin Plast Surg 1991;18:1–9
4. Zide BM. Anatomy of the eyelids. Clin Plast Surg 1981;8:623
5. Aguilar GL, Nelson C. Eyelid and anterior orbital anatomy. In: Hornblass A, ed. Oculoplastic, Orbital, and Reconstructive Surgery. Vol. 1: Eyelids. Baltimore: Williams & Wilkins; 1988
6. Jones LT. New concepts of orbital anatomy. In: Tessier P, Callahan A, Mustarde JC, et al, eds. Symposium on Plastic Surgery in the Orbital Region. St Louis: CV Mosby; 1976
7. Doxanas MT. Blepharoplasty: key anatomical concepts. Facial Plast Surg 1984;1:259
8. Nesi F, Lisman R, Levine M. Smith's Ophthalmic Plastic and Reconstructive Surgery. 2nd ed. St. Louis: CV Mosby; 1998:1–78
9. Freeman MS. Transconjunctival sub-orbicularis occlui fat (SOOF) pad lift blepharoplasty: a new technique for the effacement of nasojugal deformity. Arch Facial Plast Surg 2000;2:16–21
10. Rees TD, Jelks GW. Blepharoplasty and the dry eye syndrome: guidelines for surgery? Plast Reconstr Surg 1981;68:249
11. Jelks GW, McCord CD. Dry eye syndrome and other tear film abnormalities. Clin Plast Surg 1981;8:803
12. Sacks SH, Lawson W, Edelstein D, et al. Surgical treatment of blindness secondary to intraorbital hemorrhage. Arch Otolaryngol Head Neck Surg 1988;114:801
13. Mahaffey PJ, Wallace AF. Blindness following cosmetic blepharoplasty: a review. Br J Plast Surg 1986;39:213
14. Callahan MA. Prevention of blindness after blepharoplasty. Ophthalmology 1983;90:1047–1051
15. Beekhuis GJ. Blepharoplasty. Otolaryngol Clin North Am 1982;15: 179
16. McKinney P, Zukowski ML. The value of tear film breakup and schirmer's tests in preoperative blepharoplasty evaluation. Plast Reconstr Surg 1989;84:572
17. Holt JE, Holt GR. Blepharoplasty: indications and preoperative assessment. Arch Otolaryngol 1985;111:394
18. Bourquet J. Les hernies graisseuses de l'orbite: notre traitment chirurgical. Bull Acad Natl Med 1924;92:1270–1272
19. Perkins SW, Dyer WD II, Simo F. Transconjunctival approach to lower eyelid blepharoplasty. Arch Otolaryngol Head Neck Surg 1994;120: 172–177
20. Mahe E. Lower lid blepharoplasty: the transconjunctival approach: extended indications. Aesthetic Plast Surg 1998;22:1–8
21. Zarem HA, Resnick JI. Minimizing deformity in lower blepharopasty: the transconjuctival approach. Plast Reconstr Surg 1991; 88:215
22. McKinney P, Zukowshi ML, Mossie R. The 4th option: a novel approach to lower lid blepharoplasty. Aesthetic Plast Surg 1991;15: 293–296
23. Baylis HI, Long JA, Groth MJ. Transconjunctival lower eyelid blepharoplasty. Ophthalmology 1989;96:1027
24. Cheney ML. Facial Surgery: Plastic and Reconstructive. Baltimore: Williams & Wilkins; 1987:895–904
25. Netscher DT, Patrinely JR, Peltier M, et al. Transconjunctival versus transcutaneous lower eyelid blepharoplasty: a prospective study. Plast Reconstr Surg 1995;96:1053–1059
26. Tessier P. The conjunctival approach to the orbital floor and maxilla in congenital malformation and trauma. J Maxillofac Surg 1973; 1:3–8
27. Spira M. Blepharoplasty. Clin Plast Surg 1978;5:121
28. David LM. The laser approach to blepharoplasty. J Dermatol Surg Oncol 1988;14:741
29. Mele JA III, Kulick MI, Lee D. Laser blepharoplasty: is it safe? Aesthetic Plast Surg 1998;22:9–11
30. Mommaerts MY, Beirne JC, Jacobs WI, Abeloos JSV. Use of fibrin glue in lower blepharoplasties. J Craniomaxillofac Surg 1996; 24:78–82
31. Holt JE, Holt GR, Cortez EA. Blepharoplasty. Ear Nose Throat J 1981;60:42
32. Cook TA, Dereberry J, Harrah ER. Reconsideration of fat pad management in lower lid blepharoplasty surgery. Arch Otolaryngol 1984;110:521
33. Klatsky SA, Manson PN. Separate skin and muscle flaps in lower lid blepharoplasty. Plast Reconstr Surg 1981;67:151
34. Wolfey DE. Blepharoplasty: the ophthalmologist's view. Otolaryngol Clin North Am 1980;13:237
35. McCollough EG, English JL. Blepharoplasty: avoiding plastic eyelids. Arch Otolaryngol Head Neck Surg 1988;114:645
36. Goldberg RA, Fiaschetti D. Filling the periorbital hollows with hyaluronic acid gel: initial experience with 244 injections. Ophthal Plast Reconstr Surg 2006;22:335–341
37. Goldberg RA. Transconjunctival orbital fat repositioning: transposition of orbital pedicles into a subperiosteal pocket. Plas Reconstr Surg 2000;105:743–748; discussion 749–751
38. Trepsat F. Periorbital rejuvenation combining fat grafting and blepharoplasties. Aesthetic Plast Surg 2003;27:243
39. Adams BJS, Feurstein SS. Complications of blepharoplasty. Ear Nose Throat J 1986;65(1):11–28
40. Castanares S. Complications in blepharoplasty. Clin Plast Surg 1978; 5:149
41. Moser MH, DiPirro E, MaCoy FJ. Sudden blindness following blepharoplasty: report of seven cases. Plast Reconstr Surg 1973; 51:363
42. Anderson RL, Edwards JJ. Bilateral visual loss after blepharoplasty. Ann Plast Surg 1980;5:288
43. Loeb R. Fat pad sliding and fat grafting for leveling lid depressions. Clin Plast Surg 1981;8:757

24 Liposuction of the Face and Neck: The Art of Facial Sculpture

Russell W. H. Kridel, Paul E. Kelly, and Richard D. Castellano

Formation of a double chin, diminution of the cervicomental angle and definition of the jaw line, and the appreciation that the face and neck have become one structure rather than two, cause much consternation to the patient who has gained weight or who has aged. Plastic surgeons have attempted to redefine these natural facial angles through resuspension or removal of the ptotic or excessive soft tissue envelope. The facial and neck adiposity, however, has been a significant hurdle that over the years has thwarted achievement of the ideal surgical result. Liposuction with extraction of fatty deposits was first performed as an adjunctive procedure to facelift, significantly improving aesthetic outcomes.

In the early 1970s, Schrudde[1] discussed the concept of "lipoexeresis." The concept of fat removal continued to evolve with Fischer and Fischer[2] and Kesselring's[3] suggestion of placing a tube connected to a suction device through small incisions in a covered field to access fat deposits. Illouz described the technique of lipolysis in which he injected hypotonic saline in the proposed surgical site and then used a blunt-tipped cannula with a high vacuum for fat aspiration.[4] Today facial liposuction is used as a primary facial sculpting and/or rejuvenation procedure and in combination with other regional aesthetic operations. In contrast to earlier direct and open methods, suction lipectomy offers important advantages of minimal scarring, reduced tissue trauma, shorter recuperative periods, and hidden incisions. Some feel that liposuction has revolutionized aesthetic surgery.[5–9] The advent of smaller cannulas, the use of tumescence of the adipose tissue, the application of ultrasonic (U/S) techniques, and the use of the liposhaver are the latest advances in this field.

General Principles

Localized adiposity may be attributed to hereditary factors, hormonal imbalance, or poor dietary and exercise habits. Evenly distributed fat stores, unlike isolated facial deposits,[8–10] diminish with exercise and diet. Frequently and unfortunately, the localized deposits are the first to hypertrophy with weight gain. This isolated excess of fat is readily addressed with submental liposuction; however, patients with generalized fat deposition are best served with a weight loss program.

Illouz, one of the pioneers in liposuction, extensively studied the physiology of the human adipocyte. He was able to determine that human adipocytes multiply from birth until puberty and then are stable in number. Based on histological study, he described obese children as having a large number of adipocytes (a hyperplastic state) versus the obese adult simply having "large" fat cells (a hypertrophic state).[4] Through the incorporation of triglycerides and fatty acid deposits, the overall volume of the fat cell increases. Weight loss is a reduction not in the number of fat cells but rather in their volume.[4,11] Surgical intervention should be directed at eliminating localized fat cells, ideally in a permanent fashion.

The majority of new technological interventions, with one exception, take seed from body contouring research, which can frequently be applied to facial surgery. The use of a rigid, blunt-tipped aspiration cannula that is attached to a suction device continues to be the mainstay for suction lipectomy. Recontouring of the overlying soft tissue envelope is achieved through elimination of fat cells by suction-assisted avulsion and by subdermal contraction seen during the healing phase.

Traditional liposuction permits a relatively precise reduction in fat cell mass coupled with a low complication rate as compared with direct lipectomy.[2,7] Specifically, the tunneling technique of liposuction allows the neurovascular bundles to the skin to be preserved, resulting in a lower risk of hematoma formation, and a return of skin sensation in 3 to 8 weeks.

Recontouring takes place as healing progresses, with contraction of the subcutaneous tunnel network created by the liposuction tunneling technique. A carefully designed and evenly distributed tunnel system minimizes bulges and irregularities secondary to localized fat. Early healing irregularities may be seen but are usually fleeting.[5,8,12–14] Asymmetries, dimples, or bulges that persist beyond 6 months postoperatively are often amenable to additional liposuction, subcutaneous steroid injection, or localized fat injection.

Suction-assisted lipectomy (SAL) demonstrates numerous advantages over techniques designed for direct fat excision. SAL eliminates the need for large incisions and reduces operative and recuperative time. By selecting patients with good skin elasticity and localized adiposity and using the appropriate operative and postoperative techniques, surgeons can improve aesthetic results and create happy patients.

This chapter will outline the selection of the appropriate candidate for liposuction. It will review the physiology and technique of liposuction, highlight necessary equipment, and suggest ways to avoid complications. Finally, the most recent advances in this field will be discussed.

Patient Evaluation

Cervicofacial liposuction as an isolated procedure should be limited to those patients with good elasticity to the neck skin, lack of wrinkled or lax skin, lack of visible platysmal banding, and to those with a palpable submental fat mass. There is a degree of unpredictability for the results of submental liposuction that all patients must be aware of. Once the fat is removed, the outcome is dependent on the individual's skin to contract, in much the same way as in postpartum females, a previously stretched abdominal wall may contract totally in some and to a lesser degree in others. It may also take up to 6 months to see the final result, and no promises can be made as to what degree of change will occur.

When contemplating cervicofacial liposuction, the surgeon must consider the neck skeletal configuration, the muscular support of the neck, and the patient's body habitus, in addition to the skin elasticity and tone of the neck and face. Conley[15] showed that the position of the hyoid bone in relation to the mentum is the most significant determinant of a desirable cervicomental angle. A low, anterior hyoid position will produce a less favorable result in liposuction than will a high, posteriorly placed hyoid. Additionally, those with a retrusive chin will show less of an effect with liposuction, and in such patients, consideration should be given to concomitant chin implantation (**Fig. 24.1**). Ptotic submandibular glands may also detract from the acuity of the cervicomental angle.

Those who demonstrate localized adipose deposits that are out of proportion to the remainder of the body will benefit most from a localized fat removal procedure. Skin elasticity and muscle tone usually are good indicators of postoperative skin contraction and redraping of the soft tissue envelope; therefore, younger patients are generally more appropriate candidates. Overweight patients should be at the lower end of their usual range, with any planned weight-loss taking place several months prior to the procedure; if these patients have had dramatic fluctuations in their weight, they may have lost the needed skin elasticity for later contraction. In general, women have greater skin elasticity than men, and are better candidates for closed cervicofacial liposuction as a primary procedure (**Fig. 24.2**). Women tend to have thinner skin that contracts over the reduced subcutaneous bed. This is not to say that men are not to be considered for this procedure; simply expectations for this subset must be tempered. However, we have had older male patients exhibit significant skin retraction, and younger patients who did not, demonstrating some unpredictability to the procedure done in isolation.

Inappropriate candidates for cervicofacial liposuction are those who present with prominent wrinkling of the skin, significant ptosis to the muscular sling, and prominent platysmal bands. The shape of the neck is also determined by the position and tone of the platysmal muscle, and when a wide diastasis, prominent banding, or asymmetry is present, a formal platysmaplasty, and not isolated submental liposuction, is additionally indicated. Redundant and inelastic skin often fails to redrape appropriately after the removal of moderate to large amounts of subcutaneous fatty deposits.[5,16–20] Exceptions certainly do occur, and some patients may have remarkable results (**Fig. 24.3**). Bank et al[21] discussed 58 patients between the ages of 40 and 75, 20 of which underwent submental liposuction.

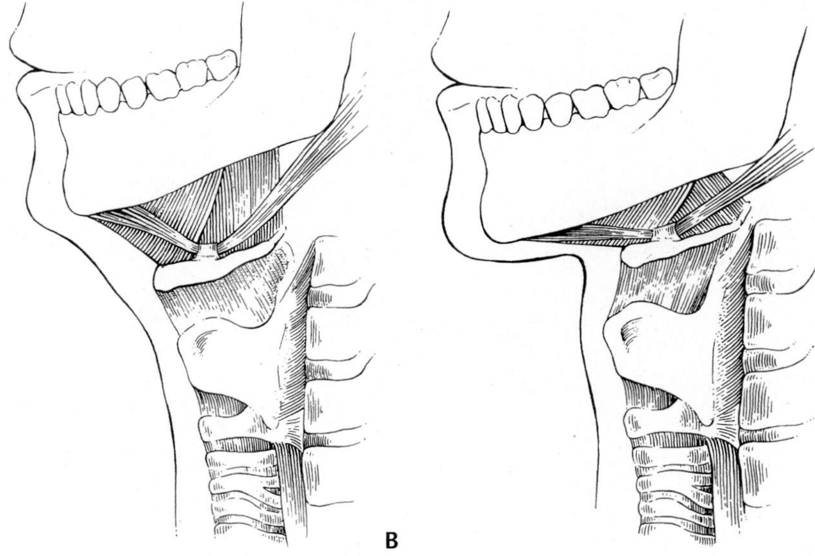

Fig. 24.1 Liposuction of the neck and submnetum produces the most well-defined cervicomental angle if the hyoid bone is positioned high and posterior (**A**). However, a low and anterior hyoid limits the desired appearance of the neck in liposuction and should be noted preoperatively and discussed with the patient as a limitation (**B**). (From Conley J. Facelift Operation. Springfield, IL: Charles C. Thomas; 1968:40-41. Reprinted by permission.)

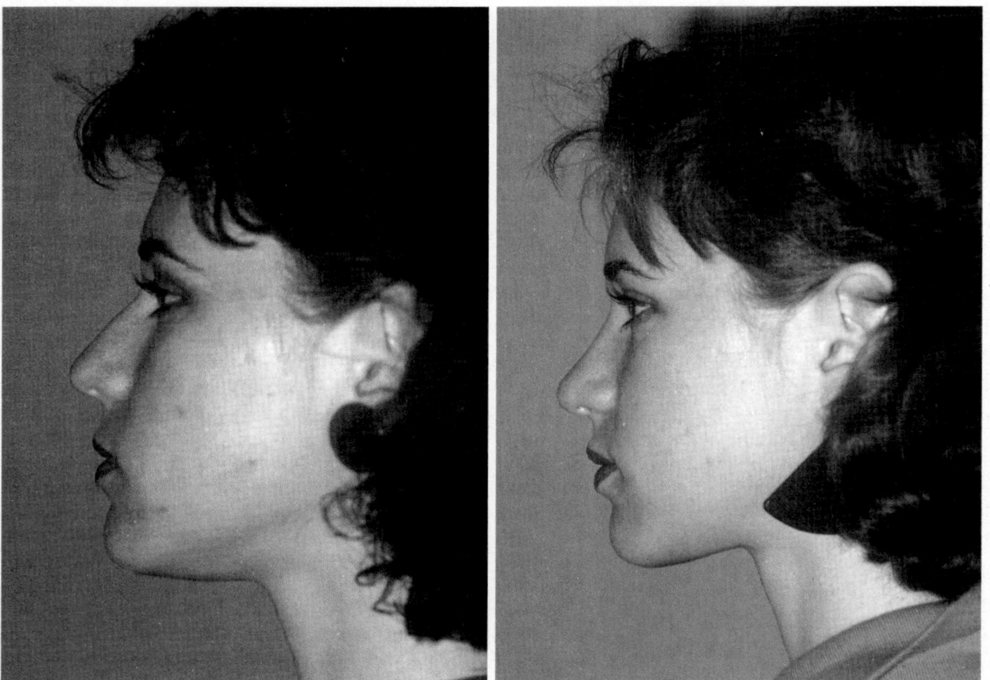

Fig. 24.2 (**A**) Preoperative. Ideal candidate with a high posterior hyoid with submental liposis and elastic healthy skin envelope. (**B**) Six months postoperatively, after submental liposuction and rhinoplasty. (Copyright © R. Kridel, MD. Reprinted by permission.)

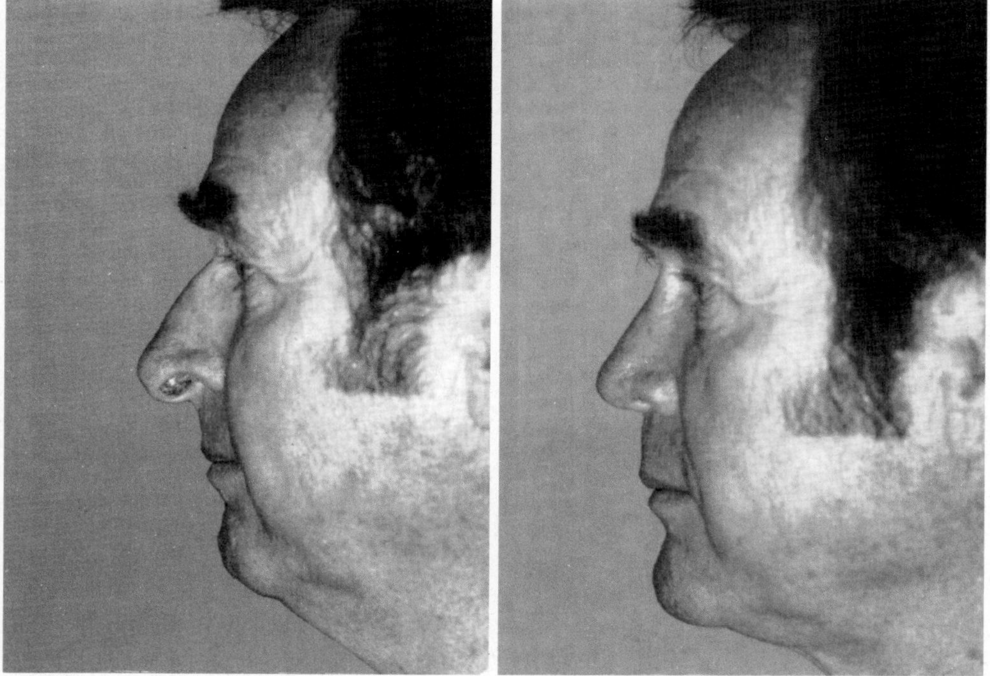

Fig. 24.3 (**A**) Preoperative. Older patient with cervicofacial fat as well as redundant skin who refused rhytidectomy. (**B**) Two months after liposuction and nasal surgery only. Excess skinfolds persist, but with dramatic cosmetic result. (From Kridel R, Buchwach K. Suction lipectomy. In: Krause CJ, Mangat DS, Pastorek N, eds. Aesthetic Facial Surgery. Philadelphia: JB Lippincott; 1991. Reprinted by permission.)

Of these 20 patients, the average age was 57 (range: 40–74), the average fat extracted was 75 mL (range: 25–125), and the average amount of lidocaine used was 4 mg/kg (range: 1.5–6). All patients were noted to have good to excellent results, no significant complications, and no problems with excess skin sagging or unfavorable skin redraping.

The problem of platysmal banding will not be eliminated with cervical liposuction and may be exacerbated by fat resection. The patient with significant submental fat may have postliposuction exposure of previously masked platysmal banding, producing a cobra deformity of the submentum. The patient with significant banding or cording should be informed preoperatively of the need for either a playtsmal plication or a full rhytidectomy for optimal results.

Finally, skin irregularities and asymmetries should be noted and shared with the patient preoperatively. With rare exceptions, neither dimpling, depressions, nor scarring will improve with liposuction alone, and perhaps may become more pronounced with a change in neck contour.

Indications

Although the focus of this chapter is the aesthetic use of liposuction in the head and neck area for removal of adiposity, liposuction as a technique may also be used to manage a variety of other surgical problems. It can be used to elevate soft tissue facelift flaps atraumatically,[9] to defat pedicled or free flaps,[22] and is also effective for removal of benign fatty tumors.[23,24]

When used in isolation as a closed technique (through a small incision) without muscle or SMAS elevation, suspension, excision, plication, or imbrication liposuction's greatest effectiveness is seen in creating contour changes in the cervicomental angle and, when used judiciously, in the jowl region. The open technique implies suction directly over fat deposits under direct vision, generally in association with rhytidectomy. The nasolabial folds and the lower jowl fat pads have both been addressed with the use of closed liposuction with less predictable results and absence of controlled long-term follow-up. Nasolabial fold prominence is usually a gravity problem and although liposuction results vary, judicious liposuction here may be helpful. The natural tendency for progressive atrophy of facial fat[5,8,17] makes midface liposuction risky. It is helpful to inquire as to the family history of facial fat changes. Some parents and grandparents have full faces throughout life, and perhaps a buccal lipectomy is indicated for the similarly shaped faces of their descendants rather than midface liposuction.

Ideal candidates for primary liposuction of the cervicofacial region exhibit sufficient skin elasticity, which will promote skin contraction. In those patients with moderate or poor skin elasticity, removal of localized adiposity may predispose to an increased appearance of sagging skin. Some erroneously promote liposuction as a procedure to reduce sagging skin,[25] whereas in our experience it can compound this problem. Dedo suggests that, after the age of 40 years, the contractile ability of skin may become unsatisfactory.[26] Others suggest age be taken into consideration, but that one should rely on actual tissue assessment as the predicting factor.[10,26] Occasionally the young patient with apparently good skin elasticity may have limited results. Again, patients should be aware that good results are not totally predictable.

Methodology and Physiology

There are several different methods to accomplish the primary goal of liposuction. When considering liposuction of the face and neck, the surgeon must be cognizant of the thinness of the facial skin, the proximity of sensory and motor nerves (i.e., the marginal mandibular branch of the facial nerve), the depth of fat to be aspirated, and the natural effects of aging on facial fat deposits.

Liposuction as it was introduced in the 1970s makes use of a rigid cannula and a suction device.[1,2] The cannula is rapidly advanced and retracted through the fatty deposits via subcutaneous tunnels. Fat cells are sharply avulsed by being drawn into the perforated cannula by the negative pressure created by the suction device. If the suction pressure is high enough, the fat cells are actually lysed and destroyed.

The addition of tumescence—the infiltration of hypotonic saline combined with local anesthetic—to the liposuction regimen is widely used for body contouring. Tumescence may be used in the head and neck in smaller volumes not only for fat aspiration, but also for tissue plane dissection. However, in the face and neck tumescence may produce distortion and make the end point more difficult to discern.[27–29]

The demand for improved results in body liposuction with low morbidity has led to the development of U/S energy, either internal or external to the fatty deposit, for fat cell disruption and facilitated aspiration. Many of the more frequent areas of localized body adiposity have a high fibrous content,[27] and advancement of the liposuction cannula with the internal or external U/S device is not only less strenuous for the surgeon, but reportedly more efficient for fat aspiration.[28–31] Some studies of body liposuction with U/S assistance also report less swelling and less bruising postoperatively.[32]

Physiologically, the U/S energy is transformed into mechanical vibrations that create a "micromechanical effect, a cavitational effect (expansion and compression cycles form microcavities in adipose tissue, which then implode, resulting in cellular destruction; that is, liquefaction of fat, and a thermal effect on fat cells)."[29] Grippaudo et al[33] utilized gas chromatography to confirm that U/S energy disrupts the adipocyte membrane, resulting in an egress of cellular contents without mechanical or enzymatic damage to triglyceride molecules.

Numerous studies show potential problems with use of subcutaneous U/S energy, such as excess heat generated by the U/S device at the skin incision site,[8,29,33,34] and the potential heat-related complications generated at more distant subdermal sites.[20,35] Use of the external U/S liposuction device is discussed less frequently in today's literature, and it is touted as having similar benefits as internal U/S in terms of surgical facilitation and recovery period.[27,28,36] Further research is indicated in this modality as the most recent literature discussing this technique is unable to offer definitive guidelines for use of the external device but rather suggests ranges of safety.[36] Cardenes-Camerana et al[37] report on an interesting series of 13 patients undergoing tumescent body liposuction assisted by external ultrasound. Histological examination of skin biopsies after liposuction with and without U/S assistance revealed only transient increases in vascular congestion, hypopigmentaiton, tissue edema, and inflammatory infiltration with ultrasound use, peaking at 1 week postoperatively, and disappearing at 6 months postoperatively. Overall, there were essentially no differences in the aesthetic result or in skin retraction.

The facial plastic surgeon should be cautious when considering use of internal U/S–assisted liposuction in the cervicofacial area second to the close proximity of neural structures. An animal based study by Howard evaluated the effects of U/S energy on neural tissue. The study results showed that low amplitude U/S energy will induce visible injury to the nerve when applied directly.[30] No functional evidence of nerve injury was noticed, however, until higher amplitude settings were reached. Our MEDLINE search did not find any controlled studies demonstrating the safety or added benefit of U/S-assisted liposuction in the face or neck as compared with the standard microcannula liposuction procedure.

The most recent addition to liposuction is the liposhaver as advocated by Gross and Becker[38,39] for direct lipectomy or for use in a closed technique in the cervicofacial area. A similar tool (the microdebrider) has made great strides in the endoscopic sinus arena[40] and a further adaptation has also been advocated by some for use in nasal dorsal rhinoplasty.[41] The liposhaver is a guarded, motorized blade that is reported to remove fat via sharp excision either under direct vision, or under a subdermal flap. Trauma is reportedly less than with standard techniques because of the excision versus avulsion principle. However, it is an interesting historic note to recognize that liposuctions, as originally proposed by Schudde,[1] made use of sharp curet-type instruments that excised rather then avulsed fatty deposits. This technique fell from favor after reports of tissue death and even loss of an extremity secondary to vascular damage.

The shaver differs from the traditional, the tumescent, and the U/S liposuction techniques in that it does not require high suction pressures, and it actively excises rather than avulses the fatty deposit.[38,39] Multiinstitutional comparison trials[39] have shown success of the device and offer it simply as an alternative to conventional liposuction with perhaps less postoperative bruising and in experienced hands precise lipolysis. Greater care must be exercised when using this device to ensure that only subcutaneous fat is excised and aspirated and that no dermal contact is made. When used in a closed procedure, the tent and superficial projection of the cannula tip—accomplished by the surgeons nondominant hand—allows even fat extraction and prevents vessel or neural injury. Concerns with seromas and hematomas may be slightly increased with use of the liposhaver as compared with the traditional liposuction method. An interesting study on 21 patients performed by Katz et al[42] showed that when compared with traditional liposuction, liposhaving resulted in faster recovery, less ecchymoses, and less surgeon fatigue when sculpting truncal and extremity fat. The only studies that exist for submental liposhaving are subjective comparisons of surgeons noting that the liposhaver is a precise alternative to conventional liposuction.[43,47]

Instrumentation

The basic tools for liposuction are few, but they have continued to evolve since their introduction in the early 1970s.[2,3] With the exception of the liposhaver, the physiological base for liposuction remains the same—subcutaneous fat is avulsed into a cannula by the back and forth motion of the instrument and the negative pressure created by a suction device.[38,39] Today the advent of the 1 mm, 2 mm, and 3 mm blunt-tipped liposuction cannulas allows for better control and precision in the art of liposculpting. Smaller cannulas do have less risk of creating contour irregularities that may be caused by larger cannula apertures, though caution must be exercised with thinner cannulas as the risk of skin perforation is greater.

Some of the innovations in cannula design include the use of lightweight metals and a variety of grip sizes. Some cannulas are equipped with a variable number of suction apertures. Cannula openings may be only on one side, allowing the surgeon to ensure that the dermis does not sustain a suction injury. However, in areas with a great volume of fat, a Mercedes tip, or openings on all sides of the cannula is helpful for expedient fat removal,

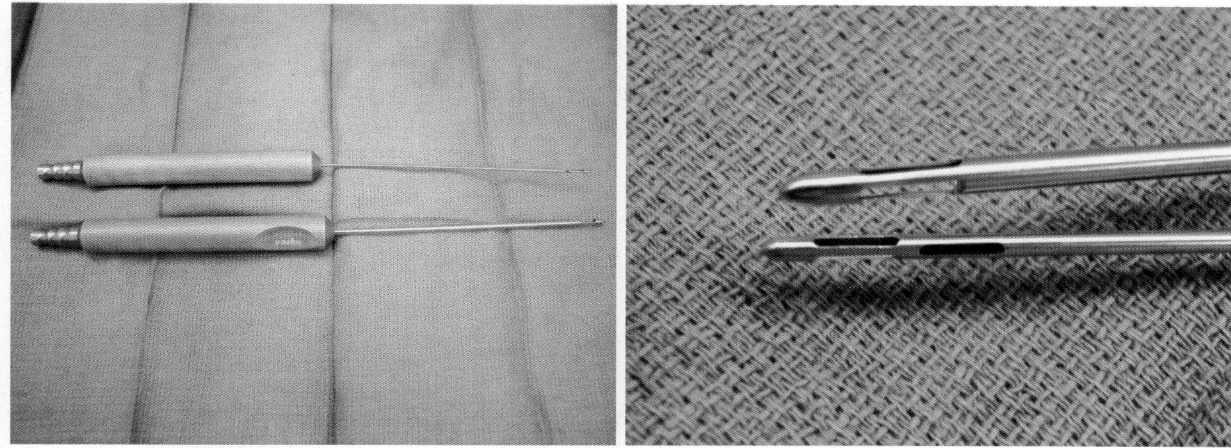

Fig. 24.4 Liposuction cannulas. (**A**) Liposuction cannulas, 6 mm (upper) and 4 mm (lower). (**B**) Note the Mercedes-type apertures on the 6 mm cannula (upper), and the multiple smaller openings on the 4 mm cannula (lower).

providing there is a buffer of tissue between the cannula and the dermis (**Fig. 24.4**). Tip designs range from sharp to the more blunted and spatulated endings. As will be explained in the technique section of this chapter, the various cannulas should be used in the different phases of liposculpting. These phases include active fat removal, sculpting, and feathering. Additionally, the tip of the cannula should be blunt so as not to perforate the skin or damage the dermis.

When liposuction is used to harvest fat for reinjection as a soft tissue filler, it is recommended to use less suction pressure to preserve adipocyte structure and increase graft survival. This is accomplished using a Luer-Lock aspiration cannula on a 10 or 20 cc syringe, and is usually performed in an area with more fat than the submentum (i.e., lower abdomen, bilateral thighs, etc). The cannula of the handheld device differs in design by being slightly smaller: ~14 to 17 gauge.[44,45]

The tumescent technique and the use of internal or external U/S energy are used less frequently in the cervicofacial regions, but they have a following.[20,35,36] Tumescent cannulas are narrow and blunt tipped and serve simply as a conduit for the rapid infusion of the hypotonic/anesthetic saline solution. The U/S equipment consists of either an external handheld device used external to the skin, or a cannula (hollow or solid bore) with an incorporated U/S system. Polyethylene sleeves are available to help decrease the risk of incision site burns, though no protection is offered for distal sites.

A basic requirement for liposuction is a suction device that is capable of generating enough negative pressure for fat avulsion and aspiration. Negative pressure in liposuction may be generated by a commercially available unit or from a handheld syringe. The electrical units may generate up to at least 1 atm of negative pressure (960 mm Hg) and a handheld syringe creates close to 700 mm Hg with initial aspiration that then drops to a stable pressure closer to 600 mm Hg.[44,45] Of note, handheld liposuction requires a closed skin environment to maintain suction pressure, whereas vacuum pressure can be used in both closed and open environments. Suction pressure should always be checked prior to initiation of the procedure to ensure pressure is not too high. Theoretically, the higher the suction pressure the greater the chance of neural or vascular structures being aspirated and avulsed (**Fig. 24.4**).

Preoperative Preparation

Preoperative Marking

Areas of submental fat and important facial landmarks, including the sternocleidomastoid (SCM) muscle, the hyoid bone, and the angle of the mandible are marked in the preoperative holding area with the patient in a sitting position (**Fig. 24.5**). Preoperative marking is helpful as fatty accumulations may shift or disappear when the patient lies supine. Submental and infralobular incision sites are also marked prior to infiltration of anesthetic solution. Patients with prominent submandibular glands should be aware that these will not be reduced in size and may be more prominent in appearance after submental and submandibular liposculpting.

In most cervical liposuction cases, the subcutaneous tunnel dissection extends to the SCM laterally, and at least to the hyoid bone inferiorly. Submental fat is generally located centrally, and so dissection and suction extending to these borders serves as more of a feathering function with the most fat aspirated in the area of greatest concern. Graduated markings should reflect the area in which the function of liposuction is to blend and not necessarily to recontour. When the jowl areas require recontouring,

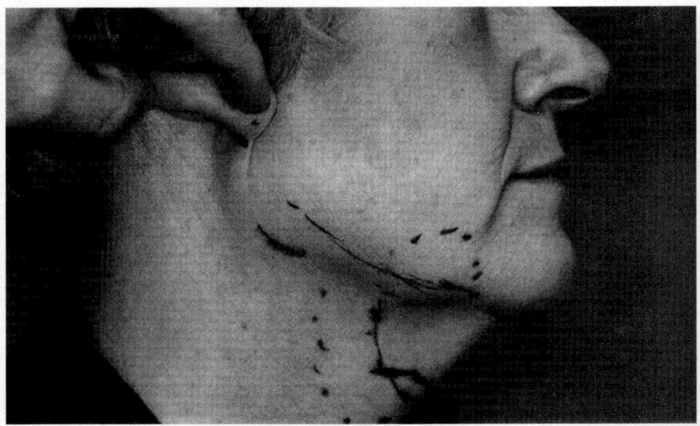

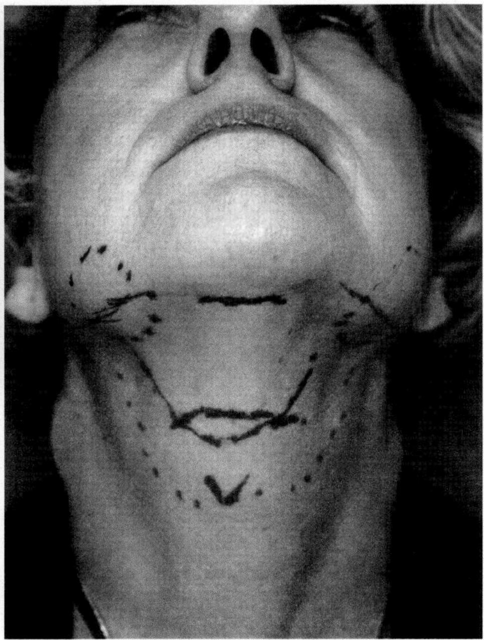

Fig. 24.5 (**A**) Preoperative. Patient on three-fourths view with submental fullness and early jowls outlined, with the posterior earlobe and submental incisions marked. (**B**) Preoperative marking on base view of the mandibular angle, border of the mandible, hyoid bone, thyroid notch, area of greatest submental liposis, and area of planned feathering.

approach to this site may be gained from an infralobular or transnasal approach, utilizing very small bore cannulas under lower pressure to avoid over suctioning or nerve damage.

Anesthesia

Cervicofacial liposuction is usually performed as an isolated procedure with local infiltrative anesthesia with or without intravenous sedation. A tumescent technique in the face and neck—although not frequently used in our practice—consists of varied mixtures of 0.5% lidocaine with 1:200,000 epinephrine and hypotonic saline. In addition to local infiltration, regional blocks with 0.25% Marcaine (bupivicaine) with epinephrine at Erb's point, in the area of the mental nerve, and circumferential to the planned treatment area will provide longer-term definitive anesthesia. Anesthesia and suitable vasoconstriction in the nontumescent technique are provided by a field block of 1% lidocaine with 1:100,000 epinephrine. It is not uncommon in the neck to infiltrate 15 to 20 cc of anesthesia, and an additional 10 cc for any areas of concern in the face proper.

Surgical Technique

The goal of liposuction regardless of methodology is to recontour areas of adiposity by precise reduction in localized collections of fat while minimizing external irregularities or scars. The technique is not difficult to perform, though several details of the procedure must be appreciated to produce smooth surface contours and minimize postoperative problems.

Underestimating the amount of fat reduction necessary to meet aesthetic goals may be the lesser of two evils—the greater evil being overaggressive fat removal with creation of an unnatural concavity, hollowing, or unmasking of plastysmal banding. If the skin fuses to the underlying musculature after removal of too much subcutaneous fat, irregularities may become obvious, requiring an open plastysmaplasty with or without facelift for correction (**Fig. 24.6**). Additionally, a masculinized appearance may result by skeletonization of the thyroid notch, where skeletonization creates a "pseudolaryngeal prominence," more characteristic of the male neck. Liposuction inferior to the hyoid bone must be done with caution as injury to the dermis in this area can result in scar band formation at the cervicomental angle.

Cervicofacial liposuction as an isolated procedure is performed in a closed fashion. When a facelift is performed, the open nature of the flaps provides access for a combination of the closed and open liposuction.

Liposuction as a Primary Procedure

Incisions in the submental crease, in the posterior lobular crease, or in the nasal vestibule, are well hidden and give excellent access to the entire cervicofacial region.

Too small an incision regardless of technique may predispose to friction burns or skin excoriation at the incision site, simply from the back and forth motion of the suction

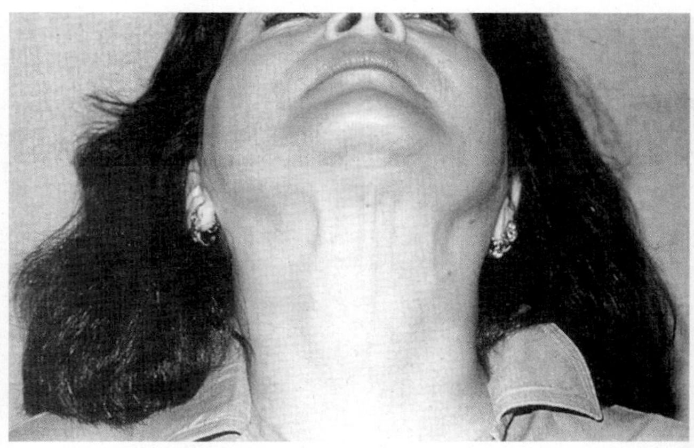

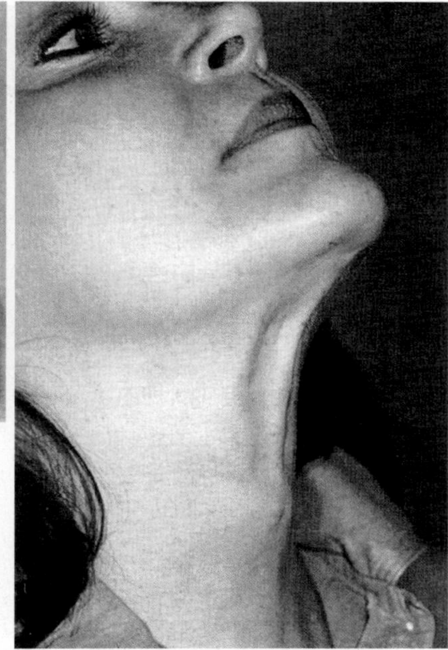

Fig. 24.6 Unmasking of the platysmal bands (**A**) and masciulinzation (**B**) of the thyroid notch after overaggressive submental liposuction. (From Kridel RWH, Pacella BL. Complications of liposuction. In Eisele D, ed. Complications of Head and Neck Surgery. St. Louis: Mosby-Year Book; 1992:791-803. Reprinted by permission.)

cannula. The incision length is generally 4 to 8 mm long. The incision should accommodate a 4 or 6 mm cannula—the largest cannula diameters suggested in cervicofacial liposuction procedures.[5,8,46] The incision is created and the immediate surrounding skin is sharply undermined with a small tenotomy scissors to allow appropriate placement of the cannula in the proper plane and to prevent postoperative irregularities at the incision site. The appropriate plane is just deep to the dermal–subcutaneous interface.

The proper plane in the fibrotic or previously operated neck is elusive and pretunneling is helpful to ensure proper dissection depth. Once the dissection is initiated, the aspiration cannula may be introduced through this site without the suction tubing attached to judge the ease of passage of the cannula. Such pretunneling is then performed until easy passage is appreciated. The suction is then attached to the cannula. A superficial tunnel is utilized by tenting the skin away from the deeper tissues with the cannula tip. The left hand (for the right-handed surgeon) is the dominant hand during this procedure. It serves to guide the cannula, direct the fat into the lumen, and maintain the correct tissue plane. The right hand is the motor, and advances the cannula through the space. Evenness of cannula motion and a fan-type pattern ensures the correct dissection plane, and even fat extraction. The suction pressure is adjusted to be enough to fill the suction tubing with fat and at the same time preserve neurovascular and lymphatic continuity between skin and deeper subcutaneous tissues.

Suction pressure should be briefly suspended each time that the cannula is removed from or inserted into the incision site to decrease the potential for entrance site injury from the suction pressure. A simple pinch of the suction tubing and release technique is adequate to stop suction and prevent entrance site injury. Entrance of the cannula lumen through the incision site is done such that the lumen opening is always directed deep toward the subcutaneous tissues away from the dermis. When performing liposuction in the cervicofacial region there are few if any indications for directing the cannula lumen aperture toward the dermal surface.[18] Vigorous suction against this surface may cause injury to the subdermal plexus with the result being scar formation and significant postoperative irregularities.

Fat is removed by directing the cannula throughout the pretunneled area in the same radially directed manner used initially. When addressing the submental liposis, the dissection will fan across the neck from jowl to jowl. The tunnels will circumscribe an arc that extends to the sternocleidomastoid muscles laterally and to the thyroid cartilage inferiorly. The radiating tunnels will center at the incision site in the submental crease (**Fig. 24.7**). The most vigorous suction should be performed in the area of greatest liposis, delineated by preoperative marks. The larger cannulas are then used here for fat volume reduction, but may be too large and are not appropriate for all patients, especially those with only minimal or moderate fat deposits. Sculpting with a blunt-tipped small lumen cannula is most appropriate for the mandibular border or jowl region. Liposuction more distal to the primary sites of concern should be aimed at blending or feathering the newly recontoured area. Feathering is best accomplished with use of a smaller lumened, less aggressive cannula having a single or double aperture. Fat extraction

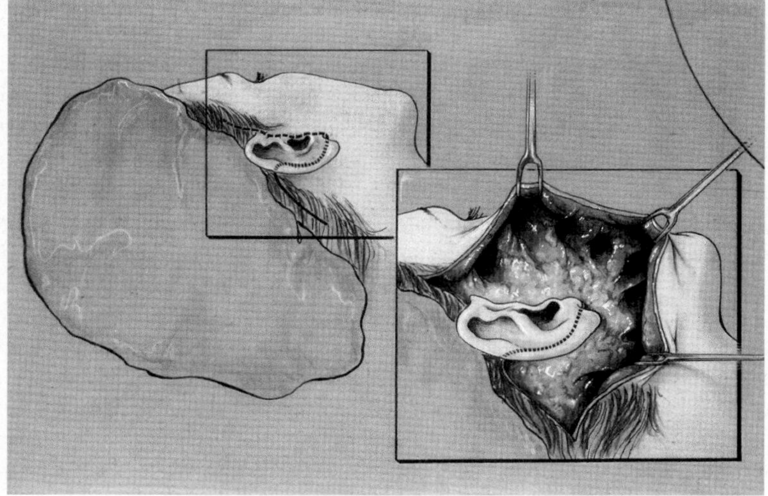

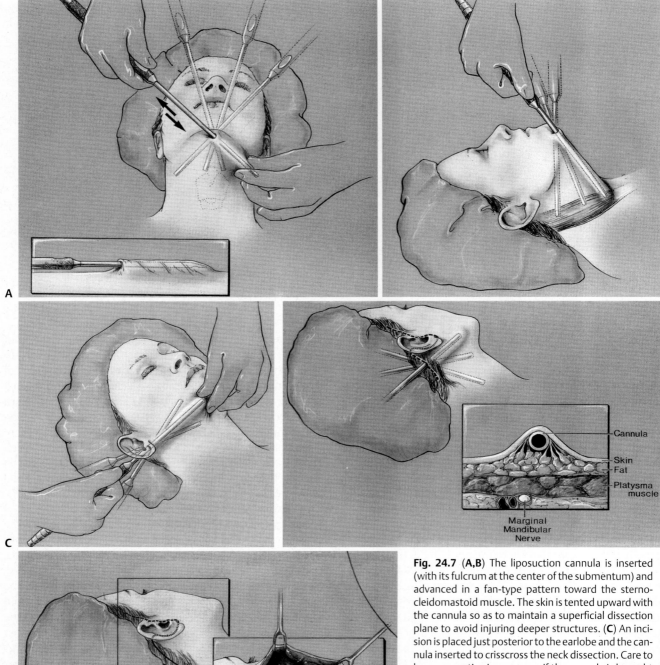

Fig. 24.7 (**A,B**) The liposuction cannula is inserted (with its fulcrum at the center of the submentum) and advanced in a fan-type pattern toward the sternocleidomastoid muscle. The skin is tented upward with the cannula so as to maintain a superficial dissection plane to avoid injuring deeper structures. (**C**) An incision is placed just posterior to the earlobe and the cannula inserted to crisscross the neck dissection. Care to be conservative is necessary if the cannula is brought over the mandibular angle to approach the jowl. (**D**) When a facelift is planned, liposuction cannulas can help dissect the flaps. Skin-flap elevation after liposuction dissection shows the creation of a network of subcutaneous tunnels. (**E**) Tunnels created by the advancement and retraction of the cannula within the submentum allow preservation of the neurovascular network. (From Kridel R, Konior R. Suction lipectomy. In: Krause CJ, eds. Aesthetic Facial Surgery. Philadelphia: JB Lippincott; 1991. Reprinted by permission.)

continues in this preplatysmal plane until the desired result is achieved.

Redefining the jaw line may necessitate two additional incisions, one behind each earlobe, hidden in the infralobular crease. These incisions should be vertically oriented, and only long enough to accommodate a 2 or 3 mm cannula. Development of the subdermal dissection plane is again initiated with use of small scissors.

The lateral infralobular approach in addition to the submental approach will allow better access to the area below the mandibular angle. This multidirectional crisscross approach creates an extensive overlapping subcutaneous tunnel network that encourages maximal contour enhancement. As the cannula is advanced into the subdermal plane, the arc and fan technique is used. Some feel that in the heavier face, the surgeon can judiciously extend the liposuction area up over the mandible with very small cannulas with caution.

Frequent inspection of the site and use of the pinch-and-roll technique helps the surgeon avoid overextraction. In this maneuver, the skin is gently pinched between the thumb and forefinger and rolled. A sufficient amount of fat has been extracted when the surgeon can feel a thin layer of adipose tissue remaining between the opposing deep surfaces. Extraction volumes vary from person to person, but most require between 10 and 100 cc.

Occasionally, fat deep to the surface of the platysmal muscle will be responsible for loss of the youthful cervicomental angle. In these cases, the cannula can be directed to the deeper plane through the submental access site. Removal of fat here poses little risk to neural structures such as the marginal mandibular nerve, but small vessel injury is possible. Cannula direction should stay within the central midline to avoid neural injury laterally. In facelift patients, the authors have often followed what was thought to be effective and aggressive neck liposuction, but with open inspection, and have found much fat still left in the midline that required direct excision.

A limitation of neck liposuction is seen in its incomplete removal of deeper midline submental fat that frequently requires direct midline excision. This procedure may be performed with scissors or with the use of the liposhaver. More definitive undermining and a slightly larger incisions are required for sharp lipectomy and neurovascular bundles are sacrificed. The undermining can be done with the facelift scissors or the suction bovie cautery on a low setting. If using the cautery to complete flap undermining, the overlying skin is tented away and protected with the Converse retractor. The plane of dissection is then developed under direct vision.

Addressing the lower fullness in the jowl area with liposuction as the primary procedure should be done cautiously. The posterior earlobe–crease incisions will allow improved access to this area. Unless the entire region between the incision site and the fat collection is to be contoured, suction should not be applied until the cannula tip enters the offending adipose deposit. Failure to observe this detail may result in an obvious linear depression between the incision site and the distant fat pocket.

Isolated liposuction of the midface alone can be disastrous if overaggressive suctioning is performed, creating marked depression and visible irregularities that are difficult to correct (**Fig. 24.8**). Conservative suctioning of full nasolabial mounds may be helpful and can be accomplished with small cannulas via an intranasal approach.

The surface contour of the neck must now be carefully inspected before concluding the procedure. Dimpling generally implies residual attachments between the subcutaneous fat and overlying skin. Release of these isolated attachments usually resolves the problem. Subtle platysmal banding that may not have been evident preoperatively may now be more noticeable. Through the submental incision these bands may be plicated with or without direct excision to prevent postoperative visibility; however, because there is no skin excision, there may be excess tissue. If the bands are anticipated preoperatively, the fat extraction may be tempered to prevent increased postoperative visualization. Lengthening of the submental incision may be necessary to allow suture approximation of the medial aspect of the platysmal muscles. Lengthening of the incision should entail a gentle lateral curve directed posteriorly so the incision does not relocate up over the mandible with healing or with the potential superolateral skin traction of a future facelift.

After the procedure is complete and final assessment (by pinching and rolling the skin between the fingers) reveals good symmetry, the incision sites are closed in layers with 6–0 stitches and then are covered with paper tape. The dissection pocket is milked to ensure no blood collections and no loose fat globules remain. In patients with larger fat volume removal, and prior to closure, irrigation of the area may be performed to remove as much loose or liquified fat as possible, preventing postoperative irritation. Closed liposuction as a primary procedure does not require suction drainage, but it does require a light pressure wrap to reduce tissue edema and to immobilize and reshape the skin over the recontoured soft tissue facial framework. More pressure should be applied if direct sharp lipectomy was also required. The skin overlying the dissection is first covered with a smooth piece of cotton or Telfa (Kendall, Mansfield, MA), and then may be wrapped with Kerlix (Johnson and Johnson, Inc., Arlington, TX) gauze. The dressing is completed with either a Coban (3M Healthcare, St. Paul, MN) elastic dressing or a facial sling. The elastic sling is comfortable, may be repositioned, and allows easy access to assess the surgical site. The patient is instructed to limit head and neck mobility for 36 to 48 hours to allow reattachment of the skin to the underlying soft tissue bed.

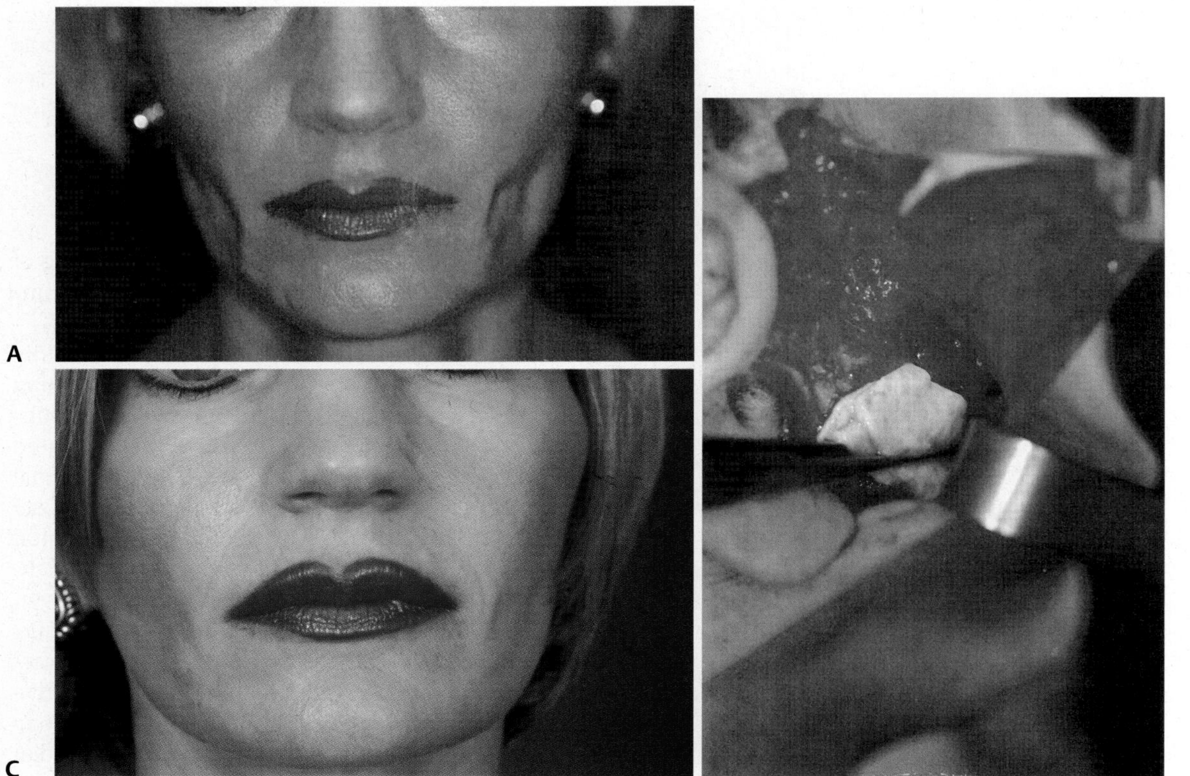

Fig. 24.8 (**A**) Overaggressive isolated liposuction of the buccal midface area caused marked depressions that necessitated a facelift with acellular dermal sheeting implants and injections for correction. (**B**) Operative intervention in the form of facelift and placement of acellular dermal grafting material, for the correction of buccal/jowl defects after liposuction. (**C**) Postoperative.

Liposuction as an Adjunctive Procedure

Choosing the appropriate candidate for liposuction may entail choosing a different primary procedure and using liposuction as a secondary or refining technique. Although a discussion of liposuction may have been the intent of the patient's visit, the surgeon may need to explain why a better avenue for facial rejuvenation may be, for example, augmentation of the chin, rhytidectomy, and/or platysmaplasty.

Liposuction Combined with Chin Augmentation

When microgenia (small chin) or retrognathia (retrodisplaced mandibular malocclusion) coexist with submental liposis, results of chin augmentation or orthognathic surgery or submental liposuction alone may be less then optimal. When combined together the result may be dramatic (**Fig. 24.9**). The overlying goal is recreation of the acuity of the cervicomental angle. Patients who have a recessed chin and/or low and anterior hyoid position are those who benefit from extraction of submental fat and increased projection of the chin.

The placement of the incisions for a combined submental liposuction and chin augmentation procedure is similar when compared with liposuction as a primary procedure, with one exception. If the chin is augmented from an external approach, the submental incision is extended slightly to accommodate the chin implant. If the surgeon prefers, a separate gingivolabial incision may be used for placement of the implant through the oral approach. In this case, care should be taken to keep the two surgical sites—the chin and the submentum—separate from one another. The tendency for intraorally placed implants is to migrate superiorly, whereas those implants placed externally are more apt to fall inferiorly creating a witches chin deformity. Suture fixation and precise pocket techniques are helpful in maintaining chin implant position.

Liposuction-Assisted Rhytidectomy

Liposuction can significantly enhance the results of rhytidectomy by removing the unwanted fat not only in the submentum, but also in the pretragal and jowl areas. The benefit is seen with the addition of this technique in its ability to recontour with little risk to underlying

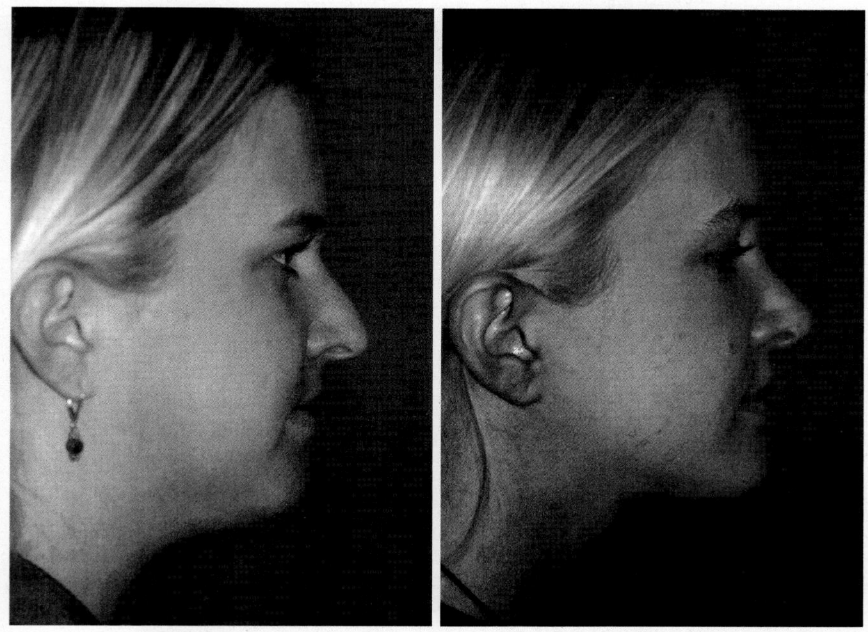

Fig. 24.9 (**A**) Preoperative. Patient with submental fullness, microgenia, and young elastic skin. (**B**) Favorable postoperative result from submental liposuction, nasal surgery, and chin augmentation.

neurovascular structures. Fat removal prior to the advent of liposuction from areas such as the jowls was either not done or looked on unfavorably because of the risk of neural injury or contour irregularity due to overaggressive suctioning or tracking. Access to the jowl region was difficult from the standard facelift incisions, and the thought of additional incisions was antithetical to the well-concealed incision techniques of established facelifting protocols.

Three key maneuvers are required to fully appreciate the benefits of liposuction during a facelift. First, closed liposuction is used to reduce the prominent facial fatty deposits with minimal bleeding. Next, the cannula with or without employment of the suction facilitates facial flap elevation, and, finally, open liposuction fully refines the region under direct visualization.

The standard closed liposuction technique is used first to remove any prominent adipose accumulations in the submental, submandibular, and jowl regions. The incision in the submentum is between 5 and 8 mm long, and the initial dissection is initiated with use of a small scissors. A 3 or 4 mm cannula may be helpful for initial fat extraction with pretunneling, but it is not absolutely necessary. Infralobular incisions and preauricular incisions allow further access to facial fatty deposits with the understanding that excess skin will be addressed in the rhytidectomy part of the procedure. While knowing this to be so, a conservative approach to fat extraction in the midface and jowl regions is still recommended. Unwanted postoperative irregularity or depressions can result from overaggressive midface liposuction (**Fig. 24.10**).

After reducing the bulk of the cevicofacial adipose accumulations with the closed technique, undermining of the facial flaps is completed with the standard scissors technique. Undermining after use of the blunt-tipped cannula in the closed liposuction technique is easy and quick. The subcutaneous bands created with the tunneling technique of liposuction are simply identified and divided, and flap elevation is finished. The relatively atraumatic nature of this blunt dissection process allows undermining to proceed up to the nasolabial fold without concern for neurovascular injury.

Once flap elevation is complete, initial flap inset incisions are created, and plication or imbrication of the SMAS or a deep plane lift is performed. Open liposuction may be used as a refining final step. A spatula-shaped tip maximizes contact between the suction cannula and the soft-tissue bed, which is required to maintain a seal with continuous suction in an open environment. Unwanted fat deposits are removed by placing the suction cannula aperture directly on the subcutaneous bed and moving it rapidly with a to-and-fro motion along the open face of the dissection pocket. Liposuction before plication or imbrication in the pretragal/preauricular area can be used to ensure less immediate postoperative fullness in the area where much of the superficial musculoaponeurotic system (SMAS) is secured with resuspension sutures. After final assessment is performed to determine whether addition liposculpting is necessary, the remainder of the rhytidectomy, including skin excision, should proceed in a routine fashion (**Fig. 24.11**). Access to the jowl fat

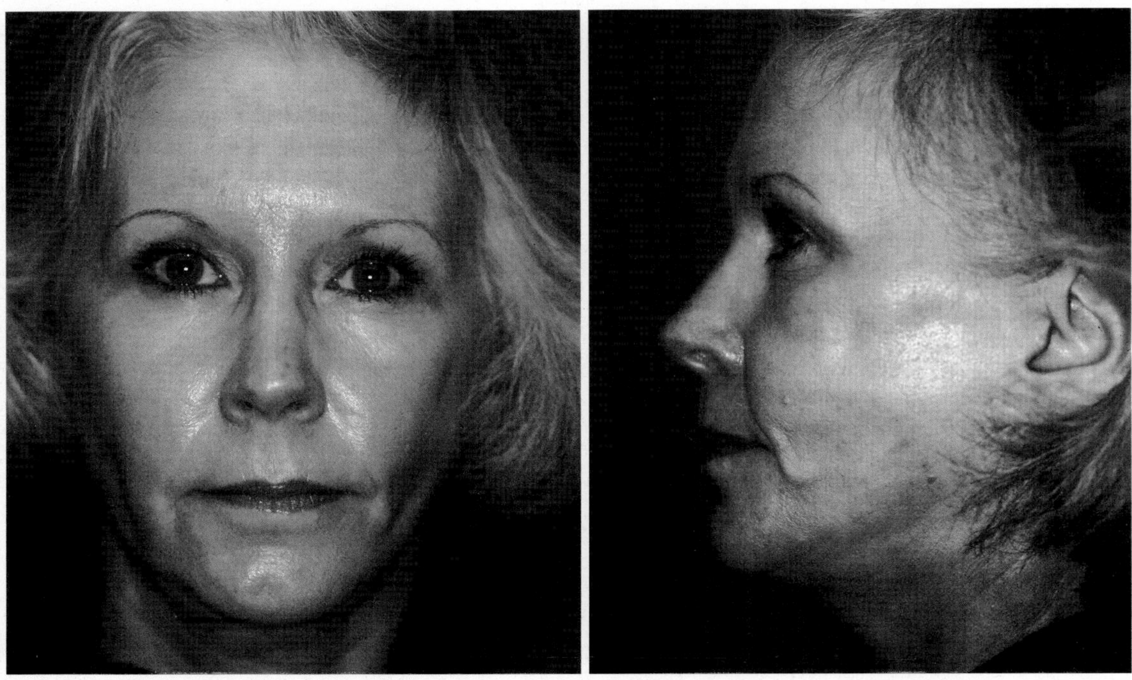

Fig. 24.10 (**A**) Postoperative result from outside institution (front view). Patient with concave deformity in the inframalar area from overaggressive midface liposuction during facelift procedure. (**B**) Postoperative result from outside institution (lateral view). Poor patient result after bilateral lower jowl liposuction with resultant concavity and laxity to skin.

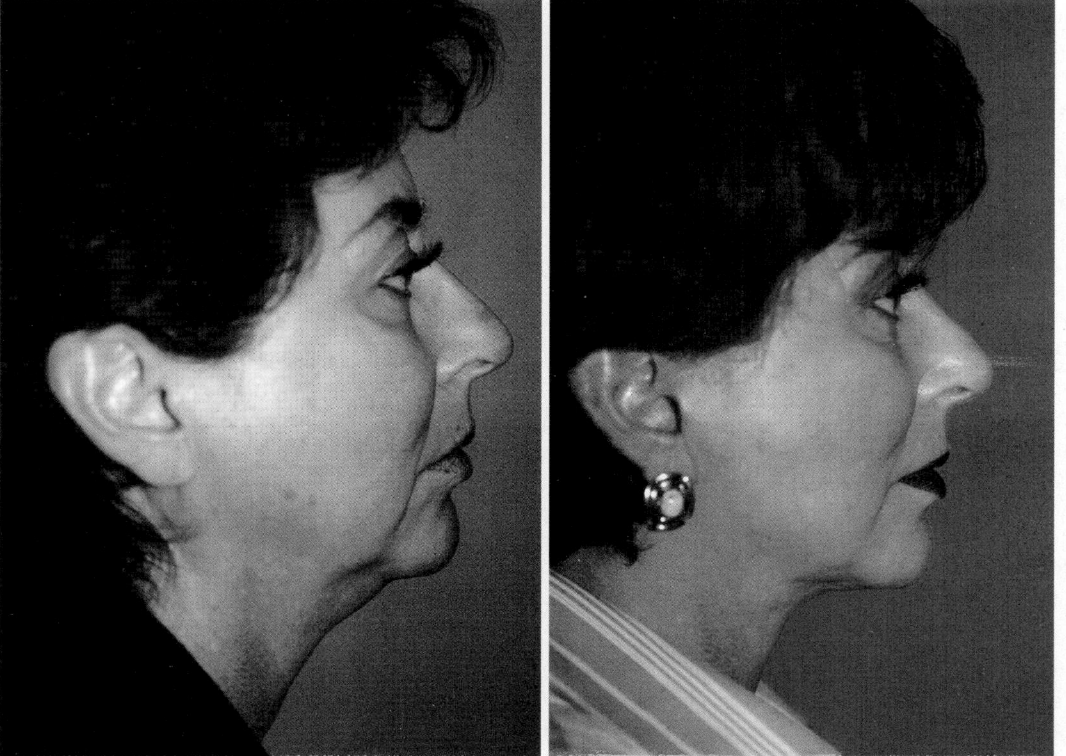

Fig. 24.11 This patient had a combination of facelift and liposuction: (**A**) before and (**B**) years postoperative.

pad is also facilitated after the routine facelift flaps are developed; a very small 1 or 2 mm cannula can be inserted under the facelift flaps directly into the jowl fat under direct visualization.

Postoperative Course

Patients should be counseled preoperatively regarding the natural postoperative changes encountered after liposuction surgery. Bruising and discoloration are variable after closed liposuction technique, and last anywhere from 7 to 21 days. Although rare, prolonged pigment changes in the form of hemosiderin deposits can occur. Postoperative edema and induration may persist for weeks to months and may be great enough to mimic the original contour problem. A wide elastic band (with padding extending over the ears, to prevent a pressure injury to the pinna) is used for 1 week, day and night, and then at night for an additional 4 weeks. This band seems to effectively limit the majority of swelling and improves irregularities. As the edema resolves, it is common to find subtle irregularities. Irregularities that become evident are usually transient and treated with reassurance, gentle massage, and the occasional need for dilute steroid injection. Short-term numbness and tingling are frequently described and always discussed in the preoperative visit. This is most important in the male who must exercise extra caution with shaving in the early postoperative period.

Postoperative discomfort after primary liposuction is variable. Most patients resume their normal activities within 2 to 3 days of the procedure. Reminders are given to the patient to refrain from active head and neck movement for 2 weeks to allow the newly undermined soft tissue envelope to readhere to the subcutaneous bed. Results with liposuction are varied and may require upward of 6 months for skin contracture and shrinkage.

Complications

Minor and transient irregularities are the rule with liposuction of the cervicofacial regions as compared with the potentially serious complications after whole body liposuction procedures. Unlike body liposuction procedures where large-volume fat reductions can cause rapid fluid shifts, blood loss, and blood pressure problems, liposuction in the head and neck rarely influences the patient's hemodynamic status. As indicated earlier, typical volumes extracted range from 10 to 100 cc of fat.

Infections are rare, occurring in less than 1% of patients.[8] Preoperative antibiotics are not required, but by and large, most surgeons in the private practice arena utilize at least one dose of perioperative intravenous antibiotic. Beeson et al[48] reported on a patient who developed a group A streptococcal fasciitis after submental liposuction and platysmaplasty. This patient was treated successfully with intravenous antibiotics and suffered no permanent sequelae. However, there are also reports of necrotizing fasciitis occurring after tumescent liposuction of trunk and lower extremities, so a high index of suspicion is warranted for any signs of infection.[49,50] Hematomas, seromas, or sialoceles are seen in less than 1% when liposuction is used as a primary procedure. Sialoceles are more common when liposuction is done over the parotid bed and treatment may require a pressure wrap, anticholinergics, Botox, and/or drainage.

Long-standing irregularities may exist in the form of saggy skin or dermal scarring. Extra sagging skin may result from unexpected, senile, or presenile skin changes, and may require a rhytidectomy for resolution. Scarring may be the result of poor healing, operative technique, or infection. Excessive thinning of the dermal fat or misdirection of the cannula lumen may contribute to this problem. Options for correction of dermal scarring are limited.

Uneven aspiration may create asymmetry and usually diminishes with surgical experience. A touch-up procedure may be accomplished in the office under local anesthesia with the syringe-assisted suction technique, coupled with a small sculpting cannula. Areas that are too small for even sculpting may be addressed with cautious injection of a 0.1 to 0.2 cc of 10 mg/mL triamcinolone acetonide solution at 4- to 6-week intervals. Overinjection or injections too frequently may result in dermal thinning, dimpling, and the formation of spider telangectasias.

Small, localized, long-term postoperative depressions may require a soft tissue filler. Autologous fat injections, submalar cheek implants, or the placement of dermal graft materials such as an acellular dermal sheeting graft (AlloDerm, LifeCell Corp., Branchburg, NJ) are all potential modalities to correct overaggressive fat removal.

Permanent injury to the marginal mandibular branch of the facial nerve is rare as is hypesthesia secondary to injury to the great auricular nerve. When paresis, paresthesias, or paralysis does occur, it is usually short-lived and resolves with time. Ensuring a dissection plane superficial to the platysmal muscle usually prevents nerve injury.

References

1. Schrudde J. Lipexeresis as a means of eliminating local adiposity. In: International Society of Aesthetic Plastic Surgery. Vol 4. Amsterdam: Springer-Verlag; 1980
2. Fischer A, Fischer GM. Revised technique for cellulitis fat reduction in riding breeches deformity. Bull Int Acad Cosmet Surg 1977;2:40
3. Kesserling UK. Regional fat aspiration for body contouring. Plast Reconstr Surg 1983;72:610–619

4. Illouz YG. Body contouring by lipolysis: a 5-year experience with over 3000 cases. Plast Reconstr Surg 1983;72(5):591–597
5. Dedo DD. Management of the platysma muscle after open and closed liposuction of the neck in facelift surgery. Facial Plast Surg 1986;4:45–56
6. Chrisman BB. Liposuction with facelift surgery. Dermatol Clin 1990;8(3):501–522
7. Daher JC, Cosac OM, Domingues S. Facelift: the importance of redefining facial contours through facial liposuction. Ann Plast Surg 1988;21(1):1–10
8. Kridel RWH, Pacella BL. Complications of liposuction. In: Eisele D, ed. Complications of Head and Neck Surgery. St. Louis: Mosby Year-Book Co.; 1992:791–803
9. Teimourian B. Suction lipectomy of the face and neck. Facial Plast Surg 1986;4(1):35–39
10. Courtiss EH. Suction lipectomy: a retrospective analysis of 100 patients. Plast Reconstr Surg 1984;73(5):780–796
11. Bloom W, Fawcett D. Histophysiology of Adipose Tissue. In: A Textbook of Histology. 9th ed. Philadelphia: W.B. Saunders Company; 1968:171–172
12. Flageul G, Illouz YG. Isolated cervicofacial liposuction applied to the treatment of aging. Ann Chir Plast Esthet 1996;41(6):620–630
13. Kamer FM, Lefkoff LA. Submental surgery: a graduated approach to the aging neck. Arch Otolaryngol Head Neck Surg 1991;117:40–46
14. Tapia A, Ferreira B, Eng R. Liposuction in cervical rejuvenation. Aesthetic Plast Surg 1987;11(2):95–100
15. Conley J. Facelift Operation. Springfield, IL: Charles C. Thomas; 1968: 40–41
16. Goddio AS. Cutaneous retraction: data from liposuction and other clinical procedures. Ann Chir Plast Esthet 1992;37(2):194–201
17. Goodstein WA. Liposhaver in facial plastic surgery [letter]. Arch Otolaryngol Head Neck Surg 1998;124:1271–1272
18. Guerrerosantos J. Liposuction in the cheek, chin, and neck: a clinical Study. Facial Plast Surg 1986;4(1):25–34
19. Hetter GP. Improved results with closed facial suction. Clin Plast Surg 1989;16(2):319–332
20. Hudson P. Recent advances in liposuction. Plastic Surgery Products 1998;Mar/April:20–22
21. Bank DE, Perez MI. Skin retraction after liposuction in patients over the age of 40. Dermatol Surg 1999;25(9):673–676
22. Hallock GG. Liposuction for debulking free flaps. J Reconstr Microsurg 1986;2:235–237
23. Coleman WP III. Noncosmetic applications of liposuction. J Dermatol Surg Oncol 1988;14(10):1085–1090
24. Wilhelmi BJ, Blackwell SJ, Mancoll JS, Phillips LG. Another indication for liposuction: small facial lipomas. Plast Reconstr Surg 1999;103(7):1864–1870
25. Williams EF. Liposuction of the face and neck. Plastic Surgery Products 1999;March:66–67
26. Dedo DD. Liposuction of the head and neck. Otolaryngol Head Neck Surg 1987;97(6):591–592
27. Cook WR. Utilizing external ultrasonic energy to improve the results of tumescent liposculpture. Dermatol Surg 1997;23:1207–1211
28. Havoonjian HH, Luftman DB, Manaker GM, Moy RL. External ultrasonic tumescent liposuction a preliminary study. Dermatol Surg 1997;23:1201–1206
29. Igra H, Satur NM. Tumescent liposuction versus internal ultrasonic-assisted tumescent liposuction: a side-to-side comparison. Dermatol Surg 1997;23:1213–1218
30. Howard BK, Beran SJ, Kenkel JM, Krueger J, Rohrich RJ. The effects of ultrasonic energy on peripheral nerves: implications for ultrasound-assisted liposuction. Plast Reconstr Surg 1999;103(3):984–989
31. Lawrence N, Coleman WP. The biologic basis of ultrasonic liposuction. Dermatol Surg 1997;23(12):1197–1200
32. Zocchi M. Ultrasonic liposculpturing. Aesthetic Plast Surg 1992;16:287–298
33. Grippaudo FR, Matarese RM, Macone A, Mazzocchi M, Scuderi N. Effects of traditional and ultrasonic liposuction on adipose tissue: a biochemical approach. Plast Reconstr Surg 2000;106(1):197–199
34. Kridel RWH, Konior RJ, Buchwach KA. Suction lipectomy. In: Krause CJ, ed. Aesthetic Facial Surgery. Philadelphia: JB Lippincott; 1991:689–705
35. Kloehn RA. Commentary on ultrasound-assisted lipoplasty. Task Force July 1996 Report to the Membership. Plast Reconstr Surg 1997;99(4):1198–1199
36. Wilkinson TS. External ultrasound—assisted lipoplasty. Aesthetic Surg J 1999;19(2):124–129
37. Cardenes-Camerana L, Cardena A, Fajhardo-Barajas D. Clinical and histopathological analysis of tissue retraction in tumescent liposuction assisted by external ultrasound. Ann Plast Surg 2001;46(3):287–292
38. Becker DG, Weinberger MS, Miller PJ, et al. The liposhaver in facial plastic surgery: a multiinstitutional experience. Arch Otolaryngol Head Neck Surg 1996;122:1161–1167
39. Gross CW, Becker DG, Lindsey WH, Park AA, Marshall DD. The soft-tissue shaving procedure for removal of adipose tissue. A new, less traumatic approach than liposuction. Arch Otolaryngol Head Neck Surg 1995;121:1117–1120
40. Gross WE. Soft-tissue shavers in functional endoscopic sinus surgery (standard technique). Otolaryngol Clin North Am 1997;30(3):435–441
41. Becker DG, Toriumi DM, Gross CW, Tardy ME Jr. Powered instrumentation for dorsal reduction. Facial Plast Surg 1997;13:291–297
42. Katz BE, Bruck MC, Coleman WP III The benefits of powered liposuction versus traditional liposuction: a paired comparison analysis. Dermatol Surg 2001;27(10):863–867
43. Becker DG, Cook TA, Want TD, et al. A 3-year multiinstitutional experience with the liposhaver. Arch Facial Plast Surg 1999;1:171–176
44. Fournier PF. Who should do syringe liposculpturing? J Dermatol Surg Oncol 1988;14(10):1055–1056
45. Fournier PF. Why the syringe and not the suction machine? J Dermatol Surg Oncol 1988;14(10):1062–1069
46. Kesselring UK. Facial liposuction. Facial Plast Surg 1986;4(1):1–4
47. Schaeffer BT. Endoscopic liposhaving for neck recontouring. Arch Facial Plast Surg 2000;2:264–268
48. Beeson WH, Slama TG, Beeler RT, Rachel JD, Picerno NA. Group A streptococcal fasciitis after submental tumescent liposuction. Arch Facial Plast Surg 2001;3:277–279
49. Gibbons MD, Lim RB, Carter PL. Necrotizing fasciitis after tumescent liposuciton. Am Surg 1998;64:458–460
50. Alexander J, Takeda D, Sanders G, Goldberg H. Fatal necrotizing fasciitis following suction-assisted lipectomy. Ann Plast Surg 1988;20:562–565

25 Dermabrasion and Chemical Peels

Stephen H. Mandy and Gary D. Monheit

Dermabrasion

Dermabrasion is a mechanical, "cold steel" method of removing the epidermis and creating a papillary to upper reticular dermal wound. The subsequent manufacture of new collagen and a resurfaced epidermis germinated from deeper, less sun damaged cells yields excellent cosmetic improvement in actinically damaged, aged, or scarred skin. The pre- and postoperative management that optimizes wound healing is well established and predictable, and morbidity and complications are encountered infrequently.

Modern dermabrasion began when Kurtin,[1] in the late 1940s, modified the technique first described by Kronmayer[2] at the turn of the century. Kurtin's development of the wirebrush technique, which was modified by Burke[3] in the mid-1950s, led to the techniques used today. The basics of a rapidly rotating wire brush or diamond fraise skillfully applied to chilled skin are recognized as effective therapy for a wide range of indications.[4,5]

Anatomy and Healing

It is essential to understand the basic macroscopic anatomy of the skin when applying the techniques of dermabrasion that yield beneficial results. For all practical purposes, the skin is divided into three layers: (1) epidermis, (2) dermis, and (3) subcutaneous tissue. Most important in dermabrasion is the dermis, which is composed of two layers: the superficial papillary layer and the deeper reticular layer. Injuries to the epidermis and papillary dermis heal without scarring, whereas injuries that extend into the reticular dermis always result in scar tissue. The purpose of dermabrasive surgery is to reorganize or restructure the collagen of the papillary dermis without injuring the reticular dermis. The thickness of these dermal layers varies greatly from one area to another, and though all areas may be dermabraded without scarring, it is the face that is ideally suited to dermabrasion. This is partly because of the manner in which dermabrasion wounds heal. Reepithelialization begins from the wound margins and from within the epidermal appendages that remain after dermabrasion. The pilosebaceous follicle is the primordial germ for this reepithelialization, and the face is richly endowed with sebaceous glands. Nelson at al[4,5] have shown that this injury results in significant increases in type I procollagen, type III procollagen, and transforming growth factor β_1 in the papillary dermis. Their results suggest that increased fibroblast activity and consequent collagen I and III synthesis underlie the clinical improvement in collagen reformation seen in dermabrasion.

The preoperative application of tretinoin 0.5% for several weeks before partial-thickness dermabrasive wounds has been shown clinically and in the laboratory to accelerate healing.[6,7] Patients placed on tretinoin at least several weeks before dermabrasion heal in 5 to 7 days. Patients without pretreatment heal in 7 to 10 days (**Fig. 25.1**). Another significant factor in promoting healing of dermabrasive wounds is the use of occlusive dressings. Since the work of Maibach and Rovee,[8] it has been understood that wounds managed with occlusive dressings heal up to 40% faster than wounds left to air-dry. This is especially true with the dermabrasive wounds covered with an appropriate biosynthetic dressing, which heal much more rapidly than those left to form crusts.[9] Furthermore, biosynthetic dressings alleviate postoperative pain almost immediately when applied after surgery. Biosynthetic dressings act to keep wounds moist, thereby allowing free epithelial migration across the surface. They also cause wound fluids, which contain growth factors that stimulate wound healing, to remain in constant contact with the wound surface. There is also increasing laboratory evidence to suggest that the presence of occlusive dressings modulates collagen synthesis and results in a cosmetically more satisfying scar.[10]

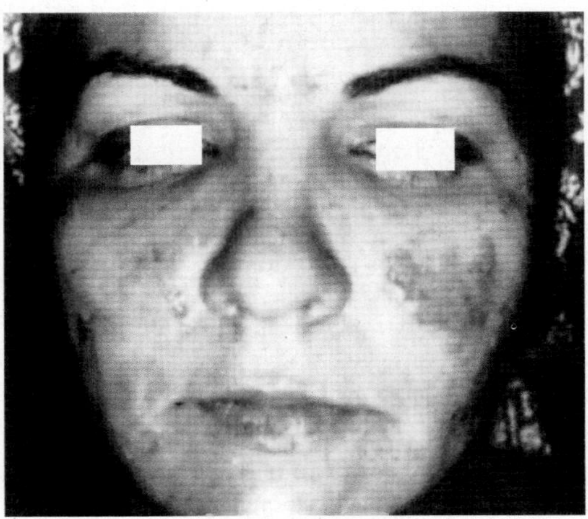

Fig. 25.1 Tretinoin applied preoperatively to the right side of the face produced prompter healing at 5 days.

Patient Selection and Indications

Among the many indications for dermabrasion, those most common today are the treatment for acne scars, facial wrinkles, premalignant solar keratoses, rhinophyma, traumatic and surgical scars, and tattoos. Acne scars represent the single greatest application of the dermabrasive technique. Dramatic improvement may be achieved with facial scars resulting from acne, but perfection is impossible. Patients must have realistic expectations of surgical results. In patients who have deep, ice-pick scarring, punch excision followed by suture closure of these scars 4 to 6 weeks before dermabrasion is most likely to yield a good result. Patients who have extensive acne scarring should be warned of the possibility of further scarring as a result of dermabrasion. Patients with dark pigmentation should be warned of the possibility of postoperative hypo- or hyperpigmentation. This is frequently transitory, and pigment returns to normal over the course of several months. Occasionally, if scarring and dermabrasion are deep, pigmentation may be altered permanently. This is especially likely in patients of Asian descent.

Dermabrasion patients have often been treated for their acne with systemic 13-*cis*-retinoic acid. This potent antiacne agent causes sebaceous gland atrophy, and from the early days of its use, concern was expressed that it might delay wound healing in dermabrasion patients. Initial reports in the literature indicated that dermabrasion patients were unaffected by previous treatment with isotretinoin (Accutane, Hoffmann-La Roche, Inc., Nutley, NJ).[11] However, later reports suggested that patients who were dermabraded after Accutane therapy exhibited atypical scarring postdermabrasion.[12,13] Subsequent to those reports, other authors have cited numerous cases of patients who had been treated with Accutane and then dermabraded without sequelae.[14] This unsettling controversy clearly has significant medical and legal implications. A clearcut cause-and-effect relationship has not been established between use of Accutane and atypical scarring. In fact, laboratory studies have failed to substantiate any abnormalities in fibroblast activity or collagen synthesis in Accutane-treated skin.[15,16] Until an answer to this question is found, it is probably prudent for physicians to suggest that patients treated with Accutane wait at least 6 months before undergoing dermabrasion.

Acquired immune deficiency syndrome (AIDS) virus has been the latest factor to consider when selecting patients for dermabrasion. Of all surgeries performed, dermabrasion is most likely to aerosolize blood and tissue products and live infective viral particles. A recent study by Wentzell et al[17] indicated that aerosolized particles produced during dermabrasion were of sufficient size for access and retention by mucosal and pulmonary surfaces. Furthermore, their study indicated that commonly used personal protection devices, such as operator masks, goggles, and scatter shields, do not prevent the respiration of these particles. In addition, the settling velocities of such small particles may extend the exposure for many hours after the procedure has been performed, thereby endangering personnel not directly involved in the procedure. Another problem of the AIDS virus is the inability to determine if a patient is in the latent period between the infection and the positive antibody test. There is also the legal implication of refusing a patient who has had a positive blood test. It is clear that there is a risk to the physician, assistants, and other personnel. Dermabrasion certainly should not be performed without a thorough history of high-risk behavior; protection of gloves, masks, goggles; and the awareness that even with protective devices a certain degree of risk remains. Similar precautions pertaining to hepatitis are also prudent.

One of the growing indications for dermabrasion is aging skin, especially that which has been actinically damaged and shows pathology such as premalignant solar keratoses. Dermabrasion has been shown to be as effective, if not more effective, than topically applied 5-fluorouracil (5-FU) in the management of precancerous skin lesions.[18] In a study of half-face planing of actinically damaged skin, Burke et al showed that precancerous lesions were substantially reduced and their future development retarded over a 5-year period.[19] These facts, combined with dramatic improvement in rhagades, makes dermabrasion a viable modality in the treatment of aging skin (**Figs. 25.2 and 25.3**). This work has more recently been corroborated by Coleman et al.[14]

Yarborough demonstrated that dermabrasions performed on traumatic or surgical scars ~6 weeks after injury often result in complete disappearance of the scars (**Fig. 25.4**).[20] In fact, surgical scars respond so well to dermabrasion that most patients who have excisional surgery are told that they may have dermabrasion 6 weeks postoperatively. Although this is usually not necessary, forewarning the patient eases its introduction. Dermabrasion is especially likely in patients who have sebaceous skin or in facial areas such as the nose where improvement after dermabrasion is most dramatic. Improvement in scars after dermabrasion is further enhanced by the postoperative use of biosynthetic dressings, which significantly affect collagen synthesis, resulting in cosmetic improvement of the surgical scar[10] (**Fig. 25.5**).

Removal of tattoos can be accomplished with superficial dermabrasion, followed by application of 1% gentian violet and a petrolatum (e.g., Vaseline) gauze dressing daily for 10 days. The gentian violet delays healing, causing pigment to leach out into the dressing and creating continued inflammation that causes phagocytosis of the

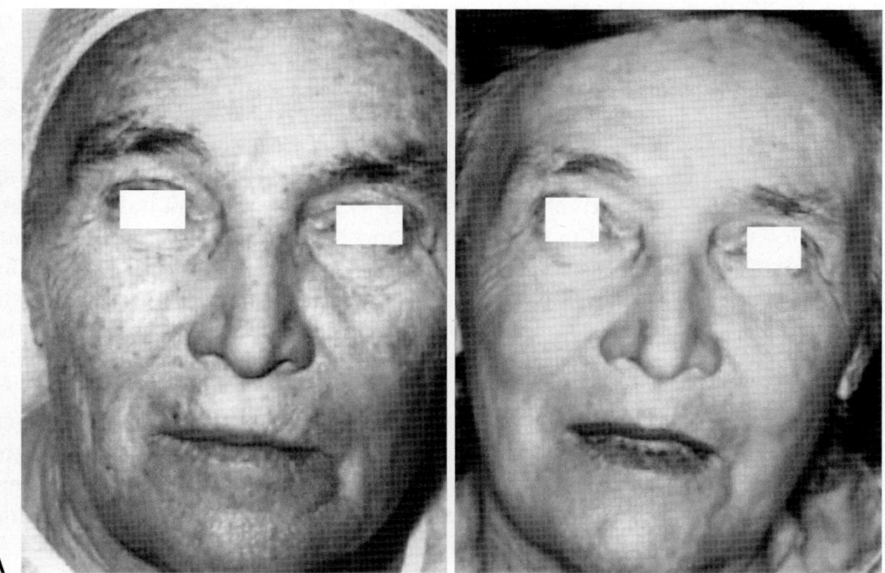

Fig. 25.2 (A) Predermabrasion for actinic keratoses. (B) Postdermabrasion.

remaining pigment. Abrading only to the upper papillary dermis avoids scarring. Do not attempt to remove the pigment by abrasion. Professional tattoos are more responsive than amateur or traumatic tattoos but all can be improved. Usually 50% resolution can be achieved with one procedure, which can be repeated every 2 to 3 months until the desired result is achieved. Tattoos are a good training procedure for the novice in dermabrasion.

Benign tumors, such as adenoma sebaceum and syringomas, may be successfully dermabraded for marked cosmetic improvement, but gradual recurrence is the rule. Dramatic improvement may also be achieved with rhinophyma when dermabrasion is combined with electrofulguration (**Fig. 25.6**).

Instrumentation

A wide variety of abrading instruments are commercially available. They vary from hand engines to cable-driven power sources and battery-operated units. More recently, air-driven "microdermabraders" that blow small aluminum or glass particles over the skin have appeared. The important consideration, in terms of the power source, is that it have the torque necessary to continue a sustained and even drive over the abrading surface, either a wire brush or a diamond fraise. Excellent reviews by Yarborough[20,21] and Alt[22] of the wire brush and diamond fraise dermabrasive techniques require little elaboration. However, it cannot be overemphasized that no article

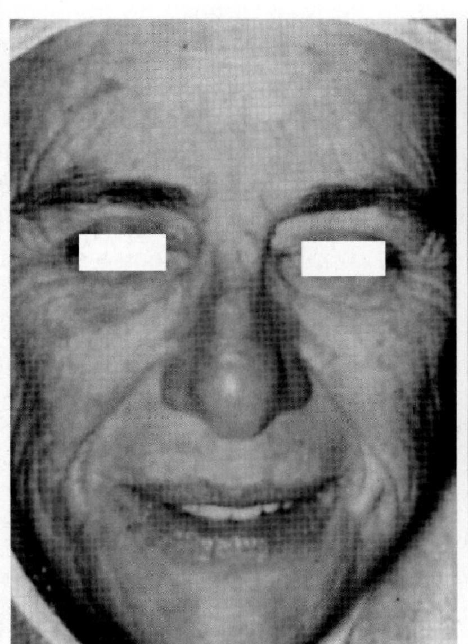

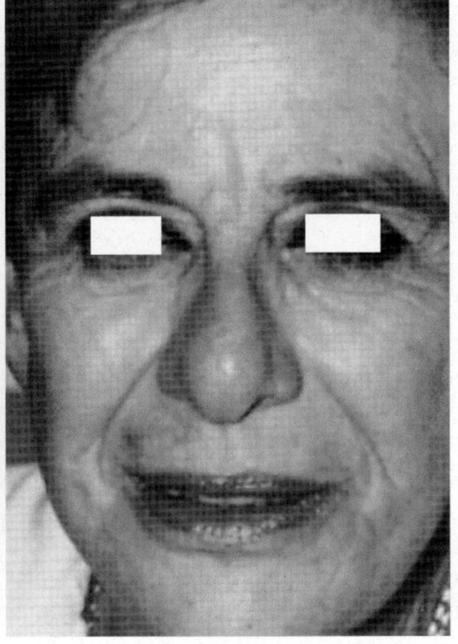

Fig. 25.3 (A) Predermabrasion for wrinkles. (B) Postdermabrasion for wrinkles.

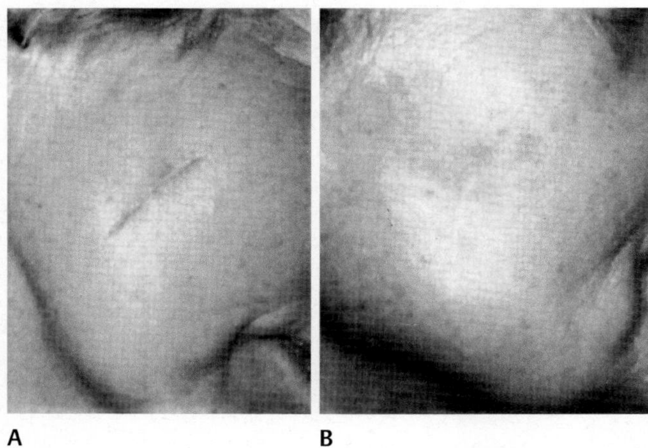

Fig. 25.4 (**A**) Predermabrasion of 6-week-old scar. (**B**) Postdermabrasion of scar.

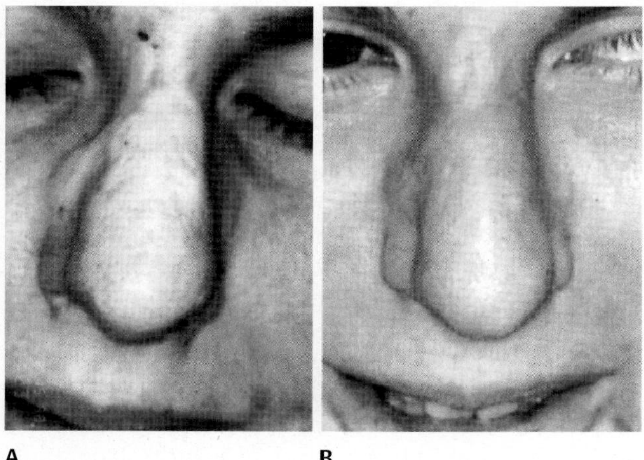

Fig. 25.5 (**A**) Scar preabrasion. (**B**) Postabrasion and biosynthetic dressings.

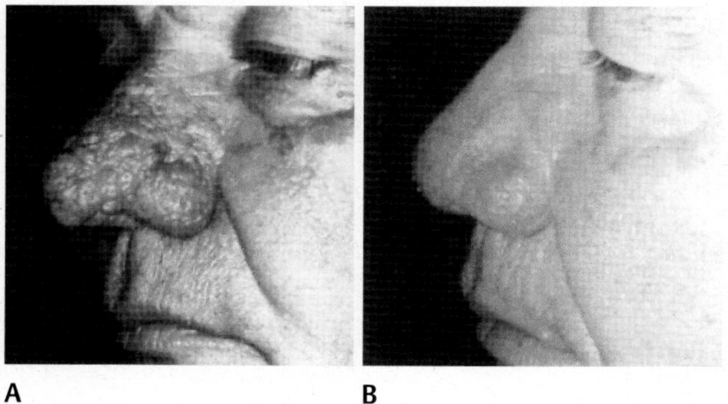

Fig. 25.6 (**A**) Predermabrasion for rhinophyma. (**B**) Postdermabrasion.

can be substituted for thorough hands-on experience in a preceptorship environment, where the student is able to watch and assist someone experienced in the art of dermabrasion. Most authors agree that the wire-brush technique requires more skill and runs a higher risk of potential injury because it involves cutting more deeply and more quickly than the diamond fraise technique. With the exception of the extracoarse diamond fraise, superior results are achieved with the wire brush.

One of the continuing controversies surrounding dermabrasive surgery is the use of preabrasive chilling of the skin. Animal and clinical work reviewing various cryanesthetic materials available to chill the skin before sanding has shown that materials that freeze the skin below −30°C, and more especially below −60°C, have the potential to cause substantial tissue necrosis and subsequent scarring.[23-25] It is necessary to freeze the skin before dermabrasion to have a rigid surface that will abrade evenly and preserve anatomical markings that might otherwise be distorted when tissue is thawed. Because thermal injury may result in excessive scarring, caution would suggest that use of cryanesthetic agents that do not freeze below −30°C is prudent and as effective as use of those that freeze more deeply. Because regulation of fluorocarbons is making cryanesthetic agents more difficult to obtain, many surgeons are employing tumescent anesthesia instead of chilling to induce turgor.

Technique

Anesthesia

Preoperative analgesia has made dermabrasion a feasible technique in the outpatient setting. Anxiolytics like Diazepam and analgetics like Hydrocodone may be administered orally ~45 minutes to an hour preoperatively, to make the patient more comfortable and less anxious. Before administering regional block anesthesia with a lidocaine–bupivacaine mixture, 1 mL of intravenously administered fentanyl or IM meperidine and midazolam gives the patient a great sense of euphoria and relieves the discomfort associated with regional anesthesia. However this may require a level 2 facility in same states. Once analgesia has taken effect, the administration of regional anesthesia to the supraorbital, infraorbital, and mental foramina usually results in anesthesia to 60 to 70% of the entire face. When this is coupled with the use of refrigerant spray, most patients can be dermabraded without pain. The use of nitrous oxide analgesia to supplement anesthesia if the patient becomes uncomfortable during the procedure allows the procedure to progress without interruption.

Sanding Procedure

Once the skin has been rendered solid by the refrigerant spray, the sanding procedure begins in areas that can be abraded in ~10 seconds or ~1- to 2-in. areas.

The dermabrasion instrument, which should be grasped firmly in the hand, should be pulled only in the direction of the handle and perpendicular to the plane of rotation. Back-and-forth or circular movements may gouge the skin. The wire brush requires almost no pressure and produces multiple microlacerations, which are a sign of adequacy of the depth of the procedure. Adequate depth is recognized by several landmarks progressing through the skin. The removal of skin pigmentation signifies passage through the basal layer of the epidermis. Advancing into the papillary dermis, the small capillary loops of the papillary dermis are identified as the tissue thaws and punctate bleeding results. As the papillary dermis is entered further, faintly visible, small parallel bands of collagen become apparent. The fraying of these parallel strands signifies that dermabrasion has been carried to the correct level. Going further may result in scarring.

Many authors suggest the use of cotton towels or cotton gloves as absorbent material for blotting instead of gauze, which may become ensnared in the dermabrading instruments. Entanglement of gauze in the instruments results in a loud flapping that frightens the patient and may compromise the function of the instrument.

It is easiest to begin the dermabrasion centrally beside the nose and work outward. Because these are usually the areas of greatest disfigurement and the greatest anesthesia, this process allows the patient the least discomfort and the surgeon the most time to proceed. Special attention must be paid to fixing the lip by traction when dermabrading the lip, which can be ensnared in the machine, causing significant laceration. Staying constantly parallel to the surface is essential, especially in areas of complex curvature such as the chin and the malar eminences. Dermabrasion should always be performed within the facial units to avoid demarcation by pigmentation. Dermabrading to just beneath the jawline out to the preauricular area and up to the suborbital areas ensures that a uniform texture and appearance will be achieved. Next, 35% trichloroacetic acid (TCA) can be applied to any unabraded skin, the eyebrows, and the first few centimeters of the hairline to blend pigmentation more effectively.

Postoperative Care

Pain relief is achieved when biosynthetic dressings are applied at the end of the procedure. Postoperatively patients are put on prednisone 40 mg/d for 4 days, which greatly reduces the postoperative edema and discomfort. One of the most important recent advances has been the use of acyclovir in patients with a history of herpes simplex virus (HSV) infection. Begun 24 hours preoperatively at a dose of 400 mg 3 times/day for 5 days, no patients on this regimen have developed postoperative HSV infection, even with a preexisting history of that problem. Many authors now recommend routine prophylaxis with acyclovir or similar derivatives in all patients, regardless of history. Most patients reepithelialize completely between 5 and 7 days postoperatively when biosynthetic dressings have been used. Some of the dressings, such as Vigilon (Bard Medical Division, Covington, GA), must be changed daily. Others may be applied at the time of dermabrasion and left intact until they peel off spontaneously. Biosynthetic dressings need to be covered initially with gauze held in place with a flexible surgical netting. After the skin is reepithelialized, daily use of sunscreens is mandatory, and the patients are usually restarted on tretinoin between 7 and 10 days postoperatively.[26] Patients with a history of pigment problems, such as melasma, are also started on topical hydroquinone at the same time as the tretinoin. If by the tenth to fourteenth day the patient shows signs of disproportionate erythema, a topical 1% hydrocortisone is begun. Patients are cautioned after surgery that it will take at least a month for their skin to return to normal appearance. However, most patients are able to return to work within 7 to 10 days of surgery if light makeup is applied.

Complications

Milia are one of the most common complications of dermabrasion and usually appear 3 to 4 weeks postoperatively. If tretinoin has been used postoperatively, milia are rarely encountered. When milia do occur, they usually respond quickly to tretinoin therapy. Acne flares are another common complication in patients who are prone to acne. If the patient has had active acne in proximity to the dermabrasion, the acne flare can often be prevented by tetracycline starting in the immediate postoperative period. When acne does occur, tetracycline usually causes its prompt resolution. Although erythema is expected after dermabrasion, persistent or unusually severe erythema after 2 to 4 weeks should be managed with topical steroids to avoid hyperpigmentation and scarring. The daily use of sunscreens should begin when healing has occurred and should continue for several months postoperatively. If hyperpigmentation begins to appear several weeks postoperatively, topical application of hydroquinone and tretinoin will cause its resolution.

Although uncommon, postoperative infection can occur as a result of dermabrasion. The most common organisms are *Staphylococcus aureus*, HSV, and *Candida*. Staphylococcal infection usually manifests itself within 48 to 72 hours of dermabrasion with unusual facial swelling and honey crusting, as well as systemic symptoms such as fever. HSV infections frequently occur if the patient was not pretreated with acyclovir and are recognized by severe disproportionate pain, usually 48 to 72 hours postoperatively. *Candida* infections usually result in delayed healing and are recognized somewhat later at 5 to 7 days with exudation and facial swelling as clinical symptoms. Appropriate treatment with a staphylococcal antibiotic, acyclovir, or ketoconazole usually results in resolution of the infection without sequelae.

Comparison with Other Modalities

All resurfacing techniques result in an upper- to middermal wound. Dermabrasion relies on mechanical cold-steel injury, acid peels result in a "caustic" injury, and lasers result in a thermal injury. Recent studies in a porcine model comparing CO_2 laser, TCA, and dermabrasion by Fitzpatrick et al[27] and Campell et al[28] have shown that histologic and ultrastructural changes seen following these procedures are comparable. Giese et al[29] revealed that when dermabrasion is compared with chemical peels, significant differences are seen in the alteration of elastic fibers in histologic and mechanical properties. At 6 months following phenol treatment, the skin was stiffer and weaker than dermabraded skin. Holmkvist[30] reported that half-face perioral dermabrasion contrasted to half-face CO_2 laser resurfacing yielded identical clinical results but that dermabrasion healed in approximately half the time and with significantly less postoperative erythema and morbidity. Similar results were obtained by Gin et al.[31] Most surgeons practicing resurfacing agree that extended postoperative erythema and delayed hypopigmentation are much more common with phenol or laser than with dermabrasion. A review by Baker[32] points out that dermabrasion equipment is inexpensive, portable, and widely available, requiring no specialized accessory equipment and posing no fire hazard in the operating room.

Conclusion

In this era of computer-generated pulsed lasers and a potpourri of acid peels, there are those who might choose to recognize dermabrasion as an archaeological curiosity. However, dermabrasion is a well-understood procedure with established pre- and postoperative protocols and a highly predictable and reproducible result. Healing is prompt, with a minimum of morbidity and few complications. Equipment is simple and the cost reasonable. Dermabrasion offers a practical means of addressing a significant number of indications with the expectation of a positive outcome.

Chemical Peels

The explosion of interest in chemical peeling and laser resurfacing on the part of cosmetic surgeons has paralleled the general public's interest in acquiring a youthful appearance by rehabilitating the photoaged skin. The public's interest has been further heightened by advertising for cosmetic agents, over-the-counter chemicals, and treatment programs that have entered the general market of products meant to rejuvenate skin and erase the marks of sun damage and age. Most of these over-the-counter do-it-yourself programs have been tried by patients who, by the time they consult their dermatologist, are ready for a more definitive procedure performed with either chemical peeling or laser resurfacing. It is the role of the physician to analyze the patient's skin type and degree of photoaging, and to prescribe the correct facial rejuvenation procedure that will give the greatest benefit with the lowest risk and morbidity. The dermatologist should make available to the patient the options of medical or cosmoceutical topical therapy, dermabrasion, chemical peeling, and lasers for selective skin destruction and resurfacing. Each of these techniques has a place in the armamentarium of the cosmetic surgeon.

Chemical peeling involves the application of a chemical exfoliant to wound the dermis and epidermis for the removal of superficial lesions and to improve the texture of skin. Various acidic and basic chemical agents are used to produce the varying effects of light to medium to deep chemical peels through differences in their ability to destroy skin. The level of penetration, destruction, and inflammation determines the level of peeling. The stimulation of epidermal growth through the removal of the stratum corneum without necrosis consists of light superficial peel. Through exfoliation the peel thickens the epidermis with qualitative regenerative changes. Destruction of the epidermis defines a full superficial chemical peel inducing the regeneration of the epidermis. Further destruction of the epidermis and induction of inflammation within the papillary dermis constitutes a medium-depth peel. Then further inflammatory response in the deep reticular dermis induces production of new collagen and ground substances, which constitutes a deep chemical peel. These have now been well classified for various conditions associated with photoaging skin based on levels of penetration.[33] Thus the physician has tools for solving problems that may be mild, moderate, or severe with agents that are very superficial, medium-depth, and deep peeling chemicals. The physician must choose the right agent for each patient and condition.

Indications and Patient Selection

Analysis of patients with photoaging skin must take into account skin color and skin type as well as degree of photoaging. Various classification systems have been available, and I will present a combination of three systems so as to simplify and to help the physician define

Table 25.1 Fitzpatrick's Classification of Skin Types

Skin Type	Color	Reaction to Sun
I	Very white or freckled	Always burns
II	White	Usually burns
III	White to olive	Sometimes burns
IV	Brown	Rarely burns
V	Dark brown	Very rarely burns
VI	Black	Never burns

the right program or therapeutic procedure for a patient. The Fitzpatrick skin typing system classifies degrees of pigmentation and ability to tan. Graded I through VI, it prognosticates sun sensitivity, susceptibility to photodamage, and ability for facultative melanogenesis (one's intrinsic ability to tan). In addition, this system classifies skin in terms of risk factors for complications during chemical peeling. Fitzpatrick divides skin types I through VI, taking into account both color and reaction to the sun.[34] Skin types I and II are pale white and freckled with a high degree of potential to burn with sun exposure. Three and four can burn but usually are an olive to brown coloration. Five and six are dark brown to black skin that rarely ever burns and usually does not need sunscreen protection (**Table 25.1**). The patient with type I or II skin with significant photodamage needs regular sunscreen protection prior to and after the procedure. However, such an individual has little risk for hypopigmentation or reactive hyperpigmentation after a chemical peeling procedure. The patient with type III through VI skin has a greater risk for pigmentary dyschromia—hyper- or hypopigmentation—after a chemical peel and may need pre- and posttreatment with both sunscreen and bleaching to prevent these complications.[35] Pigmentary risks are generally not a great problem with very superficial and superficial pigment chemical peeling, but they may become a significant problem with medium and deep chemical peeling. It can also be a significant risk when regional areas, such as lips and eyelids, are peeled with a pulsed laser, creating a significant color change in these cosmetic units. This has been classified as the "alabaster look" seen with taped deep chemical peels in regional areas. The physician must inform the patient of this potential problem (especially for the patient with skin type III through VI), explain the benefits and risks of the procedure, and plan for the appropriate techniques to prevent these unwanted changes in color.

The peeling agent is a chemical escharotic that damages the skin in a therapeutic manner. It is important that the physician understand the patient's skin and its ability to withstand this damage. Certain skin types withstand the damage to a greater degree than others, and certain skin disorders have a greater tendency to promote side effects and complications of chemical peels. Patients with extensive photodamage may require stronger peeling agents and repeated applications of medium-depth peeling solutions to obtain therapeutic results. Patients with skin disorders such as atopic dermatitis, seborrheic dermatitis, psoriasis, and contact dermatitis may find their disease exacerbated in the postoperative period or may even develop problems with postoperative healing, such as prolonged healing, posterythema syndrome, or contact sensitivity during a postoperative period. Rosacea is a disorder of vasomotor instability in the skin and may be associated with an exaggerated inflammatory response to peeling agents. Other important factors include a history of radiation therapy to the proposed facial skin as chronic radiation dermatitis decreases the body's ability to heal properly.[36] A general rule of thumb is to examine the facial hair in the area treated by radiation; if it is intact, there are enough pilosebaceous units to heal the skin properly after medium or even deep chemical peeling. However, this is not absolute and one should establish from the history the dates of radiation treatment and the dosage used in each separate treatment. Some of our patients with the greatest amount of radiation dermatitis had had acne-related treatments in the mid-1950s, but over the years the skin developed the resultant degenerative changes.

Herpes simplex can be a postoperative problem with significant morbidity. Susceptible patients should be pretreated with antiherpetic agents such as acyclovir or valcyclovir to prevent herpetic activation. These patients can be identified in the preoperative consultation and placed on appropriate therapy at the time of the chemical peel. All antiherpetic agents act by inhibiting viral replication in the intact epidermal cell. The significance of this in peeling is that the skin must be reepithelialized before the agent has its full effect. Thus the antiviral agent must be continued in deep chemical peeling for the entire 2 weeks or in medium-depth peeling for at least 10 days.[37] The authors rarely use antiviral agents in light or superficial chemical peeling because the injury pattern is not usually deep enough to activate the herpes simplex virus. The chief indications for chemical peeling are associated with the reversal of actinic changes such as photodamage, rhytides, actinic growths, pigmentary dyschromias, and acne scars.[38] The physician thus can use classification systems to quantitate and qualitate the level of photodamage and prescribe the appropriate chemical peeling combination (**Table 25.2**).

Superficial Chemical Peeling

Superficial chemical peeling is truly an exfoliation of the stratum corneum or the entire epidermis to encourage regrowth with less photodamage and a more youthful

Table 25.2 Index of Photoaging

Texture Changes	Points				Score
Wrinkles (% of potential lines)	1 < 25%	2 < 50%	3 < 75%	4 < 100%	
Cross-hatched line (% of potential lines)	1 < 10%	2 < 20%	3 < 40%	4 < 60%	
Sallow color	1 Dull	2 Yellow	3 Brown	4 Black	
Leathery appearance	1	2	3	4	
Crinkley (thin and parchment)	1	2	3	4	
Pebbly (deep whitish nodules; % of face)	2 < 25%	4 < 50%	6 < 75%	8 < 100%	
Lesions					
Freckles-mottled skin (# present)	1 < 10	2 < 25	3 < 50	4 > 100	
Lentigines (dark and irregular) and SKs (size)	2 < 5 mm	4 < 10 mm	6 < 15 mm	8 > 20 mm	
Telangiectasia–erythema flush (# present)	1 < 5	2 < 10	3 < 15	4 > 15	
AKs and SKs (# present)	2 < 5	4 < 10	6 < 15	8 > 15	
Skin cancers (# present, now or by history)	2 1 ca	4 2 ca	6 3 ca	8 > 4 ca	
Senile comedones (in cheekbone area)	1 < 5	2 < 10	3 < 20	4 > 20	
					Total Score ________

Corresponding Rejuvenation Program

Score	Needs
1–4	Skin care program with tretinoin, glycolic acid peels
5–9	Same plus Jessner peels; pigmented lesion laser and/or vascular laser
10–14	Same plus medium peels—Jessner/TCA peel; skin fillers and/or Botox
15 or more	Above plus laser resurfacing

____________________	____________________
Staff Signature Date	**Patient Signature Date**

Abbreviations: AK, actinic keratosis; SK, seborrheic keratosis; TCA, trichloroacetic acid.

appearance. It usually takes repetitive peeling sessions to obtain maximal results. These agents have been broken down into very superficial chemical peels, which will remove the stratum corneum only, and superficial chemical peels, which will remove stratum corneum and damaged epidermis as well. It is to be noted that the effects of superficial peeling on photoaging skin are subtle, and the procedure will not produce a prolonged or very noticeable effect on dermal lesions such as wrinkles and furrows. Agents used include TCA 10 to 20%, Jessner's solution, glycolic acid 40 to 70%, salicylic acid–β-hydroxy acid, and tretinoin[39] (**Table 25.3**). Each of these agents has its own characteristics and methodological requirements, and a physician must be thoroughly familiar with the chemicals, the methods of application, and the nature of healing. The usual time for healing is 1 to 4 days, depending on the chemical and its strength.

Very-light-peeling agents include glycolic acid in low concentrations, 10% TCA, and salicylic acid (a β-hydroxy acid).

Ten to twenty percent TCA produces a light whitening or frosting effect on the skin with a result of sloughing of the upper one half to one third of the epidermis. Skin

Table 25.3 Agents Used for Superficial Chemical Peeling

Agent	Concentration	Mechanism of Action
Trichloracetic acid	10–25%	Protein precipitation
Jessner's solution	Formulated	Keratolysis
Glycolic acid	Keratinocyte	Protein precipitation
Jessner's solution	Formulated	Keratolysis
Glycolic acid	40–70%	Keratinocyte dyscohesion Epidermolysis
Salicylic acid	5–15%	Keratolysis

Table 25.4 The Jessner's Solution Formula

Resorcinol	14 g
Salicylic acid	14 g
Lactic acid	14 mL
Ethanol (qs)	100 mL

preparation prior to this peel consists of washing the face thoroughly and using acetone to remove surface oils and excessive stratum corneum. TCA is applied evenly with saturated gauze or a sable brush, and it usually takes 15 to 45 seconds for the frosting to become evident. This would be categorized as a level I frosting with the appearance of erythema and streaky whitening on the surface. Level II and III frosting is seen in medium-depth and deeper peels (**Fig. 25.7**). The patient experiences stinging and some burning during the procedure, but this subsides very rapidly and the patient then can resume normal activities. There is erythema and resulting desquamation, which last for 1 to 3 days. Sunscreens and light moisturizers are permitted, and minimal care is needed in this superficial chemical peel.

Jessner's solution is a combination acid (escharotic) that has been used for more than 100 years in the management of hyperkeratotic skin disorders (**Table 25.4**). It has been used as part of acne treatment for the removal of comedones and signs of inflammation. In superficial peeling it performs as an intense keratolytic agent. The application is similar to that for superficial TCA application with wet gauze, sponges, or a sable brush, producing an erythema with blotchy frosting. Tentative applications are done on an every-other-week basis, and the levels of Jessner's solution coatings can be increased with repetitive applications. The visual end point is predictable, that is, epidermal exfoliation and regrowth. This usually occurs within 2 to 4 days and is followed by the use of mild cleansers, moisturizing lotion, and sunscreen protection.

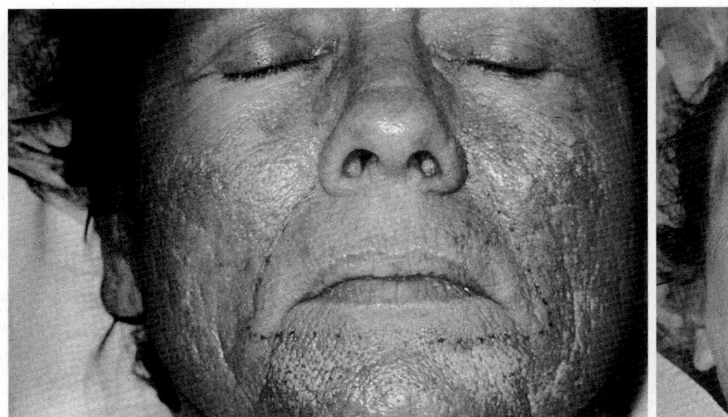
A

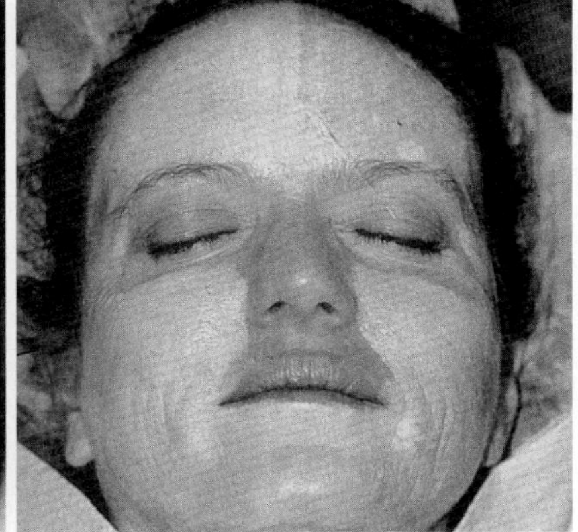
B

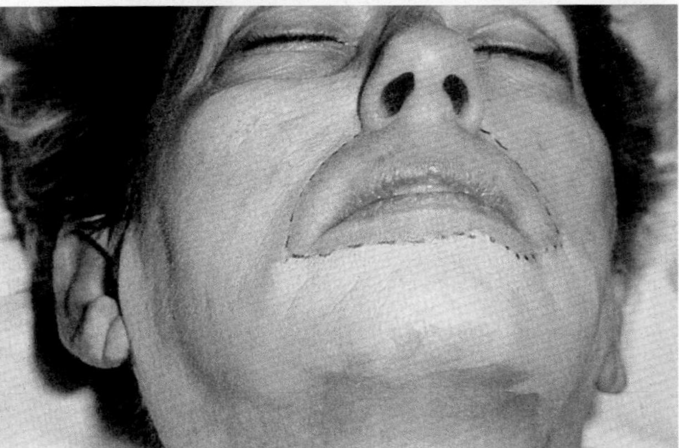
C

Fig. 25.7 Levels of frosting. (**A**) Level I—erythema with streaky frosting. (**B**) Level II—even white frosting with erythema showing through. (**C**) Level III—solid white enamel frosting.

α-Hydroxy Acids

α-hydroxy acids, specifically glycolic acid, have become the wonder drug of the early 1990s with promises of skin rejuvenation with home use and topical therapy. Hydroxy acids are found in foods (e.g., glycolic acid is naturally present in sugarcane, lactic acid in sour milk, malic acid in apples, citric acid in fruits, and tartaric acid in grapes). Lactic acid and glycolic acid are widely available and can be purchased for physician use. Glycolic acid is found in unbuffered concentrations of 50 to 70% for use as a chemical peel. Weekly or biweekly applications of 40 to 70% unbuffered glycolic acid treatments have been used for wrinkles by applying the solution to the face with a cotton swab, sable brush, or saturated gauze. The time of application is critical for glycolic acid because it must be rinsed off with water or neutralized with 5% sodium bicarbonate after 2 to 4 minutes. Mild erythema may persist for about an hour with slight stinging and minimal scaling. Wrinkle reduction and removal of benign keratoses have been reported to result from repeated applications of these peeling solutions.[40]

Superficial chemical peels can be used for comedonal acne and postinflammatory erythema or to correct pigmentation problems caused by acne, treatment for mild photoaging, and melasma.

To treat melasma effectively, the skin must be pretreated and posttreated with sunscreen, hydroquinone 4 to 8%, and retinoic acid. Hydroquinone is a pharmacological agent that blocks tyrosinase from developing melanin precursors for the production of new pigment. Its use essentially blocks new pigment formation as the new epidermis heals after a chemical peel. Thus it is needed when peeling for the treatment of pigmentary dyschromias as well as when applying chemical peels in type III to VI Fitzpatrick's skin (the skin type most prone to development of pigmentary problems).[41]

When using superficial chemical peels, the physician must understand that repetitive peeling will not summate into medium-depth or deep peels. A peel that does not affect the dermis will have very little effect on textural changes that originate from dermal damage. The patient must understand this preoperatively so as not to be disappointed with the results. On the other hand, repetitive peeling procedures are necessary for maximal benefits to be obtained with superficial chemical peeling. These are performed once a week for a total of six to eight chemical peels and enhanced by the appropriate cosmoceutical agents.

Medium-Depth Chemical Peeling

Medium-depth chemical peeling is defined as controlled damage from a chemical agent to the papillary dermis resulting in specific changes that can be performed in a single setting. Agents currently in use include combination products—Jessner's solution, 70% glycolic acid, and solid CO_2 with 35% TCA (**Table 25.5**). The hallmark for this level peel is 50% TCA. It has traditionally achieved acceptable results in ameliorating fine wrinkles, actinic changes, and preneoplastic conditions. However, because TCA itself is an agent more likely to be fraught with complications, especially scarring, in strengths of 50% or higher, it has fallen out of favor as a single-agent chemical peel.[42] It is for this reason that the combination products along with a 35% TCA formula have been found to be just as effective in producing this level of control damage without the risk of side effects.

Table 25.5 Agents for Medium-Depth Chemical Peel

Agent	Comment
1. TCA–50%	Not recommended because of risk of scarring
2. Combination–35% TCA–solid CO_2 (Brody)	The most potent combination
3. Combination–35% TCA–Jessner's (Monheit)	The most popular combination
4. Combination 35% TCA–70% glycolic (Coleman)	An effective combination
5. 89% phenol	Rarely used

Abbreviations: TCA, trichloroacetic acid.

Brody developed the use of solid CO_2 applied with acetone to the skin as a freezing technique prior to the application of 35% TCA. This appears to break the epidermal barrier for a more even and complete penetration of the 35% TCA.[43]

Monheit demonstrated the use of Jessner's solution prior to the application of 35% TCA. Jessner's solution was found to be effective in destroying the epidermal barrier by breaking up individual epidermal cells. This allowed deeper penetration of the 35% TCA and a more even application of the peeling solution.[44] Similarly, Coleman demonstrated the use of 70% glycolic acid prior to the application of 35% TCA. Its effect has been very similar to that of Jessner's solution.[45]

All three combinations have been proven more effective and safer than 50% TCA. The application and frosting are more controlled with the combination so that the "hot spots" with higher concentrations of TCA, which can produce dyschromias and scarring, are not a significant problem with lower-concentration TCA as used in this combination medium-depth peel. The Monheit version of Jessner's solution −35% TCA peel is a relatively simple and safe combination. The technique is used for mild to moderate photoaging, including pigmentary changes, lentigines, epidermal growths, dyschromias, and rhytides. It is a single procedure with a healing time of 7 to 10 days.

It is useful also to remove diffuse actinic keratoses as an alternative to chemical exfoliation with topical 5-FU chemotherapy. It significantly reduces the morbidity and gives the cosmetic benefits of improved photoaging skin.[46]

The procedure is usually performed with mild preoperative sedation and nonsteroidal anti-inflammatory agents. The patient is told that the peeling agent will sting and burn temporarily; aspirin is given before the peel and continued through the first 24 hours if the patient can tolerate the medication. Its anti-inflammatory effect is especially helpful in reducing swelling and relieving pain. If given before surgery, it may be all that the patient requires during the postoperative phase. However, for full-face peels it is useful to give a preoperative sedative (diazepam 5 to 10 mg orally) and a mild analgesic [meperidine 25 mg (Demerol, Sanofi-Aventis, Bridgewater, NJ), and hydroxyzine hydrochloride 25 mg IM (Vistaril, Pfizer Inc., New York, NY)]. The discomfort from this peel is not long lasting, so that short-acting sedatives and analgesics are all that is needed.[46]

Vigorous cleaning and degreasing are necessary to achieve even penetration of the solution. The face is scrubbed gently with ingasam (Septisol, STERIS Corp., Mentor, OH) (4 × 4 in. gauze pads) and water, then rinsed and dried. Next a masetol preparation is applied to remove residual oils and debris. It is necessary to perform a thorough degreasing for an even and fully penetrant peel. A splotchy peel is usually the result of uneven penetration of peel solution due to residual oil or stratum corneum from inadequate degreasing.

Jessner's solution is then applied with cotton-tipped applicators or 2 × 2 in. gauze. The frosting achieved with Jessner's solution is much lighter than that produced by TCA, and the patient is usually not uncomfortable. A mild erythema appears with a faint tinge of frost evenly over the face (**Fig. 25.8**).

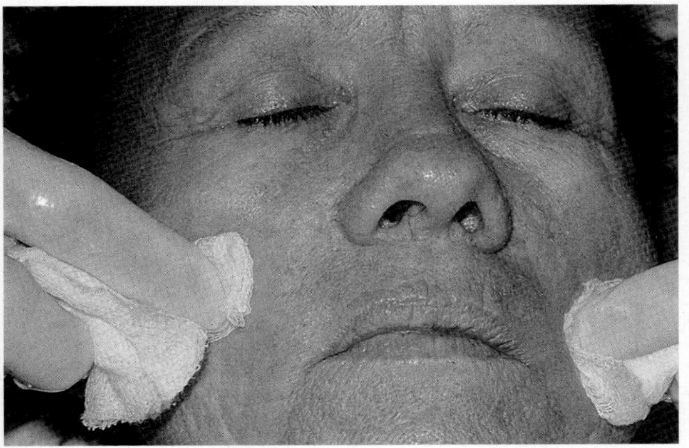

Fig. 25.8 Jessner's solution. Appearance of frosting with erythema with blotchy frosting.

TCA is then applied evenly with one to four cotton-tipped applicators that can be used on different areas with light or heavier doses of the acid. Four cotton-tipped applicators are used with broad strokes over the forehead as well as on the medial cheeks. Two mildly soaked cotton-tipped applicators can be used across the lips and chin, and one damp cotton-tipped applicator on the eyelids. Thus the dose of TCA is contingent on the amount used, and the number of cotton-tipped applicators used, and the clinician's technique. The cotton-tipped applicator is useful in controlling the amount of peel solution to be applied (**Fig. 25.9**).

White frost from the TCA application appears on the treated area after a few minutes. Even application should eliminate the need to go over areas a second or third time, but if frosting is incomplete or uneven, the solution should be reapplied. TCA takes more time to frost than Baker's formula or straight phenol, but less time than the superficial peeling agents. The surgeon should wait at least 3 to 4 minutes after the application of TCA to ensure the frosting has reached its peak. He or she can then analyze the completeness of a frosted cosmetic unit and touch up the area as needed. Areas of poor frosting should be carefully retreated with a thin application of TCA. The physician should achieve a level II to level III frosting. Level II frosting is defined as white-coated frosting with erythema showing through. A level III frosting, which is associated with penetration to the dermis, is a solid white enamel frosting with no background of erythema.[47] Most medium-depth chemical peels use a level II frosting; this is especially true for eyelids and areas of sensitive skin. Those areas with a greater tendency to scar, such as the zygomatic arch, the bony prominences of the jawline, and the chin, should only receive up to a level II frosting. Overcoating TCA increases its penetration, so that a second or third application will dry the acid further, causing more damage. One must be careful in overcoating only areas in which the take-up was not adequate or the skin is much thicker.

Anatomical areas of the face are peeled sequentially from forehead to temple to cheeks and, finally, to lips and eyelids. The white frosting indicates keratocoagulation, and at that point the reaction is complete. Careful feathering of the solution into the hairline and around the rim of the jaw and brow conceals the line demarcation between peeled and nonpeeled areas. The perioral area has rhytids that require a complete and even application of solution over the lip skin to the vermilion. This is best accomplished with the help of an assistant who stretches and fixates the upper and lower lips while the peel solution is applied.

Certain areas and lesions require special attention. Thicker keratoses do not frost evenly and thus do not pick up peel solution. Additional applications rubbed

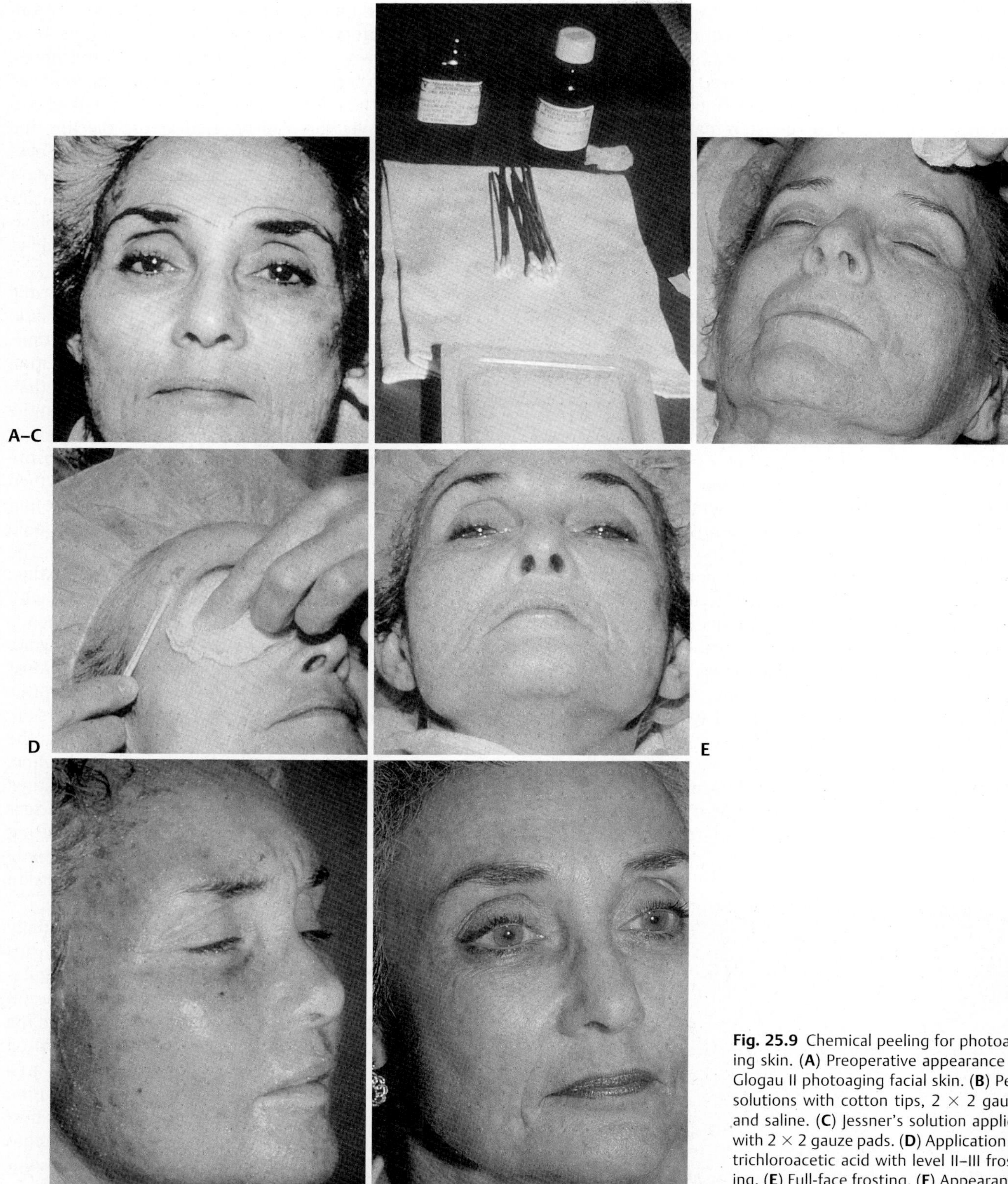

Fig. 25.9 Chemical peeling for photoaging skin. (**A**) Preoperative appearance of Glogau II photoaging facial skin. (**B**) Peel solutions with cotton tips, 2 × 2 gauze and saline. (**C**) Jessner's solution applied with 2 × 2 gauze pads. (**D**) Application of trichloroacetic acid with level II–III frosting. (**E**) Full-face frosting. (**F**) Appearance 4 days postoperative. (**G**) Appearance 6 months postoperative.

vigorously into the lesion may be needed for peel solution penetration. Wrinkled skin should be stretched to allow an even coating of solution into the folds and troughs. Oral rhytides require peel solution to be applied with the wood portion of a cotton-tipped applicator and extended into the vermilion of the lip. Deeper furrows, such as expression lines, will not be eradicated by peel solution and thus should be treated like the remaining skin.

Eyelid skin must be treated delicately and carefully. A semidry applicator should be used to carry the solution to within 2 to 3 mm of the lid margin. The patient should be positioned with the head elevated at 30 degrees and the eyelids closed. Excess peel solution on the cotton tip should be drained gently on the bottom before application. The applicator is then rolled gently on the lids and periorbital skin. Never leave excess peel solution on the lids because the solution can roll into the eyes. Dry tears with a cotton-tipped applicator during peeling because they may pull peel solution to the puncta and eye by capillary attraction (**Fig. 25.10**). The Jessner's–TCA peel procedure is as follows:

1. The skin should be cleaned thoroughly with Septisol.
2. Acetone or acetone alcohol is used to further debride oil and scale from the surface of the skin.
3. Jessner's solution is applied.
4. Thirty-five percent TCA is applied until a light frost appears.
5. Cool saline compresses are applied to neutralize the solution.
6. Healing is facilitated by 0.25% acetic acid soaks and a mild emollient cream.

There is an immediate burning sensation as the peel solution is applied, but this subsides as frosting is completed. Cool saline compresses offer symptomatic relief for a peeled area as the solution is applied to other areas. Following the peel, the compresses are placed over the face for several minutes until the patient is comfortable. The burning has subsided fully by the time the patient is ready to be discharged. By then most of the frosting has faded and a brawny desquamation is evident.

Postoperatively, edema, erythema, and desquamation are expected. With periorbital peels and even forehead peels, eyelid edema can be severe enough to close the lids. For the first 24 hours, the patient is instructed to soak four times a day with a 0.25% acetic acid compress made of 1 teaspoon white vinegar in 1 pint of warm water. A bland emollient is applied to the desquamating areas after soaks. After 24 hours, the patient can shower and clean gently with a mild nondetergent cleanser. The erythema intensifies as desquamation becomes complete within 4 to 5 days. Thus healing is completed within 1 week to 10 days. At the end of 1 week, the bright red color has faded to pink and has the appearance of a sunburn. This can be covered by cosmetics and fades fully within 2 to 3 weeks.

The medium-depth peel is dependent on three components for therapeutic effect: (1) degreasing, (2) Jessner's solution, and (3) 35% TCA. The amount of each agent applied creates the intensity and thus the effectiveness of this peel. The variables can be adjusted according to the patient's skin type and the areas of the face being treated. Therefore, the medium-depth peel is the workhorse of peeling and resurfacing in my practice because it can be individualized for most patients.

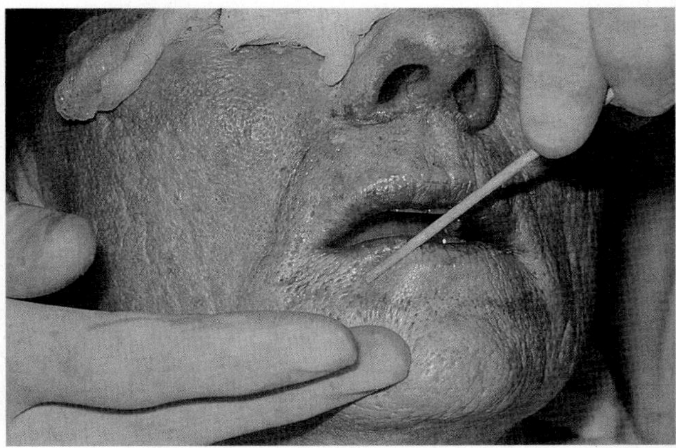
A

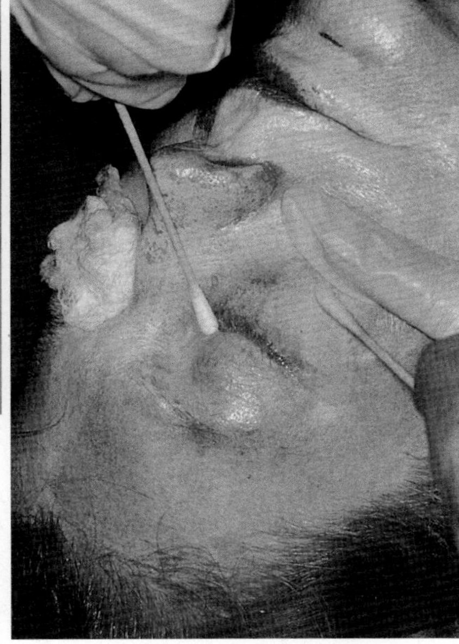
B

Fig. 25.10 (**A**) Oral rhytides are treated with wood portion of cotton tip for deeper penetration. (**B**) Eyelids are painted cautiously with damp cotton-tipped applicators; dry cotton tips are used to blot the tears.

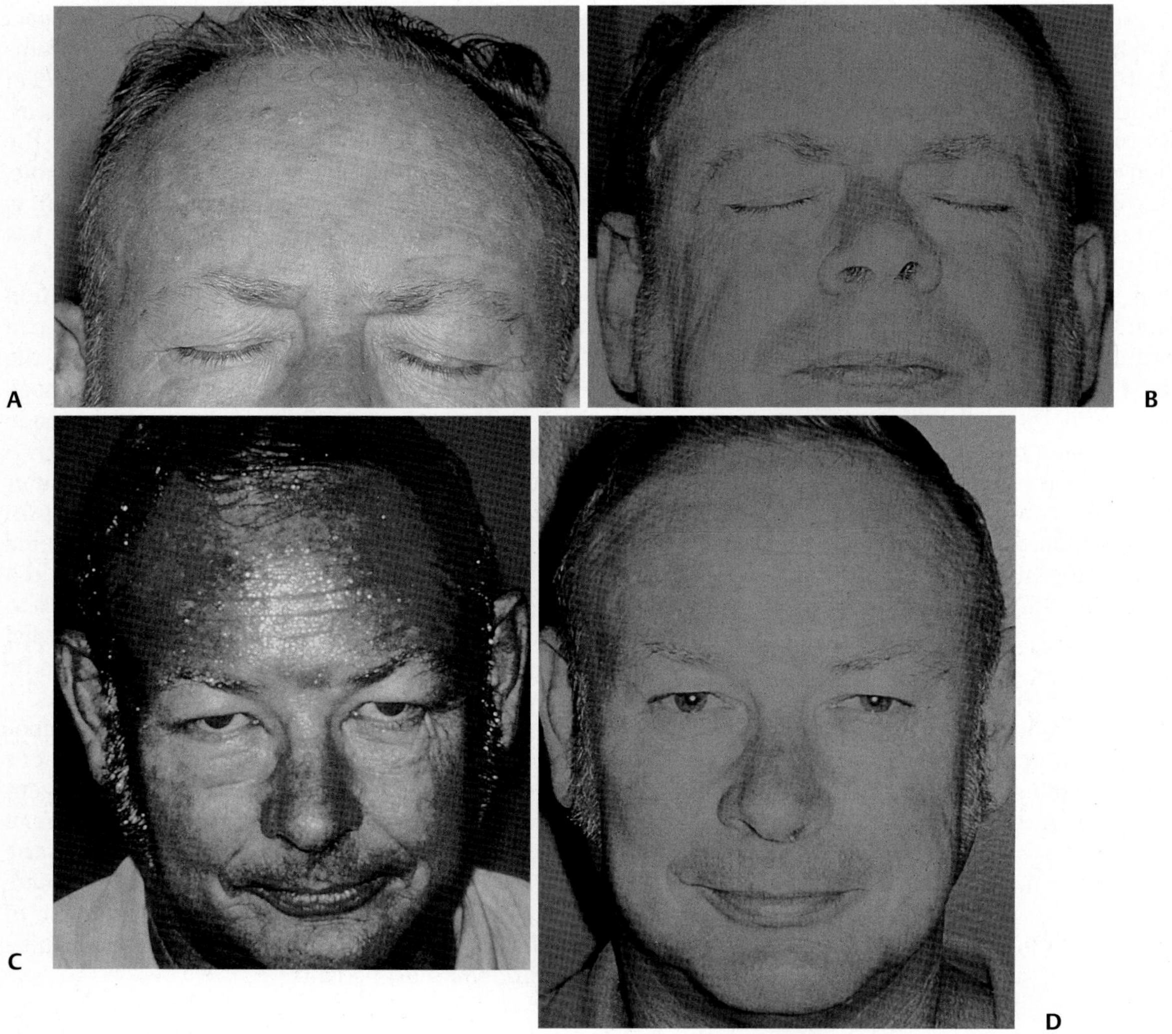

Fig. 25.11 Treatment of actinic keratoses with Jessner's 35% trichloroacetic acid (TCA) peel. (**A**) Preoperative appearance—actinic keratoses forehead and temples. (**B**) Application of Jessner's solution with 35% TCA—level II frosting. (**C**) Jessner's solution with 35% TCA, 3 days postoperative. (**D**) Six weeks postoperative.

The medium-depth chemical peel thus has five major indications: (1) destruction of epidermal lesions–actinic keratoses (**Fig. 25.11**); (2) resurfacing of the level II moderately photoaging skin (**Fig. 25.12**), (3) correction of pigmentary dyschromias (**Fig. 25.13**), (4) repair of mild acne scars; and (5) blending of photoaging skin with laser resurfacing and deep chemical peeling[48] (**Fig. 25.14**).

Deep Chemical Peeling

Level III photodamage requires deep chemical peeling. This entails the use of either TCA above 50% or the Gordon–Baker phenol peel. Laser resurfacing can also be used to reliably reach this level of damage. TCA above 45% has been found to be unreliable, with a high incidence of scarring and postoperative complications. For this reason it is not included as a standard treatment for deep chemical peeling. The Baker–Gordon phenol peel has been used successfully for more than 40 years for deep chemical peeling and produces reliable results (**Table 25.6**). It is a labor-intensive procedure that must be taken as seriously as any major surgical procedure. The patient requires preoperative sedation with an intravenous line and preoperative intravenous hydration. Usually a liter of fluid is given preoperatively and, in addition, a liter of fluid is given during the procedure. Phenol is both a cardiotoxin and a hepatotoxin, and it is nephrotoxic. For this reason, one must be concerned with the serum concentration

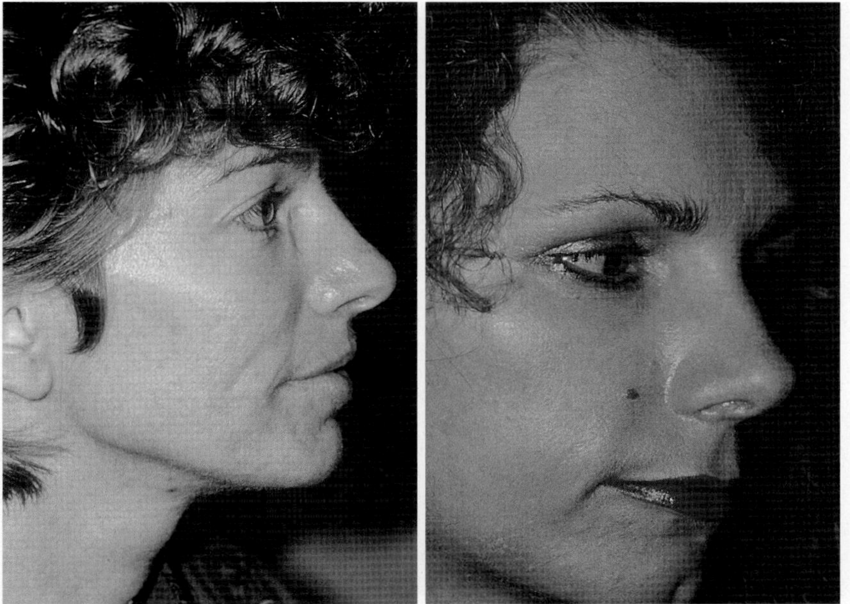

Fig. 25.12 The Jessner's +35% TCA peel for moderately photoaging skin and acne scars. (**A**) Preoperative appearance. (**B**) Six months postoperative.

of phenol through cutaneous absorption. Methods to limit this include the following:

1. *Giving intravenous hydration prior to and during the procedure* to flush the phenolic products through the serum.
2. *Extending the time of application for a full-face peel to more than 1 hour.* Cosmetic units are applied for the 15-minute wait between units. That is, the forehead, cheeks, chin, lips, and eyelids are each given a 15-minute period for a total of 60 to 90 minutes for the procedure.
3. *Monitoring of the patients.* If there is any electrocardiographic abnormality (e.g., premature ventricular contraction or premature aortic contraction), the procedure is stopped and the patient watched carefully for other signs of toxicity.
4. *Administration of oxygen.* Many physicians believe that O_2 given during the procedure can be helpful in preventing rhythm complications.

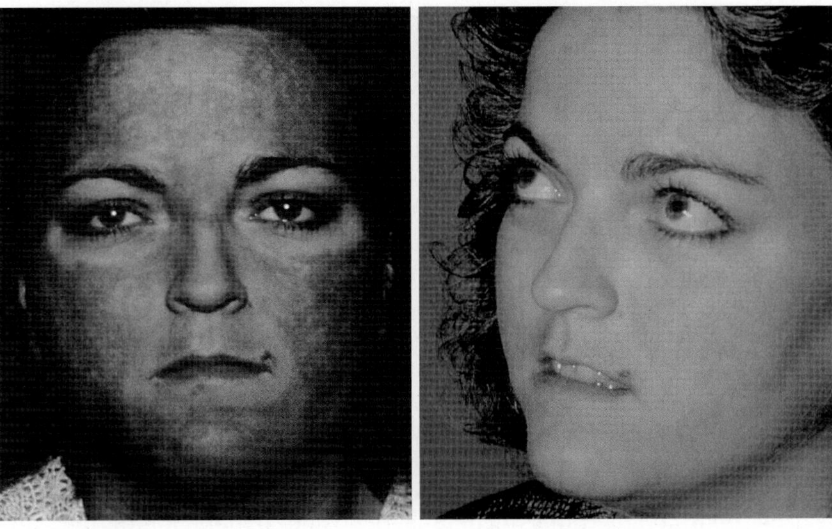

Fig. 25.13 Treatment of pigmentary dyschromias with medium-depth chemical peel and cosmoceutical treatment with tretinoin and hydroquinone 4%. (**A**) Preoperative appearance. (**B**) Postoperative appearance, 6 months.

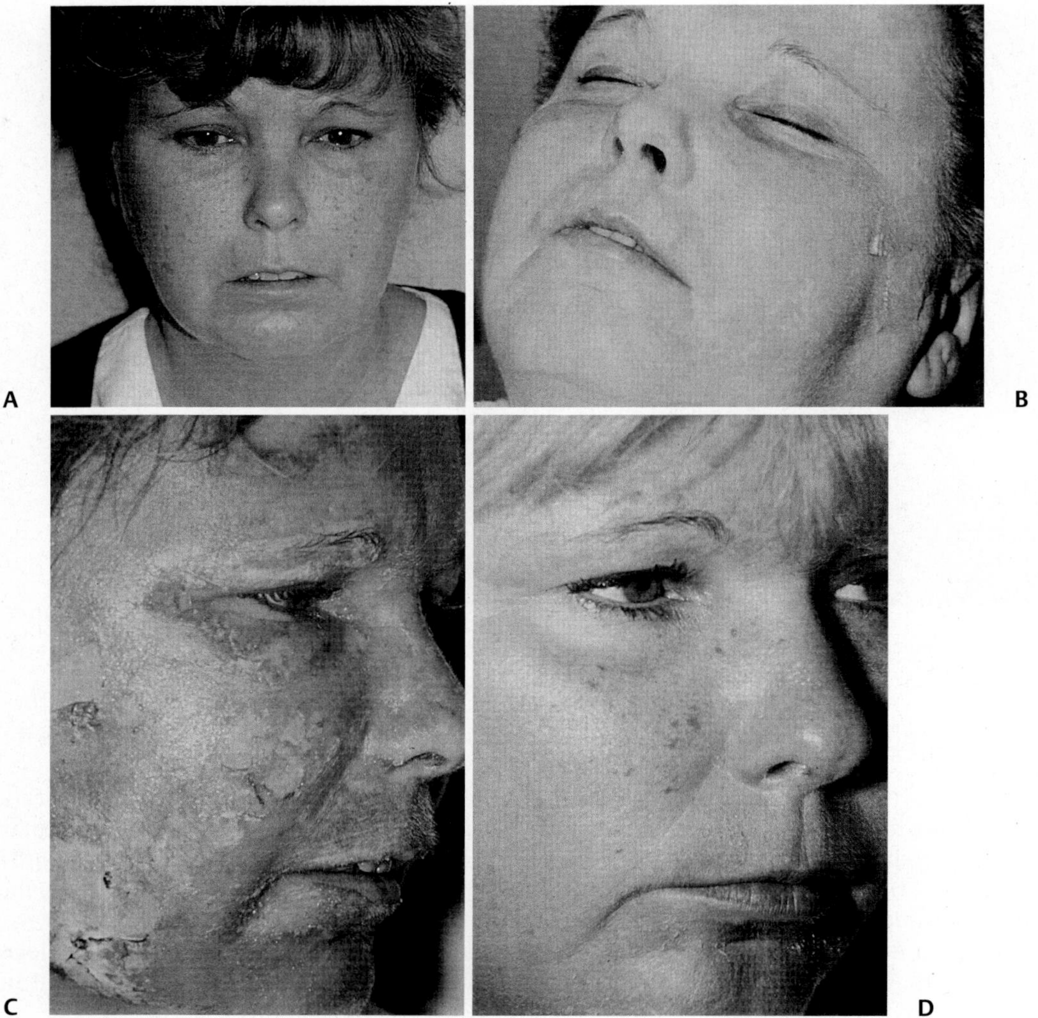

Fig. 25.14 Combination deep chemical peel—perioral area with medium-depth peel over remaining face. (**A**) Preoperative. (**B**) Peel solution applied. (**C**) Postoperative, 4 days. (**D**) Postoperative, 6 weeks.

5. *Proper patient screening.* Any patient with a history of cardioarrhythmia or hepatic or renal compromise, or who is on medications that give a propensity for arrhythmias should not undergo the Baker–Gordon phenol peel.[49]

Patients who are undergoing deep chemical peeling must recognize the significant risk factors, the increased morbidity, and possible complications involved in this procedure so that the benefits can be weighed positively against these particular factors. In the hands of those who perform this technique regularly, it is a reliable and safe way to rejuvenate severely photoaged skin that may show deep perioral rhytids, periorbital rhytids and crow's feet, forehead lines and wrinkles, as well as the other textural and lesional changes associated with the more severe photoaging process.

There are two modalities for deep chemical peeling: Baker's formula phenol unoccluded, and Baker's formula phenol occluded. Occlusion is accomplished with the application of waterproof zinc oxide tape, such as 0.5-in. Curity tape. The tape is placed directly after the phenol is applied to each individual cosmetic unit. Tape occlusion increases the penetration of the Baker's phenol solution and is particularly helpful for deeply lined, "weather-beaten" faces. A taped Baker's formula phenol peel creates the deepest damage in midreticular dermis, and this form of chemical peeling should only be performed by the most knowledgeable and experienced cosmetic surgeons who understand the risks of overpenetration and deep damage to the reticular dermis.[50] These complications include hyper- and hypopigmentation, textural changes such as "alabaster skin," and the potential for scarring.

Table 25.6 The Formula for the Baker–Gordon Phenol Peel

3 mL USP liquid phenol 88%
2 mL tap water
8 drops liquid soap (Septisol)
3 drops croton oil

The unoccluded technique as modified by McCollough and Langsdon involves more skin cleansing and application of more peel solution. On the whole, this technique does not produce as deep a peel as the occluded method.[51]

The Baker–Gordon formula for this peel was first described in 1961 and has been used with success for more than 40 years. The formula (**Table 25.6**) penetrated further into the dermis than full-strength undiluted phenol because full-strength phenol allegedly causes an immediate coagulation of epidermal keratin proteins and self-blocks further penetration. Dilution to ~50 to 55% in the Baker–Gordon formula causes keratolysis and keratocoagulation, resulting in greater penetration. The liquid soap Hibiclens (Mölynlycke Health Care Inc., Norcross, CA) is a surfactant that reduces skin tension, thus allowing a more even penetration. Croton oil is a vesicant epidermalytic agent that enhances phenol absorption. The freshly prepared formula is not miscible and must be stirred in a clear-glass medicine cup immediately before application to the patient. Although the mixture can be stored in an amber glass bottle for short periods, this is usually unnecessary. It is preferable to reformulate the mixture on a regular basis.

Techniques

Before the administration of anesthesia, the patient is seated and the face marked, noting such landmarks as the mandibular angle, the chin, the preauricular sulcus, the orbital rim, and the forehead. This is done to extend the peel thoroughly throughout the limits of the face and slightly over the mandibular rim to blend any color change. This peel does require sedation. An intravenous combination such as fentanyl citrate (Sublimaze, Akorn, Inc., Buffalo Grove, IL) and midazolam (Versed, Roche Laboratories, Basel, Switzerland) can be administered intravenously by an anesthetist while the patient is monitored and given intravenous sedation. It is helpful to use local nerve blocks along the supraorbital nerve, infraorbital nerve, and mental nerve with bupivacaine hydrochloride (Marcaine, Hospira, Inc., Lake Forrest, IL), which should provide some local anesthesia for up to 4 hours. The entire face then is cleansed and degreased with a keratolytic agent, such as hexochlorophene with alcohol (Septisol), with emphasis placed on oily areas such as the nose, the hairline, and the midfacial cheeks.

The chemical agent is then applied sequentially to six aesthetic units: forehead, perioral, right and left cheeks, nose, and periorbital areas. Each cosmetic area takes 15 minutes for application, allowing 60 to 90 minutes for the entire procedure. Cotton-tipped applicators are used with a similar technique as discussed on the medium-depth Jessner's–35% TCA peel. However, less agent is used because frosting becomes evident much more quickly. An immediate burning sensation is present for 15 to 20 seconds and then subsides; however, pain returns in 20 minutes and persists for 6 to 8 hours. The last area for the peel is the periorbital skin to which the chemical is applied with only damp cotton-tipped applicators. Great care is taken to keep the drops away from the eye and the tears off the skin, as tearing may allow the peel solution to reach the eye by capillary attraction. It is important to remember that water dilution of a chemical may increase the absorption; therefore, if the chemical does get into the eye, flushing should be done with mineral oil rather than water.

Following the full application of peel solution, the frosting becomes evident and the tape can be applied for an occluded peel. Ice packs can be applied at the conclusion of the peel for comfort; and if this is an untaped peel, petrolatum is used. A biosynthetic dressing, such as Vigilon (Bard Medical, Covington, GA) or Flexzan (Mylan Canonsburg, PA), is applied for the first 24 hours.[52] The patient is usually seen in 24 hours for removal of the tape or the biosynthetic dressing and to monitor the healing. At this time the patient is reinstructed regarding the use of compresses and occlusive ointments or dressings. It is important to keep the skin crust free.

The four stages of wound healing are apparent after a deep chemical peel. They include (1) inflammation, (2) coagulation, (3) reepithelialization, and (4) fibroplasia.[53] At the conclusion of the chemical peel, the inflammatory phase has already begun with a brawny, dusky erythema that progresses for the first 12 hours. This is an accentuation of pigmented lesions on the skin as the coagulation phase separates the epidermis, producing serum exudation, crusting, and pyoderma. During this phase it is important to use debridant soaks and compresses as well as occlusive salves. These will remove the sloughed, necrotic epidermis and prevent the serum exudate from hardening as crust and scab. These authors prefer the use of 0.25% acetic acid soaks found in the vinegar–water preparation (1 teaspoon white vinegar, 1 pint warm water) because it is antibacterial, especially against *Pseudomonas* and other gram-negative organisms. In addition, the mildly acidic nature of the solution is physiological for the healing granulation tissue, and mildly debridant because it will dissolve and cleanse the necrotic material and serum. We prefer to use bland emollients and salves such as petrolatum (Vaseline), Eucerin (Beiersdorf, Inc., Wilton, CT), or Aquaphor (Beiersdorf, Inc.,

Wilton, CT) because the skin can be monitored carefully day by day for potential complications.

Reepithelialization begins on day 3 and continues until day 10 to 14. Occlusive salves promote faster reepithelialization and less tendency for delayed healing. The final stages of fibroplasia continue well beyond the initial closure of the peeled wound and continue with neoangiogenesis and new collagen formation for 3 or 4 months. Prolonged erythema may last 2 to 4 months in unusual cases of sensitive skin or with contact dermatitis. New collagen formation can continue to improve texture and rhytides for up to 4 months during this last phase of fibroplasia.

Complications

Many of the complications seen in peeling can be recognized early on during healing stages. The cosmetic surgeon should be well acquainted with the normal appearance of a healing wound and its time frame for both medium and deep peeling. Prolongation of the granulation tissue phase beyond 7 to 10 days may indicate delayed wound healing. This could be the result of viral, bacterial, or fungal infection; contact dermatitis interfering with wound healing; or other systemic factors. A red flag should alert the physician to careful investigation, and prompt treatment should be instituted to forestall potential irreparable damage that may result in scarring.

Complications can be caused either intraoperatively or postoperatively. The two inherent errors that lead to intraoperative complications are (1) incorrect peel medication and (2) accidental solution misplacement. It is the physician's responsibility to ensure that the solution and its concentration are correct. TCA concentrations should be measured weight by volume because this is the standard for measuring depth of peel. Glycolic acid and lactic acid solutions as well as Jessner's solution must be checked for expiration date given that the potency decreases with time. Alcohol or water absorption may inappropriately increase the potency, so one must ensure that the shelf life is appropriate. The peel solution should be applied with cotton-tipped applicators, and in medium and deep peels it is best to pour the peel solution in a secondary container rather than apply the solution spun around the neck of the bottle because intact crystals may give the solution a higher concentration as it is taken directly from its container. One should be careful to apply the solution to its appropriate location and not to pass the wet cotton-tipped applicator directly over the central face where a drop may inadvertently fall on sensitive areas, such as the eyes. Saline and bicarbonate of soda should be available to dilute TCA or neutralize glycolic acid if placed in the wrong area. Likewise, mineral oil should be present for Baker's phenol peels. Postoperative complications most commonly result from local infection or contact dermatitis. The best deterrent for local infection is the continuous use of soaks to debride crusting and necrotic material. *Streptococcus* and *Staphylococcus* infections can occur under biosynthetic membranes or thick occlusive ointments. The use of 0.25% acetic acid soaks seems to deter this as does the judicious removal of ointment with each soak. *Staphylococcus, Escherichia coli*, or even *Pseudomonas* infection may result from improper care during healing and should be managed promptly with the appropriate oral antibiotic.

Frequent postoperative visits are necessary to recognize the early onset of a bacterial infection. It may present itself as delayed wound healing, ulcerations, buildup of necrotic material with excessive scabbing, crusting, purulent drainage, and odor. Early recognition allows peeling of the skin and prevents the spread of infection and scarring.

Herpes simplex infection is the result of reactivation of HSV on the face and most commonly on the perioral area. A history of previous HSV infection should necessitate the use of prophylactic oral antiviral medications. Patients with a positive history can be treated with 400 mg of acyclovir three times a day beginning on the day of the peel and continuing for 7 to 14 days, depending on whether it is a medium-depth or deep chemical peel. The mechanism of action is to inhibit viral replication in the intact epidermal cell. This would mean that the drug would not have an inhibitory effect until the skin is reepithelialized, which is 7 to 10 days in medium and deep peels. In the past, these agents were discontinued at 5 days and clinical infection became apparent in 7 to 10 days.[54]

Active herpetic infections can easily be treated with antiviral agents. When treated early, they usually do not scar.

Delayed wound healing and persistent erythema are signs that the peel is not healing normally. The cosmetic surgeon must know the normal time table for each of the healing events to occur so as to recognize when healing is delayed or the erythema is not fading adequately. Delayed wound healing may respond to physician debridement if an infection is present, to corticosteroids if due to contact allergic or contact irritant dermatitis along with a change of the offending contact agent, or to protection with a biosynthetic membrane such as Flexzan or Vigilon. When this diagnosis is made, patients must be followed daily with dressing changes and a close watch on the healing skin.

Persistent erythema is a syndrome where the skin remains erythematous beyond what is normal for the individual peel. A superficial peel loses its erythema in 15 to 30 days, a medium-depth peel within 60 days, and a deep chemical peel within 90 days. Erythema and/or pruritus beyond this period of time is considered abnormal and fits this syndrome. It may be contact dermatitis, contact sensitization, reexacerbation of prior skin disease, or a genetic susceptibility to erythema, but it may also indicate potential scarring. Erythema is the result of the angiogenic factors stimulating vasodilation, which also includes the phase of fibroplasia that is being stimulated for a prolonged period of time. For this reason, it can be accompanied by skin thickening and scarring. It should be managed promptly and appropriately with topical steroids, systemic steroids, intralesional steroids if thickening is occurring, and skin protection to eliminate the factors of irritancy and allergy. If thickening or scarring becomes evident, other measures that can be helpful include the daily use of silicone sheeting and dye-pulsed laser treatment of the vascular factors. With prompt intervention, scarring can often be averted.

Conclusion

It is the physician's responsibility to choose the appropriate modality for management of such skin conditions as photoaging, scarring, dyschromia, and neoplasia. Many modalities are available, including the three levels of chemical peel reviewed. The physician must have thorough knowledge of all of these tools so as to offer each patient the optimal treatment.

References

1. Kurtin A. Corrective surgical planing of skin: new technique for treatment of acne scars and other skin defects. Arch Dermatol Syphilol 1953;68:389–397
2. Kronmayer E. Die Heilung der Akne durch ein Neves Narben Lascs Operations ver Faren: das Stranzen. Ilustr Monatssehr. Aerztl Poly Tech 1905;27:101
3. Burke J. Wire Brush Surgery. Springfield, Il: Charles C Thomas; 1956
4. Nelson BR, Majmudar G, Griffiths CE, et al. Clinical improvement following dermabrasion of photoaged skin correlates with synthesis of collagen I. Arch Dermatol 1994;130:1136–1142
5. Nelson BR, Metz RD, Majmudar G, et al. A comparison of wire brush and diamond fraise superficial dermabrasion for photoaged skin: a clinical immunohistologic and biochemical study. J Am Acad Dermatol 1996;34:235–243
6. Mandy SH. Tretinoin in the pre- and postoperative management of dermabrasion. J Am Acad Dermatol 1986;115:878
7. Hang VC, Lee JV, Zitelli JA, Hebda PA. Topical tretinoin and epithelial wound healing. Arch Dermatol 1989;125:65–69
8. Maibach H, Rovee D. Epidermal Wound Healing. Chicago: Year Book Medical Publishers; 1972
9. Mandy SH. A new primary wound dressing made of polyethylene oxide gel. J Dermatol Surg Oncol 1983;9:153
10. Alvarez OM, Mertz PM, Eaglestein WH. The effect of occlusive dressings on collagen synthesis in the superficial wounds. J Surg Res 1983;35:142
11. Roenigk HH Jr, Pinski JB, Robinson JK, Hanke CW. Acne, retinoids, and dermabrasion. J Dermatol Surg Oncol 1985;11:396–398
12. Rubenstein R, Roenigk HH Jr, Stegman SJ, Hanke CW. Atypical keloids after dermabrasion of patients taking isotretinoin. J Am Acad Dermatol 1986;15:280–285
13. Dzubow CM, Miller WH Jr. The effect of 13-*cis*-retinoic acid on wound healing in dogs. J Dermatol Surg Oncol 1987;13:265
14. Coleman WP, Yarborough JM, Mandy SH. Dermabrasion for prophylaxis and treatment of actinic keratoses. J Dermatol Surg Oncol 1996;22:17–21
15. Moy R, Moy L, Zitelli J, Mandy S. Effects of systemic 13 cis-retinoic acid on wound healing in vivo. American Academy of Dermatology, San Antonio, Texas, 1987
16. Moy R, Zitelli J, Uitto J. Effect of 13 cis-retinoic on dermal wound healing in vivo. [abstract] J Invest Dermatol 1987;88:508
17. Wentzell JM, Robinson JK, Wentzell JM Jr, Swartz DE, Carlson SE. Physical properties of aerosols produced by dermabrasion. Arch Dermatol 1989;125:1637–1643
18. Field L. Dermabrasion versus 5 fluorouracil in the management of actinic keratoses. In: Epstein K, ed. Controversies in Dermatology. Philadelphia: WB Saunders; 1984:62–102
19. Burke J, Marascalco J, Clark W. Half-face planing of precancerous skin after 5 years. Arch Dermatol 1963;88:140
20. Yarborough JM. Dermabrasive surgery state of the art. In: Millikan LE, ed. Clinics in Dermatology, Advances in Surgery. Philadelphia: JB Lippincott; 1987;5:57–74
21. Yarborough JM. Dermabrasion by wire brush. J Dermatol Surg Oncol 1987;13:610
22. Alt T. Facial dermabrasion: advantages of the diamond fraise technique. J Dermatol Surg Oncol 1987;13:618
23. Hanke CW, O'Brien JJ, Solow EB. Laboratory evaluation of skin refrigerants used in dermabrasion. J Dermatol Surg Oncol 1985; 11:45–49
24. Dzubow LM. Survey of refrigerant and surgical techniques used for facial dermabrasion. J Am Acad Dermatol 1985;13:287–292
25. Hanke CW, Roenigk HH, Pinske JB. Complications of dermabrasion resulting from excessively cold skin refrigeration. J Dermatol Surg Oncol 1985;11:896
26. Griffiths CE, Russman AN, Majmudar G, et al. Restoration of collagen formation in photodamaged human skin by tretinoin (retinoic acid). N Engl J Med 1993;329:530–535
27. Fitzpatrick RE, Tope WD, Goldman MP, Satur NM. Pulsed carbon dioxide laser, trichloracetic acid, Baker–Gordon phenol, and dermabrasion: a comparative clinical and histologic study of cutaneous resurfacing in a porcine model. Arch Dermatol 1996;132:469–471
28. Campbell JP, Terhune MH, Shotts SD, Jones RO. An ultrastructural comparison of mechanical dermabrasion and carbon dioxide laser resurfacing in the minipig model. Arch Otolaryngol Head Neck Surg 1998;124:758–760
29. Giese SY, McKinney P, Roth SY, Zukowski M. The effect of chemosurgical peels and dermabrasion on dermal elastic tissue. Plast Reconstr Surg 1997;100:489–498
30. Holmkvist KA. Treatment of perioral rhytides: a comparison of dermabrasion and superpulsed carbon dioxide laser treatment. Delivered to the American Society for Dermatologic Surgery, Portland, Oregon, May 1998
31. Gin I, Chew J, Rau K, Amos D, Bridenstein J. Treatment of upper lip wrinkles: a comparison of the 950_sec dwell time CO_2 laser to manual tumescent dermabrasion. Dermatol Surg 1999;25:468–474
32. Baker TM. Dermabrasion as a complement to aesthetic surgery. Clin Plast Surg 1998;25:81–88
33. Stegman SJ. A comparative histologic study of effects of three peeling agents and dermabrasion on normal and sun-damaged skin. Aesthetic Plast Surg 1982;6:123–125
34. Fitzpatrick TB. The validity and practicality of sun-reactive skin types I through VI. Arch Dermatol 1988;124:869–871
35. Monheit GD. Chemical peeling for pigmentary dyschromias. J Cosmet Dermatol 1995;8:10–15
36. Wolfe SA. Chemical face peeling following therapeutic irradiation. Plast Reconstr Surg 1982;69:859
37. Monheit GD. Facial resurfacing may trigger the herpes simplex virus. J Cosmet Dermatol 1995;8:9–16
38. Glogau RG. Chemical peeling and aging skin. J Geriatr Dermatol 1994;2:30–35
39. Rubin M. Manual of Chemical Peels. Philadelphia: JB Lippincott; 1995:50–67
40. Moy LS, Murad H, Moy RL. Glycolic acid peels for the treatment of wrinkles and photoaging. J Dermatol Surg Oncol 1993;19:243–246

41. Monheit GD. Chemical peeling for pigmentary dyschromias. J Cosmet Dermatol 1995;8:10–15
42. Brody HJ. Trichloracetic acid application in chemical peeling, operative techniques. Plast Reconstr Surg 1995;2:127–128
43. Brody HJ. Variations and comparisons in medium depth chemical peeling. J Dermatol Surg Oncol 1989;15:953–963
44. Monheit GD. The Jessner's +TCA peel: a medium-depth chemical peel. J Dermatol Surg Oncol 1989;15:945–950
45. Lawrence N, Brody H, Alt T. Chemical peeling: resurfacing Techniques. In: Coleman III WP, Lawrence N, eds. Skin Resurfacing. 1st ed. Philadelphia: Williams & Wilkins; 1998:95
46. Monheit GD. The Jessner's-trichloracetic acid peel: an enhanced medium-depth chemical peel. Dermatol Clin 1995;13:277–283
47. Rubin M. Manual of Chemical Peels. Philadelphia: JB Lippincott; 1995:120–121
48. Monheit GD, Zeitouni NC. Skin resurfacing for photoaging: laser resurfacing versus chemical peeling. J Cosmet Dermatol 1997;10:11–22
49. Baker TJ, Gordon HL. Chemical face peeling. In: Surgical Rejuvenation of the Face. St. Louis: Mosby; 1986
50. Alt T. Occluded Baker–Gordon chemical peel. Review and update. J Dermatol Surg Oncol 1989;15:998
51. McCollough EG, Langsdon PR. Chemical peeling with phenol. In: Roenigk H, Roenigk R, eds. Dermatologic Surgery: Principles and Practice. New York: Marcel Dekker; 1989
52. Falanga V. Occlusive wound dressings. Arch Dermatol 1988;124:877
53. Goslen JB. Wound healing after cosmetic surgery. In: Coleman WP, Hanke CW, Alt TH, et al, eds. Cosmetic Surgery of the skin. Philadelphia: BC Decker; 1991:47–63
54. Monheit GD. Facial resurfacing may trigger the herpes simplex virus. J Cosmet Dermatol 1995;8:9–16

26 Ablative Laser Facial Skin Rejuvenation

Paul J. Carniol, Christopher B. Harmon, and Mark M. Hamilton

Current technology and techniques for facial skin rejuvenation have expanded significantly since the publication of Carniol's *Laser Skin Rejuvenation*.[1]

Laser resurfacing is only a portion of the armamentarium of most facial plastic surgeons. In addition to ablative resurfacing lasers there are now nonablative lasers and light devices that can be used to diminish epidermal lesions, stimulate neocollagen production, and tighten skin. Furthermore, as technology and techniques have improved we have been able to offer our patients a broader range of improvement, selecting the optimal available technology and setting higher standards for our results. Besides addressing texture, rhytids, and laxity, we should also address telangiectasias, vascular lesions, dyschromias, and lentigines. By addressing all of these issues we can optimize our patients' results. Acne and acne scars can be treated with ablative[2] and nonablative lasers.[3]

Laser Resurfacing

Currently, resurfacing can be performed with the carbon dioxide or erbium:yttrium-aluminum-garnet (Er:YAG) lasers. The depth of resurfacing can be varied depending on the desired result. Recently, superficial erbium laser resurfacing has become popular to reduce epidermal lesions, dyschromias, and rhytids.

Laser Biophysics

The concept of selective photothermolysis allows the surgeon to select a laser wavelength that is maximally absorbed by the targeted tissue component, the tissue chromophore. The primary chromophore for the CO_2 lasers and Er:YAG lasers is water. Whenever using a laser, one should consider other competitive chromophores that may absorb the wavelength. These competing chromophores may give additional benefit or create additional risks associated with using a particular laser wavelength.

For example, at a wavelength of 532 nm, there is absorption of laser energy by both oxyhemoglobin and melanin. Thus this type of laser can affect both vascular and pigmented lesions. The possibility of competing chromophores should be considered whenever a laser is being selected. This should also be considered whenever using an intense pulsed light device, which can produce a spectrum of wavelengths. The spectrum of emitted wavelengths will depend on the light source as well as any associated filters.

Another example of competing chromophores are the current hair reduction lasers, which exert their effect on melanin, the target chromophore. These lasers may also be absorbed by hemoglobin, which is a competing chromophore. This absorption by hemoglobin, the competing chromophore, can also result in injury to the blood vessels supplying the hair follicle, which is desirable.

Ninety percent of the epidermis is water. Consequently, water is the primary chromophore for many current resurfacing lasers. During resurfacing treatments, the intercellular water absorbs laser energy and instantly boils or vaporizes. The amount of energy that a laser delivers to the tissue and the time over which it is delivered determines the amount of tissue vaporized. For skin resurfacing, the objective is to vaporize the primary chromophore, water, while transferring a limited amount of heat to the surrounding collagen and other structures. This is because type I collagen is extremely heat-sensitive and becomes denatured at 60 to 70°C. Excessive thermal injury to the collagen can produce unwanted scarring.

The fluence of a laser represents the amount of energy (joules) that is applied to the surface area of tissue (centimeter squared). Therefore, fluence is expressed as J/cm^2. For CO_2 lasers, 0.04 J/mm^2 is the critical energy needed to overcome the tissue ablation threshold. For skin resurfacing, this is usually accomplished with 250 mJ per pulse using a 3 mm spot size. After each pulse the tissue is allowed to cool before the delivery of the next pulse. The tissue thermal relaxation time is the amount of time necessary between pulses for complete cooling to occur. With laser resurfacing, a very high energy is selected to vaporize target tissue almost instantly. This high energy allows very short pulse durations (1000 µs) to be used. Consequently, unwanted heat conduction to adjacent tissue is minimized. Power density, usually measured in watts, takes fluence, pulse duration, and treatment area into account (e.g., 60 W). A common misconception is that lower fluences or lower power densities will reduce the risk of scarring, when in reality the lower energy boils the water more slowly and causes greater nonspecific thermal injury. The water absorption is much stronger for the erbium laser. It ablates tissue with less adjacent thermal injury. Therefore, healing is faster than after resurfacing using a carbon dioxide laser. This makes superficial resurfacing with an erbium laser more acceptable to patients because there is a significantly shorter recovery time for an equal depth of resurfacing.

However, with the less adjacent thermal injury there is also less neocollagen production.

Histologic studies of biopsies taken immediately after laser resurfacing demonstrate a zone of tissue vaporization and ablation, beneath which lies a basophilic zone of thermal necrosis (**Fig. 26.1**).

The energy of the initial laser pass is absorbed by the water within the epidermis. Once the dermis has been entered, there is less water to absorb laser energy, and heat transfer contributes to more thermal injury with each successive pass (**Fig. 26.2**). So ideally, for the carbon dioxide laser a greater depth of ablation with a smaller number of passes and less thermal injury offers the least risk of scarring. Ultrastructural studies demonstrate smaller collagen fibers within larger collagen bundles in the papillary dermis (**Fig. 26.3A,B**). After laser resurfacing, wound-healing molecules, such as the glycoprotein tenascin, are expressed as new collagen that is produced in the papillary dermis (**Fig. 26.4**).

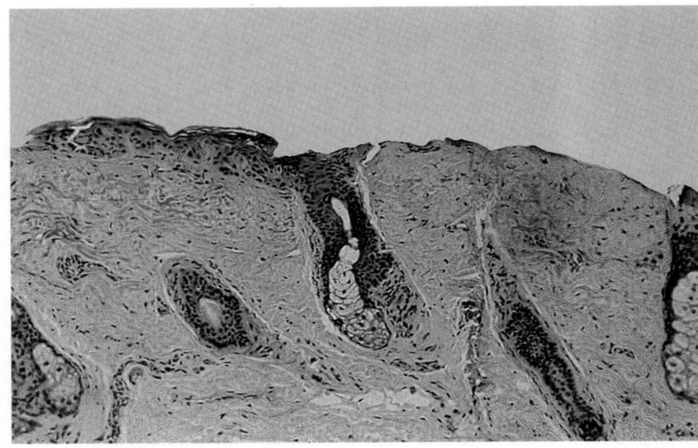

Fig. 26.1 Immediately following a single pass with the Ultrapulse laser (Coherent Medical Products, Palo Alto, CA), the epidermis has been ablated on the right half of the specimen. A thin layer of basophilic thermal necrosis can be seen beneath the ablated epidermis.

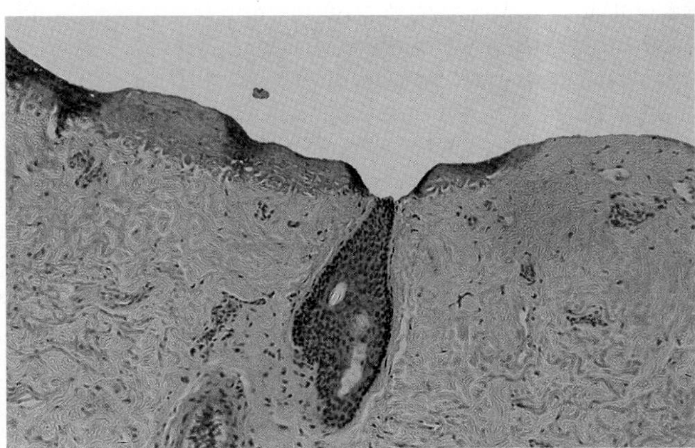

Fig. 26.2 After five passes with the Tru-Pulse (Tissue Technologies, Palomar Medical Products Inc., Lexington, MA) CO_2 laser, a broad zone of thermal necrosis can be seen beneath the ablated epidermis.

Laser Safety

The importance of proper laser safety technique cannot be overemphasized. Laser safety includes, but should not be limited to, the current standards of the Laser Institute of America (Orlando, Florida).

Protective Eyewear

The first safety issue with any laser is avoidance of eye injury. Injury can occur with visible and invisible laser wavelengths. Most of the current invisible resurfacing lasers also employ a separate simultaneous low-energy laser, usually helium–neon, which serves as an "aiming beam." This beam is visible when the laser is in use.

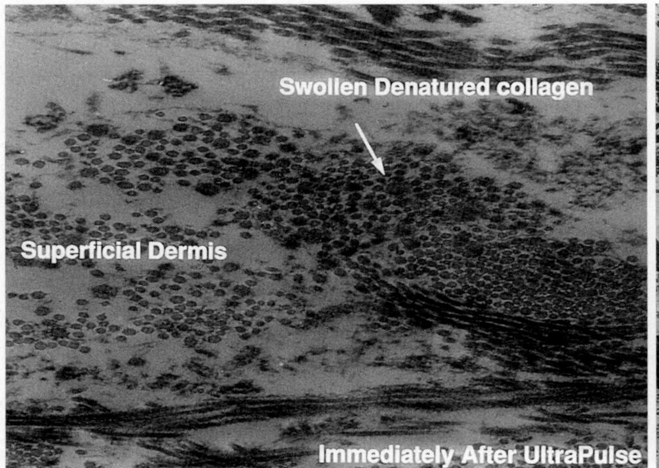

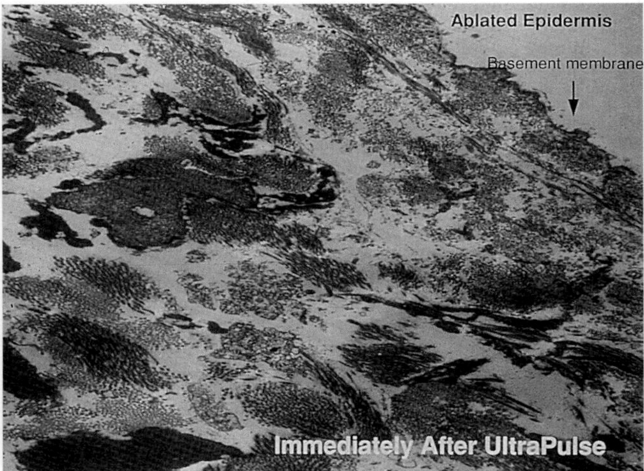

Fig. 26.3 (**A**) A scanning electron micrograph demonstrates a partially ablated basement membrane zone overlying thermally altered collagen fibers. (**B**) A higher-power electron micrograph reveals smaller denatured collagen fibers with the collagen bundles.

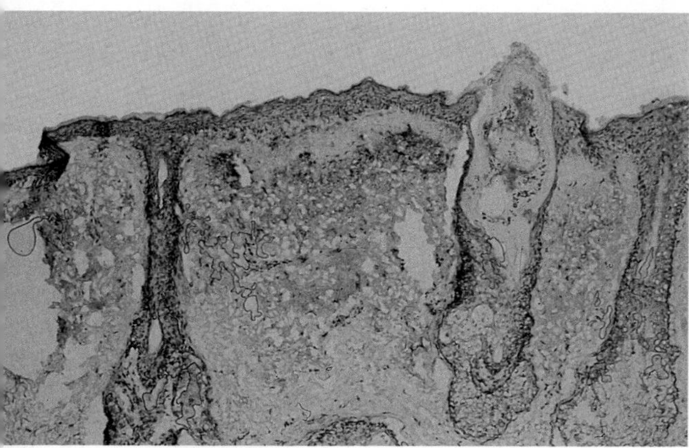

ig. 26.4 Immunoperoxidase staining demonstrates tenascin, a glycoprotein expressed during wound healing, throughout the newly egenerated papillary dermis

The eyes of the patient, laser room staff, and surgeon nust be protected from inadvertent injury. Everyone in the oom must have eye protection. The eye-protective wear nust be appropriate for the particular laser wavelength. The optical density (OD) and wavelength for which the yewear is protective should be printed on the eyewear rame. In general laser protective glasses or goggles should have an OD of at least 5. The OD scale is exponential. Thus an OD of 5 means that, for the specified wavelength noted on the side of the glasses or goggles, only one tenhousandth of the laser energy will get through the lenses. Patients should either have protective eyewear, or keep heir eyes closed and have wet eye pads over their closed ids when either the erbium or CO_2 resurfacing lasers are n use. When the surgeon is working on the thinner eyelid kin inside the osseous orbital margin, the eyes should be protected with nonreflecting metal eye shields.

Nonflammable Drapes

For resurfacing lasers, which have the greatest associated risk of laser fire, wet drapes or crinkled reflective foil will reduce the risk of spark-induced combustion.

Skin Preparation

All makeup and moisturizers must be removed before reatment is initiated. Alcohol-based skin preparations hould be avoided because these can create a fire hazard. t is safer to use aqueous-based solutions. Proper precauions must be taken for all skin cleansers.

Smoke Evacuator

Smoke evacuators with specifically designed laser filters o trap laser plume contents should be used.

Laser Masks

During a resurfacing procedure each person in the operating room should use a laser mask, which effectively filters infectious particles in the laser plume. These masks have a 0.1 mm filter pore size.

Anesthesia

Resurfacing can be performed under topical, local, regional, intravenous, or general anesthesia. The first author (PJC) uses topical anesthetic for superficial erbium laser resurfacing. Any additional passes will require additional anesthesia. Topical anesthesia alone is not adequate for carbon dioxide resurfacing. It is important not to exceed safe levels of local or topical anesthesia.

For resurfacing, the depth must be evaluated carefully. Care should be taken not to resurface too far into the reticular dermis. If too much epinephrine is used, the pink color that heralds entry into the papillary dermis may not be seen after an initial laser pass. Likewise, excessive epinephrine can obscure the pinpoint bleeding produced by erbium passes into the papillary dermis. Other skin landmarks can also be used to identify the resurfacing depth besides the vascular blush and the appearance of papillary dermal vessels. If needed, local anesthesia can be supplemented with intravenous anesthesia.

When general anesthesia is used, there is a greater risk of fire associated with the use of oxygen and an endotracheal tube. There are now metal endotracheal tubes, foil wrappings for plastic endotracheal tubes, and endotracheal tubes that are designed specifically to be used with lasers. This is important to prevent endotracheal tube ignition and a possible airway fire.

Skin Type Classification

It is important to consider skin type classification whenever considering laser or intense pulsed light therapy. The classification system is based on the response to ultraviolet light. In general, it also varies directly with the amount of melanin in the skin.

After laser resurfacing, possible problems with dyschromia depend on several factors, including the following: Fitzpatrick skin type classification; depth of resurfacing; type of laser used for resurfacing, which affects the amount of adjacent thermal injury; and any possible healing problems.

The Fitzpatrick skin classification system can be described as follows

Class I. Very fair skinned, always burn, never tan
Class II. Fair skin, burns, possible mild tan
Class III. Medium skin tone, sometimes burns, tans

Class IV. Darker medium skin tone, rarely burns, tans readily
Class V. Darker skin tone, rarely burns, intensely tans
Class VI. Darker skin tone, never burns, intensely tans

Due to potential problems with dyschromia, with current technology, the first author (PJC) does not routinely perform CO_2 laser resurfacing on patients with skin types IV, V, and VI.

Carbon Dioxide Laser Resurfacing

The CO_2 laser was invented in 1964 by Patel.[4] In the mid-1980s, CO_2 lasers were used by some physicians for the removal of exophytic skin lesions and limited cutaneous skin resurfacing. The usefulness of the continuous-wave CO_2 laser (10,600 nm) was limited by its long pulse duration, which had the potential to produce unwanted adjacent thermal damage and scarring.[5–8] As laser technology improved, higher-energy laser systems were developed that offered much shorter pulse durations more suitable for resurfacing. One of the first reported resurfacing treatments with a pulsed CO_2 laser was performed by David.[9] In 1993, Fitzpatrick reported use of the Ultrapulse CO_2 (Coherent Medical Products, Palo Alto, CA), which produced relatively high fluence and much shorter pulse duration (1000 µs) than earlier pulsed or superpulsed CO_2 lasers. This combination provided relatively clean vaporization with a limited zone of adjacent thermal injury. This was the first CO_2 laser that could be predictably used for the removal of superficial skin tumors and for cutaneous resurfacing.[10]

Initially, in describing CO_2 laser resurfacing it was recommended that resurfacing be performed until a "chamois" appearance of the tissues was achieved. In 1995, Carniol recommended the first modification of this technique to decrease postresurfacing complications and facilitate healing.[11] Other pulsed and scanned lasers, such as Silktouch and Feathertouch (Sharplan Lasers, Allendale, NJ) and Paragon (Laser Sonics, Leichhardt, Australia), were also developed for facial resurfacing. Most of these lasers utilize a 900 to 1000 µs pulse duration or a rapid scan that created a relatively similar fluence and energy exposure duration. Many laser systems employ a computerized scanner, which allows larger surface areas to be treated in a very systematic, predictable fashion.[12]

Preoperative Preparation

Patients who undergo deep resurfacing require intensive management. There is still controversy over whether skin preparation is needed for resurfacing. Some surgeons advocate pretreatment with hydroquinone, isotretinoin, or glycolic acids.[13–15] Other physicians do not use any formal preparation before the procedure. Most surgeons agree that avoidance of sun before resurfacing is important. Exposure to the sun before resurfacing can activate the melanocytes and predispose the patient to hyperpigmentation. The importance of prophylactic antivirals for all patients undergoing deep resurfacing has been well documented.[16] Treatment is initiated 2 days prior to resurfacing for those with a history of herpetic outbreak and 1 day prior for all other patients. This antiviral therapy should be continued for 10 to 14 days until all reepithelialization is complete.

The use of prophylactic antibiotics is much less universal. Many surgeons give antibiotics before and after the procedure to diminish the incidence of bacterial infection with prolonged or closed-mask dressings. Some physicians believe that prophylactic antibiotics do not diminish the chance of postresurfacing infection.[17] Physicians who use prophylactic antibiotics frequently give prophylactic antifungal medication to prevent yeast infections underneath the dressings.[18]

Intraoperative Techniques

Prior to resurfacing treatments, patients can be marked if needed, and cosmetic units outlined. It is particularly important to mark the patient's mandibular margin while he or she is sitting up because the skin moves when the patient is supine. Supine marking can cause an error in marking. Care must be taken not to place any marks on denuded skin because of the risk of permanent tattooing. Partial resurfacing treatments should be feathered along the boundary of a given cosmetic unit (i.e., orbital rim, nasolabial folds). The margin of a full-face treatment should be feathered along the mandible to produce a natural transition to the untreated skin of the neck (**Fig. 26.5A,B**).

In monitoring the depth of treatment with each pass, the laser energy and power settings are much less important than the clinical end points. With CO_2 laser resurfacing, a pink color can be seen as one enters the papillary dermis. As resurfacing progresses, this color changes to a yellow chamois within the reticular dermis. Most surgeons use saline gauze to remove vaporized tissue between each CO_2 pass to prevent thermal stacking.

Because of the hourglass shape of the pilosebaceous unit, the diameter of the pores enlarges as the level of ablation deepens. This can also be used as a resurfacing depth indicator. Furthermore, variation of skin thickness from one cosmetic unit to another calls for an adjusted number of laser passes and settings. Obviously, less tissue penetration is tolerated in the thinner skin of the eyelid than the thicker, appendage-abundant skin of

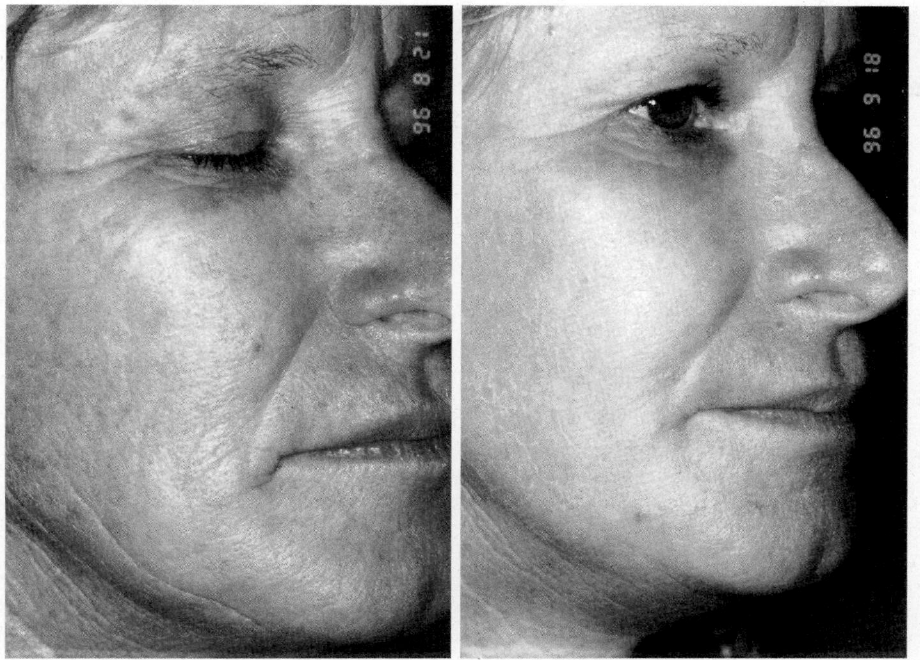

Fig. 26.5 (**A**) Extensive photodamage prior to full-face CO_2 resurfacing. (**B**) One month after full-face resurfacing, a natural transition from the treated skin of the cheek to the untreated skin of the neck is created by feathering along the mandibles.

the midcheek (**Fig. 26.6A,B**). Likewise, individual variation between patients requires less aggressive passes on thin, dry skin as opposed to deeper ablation on thicker, sebaceous skin. For example, the photodamaged thin skin of a 65-year-old female patient (**Fig. 26.7A,B**) will tolerate less laser energy than the skin of a 25-year-old male patient with acne scars. Many times the pathology (i.e., rhytids or scars) extends beyond the safety zone of treatment. The other important end point of laser resurfacing, which usually precedes entry into the reticular dermis, is the disappearance of photodamage, rhytids, or further tissue tightening.

Postoperative Care

As recognized by previous dermabraders, semiocclusive wound dressings have decreased the time of reepithelialization to as short as 5 to 7 days by maintaining an environment of critical humidity for epithelial cell migration.[19] After resurfacing more rapid healing, less pain, less scarring, and less erythema are seen with these dressings than with open or desiccated wounds. Most surgeons change these dressings daily for 3 to 5 days. Open wound care with occlusive ointments can also be used.

Once reepithelialization is complete, strict sun avoidance is critical until all postoperative erythema has subsided (usually 2 to 3 months). This decreases the chances of postinflammatory hyperpigmentation. Fragrance-free moisturizers will improve skin hydration while avoiding contact sensitization. Some physicians use class I and II topical steroids to reduce postoperative edema. The first author (PJC) does not use these routinely. They should only be used for brief periods. Hypoallergenic, noncomedogenic makeup can be used once reepithelialization is complete to camouflage residual redness. Typically, green- or yellow-based foundations will neutralize the red postoperative erythema. There is significantly less erythema after erbium resurfacing than after carbon dioxide resurfacing.

Complications

Transient postinflammatory hyperpigmentation occurs frequently at 2 to 6 weeks postoperatively. This darkening is sun induced and usually clears nicely with sun avoidance, hydroquinones, retinoic acid, and mild topical steroids.

Hypopigmentation, on the other hand, is permanent and unpredictable. This complication usually has a delayed onset of several months. It occurs in 10 to 30% of patients after deep carbon dioxide resurfacing.

Scarring is the most feared problem, beginning with persisting hyperemia that becomes indurated and nodular. Treatment with intralesional steroids, steroid

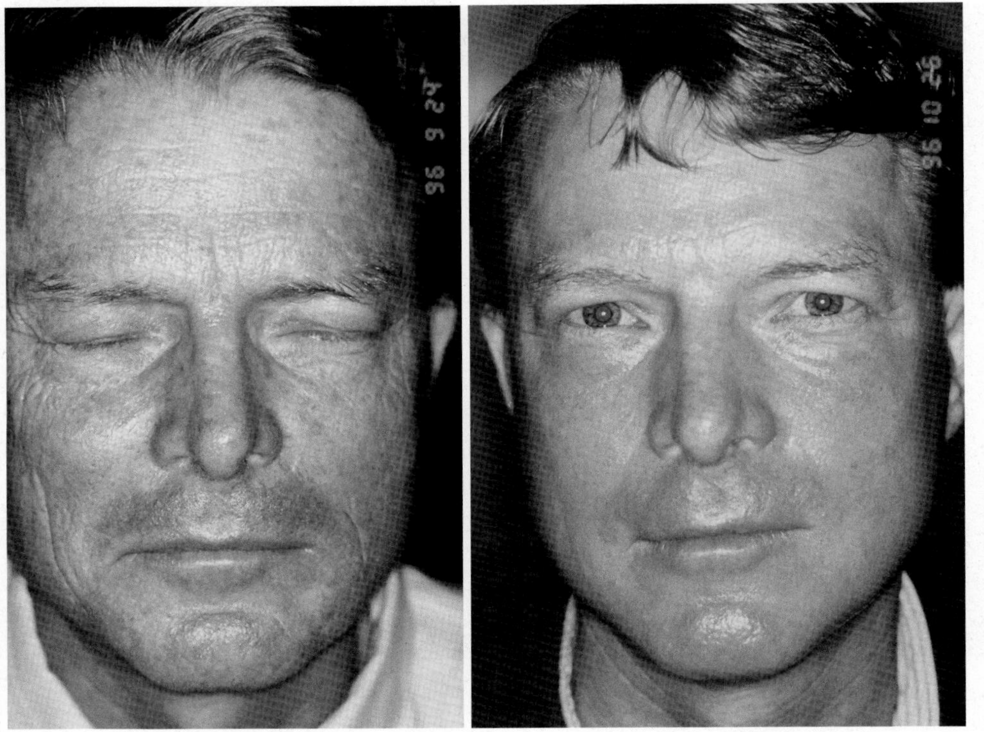

Fig. 26.6 (**A**) Preoperative photoaging and rhytids can be seen extending onto the lateral lower eyelids. The eyelid skin will be treated with one or two fewer passes than the lower face. (**B**) Following full-face laser surgery, a smaller number of passes over the eyelids prevents unwanted scarring or ectropion.

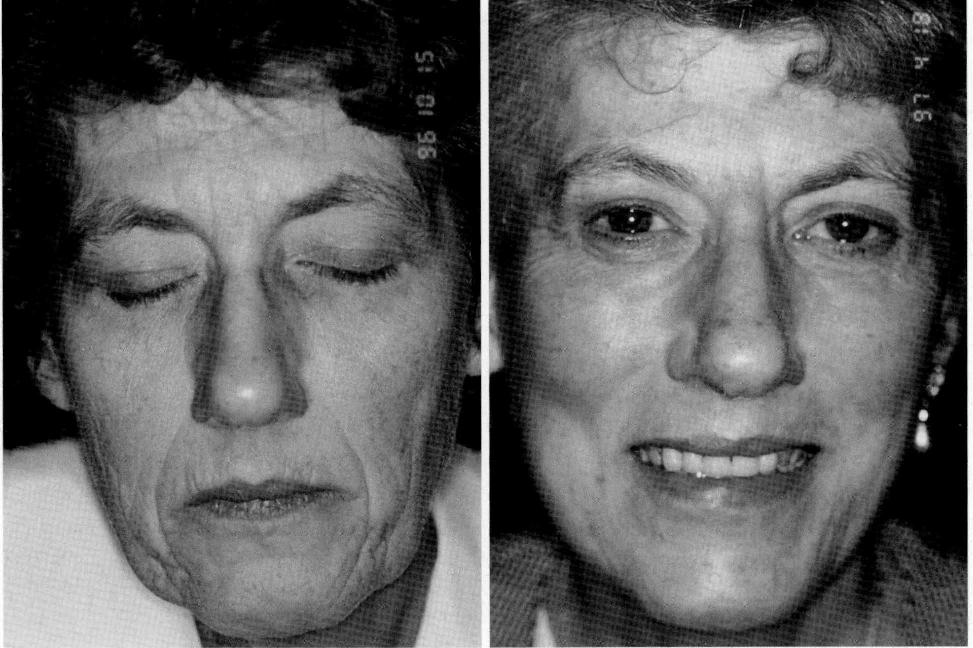

Fig. 26.7 (**A**) Rhytids and photoaging in a thin-skinned 65-year-old woman. (**B**) Six months following full-face resurfacing, rhytids and photodamage have improved but postoperative erythema persists over the malar prominence.

impregnated tape, or topical steroids is highly successful. Vascular lasers can also be used to reduce scar hypertrophy. Certain areas of the face, such as the malar prominence, upper lip, and mandible are prone to hypertrophic scarring. Frequently these scars can be avoided with optimal management as described in other texts such as *Laser Skin Rejuvenation*.[1]

Viral infections are heralded by intense pain and can occur despite the use of antiviral prophylaxis. They are usually seen 7 to 10 days following surgery as reepithelialization is concluding. A herpetic breakthrough should be treated aggressively with zosteriform dosages of medication.

Bacterial infections can also produce postoperative pain and greatly increase the risk of scarring. Furthermore, secondary fungal infections can occur when dressings are worn for more than 24 hours without being changed, or when tissue debridement and exudate removal are inadequately performed with dressing changes.

A much higher incidence of contact dermatitis occurs following laser resurfacing to ointments such as Neosporin (Johnson & Johnson Consumer Companies, Inc., New Brunswick, NJ), Polysporin (McNeill-PPC, Inc., Fort Washington, PA), and even petrolatum. Discontinue the use of the offending agent and treat with midpotency topical steroids, as well as systemic steroids.

Careful attention to the patient's skin type, areas of treatment, and laser parameters can greatly maximize surgical benefits while minimizing potential side effects. Some physicians advocate single-pass carbon dioxide laser resurfacing to minimize the associated risks.[20] Furthermore, close and attentive follow-up during the postoperative period will anticipate and reverse nearly all untoward outcomes and complications. The most important postoperative routine is constant encouragement and patient handholding.

Erbium Laser Resurfacing

The development of the Er:YAG laser for resurfacing arose out of the desire to develop a laser with a higher margin of safety and control. The Er:YAG laser has a wavelength of 2940 nm. This wavelength has a much higher water absorption coefficient than the CO_2 (10,600 nm).[21] This difference results in a 10-fold greater absorption of the erbium laser in skin as compared with the CO_2. This greater absorption leads to thinner more precise tissue removal with less adjacent thermal injury.

Because of these differences, erbium lasers are associated with shorter recovery times, less postoperative erythema, less risk of hypo- and hyper-pigmentation, and less scarring. Because there is less adjacent tissue thermal effect there is also less associated tissue tightening. Unlike the carbon dioxide laser the erbium laser is not hemostatic. Many laser surgeons reserve the erbium laser for superficial resurfacing, although similar results on deep rhytids have been reported.[18]

Advancements with erbium technology have moved in two directions. One type of advancement tries to balance the benefits of the erbium laser while trying to add some of the benefits of the CO_2 laser. Some systems have actually combined both wavelengths.[22,23] One of the current erbium lasers can use two erbium lasers simultaneously. One of these can be adjusted to cause greater adjacent tissue injury to produce greater tissue tightening. This laser achieves the greater thermal injury by increasing the pulse duration and therefore heats the tissues more slowly. Alternatively, too much energy can cause a deeper level of vaporization than is desired. With current lasers, collagen is affected by the heat that is generated with resurfacing. The greater the thermal injury, the more new-collagen synthesis. In the future, resurfacing lasers that are well absorbed by water and collagen[24] may be used clinically. The technique for erbium laser resurfacing is very similar to that of the CO_2 laser.[25]

Superficial Er:YAG laser resurfacing can be performed using topical anesthesia. Deeper resurfacing will require at least local anesthesia. As for the carbon dioxide laser some patients will require sedation for more aggressive resurfacing. Fluences are altered based on the areas that are treated. The absolute depth of resurfacing varies depending on the skin thickness. Areas of thin skin or increased risk of scarring such as the eyelids and mandibular margin are treated with more superficial resurfacing. At all times care must be taken not to resurface too deeply. Because thermal stacking is not typically an issue with erbium resurfacing, overlap of pulses can be used to avoid any pattern effect. Removal of vaporized tissue residual between passes is important to minimize excessive adjacent tissue thermal injury. The end point is determined by removing the visible pathology or by the clinical signs of resurfacing depth, which include pore size and bleeding. Care should be taken not to resurface too deeply into the reticular dermis because this can result in scarring.

The other advancement is erbium lasers that are designed for superficial resurfacing (FriendlyLight Laser Corp., Tarrytown, NY). Superficial resurfacing can often be performed with topical or local anesthesia. The goal of this technique is too remove epithelial lesions and superficial rhytids and to lessen deeper rhytids. This creates the least adjacent thermal injury. Most patients will have some pinkness for 3 to 7 days. Depending on the depth of superficial erbium resurfacing, patients may be able to resume their regular activities as soon as 3 days after the procedure is performed. Patients should be reminded of the need for sun precautions to minimize the potential for postinflammatory hyperpigmentation.

Postoperative care is similar to that after CO_2 laser resurfacing. The wound surface should be kept moist to optimize epithelialization. This can be achieved with a topical ointment such as Aquaphor (Beiersdorf, Inc., Wilton, CT). Starting 24 hours after the procedure the wound should be gently cleaned twice a day with saline or water to remove all superficial serum and debris. Topical ointment is discontinued when the area has reepithelialized. This occurs much quicker than with the CO_2 laser. For superficial erbium resurfacing this can occur within 48 to 72 hours. For deeper resurfacing this may take up to 1 week. Postinflammatory hyperpigmentation occurs less often. Unless deep resurfacing is performed delayed hypopigmentation is rare.

Nonablative Rejuvenation

Nonablative rejuvenation has become popular as new technology and procedures for facial rejuvenation. Nonablative rejuvenation refers to the ability of a laser or light energy source to selectively create selective thermal injury to the underlying dermis with minimal effect on the epidermis. This area of facial skin laser treatment is continuing to expand due to strong patient demand. Many patients prefer the minimal recovery associated with nonablative treatments even though the final result may not be as dramatic as can be obtained with laser resurfacing or a deep phenol peel.

Of these devices, many cool the overlying epidermis to protect the skin from the emitted energy. This is achieved with a cooled handpiece or dynamic cryogen device delivering a cooling spray. These devices include the 532 nm laser, the 585 nm pulsed dye laser, 1064 nm Q-switched neodymium(Nd):YAG laser, the 1320 nm long pulsed Nd: YAG with a coolant spray, the 1450 nm diode with a coolant spray, the 1540 nm erbium:glass, and a broadband light source or intense pulsed light (IPL), which emits a continuous spectrum of 515 nm to 1200 nm.

Several factors can affect the results of treatment. In general the longer the wavelength the greater the depth of penetration.

Selective absorption by chromophores includes hemoglobin, water-containing tissue (collagen), and melanin. This absorption can induce neocollagenesis.[26] The prospect of dermal remodeling without the morbidity of traditional ablative surgery is appealing, although there have been many recent studies documenting the efficacy of these devices in improvement of wrinkles.[27–30]

532 nm Laser Resurfacing

The frequency-doubled Nd:YAG laser has been studied as a potential nonablative laser with mixed results. Both the Versapulse laser (Lumenis, Inc., Santa Clara, CA) and the Diolite laser (Iridex, Mountain View, CA) allow nonablative resurfacing at this wavelength. Treatments result in minimal erythema, which resolves within 24 hours. Pain is minimal. Multiple treatments are recommended. Studies have demonstrated improvement with both systems.[31,32]

1320 nm Nd:YAG Laser

The 1320 nm wavelength is within the optimal range to target the dermis and it has been associated with more success than the 1064. In addition, with the Cooltouch system (New Star Lasers, Roseville, CA) a cryogen spray has been added to protect the epidermis during treatment. A second-generation device has been introduced that is equipped with a thermal sensing device to assure optimal epidermal temperature. This was added in attempts to minimize occasional pitting and scarring seen with the first device. Both systems have proven effective in wrinkle reduction as well as in acne scar treatment.[33] A new third-generation device has been added with pre- and posttreatment cooling to enhance comfort.

1450 nm Diode Laser

The 1450 nm wavelength, like the 1320 nm, offers excellent dermal penetration and is well absorbed by water. The Smoothbeam (Candela Corp., Wayland, MA) combines this wavelength with a cryogen spray for epidermal protection. Studies using this wavelength have demonstrated modest improvements in rhytid reduction.[34,35] A second study by Tanzi and others compared the 1450 nm with the 1320 nm in the treatment of atrophic facial scars.[36] The 1450 nm diode demonstrated superior clinical scores but also had more prolonged posttreatment erythema as well as a higher incidence of hyperpigmentation. A series of treatments with this laser followed by trichloroacetic acid chemical peels resulted in a significant improvement in rolling and boxcar type acne scars.[36]

Fraxel

The fraxel laser (Reliant Technologies, Inc., Palo Altos, CA) is based on a different method of performing nonablative treatments called fractional photothermolysis. This laser emits a 1500 nm wavelength, which is highly absorbed by water. The laser creates hundreds of microscopic areas of thermal injury called microthermal zones. Surrounding each of these zones is uninjured tissue which allows rapid reepithelialization, typically within 24 hours. Patients will experience mild erythema, which resolves within a week. Multiple treatments are required. Initial studies have been positive demonstrating rhytid reduction as well as improved skin texture and skin tightening.[37]

Other Devices and Uses of Nonablative Rejuvenation

A variety of devices are available for the treatment of facial telangiectasias and dyspigmentation seen in photoaging. The IPL device, emitting a broad spectrum of 515 nm to 1200 nm, has been effective in the treatment of both these conditions.[38] Poikiloderma on the neck has also been successfully treated with the IPL device.[39] Other vascular lasers that target the chromophore oxyhemoglobin include the 532 nm KTP, the 595 nm pulse dye, the 755 nm alexandrite, the 800 nm diode, the 940 nm diode,[40] and the 1064 nm Nd:YAG.

The solar lentigo is the most frequently encountered pigmented lesion in photoaging. The chromophore in solar lentigines is melanin. Melanin can also be successfully treated with some of the vascular lasers, including the 532 nm, 595 nm pulse dye, 694 nm ruby, 755 nm alexandrite, 800 nm diode, and 1064 nm Nd:YAG. As a general rule, in selecting a laser, the longer wavelength penetrates deeper, making it effective for deeper targets; the shorter wavelengths are better suited for more superficial targets.

Another new technology that uses radiofrequency waves as the energy source for nonablative tissue tightening has recently been developed. Like other nonablative modalities simultaneous cooling is used to help protect the overlying epidermis from burning. In contrast to traditional nonablative laser and IPL devices, which use light, the radiofrequency device (Thermage, Hayward, CA) uses radio waves to generate heat in dermal tissue. In a small study of 15 patients, 14 showed some improvement of nasolabial folds, cheek contour, and mandibular and marionette lines.[41]

A filtered, pulsed infrared light, with a chilled tip (Titan, Cutera, CA) is also being used for nonablative tissue tightening. This light is used to heat the dermal tissues to stimulate tissue contraction and tightening. These treatments have minimal associated discomfort and are very well tolerated.

Currently, there is a strong patient demand for nonablative rejuvenation, with its minimal associated downtime. Most patients cannot take the time from their busy lives required for the recovery from a deep resurfacing procedure. These are new and evolving modalities that may in time produce more dramatic results.

References

1. Carniol PJ, ed. Laser Skin Rejuvenation. Philadelphia: Lippincott-Raven; 1998
2. Carniol PJ. Feathertouch, Silktouch. In: Carniol PJ, ed. Laser Skin Rejuvenation. Philadelphia: Lippincott-Raven; 1998
3. Carniol PJ, Vinatheya J, Carniol ET. Evaluation of acne scar treatment with a 1450 nm mid infrared laser and 30% trichloroacetic acid peels. Arch Facial Plast Surg 2005;7:251–255
4. Stellar S, Polanyi TG. Lasers in neurosurgery: a historical overview. J Clin Laser Med Surg 1992;10:399–411
5. Walsh JT Jr, Flotte TH, Anderson RR, et al. Pulsed CO_2 laser tissue ablation: effect of tissue type and pulsed duration on thermal damage. Lasers Surg Med 1988;8:119–124
6. Lanzafame RJ, Naim JO, Rogers DW, et al. Comparison of continuous wave, chop wave, and superpulse laser wounds. Lasers Surg Med 1988;8:119–124
7. Welch AJ. The thermal response of laser irradiated tissue. IEEE J Quantum Electron 1984;20:147
8. Kuo T, Speyer MT, Ries WR, Reinisch L. Collagen thermal damage and collagen synthesis after cutaneous laser resurfacing. Lasers Surg Med 1998;23:66–71
9. David LM. Laser vermillion ablation for actinic cheilitis. J Dermatol Surg Oncol 1985;11:605–608
10. Fitzpatrick RE. The Ultrapulse CO_2 laser: selective photothermolysis of epidermal tumors. Lasers Surg Med Suppl 1993;5:56
11. Carniol PJ. Master's seminar: Laser Resurfacing. Annual Meeting of the American Academy of Facial Plastic and Reconstructive Surgery, Sept. 1995, New Orleans
12. Weinstein C. CO_2 laser resurfacing. In: Coleman WP, Hanke CW, Alt TH, Asken S, eds. Cosmetic Surgery of the Skin: Principles and Techniques. St Louis: Mosby Year-Book, Inc.; 1997:112–177
13. Kligman AM, Grove GL, Hirose R, et al. Topical tretinoin and epithelial wound healing. Arch Dermatol 1986;15:836–839
14. Hung VC, Lee JY, Zitelli JA, et al. Topical tretinoin and epithelial wound healing. Arch Dermatol 1989;125:65–69
15. Mandy SLH. Tretinoin in the preoperative and postoperative management of dermabrasion. J Am Acad Dermatol 1986;15:878–879
16. Perkins SW, Sklarew EC. Prevention of facial herpetic infections after chemical peel and dermabrasion: new treatment strategies in the prophylaxis of patients undergoing procedures in the perioral area. Plast Reconstr Surg 1996;98:427–433
17. Perkins SW, Sklarew EC. Prevention of facial herpetic infections after chemical peel and dermabrasion: new treatment strategies in the prophylaxis of patients undergoing procedures in the perioral area. Plast Reconstr Surg 1996;98:427–433
18. Walia S, Alster TS. Cutaneous CO_2 laser resurfacing infection rate with and without prophylactic antibiotics. Dermatol Surg 1999;25: 851–861
19. Pianski JB. Dressings for dermabrasion: new aspects. J Dermatol Surg Oncol 1987;13:673
20. Ruiz-Esparza J. One-pass carbon dioxide laser resurfacing. In: Carniol PJ ed. Facial Rejuvenation. New York: Wiley-Liss; 2000:305–311
21. Jasin M. Achieving superior resurfacing results with erbium:YAG laser. Arch Facial Plast Surg 2002;4:262–266
22. Tiekmeier G, Goldberg DJ. Skin resurfacing with the erbium:YAG laser. Dermatol Surg 1997;23:685–687
23. Kye YC. Resurfacing of pitted facial scars with a pulsed Er:YAG laser. Dermatol Surg 1997;23:880–883
24. Payne BP, Nishioka NS, Mikic BB, Venugopalam V. Comparison of pulsed CO_2 laser ablation 10.6 microns and 9.5 microns. Lasers Surg Med 1998;23:1–6
25. Caniglia RJ. Erbium:YAG laser skin resurfacing. Facial Plast Surg Clin North Am 2004;12:373–377
26. Nelson JS, Majaaron B, Kelly KM. What is nonablative photorejuvenation of human skin? Semin Cutan Med Surg 2002;21: 238–250
27. Zelickson BD, Kilmer SL, Bernstein E, et al. Pulsed dye laser therapy for sun damaged skin. Lasers Surg Med 1999;25:229–236

28. Fournier N, Dahan S, Barneon G, et al. Nonablative remodeling: clinical, histologic, ultrasound, imaging, and profilometric evaluation of a 1540 nm Er:glass laser. Dermatol Surg 2001;27:799–806
29. Goldberg DJ. Full-face nonablative dermal remodeling with a 1320 nm Nd:YAG laser. Dermatol Surg 2000;26:915–918
30. Bitter PH. Noninvasive rejuvenation of photodamaged skin using serial, full-face intense pulsed light treatments. Dermatol Surg 2000;26: 835–842
31. Bernstein EF, Ferreira M, Anderson D. A pilot investigation to subjectively measure treatment effect and side effect profile of nonablative skin remodeling using a 532 nm, 2 ms pulse duration laser. J Cosmet Laser Ther 2001;3:137–141
32. Carniol PJ, Farley S, Friedman A. Long pulse 532 nm diode laser for nonablative facial skin rejuvenation. Arch Facial Plast Surg 2003;5: 511–513
33. Goldberg DJ. Full face nonablative dermal remodeling with a 1320 nm Nd:YAG laser. Dermatol Surg 2000;26:915
34. Tanzi EL, Williams CM, Alster TS. Treatment of facial rhytids with nonablative 1450 nm diode laser: a controlled clinical and histologic study. Dermatol Surg 2003;29:124–128
35. Carniol PJ, Vynatheya J, Carniol E. Evaluation of acne scar treatment with a 1450 nm midinfrared laser and 30% trichloroacetic acid peels. Arch Facial Plast Surg 2005;7:251–254
36. Ross EV, Hardaway C, Barnette D, Keel D, Paithankar DY. Nonablative skin remodeling with a 1450 nm diode laser. Proceedings of the 20th annual meeting of the World Congress of Dermatology; Paris, France
37. Manstein D, Herron GS, Sink RK, Tanner H, Anderson RR. Fractional resurfacing: a new concept for cutaneous remodeling using microscopic patterns of thermal injury. Lasers Surg Med 2004;34:426–438
38. Weiss RA, Weiss MA, Beasley KL. Rejuvenation of photoaged skin: 5-years results with intense pulsed light of the face, neck, and chest. Dermatol Surg 2002;28:1115–1119
39. Weiss RA, Goldman MP, Weiss MA. Treatment of poikiloderma of Civatte with an intense pulsed light source. Dermatol Surg 2000;26:823–827
40. Carniol PJ, Price J, Olive A. Treatment of telangiectasias with the 532-nm and the 532/940 nm diode laser. Facial Plast Surg 2005;21: 117–119
41. Ruiz-Esparza J, Gomez JB. The medical face lift: a noninvasive, nonsurgical approach to tissue tightening in facial skin nonablative radio frequency. Dermatol Surg 2003;29:325–332 discussion 332

27 Nonablative Facial Skin Rejuvenation

R. James Koch

It is generally agreed that we have excellent modalities to resurface or peel the superficial layers of skin. This may be accomplished by the use of ablative lasers or by other modalities such as chemical peels and dermabrasion.[1,2] Nonablative skin rejuvenation would certainly be desirable when there is no indication for superficial skin peeling, for example, if there was no actinic damage, pigment irregularities, or texture problems. In addition, leaving the epidermis and upper dermis intact would reduce the healing process.

Collagen contraction begins to occur at ~55°C. This can be observed immediately and is well known to those who have used the pulsed carbon dioxide (CO_2) laser. New collagen may then be produced as part of a controlled wound-healing response. Most of the nonablative devices that are currently available are simply different ways to heat tissue at a desired depth to initiate the foregoing.

This chapter presents an overview of the main currently available nonablative devices, with special emphasis on the ThermaCool TC System (Thermage, Inc., Hayward, CA) because of the impact it has had in this area.

1320 nm Nd:YAG Laser System

The CoolTouch CT3 (New Star Lasers, Roseville, CA) is a 1320 nm neodymium:yttrium-aluminum-garnet laser (Nd:YAG) (**Fig. 27.1**). The CoolTouch 1 was the first commercially available system designed exclusively for selective dermal heating, and it has evolved over the years.

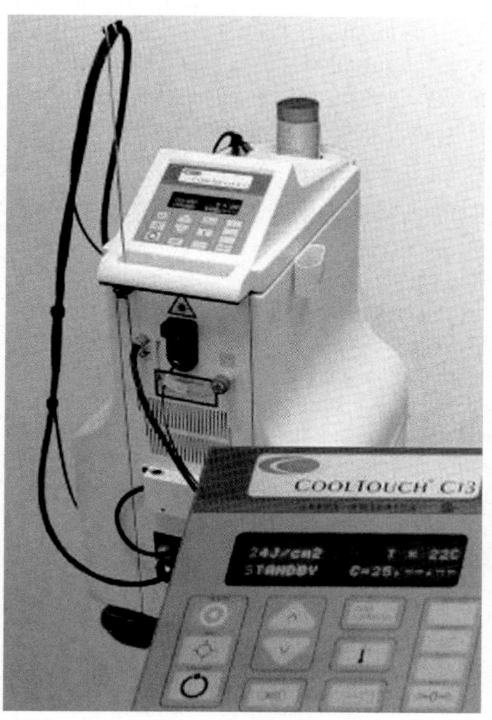

Fig. 27.1 The CoolTouch CT3 (New Star Lasers, Roseville, CA) is a 1320 nm neodymium:yttrium-aluminum-garnet laser.

The 1320 nm irradiation is nonspecifically absorbed in the human dermis. When coupled with cryogen cooling of the epidermis, a dermal wound can be created with little risk of epidermal damage. A noncontact dynamic cooling agent (tetrafluoroethane) is sprayed onto the skin for 30 msec, with a delay of 40 msec before each laser pulse (precooling modality). This cooling protects the superficial 50 to 100 mm of epidermis and allows adequate heating of the subsurface layers to stimulate fibroblasts, which will create new collagen. A thermal sensor within the laser handpiece monitors pretreatment skin temperatures as well as peak therapeutic temperatures.

The CoolTouch CT3 has been cleared for acne, acne scar, and wrinkle treatments on all skin types. Overall patient satisfaction has been reported in the subjective improvement of skin texture. Histological increases in collagen concentration in 50% of subjects do not necessarily correlate with clinical improvement. Slight but statistically significant improvement occurs in patients with Fitzpatrick skin types I or II and mild, moderate, or severe rhytids.[3]

1064 nm Q-Switched Nd:YAG Laser System

This group includes the Medlite C6 (HOYA Conbio, Fremont, CA). The chromophores for the 1064 nm radiation are, in decreasing order, melanin, hemoglobin, and water. Water weakly absorbs laser energy at this wavelength and is gently heated over the optical penetration depth of the beam (~5 to 10 mm); however, severe heating remains localized to hemoglobin and melanin.[3] It is believed that the absorbed laser energy causes the localized rupture of capillaries and melanosomes, giving rise to a partially devitalized epidermis and subsequent skin repair. Clinical indications for the 1064 nm Q-switched Nd:YAG laser include facial telangiectasia, acne rosacea, and mild solar-damaged skin. Mild improvement has been reported in 97% of class I rhytids, and some improvement has been seen in class II wrinkles.[3]

1100 nm to 1800 nm Spectrum

The Titan (Cutera, Inc., Brisbane, CA) uses an infrared light source to tighten skin (**Fig. 27.2**). It claims to heat the dermis to cause collagen contraction while preserving the epidermis through continuous cooling. In addition, it claims to stimulate long-term collagen rebuilding that leaves patients with younger-looking skin. At the time of this writing, the U.S. Food and Drug Administration (FDA) has cleared the Titan for topical heating, for the purpose of elevating tissue temperature for a temporary increase in local circulation where applied.

It operates between 1100 nm and 1800 nm, and the light source outputs from 30 J/cm^2 to 65 J/cm^2. Based upon the area being treated this results in heating at depths from 1 to 3 mm. The epidermal temperature is kept at a safe level of below 40°C by pre-, during, and post-cooling of the epidermis by a clear sapphire tip

Fluences of 36 to 46 J/cm^2 are typically used over soft tissue areas such as cheeks and the submental area. Fluences are based on patient tolerance. (Patients should be able to tolerate the treatment with no more than a moderate level of discomfort.) Two to three treatment sessions are commonly performed at monthly intervals. At the time of this writing I could not locate any published clinical studies that utilized the Titan.

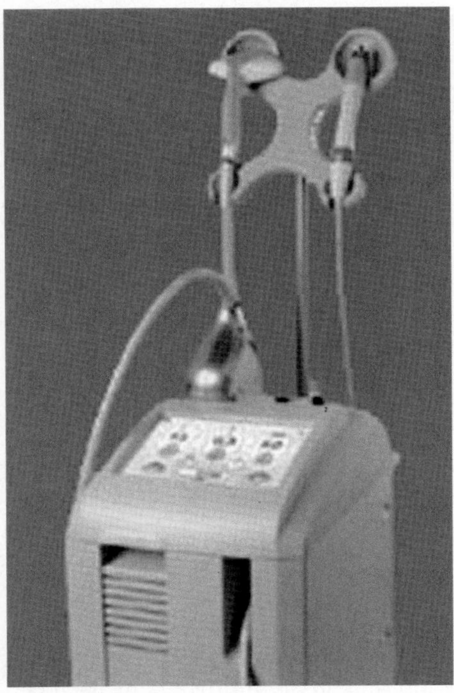

Fig. 27.2 The Titan (Cutera, Inc., Brisbane, CA) uses an infrared light source (1100 nm to 1800 nm).

Intense Pulsed Light

Intense pulsed light (IPL) devices include the Quantum SR (Lumenis, Santa Clara, CA), Estelux (Palomar, Burlington, MA), Prolite (Alderm, Irvine, CA), and Aurora (Syneron, Yokneam, Israel). IPL is a nonlaser light source that emits a broad, continuous spectrum of electromagnetic radiation ranging from 500 to 1200 nm. With cutoff filters, shorter wavelength portions of the spectrum can be blocked. Depending on the filter used, the longer portion of the transmitted spectrum targets hemoglobin, melanin, and water to varying degrees (shorter filters favor hemoglobin and melanin heating).[3] The effect on dermal collagen is presumably caused by heat diffusion from the vasculature and the secretion of inflammatory mediators induced by direct vessel heating. Tissue water is also directly heated to a lesser degree.

IPL devices are effective in the treatment of small vessel vascular and pigmented lesions. Vascular problems such as rosacea, telangiectasia, and postlaser erythema respond well to IPL therapy. Pigmentary problems such as hyperpigmentation, melasma, lentigines, postinflammatory hyperpigmentation, and lines of demarcation after laser/chemical peels are also treatable with IPL therapy.[4] The device is reportedly useful in the treatment of class I or II facial rhytids.

Radio Frequency

The ThermaCool TC System has been cleared by the FDA for the noninvasive treatment of facial rhytids. Currently all other uses are investigational. In brief, it works by using radio frequency (RF) energy to heat the skin. Concurrent cooling protects the epidermis during the treatment, and because of this one can deliver up to 144 J/cm^2 of energy to a treatment site. Because of its capacitive coupling treatment tip, it heats a uniformly large volume of tissue. The clinical effects of this are tightening or lifting of the treated tissue. The mechanisms for these effects are twofold: (1) immediate contraction of existing collagen fibrils, and (2) a delayed wound healing response, which most likely entails neocollagen production by stimulated fibroblasts.[5]

It consists of three principle components: the RF Generator, Cooling Module, and Handpiece Assembly (consisting of a handpiece and treatment tip) (**Fig. 27.3**). The generator supplies RF power while continuously monitoring and displaying output current, output energy, treatment duration, and measured impedance. The return path for the electric current is through a return pad. The generator also controls the cooling module which circulates coolant through the handpiece assembly. Canisters of coolant are utilized in the cooling module. The handpiece assembly delivers RF energy while cooling tissue by conduction. Inside the handpiece, there is a force sensor that ensures that the tip is in contac

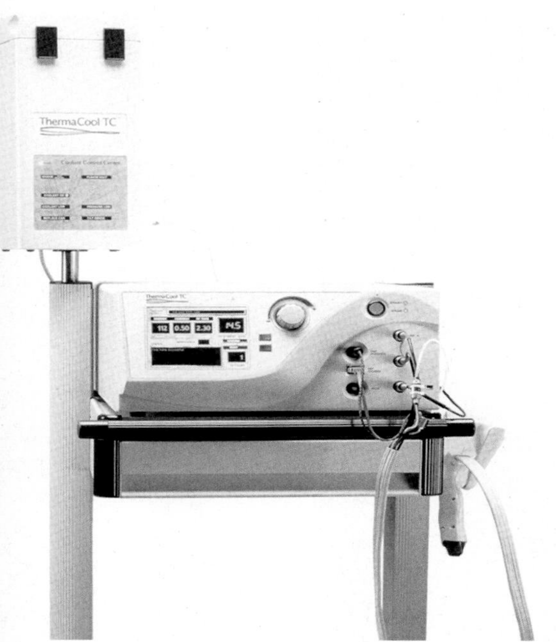

Fig. 27.3 The ThermaCool TC System (Thermage, Inc., Hayward, CA) consists of three principle components: the RF Generator, Cooling Module, and Handpiece Assembly (consisting of a handpiece and treatment tip).

with the patient, and that not too much or too little contact force is applied. Each tip contains a memory chip called an EPROM, which stores information on its size, model, and heating and cooling parameters. There are four thermistors, one in each corner, to detect the temperature of the tip and ensure that proper cooling is delivered to protect the epidermis.

Radiofrequency is a form of alternating current (AC). Most medical RF devices like electrosurgery units operate at 500 kilohertz or more. The ThermaCool operates at 6 megahertz. Electrical fields are created between two electrodes, which causes molecules to rotate or move. At the surface of the skin, the charge is changing polarity from positive to negative, alternately attracting and repelling electrons and charged ions. Polar molecules are induced to rotate back and forth, vibrating at 6 million times per second. It is the resistance to this movement that creates heat in the tissue.

Similar to a monopolar electrocautery or "Bovie" unit, an electric circuit is created by the device, and the patient becomes part of this circuit. The current flows out of the RF generator, through the handpiece cable, through the treatment tip, and into the skin. Then the current flows through the patient's body and is collected with a return pad on the patient's back. It then flows through the return cable and back to the generator.

With the current 1.5 cm^2 medium depth tip, patients can expect modest brow elevation (**Fig. 27.4**), improvement of malar bags, "minifacelift" type effects, modest neck tightening, and improvement of shallow acne scars. Our impression is that it is most effective in the jowl and submental regions (**Fig. 27.5**). Approximately 80% of our patients see these changes, which can range from subtle to

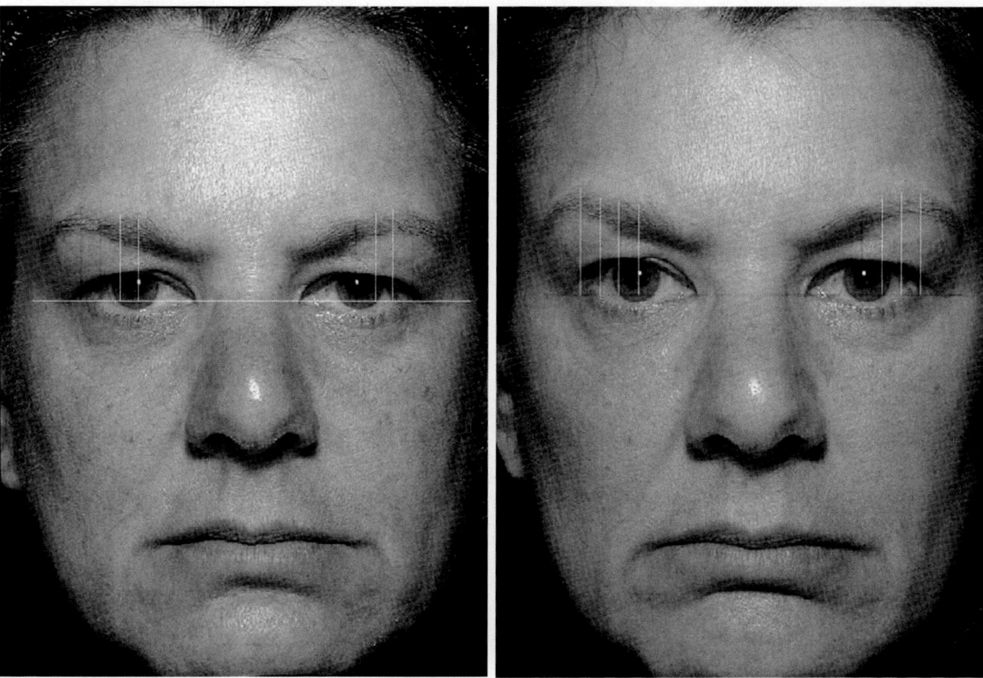

Fig. 27.4 A patient who underwent forehead and periorbital ThermaCool (Thermage, Inc., Hayward, CA) treatments. (**A**) Pretreatment. (**B**) Six months after treatment. Patient measured a 1.93 mm brow elevation on the right, and 2.25 mm elevation on the left.

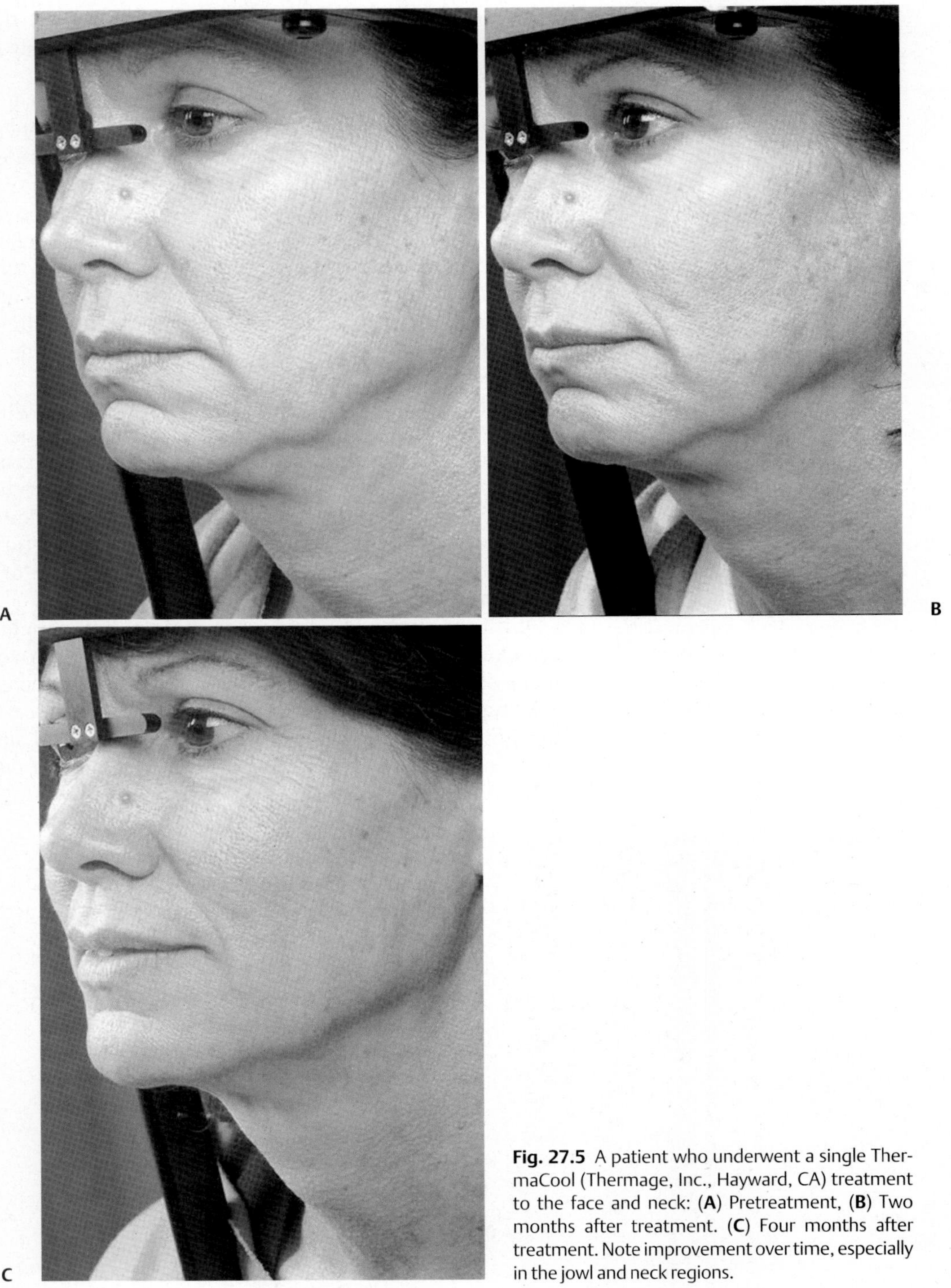

Fig. 27.5 A patient who underwent a single ThermaCool (Thermage, Inc., Hayward, CA) treatment to the face and neck: (**A**) Pretreatment, (**B**) Two months after treatment. (**C**) Four months after treatment. Note improvement over time, especially in the jowl and neck regions.

significant. There may also be a place for maintenance treatments with prior-treated patents getting annual treatments, or for touch-ups following facelift, for example. Several other tips are being tested that target different depths and therefore different applications (e.g., shallow tip for fine wrinkles, and deep for fat). Contraindications to the procedure are pacemaker or cochlear implants, sys temic corticosteroid use, and connective tissue disorder.

The procedure itself has evolved over the years, and th current treatment algorithm is based upon clinical finding and histological data. Clinical trials using low to moderat energies and applied in multiple passes demonstrate improved subjective and objective outcomes over previous techniques, which used a single-pass, high-energy approach.[6] Histology has shown immediate collagen denaturation or shrinkage with multiple passes, with the effects being greater in the deeper dermis (1 to 2 mm below surface) than in superficial dermis (0 to 1 mm). In addition, studies have shown that there is selective fibrous septae heating, which explains the three-dimensional contouring effects that are seen.[7] A side benefit of the algorithm advancement is that discomfort from the heat buildup is no longer a major factor in the procedure.

With regard to the actual procedure, our practice is to have the patient come in to the clinic 1 hour before the procedure. After jewelry is removed, topical 5% lidocaine cream (ELA-Max 5, Ferndale Laboratories, Ferndale, MI) is applied to the area to be treated for 1 hour and occluded. The patient may opt instead for oral sedatives and analgesics, which lessen the discomfort but then they lose the ability to drive home. As already noted, there is much less discomfort associated with the procedure using the current treatment algorithm but there is still significant heat perception.

It is very important to use the level of heat perception as a guide during treatment. An internal study showed that patients' stated heat perception directly correlated with their local tissue impedance; something that the device cannot currently tell you. Once the energy setting is selected based upon facial region and tissue thickness, a patient's heat perception is used to ensure that there is not excessive heat buildup. We maintain the patient at a 2 on a 4-point heat perception scale to balance efficacy, patient comfort, and safety. This sensation has been described as a building heat intensity that then dissipates. Because heat sensation feedback is so important for safety, it is strongly recommended that one avoids the use of regional nerve blocks, intravenous (IV) sedation, or general anesthesia. It is appropriate to take some of the sting out of the procedure with the foregoing measures, but patients need to be able to communicate how much heat is building up in their tissues (and hence their local impedance).

After placement of the return pad, the skin marking paper is used to temporarily mark the treatment area. The coupling fluid is used liberally to facilitate contact between the skin site and treatment tip. There is usually no change in the surface appearance of the treated skin, and any occurrences of local erythema and edema are usually resolved in 2 to 4 days. Because it is a nonablative procedure, there is no need for antibiotics, wound dressings, or ointments. We have treated all Fitzpatrick sun-reactive skin types without hyper- or hypopigmentation, and have not experienced any known complications to date.

ThermaCool treatments are not a replacement for current surgical procedures, but a noninvasive option for patients to consider. Our current practice is to offer appropriate invasive (i.e., surgical), minimally invasive, and noninvasive treatment options. An example of this for a patient with facial ptosis and jowling would be facelift, minifacelift, and ThermaCool treatments, respectively. As one looks across this continuum, efficacy is generally highest with invasive but with that usually comes the highest complication rate, cost (considering operating room and anesthesia fees), and recovery period. Patients are educated about the pluses and minuses of the different options, and they make their own choice. Treatment does not appear to preclude future surgical treatment because the author has had no problems in performing such procedures in previously treated regions. Because we do not yet have the profile of the optimal candidate, patient expectations need to be managed.

Radio Frequency and Laser

The Polaris WR (Syneron Medical Ltd, Yokneam, Israel) combines RF and diode laser energies (termed electro-optical synergy or ELOS) to address both facial wrinkles and skin laxity (**Fig. 27.6**). At the time of this writing, the FDA has granted 510K marketing clearance to the device for noninvasive wrinkle treatment. It delivers RF energy ranging from 10 J/cm^3 to 100 J/cm^3 and optical energy (910 nm diode) ranging from 10 J/cm^2 to 50 J/cm^2 in a sequential manner. Thermoelectric cooling at 5°C provides epidermal protection throughout the pulse sequence. It works on the theory that two energy sources are better than one: the RF energy will penetrate the skin and cause heating of the deeper tissue with neocollagen formation, whereas the laser energy

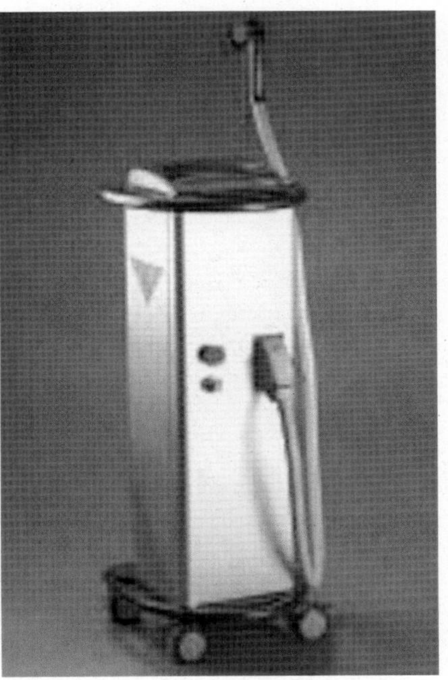

Fig. 27.6 Polaris WR (Syneron Medical Ltd, Yokneam, Israel) combines radio frequency and diode laser energies.

will be synergistic with this effect and will also address the more superficial problems of unwanted pigmentation and vascularity without epidermal injury.

A recent study reported that modest improvement in facial wrinkles was observed in the majority of patients as evidenced by investigator and independent assessor evaluations.[8] Side effects were mild and limited to transient erythema and edema. No scarring or pigment alterations were seen. The system used in this study delivered ~70 msec of RF energy and delayed diode energy. This sequence permits heating to a maximal dermal depth of 2 mm.

A limitation of this device lies in its electrode design. The bipolar, conductive coupling electrode results in concentration of the energy at the edges. This is useful for creating a very intense, shallow electric field, and is commonly used for ablating tissue. It, however, does not heat to a significant depth, and thermography has shown minimal RF effect except for superficial heating close to the bipolar electrode edges.

Conclusions

Many patients do not want the cost, risk, and downtime associated with surgical procedures, and nonablative devices give them an alternative. Minimally and noninvasive procedures have evolved as technology has advanced alongside more knowledgeable patients. We have always attempted to reduce the telltale signs of surgery, but there is now a patient-driven trend to avoid an "operated" look.

References

1. Koch RJ. Laser skin resurfacing. Facial Plast Surg Clin North Am 2001;9:329–336
2. Utley DS, Koch RJ, Egbert BM. Histologic analysis of the thermal effect on epidermal and dermal structures following treatment with the superpulsed CO_2 laser and the erbium:YAG laser: an in vivo model. Lasers Surg Med 1999;24:93–102
3. Hardaway CA, Ross EV. Nonablative laser skin remodeling. Dermatol Clin 2002;20:97–111
4. Sadick NS, Weiss RA. Intense pulsed-light photorejuvenation. Semin Cutan Med Surg 2002;21:280–287
5. Nowak KC, McCormack MC, Koch RJ. The effect of superpulsed carbon dioxide laser energy on keloid and normal dermal fibroblast secretion of growth factors: a serum-free study. Plast Reconstr Surg 2000;105:2039–2048
6. Koch RJ. Radiofrequency nonablative tissue tightening. Facial Plast Surg Clin North Am 2004;12:339–346
7. Abraham MT, Ross EV. Current concepts in nonablative radiofrequency rejuvenation of the lower face and neck. Facial Plast Surg 2005;21:65–73
8. Doshi SN, Alster TS. Combination radiofrequency and diode laser for treatment of facial rhytides and skin laxity. J Cosmet Laser Ther 2005;7:11–15

28 Neuromodulators and Injectable Soft Tissue Substitutes

Corey S. Maas, Kenneth C. Y. Yu, and Kristin K. Egan

Attitudes on the use of injectable agents for rejuvenation of the face have changed dramatically over the past decade. This is particularly true for the upper third of the face, where the impact of botulinum neuromodulator had its first application. In the senior author's (CSM) opinion, no technique, device, or pharmaceutical has had a greater impact on aesthetic surgery than the now widely employed use of botulinum neuromodulator as an injectable agent. Botulinum neuromodulator, while widely used in cosmetic indications over the past decade, received approval for a single cosmetic indication in 2002 and has become both an "entry level" treatment and a mainstay of therapy in cosmetic surgery.

Soft tissue augmentation holds a significant role in addressing treatment options for aging effects and camouflaging scars, in particular for the mid- and lower face. The past decade has witnessed a tremendous increase in consumer, professional, and corporate interest in injectable agents capable of eliminating or reducing the signs of aging and undesirable facial expression. The resultant advances in filler agents have expanded the options available for achieving soft tissue augmentation.

Until the past few years, the injectable fillers approved by the U.S. Food and Drug Administration (FDA) were limited to the collagen family of products. These included the bovine collagen products Zyderm and Zyplast (McGhan Medical, Santa Barbara, CA) and, more recently, human-derived recombinant products (Cosmoderm and Cosmoplast, Inamed, Santa Barbara, CA). Recent action by the FDA and keen corporate interest in capturing part of what is considered to be well in excess of a billion dollar market have led to the development of a series of new products. These include biological nonpermanent implants (i.e., hyaluronic acid gels, human recombinant collagen, micronized acellular human cadaveric dermis, preserved connective tissue) and the permanent alloplastic implants (i.e., silicone, Gore-Tex, W. L. Gore & Associates Inc., Flagstaff, AZ). The biological products offer the advantages of selective bioactivity, ease of use, and greater longevity than currently available collagen-based products.

Selective bioactivity is, in the authors' opinion, the central characteristic of successful injectable biomaterials. Selective bioactivity can be characterized by limited and/or selective inflammatory response, a measurable and predictable effective half-life or reversibility, and biocompatibility. Biocompatibility is defined as noncarcinogenic, nontoxic, and nonimmunogenic. Nonimmunogenic can be considered a misnomer because any injected material elicits some inflammatory (and thus immunogenic) response. The pressure to market various new fillers led some companies not to apply for the standard FDA "device" approval process; soft tissue fillers are considered devices and not pharmaceutical agents. Instead, some companies sought clearance by defining their products as transplantable devices. Examples of such "transplant devices" include Cymetra (LifeCell Corp., Branchburg, NJ), Fascian (Fascia Biosystems, Beverly Hils, CA), and Dermalogen (Collagenesis Inc., Beverly, MA).

This chapter reviews the currently available neuromodulators (**Table 28.1**) and soft tissue fillers (**Table 28.2**), their mechanisms of action, techniques for use, and clinical characteristics. Also discussed are current data on certain products under FDA review for these applications. Although this family of products has grown, there are still limitations to available filler agents, as well as those undergoing clinical investigation and the FDA approval process. Although there are several ways to classify these soft tissue augmentation materials and neuromodulators, we employ a system that is based on selective bioactivity.

Botulinum Neuromodulators

First employed by Dr. Allen Scott of San Francisco in the 1980s, botulinum neuromodulator showed promise in laboratory chick models for selective weakening of treated muscles and soon thereafter was used in the management of strabismus.[1] Under the trade name Oculinum this product was picked up by Allergan, Inc. (Irvine, CA), primarily an ophthalmic pharmaceutical company, for this and other neuromuscular disorders around the eye.

Table 28.1 Botulinum Neuromodulators

1. Botulinum toxin type A
    a. Botox
    b. Purtox
    a. Reloxin
2. Botulinum toxin type B
    a. Myobloc

Table 28.2 Soft Tissue Fillers

1. Biological materials
   a. Tissue-derived injectable
      i. Bovine collagen (Zyderm, Zyplast)
      ii. Porcine collagen (Evolence)
      iii. Human collagen (Dermalogen)*
      iv. Avian hyaluronic acid (Hylaform)
      v. Human particulate "dermal matrix" (Cymetra)*
      vi. Human particulate connective tissue (Fascian, Tutoplast)
      vii. Cultured autologous fibroblasts (Isologen)
   b. Synthesized injectable
      i. Hyaluronic acid (Restylane, Perlane, Juviderm, Captique)
      ii. Collagen (Cosmoderm, Cosmoplast)
   c. Implantable soft tissue fillers
      i. Human acellular dermis (AlloDerm)
      ii. Porcine acellular dermis (Surgisis)
   d. Autologous tissue transfer materials
      i. Fat
      ii. Dermal fat grafts
      iii. Fascia
2. Synthesized selective bioactive (resorbable) injectable materials
   a. Calcium hydroxyapatite particles (Radiesse)
   b. Polylactic acid particles (Sculptra)
3. Synthesized nonresorbable injectable polymers
   a. Silicone (Silkon)
   b. Polymethylmethacrylate (PMMA) (Artecoll, Artefill)*
   c. Others *(over half of the 63 "regulated" fillers worldwide are microparticulate synthetic polymers)
4. Implantable synthetic polymers
   a. Extruded polytetrafluoroethylene (ePTFE)—solid (Advanta, Gore-Tex) Ultrasoft)
   b. Extruded polytetrafluoroethylene (ePTFE)—tube (Softform, UltraSoft)

*Unavailable or U.S. Food and Drug Administration trials ongoing.

Botulinum neuromodulator is found in nature in seven serotypes (A through G) defined by their specific biological action in cleaving the particular proteins in the active transport of acetylcholine into the neurosynaptic cleft responsible for muscle contraction (and other autonomic functions).[2] These naturally occurring proteins were originally described as toxins due to the illness botulism, which is associated with ingestion of large amounts of *Clostridium botulinum*–contaminated food. They are better described, with respect to their now widespread medical use, as *neuromodulators*. Their distinct beneficial action is selective weakening, relaxation, or paralysis of treated muscles or muscle groups. By selective weakening of certain hypertrophic muscle groups in the face and neck, unwanted lines and facial expressions can be suppressed or even eliminated.

Although the B serotype neuromodulator (Myobloc, Solstice Neurosciences, San Francisco, CA) has demonstrated benefit in the treatment of hyperfunctional frown lines (HFLs), its benefit under current formulations is limited by the shorter duration of effect of the product.[3,4]

The A serotype has demonstrated the longest duration of effect (90 to 120 days) and least discomfort with injection. The standard for neuromodulators has been set by Botox (BTX) (Allergan, Inc., Irvine, CA), which has demonstrated a safety and efficacy record of over 15 years. The techniques and dosages described herein are in reference to the use of this medicinally original botulinum neuromodulator.

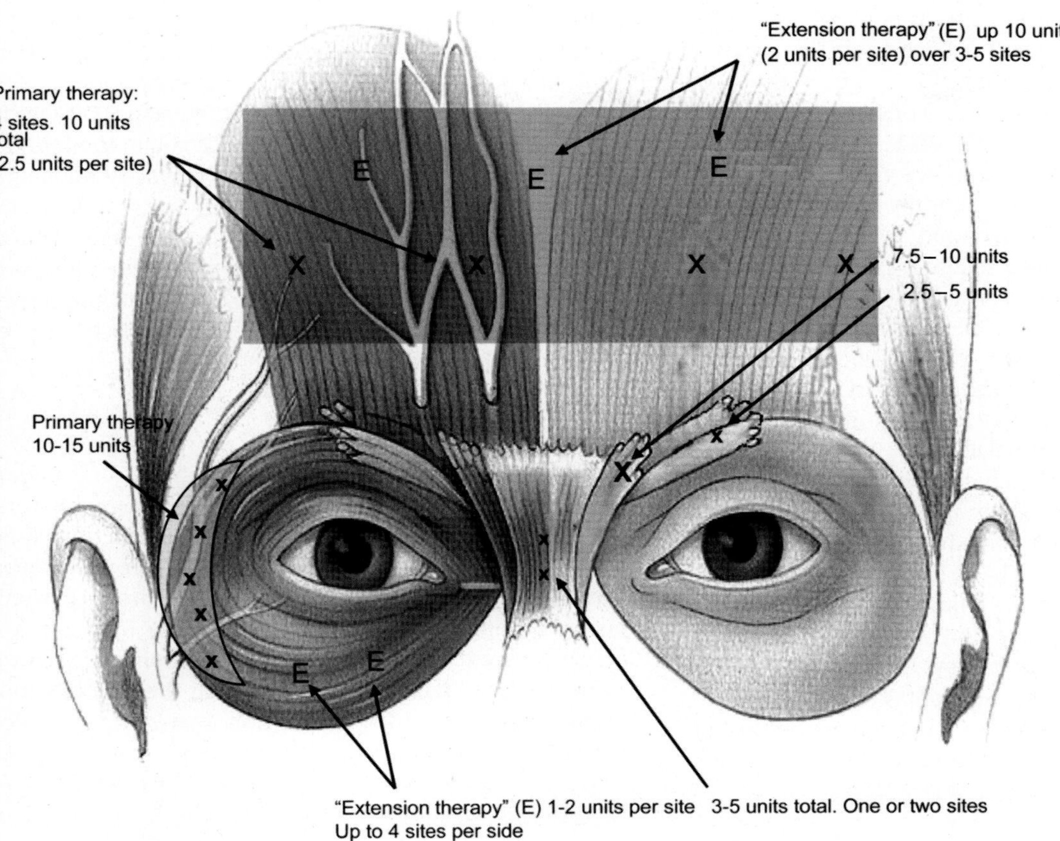

Fig. 28.1 Anatomy of face demonstrating recommended injection sites and dosages.

Reloxin (Inamed, Inc., Santa Barbara, CA), known as Dysport in Europe, is in current phase III FDA clinical trials and shows promise, as does Purtox (Mentor Corp., Santa Barbara CA), which is in its early-phase FDA trials.

An understanding of how to use BTX relies on a clear understanding of the facial muscular anatomy (**Fig. 28.1**). Although many techniques and surface points of injection have proven effective, it is clear that optimal response with minimal effective dosages requires precise placement in the selected muscle or muscle group.

The senior author has demonstrated the upper facial anatomy in controlled, large-population anatomical studies.[5] The interest in lower facial applications reinforces the need for a fundamental understanding of this muscular anatomy.[6] It is clear, however, that due to diffusion effects and the relative safety of BTX, the variability in points of injection and dosages has not significantly reduced the product's overall satisfactory clinical results. In the opinion of the senior author, required dosages for a given anatomical area can be reduced by precise localization and direct injection into the targeted muscle or muscle groups. Diffusion is helpful for those who lack a solid understanding of muscle location and general anatomy. In some cases, this has been perpetuated by inaccurate published anatomical drawings.

It is imperative that one keep in mind not only the specific muscle locations when providing neuromodulator treatment but also the functional interrelationships of the muscle action. Many of these act as antagonist-protagonists in the position of the brow (**Fig. 28.1**). The use of BTX in general has evolved with experienced and thoughtful injectors from a simple wrinkle treatment to means of reshaping, contouring, and softening the facial features associated with aging and the stigmata of the frowning, angry, or worried facial form.

The Glabellar Complex

Furrows created at the base of the nose (radix) are created by the procerus muscle, which is statistically larger in women than in men. Although this muscle has limited action as a brow depressor, it is a powerful "wrinkler" of the nose, which with chronic activity creates deep furrows. Many patients seeking treatment for vertical glabellar furrows have very limited procerus activity and do not require concurrent treatment. It is safe to say that not all patients are the same and thus treatment formulas that are universal are wasteful and unnecessary. Three to five units placed in one or two aliquots in the area of the radix are sufficient for most patients to achieve a satisfactory reduction in procerus activity (**Fig. 28.1**).

The corrugator supercilii and its accompanying depressor orbicularis oculi muscle are clinically indistinguishable. Their anatomy is poorly understood as it relates to that position. In contrast to many schematic and/or figurative diagrams showing the tail (or insertion) of the corrugator muscle 1 cm above the brow, the corrugator in the vast majority of patients follows the course of the eyebrow and delicately interdigitates with the orbicularis oculi muscle laterally and the frontalis muscle superiorly. Thus injections well above the midpupillary brow are of little value in targeting corrugator function and primarily disable the lower portions of the frontalis muscle. Such injections would be expected to result in medial brow ptosis.

Proper targeting requires the bulk of dosing for the corrugator at the clubhead of the eyebrow. We employ a minimum of 7.5 units in this area and 2.5 units in the scant muscle of the lateral brow to address "recruitment" of this lateral portion and some of the horizontally oriented orbicularis. These injections are directed at or slightly (within 1 or 2 mm) above the level of the eyebrow as the musculature descends with the aging ptotic brow (**Fig. 28.1**).

The Lateral Orbital Region

The orbicularis oculi (O.o.) muscle and the "crow's feet" are seemingly poorly understood. Although primary emphasis is focused by many on the softening of lines in this area, the lateral O.o. is the most powerful depressor of the brow and, as such, has the greatest potential with neuromodulation to reshape the upper face. The emphasis on the lateral orbicularis muscle is paramount because the muscle is a sphincter, and its superior and inferior portions create vectors of force that are in the horizontal plane. Treating these regions provides for softening vertically oriented supraorbital lines and "crepey" lines in the infraorbital region. Contrary to popular belief, the treatment of these areas has limited impact on horizontal brow position, in the senior author's opinion.

Treatment strategies therefore are stratified (although not mutually exclusive) around treatment of hypertrophic lines and reshaping the brow. Although single-point limited dosing at the lateral brow margin may provide some benefit in elevating brow position, it is advisable to keep in mind that the entire lateral O.o. is responsible for brow depression and, as shown in the senior author's previous work,[7,8] treatment of this large and powerful depressor can have a profound impact on brow position. In contrast, the supra- and infraorbital lines of expression can be substantively impacted by small doses in these regions. Concerns about effects on extraocular movements and the elevators of the lip have not proven problematic in our experience where lower eyelid injections are targeted outside the orbital rim and in the immediate subcutaneous plane.

Starting doses for the lateral orbital region (LOR) are in the range of 10 units per side, and one can quite comfortably go as high as 20 units per side in our experience without impact on sphincteric function. Small (2.5 units) aliquots are placed at roughly 1 cm intervals in a "half-moon" configuration from the infralateral brow to the inferior extent of horizontally oriented lines (**Fig. 28.1**). Extension for the crepey skin in the infraorbital region is easily done up to the area of the nasojugal groove.

The Forehead

The forehead is probably the most variably and poorly treated region of the upper face with neuromodulators. Injectors must balance the benefit of hyperfunctional line improvement with relaxation of the only brow elevator, the frontalis, and attendant ptosis of the brow that will occur. Dosages exceeding 20 units in the forehead are rarely warranted, in the senior author's opinion, because complete line effacement is not worth the side effect of noticeable brow ptosis. In addition, many strategies for treating the forehead region leave lateral frontalis muscle action unattenuated, resulting in a "Mr. Spock–like" forehead deformity (**Fig. 28.2**) that is both a hallmark of

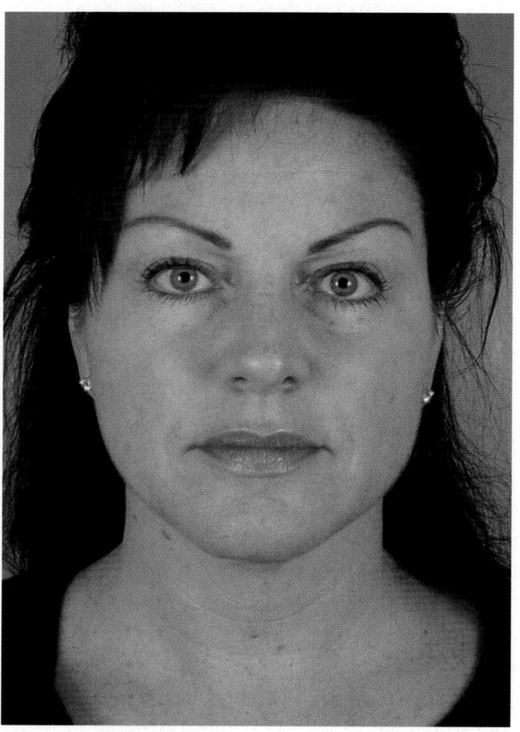

Fig. 28.2 Excessive dosage of botulinum neuromodulator in the forehead can result in the "Dr. Spock–like" deformity.

treatment and unattractive. The key to success in forehead treatment is modest dosing (enough to soften the lines with minimal impact on brow position) and uniform distribution of injections to avoid asymmetries and an artificial appearance of brow position.

Typical starting doses are around 5 units per side in four or five 2.0- to 2.5-unit aliquots (**Fig. 28.1**). Extension areas (E) may also be treated with similar dosing strategies deposited just through the galea aponeurosis. This layer can be "felt" as a gentle pop of the needle with insertion and is well above the frontal periosteum.

Perioral Lip Lines

Historically, fillers have been the primary therapy for perioral lip lines and, along with resurfacing for longer-term results, remain the mainstay for treatment of these dynamic lines. The lines, often referred to as "smoker's lines," are the result of repetitive muscle action of the orbicularis oris muscle and photoaging. With the etiology of these lines of facial expression in mind, one can use sparing amounts of BTX to suppress pursing expressions. Generally, 4 to 6 units of Botox are placed with precise symmetry at the vermillion border in four to six 1-unit aliquots for the upper and lower lips. Beyond these doses, one risks significant early problems with dysarthria and oral competence.

Marionette Lines

The depressor anguli oris (DAO) arises from the oblique line of the mandible, and inserts, by a narrow fasciculus, into the angle of the mouth (**Fig. 28.3**). At its origin, it is continuous with the platysma; at its insertion, it is continuous with the orbicularis oris. Contraction of this muscle over time results in melomental folds, or "marionette lines," which may be treated by injecting botulinum toxin directly into the DAO muscle at one location. Typically, 3 U are injected into each muscle, located where the nasolabial fold intersects the mandible. One must take care to avoid injecting the lip depressors.

Dimpled Chin

The mentalis muscle originates from the mandible, covers the chin, and inserts into the skin below the lower lip. Its action can cause wrinkles and dimpling (**Fig. 28.4**). A dose of 2 to 5 U is injected into one or more sites. The injection is targeted low or just below the prominence of the chin. After injecting, the muscle is massaged in a lateral direction. One should take care not to inject too high or risk weakening the orbicularis oris, causing lower lip incontinence and possible drooling. One must also avoid injecting the depressor labii, which can cause the lower lips to depress.

Platysmal Bands and Neck Contouring

Hypertrophic or flaccid platysmal muscle can be one etiology of the aging neck. Other potential causes include lipodystrophy, ptotic submandibular glands, or excess skin. Consequently, proper patient selection for BTX is critical and the greatest challenge. Using BTX to address platysmal bands works best for younger patients with good skin elasticity or postoperative residual bands.[9] Number of injections and injection dosages vary among practitioners; from three to five sites per band and dosages varied from 6 to 40+ U total doses per band. The senior author prefers to inject 10 U per band and targets those bands at the cervicomental area. Usually two bands are treated in one session, and repeat treatments typically occur after 3 to 4 months (**Fig. 28.5**).

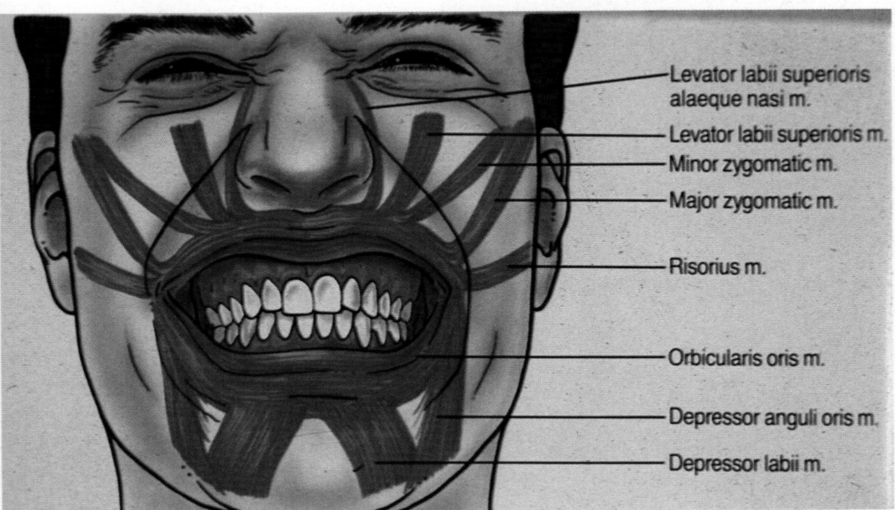

Fig. 28.3 Lower facial musculature pertinent to treatment of the marionette lines.

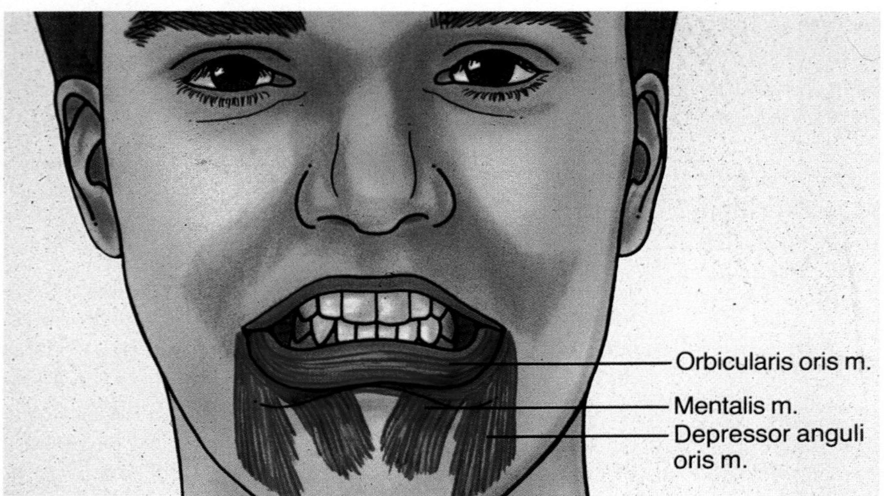

Fig. 28.4 Lower facial musculature pertinent to dimpled chin treatment.

When injecting the platysmal bands, care must be taken to avoid the strap muscles.[10] Complications may include ecchymosis, headaches, dyspnea, and neck weakness.[11] Although BTX can produce temporary satisfactory results, the optimal and longest-lasting results can only be achieved through surgery.[12] BTX will not correct skin laxity or fat deposits.[9] There is general consensus that BTX should be limited to patients who are poor surgical candidates.[10,12]

Soft Tissue Fillers

Historically, soft tissue fillers, namely Zyderm (Inamed Corporation, Santa Barbara, CA), were the only available injectable agents for management of the aging face. This legacy has largely been supplanted by the use of BTX. However, there is still a role for the use of these materials in upper as well as lower facial rejuvenation. Despite BTX's excellent results and established track record, there remain shortcomings to the use of BTX alone in the upper face, especially the inability to correct dermal resting lines, particularly deeper lines and those in older patients. The predominant use of fillers in upper portions of the face is in the management of fine dermal lines, commonly in combination with BTX. Historically, Zyderm was used to treat crow's feet, horizontal forehead lines, and glabellar lines. The effectiveness of BTX in management of these regions has largely limited the use of fillers to deep dermal lines in the glabellar area refractory to the muscle atony induced by BTX.

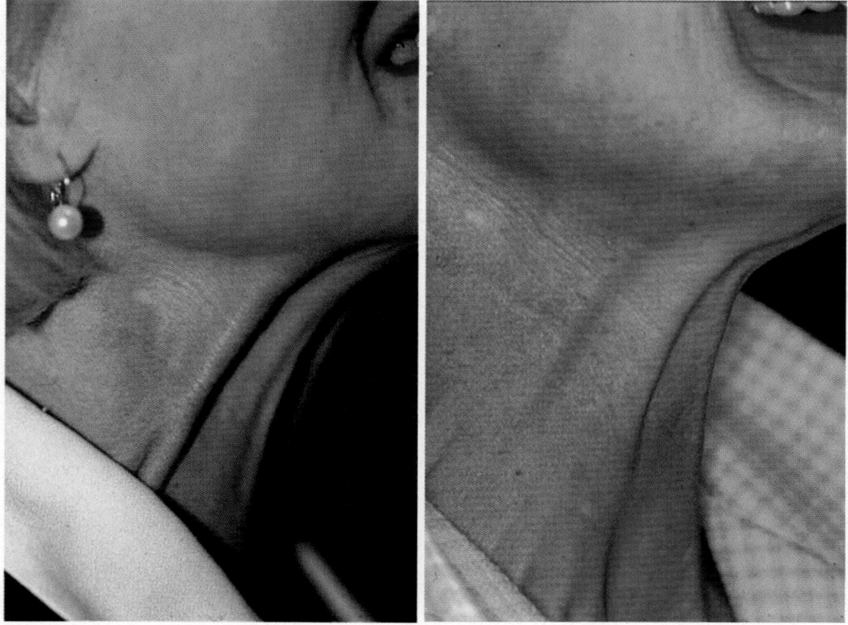

Fig. 28.5 (**A**) Before and (**B**) after photos of platysmal bands treated with Botox injections.

Soft tissue fillers hold a more useful role in rejuvenating the mid- and lower thirds of the face. Increased nasolabial and melolabial folds are commonly seen during the aging process. In addition, loss or contracture of tissue resulting from surgery, trauma, or acne can be improved with fillers. The hypoplastic lip is another common cosmetic concern that can be treated with soft tissue fillers.

Historical Background

The ideal filler agent is one that is easy to use and creates reproducible, long-lasting results. It is biocompatible, nonallergenic, noncarcinogenic, and nonmigratory. In addition, it can be transported and stored at room temperature and has a long shelf life. The search for an ideal soft tissue augmentation product has been continuing with varying degrees of success since the end of the nineteenth century. Autologous fat was first reported as a soft tissue filler by Neuber in 1893.[13] Paraffin was later used, but the high incidence of inflammatory reaction and foreign body granuloma formation made it unsafe, and paraffin's use was abandoned around the time of the First World War.[13,14] The ensuing years brought the use of vegetable oils, mineral oil, lanolin, and beeswax; however, all of these exhibited problems that continue to be associated with the fillers in use today, namely, chronic inflammation, infection, and migration.[15–18]

In the 1960s, interest turned to new, highly purified polymers and their potential application for soft tissue augmentation. Pure injectable liquid silicone was embraced as ideal among these synthetic polymers. Despite caution suggested in several reports, silicone became widely used to augment many soft tissue defects by direct injection.[19,20] Severe complications can occur with large-volume injections. For instance, late-term granulomas are not uncommon, and large-volume injection (greater than 0.5 mL), particularly in the lips, can have irreversible consequences. Yet, controversy persists regarding the efficacy and safety of the so-called microdroplet injection technique popularized by Orentreich and Orentreich and Webster et al.[21,22] They argue that silicone is both effective and safe when used in limited amounts mandated by the microdroplet technique. If limited siliconoma develop, corticosteroids may be helpful.[23] Another synthetic polymer, polytetrafluoroethylene (Teflon) paste, was initially thought to be a useful soft tissue filler. However, the technical difficulties encountered when injecting this thick paste, as well as an exaggerated inflammatory reaction, prevented its widespread use.[24]

Over the next 4 decades, investigations and development produced many alternative materials such as injectable collagen, human acellular dermis, and synthetic selective bioactive materials. In just the past 2 years we have witnessed the introduction of an extraordinary number of soft tissue augmentation fillers in response to the public's ever-increasing demand for minimally invasive cosmetic procedures. **Table 28.2** summarizes the current most popular soft tissue fillers.

Biological Materials

The use of biological materials for injection is, in general, advantageous because infection rates are lower than with synthetic materials, which, regardless of biocompatibility, are foreign bodies. However, infection has not been eliminated altogether, and biological fillers are, without exception, subject to variable degrees of either or both remodeling and resorption. The rates of biological degradation of these materials are determined by several factors and have been fairly clearly characterized for certain biological fillers. Historically, manufacturers of commercially available products have exaggerated the duration of clinical effect, leaving physicians with difficulty with patient expectations. Hypersensitivity responses are generally uncommon and well described for bovine collagen products.

Bovine Collagen

Bovine collagen was the first material approved by the FDA for use as an injectable soft tissue filler in 1981.[15] Injectable collagen is a reconstituted, purified, enzyme-digested, bovine dermal collagen suspended in a phosphate buffered saline with 0.3% lidocaine.[25] Commercial products include Zyderm I, Zyderm II, and Zyplast (Inamed Corp., Santa Barbara, CA). Zyderm I was the first approved agent for use as a soft tissue filler in the United States in 1981.[26] Zyderm I contains a collagen concentration of 35 mg/mL and is made up of 95% type I collagen and 5% type III collagen.[27] The processing of Zyderm removes the immunogenic telopeptide regions of the molecule without disrupting the natural helical structure. Zyderm II is similar to Zyderm I but contains a higher concentration of collagen (65 mg/mL).[27] Zyplast differs from Zyderm in that it contains glutaraldehyde cross-linked collagen, making it less susceptible to collagenase degradation and less immunogenic.[27] Patients considering bovine collagen injection must be skin tested prior to treatment. The material is injected subdermally, in a dose of 0.1 mL, in the volar forearm area. The site is examined after 48 to 72 hours and at 1 month. A positive test, exhibited by erythema and/or induration, is a contraindication to use this product. Three to 3.5% of the population demonstrate a hypersensitivity to bovine collagen, and after one negative skin test, 1% (or less) of patients will demonstrate hypersensitivity to a second challenge.[28] Consequently, a repeat test in 2 to 4 weeks is usually recommended, and treatment may proceed after a second negative skin test.

Zyderm and Zyplast have a good safety record and come prepackaged in a 1 mL syringe. Zyderm I has very favorable flow characteristics and as such is excellent for treating fine lines. The duration of effect with bovine collagen is highly variable (generally 3 months) and is dependent on the injection site and the patient's metabolism. Disadvantages include the need for refrigeration, possibility of allergic reaction, and the short duration of improvement, and treatment can be expensive if increased amounts must be injected for older patients.[29]

Zyderm and Zyplast are injected intradermally, and the effects are immediate. Results with the use of Zyderm and Zyplast are good but can be modified by delayed hypersensitivity. Zyderm is infiltrated into the superficial papillary dermis, and its effect makes it an excellent filler for addressing fine lines. Zyplast is placed into the midreticular or deep reticular dermis at the dermal subcutaneous interface. Zyplast should not be injected into the superficial papillary dermis or in areas of thin skin because it can form beads on placement.[27] Because Zyplast is injected into the deep reticular dermis, it can be used to address deep folds and wrinkles as well as augmenting the lips. Provided the patient has been skin tested, Zyplast is an excellent option for those who desire a quick enhancement prior to a social event. Zyderm and Zyplast contain lidocaine for more comfortable administration; however, additional topical anesthetic may be useful.

Human Collagen

The success of injectable bovine collagen led to the development of a myriad of alternative injectable biological fillers, including, in the United States, Autologen and Dermalogen (Collagenesis, Inc., Beverly, MA). These products gained limited popularity and are mentioned for historical purposes. Autologen was an injectable autologous human tissue matrix processed from skin harvested during skin excision surgery (i.e., rhytidectomy, blepharoplasty). For theoretical long-term results, at least three injections were required spaced 2 weeks apart to satisfactorily augment a soft tissue defect. With autologous tissue there was little risk of disease transmission or allergic reaction; however, the results were not shown to last longer than those achieved with bovine collagen. Because Autologen was material harvested from the patient's own body, the time, expense, equivocal duration, and delayed treatment doomed Autologen to failure in the filler marketplace.

Dermalogen was developed to overcome the obstacle of surgical harvesting and used cadaveric banked tissue, which had been aseptically processed, was acellular, and was structurally similar to Autologen.[30] The cosmetic results of both Autologen and Dermalogen demonstrated a natural, softer appearance like the result seen with bovine collagen. One study by Sclafani et al[31] evaluated a direct comparison of Dermalogen and Zyplast in 20 patients over a 12-week period. It demonstrated that the clinical persistence and histological behavior of Dermalogen was comparable to Zyplast. The product is no longer available.

Human Recombinant Collagen (Cosmoderm and Cosmoplast)

The delay time from presentation to treatment and measurable delayed hypersensitivity response seen with bovine collagen led to the development of a human-derived "tissue engineered" collagen product. The emphasis on this technology was underscored by diminishing sales of bovine-based products, particularly in Europe, where bovine spongiform encephalopathy (BSE) or "mad cow disease" left much of the public concerned about transmissibility of this disease through bovine collagen injections. No such cases have been reported. CosmoDerm I/II and CosmoPlast (Inamed, Santa Barbara, CA) are the only currently available dermal fillers made from natural human collagen grown under controlled laboratory conditions. They contain purified collagen derived from cell cultures of human fibrocytes. The cell lines are obtained from the foreskin of a newborn and are screened for viruses, tumerigenicity, and other potential pathogens. Because these products contain the basic human collagen molecule stripped of antigenic determinants, no skin testing is required. This is an advantage over Zyderm and Zyplast, allowing one to inject this product at the initial consultation. The disadvantages are similar to Zyderm and Zyplast: need for refrigeration, cost, and duration of effect.

Human Particulate "Connective Tissue"

Fascian (Fascia Biosystems, Beverly Hills, CA) and Tutoplast (Tutogen Medical, Inc., Alachua, FL) are preserved, irradiated human cadaver fascial tissue in particulate form that can be injected for soft tissue augmentation.[32] They are supplied in various particle sizes and must be rehydrated with lidocaine or saline before injection. The implant is injected subdermally with a 16- to 26-gauge needle, depending on the particle size selected. Fascian should not be injected into the dermis because inflammation with lumpiness can occur.

The promoted advantages of fascial tissue are that they may last longer than collagen, it can be stored at room temperature, and no skin testing is required. Disadvantages include the requirement for rehydration prior to use, the need for local anesthetic, and the fact that it is contraindicated in patients with allergies to polymyxin sulfate, bacitracin, or gentamicin because there may be trace amounts of these substances in these implants. These products are not useful for superficial lines. Clinical reports with these products have been limited and in general have been reported by company principles. The general impression of the clinical and academic community is that this product is similar to Cymetra in that it causes swelling and is of short duration).

Hyaluronic Acid Derivatives

Hyaluronic acid (hyaluronan, sodium hyaluronate; HA) is a natural biopolymer of glycosaminoglycan chains that coil in on themselves, resulting in an elastic and viscous matrix. It exhibits no species or tissue specificity and its chemical structure is uniform throughout nature. Thus there is limited potential for immunogenicity. It is found naturally in the dermis and has a high affinity for water, thereby serving to hydrate the skin.[33] The loss of HA as we age leads to dermal dehydration and the formation of rhytides.[34] Cross-linking can serve to lengthen the half-life of HA but cannot eliminate its degradation. Current FDA-approved HA fillers are limited to Hylaform (Biomatrix, Inc., Ridgefield, NJ), Restylane (Q-Med, Uppsala, Sweden) and Captique (Inamed Corp., Santa Barbara, CA). Hylaform is a xenogenic variety derived from rooster combs. Restylane and Captique are partially cross-linked and processed from *Streptococcus* fermentation.[33] Restylane and Captique, nonanimal products, have a theoretical lower risk of delayed hypersensitivity reaction. In side by side comparison with Restylane, Hylaform showed a higher incidence of skin reaction.[35] Both forms are reabsorbed, albeit at a slower rate than the collagen products. It has been reported that effects last up to 6 months.[36]

Restylane, Captique, and Hylaform do not require skin testing; although early studies did not demonstrate hypersensitivity or allergic reactions, several case series have reported delayed reactions.[37,38] A study of 709 patients over 4 years showed positive skin testing in patients who developed delayed skin reactions to these materials. The manufacturer does not recommend skin testing for these materials but these reports may suggest otherwise.[39] Case reports have also shown the potential for granuloma formation with the use of HA derivatives.[40] Positive skin tests have demonstrated chronic inflammatory reactions at up to 11 months and serum immunoglobulin G (IgG) and IgE antibodies to HA; however, these reactions are quite rare.[38] HA is contraindicated in patients with severe allergies manifested by history of anaphylaxis or history of multiple severe allergies. Restylane, Captique, and Hylaform are contraindicated for breast augmentation and implantation into bone, tendon, or ligament. It must not be injected in blood vessels because it may occlude vasculature, leading to infarction or embolism.

Restylane is approved for mid- to deep dermal injections and can be used in all areas of the face. The most commonly treated areas include the lips and nasolabial folds, although perioral areas (e.g., marionette lines, oral commissure), glabellar complex, and brows are also potential targets. Olenius and Duranti et al demonstrated encouraging results, with the majority of patients reporting good results for up to 8 months.[41,42] A randomized study of 138 patients comparing Restylane and Zyplast on the correction of nasolabial folds (**Fig. 28.6**) demonstrated that a more durable aesthetic improvement was found with Restylane.[43] Less injection volume was required with Restylane, and it was superior to Zyplast in retaining its shape. A comparison of Restylane with and without the addition of Botox (Allergan, Inc., Irvine, CA) demonstrated that glabellar rhytides responded better to the combination of Restylane and Botox.[44] Those patients who present with deep vertical glabellar lines at rest may not be able to achieve the elimination of those lines with the use of Botox alone. Restylane can serve to fill the resting lines, and the addition of Botox delays the deformation of the filler residing in the dermis, thereby performing a protective function. Restylane is also well

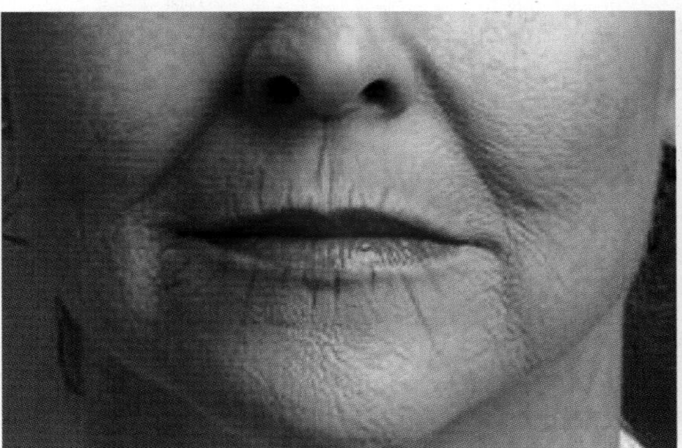

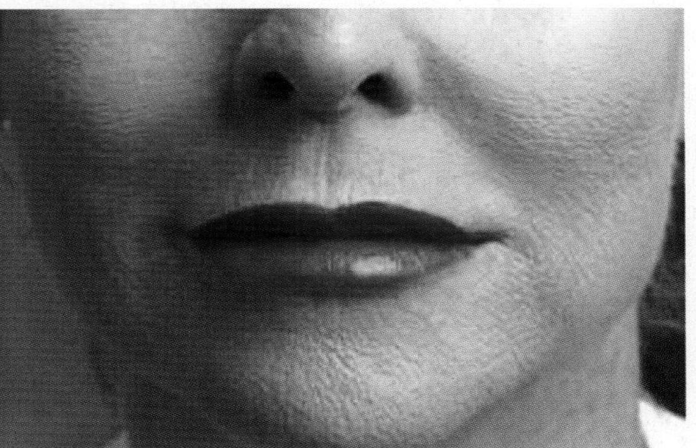

Fig. 28.6 (**A**) Before and (**B**) after photos of nasolabial folds injected with Restylane.

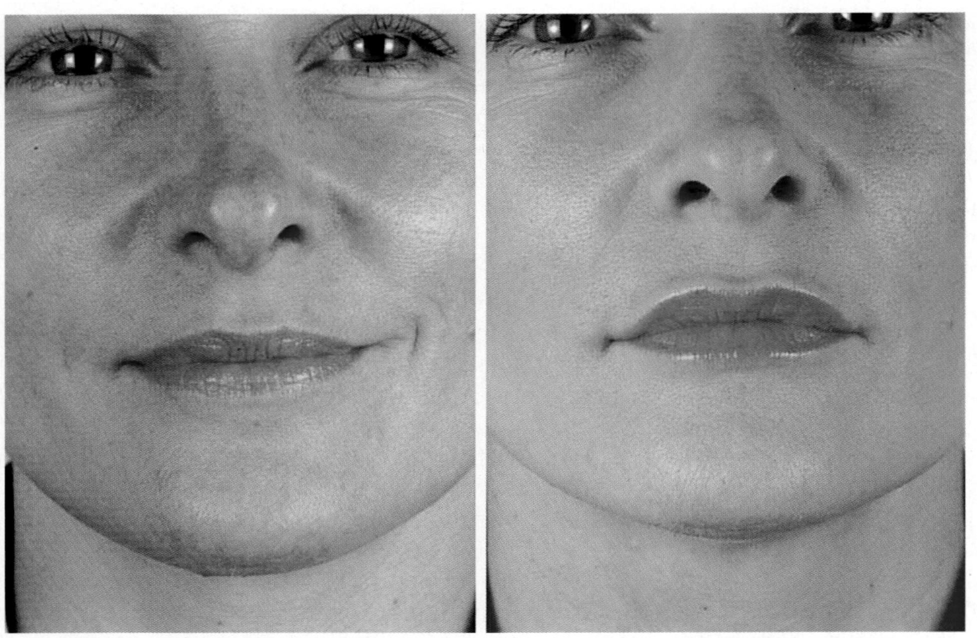

Fig. 28.7 (A) Before and (B) after photos of microchelia treated with Restylane injection.

used as a soft tissue filler for microchelia (**Fig. 28.7**). Finally, Restylane is being used more and more as a soft tissue filler in areas such as the submalar areas, temporal areas, and the nasal jugal groove (**Fig. 28.8**). The rationale behind using Restylane to replace or enhance volume is based on injecting into the *subdermis* area. There is a growing sense that Restylane in this area may last longer (the duration of effect may not even be an issue) and is possibly safer. HA fillers such as Restylane are not ideal in addressing the perioral fine lines due to visible ridges and a bluish tint (Tindel effect) (**Fig. 28.9**).

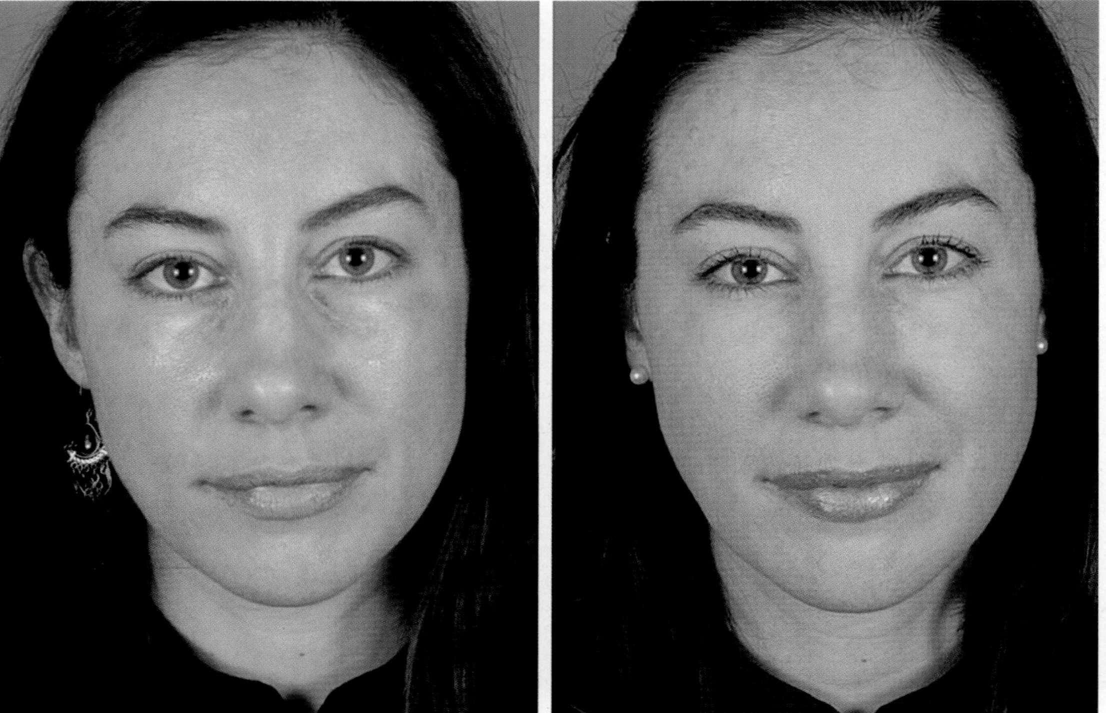

Fig. 28.8 (A) Before and (B) after photos of Restylane injection of the nasal jugal groove area.

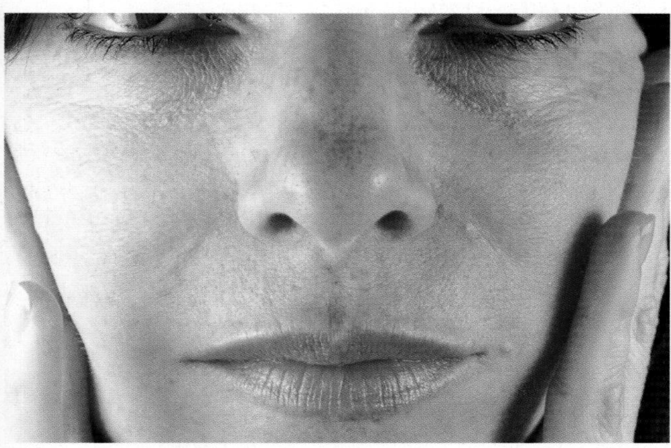

Fig. 28.9 Unpleasant bluish tint (Tindel effect) seen in the nasolabial folds from Restylane injection.

These fillers also have the potential for reabsorption and may require repeat injections at 2 to 4 weeks.[33] Restylane is more viscous than Hylaform, and it has been postulated that a decreased concentration may allow the material to absorb more water and lead to a more long-term correction. None of the HA fillers contain lidocaine, and preinjection with local anesthetic is recommended. No overcorrection is necessary. These fillers can be stored at room temperature for at least a year but must be used within 24 hours when opened. Restylane has demonstrated excellent clinical results with softness, durability, and patient acceptance since its introduction in the U.S. market. These features and an admirable marketing campaign have resulted in Restylane capturing some 50% of the total injectable filler market. In contrast, the limited duration of effect seen with other HA fillers has limited their success.

Juvederm (Allergan, Inc., Irvine, CA) is in FDA trials in the United States and is another HA in the form of viscoelastic gel, which is transparent and homogeneous and which has four major benefits. It is obtained by biosynthesis, is of nonanimal origin, and does not require any prior skin testing. Also, the molecule is highly biocompatible and is obtained by bacterial fermentation. Juvederm is presented in the form of a prefilled syringe, containing a viscoelastic, transparent HA gel and is available in three different concentrations, their use depending on the nature of the depression needing correction. Juvederm 18 is used for fine wrinkles such as perioral wrinkles. Juvederm 24 is for glabellar lines, mild to moderate nasal furrows, and cheek wrinkles. Juvederm 30 is used for deep nasolabial folds and lip volume. Data from European and other experience suggest that Juvederm compares favorably with Restylane in ease of use and patient satisfaction.

Cultured Autologous Fibroblasts

Isolagen (Isolagen Tech., Metuchen, NJ) is currently under FDA investigation. It consists of injectable autologous fibroblasts derived from an autologous source. It has been advocated for the treatment of facial rhytids, nasolabial folds, glabellar furrows, scars, and hypoplastic lips. Recommended treatment consists of three to four injections over a 3- to 6-month period. Theoretically, Isolagen has the advantage of low immunoreactivity; there has been no report of major complications or hypersensitivity reactions. Isolagen's manufacturer attempted several years ago to achieve approval as a transplant material; it was temporarily on the market but was subsequently required to perform standard FDA device clinical research. Currently, this research is ongoing and Isolagen remains under clinical investigation.

Human Acellular Dermis

AlloDerm (LifeCell Corp., Branchburg, NJ) is an acellular, freeze-dried dermal graft harvested from screened cadavers. AlloDerm is processed from cadaveric skin, preserving the basement membrane and dermal collagen matrix. After the fibroblasts are extracted, the material is cryoprotected, enabling it to be freeze dried in a two-step procedure. Like all other materials harvested from cadavers, AlloDerm is screened for contaminants before it is shipped. To date, no reported cases of disease transmission exist. It is stable for 2 years under refrigeration and must be rehydrated for 10 to 20 minutes in normal saline or lactated Ringer's solution immediately prior to use. The various sizes and thicknesses available make it an excellent material for repairing large tissue defects. If infection occurs, it may not be necessary to remove the implant, only to treat the infection.[28] Zyplast was studied in direct comparison with AlloDerm with follow-up at 1 year by Sclafani et al. Superior results were seen with AlloDerm, which stabilized in resorption at 6 months, whereas Zyplast was progressively absorbed.[45] Unfortunately, AlloDerm does not appear to last as long or be as consistent as originally described. The reduced duration of effect and its high cost have decreased its use and popularity.

Cymetra (LifeCell) is micronized AlloDerm designed as an injectable soft tissue filler. Cymetra must be reconstituted with 1 mL of lidocaine before injection and used within 2 hours. Some reports suggest that Cymetra does not reabsorb as Zyplast is observed to do, and therefore repeated treatments are more effective.[46] In addition, Cymetra carries an increased incidence of inflammatory reactions and has not shown to last longer than Zyplast. It also requires mixing with 1 or 2% lidocaine; the resultant thick paste can be difficult to inject. The senior author's experience with Cymetra has been variable, but the marked swelling and shorter than advertised duration of effect have limited the clinical use of this product.

Porcine Acellular Dermis

Surgisis (Cook Biotech, Inc., West Lafayette, IN) is a sterile acellular graft material extracted from the small intestine submucosa of pigs. The submucosa is processed to retain the natural composition of matrix of collagen (type I, III, VI), glycosaminoglycans (HA, heparin, heparin sulfate, and chondroitin sulfate), proteoglycans, and fibronectin. The material acts as a natural extracellular matrix, which acts as a scaffold for host tissue remodeling. The manufacturing process is also carefully validated to ensure any potential virus in host animals is inactivated. Like AlloDerm, it must be hydrated in sterile normal saline or lactated Ringer's prior to use. Surgisis has a long shelf life (~18 months) and can be stored at room temperature. Its main use continues to be for nasal reconstructive surgery, but increasing experience may broaden its applications.

Autologous Fat Injection

Since Neuber first introduced free fat autografts in 1893, the use of fat as a filler agent has fallen in and out of favor due to its high resorption rate and unpredictability. In 1950, Peer reported an average loss of 45% in the weight of the free fat implant by 1 year.[48] The arrival of liposuction has renewed interest in autologous fat injection.[49]

Fat is harvested aseptically into a sterile container, using local anesthesia and tumescent technique with a blunt-tipped microcannula or a syringe. Donor site choices include the submental, lateral thigh, hips, or umbilical regions. The harvested fat can also be frozen in liquid nitrogen for future use. The harvested fat is then washed with sterile saline, although some believe that washing the fat can lead to increased mechanical trauma and decreased fat survival.[50] Currently there is no gold standard for autologous fat injection.[51] The fat is injected into the subcutaneous tissue with a large-bore needle (i.e., 16- or 18-gauge needle). After injection, the area is massaged so that the fat fills the injected fields smoothly. Fat injection may be used to address nasolabial and melolabial folds, glabellar furrows, lips, and hemifacial atrophy. Due to the expected resorption, overcorrection of 30 to 50% is usually recommended. The role of fat transplantation, like many fillers, has changed over the past decade. Its primary role is now well established as a volume restoration product in the brow, midface, and lower facial areas. In these areas, the variable results that are often described when filling lines and borders are largely eliminated. Fat has truly found its role due to the work of Coleman and others in volume restoration.

Autologous fat injection offers certain advantages. Because it is from the patient's own body, there is no risk of allergic reaction. Fat is abundant in the body, making it versatile (able to fill large and small areas over much of the body).[29] Disadvantages include donor site morbidity, and the unpredictable resorption rate.

Synthetic Selective Bioactive Injectable Fillers

Calcium Hydroxyapatite Particles

Radiesse, formerly Radiance FN (Bioform, Inc., Franksville, WI), is composed of microscopic calcium hydroxyapatite particles (ranging in size from 25 to 40 μm) suspended in a carboxymethyl-cellulose gel. The mechanism of action by Radiesse is both in volume restoration and to act as a framework for fibroblastic ingrowth in soft tissue. Radiesse is FDA approved and has been used for years in dental reconstruction, as well as bone, bladder, and neck implants, and is also approved for oral-maxillofacial defects.

Radiesse also does not require skin testing because it contains no animal products. Its effects are reported to last from 2 to 5 years in urological studies. In facial applications its duration is in the range of 6 to 12 months depending on the site of the injection and the technique used. In the senior author's and others' experience, Radiesse looks and feels quite natural.[29]

In histological studies, Radiesse microspheres were gone at 9 months but they stimulated almost no foreign body reaction.[52] Few macrophages were visualized surrounding the microspheres of Radiesse, suggesting that they are degraded by enzymatic rather than cellular processes.

Radiesse is in late-phase clinical trials for cosmetic indications, namely, the nasolabial fold where side by side comparisons with an HA control demonstrated patient and physician preference for Radiesse. This product may well have a significant impact our choices and methodologies when using fillers with FDA approval.

Radiesse can produce excellent results for deeper folds, wrinkles, and lip enhancement, when used judicially, but should not be used for superficial lines.[29] Its application, too, has expanded into the role of volume enhancement. More and more practitioners are using Radiesse to enhance nasolabial folds, the nasojugal groove, and inframalar areas. The attraction of Radiesse is its longer duration of effect (8 to 18 months) and hypoallergenic characteristics. Although Radiesse has been used in the lip, we do not recommend its use in lip augmentation because the microspheres will be compressed into strands during the act of mastication. Others have also noted problems with its use in the lip.[53] Injections with Radiesse are painful and require local anesthesia. Swelling can occur for 2 days after injection.

Polylactic Acid Particles (Sculptra)

Sculptra (Dermik Aesthetics, Berwyn, PA) is an injectable form of poly-L-lactic acid, a compound that has been used in absorbable suture material for over 40 years. It is a nontoxic, synthetic, immunologically inactive, biodegradable lactic acid polymer. It is approved in Europe for the treatment of scars and wrinkles and was recently approved by the FDA for treating facial lipoatrophy associated with human immunodeficiency virus (HIV) disease. Sculptra comes in powdered form and must be reconstituted with sterile water with or without lidocaine. The reconstituted form must then sit for 2 hours to ensure complete hydration of the product. It requires a 26-gauge or larger needle for injection and must be used within 72 hours. Theoretically, Sculptra can be injected into the deep dermis or subcutaneous tissue. In the senior author's experience, however, this product must be placed in deep subcutaneous tissue to avoid the reported complications of visible and palpable granulomas and draining fistulas. Multiple sessions at 2-week intervals are needed for significant improvement. Initial studies demonstrated skin thickness increase as early as 6 weeks after injection, which remained for up to 96 weeks.[54]

Advantages of Sculptra are that it does not require refrigeration and no skin test is necessary. However, it must be reconstituted 2 hours before injection, and a local anesthetic is usually required. In Europe, the current opinion of Sculptra is variable. Although it may produce some improvement initially, the fluid is absorbed after a week, and the effect is diminished. Multiple repeat injections are required to stimulate the proposed collagen growth before the desired effect is achieved, which may take up to 3 to 4 months. The advertised duration of months to years must be interpreted with caution because many injections spaced months apart are necessary to achieve this. Finally, granulomas, nodule formation, and drainage have all been reported, and these complications can be difficult to manage.

Synthetic Nonresorbable Injectable Polymers

Silicone

Silicone is a polymer of dimethylpolysiloxane that can come in various forms, ranging from liquid to solid.[55] Silicone may be used off label, but because it is classified as a device and not a drug, it may not be advertised in the office, phone book, Internet, or other media.

Silicone is injected through a 30-gauge needle in microdroplets of 0.01 mL into the subdermis.[55,56] Serial injections should be separated by 1 to 2 mm of tissue. Each microdroplet produces augmentation via a fibroblastic response; a fibrous capsule forms around each capsule of silicone. This process takes several weeks. One should inject microamounts and undercorrect.[55] When considering injectables, there are basically three techniques used to deliver material to the deep dermis or subcutaneous level: linear threading, serial puncture, and droplet (**Fig. 28.10**). Linear threading is a technique by which an agent is delivered in a uniform fashion while the needle is slowly withdrawn from the tissue. The linear threading is a technique that is particularly effective when performing lip augmentation along the mucocutaneous border. The serial puncture technique is used to deliver small aliquots of filler at multiple spots to achieve even distribution over a two-dimensional area. Finally, the droplet technique is used in a manner similar to that in linear threading. However, instead of an even distribution of filler as the needle is withdrawn, microdroplets of filler are delivered into the tissue by gentle pumping on the syringe as the needle is withdrawn. The droplet technique has been advocated for use when injecting silicone. The depth of injection, however, is dependent on the injectable used. Multiple treatments may be necessary and should be performed at intervals of 6 or more weeks.

Silicone is permanent, does not require skin testing (there are no antibodies to liquid silicone), can be stored at room temperature, does not support bacterial growth, and can be used to treat many areas. However, its disadvantages are numerous, including inflammation, induration, discoloration, ulceration, migration, and formation of silicone granulomas.[55] Silicone is also very difficult to remove after it is injected into soft tissue. There are those who believe the complications seen with silicone are caused by improper injection technique, injecting too much silicone, or the quality of silicone.[25,56]

Polymethylmethacrylate

Artecoll (Artes Medical, Inc., San Diego, CA) is a suspension of polymethylmethacrylate (PMMA) microspheres 30 to 40 μm in diameter in 3.5% bovine collagen solution and is the most advanced synthetic permanent injectable. Artecoll works by microgranuloma formation, which may not be controllable. This product produces immediate correction with collagen and also permanent replacement with new collagen produced as part of the inflammatory response.[28] Artecoll, unlike the other microspheres, does not become reabsorbed, and histologically new collagen deposits are visible at 1 month.[52]

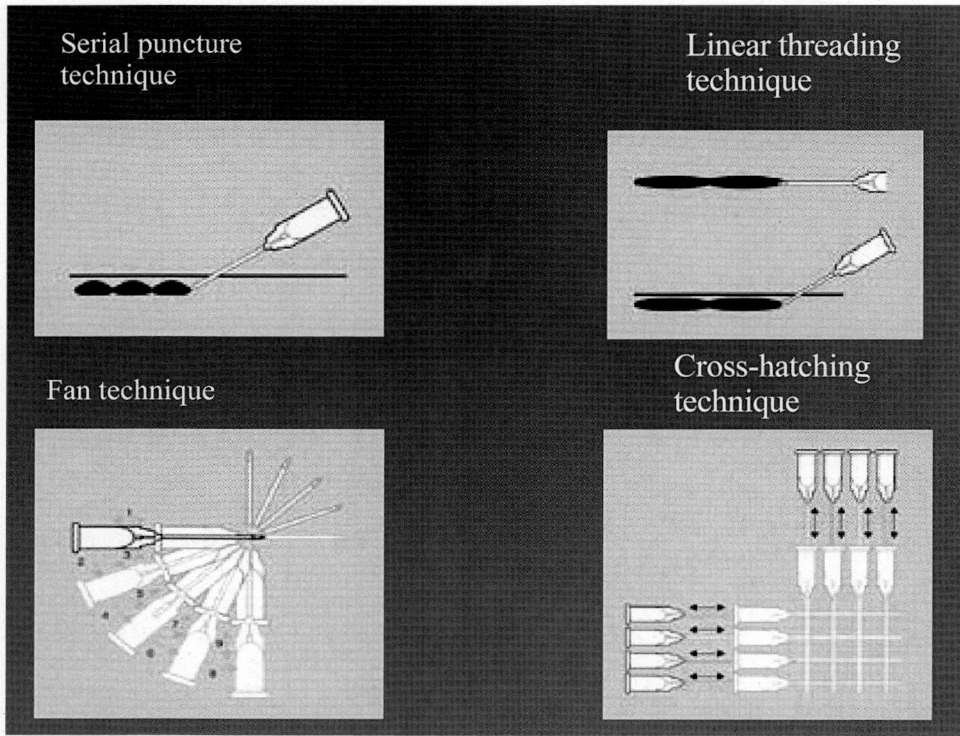

Fig. 28.10 Various injection techniques.

The smooth surface of the microsphere decreases a foreign body reaction, and its size prevents migration and phagocytosis.[57] It should not be used in areas of fine skin because the implants may be more visible and should be avoided in those prone to keloids given that any foreign material may serve to increase the incidence of keloids. However, Artecoll demonstrates a much lower incidence of immunological response (0.06%) as compared with Zyderm, which has an incidence of 3%.[52] A concern with the use of permanent filler is the potential for migration to other areas outside of the injection site, which can lead to potential deformities. Migration has only been observed when the material is injected into the dermis in trials with guinea pigs and has not been observed with correct placement of the material.[58] Granulomas may also occur, and, although it is impossible to predict which patients may face this consequence, those fillers that are composed of microspheres with a smooth surface, such as Artecoll and New-Fill (Dermik Laboratories, Berwick, PA), are less likely to cause this reaction than fillers with irregularly surfaced microspheres, such as Dermalive.[14] Reviderm (Rifol Medical International, Netherlands), available in Europe, is a suspension of 2.5% dextran microspheres of 40 μm in 2.0% hyaluronic acid. The microspheres of Reviderm produced the greatest amount of granulation tissue but were also disintegrated at nine months.

Artecoll may be used to treat facial rhytids or scars. We do not advocate its use in lips due to the potential development of granulomas, which are difficult to remove. In addition, thin skin areas (i.e., crow's feet) should be avoided because the implant may be visible or palpable; hence, the implant should not be injected into the dermis. Artecoll is injected into the subdermis with a 27-gauge needle under constant pressure using the needle to create tunnels. The patient is also encouraged to massage the area for 3 to 5 days.[57] Slight overcorrection is recommended and repeat injections may be performed one to three months later.

Combinations of materials are also available outside the United States, including Dermalive and Dermadeep (Dermatich, Paris, France). Dermalive, a 40% HA, and Dermadeep, a 60% HA, are combinations of HA and the active constituent acrylic hydrogel (contact lens material), which have been studied in Europe. They, along with over 50 other permanent microparticulate synthetic products worldwide, were developed for sustained irreversible soft tissue augmentation. The tolerance for Dermalive, like silicone or PMMA beads in patients who demonstrate no early or late-term chronic inflammatory response to the acrylic polymer, is good and it has been supplemented with injections of Juvederm or Restylane for fine line and superficial defects.[59] A 3-year study of this combination therapy in 455 patients demonstrates an 88% patient satisfaction rate with limited side effects.[59] Experience with these permanent bead products demonstrates a measurable incidence of deforming side effects requiring surgical intervention.

Implantable Synthetic Polymers

Expanded Polytetrafluroethylene

Implantable expanded polytetrafluoroethylene (e-PTFE) (W.L. Gore and Associates, Flagstaff, AZ) has been used in the field of vascular surgery for over 30 years, a testament to its safety and reliability.[60] Tissue in-growth is marginal into the material, but when shaped into a tube, longitudinal growth occurs. This serves to strengthen the filler and secure it to the site of implantation.[61] The tubular form, marketed under the name SoftForm (Collagen Corp., Palo Alto, CA), was used as a soft tissue filler for lip augmentation. There still exists a risk of extrusion or exposure of the ends of the material at the entrance wound where the implant is delivered. SoftForm showed wall stiffening due to the abundance of ePTFE and will shorten and harden with time. This can create an "accordion effect." The risk of extrusion at the insertion sites creates a·potential source of infection. If complications do arise, the implant is always removable. Because of these limitations, SoftForm has been improved and is now marketed under the new name Ultrasoft, a thinner and softer form.

Ultrasoft is dispensed alone or within an included trocar. A stab incision is made where the implant is to be inserted after obtaining local anesthesia. The implant is tunneled parallel to the defect at the level of the deep reticular dermis or subdermis. The implant is cut at the remaining end and the entrance wound is closed in layers. Careful attention is paid to insure symmetric and even soft tissue distribution over the implant prior to removing the tunneling trocar.

Techniques to Deliver Soft Tissue Fillers

When considering injectables, there are basically four techniques used to deliver material to the deep dermis or subcutaneous level: linear threading, serial puncture, and the subcutaneous techniques of fanning and cross-hatching (**Fig. 28.10**).

Linear threading is a technique by which an agent is applied in a uniform fashion while the needle is slowly advanced or withdrawn from the tissue. Uniformity in the depth of deposition is the challenge when placing products intradermally using this technique. Subcutaneous or deep intradermal applications, however, can be reliably performed using linear threading. This technique is commonly employed (along with fanning) for nasolabial fold and oral commissure augmentation as well as volume enhancement and contouring. The HA fillers and Radiesse are commonly applied using this technique.

Linear threading is a particularly effective technique when one is performing lip augmentation along the mucocutaneous border. By placing the needle in the proper plane along the vermillion border and applying steady and light plunger pressure the injector can achieve an effective and uniform placement of the product effectively by hydrodissection. The anatomical plane filled employing this technique can provide a natural lip roll and substantial natural augmentation.

The serial puncture technique is used to deliver small aliquots of filler at multiple spots to achieve even distribution over a two-dimensional area. It is particularly effective in accurately delivering product at the more superficial levels of the mid- to upper dermis and thus is ideal for correcting fine lines. The flow characteristics and color of Cosmoderm I and Zyderm I make these products more suitable for this technique, although some authors have reported success using fine (30-gauge) needles and HA products for fine lines. The skin is punctured superficially and gentle plunger pressure is applied to achieve a visible blanching effect that elevates the line and spreads circumferentially beyond its confines. Four to 8 mm of wheal are thus created, and the needle is withdrawn and topographically reinserted at approximately the radius of the previous wheal. The linear defect is followed as such to achieve complete correction. In general, although HA products are theoretically designed and approved for intradermal injection, many expert providers are injecting these products subdermally and demonstrating excellent results and longevity. Examples of applications where subdermal injections are required and have shown good results and longevity include the tear trough deformity, mandibular border, lips, and even the nasolabial fold.

The senior author has witnessed many "expert" demonstrations of injection in which the instructor represented that the injections were in the "deep dermis" while plunging the needle 5 to 8 mm or more below the skin surface. Although anatomically incorrect in the description of placement, subdermal injections may be an ideal level for many areas. It is understandable that companies cannot promote off-label use of products, however, as practitioners we should take care to more accurately represent the level of place, which in the case of HA products, may not need to be placed in the dermis to provide excellent and lasting cosmetic effect.

As such, when using HA products we use both a topical and nerve block anesthesia to achieve high levels of patient comfort. After proper anesthesia the skin is prepared with topical alcohol. The patient is generally in the lounge chair position, although for gravity-dependent areas such as the nasolabial fold, one may need to place the patient more upright for accuracy. A linear threading technique is used in the deep dermal–subcutaneous junction for nasolabial folds starting inferiorly and moving superomedially. The lips are injected from lateral to medial in the subcutaneous plane along the vermilion border by gentle pressure and "hydrodissection." Upper and lower lips are treated similarly with focus on the central one third of the lower lip. Further plumping and eversion can be achieved by everting the lip and placing several linear "beads" caudal to the wet lip border.

The mandibular border and tear trough deformity are treated in the deep subcutaneous tissues with linear threading and serial point and aggressive massage. Care must be taken and consent given for the potential risk of periorbital vascular occlusion. Although the author is not aware of intracranial or intraorbital occlusion complications, such complications have been reported with steroid injections and are theoretically possible.

One unique benefit of the HA products is the immediate reversibility or correction of this product with hyaluronidase. Using 25 to 150 units of hyaluronidase injected directly into the irregularity can improve contour within 24 hours in the authors' experience.

Collagen Products

In contrast to HA products, the collagen products should be used intradermally because they have in general very short effective half-lives when placed subcutaneously. Zyderm and Cosmoderm remain the most effective fine line fillers in the authors' opinion and as such play a large role in minimally invasive cosmetic enhancements. For fine line treatments they are injected using a 30-gauge needle placed at 30 to 45 degrees to the skin surface and injected slowly in a serial point fashion along the generally linear defects. A blanching effect is seen as the collagen slowly expands in the mid- to upper dermis with an overcorrection of 150 to 200% recommended. Standard recommendations urge against overcorrection when using Zyplast or Cosmoplast; however, reports show better results with slight overcorrection.[51]

An emerging strategy gaining popularity is utilizing CosmoDerm in conjunction with other fillers such as HA. An HA filler such as Restylane can be used to address deeper lines and enhance volume, whereas CosmoDerm is used to treat the more superficial lines.[62]

Calcium Hydroxyapatite Particles (Radiesse)

Calcium hydroxyapatite is injected subcutaneously using a linear threading or fanning technique. The deeper placement provides a softer feel and does not seem to impact the longevity, which is generally seen to be in the 6- to 12-month range. Slight overcorrection is recommended because the carboxymethylcellulose carrier will resorb over a short period.

Summary

The introduction of the botulinum neurotoxin, injectable fillers, and other minimally invasive techniques has changed the treatment paradigm for the aging face. The choice of which to use can be based on several factors, including desires of the patient, cost to the patient, and experience of the clinician. Caution must be exercised, however, when considering the use of newly introduced "permanent" soft tissue fillers that have not undergone long-term observation and study. The new fillers work well alone, but the current trend seems to be toward using them in combination and in particular with botulinum toxin for relaxation of hyperfunctional muscles and dynamic lines, volume restoration, and line and border filling.

Results with this combination of products can be remarkable, even stunning, and the technique provides a true alternative to surgical intervention in many selected patients.

Although the products and technologies for rejuvenation and contouring are rapidly evolving, it is advisable to employ comprehensive management and approaches that include combinations of the available injectable agents.

References

1. Scott AB. Botulinum toxin injection into extraocular muscles as an alternative to Strabismus surgery. J Pediatr Ophthalmol Strabismus 1990;17:21–25
2. Schantz EJ, Johnson EA. Persp Biol Med. 1997; 40:317–327. Schantz EJ, Johnson EA. In: Jankovic J, Hallet M, eds. Therapy with Botulinum Toxin. 1994
3. Ramirez AL, Reeck J, Maas CS. Preliminary experience with botulinum toxin type B in hyperkinetic facial lines. Plast Reconstr Surg 2002;109:2154–2155
4. Ramirez AL, Reeck J, Maas CS. Botulinum toxin type B (Myobloc) in the management of hyperkinetic facial lines. Otolaryngol Head Neck Surg 2002;126:459–467
5. MacDonald M, Spiegel J, Maas CS. Glabellar anatomy: the anatomic basis for BoTox therapy. Arch Otolaryngol Head Neck Surg 1998; 124:1315–1320
6. Loos BM, Maas CS. Relevant anatomy for botulinum toxin facial rejuvenation. Facial Plast Surg Clin North Am 2003;11:439–443
7. Ahn M, Catten M, Maas CS. Temporal browlift using botulinum toxin: plastic and reconstructive surgery. Plast Reconstr Surg 2000; 105:1129–1135
8. Maas CS, Kim EJ. Temporal brow lift using botulinum toxin A: an update. Plast Reconstr Surg 2003; 112(5, Suppl)109S–112S
9. Carruthers J, Fagien S, Matarasso SL. Consensus recommendations on the use of Botulinum toxin type A in facial aesthetics. Plast Reconstr Surg 2004; 114(6, Suppl)1–22

10. Matarasso A, Matarasso SL. Botulinum A exotoxin for the management of Platysmal bands. Plast Reconstr Surg 2003; 112(5, Suppl)138–140
11. Matarasso SL. Complications of botulinum A exotoxin for hyperfunctional lines. Dermatol Surg 1998;24:1249
12. Guyuron B. Nonsurgical treatment of platysmal bands with injection of botulinum toxin A. Plast Reconstr Surg 2003; 112(5, Suppl)123–124
13. Neuber F. Fat grafting. Cuir Kongr Verh Otsum Ges Chir. 1893;20:66
14. Ersek RA, Beisang AA III. Bioplastique: a new biphasic polymer for minimally invasive injection implantation. Aesthetic Plast Surg 1992; 16:59–65
15. Bailin PLBM. Collagen implantation: clinical applications and lesion selection. J Dermatol Surg Oncol 1988;14:49
16. Castrow FF II, Krull EA. Injectable collagen implant—update. J Am Acad Dermatol 1983;9:889–893
17. Maas CS, Papel ID, Greene D, Stoker DA. Complications of injectable synthetic polymers in facial augmentation. Dermatol Surg 1997; 23:871–877
18. Newcomer VD, Graham JH, Schaffert RR, Kaplan L. Sclerosing lipogranuloma resulting from exogenous lipids. AMA Arch Derm 1956;73:361–372
19. Ben-Hur N, Neuman Z. Siliconoma: another cutaneous response to dimethylpolysiloxane: experimental study in mice. Plast Reconstr Surg 1965;36:629–631
20. Achauer BM. A serious complication following medical-grade silicone injection of the face. Plast Reconstr Surg 1983;71:251–253
21. Orentreich DS, Orentreich N. Injectable fluid silicone. In: Roenigk RK, Roenigk HH Jr, eds. Dermatologic Surgery: Principles and Practice. New York: Marcel Dekker; 1989:1349–1395
22. Webster RC, Fuleihan NS, Gaunt JM, et al. Injectable silicone for small augmentations: twenty-year experience in humans. Am J Cosm Surg 1984;1:1–7
23. Bigata X, Ribera M, Bielsa I, Ferrandiz C. Adverse granulomatous reaction after cosmetic dermal silicone injection. Dermatol Surg 2001; 27:198–200
24. Landman MD, Strahan RW, Ward PH. Chin augmentation with Polytef paste injection. Arch Otolaryngol 1972;95:72–75
25. Clark D, Hanke W, Swanson N. Dermal implants: safety of products injected for soft tissue augmentation. J Am Acad Dermatol 1989; 21:992–998
26. Cooperman LS, Mackinnon V, Bechler G, Pharriss BB. Injectable collagen: a 6-year clinical investigation. Aesthetic Plast Surg 1985; 9:145–151
27. Skouge JW, Diwan RV. Soft tissue augmentation with injectable collagen. In: Papel ID, Nachlas NE, eds. Facial Plastic and Reconstructive Surgery. St. Louis, Mosby Year Book; 1992:208
28. Ashinoff R. Overview: soft tissue augmentation. Clin Plast Surg 2000; 27:479–487
29. Narins RS, Bowman PH. Injectable skin fillers. Clin Plast Surg 2005; 32:151–162
30. Fagien S. Facial soft-tissue augmentation with injectable autologous and allogeneic human tissue collagen matrix (autologen and dermalogen). Plast Reconstr Surg 2000;105:362–375
31. Schell JJ. Polytef injection for nasal deformity. Arch Otolaryngol 1970; 92:554–559
32. Burres S. Preserved particulate fascia lata for injection: a new alternative. Dermatol Surg 1999;25:790–794
33. Krauss MC. Recent advances in soft tissue augmentation. Semin Cutan Med Surg 1999;18:119–128
34. Duranti F, Salti G, Bovani B, Calandra M, Rosati ML. Injectable hyaluronic acid gel for soft tissue augmentation: a clinical and histological study. Dermatol Surg 1998;24:1317–1325
35. Lowe NJ, Maxwell CA, Lowe P, Duick MG, Shah K. Hyaluronic acid skin fillers: adverse reactions and skin testing. J Am Acad Dermatol 2001;45:930–933
36. Maas CS. Characteristics of implant materials. Arch Facial Plast Surg 2000;2:67
37. Lowe NJ, Maxwell A, Lowe P, et al. Hyaluronic acid fillers: adverse reactions and skin testing. J Am Acad Dermatol 2001;45:930–933
38. Micheels P. Human antihyaluronic acid antibodies: is it possible? Dermatol Surg 2001;27:185–191
39. Lemperle G, Morhenn V, Charrier U. Human histology and persistence of various injectable filler substances for soft tissue augmentation. Aesthetic Plast Surg 2003;27:354–366 discussion 367
40. Fernandez-Acenero MJ, Zamora E, Borbujo J. Granulomatous foreign body reaction against hyaluronic acid: report of a case after lip augmentation. Dermatol Surg 2003;29:1225–1226
41. Olenius M. The first clinical study using a new biodegradable implant for the treatment of lips, wrinkles, and folds. Aesthetic Plast Surg 1998;22:97–101
42. Duranti F, Salti G, Bovani B, et al. Injectable hyaluronic acid gel for soft tissue augmentation: a clinical and histological study. Dermatol Surg 1998;24:1317–1325
43. Narins RS, Brandt F, Leyden J, Lorenc ZP, Rubin M, Smith S. A randomized, double-blind, multicenter comparison of the efficacy and tolerability of Restylane versus Zyplast for the correction of nasolabial folds. Dermatol Surg 2003;29:588–595
44. Carruthers J, Carruthers A. A prospective, randomized, parallel group study analyzing the effect of BTX-A (Botox) and nonanimal sourced hyaluronic acid (NASHA, Restylane) in combination compared with NASHA (Restylane) alone in severe glabellar rhytides in adult female subjects: treatment of severe glabellar rhytides with a hyaluronic acid derivative compared with the derivative and BTX-A. Dermatol Surg 2003; 29:802–809
45. Sclafani AP, Romo T III, Jacono AA. Rejuvenation of the aging lip with an injectable acellular dermal graft (Cymetra). Arch Facial Plast Surg 2002;4:252–257
46. Sclafani AP, Romo T III, Parker A, McCormick SA, Cocker R, Jacono A. Homologous collagen dispersion (dermalogen) as a dermal filler: persistence and histology compared with bovine collagen. Ann Plast Surg 2002;49:181–188
47. Castor SA, To WC, Papay FA. Lip augmentation with AlloDerm acellular allogenic dermal graft and fat autograft: a comparison with autologous fat injection alone. Aesthetic Plast Surg 1999;23:218–223
48. Peer LA. Loss of weight and volume in human fat grafts. Plast Reconstr Surg 1950;5:217
49. Illouz Y. The fat cell "graft": a new technique to fill depressions. Plast Reconstr Surg 1986;78:122–123
50. Coleman S. Facial contouring with lipostructure. Clin Plast Surg 1997;24:347–367
51. Cheng JT, Perkins SW, Hamilton MM. Collagen and injectable fillers. Otolaryngol Clin North Am 2002;35:73–85
52. Lemperle G, Kind P. Biocompatibility of Artecoll. Plast Reconstr Surg 1999;103:338–340
53. Kanchwala SK, Holloway L, Bucky LP. Reliable soft tissue augmentation: a clinical comparison of injectable soft-tissue fillers for facial-volume augmentation. Ann Plast Surg 2005;55:30–35
54. Valantin MA, Aubron-Olivier C, Ghosn J, et al. Polylactic acid implants (New-Fill) to correct facial lipoatrophy in HIV-infected patients: results of the open-label study VEGA. AIDS 2003;17:2471–2477
55. Spira M, Rosen T. Injectable soft tissue substitutes. Clin Plast Surg 1993;20:181–188
56. Pollack S. Silicone, fibril, collagen implantation for facial lines and wrinkles. J Dermatol Surg Oncol 1990; 16:957–961
57. Lemperle G, Hazan-Gauthier N, Lemperle M. PMMA microspheres (Artecoll) for skin and soft-tissue augmentation, II: Clinical investigations. Plast Reconstr Surg 1995;96:627–634
58. McClelland M, Egbert B, Hanko V, Berg RA, DeLustro F. Evaluation of Artecoll polymethylmethacrylate implant for soft-tissue augmentation: biocompatibility and chemical characterization. Plast Reconstr Surg 1997;100:1466–1474
59. Bergeret-Galley C, Latouche X, Illouz YG. The value of a new filler material in corrective and cosmetic surgery: DermaLive and DermaDeep. Aesthetic Plast Surg 2001;25:249–255
60. Costantino PD. Synthetic biomaterials for soft-tissue augmentation and replacement in the head and neck. Otolaryngol Clin North Am 1994;27:223–262
61. Ahn MSMN, Maas CS. Soft tissue augmentation. Facial Plast Surg Clin North Am 1999;7:35–41
62. Bauman L. CosmoDerm/CosmoPlast (Human Bioengineered Collagen) for the aging face. Facial Plast Surg 2004;20:125–128

29 Complementary Fat Grafting

Mark J. Glasgold, Samuel M. Lam, and Robert A. Glasgold

Facial volume loss has become increasingly recognized as an important if not primary mechanism by which the aging process occurs. Interest in facial fat grafting for volume restoration has been increasing due to recent advances in technique that have proven beneficial in achieving consistently excellent cosmetic results while at the same time reducing morbidity. A simplified analogy can be used to understand the effects of aging secondary to volume depletion: the face is like a grape in youth that over time becomes a raisin. The question then is why should the redundant skin that arises be lifted, pulled, and cut away so that what is left no longer resembles the grape of youth but appears more like a truncated pea. Instead, we should fill and restore the depressed facial zones as needed to achieve the highlights, contours, and convexities that define youth. The reductionist philosophy espoused here does not truly reflect the authors' opinion entirely because we recognize the complexity of the aging process that can be made up of volume loss, volume gain, gravitational descent, and dermatologic changes. Nevertheless, what may have been perceived in the past as only gravity or skin redundancy should be reinterpreted as possibly arising from tissue deflation that could be corrected with facial fat grafting.

How can we determine what would be the best course of action to rejuvenate an individual seeking to restore a youthful countenance? One answer can be found in photographs of patients when they were younger. These images, or alternatively photographs of attractive youthful faces, help us understand what the aesthetic goal should be. Too often the surgical procedure dictates the aesthetic goal, rather than the aesthetic goal dictating the procedures we use. For example, browlifts, in our opinion, have been overused for upper face rejuvenation, and often create an unnatural skeletonized superior orbital rim and an unattractive elongated face. This type of result is not natural and is often not consistent with the way the patient appeared at a younger age. By using old photographs as a guide, judicious combination of fat grafting, liposuction, blepharoplasty, facelifting, skin therapies, and so forth, can be used to achieve a result that more closely approximates the image of one's former self. We have entitled this combination approach toward fat grafting "complementary fat grafting," because we see the value in fat grafting not necessarily as a stand-alone procedure in every case but as complementary to traditional procedures.[1] This integrated strategy allows the surgeon to select a combination of procedures that can be tailored to an aesthetic goal (**Fig. 29.1A,B**).

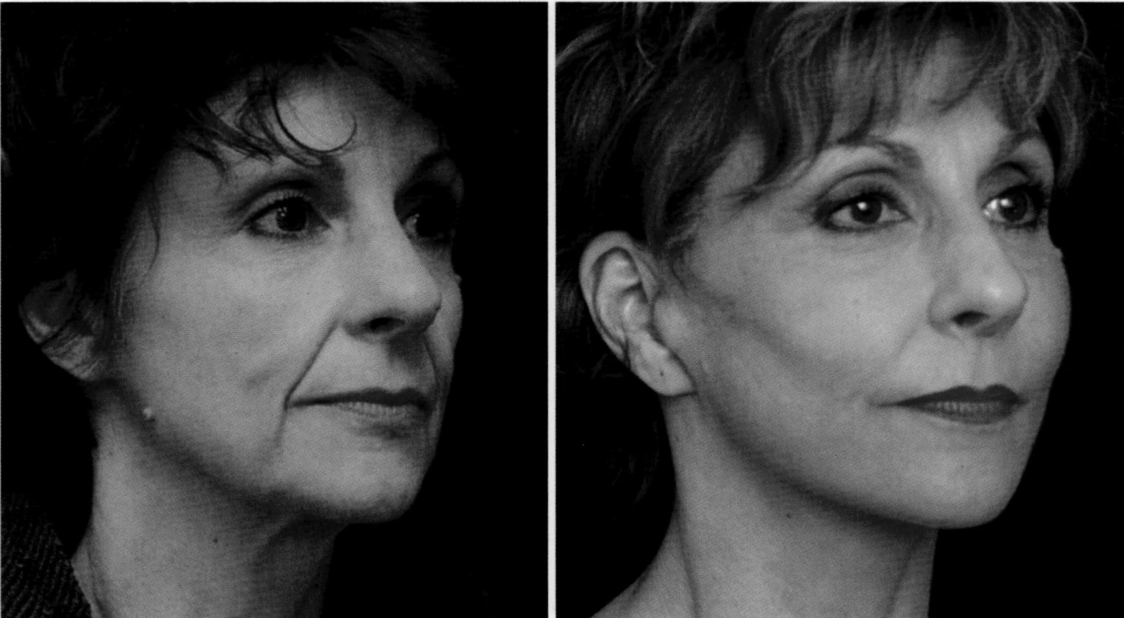

Fig. 29.1 (**A**) Preoperatively this patient displays changes related to both volume loss and tissue descent. (**B**) Five years following a facelift and midface and periorbital fat transfer. (From Lam SM, Glasgold MJ, Glasgold RA. Complementary Fat Grafting. Philadelphia: Lippincott Williams & Wilkins; 2007. Reprinted by permission.)

History

The recent interest in facial fat grafting, evidenced in that this third-edition book is the first to include any mention of the technique, may seem to indicate that fat grafting has been around for only a short time. In fact, the first clinical case of fat transfer can be traced back to Neuber in 1893, who described the use of fat grafting to restore a facial defect that arose from tuberculous osteitis.[2] Two years later, Czerny discussed reconstruction of a breast defect left behind by removal of a benign mass by implanting an excised lipoma.[3] In 1910 Lexer used larger parcels of transplanted fat to improve fat survival,[4] followed the next year by Bruning who restored a postrhinoplasty defect successfully with fat grafting[5] and Tuffier who implanted fat into the extra-pleural space to ameliorate certain pulmonary conditions.[6] In 1932 Straatsma and Peer closed a fistula following frontal sinus surgery using autologous adipose tissue.[7] Two years later Cotton morcellized and placed fat to improve various contour defects.

The advent of liposuction in 1974 stimulated the interest in employing the removed fat as grafting material.[8] In 1982, Bircoll described using liposuctioned fat to correct a host of contour problems.[9] Illouz,[10] Krulig,[11] and Newman[12] continued the trend in using aspirated fat to recontour the face and body during the 1980s. The two proponents that have substantially influenced the current resurgence in autologous fat transfer are Sydney R. Coleman of New York[13] and Roger Amar of France,[14] who have advocated using low pressure hand (rather than machine) suction for fat harvesting, followed by centrifugation to purify the fat cells, and injection of only tiny parcels of fat using blunt cannulas. Placing only very small amounts (0.05 to 0.1 mL per pass of the cannula) has been advocated to facilitate a smoother result and at the same time to improve long-term transplant survival owing to the enriched blood supply that surrounds each microparcel of fat.

Preoperative Considerations

Conveying to a patient the potential benefits of fat grafting may initially be more difficult than convincing him or her of the merits of a facelift. Most plastic surgeons, the media, and one's peers are familiar with what a facelift does and it is not uncommon for patients to come through the door holding their face up with two fingers to indicate the desired changes. However, correcting the effects of gravity may not be the only beneficial course of action or may not be needed at all, especially in the younger individual. Oftentimes, a younger person in his or her thirties and early forties may only exhibit volume loss, which will not be improved by a lifting procedure (**Fig. 29.2A,B**).

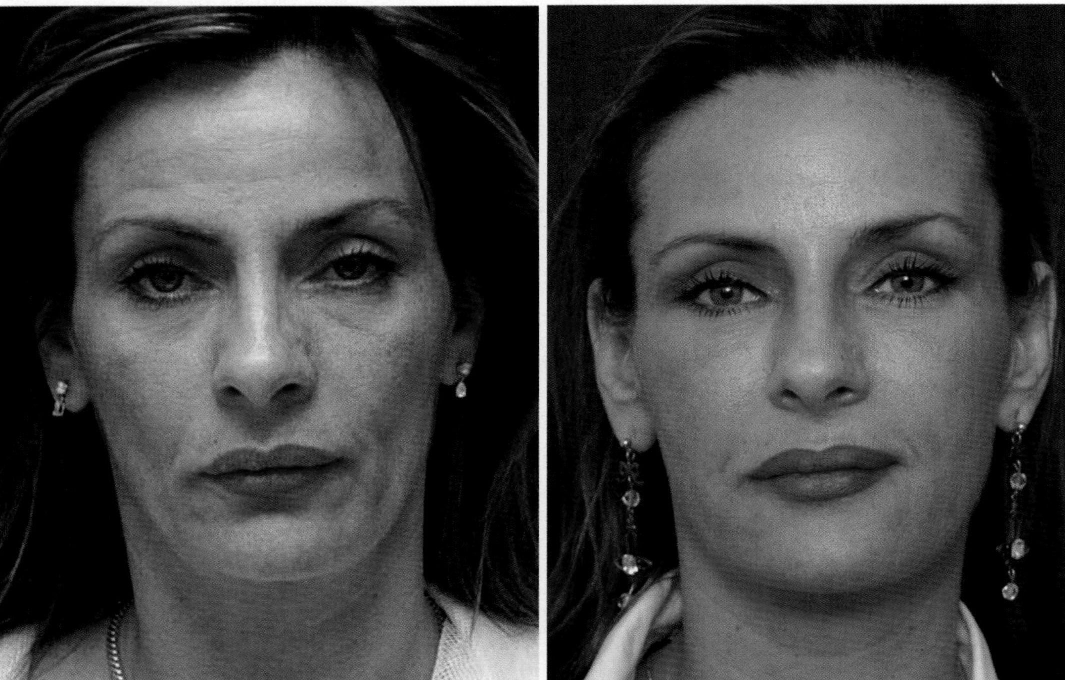

Fig. 29.2 (**A**) Preoperative view of a patient who desired a facelift, but who needed volume replacement. (**B**) Full face fat transfer without a facelift produced a natural, more youthful appearance. (From Lam SM, Glasgold MJ, Glasgold RA. Complementary Fat Grafting. Philadelphia: Lippincott Williams & Wilkins; 2007. Reprinted by permission.)

If one reflects for a moment how an observer can tell that another individual is a teenager, twentysomething, or thirtysomething even before acknowledging the influence of clothing styles or mannerisms, the answer lies in the volume changes of the face, more specifically the ongoing loss of what is known colloquially as "baby fat." In fact, some women and men would not like to go back to the exuberant fullness that characterizes a teenager or a twentysomething. Using old photographs can help establish dialogue about the evolution of aging that is witnessed in that particular individual and the specific goals for facial rejuvenation.

There are three general concepts useful for facial analysis in terms of volume depletion. These include facial volume and shape, highlights and shadows, and the importance of framing the eyes. As an individual ages, their facial shape progresses from a youthful heart shape, or triangle, to a more rectangular appearance. The apices of the youthful triangle are the malar prominences and the chin, all of which are full and convex. With age, volume loss in the malar regions and mentum combine with volume contraction in the prejowl sulcus and soft tissue ptosis in the jowl, to change facial shape. The result of a narrowed upper face and a widened lower face is a rectangular, and aging, facial shape. One of the principle goals of facial rejuvenation is to reconstitute the idealized triangle, or heart shape, that defines youth (**Fig. 29.3A,B**). The malar region and mentum/prejowl sulcus can be augmented with facial fat grafting, whereas the jowl can be reduced by selective microliposuction with or without a facelift as needed. In a patient with a heavy jowl or a very obtuse cervicomental angle, fat grafting alone will often fail to achieve the desired aesthetic result. In these cases, a combination of fat grafting together with a facelift will yield superior results.

The volume and shape of a face are what first give an impression of facial age and are the most important factors to control in achieving a youthful aesthetic result. Many women evaluate their own faces using a magnifying mirror and bright illumination while applying their makeup. As a result they tend to focus on minor imperfections. However, most onlookers do not see these minor cutaneous flaws that the individual is complaining of because they are often not visible to others at a normal conversational distance. To help patients appreciate this apparent contradiction it is useful to review current photographs of the patient, and if available look at photos of them at a younger age. In addition, showing examples of patients with similar facial aging changes, both before and after correction with fat transfer, is particularly enlightening for prospective patients. Review of these photos will help patients visualize the shadows that develop with aging, which include the depressed brow, temple, inferior orbital rim, anterior malar septum, submalar and buccal hollow, and prejowl sulcus.

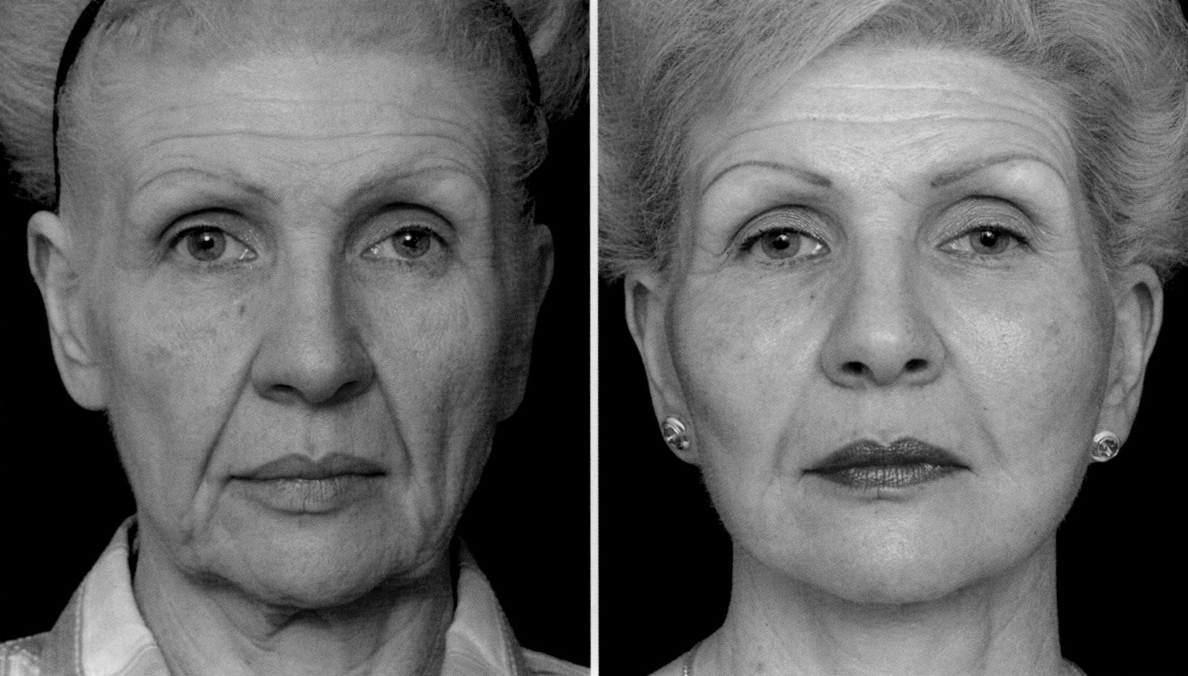

Fig. 29.3 (**A**) Volume changes typical of the aging process create a rectangular, elongated facial shape. (**B**) Restoring the heart shape through facelift and midface fat transfer creates a more youthful facial shape. (From Lam SM, Glasgold MJ, Glasgold RA. Complementary Fat Grafting. Philadelphia: Lippincott Williams & Wilkins; 2007. Reprinted by permission.)

Appreciating the dominance of shadows that develop with age emphasizes the role of fat grafting in the elimination of senescent shadows and creation of youthful highlights. Some of the important youthful highlights include the lateral brow highlight, the anterior and lateral cheek highlights, and the chin highlights. Reducing the shadowed demarcations that divide the face and creating more youthful highlights can dramatically transform a tired, older face into a more vibrant, youthful one (**Fig. 29.4A,B**).

The concept of providing an adequate frame for the eyes is critical in patient evaluation for fat grafting. The eyes are perhaps the most important area to rejuvenate because they are the focal point of the face. Traditional blepharoplasty relies on the removal of skin and fat and has a tendency to exacerbate already hollow and aged eyes. In emphasizing volume we are not dismissing the role of skin excision, but feel that volume loss along the orbital rim and brow contributes to the development of skin redundancy and needs to be addressed with volume replacement. In practice this has translated into an approach to the upper lid where we perform a conservative skin excision with fat reduction, only when there is a significant medial fat prominence, in conjunction with fat transfer to the superior orbital rim. Addressing the lower lid will include a transconjunctival blepharoplasty to conservatively reduce medial, central, or lateral fat, if they are prominent, combined with fat transfer to the inferior orbital rim and cheek (**Fig. 29.5A,B**). The cheek should be thought of as an extension of the lower eyelid subunit. An ideal youthful face will not have a demarcation between the lower lid and cheek, but instead will have a single convexity from lid to cheek. Creating the appropriate frame for the eye includes smoothly contouring the lid into the cheek (**Fig. 29.6A,B**).

Men typically like the increasingly sculpted appearance as facial volume loss occurs and generally present for correction at a later stage of volume loss. In contrast, women will often be more acutely aware and bothered by these changes at an earlier stage because the volume changes tend to masculinize the female face. Accordingly, facial fat grafting can truly feminize the face and restore the luster of feminine youth. The anterior cheek in particular when accentuated can be very feminizing. This is one of the areas where the goal of rejuvenation is gender specific, in that too much anterior cheek fullness will impart a feminine appearance to a man's face.

Patients can also be encouraged to review the facial features that attractive, youthful models exhibit in popular

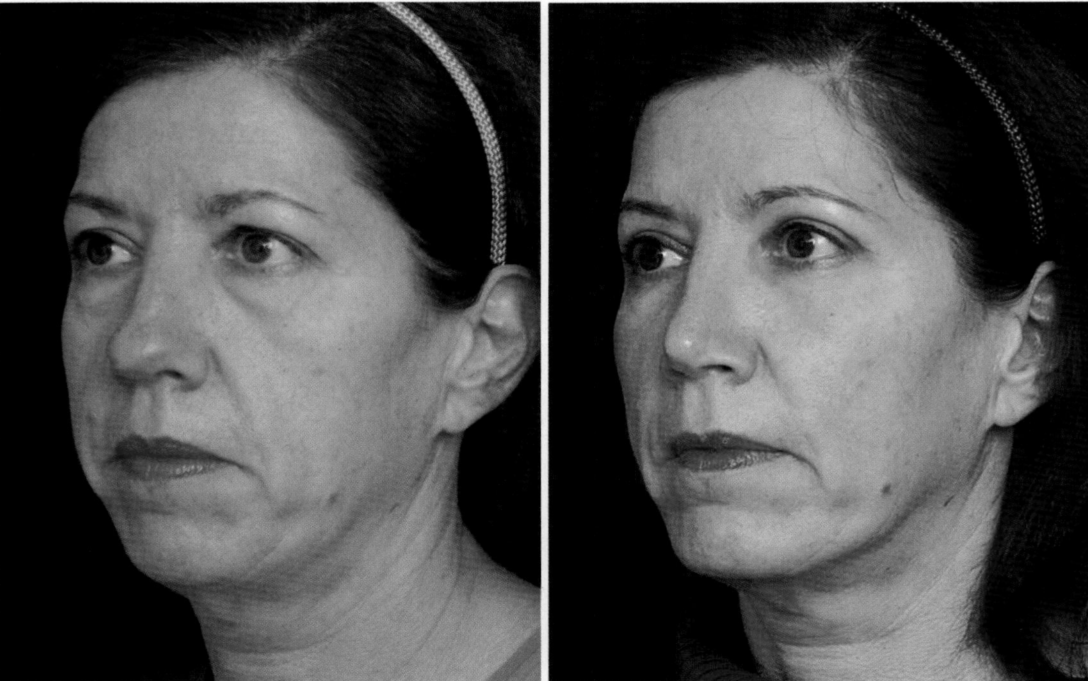

Fig. 29.4 (**A**) The shadows of the inferior orbital hollow and the malar depression are typical of the aging face. (**B**) Periorbital and midface fat transfer (combined with skin only upper lid blepharoplasty, conservative transconjunctival lower lid blepharoplasty, and chin implant) recreates youthful facial highlights. (From Carniol and Sadick. Clinical Procedures in Laser Skin Rejuvenation. Informa Healthcare; 2007. Reprinted by permission of Informa Healthcare.)

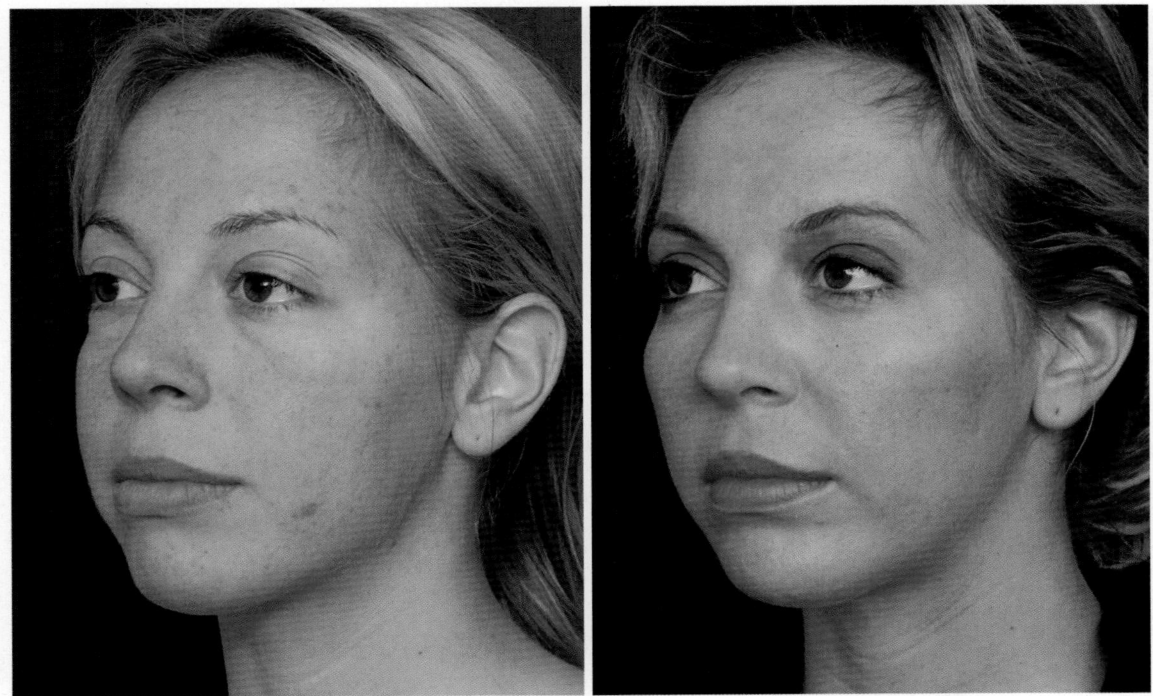

Fig. 29.5 (**A**) Patient with a poor periorbital frame has a prominent appearing eye due to inadequate volume in the superior and inferior orbital rim. (**B**) The eye is attractively framed following periorbital and midface fat transfer and conservative transconjunctival lower lid blepharoplasty. (From Lam SM, Glasgold MJ, Glasgold RA. Complementary Fat Grafting. Philadelphia: Lippincott Williams & Wilkins; 2007. Reprinted by permission.)

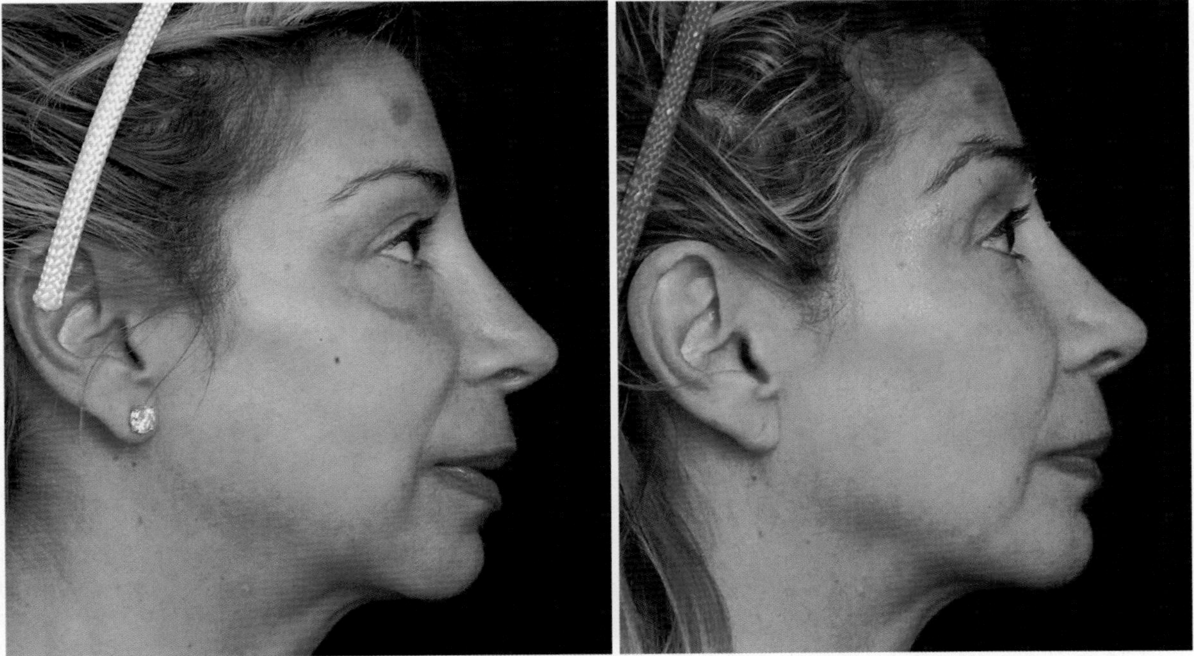

Fig. 29.6 (**A**) Inferior orbital rim volume loss creates a demarcation between the lower lid and cheek. (**B**) The youthful single convexity in which there is a smooth transition from the lower lid to cheek is restored with fat transfer. (From Lam SM, Glasgold MJ, Glasgold RA. Complementary Fat Grafting. Philadelphia: Lippincott Williams & Wilkins; 2007. Reprinted by permission.)

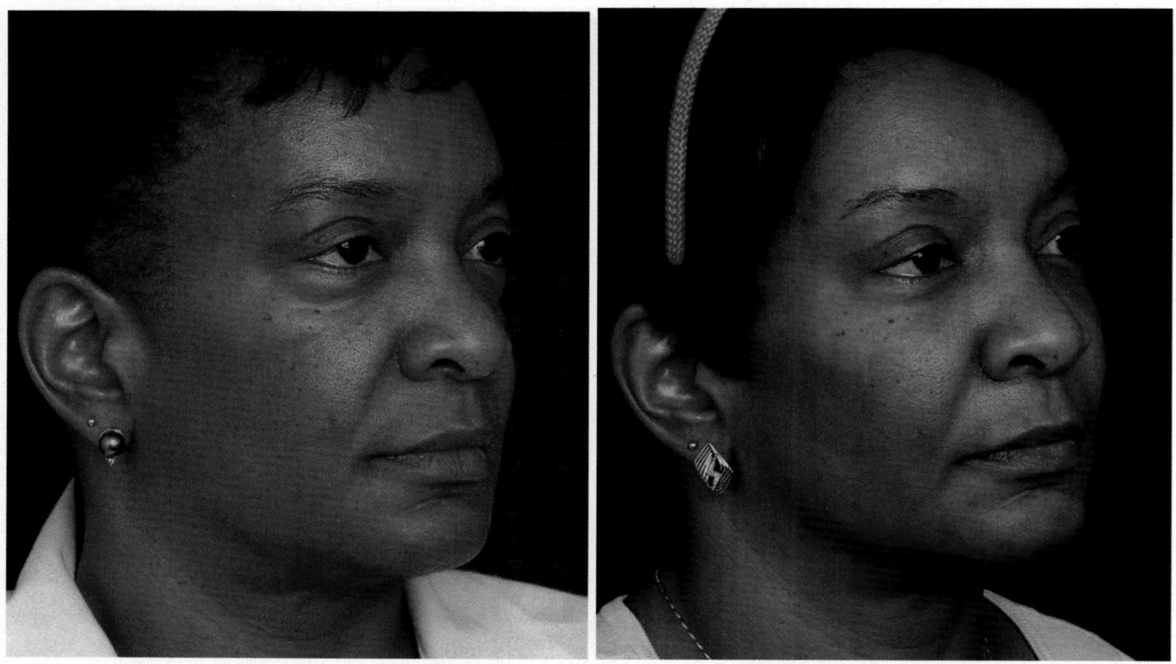

Fig. 29.7 Volume restoration for midfacial rejuvenation. (**A**) Preoperative. (**B**) Postoperative, following periorbital and midface fat transfer. (From Lam SM, Glasgold MJ, Glasgold RA. Complementary Fat Grafting. Philadelphia: Lippincott Williams & Wilkins; 2007. Reprinted by permission.)

fashion magazines in order for them to understand more convincingly the role that volume restoration has on a youthful countenance. For individuals who have undergone prior facial procedures, asking them to remember when they were just slightly swollen (not grossly distorted) in the immediate postoperative setting can help them understand the attraction that volume restoration carries during this so-called phase of "honeymoon swelling."

Fat grafting has proven to be a useful rejuvenative tool across all racial divides.[15] Many individuals of darker complexion may be more recalcitrant to photodamage and gravity than those with a very fair complexion. Accordingly, facial fat grafting has been a principal mechanism for facial rejuvenation in all skin types, as every race suffers from volume loss in high measure (**Fig. 29.7A,B**).[16]

Surgical Techniques

This section is structured in chronological order, as the surgeon would proceed on the day of the procedure: marking the recipient sites, selection of donor site, anesthesia, donor-site harvesting, processing the fat, injection techniques, and immediate postoperative care.

Marking the Recipient Sites

The patient should be in an upright position so that all the folds and depressions can be easily visualized. All of the areas to be augmented with fat are outlined. These will generally include the brow, temple, inferior orbital rim, tear trough, anterior cheek, lateral cheek, buccal hollow, precanine fossa, nasolabial fold, and prejowl sulcus (**Fig. 29.8**).

Selection of Donor Site

The donor site selection is based on fat availability and ease of harvesting relative to patient positioning. Asking the patient where their most abundant adipose reserves are located is perhaps the easiest method in selecting a favorable donor site for fat harvesting. The lower abdomen serves as a good source in many individuals and is a site that can be easily accessed without patient repositioning. Although men carry their extra fat stores almost exclusively in a truncal distribution, women can be either truncal or extremity dominant in terms of their fat stores. When evaluating the lower abdomen as a potential donor site, patients should be examined to rule out the presence of abdominal hernias. In men an alternative donor site is the hip but requires intraoperative patient repositioning. In women the inner and outer thighs are very good

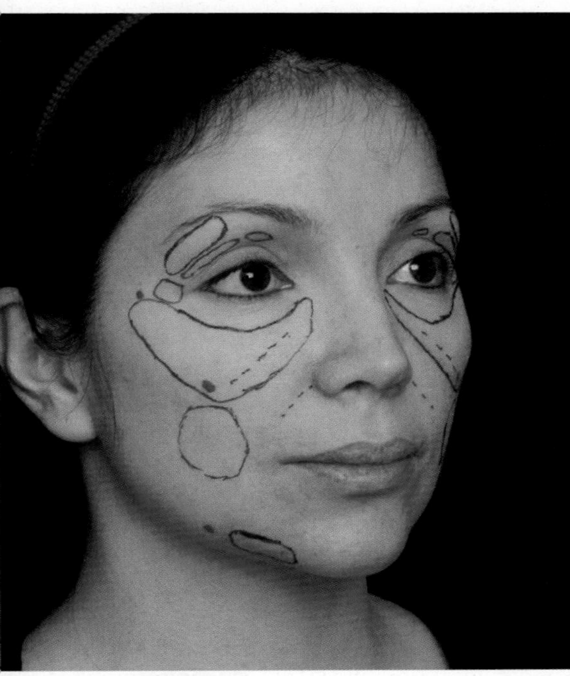

Fig. 29.8 The areas for volume augmentation with fat are delineated preoperatively. The red marks show the planned location of the three major entry sites for injections, located in the midcheek, lateral canthus, and lateral to the prejowl sulcus. (From Lam SM, Glasgold MJ, Glasgold RA. Complementary Fat Grafting. Philadelphia: Lippincott Williams & Wilkins; 2007. Reprinted by permission.)

alternatives for fat harvesting, with the inner thigh having the advantage of not requiring patient repositioning.

Anesthesia and General Considerations

Fat grafting can be undertaken with almost any level of anesthesia, from straight local anesthesia to general anesthesia. We prefer moderate intravenous sedation to achieve the best balance of patient comfort and patient cooperation for repositioning during fat harvesting. The patient's donor and recipient sites are prepared in a sterile fashion using povidone-iodine solution and sterile drapes. If other procedures are being performed concurrently we recommend completing fat harvesting before proceeding to the other procedures.

Donor-Site Harvesting

The donor site is anesthetized once the patient achieves an appropriate level of sedation. An injection of 20 mL of 0.25% lidocaine with 1:400,000 epinephrine is infiltrated with a 7-inch 22-gauge spinal needle placing half in the superficial aspect of the fat pad (the immediate subcutaneous plane) and the other half in the deep aspect of the fat pad. The 20 mL mixture of anesthetic solution can be constituted by mixing 15 mL of normal saline with 5 mL of 1% lidocaine with 1:100,000 epinephrine. For individuals who are under lighter sedation or straight local anesthesia, a 50/50 mix of 10 mL of normal saline and 10 mL of 1% lidocaine with 1:100,000 epinephrine can be used instead. A total of 20 mL of anesthetic mixture can be used for the entire lower abdomen, whereas 20 mL per extremity donor site is preferred.

After appropriate time for anesthesia has elapsed, a 16-gauge Nokor needle is used to create a stab incision through which the harvesting cannula can be inserted. All fat harvesting is undertaken with a blunt bullet-tip cannula (Tulip Medical, Inc., San Diego, CA) attached to a Luer-Lok 10 mL syringe (**Fig. 29.9**). Harvesting is performed with gentle hand suction, retracting on the plunger with ~2 mL of negative pressure to minimize trauma to the adipocytes. As the surgeon traverses the fat pad during harvesting, it is imperative not to dimple the skin but to remain in the middepth of the fat pad. The nondominant hand can be used to stabilize the fat pad but should not pinch or tent the skin, which can lead to uneven fat harvesting. When harvesting from the inner thigh, the contralateral (nonharvested leg) should be frog-legged while the leg to be harvested should remain straight. To avoid a contour deformity in the inner thigh, the cannula should pass through an initial fascial layer that can be recognized by the feel of a release as the cannula passes through this layer. In general, the surgeon should also ensure that the same area of the fat pad is not being overharvested. After the cannula is passed back and forth in a small area, the surgeon should retract the cannula back almost to the entry site before redirecting the cannula into a fresh adjacent site. This maneuver ensures that there is uniform harvesting over the entire donor area and prevents iatrogenic contour irregularity. In estimating the amount of fat that needs to be harvested, on average half of the collected syringe will consist of injectable fat. The remainder of the syringe consists of blood, lysed fat cells, and lidocaine, which will be separated out during the centrifugation process. (For recommended volumes of injection, please consult the following section on Injection Techniques.)

Processing the Fat

After the fat has been harvested into 10-mL Luer-Lok syringes (Becton Dickinson, Franklin Lakes, NJ), it is spun in a centrifuge. Fat processing is performed on a sterile field. Although the centrifuge is off of the sterile field, sterile sleeves within which the 10 mL syringes sit are used to maintain sterility. A dedicated plug and cap (Miller Medical, Inc., Mesa, AZ) must be attached to each syringe to avoid spillage of contents during the centrifugation process. It is imperative not to use the tiny plastic Luer-Lok cap that comes packaged with the 10 mL Luer-Lok syringe because it will allow the contents of the syringe to leak during centrifugation. Many centrifuge models exist that can accommodate sterile sleeves or entire insertable rotary trays to maintain the sterile environment of each syringe (Miller Medical Inc.; Byron Medical Inc., Tucson, AZ). The syringes are inserted into the centrifuge in a balanced distribution and spun at ~3000 rpm for 3 minutes. Upon removal, the supranatant (on the non–Luer-Lok side) containing the lysed fatty acids is poured off first into a waste basin. Only after the supranatant is poured off should the bloody infranatant be drained from the Luer-Lok side. Inadvertently draining the infranatant first will predispose the column of fat to slide out of the other side of the syringe when draining the supranatant. The syringe, now containing only a column of purified fat, is placed into a test tube rack. A noncut 4 × 4 cotton gauze or cotton neuropaddie is inserted into the syringe in contact with the fat to wick away the excess supranatant for a 5- to 10-minute period.

The contents from several 10 mL syringes are then transferred to an empty 20 mL syringe from the open non–Luer-Lok to the open non–Luer-Lok side. To facilitate fat preparation the 20 mL syringe should not be filled with more than 15 mL of fat. The plunger is then inserted into the back of the 20 mL syringe, and the contents are then transferred using a Luer-Lok transfer hub into individual 1 mL Luer-Lok syringes. Fat injections are done from the 1 mL syringe using a 0.9 or 1.2 mm blunt spoon tip cannula (**Fig. 29.9**).

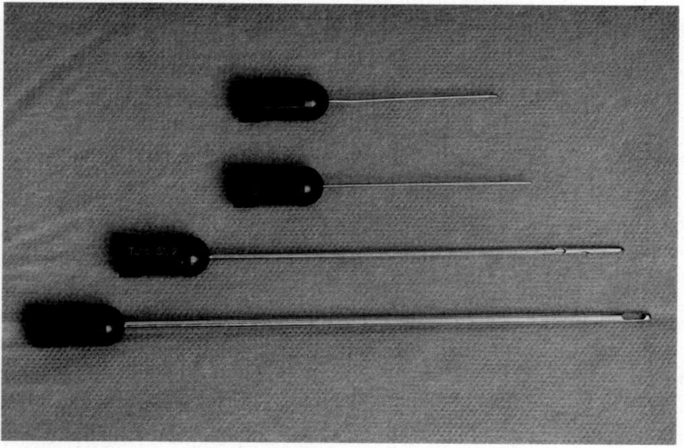

Fig. 29.9 The Glasgold Fat Transfer Set (Tulip Medical, Inc., San Diego, CA): 0.9 mm × 4 cm blunt spoon tip infiltration cannula; 1.2 mm × 6 cm blunt spoon tip infiltration cannula; 2 mm × 12 cm multiport harvesting cannula; 3 mm × 15 cm bullet tip harvesting cannula. (From Lam SM, Glasgold MJ, Glasgold RA. Complementary Fat Grafting. Philadelphia: Lippincott Williams & Wilkins; 2007. Reprinted by permission.)

Injection Techniques

General Principles

To increase the likelihood of fat survival, only small parcels of fat (0.05 to 0.1 mL) are infiltrated per pass of the cannula across multiple tissue planes. The three tissue planes that will be referred to in the following section are deep, middle, and superficial, corresponding respectively with a supraperiosteal plane, a midfascial to deep subcutaneous plane, and a superficial subcutaneous plane. Although these are clearly not distinct visualized planes, their importance is for guiding fat placement in such a way that fat survival can be maximized and contour problems minimized.

The amount of fat injected per pass of the cannula varies from 0.05 to 0.1 mL depending on the area treated. There are three basic cannula entry sites, referred to as entry site A, B, and C. Entry site A is located at the midcheek approximately at the base of the malar depression. Entry site B is ~2 cm lateral to the lateral canthus, and entry site C is situated posterior to the prejowl sulcus at the anterior border of the jowl (**Fig. 29.8**). These are approximate locations and are a starting point for the procedures. Other entry sites can be made as needed to better address an area. The entry sites are made with a standard 18-gauge needle through which the blunt infiltration cannula can be inserted.

Prior to fat infiltration the entry and recipient sites need to be anesthetized with 1% lidocaine with 1:100,000 epinephrine. The entry sites and field blocks are done with a 30-gauge and 27-gauge needle, respectively. The recipient sites are also infiltrated diffusely with the same anesthetic using a blunt infiltration cannula. Use of a blunt infiltration cannula (the same used for fat infiltration) can minimize the likelihood of developing ecchymosis. In general, 5 to 10 mL of lidocaine is sufficient to achieve adequate anesthesia per side of the face.

Site-Specific Fat Infiltration

Inferior Orbital Rim (from port A)

The inferior orbital rim stands as the most technically difficult area to achieve a consistently excellent result. Care must be taken not to place the fat with too large a bolus per cannula pass, into the wrong plane, or with too large a total volume—all of which can lead to a complication that is not easy to rectify. From past experience we have found that approaching the inferior orbital rim from a lateral canthal entry point with placement of fat in a parallel orientation to the inferior orbital rim can predispose toward the development of contour irregularities. Placement of fat should be approached so that the cannula is directed at the inferior orbital rim from a perpendicular direction (i.e., from entry point A).

As the cannula is directed toward the eye, the index finger of the nondominant hand is used to protect the globe during fat infiltration. The nondominant hand also provides tactile feedback to ensure the cannula tip is in the immediate supraperiosteal plane (the deep plane) (**Fig. 29.10A,B**). The cannula tip should pass back and forth across the inferior orbital rim against the periosteum placing 0.03 to 0.05 mL per cannula pass. If the cannula tip becomes clogged, it is important that the cannula be removed from the patient before forcibly clearing it to avoid injection of too large a bolus in this very sensitive area. During the learning phase of fat grafting 2 mL of fat should be placed deeply along the inferior orbital rim. As experience is gained, greater volumes of fat can be placed more superficially along the inferior orbital rim. This is particularly necessary in individuals with more significant volume depletion along their inferior orbital rim. As a general rule we caution against injection of more than 4 mL per inferior orbital rim to minimize the risk of overfilling or contour problems. It is always better to attempt a more conservative approach, especially when addressing the inferior orbital rim, because placing additional fat is a very easy task, whereas removal of excessive fat is a difficult venture. The general philosophy that it is better to "hit doubles" than "hit a homerun" is particularly apropos with fat grafting.

Nasojugal Groove (from Port A)

The bony nasojugal groove is the triangular bony fossa bordered superiorly by the medial inferior orbital rim and medially by the nasal sidewall. For the purposes of fat injection we make a distinction between the nasojugal groove, defined by the bony landmarks, and the tear trough, which is a superficial visible depression (in some patients these two areas directly correlate). Nasojugal groove injection is done in a deep supraperiosteal plane using the bony landmarks as a guide. In contrast, filling of the tear trough is done in a more superficial plane, but still below the orbicularis oculi muscle (we do not recommend any periorbital fat injections be done superficial to the orbicularis oculi muscle). The decision as to whether to add tear trough filling to the surgical plan is dictated by the presence of a visible depression and the surgeon's experience. Filling of the nasojugal groove can be done through entry point A with 1 to 2 mL of fat, placing 0.1 mL per pass.

Lateral Brow (from Port B)

The brow is defined as the soft tissue that resides principally inferior and deep to the hair-bearing portion of the eyebrow and superior to the upper eyelid itself. With advancing age, the brow deflates, revealing a more skeletonized superior orbital rim. Placement of fat into the lateral brow can restore the youthful convexity and

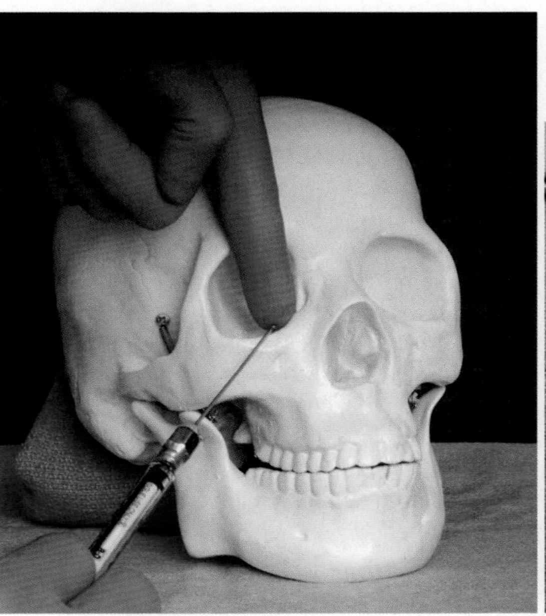
A

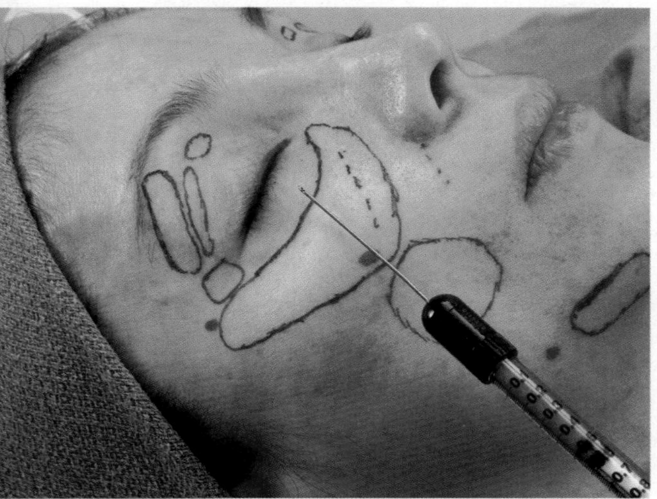
B

Fig. 29.10 Technique of injecting inferior orbital rim. (**A**) Demonstration of the use of the index finger on the orbital rim to protect the globe. (**B**) Intraoperative photograph showing the orientation of the cannula during injection. (From Lam SM, Glasgold MJ, Glasgold RA. Complementary Fat Grafting. Philadelphia: Lippincott Williams & Wilkins; 2007. Reprinted by permission.)

highlight in this area. From entry point B, the cannula can be passed into the lateral brow along a plane of least resistance, fanning across this area to achieve the desired convexity. In contrast to the inferior orbital rim, fat can be placed from a lateral entry site passing parallel to the orbital rim. Approximately 2 mL of fat can be injected with 0.1 mL per pass.

Lateral Canthus (from Port B)

At times a small depression remains visible, or becomes exaggerated, at the lateral canthus following superior and inferior orbital rim injections. Approaching this area with the smaller 0.9 mm spoon tip cannula (Tulip Medical, Inc., San Diego, CA) facilitates placement of fat into the lateral canthus where tenacious retaining fibers traversing the lateral canthus create more resistance to injection. Only 0.5 mL should be placed into the lateral canthus with 0.05 mL fat per pass.

Anterior Cheek (from Port B)

The focus of anterior cheek augmentation is along the soft tissue, linear depression that runs from superomedial to inferolateral corresponding with the malar septum (**Fig. 29.11**). Approaching the anterior cheek from entry port B allows for fat injection perpendicular to the malar septum. The cannula is passed back and forth across the malar septum filling the entire cheek with an emphasis on the malar depression, which is usually the area of greatest volume loss. In most patients some resistance may be encountered as the cannula passes through the malar septum. It is important that the cannula be pushed through the septum layering fat medial to and across it. A total of 3 mL of fat on average should be placed with 0.1 mL per pass. Fat is infiltrated into all three tissue planes (deep, middle, and superficial), crossing gradually from one tissue plane to the next so that it is equally distributed. By placing small aliquots of fat across the entire malar depth, the surgeon can ensure that each parcel of fat has maximal contact with the surrounding tissue for optimal nourishment/blood supply that can translate into improved viability of the transferred adipocytes.

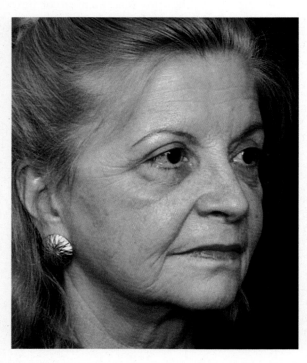

Fig. 29.11 Patient demonstrates the malar depression of the anterior cheek along the malar septum. (From Lam SM, Glasgold MJ, Glasgold RA. Complementary Fat Grafting. Philadelphia: Lippincott Williams & Wilkins; 2007. Reprinted by permission.)

Lateral Cheek (from Port A)

The lateral cheek is centered over the bony zygomatic arch, which can be palpated with the nondominant hand to guide placement. The lateral cheek is approached from entry port A and filled across all three tissue planes with the same technique outlined for anterior-cheek augmentation, placing 0.1 mL per pass in a progressive fashion from deep to superficial. One to 3 mL of fat can be placed depending on the aesthetic end point desired. When necessary, based on patient evaluation, lateral cheek filling should be tapered into the submalar region.

Buccal (from Port A)

The buccal region tends to be more important to fill in the very gaunt individual. If a facelift is being performed in which dissection will extend out to the buccal region concurrent fat grafting cannot be performed. The buccal region is forgiving and it is unlikely to show contour deformities. As a baseline, for mild buccal hollowing, 3 mL of fat should be placed per side. The fat is placed in a deep subcutaneous plane and is layered with 0.1 mL per pass. In patients who have significant buccal volume loss, up to 7 mL of fat may be placed per side. In patients with a thin face, even if the buccal region does not appear deficient, be conscious of the fact that as fat is placed in the adjacent areas (cheek, submalar, and jawline) buccal hollowing will be accentuated.

Prejowl Sulcus/Anterior Chin (from Port C)

The prejowl sulcus is defined as the depression immediately anterior to the jowl. This is an important area to fill both in younger patients with a minimal jowl as well as in older patients who will be undergoing concurrent facelifting. In the younger patient, volume restoration to the prejowl sulcus is often sufficient for masking the jowl and recreating a youthful jawline (**Fig. 29.12A,B**). In patients with more advanced signs of aging where a facelift is the primary treatment for the jowl, filling the prejowl sulcus will produce a more ideal result. Microliposuction of the jowl with an 18-gauge Klein-Capistrano cannula is a simple, adjunctive procedure that can further enhance the overall aesthetic outcome. When addressing the prejowl sulcus, 3 mL of fat is injected from entry point C anteriorly into the prejowl sulcus with 0.1 mL per pass. The fat should be layered in multiple planes from supraperiosteal to subcutaneous. Volume loss in the prejowl sulcus should be thought of as a process of radial contraction resulting in a deficiency on the lateral and inferior border of the mandible. Correction of this to reestablish a smoothly contoured jawline requires layering of fat along the arc of contraction, from lateral to inferior mandibular border.

Individuals with a mild degree of microgenia can obtain increased anterior projection with fat grafting to the mentum. This is a viable alternative for patients needing minimal projection and who are undergoing fat transfer to other areas. In the patient whose primary need is anterior chin projection alloplastic implants provide a more predictable and effective correction.

Immediate Postoperative Care

At the conclusion of the procedure, there is no need to suture any of the entry sites used for harvesting or injecting. The entry sites for harvesting through which the larger cannulas pass may remain hyperpigmented for months, and patient counseling regarding this possibility should be done preoperatively. There is no need for dressings or bandages on the harvest or recipient sites following isolated fat grafting procedures. Head elevation and icing for 48 to 72 hours after surgery will reduce and expedite resolution of postoperative edema. Beyond the first few postoperative days the cheek area may feel a bit flushed or sore, and ice packs can be applied to alleviate these symptoms. Patients generally have very little discomfort in the face other than a tight sensation and are more apt to be aware of soreness and pain at the harvest sites.

Patients are encouraged to rest the week following fat grafting and not engage in any excessive activities that require Valsalva or bending over, including gardening or housework. Isometric exercise can be initiated in the first postoperative week but patients should be aware this may exacerbate facial edema. There is no contraindication to engaging in exercise of the harvest areas, as tolerated, with the exception of not performing abdominal crunches that will raise intrathoracic pressure

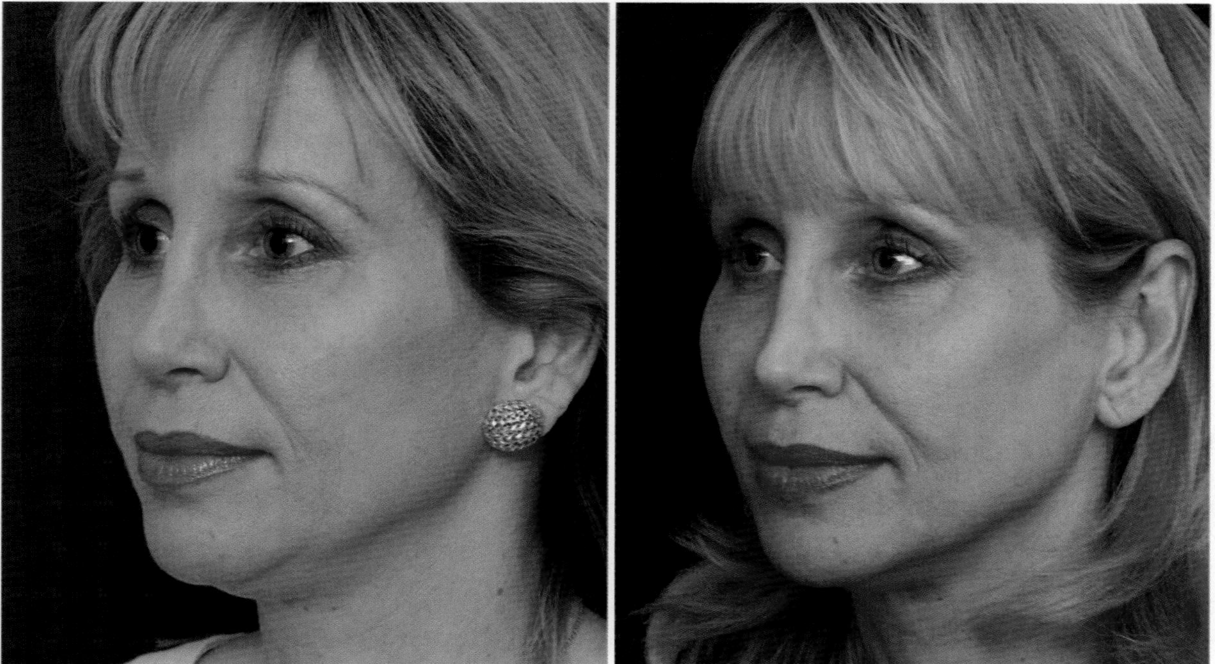

Fig. 29.12 (**A,B**) Patient demonstrating improved jawline contour following isolated prejowl sulcus augmentation. (From Lam SM, Glasgold MJ, Glasgold RA. Complementary Fat Grafting. Philadelphia: Lippincott Williams & Wilkins; 2007. Reprinted by permission.)

and worsen edema. Reducing dietary salt can minimize edema, especially during the critical first postoperative week. Patients should understand that edema takes several weeks to months to fully resolve. Reviewing photographs of other patients who have undergone fat grafting during their recuperative phase can be instructive. Although there is almost no postoperative care that the patient must perform and very few care instructions that the physician need relate to the patient, the physician should see the patient as often as the patient should desire to alleviate any uncertainty regarding the patient's swelling.

Complications

With a conservative and precise methodology outlined in this chapter, the physician should encounter few complications. Treatment strategies are predicated on identification of the correct pathology. This section is intended to enumerate a classification of unique complications following fat grafting that include lumps, bulges, overcorrection, undercorrection, and entry-site divot.

Contour Irregularity

Lumps

A lump refers to a discrete focus of excessive fat. Although rare, the inferior orbital rim is the most susceptible to this problem. It is likely due to infiltration of too large a bolus in a superficial plane in an area with thin overlying skin. Although steroid injections may seem like a reasonable option, they tend not to work on discrete lumps and risk the potential side effects of steroids. The treatment that has been most effective and precise is excision of the lump through a discreet incision situated along inferior orbital rim at the junction of the thin lower lid skin and the thicker cheek skin (**Fig. 29.13A to D**).

Bulges

A bulge describes a wider contour irregularity, characterized by palpable induration or thickening. This has primarily been observed as an oval-shaped elevation with palpable induration oriented parallel to the inferior orbital rim. The etiology of this is uncertain but in our experience has only been seen in patients whose inferior orbital rim was injected with fat from a lateral canthal entry point through which fat was layered parallel to the orbital rim. This problem has been avoided by performing all fat infiltration of the inferior orbital rim through a midcheek entry point laying the fat across the bony rim in a perpendicular orientation. Triamcinolone acetonide is extremely effective in resolving this problem. Increasing doses in concentrations from 10 mg/mL to 40 mg/mL repeated every 1 to 2 months will oftentimes take care of the problem. Direct liposuction has not proven to be useful for correcting a bulge. When steroid injections are not successful, directly excising the indurated tissue through an inferior orbital rim incision is undertaken.

Overcorrection

As mentioned, a conservative strategy for autologous fat transfer should be instituted to prevent this problem from arising. Correction of this entity involves microliposuction of the areas perceived to be overcorrected using an 18-gauge Klein-Capistrano microliposuction cannula in a cross-hatched pattern. At times overcorrection can arise due to excessive weight gain, usually over 25 lb. The best solution to correct this problem is weight loss. Patients are commonly concerned about overcorrection in the early postoperative period. It is important to delay treatment of overcorrection for at least 6 months to allow swelling to completely resolve.

Undercorrection

Undercorrection is the best complication to encounter, as additional fat grafting can be easily undertaken to arrive at the desired level of patient satisfaction. The espoused aphorism that "hitting doubles" (i.e., being more conservative with fat grafting, especially early in a surgeon's experience with fat grafting), should always be heeded. Due to the variable survival of transferred adipocytes, we counsel all patients preoperatively of the possible need for a touchup procedure to achieve the desired end point. Additional fat transfer procedures are more likely in patients who require significant volume augmentation (as may be needed in the cheek or lateral jawline) or when striving for a very precise correction of orbital rim hollowing. Undercorrection of the orbital rim is much easier for both the patient and the surgeon to tolerate than having to deal with overcorrection.

Entry-Site Divot

Tethering or divoting at the entry site is a very rare occurrence and usually manifests as a dimple at the entry site during facial animation. This complication can be easily rectified by limited subcision using a 20-gauge needle under the scar band.

Conclusions

The revolution of facial fat grafting has arrived and is here to stay. The new paradigm that emphasizes volume changes as a vital component of the aging process has altered our evaluation of patients and our approach to facial rejuvenation. Alternative techniques with dermal fillers to create volume and the advent of a dedicated injectable agent to restore volume have provided nonsurgical, approximate substitutes for facial fat grafting but underscore our awakened appreciation to the importance of volume in facial rejuvenation.[17]

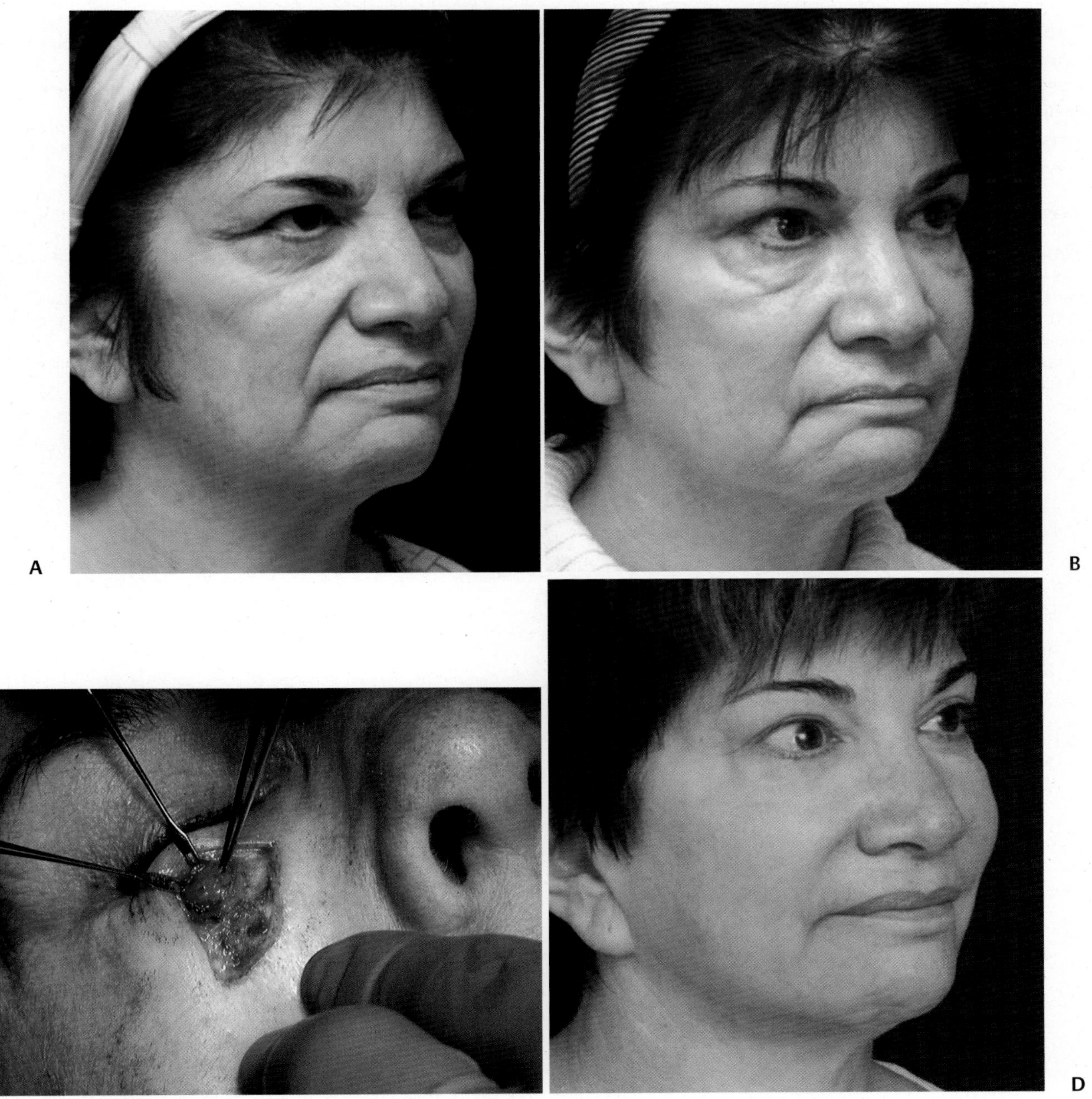

Fig. 29.13 (**A**) Preoperative photograph. (**B**) Following upper lid blepharoplasty and periorbital fat transfer the patient presented with visible lumps in the inferior orbital rim. (**C**) Direct excision of transferred fat to correct contour. (**D**) Postoperative photograph showing correction of the complication. (From Lam SM, Glasgold MJ, Glasgold RA. Complementary Fat Grafting. Philadelphia: Lippincott Williams & Wilkins; 2007. Reprinted by permission.)

The strategy outlined in this chapter does not conform to a purist doctrine that only fat grafting is an acceptable treatment modality for facial rejuvenation. Instead, fat grafting is perceived as a complement to traditional lifting procedures and skin therapies so as to achieve a natural, appropriate, balanced, and global rejuvenation of the face.

Besides merely yielding contour benefits, fat grafting has also been shown, albeit anecdotally, to improve the texture and tone of the skin along with diminution of scars.[18] Although a definitive mechanism for this improvement has yet to be firmly established, this ancillary advantage may provide a fascinating avenue of further research and increase overall patient satisfaction as well.

References

1. Lam SM, Glasgold MJ, Glasgold RA. Complementary Fat Grafting. Philadelphia, PA: Lippincott, Williams, & Wilkins; 2006
2. Neober F. Frettransplantation. Chir Kongr Verh Dtsch Ges Chir 1893;22:66
3. Czerny M. Plastscher ersatz der brusterluse durch ein lipom. Verh Dtsch Ges Chir Zbl Chir 1985;27:72–75
4. Lexer E. Freie Fettransplantation. Dtsch Med Wochenschr 1910;36:640
5. Bruning P. Cited by Broeckaert TJ, Steinhaus J: Contribution e l'etude des greffes adipueses. Bull Acad R Med Belg 1914;28:440
6. Tuffier T. Abces gangreneux du pouman ouvert dans les bronches: hemoptysies repetee operation par decollement pleuro-parietal; guerison. Bull Mem Soc Chir Paris 1911;37:134
7. Straatsma CR, Peer LA. Repair of postauricular fistula by means of a free fat graft. Arch Otolaryngol 1932;15:620–621
8. Shiffman MA, ed. Autologous Fat Transplantation. New York: Marcel Dekker; 2001
9. Bircoll M. Autologous fat transplantation. The Asian Congress of Plastic Surgery, Singapore, February, 1982
10. Illouz YG. The fat cell graft: a new technique to fill depressions. Plast Reconstr Surg 1986;78:122–123
11. Krulig E. Lipo-injection. Am J Cosmet Surg 1987;4:123–129
12. Newman J, Levin J. Facial lipotransplant surgery. Am J Cosm Surg 1987;4:131–140
13. Coleman SR. Structural Fat Grafting. St. Louis: Quality Medical Publishing; 2004
14. Amar RE. Adipocyte microinfiltration in the face or tissue restructuration with fat tissue graft. Ann Chir Plast Esthet 1999;44:593–608 French
15. Shu T, Lam SM. Liposuction and lipotransfer for facial rejuvenation in the Asian patient. Int J Cosmet Surg Aesthetic Dermatol 2003;5: 165–173
16. McCurdy JA Jr, Lam SM. Cosmetic Surgery of the Asian Face. 2nd ed New York: Thieme; 2005
17. Lam SM, Azizzadeh B, Graivier M. Injectable poly-L-lactic acid (Sculptra): technical considerations in soft-tissue contouring. Plast Reconstr Surg 2006;118:55S–63S
18. Coleman SR. Structural fat grafting: more than a permanent filler. Plast Reconstr Surg 2006;118:108S–120S

30 Botulinum Toxin for Facial Wrinkles

Tanya K. Meyer and Andrew Blitzer

Botulinum exotoxin (BTX), produced by the bacterium *Clostridia botulinum*, is a potent neurotoxin that exerts its effect at the neuromuscular junction through inhibition of exocytotic neurotransmitter release causing a flaccid paralysis.[1,2] Clinical use for muscular hyperfunction was pioneered by Alan B. Scott in the 1970s, and in 1989 the U.S. Food and Drug Administration (FDA) approved the use of botulinum toxin serotype A (BTX-A) for strabismus and blepharospasm. Clinical use expanded to the treatment of other hyperfunctional muscular disorders, including craniofacial and laryngeal dystonia. In treating these patients, we noticed a cosmetic benefit, and often patients who were receiving unilateral toxin injections for dystonia or hemifacial spasm would return asking to have their contralateral side injected to give them a more youthful appearance.[3] In 2002, BTX-A was approved for the treatment of glabellar rhytids.

Botulinum toxin improves the cosmetic appearance by decreasing or eliminating the hyperfunctional facial lines caused by skin pleating due to contraction of the underlying mimetic musculature.[4] The loss of facial hyperfunctional lines resulting in a smooth skin surface is evident in conditions that cause facial weakness, such as facial nerve injury, Bell's palsy, or stroke. BTX does not address skin lines unrelated to muscular hyperfunction, such as actinic damage, loss of dermal elastic fibers, or skin atrophy. These changes may be best managed with chemical peels, laser resurfacing, or injection of filler materials. The senior author (AB) has used BTX for more than 21 years and reported it for the correction of hyperfunctional lines of the face, including glabellar lines, horizontal forehead lines, lateral orbital lines (crow's feet), platysmal bands, and hyperactive mentalis muscles.[5] Carruthers and Carruthers reported similar results of BTX injections for the correction of hyperfunctional facial lines.[6]

History and Biology

Botulism historically occurred after the consumption of spoiled food.[1,2,7] During the Napoleonic Wars, smoked sausages were identified as the problematic agent, and the contamination was termed sausage poison (*botulus* in Greek means blood sausage). Symptoms included blurred vision, dry mouth, dizziness, and nausea, and could progress to a deadly flaccid paralysis. In 1895, the Belgian scientist Emile Pierre van Ermengem identified the bacterium that produced the toxin and named it *Bacillus botulinus*, which was later renamed *Clostridium botulinum*. In the 1920s a crude form of the toxin was first isolated by Dr. Herman Sommer at the University of California, San Francisco, and in 1946 a crystalline form was purified by Dr. Edward Schantz. As already mentioned, clinical applications for BTX were pioneered by Alan B. Scott in the 1970s, and BTX-A* received FDA approval in 1989 for the treatment of strabismus and blepharospasm. Approval was granted in 2000 for use in cervical dystonia to decrease the severity of abnormal head position and associated neck pain. In 2002, BTX-A was approved for the treatment of glabellar rhytids. Most recently, in 2004, BTX-A was approved for the treatment of axillary hyperhydrosis not responsive to topical management. Botulinum toxin B (BTX-B) was FDA approved for the treatment of cervical dystonia in 2000.

Clostridium botulinum is an anaerobic, spore-forming, gram-positive rod, which is commonly found in water and soil. Disease is naturally caused by (1) inoculation of a wound with local proliferation of the bacterium and systemic spread of the toxin, (2) ingestion of the spores in improperly cooked food, with germination and growth in the gut and absorption of the toxin, or (3) ingestion of preformed toxin in improperly cooked foods with systemic absorption. The toxin is heat labile and can be inactivated by boiling for several minutes.

There are seven serotypes (A through G), which exert their paralytic effect by inhibiting the exocytotic release of acetylcholine at the neuromuscular junction. The toxins are composed of a heavy and light chain. The heavy chain is responsible for neuron-specific binding and internalization, and the light chain is a metalloproteinase, which cleaves one of the fusion proteins responsible for vesicle docking thus preventing neurotransmitter exocytosis. Specific serotypes target different docking proteins, BTX-A and E target SNAP-25; BTX-B, D, F, and G target synaptobrevin; and BTX-C targets syntaxin.

When neuromuscular transmission is initially interrupted, the axon responds by creating sprouts to establish new junctions. These new junctions allow weak stimulation at about 1 month. At ~60 to 90 days, the original terminals regain activity through regeneration of docking proteins, resulting in regression of the sprouts.

*Please note that in the United States, the only current FDA-approved BTX-A formulation is BOTOX (Allergan, Inc., Irvine, CA), and the FDA-approved BTX-B formulation is Myobloc (Solstice Neurosciences, Inc., South San Francisco, CA). Other commercial BTX preparations are available in Europe and Asia.

The specific clinical characteristics of each serotype are determined by the formulation, size of the neurotoxin complex, and the targeted docking protein. BTX-A has a pH of ~7, a larger neurotoxin complex size, and targets SNAP-25. BTX-A closely associates with the hemagluttins in its neurotoxin complex, which is felt to delay the contact of the toxin to the target docking protein and thus account for the onset of 2 to 3 days. Because of the larger size, BTX-A has minimal diffusion and distant effect. The duration of BTX-A is ~3 months, which is felt to correlate with the time for regeneration of SNAP-25. In comparison, BTX-B is stored at a lower pH of 5.6 resulting in a rapid dispersion of the neurotoxin complex after injection, giving an onset of less than 24 hours. BTX-B has a smaller neurotoxin complex size, which facilitates diffusion and may account for an increased incidence of distant effects (such as dry mouth). The duration of BTX-B is ~2 months, which is felt to correlate with the time for regeneration of synaptobrevin.

Botulinum toxins are measured in units of biological activity [for BOTOX, one unit is defined as the dose that, when administered intraperitoneally into a group of mice, is lethal to 50% of the animals injected (LD50)]. Differences in animal model, formulations, and serotypes impart unique efficacy and safety profiles, which make it difficult to derive a simple dose ratio conversion between products. In general, for the doses used in cosmetic human therapy, one unit of BOTOX (Allergan, Inc., Irvine, CA) is considered equivalent to 3 to 4 units of Dysport (BTX-A used in Europe; Ipsen Pharmaceuticals, Berkshire, UK) and to 50 to 100 units of Myobloc (Solstice Neurosciences, Inc., South San Francisco, CA). The LD50 in humans is estimated to be ~3500 units of BOTOX.[8]

Individuals can form neutralizing antibodies, which appear to cause no harm in terms of anaphylactic reactivity, but do render the patients resistant to the paralytic effect of the toxin. Individuals immunoresistant to one form of toxin usually receive benefit from switching to another form. To avoid antibody formation, it is recommended that the lowest effective dose is used at the longest inter-injection interval to minimize toxin protein exposure to host immune surveillance.

Storage and Reconstitution

Unreconstituted BOTOX is stored in a standard refrigerator at 2 to 8°C for up to 24 months. Each vial contains 100 units of vacuum-dried, purified botulinum toxin A. Although the package insert recommends reconstitution with preservative-free saline, we have found that there is no decrease in efficacy with the use of saline preserved with 0.9% benzyl alcohol. Additionally, patients report that injections with preserved saline used as the diluent are less painful. Use of preserved saline also allows storage of the toxin in a refrigerator for several weeks without diminution in efficacy.[9] We use two standard dilutions: 4 mL of saline added to a vial containing 100 units of toxin yielding 25 units/mL (2.5 units in 0.1 mL) and 2 mL saline to 100 units of toxin yielding 50 units/mL (5 units in 0.1 mL).

Although Myobloc (BTX-B) is less commonly used for cosmetic purposes, we do use it for therapeutic treatment of individuals with dystonia or spasm if they become resistant to BTX-A. Myobloc is distributed as a reconstituted solution in multiuse vials at a concentration of 2500 and 5000 units BTX-B/mL and has a shelf life of up to 21 months refrigerated.

Preprocedure Evaluation

The patient's facial lines are photographed for documentation and posttreatment comparison. The photographs should show the patient's face at rest and with activity producing the undesirable facial lines. A detailed analysis of the facial lines will decipher which lines are functional (dynamic wrinkles amenable to BTX treatment) and which are caused by actinic or age-related changes in the skin (static wrinkles). Deeper lines in the brow and lower face may require both BTX and a dermal filler for an optimal cosmetic result. A careful medical history is taken, with particular attention to prior cosmetic surgery and facial treatments, prior trauma, bleeding tendency, current medications, sensitivity to drugs, propensity to scarring, or hypo-/hyperpigmentation.

Despite the paucity of data, patients who are pregnant or lactating should not be injected because the effects of toxin on the fetus are unknown. We recommend cautious treatment of patients with underlying neuromuscular disease, such as Eaton-Lambert syndrome, myasthenia gravis, and motor neuron disease. Aminoglycoside antibiotics may interfere with neuromuscular transmission and potentiate the effect of a given dose of BTX; therefore, we do not recommend administering BTX to a patient undergoing aminoglycoside treatment.[10]

Technique

Patients should be carefully counseled regarding the nature of their wrinkles (dynamic vs static) and potential response to toxin therapy to ensure that they have realistic expectations for the treatment results. After discussion of the injection procedure and potential complications informed consent is obtained. The site of each injection is marked, allowing a 1.0 to 1.5 cm radius for diffusion of toxin. Care is taken to place toxin such that hyperfunctional muscles are targeted without causing undesirable weakness in adjacent muscles. A diagram of the injection sites with the corresponding dose should be kept as part of the patient record.

When the marking is complete, the area of interest can be iced or treated with topical anesthetics to decrease the discomfort associated with injection. The toxin is then drawn up in a tuberculin syringe, and a 30-gauge needle is used. We find that a volume of 0.1 mL works well at each injection site. If a larger dose is needed in a given area, either a larger volume or an increased concentration in the same volume can be given. Increasing the volume may lead to diffusion of toxin to adjacent muscles, causing unwanted weakness.

In general, electromyographic (EMG) guidance is not necessary due to the superficial nature of mimetic musculature. Most superficial facial muscles are adequately accessed by subcutaneous placement of toxin. Care should be taken to avoid injuring the periosteum, which will result in postinjection pain. Individuals with poor results or treatment of deeper muscles used in facial rebalancing (such as the platysma, or the zygomaticus and depressor anguli oris after facial nerve paresis/paralysis) benefit from EMG guidance (**Fig. 30.1**).

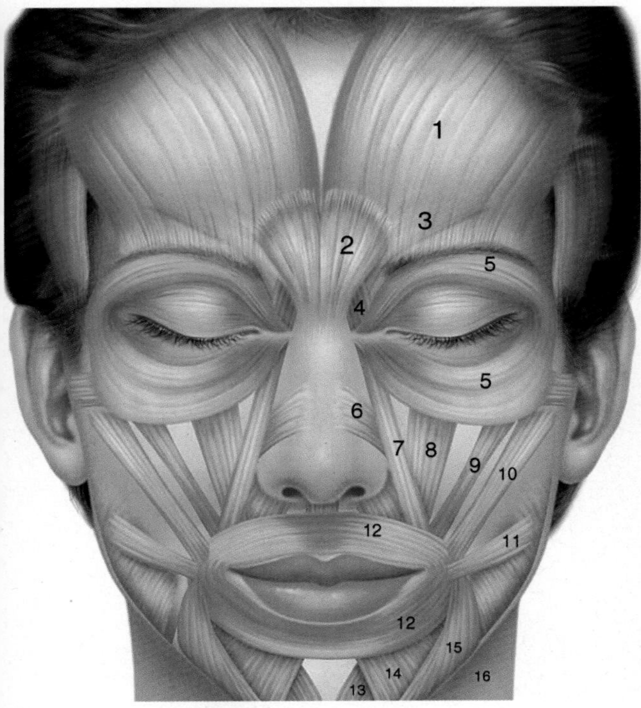

Fig. 30.1 Facial mimetic musculature. 1, frontalis; 2, procerus; 3, corrugator; 4, depressor supercilii portion of the corrugator; 5, orbicularis oculi; 6, transverse nasalis; 7, levator labii superioris alaeque nasi; 8, levator labii superioris; 9, zygomaticus minor; 10, zygomaticus major; 11, risorius; 12, orbicularis oris; 13, mentalis; 14, depressor labii inferioris; 15, depressor anguli oris; 16, platysma. (Image courtesy of Allergan.)

After the injection is performed, gentle pressure can be applied to the needle site to avoid ecchymosis and encourage toxin diffusion to the desired area. The patient is asked not to rub or massage the injected area for 6 hours to avoid inappropriate diffusion to adjacent muscles.

Note: All doses cited in the following text are for BOTOX (Allergan), the FDA-approved formulation of BTX-A. The only FDA-approved cosmetic indication for BOTOX, as of the writing of this text, is for injection of the glabellar complex. All other uses are off-label.

Glabellar Injections

Glabellar injections (**Fig. 30.2**)[5,11–14] control the hyperactivity of the corrugator and procerus muscles, which are responsible for producing scowl lines. In our series, we have injected 7.5 to 25 units in this area to control the muscle contractions producing the glabellar lines. We usually start with 2.5 to 5 units per 0.1 mL in each corrugator muscle (at the medial superior aspect of the eyebrow hair) and 2.5 to 5 units per 0.1 mL into the procerus (centrally at the glabella). Massage of the glabellar injection will allow diffusion to the depressor supercilii portion of the corrugators, which will allow some elevation of the medial eyebrow. The total dose depends on the preinjection assessment of the size of the muscle. Men generally have larger muscles and require larger doses. The injection of the corrugator muscle should extend laterally enough to encompass the length of the muscle without passing the midpupillary line and staying ~1 cm above the orbital rim. Too much lateral extension too close to the brow may lead to weakness of the levator muscles of the upper lid and produce ptosis.

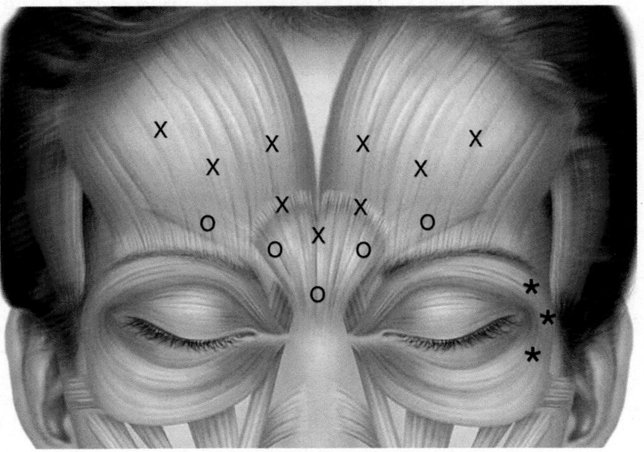

Fig. 30.2 Location of injections for brow and orbit. See text for details. O, glabellar complex (procerus and corrugator); X, frontalis; *, orbicularis oculi.

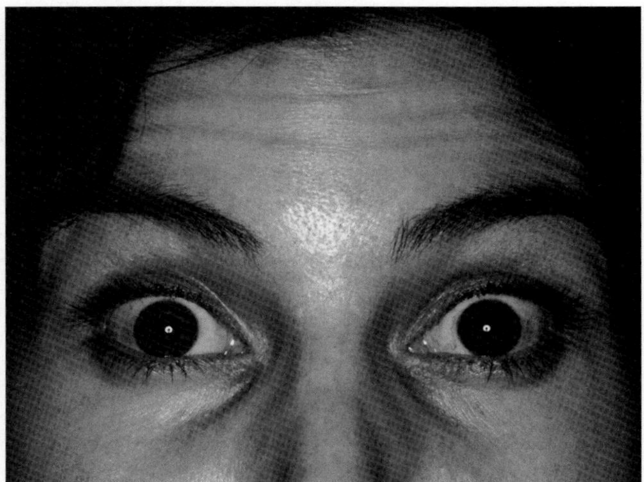

Fig. 30.3 Patient demonstrating hyperfunctional forehead lines prior to injection.

If ptosis is produced, the patient can be treated with apraclonidine 0.5% eye drops (Iopidine, Alcon, Inc., Fort Worth, Texas). This drop stimulates the Müller muscle (adrenergic muscle), which is below the levator muscle. Treatment usually produces a 1 to 2 mm elevation of the lid margin.

Frontalis Injections

The frontalis muscle pulls in a vertical direction, creating horizontal pleats in the forehead skin (**Figs. 30.2, 30.3, and 30.4**).[5,11–14] Toxin should not be injected within 1 cm of the orbital rim because this may cause brow ptosis or even levator ptosis. We like to raise the injection site progressively away from the brow with the lateral injections to leave some functional frontalis, thereby maintaining expressive function to the lateral brow while eliminating central forehead wrinkles. Most of our patients prefer to have some residual mimetic function of the brow. If there are multiple horizontal forehead lines, several rows of injections can be made to encompass the lines. Injection sites are marked at 1.0 to 1.5 cm intervals to ensure that all desired areas of weakness are included in the injection plan. We generally inject 2.5 units per 0.1 mL at each mark over the forehead. Our dose range is 10 to 30 units. If there is a particularly hyperactive area near the brow, we will use a more concentrated solution in that area.

Brow Adjustment

The final position of the brow is determined by the relative pull of the various muscles of the forehead and orbit (**Fig. 30.5**).[15] The frontalis acts as a brow elevator, the orbicularis oculi as a lateral depressor, the depressor supercilii as a medial depressor, and the corrugator and procerus as medializers. Often, weakening the glabellar and medial frontalis muscles causes an upward arching of the lateral brow (the "Dr. Spock" appearance) if the

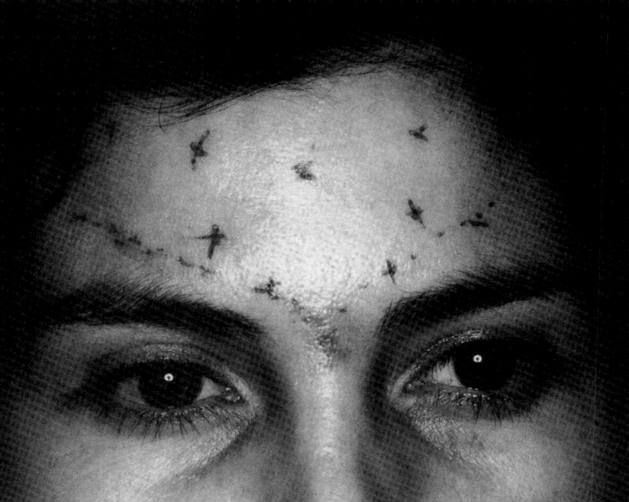

Fig. 30.4 We mark the injection site location in all patients. To guard against unwanted areas of weakness that can occur with forehead injections, the "allowed" area of injection is outlined first. One mark is placed between the medial aspect of the brows and 1 cm above the brows bilaterally at the midpupillary line. A triangle is then drawn. The toxin injections are all given above these lines. This prevents migration of toxin to the levator muscle and also preserves the mimetic function to the lateral brow. Marks are then made ~1.5 cm apart across the forehead lines to encompass the hyperfunctional areas within the triangle.

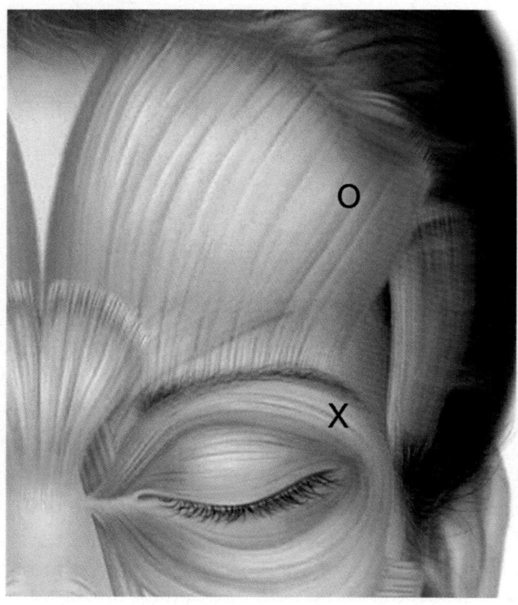

Fig. 30.5 Brow adjustment. Injection into the lateral frontalis (O) will drop the brow. Injection into the superior lateral portion of the orbicularis oculi (X) just outside the orbital rim will raise the brow. See text for further details.

lateral frontalis fibers are not treated. Conversely, excessive lateral frontalis weakening can cause brow ptosis. If too much arching is produced, a small amount of toxin (1 unit per 0.1 mL) can be injected into the lateral frontalis to drop the brow slightly. If not enough brow elevation was achieved, a similar dose injected at the juncture of the orbital rim and temporal line will weaken the attachment of the orbicularis oculi and allow for more pull by the frontalis to elevate the lateral brow. Elevation of the medial brow is achieved by treatment of the depressor supercilii, the most inferior slips of the corrugator muscle.

Crow's Feet Injections

Lateral orbital lines or crow's feet result from hyperactivity of the lateral portion of the orbicularis oculi muscle (**Figs. 30.2, 30.6, 30.7A,B, 30.8, and 30.9**).[5,11–14,16] This muscle functions in eye closure, blinking, and squinting. Small amounts of BTX can weaken the lateral aspect of this muscle and thereby decrease skin wrinkling without interfering with eye blink or eye closure. The first injection site is marked at the orbital rim, at least 1 cm from the lateral canthi. The patient is asked to squint, and hyperfunctional lines above and below this mark are also addressed with additional injections. Each site is placed ~1 cm apart and generally lateral to a vertical line drawn through the lateral canthus. Although injections can be extended judiciously along the inferior orbital rim to the midpupillary line, these can interfere with tear pumping and cause epiphora. It is important not to inject inside of the orbital rim because this may cause delayed eye closure, decreased blink, epiphora, mild ectropion, or possible diplopia.

Our starting dose is generally 2.5 units per 0.1 mL in each site with a total dose of 7.5 to 15 units per side. The needle is inserted so that the toxin is infiltrated away from the globe, and gentle pressure is applied in a lateral direction to prevent medial diffusion of toxin. The patients are reminded not to massage or rub their eyes for 6 hours.

Nasal Scrunch (Bunny Lines) and Nasal Flare

Excessive contracture of the transverse nasalis muscle with smiling will cause radial lines along the lateral nasal dorsum (**Fig. 30.10**).[11,14] Chemodenervation of the transverse nasalis will soften this appearance. We usually use 2.5 or 5 units on each side.

Some patients have excessive and bothersome flaring of the nasal alae due to excessive contraction of the alar portion of the nasalis muscle. We have utilized a technique described by Carruthers in which 5 units per 0.1 mL is injected at the rim of the nostril bilaterally.

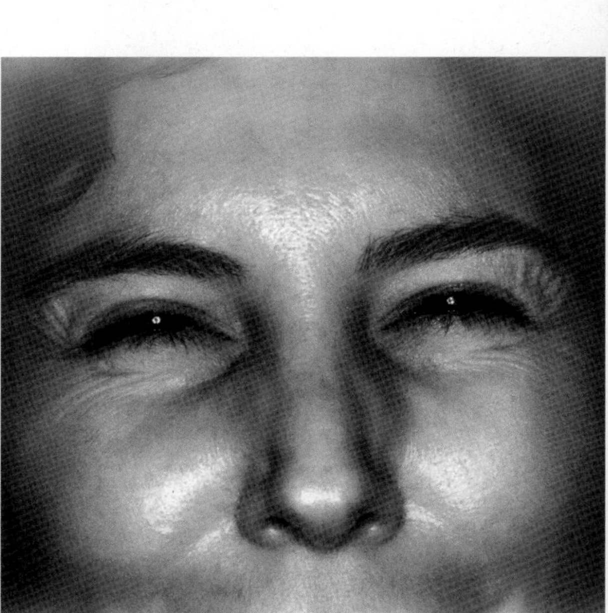

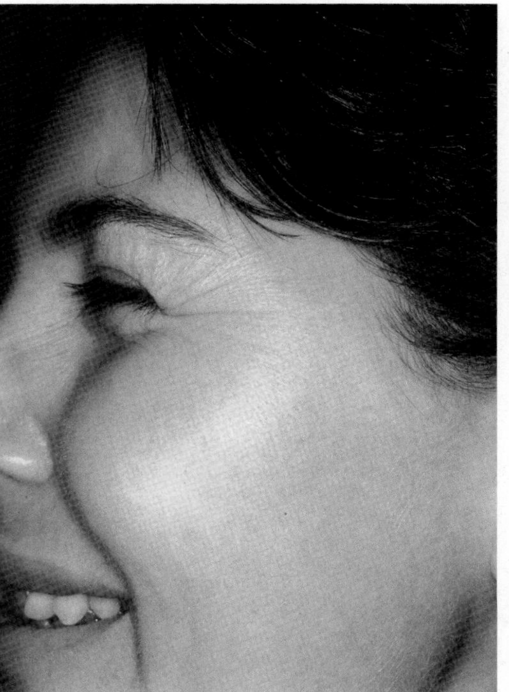

Fig. 30.6 Patient before injection with excessive squint lines (crow's feet) around the lateral and inferior orbital area.

This has produced excellent results if used in small volumes to avoid diffusion to the lip elevator muscles.

Lower Face Injections

The mentalis muscle originates on the mentum and extends multiple fibrous dermal insertions to create a "peau d' orange" or popply chin appearance with facial animation (**Fig. 30.10**).[5,10–12,14,17,18] This phenomenon can be exacerbated after chin implants or orthognathic surgery. Small amounts of toxin (2.5 to 5 units) on each side may be used to prevent this overactivity and improve the skin's appearance. The injections are placed 1 cm lateral to midline ~1 cm from the edge of the mandible to prevent weakening the depressor labii inferioris.

The depressor anguli oris originates from the mandibular border and inserts at the corner of the mouth. Contraction of this muscle turns down the corner of the mouth with frowning or displeasure resulting in "marionette lines." Weakening of this muscle can subtly elevate the corner of the mouth and create a more joyful and energetic appearance. The patient is asked to show the lower teeth, and the muscle contraction is felt and visualized. Injections (2.5 to 5 units) are placed inferolateral to the corner of the mouth 1 cm above the mandibular boarder. Side effects of this injection include food trapping in the gingiolabial suclus, subjective dysarthria, and incompetence of the lower lip. It is important to keep the injections low to prevent weakness of the orbicularis and the depressor labii inferioris. We often combine weakening of the depressor anguli oris with soft tissue fillers to create a "strut" to support the corner of the mouth, with excellent patient satisfaction.

Deep nasolabial folds can be softened with injection at the connection between the orbicularis oris and the levator muscles (zygomaticus major and minor and levator anguli oris). Electromyography (EMG) guidance is essential to determine the precise location and depth of injection. However, weakening these muscles changes the character of the patient's smile and can elongate the upper lip, which is unacceptable to most people. This treatment is most often used in facial rebalancing after seventh nerve damage when the normal side is weakened to create symmetry with the paralyzed side. For age-related deepening of the nasolabial folds, the use of filler materials produces better results.

Some individuals have excessive upper lip retraction and gingival exposure with smiling. This "gummy smile"

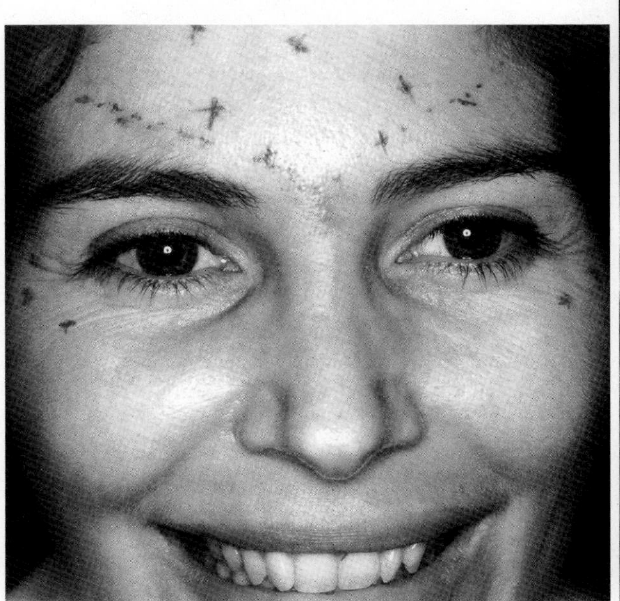

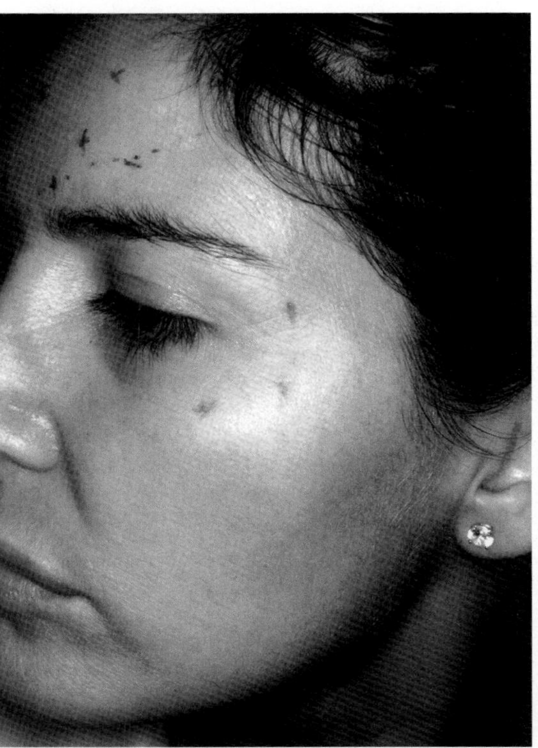

Fig. 30.7 (**A**) The crow's feet lines are marked while the patient is smiling. The first mark is made 1 cm lateral to the lateral canthal ligament and on the plane of the lateral canthus. If there are lines above this area, a second mark is made above. A third or forth mark is made over the inferior wrinkles following the orbital rim. These are marked bilaterally and then injected. (**B**) A lateral view showing the crow's feet marks for injection.

is due to contraction of the levator labii superioris alaeque nasi, which retracts and shortens the upper lip. Botulinum toxin to this muscle placed in the most superior medial portion of the nasolabial fold at the pyriform aperture will lengthen the lip during smiling and decrease the depth of the fold in this area. We recommend starting conservatively (1 unit to each side) with readjustment if necessary in 2 weeks because patients often need to accommodate to changes in their upper lip function.

Lipstick or smoker's lines are annoying rhytids that radiate from the vermillion border and are due to activity of the orbicularis oris from lip pursing. If enough weakness is created to eliminate the lines, the lips become incompetent with consequent drooling of liquids and interference with plosive and fricative speech elements. Small amounts of toxin (1 unit in two to four locations in the upper lip) can be gingerly applied in combination with an injectable filler to achieve satisfactory results.

Platysmal Band Injections

Prominent platysmal bands can be softened with chemodenervation.[14,19] We perform these injections by first marking the anterior and posterior edges of the muscle bilaterally and drawing horizontal lines ~2 cm apart over the region of the excessive platysmal banding. Generally three horizontal lines are sufficient. The muscle is "skewered" using EMG guidance on a 1.5 in. needle passed perpendicularly to the muscle fibers, and toxin is injected on withdrawal of the needle. The muscle is generally injected with 2.5 to 5.0 units per 0.1 mL per site with three sites per side. The dose range in our series is 7.5 to 20 units per side. One needs to keep the volume and dose small to prevent diffusion to the strap muscles of the anterior neck, which can cause dysphonia or dysphagia if weakened. If the toxin diffuses to the cricothyroid muscles, changes in voice pitch will occur, which may be very noticeable in singers.[20]

Adjunctive BTX Injections

Relaxation of the underlying facial musculature can enhance the results of laser resurfacing and the effects of dermal fillers such as collagen or hyaluronic acid. The best results are staged, starting with BTX injections and having the patient return after 1 to 2 weeks for the second procedure.[21,22] If the patient is having laser resurfacing, softening the wrinkles allows proper reorientation of the collagen fibers to give optimal and durable results. The skin will heal without the wrinkle, until the muscular

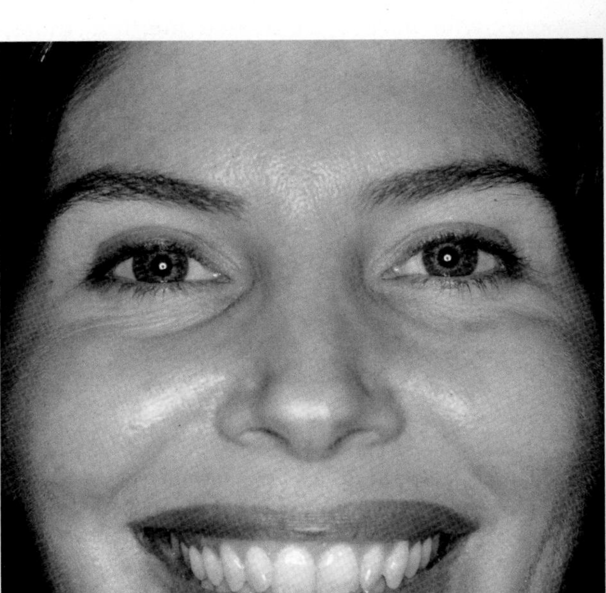

A

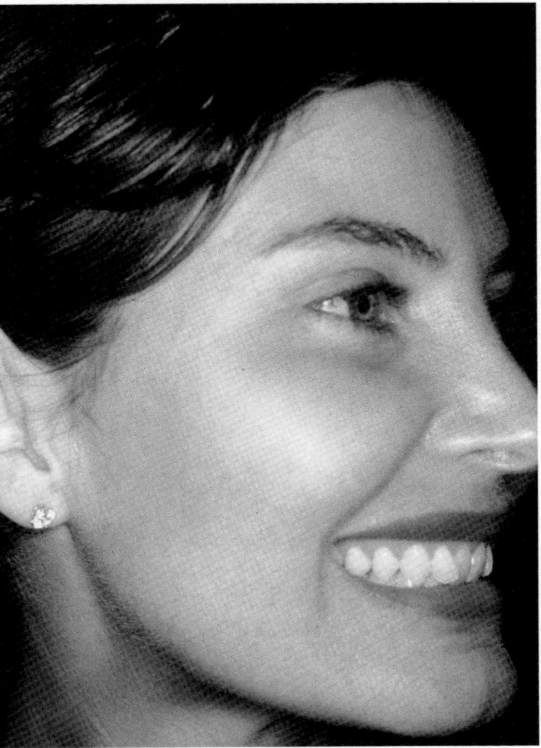

B

Fig. 30.8 Patient 2 weeks postinjection. (**A**) Note the loss of lines in the forehead area and a diminution of the crow's feet lines. (**B**) Note the pleasing contour of the periorbital skin.

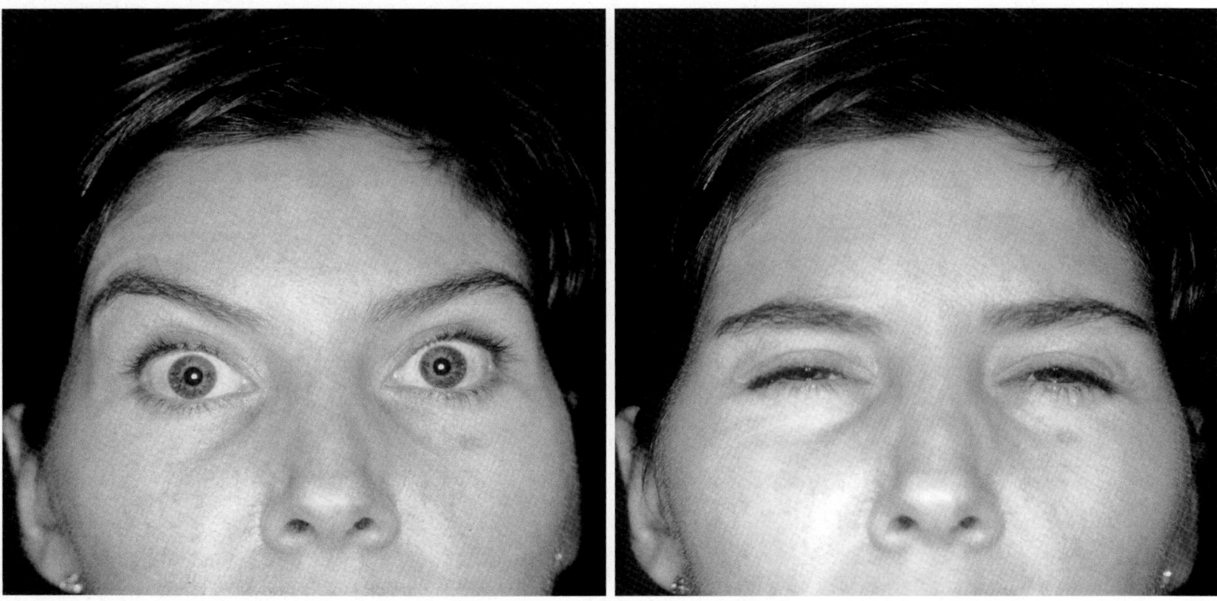

Fig. 30.9 Patient 2 weeks post injection. (**A**) Note the flat forehead with preservation of lateral brow expressivity. (**B**) Note the minimal number of lateral orbital lines with squinting.

strength returns at 4 months, at which time BTX injections may need to be repeated.

BTX can relax the skin lines and therefore minimize the amount of collagen or other filler needed to enhance the cosmetic result. Once the persistent furrow is filled, the material seems to last much longer without the constant muscular squeezing effect. Therefore, less material is needed to correct the line, and the material lasts longer when used in conjunction with BTX.

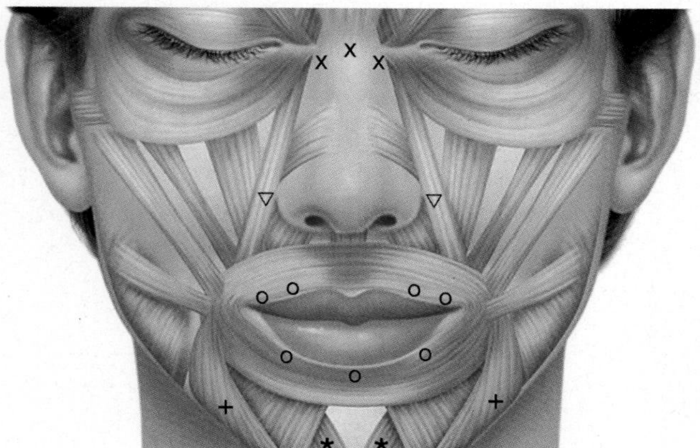

Fig. 30.10 Location of injections for the middle and lower face. See text for details. X, bunny lines (transverse nasalis); O, lipstick lines (orbicularis oris); *, popply chin (mentalis); +, marionette lines (depressor anguli oris); ∇, gummy smile (levator labii superioris alaeque nasi).

Follow-Up

Patients are reevaluated at 2 weeks postinjection. If the hyperfunctional lines remain, additional toxin may be injected. The patient is instructed to return in 4 to 6 months when the facial lines again become prominent and bothersome. We discourage reinjection before a 4-month interval to prevent immunoresistance. In some patients who have been treated multiple times, the BTX effect seems to last for longer and longer periods, perhaps related to behavior modification.

Complications

Complications of BTX injections include mild bruising or local pain at the site of injection, and rarely a mild headache and/or "flulike" syndrome for several days after the injection.[14,23,24] There may also be transient weakness of adjacent muscles related to diffusion of the toxin, although this is technique and dose-related.

There have been no long-term complications or hazards of BTX use. Muscle biopsies taken from patients after repetitive injections have not shown any permanent atrophy or degeneration. Some patients receiving high doses (300 units or more, such as for torticollis) may develop antibody to toxin. Although these antibodies have not produced hypersensitivity reactions or anaphylaxis, they do block the effect of the toxin, making the patient resistant to further therapy.

To minimize the chance for immunoresistance we recommend using the smallest possible effective dose and extending the interval between treatments for a long as possible to minimize the number of exposures.[1]

Over the past 17 years, we have found BTX injections for hyperfunctional facial lines to be extremely safe and useful. The injections may be used alone or in combination with peels, resurfacing, or filling techniques. Patient satisfaction is extremely high.

References

1. Blitzer A, Sulica L. Botulinum toxin: basic science and clinical uses in otolaryngology. Laryngoscope 2001;111:218–226
2. Rohrer TE, Beer K. Background to botulinum toxin. In: Carruthers A, Carruthers J, eds. Botulinum Toxin. Philadelphia: Elsevier; 2005:9–17
3. Blitzer A, Brin MF, Keen MS, Aviv JE. Botulinum toxin for the treatment of hyperfunctional lines of the face. Arch Otolaryngol Head Neck Surg 1993;119:1018–1022
4. Keen M, Blitzer A, Aviv J, et al. Botulinum toxin A for hyperkinetic facial lines: results of a double-blind, placebo-controlled study. Plast Reconstr Surg 1994;94:94–99
5. Blitzer A, Binder WJ, Aviv JE, Keen MS, Brin MF. The management of hyperfunctional facial lines with botulinum toxin: a collaborative study of 210 injection sites in 162 patients. Arch Otolaryngol Head Neck Surg 1997;123:389–392
6. Carruthers A, Carruthers J. Aesthetic indications for botulinum toxin injections. Plast Reconstr Surg 1995;95:427–428
7. Hambleton P, Moore AP. Botulinum neurotoxins: origin, structure, molecular actions, and antibody. In: Moore AP, ed. Handbook of Botulinum Toxin Treatment. Oxford: Blackwell Scientific; 1995:1–27
8. Meyer KF, Eddie B. Perspectives concerning botulism. Z Hyg Infektionskr 1951;133:255–263
9. Hexsel DM, De Almeida AT, Rutowitsch M, et al. Multicenter, double-blind study of the efficacy of injections with botulinum toxin type A reconstituted up to 6 consecutive weeks before application. Dermatol Surg 2003;29:523–529 discussion 529
10. Blitzer A, Binder WF, Brin MF. The use of botulinum toxin for the management of hyperfunctional lines and wrinkles. In: Blitzer A, Pillsbury HC, Jahn AF, Binder WJ, eds. Office-Based Surgery in Otolaryngology. New York: Thieme; 1998
11. Carruthers A, Carruthers J. Clinical indications and injection technique for the cosmetic use of botulinum A exotoxin. Dermatol Surg 1998;24:1189–1194
12. Binder WJ, Blitzer A, Brin MF. Treatment of hyperfunctional lines of the face with botulinum toxin A. Dermatol Surg 1998;24:1198–1205
13. Lowe NJ. Botulinum toxin type A for facial rejuvenation: United States and United Kingdom perspectives. Dermatol Surg 1998;24:1216–1218
14. Carruthers J, Fagien S, Matarasso SL. Consensus recommendations on the use of botulinum toxin type a in facial aesthetics. Plast Reconstr Surg 2004; 114(6, Suppl)1S–22S
15. Carruthers JD, Carruthers JA. Treatment of glabellar frown lines with C. botulinum-A exotoxin. J Dermatol Surg Oncol 1992;18:17–21
16. Fagien S. BOTOX for the treatment of dynamic and hyperkinetic facial lines and furrows: adjunctive use in facial aesthetic surgery. Plast Reconstr Surg 1999;103:701–713
17. Blitzer A, Binder WJ. Current practices in the use of botulinum toxin A in the management of facial lines and wrinkles. Facial Plast Surg Clin North Am 2001;9:395–404
18. Lowe NJ, Yamauchi P. Cosmetic uses of botulinum toxins for lower aspects of the face and neck. Clin Dermatol 2004;22:18–22
19. Kane MA. Nonsurgical treatment of platysma bands with injection of botulinum toxin a revisited. Plast Reconstr Surg 2003;112(5, Suppl) 125S–126S
20. Matarasso A, Matarasso SL, Brandt FS, Bellman B. Botulinum A exotoxin for the management of platysma bands. Plast Reconstr Surg 1999;103:645–652 discussion 653–645
21. Yamauchi PS, Lask G, Lowe NJ. Botulinum toxin type A gives adjunctive benefit to periorbital laser resurfacing. J Cosmet Laser Ther 2004; 6:145–148
22. Carruthers J, Carruthers A. The adjunctive usage of botulinum toxin. Dermatol Surg 1998;24:1244–1247
23. Matarasso SL. Complications of botulinum A exotoxin for hyperfunctional lines. Dermatol Surg 1998;24:1249–1254
24. Klein AW. Contraindications and complications with the use of botulinum toxin. Clin Dermatol 2004;22:66–75

31 Aesthetic Mandibular Implants

Harry Mittelman and Albert Jen

The use of alloplastic materials to augment the central mentum dates back more than 40 years. Recently the popularity of this procedure has increased substantially due to a better understanding of the anatomy and aging process of the mandible as well as an increase in diversity of alloplastic implants, which have been more artistically designed for fit, form, and function. An appreciation of the indications for augmentation of the central mentum and midlateral mandible is rooted in an understanding of the aesthetic facial proportions and the anatomy of both the young and the aging mandible.

One of the prerequisites for beauty in today's ever-growing fashion industry is a balanced proportion of the chin in its central mentum and a straight, youthful, full jawline as the central mentum transitions into the midlateral mandible. The beauty of a strong jawline has been depicted by some of the great artists of the past as well. Although a variance exists between the "strong" chin of a man and of a woman, both give the illusion of power, strength, confidence, assertiveness, aesthetic balance, and beauty. A receding chin often conveys an illusion of negative attributes, such as weak character, combined with a lack of proper facial proportions, resulting in a lack of optimal beauty.

It may seem at first glance that chin augmentation is a relatively minor procedure. When one understands the anatomy of the balanced optimal mandible as well as the genetic differences in mandibles, and particularly the aging process of the mandible, the actual surgical procedure can be straightforward. However, the quality of the result is based on the proper selection of the implant to be used. That selection process is difficult unless the surgeon is aware of the different options and how to choose among them. The number of alloplastic implants available can sometimes be confusing, but it is possible to fulfill 98% of the facial aesthetic surgeon's needs using a relatively small armamentarium of alloplastic extended mandibular implants. The surgeon who understands the anatomy and aging process of the mandible to be augmented can achieve optimal surgical results. Although there are various alloplastic implants, it is important to understand that essentially the same procedure can be used to treat the genetically imperfect mandible, the traumatized mandible, and the aging process of the mandible and its overlying soft tissue. No aesthetic surgical procedure in the authors' armamentarium yields as much aesthetic benefit for as little time and effort as is involved in augmenting the mandible with the properly chosen alloplastic implant.

Analysis of the Lower Jaw

The most common indication for chin augmentation is the presence of a hypoplastic mentum. The basic tenets of facial aesthetic proportions have been summarized by Powell and Humphreys and include both a frontal and a lateral assessment.[1] The frontal view of the face may be divided into thirds, with the lower third extending from the subnasale to the menton. This lower third can be subdivided so that the upper third is occurring from the subnasale to the stomion superiorus and the lower two thirds occurring from the stomion inferiorus to the menton. There is loss of the vertical height and anterior projection of the mandible with advancing age, resulting in a loss of the ideal proportions. Simultaneously, during this aging process, the soft tissues covering the mandible often display some atrophy as well as laxity. On lateral view, the method of Gonzales-Ulloa[2] may be applied to define a hypoplastic mentum. In this technique, a line is dropped from the nasion perpendicular to the Frankfort horizontal plane. The ideal chin projection should be at this line. However, when the chin is posterior to this line and the patient has a class I occlusion, then a hypoplastic mentum is present. Another frequently used method is to simply drop a line from vermilion of the lower lip perpendicular to the Frankfort horizontal plane. Once again, the ideal chin projection should be at this line and a chin posterior to this line with class I occlusion is considered hypoplastic. A hypoplastic mentum may be a result of microgenia, which is a small chin that results from underdevelopment of the mandibular symphysis, or from micrognathia, which is a result of hypoplasia of various parts of the jaw. Mandibular augmentation is generally done for microgenia or mild cases of micrognathia. As noted above, a hypoplastic mentum and prejowl sulcus is quite frequently a result of the aging process of the soft tissue and bony mandible. Critical in evaluation of these patients is the dental occlusion, with augmentation considered in those individuals with normal or near-normal occlusion.

Although congenital factors contribute to the presence of a hypoplastic mentum, the development of a prejowl sulcus is due primarily to the aging process. Loss of elasticity of the skin of the eyes, face, neck, and submental wattles are the most obvious and commonly observed effects of aging. A subtle change also occurs in the configuration of the area just anterior to the jowl, which can have an important effect on facial appearance. As a result of progressive atrophy of soft tissue in the area between the chin and jowl as well as gradual bone reduction of the mandible in this same area, a patient may develop a groove between the chin and the remainder of the body of the mandible, an area known as the prejowl sulcus[3] (**Fig. 31.1**). During aging, there are two major contributing factors to the formation of the prejowl sulcus. One is bony resorption of the mandible at the junction of the central mandible (mentum) and the midlateral mentum. This area, below the mental foramen, has been shown in anatomy books to develop bony resorption and a concavity.[4] Referred to and named by the senior author as the anterior mandibular groove, this area may be reflected on the external surface of the soft tissue jawline as an indentation between the jowl and the chin, which is then referred to as the prejowl sulcus. The other major contributing factor to the formation of the prejowl sulcus is soft tissue atrophy, which occurs between the chin and the jowl during the aging process. With time this can become part of the commissure mandibular "marionette line" or "drool line." In most individuals who form a prejowl sulcus with aging, it is frequently due to a combination of both soft tissue atrophy and bony resorption.

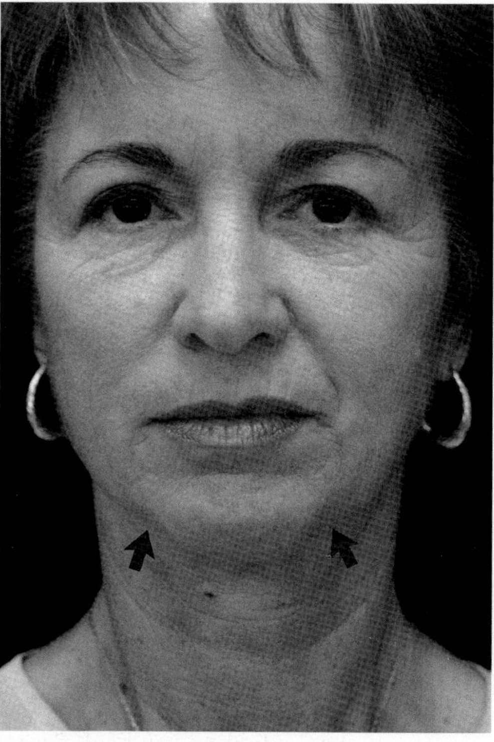

Fig. 31.1 Example of the prejowl sulcus (*arrows*) due to aging of the underlying mandible and soft tissues in an adult woman.

Relevant Anatomy of the Mentum

Although the basic anatomy of the mandible is familiar to the aesthetic surgeon, some points are worth emphasizing. The position of the mental foramina is somewhat variable but is usually found below the second premolar tooth. An anatomical study has been described showing that in 50% of cases the mental foramen is at the level of the second premolar, in 25% it is found between the first and second premolars, and in the remaining 25% it is posterior to the second premolar.[5] In the young adult mandible, the mental foramina generally lies midway between the alveolar ridge and the inferior border of the mandible and ~25 mm lateral to the midline, with the distance varying between 20 to 30 mm. In children, it is lower on the mandible and more anterior, whereas during the aging process, because of the atrophy of the alveolar ridge, the mental foramen is closer to the alveolar ridge while maintaining a fairly constant distance from the inferior border of the mandible. Thus its relative position is higher. Even in the aging mandible, there seems to be a distance of more than 8 mm between the mental foramen and the inferior border of the mandible at the site of the muscle attachments. The neurovascular bundle exits the mental foramen in a superior direction and has a tough sheath surrounding it.

The importance of the anatomy of the mental foramina in the aging mandible relates directly to the comfort level that the aesthetic surgeon has in the technique used for placement of extended mandibular implants. This anatomy clearly indicates that the surgeon must dissect carefully in creating a pocket for the implant that is below the mental foramen yet above and down to the level of the insertion of the muscle in the inferior border of the mandible. Generally, one has at least 8 to 10 mm of space in that area. Properly designed implants should have a height in this area of around 6 to 8 mm. Because of the upward direction and durable sheath of the neurovascular bundle of the mental foramen, the use of an elevator in this 8 to 10 mm space may touch the sheath and even stretch it to some degree, but it would be difficult to transect it. Although the surgeon has a greater safety factor because of the nature of this anatomy, at the same time he or she must use caution in the technique of elevating this pocket.

Implant Selection

Factors involved in selecting an implant include the type of material from which the implant is made, as well as the particular shape of implant that meets the needs of the patient's aesthetic imperfections. The ideal material for mandibular implants should have the right consistency, flexibility, firmness, nonreactivity, resistance to infection, stability, removability, changeability, and ease of manufacture, and should be harmless to the surrounding tissue.[6] The only alloplastic implant that meets almost all of these criteria is solid but flexible silicone elastomer rubber (Silastic, Dow Corning, Midland, MI).

Silastic is made of a polymer that can be varied to provide the proper consistency in terms of softness as well as flexibility. The body accepts the material, forming a fibrous capsule around the implant without distorting the implant itself. Fenestrated Silastic implants can be further stabilized with fibrous tissue ingrowth. The material can be commercially machined to different sizes and shapes with the help of computer-aided design technology. These preformed implants can be customized by trimming with conventional instruments and blades in the operating room as indicated. Expanded polytetrafluorethylene (Gore-Tex, W. L. Gore & Associates, Inc., Flagstaff, AZ) is another material available for mandibular implants. The senior author feels that there is limited tissue ingrowth with Gore-Tex implants, which can make removal of the implant, if necessary, more difficult than removal of Silastic implants, but still very acceptable. Another available material is polyethylene or Medpore (W. L. Gore & Associates, Inc., Flagstaff, AZ). This material is rigid, difficult to shape, and permits extensive fibrous tissue ingrowth, which would make removal of the implant very difficult. Also, due to the rigid nature of polyethylene, each side of the implant needs to be placed separately and then connected in the midline in order for the implant to be placed in an incision of acceptable size.

Selection of one of the many commercially available Silastic mandibular implants can be confusing. The first decision must be the use of an extended mandibular implant rather than a central chin implant. Central chin implants result in an unnatural, nonanatomical augmentation of the central mentum, with a pointed-looking chin and undefined jawline. Properly designed extended mandibular implants have a smooth transition from the central mentum to the lateral mandible with preservation and enhancement of the natural jawline. The three best researched and most commonly used extended mandibular implants are the extended anatomical mandibular implant (four sizes), the variety of Flowers chin implants (standard, vertical, anterior tilt, and posterior tilt), and the Mittelman prejowl-chin implants (four sizes) (**Fig. 31.2**). All three of these implant types provide a slightly different configuration and philosophy but give very good results. The extended anatomical mandibular implant provides varying chin augmentation, depending on the need of the patient, but the extension of the implant beneath the mental foramen is of approximately the same size no matter what size augmentation is in the area of the mentum itself. In other words, augmentation in the area of the prejowl sulcus stays almost the same regardless of the size of the augmentation in the area of the mentum. The Flowers mandibular implant provides for a variation in the tilt of the Silastic implant at the central mentum with a tapered extension along the mandible beneath the mental foramen.

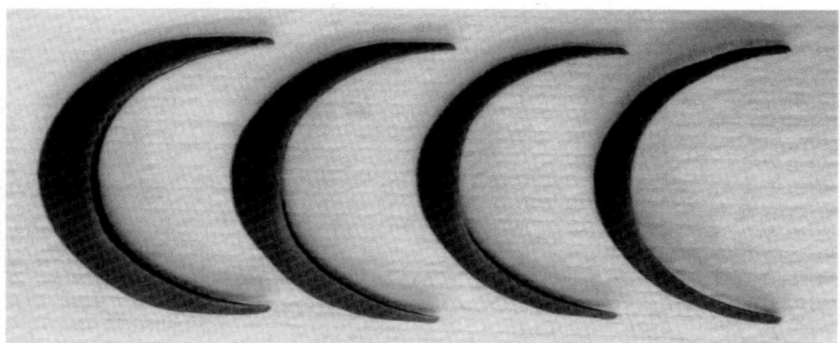

Fig. 31.2 Complete set of sizers for chin–jowl implants (XL, L, M, S).

The Mittelman prejowl-chin implant provides four variations in augmentation of the mentum combined with a comparable four variations of the extension of those implants into the area of the prejowl sulcus. It is intended to provide four different sizes of augmentation in the prejowl sulcus at the same time that the surgeon is providing four different sizes of augmentation of the mentum. In addition to this, there is an extended mandibular implant that provides no augmentation in the mentum itself, providing augmentation only of the prejowl sulcus (**Fig. 31.3**). This implant becomes an extremely important adjunct for the facelift patient who has adequate chin augmentation but who so frequently has a prejowl sulcus. There has been another modification of the extended chin implant by Terino[7] whereby a more squared anterior projection has been designed that is particularly helpful in achieving a more prominent anterior projection, especially suitable for some males.

The Silastic implants described here can be of varying durometers or firmness. The softer solid implants are more flexible and can be more easily placed through smaller incisions. They are also more conforming to the mandible and may cause less bony resorption. We utilize Silastic implants manufactured with a durometer of 10 for mandibular augmentation. Most of the extended mandibular implants and all of the prejowl implants have multiple fenestrations, which can help with fixation of the implant to the periosteum or soft tissue of the mentum. These extended implants are very stable and do not displace postoperatively in the senior author's vast experience. There is

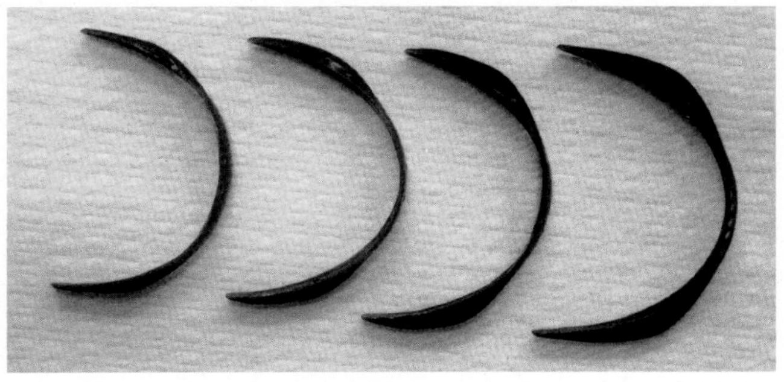

Fig. 31.3 Complete set of sizers for prejowl implants (S, M, L, XL).

no standardization of the implant sizes (e.g., the mentum size of one manufacturer vs that of another). However, there is some consistency among different designed implants of the same manufacturer. Physician judgment is made easier by the availability of "sizers" by the established manufacturers. The sizers can be inserted until the surgeon feels satisfied with the result. Then the sizer is removed and the actual implant of that size is placed into the pocket.

Surgical Technique

The chin implants described here can be placed either intraorally or through a submental incision. The intraoral approach avoids an external scar, but implant placement is less precise, with a greater chance of implant malpositioning. The senior author feels that the submental incision is well hidden and the benefits of precise placement from this approach far outweigh the small, well-camouflaged scar. The essential setup includes a Bernstein retractor, narrow but blunt, slightly curved dissectors, straight clamps, and a gentamicin saline solution (40 mg gentamicin in 100 mL normal saline) to bathe the implant and instruments prior to placement (**Fig. 31.4**). The submental incision is generally placed just anterior to the submental crease; placement of the incision in the submental crease may occasionally result in a more depressed scar. In the aging patient with a significant submental crease, the skin is undermined slightly posteriorly to free the fibrous skin attachments at the submental crease, which usually results in some bleeding that is easily controlled with bipolar cautery. This is done because release of the fibrous attachments results in the desired blunting of the submental crease during the healing process. The dissection is now undermined anterior to the incision and carried down through the soft tissue, muscle, and periosteum at the level of the inferior border of the mandible. Care is taken to ensure that the scalpel blade is perpendicular to the tissues and not beveled, which would lead to incising the periosteum too high or too low

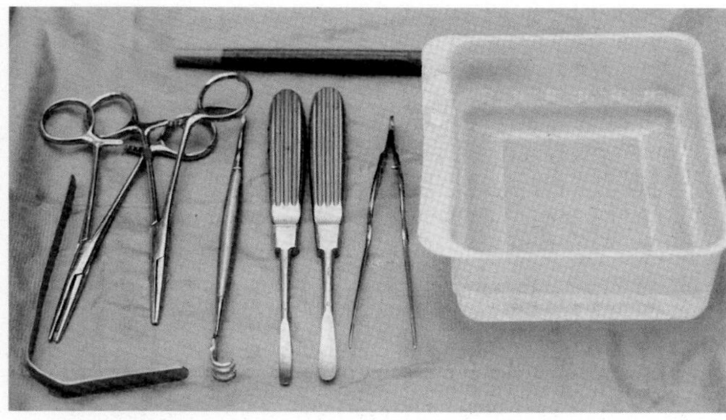

Fig. 31.4 Instruments used for aesthetic chin augmentation. Note the basin of gentamicin saline solution.

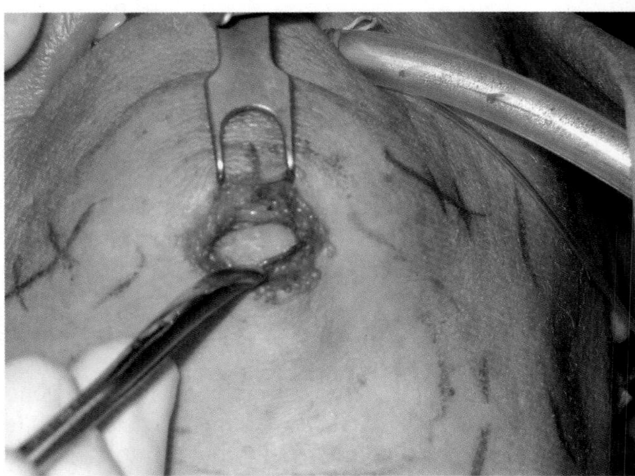

Fig. 31.5 Exposure of the central mentum after skin, subcutaneous tissue, and periosteum have been divided.

(**Fig. 31.5**). The periosteum is then dissected free for a few millimeters inferiorly and ~2 cm above the inferior border of the bony mentum superiorly, exposing the central mentum. Dissection is then performed in the subperiosteal plane with the right hand holding the dissector and the left "smart" hand guiding the instrument externally (for a right-handed surgeon), thus protecting from any excursions above the intended dissection pocket (**Fig. 31.6**). The lateral pockets should be dissected ~6 cm from the midline and remain below the level of the mental foramen for proper positioning. After the pockets are developed, the implant is removed from the gentamicin solution and placed in the pocket with the help of a clamp. After the right half of the implant is placed in the right subperiosteal pocket, the left half of the implant is guided with clamps and a retractor into the left pocket by folding it acutely onto

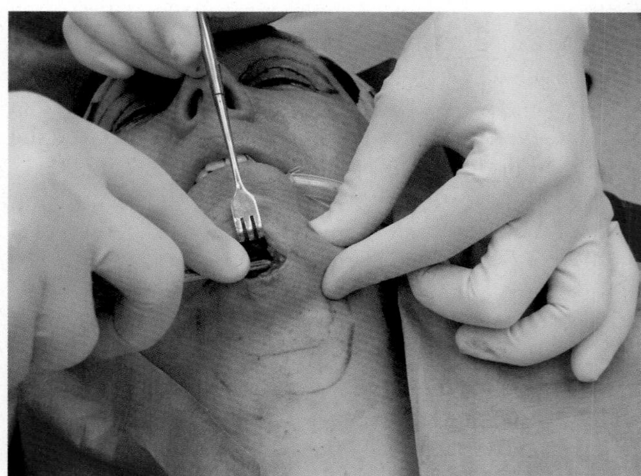

Fig. 31.6 Dissection of the lateral pocket for insertion of the Silastic (Dow Corning, Midland, MI) implant. Note the noninstrument "smart" hand guiding the path of dissection along the inferior border of the mandible.

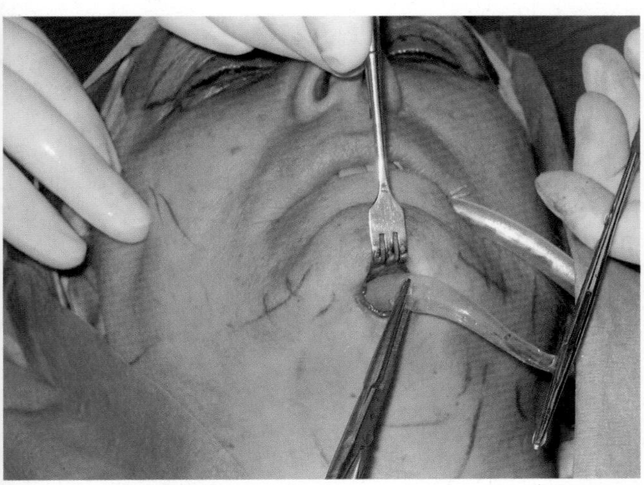

Fig. 31.7 Placement of the Silastic (Dow Corning, Midland, MI) implant into the right half of the dissected pocket with guidance using straight clamps.

itself (**Figs. 31.7 and 31.8**). In cases in which an extra large or large implant is placed, it is not uncommon to have to cut the implant in half and place each side separately because the large anterior projection prevents the acute folding of the implant. The two halves are then sutured together after individual placement. Also periosteum can be left intact centrally and elevated laterally with placement of the central portion of the implant on periosteum and the lateral portion on bone. The theoretical advantage is that by leaving the periosteum centrally, bone resorption due to the implant is minimized. However, the senior author feels that elevating the periosteum centrally as well as laterally enables more precise placement and that the resorption that occurs is minimal and actually allows the implant to better conform to the mandible. After placement, the

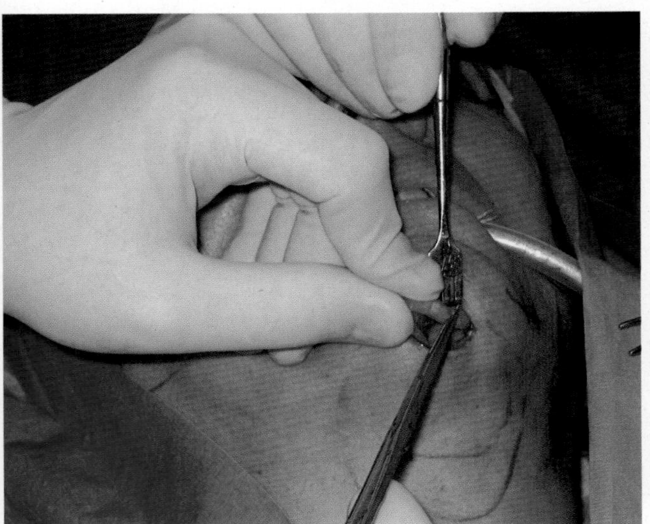

Fig. 31.8 Folding of the Silastic (Dow Corning, Midland, MI) implant acutely to facilitate passing into the contralateral dissection pocket.

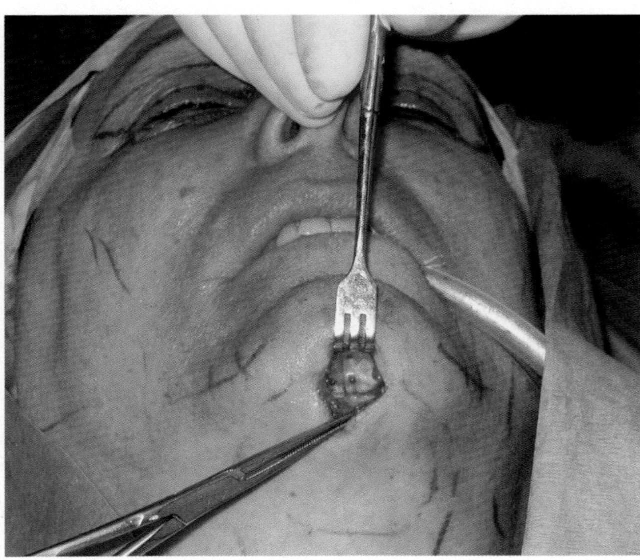

Fig. 31.9 Implant has been placed and is checked for alignment. Note the midline blue mark of the implant.

implant is checked for smoothness against the mandible and absence of lateral fullness from the implant's most lateral extensions folding or "curling" (**Fig. 31.9**). The implant has multiple fenestrations and a central blue marking that designates the middle of the implant. The fenestrations within the implant allow for tissue ingrowth and stability of the implant. The blue mark in the implant assists the surgeon in placing the implant symmetrically. Prolene sutures (Ethicon, Inc., Somerville, NJ) secure the implant to the periosteum, and the overlying soft tissue and muscle are then closed over the implant (**Figs. 31.10 and 31.11**). A meticulous closure of the muscle and subcutaneous tissue is then performed, followed by a separate skin closure. The results of chin augmentation can be appreciated on both lateral and oblique views (**Figs. 31.12–31.15**).

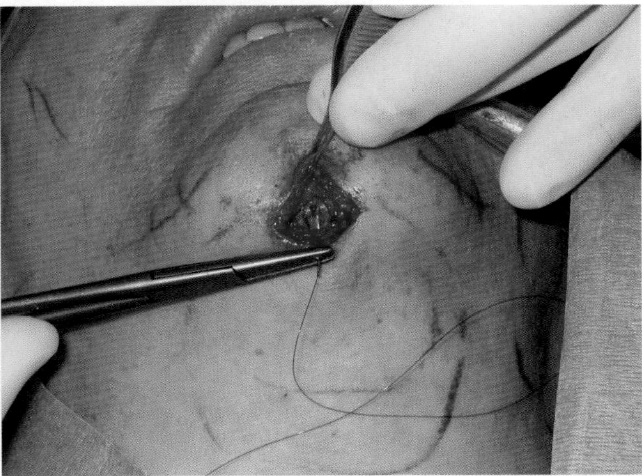

Fig. 31.10 Securing the implant with a fixation suture through the periosteum, soft tissues, and fenestrations of the implant.

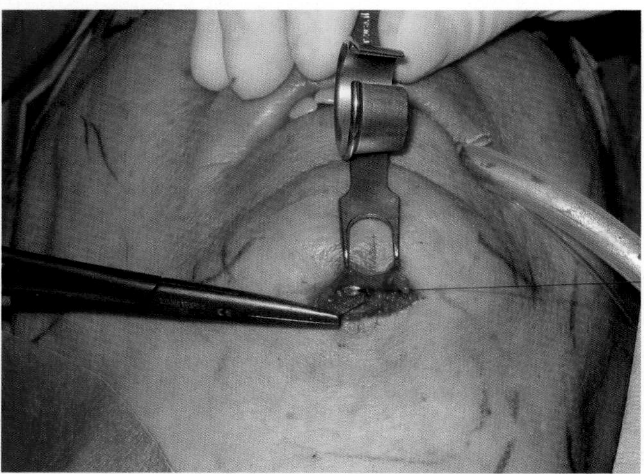

Fig. 31.11 Closure of the periosteum and soft tissue over the implant with Prolene suture (Ethicon, Inc., Somerville, NJ).

Postoperative Considerations and Complications

Although a long list of complications can be listed with any procedure, the incidence of these problems in the case of mandibular augmentation is often low and almost always temporary. When complications occur, they are easily treatable, and in the case of proper implant selection or patient preference, the procedure is reversible and changeable to suit the postoperative desires of the patient or the surgeon.

The old literature suggests that infection with the use of alloplastic implants occurs in ~4 to 5% of procedures. However, this incidence is lowered dramatically by the use of intraoperative gentamicin solution to soak the implant and irrigate the surgically created pockets. Hematoma is very uncommon. Asymmetry does not occur with extended anterior mandibular implants unless one or both of the pockets are placed above the mental foremen.

However, sensory alterations occur in 20 to 30% of patients with chin implants, though on a temporary basis. This hypesthesia should be expected and discussed preoperatively. This occurs far more often than with central mandibular implants but should not dissuade the aesthetic surgeon from using extended mandibular implants. Migration or extrusion of the implant has not been experienced with extended mandibular implants. Also, skin necrosis from the external approach and allergy to the Silastic extended mandibular implants has not been experienced.

Bone resorption under chin implants has been reported since the 1960s, but without significant clinical effects.[8] Implants placed too high over the suprapogonion erode through the thin cortex more easily. The

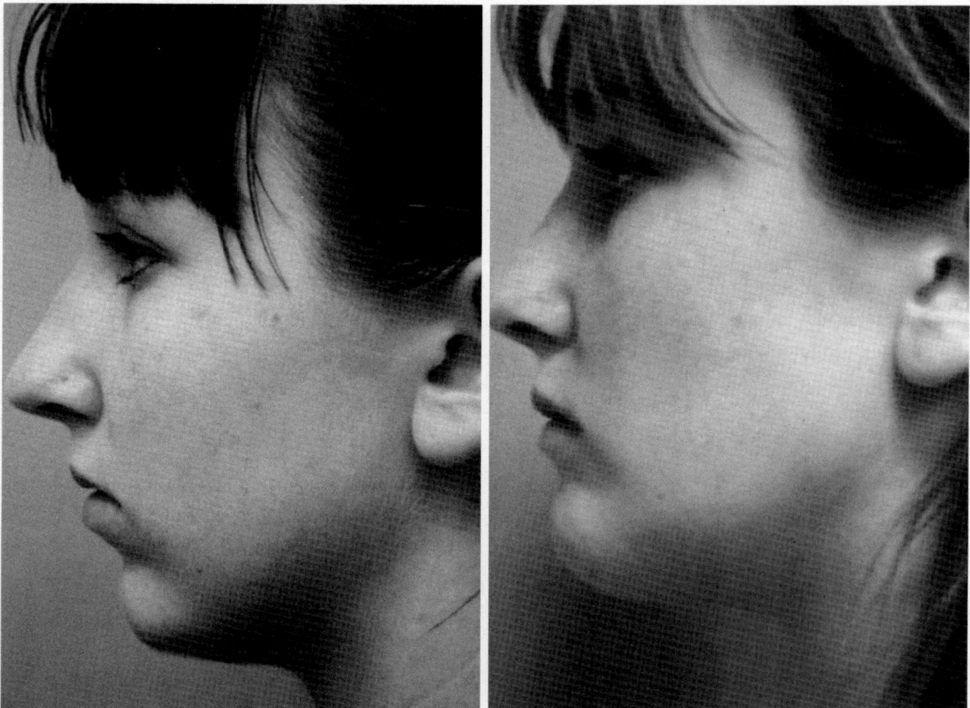

Fig. 31.12 (**A**) Preoperative lateral view of an adolescent woman with a hypoplastic mentum. (**B**) Postoperative lateral view of the same patient after aesthetic chin augmentation.

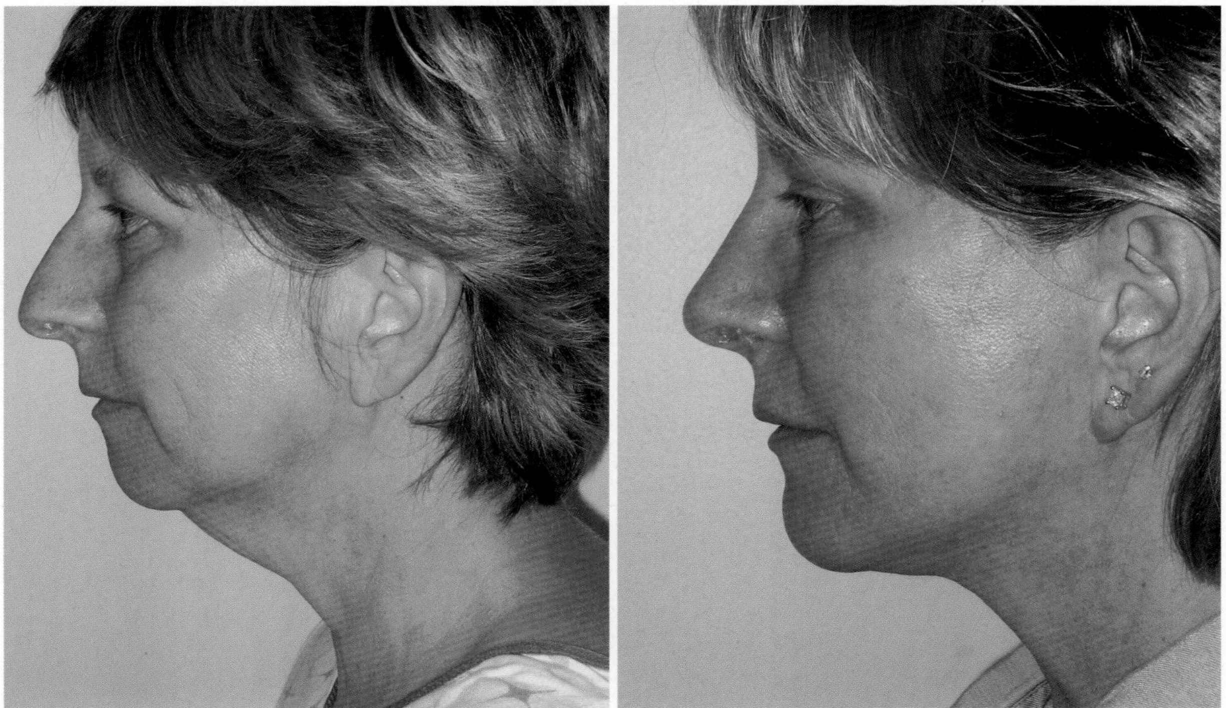

Fig. 31.13 (**A**) Preoperative lateral view of a woman with a hypoplastic mentum and aging changes of the face. (**B**) Postoperative lateral view of the same patient after aesthetic chin augmentation combined with rhinoplasty, face/neck lift, and submentoplasty.

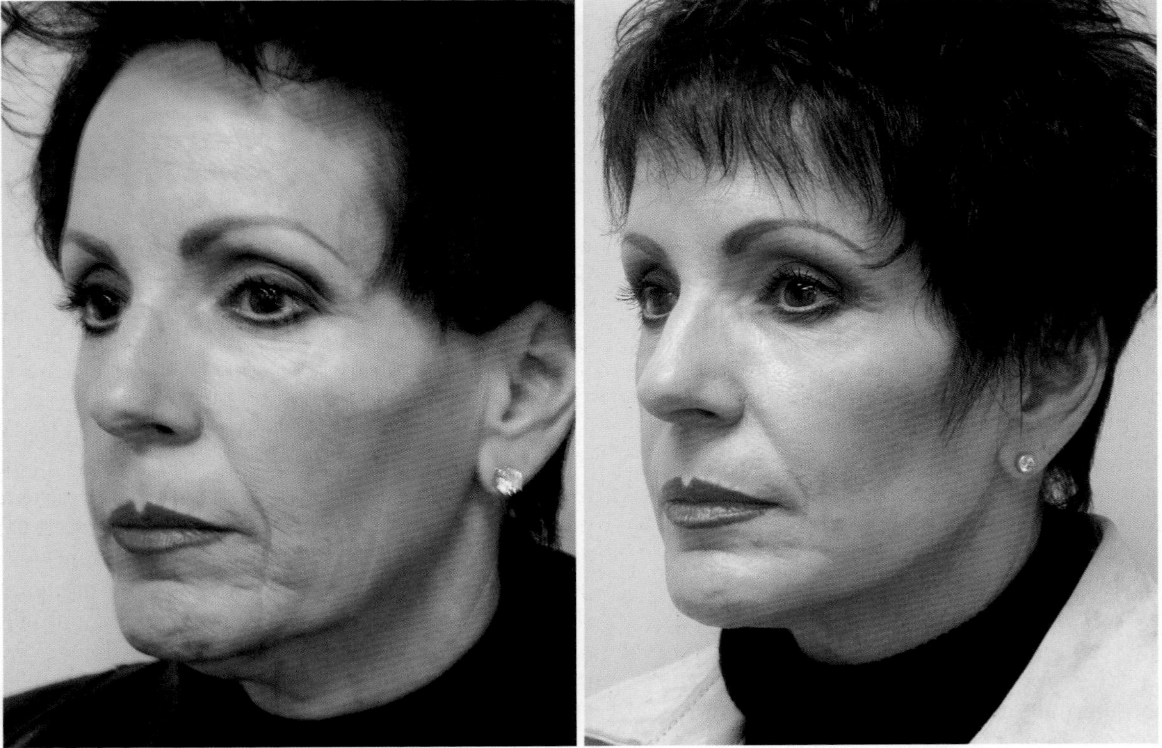

Fig. 31.14 (**A**) Preoperative oblique view of a woman with a hypoplastic mentum and aging changes of the face. (**B**) Postoperative lateral view of the same patient after aesthetic chin augmentation combined with face/neck lift and submentoplasty.

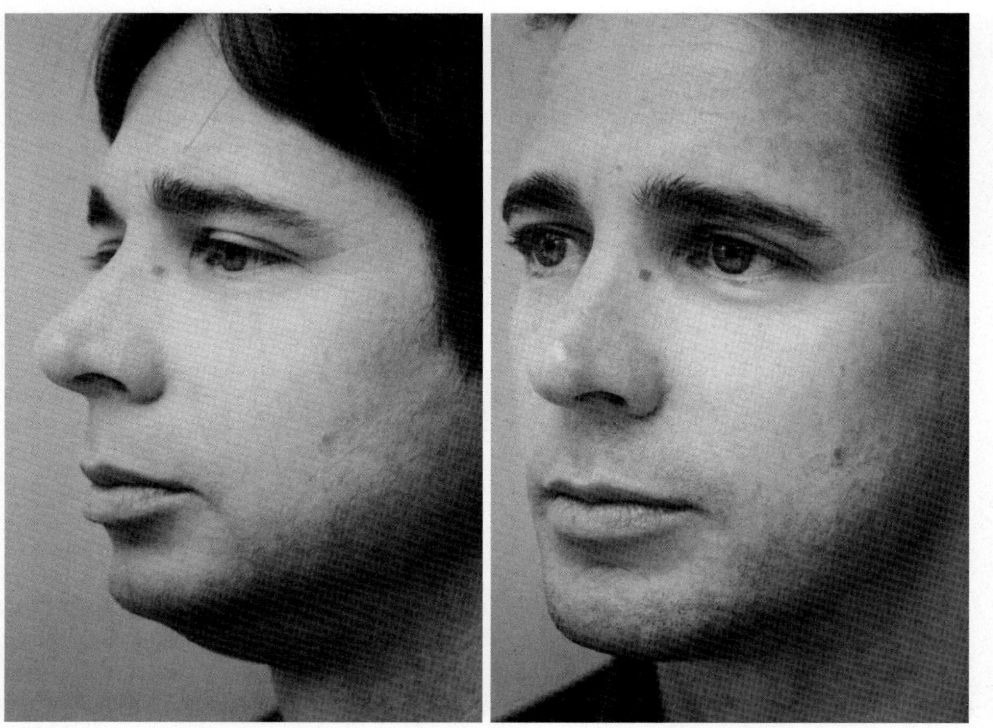

Fig. 31.15 (**A**) Preoperative oblique view of an adult male with a hypoplastic mentum. (**B**) Postoperative oblique view of the same patient after aesthetic chin augmentation.

absorption over the thicker cortical bone of the mental protuberance and the pogonion is less and is clinically less significant. The extended mandibular implants that by virtue of the mental foramen keep it from riding up higher, and the muscle attachments that keep it from riding inferiorly, provide ideal stability at the proper level of the chin. The softer solid Silastic implants tend to resorb less bone than the harder implants. The larger implants may cause greater resorption due to a greater degree of tension/pressure between the periosteum, muscle, and bony cortex. Absorption seems to occur in the first 6 to 12 months and is self-limiting if the implant is properly positioned. It is possible that a small portion of the resorption actually stabilizes the implant over the following years. The soft tissue profile of the chin seems to remain fairly stable despite this process. No pain or dental erosion has been experienced as a result of this. If the implant is removed, the bony resorption area may regenerate.

Visual or palpable projections of the lateralmost portion of the extended implants does occasionally occur, possibly as the result of the capsular formation buckling the feathered edges upon themselves. This is especially true with the extremely thin, very pliable edges of the extended anatomical chin implants. Frequently, palpation and massaging of these edges expand the capsule in that area and eliminate this palpable projection, making it clinically insignificant. Rarely the implant has to be removed, the pocket expanded, and the implant repositioned. A pocket that is initially too small will also cause a buckling of the feathered edges, creating this type of imperfection within the first few weeks after surgery. The projection that is due to capsular contraction frequently occurs after 6 weeks.

The smile may be temporarily altered as a result of muscle injury or swelling of the lower lip that can only be evidenced on smiling but not in the resting position. A portion of one lower lip may appear to be weaker by not retracting inferiorly as much as the lateral portion of the lip due to a temporary injury of the depressor muscles. This occurs more often with the intraoral approach.

Although asymmetry secondary to proper placement of an implant may not occur, poor preoperative planning for a preoperative asymmetrical mandible may be evident postoperatively. Any preoperative asymmetry must be discussed with patients so that they understand that any postoperative asymmetry is a result of the preoperative status and not caused by the implant or implantation technique. A very small percentage of patients exhibit a temporary speech impediment, usually lisping, secondary to the effects of swelling or dissection on the depressor muscles of the lip. Enough of an effect on the depressor muscles or the mentalis combined with hypesthesia can occasionally cause temporary drooling and slight slurring of speech.

Motor damage to the branches of the marginal mandibular nerve is rare and temporary if it occurs. Preoperative chin clefts or dimples may change to some degree postoperatively. Although the list of potential problems listed here is long, actual experiences with problems other than hypesthesia and bony resorption have been uncommon and temporary.

References

1. Powell N, Humphreys B. Proportions of the Aesthetic Face. New York: Thieme-Stratton; 1984
2. Gonzalez-Ulloa M. A quantum method for the appreciation of the morphology of the face. Plast Reconstr Surg 1964;34:241–246
3. Mittelman H. The anatomy of the aging mandible and its importance to facelift surgery. Facial Plast Surg Clin North Am 1994;2:301–311
4. Anderson JE. Grant's Atlas of Anatomy. Baltimore: Williams & Wilkins; 1983
5. Hollinshead WH. Anatomy for Surgeons: The Head and Neck. Philadelphia: Harper & Row; 1982
6. Binder W, Kamer F, Parkes M. Mentoplasty: a clinical analysis of alloplastic implants. Laryngoscope 1981;91:381–391
7. Terino EO. Alloplastic facial contouring by zonal principles of skeletal anatomy. Clin Plast Surg 1992;19:487–493
8. Lilla JA, Vistnes LM, Jobe RP. The long-term effects of hard alloplastic implants when put on bone. Plast Reconstr Surg 1976;58:14–18

32 Aesthetic Facial Implants

William J. Binder, Babak Azizzadeh, and Geoffrey W. Tobias

Over the last 2 decades, the marked improvement in biomaterial and the design of facial implants have expanded their use in aesthetic surgery. Alloplastic implants offer a long-term solution to augment skeletal deficiency, restore facial contour irregularity, and rejuvenate the midface. Common implant procedures include cheek augmentation to balance the effects of malar hypoplasia; mandibular augmentation to create a stronger mandibular profile and better nose–chin relationship; mandibular prejowl and angle implants to augment traditional cervicofacial rhytidectomy; submalar and midfacial implants to augment the hollowness that occurs during the aging process; nasal implants for dorsal augmentation; and premaxillary implants to augment a retrusive midface. Computer-assisted custom-designed implants now provide solutions for more complex facial defects due to trauma, congenital deformities, and human immunodeficiency virus (HIV) lipoatrophy.[1,2]

The concept of facial contouring implies a change in the shape of the face. The surgeon can produce substantive contour changes by judiciously altering mass and volume in different anatomical regions and redistributing the overlying soft tissue. Accurate facial analysis is critical to the success of using facial implants. The appropriate implant will depend on the relationship between different bony promontories and the surrounding soft tissue. The individual configuration of the nose, malar–midface area, and mandible–jawline determine the fundamental architectural proportions and contour of the face. Balance between these structures and the constant distribution of the overlying soft tissue structures determines facial beauty and harmony. Modern hallmarks of beauty are distinguished by bold facial contours that are accentuated by youthful convex malar–midface configurations and a sharp, well-defined jawline. Any of these promontories that are too small or too large affect the aesthetic importance of the others. For example, reducing the nasal prominence causes both the malar–midface and the mandibular–jawline volume and projection to appear relatively more distinct. In the same manner, enhancement of the mandibular or malar–midface volumes makes the nose appear smaller and less imposing. Typically, when augmentation is the desired goal, it is accomplished through selecting implants with the proper shape and design while controlling their position over the facial skeleton and soft tissue. As a result alloplastic facial contouring can be utilized to augment bony or soft tissue anomalies.

Implants and Biomaterials

All implant materials induce the formation of fibroconnective tissue encapsulation, which creates a barrier between the host and the implant.[3,4] Adverse reactions are a consequence of unresolved inflammatory response to implant materials. The behavior is also a function of configuration characteristics of the site of implantation such as the thickness of overlying skin, scarring of the tissue bed, and underlying bone architecture that would tend to create a condition for implant instability. For example, implants that are more deeply placed with thicker overlying soft tissue rarely become exposed or extrude. Other important factors such as prevention of perioperative hematoma, seroma, and infection can significantly reduce host–implant interaction and thereby improve implant survivability.

The Ideal Implant

The ideal implant material should be cost-effective, nontoxic, nonantigenic, noncarcinogenic, and resistant to infection. It should be inert, easily shaped, conformable, placed effortlessly, and able to permanently maintain its original form. The implant should be easy to modify and customize to the needs of the recipient area during the surgical procedure without compromising the integrity of the implant and should be easy to autoclave without degradation.

Favorable surface characteristics are important for implant placement and stabilization, and, paradoxically, equally important to facilitate easy removal and exchangeability without causing injury to surrounding tissues. Implant immobilization is related to their ability to be fixed in place for the lifetime of the patient. The characteristics of implant materials such as silicone elastomer induce the formation of a surrounding capsule that maintains implant position, while expanded polytetrafluoroethylene (ePTFE) (W. L. Gore & Associates, Inc., Flagstaff, AZ) which encapsulates to a lesser degree, provides fixation with minimal tissue ingrowth. Each material–host interaction provides certain advantages in different clinical settings. Materials that cause significant tissue ingrowth and permanent fixation are often undesirable, particularly if the patient desires to change augmentation characteristics in later years. The natural encapsulation process of silicone and the minimal surface

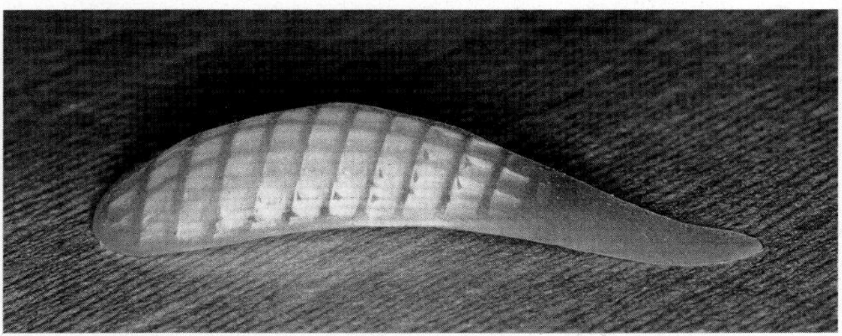

Fig. 32.1 The Conform type of implant (Implantech Associates, Ventura, CA) is made from a softer silicone material and has a grid design on the posterior surface of the implant that reduces its memory to more easily adapt to the underlying bone surface. The grid feature also reduces the chances of implant slippage and prevents displacement.

ingrowth in ePTFE products insure immobility yet provide exchangeability without damage to surrounding soft tissue.

The ideal implant design should have tapered margins that blend on to the adjacent bony surface to create a nonpalpable and smooth transition to the surrounding recipient area. An implant that is malleable and readily conforms to the underlying structures further reduces mobility, whereas the anterior surface shape should imitate the desired natural anatomical configuration. Newer silicone implants are currently being engineered for enhanced conformability to the underlying bony surface and surrounding soft tissue. For example, Conform implants (Implantech Associates, Ventura, CA) with a new type of grid backing reduces the memory of the silicone elastomer and improves flexibility. Greater adaptability to irregular bony surfaces reduces chances of movement and prevents posterior dead space from occurring between the implant and underlying bone (**Fig. 32.1**). Renewed interest in research and development in biomaterial engineering has developed a composite implant (using both silicone and ePTFE) that promises to combine the advantages two biomaterials for future use in facial implants.[5]

Implant Biomaterials

Polymeric Materials/Solid Polymers

1. *Silicone polymers.* Since the 1950s, various forms of silicone have been clinically used with an excellent safety-efficacy profile. Silicone is polymerized dimethylsiloxane that can be solid, gel, or liquid depending on its polymerization and cross-linkage. Solid silicone products tend to be more stable. The gel form of silicone can potentially over time leak some of its internal molecular substances. However, the most recent studies on breast implant gel silicone have shown no objective cause and effect for silicone in producing scleroderma, lupus, collagen vascular, or other autoimmune diseases.[6,7] Solid silicone elastomer has a high degree of chemical inertness. It is hydrophobic and extremely stable without any evidence of toxicity or allergic reactions.[8] Tissue reaction to solid silicone implants is characterized by a fibrous tissue capsule without tissue ingrowth. When unstable or placed without adequate soft tissue coverage, the implants are subject to moderate ongoing inflammation and possible seroma formation. Capsular contracture and implant deformity rarely occurs unless the implant is placed too superficially or if it migrates to the overlying skin.
2. *Polymethacrylate (acrylic) polymers.* This is supplied as a powdered mixture and catalyzed to produce a very hard material. The rigidity and hardness of the acrylic implants cause difficulty in many of the applications for using large implants inserted through small openings. In the preformed state, there is difficulty in conforming the implant to the underlying bony contour.
3. *Polyethylene.* Polyethylene can be produced in a variety of consistencies, now most commonly used in a porous form. Porous polyethylene, also known as MEDPOR (Porex Surgical, Inc., Newnan, GA) causes minimal inflammatory cell reaction. The material, however, is hard, and difficult to sculpt. The porosity of polyethylene permits extensive fibrous tissue ingrowth that provides an advantage for enhanced implant stability but makes it extremely difficult to remove.
4. *Polytetrafluoroethylene.* Polytetrafluoroethylene comprises a group of materials that have had a defined history of clinical application. The known brand name was Proplast, which is no longer made in the United States because of the related complications of its use in temporomandibular joints. Under excessive mechanical stress, this implant material was subject to breakdown, intense inflammation, thick capsule formation, infection, and ultimate extrusion or explantation.
5. *Expanded polytetrafluoroethylene.* ePTFE was originally produced for cardiovascular applications.[9,10] Animal studies showed the material to elicit limited fibrous tissue ingrowth without capsule formation and minimum inflammatory cell reaction. The reaction seen over time compared favorably with many of the materials in use for facial augmentation. The material has found acceptable results in subcutaneous tissue augmentation and for use as preformed implants. Due to lack of significant tissue ingrowth, ePTFE offers advantages in subcutaneous tissue augmentation because it can be modified secondarily and removed in the event of infection.
6. *Mesh polymers.* The mesh polymers, which include Marlex (Chevron Phillips Chemical Company, The Woodlands, TX), Dacron (Unifi, Inc., Greensboro, NC), and Mersilene (Ethicon, Cincinnati, OH), have similar advantages of being able to be folded, sutured, and shaped with relative ease, but they also promote

fibrous tissue ingrowth causing difficulty with secondary removal. Supramid (Resorba Wundversorgung, Nürnberg, Germany) is a polyamide mesh derivative of nylon that is unstable in vivo. It elicits a mild foreign body reaction with multinucleated giant cells, and over time causes implant degradation and resorption.[11]

Metals

Metals consist essentially of stainless steel, vitallium, gold, and titanium. Except for use of gold in eyelid reanimation and dentistry, titanium has become the metal of choice for long-term implantation. The advantages of titanium include high biocompatibility, corrosion resistance, strength, and minimal x-ray attenuation during computed tomographic scanning or magnetic resonance imaging. Titanium is primarily used in craniofacial reconstruction and has no use in facial augmentation.

Calcium Phosphate

Calcium phosphate or hydroxyapatite materials are not osteoconductive but do provide a substrate into which bone from adjacent areas can be deposited.[12] The granule form of hydroxyapatite crystals is used in oral and maxillofacial surgery for augmenting the alveolar ridge. The block form has been used as interpositional grafts in osteotomies.[13] However, they have been shown to be of less value as an augmentation or onlay material due to its brittleness, difficulty in contouring, and inability to adapt to bone surface irregularities and mobility.

Autografts, Homografts, and Xenografts

Autografts, available as autogenous bone, cartilage, and fat are limited by donor site morbidity and limitation of available donor material. Processed homograft cartilage has been used in nasal reconstruction, but eventually succumbs to resorption and fibrosis.

Tissue-Engineered Biocompatible Implants

During the past several years, tissue engineering has emerged as an interdisciplinary field. Properties of synthetic compounds are manipulated to enable delivery of an aggregate of dissociated cells into a host to re-create new functional tissue. The field of tissue engineering has evolved by combining scientific advances in multiple fields, including material science, tissue culture, and transplantation. These techniques facilitate the seeding of cells into a suspension that provides a three-dimensional environment that promotes matrix formation. This structure anchors cells and permits nutrition and gas exchange with the ultimate formation of new tissue in the shape of a gelatinous material.[14] Several tissue-engineered cartilage implants have previously been generated based upon these new principles. This includes joint articular cartilage, tracheal rings, and auricular constructs. Tissue engineering offers the potential to grow cartilage in a precisely predetermined shape, and presently is in the developmental stage of generating various types of contoured facial implants consisting of immunocompatible cells and matrix.[15] Once employed on a commercial basis, these techniques would require minimal donor site morbidity and, like alloplastic implants, reduce operative time.

Surgical Considerations for Alloplastic Implants

General

Patients endowed with strong, well-balanced skeletal features will best endure the negative effects of aging.[16] Analysis of the faces of teens reveals an abundance of soft tissue that provides the underlying framework for the harmonious composite of youthful facial form. Full cheeks with smooth, symmetrical contours and free of sharp, irregular projections, indentations, rhytids, or dyschromias commonly embody these youthful qualities.[17] Facial aging is influenced by genetic factors, sun exposure, smoking, underlying diseases, gravity, and the effects of muscular action, which produce hyperfunctional lines of aging.[18]

Depending upon the underlying skeletal structure, involutional soft tissue changes associated with the aging process bring about definable configurations of the face that appear progressively more obvious and pronounced with time. Recognizing these various defects and configurations is an integral part of determining if a patient is a candidate for facial contouring procedures. Facial involutional changes contribute to the flattening of the midface, thinning of the vermillion border of the lips, development of deep cavitary depressions in the cheek, and formation of deep skin folds and rhytides.[19] Other specific soft tissue configurations include the prominence of the nasolabial folds, flattening of the soft tissue button of the chin, and formation of the prejowl sulcus[20,21] (**Fig. 32.2**).

The ability to permanently replace soft tissue volume in sufficient quantity is one of the most elusive aspects of facial rejuvenation. The recent popularity of fat transplantation has reemphasized tissue replacement as a key component of the rejuvenation process. Alloplastic augmentation techniques are able to permanently address these problems by softening sharp angles or depressions, reexpanding the underlying surface to reduce rhytids as well as enhance inadequate skeletal structure.[22–24]

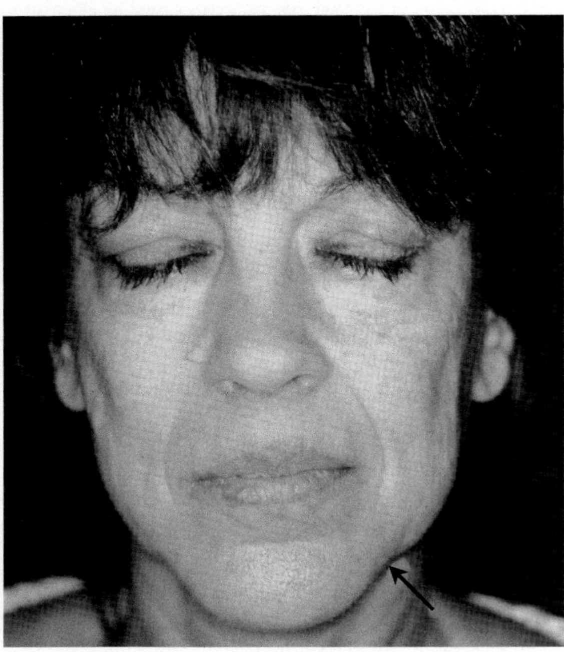

Fig. 32.2 Resorption of bone within the anterior mandibular groove, coupled with relaxation of the soft tissue causing progressive encroachment of the jowl, creates the prejowl sulcus and contributes to the development of the marionette lines (*arrow*). In these conditions, the prejowl implant is used to augment and help correct this specific deficiency and assist the rhytidectomy to achieve the desired straight mandibular line and prevent recurrence of the jowl. (From Binder WJ. A comprehensive approach for aesthetic contouring of the midface in rhytidectomy. Facial Plastic Surgery Clinics of North America, Elsevier, 1993;1:231–255.)

Nasal Augmentation

The relatively thin skin overlying the nasal dorsum often fails to provide adequate camouflage for poorly contoured replacement tissue. Nasal augmentation has been performed using many different materials. Effective long-term dorsal nasal reconstruction has continued to remain problematic despite extensive efforts to use a wide variety of autografts, allografts, and alloplastic materials. A suitable replacement implant to reconstruct the original nasal profile must possess several unique characteristics. Its shape must be of adequate length, consistent curves, thickness, and tapered edges so that it can fit well over the nasal bridge and blend in with the surrounding soft tissues and bone. It must also possess a high degree of malleability, flexibility, and compliance so that the implant can endure long-term stress and trauma.

Autogenous tissues such as calvarial bone grafts as well as septal, conchal, and costal cartilage are always preferred. However, septal and conchal cartilages often do not provide adequate volume. Costal cartilage and calvarial bone grafts have additional donor site morbidity. Costal cartilage also has the potential to warp if not carved properly. Homograft cartilage has also been utilized for nasal reconstruction but has a high percentage of resorption. Currently, the most commonly used alloplastic implants for nasal augmentation consist of silicone, ePTFE (Gore-Tex) and polyethylene (MEDPOR). Silicone can eventually produce overlying skin atrophy and must be anchored to prevent movement. Silicone and ePTFE have the potential for infection but are easily removed and replaced. Polyethylene implants, as with any other implant that promotes significant tissue ingrowth, have the potential for major soft tissue damage to the overlying skin if removal becomes necessary. Currently, silicone is the most commonly used alloplastic implant in Asian rhinoplasty, whereas ePTFE is favored for non-Asian augmentation.

The use of autogenous tissue avoids the problem of incompatibility but sometimes fails to provide necessary volume to provide the size and shape. A more ideal substitute to replace deficient skeletal structure, particularly over the nasal dorsum, would be a neocartilage graft reproduced from one's own cells that closely mimics the original skeletal contour. This cartilage implant can be synthesized through the process of tissue engineering.[25] The concept involves use of donor septal cartilaginous tissue that is harvested and then broken down into its cellular components. The cells are cultured in vitro, permitting them to multiply. A synthetic alginate scaffold is created in the shape of a dorsal nasal implant through a molding process. The cells are impregnated into the gelatin scaffold, which is placed subcutaneously into mice and permitted to evolve in vivo into a final shape. It is during this phase that the alginate scaffold slowly dissolves and is replaced by viable hyaline cartilage. The cartilage is then harvested as an autogenous implant. This process has the potential of becoming a valuable addition to nasal and facial augmentation in the near future.[26]

Midface Augmentation

Rhytidectomy has become just one component of facial rejuvenation. Midfacial augmentation, midface lifts, and resurfacing techniques all must be considered when customizing a surgical plan for the patient. The pathophysiology of the aging process is a key factor in determining the correct surgical treatment. It is now well understood that the aging process not only results in the descent of the midface but also in the atrophy of the soft-tissue in multiple facial planes. Midface rejuvenation can therefore be achieved not only through suspension techniques, but also by the augmentation of the soft tissue and skeletal foundation. Alloplastic augmentation is an effective way to alter the midface appearance in appropriate candidates. Midface augmentation is straightforward, long-lasting, and relatively low-isk surgical option that can consistently and predictably nprove midface aesthetics. It has the ability not only o replace lost facial soft tissue volume but also to ıcrease the anterolateral projection of the area thereby nproving midface laxity and decreasing the depth of he nasolabial folds. Implants are readily reversible nd can be combined with standard rhytidectomy rocedures. The net effect is softening of the sharp ngles and depressions of the aged face resulting in a atural “unoperated” look. In appropriate candidates, ıoderate facial rejuvenation can be achieved sim-ly with the placement of submalar midface implants /ithout concomitant rhytidectomy.

Midface augmentation can also facilitate rhytidec-omy in several ways. The skin and soft tissue can be raped over a broader, more convex midface region after nplant augmentation. There is also minimal traction n the perioral tissues and lateral commissure if placed rior to the rhytidectomy, which can help to avoid an overpulled” appearance. Many patients who present for evision rhytidectomy that require volume restoration an also be improved by expanding the midface region, /hile decreasing downward vertical traction forces on ıe lower eyelid.

Specific criteria are available for determining regions f aesthetic deficits and their corresponding alloplastic olutions.[27,28] In addition, other regions that contribute) the midfacial appearance must be carefully consid-red during patient evaluation. In the periorbital region, ıe aging process results in the weakening of the orbital eptum and herniation of the periorbital fat, causing ıfraorbital bulges. The orbicularis muscle becomes totic, especially in its most inferior aspect. The use of onventional blepharoplasty will tend to exacerbate xity of the lower canthal ligament, which can contrib-te to the formation of the “tear-trough” deformity and wer lid malposition.[29,30] Attendant with aging is sub-utaneous tissue atrophy, which has more damaging ffects on the very thin infraorbital skin accounting for e hollowness of the eyes with advanced aging. Skel-tal insufficiency and imbalances are usually caused rimarily by the hypoplastic development and inherent ony imbalances of the facial skeleton that are exacer-ated by the aging process. Midfacial descent involves tosis of the infraorbital subcutaneous tissues, malar t pad, suborbicularis oculi fat (SOOF), and orbicu-ris muscle. The SOOF is the transition tissue between ıe orbital septum and the malar fat pad. This is a thin yer of granular fat present under the lower orbicularis bers. It is *not* connected with the periorbital fat, which emains separated from the SOOF by the orbital sep-ım and its insertion onto the inferior orbital rim at the rcus marginalis.

As the cheek falls and collects on the upper nasolabial fold, the thicker tissues of the malar fat pad descend and leave the infraorbital region exposed to thin soft tissue covering. Thus the nasojugal/tear trough region becomes prominent, the lower eyes appear hollow, and the infraorbital rim becomes more prominent. The loss of subcutaneous tissues occurs throughout the body, but in particular affects midfacial tissues more severely, including the buccal fat pad, the malar fat pad, and the SOOF. As these tissues continue to lose volume and descend, different patterns of midfacial aging develop in the infraorbital and cheek regions.

In the midface, most soft tissue deficiencies are found within the recess described as the “submalar triangle.”[31] This inverted triangular area of midfacial depression is bordered above by the prominence of the zygoma, medially by the nasolabial fold, and laterally by the body of the masseter muscle (**Fig. 32.3**). The aging process is exaggerated when severe soft tissue involutional changes are associated with deficient underlying bone structure. Facial depressions can also become apparent in individuals who have prominent cheek bones combined with thin skin lacking subcutaneous or deep supporting fat. This type of pattern causes a gaunt appearance in an otherwise healthy person. The severe form of this midfacial pattern can be seen in anorexia nervosa, starvation, or HIV-associated lipoatrophy. In combination with the primary disease process, protease inhibitors and other

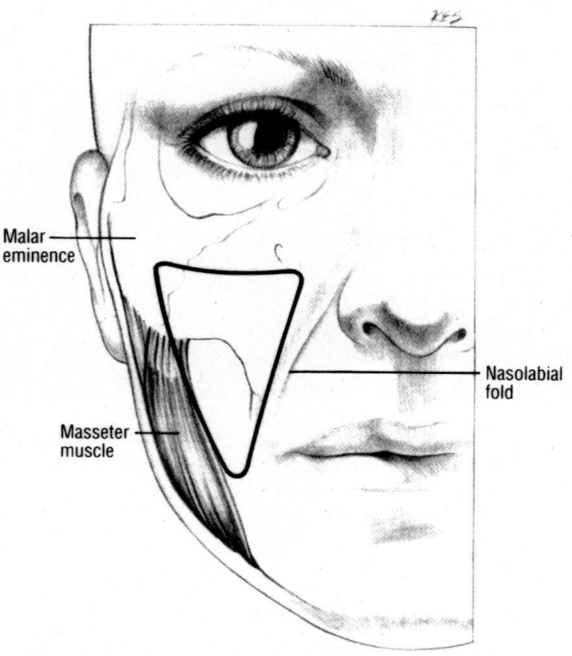

Fig. 32.3 The inverted submalar triangle is an area of midfacial depression bordered medially by the nasolabial fold, superiorly by the malar eminence, and laterally by the main body of the masseter muscle.

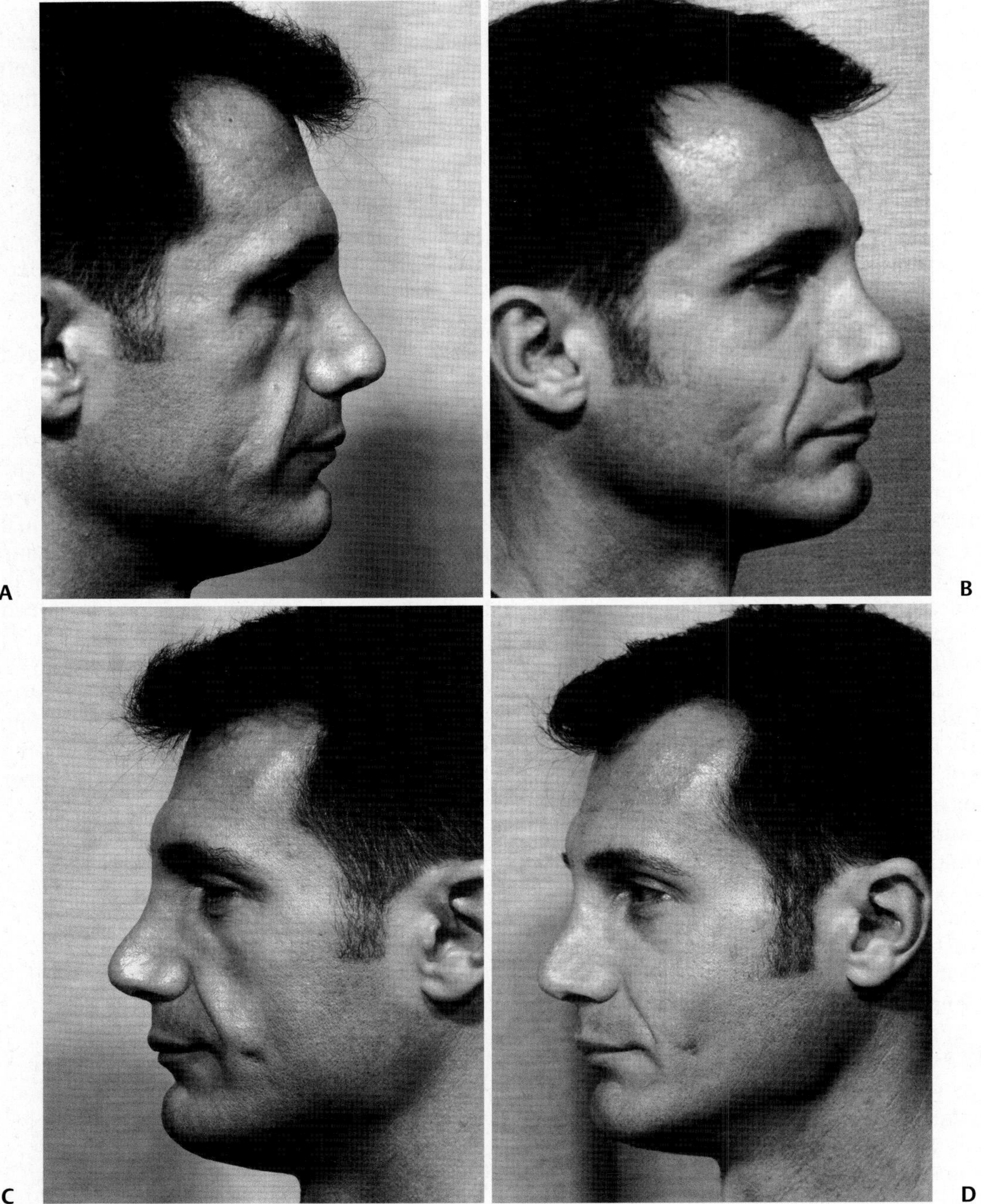

Fig. 32.4 (**A,C**) Preoperative photographs of a human immunodeficiency virus (HIV) patient who has been treated with protease inhibitors for a prolonged period of time. Many patients eventually develop complete erosion of the midfacial fat and the buccal fat pad leaving a particularly deep cavitary depression in the midface. (**B,D**) At 1 year postsurgery, the condition was successfully treated with computer-assisted, custom-designed midfacial implants.

newer-generation HIV therapies have a predilection for erosion of the midfacial fat and the buccal fat pad (**Fig. 32.4**).[1,2] These conditions of volume loss that are also associated with the aging process often preclude rhytidectomy, alone, to completely rejuvenate the face and are currently being successfully treated with the use of computer-assiste custom-designed facial implants.[32]

For successful rejuvenation of the midface, a three dimensional approach must be utilized. The descen and volume loss of the midface must be camouflage corrected, or replaced. The surgeon must therefore approach facial rejuvenation using a multilevel as well as a multimodality method. Camouflage techniques such as lower blepharoplasty with fat repositioning can result in the blunting of the nasojugal groove/tear trough region by securing the infraorbital fat past the arcus marginalis.[33] Midface cheek lift techniques reverse midfacial descent by lifting the midfacial tissues and anchoring them in a more superior-lateral direction.[34,35] Alloplastic or autogenous augmentation techniques reverse the effects of midfacial descent by replacing midfacial volume loss and providing soft tissue support at the deepest plane. Acknowledging the many elements of structural deficiency and phenomena of aging, multimodality treatments are necessary to restore the face to a more youthful appearance.

Preoperative Analysis for Facial Contouring

General

Facial augmentation is a three-dimensional procedure that exponentially increases the variability of structural diagnosis and treatment. A good understanding of skeletal anatomy and the ability to identify specific types of topographical patterns guide the surgeon in making the final determination for optimal implant selection and placement. Evaluation of the face for contouring procedures starts with an understanding of specific zones of skeletal anatomy and identifying distinctive and recognizable configurations of facial deficiency. Correlating these elements of structural and topographical variations is essential for choosing the optimal implant shape, size, and position to obtain the best results in facial contouring.

Mandibular Contour Defects

Chin projection is one of the most important features of the face. Appropriate chin projection and shape can provide an advantageous anatomical feature for facial rejuvenation as well as rhinoplasty. Poor chin projection can exaggerate the appearance of the nose. Prejowl sulcus can develop in the setting of soft tissue atrophy and bony erosion in the symphyseal region. After dental occlusion evaluation, the chin position can be assessed from the lateral view. Gonzalez-Ulloa developed a simple method based on the Frankfort line to analyze facial and chin projection. The Frankfort plane is a straight horizontal line drawn between the supratragal notch and the infraorbital rim. A perpendicular line, designated as the 0° meridian, is then drawn from the Frankfort plane at the level of the nasion to determine the amount of chin projection. If the pogonion is posterior to this line, the patient has microgenia. In women, the 0° meridian is generally 1 to 2 mm anterior to the pogonion.

Delineation of zonal principles of anatomy within the premandible space allows the surgeon to create specific chin and jawline contour.[27] Traditionally, chin implants were placed over the area between the mental foramina. This familiar location constitutes only one segment or zone of the mandible that can be successfully altered. Implants placed in the central segment alone and without lateral extension often produce abnormal round protuberances that are unattractive. A midlateral zone within the premandibular space can be defined as the region extending from the mental foramen posteriorly to the oblique line of the horizontal body of the mandible. Augmentation of this zone in addition to the central mentum results in a widening of the anterior jawline contour. This is the basis for the development of the extended anatomical and prejowl chin implants (**Fig. 32.5**). The posterior lateral zone is the third zone of the premandibular space, which encompasses the posterior half of the horizontal body, including the angle of the mandible and the first 2 to 4 cm of the ascending ramus. This zone can be modified with a mandibular angle implant that will either widen and/or elongate the posterior mandibular angle to produce a stronger posterior jawline contour. This area should be approached with extreme caution by the novice surgeon.

Midfacial Contour Defects

We have modified our previous midface deformity classification to simplify the analysis of the area during the consultation (**Table 32.1, Fig. 32.6**). It is prudent to separately evaluate the bony malar region and the soft tissue submalar area to best determine the appropriate surgical procedure. Patients with type I deformity have primary malar hypoplasia with adequate submalar soft tissue. This defect is best addressed with malar shell implants that cover the bony midface and project the cheek in a lateral direction (**Fig. 32.7**). Type II deficiency occurs in individuals who have submalar soft tissue deficiency with normal malar skeleton. This is the most common deficiency found in the aging population. Inferior descent and soft tissue atrophy of the submalar soft tissue leaves a flat and hollowed appearance to the midface. Type II deficiency is best treated surgically with submalar implants, which restore midface convexity and provide greater anterior projection to the flattened face (**Figs. 32.8 and 32.9**). Submalar implants can be used alone or in combination with rhytidectomy for facial rejuvenation. Type III deformity occurs when there is a combined bony malar hypoplasia and soft tissue paucity. These patients can undergo exaggerated effects of aging because ptotic soft tissues have little bony support and readily descend along the nasolabial folds

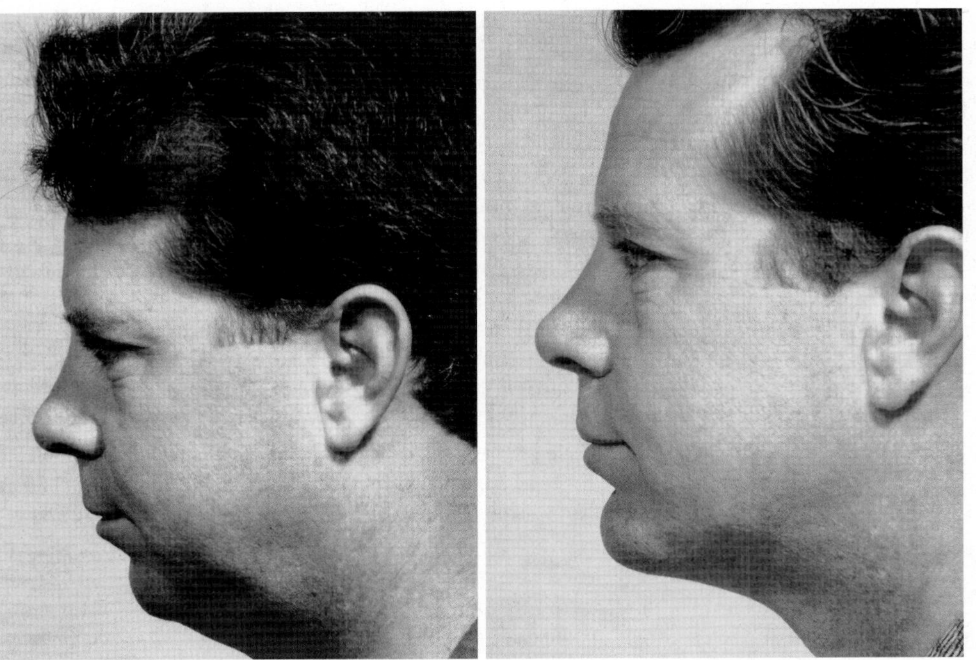

Fig. 32.5 (**A**) Preoperative and (**B**) postoperative photographs of a patient who underwent an extended mandibular implant combined with submental liposuction.

and oral commissure. Rhytidectomy alone would provide suboptimal results in these patients because they have limited underlying skeletal support with which to resuspend the skin and soft tissue. Combined malar–submalar implants can significantly improve the overall appearance of type III patients (**Fig. 32.10**).

Surgical Procedure

General Guidelines for Facial Implants

The basic principles for augmenting the malar, midfacial, premandibular spaces or nasal augmentation are identical, while controlling the shape, size, and positioning of the implant will determine the overall final facial contour. The surgeon must be prepared to have all anticipated designs, shapes, and/or materials available and be prepared to modify the implant intraoperatively. Since all faces are different, it should be the rule, rather than the exception, that implants require modification. Therefore failure to have the right implant for a particular patient can only yield a suboptimal result.

The day prior to surgery, patients are started on broad-spectrum antibiotics, which will be continued for 5 days after surgery. Intravenous antibiotics and dexamethasone are also administered perioperatively. Before starting anesthesia, the patient must be in an upright position while the precise area to be augmented is outlined with a marking pen. This initial outline that is drawn on the

Table 32.1 Pattern of Midfacial Deformity and Type of Implant for Correction

Deformity Type	Description of Midfacial Deformity	Type of Augmentation Required	Type of Implant Predominantly Used
Type I	Primary malar hypoplasia; adequate submalar soft tissue development	Requires projection over the malar eminence	Malar Implant: "shell-type" implant extends inferiorly into submalar space for more natural result
Type II	Submalar deficiency; adequate malar development	Requires anterior projection; implant placed over face of maxilla and/or masseter tendon in submalar space; also provides for midfacial fill	Submalar Implant (New Conform type (Implantech Associates, Ventura, CA) or Generation I Submalar Implant)
Type III	Malar hypoplasia and submalar deficiency	Requires anterior and lateral projection; "volume replacement implant" for entire midface restructuring	"Combined" Submalar-Shell Implant; lateral (malar), and anterior (submalar) projection; fills large midfacial void

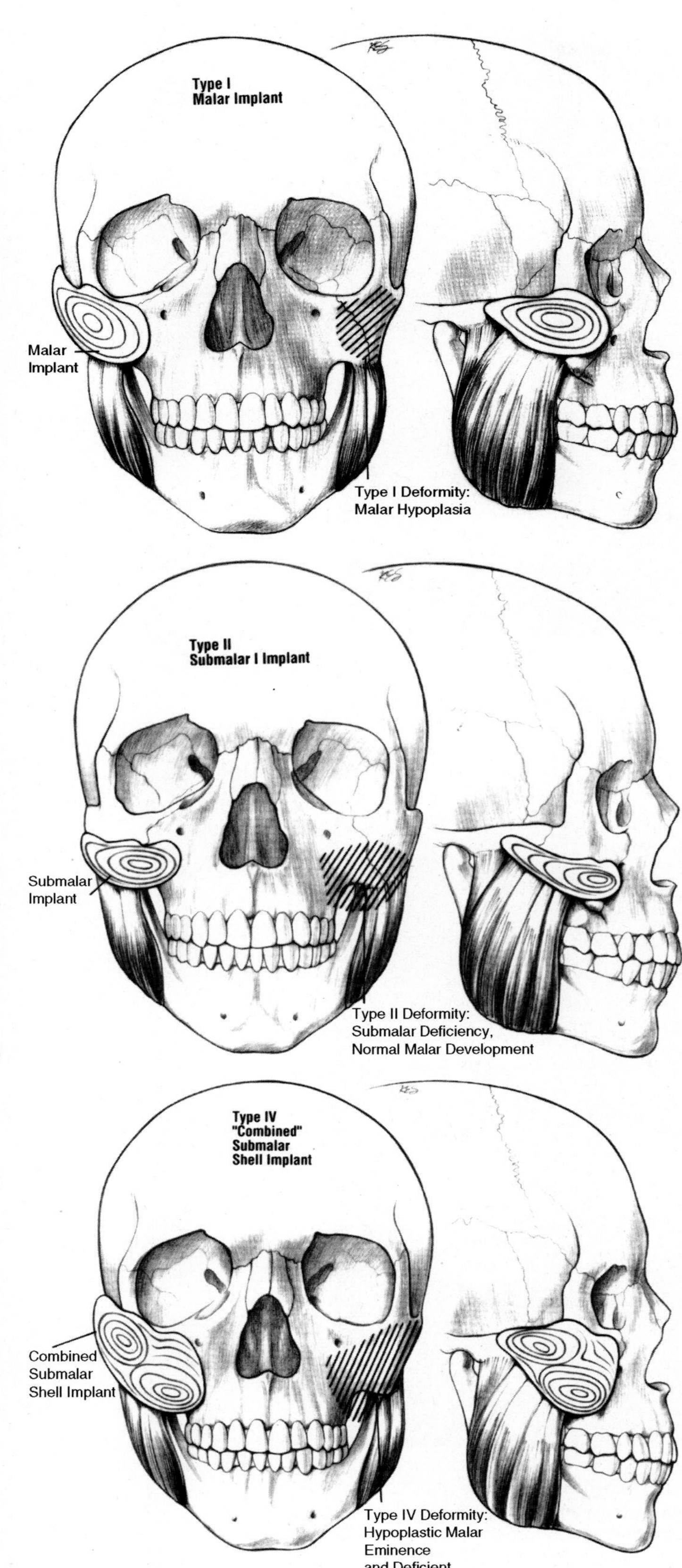

Fig. 32.6 Frontal and lateral drawings illustrate the anatomical areas of the midface and three distinctive topographical patterns of midfacial deformity. Specific implants that are directly correlated with and used to correct these specific patterns of midfacial deformity are selected (Table 32.1).

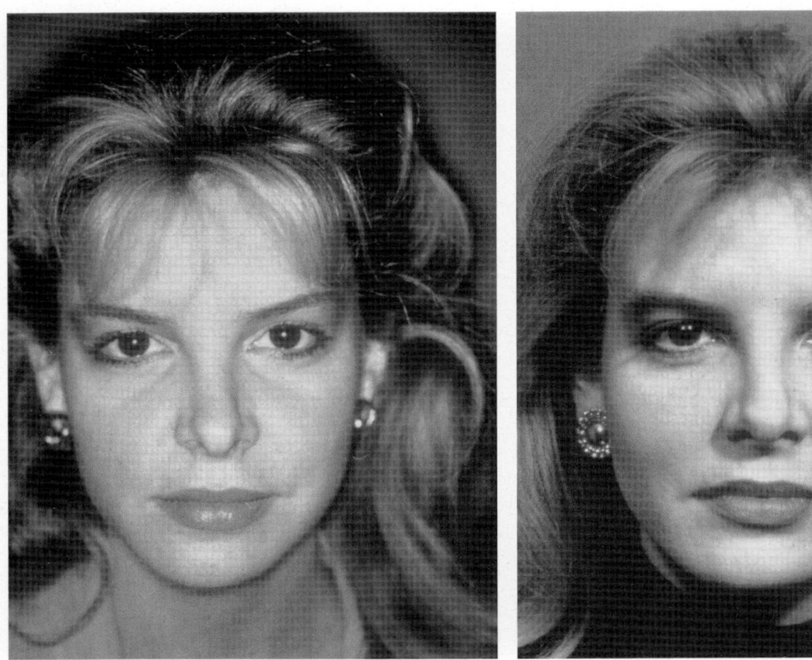

Fig. 32.7 (**A**) Preoperative example of malar hypoplasia (type I deficiency). (**B**) Eight months after malarplasty using a malar shell implant. Augmentation of a greater surface area and extension inferiorly into the submalar space produces a more natural high cheekbone effect.

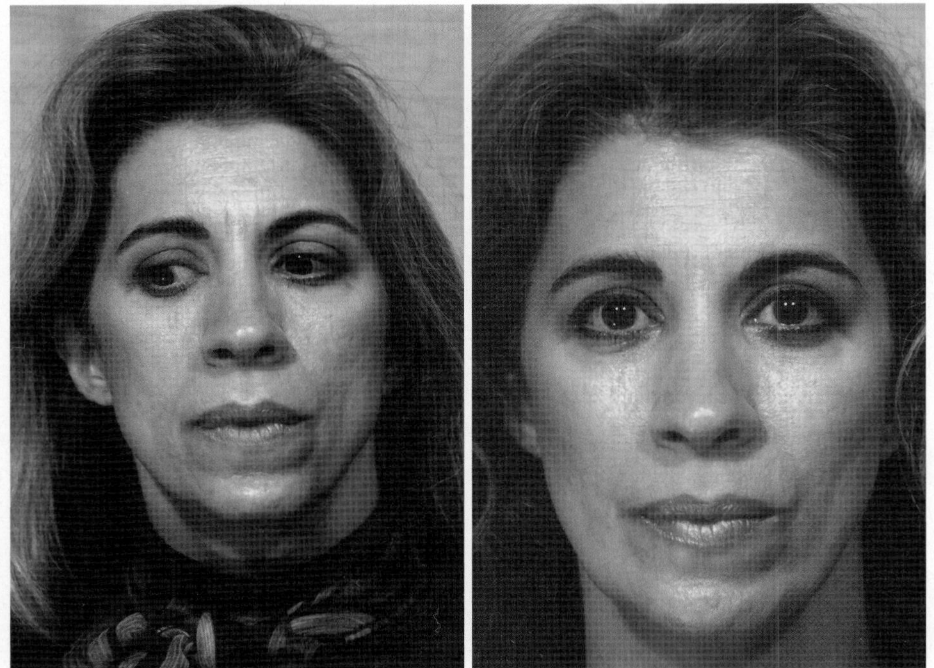

Fig. 32.8 (**A**) Preoperatively, this patient has a relatively good malar bone structure but was complaining of early flatness to the midface (type II deformity) in addition to a mandibular parasymphyseal depression caused by an earlier performed genioplasty. (**B**) Submalar augmentation restored the anterior projection to the midthird of the face, providing a more youthful expression as well as reducing the depth of the nasolabial folds, while a custom implant was used to fill in the parasymphyseal depression.

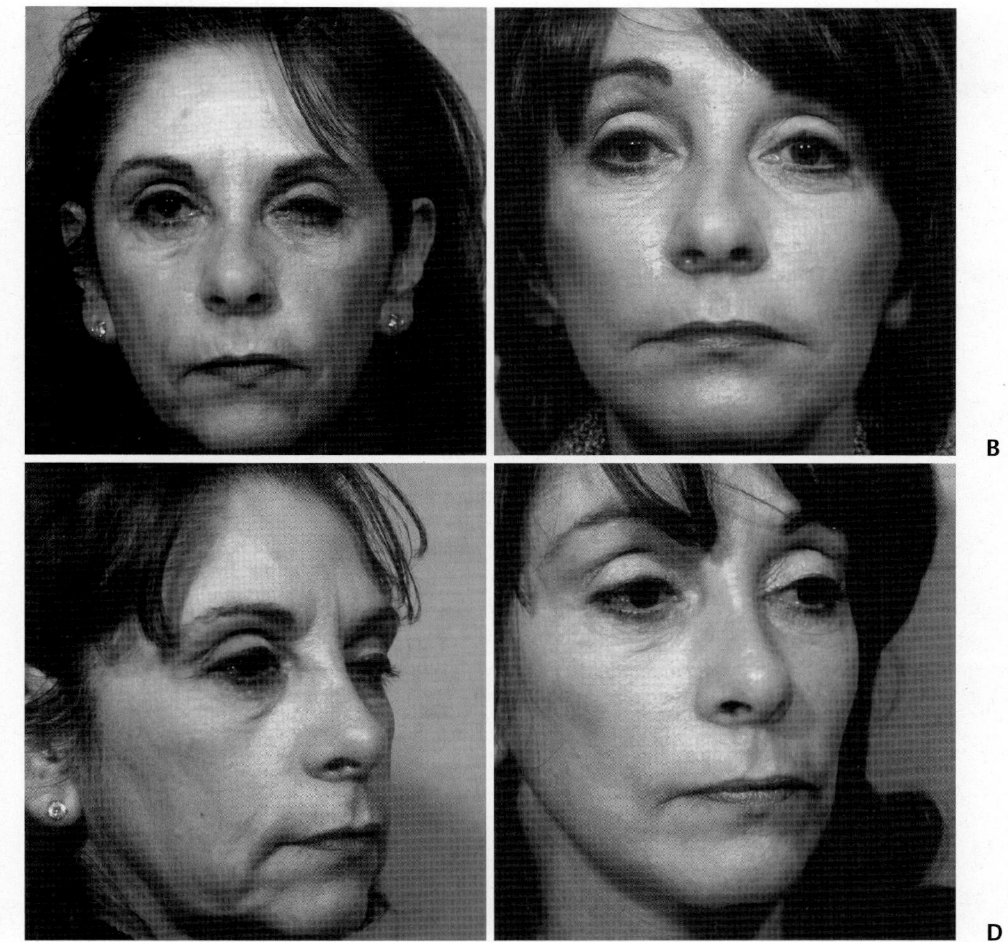

Fig. 32.9 (**A,C**) Preoperative. (**B,D**) Six months postoperative. In conjunction with rhytidectomy, lower blepharoplasty, and brow lift, a Conform submalar implant (Implantech Associates, Ventura, CA) was used as adjunctively to help restore volume and structure and to establish the basis for a greater longevity to the facelift operation.

skin is then explained to the patient so that a cooperative effort is made to finalize both the surgeon's and the patient's perception of implant shape, size, and position to optimize their mutual goals (**Fig. 32.11**).

Surgical Technique for Mandibular Augmentation

Anterior Mandibular Implants

Either an intraoral or an external route can accomplish access to the premandibular space. The intraoral route provides the obvious advantage of leaving no external scars. The entry wound for the intraoral route is a transverse incision made through the mucosa. The mentalis muscle is divided vertically in the midline raphe to avoid transection of the muscle belly or detachment from the bony origins. This midline incision provides adequate access inferiorly to the bone of the central mentum and eliminates potential muscle weakness that may occur if transected. Lateral dissection requires identification and retraction of the mental nerves. The external route utilizes a 1.0 cm to 1.5 cm incision in the submental crease. The advantages of the external route include avoidance of intraoral bacterial contamination, direct access to the inferior mandibular border where cortical bone is present, limited retraction of the mental nerve, and easy fixation of the implant to the inferior mandibular periosteum. Fixation of the implant prevents side-to-side or vertical slippage of the implant.

Basic technical rules should be followed for safe and accurate mandibular augmentation. (1) The dissection should stay on bone. Placement of implants in the subperiosteal plane creates a firm and secure attachment of the implant to the bony skeleton. Strong adherence of periosteum along the anterior-inferior border of the

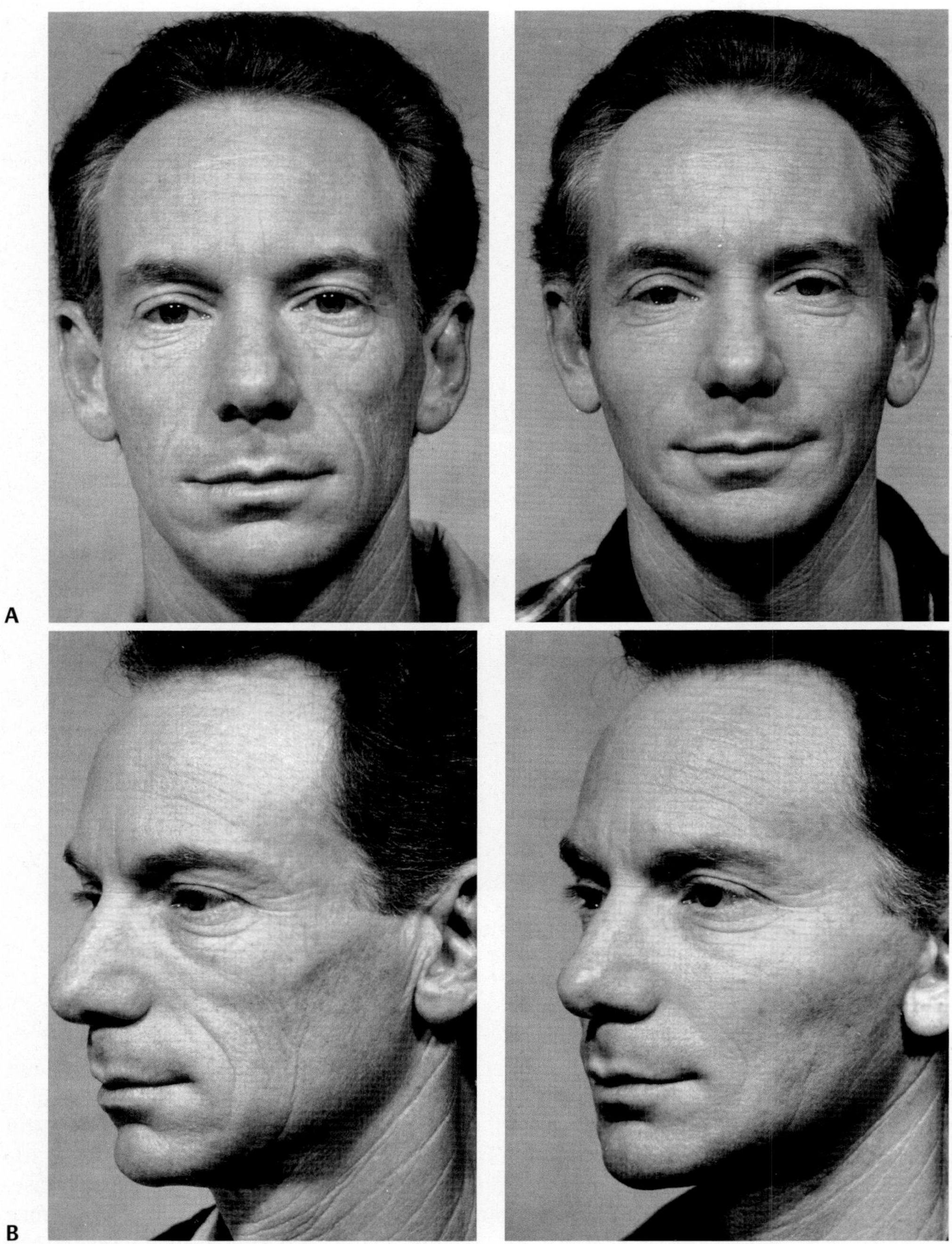

Fig. 32.10 (**A**) Frontal; (**B**) oblique. *Left:* Preoperative analysis of the facial configuration in this 40-year-old patient reveals the presence of severe deficiency in both skeletal structure and soft tissue volume contributing primarily to the excessive wrinkling of the skin in the area of the midface. *Right:* Seven months postoperative; performed concurrently with rhytidectomy, the combined submalar-shell implants were used to restructure the entire midface, and a prejowl implant was used to add width to the mandible. In this patient, these augmentation procedures were essential for the structural and volumetric enhancement required for the facelift procedure to provide a meaningful, long-term improvement. (From Binder WJ. A comprehensive approach for aesthetic contouring of the midface in rhytidectomy. Facial Plastic Surgery Clinics of North America, Elsevier, 1993;1:231–255. Reprinted by permission.)

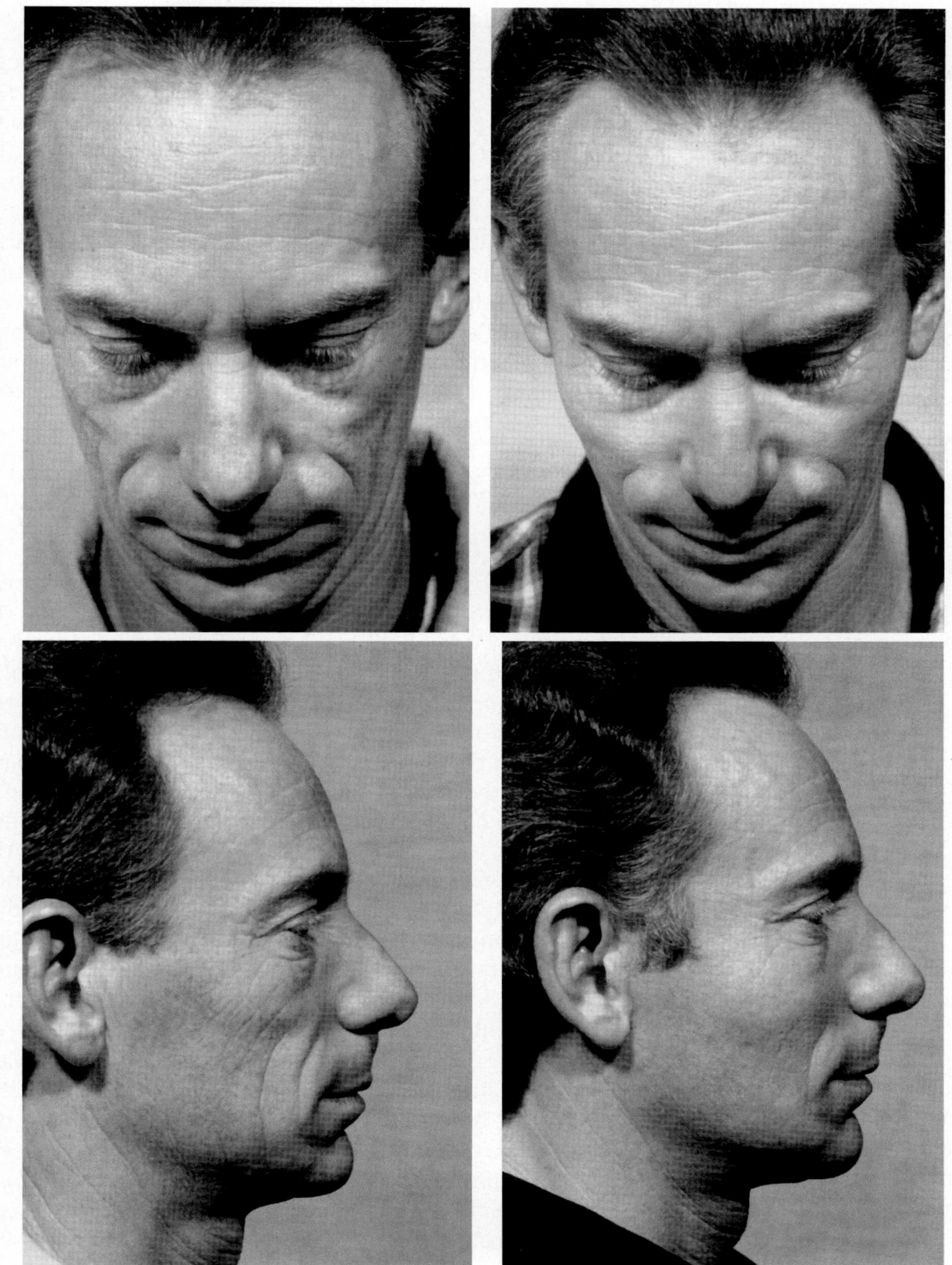

Fig. 32.10 (*Continued*) (**C**) head down; (**D**) lateral.

mandible comprises the origins of the anterior mandibular ligament, which defines the prejowl sulcus at the inferior aspect of the aging marionette crease. It is often necessary to incise these ligamentous attachments to allow dissection to continue along the inferior segment of the mandible. (2) The dissection must be adequately expanded to accommodate the prosthesis comfortably. A sharp dissecting instrument may be used centrally, but only blunt instruments are used around the nerves and adjacent to soft tissues. (3) The mental nerve should be avoided. This is accomplished by compressing the tissues around the mental foramen with the opposite hand that helps to direct the elevator away from the nerve and along the inferior border of the mandible. A dry operative field

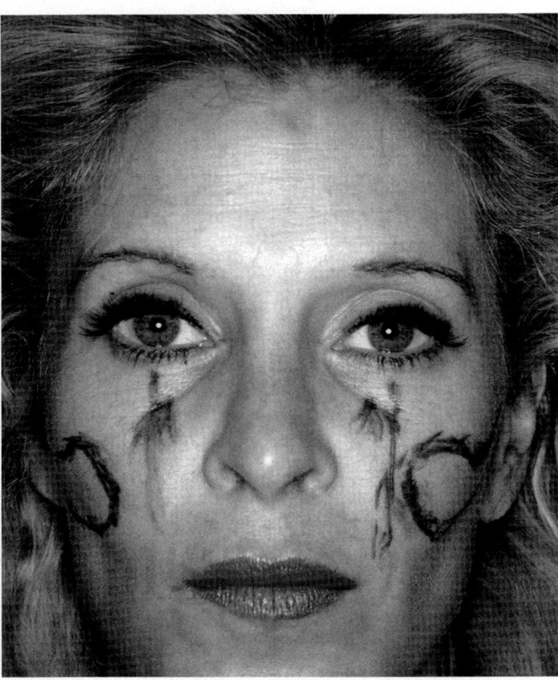

Fig. 32.11 Prior to infiltration of local anesthetic, the areas requiring augmentation are specifically outlined with the patient sitting in the upright position. In the majority of cases, the medial border of submalar or malar implants is placed lateral to the infraorbital foramen corresponding approximately to the midpupillary line. (From Binder WJ. A comprehensive approach for aesthetic contouring of the midface in rhytidectomy. Facial Plastic Surgery Clinics of North America, Elsevier, 1993;1:231–255. Reprinted by permission.)

is essential for accurate visualization, precise dissection, proper implant placement, and the prevention of postoperative hematoma or seroma.

A Joseph's or 4 mm periosteal elevator is used to perform the dissection along the inferior mandibular border. Once the pockets are large enough, one side of the implant is inserted into the lateral portion of the pocket on one side and then folded upon itself whereby the contralateral portion of the implant is inserted into the other side of the pocket. The implant is then adjusted into position. If the implant material does not allow flexibility, then the incision either must be made larger or the procedure must be performed through an intraoral incision. Implants expanding into the midlateral or parasymphyseal region accomplish anterior widening of the lower third of the facial segment. The average central projection necessary is between 6 and 9 mm for men and 4 to 7 mm for women. Occasionally, in a patient with severe microgenia, implants measuring 10 to 12 mm in projection or greater may be necessary to create a normal profile and a broader jawline.

Mandibular Angle Implants

Access to the angle of the mandible is achieved through a 2 to 3 cm mucosal incision at the retromolar trigone. This gives direct access to the angle of the mandible. Dissection is performed on bone and beneath the masseter muscle to elevate the periosteum upward along the ramus and then anteriorly along the body of the mandible. A curved (90 degree) dissector is used to elevate the periosteum around the posterior angle and ramus of the mandible. This permits accurate placement of the angle implants that are specifically designed to fit the posterior bony border of the ascending ramus and enhance angle definition. These implants are secured with a titanium screw.

Surgical Techniques for Malar and Midface Contouring

The primary route for entering the malar–midfacial areas is the intraoral approach. Other approaches include the subciliary (via lower blepharoplasty), transconjunctival, rhytidectomy, zygomaticotemporal, and transcoronal routes. The intraoral route is the most common and the preferred route for most midfacial implants. After infiltration of the anesthetic solution, a 1 cm incision is made through the mucosa and carried directly down to bone in a vertical oblique direction above the buccal–gingival line and over the lateral buttress (**Fig. 32.12A**). Because the mucosa will stretch and allow complete visual inspection of the midfacial structures, a long incision through adjacent submucosal or muscular layers is not necessary and is discouraged. The incision should be made high enough to leave a minimum of 1 cm of gingival mucosal cuff. If the patient wears dentures, this incision must be placed above the dentures' superior border. Dentures can be left in place after the procedure, and in our experience they have not been found to cause extrusion or increase the incidence of complications. A broad Tessier-type elevator (10 mm wide) is directed through the incision onto the bone in the same orientation as the incision. A broad rather than narrow elevator helps to facilitate the dissection safely and with relative ease within the subperiosteal plane (**Fig. 32.12B**). While keeping the elevator directly on bone, the soft tissues are elevated obliquely upward off the maxillary buttress and the malar eminence. The elevator is kept on the bone margin along the inferior border of the malar eminence and the zygomatic arch. The external or free hand is used to help guide the elevator over the designated areas. For routine malar–submalar augmentation procedures, no attempt is made to visualize or dissect within the vicinity of the infraorbital nerve unless an implant is intended for this area. If necessary, the infraorbital nerve is easily visualized in a more medial location.

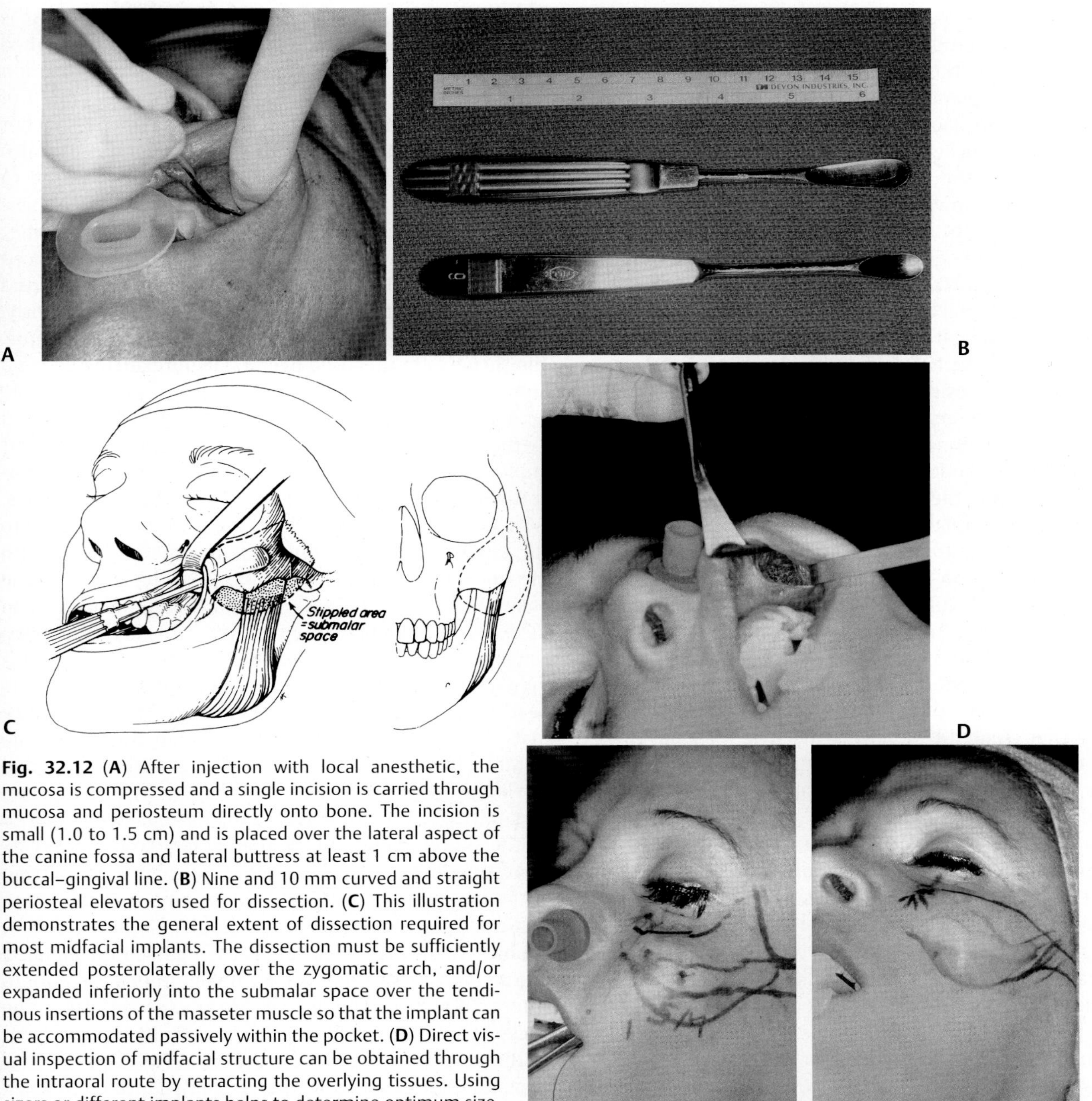

Fig. 32.12 (**A**) After injection with local anesthetic, the mucosa is compressed and a single incision is carried through mucosa and periosteum directly onto bone. The incision is small (1.0 to 1.5 cm) and is placed over the lateral aspect of the canine fossa and lateral buttress at least 1 cm above the buccal–gingival line. (**B**) Nine and 10 mm curved and straight periosteal elevators used for dissection. (**C**) This illustration demonstrates the general extent of dissection required for most midfacial implants. The dissection must be sufficiently extended posterolaterally over the zygomatic arch, and/or expanded inferiorly into the submalar space over the tendinous insertions of the masseter muscle so that the implant can be accommodated passively within the pocket. (**D**) Direct visual inspection of midfacial structure can be obtained through the intraoral route by retracting the overlying tissues. Using sizers or different implants helps to determine optimum size, shape, and position of the final implant selected. (The stippled area represents a sizer that has been placed within the pocket.) (**E**) *Left*: The external drawings made on the skin delineate the malar bone and submalar space below. *Right*: The shape and size of the superimposed implant should roughly coincide with the external topographical defect demarcated prior to surgery. In this case the inferior aspect of the implant extends downward to occupy the submalar space. (From Binder WJ. A comprehensive approach for aesthetic contouring of the midface in rhytidectomy. Facial Plastic Surgery Clinics of North America, Elsevier, 1993;1:231–255. Reprinted by permission.)

The submalar space is created by elevating the soft tissue inferiorly over the masseter muscle below the zygoma (**Fig. 32.12C**). One is able to discern the correct plane of dissection by the glistening white fibers of the masseter tendons by direct vision. It is important to note that these masseteric attachments are not cut and are left completely intact to provide a supporting framework upon which the implant may rest. As the dissection moves posteriorly along the zygomatic arch, the space becomes tighter and is not as easily enlarged as the medial segment. However, gently advancing and elevating the tissues with a heavy, blunt periosteal elevator can open part of this space. It is of utmost importance that the dissection is extended sufficiently so that the implant fits passively within the pocket. A pocket that is too small will force the implant toward the opposite direction, causing implant displacement or extrusion. Under normal conditions, the pocket is estimated to collapse and obliterate most of the space around the implant within 24 to 48 hours following surgery. Implant selection is aided by observing the actual topographical changes produced by placement of the different implant "sizers" into the pocket (**Fig. 32.12D**).

Final implant placement must correspond to the external topographical defects outlined on the face preoperatively (**Fig. 32.12E**). In *submalar* augmentation, the implant may reside below the zygoma and zygomatic arch, over the masseter tendon, or it may overlap both bone and tendon. *Malar* implants reside primarily on bone in a more superior and lateral position and may extend partly into the submalar space. The combined *malar–submalar* implants will occupy both areas. Any implant placed in patients with noticeable facial asymmetry, thin skin, or an extremely prominent bone structure may require modification to reduce its thickness or length to avoid abnormal projections. Among the advantages of silicone elastomer midfacial implants is flexibility enabling large implants to be compressed through small openings, which are then able to reexpand within the larger pocket created beyond the incision.[36] This avoids having to make larger incisions required for more rigid implants and allows for ease of implant insertion and removal during the selection process.

The most difficult task in achieving successful results in facial contouring is the management of facial asymmetry. During the preoperative consultation, a thorough discussion regarding this problem is essential because most patients are usually unaware of the qualitative or quantitative presence of their own facial asymmetry.[37] Meticulous attention to detail is required to visualize, perceptually integrate, and then make procedural adjustments to accommodate existing three-dimensional discrepancies. It is not unusual to find adequate malar development and a well suspended soft tissue pad with good external contour on one side of the face, and a hypoplastic malar eminence along with relative atrophy of the soft tissues and greater wrinkling of the skin on the other side. In these cases, it is essential to have an adequate selection of implants available and to anticipate carving or altering the implants to adjust to the differences in contour between the two sides. Unusual asymmetries may also require using different implants for each side or shims that can be carved from a silicone block and sutured to the posterior surface of the implant to increase the projection of a particular segment of the implant.

Once the implant position has been established, it is usually necessary to secure it. This can be accomplished by several different methods. Internal suture fixation relies on the presence of an adjacent stable segment of periosteum or tendinous structure upon which to anchor the implant. Stainless steel or titanium screws can also be used. External fixation sutures can also be used to stabilize midfacial implants. The *indirect lateral suspension technique* uses 2–0 Ethilon sutures (Ethicon, Inc., Somerville, NJ) wedged on large Keith needles and placed through the implant tail. These needles are then inserted through the pocket, directed superiorly and posteriorly, to exit percutaneously posterior to the temporal hairline. The sutures are then tied over a bolster exerting traction on the tail of the implant. This technique is more suitable for malar implants. *Direct external fixation* is the preferred method for submalar and combined malar–submalar implants to prevent slippage in the immediate postoperative period and to obliterate the anterior dead space. With this method, the implants are positioned directly to correspond with marks on the skin, which coincide with the two most medial fenestrations of the implant. The position of the medial fenestration should be marked on the external skin while the implant is inside the subperiosteal pocket. Locating these holes can be achieved with a right angle clamp that pushes the implant upward, underneath the fenestration, causing an external protuberance that can be marked on the external skin. Measuring the distance from the midline to both right and left medial markings ensures symmetric placement of the implants (**Fig. 32.13A**). The implants are then removed and placed on the skin by lining up the medial fenestration over its corresponding mark. The position of the lateral portion of the implant is then decided by placing a second mark corresponding to the adjacent implant fenestration. A double-armed 2–0 silk suture is then passed through the two medial fenestrations of the implant from a posterior to anterior direction. The needles are advanced through the pocket, passed perpendicularly through the skin, and exit at the respective external markings (**Fig. 32.13B**). The implant, following the needles, is guided into the pocket. The implant is then secured in place by tying the sutures over bolsters consisting of two dental roles (**Fig. 32.13C**).

Complications

Complications of implants in facial augmentation include bleeding, hematoma, infection, exposure, extrusion, malposition, displacement or slippage, fistula, seroma, persistent edema, abnormal prominence, persistent inflammatory action, pain, and nerve damage.[38] However, in most of the complications listed, very few are due solely to the implant material itself. It is extremely

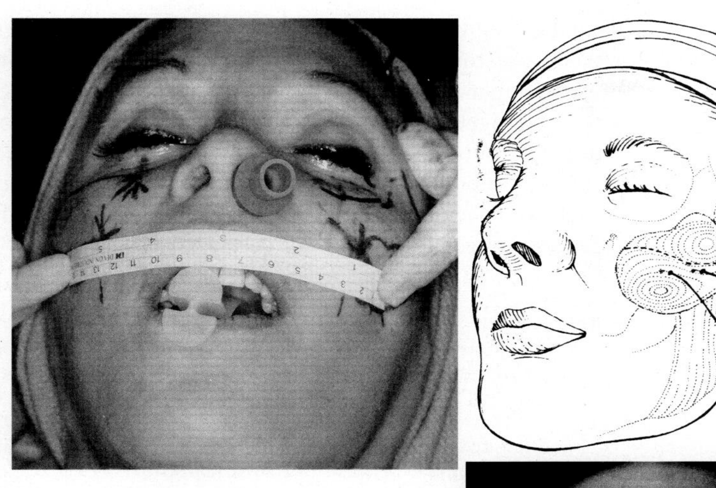

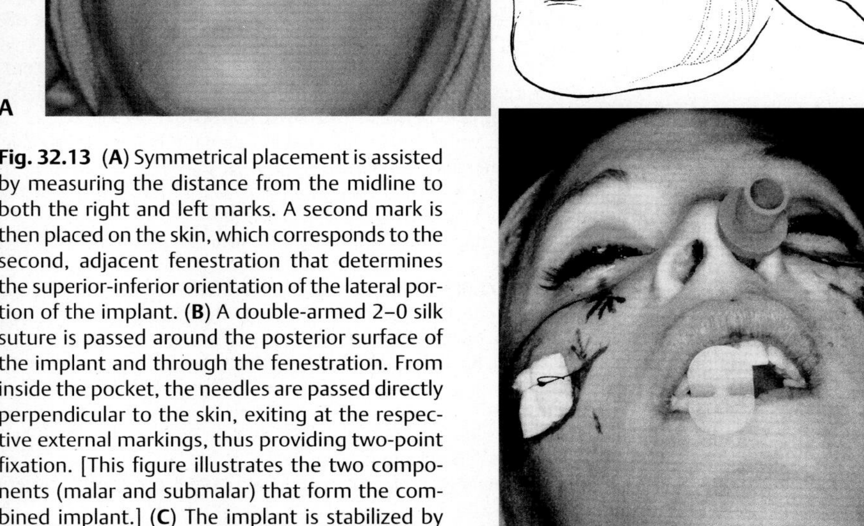

Fig. 32.13 (**A**) Symmetrical placement is assisted by measuring the distance from the midline to both the right and left marks. A second mark is then placed on the skin, which corresponds to the second, adjacent fenestration that determines the superior-inferior orientation of the lateral portion of the implant. (**B**) A double-armed 2–0 silk suture is passed around the posterior surface of the implant and through the fenestration. From inside the pocket, the needles are passed directly perpendicular to the skin, exiting at the respective external markings, thus providing two-point fixation. [This figure illustrates the two components (malar and submalar) that form the combined implant.] (**C**) The implant is stabilized by tying the suture directly over an external bolster (consisting of two cotton rolls). The suture and bolster are removed by the third postoperative day. (From Binder WJ. A comprehensive approach for aesthetic contouring of the midface in rhytidectomy. Facial Plastic Surgery Clinics of North America, Elsevier, 1993;1:231–255. Reprinted by permission.)

difficult to separate out the surgical technique, the surrounding circumstances of the individual operation, as well as the individual patient risk factors that are not associated with the implant.

Extrusion should not occur if the technical rules outlined have been followed. The extended surface area of the larger or extended implants that fit along the midface and mandibular contours minimizes malposition and malrotation. Adequate dissection of the subperiosteal space large enough to create midlateral and posterolateral tunnels in the mandible and the desired pockets in the midface will maintain the implant in proper position. In mandibular augmentation, the mandibular branch of the facial nerve passes just anterior to the midportion of the mandible in the midlateral zone. It is important not to traumatize the tissues that overly this area. The course of the mental nerve is anatomically directed superiorly into the lower lip, which also helps to protect it from dissection trauma. Temporary hypesthesia of the mental nerve can occur for several days to several weeks after surgery. Permanent nerve damage is extremely rare and in one study represented less than 0.5% of a statistically large number of cases.[39] If encroachment on the nerve by the implant is detected due to misplacement or malrotation, then the implant should be repositioned below the nerve as early as possible.

The frontal branch of the facial nerve passes posterior to the mid aspect of the zygomatic arch and care must also be exercised when dissecting in this area. Infection can be minimized by irrigation of the pocket at the end of the procedure with either normal saline or bacitracin, 50,000 units per liter of sterile saline. Soaking the porous implants in antibiotic solution is advised. Drainage techniques are not ordinarily necessary in mandibular augmentation but may be used in midfacial augmentation if there is more than the normal amount of bleeding. We have found that immediate application of pressure over the entire midface by using a full face compression garment considerably reduces the risk of hematoma, seroma, and swelling, and consequently the

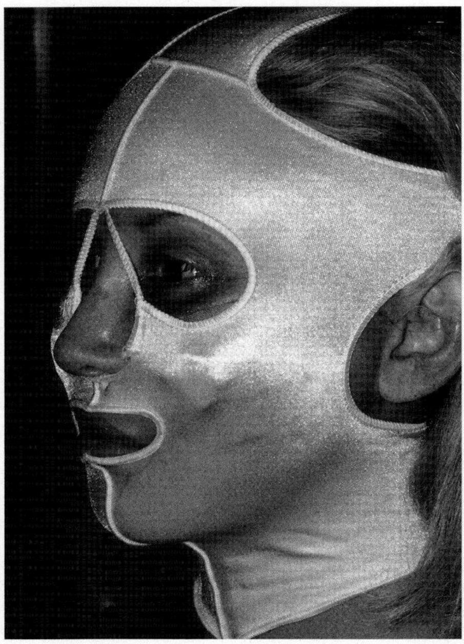

Fig. 32.14 The immediate application of some pressure over the entire midface by using a full-face compression garment has been found to considerably reduce the risk of hematoma, seroma, and swelling.

postoperative complications related to fluid accumulation within the pocket (**Fig. 32.14**).

Bone resorption is more commonly found in mandibular augmentation than in other alloplastic implant procedures. Findings of bone erosion following chin implants were reported in 1960. However, since these early reports, there have not been reports of clinical significance after surveying large populations of surgeons.[39] As long as the implant is in the correct position over cortical bone, the condition appears to stabilize without the loss of any substantial projection or prior cosmetic enhancement.

Conclusion

Facial contouring is extremely predictable when the surgeon understands the principals of facial topography and anatomy as well as pays careful attention to the basic surgical techniques. Critical facial analysis with appropriate communication between the surgeon and patient will lead to optimal patient satisfaction. Many different types of facial implants are available for the surgeon to create a variety of contours to fulfill most needs. Reconstructing more complex contour defects can be accomplished by using three-dimensional computer imaging and computer-aided design and manufacturing (CAD/CAM) technology to manufacture custom implants.[27]

Facial implant procedures provide an excellent long-term solution for the facial plastic surgeon. Midface implants can be used to correct underlying skeletal abnormalities as well as restore a youthful appearance. Chin augmentation with alloplastic implants provide a safe alternative to correct microgenia. It can also be used with excellent outcome in facial rejuvenation for patients with prominent prejowl sulcus. Although challenging, there are very few procedures that can provide the major rewards that facial contouring procedures can offer.

References

1. Carr A, Samaras K, Burton S, et al. A syndrome of peripheral lipodystrophy, hyperlipidemia, and insulin resistance in patients receiving HIV protease inhibitors. AIDS 1998;12(7):F51–58
2. Kotler DP, Rosenbaum K, Wang J, Pierson RN. Studies of body composition and fat distribution in HIV-infected and control subjects. J Acquired Immund Deficiency & Human Retrovirology 1999;20:229
3. Anderson JM, Miller KM. Biomaterial biocompatibility and the macrophage. Biomaterials 1984;5:5
4. Ziats NP, Miller KM, Anderson JM. In vitro and in vivo interactions of cells with biomaterials. Biomaterials 1988;9:5
5. Personal communication. Implantech Associates, Inc., and W.L. Gore, Inc. Jan. 1999
6. Gabriel SE, O'Fallon WM, Kurland LT, Beard CM, Woods JE, Melton LJ III. risk of connective-tissue diseases and other disorders after breast implantation. N Engl J Med 1994;330:1697
7. Park AJ, Black RJ, Sarhadi NS, Chetty U, Watson ACH. Silicone gel-filled breast implants and connective tissue diseases. Plast Reconstr Surg 1998;101:261
8. Park JB, Lakes RS, eds. Polymeric materials. In: Biomaterials: An Introduction. New York: Plenum; 1994:164
9. Soyer T, Lempier M, Cooper P, et al. A new venous prosthesis. Surgery 1972;72:864
10. McCauley CE. A 7-year follow-up of expanded polytetrafluoroethylene in femoropopliteal bypass grafts. Ann Plast Surg 1984; 199:37
11. Brown BI, Neel HB III, Kern EB. Implants of Supramid, Proplast, Plastipore, and Silastic. Arch Otolaryngol Head Neck Surg 1979;105:605
12. Alexander H. Calcium-based ceramics and composites in bone reconstruction. CRC Crit Rev Biocompat 1987;4:43
13. Salyer KE, Hall CD. Porous hydroxyapatite as an onlay bone graft substitute in maxillofacial surgery. Plast Reconstr Surg 1989;84:236
14. Rodriquez A, Vacanti CA. Characteristics of cartilage engineered from human pediatric auricular cartilage. Plast Reconstr Surg 1999;103:1111
15. Langer R, Vunjak G, Freed L, et al. Tissue engineering: biomedical applications. Tissue Engin 1995;1:151
16. Romm S. Art, love, and facial beauty. Clin Plast Surg 1987;14:579
17. Broadbent TR, Mathews VI. Artistic relationships in surface anatomy of the face. Application to reconstructive surgery. Plast Reconstr Surg 1957;20:1
18. Blitzer A, Binder WJ, Aviv JE, Keen MS, Brin MF. The management of hyperfunctional facial lines with botulinum toxin: a collaborative study of 210 injection sites in 162 patients. Arch Otolaryngol Head Neck Surg 1997;123:389–392
19. Gonzalez-Ulloa M, Stevens EF. Senility of the face: basic study to understand its causes and effects. Plast Reconstr Surg 1965;36:239
20. Mittelman H. The anatomy of the aging mandible and its importance to facelift surgery. Facial Plast Surg Clin North Am 1994;2:301
21. Binder W. Submalar augmentation: an alternative to facelift surgery. Arch Otolaryngol 1989;115:797
22. Belinfante LS, Mitchell DL. Use of alloplastic material in the canine fossa-zygomatic area to improve facial esthetics. J Oral Surg 1977;35:121
23. Binder W. Submalar augmentation: a procedure to enhance rhytidectomy. Ann Plast Surg 1990;24:200

24. Binder W, Schoenrock L, eds. Facial Contouring and Alloplastic Implants. Philadelphia: Saunders; 1994
25. Cao Y, Vacanti JP, Paige KT, Upton J, Vacanti CA. Transplantation of chondrocytes utilizing a polymer-cell construct to produce tissue-engineered cartilage in the shape of a human ear. Plast Reconstr Surg 1997;100:297–302
26. Personal communication. Tobias G. Mount Sinai School of Medicine, New York, New York; Sept. 1999
27. Terino EO. Alloplastic facial contouring by zonal principles of skeletal anatomy. Clin Plast Surg 1992;19:487
28. Binder WJ. A comprehensive approach for aesthetic contouring of the mid-face in rhytidectomy. Facial Plast Surg Clin North Am 1993;1:231–255
29. Flowers RS. Cosmetic blepharoplasty, state of the art. In: Advances in Plastic and Reconstructive Surgery, vol 8. St. Louis: Mosby Year Book; 1992:31
30. Flowers RS. Tear trough implants for correction of tear trough deformity. Clin Plast Surg 1993;20:403
31. Tobias GW, Binder WJ. The submalar triangle: its anatomy and clinical significance. Facial Plast Surg Clin North Am 1994;2:255
32. Binder WJ, Kaye A. Reconstruction of posttraumatic and congenital facial deformities with 3-D computer assisted custom-designed implants. Plast Reconstr Surg 1994;94:775
33. Hoenig JA, Shorr N, Shorr J. The suborbicularis oculi fat in aesthetic and reconstructive surgery. Int Ophthalmol Clin 1997;37:179
34. Moelleken B. The superficial subciliary cheek lift, a technique for rejuvenating the infraorbital region and nasojugal groove: a clinical series of 71 patients. Plast Reconstr Surg 1999;104:1863
35. Schoenrock LD, Chernoff WG. Subcutaneous implantation of Gore-Tex for facial reconstruction. Otolaryngol Clin North Am 1995;28:325
36. Schultz RC. Reconstruction of facial deformities with alloplastic material. Ann Plast Surg 1981;7:434
37. Gorney M, Harries T. The preoperative and postoperative consideration of natural facial asymmetry. Plast Reconstr Surg 1974;54:187
38. Courtiss E. Complications in aesthetic malar augmentation-discussion. Plast Reconstr Surg 1983;71:648
39. Terino EO. Complications of chin and malar augmentation. In: Peck G, ed. Complications and Problems in Aesthetic Plastic Surgery. New York: Gower Medical; 1991

33 Hair Replacement Techniques

Daniel E. Rousso, Sandeep Sule, Dow Stough, and Jeffrey M. Whitworth

Baldness has afflicted humans for so long that its origins are lost in the mists of prehistory. It is useful to consider the fact that some primates, such as chimpanzees and certain monkeys, also exhibit maturity-related alopecia.[1]

The imaginative remedies for baldness over the course of time are legion, ranging from camel dung to stump water to even less appealing substances. The record of such remedies starts with ancient papyri dating back 5000 years.[1] The Bible sympathized with those who had bald pates but could offer no remedy.

The first descriptions of hair transplantation date to the 1930s with Okuda. However, surgical transplantation did not gain widespread acceptance until Orentreich described his work and techniques. Since this time, multiple new techniques and refinements have been developed. Currently there are delicate and effective surgical techniques for hair transplantation, and they do provide a remedy. These new techniques incorporate the following refinements and advances: the mixing of various sizes of smaller grafts, attention to minute detail in graft preparation and placement, an appreciation of the ramifications dictated by hair quality, and the customizing of procedures to each individual patient.

New techniques have virtually revolutionized hair replacement surgery. As a consequence of advances that have been made, results in males with pattern alopecia have reached a surprising level of excellence, efficacy, and patient acceptance. Today's methodology demands a high degree of expertise in planning and execution.

Anatomy and Physiology

The scalp consists of five distinct layers: skin, loose connective tissue, epicranium aponeurosis, loose areolar tissue, and periosteum. The scalp is extremely vascular, supplied in the preauricular region by the supratrochlear, supraorbital, and superficial temporal arteries, and in the postauricular region by the posterior auricular and occipital arteries. An extensive collateral system exists between these vessels. A complex venous system drains the scalp. The anterior scalp is drained by the supratrochlear and supraorbital veins, which communicate with the ophthalmic vein and the cavernous sinus. Additionally, there are numerous communications with emissary veins to the intracranial venous sinuses.

Hair follicles are derived from both ectoderm and mesoderm. The hair shaft is lined by epidermal cells. One or more sebaceous glands are associated with each hair follicle, making up the pilosebaceous unit. At the base of each follicle is the papilla. The papilla, combined with the surrounding epidermal cells, makes up the hair bulb. The hair bulb is the site of hair shaft formation as cells multiply. Melanocytes in the hair bulb synthesize melanosomes, which are then transferred to cells of the hair shaft for hair color. Follicular units are naturally occurring groups of one to four terminal hairs that are present in the scalp. Each group also contains sebaceous glands, a neurovascular plexus, and an erector pilorum muscle. This is surrounded by collagen called the perifolliculum

Hair growth is cyclical. The anagen phase, which can range from 2 to 6 years, is the main growth phase. Scalp hair grows ~1 mm every 3 days. Following the anagen phase is the transition involutionary catagen phase. The catagen phase typically lasts ~2 to 3 weeks. The hair then enters telogen, the resting phase. The telogen phase usually lasts ~3 months.

Male Alopecia

Etiology

There are multiple causes of hair loss. By far the most common is androgenic alopecia. This can present as male pattern androgenic alopecia, female pattern androgenic alopecia, or diffuse androgenic alopecia. Hair loss susceptibility is inherent in each hair follicle and is controlled by both genetic factors and circulating androgens. Circulating androgens target cells in the hair papilla and control the genetic potential of hairs. The effect of 5-dihydrotestosterone (DHT) on susceptible hair follicles leads to androgen-induced alopecia.[2]

In addition to androgenic alopecia, there are many infectious and inflammatory etiologies for alopecia. Some of the more common infectious causes include dermatophytes and syphilis. Both of these usually present with patchy, "moth-eaten" alopecia scattered throughout the scalp.[3] When the hair loss is severe, destruction of the hair follicle with subsequent scarring may occur. Inflammatory etiologies include seborrheic dermatitis, psoriasis, and pityriasis amiantacea. Again, these forms of alopecia present with patchy hair loss along with associated scalp changes (i.e., scales, erythematous papules). Finally, other causes of alopecia include radiation, drugs, autoimmune disorders (i.e., scleroderma, lupus), granulomatous disorders (i.e., sarcoid), and even developmental/hereditary causes.

Medical Treatment

An extensive discussion of medical alopecia treatment is beyond the scope of this chapter. However, there are several treatments of androgenic alopecia worth mentioning. Minoxidil is a piperidinopyrinidine derivative that functions as a vasodilator initially used for cardiac purposes. A side effect of the oral medication was hypertrichosis, seen in ~70% of patients. Therefore, a topical preparation was developed to utilize this hair growth. The exact mechanism of action for minoxidil is unknown.[4] It does not appear to be antiandrogen. The efficacy of topical minoxidil in men and women is undisputed. Initial studies of efficacy [on patients with Norwood (III to VI)] involved 2% and 3% topical minoxidil. Currently a 5% topical is also available. Significant hair growth is seen with continuous use in 4 to 6 months.[5] Discontinuation of 2% minoxidil leads to loss of gained hair over 3 to 4 months.[6] In general, patients should be advised to use a 1-year trial of twice daily minoxidil, although improvement can be seen in 6 months. Patients should also be warned that initial hair shedding may actually increase over the first months of treatment, as hairs are induced into anagen, and telogen hairs are shed.

Finasteride is a potent 5-α-reductase inhibitor without any steroid activity. As stated in the prior section, 5-α reductase is important in the conversion of serum testosterone into DHT. Finasteride in doses of 0.2 mg, 1 mg, and 5 mg were tested in initial studies with data favoring 1mg usage.[7] Hair counts in men (with Norwood classification II to V) using 1 mg finasteride typically increase significantly within a 1-year time period. After 1 year of use, patients have a plateau of hair growth, but continued decline in hair loss. The use of finasteride in women is controversial. Because of the risk of teratogenicity, finasteride is contraindicated in premenopausal women. Studies of efficacy in postmenopausal women showed no significant difference in hair counts after 1 year of treatment. However, the role of finasteride in these postmenopausal women remains to be determined.[8]

Surgical Treatment and Techniques

There are many factors and variables to consider when planning for the establishment of a hairline and the reconstruction of hair over the scalp. The following list contains some of the most important considerations:

1. Classification of baldness
2. Classification of hair quality
3. Color similarity between hair and skin
4. Future hair loss expectation
5. Age of patient
6. Motivation, expectations, and desires of patient

Consultation and Patient Selection

In the initial consultation, we judge who will be and who will not be a good candidate for hair restoration surgery. In our assessment, we look at five qualities: patient age, a definitive bald area, skin-to-hair color match, hair curl, and density of the donor area.[9] If a patient is felt to be an acceptable candidate, a discussion of risks and benefits of surgery follows, along with arrangements for preoperative laboratory work and medications. This is also the time for discussion of the general medical history of the patient, including current medications and drug allergies.

Classification of Baldness

The Norwood system for the classification of baldness[10] is the most widely used today. It describes and diagrams male pattern baldness stages I through VII, plus the type of variation in those stages. Stage I is the least severe, showing minor to no temporal recession and no crown balding. Stage VII is the most severe, with only the classic horseshoe-shaped band of hair remaining. Stages II to VI represent the progressive stages of hair thinning. The system is similar to that devised by Hamilton[11] and yields similar results. A new view of alopecia suggests that these classifications may be useful primarily as a means of defining populations for clinical trials rather than as a determinant of treatment.

Classification of Hair Quality

The term *hair quality* includes considerations of density, texture, curl, and color. Broad criteria have been previously defined for the grading of hair quality.[12] The various grades of hair quality may overlap, and each can be subdivided more specifically.

Hair of coarse texture and above-average density is rated "A" or highest in donor quality, and hair that is fine and sparse in density is rated "D" or lowest in donor quality. There are two intermediate ratings, "B" and "C" that cover the range in between. In general, individuals with hair color that matches the skin color can expect better results than those who have a color contrast between skin and hair. Curliness of hair is also an advantage.

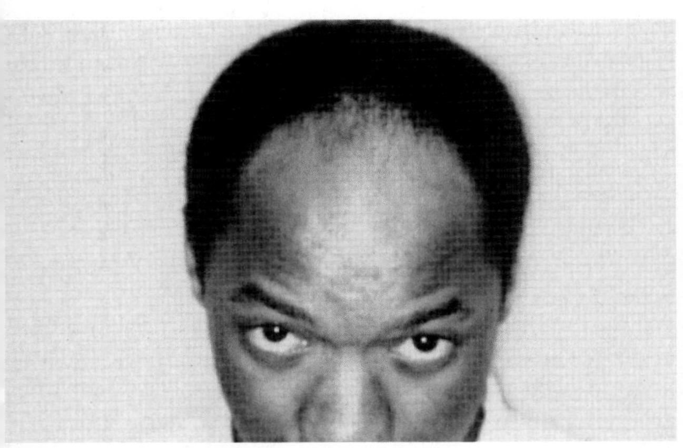

Fig. 33.1 Patient shown before transplantation. Good results can be expected with standard round grafts or with incisional-slit grafting because this patient has an excellent match of skin and hair color.

Color Similarity between Hair and Skin

Hair color and texture are important considerations as well. The more contrast there is between hair color and skin color, the more noticeable the hair transplants will be. The hair colors that are best suited for transplantation procedures include blonde, red, gray, and the salt-and-pepper combination. The colors of black and dark brown present more of a challenge, especially in individuals with straight hair. Individuals who have dark hair color and light skin may be less suitable candidates for transplantation because it is difficult to camouflage. The final appearance after transplantation is significantly affected by the degree to which hair color and skin color match. Matching minimizes visual contrast.

The most propitious combination is dark skin combined with dark, curly hair (**Figs. 33.1 and 33.2**). At the other end of the scale is the combination of light, pale skin and dark, straight hair. In the latter combination, the degree of visual contrast increases the visibility of any transplantation undertaken. There are innumerable combinations on the scale between these two extremes, and hair color differences between the vertex area and the occipital area may occasionally be seen in an individual (**Figs. 33.3 and 33.4**).

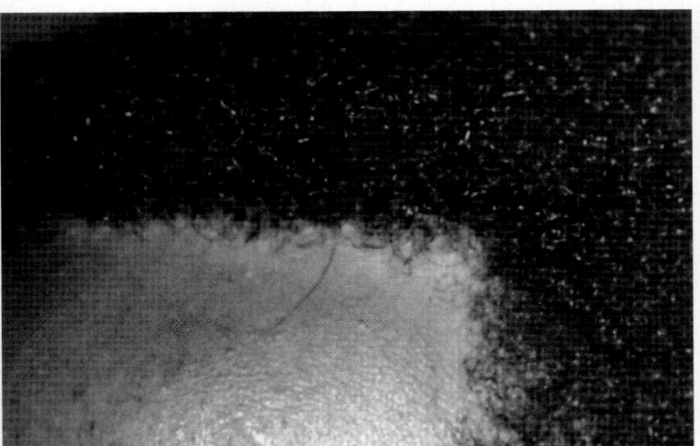

Fig. 33.2 The same patient as in **Fig. 33.3** after hair transplantation. Incisional slit grafting was used primarily. Some round grafts were placed in the vertex posterior to the hairline area.

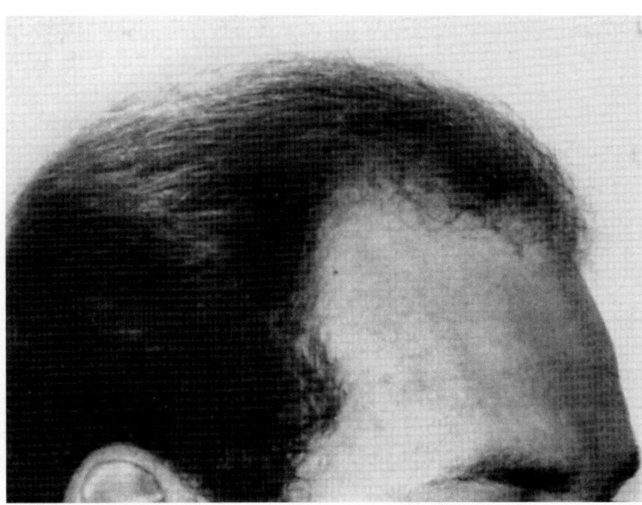

Fig. 33.3 This man is shown before transplantation. The hair present in the frontal forelock is of sparse density and light color.

Expected Future Hair Loss

Because androgenetic alopecia is genetically controlled and therefore inherited, expectation of future hair loss can be

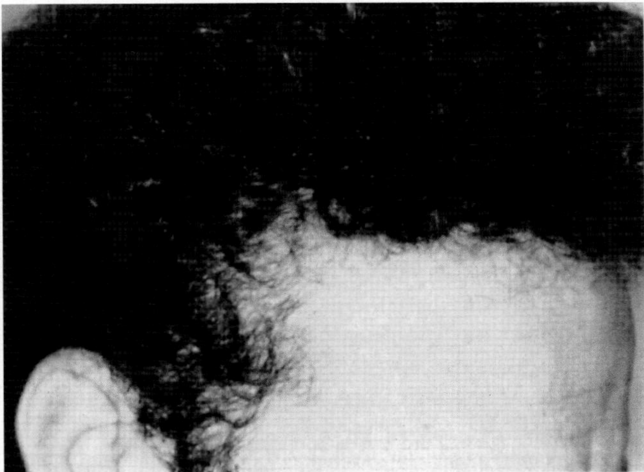

Fig. 33.4 The same patient as shown in **Fig. 33.5** after transplantation. This patient's occipital (donor) hair was darker in color than the original frontocentral hair. Both incisional slit grafts and standard round grafts were used.

roughly estimated by referring to a carefully drawn family history. The propensity for alopecia can be passed from both maternal and paternal sides. Information on close family members should be gathered during initial interviews and used in conjunction with other factors such as age and present stage and pattern of hair loss to arrive at an estimate of expected future hair loss. It is impossible to predict future hair loss with absolute accuracy, and patients should be warned of this uncertainty.

Age of Patient

Androgenetic alopecia is an ongoing process (i.e., it usually occurs over an extended portion of the individual's lifetime). Patient age indicates an individual's place on the alopecia continuum. Knowledge of whether one is at the beginning of the process or the end point allows planning judgments to be made more appropriately. It is true that with today's techniques virtually everyone can experience a satisfying improvement in appearance, but it is also true that those who have unrealistic expectations should be discouraged.

A consideration of patient's age also allows an assessment of the appropriate position and contour for the hairline. Patients aged 20 or younger are generally discouraged from undergoing transplantation because it is too difficult to predict what form and course future alopecia will take. Exceptions are made when the patient understands that the extent of future hair loss is an unknown and therefore an accurate prediction of its course impossible and still wishes to proceed.

Motivation and Expectations

Discussion of the patient's expectations should enlighten the surgeon about the degree of patient motivation present and the patient's perception of the anticipated improvement. The patient should be well informed, must be highly motivated, and should be advised realistically about the expected results of the anticipated procedures. A hairline that complements the facial structures and that represents the surgeon's considered approach to anticipated work should be drawn and discussed with the patient. It is important that each patient have a thorough understanding of the anticipated cosmetic effect before starting procedures, and some believe it is advisable to underrepresent potential benefits. This can serve to guard against unrealistic expectations and avoid future dissatisfactions.

Placement of the Hairline

In determining the placement of the hairline so that it creates balance and compensates for facial inequalities, the surgeon should visualize the face divided by imaginary horizontal planes into three segments of approximately equal vertical depth. The anthropometric demarcations for the three segments are (1) chin to columella; (2) columella to glabella; and (3) glabella to frontal hairline or proposed hairline. The position where the upper boundary of the upper segment falls can serve as a general guide for determining the appropriate height for placement of the hairline.

Caution must be exercised in using this measurement alone because doing so would often result in the hairline being placed too low. As a matter of practice, hairlines are generally placed between 7.5 and 9.5 cm above the midglabellar area. This is a general guide and should not be taken as an absolute or rigid parameter.

The hairline must be placed and designed so that it will indicate an appropriate level of maturity as the years go by, rather than perpetuate a youthful, free-of-recession look that will become inappropriate and possibly even unattractive. In many cases, it will be necessary to place the margin of the future hairline somewhat posterior to the remnant original hairline. This conservative approach will allow an optimum use of donor hair and is more likely to provide adequate coverage. A low, wide hairline will often lead to inadequacies in donor hair, resulting in sparse coverage and poor cosmesis.

All transplanted, re-created hairlines should look natural, but not all natural hairlines are the most aesthetically pleasing in appearance. In other words, the hairline should not be "abnormally young."[12] Because the contours of design will be more or less permanent, their overall effect should be acceptable to the patient throughout a lifetime. It is best to establish a natural but mature hairline. The low hairline of youth may look quite natural at certain ages but could also begin to look inappropriate as years pass. The frontotemporal angle, which constitutes the area in which male pattern baldness begins, is most critical to the design and final appearance.

Over the past 30 years, most transplant surgeons have created sharp symmetric hairlines. There has been a general tendency among surgeons to line up the grafts uniformly along the most anterior portion of the hairline. The results from this symmetric approach can appear artificial. Hairlines in their natural state are not symmetric, nor are they carefully edged like a well-groomed lawn. They exist in an irregular fashion, with hairs scattered up to 1 cm in front of the area where the eye actually begins to perceive the hairline.

Styling preferences particular to certain fashion statements in vogue at any given time should not dictate the design of the hairline because these are fads and sure to change. Of historical interest, it is sometimes possible to gauge the year of previous transplant work by observing the configuration of the hairline. The widow's peak is now rarely employed, and its presence probably indicates a transplant performed in the 1960s.

Incisional Slit Grafting

A transition zone of single hair grafts can be utilized, which were placed in an intentionally irregular though not exaggerated pattern. These single hairs were used to construct the transition zone into the more densely transplanted scalp. The results were cosmetically pleasing but still lacked the degree of irregularity of a natural hairline. Observations of our own cases have now led us to conclude that when constructing a hairline a much more exaggerated pattern should be employed to achieve the most undetectable result. We now refer to this as a zigzag pattern.[13]

The shape of the hairline is drawn into position on the patient prior to making recipient sites. After the general outline has been made, marking pens are used to create an undulating or zigzag line. With this method, the original marked hairline is used for positioning and then transformed into a waving irregular shape. Recipient sites are placed using the undulated line as the true border. Densities within this zone can be varied. This irregular template has been referred to as a sawtooth, snail track, or zigzag pattern. Posterior to this, larger follicular unit grafts of up to four hairs are transplanted to provide a more concentrated density[13] (**Figs. 33.5 and 33.6**).

Separated Needle Stick and Graft Placement Technique

Donor Strip Harvesting

Improvements in donor area harvesting have revolutionized what can be accomplished with transplantation.

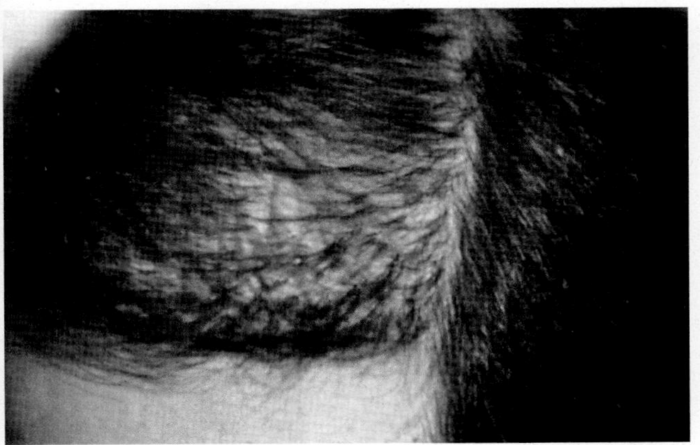

Fig. 33.5 The combination of round grafts with incisional slit grafting can be effective. An intermediate stage in this process is shown after round grafts have been placed but before incisional slit grafting.

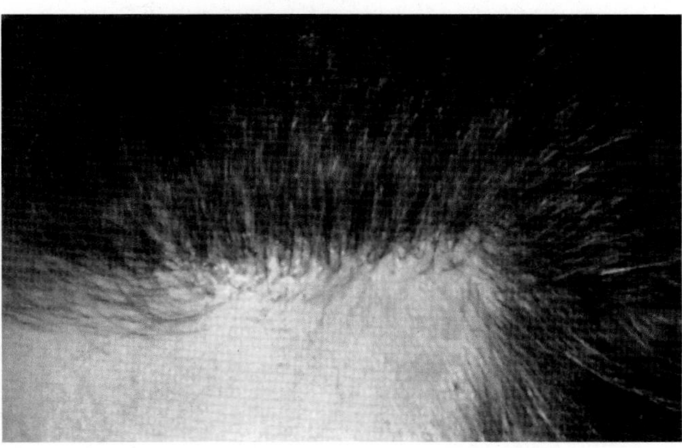

Fig. 33.6 The same patient as in **Fig. 33.1**, after incisional-slit grafting refinement and the development of a feathering zone hairline.

Assessment of donor area boundaries encompasses hairs that are permanent in their original site. This allows for these transplanted hairs to be permanent in their new sites. The anterior border of the donor site is usually thought of as vertically superior to the external auditory meatus. This area then extends posteriorly over the occipital protuberance. This, in general, is ~69 mm high in the midline from the inferior hairline limit.

On the day of surgery, the patient is brought into the surgical suite, a series of standardized preoperative photographs are taken, and the area for donor site harvesting is marked, shaved, and prepared with tumescent anesthesia for excision (**Fig. 33.7**). An elliptical donor harvest using a multibladed knife is employed. The donor site is then closed using a running 2–0 Prolene suture (Ethicon, Inc., Somerville, NJ) (**Fig. 33.8**).[14] Immediately after removing the donor strip from the patient, the tissue is given to a team of three or four

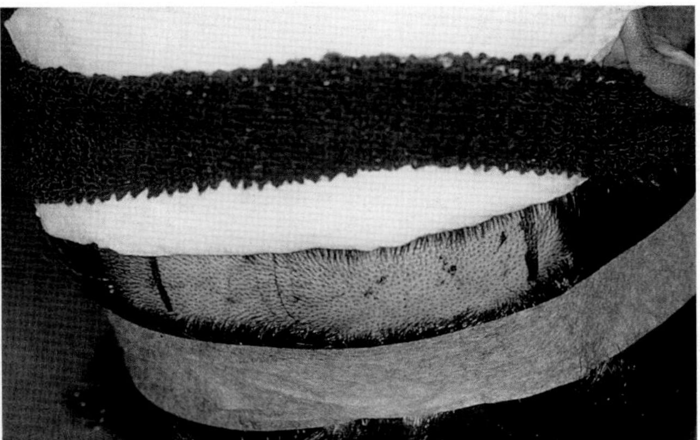

Fig. 33.7 The donor area is prepared for donor site harvesting. The area is marked, shaved, and injected for tumescence. The gauze padding and headband are placed into position prior to harvesting the strip. Afterward they will be pulled over the incision site.

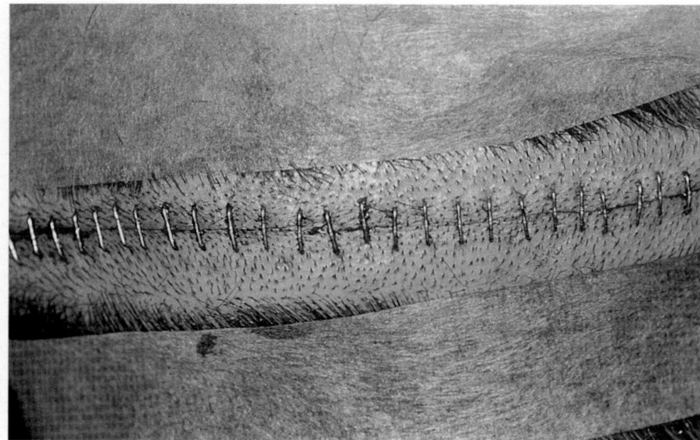

Fig. 33.8 Elliptical donor harvesting is employed using a double-bladed knife. The donor site is then closed with staples.

technicians who subsection it using dissection with back-lighting (**Fig. 33.9**). Subsectioning is achieved by initially slivering the donor tissue into thin slivers, one follicular unit in width, then by dissecting individual follicular units from each sliver[9] (**Figs. 33.10 and 33.11**).

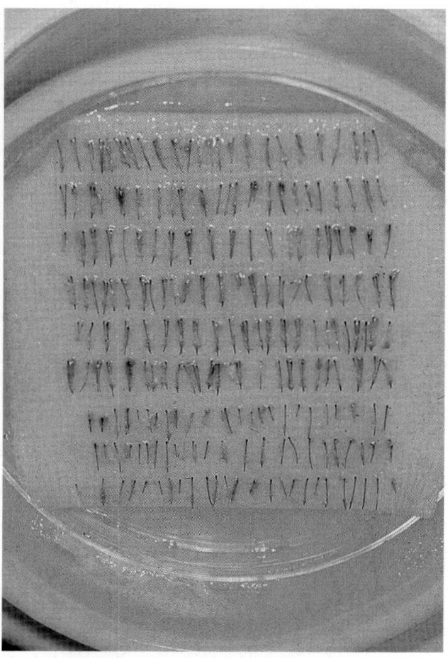

Fig. 33.10 Individual follicular units are produced under careful stereomicroscopic dissection.

Recipient Site Creation

Following donor strip harvesting, the patient is turned from the prone position to the reclined sitting position. Anesthesia of the area is administered first with blocks of the supraorbital and supratrochlear nerves.[15] Epinephrine in a concentration of 100,000 is infiltrated throughout the entire recipient area in a superficial dermal location. Following this, recipient sites are made using 18-gauge needles for smaller follicular unit grafts and 19-gauge needles for single-hair grafts at the frontal hairline. Needles are inserted at 30 to 40 degrees from the scalp surface, so that transplanted grafts will be gently angled anterior toward the patient's nose. This allows the patient the most versatility in hair styling options. After all recipient sites have been made, the follicular unit grafts are inserted. Thus the technique is termed separated needle stick and graft placement because recipient site creation with needles is separated in time from graft insertion. This is an important distinction from the simultaneous needle stick and graft placement techniques. Both methods have their advantages and proponents.[9]

Graft Insertion

Grafts are then inserted using jeweler's forceps. This can be done using two people to reduce surgical time. There

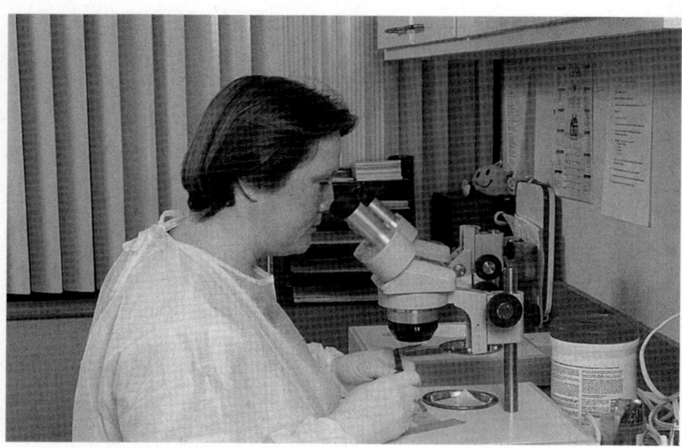

Fig. 33.9 A technicians subsectioning donor tissue using stereomicroscopic dissection with back-lighting.

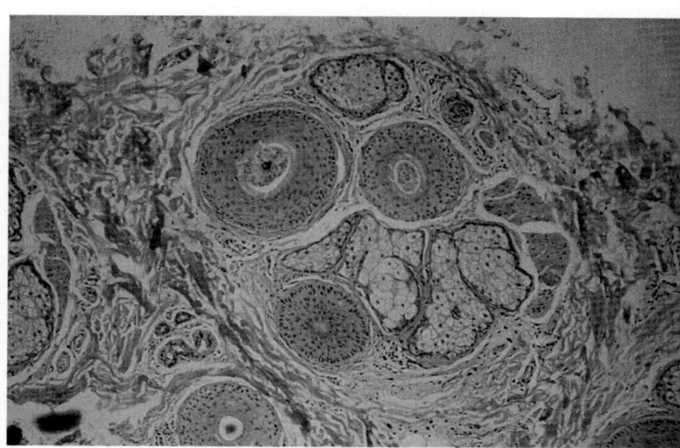

Fig. 33.11 The follicular unit anatomy is demonstrated showing a single unit enveloped by a fibrous stroma enclosing hair shafts, sebaceous glands, and erector pili muscles.

are several complications that can occur with graft insertion. First, prolonged exposure to dry, dehumidified air can reduce graft survival. Additionally, prolonged time outside the body can reduce graft survival. Limmer showed a graft survival rate of 92% for grafts kept out of the body for up to 6 hours. This rate decreases ~1% per hour for every hour beyond 6 hours.[16] Furthermore, physical trauma, such as squeezing the graft between the tips of forceps or crushing grafts between the forceps and insertion site, can lead to failed transplants. Overly deep placement below the level of the epithelium can cause epithelial inclusion cysts and ingrown hairs to form. Finally "popping" can occur when previously inserted grafts are displaced by the lateral or inferior forces of newly inserted grafts. This can occur from large graft size, shallow recipient sites, scar tissue at recipient sites, and bleeding.[16]

Following graft insertion, the hair is wrapped in a nonadherent (i.e., Telfa) dressing with firm pressure for 24 hours. This dressing is removed on postoperative day 1, and gentle shampooing is started to remove any scabs. Patients may return to work as soon as postoperative day 2.

Posttransplant, all hair will go into the telogen phase of growth. The hair will temporarily fall out and new hair will generate from the follicle in ~3 to 4 months. Sequential stages of transplantation can usually be done in 3 to 6 months. This allows for growth from the previous stage to develop. For microminigrafting, natural results can be seen in two to three sessions, depending on hair texture and color (**Fig. 33.12**).

Discussion

The separated needle stick and graft placement technique allows for a 1000-graft procedure to be completed in less than 5 hours on average. Those patients with minimal bleeding and excellent donor tissue characteristics can be completed in considerably less time. The advantages of this technique include the physician having complete control of hairline placement, as well as the positioning and the direction of each graft. The use of stereomicroscopic dissection limits follicular transection, which may contribute to superior quality of transplanted hair. Also, there are several other reported advantages of follicular unit transplantation. These include maintaining and creating a more natural hairline, maximizing oxygen diffusion, minimizing interruption of blood flow, placing hair units more densely, and distributing hair in a natural pattern.[17] In addition to these benefits, once the physician is finished making recipient sites, he or she is free to engage in other patient care activities. The disadvantages of this technique include the necessity for training in the use of stereomicroscopes for slivering the donor tissue and dissecting the grafts.

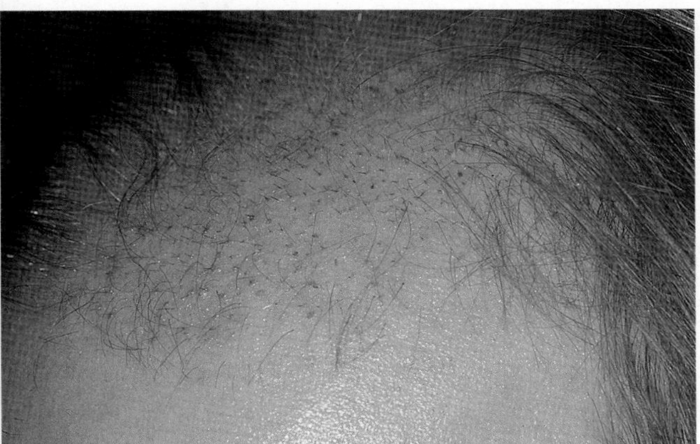

Fig. 33.12 One day after surgical placement of 650 follicular unit grafts.

Though there are a few proponents of techniques that use larger, standard round grafts or a combination, these techniques are no longer commonly employed because the cosmesis of the finished product is less than natural. Follicular unit transplanting does create a result that most closely resembles the natural state (**Figs. 33.13 and 33.14**).

Scalp Reductions

Another important technique in hair replacement surgery is scalp reduction. Scalp, or alopecia reduction is a technique in which balding scalp, usually in the vertex/crown area, is excised. Patients with exclusive crown alopecia are good candidates for this surgery as are patients over age 40 years with stable hair recession.[3]

Scalp reductions are usually designed on an individual basis to fit a particular area of baldness. Numerous shapes have been used (e.g., straight, paramedian, mercedes, and double or triple rhomboid). The straight ellipse, the Y, the T, the S, and the crescent have predominated in actual usage. Variations and permutations of these may also be used.

The straight ellipse is the simplest type of reduction. Although technically the easiest of the configurations, it is best to substitute a paramedian approach when possible. The paramedian is less cosmetically obvious and has other inherent benefits when the hair is styled.

The procedure of scalp reduction is performed under local anesthesia (ring block) and clean conditions. The midlines and proposed outer boundaries of the areas intended for excision are marked. The first incisions proceed along an outer margin of a marked area. The use of a Shaw scalpel (hot blade) can aide in establishing a dry

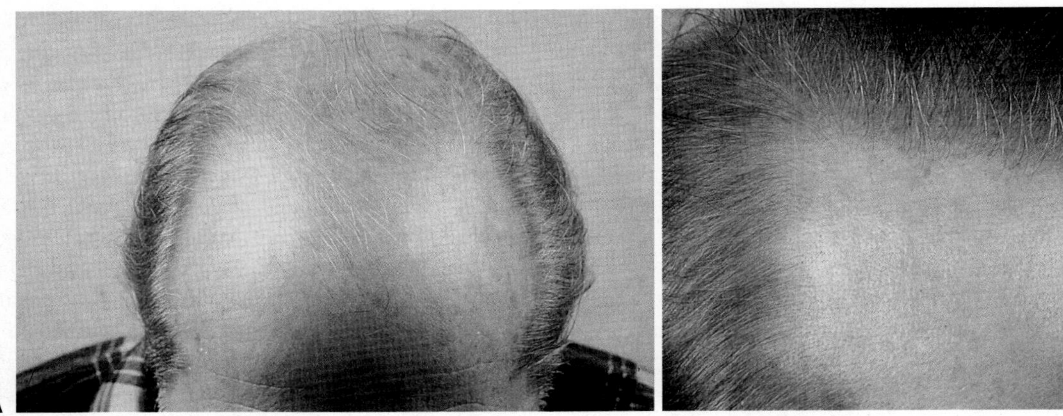

Fig. 33.13 (**A**) A 55-year-old white man prior to transplantation. This patient was classified as having Norwood VI male pattern alopecia. (**B**) Same patient after five sessions of transplantation. Each session averaged ~600 grafts.

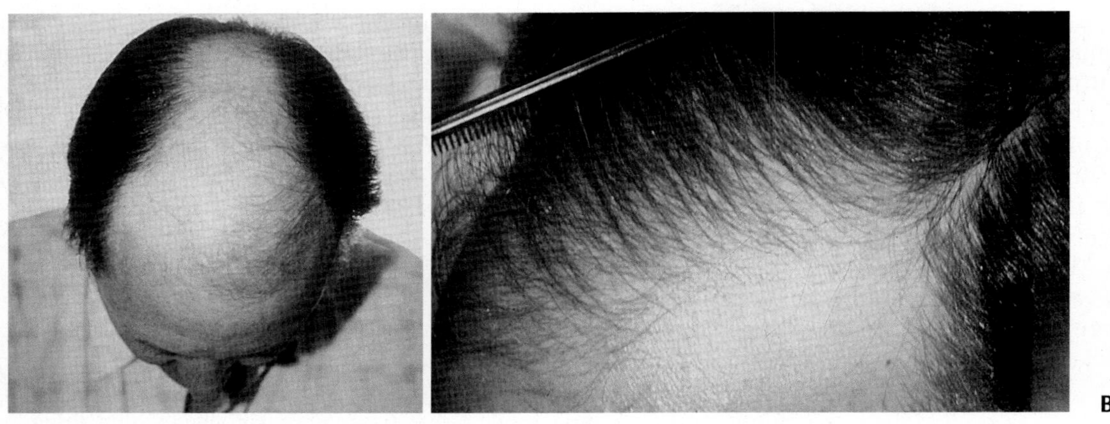

Fig. 33.14 (**A**) A 50-year-old white man with Norwood V male pattern alopecia shown prior to transplantation. (**B**) The same patient shown after follicular unit transplantation averaging 500 grafts per session. Note that the density is marginal due to the thin, fine-caliber hair shafts. The final density of a transplant is dependent on the starting caliber of the donor area hair.

field and reduces the actual operative time because this instrument has the dual function of excision and cautery (**Fig. 33.15**).

Undermining is performed for a distance of ~7 to 10 cm on each side of an incision. After undermining has been accomplished, a determination must be made regarding the actual width of the tissue to be excised. Generally, this can be accomplished by manually overlapping one incision edge with another and cutting off the redundant or overlapping segment.

Some judgment must be made regarding the degree of tension that will be placed on the galeal closing. An aggressive approach to reduction would call for removal of a relatively larger amount of scalp, increasing tension on the galeal closure. A conservative approach would dictate a less ambitious excision of tissue, minimizing

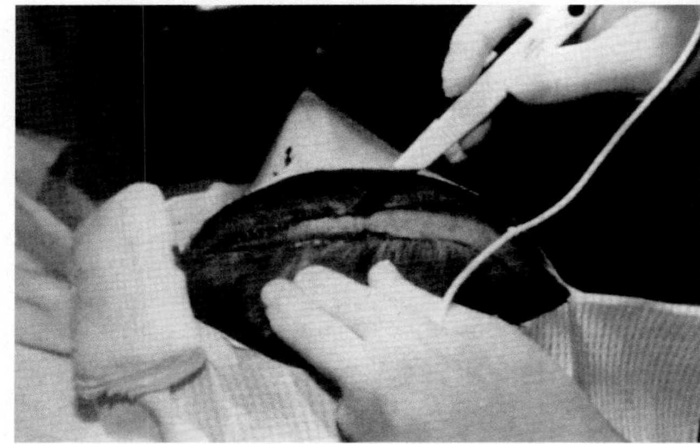

Fig. 33.15 Bleeding during a scalp reduction is controlled with the use of a Shaw hot blade.

tension placed on the galeal closure. There are advantages and disadvantages to both approaches.

The aid of intraoperative scalp expanders (**Fig. 33.16**) to stretch the denser hair–bearing regions of tissue may be employed. Caution is advised in attempting reductions on patients with thin, tight scalps because these patients are less suitable candidates than those with thick, elastic scalps.

After excision of scalp tissue has been completed, the galea is closed first, usually with 2–0 PDS sutures. When closure of the galea has been completed, the skin is closed with staples.

The actual configuration of the patterns used in scalp reduction is frequently modified to avoid leaving scars that are cosmetically apparent. It is often feasible to curve or otherwise adapt various segments of reduction patterns so that the scar can be more easily covered. A Z-plasty procedure should be performed on the posterior segment of scalp reductions to further camouflage this sensitive area.

Scalp reductions are almost always followed by hair transplantation procedures to complete the restoration and to provide cover for the reduction procedure scars.

Crown Balding

For the correction of crown balding, reductions are generally preferred to grafts. Again, patients with thick, loose scalps are much better candidates than those with thin, tight scalps. Small grafts are later placed in the scar area for camouflage. The use of grafts larger than 2 mm in the crown area may lead to the development of a stalked appearance. Only quarter grafts should be used in this area. Also, care must be taken not to place the grafts too close to each other along the edge of the scar because this may produce a zipper effect and thus preclude a natural appearance in the final result.

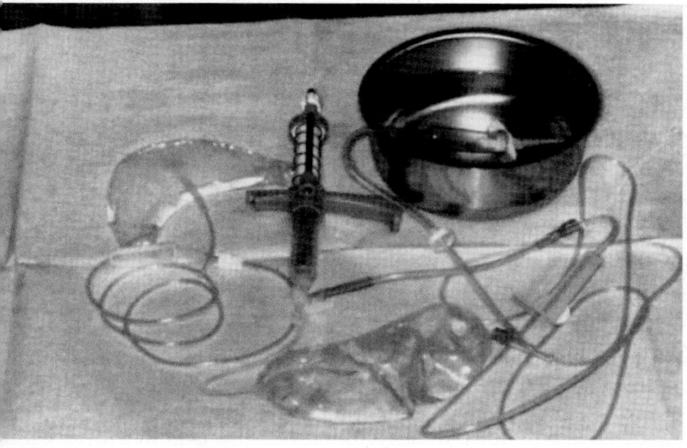

Fig. 33.16 The use of intraoperative scalp expanders allows for maximum removal of tissue. These are most useful when dealing with tight scalps.

Exceptions to the rule of treating crown balding with reductions preferentially are made for patients with extremely thin or extremely tight scalps and for those who fear scalp reductions in the belief that the procedure will be too painful. However, most patients are surprised to find that the procedure is comparable with a graft session, and a fair percentage of patients actually prefer a scalp reduction session over a transplant session.

Most patients will require more than one scalp reduction. The limiting factors are scalp thickness and elasticity. All patients should be advised that the resulting scar must be covered with grafts in subsequent transplant procedures.

Scalp Flaps

Previously a mainstay of hair replacement techniques, scalp flaps are now less commonly utilized or indicated. Still, there are advantages of scalp flaps over hair transplantation. The major difference involves maintaining the blood supply to hair follicles, thereby preventing hairs from entering the telogen (resting) phase. The hair is not trimmed and does not fall out (as in transplants) and therefore patients have stylable hair that continues to grow immediately after the procedure. Hair density is maximized with the results of scalp flaps being seen instantaneously, in contrast to the delayed, stepwise fashion of hair transplants.[3]

As with any surgical procedure, appropriate patient selection is critical. Patients with alopecia restricted to the frontal area are the ideal candidates for scalp flaps. Multiple scalp flaps have been described, including the Juri flap, and shorter flaps, such as the Dardou and temporoparietal flap.

The Juri flap is an axial flap following the superficial temporal artery. The flaps can be between 3 to 4 cm wide and 25 cm long. This allows for the entire frontal hairline to be bridged with one flap. This does, though, require a delay procedure to aid in the survival of this long and narrow flap. Mayer and Fleming further refined the Juri flap, advocating an irregular, trichophytic hairline to yield an undetectable frontal scar.[18]

Random scalp flap procedures, such as Dardour and Nataf, allow for a natural appearance to hair growth. However, because of the random nature of these flaps, the blood supply is not as predictable as with axial flaps, potentially leading to early telogen or tip necrosis.

A thorough discussion of scalp flaps is beyond the scope of this text. Readers interested in more information on scalp flaps are directed to the reference *Aesthetic and Reconstructive Surgery of the Scalp* by Toby Mayer and Richard Fleming.

Grooming

The need to attend to the aesthetics of hair transplantation does not end with the design of the frontal hairline and other areas but extends to providing the patient with proper advice concerning grooming. As soon as patients commit themselves to hair replacement surgery, the requirement for ongoing styling and grooming must be addressed. Proper advice and the recommendation of grooming aids are necessary to maximize the effectiveness of the transplant and the satisfaction of the patient.

There are many reliable grooming aids on the market that enrich the texture of the hair and give an appearance of greater thickness. A hairstyling blow-dryer is essential for achieving the full effect. In patients with thin, straight hair, a permanent body treatment may be desirable. Although many men are reluctant to visit a stylist, this reluctance is misplaced and should be overcome. It may be necessary for the physician to propose or even insist on a permanent, especially in patients with grade C or D hair quality.

Some patients may benefit additionally from fogging the scalp with a Couvré scalp cover or by using a scalp camouflage cream. These types of products deflect light in thin areas and render them less obvious. The proper length of the hair should be determined for the individual, and it is helpful to routinely enlist the aid of an expert stylist in this matter.

It is the hair replacement surgeon's obligation to counsel and direct patients in these areas because the patient's ultimate appearance is a critical factor in the overall success of treatment.

Complications of Transplant Procedures

Syncope

During the initial visit, syncope may occur following injection of the first few milliliters of anesthetic. It also occurs rarely in the latter stages of the procedures. Placing the patient in a horizontal position initially will ordinarily prevent this condition.

Bleeding

The occipital region is most commonly the area of arterial bleeding. This bleeding is best controlled with sutures. Pressure is often essential for adequate hemostasis. For this reason elastic bandages are routinely used to apply a moderate, persistent pressure to the donor area for 15 to 20 minutes after harvesting the grafts and closing the wound. After completion of the entire session, a pressure bandage is put in place and maintained for the following 8 to 12 hours. If bleeding develops after the patient has left the physician's office, the patient is advised that persistent manual pressure with a clean bandage or handkerchief may be necessary. When hemostasis is not achieved by this method, a ligature is indicated. If bleeding occurs in the recipient spaces while implants are being inserted, it may be necessary to remove the graft and control the bleeder. After healing, a small scar will usually remain that can later be excised and replaced with a small graft if necessary.

Edema

Postoperative edema over the scalp and forehead is common, especially if extensive grafting has been performed. This may be reduced by use of oral prednisone during the first week postoperative. It will subside as healing takes place.

Infection

Infection occurs in less than 1% of cases but should nevertheless be guarded against and treatment instituted should it develop. The use of a prophylactic, broad-spectrum antibiotic (cephalexin 500 mg b.i.d.) is routinely employed postoperatively.

Scarring

Scarring resulting from small-graft hair transplantation is rarely of sufficient scope to be a matter of serious concern. In blacks, keloids may sometimes be observed. When a patient's history indicates a possibility of keloid development, there should be a waiting period of 3 months after the initial session. This will allow adequate time for any possible keloid development, and a decision can then be made regarding the advisability of continuing treatment.

Poor Hair Growth

Ischemia, poor hair survival, or even sloughing of grafts may result from crowding recently placed implants. Some patients with fine hair may show marginal growth of transplanted hair, regardless of the transplant method used.

Miscellaneous

Occasionally, individuals may undergo varying degrees of spontaneous effluvium over the scalp. In patients with only a limited number of transplants and normally thinning hair the temporary loss of hair may be distressingly apparent, but the patient should be reassured that regrowth is imminent. Arteriovenous fistulas may occasionally be encountered in the occipital region. Simple dissection and ligature of the fistula are indicated.

Poor Outcomes

What many laypersons interpret as a poor outcome is often an incomplete transplant or a case of inadequate grooming. Statistics based on 25 years of experience indicate that 85% of hair replacement patients were happy and would repeat the procedure. Of the 15% who would not repeat the procedure and were not totally satisfied, ~90% did not complete the procedure as prescribed. Thus the vast majority of unhappy patients were those who failed to complete a minimum of work. With the advent of new techniques, a higher percentage of patients are satisfied, and the realm of treatable disorders has been extended.

Future Developments

Concerns about donor site morbidity (such as a widened scar), especially with the advent of short haircut styling, have led to the development of techniques to improve or eliminate donor area scars. Follicular unit extraction (FUE) was first described by Inaba in 1988. Multiple 1 mm punches are used to harvest hair in the occipital area. Using the small (1 mm) punches to remove individual follicular units in an irregular, diffuse fashion leaves donor defects so small that the resulting scars are undetectable. This affords patients the ability to trim the donor hair as short as desired, avoiding the donor defect scar that is a result of strip harvesting. The FUE defects heal spontaneously without any sutures. Drawbacks of FUE include increased operative time, limited number of obtained grafts (compared with conventional strip harvest), and increased potential for transection of follicles with reduced survival of grafted hair. FUE can be very time consuming, requiring up to 4 hours to harvest 1000 follicles.[19]

Suitable patients for follicular unit extraction include those desiring to keep a shaved or "buzz" donor area style haircut, those with a predisposition for widened scars, and those with tight scalps.

Recent attention has been directed toward improving and refining the resulting scar after conventional strip or block donor harvesting. The trichophytic incision technique can help minimize donor scar width by allowing hairs to grow through the residual scar thereby adding to the camouflage effect. After excising the donor strip, a small strip of superficial skin is excised from one side of the incision that only removes the top one third of the hair shaft. The deep, remaining bulbs will then grow through the new scar and yield a more inconspicuous, narrow scar.[20] This technique employs the same trichophytic concept that has been advocated to minimize the scar along the frontal hairline in the Mayer-Fleming flap as well and during brow lifting procedures.

Female Alopecia

Although male pattern alopecia continues to dominate the lay press and medical literature, female alopecia is commonly encountered by dermatologists.[13] There are three recognized patterns of hair loss. The first is a caudal and centrifugal pattern in which the frontal hairline is maintained. The second pattern closely resembles the "male" pattern of Norwood class III and IV. Finally, a "Christmas tree" pattern in which hair loss starts as a widened hair part but evolves into a zone of hair loss that is widest at the anterior and narrows in the posterior direction.[21] The most common presentation of female baldness is in the form of diffuse frontovertical thinning.[3] Women with a strong family history of alopecia may develop either the diffuse thinning or a male pattern loss. In this genetically predisposed subset, varying degrees of baldness may occur even when androgen levels are normal.

Women with scalp hair loss should always be evaluated with a thorough history and physical examination. Endocrine abnormalities should be investigated. Stress and emotional factors can also lead to temporary hair loss. However, the majority of women have no identifiable reason for the hair loss. If the woman has adequate donor density in the occipital area, hair transplantation can be utilized. Hair transplantation is especially useful to fill in vertex and frontovertex areas.

Recently, it has become feasible to treat females who have diffuse alopecia provided that they have adequate donor hair density in the occipital area. The use of smaller grafts in female pattern baldness has become a useful and effective method for increasing the apparent density of hair in females, particularly in the vertex and frontovertex areas (**Figs. 33.17 and 33.18**). Follicular unit grafts are interspersed between existing hairs, and the end result appears as an increase in density. With the technique of

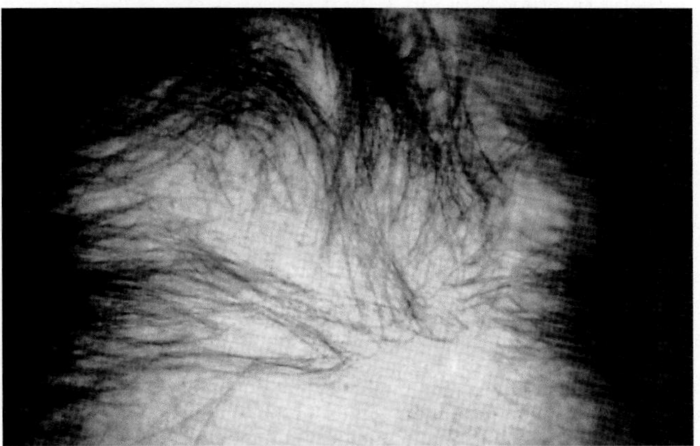

Fig. 33.17 Typical female pattern alopecia.

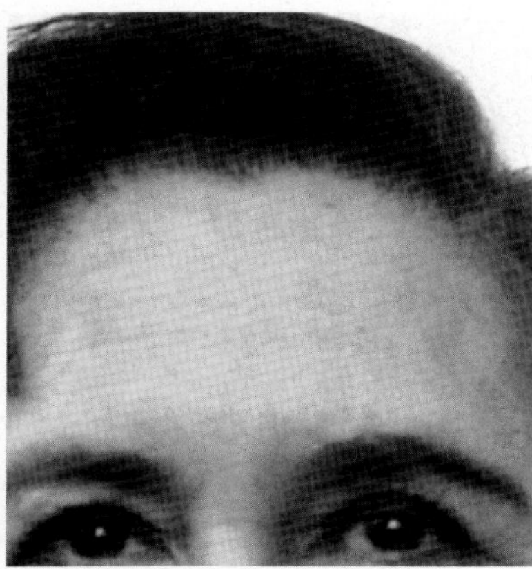

Fig. 33.18 The same patient as in **Fig. 33.17** after six sessions of incisional slit grafting.

incisional slit grafting, which removes no recipient bed tissue, there is maximum preservation of existing hairs.

In females with male pattern hair loss, the treatment and transplant approaches and objectives are the same or similar to those developed for male patients.

Summary

There has been a revolution in the field of hair transplantation. The older approaches that used large round grafts without attention to hair quality are now archaic. As a result of technological advances, treatment may now be provided for a wider range of hair loss etiologies and patterns. With today's techniques and sufficient attention to detail, hair restoration can approach its goal of the perfect transplant: a natural hairline and an overall appearance that offers little discernible evidence of surgical intervention.

References

1. Micheli-Pelligrini V. The history of hair. Facial Plast Surg 1985;2:167
2. Rousso DE. Hair replacement surgery and transplantation. Curr Opin Otolaryngol Head Neck Surg 1997;5:209–213
3. Olsen EA. Infectious, physical, and inflammatory causes of hair and scalp abnormalities. In: Disorders of Hair Growth: Diagnosis and Treatment. New York: McGraw-Hill 2003:87–123
4. Uno H, Cappas A, Schlagel C. Cyclic dynamics of hair follicles and the effect of minoxidil on the bald scalps of stump-tailed macaques. Am J Dermatopathol 1985;7:283
5. Olsen EA, Dunlap FE, Funicella T, et al. A randomized clinical trial of 5% topical minoxidil vs. 2% topical minoxidil and placebo in the treatment of androgenetic alopecia in males. J Am Acad Dermatol 2002;47:377–385
6. Olsen EA, Weiner MS. Topical minoxidil in male pattern baldness: effects of discontinuation of treatment. J Am Acad Dermatol 1987;17:97–101
7. Price VH, Menefee E, Sanchez M, et al. Changes in hair weight and hair count in men with androgenetic alopecia after treatment with finasteride 1 mg daily. J Am Acad Dermatol 2002;46:517–523
8. Fruzzetti F, de Loorenzo D, Parrini D, Ricci C. Effects of finasteride, a 5-alpha reductase inhibitor, on circulating androgens and gonadotropin secretion in hirsute women. J Clin Endocrinol Metab 1994;79:831–835
9. Stough D, Whitworth JM. Methodology of follicular unit hair transplantation. Dermatol Clin 1999;17:297–306
10. Norwood OT, Shiell RC. Hair Transplant Surgery. 2nd ed. Springfield, IL: Charles C Thomas; 1984
11. Hamilton JB. Patterned loss of hair in man: types and incidence. Ann N Y Acad Sci 1951;53:708
12. Stough DB, Abramson LJ, Strange P. A contemporary approach to male pattern alopecia. J Dermatol Surg Oncol 1987;13:756
13. Stough DB, Whitworth JM. Constructing the zig-zag hairline: architectural considerations. Poster presented at the International Society of Hair Restoration Surgery, October 1999
14. The donor site. In: Stough DB, Haber RS, eds. Hair Replacement: Surgical and Medical. St. Louis: Mosby; 1995:134
15. Anesthesia: nerve block anesthesia of the scalp. In: Stough DB, Haber RS, eds. Hair Replacement: Medical and Surgical. St. Louis: Mosby; 1995:89–93
16. Recipient site grafts and incisions. In: Unger WP, Shapiro R, eds. Hair Transplantation. New York: Marcel Dekker; 2004:383–533
17. Bernstein RM, Rassman WR, Stough D. In support of follicular unit transplantation. Dermatol Surg 2000;26:160–162
18. Flap F-M. (Modified after Juri). In: Mayer T, Fleming RW. Aesthetic and Reconstructive Surgery of the Scalp. St. Louis: Mosby; 1992: 122–123
19. Rassman WR, Bernstein RM, McClellan R, et al. Follicular unit extraction: minimally invasive surgery for hair transplantation. Dermatol Surg 2002;28:720–728
20. Straub P. How to make fine donor scars all the time. ESHRS 2004;4: 8–10
21. Venning VA, Dawber RPR. Patterned androgenic alopecia in women. J Am Acad Dermatol 1988;18:1073

34 Otoplasty

Nathan E. Nachlas

The plethora of otoplasty techniques that have appeared in the literature over the past century makes it a unique study in our field. More than 200 techniques to correct the lop-ear deformity have appeared since Ely's description of this procedure in 1881.[1] As with all facial plastic surgical techniques, the modern themes of conservatism and minimalism have dominated recent studies.

Otoplasty is the surgical correction of the lop-ear deformity. Analogous to rhinoplasty, achieving the optimal result begins with a three-dimensional analysis of the deformity. Surgical correction requires relating the components of the auricle to the underlying bony skeleton. Furthermore, these components—the helix–antihelix, concha, tragus–antitragus, and lobule—must be evaluated preoperatively and placed in harmony intraoperatively to maintain a natural auricular appearance.

Historical Overview

Deformities of the auricle have inspired much creative analysis over the years. In fact, certain characteristics (e.g., prominent Darwin's tubercles and flattened helical margins) have been suggested as predisposing to criminal behavior.[2] The particular deformity addressed in this chapter is actually a group of deformities that have a common overall appearance of the prominent auricle. This may result from the classic absence of the antihelix, from overprojection of the concha, or from a combination of these deformities. Less frequently a twisted or overprojected lobule may exacerbate the deformity.

Since the nineteenth century, techniques have been described to restore the normal relationship of the auricle to the scalp and underlying mastoid bone. The first written description of otoplasty is attributed to Ely, who reduced a prominent ear by excising a through-and-through piece of auricle consisting of anterior auricular skin, auricular cartilage, and posterior auricular skin.[1] Similar techniques followed (Haug, Monks, Joseph, Ballenger, and Ballenger), all involving a reduction approach to otoplasty that attempted to reduce prominent ears by the removal of skin or cartilage.

In 1910, Luckett correctly attributed the classic lop-ear deformity to the absence of the antihelical fold.[3] This new revelation as to the correct anatomical defect enabled him and subsequent authors to devise correction techniques. Earlier techniques involved incisions in the auricular cartilage anterior and posterior to the desired antihelix position. In Luckett's technique, a crescent-shaped excision of skin and cartilage was performed at the site of the intended antihelix. The remaining cartilage edges were then sutured. Becker's technique also included anterior and posterior incisions around the intended antihelix. He then formed the new antihelix with fixation sutures and posterior abrasion.[4] A further variation is seen in the technique of Converse, whereby the anterior and posterior incisions were followed by suturing the antihelical segment to form a tunnel.[5]

Modern techniques stress the importance of avoiding the surgical appearance. Visible edges of cartilage are to be avoided, and a smooth, pleasantly shaped auricle in normal relation to the skull is desired. We discuss the pertinent anatomy and embryology and then outline the two basic approaches to otoplasty—cartilage suturing and cartilage sculpting—and the multiple variations that have been developed for both techniques.

Anatomy and Embryology

The external ear is a cartilaginous structure except for the lobule, which contains no cartilage (**Fig. 34.1**). This flexible elastic cartilage is covered with skin, which is closely adherent anteriorly and more loosely attached posteriorly. The plate of cartilage has a definite shape and may be described as a combination of ridges and hollows incompletely surrounding the bony external auditory canal.

The normal auricle protrudes 20 to 30 degrees from the skull (**Fig. 34.2**). When measured from the lateral edge of the helix to the mastoid skin, this distance is usually 2.0 to 2.5 cm. When analyzed from a superior viewpoint, the angulation is seen to result from a combination of a conchomastoid angle of 90 degrees and a conchoscaphalic angle of 90 degrees. The average length and width of the male auricle are 63.5 and 35.5 mm, respectively. Corresponding measurements in the female are 59.0 and 32.5 mm.[6,7]

Analysis of the convolutions of the normal auricle begins with the helix and antihelix. They begin inferiorly at the level of the tragus and diverge as they extend superiorly. They are separated through their course by the scaphoid fossa. As the antihelix is followed superiorly, it divides into a smoother, wider superior crus and an inferior crus, which characteristically is narrower and sharper. The fossa triangularis lies between the superior crus and the inferior crus. From the frontal viewpoint, the helix forms the most

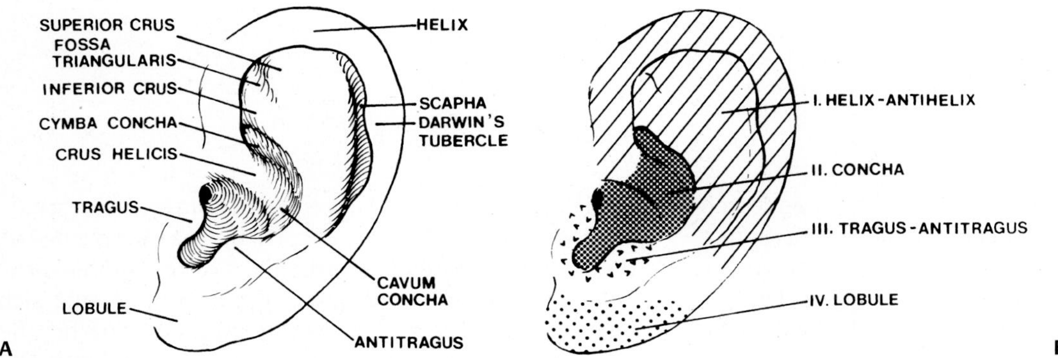

Fig. 34.1 (**A**) Landmarks of the normal auricle. (**B**) Four components of the auricle.

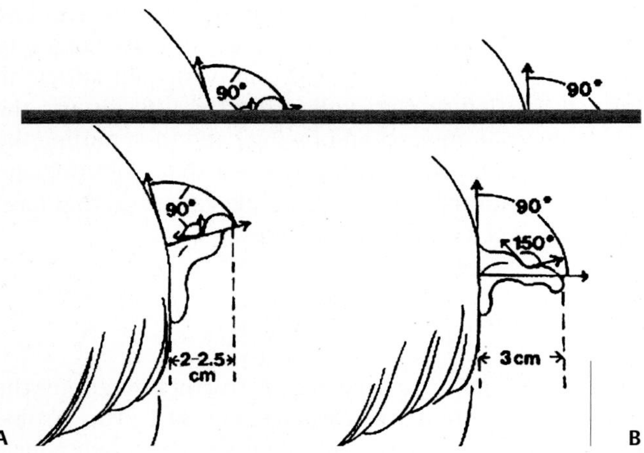

Fig. 34.2 Relationship of auricle to scalp. (**A**) Axial view of the normal ear demonstrating the relationship of the auricle to the scalp. The conchomastoid angle of 90 degrees is combined with the conchoscaphalic angle of 90 degrees. This produces the auriculomastoid angle of 30 degrees. (**B**) Analogous angles demonstrated in the lop ear with conchoscaphalic obtuse angle of 140 to 150 degrees.

lateral extent of the auricle superiorly and should be just visible behind the antihelix and superior crus.

The cartilage is attached to the skull by three ligaments. The anterior ligament attaches the helix and tragus to the zygomatic process of the temporal bone. The front portion of the cartilaginous external auditory canal is free of cartilage but is bridged by a ligament passing from the tragus to the helix.

The ear has both intrinsic and extrinsic muscles supplied by the seventh cranial nerve. These small muscle masses form in definite areas and create soft tissue thickness with an associated increase in blood supply. These muscles have essentially no function, although some people can wiggle their ears.

Fig. 34.3 depicts the arterial blood supply of the auricle. Contributions are primarily from the superficial temporal artery and the posterior auricular artery, although some branches also feed from the deep auricular artery. Venous drainage is via the superficial temporal and posterior auricular veins. Lymphatic drainage is to preauricular and superficial cervical nodes.

Sensory innervation to the external ear is derived from multiple sources (**Fig. 34.4**). The auriculotemporal

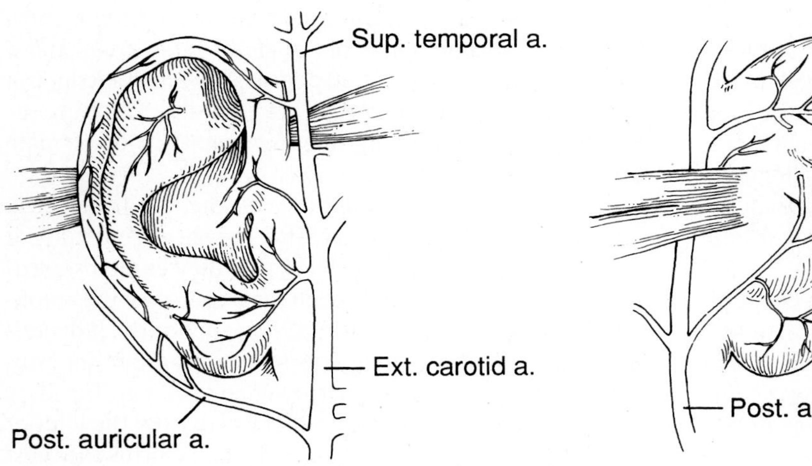

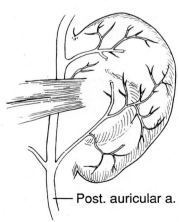

Fig. 34.3 Arterial blood supply of the external ear.

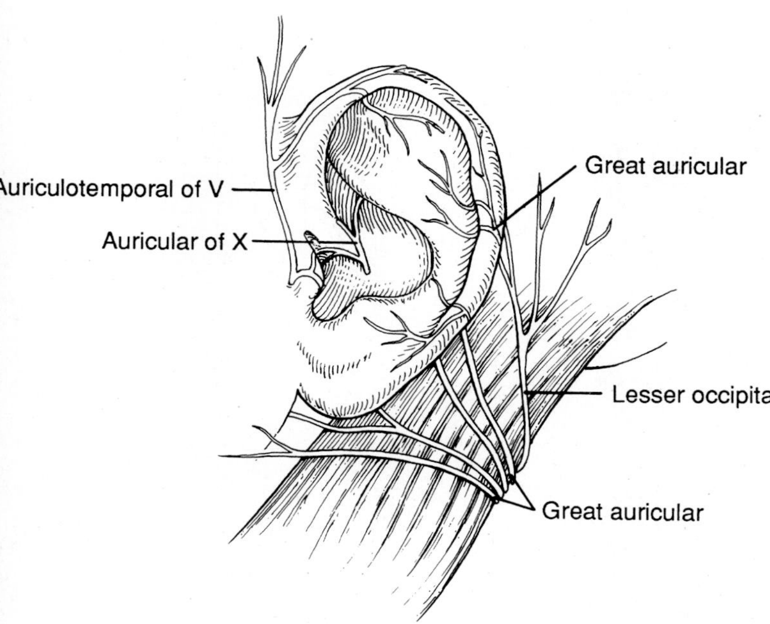

Fig. 34.4 Nerve distribution to the external ear.

branch of the mandibular division of the fifth cranial nerve supplies the anterior limb of the helix and part of the tragus. The remainder of the anterior auricle is supplied chiefly from the greater auricular nerve, whereas the posterior surface receives its innervation from the lesser occipital nerve. Minor contributions are also made from the seventh, ninth, and tenth cranial nerves.

The *hillocks of His* refers to a description by that author of six visible protruberances in the 39-day embryo that develop into the auricle. Although His originally traced the origin of the first three hillocks to the first branchial arch and that of the second three hillocks to the second branchial arch, subsequent studies have challenged this theory. It now appears that only the tragus may be traced to the first branchial arch and that the remainder of the auricle is derived from the second branchial arch (**Fig. 34.5**). This is supported by the location of congenital preauricular pits and fistulae located along the anterior incisura and incisura intertragica. Because these regions anatomically represent the dividing line between the first and second branchial arches, these anomalies would therefore arise from the first pharyngeal depression.[2,8,9] The majority of auricular deformities are inherited in an autosomal dominant pattern.[10] Similar inheritance patterns are also seen in preauricular pits and appendages.

Function

The function of the auricle in lower animals has been extensively studied.[4] Sound localization and protection against water entry are two of the documented functions. Water protection is afforded by apposition of the tragus and antitragus. These physiological functions are not documented in humans.

Preoperative Evaluation

Like all facial plastic surgical procedures, otoplasty requires precise preoperative evaluation and analysis. Each ear must be evaluated separately because the deformity or deformities present may be very different between the two ears. The auricle should be evaluated as to its size, its relationship to the scalp, and the interrelationship between its four components (helix, antihelix, concha, and lobule). Typical measurements recorded during the preoperative examination include the following:

1. The mastoid–helical distance as measured at the superior aspect of the helix
2. The mastoid–helical distance as measured at the level of the external auditory canal
3. The mastoid–helical distance as measured at the level of the lobule

Additional measurements included by some authors are the distance from the top of the helical rim to the junction of the inferior and superior crus, and the distance from the helical rim to the antihelix (**Fig. 34.6**).

Preoperative photographs include an anterior full-face view, a posterior full-head view, and close-up photographs of the involved ear(s) with the head positioned so that the Frankfort plane is parallel to the floor.

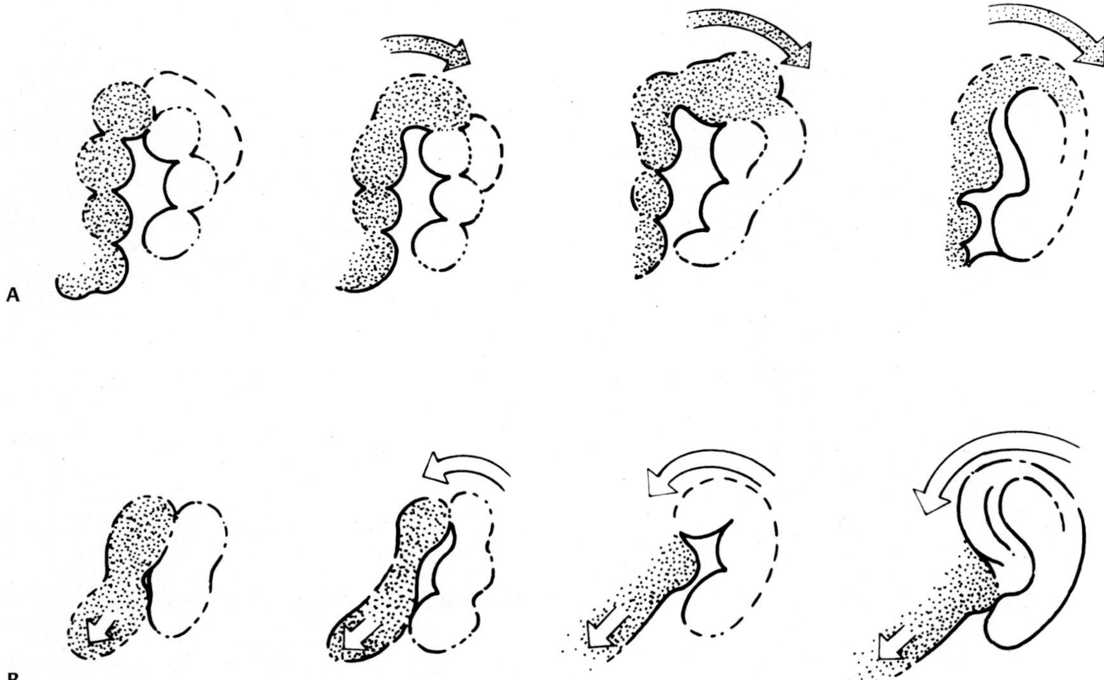

Fig. 34.5 Embryology of the auricle. (**A**) In the original description by His, the auricle is derived equally from the first and second branchial arches. In this theory, the first three hillocks were derived from the first branchial arch, whereas hillocks four through six were derived from the second branchial arch. This would place the division between the first and second branchial arches at the tuberculum auriculae. (**B**) Current embryologic theory as described by Wood-Jones and I-Chuan.[9] In this description, the first branchial arch contribution is limited to the tragus. In this theory, the separation between the first and second arch contributions would lie along the anterior incisure and the intertragic incisure.

The abnormality most commonly observed in the protruding ear is the overgrowth or protrusion of the conchal cartilage. Such deformities are not corrected by otoplasty techniques designed to re-create the antihelix. These ears require an alteration of the relationship between the concha and the mastoid cortex. Protuberan lobules may be the only deformity present in an other wise normal ear. This may be secondary to an abnormall shaped cauda helicis (**Fig. 34.7**).

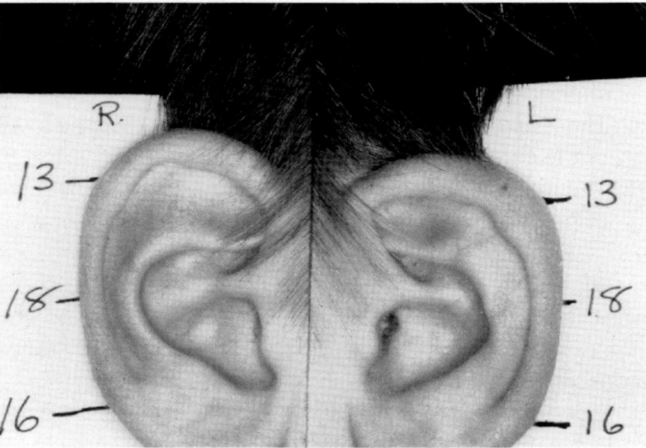

Fig. 34.6 Right and left normal ears, showing distances in millimeters from the mastoid skin to the anterior surface of the ear at the top, midportion, and lobule. (Courtesy of Smith and Keen.)

Surgical Techniques

The typical patient for otoplasty is a young child, age 4 t 5 years, who is referred by the pediatrician or parents fo overprojecting auricles. This is the ideal age for correctio because the auricle is fully developed, and the child ha not yet entered school where he or she would be subjec to peer ridicule.

In the young child, general anesthesia is most ofte utilized. In older children and adults, intravenous seda tion is preferred. The patient is placed on a headrest wit both ears exposed during the procedure.

The surgical techniques used in correction of th lop-ear deformity are dependent on the preoperativ analysis. Often conchal protrusion is present, either as th lone deformity or, more commonly, associated with a antihelical deformity.

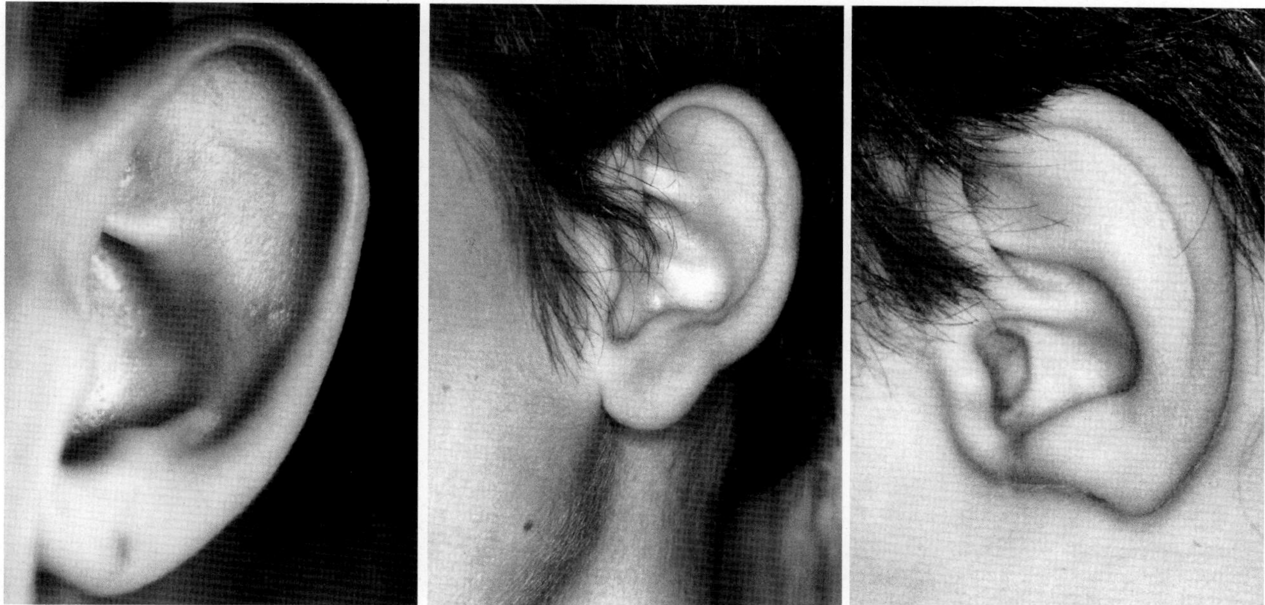

Fig. 34.7 Examples of prominent ears. (**A**) Classic lop ear. The concha and lobule are normal in appearance. (**B**) Combined conchal-antihelical deformity. Correction requires conchal setback followed by antihelical correction. (**C**) An example of congenital lobule deformity, which requires primarily soft tissue techniques for correction.

Conchal Setback

Returning the concha to its correct anatomical position with respect to the mastoid bone is accomplished with sutures, with or without concomitant trimming of the lateral aspect of the concha cavum. The traditional conchal setback technique as originally described by Furnas[11] remains the technique of choice for conchal protrusion. This technique involves wide exposure of the posterior auricular surface as well as the mastoid periosteum. Permanent sutures (author's preference 4–0 Mersilene, Ethicon, Inc., Somerville, NJ) are placed through the conchal cartilage and then through the mastoid periosteum in such a manner as to fix the concha in a posterior and medial direction. Care must be taken not to place the mastoid periosteal suture too far anteriorly or the external auditory canal may be compromised (**Fig. 34.8**). Additional correction of conchal protuberance may be achieved by removing a lateral strip of conchal cartilage. By delineating the lateral extent of the conchal cartilage with anteriorly placed 25-gauge needles tattooed with methylene blue, an incision may be made in the lateral extent of the conchal bowl. An elliptical wedge of conchal cartilage may then be removed to allow additional medialization of the auricle.

An alternative conchal procedure is described by Spira and Stal.[12] In this lateral flap technique, a laterally based flap of conchal cartilage is developed and subsequently sutured posteriorly to the mastoid periosteum (**Fig. 34.9**). Proponents suggest that this decreases the likelihood of compromise of the external canal.

Antihelix Deformities

The plethora of procedures described to re-create a missing antihelix underscores the lack of total satisfaction with any one technique. As otoplasty techniques were developed in the middle of the twentieth century, two schools of thought emerged. The first, following the teachings of Mustarde,[13] performed the procedure using sutures to re-create the antihelix. The second group of techniques all involved surgical alteration of the cartilage, whether through incisions, dermabrasion, or scoring. Most current techniques represent a combination of the two, using sutures to fix the final position of the antihelix but adding a cartilage-modifying technique to lower the risk of reprotrusion.

Suture Techniques

For most otoplasty procedures, the exposure and landmark identification are similar. A postauricular incision is made and wide undermining performed in the supraperichondrial plane. The area of intended neoantihelix may be demarcated by placing 25-gauge needles through the anterior auricular skin at the intended site of antihelix creation and bringing the

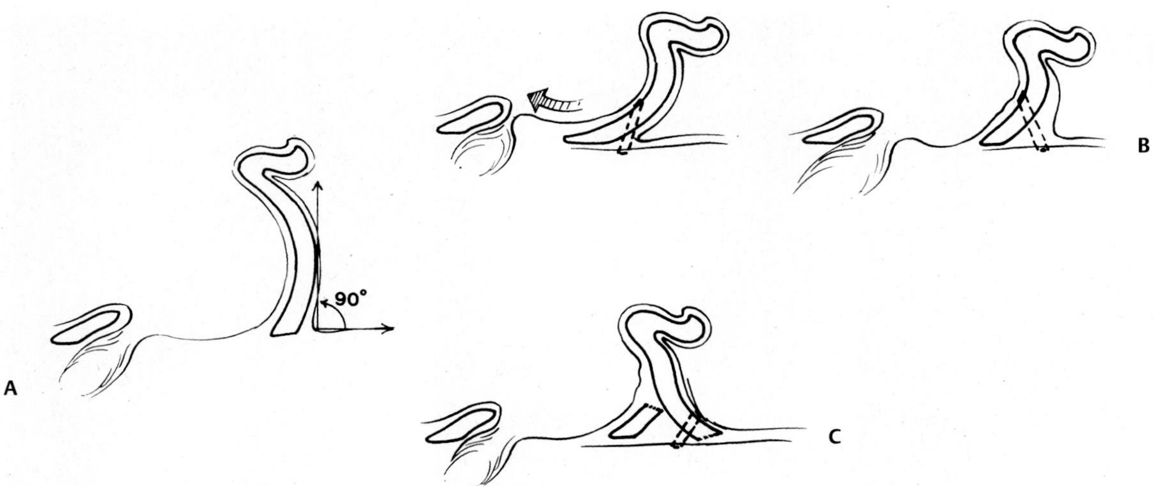

Fig. 34.8 Conchal setback techniques. (**A**) The conchal suture technique as described by Furnas.[11] This demonstrates improper suture technique, where the mastoid periosteal suture is placed too far anteriorly and the external auditory canal is compromised. (**B**) Correct suture placement in the Furnas technique. The mastoid periosteal suture is placed far enough posteriorly to provide adequate correction without compromise of the external canal. (**C**) The lateral flap technique as described by Spira and Stal.[12] In this technique, a laterally based conchal cartilage flap is developed and sutured to the posterior mastoid periosteum.

needle out posteriorly. The cartilage is then marked with methylene blue.

The Mustarde procedure consists of inserting three or four horizontal placement sutures to permanently recreate the antihelix. We have found 4–0 Mersilene to be most suited for this purpose, but a wide variety of sutures have been reported. The suture placement

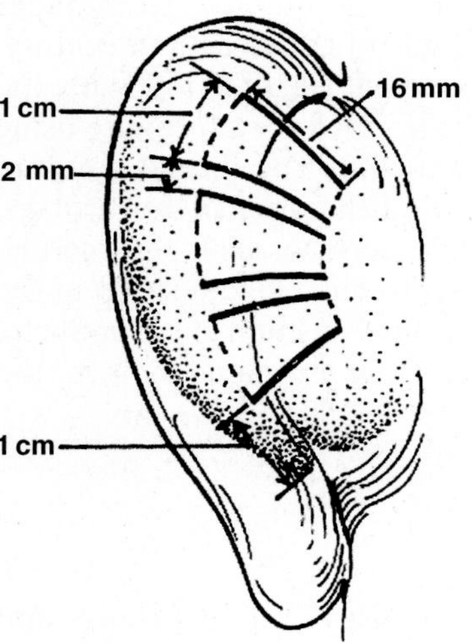

Fig. 34.9 Mustarde's suture otoplasty technique. Posterior view of the auricle demonstrating suture placement in the mattress suture technique of Mustarde. The sutures must be placed through cartilage and anterior perichondrium but not through the anterior skin. They should be placed close enough together that the ear does not buckle when they are secured. Dimensions cited are from Bull and Mustarde.[14]

is critical to achieve smooth correction and to avoid buckling of the superior auricle.[14] The suture is placed through the cartilage and anterior perichondrium but not through the anterior skin. If the suture does not incorporate the anterior perichondrium, then there is the risk of pulling through the cartilage. If the suture is placed too far anteriorly, then it may catch the underside of the anterior auricular dermis and an ulceration at the insertion site may result.

Suture placement should mimic the suggestions by Bull and Mustarde[14] as closely as possible. The sutures must be placed close enough to each other to avoid buckling. If placed too closely, then the cartilage may weaken between suture sites. Furthermore, if the outer bite of the suture is too close to the auricular summit, then a postlike deformity may result. The measurements in **Fig. 34.8** are from Bull and Mustarde.[14] They propose outer cartilage bites of 1 cm separated by 2 mm. The distance between outer and inner cartilage bites is 16 mm. The most inferior stitch should be placed to allow retrodisplacement of the cauda helicis. In some cases, this is actually trimmed.

The technical challenges in the standard Mustarde otoplasty all relate to accuracy of suture placement. Securing the sutures is often done blindly, with the surgeon gauging the appropriate tightness of the suture by observing the folding of the antihelix from the anterior aspect of the auricle. All sutures should be placed prior to final tightening. Several authors have described a technique using temporary sutures placed anteriorly to fix the desired antihelix into place while the posterior sutures are being secured.[15–17] Burres described the "anterior–posterior" technique whereby the conchal setback is performed through a posterior incision but the helical sutures are placed anteriorly through a series of anterior stab incisions.[15] Alternatively, these sutures may be placed externally but buried through small stab incisions.[18] The scores of adjunctive procedures described since Mustarde's original paper[13] mostly address the tendency of the auricle to reprotrude over time. This results from several factors. First, incorrect placement of the suture whereby it does not include an adequate bite of cartilage results in tearing of the cartilage and reprotrusion. Second, failure to include perichondrium in the suture promotes cartilage tearing. Assuming that great care is taken to assure correct suture placement, the most common reason for reprotrusion is resilience of the cartilage. Therefore different maneuvers have been described to lessen this memory. Adhering to physiological principles, scoring of the anterior surface of the auricle would promote bending of the cartilage in the desired direction. The original studies for this derive from the work of Gibson and Davis,[19] who showed that scored rib cartilage would bend in the opposite direction. Using rib cartilage, they demonstrated that if one side of the rib was denuded of perichondrium, then the cartilage would bow to the side with the perichondrium intact. When attempting to create a new antihelix from a flat piece of auricular cartilage, weakening the anterior surface of the cartilage produces bowing with a convex anterior surface. Scoring the anterior surface of the auricular cartilage at the site of the new antihelix may be done with a needle, an abrader, or a burr. Care must be taken not to be overly aggressive in this maneuver or sharp edges could be evident. Exposure to the anterior surface may be achieved by an anterior auricular incision, undermining around the helical rim through a postauricular incision, or in the technique described by Spira, scoring the cartilage with a needle introduced by a stab incision anteriorly. Spira describes his modification in more than 200 otoplasty cases with minimal complications.[20]

Burring down the posterior surface of the auricle is technically simpler than the anterior techniques because the exposure has already been accomplished. Physiologically, the cartilage will have a tendency to bend in the direction opposite to that desired for the neoantihelix, but the suture placement readily overcomes this. More than 300 otoplasties were performed by Pilz and associates, with reported excellent results.[21]

Cartilage Sculpting Techniques

The cartilage sculpting techniques date back to the very first otoplasty procedures.[1] They have in common a reshaping of the auricular cartilage. If done successfully, these procedures do not require permanent suture placement. This lessens the foreign body–related risks associated with Mustarde procedures.

The cartilage-splitting otoplasty technique was originally described by Nachlas and associates in 1970.[22] Based on earlier work by Cloutier,[23] this procedure utilizes the Gibson and Davis principle to form the new antihelix. The incision is a standard postauricular incision, whose placement is determined following the placement of 25-gauge needles tattooed with methylene blue through the intended neoantihelix (**Fig. 34.10**). An elliptical piece of skin is usually excised. Sometimes an hourglass-shaped excision is performed if there is a prominent earlobe. The needles are then withdrawn. Standard wide postauricular undermining is then performed, exposing the cauda helicis, fossa antihelicis scapha, and conchal cartilage. An incision through the auricular cartilage is then made with a Cottle knife. This incision should be made ~5 mm anterior to the tattoo marks indicating the apex of the neoantihelix. The incision will be curvilinear, parallel to the helical rim, and extend from ~5 mm from the superior aspect of the helical rim to the cauda helicis. Resection of the cauda helicis helps to eliminate postoperative bowing of the lobule. Triangular wedges are removed perpendicular to the superior and inferior edges of the cut. At this point in the dissection, the lateral segment of cartilage is attached to its medial counterpart only at the superior rim. The perichondrium is dissected off of the anterior surface of the cartilage for a distance of 1 cm. The anterior surface of the medial cartilage is then burred, using a diamond burr, until a round smooth neoantihelix and superior crus is formed. The anterior surface of the lateral cartilage is also beveled. The medial beveled cartilage is placed anterior to the lateral cartilage, restoring the normal contour of the ear. No sutures are placed in the cartilage. The skin is closed using a running subcuticular closure.

In the cartilage-splitting otoplasty technique, the cut edges of cartilage are facing posteriorly; the only cartilage surface visible on the anterior aspect of the auricle is the smooth convexity of the new antihelix. A modification of the technique was described by Schuffenecker and Reichert utilizing a large V-shaped cartilaginous flap at the site of the intended antihelix.[24] Instead of the single curved cartilage incision at the site of the new antihelix, they elevate a flap of cartilage hinged superiorly. The desired convexity is then achieved by scoring the anterior surface with a blade.

Choosing the right otoplasty technique depends on the surgeon's comfort level and experience with any one procedure. For the beginning otoplasty surgeon, the Mustarde technique is the most straightforward. Weakening

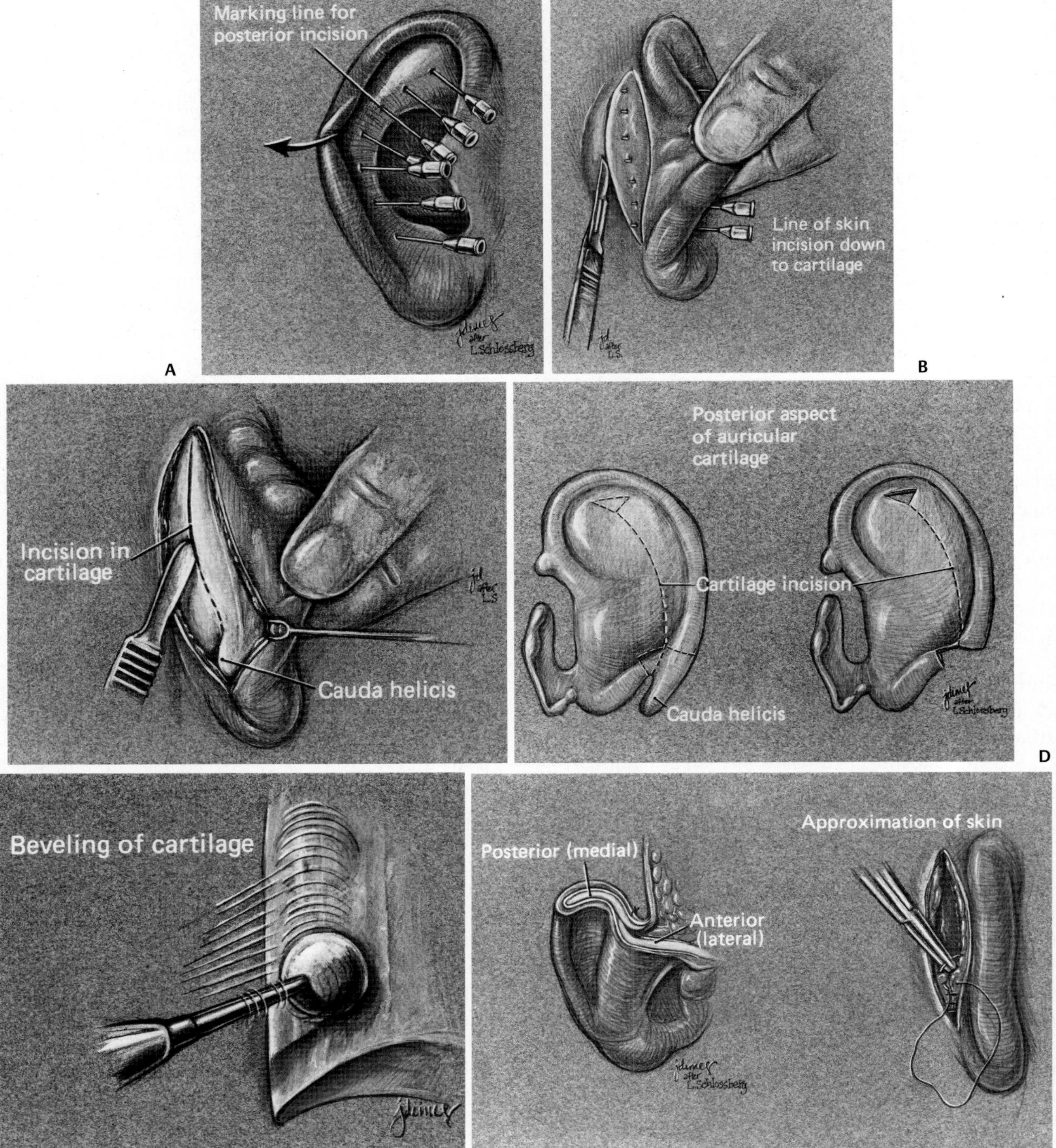

Fig. 34.10 Cartilage-splitting otoplasty. (**A**) The ear is folded in a normal position. Using 25-gauge needles, the auricle is penetrated from an anterior to posterior direction at the line of the proposed new antihelix. The needles are then tattooed with methylene blue. This tattoos both the posterior skin and the auricular cartilage. (**B**) On an elliptical piece of skin is placed a mark ~1 cm in width. This may be altered to an hourglass incision if there is a prominent ear lobe. (**C**) The posterior aspect of the auricular cartilage, showing the incision in the cartilage following wide undermining. The incision should be ~4 mm laterally to the previous cartilage tattoo marks. (**D**) The relationship of the cartilaginous incision to the auricular cartilage landmarks. Note the resection of the caudal helicis. Also note the inverted triangle at the superior aspect of the cartilaginous incision. This allows overlapping of the segments later without buckling. (**E**) Beveling of the anterior aspect of the lateral and medial cartilaginous flaps. Beveling is accomplished using a diamond bur. Beveling is done until the cartilage assumes a gradual convexity approximating the appearance of a normal antihelix. (**F**) Overlapping of the lateral segment over the medial segment of cartilage is done, restoring the normal contour to the ear. No sutures are placed in the cartilage. The skin is closed with a running subcuticular stitch.

the posterior cartilage with the diamond abrader adds little difficulty to the procedure and greatly lowers the risks of reprotrusion. In more demanding cases, the cartilage-splitting otoplasty in this author's hands allows more predictable results while avoiding suture complications associated with the Mustarde techniques.

Irrespective of the otoplasty technique utilized, proper dressing of the ears is critical in maintaining position of the auricles without undue stress. Cotton soaked in mineral oil is placed in the grooves of the auricle to prevent postoperative anterior edema. Kerlix fluffs (Tyco Healthcare, Chicopee, MA) followed by a Kerlix wrap, followed by Coban taping (3M Health Care, St. Paul, MN) is routinely performed. The use of drains is recommended. The ears are inspected on the first postoperative day. The patient is instructed to bring a tennis headband to the office at the time of the first dressing change. The surgeon positions this headband after removal of the dressings, and it is left in place until suture removal 1 week later. The patient is instructed to wear the headband at night for 2 months following the procedure to avoid inadvertent distraction of the auricle.

Results

Otoplasty in general is a highly satisfying operation both to the patient and to the surgeon. Achieving symmetry between the ears and producing ears with smooth convolutions and grooves are the goals of otoplasty (**Figs. 34.11–34.15**). Because these results may be achieved with any of several techniques, it becomes increasingly important to select a technique that is associated with the fewest complications and the best long-term results. Many authors have satisfactory results with a large variety of techniques, so the selection of the particular technique is probably not as critical as facility with that technique.

Complications

Early Complications

The most feared early complications of otoplasty are hematoma and infection. Cartilage necrosis may result from the excess pressure placed on the auricular cartilage by a hematoma. Infection may lead to perichondritis and suppurative chondritis, with resulting necrosis and deformity of the auricular cartilage. The incidence of hematoma is around 1%. In a series of 3200 ears treated with a cartilage sculpting technique, Schuffenecker and Reichert reported two incidences of hematoma.[24]

Avoiding hematoma formation begins with a careful preoperative documentation of bleeding or bruising tendencies. In the absence of clinical or family history suggestive of a bleeding disorder, coagulation studies are not performed routinely. Intraoperatively, a bipolar cautery is used to avoid necrosis of the auricular cartilage. In cases of bilateral otoplasty, the first ear must be treated with a conforming soaked-cotton dressing before the contralateral side is treated. After the contralateral otoplasty is performed, the initial ear must be reexamined

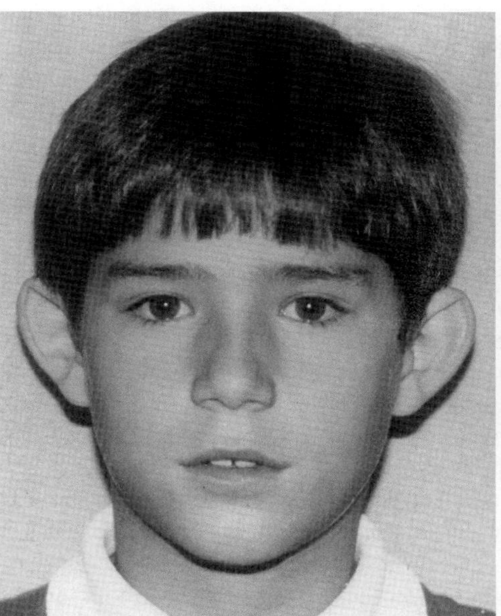
A

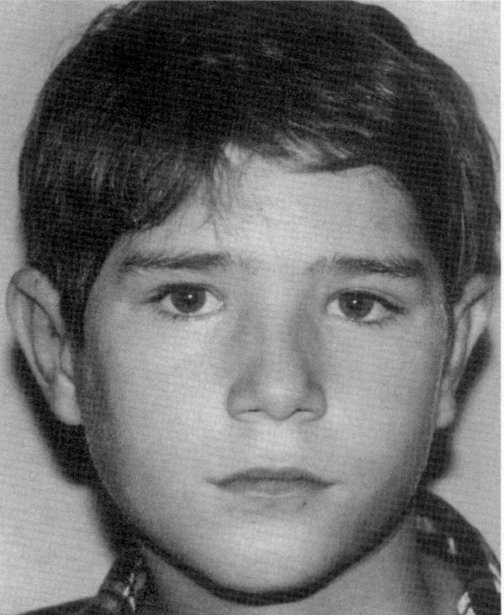
B

Fig. 34.11 A 10-year-old boy with bilateral auricular deformity. (**A**) Preoperative and (**B**) postoperative frontal view following cartilage-splitting otoplasty.

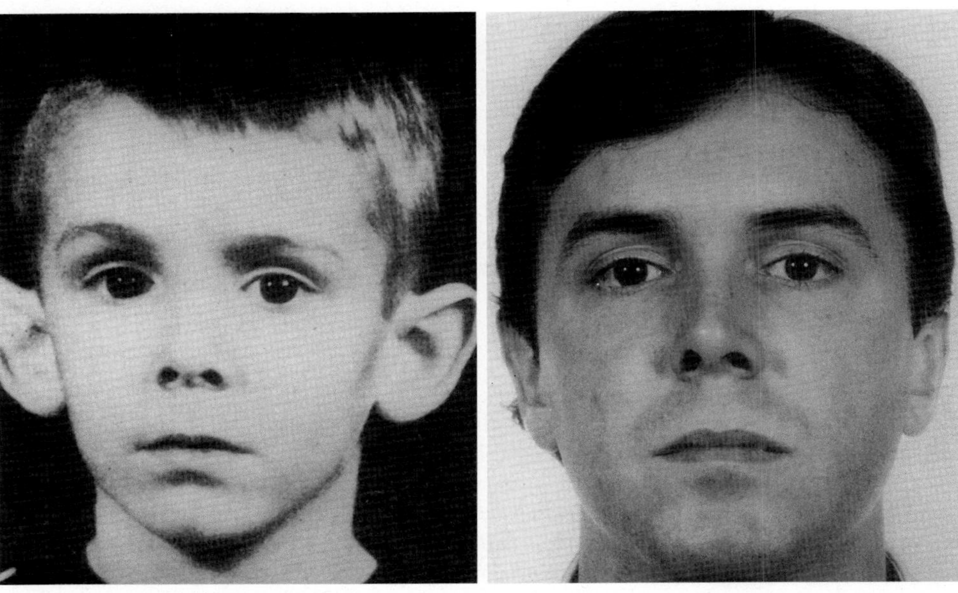

Fig. 34.12 A 5-year-old boy with bilateral auricular deformity. (**A**) Preoperative and (**B**) 18-year follow-up showing maintained correction following cartilage-splitting otoplasty.

to ensure that no hematoma has formed. A small rubber-band drain is left in the postauricular sulcus and is brought out through the incision until the first dressing change.

Unilateral pain is the earliest warning sign of developing hematoma. In general, the otoplasty patient is in minimal discomfort during the first 48 hours after surgery. Any unusual discomfort should be investigated by removing all bandages and inspecting the wounds. The presence of a hematoma necessitates reopening the wound, controlling the bleeding, irrigating with an antibiotic solution, and reapplying the dressing.

Wound infections usually manifest on postoperative day 3 or 4. Erythema of the wound with pustular drainage may be present in the absence of significant pain. Wound infection must be treated aggressively before perichondritis or chondritis occurs. Administration of systemic antibiotics, including coverage for *Pseudomonas aeruginosa*, is required in these cases. Suppurative chondritis is a rare but serious complication in which the infection has spread into the cartilage, with resulting necrosis and resorption. The heralding sign is pain, and it is deep and boring in nature. The physical findings are often unimpressive compared with the symptoms. The diagnosis is established after conservative methods have failed to control wound infection. Treatment principles include systemic antibiotics, again covering for *Pseudomonas*, debridement, and wide drainage. Repeated conservative debridements are usually required. Resolution of the infection is evidenced by amelioration of the pain and improvement in wound appearance. Long-term sequelae of chondritis can be devastating. Cartilage necrosis leads to permanent auricular deformity.

Late Complications

Late complications after otoplasty include suture extrusion and aesthetic complications. Suture extrusion is not uncommon following Mustarde procedures and may occur at anytime in the postoperative period. It may result from incorrect suture placement, from excess tension on the auricular cartilage, or from infection. Treatment is the removal of the offending suture(s). Early suture extrusion requires revision surgery to restore the correction. Later extrusions may not require revision surgery because the auricle may retain the corrected shape.

Aesthetic complications include abnormalities in the relationship of the auricle to the scalp and distortion of the auricle itself. The former category includes inadequate correction of the protruding ear, reprotrusion, and overcorrection. Distortions of the auricle include telephone deformity, reverse telephone deformity, auricular buckling, visible cartilage edges, and bowstringing of sutures.

Inadequate correction may result from error in diagnosis. Ears whose main deformity is conchal protrusion will not be corrected by techniques designed to re-create the antihelix. Accuracy of preoperative and intraoperative measurements is critical in achieving the degree of correction desired. Other possible factors include suture extrusion and loosening of sutures. Some degree of reprotrusion secondary

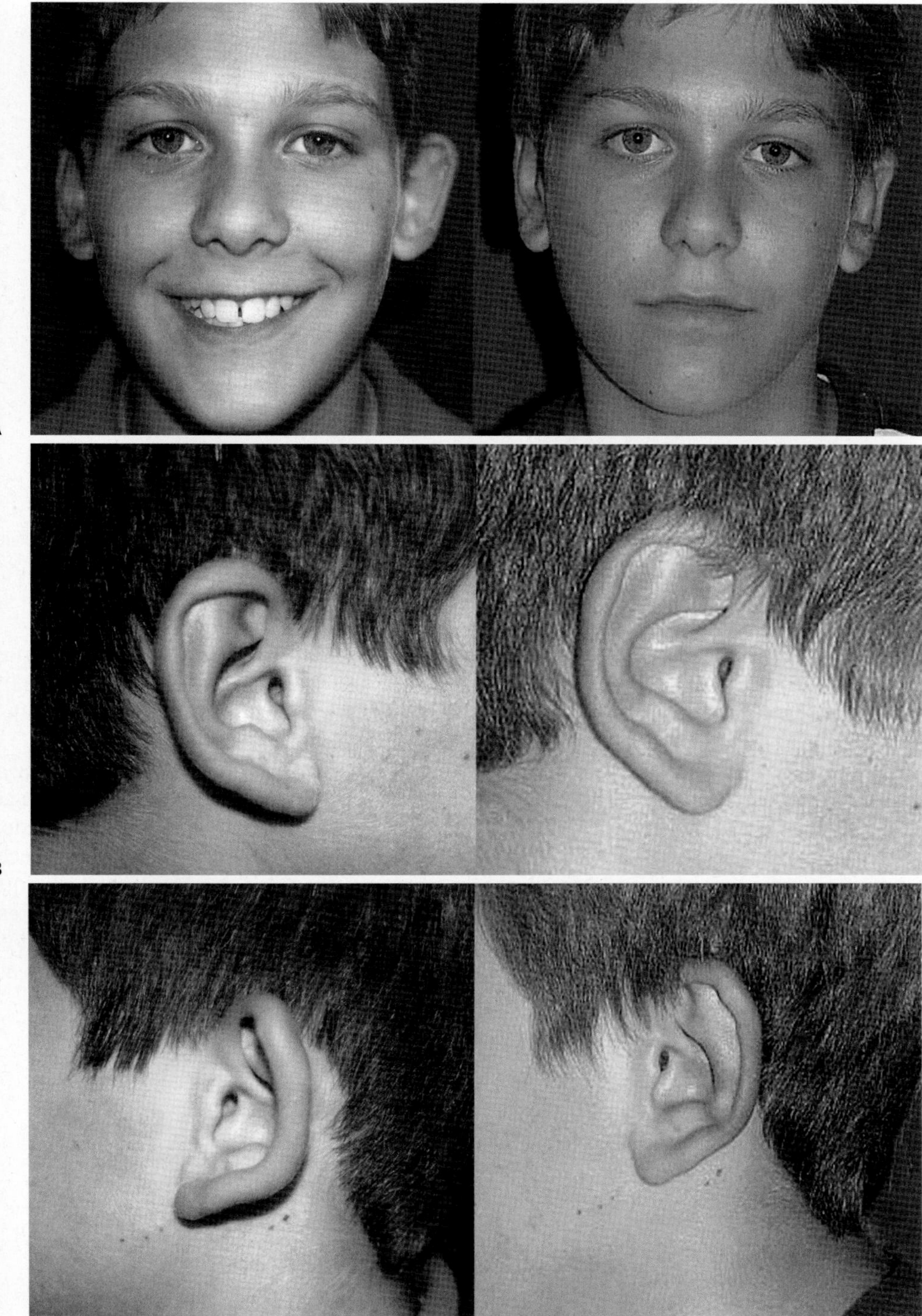

Fig. 34.13 A 10-year-old boy with asymmetric auricular deformity. Left auricle demonstrates marked auricular and conchal deformity. The right auricle was over protruding secondary to conchal deformity. Bilateral conchal setbacks were performed. The left ear also had a modified Mustarde procedure with posterior cartilage abrasion. (**A**) to (**C**) Preoperative (left) and postoperative (right) frontal, right auricle, and left auricle views.

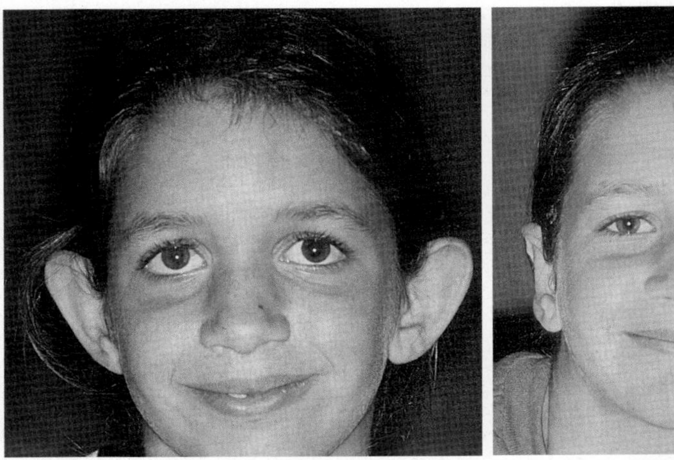

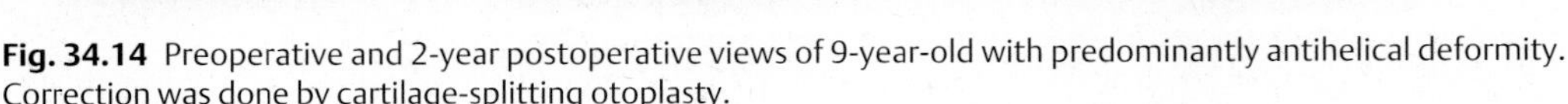

Fig. 34.14 Preoperative and 2-year postoperative views of 9-year-old with predominantly antihelical deformity. Correction was done by cartilage-splitting otoplasty.

to cartilage memory is reported in most ears corrected by a suture-only technique. Stal and Spira[25] report some degree of reprotrusion in all cases, most noticeably in the upper pole. Overzealous correction of the protruding ear can lead to flattening of the ear against the scalp. This is often more worrisome to the surgeon than to the patient but nevertheless can be avoided by careful intraoperative measurements.

The telephone deformity of the auricle describes an unnatural result where the middle third of the auricle is overcorrected with respect to the superior and inferior poles. This is often seen following an aggressive conchal setback where the superior pole is undercorrected. An undertreated protuberant cauda helicis may also contribute to telephone deformity. Reverse telephone deformity occurs when the midauricle protrudes after adequate or overcorrection of the superior pole and lobule. This may result from an untreated conchal protrusion. Secondary correction of either deformity may lead to excessive setback of the auricle.

Buckling of the auricular cartilage is seen with suture techniques where the sutures are placed too far apart. This may be avoided by adhering to the recommended measurements for this technique.[14]

Unsightly postauricular scars range from bowstringing of the sutures to keloid formation (**Fig. 34.16**). Bowstringing is seen only in suture otoplasty, where excess suture tension causes draping of the skin around the sutures. This produces an unsightly postauricular scar. Any otoplasty technique where the postauricular incision is closed under excess tension may result in hypertrophy of the scar. Keloid formation is unusual, although its incidence in black patients

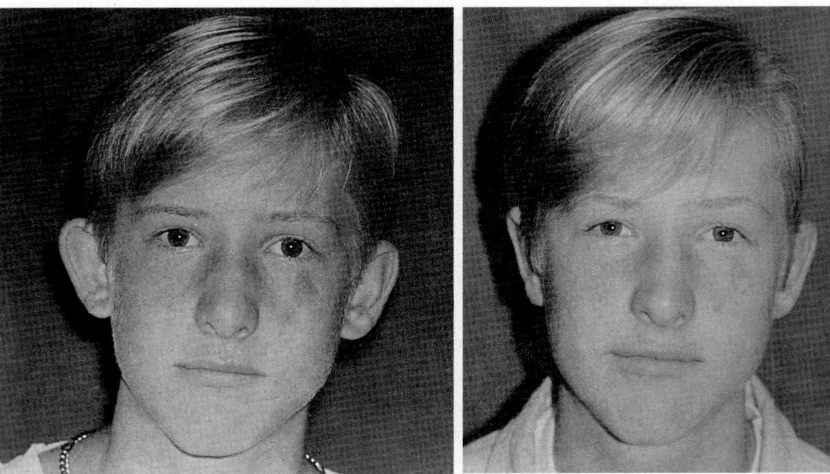

Fig. 34.15 Preoperative and 2-year postoperative views of adolescent with antihelical deformity corrected with cartilage-splitting otoplasty.

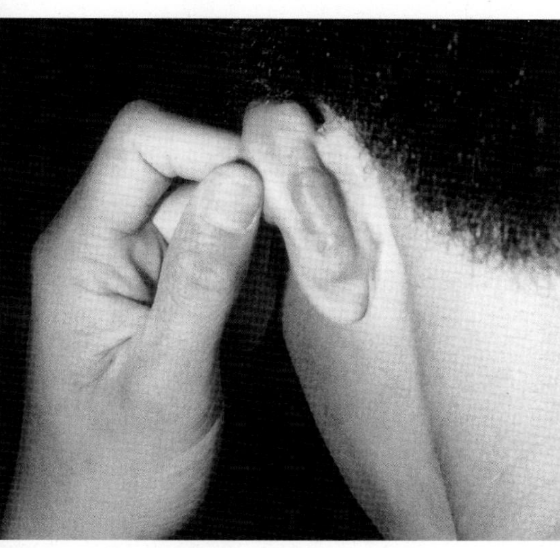

Fig. 34.16 Keloid formation following otoplasty.

is higher. In a large series reported by Baker and Converse, the incidence of postoperative keloid formation is 2.3%.[26] Treatment of keloids is initially conservative, with injections of triamcinolone acetonide (10, 20, or 40 mg/mL) every 2 to 3 weeks. The mechanism of action of steroids appears to be to decrease collagen activity and enhance collagen breakdown.[27] If surgical excision is required, a conservative excision using the carbon dioxide laser is used. Some authors advocate leaving a rim of the keloid tissue to prevent restimulation of keloid production.[28] Steroid injections are used in the postoperative period, as are pressure earrings in female patients. Low-dose radiation therapy has also been reported with some success in the management of recurrent keloids.

Summary

Otoplasty is one of the most challenging and rewarding procedures in facial plastic surgery. Emphasis is placed on precise preoperative analysis and measurements, predictable operative techniques, and the avoidance of a surgical appearance of the ear. Although no surgeon can be versatile in all otoplasty techniques, a fundamental knowledge of the principles of otoplasty will permit correction of a wide variety of deformities with any given approach.

References

1. Ely E. An operation for prominence of the auricles. Arch Otolaryngol 1981;10:97–99
2. Rogers BO. Mirotic, lop, cup, and protruding ears. Plast Reconstr Surg 1968;41:208–231
3. Luckett W. A new operation for prominent ears based on the anatomy of the deformity. Surg Gynecol Obstet 1910;10:635
4. Becker OJ. Surgical correction of the abnormally protruding ear. Arch Otolaryngol 1949;50:541–560
5. Converse JM, Wood-Smith D. Technical details in the surgical correction of the lop ear deformity. Plast Reconstr Surg 1963;31:118–128
6. Farkas LG. Anthropometry of normal and anomalous ears. Clin Plast Surg 1978;5:401–412
7. Weerda H. Embryology and structural anatomy of the external ear. Facial Plast Surg 1985;2:85–91
8. Streeter GL. Development of the auricle in the human embryo. Contrib Embryol 1922;69:111
9. Wood-Jones F, I-Chuan W. Development of the external ear. J Anat 1934;68:525–533
10. Potter E. A hereditary ear malformation. J Hered 1937;28:255
11. Furnas DW. Correction of prominent ears by conchamastoid sutures. Plast Reconstr Surg 1968;42:189–193
12. Spira M, Stal S. The conchal flap: an adjunct in otoplasty. Ann Plast Surg 1983;11:291–298
13. Mustarde JC. Correction of prominent ears using simple mattress sutures. Br J Plast Surg 1963;16:170–178
14. Bull TR, Mustarde JC. Mustarde technique in otoplasty. Facial Plast Surg 1985;2(2):101–107
15. Burres S. The anterior-posterior otoplasty. Arch Otolaryngol Head Neck Surg 1998;124:181–185
16. De la Torre J, Tenenhaus M, Douglas BK, Swinburne JK. A simplified technique of otoplasty: the temporary Kaye suture. Ann Plast Surg 1998;41:94–96
17. Hilger P, Khosh MM, Nishioka G, Larrabee WF. Modification of the Mustarde otoplasty technique using temporary contouring sutures. Plast Reconstr Surg 1997;100:1585–1586
18. Connolly A, Bartley J. "External" Mustarde suture technique in otoplasty. Clin Otolaryngol 1998;23:97–99
19. Gibson T, Davis WB. The distortion of autogenous cartilage grafts: its cause and prevention. Br J Plast Surg 1958;10:257
20. Spira M. Otoplasty: what I do now—a 30-year perspective. Plast Reconstr Surg 1999;104:834–841
21. Pilz S, Hintringer T, Bauer M. Otoplasty using a spherical metal head dermabrador to form a retroauricular furrow: five-year results. Aesthetic Plast Surg 1995;19:83–91
22. Nachlas NE, Duncan D, Trail M. Otoplasty. Arch Otolaryngol 1970;91:44–49
23. Cloutier AM. Correction of outstanding ears. Plast Reconstr Surg Transplant Bull 1961;28:412–416
24. Schuffenecker J, Reichert H. A scoring and V-Y plasty technique. Facial Plast Surg 1958;2:119
25. Stal S, Spira M. Long-term results in otoplasty. Facial Plast Surg 1985;2:153–165
26. Baker DC, Converse JM. Otoplasty: a twenty-year retrospective. Aesthetic Plast Surg 1979;3:36
27. Cohen IK, McCoy BJ. Keloids and hypertrophic scars. In: Rudolph R, ed. Problems in Aesthetic Surgery. St. Louis: CV Mosby; 1986
28. Peacock EE, Madden JW, Trier WE. Biologic basis for the treatment of keloids and hypertrophic scars. South Med J 1970;63:755–760

35 Cosmetic Surgery of the Asian Face

John A. McCurdy Jr.

In surgical parlance, the term *Asian* is currently applied as a designation for individuals belonging to the Mongoloid race of peoples. It should be noted, however, that consistent with the geographic immenseness of the Asian continent, its native inhabitants demonstrate racial diversity exceeding that of Europe, Africa, and the New World. The indigenous people of western Asia are essentially Caucasian, whereas those of southern Asian regions are largely Indo-Pakistani or Malay. The surgical appellation "Asian" applies to the population of eastern Asia, a region historically termed the Orient. Thus, although technically a misnomer, the term *Asian*, when used in this chapter will, in the interest of conforming to contemporary surgical linguistics, refer to the group of people originating in east Asia who have been previously known as Oriental.

Although the physical characteristics of the Asian face differ substantially from those of the Caucasian, justifying separate discussion of the unique surgical approaches devised for aesthetic modification, it should be noted that, as in the Caucasian face, considerable individual variation exists as a result of alteration of the gene pool by centuries of migration and intermarriage. The most common of the anatomical features for which surgical manipulation requires formulation of distinctly different approaches are the eyelids, the nose, and the maxillary (midfacial) region, and the majority of this chapter will focus on these areas. Surgical procedures designed to modify other components of the face are essentially comparable to their counterparts in the Caucasian patient, and discussion of these procedures will be limited to a few specific observations and technical considerations, which may facilitate such operations.

The past 3 decades have witnessed an exponential increase in the incidence of cosmetic surgery of the Asian face, a situation attributable to increasing influence of and immigration to the West as well as general affluence in developing Asian nations. It is essential to understand, however, that the nature of requests for cosmetic facial surgery has changed dramatically since the 1960s and 1970s when a predominant desire was for "westernization." In contemporary times, however, Asian patients seldom request westernization, desiring instead relatively conservative modifications that improve facial balance and harmony while maintaining ethnic identity. It has been my distinct observation that patient dissatisfaction following surgery performed by Western surgeons is often related to overly aggressive surgery, whereas dissatisfaction following surgery performed in the Orient is more likely related to an overly conservative approach.

Planning Cosmetic Surgery of the Asian Face

General Considerations

As in Caucasians, skin texture and pigmentation of Asians exhibit substantial individual variation. In general, those individuals originating from more southerly latitudes show darker pigmentation, whereas a substantial percentage of natives of central and northern East Asia (i.e., Northern Chinese, Koreans, Japanese) have more lightly colored, even milky white skin pigmentation often described as exhibiting a yellowish hue. This yellow tint of Asian skin is largely a consequence of the number and distribution of melanin granules rather than differences in the structural skin lipoproteins themselves.

Regardless of the extent of skin pigmentation, Asians generally demonstrate thicker dermis than equivalently pigmented Caucasians. A consequence of greater collagen density, this situation is associated with a tendency toward a more vigorous fibroplastic response during wound healing, which may result in hypertrophic scarring and prolonged redness during scar maturation in an incidence worthy of note even in lightly pigmented Asians. Clinically, hypertrophic scarring is most common in the epicanthal region and the postauricular (and occasionally temporal) incisions following rhytidectomy. For unknown reasons, hypertrophic scarring rarely if ever occurs on the lower eyelids or following alar base excision. In spite of the fact that hypertrophic scarring is common in the noted areas, frank keloid formation is rare, occurring most commonly in the ear lobule after piercing.

Increased dermal thickness may account for a substantially lower incidence of fine facial rhytides in both darker and fair Asians as compared with Caucasians of equivalent age. On the other hand, Asian skin tends to respond to sun exposure and the aging process with an accelerated development of pigmented dermatoses (lentiginous actinic keratoses, seborrheic keratoses, etc.) as compared with Caucasian skin. However, skin malignancies of all types are markedly less common in Asians than in Caucasians.

Cultural Considerations

An understanding of cultural differences among Asian nationalities is perhaps as important in achieving optimal surgical results as thorough comprehension of anatomical factors. Effective communication between patient and surgeon is of utmost importance in preoperative planning as well as in management decisions during the postoperative healing period. Appreciation of cultural and personality characteristics facilitates precise interpersonal communication. Miscommunication predicated on failure to understand such differences is all too often the basis for inappropriate surgical decisions and manipulations (initial or corrective).

In spite of the significant influence of the Western world on the East, the tremendous differences between Western and Eastern cultures soon becomes obvious to Westerners who associate with native Asians. These differences may exert significant effects on patient perceptions about surgery (and the surgeon), as well as expectations and behavior during the postoperative period. Although cultural differences are less defined in the generations descended from the immigrant populations, certain powerful cultural influences often persist, and these may exert significant effects on attitudes concerning (or behavioral reactions following) cosmetic surgery. As stressed previously, a basic appreciation of these cultural factors is of great assistance in providing insight into the psychological makeup of the diverse Asian nationalities and will enable the surgeon to communicate more effectively with, and respond more appropriately to, the concerns and desires of Asian patients.

One of the basic foundations of Asian philosophy is a strong belief in fate, destiny, and the importance of luck, both good and bad, in daily affairs. Many Asians have strong beliefs in certain maxims, proverbs, and superstitions and apply these beliefs and superstitions to important situations encountered in their daily lives.

Asian cultures also place great significance on physiognomy—the relationship of physical traits or characteristics to behavior and personality, as well as to prospects for success in business, friendship, marriage, and other human relationships.

Most Asians exhibit great respect for higher education and for persons in a position of authority. This degree of respect may result in a deference to surgeons that may impair effective communication. Questioning the physician is considered to be a sign of disrespect; thus, patients may be reluctant to request clarification of matters that they do not understand completely.

Asian patients frequently feel that their surgeon will automatically know (and do) what is best. However, an unsatisfactory result frequently fragments this patient–physician bond, unleashing emotions and behavioral forces that could have been attenuated by effective preoperative communication.

Importance of Beauty

Physical beauty is particularly important to Asian women, as in Oriental cultures it is generally considered that a major duty of a wife is to maintain attractiveness so that she can be a source of pride to her husband and family. There is a general cultural belief that if a woman does not remain attractive to her husband, he has every right to wander in search of other sources of affection. Before the advent of cosmetic surgery, a fatalistic attitude toward appearance was predominant, a stance that to a large extent—at least in more urbanized areas—has been supplanted by a strong desire to undergo surgery for improvement in appearance. Submission to cosmetic surgery, however, often results in subconscious feelings of guilt that in some cases may complicate the healing period. A major source of such guilt is a strong attachment to family and the belief that it is disrespectful to one's parents to alter physical characteristics that were "given" to an individual by the parents. The strong belief in the importance of beauty and its relationship to personal success has, to a large extent, superseded this cultural tradition.

Alternatively guilt over having undergone cosmetic surgery may result in withdrawal ("hiding") from family and friends. Such self-imposed isolation may rob the patient of much needed emotional support during the critical postoperative period that may contribute to obsessive or delusional concerns. The surgeon must be cognizant of these potential disruptive forces during the early postoperative healing period and firmly resist requests for premature or inappropriate revision procedures. One prominent Vietnamese surgeon admonishes his patients in printed informational material, "Please do not look in the mirror for you will surely be disappointed!"

The Asian appreciation for harmony and symmetry, the basic elements of beauty, as well as an eye for detail are manifested in the precision of Oriental craftsmanship. However, this appreciation for perfection may translate to unrealistic anxiety about postoperative asymmetry and other minor imperfections during the healing period, requiring considerable patience and understanding on the part of the surgeon. Asian patients, in contrast to the average Westerner, openly discuss cosmetic surgery with their acquaintances and often solicit the opinions of family and friends about their appearance during the early postoperative period, being very susceptible to unflattering comments during this stage. Such behavior is a common source of early postoperative unhappiness and dissatisfaction, and the surgeon must firmly resist requests for inappropriate revision procedures during this time.

National Characteristics

Although many of the basic cultural nuances noted previously are common to all Asian cultures, each ethnic group shares certain common behavioral and personality traits and attitudes that, while certainly not universal, tend to characterize and distinguish members of these nationalities.

The concept of "national identity" is certainly familiar to Westerners. The British, for instance, are often characterized as polite but formal, having a "stiff upper lip," and Germans are stereotyped as stern, diligent, and perfectionistic. In the United States, the characteristics of citizens from different regions provide a basis for similar stereotyping. Texans, for example, are characterized as friendly and relaxed with a tendency toward exaggeration, whereas New Yorkers are often thought of as impatient, blunt, and sarcastic.

In the same manner, Asian nationalities recognize certain typical characteristics among themselves and stereotype various nationalities according to commonly observed traits. Whenever I lecture on surgery in Asian patients, without exception, one of the most common questions asked is, "I just can't seem to get through to my Asian patients. How do you communicate with them effectively?" An understanding and appreciation of ethnic differences and stereotypical traits of the many Asian nationalities may be helpful in this endeavor.

Interacting with the Asian Patient

As a group, Asian patients tend to be reserved and self-effacing, necessitating open-ended, somewhat probing discussions to extract pertinent information and encourage formation of realistic expectations, both before and after surgery. The surgeon should (1) encourage the patient to communicate any fears, worries, or disappointments honestly and (2) be, likewise, frank and straightforward when discussing expectations, likely results, and possible complications.

Blepharoplasty in the Asian Eyelid

General Considerations

Surgical modification of the upper eyelid has become increasingly popular in Asia since World War II and is currently the most commonly performed aesthetic operation in the Far East. Although surgery of the Asian eyelid is similar to blepharoplasty in other ethnic groups, important anatomical and technical differences do exist, and the surgeon must be familiar with these variations to maximize aesthetic results.

As a group, ~50% of Asians exhibit a "single eyelid," so-called because in the absence of a superior palpebral fold the lid hangs like a curtain from the supraorbital ridge. Creation of a palpebral sulcus divides the lid into well-defined pretarsal and palpebral segments, producing the "double eyelid" desired by many Asian women as well as an increasing number of men.

The incidence of the single eyelid, of course, is higher in Asian populations that have remained homogeneous (i.e., Japanese, North Koreans), whereas double eyelids are more common in heterogeneous populations (i.e., Vietnamese, South Koreans, Southeast Asians, and Filipinos). However, most Asians with natural double eyelids exhibit a small fold accompanied by abundant periorbital and submuscular fat as well as excess upper eyelid skin that exhibits considerable pretarsal laxity.

It would be erroneous to assume that the popularity of the double-eyelid operation is related solely to Western influence. Asian cultures have long regarded the bright-eyed look associated with the double eyelid as an aesthetically desirable feature. Many Oriental women produce double eyelids by using various tapes and glues to encourage temporary adherence of the pretarsal upper lid skin to preseptal skin, resulting in a palpebral fold. Because such rituals are time consuming and temporary, surgery is frequently requested after a girl has reached the age of 15 or 16.

Given the fact that many Asian cultures regard the double eyelid as an aesthetically desirable facial feature, it is important that the surgeon understand that a request for surgical modification of the single eyelid is generally not a request for westernization of the lid. Many patients, particularly those who have been born in North America, simply desire a small double eyelid while maintaining ethnic character.

Westernization of the eyelid, on the other hand, requires reduction of the characteristic puffiness of the Asian lid via removal of excess skin and fat and, in many cases, modification of an epicanthal fold. In general, recent immigrants to Western countries tend to request creation of a large eyelid (i.e., higher palpebral fold), whereas individuals born or raised in Western society usually request a more "natural" lid with preservation of their ethnicity.

Anatomical Considerations

Despite the popularity of the double-eyelid operation, controversy exists among surgeons regarding the precise anatomical basis for the supratarsal fold and thus the most effective method for creation of a natural and durable crease.

The most commonly proposed anatomical explanation of the differences between single and double eyelid is as follows: In the Caucasian eye, filaments of the levator expansion penetrate the orbital septum and orbicularis muscle and attach to the overlying dermis, creating a superior palpebral fold when the eye is opened. In the Asian lid, the levator aponeurosis does not penetrate the orbital septum of the orbicularis muscle but terminates on the superior margin of the tarsus. It must be noted, however, that the levator filaments postulated to be responsible for formation of the double eyelid have never been conclusively demonstrated in gross or histological studies.

Moreover, recent studies, suggest that the anatomical basis for formation of the superior palpebral fold is somewhat more complex. Rather than attaching directly to the dermis, filaments of the levator aponeurosis appear to extend inferiorly into the pretarsal portion of the lid, interdigitating with fibrous septa coursing from the tarsus (penetrating the pretarsal orbicularis) to the pretarsal skin, thus producing adherence between the pretarsal skin, orbicularis muscle, and tarsus. The actual mechanism of lid fold creation appears to relate to this adhesion of pretarsal skin, orbicularis, and tarsus. The preseptal skin, in contrast, is nonadherent to the preseptal muscle and thus relatively mobile. As the levator contracts, the mobile preseptal skin folds over the relatively rigid pretarsal lid (skin, orbicularis, and tarsus) that is elevated as a unit, thus forming the fold; or, stated in another way, the components of the pretarsal lid are retracted together in a boardlike fashion posterior to the mobile preseptal skin on levator contraction. This concept is consistent with the fact that in eyelids without a well-defined palpebral fold, the pretarsal skin is redundant because it lacks attachments to the pretarsal muscle and tarsus. Surgical procedures that create a superior palpebral fold can be used to achieve this goal by virtue of the fact that the process of supratarsal fixation effectively produces an adhesion between the pretarsal skin and the lid-opening mechanism, thus allowing its elevation and invagination posterior to preseptal skin as a single unit on levator contraction. This modified understanding of the anatomical basis for the lid fold has clinical implications in double-eyelid surgery because a more stable adhesion in the pretarsal lid and tightening of the pretarsal skin can be achieved by undermining the pretarsal skin for several millimeters prior to placement of fixation sutures.

Furthermore, the lack of adherence between pretarsal skin, orbicularis, and tarsus allows a wedge of periorbital fat (bounded anteriorly by the levator aponeurosis and posteriorly by the orbital septum) to descend inferiorly, anterior to the tarsal plate, producing the characteristic puffiness of the pretarsal lid. An abundant layer of suborbicularis fat is often present in the Asian lid, contributing to fullness in the pretarsal area. Interestingly, the location of the palpebral fold in all ethnicities appears to coincide with the point of fusion between the levator aponeurosis and orbital septum, with the descending wedge of fat bounded by these structures acting as a barrier preventing adherence of pretarsal skin, orbicularis, and tarsus. Clinically, this barrier of fat must be surgically excised inferior to the point at which the palpebral fold is created to create permanent adhesion of pretarsal tissue layers. Failure to adequately remove this tissue is frequently the cause of "falling out" of the surgically created fold (i.e., postoperative fold failure) and occurs most commonly in the lateral aspect of the eyelid.

Preoperative Evaluation and Counseling

The major objective of blepharoplasty in the Asian upper lid is creation or enhancement of a crisp, well-defined, and natural palpebral fold. Because of the many possible variations in achieving this goal (i.e., the level of the palpebral fold, the depth of the palpebral sulcus, as well as the appearance of the epicanthal region) that can be controlled by modifications of surgical technique, careful preoperative evaluation and counseling of each prospective patient are mandatory when planning this operation. Many patients desire only the creation of a palpebral fold and wish to retain the other characteristics of the Asian eyelid. Others, however, prefer a less conservative transformation or even a westernization procedure that requires modification of the epicanthal fold as well as reduction of lid puffiness by removal of large volumes of redundant skin and fat.

Several methods assist the surgeon and patient in selecting the type of eyelid transformation desired. In my practice, patients are advised that three basic decisions are necessary: (1) size of the "new" eyelid, (2) shape of the new eyelid, and (3) disposition of the epicanthal fold. For purposes of counseling, double eyelids are arbitrarily divided into small, medium, and large, depending on the amount of visible pretarsal skin and the depth of the palpebral sulcus. Likewise, eyelids are classified as having one of two shapes: round or oval. Patients are then shown pre- and postoperative photographs illustrating the various sizes and shapes of eyelids (**Fig. 35.1**). In many patients, it is possible to demonstrate the approximate size and shape of the lid (while the patient is looking into a mirror) by manipulating the eyelid skin with a bent paper clip or forceps. In discussing the epicanthal region, differences between the so-called inside and outside folds are demonstrated with pre- and postoperative photographs, facilitating a more rational discussion of possible variations (**Fig. 35.2**).

Some patients bring pictures of magazine models to their consultations, and though it must be stressed that a surgeon cannot construct an eyelid to the patient's exact specifications, examining these pictures in conjunction with pre- and postoperative photographs is often helpful in assisting the surgeon to determine the general size and shape of eyelid that an individual desires.

Anesthesia

The operation is performed under local anesthesia using anesthetic solution with fresh, unbuffered epinephrine (0.5 bupivacaine or 1% lidocaine with epinephrine 1:50,000) with intravenous sedation. To minimize intraoperative bleeding (which slows surgery, interferes with judgment of symmetry, and increases edema and ecchymosis, prolonging the healing period), anesthetic solution with fresh, unbuffered epinephrine (0.2 cm^3 epinephrine 1:1000 per 10 cm^3 plain 1% lidocaine) is prepared prior to each procedure. The vast majority of cases are performed as outpatient procedures in an office surgical facility. Because frequent opening and closing of the eyes during surgery is helpful in the evaluation of symmetry, general anesthesia is not recommended. For the same reason, the level of sedation during surgery should be light. Diazepam and midazolam are best avoided because both agents frequently interfere with lid opening. Methohexital or propofol is an excellent agent for eyelid surgery because the rapid onset and brief duration of action allow for painless anesthetic infiltration and a comfortable and reasonably cooperative patient intraoperatively.

Surgical Procedure

The key to success in upper lid blepharoplasty in Asian patients is to perform each step (from preoperative marking to final suturing) with the goal of achieving eyelid symmetry. The sequence for preparation and surgical intervention is as follows:

1. Proper preoperative markings (**Fig. 35.3**) are of the utmost importance and are determined by the size (small, medium, large) and shape (round, oval) of the desired eyelid transformation. The most important factor in determining the level of the superior palpebral fold is the distance from the ciliary margin at which the inferior lid incision is drawn. This distance ranges from 6 to 10 mm.
   a. For creation of a small double eyelid, the incision is placed 6 to 7 mm above the ciliary margin, whereas in patients desiring a medium-sized lid, the incision is placed 8 mm above the ciliary margin. For a large eyelid, the incision is marked 9 to 10 mm above the ciliary margin.
   b. Prior to marking, it is important to tense the pretarsal skin to the point of lash eversion. An initial mark

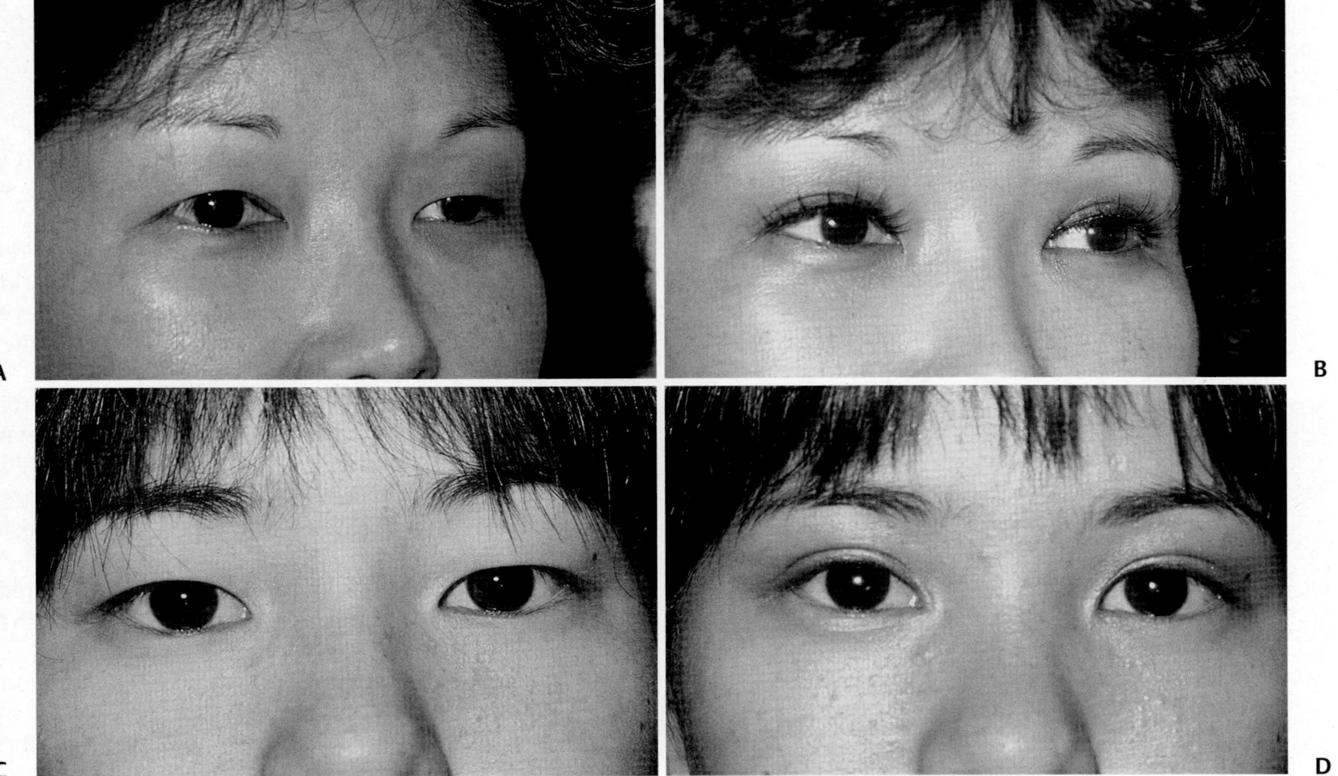

Fig. 35.1 (**A**) Pre- and (**B**) postoperative photographs showing surgical creation of a small double eyelid that is round in configuration with an inside fold. (**C**) Pre- and (**D**) postoperative photographs of surgical creation of a double eyelid that is oval in configuration with an inside fold.

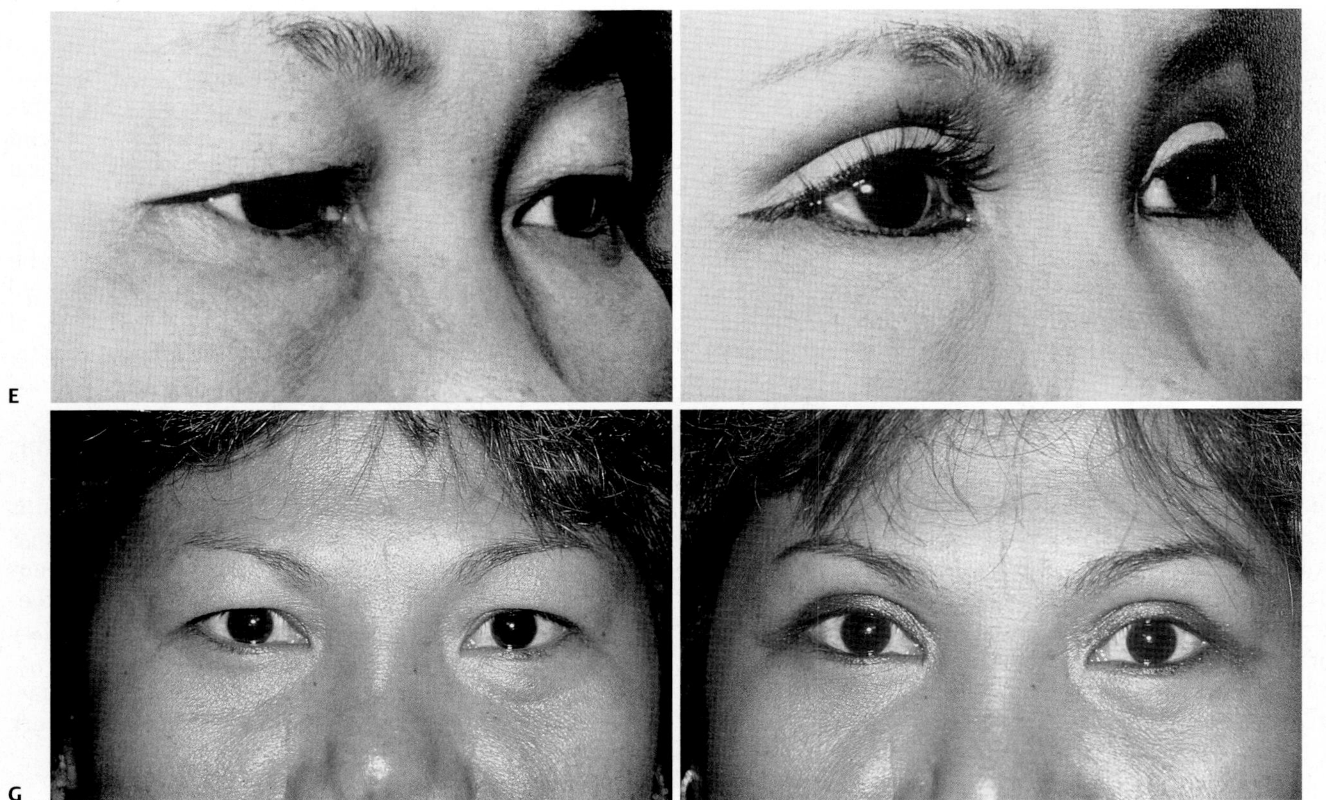

Fig. 35.1 (*Continued*) (**E**) Pre- and (**F**) postoperative photographs showing surgical creation of a large double eyelid with an outside fold. (**G**) Pre- and (**H**) postoperative photographs showing surgical creation of a medium-sized double eyelid with an outside fold.

is placed at the desired height at the level of the lateral limbus, following which the entire inferior incision is drawn.

i. To create an eyelid with an oval shape, the incision is configured so that it is 1 to 2 mm more inferior when it reaches the medial canthus while remaining at approximately the same level at the lateral canthus as in the center of the lid. The incision is then extended slightly superiorly and laterally so that it will fall in a periorbital line.

ii. If a round eyelid is desired, the lateral aspect of the incision is drawn so that it is ~2 mm more inferior at the level of the lateral canthus than at the level of the lateral limbus (also being 2 mm more inferior medially).

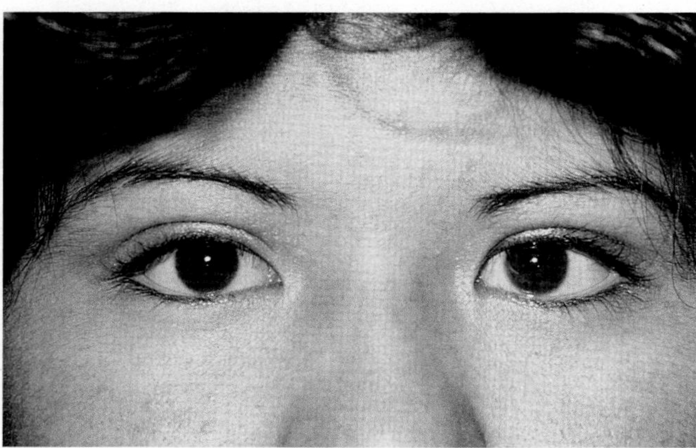

Fig. 35.2 The left eye exhibits an outside fold, whereas the right eye exhibits an inside fold, maintaining the epicanthus.

c. Individual desire regarding management of the epicanthal region determines the location of the lid incision in this area.

i. If an inside fold (i.e., no epicanthal modification) is requested, the incision is drawn lateral to the existing epicanthus (**Fig. 35.3A**).

ii. If an outside fold (epicanthal effacement) is desired, the incision terminates medial to the epicanthal web (**Fig. 35.3B,C**).

2. The level of the superior incision, which determines the amount of skin to be excised, is determined by pinching the skin with forceps and asking the patient to open and close the eyes as in a standard blepharoplasty procedure. The average amount of skin excised is 3 to 10 mm, depending on the age of the patient and the type of eyelid desired. It is important to individualize

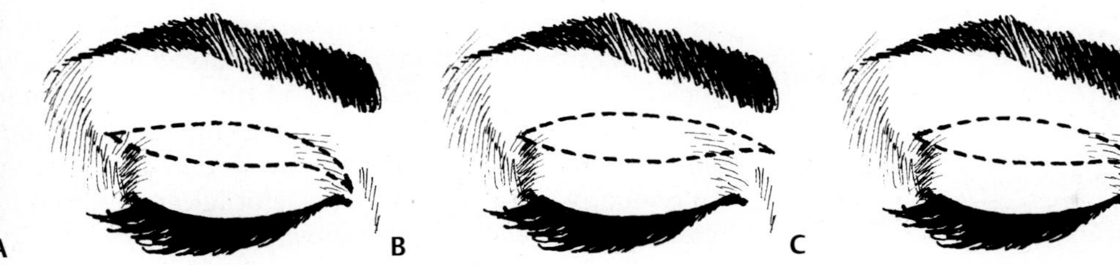

Fig. 35.3 Incisions used for the creation of (**A**) an inside fold, (**B**) an outside fold, and (**C**) a fold terminating on the origin of a small epicanthus.

the amount of skin removed according to the size of eyelid requested because this factor is important in determining the amount of pretarsal "show."

a. In the patient who desires a small double eyelid, only 2 to 3 mm of skin is excised.
b. For creation of a medium-sized lid, half of the maximal amount of skin that can be removed (as determined by forceps pinching) is actually removed; that is, if 12 mm of skin can be maximally removed, the incision is placed 6 mm above the level of the inferior skin incision.
c. If a large, westernized lid is desired, 2 to 3 mm less than the maximum amount of skin that could be removed as determined by forceps pinching is actually excised. The superior incision is marked so that it courses parallel to the previously marked inferior incision, joining it at the medial and lateral canthal areas.

3. Following infiltration of local anesthetic, skin and subcutaneous tissues are excised exposing the orbicularis muscle.
   a. A 3 to 5 mm strip of orbicularis is excised above the tarsal plate.
   b. The orbital septum is then incised, exposing periorbital fat.
      i. If a deep "Western" palpebral sulcus is desired, removal of all visible fat in the central and lateral compartments is performed so that the levator expansion is completely cleared.
      ii. Removal of medial fat is more conservative because creation of a deep hollow in the medial aspect of the lid does not produce the aesthetically desirable effect that often results from sculpturing this area in the Occidental eye. Excessive fat removal medially also predisposes to hypertrophic scarring because more tension is placed on the skin closure.
      iii. Little or no fat in any compartment is excised if a small double lid is desired; in such cases, the fat is carefully separated so that the levator expansion can be identified.
4. Prior to placement of fixation sutures, a 2 to 3 mm strip of muscle is removed from beneath the skin at the level of the inferior skin incision (**Fig. 35.4**). This maneuver effectively undermines the skin 2 to 3 mm, providing a wider base of adhesion for formation of the palpebral fold, and allows tightening of pretarsal skin during fixation.
5. Fixation sutures of 5–0 nylon are then placed, incorporating the skin edge of the inferior incision, the levator aponeurosis, and the superior skin incision (**Fig. 35.5**).
   a. Buried "internal" fixation sutures of permanent or absorbable suture incorporating only the inferior skin edge and levator may be substituted for the "external" fixation suture, but including the upper skin edge in the fixation enhances interoperative determination of symmetry as the extent of "hooding" contributed by the suprafold tissues is more easily determined.
   b. Three fixation sutures are utilized: laterally at a point approximately one half the distance between the lateral canthus and lateral limbus, centrally at the midpupillary level, and medially at the level of the medial limbus.
      i. The lateral fixation suture is placed initially, followed by the middle and medial sutures.
      ii. Assessment of symmetry is enhanced if the sutures are placed sequentially in the right and left eyelids (i.e., the lateral fixation suture is placed in the right eyelid following which lateral fixation suture placement is performed in the left lid). With the eyes open, symmetry is assessed by inspection and direct measurement,

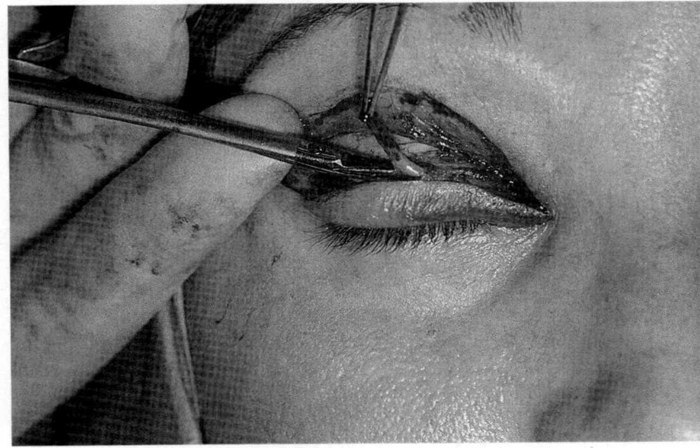

Fig. 35.4 Excision of a 2 to 3 mm strip of muscle beneath the skin at the level of the inferior skin incision.

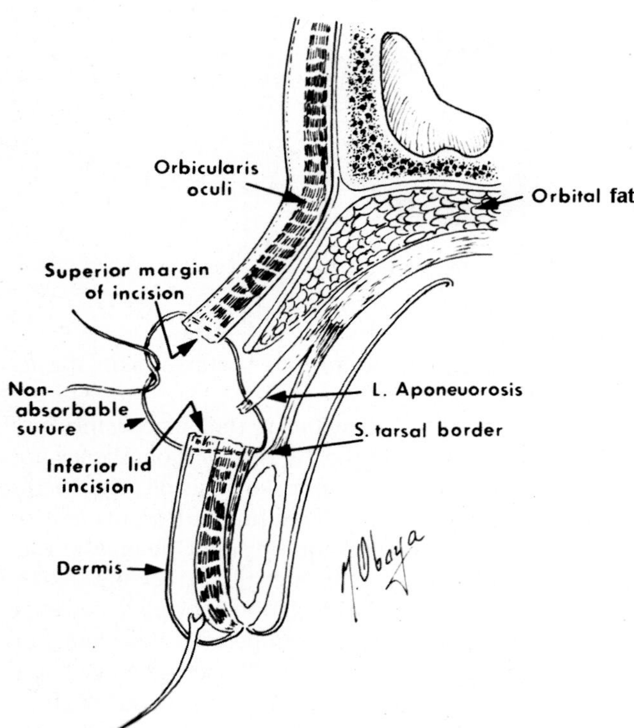

Fig. 35.5 Placement of an external fixation suture (5–0 nylon).

following which the middle fixation sutures are placed.

iii. One or two additional medial fixation sutures are often placed in the medial aspect of the lid to efface the epicanthal fold if desired. On occasion, more advanced techniques of epicanthoplasty are necessary.

6. The entire incision is then approximated with a running suture of 6–0 nylon. Both fixation sutures and the running cuticular suture are removed in 7 days.
7. To minimize the incidence of hypertrophic scar formation in the medial canthal region, 0.2 cm^3 triamcinolone (10 mg/cm^3) is routinely injected into the subdermal tissues of this area. In addition to causing a marked decrease in hypertrophic scarring, this procedure results in healing with considerably less palpable induration that may produce local distortion of the palpebral fold.

Postoperative Course

The early postblepharoplasty period is characterized by marked edema of the pretarsal portion of the lid as well as by variable degrees of blepharoptosis. The extent and duration of this ptosis are directly related to the level of fixation as well as the amount of skin and fat excised, being more significant if a larger lid is created. Blepharoptosis is generally not objectionable following removal of the fixation sutures on the seventh postoperative day but may occasionally cause persistent concern because of resultant asymmetry if it is more marked unilaterally. Slowly resolving asymmetrical ptosis is often related to hematoma or edema of the Müller muscle. Occasionally, residual pretarsal edema may be detectable for up to 6 months but is usually satisfactorily camouflaged by cosmetics following suture removal.

Complications

Perhaps the most common source of dissatisfaction in Asian patients undergoing upper lid blepharoplasty is postoperative asymmetry of the lid folds. This problem occasionally occurs even in the hands of the most experienced surgeon.

Postoperative asymmetry is more likely to occur when lid or brow asymmetry exists preoperatively, and each prospective candidate for upper lid blepharoplasty must be carefully evaluated in this regard. Minimal ptosis, often unnoticed preoperatively, also predisposes to postoperative asymmetry. If asymmetry exists, it must be carefully pointed out to the patient, with the explanation that exact postoperative symmetry will be more difficult to achieve. Preoperative asymmetry, of course, must be carefully documented in the medical record as well as by preoperative photographs.

Strict adherence to certain technical points minimizes the occurrence of postoperative asymmetry:

1. The preoperative markings on the upper eyelid must be performed while the skin is stretched cephalically. The skin is tensed until the eyelashes begin to evert—a checkpoint that will facilitate symmetrical placement of the preoperative marks bilaterally.
2. After completion of the markings, they are rechecked for symmetry using a ruler prior to infiltration of anesthetic. On rechecking the incisions, it will be surprising how often a millimeter of asymmetry is discovered, allowing appropriate correction before beginning the operation.
3. After placing the initial fixation suture (usually at the lateralmost fixation point), a corresponding fixation suture is placed in the opposite lid, following which the patient is asked to open the eyes so that they can be inspected for symmetry. The height of both sutures above the ciliary margin is also carefully measured. In placing this initial suture as well as subsequent fixation sutures, the pretarsal skin is stretched to the point where the eyelashes begin to evert—a visual check also utilized in preoperative marking as described previously. If a difference of even 1 mm is noticed on measuring the height of the initial fixation sutures, or asymmetry is noted on inspection of the opened eyes, it must be corrected at this time. Following placement of subsequent fixation sutures, a similar measurement coupled with inspection of the

opened eyes is performed, allowing prompt replacement of these sutures if necessary.

4. Avoid excessive sedation during the operative procedure because it may interfere with voluntary lid opening, making it more difficult to assess the symmetry following placement of fixation sutures. Use of an external fixation suture that incorporates both upper and lower skin incisions facilitates intraoperative assessment of the palpebral fold because the contribution of the upper skin segment to the final eyelid size and shape can be visually assessed during actual construction of the fold, as described previously. Slight asymmetry in the early postoperative period is very common because of differential swelling of the eyelids as well as the mild ptosis that may temporarily follow fixation procedures. Although many patients are concerned about this asymmetry, the surgeon should carefully explain the problem and firmly refuse to consider revision until edema has resolved. Occasionally more marked lid asymmetry due to obvious failure of one or more fixation sutures deserves earlier correction, with repair easily being accomplished by replacement of the failed suture through a small incision in the area of failure.
5. Measure, remeasure, then measure again!

Other possible complications of the double eyelid operation are the same as those in standard upper lid blepharoplasty. Because the skin of the Asian eyelid tends to be thicker than that of the Caucasian lid, the incidence of prolonged induration and erythema is somewhat higher. However, frank scar hypertrophy is unusual except in the biologically predisposed medial canthal region. As noted previously, uncomplicated healing in this area is greatly enhanced with the routine use of intraoperative triamcinolone.

Management of the Epicanthus

Although ~90% of Asians exhibit an epicanthus, the size of the fold, although varying widely among individuals, is usually relatively small; thus aesthetically successful effacement only rarely requires complex procedures that have been described for management of this condition in the Caucasian eye. A major reason for the relative ease in managing the Asian epicanthal fold is that, in contrast to epicanthus encountered in Caucasians in which a vertical shortage of skin is problematic, the epicanthal fold in the Asian lid is usually associated with skin redundancy of the entire upper lid. This can be demonstrated by medial displacement of the skin with a cotton-tipped applicator. Successful effacement of the fold can thus be conceptualized as a medial advancement of the epicanthal web. The goal of this advancement, in addition to removal of the fold itself, is to elongate the entire palpebral fold in a medial direction. Further benefits of this maneuver are the illusion of an enlarged eye and eyelid and a narrowing of the nasal bridge, a wide bridge, and small widely separated eyes being concerns of many individuals with prominent epicanthal folds.

Patient Evaluation and Counseling

In many patients, no specific intervention in the epicanthal area is necessary. This group includes those who desire an inside fold as well as other patients with a small, almost rudimentary epicanthus in whom the surgical approach used to create the palpebral fold results in sufficient medial advancement of the epicanthus to achieve satisfactory effacement.

The major advantage, of course, in minimizing surgery in the medial canthal region is the reduced risk of hypertrophic scarring. This region exhibits a biological predisposition to hypertrophic scar formation, and thus even the most meticulously performed procedure in this area may be complicated by the presence of an aesthetically unpleasant scar.

In keeping with the known propensity for scar formation in the medial canthal area, it is best to encourage patients who are either unaware of their epicanthal folds or uncertain if they really desire modification of this region to defer epicanthaplasty at the time of primary surgery. Such patients are counseled that epicanthal modification can be performed as a secondary procedure should they so decide.

Always inform patients about asymmetry that exists preoperatively in the eyelids, epicanthal region, and palpebral fissures because usually it will persist or become more apparent postoperatively. Patients must understand that differences in postoperative edema between the two eyelids frequently translate to postoperative asymmetry and that judgment regarding final symmetry may be unreliable for 6 months or more postoperatively. Preoperative counseling must stress proposed management of the epicanthal fold, and if a patient is uncertain as to whether modification of the fold is desired, epicanthoplasty may be best performed as a secondary procedure. Patients must understand that once the epicanthal fold is removed, it can never be reconstructed. It is helpful to inform patients that, in general, effacement of the epicanthus produces a more westernized appearance, whereas preservation or slight modification of the fold preserves the Asian characteristics of the eye.

Surgical Procedure

Epicanthaplasty, if desired or indicated, is usually performed in conjunction with upper lid blepharoplasty. One of three

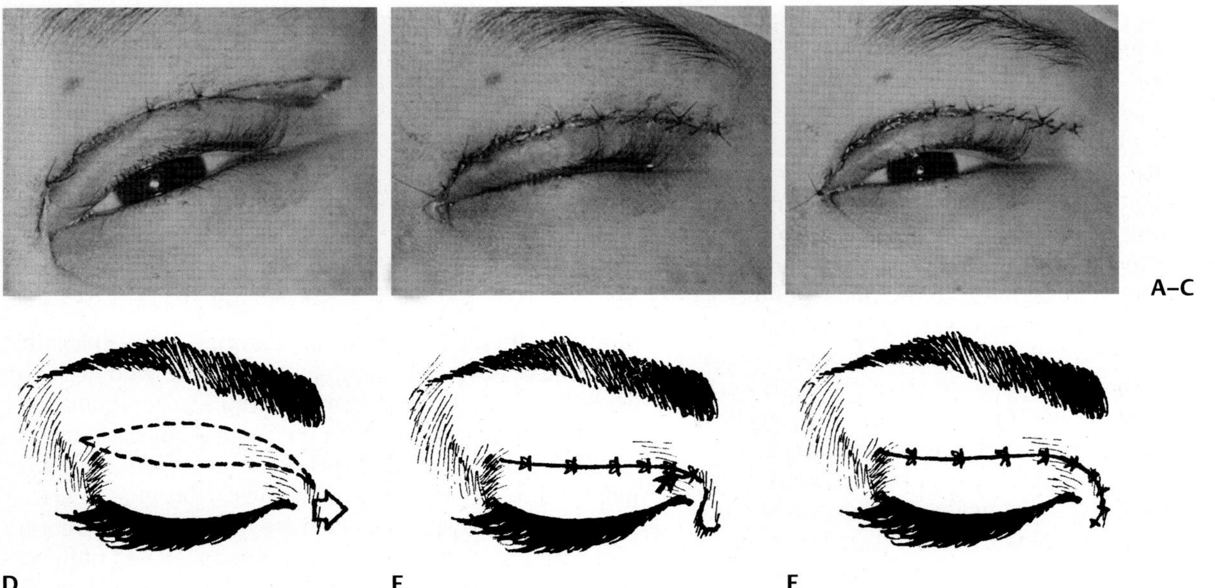

Fig. 35.6 Effacement of a small epicanthus by medial fixation sutures combined with excision of a small "dog ear." (**D–F** from McCurdy JA. Cosmetic Surgery of the Asian Face. New York: Thieme; 1990. Reprinted by permission.)

approaches is used to efface the epicanthus, depending on the size of the fold requiring modification. Each procedure is based on the general principle that effacement can be successfully accomplished by medial advancement of the existing fold.

1. Advancement of a small fold is performed in conjunction with the incisions used for creation of the palpebral fold. These incisions are carried medially and inferiorly to the level of the lacrimal caruncle. The pretarsal skin in the area of the epicanthus is undermined to within 1 to 2 mm of the ciliary margin. Underlying soft tissue, including orbicularis muscle, is excised. The skin is then advanced medially and secured by placement of one or two external fixation sutures (**Fig. 35.6**). If a small dog ear develops, it is excised in the direction of the skin fold, occasionally extending onto the medial aspect of the lower eyelid. A result achieved using this technique is depicted in **Fig. 35.7**.
2. If additional advancement is required, a half Z-plasty is utilized (**Fig. 35.8**). The epicanthal fold is incised near the medial terminus of the palpebral wound, creating a triangular flap that is undermined and advanced nasally into the triangular defect previously created. The resulting dog ear is trimmed in the direction of the skin lines as described previously. **Fig. 35.9** illustrates pre- and postoperative results.
3. Effacement of a larger epicanthus may require a greater medial advancement than is possible with Z-plasty techniques. Such a fold often terminates on the medial aspect of the lower lid, necessitating modification in this area as well. An excellent aesthetic result is generally achieved by a W-plasty advancement procedure.

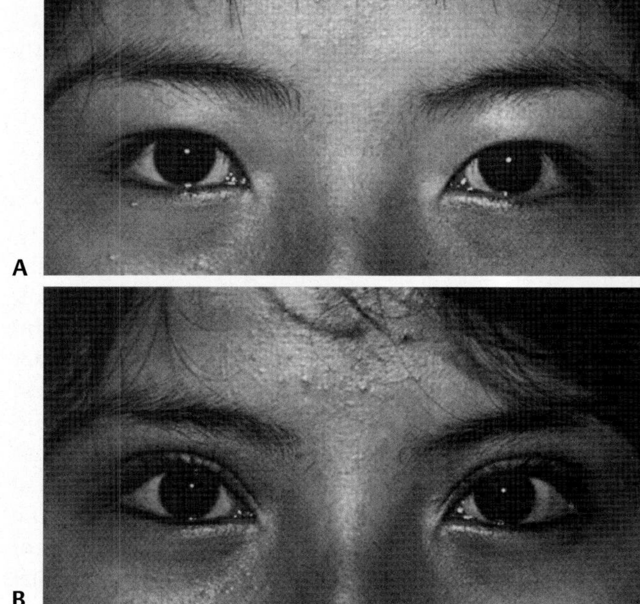

Fig. 35.7 Effacement of the epicanthal fold by advancement in conjunction with creation of an "outside fold."

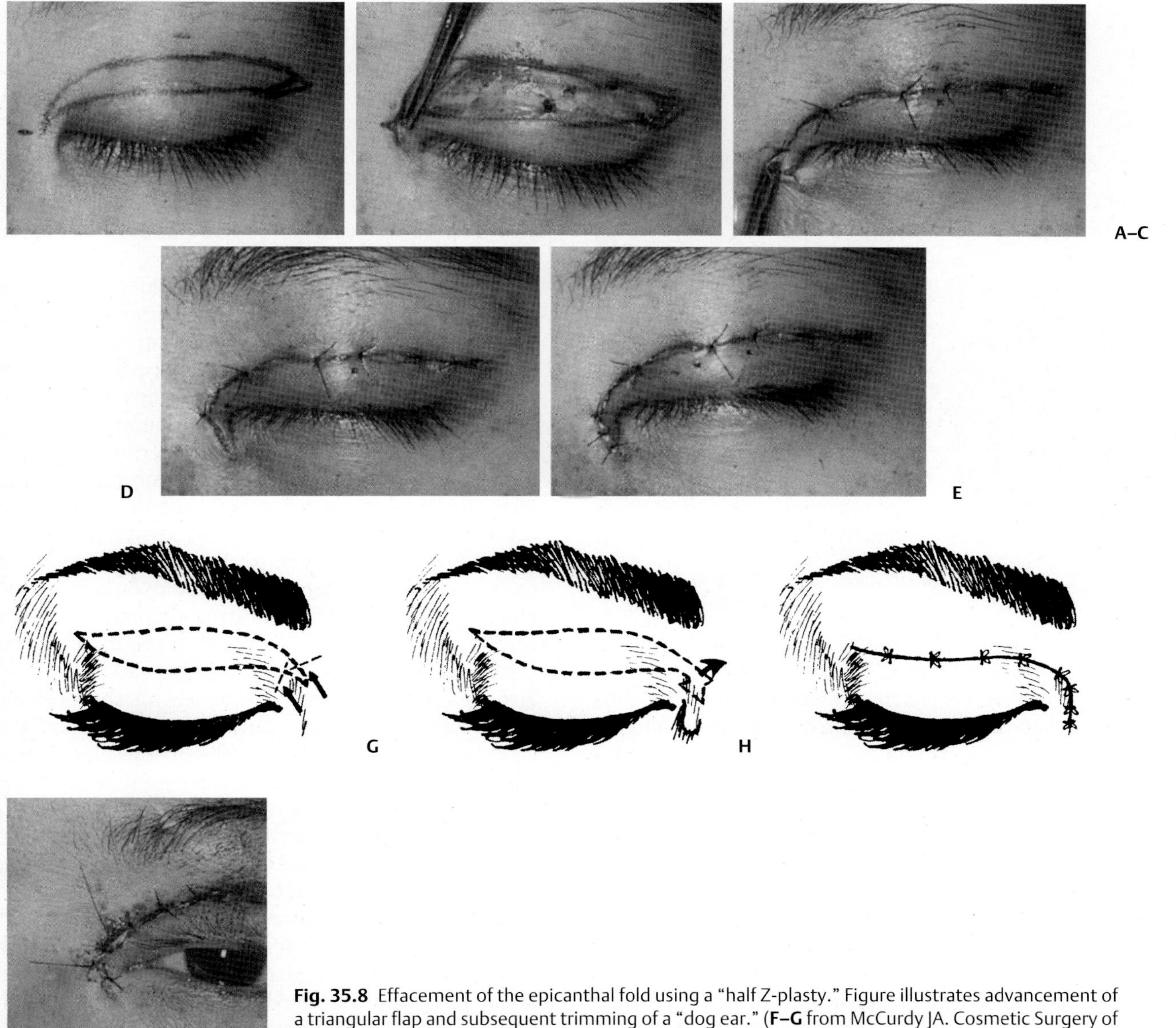

Fig. 35.8 Effacement of the epicanthal fold using a "half Z-plasty." Figure illustrates advancement of a triangular flap and subsequent trimming of a "dog ear." (**F–G** from McCurdy JA. Cosmetic Surgery of the Asian Face. New York: Thieme; 1990. Reprinted by permission.)

The desired position of the inner canthus is marked (this is a point ~2 mm medial to the desired position of the inner canthus), following which two V-shaped flaps, forming a W, are outlined. The triangular flaps have their bases on the segments of the epicanthus located on the upper and lower lids (**Fig. 35.10**).

The outlined W is incised and the triangular flaps are undermined toward the inner canthus, following which the flaps are advanced and sutured with 6–0 nylon. **Fig. 35.11** shows pre- and postoperative results.

In addition to improving facial balance by elongating "small eyes," epicanthaplasty improves the appearance of the nose because the nasal bridge may appear excessively wide when the lateral dimension of the eyes is decreased by a large epicanthal fold (**Fig. 35.11**).

Lower Lid Blepharoplasty

General Considerations and Patient Evaluation and Counseling

As in the upper eyelid, the Asian lower lid characteristically exhibits a considerable volume of periorbital fat that frequently produces a puffy appearance even at an early age. In many patients, considerable fat is also present in

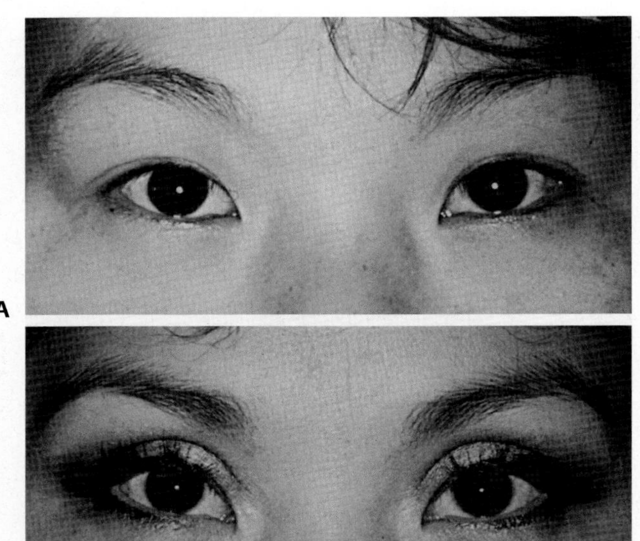

Fig. 35.9 Epicanthoplasty with the half Z-plasty procedure.

the pretarsal plane (superficial to the orbital septum), accentuating eyelid fullness.

Although a wide spectrum exists, Asian skin is generally thicker than Caucasian skin, and deeply etched rhytides extending laterally (i.e., laugh lines or crow's feet) occur less frequently. Eccrine syringomas occur on the lower eyelid skin in some individuals, and such patients must understand that these blemishes will not be eliminated by blepharoplasty. Pigmented lesions (seborrheic keratoses, lentigines, etc.) are also common on the lower lid.

Hypertrophy of the orbicularis muscle is particularly common in the Asian lower lid, often producing an unaesthetic infraciliary bulge at an early age. Such patients must be counseled regarding the differences between puffiness caused by fat protrusion and orbicularis hypertrophy, as well as the aesthetic and technical limitations of partial muscle resection.

The puffiness of the Asian lower lid may tempt the surgeon to recommend a transconjunctival approach. However, many if not most Asian patients are firmly convinced that "too much skin" is a component of their problem, and thus dissatisfaction often follows with an operation that does not remove skin. This observation, coupled with the fact that transconjunctival blepharoplasty does not allow modification of orbicularis hypertrophy, makes the skin/muscle flap approach the procedure of choice for most patients, except perhaps the very young patient with no concern about skin excess or men whose only request is elimination of "bags" resulting from periorbital fat protrusion.

To achieve maximum aesthetic results in skin/muscle flap blepharoplasty, the surgical plan must address all components of the lower lid "deformity," that is, skin excess and laxity, orbicularis hypertrophy, periorbital fat protrusion, and, occasionally, bone (prominence of the infraorbital rim) as determined by preoperative analysis. The skin/muscle flap approach provides excellent access to all eyelid components, the relative importance of which varies from patient to patient, necessitating individualization of the procedure.

Perhaps the most important consideration in lower lid blepharoplasty is preservation (or reinforcement) of the structures that provide critical support for the lid. Even the most accomplished and experienced surgeon must deal with the problem of lower lids whose posture was normal in the immediate postoperative period but descend relentlessly into a more inferior, aesthetically unattractive position as the healing process continues. Such lower lid malposition is frequently referred to as *ectropion*, which is attributed to excessive skin excision. However, the majority of such situations are a consequence of a process termed retraction (or vertical shortening) of the lower lid. The true pathological basis of retraction is fibrosis in the plane of the middle lamella (orbital septum and capsulopalpebral fascia, often also involving the posterior aspect of the orbicularis oculi). This results in scar contracture and vertical shortening of this plane that overwhelm the often tenuous supporting structures of the lower eyelid, which are further compromised by the surgical procedure. In contrast, frank ectropion is related to shortening (whether by scar contracture or, more commonly, overzealous tissue resection) of the anterior lamella (skin and orbicularis oculi). Of course, retraction and ectropion may coexist.

The lower eyelid derives support from both static and dynamic mechanisms. Static support is provided by the tarsal plate and associated medial and lateral canthal tendons, whereas the dynamic component consists of the action of the pretarsal component of the orbicularis oculi that is firmly attached to the tarsus. Lower lid position is determined by the balance (**Fig. 35.12**) between the supporting structures and the forces tending to displace the eyelid inferiorly (i.e., gravitational and cicatricial forces subsequent to surgery or trauma). The surgeon must be cognizant of the fact that the static supporting mechanism is gradually attenuated by the aging process, whereas dynamic lid support is easily compromised during surgery. The key to success in lower lid blepharoplasty, therefore, is to incorporate measures designed to preserve and reinforce or reconstruct lower lid support into each and every blepharoplasty procedure. A five-point program for lower lid blepharoplasty is a valuable concept in this regard and has proven a reliable method of reducing the incidence of lower lid retraction.

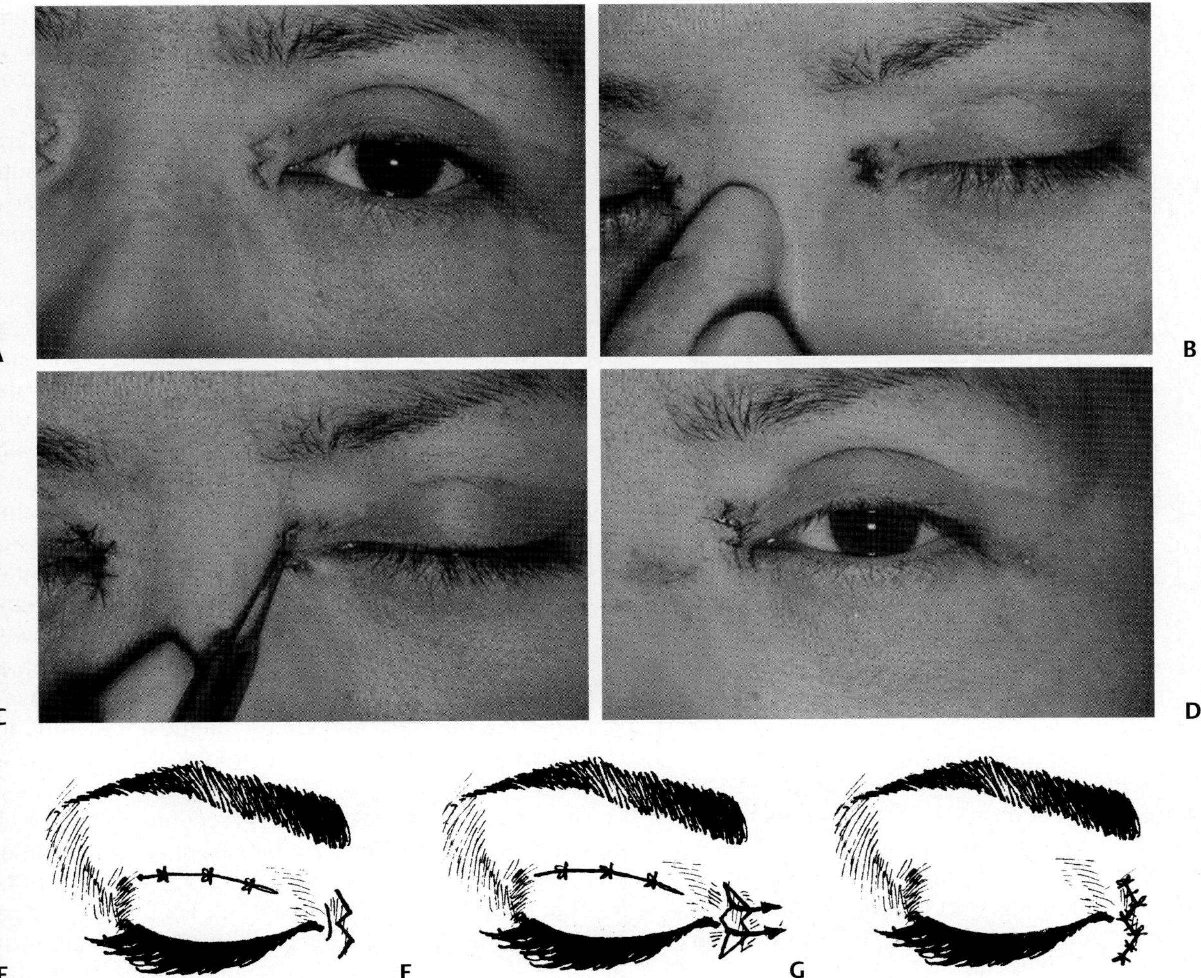

Fig. 35.10 Epicanthoplasty with the W-plasty advancement procedure (see text). (**E–G** from McCurdy JA. Cosmetic Surgery of the Asian Face. New York: Thieme; 1990. Reprinted by permission.)

Surgical Technique

The five-point operative plan for skin/muscle flap lower lid blepharoplasty is as follows:

1. The lateral extensions of the skin incisions should be placed as horizontally as possible (in a horizontal periorbital line, i.e., not inclined inferiorly) to minimize the tendency for lateral canthal rounding and inferior displacement that may result from postoperative scar contracture in this area.
2. Because the pretarsal segment of the orbicularis muscle, which is adherent to the tarsal plate, provides an element of dynamic support for the lower lid, the surgeon should ensure that a generous strip of this muscle remains adherent to the tarsus. This can be accomplished by completely undermining the skin/muscle flap via the lateral aspect of the lower lid incision. The infraciliary portion of the incision is then completed and a 3 to 4 mm skin flap is developed. This abbreviated skin is then connected with the skin/muscle flap by incising the orbicularis muscle with a diagonally oriented scissors, thus preserving an adherent muscle strip on the tarsus.
3. When determining the amount of tissue to be excised from the skin/muscle flap, the flap is draped over the ciliary margin in a superior and medial direction, as opposed to the superior and lateral direction usually recommended. This offers several advantages, perhaps the most important of which is the absence of concentrated tension in the lateral aspect of the wound. A concentration of tension in this area creates force vectors that predispose to inferior and medial displacement postoperatively, resulting in intercanthal shortening producing the "sad eye" or "hound dog" look. This is of particular importance in patients in whom the lateral canthal tendon and

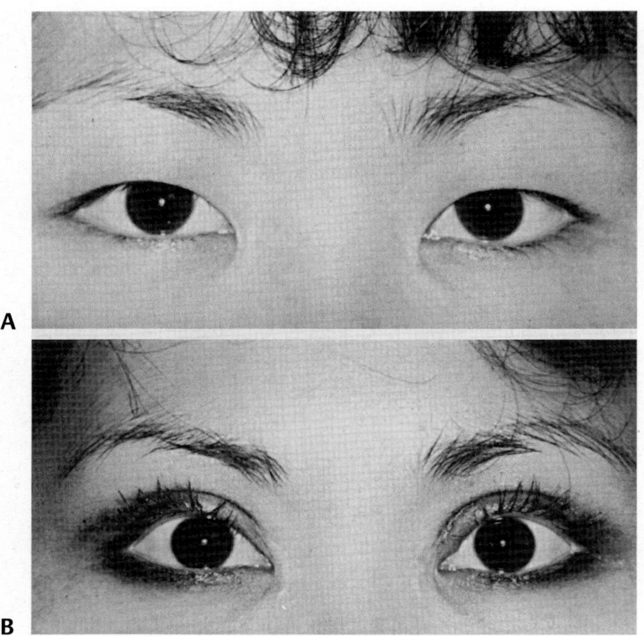

Fig. 35.11 Effacement of an epicanthal fold using the W-plasty advancement procedure.

tarsus have been attenuated by the aging process. Laterally directed traction of the flap may also contribute to the accentuation of lateral periorbital lines often noted following blepharoplasty. An additional advantage of medial draping of the flap is minimization of the length of the lateral aspect of the incision because it is not necessary to "chase a dog ear" laterally.

4. Prior to skin closure, a permanent suspension suture of 5–0 nylon is placed between the deep surface of the orbicularis muscle and lateral orbital periosteum. It is important to suspend the muscle at the level of the lateral canthus and to avoid excessive tension on the flap that might cause buckling of the tarsus or suture failure due to tearing through the orbicularis muscle. Orbicularis suspension reinforces static support of the lower lid and assists in resisting cicatricial forces that produce inferior lid displacement postoperatively.
5. Prior to skin closure, 0.2 cm^3 of triamcinolone (10 mg/cm^3) is infiltrated into the plane of the orbital septum (middle lamella) prior to skin closure. This has proven to be of considerable benefit in combating the forces of contracture and greatly reduces the incidence of postoperative induration that generally precedes the onset of clinical lower lid retraction. Perhaps the most persuade argument for routine use of steroid in lower lid blepharoplasty relates to the observation that accumulation of small amounts of blood in the middle lamellar plane are a common etiologic factor in the pathogenesis of lower lid retraction, blood being a potent precipitator of fibrosis. Such blood accumulation may develop even following the most meticulous hemostasis; thus it occurrence is entirely unpredictable.

The five-point operative plan is recommended for all patients undergoing lower lid blepharoplasty who demonstrate no preoperative risk factors predisposing to postoperative lower lid malposition. Those with preexisting lid laxity (a condition noted much less frequently in the Asian than in the Caucasian lid) are candidates for other ancillary techniques (i.e., tarsal suspension etc.) performed in conjunction with the blepharoplasty procedure.

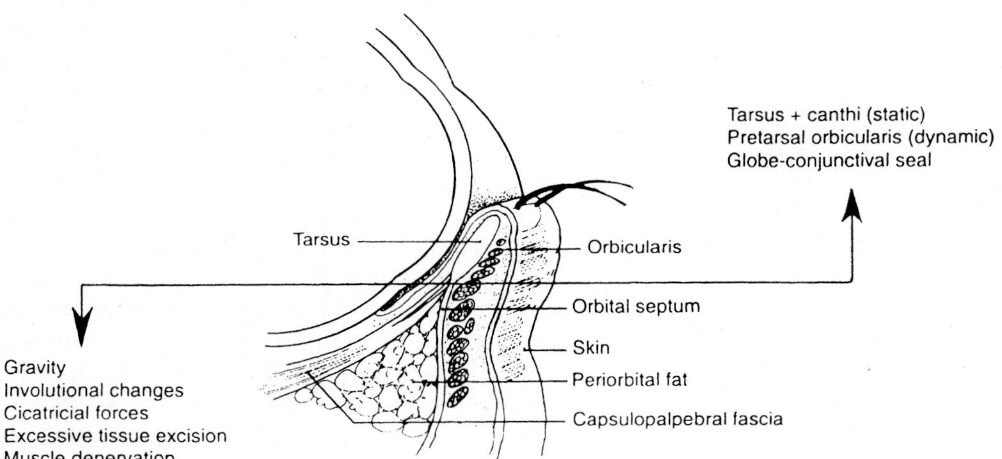

Fig. 35.12 Opposing forces that determine lower lid position. (From McCurdy JA. Cosmetic Surgery of the Asian Face. New York: Thieme; 1990. Reprinted by permission.)

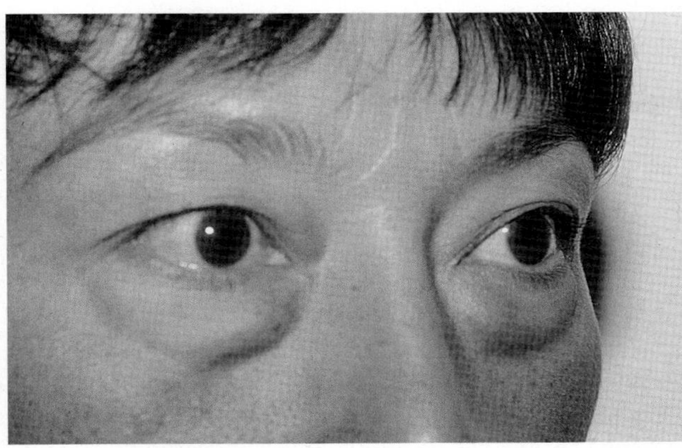

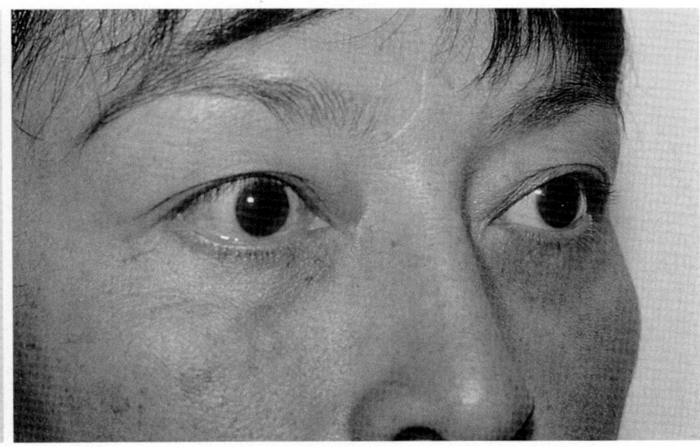

Fig. 35.13 Lower lid blepharoplasty. (**A**) Preoperative and (**B**) postoperative views.

Although a thorough understanding of structural and functional anatomy and meticulous attention to detail during the operative procedure are the keys to success in all facial plastic surgery, they are of particular importance in eyelid operations because a myriad of structures having both functional and aesthetic significance are densely packed into a small area. Surgical intervention in the eyelids must be precise and deliberate if the beauty and expressiveness of the eyes are to be enhanced, preserved, or reconstructed (**Fig. 35.13**).

Augmentation Rhinoplasty

General Considerations

The goal in aesthetic rhinoplasty of the Asian nose is similar to that in Occidental rhinoplasty: creation of a strong, smooth, natural dorsum exhibiting a prominent origin at the nasion but not competing with the tip as the leading point of the nasal profile. A delicate, well-defined, refined lobule with definite columellar "show" and an oblique anteroposterior orientation of the nares constitute an equally important but seldom emphasized goal.

The characteristic anatomy of the Asian nose requires that the surgeon plan an augmentation procedure rather than reduction rhinoplasty, and augmentation rhinoplasty is requested with increasing frequency in areas with large Asian populations. Although it might be assumed that the popularity of this operation reflects a desire for westernization, it should be noted that in many Asian cultures, the high, narrow nasal bridge is an aesthetically desirable feature, a fact of which the surgeon must be cognizant in preoperative counseling and planning.

Historically, many materials have been employed to augment the Asian nose. At the present time, Western surgeons tend to prefer autogenous material, whereas in the Orient, use of silicone implants predominates. Many Western surgeons preach against the use of alloplastic nasal implants with evangelical fervor, apparently ignoring the fact that the long-term results using this material in the Asian nose have been excellent. The incidence of infection, displacement, or extrusion is substantially lower than would be expected on the basis of experience in augmentation of the non-Asian nose with solid implants. The reasons for this tolerance are unknown but may be related to greater thickness of skin and subcutaneous tissue generally noted in the Asian nose. As with other cosmetic procedures, complications are usually attributable to technical error rather than an inherent problem with the operation and implant composition itself. Although the basic principle that autogenous material, when available, is preferable to alloplastic implants is valid, many Asian patients are unhappy with the results of nasal augmentation using autogenous cartilage and bone because satisfactory sculpturing of the lobule is often not achieved. Techniques of tip rhinoplasty that are highly successful in the Caucasian nose are frequently unsatisfactory in the Asian because the attenuated lower lateral cartilages alone are not strong enough to accentuate tip projection and support, and the lobular skin and subcutaneous tissue are too thick to reflect sculpturing of the delicate cartilage. Thus, if tip projection is to be enhanced, the surgeon must reinforce or buttress lobular cartilage with cartilage grafts.

Asian craftsmanship, renowned throughout the world, is characterized by a pragmatic concern for function coupled with a keen eye for beauty and symmetry along with meticulous attention to detail. Augmentation rhinoplasty using silicone implants has been refined by conscientious, experienced, and well-trained Asian surgeons, and any temptation to label such procedures as inherently dangerous or unreliable should be tempered with respect for the experience and accomplishments of our colleagues in the East. Evolution in the technology of silicone implants has continued as softer grades of silicone elastomer have become available for implant fabrication. Softer implants are inherently more flexible, resulting in reduced tension at the implant–tissue interface, which translates to a substantial reduction in problems that may develop as a consequence of pressure on the nasal skin.

Although frustration over the dissatisfaction of Asian patients with the results of tip-plasty using techniques that produced excellent results in the Caucasian nose led me to begin exploration of the possibilities of alloplastic implants in sculpturing the entire nose as opposed to the dorsum alone, there is no question that in some noses only subtle augmentation of the dorsum is required. In such cases, autogenous cartilage or alloplastic materials, such as Mersilene mesh (Ethicon, Inc., Somerville, NJ) or Gore-Tex (W. L. Gore & Associates, Inc., Flagstaff, AZ), are viable alternatives to silicone implants in these patients. The decision to use autogenous or alloplastic material is individualized according to the desires of each patient with regard to the extent of lobular sculpturing and dorsal augmentation. Anatomical factors, such as skin thickness and configuration of the lower lateral cartilages, assist in determining the type of procedure to be employed. Thin lobular skin constitutes a relative contraindication to the use of silicone implants. Given the current social and medicolegal environment, feelings of individual patients regarding use of foreign materials in the body must be factored into the equation.

In the final analysis, surgeons experienced in augmentation of the Asian nose generally conclude that contemporary silicone implants provide the best aesthetic solution for most patients who desire increased lobular definition or tip projection in conjunction with dorsal augmentation.

Preoperative Evaluation and Counseling

It is of the utmost importance that the candidate for augmentation rhinoplasty completely and carefully communicate the specifics of the nasal transformation that is desired. Many Asian patients assume that the surgeon knows best and will automatically adapt to the surgeon's specifications. If communication between patient and surgeon is unclear or imprecise, disappointment may ensue regarding such matters as dorsal height, lobular configuration, and tip projection. The surgeon must determine whether the patient wants the tip to be narrow or relatively broad. Is the desired nasion wide or narrow? Does the patient wish the dorsal profile to be straight or slightly convex? Pre- and postoperative photographs of various augmentation rhinoplasty procedures are often helpful in this regard. It should be stressed to the patient, however, that a surgeon cannot promise to construct the nose to exact specifications or guarantee that the nose will demonstrate the precise configuration of a photograph.

The goals, limitations, and possible complications of surgery are thoroughly discussed. Language barriers and preconceived notions on the part of the patient regarding the goals and limitations of the procedure should be recognized and addressed during preoperative consultation.

Surgical Technique for Alloplastic Implants

Augmentation rhinoplasty is generally performed under local anesthesia in an office operating suite. An oral cephalosporin or its equivalent is initiated on the evening prior to surgery and antibiotic prophylaxis is continued for 3 days postoperatively.

1. Access to the dorsum and lobule is obtained via a marginal incision that extends into the columella (**Fig. 35.14**). Dissection of a precise midline pocket is facilitated by initiating the dissection via the columellar portion of the incision. The lower lateral cartilages are freed from the lobular skin but are not otherwise modified because the implant will rest on their anterior surfaces.
2. The silicone implant is not premeasured but is individually tailored at the time of surgery. This tailoring is accomplished by placing the implant into the dorsum, determining its effect, and then removing it for modification as indicated by the desires of the patient as well as the aesthetic sense of the surgeon.
3. A columellar strut is always utilized because it stabilizes the proximal portion of the implant in the midline, thus decreasing the incidence of postoperative instability or "wobbling" and resultant asymmetry. It is important to understand that the function of the columellar strut is not to thrust the tip anteriorly; thus

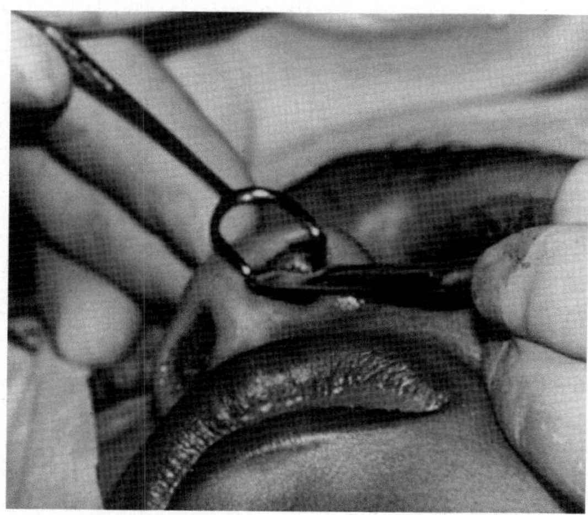

Fig. 35.14 Marginal incision used for augmentation rhinoplasty.

the strut does not extend to the nasal spine. Overzealous attempts to enhance tip support with a strut are ill-conceived maneuvers that markedly increase the incidence of implant extrusion.

4. The distal end of the dorsal implant terminates at a point halfway between the interbrow and intercanthal lines and should be sculptured to blend inconspicuously with the nasion so that it is not readily palpable. The nasofrontal angle must be preserved.
5. If the surgeon experiences difficulty freeing both lower lateral cartilages via a single marginal incision, a similar incision should be made on the opposite side to ensure symmetrical placement of the implant in the lobular area. The subcutaneous pocket should be of generous size. If resistance is encountered on placing the implant, the pocket is too small and should be enlarged to prevent excessive tension on the nasal skin. If a small dorsal hump is present, it is generally easier to rasp the dorsum than to modify the implant to accommodate this hump.
6. Following satisfactory placement of the implant, the nasal alae are analyzed and, if necessary, an alar reduction procedure is performed.
7. Some patients may benefit from narrowing of the nasal pyramid achieved by lateral osteotomy.
8. Occasionally, a nose may require reduction of lobular bulk by excision of lower lateral cartilage and lobular subcutaneous tissue. If indicated, this is best performed via a separate cartilage-splitting incision executed following implant placement and suturing of the marginal incision.

Implant Configuration

The nasal implant that I recommend for routine use differs from other commercially available implants primarily in its columellar aspect (**Fig. 35.15**). The columellar strut has two functions: (1) stabilization of the proximal segment of the implant in the midline, which results in resistance to displacement and subsequent malposition; and (2) sculpturing the columella; that is, displacement of the typically retracted columella inferiorly, thus increasing its "show." If hard elastomer is utilized for the columellar strut, it can be relatively short and thin because the firm material is resistant to deformation by columellar tension. The fibrous capsule that naturally forms around the implant often exerts a rotational force on the implant, resulting in lateral displacement of the strut with resultant perforation in the vestibular aspect of the columella, that is, the incision (the most common site of implant extrusion). These rotational forces are less likely to be transmitted to a columellar strut fabricated from a soft elastomer because of the flexibility at the lobular–columellar junction of the implant. However, this flexibility results in superior deformation of the strut (by columellar tension) unless the strut has sufficient breadth to allow it to be wedged between the caudal septal cartilage and columellar skin. During surgery, the flared columellar strut is carefully trimmed so that it is wedged between the skin and caudal septum at the most anterior point that allows aesthetically sufficient inferior displacement of the columella (producing columellar show).

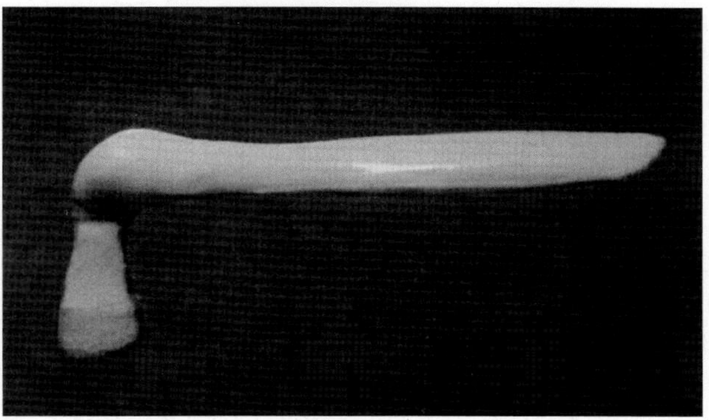

Fig. 35.15 Design of a silicone nasal implant (see text).

The inferior inclination (angulation) of the columellar strut with respect to the dorsal component assists in achieving this goal. (Other commercially available nasal implants are constructed so that the columellar strut projects at a 90-degree angle from the dorsal component.)

Following final trimming, the columellar strut never extends posteriorly for a distance greater than 75% of the length of the columella. Allowing the strut to contact the nasal spine results in a "tent pole" effect—an invitation to disaster in the form of implant extrusion secondary to pressure necrosis of the lobular skin. Always remember that the function of the columellar strut is not to project the lobule in a tent pole fashion. Lobular projection is achieved by the sheer volume of the rounded, slightly elevated (i.e., mound) lobular component, in a fashion similar to the cantilever effect of bone grafts utilized for total nasal reconstruction.

Because of complaints that clear silicone implants may be visible through the nasal skin under bright indoor lighting, the implant should be a neutral color (e.g., beige). Like other commercially available implants, soft elastomer is used for fabrication of the implant described previously.

Complications

Asymmetry as a consequence of improper placement of the implant or subsequent displacement of its distal aspect is the most common complication of augmentation rhinoplasty in the Asian nose. In the early postoperative period, apparent asymmetry may merely be the result of edema. Slight asymmetry is often successfully managed by instructing the patient in manipulation of the distal aspect of the implant. If noticeable asymmetry persists, however, correction can only be effected by removal and replacement of the implant.

Infection requires immediate removal of the prosthesis. Antibiotic therapy is initiated and continued according to the results of culture and sensitivity studies. The infection resolves rapidly, following which subsequent augmentation with the same implant can be performed. Although many surgeons recommend deferring revision surgery for 6 to 12 weeks, if thinned, stretched skin in the lobular region is not supported within 2 weeks of implant removal, contraction will commence, resulting in a cutaneous dimple that is difficult to efface. Support of the thinned skin is often best achieved by interposition of morcellized autogenous cartilage between the prosthesis and the dermis.

Delayed extrusion is the most worrisome complication of augmentation rhinoplasty in the Asian nose. The incidence of this complication is extremely low and is generally a consequence of technical error. Perhaps the most common reason for delayed extrusion is excessive tension in the lobular region secondary to ill-conceived attempts to enhance tip projection with a columellar strut. The surgeon must be conservative in attempts to increase tip projection and explain the reasons for this conservatism to each patient. The incidence of delayed extrusion is also reduced by ensuring that the implant does not fit too snugly in the dorsum, thus reducing tension at the host–prosthesis interface. Extrusion is also reduced by the presence of a columellar strut because this reduces instability or postoperative wobbling of the proximal aspect of the implant.

Impending extrusion is suggested by progressive thinning of the lobular skin. If recognized at an early stage, salvage of the implant can often be achieved by prompt removal. The implant is sculptured to a smaller size; a dermal, temporalis fascia, or crushed cartilage graft is secured over the lobular component; and the implant is replaced in the existing nasal pocket.

Remember that the major goals of rhinoplasty in the Asian nose include augmentation of the nasal dorsum in conjunction with refinement of the lobule. Although various materials, as noted previously, may be used to achieve these goals, individually sculptured solid silicone implants are presently the most commonly used prostheses. Some surgeons currently advocate the use of cartilage grafts to enhance tip projection while continuing the use of silicone implants for dorsal augmentation. Although I remain firmly convinced of the advantages of silicone implants because of their proven efficacy and reliability (as well as for their cost to benefit ratio), I applaud the efforts of those surgeons exploring the possibilities of more successful use of autogenous materials in the Asian nose. Although recent reports suggest that long-term survival of cartilaginous grafts of the onlay type in the nose is excellent, consider that the fate of columellar struts, which are subjected to stresses of a different magnitude, may well be different. Is it significant that proponents of such grafts recommend "overcorrection"?

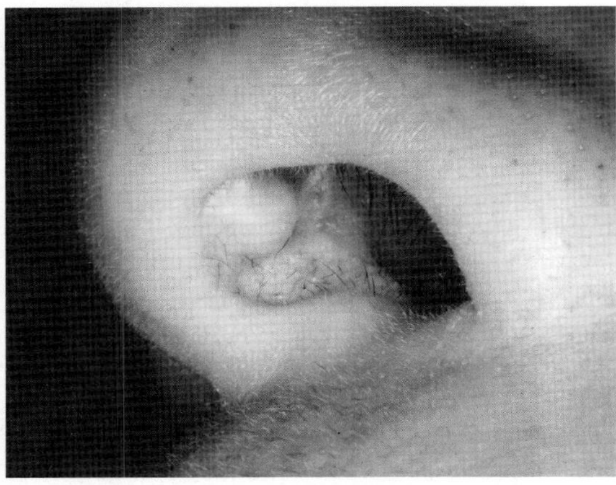

Fig. 35.16 Impending exposure of columellar strut.

The surgeon should be conservative in selection of implant size, remembering that subtle enhancement often produces substantial aesthetic benefit. Conservatism is of the utmost importance in attempts to enhance tip projection as excessive tension on the lobular skin is a prime factor in delayed extrusion of alloplastic implants. Infection is a secondary cause of implant extrusion; such abscesses most commonly develop in the columellar region (**Fig. 35.16**) but can occur over any portion of the implant.

Successful aesthetic rhinoplasty in the Asian nose requires knowledge of anatomical variables, appreciation of nasal aesthetics and social and cultural concerns, thorough preoperative evaluation and patient counseling, along with careful attention to detail.

Careful and considered use of silicone implants in augmentation rhinoplasty offers facial plastic surgeons an opportunity to utilize their aesthetic senses to the fullest extent, enabling them to produce dramatic changes in nasal appearance (**Fig. 35.17**). When such surgery is properly planned and executed, the incidence of complications is low. It must be reemphasized that complications following augmentation rhinoplasty with alloplastic implants are usually the result of technical errors and are not due to inherent deficiencies in the operation or implant composition per se. A thorough understanding of the basic principles and important safeguards when using such materials in the nose is essential for successful surgery.

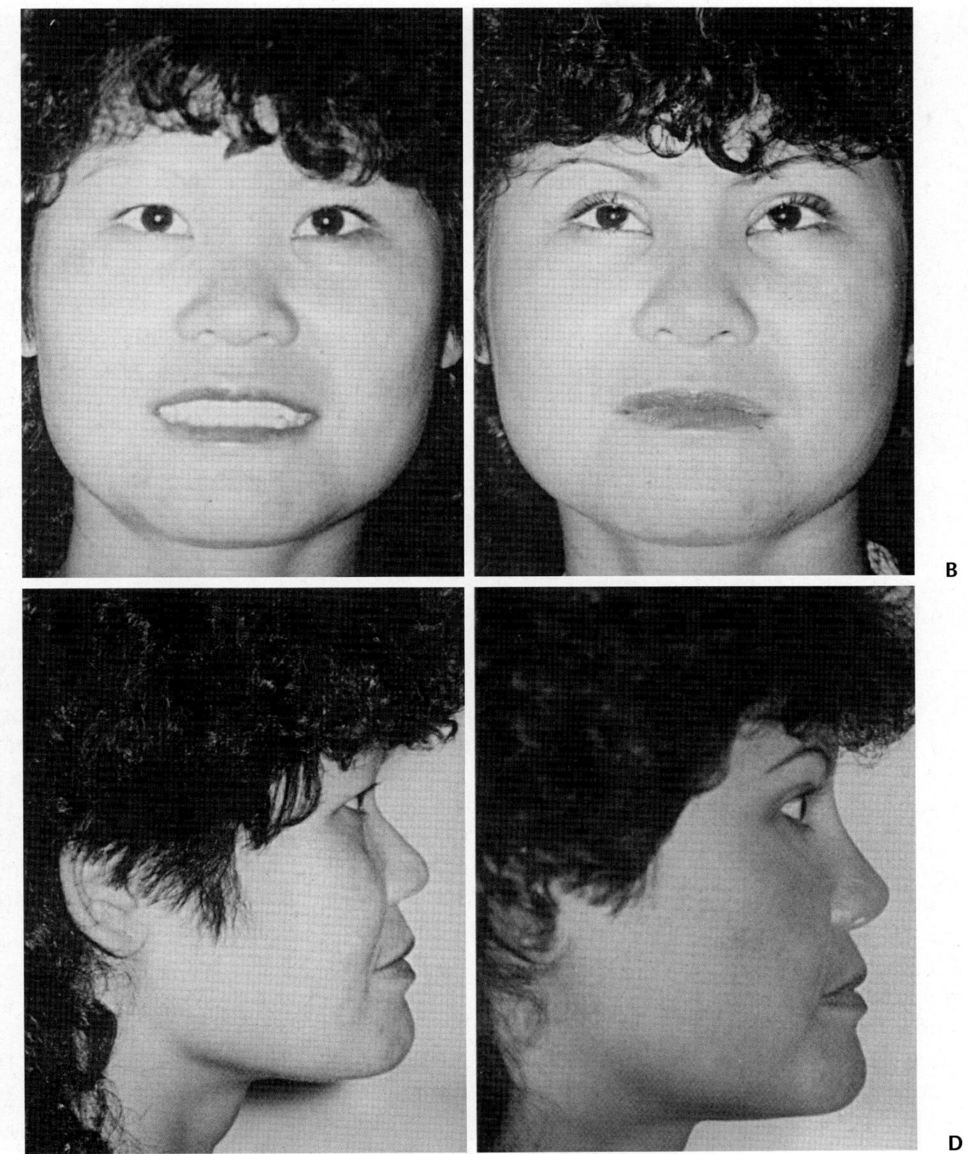

Fig. 35.17 Pre- and postoperative photographs demonstrating the results of augmentation rhinoplasty using a silicone implant.

Maxillary Implants

Bimaxillary protrusion resulting in relative depression of the midfacial region is a relatively common characteristic of the Asian face, often being accentuated by an anterior inclination of the maxillary incisors. With increasing age, such a midfacial configuration tends to be associated with deepening of the nasolabial folds.

Although correction of this facial disproportion is an aesthetically rewarding procedure, the number of patients who are willing to undergo a relatively simple corrective operation is amazingly small.

Correction of midfacial retrusion can be effected by using either silicone or Mersilene mesh implants. Mesh implants can be placed via an intranasal approach for correction of small degrees of retrusion, but the intraoral approach affords better visualization for correction of larger "deformities."

The implant is placed in a supraperiosteal plane via a vertical transfrenular sublabial incision. When mesh implants are utilized, the lateral aspect of augmentation extends beneath the origin of the nasolabial fold.

Preformed silicone premaxillary implants (Guinta design) are available in two sizes. Regardless of the size selected,

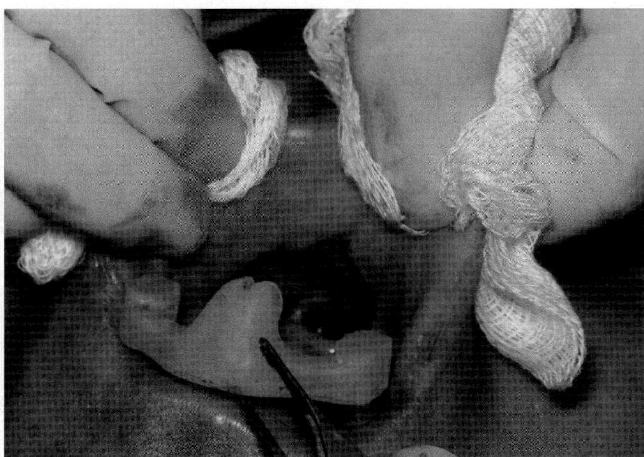

Fig. 35.18 Preformed silicone premaxillary implant (Guinta design) placed via a sublabial approach.

these implants usually require further sculpturing to fit individual facial anatomy (**Figs. 35.18 and 35.19**).

Cervicofacial Rhytidectomy

Anatomical Considerations

Although the goals of facial rejuvenation are identical in both Caucasians and Asians, anatomical variations as well as differences in the aging process justify some modification in the planning and execution of the operative procedures utilized to achieve these goals. Differences between the Caucasian and Asian face are manifested in skin thickness and texture, patterns of fat accumulation, and, perhaps most importantly, skeletal structure. When considering these anatomical differences, it is important to note that just as in the Caucasian, considerable individual variations in anatomy exist among the various Asian populations.

Skin

A wide variation in skin texture and thickness exists among Asians, the dermis being thicker and more fibrous in individuals with darker pigmentation. This greater collagen density is manifested in a tendency to more vigorous fibroplasia during wound healing, which may result in hypertrophic scarring or prolonged erythema during scar maturation. This observation also applies to more lightly pigmented Asian faces. In surgery for facial rejuvenation, hypertrophic scarring is most common in the postauricular regular region and occurs occasionally in the inferior aspect of the temporal incision. Frank keloid formation is unusual.

Fat

During the aging process, the Asian face typically accumulates a greater volume of fat than the Caucasian face. Such fat accumulation tends to be concentrated in the jowl, cheek (nasolabial mound), and buccal regions. The clinical significance of such fat accumulation is often enhanced by skeletal deficiency of the midface, accentuating the "cheeky" appearance. However, fat accumulation in the neck producing the so-called double chin is less common in younger Asians than in their Caucasian counterparts but becomes more common in the aging Asian face.

Platysma Muscle

Although the platysma muscle is generally thicker in the Asian neck than in the Caucasian, the incidence of diastasis

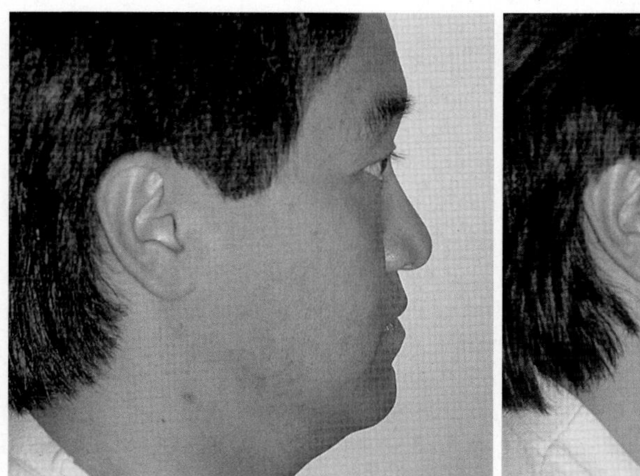

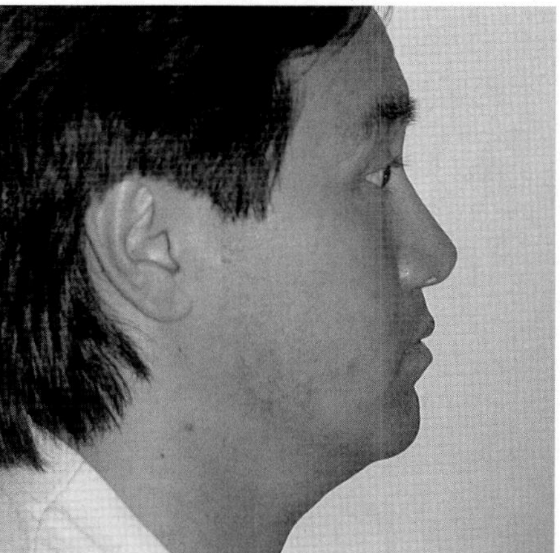

Fig. 35.19 (**A**) Pre- and (**B**) postoperative photographs illustrating the results of maxillary augmentation using a silicone implant.

s considerably less, occurring in ~30% of patients who ındergo cervicofacial rhytidectomy as compared with ~60% of Caucasians undergoing the procedure.

̧Skeletal Structure

'erhaps the most significant anatomical differences between the Caucasian and the Asian face are related to skeletal structure. The Asian face is characterized by prominent malar eminences associated with relative deficiency of he maxillary region, resulting in shallowness of the midacial area. Wide, prominent mandibular angles are often noted, contributing to a square, fat appearance of the face. Microgenia is less common than in the Caucasian face, as is he cervical deformity attributed to low hyoid placement.

Cervicofacial Rhytidectomy

The basic procedure for cervicofacial rhytidectomy is essentially the same for both the Asian and the Caucasian. However, special attention, must often be directed to he midface. As a consequence of fat accumulation and skeletal deficiency, ptosis of the malar fat pad of the midace produces especially prominent nasolabial mounds and deep nasolabial folds. Although any recent innovative surgical procedure designed to correct midfacial ptosis can be utilized, I have found that a direct approach to subperiosteal dissection of the midface that can be performed via the exposure of a standard cheek flap (i.e., obviating the necessity to initiate subperiosteal dissection through a coronal approach) allows excellent, often dramatic rejuvenation of the face (**Fig. 35.20**).

Surgical Technique for Direct Subperiosteal Dissection of the Midface

If subperiosteal dissection of the midface is to be performed, the temporal aspect of the incision is extended superiorly to a level superior to the lateral brow. Skin undermining begins in the temple in the subdermal plane at a level sufficiently deep to preserve hair follicles. Dissection at this level (i.e., superficial to the superficial layer of temporal fascia rather than deep to this fascial layer) provides additional protection for the temporal branch of the facial nerve. Undermining extends anteriorly to the lateral aspect of the brow, the lateral temporal region, and 1 cm anterior to the anterior border of the masseter muscle. The dissection then extends over the mandibular margin to join the cervical flap.

Attention is then directed to the midfacial region. The anatomical foundation of this simplified approach to subperiosteal dissection of the malar fat pad/zygomatic muscle complex relates to the constant relationship between the temporal and zygomatic branches of the facial nerve in this region (**Fig. 35.21**). Initiation of the subperiosteal dissection just posterior to the junction of the zygomatic body and frontal process of the zygoma ensures

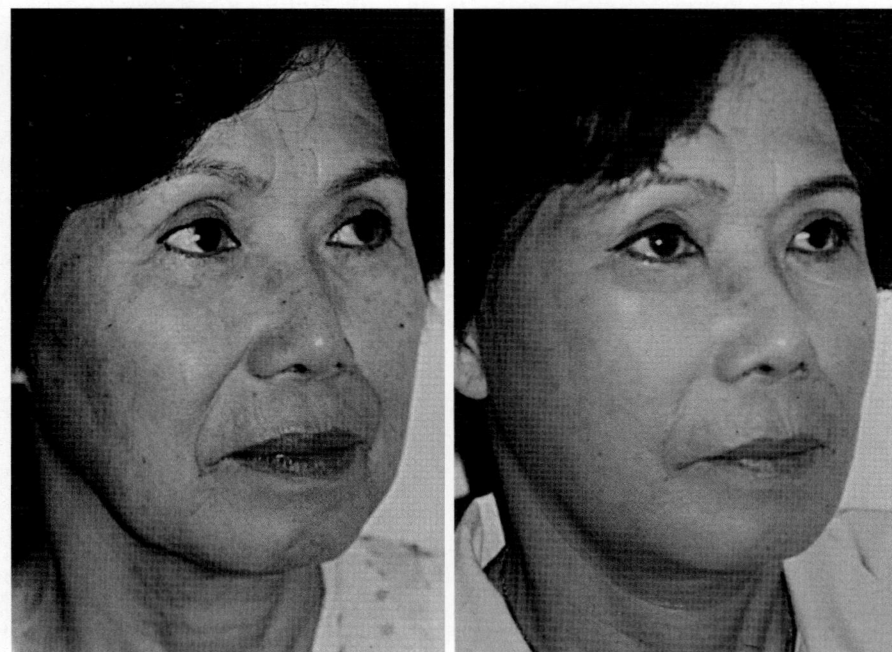

Fig. 35.20 Cervicofacial rhytidectomy. (**A**) Preoperative; (**B**) postoperative.

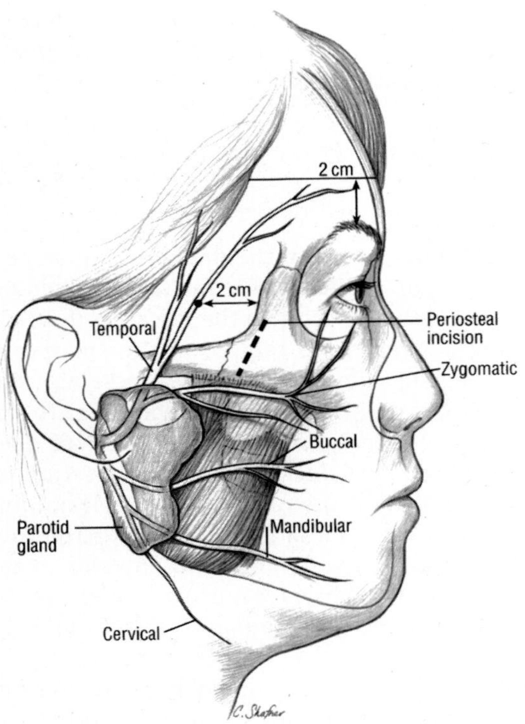

Fig. 35.21 Constant anatomical relationships of the temporal and zygomatic branches of the facial nerve.

that both branches are protected. The subperiosteal dissection proceeds inferiorly and medially into the canine fossa toward the pyriform aperture beneath the nasolabial fold. The key to successful mobilization and elevation of these tissues is release of this composite flap (**Fig. 35.22**) from its attachments to the tendinous anterior aspect of the masseter, easily and safely accomplished by blunt dissection. Should flap mobilization prove difficult, the tendency on the part of the inexperienced surgeon would be to extend dissection medially. Such dissection, however, proves fruitless. Additional flap mobilization can only be obtained by dissection more posteriorly along the zygoma and inferiorly along the tendinous portion of the masseter muscle. Additional subperiosteal section along the body of the zygoma ensures that all fibers of the zygomatic ligament are released. Approximately 1 to 1.5 cm of posterosuperior, composite flap advancement is then possible, resulting in effacement of the nasolabial fold and repositioning of the malar fat pad in a more youthful position (**Fig. 35.23**). The flap is imbricated, being fixed to the superior aspect of the original flap incision (to avoid strangulation of more superiorly located facial nerve branches) with two or three sutures of 3-0 nylon (to provide "permanent" fixation) supplemented with 4–0 polydioxanone.

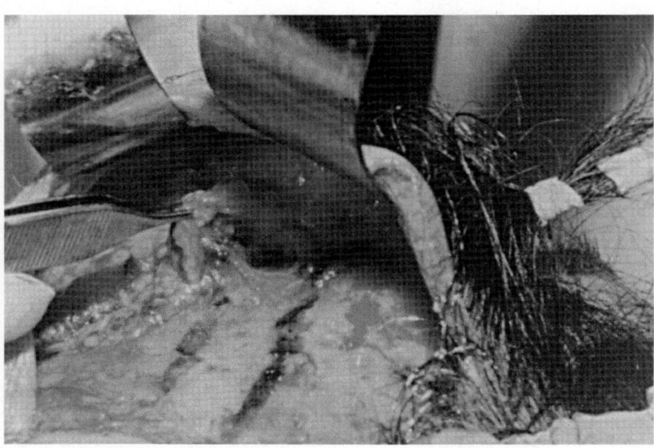

Fig. 35.22 Dissection of the subperiosteal malar flap.

Because of the extensive mobilization and elevation of the midfacial region, the skin flap must be dissected to the level of the orbital rim to avoid bunching. Such dissection allows exposure and modification of the orbicularis muscle, if indicated. In some patients, the midfacial skin is dissected over the malar region and to the nasolabial fold to enhance draping of the skin flap. Although subperiosteal dissection of the midface may benefit by this increased skin undermining, tension on the skin flap is actually reduced by prior advancement or suspension of the composite flap. This is in marked contrast to the extraordinary tension placed on the skin flap by advocates of the deep-plane or composite facelift operations who utilize the skin as a vehicle for advancement of the malar fat pad.

Because the nasolabial fold has been effaced by the composite malar flap, wide superficial musculoaponeurotic system dissection toward the central face is unnecessary.

Considerable improvement to the jowl region is often achieved by spot liposuction of jowl fat via a stab wound in the labiomental fold utilizing a 14-gauge needle cannula (**Fig. 35.24**). Maximal effacement of the jowl may require skin flap elevation to the oral commissure to reduce the tethering effect of the mandibular ligaments.

Segmental Operations for Correction of Cheek and Temple Ptosis

Many Asian patients demonstrate manifestations of aging in the facial area that are not associated with the problems in the cervical region. Management of cheek ptosis and fat accumulation without associated neck fullness or redundancy can be managed successfully with a cheeklift operation, the incisions for which are illustrated

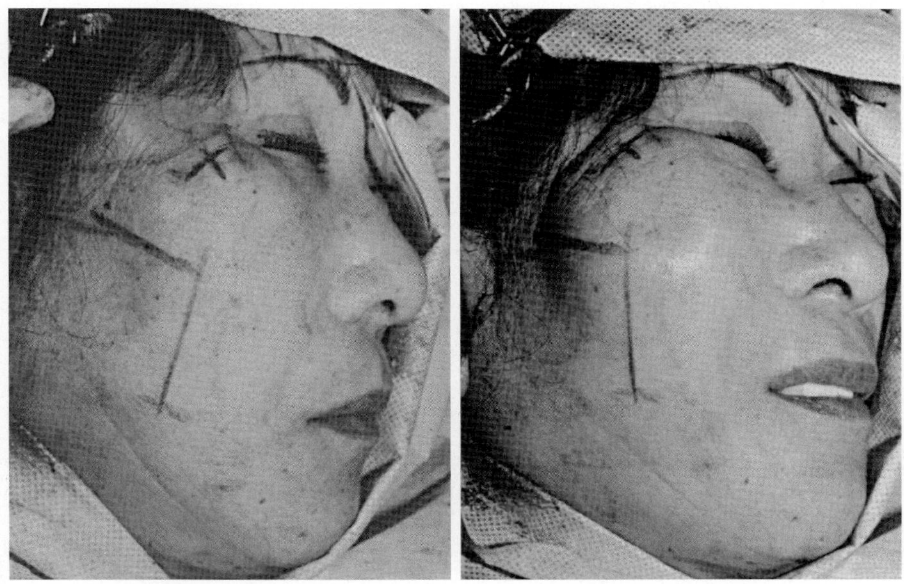

Fig. 35.23 Interoperative traction on the subperiosteal malar flap demonstrating the extent of cheek mobility possible.

in **Fig. 35.25**. This procedure is not a "minilift" because it involves considerable skin undermining, most often accompanied by subperiosteal dissection of the midface described previously. The results of such procedures (**Fig. 35.26**) are often enhanced by spot liposuction of the jowl and nasolabial mound using a syringe technique (**Fig. 35.24**).

If indicated, the temporal aspect of the cheeklift incision can be extended superiorly, resulting in another segmental operation termed the cheek/temple lift.

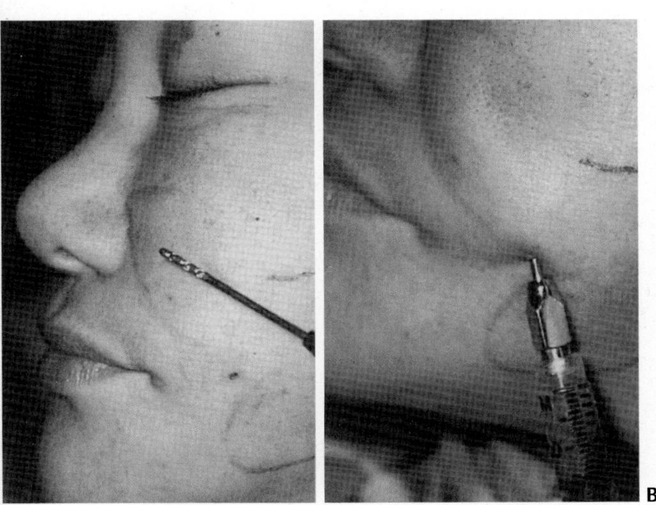

Fig. 35.24 Spot liposuction of the jowl and nasolabial mound.

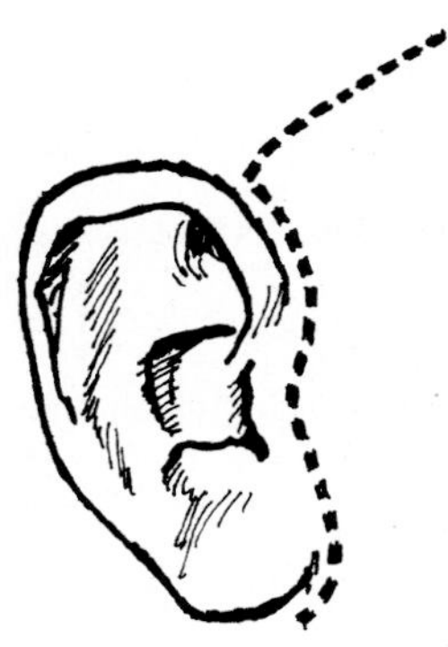

Fig. 35.25 Cheeklift incision.

Complications

Complications of these operations are identical to those occurring after surgery in the Caucasian face (i.e., bleeding, hematoma, infection, scar formation, flap necrosis, hair loss, nerve injury, and asymmetry). Older Asian patients tend to exhibit a high incidence of hypertension; thus the surgeon should ensure that adequate control of blood pressure has been obtained preoperatively. As is true in Caucasians, hematoma is more common following facelift procedures in men. Flap necrosis is somewhat less common in Asians because of the increased thickness of their skin. The incidence of hypertrophic scarring is, however, higher in this group. Such scars occur most commonly in the postauricular region but occasionally

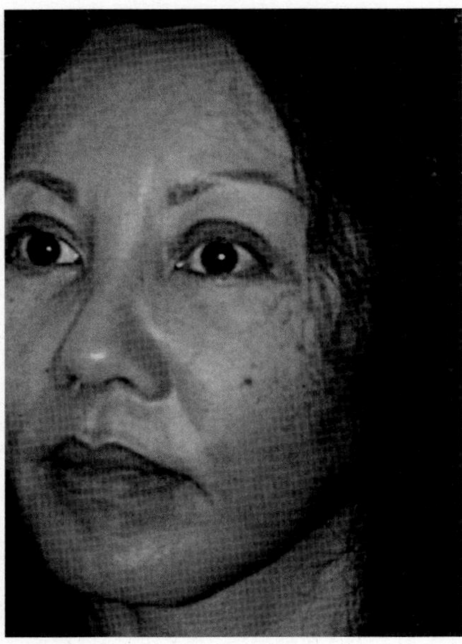
A

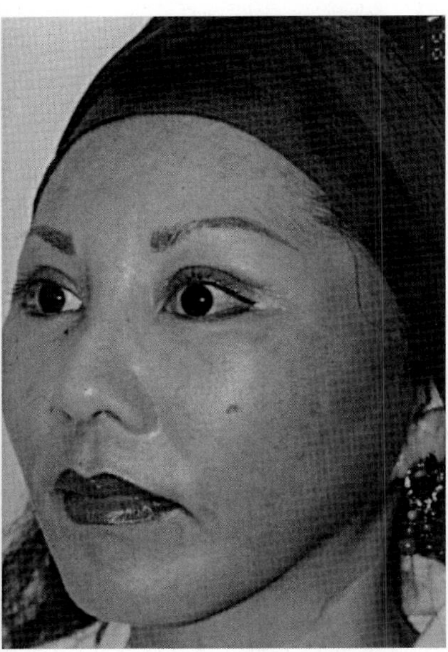
B

Fig. 35.26 Cheeklift. (**A**) Preoperative; (**B**) Postoperative.

manifest themselves in the preauricular and temporal areas. In most cases, satisfactory management of hypertrophic scarring is achieved with intralesional steroid injections.

Suggested Readings

Boo-chai K. Plastic construction of the superior palpebral fold. Plast Reconstr Surg 1963;31:74–78

Boo-chai K. Sculpturing the nasal tip and lobule region. Clin Fac Plast Surg 1996;4:103–116

Cheu MT, Lu SY. Secondary blepharoplasty for Oriental eyelid. Clin Fac Plast Surg 1996;4:49–54

Fernandez LR. Double eyelid operation in the Oriental in Hawaii. Plast Reconstr Surg 1960;25:257–264

Flowers RS. The art of eyelid and orbital aesthetics: multiracial considerations. Clin Plast Surg 1987;14:703–721

Giunta SX. Premaxillary augmentation in Asian rhinoplasty. Fac Plast Surg Clin 1996;4:93–102

Hin LC. Oriental blepharoplasty: a critical review of technique and potential hazards. Ann Plast Surg 1981;7:362–374

Hin LC. Unfavorable results in Oriental blepharoplasty. Ann Plast Surg 1985;14:523–534

Hiraga Y. Complications of augmentation rhinoplasty in the Japanese. Ann Plast Surg 1980;4:495–499

McCurdy JA Jr. Augmentation rhinoplasty: implant selection and design. Fac Plast Surg Clin 1996;4:87–92

McCurdy JA Jr. Lower lid blepharoplasty. Clin Fac Plast Surg 1996;4:41–47

McCurdy JA Jr. Management of the epicanthal fold. Clin Fac Plast Surg 1996;4:25–33

McCurdy JA Jr. Cosmetic Surgery of the Asian Face. New York: Thieme 1990

Yang HH, Peterson RL. Asian blepharoplasty: suture technique. Fac Plast Surg Clin 1996;4:35–40

36 Aesthetic Surgery of the Lip

Brian P. Maloney

Voluptuous lips are not just for Valentine's Day. Lips not only serve a very significant functional role, such as in speaking and eating; they are an important aesthetic feature of the face. Full lips imply youth, health, and strength. Because of society's quest for these attributes, the number of lip procedures has increased dramatically as people strive to achieve these goals. Cosmetic surgeons now have the ability to enlarge, reduce, refine, shorten, and lengthen lips in accordance with patients' goals. This chapter reviews the embryology, anatomy, aesthetics, and goals of lip surgery. The chapter concludes with a description of many contemporary lip procedures.

Embryology and Anatomy

An understanding of the embryology of lips serves as a foundation for understanding the basis behind the multitude of lip surgeries currently performed. The upper lip forms during development from two distinct pairs of structures: maxillary swellings and medial nasal swellings.[1] The lateral maxillary swellings fuse with the paired medial nasal swellings to form the upper lip. Thus the characteristic undulations of the philtral ridge and cupid's bow reflect the union of these different structures (**Fig. 36.1**). The lower lip forms from the merger of the paired mandibular swellings, resulting in a simpler and less defined structure. Because of the embryological difference, the upper and lower lips function very differently from one another. The upper lip tends to be much more mobile than the lower lip.[2]

The defining points of the upper lip rest in the central cupid's bow complex. This complex is formed by the two high points of the vermilion lying along each philtral ridge with a V-shaped depression between them (**Fig. 36.2**). The greatest vermilion show of the lower lip lies on parallel points to the upper lip with no central depression. Another characteristic feature of the lips is the presence of the white line or roll.[3] This structure is a raised line of skin, which separates the vermilion from the cutaneous portion of the upper and lower lip. Its function is unknown; however, Giles hypothesized that the white roll serves as a reservoir of skin that allows the lip to perform its many complex motions, such as puckering, smiling, talking, and eating.

The cutaneous portion of the skin contains hair, sebaceous glands, and eccrine glands. The vermilion of the lips is red due to a lack of keratinization and the underlying capillary plexus. The lip vermilion is composed of a dry and a wet portion. The dry mucosa is exposed to the air and is generally the visible vermilion of the lip. It borders the cutaneous portion of the lip anteriorly and is separated from the wet mucosa posteriorly by the wet line.

The bulk of the lip consists of the orbicularis muscle. The vermilion and adjacent cutaneous portion are separated from the underlying muscle by a thin fascial layer. In the center of the upper lip the orbicularis fibers decussate and insert into the contralateral philtral ridge. The commissure of the lips represents a complex area where the orbicularis muscle decussates and the lip elevators, lip depressors, and the buccinator muscle join.

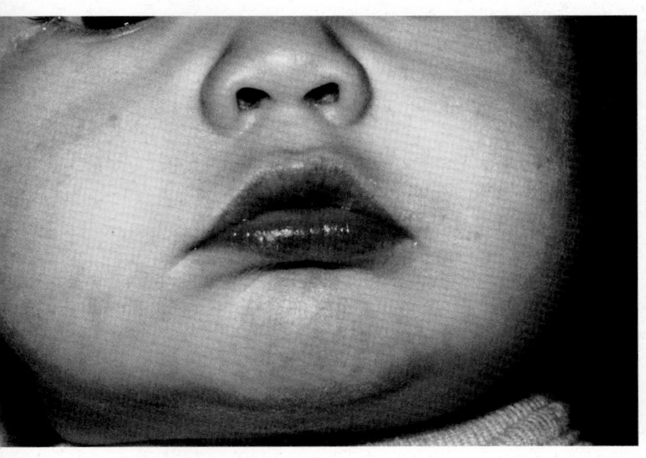

Fig. 36.1 A 6-month-old child highlights the embryological difference between the upper and lower lip.

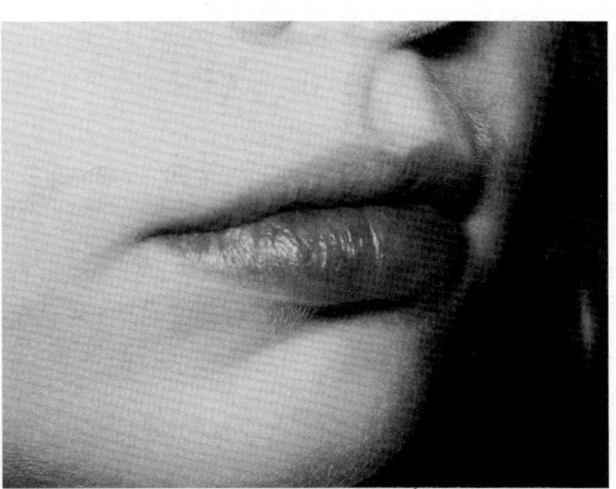

Fig. 36.2 Oblique view of the lips showing a well-defined white roll, central tubercle, and cupid's bow area.

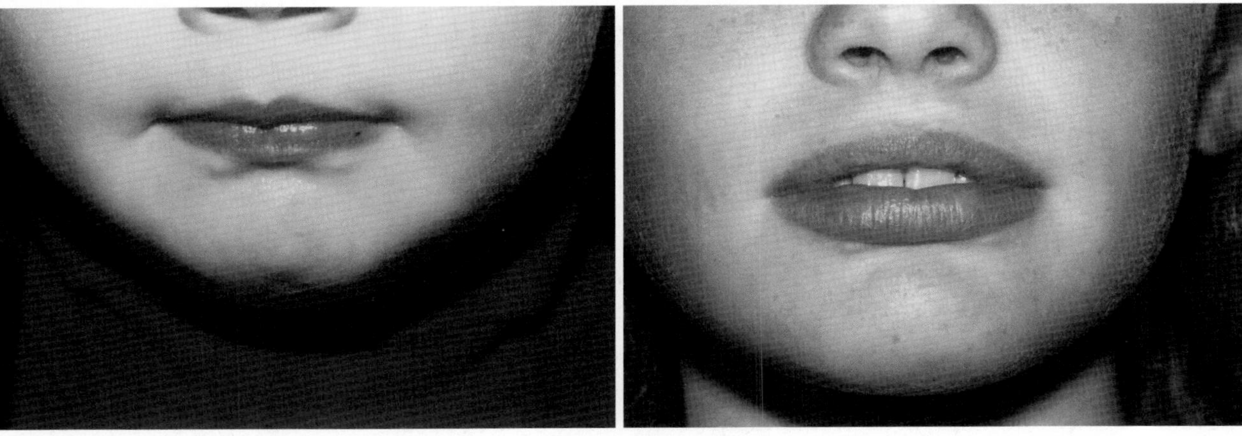

Fig. 36.3 (**A**) A 3-year-old girl showing well-defined lip shape. (**B**) Same child 6 years later showing the hypertrophy of the lip tissues resulting in aesthetically full lips.

Aesthetics

There is no ideal standard for the perfect lip. Everyone has a different concept of what constitutes a beautiful lip. Many people like a fuller lower lip, whereas others prefer a more projecting upper lip. Despite individual preferences, there are some fundamental proportions and anatomical features that contribute to attractiveness.

The distance from the menton (the lowest point of the chin) to the subnasale (the point where the columella meets the upper lip) should be one third of the distance from the menton to the hairline. If a patient has a high forehead the former measurement should equal the distance from the subnasale to the glabella (the most prominent point on the forehead). Within the lower one third of the face, the upper lip should contribute one third and the lower lip two thirds of the distance.

On the profile, a line from the subnasale to the soft-tissue pogonion (the most prominent point of the chin) can be used to assess lip projection. Previously, some authors, such as Burstone, cited guidelines (e.g., "the upper lip should lie 3.5 mm anterior to this line and the lower lip 2.2 mm").[4] However, due to variances in individual aesthetic ideals, it is generally difficult to cite specific measurements for projection of the lips. A crucial point in evaluating projection of the lips is to consider the position of the teeth. The lips drape over the teeth, and therefore lip under- or overprojection can reflect underlying dental malposition.

Effects of the Aging Process

Thin, poorly defined lips can result from genetics, trauma, or the aging process. The aging process is a reflection of two distinct factors. The first factor responsible for aging is directed in large part by heredity, resulting in intrinsic aging. Lip size appears to increase until puberty due to hypertrophy of the muscular and glandular components (**Fig. 36.3**) and then begin a gradual decline. The second component consists of extrinsic factors, such as sun exposure and cigarette smoking, which can accelerate the aging process. The senile transition of lips reflects changes not only in the skin but in the supporting tissues (muscle, fat, teeth, bone). Over time the well-defined raised white roll that surrounds the upper and lower lip begins to flatten (**Fig. 36.4**). As this happens, there is blunting of the cupid's bow and a decrease in vermilion show. As the subcutaneous layer begins to thin and the muscles begin to lose their tone, there is a loss of lip projection. These processes also

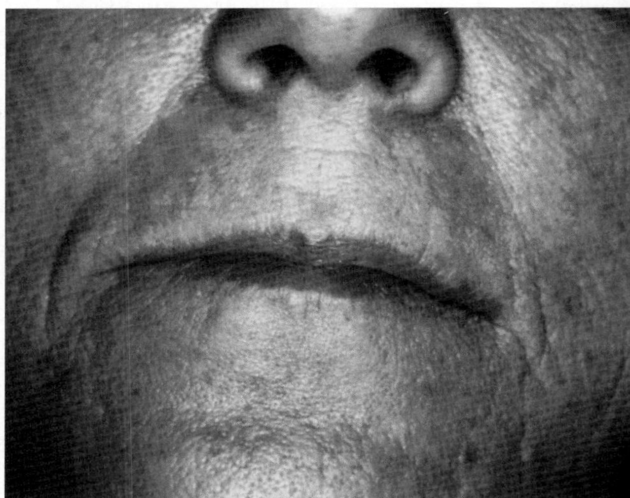

Fig. 36.4 Patient showing aging-related changes to the lip: lengthening of the upper lip, blunting of central defining points and philtrum, flattening of the white roll, decreased vermilion show, rhytids, downturning of the commissures, and decreased lip projection.

result in a downturning of the corners of the mouth. Because of the combination of loss of volume of the supporting elements of the lip and the loss of skin tone rhytids develop in both the vermilion and the cutaneous skin. Thus the end-stage result is a long, poorly defined lip with little vermilion show and minimal projection.

Lip Surgery

Preoperative Evaluation and Goals

Many patients come in with very specific ideas about their purpose in having the surgery. Others come in with less precise goals and more generalized concepts. During the consultation period, it is very important for the surgeon to identify any expectations the patient has regarding the lip surgery. That is, is the patient concerned about the length of the lip, definition of cupid's bow area, the amount of vermilion show, the amount of projection, presence of rhytids in the vermilion and cutaneous areas, downturning of the corners of the mouth, or possibly the lack of definition along the white roll or the philtral ridges? It is very helpful to have the patient sit in front of the mirror and point to specific areas of concern, thus allowing patient and surgeon to come to a common understanding.

The review of the patient's history should include any history of previous lip treatments, surgeries, or trauma. This should include previous collagen injections, which can result in some fibrosis of the lip area, as well as a history of herpes simplex, allergies, or other significant medical conditions.

Physical examination of the lips should occur with the patient's face in a resting state. Following is an outline of the physical examination process.

1. Assessment of the underlying dental occlusion
2. Analysis of the facial proportions: examining the vertical one third and documenting the length of the upper and lower lip
3. Degree of cupid's bow definition
4. Definition of the philtral ridges
5. White roll definition around both upper and lower lip
6. Vermilion show of the upper lip and lower lip
7. Amount of dental show (younger patients will have several millimeters of central tooth visible, but as the lip lengthens with age this becomes less visible)[5]
8. Position of the corners of the mouth
9. Condition of the vermilion epithelium
10. Condition of cutaneous lip epithelium
11. Evaluation of lip projection
12. Chin position (microgenia can make full lips look even larger)

By following these detailed steps, the surgeon should be able to identify existing conditions that contribute to the patient's underlying concerns. The proper diagnosis of these conditions will serve as a cornerstone for a successful outcome.

Photography

Photography has a very important roll in all cosmetic surgery. With regard to lips, it allows the surgeon to identify and confirm asymmetries preoperatively for planning purposes. It also allows patients to refer back to their preoperative condition after they have undergone the procedure(s) to identify changes that have been achieved. Photographs should be taken with the patient wearing no lipstick or makeup of any kind. The superior border of the lip series should run from the infraorbital rim superiorly to the hyoid bone inferiorly. Frontal, right and left oblique views, and right and left profile views with lips at rest and with frontal smiling and puckering views will generally suffice.

Anesthesia

The upper and lower lip area can be anesthetized very easily with regional blocks. Four percent lidocaine (Xylocaine, Abraxis Pharmaceutical Products, East Schaumburg, IL) jelly is applied to the mucous membranes of the upper and lower lips (**Fig. 36.5**). Regional blocks consisting of 0.5% bupivacaine, 1:200,000 epinephrine mixed with an equal volume of 1% lidocaine with 1:100,000 epinephrine can be placed through the oral mucous membranes to reach the mental nerves, infraorbital nerves, and greater palatine branch. When regional blocks are accomplished,

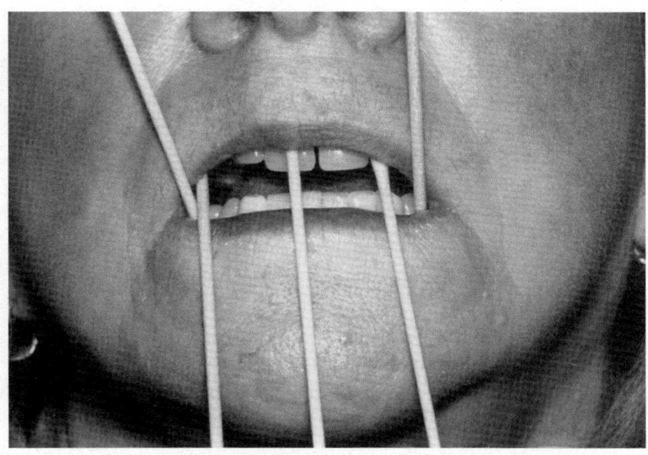

Fig. 36.5 Cotton swabs with a topical anesthetic placed in appropriate locations of upper and lower lip prior to placement of lidocaine regional blocks.

the lips can be injected locally with 1% lidocaine, 1:100,000 epinephrine, and hyaluronidase mixed in a ratio 10 mL to 1 mL, respectively. This mixture is injected along the lips in the plane of dissection. The volume of anesthetic material is limited so as to help reduce possible distortion of the lip. The wydase is not used when dermal matrix grafts are used to reduce the possibility of graft breakdown. Depending on patient sensitivities and whether or not additional procedures are going to be performed, additional anesthesia ranging from oral diazepam 20 mg, or hydrocodone bitartrate (Lortab) 15 mg, to the twilight or general anesthetic may be appropriate.

Treatment of the Lip Cutaneous Skin and Vermilion

Rhytids appear around the perioral region as a result of aging, and the process is accelerated by exposure to sunlight and cigarette smoking. Often these changes reflect damage both in the dermal layer of the skin and in the subcutaneous layer, with a loss of volume of the lip vermilion. This process is exacerbated by frequent puckering, such as cigarette smoking and use of straws. Because superficial fibers of the orbicularis insert into the perioral skin, vertical lines appear around the mouth. These lipstick lines can be treated with botulinum toxin. One to two units can be placed in the middle of the rhytid immediately beneath the skin at several points along the lip. Care should be exercised in a patient with a very thin lip because the thinner muscle mass may result in unwanted motor impairment of the lip.

Other short-term treatments of cutaneous rhytids involve injection of a filler into the perioral lines. Historically bovine collagen was the most common lip filler. However, because of the dynamic nature of the area, collagen may last for as little as 2 weeks. Due to its short duration for most and potential for allergic reactions, hyaluronic-based products have become popular for this purpose. Hyaluronic acid is found naturally in our skin as the glue between the cells. Two common genetically engineered preparations are Juvéderm (Corneal, Paris, France) and Restylane (Medicis, Scottsdale, AZ). Both have a longer chain and are reported to last from 4 to 6 months for most patients. These products are injected with a 30-gauge needle into or just below the dermis, depending on if one is treating a superficial rhytid or furrow, respectively. Sometimes fillers will be combined with botulinum toxin injections as previously described to achieve a longer-lasting result.

Longer-term treatments involve resurfacing of the perioral skin. In the past dermabrasion and phenol-based chemical peel solutions were performed on the perioral rhytids. More recent resurfacing tools include power peeling for very superficial rhytids to chemical peels and carbon dioxide laser resurfacing for deeper rhytids. Nonresurfacing laser technology is evolving and may provide a larger benefit in the future. The deepest rhytids can oftentimes be pretreated with acetone followed by the application of a phenol-based Baker's chemical peel solution with a wooden end of a cotton swab. This peel solution can be applied to the dry vermilion of the lip as well. CO_2 laser resurfacing up to the vermilion surface is then performed, including the previously spot-peeled areas. This results in a softening of the lip rhytids with the effect of increased vermilion show (**Fig. 36.6**). For less severe rhytids patients may not require the pretreatment with the chemical peel solution. Deep lines in the vermilion are often a result of loss of substance of the lip, very similar to a balloon losing some of its air. By restoring some of the bulk to the

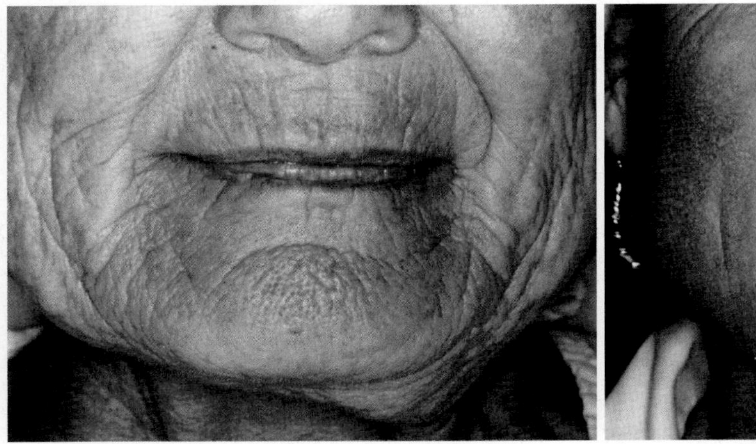

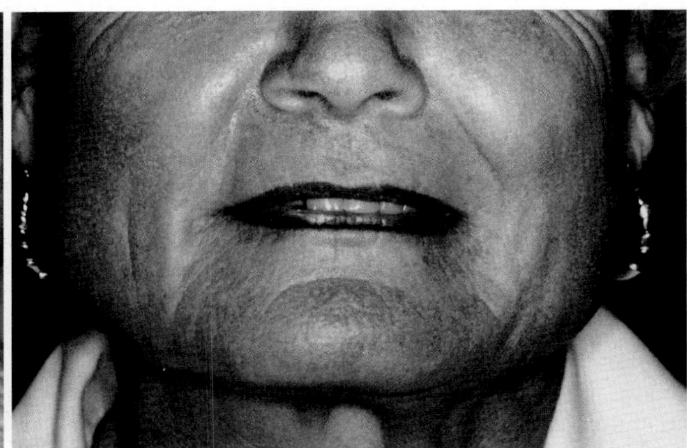

Fig. 36.6 (**A**) Patient showing classic signs of aging. (**B**) After full-face carbon dioxide laser treatment. Pretreatment of the deeper lines with Baker's peel solution was performed.

lip with current augmentation materials, the vermilion rhytids will be softened.

Procedures That Lengthen the Lip

Augmentation

Augmentation of the upper and lower lip has been reported with autologous materials, such as dermis, fat, fascia, superficial muscular aponeurotic system (SMAS), or material such as AlloDerm (LifeCell Corp., Branchburg, NJ) (acellular human dermal matrix grafts), Gore-Tex (W. L. Gore & Associates, Inc., Flagstaff, AZ), silicone, and a variety of other fillers.

The basic principles of augmentation involve either increasing the vertical length of the lip or increasing the projection of the lip. The goal one is trying to achieve determines the placement of the implant material (**Fig. 36.7**). When lengthening the lip is the goal, the implant material is generally placed in a submucosal plane or in a tunnel along the inferior aspect of the upper lip and superior aspect of the lower lip. If one is trying to achieve an increase in projection, the implant is either deposited in the submucosal along the anterior surface of the lip or in a tunnel along the anterior surface. Because of the dynamic nature of the lips, it can be a challenge to maintain implant materials in the lip for any length of time.

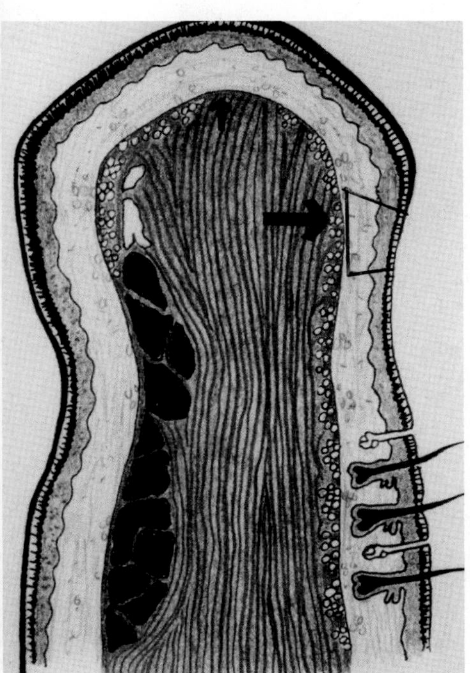

Fig. 36.7 Cross-section of lip, with small arrow showing tunnel for lengthening of lip and larger arrow showing plane for increasing projection of lip. Solid line to indicate plane of dissection for lip advancement, which can be performed separately or conjointly.

Autologous materials are generally readily available; however, they involve morbidity of a second site. Fat historically has survived in an unpredictable fashion, often resulting in an unevenness of the lip surfaces.[6] However, the success of fat survival has increased dramatically with improved harvesting and microdroplet placement, thus making fat an exciting lip filler with greater reliability than the past. Fat transplantation requires a sterile environment due to the multiple stages, and specialized equipment.

Dermal grafts as well as SMAS grafts have not generally survived for very long in the lip as a result of the dense cellular nature of these graft materials. Temporalis fascia is generally very thin and does not offer a significant amount of augmentation material for most patients.

Hyaluronic acid fillers have the flexibility of allowing one to inject along the white roll, along the filtrum, and along the vermilion. A small percentage of patients may exhibit an allergic reaction to components of the material. This can generally be treated with systemic antihistamines and topical steroid preparations. In the lip area, hyaluronic acid products may last from 4 to 6 months for most patients. Patients are advised to gently squeeze the lip between their fingers three to four times a day for 2 days to help minimize lumpiness. Massage past the second day seems to break down the material, resulting in a shorter aesthetic effect.

I personally do not recommend certain fillers to my patients because they may have a tendency to make the lips hard. Calcium hydroxyapatite and methylmethacrylate beads are two such implants that have been used in the lips. The thin mucosal covering of the lip may result in visible lumps as well as firmness. Some patients are not bothered by this and like the potential longer aesthetic effect.

AlloDerm

Acellular human dermal matrix grafts were originally developed for the covering of large burned areas; however, they have been used successfully for lip implants.[7] The graft material is procured from an accredited tissue bank. Following chemical removal of the cells within the dermis, the material is freeze-dried. This results in an acellular matrix that allows for tissue ingrowth and repopulation of the matrix (AlloDerm). Because of the constant rebuilding of one's body, by the end of a year the AlloDerm is no longer present and has been entirely replaced with the patient's tissues. This is an exciting concept of placing a temporary scaffold into one's body to encourage new tissue growth. AlloDerm can be inserted into the lips after they have been anesthetized with regional blocks through incisions in the commissure. A submucosal tunnel is created with a tendon passer along either the anterior or the inferior aspect of the lip,

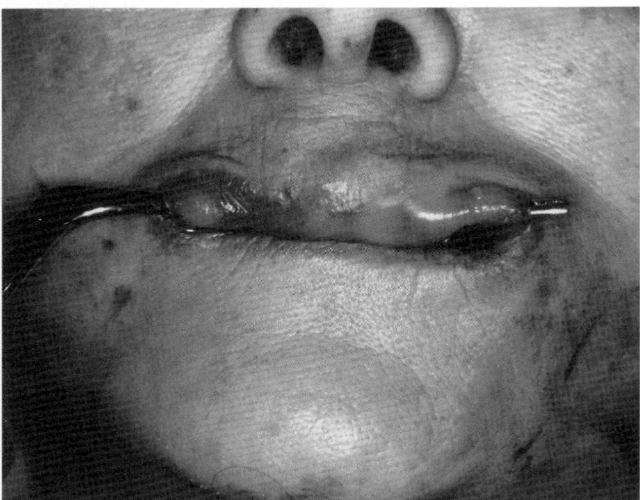

Fig. 36.8 Straight-tendon passer being used to create a tunnel along the superior lip border. The incisions are placed in the commissure so that the same incisions can be used to augment both upper and lower lips.

depending on one's goals for the procedure (**Fig. 36.8**). After the instrument is passed through to the opposite side, the appropriate-sized piece of AlloDerm is then pulled into the pocket. When using this material, the surgeon must remember that the swollen rehydrated form will be compacted in the host's tissues back to a size more comparable to the dry state. Therefore the surgeon should estimate the amount of augmentation desired with the dry AlloDerm as opposed to the rehydrated form. Commonly, two thirds of a 3 × 7 cm sheet can be placed in the upper lip and one third in the lower lip (**Fig. 36.9**). However, it is often possible to place an entire sheet in each lip. The tunnel should be placed submucosally or sufficiently submucosally to avoid seeing any of the whitish implant through the lip material. If a small area of material is exposed in the commissure or vermilion surface postoperatively, the exposed material may be trimmed back generally without consequence. Injectable AlloDerm is available; however, the long-term effectiveness does not appear to be as good as the sheets. Because of the particle size it is used as a subcutaneous implant, in contrast to other fillers A 2-in. 25-gauge needle is inserted

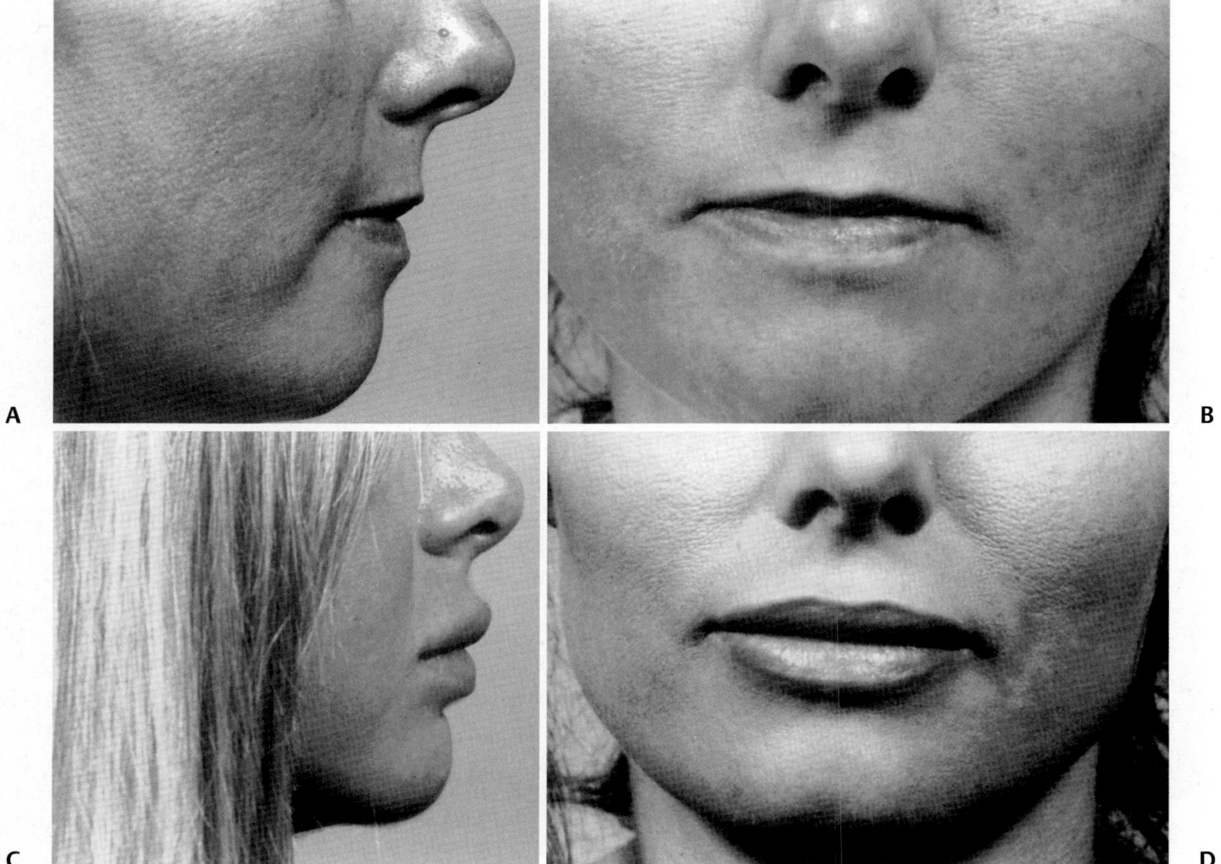

Fig. 36.9 Upper and lower lip. AlloDerm augmentation (**A,B**) before and (**C,D**) after.

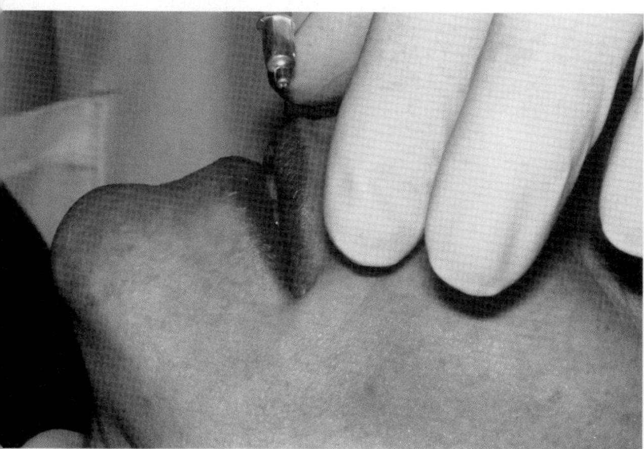

Fig. 36.10 Injectable AlloDerm can be placed into the lips through a central incision, followed by threading the material in the desired plane from the commissure to the midline and then similarly on the opposite side.

at the midline and threaded through the lip in the desired plane (the same plane if one were inserting sheets of AlloDerm). Micronized AlloDerm is evenly deposited on withdrawal of the syringe (**Fig. 36.10**).

Expanded Polytetrafluoroethylene

Expanded polytetrafluoroethylene (ePTFE, Gore-Tex) has been used extensively over the years as a lip augmentation material.[8] This implant material is not subject to reabsorption. However, when placed in the lip it does develop a capsule fibrosis around it, which can result in tightening and firmness of the lip. The other disadvantage is that patients can generally feel ePTFE in the lip. The complex motions of the upper lip make it very difficult for the upper lip to maintain ePTFE within it, and extrusion is not uncommon in the upper lip. The manufacturers have attempted to increase the flexibility of larger pieces of ePTFE by changing it to a multistranded implant (**Fig. 36.11**). This seems to work well in the lower lip; however, it has not been tolerated in the upper lip, in the author's experience. Manufacturers are making ePTFE softer and softer. As this occurs its role in lip augmentation may change.

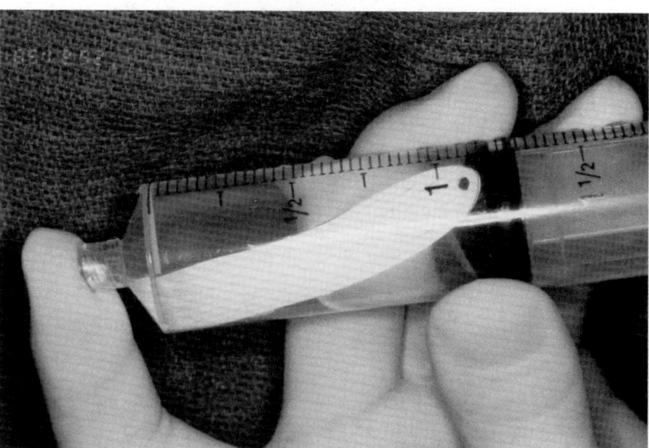

Fig. 36.11 Multistrand Gore-Tex lip implant being impregnated with an antibiotic solution via a vacuum in the syringe.

Silicone

Microdrop silicone is a possible lip augmentation material that was used extensively in the past. However, because of its current Food and Drug Administration (FDA) standing, microdrop silicone is not generally used by many physicians. Occasional reactions to the microdroplet could be seen, and this is possibly related to impurities within the silicone itself. A liquid silicone has recently been FDA approved for orbital reconstruction. Its use as an "off-label" filler may reappear because of this. Great care should be exercised because quite often lips seem to adopt a fleshy look with silicone injections.

V-Y Advancement

V-Y advancement or augmentation cheiloplasty, a technique that has been around for many years and was initially used to treat the whistle-lip deformity, involves use of a V-Y closure technique at the mucosa (**Fig. 36.12**).[9–11] The entire mucosa can be brought forward by placing two

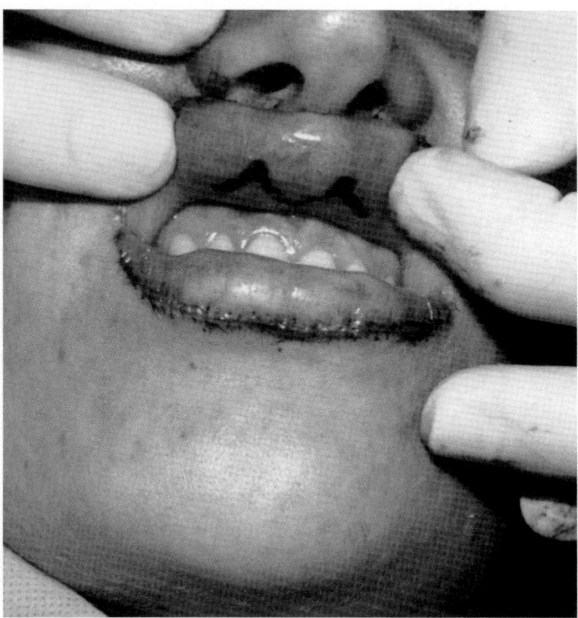

Fig. 36.12 Patient who has undergone upper and lower lip V-Y advancement. The goal of the V-Y advancement was to increase the projection and bulk of the central lip. If more lateral fullness was desired the V-Y advancement would extend to the commissures.

Vs next to each other in a W fashion and advancing these in V-Y fashion. The exact amount of augmentation desired can be slightly unpredictable. To advance the lateral vermilion, it is necessary to extend the W-plasty to the commissures. The flaps are elevated and the incisions closed with a V-Y advancement technique. Scarring does not appear to be significant or create much firmness for the patient.

Procedures That Shorten the Lip

Lip Advancement or Vermilion Advancement

Lip or vermilion advancement was originally described by Gilles and later refined by other surgeons.[12,13] It involves the removal of an ellipse of cutaneous skin adjacent to the vermilion of either the upper or lower lip. In the case of a long upper lip with little cupid's bow definition, the technique can be used to restore the central defining points. It is often handy to have patients draw with the marking pen on the upper and lower lips to show the shape and size they would like to achieve. This can be done with them sitting in front of a mirror and allows for better physician–patient understanding of the surgical goals (**Fig. 36.13**). Care is to be taken to note and discuss any preoperative asymmetries. After the areas are marked, an additional 1 mm should be excised to accommodate for some lip recoil. The ellipse of skin is excised in the fascial plane, immediately beneath the skin and above the muscle (**Fig. 36.14**). This will help to re-create the white-roll fullness adjacent to the vermilion. Care is taken not to go beneath this facial plane because scarring and tightness may result. The defining points of the upper lip are brought together with vertical mattress sutures without any undermining of the adjacent edges. Final wound closure can be performed with a running subcuticular 5–0 Prolene suture (Ethicon, Inc., Somerville, NJ) and reinforced with absorbable sutures as necessary (**Fig. 36.15**).

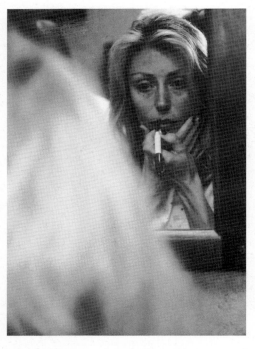

Fig. 36.13 Allowing patients to draw their desired lips in the mirror can facilitate physician–patient communication regarding the goals of surgery.

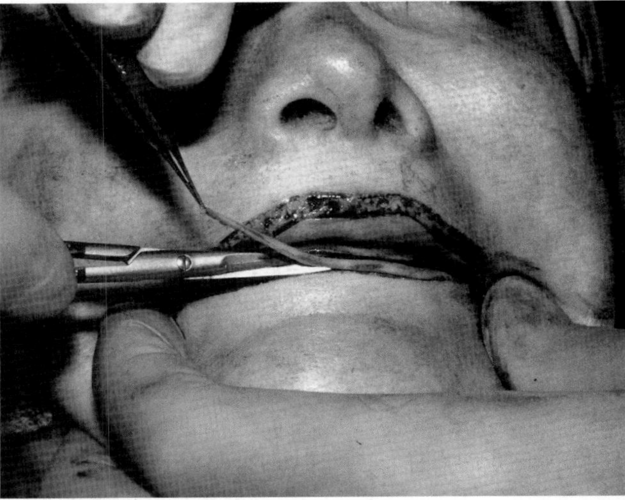

Fig. 36.14 The boundaries of the areas to be excised are first scored with a no. 15 knife blade. Removal of the areas in a superficial plane can be accomplished with sharp scissors as shown. Note that the plane of dissection is superficial to the muscle.

Nasal Base Resection

Nasal base resection is an excellent procedure for patients with a long upper lip, and a well-defined cupid's bow area, and a well-defined nasal base.[14] The ellipse of skin at the base of the nose should follow in a seagull fashion the contours of the base of the nose. Depending on the anatomy of the nasal sill, the incision can extend into this area. A parallel line is drawn inferior to this, thus creating the ellipse of skin to be excised. The skin is excised in the subcutaneous plane, and wound closure is accomplished in a two-layer fashion (**Fig. 36.16**). It is reported by Millard[15] that the distance from the philtrum origin at the nasal sill to the insertion at the vermilion varies from 18 to 22 mm. If the lip exceeds this measurement or is longer than the relative proportions of the face, the nasal base resection may be an appropriate procedure for the patient.

Cheiloplasty

Cheiloplasty, or vermilion reduction, can be performed by excising an equal amount of the vermilion on each

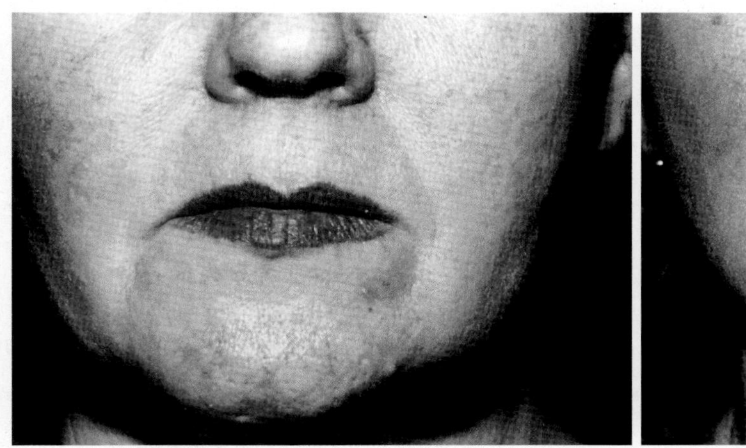
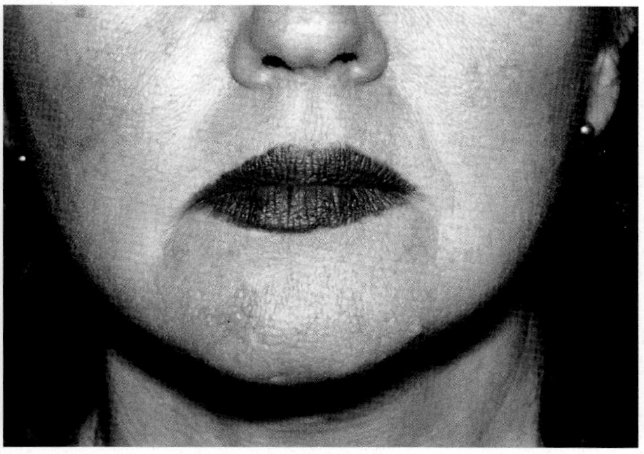

Fig. 36.15 (**A**) Preoperative view of patient with significant asymmetry between the two sides of her lips. (**B**) After upper and lower lip advancement.

side of the wet line of the lip. The goal is to maintain the incision at or slightly behind the wet line of the lip. This incision may involve more than just the mucosa, depending on the bulk of the lip to be reduced. The incisions are then closed with absorbable sutures. Generally overresection of the lip is necessary to accommodate postoperative recoiling of the lip. Reduction cheiloplasty must address each component of lip enlargement, including increased anterior projection, vertical lip height, and wet-vermilion show. To help minimize overresection of the mucosa one can incise one side of the ellipse first, then undermine the mucosa and hypertrophic glandular tissue and retract this posteriorly, excising the excess tissue. Care should be taken to preserve the height of the lower lip at the level of the lower incisors.

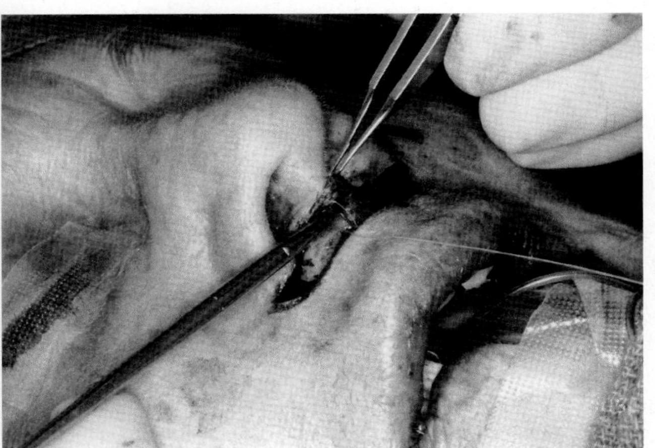

Fig. 36.16 Photograph of the nasal base resection showing removal of skin from the upper lip and closure of subcutaneous tissues.

Postoperative Care and Recovery

Following lip procedures of almost any type, patients report that their lips feel "tight," as well as abnormal when smiling, for ~6 to 8 weeks. Although their lips may not appear abnormal, patients may feel uncomfortable during this period. Following surgery, patients are instructed to rest the lips for ~2 weeks. They are also instructed to avoid smoking. Patients are generally placed on an antiviral agent pretreatment if there is a history of herpes simplex. If an outbreak occurs in a patient who has undergone augmentation, the patient should exercise caution. The inflamed tissues may be more friable and therefore susceptible to graft exposure. A broad-spectrum antibiotic is also routinely used in patients who undergo any autologous fillers or surgical lip procedures.

Additional Refinements

Use of permanent cosmetics or dermal pigmentation can help highlight the lip shape or possibly balance out postoperative asymmetries. This procedure can be performed in the office under regional anesthetic block.

Complications

Infection and bleeding are potential complications of any surgical procedure. Because of the complex anatomy of the perioral region, it is very important to identify preoperative asymmetries because some of these may persist postoperatively. Whereas some procedures lend themselves to the correction of minor asymmetries, other lip procedures described will not correct these asymmetries and could potentially accentuate them. Significant postoperative asymmetries may be attributed to localized edema and can be treated with diluted steroid injections. Paresthesia of the lip may persist for up to 6 months.

Small extrusions of implant material may be treated by removing the exposed material, followed by local wound care. Larger extrusions or infections of the augmentation material generally require removal of the graft material. Following removal of the implant the potential space from which it came can fill with scar tissue, resulting in tightness of the lip. To minimize tightness of the lip, dilute triamcinolone injections are performed weekly or biweekly. Patients are instructed to massage and stretch the lips 6 to 10 times daily. This routine is performed for 10 to 12 weeks until the lips relax.

Conclusion

Lip procedures are becoming increasingly popular. The cornerstone to a successful outcome is for both the patient and the surgeon to have a solid understanding of the patient's goals and starting point. Once the surgeon has made an appropriate diagnosis, there are many tools available to help achieve the desired outcome.

References

1. Latham RA, Deaton TG. The structural basis of the contour of the vermilion border: a study of the musculature of the upper lip. J Anat 1976;121:151–160
2. Mortegi K, Yamazato S. The relationship between cleavage lines and postoperative scars after repair of cleft lip. J Fac Surg 1985;13: 183–184
3. Binnie WH, Lehner T. Histology of the mucocutaneous junction at the corner of the human mouth. Arch Oral Biol 1970;15:777–786
4. Burstone CJ. Lip posture and its significance in treatment planning. Am J Orthod 1967;53:262–284
5. Vig RG, Brundo C. The kinetics of anterior tooth display. J Prosthet Dent 1978;39:502–504
6. Leaf N, Zarem HA. Correction of contour defects of the face with dermal and dermal fat grafts. Arch Surg 1972;105:715–719
7. Maloney BP. Soft tissue contouring using acellular dermal grafts. Am J Cosmet Surg 1998;15:369–380
8. Shoenrock LD, Reppucci AD. Gor-Tex in facial plastic surgery. MJ Aesth Restor Surg 1993;1:63–68
9. Lassus C. Thickening the thin lips. Plast Reconstr Surg 1981;68:950–952
10. Robinson DW, Ketchum LD, Masters FW. Double V-Y procedure for whistling deformity and repair of cleft lips. Plast Reconstr Surg 1970;46:241–244
11. Aiache AE. Augment cheiloplasty. Plast Reconstr Surg 1991;88:223–226
12. Rozner L, Isaacs GW. Lip lifting. Br J Plast Surg 1981;34:481–484
13. Maloney BP. Cosmetic surgery of the lips. Facial Plast Surg 1996;12: 265–278
14. Austin HW. The lip. Plast Reconstr Surg 1986;77:990–994
15. Millard DR Jr. Cleft Craft: The Evolution of Lip Surgery. Vol 1. The Unilateral Deformity. Boston: Little, Brown; 1976

37 Advances in Aesthetic Dentistry

Garrett B. Lyons Jr. and Roger P. Levin

The concept of aesthetic dentistry has evolved to become an underlying principle in all of the dental disciplines. The past decade has heralded tremendous technological advances, allowing patients to expect and to receive optimal aesthetic treatment from their dentist.

We live in a beauty-conscious society. The American advertising community has pushed the idea that "beautiful is better." Self-improvement is no longer the exclusive domain of the rich and famous, nor is it considered a sign of self-indulgence. Today, taking steps to improve one's appearance is considered an investment in health and well-being and is as socially acceptable as it is personally gratifying. It all begins with a smile.

In addition to expecting technical competence, American consumers expect their dentist and staff to be caring and concerned. Dentists enjoy the satisfaction that comes from delivering treatment that is both functionally gratifying and aesthetically pleasing, and that gives the patient a sense of well-being and satisfaction. Recent advances in aesthetic dentistry have changed modern dental practice dramatically. Aesthetic improvements once considered to be impossible are now considered routine. First, dentists should facilitate patient selection of the most appropriate treatment alternative. Aesthetic improvements must also encompass periodontal health, occlusion, and proper positioning and alignment of teeth, not just a postoperative appearance of a smile viewed in the mirror. Dentists must accurately inform patients of the advantages, disadvantages, and necessary precautions associated with the aesthetic treatment procedure. Dentists must maintain a high level of technical quality because there is no substitute for excellence. Cosmetic dentistry requires problem-solving whereby the practitioner determines the diagnosis, formulates a treatment plan, and selects the appropriate instruments and materials. Treatment must then be dispatched in an orderly fashion with the understanding of proper technique and specific material manipulation.

Color in Treatment of Discolored, Diseased, or Damaged Teeth

Color Analysis of Teeth

The emergence of new techniques to improve patient appearance and enhance the aesthetic restoration of posterior teeth increases the complexity of color selection. Some materials available for aesthetic composite–resin bonding procedures are available in more than 15 shades. The aesthetically oriented dentist must be able to do the following:

1. Identify color patterns and shades of natural teeth
2. Understand the color relationships of enamel, dentin, and cementum
3. Understand the ideal, natural tooth colors, including translucency near the incisal edge of anterior teeth
4. Relate natural tooth colors to shade guides of the various materials available to enhance aesthetics
5. When necessary, diagnose and communicate aesthetic color needs to laboratory technicians
6. Evaluate case results and troubleshoot problems
7. Custom-stain in aesthetic cases
8. Meet patient expectations expressed during consultation and treatment planning

There are three basic parameters of color that are useful to the aesthetically oriented dentist

1. *Hue.* The quality of color that distinguishes one from another. Examples are blue, yellow, and green.
2. *Chroma.* Reflects the intensity of the hue. An example is light blue versus dark blue.
3. *Value.* The light-to-dark aspect of hue. White is the highest value, black the lowest.

Aesthetically oriented dentists can use three factors to analyze and select color. A good shade guide will reflect all three of the previous factors.[1]

Treatment of Color in Discolored, Diseased, or Damaged Teeth

Bleaching

Vital bleaching is becoming a viable treatment option with discolored teeth. Bleaching alone can significantly change the appearance of teeth, sometimes as a result of only one office visit, and almost always less invasively and less expensively than procedures such as crown and bridge, bonding, or veneering. Moreover, bleaching can be used as an adjunctive treatment. For example, it can improve the effect of another procedure for restoration or change of coloration and lessen the number of teeth involved in that procedure, or it may make it possible to restore affected teeth with a lighter shade than would otherwise be possible. The earliest efforts to bleach discolored teeth occurred more than a century ago, but bleaching did not become a vital part of aesthetic dentistry until past decades when the technique gained widespread use for tetracycline-stained vital teeth (**Figs. 37.1 and 37.2**).

Although the mechanisms by which bleaching removes discoloration are not fully understood and may differ, the type of stains the basic process removes almost always involve oxidation, at which time the molecules causing the discolorations are released.[2] Consequently, the success of the technique is dependent on the ability of the bleach to penetrate to the source of the discoloration and remain there long enough to overcome the stain (**Figs. 37.3–37.6**).

In the field of resins it is interesting to note the diversity of the resins and their clinical applicability. The hybrid resins are made of glass and silicon dioxide. They are of high

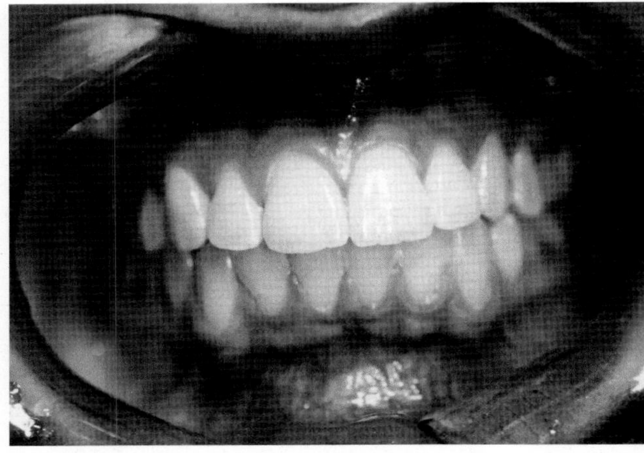

Fig. 37.3 Preoperative photo before bleaching.

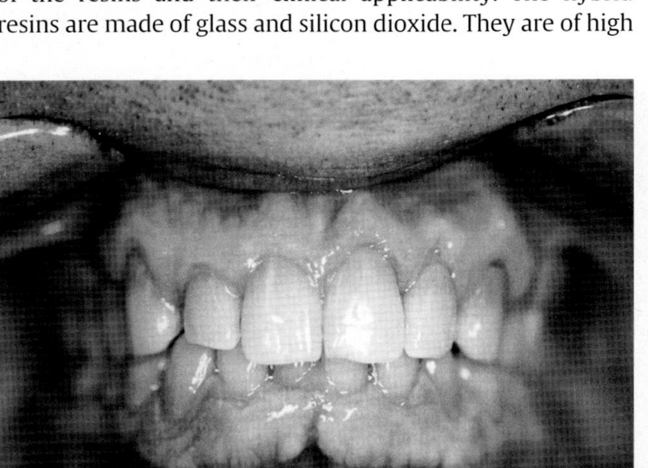

Fig. 37.1 Preoperative photo of tetracycline-stained teeth.

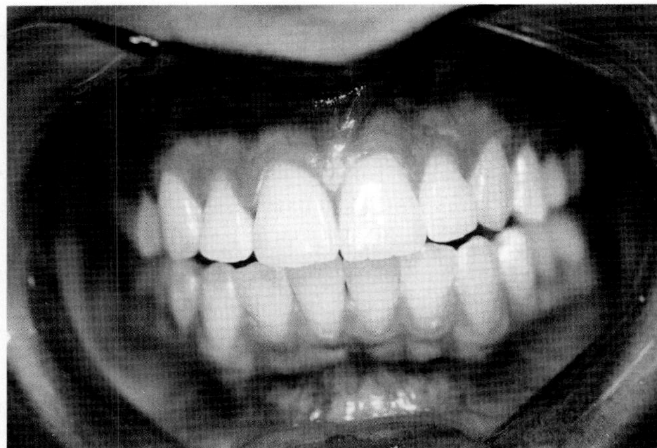

Fig. 37.4 Postoperative photo of bleached teeth.

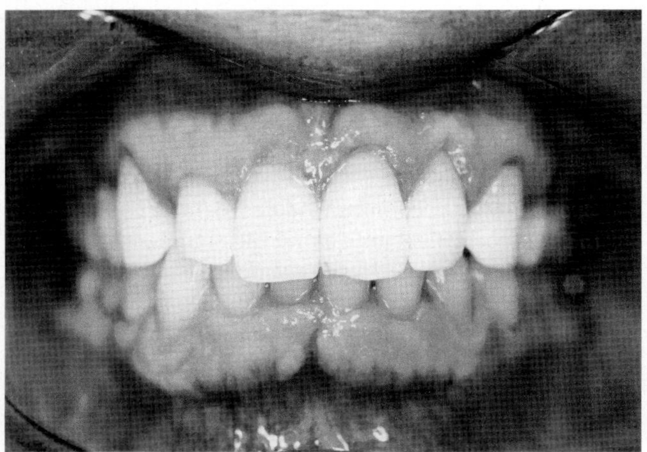

Fig. 37.2 Postoperative photo of bleached teeth at 8 months.

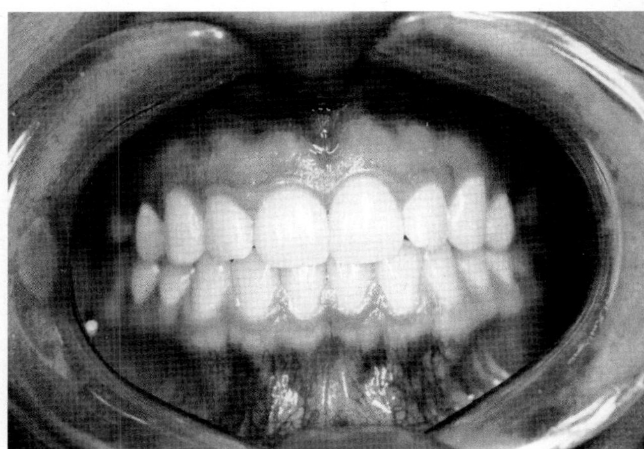

Fig. 37.5 Preoperative photo before bleaching.

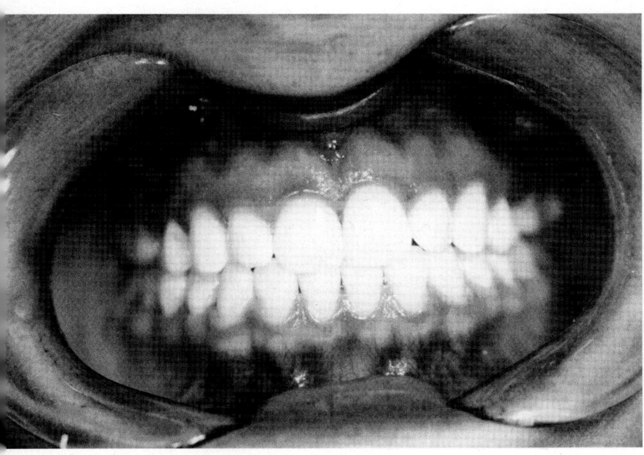

Fig. 37.6 Postoperative photo of bleached teeth.

strength and low expansion and contraction and are associated with low polymer shrinkage. Their strength is the ease of finishing with unfortunate high wear. The microfil resins are also silicon dioxide filled (~50%). Their main use is in anterior applications, and they are noted for smoothness, translucency, and low wear, though not as strong as a hybrid. They are used many times as a veneer over a hybrid in class III and IV applications. Other hybrid resins used for posterior restorations are materials that have a low wear but are less than perfect aesthetically. They are not as strong as some of the other hybrid resins but are best used under hybrids.

Sealants are promoted as unfilled resins. They tend to be used with increasing amounts of filler content. However, they are now being replaced by flowable composites. The flowable resin composites are not very different from sealants. They are hybrid resins with lower viscosity and lower filler content than conventional restorative resin-based composites. They are used in class I restorations of pits and fissures, and sometimes they are the original material placed in a proximal box of class II resins. They have very low strength and are the most wearing of all the composites.

The packable resin-based composites today are condensable; they come compacted but not condensed. These materials are used because of inadequate development of contacts on class II restorations. They are analogous to the spherical amalgams and contain large filler particles.

The last category is the superficial sealing microfils. These contain 50% silicon dioxide and are filled with clear resin-based composites. They resemble a superficial skin that is placed over a composite resin restoration. The way they are used is by being acid-etched over the top of the composite material and made to fill in voids and margins; however, their long-term significance is doubtful.

Indirect resins such as polyglass or polymer ceramic restorations have begun to experience increased usage. These materials are the relatives of in-office direct composites. All of these indirect composite restorative systems are actually modifications of existing tooth resin composites. Their chemistry is similar, though their strength, durability, filler content, and method of curing may be enhanced. Indirect composites are becoming very popular due to the fact that patients are demanding more and more metal-free restorations or metal-free dentistry. The indirect composite resins have a more lifelike appearance. A composite can reflect light in much the same way that a natural tooth structure does. In addition, composites may offer more optimal shade matching than porcelain. There are two main reasons for using an indirect composite resin: (1) the size of the cavity and (2) the function of the force to which the restoration is subjected. These indirect composite resins can be made to fit very well, have terrific aesthetics, and even have low wear to opposing natural tooth and high-wear resistance to function. These materials can also be repaired in the mouth (**Figs. 37.7 and 37.8**).

In 1993, the porcelain laminate veneer was introduced. It combined the aesthetics and positive tissue response of porcelain with the adhesive strength of acid-etched restorations and the convenience of laboratory-fabricated restorations. Aesthetic improvement of acceptably shaped or discolored teeth by chemical means is highly desirable because of its conservative nature. The chemical agents and specific procedures used depend on several factors, including the type, intensity, and location of the discoloration. Porcelain veneers were introduced by Dr. Charles Pincus in Hollywood in the 1930s to enhance an actor's appearance for movie close-ups. Dr. Pincus attached these thin veneers temporarily with a denture-adhesive powder. Indirect veneering did not progress until the 1970s, when Dr. Franck Faunce described a prefabricated acrylic resin veneer that integrated the adhesion principles of Buonocore and Bowen with an indirect

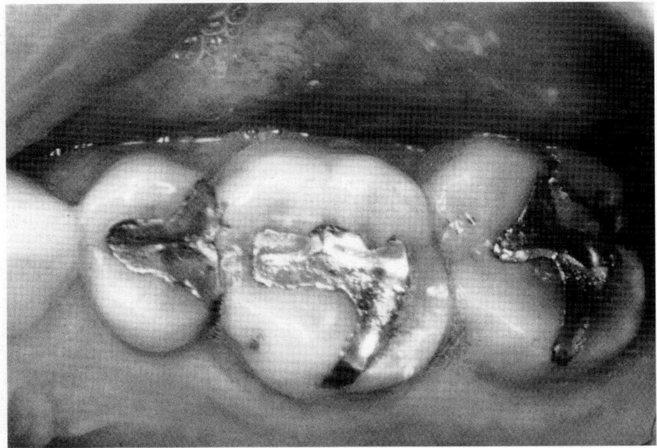

Fig. 37.7 Preoperative photo of amalgam due to be replaced with induct restorations.

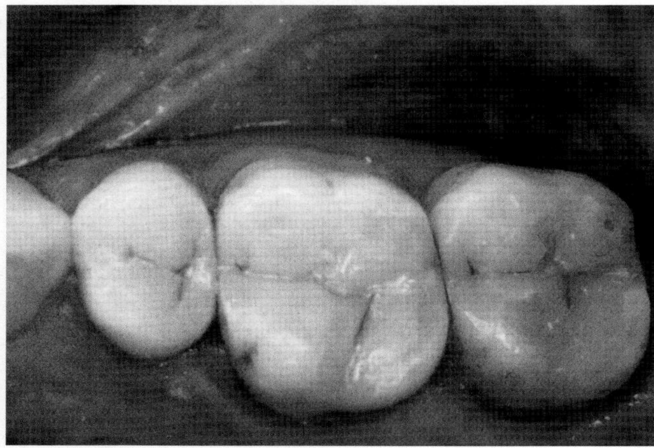

Fig. 37.8 Postoperative photo of indirect tooth-colored restorations.

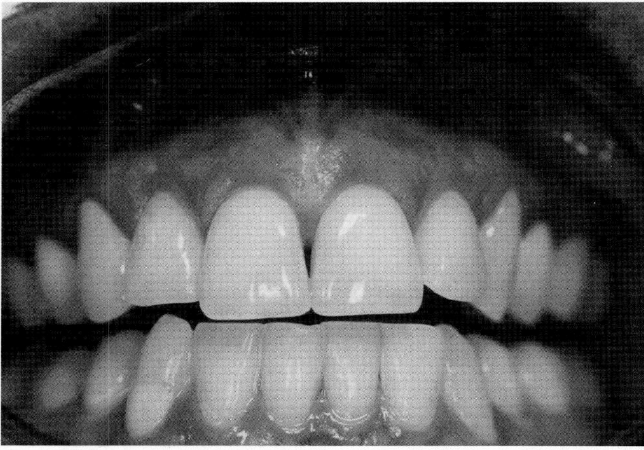

Fig. 37.9 Preoperative photo of teeth to be laminated with veneers.

veneer alternative to porcelain. These veneers were primed with an ethyl acetate or methylene chloride liquid and luted to the etched tooth with a composite resin.[3] The advent of the etched portion of the laminate veneer represents the progress of several decades of research culminating in the synthesis of the acid etch technique and dentistry's most time-honored aesthetic material, porcelain (**Figs. 37.9 and 37.10**).

Glazed porcelain or ceramics often offers abrasion resistance, biocompatibility with gingival tissues, and long-term color stability. The inorganic filler component of composite resins is responsible for its improved physical properties, as opposed to the older unfilled silicates and acrylics. It is composed of quartz, silica, and glass composite fillers, which tend to be hard and similar to tooth structure in terms of translucency and refractive index. Many physical properties, notably fracture and wear resistance, along with polymerization shrinkage, are enhanced as the amount of filler in the composite material increases.

In 1983, Dr. Horn introduced a method to bake the ceramic laminate veneer on a platinum matrix and then etched the inside of the veneer with hydrochloric acid. A coupling agent was applied to the veneer and bonded to the tooth using a light cured composite resin. Composite resin to unetched ceramic was only 230 psi and the strength was increased to 670 psi when the ceramic was etched. It was found that by using a silane coupling agent to increase the bond strength between the ceramic and the composite resin, the strength was increased to 2080 psi. The technique of etching the ceramic veneer surface using a low concentration of hydrochloric acid made possible the development of the ceramic laminate veneers (**Figs. 37.11 and 37.12**).

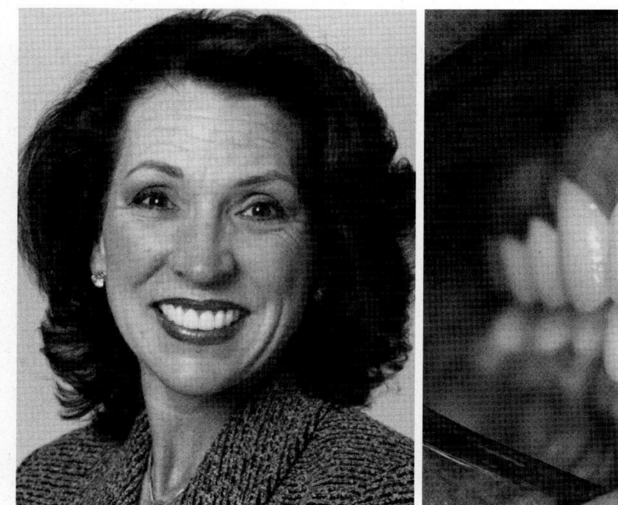

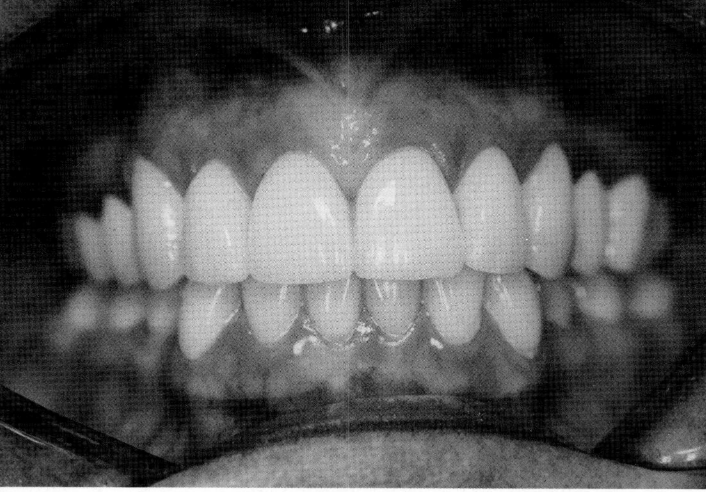

Fig. 37.10 (**A**) A satisfied patient. (**B**) Postoperative photo of laminate veneers.

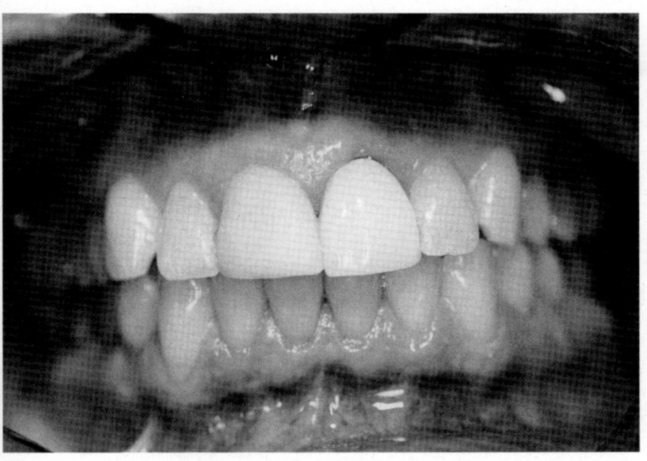

Fig. 37.11 Preoperative photo of teeth to be laminated with veneers.

Minimally invasive dentistry has emerged as a new concept. The earlier a dentist can intervene in a diverse process and the healthier the tooth structure encountered, the closer we can come to the statement, "First do no harm." Despite the role of fluoride in reducing common surface cavities, fluoride has had one unexpected effect. When strengthened by fluoride, enamel undermined by decay is much less likely to collapse. This result is that caries in pits, fissures, and grooves cannot be reliably directly detected with an explorer.

There is a preponderance of evidence that diagnosis of caries with only exploring x-rays will continue to result in nondetection of decay. Air abrasion dentistry now represents a new standard of care. In air abrasion, two powders are commonly used: 27 μm for all cavity preparations and 50 μm for adjunctive bonding enhancement and application. As far as fracturing the tooth structure and using air abrasion under scanning microscopy, studies show that microfracturing and chipping of the enamel prepared with a handpiece does not occur when a tooth is treated with air abrasion. It is overkill to destroy almost a third of the tooth surface with a bur, penetrating the dentin and causing histological changes in the pulp, creating microfractures and then placing an ugly amalgam that can promote recurrent decay and loss of tooth structure. In contrast, treatment with air abrasion and restoration with composite causes none of the histological changes, microfracturing, or excessive loss of tooth structure to which we are subject as a result of our previous decision to withhold or delay treatment. As we move forward, minimally invasive dentistry will be increasingly associated with a desirable restorative result. Minimally invasive preparations do not have the architectural beauty of the line angles and bevels of which we are inordinately proud; their beauty is in the healthy tooth structure left untouched. Although occlusal surfaces constitute only 12% of the total permanent dentition surface areas, they are the sites for the development of more than 50% of the caries reported in most school-aged children. Both permanent and primary teeth are in the pit and fissure surfaces in the molars. This constitutes over 90% of the caries detected in areas where the water is fluoridated. When a pit or fissure has been determined to be caries, air abrasion is used to access and remove the decay. Short bursts of 27 μm particles at 140 to 160 psi are used to carefully widen the grooves. After access to the decay is established, the pressure may reduce to 80 or 100 psi. This enables more control, with removal of decay and greater comfort for the patient. It has been found that the decay follows unusual paths, sometimes going in a lateral direction and reversing course and proceeding seemingly unaffected toward the nerve. It is not necessary to use anesthesia when treating teeth solely with air abrasion. Patients feel either nothing or a mild tingling sensation. Most sealants fail at a rate of ~10% per year.[5] Most of the pathogenic bugs in the mouth are negative anaerobes. Most bacteria that live in the cracks of the fissures of teeth are *Streptococcus mutans* organisms. When restoring such teeth with air abrasion, the common name used is "sealant fillings."

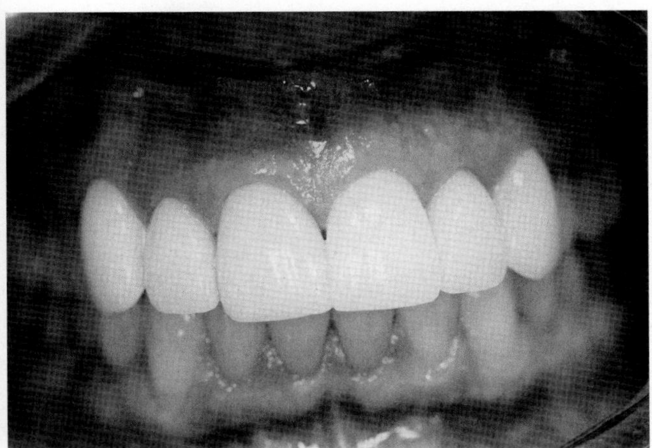

Fig. 37.12 Porcelain laminates.

Dentistry has taken the lead in the preventive approach to dealing with pathology. Noninvasive, nonmutilative tooth preservation has enabled dentists to enjoy what many refer to as the reemergence of the "golden days of dentistry."

References

1. Levin RP. Advances in aesthetic dentistry. In: Papel ID, Nachlas NE, eds. Facial Plastic and Reconstructive Surgery. St. Louis: Mosby Year Book; 1992:248–254
2. Goldstein RE. Bleaching teeth: new materials–new role. J Am Dent Assoc 1987;Spec No: 44E–52E
3. Calamia JR. Clinical evaluation of etched porcelain veneers. Am J Dent 1989;2:9
4. Christiansen G, Christiansen R. CRA status report: air abrasion for caries removal. CRA News 1996;20:3–4
5. Rosenberg S. Air abrasion: the new standard of care. Dent Today 1996;15:78, 80–83

III

Functional and Aesthetic Surgery of the Nose

38 Facial Analysis of the Rhinoplasty Patient

Kofi D. O. Boahene, Steven S. Orten, and Peter A. Hilger

The standards of facial beauty vary in different cultures and are known to change over time, eluding objective definition. Facial beauty may be characterized by a combination of factors that involve symmetry and aesthetically pleasing proportions and relationships. For centuries Greek artists highlighted their personal sense of facial proportion in their drawings often using them to reflect their subject's temperament. Modern-day anthropometric measurements of fixed skeletal and soft tissue points have allowed a more objective and quantitative analysis of the face in the form of ratios, lengths, and angles. In the last decade mathematicians and computer scientists have attempted to define facial beauty using fractal geometry and digital analysis.[1,2] One conclusion has been that facial beauty correlates with simplicity relative to the subjective observer's way of encoding and memorizing it. In other words, "beauty is in the eye of the beholder" and any attempts to quantify facial beauty has to take the observer into account. Even so, facial beauty appears to universally esteem certain geometric rules of proportions, angles, symmetry, and balance. A comprehensive understanding of these proportions, angles, measurements, and relationships that are considered to be the standard for the attractive face is requisite to identifying deviations from the ideal. Although the aesthetic analytical ideals for Caucasian patients are well categorized, ethnic variations from these standards have not been well characterized. Thus attempts to transpose uniform standards on diverse ethnic facial platforms have often resulted in gross disharmorny and dissatisfied patients. Successful rhinoplasty absolutely depends on accurate and thorough analysis of both the nose and the surrounding facial features with an in-depth appreciation for set analytical standards, ethnic variations, and the patient's desires. The purpose of this chapter is to present clinically applicable aesthetic concepts of the nose and the face that are helpful in evaluating a patient for rhinoplasty. It will focus on the analytic details for the Caucasian patient but highlight the anatomical variants in non-Caucasian patients.

Nasal–Facial Analysis

Analysis of the patient prior to rhinoplasty begins with the assessment of nasal–facial relationships. Although there is great variety in nasal and facial appearances, general guidelines regarding attractive nasal–facial proportions have been developed.[3] There have also been many different methods for analyzing facial proportions, some of which involve intricate and confusing measurements that are difficult to apply. The following diagrams provide some basic guidelines that are easy to apply both pre- and intraoperatively for the rhinoplasty patient.

The face has classically been divided by horizontal lines into thirds (**Fig. 38.1**). The forehead hairline (trichion) to the glabella, the glabella to the nasal base (subnasale), and the nasal base to the chin (menton) are approximately equal thirds. Powell and Humphrey noted that because of the variable position of the hairline the "upper third" portion was not significant except in procedures such as forehead lifts.[3] Accordingly, they redefined the evaluation of facial heights with the middle third originating from the nasion and extending to the subnasale. With these redefined boundaries, the middle third approximated 43% and the lower third 57%, respectively, of the distance from the nasion to the menton. The lower third of the face may be further subdivided into thirds, with the upper lip being one third and the lower lip and chin two thirds. The nose

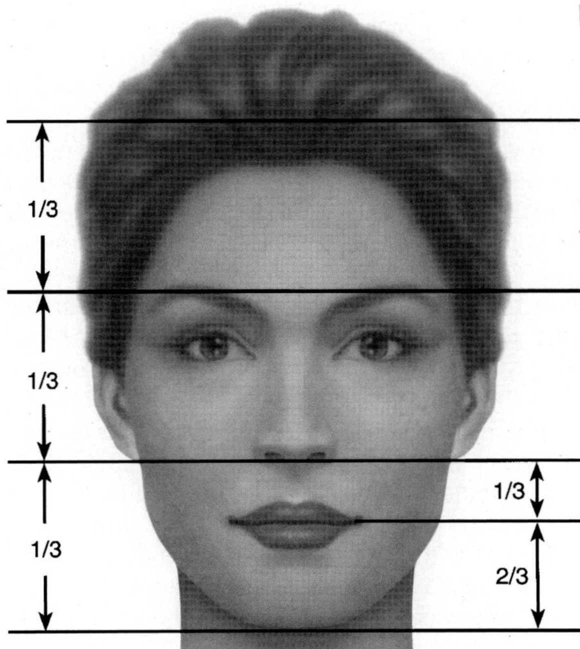

Fig. 38.1 The face is divided into vertical thirds by horizontal lines. The upper third extends from the hairline to the glabella, the middle third from the glabella to the subnasale, and the lower third from the subnasale to the menton.

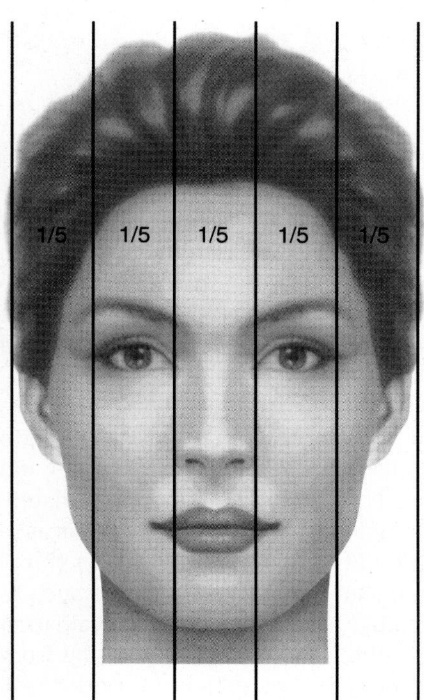

Fig. 38.2 The face may be divided by vertical lines into facial fifths, with the nasal base width equal to the intercanthal distance and the width of the palpebral fissure.

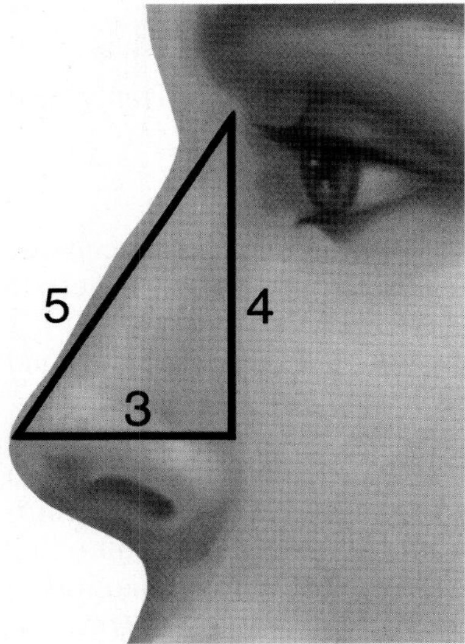

Fig. 38.3 Nasal projection and length illustrated as a 3–4-5 triangle. The ratio of projection to length is represented by the ratio of 3:5, making nasal projection 60% of nasal length.

and face may be divided by vertical lines into horizontal facial fifths, with the nasal base width equal to the intercanthal distance and the width of each eye (**Fig. 38.2**).

When viewed in profile, the nose should project from the face with the proportions of a 3–4-5 right-angle triangle with the nasal projection being 60% of the nasal length (**Fig. 38.3**).[4] The nasofrontal angle begins approximately at the level of the supratarsal crease, and the chin should approximate the lower lip in its anterior projection.

Within these general aesthetic guidelines variations exist due to individual or ethnic differences. African American, Asian, and Latino noses often deviate from the classic desription of vertical fifths and horizonatal thirds. The nasal base width among these ethnic groups is often wider than the intercanthal distance. The middle third from the nasion to the subnasale in the Middle Eastern patient is frequently longer than the lower third but is shorter in Asian and African American patients.

Most patients have facial and nasal asymmetries that should be discussed in the preoperative consultation. This is best demonstrated by using computer formatting of digital photographs to create two faces from different facial halves (**Fig. 38.4**). These asymmetries may not be noticed by the patient preoperatively; however, there is an increased likelihood that the patient will be hypervigilant to irregularities after surgery. Moreover, skeletal asymmetry, as in the case of a crooked nose resting on a deviated nasal spine and philtral column, may compromise the final result if not recognized and appropriately addressed.

Nasal Evaluation

Nasal Skin

The evaluation of the rhinoplasty patient should take into account the skin and soft tissue covering of the nose. Nasal skin that is thick and sebaceous does not drape well to reveal subtle changes that have been made in the bony cartilaginous framework. Thus reduction rhinoplasty in patients with thick skin may produce a smaller but poorly defined nose, whereas less aggressive reduction combined with judicious placement of cartilage grafts will result in a more balanced and refined appearance with preservation of airway. Many surgeons feel that edema takes longer to subside before the final results are apparent when thick, sebaceous skin is present. However, thin skin may drape too well, showing any minor deformities and irregularities underneath.

Nasal skin is generally thicker at the nasofrontal angle and becomes thinner over the rhinion (**Fig. 38.5**). From the rhinion to the supratip the skin becomes thicker again, with an increase in sebaceous glands. Over the nasal tip the skin may vary considerably from thin skin that outlines the underlying nasal tip cartilages to thicker skin that contributes to the bulbosity of the tip.

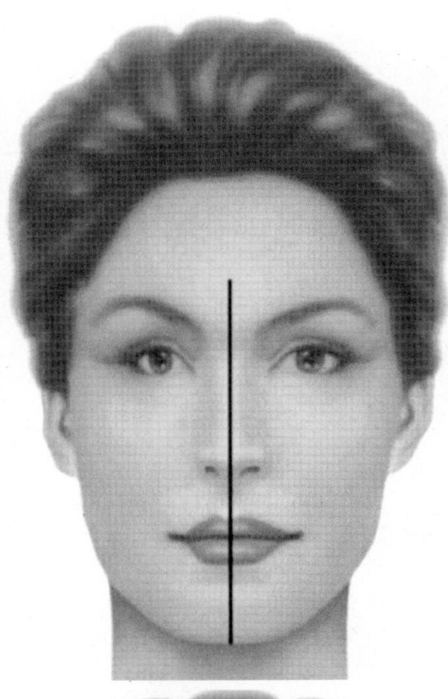

A

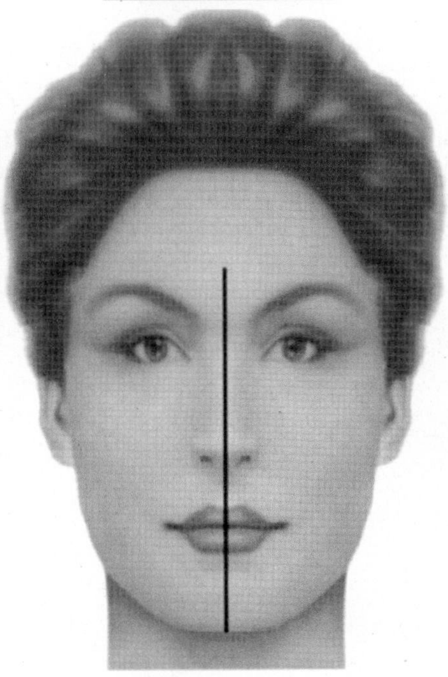

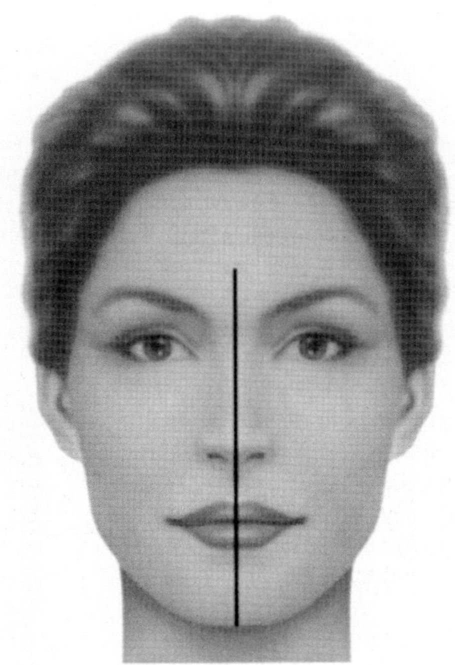

B

Fig. 38.4 (**A**,**B**) Subtle facial asymmetry becomes clearer by using computer formatting to generate two faces from different facial halves.

The alar lobule skin is also thick, with a greater density of sebaceous glands, whereas the skin of the columella is generally thinner than any area of the nose.

The presence of previous scars (chicken pox, traumatic, etc.) should be noted as they may affect how the soft tissue redrapes and may require camouflaging techniques. Signs of acne rosacea should prompt pretreatment or referral to a dermatologist because it may become exacerbated postoperatively with persistent erythema.

Framework Strength

Palpation of the bony and cartilaginous framework is an essential part of rhinoplasty analysis. For example, the stiffness of the lower lateral cartilages will influence rhinoplasty technique. Weak cartilage may require more conservative trimming or augmentation to achieve the desired contour and offset the contractive forces of healing. Conversely, stiff cartilage may require more

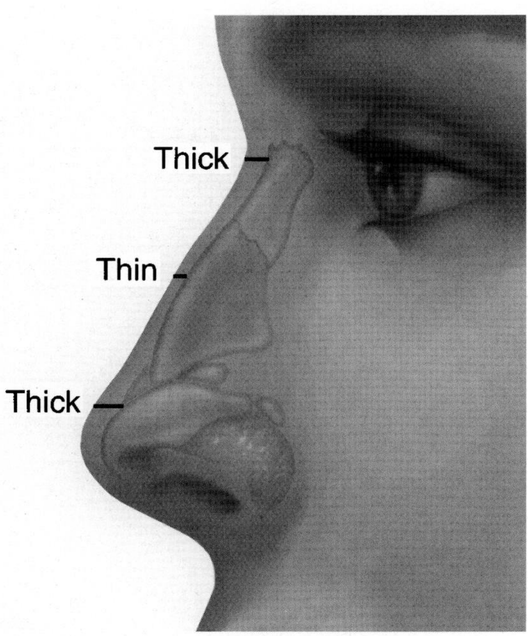

Fig. 38.5 Nasal skin thickness varies over the dorsum of the nose. The thickest skin is usually at the nasal tip, whereas the thinnest skin is at the rhinion.

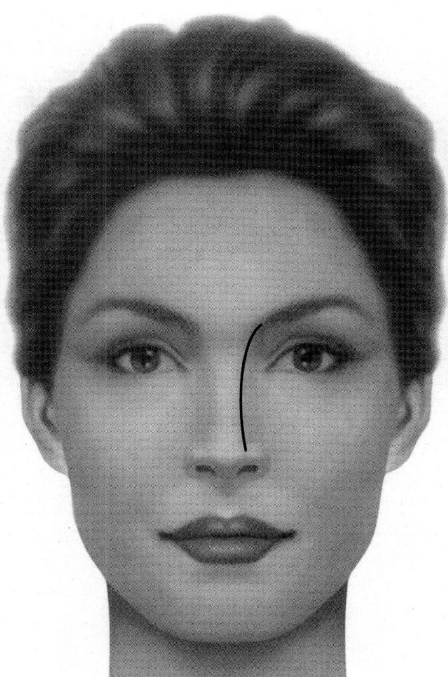

Fig. 38.6 The nasal dorsum should follow a gentle curving line from the medial brow to the nasal tip.

aggressive modification. Short nasal bones likewise will alter the surgical approach. Preservation of the structural support of the airway is mandatory. Aesthetic enhancement at the cost of physiological compromise will not benefit the patient.

Frontal View

On frontal view the symmetry of the nose can be evaluated. A curved unbroken line can be viewed sweeping from the medial brow to the ipsilateral nasal tip defining point (**Fig. 38.6**).[5] A line from the midglabella to the menton should bisect the nasal bridge and tip (**Fig. 38.7**). Any deviation or twist of the external nose should be readily apparent from this view.

The width of the nasal dorsum and alar base can best be assessed from a frontal view. The width of the alar base should be approximately the same width as the intercanthal distance (**Fig. 38.8**). If the alar base is significantly wider than the intercanthal distance, alar base modification can be considered. The width of the bony sidewall of the nose should be 75 to 80% of the normal alar base (**Fig. 38.9**). If the bony base exceeds this dimension, narrowing can be accomplished at the time of lateral osteotomy. If the width of the bony base is within the normal range but the bony dorsum is wide, mobilization of the nasal bones will be required while keeping the bony base width the same.

On frontal view, the nasal tip has two tip-defining points that represent light reflection from the skin overlying the domes of the lower lateral cartilages (**Fig. 38.10**). Asymmetries in the domes of the lower lateral cartilage

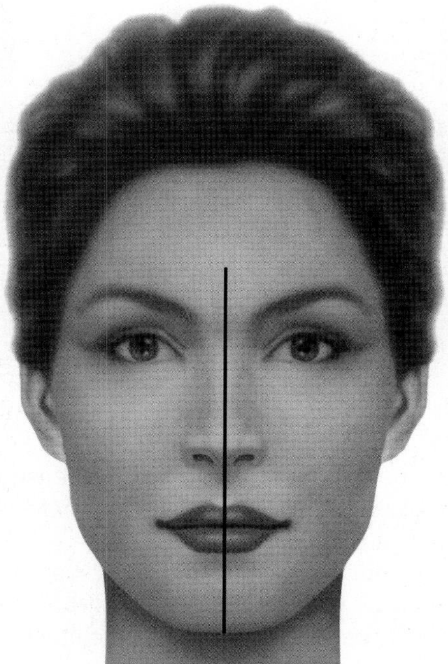

Fig. 38.7 Nasal deviation is apparent when a line is drawn vertically from the midglabella to the menton.

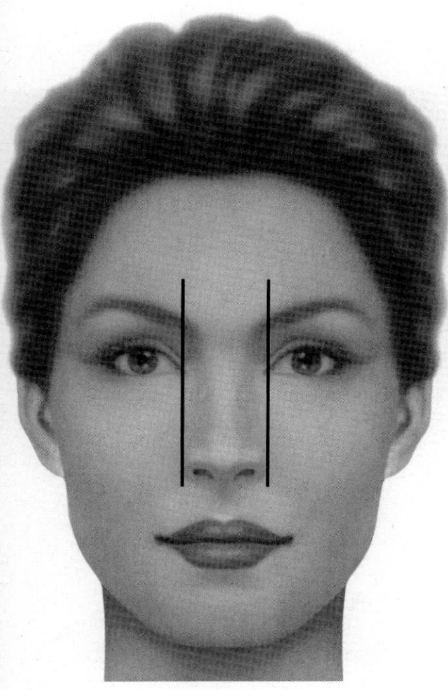

Fig. 38.8 The alar base width is equal to the intercanthal width.

will be seen as tip asymmetries on frontal view that may require tip modification during surgery. Bulbosity of the nasal tip should be noted and potential causes delineated. A bulbous, ill-defined tip may result from several

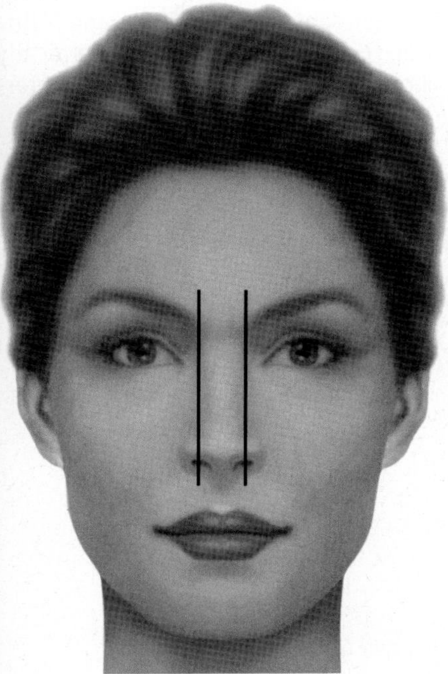

Fig. 38.9 The width of the base of the bony sidewall of the nose is ~75% of the width of the alar base.

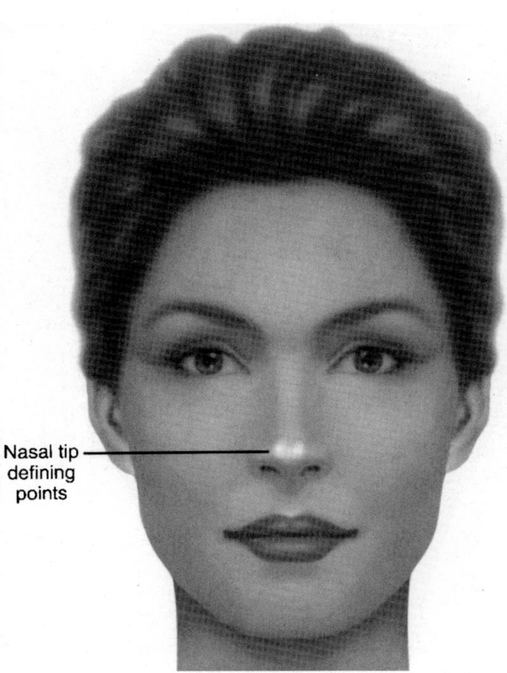

Fig. 38.10 The nasal tip-defining points are seen as two light-reflecting points of the nasal tip.

variations including: overly widened lateral alar crura, very thick sebaceous skin draping over normal cartilages, divergent interdomal angle, wide intradomal angle, and lateral crural cephalic malposition. The technique employed to achieve tip definition relies on accurate analysis of these contour-defining characteristics of the nasal tip and alar lobule. If an excessive distance is found between the tip-defining points, the domes of the lower lateral cartilage may be brought closer together at surgery by a variety of techniques, including interdomal and intradomal suturing. It is particularly important to identify the malpositioned lateral crus because ill-conceived attempts at tip definition with cephalic trimming without appropriate compensatory measures may result in delayed pinching and valve collapse. The normal angulataion of the lateral crus is 15 degrees, whereas in cephalic malpositioning the slant could be up to 60 degrees, bestowing the nose the "parenthesis" appearance.

The columella is seen to hang just inferior to the alar rims, giving the infratip lobule a gentle "gull in flight" appearance on frontal view (**Fig. 38.11A**).[6] Excessive dependence of the columella on frontal view most often indicates a protruding or hanging columella, which may require reduction. Lack of this columella contour on frontal view signifies a retracted columella, which will need augmentation. Nostril show should not be excessive indicating the nasal tip is overly rotated. Any asymmetries of the alar rim or its attachment at the alar base should be noted at this time. Lateral hooding of the alar

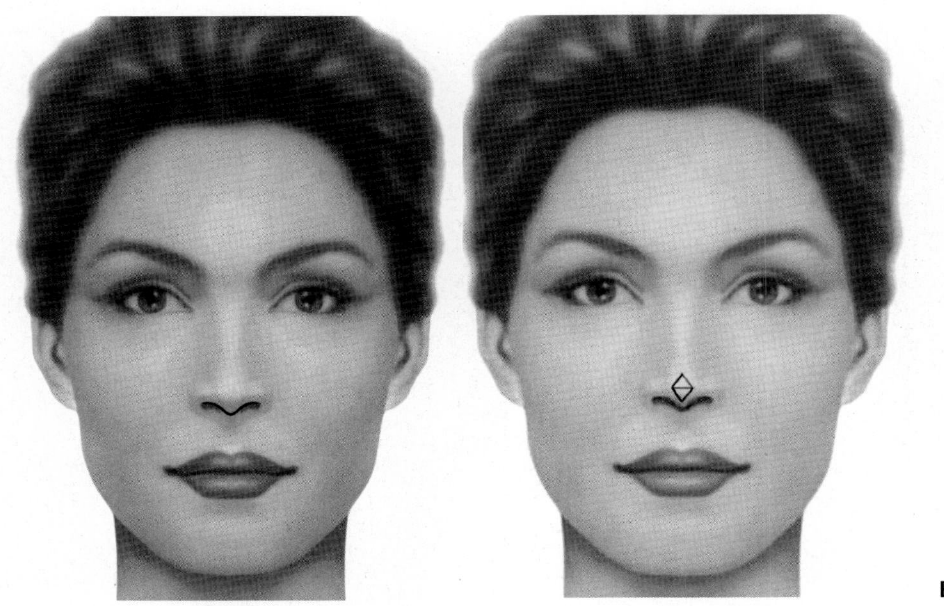

Fig. 38.11 (**A**) The "gull in flight" shape of alar rims and columella can be seen on frontal view. (**B**) The relationship between the supratip break, tip-defining points, and the infratip break can be represented by two imaginary equilateral triangles.

rim is best seen on the frontal veiw and may be addressed with specific techniques to provide tip harmony.

On frontal veiw, the refined tip reflects the double-break appearance of the the supratip and infratip. The supratip is defined by the junction of the nasal dorsum and the nasal tip, and the infratip by the junction of the tip and columella. The relationship between the infratip break, the tip-defining points, and the supratip dip can be delineated by two imaginary equilateral triangles (**Fig. 38.11B**).

A discussion of guidelines regarding proper dimensions on frontal view must be tempered by evaluation of the nose from other projections as well as consideration of harmony with other facial proportions and ethnic variations. For example, if the middle third of the face is long and the intercanthal distance is narrow, narrowing the alar base to match the intercanthal distance may cause the nose to appear excessively long and draw additional attention to the long midface. Likewise, attempts to narrow the nasal base in some ethnic noses to match the intercanthal distance may result in an unnatural appearance and functionally compromised stenotic nostrils. Recognition of these nuances and the ability to modify surgical technique to accommodate them differentiates the superior rhinoplasty surgeon from the average.

Profile View

The profile veiw allows the assessment of anterior prominences of the facial profile. Here, the maxim "small and large manifest each other" becomes central. The overall relationship between the glabella, nose, maxillar, malar eminence, lips, and chin should be appraised. From the profile view, the nasofrontal angle connects the brow with the nasal dorsum. The deepest point of the nasofrontal angle is the nasion and should lie at the level of the supratarsal crease. The nasofrontal angle is formed by a line from the nasion tangent to the glabella and a line tangent to the nasal tip (**Fig. 38.12**). This angle is typically 115 to 130 degrees. There are no well-established parameters

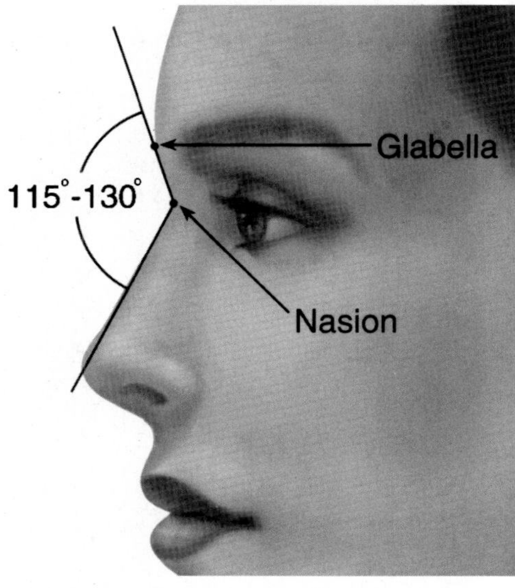

Fig. 38.12 The nasofrontal angle is typically 115 to 130 degrees.

for determining the correct depth of this angle; therefore, one must use aesthetic judgment to determine whether it is too shallow or deep in a given patient. For example, a deep nasofrontal angle combined with a strong forehead and brow will create a more masculine appearance.

Nasal tip projection is determined from the profile and is measured most simply by a 3–4-5 triangle as described by Crumley and Lancer (**Fig. 38.3**).[4] A line from the nasion to the tip is the hypotenuse of this right angle triangle. Nasal projection as measured from the alar–facial crease perpendicular to the Frankfort horizontal plane to the nasal tip should be 60% of the nasal length. Nasal projection may also be evaluated based on its relationship with the upper lip. Adequate nasal projection is present when 50 to 60% of the horizontal projection of the nose lies anterior to the upper lip (**Fig. 38.13**). If more than 60% of the nose lies anterior to the lip, the nose is considered to be overprojected. If less than 50% of the nose is anterior to the vertical lip line, it is underprojected. Simons related nasal projection to upper lip length.[7] Tip projection by this method is considered appropriate if the distance from the base of the columella (subnasale) to the nasal tip is in a 1:1 ratio with the height of the upper lip from the subnasale to the upper lip vermilion border. This last method of determining tip projection assumes the lip length is appropriate. As noted previously, balance with other facial structures is important. For example, maxillary hypoplasia will increase the perception of nasal projection. Chin and brow contours will have an even greater effect of perception and will be discussed separately.

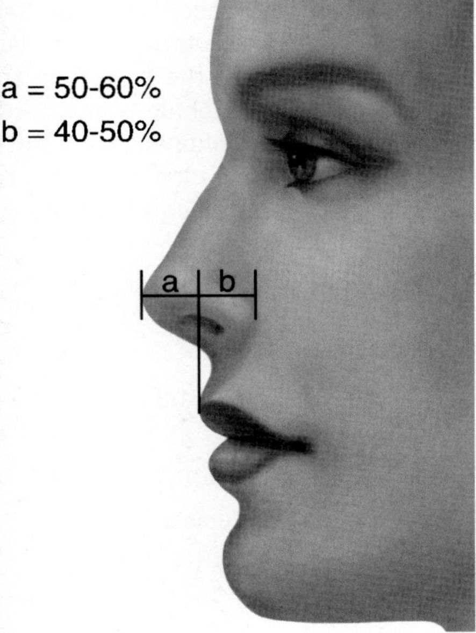

Fig. 38.13 Fifty to 60% of the nasal projection should be anterior to the upper lip.

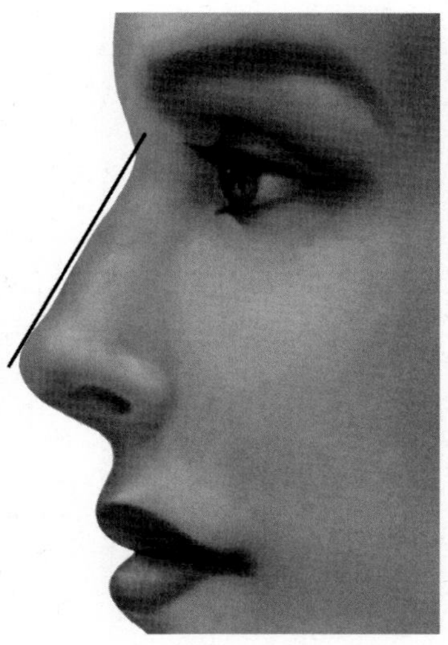

Fig. 38.14 The nasal dorsum should lie at or slightly posterior to (1–2 mm) a line drawn from the nasion to the nasal tip.

With the desired tip projection determined, the nasal dorsum can be evaluated. When a line is drawn from the nasion to the desired tip projection, the nasal dorsum should lie at or slightly (1 to 2 mm) posterior and parallel to this line (**Fig. 38.14**). If the nasal dorsum lies significantly posterior to this line, augmentation will be required. If it is anterior to this line, reduction is indicated. The projection of the nasal dorsum should also be assessed relative to the position of the radix. A low radix may lead to over estimation of the degree of dorsal projection. In addition, the length of the nasal bones should be determined. The presence of short nasal bones should be approached with caution when performing osteotomies. A slight supratip break of the dorsum gives the nose more definition and helps distinguish the dorsum from the tip. In males, a straight dorsal profile without a suprtip break is ideal.

Nasal tip rotation is best assessed in the profile view. Rotation may be thought of as the inclination of the protruding nasal tip from the anterior facial plane. The nasolabial angle, a measure of tip rotation, is determined by drawing a line from the most anterior and posterior point of the nostril on lateral view (**Fig. 38.15**). The angle this line makes with a vertical line dropped along the upper lip is the nasolabial angle. The ideal nasolabial angle differs between men and women. The ideal angle for men is 90 to 95 degrees and for women 95 to 115 degrees. This angle is again variable among non-Caucasian noses and at times could be very acute requiring premaxillary grafting. In practice, most surgeons do not measure these angles intraoperatively but make a subjective assessment based on their eye for aesthetic balance. Greater superior rotation is acceptable in shorter individuals as compared with their taller counterparts. A more projected nose tolerates less rotation.

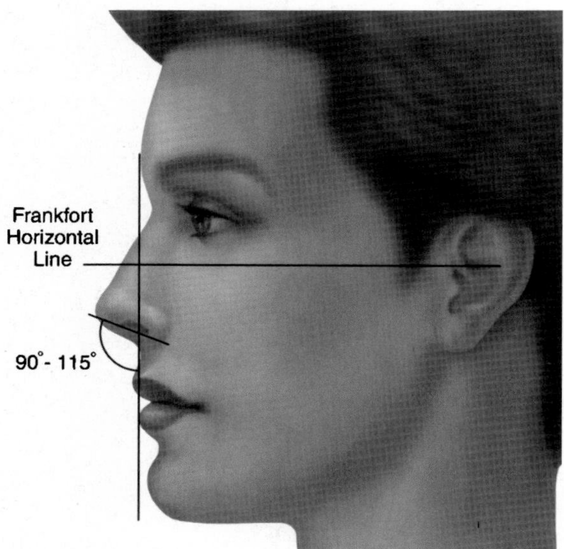

Fig. 38.15 The nasolabial angle should be 90 to 95 degrees in men and 95 to 115 degrees in women.

On lateral view, the alar–columellar relationship should be evaluated. Two to four millimeters of the columella should be visible below the alar margin on profile (**Fig. 38.16**). More than 4 mm of columella show is considered to be excessive and may be a result of a retracted alar lobule or a hanging caudal septum. Too much show below a line bisecting the ovoid created by the columella and alar margin suggests a prominent caudal septum or a large medial crura of the lower lateral cartilage. Alar retraction will be evident if the distance above this line is excessive. Inadequate columella show is usually due to columellar retraction or a heavy dependent alar lobule. From the profile veiw, the columella is seen to have a double break (**Fig. 38.17**). The first break is defined as the point at which the tip of the nose turns posterior-inferiorly onto the infratip lobule. The second break occurs at the midcolumella, where the columella takes a more horizontal course and extends posteriorly to the subnasale. This latter point usually corresponds to the junction of the medial and intermediate crura.

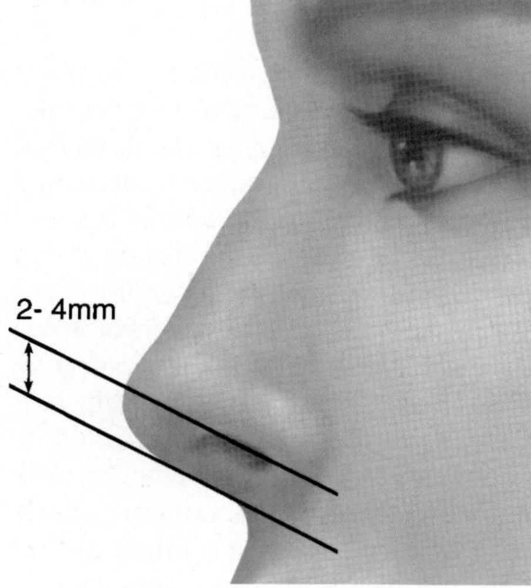

Fig. 38.16 Two to 4 mm of columellar show should be visible from the profile.

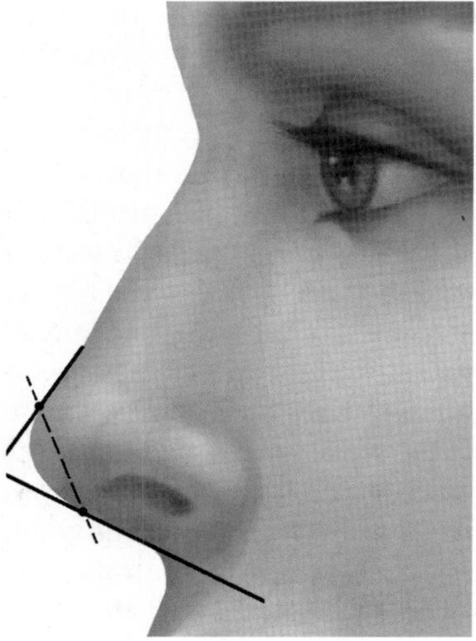

Fig. 38.17 Lateral view of the nose. Note the double break between the columella and nasal tip.

Base View

Preoperative evaluation of the base of the nose should include the size, shape, orientation, and symmetry of the nostrils, the width and length of the columella, the height of the lobule, and the size and contour of the alar lobule. When the nose is viewed from the base view an isosceles triangle is seen.[8] Ideally the lobule is one third of the height of the triangle, with the columella contributing the remaining two thirds (columella:lobule ratio 2:1) (**Fig. 38.18**). The anterior-posterior projection of the alar

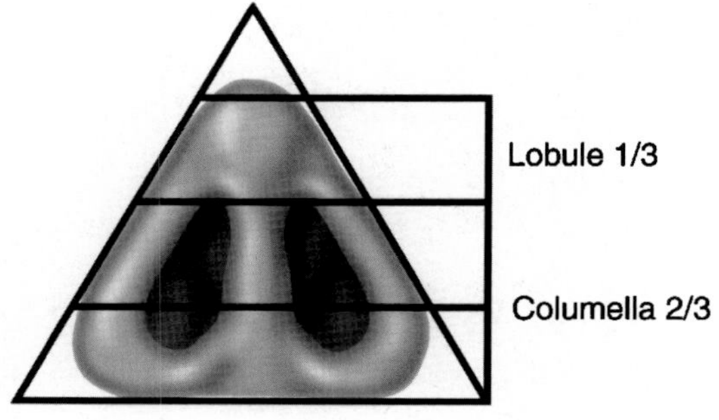

Fig. 38.18 Basal view of the nose. Resembles an isosceles triangle with the infratip lobule making up one third and the columella and nostrils two thirds.

obule should be ~50% of the total tip projection. The nos-rils should be symmetrical and are seen as pear- or tear drop-shaped, with the widest portion at the nostril sill. The width of the nostrils should be about the same as the width of the columella, with their long axis oriented at a 45-degree angle to the columella in the leptorrhine nose. The columella can be seen to flare near its base, conforming to the flare of the medial crural feet of the lower lateral cartilage. The columella is narrowest at its midportion and flares anteriorly as it meets the infratip lobule. The width of the alar base is best assessed in the basal veiw. It is measured as the distance between the alar-facial junction, which ideally should equal the intercanthal distance in Caucasians. The deviation from this ideal among non-Caucasian noses has previously been note. The columella: tip lobule ratio among African Americans, Asians, and Latinos has a range of 1–1.5:1–1.3 reflecting a relatively deprojected tip compared with Caucasian noses.[9–13] Similarly, the alar lobule proportion in these ethnic groups is greater than 50% of the total projection. A distinction between wide alar base distance and alar flaring should be made because the technique for their correction differs. Alar flare refers to the curvature of the alar lobule, which may extend beyond the alar–facial junction. A firm impression of the domal relationship should be established and any paradoxical recurvature of the lateral crura noted.

Intranasal Exam

The examination is not complete without inspection of the inside of the nose for adequacy of the airway, position of the septum, nasal valve competence, and condition of the mucosa and inferior turbinates. Palpation of the septum with a cotton-tipped applicator may be indicated to determine if septal cartilage is present in a revision rhinoplasty if cartilage grafting material will be required.

Nasal–Chin Relationship

Frequently the patient's and surgeon's attention is directed to the nose alone and the relationship of the nose to the rest of the face is neglected. Failure to address the relationship of the nose to the chin is a common error in the preoperative evaluation of the rhinoplasty patient. In patients with deficient projection of the menton the nose appears disproportionately large even though projection may be appropriate for nasal length. Several methods have been proposed for defining sagittal projection of the chin, none of which is uniformly flawless. Gonzales-Ulloa and Stevens described the appropriate chin position by dropping a line from the nasion perpendicular to the Frankfort horizontal plane (**Fig. 38.19**).[14] The adequately projected chin, assuming a normal facial height, midface projection, and class I occlusion, should approximate this line within 2 mm. A simpler method is to drop a perpendicular line from the vermilion of the lower lip and evaluate chin projection in relation to this line (**Fig. 38.20**).[15] In male patients the chin should meet or closely approximate this line. Another technique to evaluate projection utilizes a line that

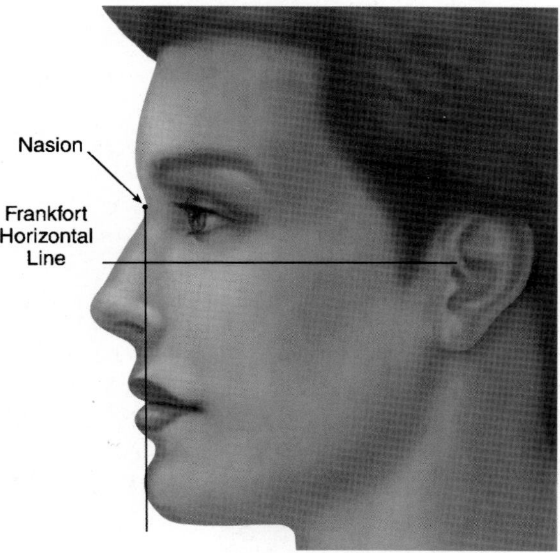

Fig. 38.19 Gonzales-Ulloa and Stevens[14] describe the appropriate chin position in relation to a vertical line dropped from the nasion perpendicular to the Frankfort horizontal plane.

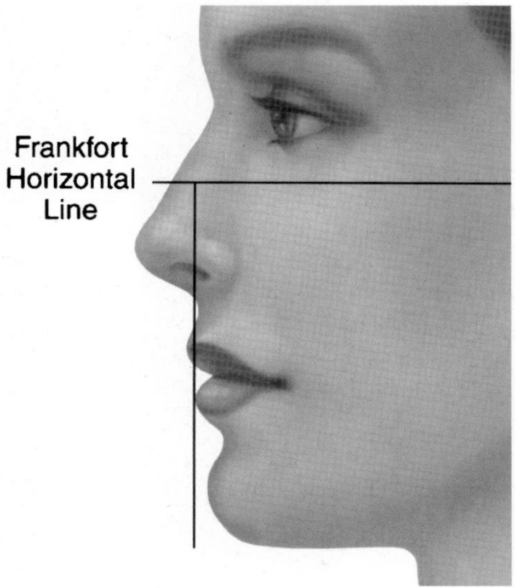

Fig. 38.20 The chin should approach a vertical line dropped from the vermilion border of the lower lip.

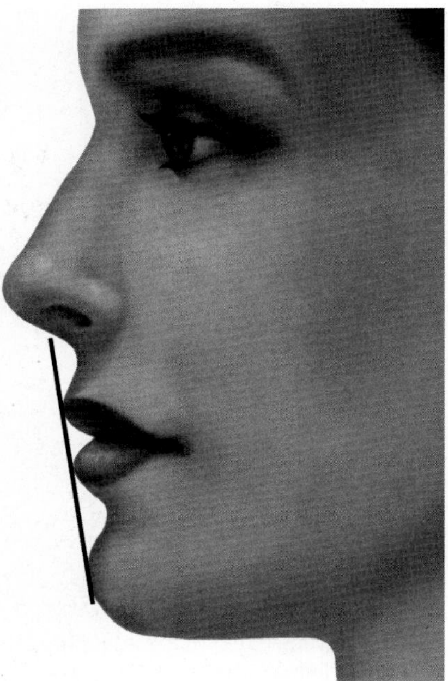

Fig. 38.21 Some authors recommend that appropriate chin projection be determined by drawing an oblique line across the most projecting portions of the lips. Inferiorly the line should touch the menton.

touches the most projecting portion (the lips and chin) (**Fig. 38.21**). Chins of female patients should be within 2 to 3 mm of this line. Computer imaging greatly facilitates communication of this important relationship to patients.

If chin projection is inadequate, it is important to determine whether the patient has microgenia (underdeveloped mental portion of the mandible), micrognathia (underdeveloped mandible with class II occlusion), or retrognathia (mandible is normal in size but retruded with class II occlusion). In the case of micrognathia or retrognathia it is important to discuss the occlusion with the patient in the event that orthognathic surgery is desired. If the patient has microgenia or does not desire orthognathic surgery for the occlusal problem, augmentation mentoplasty or osseous genioplasty may be a consideration. Besides determining the presence of sagittal deficiencies in chin projection, the vertical height of the lower third should be examined for any vertical excess or deficiency.

Nasal–Brow–Forehead Relationship

The shape of the forehead influences the perception of nasal appearance. There are essentially three fundamental forehead contours: protruding, flat, and sloping.[3] A forehead that slopes posteriorly from the brow to the hairline tends to exaggerate the appearance of nasal length and projection, whereas a flat, vertically oriented, or protruding forehead diminishes the appearance of nasal length. Similarly, the brow or frontal bar influences the perception of the nose (**Fig. 38.22**). Lowering the nasal dorsum and deprojecting the nose should be approached with caution in the patient with frontal bossing if the upper and middle third of the face are to be kept in harmony. Furthermore, a prominent brow alters our perception of the nasofrontal angle, making it appear deeper and more acute and giving the nose the appearance of greater projection.

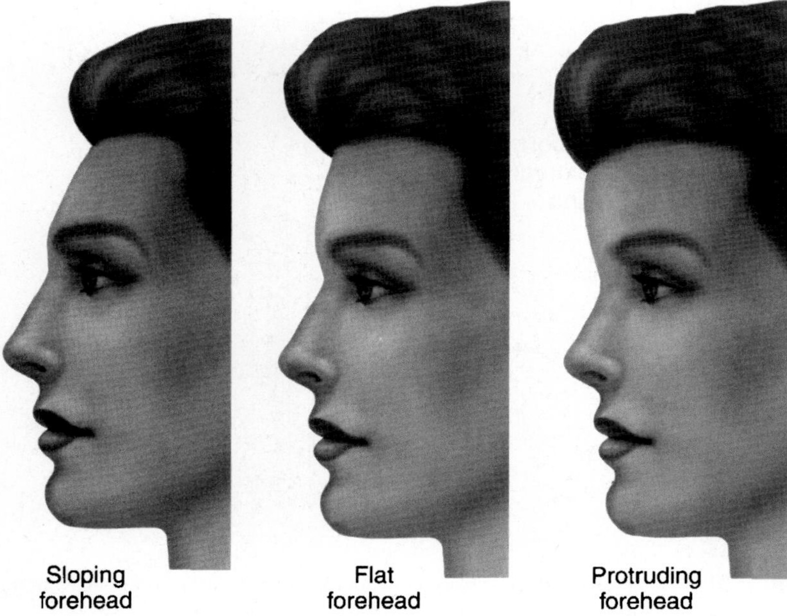

Fig. 38.22 The forehead contour influences the perception of the nose. A retrusive forehead tends to accentuate the nose, whereas a prominent forehead diminishes its appearance as seen on these images in which the forehead contour is the only feature changed.

hotography

ligh-quality photographs taken consistently with tandard views are essential for comparing pre- and ostoperative results, for teaching, and for medicole- al documentation, as well as to facilitate communi- ation with the patient. Consistency is the key in tak- ng adequate nasal photographs. Larrabee provided nformation regarding standardization of photographic quipment, background, magnification, lighting, and iews, so that pre- and postoperative photographs are omparable.[16] For the rhinoplasty patient standard views nclude the frontal, both lateral, both oblique, and basal iews. The sky or "bird's eye" view may be advantageous n some circumstances, such as in demonstration of exter- ıal nasal deviation from the midline. In addition, a lateral hotograph with the patient smiling may reveal aesthetic roblems in the lower third of the nose that are not evi- lent in repose. Before the operation, the surgeon and atient should examine the photographs and discuss the lesires and goals of the procedure. Independent study of ood photographs often reveals subtle additional features ıot evident when examining the patient.

omputer Analysis

omputer imaging systems that allow the surgeon to apture and alter the patient's image on the screen can nhance communication between surgeon and patient. esthetic concepts that are difficult to articulate can be asily visualized during office consultations. Imagers ıse video or digital cameras to display the patient's image n a monitor. Patient and surgeon can then discuss what s seen on the image in a more objective fashion. The mage can be altered with various software programs to chieve the desired surgical results. The image may be rinted on photographic paper or stored in a computer ile for later retrieval in an effort to remind the surgeon r patient about the goals of surgery. Caution is advised or those considering acquisition of this technology. Do ot "overimage." Both surgeon and patient benefits from onservative imaging.

Summary

Rhinoplasty more than any other operation in facial plastic surgery requires a thorough knowledge of facial anatomy, physiology, and aesthetics. An appreciation of facial proportions, measurements, and relationships and a keenly developed aesthetic judgment will assist the surgeon in preoperative planning and establishing the goals of surgery. Sensitivity to ethnic variations will allow the astute surgeon to refine his or her techniques to achieve results that ensure balance and harmony. The appropriate use of photography and computer imaging can be valuable tools in pre- and postoperative analysis, formulating surgical goals, and facilitating communication of aesthetic concepts between patient and surgeon.

References

1. Schmidhuber J. Facial beauty and fractal geometry. IDSIA; 1998. Available at: http://www.idsia.ch/~juergen/loco/newlocoface.html
2. Perrett DI, May KA, Yoshikawa S. Facial shape and judgments of female attractiveness. Nature 1994;368:239–242
3. Powell N, Humphrey B. Proportions of the Aesthetic Face. New York: Thieme-Stratton; 1984
4. Crumley RL, Lancer R. Quantitative analysis of nasal tip projection. Laryngoscope 1988;98:202–208
5. Sheen JH. Aesthetic Rhinoplasty. St. Louis, MO: CV Mosby; 1978
6. Rees TD. Aesthetic Plastic Surgery. Philadelphia, PA: WB Saunders; 1980
7. Simons RL. Nasal tip projection, ptosis, and supratip thickening. Ear Nose Throat J 1982;61(8):452–455
8. Bernstein L. Aesthetics in Rhinoplasty. St. Louis, MO: CV Mosby; 1978
9. Farkas LG. Anthropometry of the Head and Face. New York: Raven Press; 1994
10. Porter JP, Olson KL. Anthropometric facial analysis of the African American female. Arch Facial Plast Surg 2001;3:191–197
11. Ofodile FA, Bokhari FJ, Ellis C. The black American nose. Ann Plast Surg 1993;31:209–218
12. Sim RST, Smith JD, Chan AS. Comparison of the aesthetic facial proportions of southern Chinese and white women. Arch Facial Plast Surg 2000;2:113
13. Milgrim LM, Lawson W, Cohen AF. Anthropometric analysis of the female latino nose: revised aesthetic concepts and their surgical implications. Arch Otolaryngol Head Neck Surg 1996;122:1079
14. Gonzales-Ulloa M, Stevens E. The role of chin correction in profile plasty. Plast Reconstr Surg 1966;41:477–486
15. Simons RL. Adjunctive measures in rhinoplasty. Otolaryngol Clin North Am 1975;8:717–742
16. Larrabee WF. Facial analysis for rhinoplasty. Otolaryngol Clin North Am 1987;20:658–674

39 Rhinology in Rhinoplasty

Holger G. Gassner, David A. Sherris, and Oren Friedman

The nose is a prominent facial feature and is therefore a major determinant of facial aesthetics. When the shape of the nose is in harmony with the balanced features of an aesthetically pleasing face, attention is directed to the beauty of the eyes. In contrast, an unfavorable nasal shape draws attention away from the eyes, and the face may appear displeasing.

Fascination with the nose in the worlds of art, anatomy, and surgery explains the great interest in rhinoplasty. The nose's importance in defining facial beauty, its anatomical complexity, the considerable potential for functional deficits, and the important psychological implications associated with nasal deformities make rhinoplasty the most difficult and, at the same time, the most rewarding operation in facial plastic surgery.

The nose also serves important physiological functions that must be preserved or, at times, reconstituted if they have been compromised. Basic nasal functions include respiration, air conditioning, filtration, immune defense, and olfaction. An often underappreciated aspect of the nose's respiratory function is the airway resistance it provides. Comfortable breathing requires a certain amount of resistance to the inspired air. The air-conditioning function is responsible for warming and humidification of the inspired air, thus making it suitable for the pulmonary airways. The nose also acts as an effective barrier against airborne particles and pathogens. Several specific and nonspecific mechanisms contribute to the immune defense of the nasal mucosa and protect humans from external pathogens. The sense of olfaction is best appreciated when it is lacking. Recognition of potentially harmful inhalants can be lifesaving, and the joy of smells and flavors greatly enhances the quality of life.

Anatomical Considerations

Detailed knowledge of nasal anatomy is crucial to appreciate, identify, and correctly use the surgical planes of the nose. The nose is built in layers. Exact dissection of the anatomical tissue planes allows for atraumatic surgery with minimal bleeding and postoperative scarring.

The Skin–Soft Tissue Envelope

Nasal skin quality differs from individual to individual. Thin skin tends to unveil even minor irregularities over the tip and the dorsum, sometimes showing these irregularities years after an initially pleasing result. Thicker skin frequently limits the creation of a precisely defined tip, even after resection of subcutaneous tissue. The quality of the nasal skin also varies within the same individual. Although the thinner skin over the bony and cartilaginous dorsum is nearly devoid of subcutaneous tissue, the more sebaceous skin of the nasal tip, supratip, and nasofrontal angle is supported by abundant underlying tissue.

The superficial musculoaponeurotic layer of the face is a crucial landmark in cosmetic and reconstructive facial surgery. It extends as a distinct layer superficial to the facial muscles into the nose. Tardy[1] portrayed the muscles of the nose as encased and interconnected by the superficial musculoaponeurotic layer. The nasal muscles have been categorized into different groups on the basis of their functions (**Fig. 39.1**).[2] The nasal musculature has important implications for both the cosmetic and the functional aspects of rhinoplasty. Overactivity of the depressor muscle group, including the depressor muscle of the nasal septum, lowers the tip and results in the unfavorable appearance of a rounded and lengthened tip. This so-called U phenomenon is addressed during rhinoplasty by transecting the insertions of these muscles at the base of the columella.

Evidence is accumulating that voluntary and involuntary activity of the nasal muscles has a profound effect on nasal airway resistance. Knowledge of the microanatomy of the nasal musculature is incomplete. Detailed microscopic studies of the insertions, origins, and orientation of the individual muscle groups would help elucidate the potential effects of surgical maneuvers on nasal muscle function. The surgeon should use extra caution to preserve the anatomical integrity and neurovascular supply of these structures to minimize the potential for functional deficits.

The Structural Skeleton

The Valves

Proper postoperative function of the nasal valves determines, to a large degree, the success of rhinoplasty. The nasal valves represent the narrowest portion of the entire airway and account for half the total nasal airway resistance. The nomenclature of the nasal valves has been variable, confusing, and, at times, incorrect.

Distinguishing between the internal valve and the external nasal valve is important because these represent

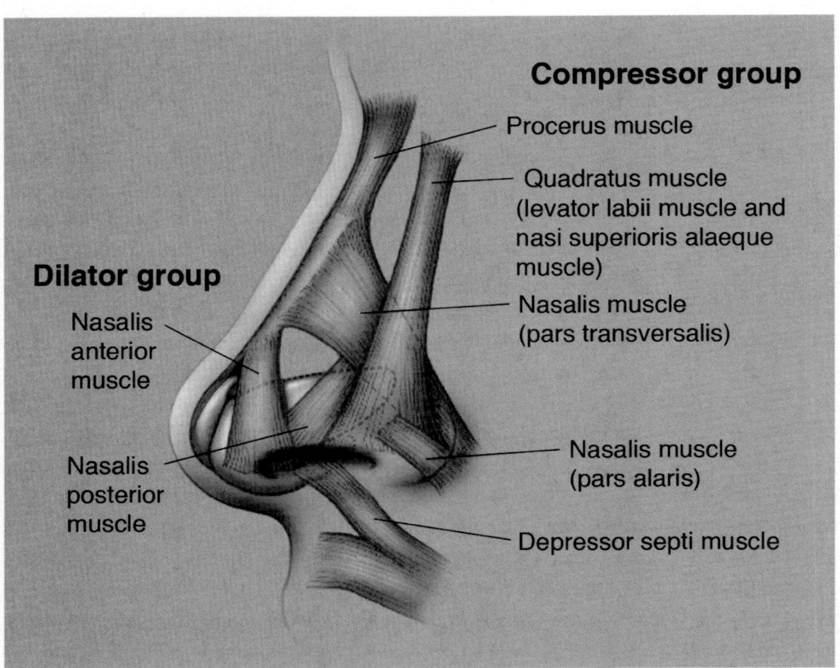

Fig. 39.1 The nasal musculature comprises two functional groups, the compressor group and the dilator group.

distinct anatomical and functional entities. The nasal valve area represents the area bound by the caudal end of the septum, the returning portion of the upper lateral cartilage, the lateral nasal wall, the floor of the nose, and sometimes the head of the inferior turbinate. The internal nasal valve proper is the slitlike portion between the caudal end of the upper lateral cartilage and the nasal septum (**Fig. 39.2**).

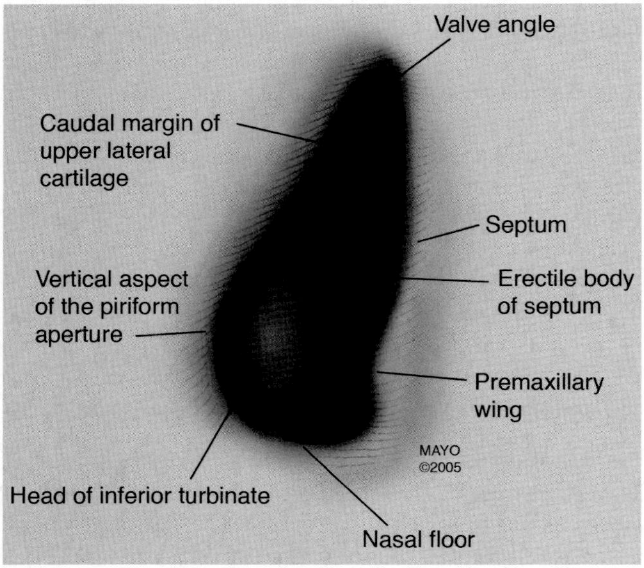

Fig. 39.2 The internal nasal valve area is formed by the caudal end of the upper lateral cartilage, the nasal septum, the nasal floor, and the head of the inferior turbinate. (Reprinted by permission of Mayo Foundation for Medical Education and Research.)

These cartilages define the valve angle, which should measure 10 to 15 degrees. Cole[3] described four functional components of the internal nasal valve area (**Table 39.1**).

The external nasal valve is supported by the alar sidewall and is delineated by the nostril rim. It is defined medially by the medial crus of the alar cartilage and inferiorly by the nasal spine and the soft tissues over the nasal floor.[4] The alar sidewall is referred to in the literature as the "fibrofatty tissues of the ala." As discussed in the section "Objective Measurement of Nasal Function," the alae display considerable muscular activity. Phylogenetically, the nasal inlet is a derivative of a muscular sphincter, and a considerable proportion of the structural support of the external nasal valve is likely derived from alar musculature. As Murakami (Murakami CS, personal communication, 2005) points out, the term *fibromuscular* appears more appropriate than "fibrofatty" to describe

Table 39.1 The Four Functional Components of the Nasal Valve*

Segment	Description
I	Internal nasal valve angle
II	The bony piriform aperture
III	The anterior head of the inferior turbinate
IV	The erectile body of the septum

*As described by Cole.[3] Segments I and II represent the structural segments, and segments III and IV the mucovascular segments of the nasal valve.

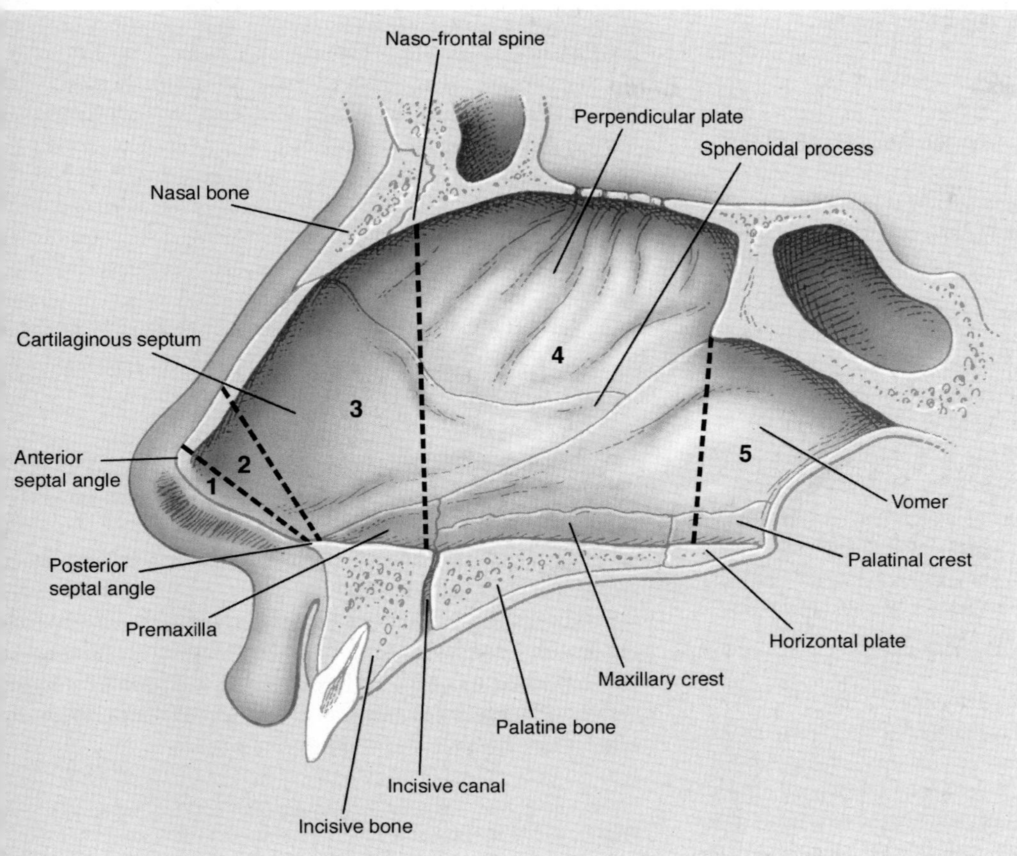

Fig. 39.3 Cottle areas of the nasal septum: area 1, nasal vestibule; area 2, internal nasal valve; area 3, attic, space enclosed by the external cartilaginous and bony pyramid; area 4, septum between the level of the bony pyramid and the choanae; and area 5, septum separating the choanae.

the anatomical and functional properties of the alar soft tissues.

The Septum

Posteriorly the bony nasal septum is formed by the perpendicular plate of the ethmoid bone and the vomer. Anteriorly the quadrangular cartilage forms the cartilaginous septum, which is contiguous with the upper lateral cartilages. The five areas of the nasal septum are shown in **Fig. 39.3**. For nasal surgery, areas 1 and 2 are of particular importance.

The Alar and Upper Lateral Cartilages

The alar cartilages determine the form and function of the nasal tip. Of surgical importance are the tip-defining points, typically the anterior-most projection of the domes, which are represented by two distinct light reflexes on the skin of the nasal tip. The interrelation of the cephalic margin of the alar cartilage with the caudal border of the upper lateral cartilage also deserves attention. In younger patients, the alar cartilage overrides the caudal end of the upper lateral cartilage, which typically curls cephalically to varying degrees.[5] The insertion of the medial crural feet into the nasal septum represents a major tip support mechanism. The lateral aspect of the lateral crus is connected to the piriform aperture by fibromuscular tissue, which frequently harbors the sesamoid cartilages and provides support to the nasal ala.

The Bony Skeleton

The nasal bones articulate with the frontal process of the maxilla laterally and with the frontal bone at the nasofrontal suture line superiorly. Asymmetries and deviations of the nasal bone result in various nasal dorsal deformities.[6] Inferoposteriorly, the nasal bones fuse with the perpendicular plate of the ethmoid bone. The internasal suture line insinuates the periosteum in the midline and may require sharp dissection to complete the elevation of the periosteum from the nasal dorsum.

Table 39.2 Major and Minor Tip Support Mechanisms*

Major
1. Size, shape, and resilience of the medial and lateral crura
2. Medial crural footplate attachment to the caudal border of the quadrangular cartilage
3. Attachment of the upper lateral cartilages (caudal border) to the alar cartilages (cephalic border)
Minor
1. The ligamentous sling spanning the paired domes of the alar cartilages
2. The cartilaginous septal dorsum
3. The sesamoid complex extending the support of the lateral crura to the piriform aperture
4. The attachment of the alar cartilages to the overlying skin and musculature
5. The nasal spine
6. The membranous septum

*This division may not be accurate in patients with anatomical variations.

The Tip Support Mechanisms

The tip support mechanisms have been described to aid in comprehending the important anatomic relationships that maintain the structural resilience of the nasal tip (**Table 39.2**). Although describing the difference between the major and minor support mechanisms has didactic value, the importance of these mechanisms varies among individuals.

The Turbinates

The arteries of the nasal mucosa branch off to capillary vessels, which drain into the venous sinusoids of the erectile tissues of the mucosa. On a volume basis, a major component of the mucosa is formed by erectile tissues, which are especially well developed at the anterior part of the inferior turbinate and on the nasal septum. When the sinusoids are filled, they form a vascular cushion and act as a radiator, which warms and humidifies inspired air. The nasal mucosa with the underlying erectile tissues has been termed the *organ of the nose* because these specialized tissues perform several physiological functions.[7]

Histology of the Endonasal Epithelium

Various types of epithelia line different aspects of the nasal cavity. In the vestibule, moderately keratinized squamous epithelium predominates. Immediately posterior, a transition zone ~1 cm wide may be lined with squamous epithelium, transitional epithelium, or pseudostratified columnar epithelium, followed by the typical pseudostratified, ciliated, columnar epithelium with goblet cells of the middle and posterior third of the nasal cavity. The cilia beat with a frequency of 10 to 20 Hz to move the mucous blanket with variable velocity between 2.3 and 23.6 mm/minute.[1] The olfactory cleft is covered by olfactory mucosa, an area of ~200 to 400 mm^2 and much thicker than the surrounding respiratory epithelium. The olfactory epithelium is pseudostratified and columnar and contains the bipolar olfactory sensory neurons. The four main cell types identified in the olfactory mucosa are ciliated olfactory receptors, microvillar cells, sustentacular cells, and basal cells.

The Paranasal Sinuses

A thorough discussion of the anatomy of the paranasal sinuses is beyond the scope of this chapter. However, for successful rhinoplasty, it is essential to be able to accurately diagnose and treat concomitant paranasal sinus pathology. A complete review is available in the excellent texts by Stammberger et al,[8] Wigand,[9] Stamm and Draf,[10] and Orlandi and Kennedy.[11]

Nasal Physiology

Nasal Cycle

Without a thorough understanding of the nasal cycle, the clinician may be easily misled in the diagnostic workup of nasal obstruction. The nasal cycle was described by Kayser in 1895 and is present in 72 to 80% of the human population. With remarkable regularity, cyclical changes in the cross-sectional lumen of the nasal cavities reciprocate approximately every 3 to 4 hours. These changes generally are unnoticed because the combined nasal airway resistance of both sides remains constant.[12] The function of the nasal cycle has been hypothesized to allow for regeneration of the nasal mucosa on the obstructed side. This would suggest that warming, humidification, and other functions challenge the nasal mucosa so greatly that these functions cannot be maintained in an uninterrupted manner. Unfortunately, no data are available to quantify the functional residual capacity of the nose. It is therefore unknown how much mucosa can be lost before function of the nose is compromised. Further research is needed to better elucidate this important issue as well as the purposes and meaning of the nasal cycle. It is important to understand that the nasal cycle may result in near-total unilateral nasal obstruction on inspection or imaging, a finding that must not be confused with pathological nasal obstruction.

Olfaction

The sense of olfaction combines neural input from the olfactory, trigeminal, glossopharyngeal, and vagus nerves. For a particular odorant to stimulate the olfactory nerve, it must be transported by endonasal airflow toward the olfactory cleft. This transport appears to be enhanced during sniffing, as inspired airflow is increased and may be directed better to the olfactory epithelium. Retrograde airflow is also suitable to transport airborne molecules derived from food in the pharynx toward the olfactory epithelium. Thus, the sense of olfaction can contribute to the flavor of food.

Filtering Function

The nasal mucosa efficiently protects the lower airways from inhalation of particulate matter. Multiple studies have investigated both deposition (uptake, absorption, retention) and regional distribution in the nose.

Particle size, shape, specific weight, and aerodynamic properties determine the degree of particle deposition on the nasal mucosa. About 60% of particles 1 μm in diameter are deposited in the nasal cavity, and the deposition of larger particles is more complete.[13]

Two major deposition sites have been identified in the nose. As a result of the transition from laminar to turbulent flow, particles are deposited on the mucosa posterior to the nasal valve. The direction of the endonasal airflow subsequently directs particles to the second site of predominant deposition, the anterior aspect of the middle turbinate.[14] The endonasal distribution of tumors has been correlated with these particle deposition patterns.

Humidifying Capacity

The relatively small surface area of the nasal mucosa (120 cm^2) is faced with the formidable task of humidifying and warming ~14,000 L of inspired air that pass through the nasal cavities of a normal, active adult in a day. Air is heated by conduction, convection, and radiation. The heat exchange is efficient because the blood flow is in the opposite direction to the incoming airflow. In comfortable room conditions, ~280 kJ of energy are required to warm the air to 32°C in the rhinopharynx. To saturate this volume of inspired air with humidity, 1400 kJ of energy and 600 g of water are expended. On expiration, a considerable proportion of warmth and humidity are extracted from the air to conserve energy.[15–17]

Airflow, Resistance, and Its Regulation

The nose acts as a dynamic resistor to inspired air. The speed of the inspired air at the entrance of the nasal cavity is ~2 to 3 m/s and rises to ~12 to 18 m/s at the internal nasal valve. Here, the airflow makes an upward angulation of ~60 degrees, hence the term *upstream resistors* to describe the area of the nasal valve. Posterior to the nasal valves the speed diminishes to 2 to 3 m/s, and the flow becomes more horizontal and eventually tilts downward toward the choanae. More air passes through the middle meatus than the inferior meatus. As the airflow becomes turbulent, warming and humidifying of the inspired air is enhanced. When entering the rhinopharynx, the airflow tilts downward, becomes laminar, and increases in velocity to 3 to 4 m/s. These generalizations of intranasal airflow have been concluded from predominantly static models. It is important to understand that the regulation of nasal resistance is a dynamic process.

A liquid or gas flowing through a tube increases its velocity and diminishes the transmural pressure at an area of constriction. This phenomenon, referred to as the Bernoulli theorem, explains the observation that the nasal valve collapses to varying degrees on inspiration. Kern[18] regards the collapsibility of the valve as one of its physiological functions, limiting the nasal airflow when inspiratory airflow becomes excessive. When nasal valve collapse becomes premature, pathological airway obstruction ensues. Its cross-sectional area and structural resilience are major determinants of the collapsibility of the nasal valve. A nasal valve with a arge cross-sectional area is subject to lower transmural pressures and remains patent more easily, and a small valve is subject to higher transmural pressures and tends to collapse. The structural resilience of the nasal valve tissues determines how well the valve can withstand negative transmural pressures. This structural resilience is provided by the tissues of the ala and adjacent areas. Recent studies have provided normative resilience values of the nasal tip (**Fig. 39.4**).

Figure 39.4 indicates that the alae represent the softest locations of the nasal tip, followed by the columella, interdomal region, and the anterior septal angle.[19] Further studies have shown that the nasal muscles profoundly influence the structural resilience of the nasal valve. An involuntary resting tone adds stiffness to the ala, and this is further increased by voluntary activation of the nasal musculature (flaring). As evidenced by rhinomanometric measurements, the involuntary (resting) muscle tone decreases nasal airway resistance. Voluntary flaring further opens the nasal airway.[20]

Immune Defense

The mechanisms that protect the nose against irritants, microorganisms, and allergens can be described as nonspecific and specific systems. The nonspecific system includes

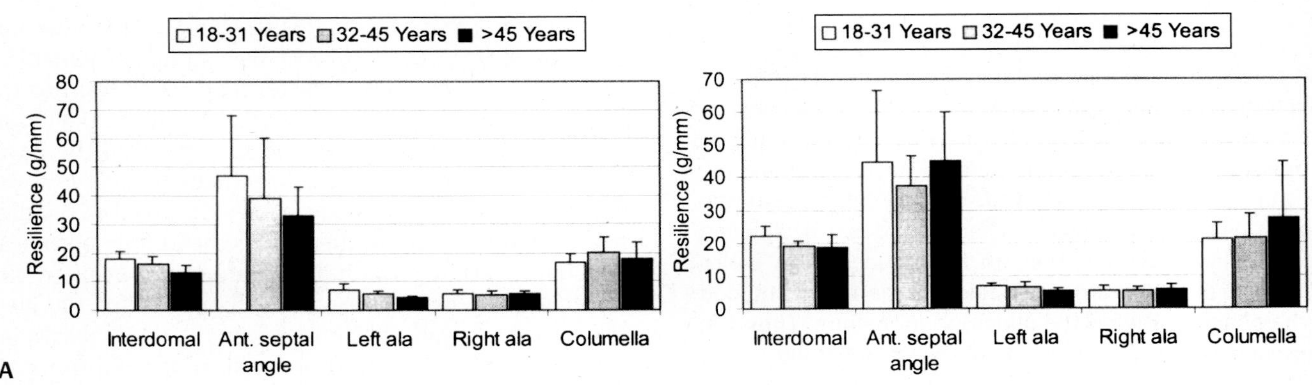

Fig. 39.4 Normative data of nasal tip tissue resilience over the interdomal region, anterior septal angle, alae, and columella, as determined by rhinoresiliography for women (**A**) and men (**B**). Error bars indicate 95% confidence intervals (±2 SEs). (Adapted from Gassner et al.[19] Reprinted by permission.)

the filtering function of the nose with the mucociliary transport system. The mucous blanket is produced by the goblet cells and is driven by ciliary movement toward the lateral pharyngeal walls for ingestion. The mean velocity of the mucous flow and particle transport is ~6 mm/min in normal conditions. Inspired microorganisms, irritants, and allergens are trapped. The specific defense mechanisms include the various immunologic, humoral, and cellular responses.

Objective Measurement of Nasal Function

Rhinomanometry

Rhinomanometry is the most commonly used objective test of the nasal airway. Various methods exist. Anterior, posterior, and postnasal rhinomanometry are distinguished by the location of the pressure sensor (**Fig. 39.5**). Active and passive rhinometry are distinguished by whether the nasal air stream is driven by the patient's respiration (active) or by an external pump (passive). Anterior active rhinometry is the clinically most commonly used method. It was developed in the beginning of the 20th century and further advanced by Masing,[21] Kern,[22] and others.

The principle is to measure airflow as a function of air pressure for each nasal cavity separately. To isolate one nasal cavity, the contralateral naris is occluded. The occluding plug or tape contains a pressure sensor, which provides a good approximation of the pressures in the contralateral nasal cavity. The nasal airflow through the unoccluded nasal cavity is quantified by a flow sensor embedded in a tight-fitting face mask. Care must be taken not to distort the anatomy of the nasal tip and nasal valve with the occluding plug or tape. Pressure and flow data are typically plotted in a diagram. The resulting graph, common to many biological processes, is a sigmoid-shaped loop or hysteresis (**Fig. 39.6**). Vogt (Vogt K, personal communication, 2003) points out that most commercially available rhinomanometry devices average data over several respiratory cycles, and as a result, differences between inspiration and expiration are lost.

Despite widespread interest and considerable research, optimal utility of rhinomanometry has not been achieved. Normative data to allow differentiation of physiological from pathological nasal airway resistance have not been standardized. Interpretation of rhinomanometry requires assessment by an experienced investigator who can analyze the acquired data in context with the clinical findings. Rhinomanometry has several shortcomings, including its inability to sufficiently assess the function of the nasal valve under the dynamic conditions of respiration. In the nondecongested state, the alternating mucosal engorgement of the nasal cycle appears to introduce a variability too marked for reproducible measurements. In the decongested state, the transmural pressures of the nasal valves are reduced and decrease the propensity for nasal valve collapse. Moreover, the attenuation of nasal airway resistance by voluntary and involuntary nasal muscle activity is not controlled with rhinomanometry. Even though rhinomanometry has contributed enormously to our understanding of nasal airway physiology, further research is needed to develop a more useful tool to determine the exact location and to quantify the degree of nasal airway obstruction.

Acoustic Rhinometry

Acoustic rhinometry is the second most commonly used objective measurement of the nasal airway. This method

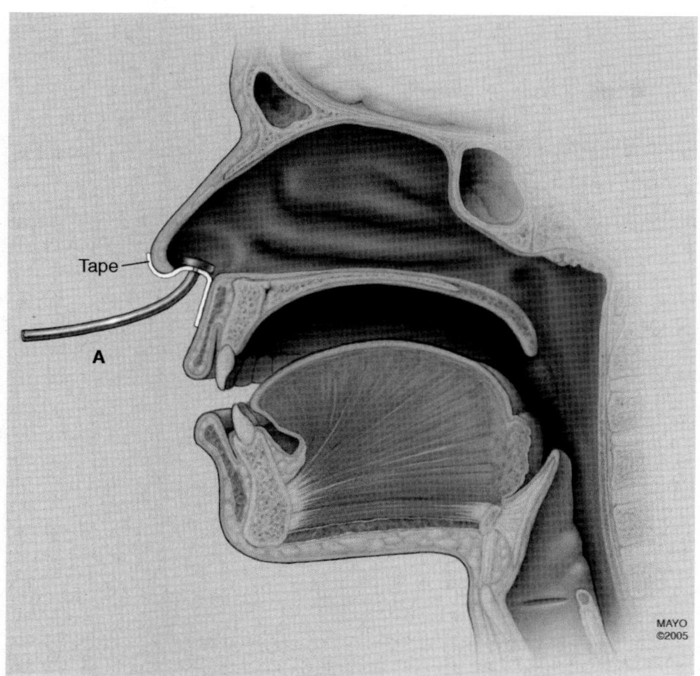

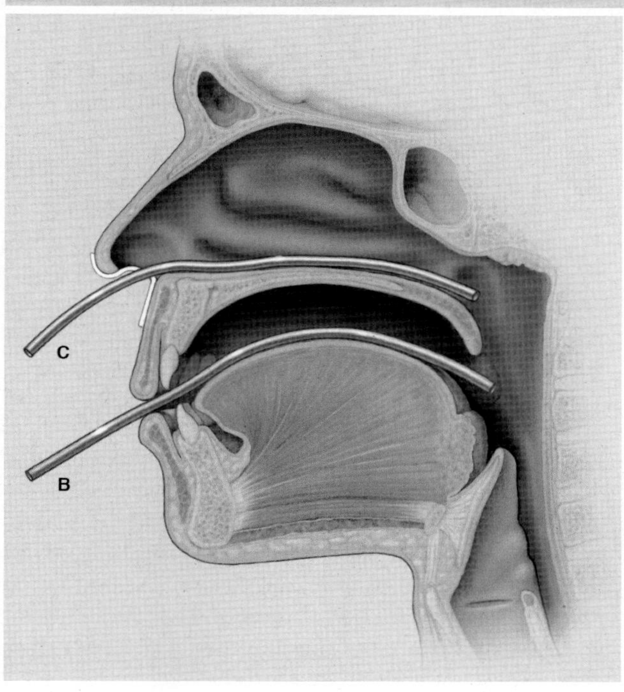

Fig. 39.5 (**A**) For anterior rhinomanometry, the pressure sensor is introduced into the contralateral nostril. (**B**) For posterior rhinomanometry, the pressure sensor is introduced into the oropharynx. (**C**) For postnasal rhinomanometry, the pressure sensor is introduced transnasally into the nasopharynx. (Reprinted by permission of Mayo Foundation for Medical Education and Research.)

was developed by Hilberg et al[23] in 1989. An acoustic rhinometer consists of a tube that harbors a sound generator and a microphone. It generates sound reflections that allow plotting of a two-dimensional profile of the endonasal anatomy. The device is coupled to the patient's nose through a flexible silicon tube and gel (Fig. 39.7).

Acoustic rhinometry gives a relatively accurate assessment of intranasal volume and monitors dimensional changes over short periods. The measurements are typically displayed as a graph indicating the integral of nasal volume over distance from the nosepiece. A physiological measurement is depicted by an ascending graph that is interrupted by two downsloping notches, creating a so-called W-pattern. The first notch results from the constriction of the valve angle and is termed the *I notch* (isthmus), and the second notch results from the anterior head of the inferior turbinate and is termed

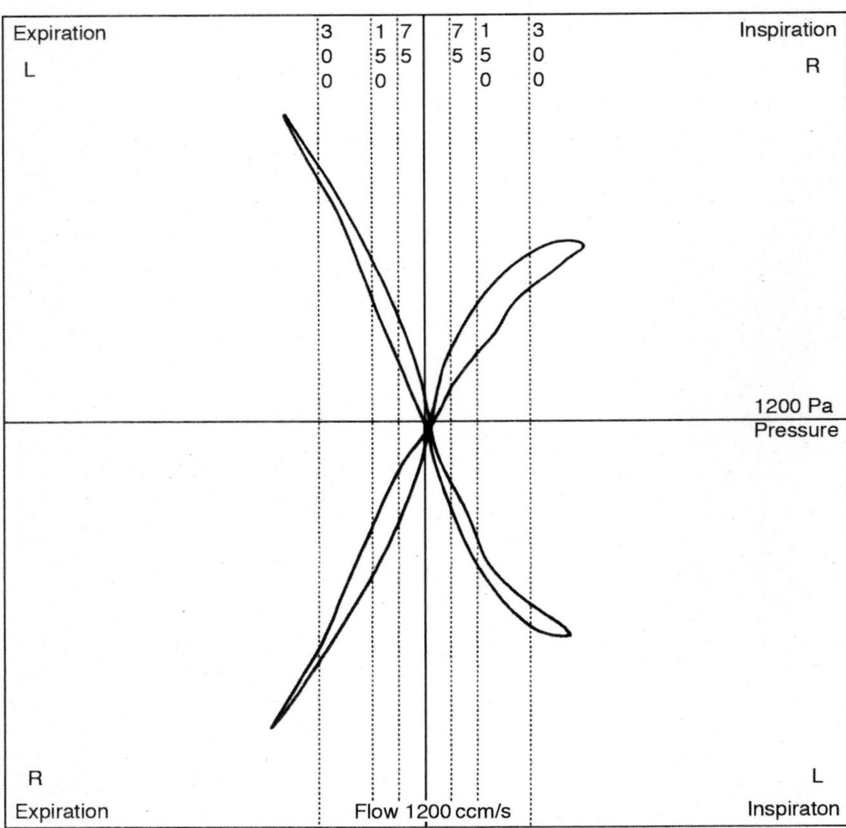

Fig. 39.6 High-resolution rhinomanometry results in a hysteresis. This type of curve is common to many biological processes and delineates changes in airway resistance between inspiration and expiration. Sigmoid-shaped curve resulting from data averaging over multiple respiratory cycles.

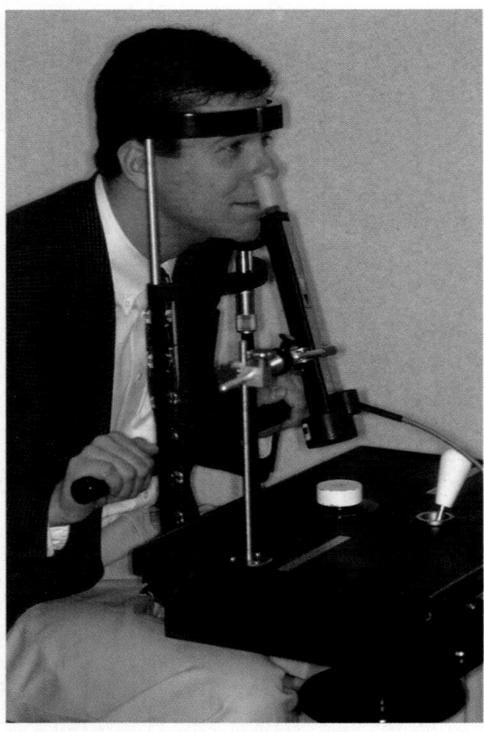

Fig. 39.7 The acoustic rhinometer is coupled to the patient's nose through a flexible silicon tube and clear gel. We prefer to use a head frame with chin rest to minimize motion artifacts.

the *C notch* (concha) (**Fig. 39.8**). Accordingly, the I notc is relatively stable, whereas the C notch is elevate with mucosal decongestion and depressed with muco sal congestion. Acoustic rhinometry also measures th size and location of the minimal cross-sectional are and the total endonasal volume.

Acoustic rhinometry has shown variations within th same subject of 10 to 16%, indicating clinically usefu reproducibility with the head, sound tube, and adapte in a fixed position.[24] Some skillful operators may attai acceptable reproducibility using a handheld device, bu attention must be paid not to distort the anatomy of th tip with the nasal adapter and to keep the sound tube a the proper angle for measurement. The further distal th measurements are obtained in the nasal cavity, the les likely these data are to be reproducible.

Like rhinomanometry, acoustic rhinometry has bee mainly used for investigational purposes. In the hands of a experienced user, it can provide useful information abou the anterior airway geometry and the responsiveness o the anterior mucovascular structures of the nose.

Rhinoresiliography

The structural support of the nasal tip is of great impor tance for nasal airway function. Rhinoresiliography (RSG measures the structural resilience and recoil of tissue a

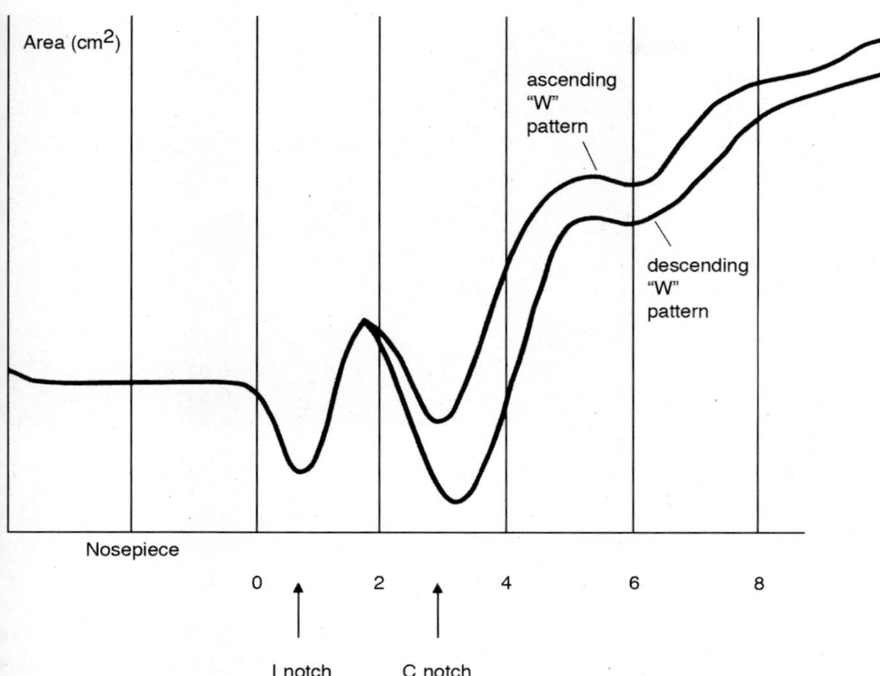

Fig. 39.8 Ascending (*curve 1*) and descending (*curve 2*) W-shaped configuration of an area-distance curve obtained with acoustic rhinometry.

a function of force over distance.[19] The device consists of a force transducer mounted on a linear potentiometer. The sensors allow acquisition of data with high resolution. A computer is used to store and display the data. Resilience is the resistance a tissue mounts to a displacing force, such as a fingertip, depressing the nasal tip. Recoil is the degree of force the previously distorted tissue exerts to reestablish its previous shape and position. The resulting graph of such a measurement is a coop or hysteresis. The loop results from the difference between resilience and recoil. The force needed to displace and deform tissue (resilience) is greater than the force the tissue mounts to regain its original shape and position (recoil). This difference between resilience and recoil may be considerable, as it depicts the ability of the nasal airway to reopen after dynamic collapse.

Data are available to describe normative values of nasal tip resilience in adults. These values were established in five anatomical areas, as shown in **Fig. 39.4**. Resilience measurements are available from only two institutions[19,25] and have been acquired with different devices. Further research is needed to better investigate disorders of nasal tip support. RSG is able to measure only one aspect of nasal airway function. As with rhinomanometry and acoustic rhinometry, this limitation reduces its usefulness in the clinical setting. Continued research may allow simultaneous measurements of various parameters, such as airflow, geometry, and recoil. Ideally, a single measurement would characterize the nature, location, and severity of nasal airway obstruction.

Olfactory Testing

Olfactory testing addresses the ability to identify odors and their detection thresholds. Modern methods allow quantitative and reproducible testing and documentation. Measurement of the detection levels can be achieved by offering the subject a series of two applicators, one with and one without the odorant. Test batteries that have proven useful in clinical practice include the Sniffin' Sticks test (Heinrich Burghart Elektro- und Feinmechanik GmbH, Weiden, Germany) and the T&T olfactometer (Takasago International Corp., Tokyo, Japan). Both these tests can be completed within 10 minutes and allow accurate quantitative documentation of the results.[26] Olfactory testing is a useful adjunct in the preoperative evaluation of candidates for nasal surgery, especially when a patient's history indicates prior olfactory symptoms.

The sense of smell and the sense of taste overlap. For test purposes, purely trigeminal stimuli can be presented to the nose and purely olfactory stimuli to the mouth. Nonrecognition of the trigeminal stimulus in the nose or recognition of the olfactory stimulus through the mouth can unmask functional anosmia.

Objective olfactory testing by electrophysiological methods is available in a few centers worldwide. Kobal and Hummel[27] have shown that pure olfactory stimuli generate olfactory-evoked potentials in the parietal area. At present, the cost and limited availability have restricted objective olfactory testing largely to research in major medical academic centers.

Other Measurements

Other measurements indicative of functions of the nose include mucociliary transport times, assessment of basal secretions for immunoglobulins and other important secretory substances, and measurement of intranasal air temperature, humidity, and particle deposition.

Pathophysiology

Nasal Obstruction

A complete discussion of the numerous potential causes of nasal airway obstruction is beyond the scope of this chapter. The interested reader is referred to the pertinent literature.[28] Causes of nasal obstruction with particular relevance for the rhinoplasty surgeon are discussed in the following sectionss.

On critical review of the literature, more easily addressed entities such as posterior septal deviations and presumed turbinate hypertrophy appear to be overdiagnosed, and nasal valve disorders underdiagnosed. Nasal valve obstruction has been diagnosed in up to 64% of patients complaining of nasal obstruction after reduction rhinoplasty.[29] According to Kern (personal communication, 2005), 90% of more than 8000 patients who presented with nasal airway obstruction at Mayo Clinic were diagnosed as having abnormalities of the nasal valve.

During anterior rhinoscopy, valve disorders are frequently overlooked because the blades of the speculum obscure and distend the nasal valve area. Numerous patients presenting with nasal obstruction report marked airway improvement when the nasal valve area is distended bilaterally with a speculum or the wooden end of a cotton-tipped applicator. The Cottle maneuver (**Fig. 39.9**) allows reliable identification of the site or sites of potential nasal valve disorders.

Kern[18] grouped causes of nasal valve obstruction according to the affected functional component of the valve (**Fig. 39.10**). Valve obstruction may be fixed or dynamic, and it may result from previous surgery, trauma, senile changes, congenital anomalies, or a combination of these factors.

Paradoxical Obstruction

Paradoxical nasal obstruction may result when a patient has severe unilateral structural obstruction, such as septal deviation. The patient is habituated to the fixed obstruction, e.g., in the left nasal cavity, and only notices the recurrent contralateral (right-sided) obstruction when the nasal cycle shifts to the right side. The patient therefore senses the obstruction on the side contralateral to the actual

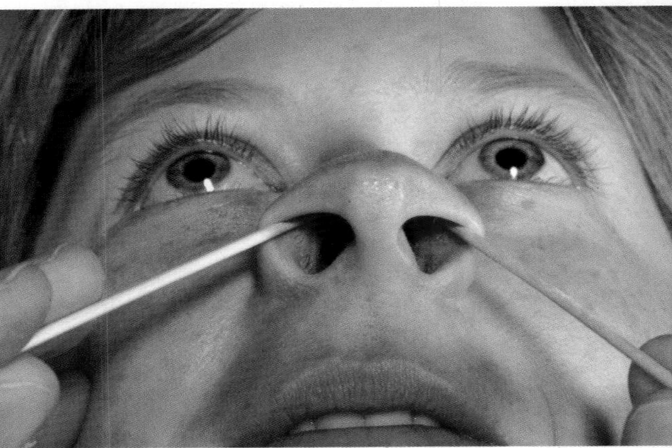

Fig. 39.9 Distention of the nasal valve area differentiates anterior (valve area) and posterior (septal areas 3–5) nasal obstruction. If this test results in substantial relief of nasal obstruction, nasal valve pathology is likely present, and posterior septal and turbinate anatomy is unlikely to contribute to obstruction.

obstruction, hence the descriptor "paradoxical." This form of obstruction can typically be corrected surgically by valve repair or septoplasty.

Another form of nasal airway impairment is also considered paradoxical obstruction. This form occurs when excessive turbinate resection results in too large a nasal cavity. The excessive reduction of nasal airway resistance causes the perception of impaired nasal breathing. This form of paradoxical obstruction and its associated symptoms are particularly difficult to treat.

We believe that better nomenclature to differentiate between these two forms of paradoxical obstruction should be proposed.

Rhinitis and Rhinosinusitis

The term *rhinosinusitis* comprises various inflammatory conditions of different causes, symptoms, duration, and clinical presentation. According to the task force for defining adult chronic rhinosinusitis, rhinosinusitis is regarded as a symptom complex or syndrome without regard to underlying pathogenesis. The duration of symptoms differentiates acute, subacute, chronic, and recurrent acute rhinosinusitis.[30] Regardless of duration, rhinosinusitis may result in nasal obstruction, which must be recognized and adequately treated, especially when a septoplasty or septorhinoplasty is planned for functional or cosmetic purposes.

Although acute rhinosinusitis is usually infectious in nature, the cause of chronic rhinosinusitis remains largely elusive. Controversy exists as to whether a single unidentified cause is responsible or rather a combination of overlapping factors is the cause.

A particularly intriguing hypothesis about the etiology of chronic polypoid rhinosinusitis has been proposed by

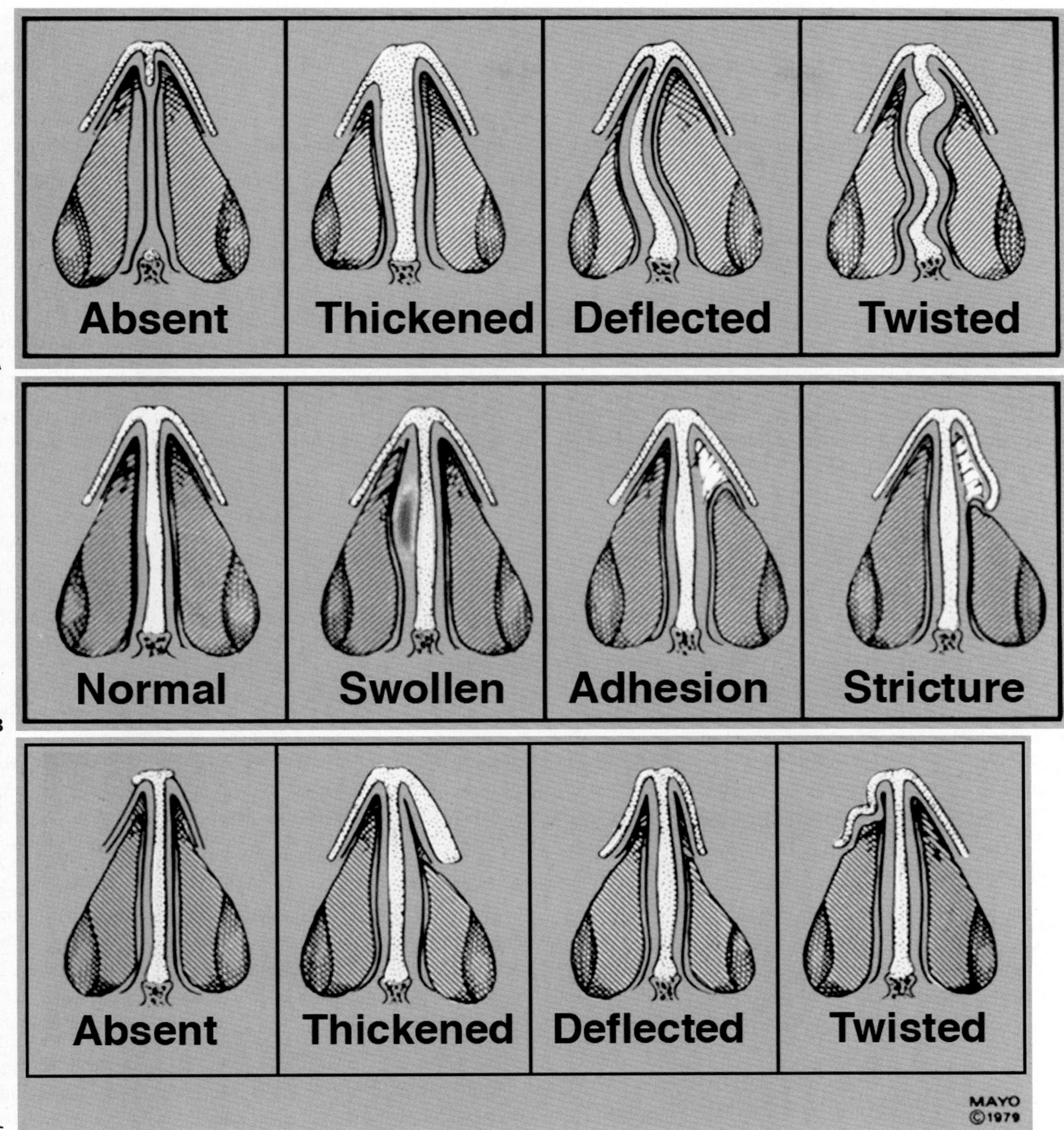

Fig. 39.10 Nasal valve pathology. (**A**) Septal pathology. (**B**) Mucocutaneous pathology. (**C**) Upper lateral cartilage pathology. (Reprinted by permission of Mayo Foundation for Medical Education and Research.)

Ponikau et al.[31] This group of investigators suggests that certain individuals mount an eosinophilic immune response to colonizing fungi. This response entails transmucosal migration of eosinophils into the nasal mucin and degranulation of the eosinophils with deposition of toxins onto the fungal elements in the mucin. The resultant chronic chemical inflammation of the mucosa leads to eventual polyp formation. Ponikau et al[31] as well as other groups[32,33] have published a considerable body of evidence that supports this hypothesis.

Chronic atrophic rhinitis is a similarly debated entity. This multifactorial disease has historically been attributed to bacterial causes. With the advent of modern antibiotics, other causes of chronic atrophic rhinitis have been recognized. The hallmarks of this disease are atrophy and loss of function of the nasal mucosa. Humidification is compromised with resultant drying, crusting, and pain. Bacterial colonization results in purulent secretions and odor. Atrophy of the intranasal tissues leaves too much space in the nose, and paradoxical obstruction ensues. Debate about this entity has resulted from a lack of data regarding the manifestation, progression, diagnosis, and etiology of the disease. Causes of chronic atrophic rhinitis include reductive turbinate surgery, radiotherapy, infection, and other destructive measures. Dry mucosa, crusting, and pain have been proposed as diagnostic criteria, but these identify only the terminal stages of the disease. Long delays between turbinate surgery and manifestation of end-stage chronic atrophic rhinitis have been reported in the literature.[34] No good test or established criteria exist to diagnose early changes of chronic atrophic rhinitis or to document its progression.

Vasomotor rhinitis represents a dysregulation of the autonomous neural network of the intranasal vasculature. Clinical manifestations include mucosal hypertrophy with nasal obstruction and clear rhinorrhea. Typically a diagnosis of exclusion, this disease responds well to topical intranasal application of albuterol.

Rhinitis medicamentosa results from overuse of decongesting nasal sprays. Typical agents are phenylephrine and oxymetazoline. Extended use of these sympathomimetic agents causes resistance to their vasoconstrictive properties, rebound vasodilation, and congestion of the nasal mucosa with obstruction. The diagnosis is established by history, and weaning of the medication is typically curative.

Medical Treatment

This brief discussion of medical treatment options for sinonasal disease focuses on the most frequently used pharmacological agents, such as oral antihistamines, topical and systemic corticosteroids, systemic antibiotics, and topical antifungals.

Antihistamines

The first generation of oral antihistamines (diphenhydramine, chlorpheniramine, and brompheniramine) was effective in the treatment of allergic rhinitis, but these drugs have been associated with sedative effects. These agents were followed by a generation of nonsedating antihistamines, such as fexofenadine, loratadine, and desloratadine. Several studies[35] have shown marked improvement in symptoms on the basis of outcome data in patients with allergic rhinitis compared with the placebo group. The low adverse-effect profile of these agents supports their use as first-line therapy for mild to moderate allergic rhinitis, especially in patients with intermittent symptoms and in children.[35] For chronic rhinosinusitis, no convincing data are available to show treatment efficacy.

Intranasal Corticosteroids

Topical corticosteroid sprays are indicated predominantly for the treatment of allergic rhinitis. Currently US Food and Drug Administration–approved agents are beclomethasone dipropionate, budesonide, flunisolide, fluticasone propionate, mometasone furoate, and triamcinolone acetonide. These agents have been shown to treat symptoms of allergic rhinitis more effectively than do oral antihistamines and are used as an alternative to or in combination with antihistamines in more severe cases of allergic rhinitis. The more recently introduced agents beclomethasone, budesonide, triamcinolone, fluticasone, and mometasone have been compared in several trials.[36–38] The symptom-based outcomes of these studies did not appear to clearly favor one agent over another.[36–38] The overall adverse-effect profile of intranasal corticosteroids is favorable and includes minor symptoms, such as dryness, stinging, or burning. Epistaxis is the most frequent major complication, occurring in ~5% of patients. The risk of septal perforation and epistaxis may be reduced by instructing the patient to direct the spray tip away from the septum toward the lateral nasal wall. Adverse effects such as suppression of the hypothalamic-pituitary axis and growth retardation have become rare with contemporary agents. An increasing body of data appears to indicate that mometasone and fluticasone are safe to use in children. Although off-label use of intranasal corticosteroids is widespread in the treatment of chronic polypoid rhinosinusitis, only mometasone has been approved by the US Food and Drug Administration for the treatment of nasal polyps.

Systemic Corticosteroids

Systemic corticosteroids are typically administered intramuscularly or orally. Intramuscular agents include betamethasone dipropionate, methylprednisone acetate, betamethasone phosphate, and triamcinolone acetonide. Systemic corticosteroids are third-line agents when antihistamines and intranasal corticosteroids have failed. These agents suppress endogenous cortisol production to a variable degree for 12 days to 3 weeks but are highly effective. Axelsson and Lindholm[39] showed symptomatic improvement in 16 of 17 patients with allergic rhinitis after administration of a single dose of triamcinolone acetonide, whereas only 2 of 21 patients improved in the placebo group. This relief can last throughout the allergic season.[39,40] Few data are available to compare oral with intramuscular corticosteroids. One study[41] showed plasma cortisol levels to be suppressed beyond 3 weeks with oral prednisolone, 7.5 mg daily, but not with intramuscular corticosteroids. With adequate screening of patients for diabetes mellitus, glaucoma, hypertension, and osteoporosis, use of systemic corticosteroids such as intramuscular triamcinolone acetonide has become an important and safe treatment of chronic inflammatory nasal disease.

Antibacterial Agents

As previously discussed, acute rhinosinusitis is a clinical diagnosis based on duration of symptoms. It is typically preceded by a viral upper respiratory tract inflammation, and in the absence of purulent nasal discharge and pathological culture results, the diagnosis of bacterial rhinosinusitis is challenging. Sinus aspirations acquired from patients with symptoms suggestive of acute bacterial sinusitis reveal pathological organisms in only 34 to 65%.[42,43] Recommendations regarding the indications, duration, and choice of agent for appropriate antibacterial treatment are evolving. Bacterial sinusitis may be suspected when acute symptoms persist for 10 days or worsen after 5 to 7 days.

According to a consensus report by the Sinus and Allergy Health Partnership,[44] a joint effort of several societies concerned with the treatment of sinusitis, recent administration of antibiotic treatment and failure of current therapy are important factors that influence outcome. Thus patients can be stratified on the basis of these factors into different treatment groups and receive different classes of antibiotics.[44]

Antifungal Therapy

The treatment of chronic rhinosinusitis is a particular challenge to the treating physician. A combination of surgical treatment, topical and systemic corticosteroids, and antifungal agents is frequently used for symptomatic relief and disease control. As discussed above, Ponikau et al[45] have produced a considerable body of data suggesting that fungi play an instrumental role in the pathophysiology of chronic rhinosinusitis. On the basis of these data, patients have been treated with long-term topical antifungal nasal washes.

Effects of Surgical Intervention on Nasal Physiology

Septal Surgery

The techniques of septoplasty are discussed in detail in Chapter 50. Some critical aspects as they relate to the preservation of nasal physiology are highlighted in the following section. Standard swinging-door septoplasty techniques effectively correct extensive posterior deformities. However because the posterior aspects of the nasal cavities are more spacious, such deviations need to be very marked to cause symptomatic obstruction. Appreciation of deviations of the caudal end and the interrelation of the dorsal septum with the upper lateral cartilages is critical. These areas require more complex maneuvers for correction. A common mistake is attempting to preserve a deformed L-shaped strut or overresecting the strut. This may result in tip ptosis, saddle nose deformity, and nasal valve obstruction. Caudal end deformities frequently require caudal end transplantation.[46] Marked deformities of the transition of the septum to the upper lateral cartilages may require separation of upper lateral cartilages from the septum. When the caudal septum is severely deformed or deficient, posterior septum, rib cartilage, or other material is grafted.[47] In addition, placement of grafts is often needed to prevent a narrow middle third of the nasal dorsum.

Another important location of septal pathology is the membranous septum. An elongated membranous septum is observed in senile tip ptosis. This deformity frequently results in bilateral nasal valve obstruction. The patient may indicate that the obstruction is relieved by pushing the nasal tip up with the finger. In addition to repositioning the sagging skin–soft tissue envelope over the dorsum and correcting middle vault pathologies, recreation of a physiological relationship between the columella and the caudal septum is important to correct this deformity.

Valve Surgery

Correction of nasal valve obstruction is the most challenging task in rhinoplasty, and accurate diagnosis of the nature and location of the pathology is paramount for successful repair. Without good structural integrity of the central pillar of the Anderson tripod (the medial crura, membranous septum, and caudal end of the septum), reconstruction of the remainder of the nasal valve is likely to fail. Advancement of the columella on a straight septum (tongue-in-groove technique), placement of a caudal end extension graft or of a well-fixated columellar strut graft, and caudal end transplantation are effective maneuvers in appropriate cases. Obstruction of the valve angle may be secondary to a large returning portion of the upper lateral cartilage and redundant vestibular mucosa. The M-plasty described by Schulte et al[48] is an excellent technique to correct valve obstruction resulting from such pathology.

If the interrelation of the upper lateral cartilages with the septum is appropriate, the lateral aspect of the valve is addressed. Structural weakness of the transition of the upper lateral cartilage to the alar cartilage is often the result of previous resection of the cephalic border of the

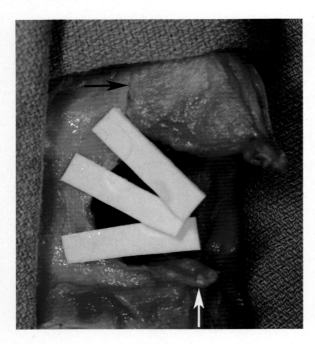

Fig. 39.11 White indicators simulate placement of batten grafts in different locations over the pyriform aperture. A higher, more vertical placement results in more effective lateralization of the lateral nasal wall (*black arrow*: nasomaxillary suture line; *white arrow*: nasal spine).

alar cartilage or of dome division. Placement of an alar batten graft, lateral crural strut graft, or alar replacement graft can contribute to the correction of these deficiencies. The shape and strength of the grafts are crucial for successful repair. The alar batten graft should be placed lateral to the piriform aperture and may be fixated with mattress sutures to the upper lateral cartilage. In the authors' experience placement of batten grafts in a more vertical direction results in more effective lateralization of the lateral nasal wall, as depicted in **Fig. 39.11**. One limitation of the batten grafts is that they cannot correct valve obstruction associated with severe deformities of the middle vault and valve angle. If such obstruction exists, the middle vault must be addressed.

Figure 39.12 shows how the integrity of the middle vault is critical for nasal breathing. The insertions of the upper lateral cartilages into the septum typically form a rounded arch that shapes the nasal valve angle at its caudal margin. After separation of the upper lateral cartilages, spreader grafts are frequently inserted. However, the placement of spreader grafts alone may be insufficient for nasal valve correction. Physiologically the typical rectangular spreader graft widens the valve area by lateralizing the upper lateral cartilage but may narrow the valve angle. A spreader graft with a trapezoidal cross-section and an angle of more than 15 degrees between the lateral surfaces is better suited to reconstruct and potentially widen the nasal valve angle. A spreader graft of this shape can be fashioned from the thicker septal cartilage located at the insertion into the nasal floor.

Alsarraf and Murakami[49] have described another technique to reconstruct the middle vault. These authors use a dorsal onlay graft sutured to the edges of the upper lateral cartilages to widen the nasal valve (**Fig. 39.12E**).[49] In the case of a deviated or asymmetric middle vault, spreader grafts need to provide rigidity and symmetry. Sherris[46] described the use of ethmoid bone spreader grafts to prevent recurrent deviations of the dorsal and caudal septum and the placement of unilateral spreader grafts to correct asymmetries. Another method that allows for excellent functional and cosmetic results is the placement of a longitudinal graft on top of the septum. In preparation, the upper lateral cartilages are separated from the septum, and the septum is reduced in height by ~2 mm. The upper lateral cartilages are then sutured along their entire length to the undersurface of the graft. This technique allows simultaneous creation of a smooth dorsal contour and widening with outward rotation of the upper lateral cartilages in cases of marked pathology of the middle vault. This type of graft can be extended to cover both the bony and the cartilaginous dorsum (**Fig. 39.12F**).

Placement of a shield-type tip graft sutured to the alar cartilages and alar rim grafts are useful techniques to address disorders of the external nasal valve. Severe saddle nose deformities, as they occur after trauma or with Wegener granulomatosis, result in marked nasal valve obstruction. Extensive grafting, usually of rib bone and costal cartilage, is required to reconstruct deficient aspects of the nasal skeleton and to rebuild the nasal airway in these cases.

Some authors advocate suture techniques to repair nasal valve disorders. The flaring suture across the upper lateral cartilage may be a useful adjunct to other techniques of valve repair. Paniello[50] popularized the suspension suture technique. This simple and quick technique allows elevation of the upper lateral cartilage and correction of valve collapse, but does not respect the important surgical principle that tissue must be dissected, mobilized, and fixated to achieve effective repositioning. This technique is an alternative to definite anatomical repair for patients who are poor candidates for rhinoplasty.

Osteotomy

Several modifications have been developed since Jacques Joseph popularized the osteotomy in rhinoplasty.[51] These techniques are described in detail elsewhere in this book. Some aspects of nasal osteotomies as they affect the function of the nose are highlighted in this section.

Inadequate lateral osteotomies after removal of a dorsal hump may result in the open roof deformity, which

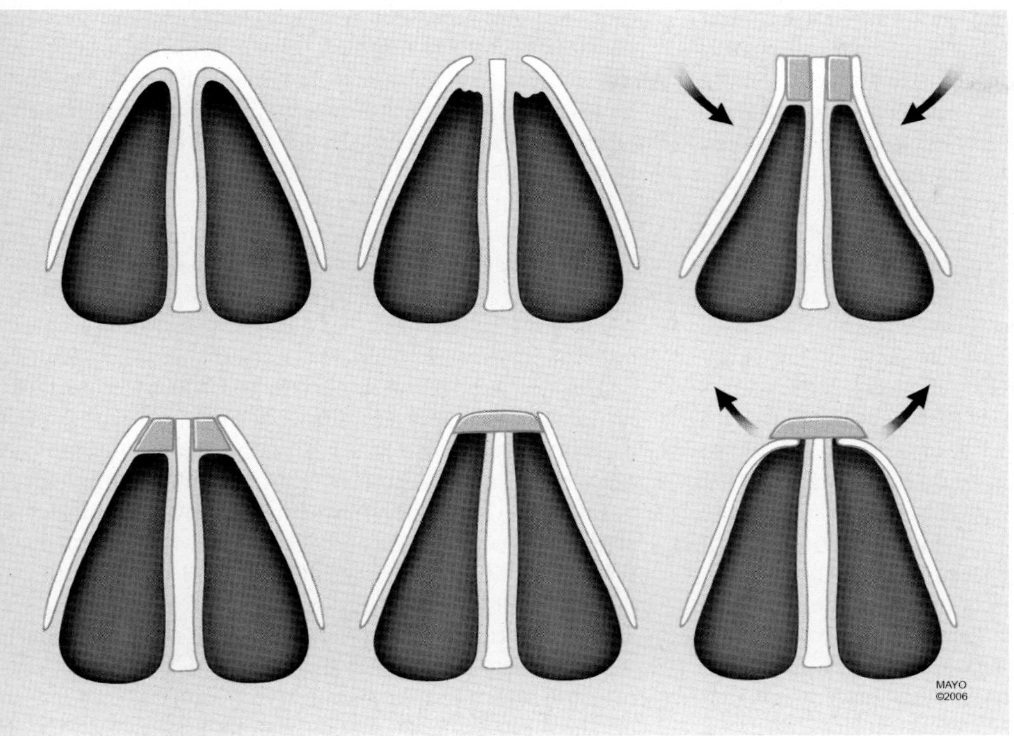

Fig. 39.12 (**A**) The transition of the septum to the upper lateral cartilages forms a rounded arch that supports the middle vault and maintains the nasal valve area. (**B**) Separation of the transition from the upper lateral cartilages to the septum destroys the skeletal support of the nasal valve and the middle vault. (**C**) Insertion of spreader grafts lateralizes the upper lateral cartilages (*arrowheads*) to a variable degree but also may pinch the nasal valve angle (*arrows*). (**D**) Spreader grafts with trapezoidal cross-sections allow more physiological reconstruction of the middle vault and nasal valve area. (**E**) The dorsal onlay graft spreads the upper lateral cartilages and nasal valve angle. (**F**) Placement of a graft on the septum. The septum is reduced in height to compensate for the addition of the graft. The upper lateral cartilages are suture fixated to the undersurface of the graft. This allows simultaneous widening and outward rotation of the nasal valve (*arrows*) as well as creation of a smooth dorsal contour. (Reprinted by permission of Mayo Foundation for Medical Education and Research.)

is a bony defect over the dorsum that is associated with pain, skin changes, and cosmetic deformities. The deep, straight lateral osteotomy follows the nasofacial groove and inserts low in the piriform aperture. Although this approach is adequate to correct nasal skeletal deformities and to close an open roof, nasal valve obstruction has been observed with the deep, straight lateral osteotomy. Webster[52] showed that the risk of nasal valve obstruction could be reduced by initiating the lateral osteotomy higher on the piriform aperture. Preservation of a triangular piece at the edge of the piriform aperture prevents medial displacement of the fibromuscular tissues of the ala and, in some cases, of the head of the inferior turbinate. Guyuron[53] found that the effect of high versus low osteotomy on nasal airway patency varies and depends on the length of the nasal bones and other anatomical factors. These data emphasize the importance of accurate, individualized preoperative assessment to determine the appropriate osteotomy for each patient.

Some patients require lateral outfracture rather than infracture to correct a medially displaced sidewall. Byrne et al[54] described the elegant method of inside-out osteotomies that preserve the integrity of the lateral periosteum by placing the guard of the osteotome on the inside of the pyramid.

Another complication following dorsal hump removal is the inverted-V deformity. Patients with short nasal bones are especially prone to development of an overly narrow middle third of the nose after hump removal and lateral osteotomies. This deformity may occur years after the osteotomy and may be prevented by exact placement of spreader grafts.

Reductive Turbinate Surgery

Turbinate hypertrophy has not been well defined and is poorly understood and researched. Tests are lacking to distinguish physiological engorgement from pathological enlargement. The exact endonasal localization of nasal obstruction relies predominantly on the surgeon's careful clinical examination. Posterior septal or turbinate pathology needs to be extensive to cause obstruction of the more spacious posterior aspects of the nasal cavity. Accordingly, obstructions of the nasal valve area occur more commonly than posterior obstructions. Before nasal obstruction is attributed to turbinate hypertrophy, the integrity of the nasal valve should be verified. When dilation of the nasal valve with specula or cotton-tipped applicators results in subjective nasal airway improvement, the cause of the obstruction is likely not turbinate hypertrophy. Turbinate hypertrophy should be refractory to anti-inflammatory medical therapy before surgical intervention is considered.

Various surgical techniques of turbinate reduction are used. Passali et al,[55] in the most comprehensive study to date, showed, in a randomized prospective fashion, that submucous resection with or without lateralization of the inferior turbinate results in longer-lasting reduction of nasal airway resistance, when compared with turbinectomy, laser cautery, electrocautery, or cryotherapy. These authors quantified secretory IgA concentrations and mucociliary clearance as a measure of physiological nasal function. Of note, all turbinate reduction techniques were associated with marked impairment of these physiological functions over the first 3 years of follow-up. At 6 years of follow-up, only submucosal resection regenerated these functions to approximately normal levels. However, follow-up data were available for only 24% of the study patients. Interestingly, crusting was reported in 8% of patients with submucous resection and in 76% of patients with turbinectomy.

In 214 of 242 Mayo Clinic patients with atrophic rhinitis reviewed by Moore and Kern,[35] biopsy confirmed the clinical diagnosis. Symptoms included nasal congestion, crusting, dryness, facial pain, anosmia, and depression. Chronic atrophic rhinitis developed in 166 patients secondary to nasal surgery, and 95% of these patients had undergone turbinectomy. Crusting of the lateral nasal sidewall occurred in all patients. Hence the patients included in this study appear to represent only the terminal stage of a disease that seems highly underdiagnosed in its early stages. Criteria for the diagnosis of atrophic rhinitis have included crusting and mucosal dryness on examination. However, crusting and dryness indicate complete decompensation of the crucial humidifying function of the nasal mucosa. When this has occurred, the remaining functions of the nose are likely also severely compromised. As Moore et al[56] noted, the time between reductive turbinate surgery and diagnosis of atrophic rhinitis is at least 3 to 5 years.

Early clinical signs and symptoms include pain associated with dry and cold air, the feeling that the undiverted inspired air stream hits the nasopharyngeal mucosa with resultant irritation and chronic cough, headaches, and decreased olfaction. Although these symptoms often are unnoticed before a diagnosis is established, the patients become focused on their nasal symptoms, frustrated by the discrepancy between objective findings and subjective symptoms, and eventually depressed. Lindemann et al[57] have shown that turbinate resection results in decreased humidifying capacity of the nasal mucosa. Future improvements in the measurements of humidification and warming of inspired air may be suitable to detect changes consistent with atrophic rhinitis at an earlier stage. Currently no test is available to reliably measure the site of nasal obstruction, the presence and degree of turbinate pathology, and the presence or absence of nasal valve obstruction. More importantly, no data are available on the long-term functional residual capacity of the nose. Thus it is unknown whether and how much the turbinates contribute to pathological nasal airway resistance. More importantly, it remains elusive how much mucosa and submucosa can be destroyed without compromising the physiological functions of the nose in the long term. Until such data are established, we advocate a turbinate- and mucosa-preserving approach to the management of nasal obstruction. Lateral outfracture and selective submucous resection of bone appear to be the only surgical maneuvers that allow reduction of the impact of the turbinates on nasal resistance without destruction of their physiological function. We feel that these maneuvers adequately address presumed turbinate pathology in the majority of cases when the remainder of the nasal skeleton has been adequately rebuilt.

Combination of Septorhinoplasty and Functional Endoscopic Sinus Surgery

The transition from headlight illumination to magnified endoscopic and microscopic techniques has greatly enhanced the quality of sinus surgery. Careful endonasal injection of vasoconstrictive agents and continuous visualization of every surgical maneuver allow for safe and nearly bloodless surgery with a very low complication rate in experienced hands.

Refinements in atraumatic surgical technique with meticulous attention to detail have also resulted in substantial improvements in functional and cosmetic rhinoplasty techniques. The shorter postoperative recovery times and more predictable results have generated an increased demand for these procedures. Both sinus surgery and rhinoplasty are routinely performed on an outpatient basis.

Patients ordinarily request combining rhinoplasty with functional endoscopic sinus surgery, when indicated, to shorten the postoperative recovery time and reduce the anesthesia risk and the cost of a staged approach.

Traditionally, surgery aimed at eradication of chronic sinus disease was thought to be associated with the risk of spreading infection. However, an increasing body of evidence indicates that chronic rhinosinusitis is not the result of a bacterial infection and may represent a dysregulation of the immune system. The risk of spreading infection from one surgical field to the other is more theoretical than real in the absence of an acute bacterial superinfection.

Several authors have reported on their experience with combined endoscopic sinus surgery and predominantly endonasal rhinoplasty procedures.[58] Toffel[59] observed a low overall complication rate in 122 patients. This author aborted the rhinoplasty portion when gross purulence or mycosis was present in the sinuses. Rizk et al[60] selected patients with mild to moderate sinus disease for concurrent intervention. Lee et al[61] reviewed the Mayo Clinic series of concurrent endoscopic sinus surgery and open septorhinoplasty procedures.[61] Their results mirror those of other authors who found no increase in complications or other adverse effects from the combination of closed rhinoplasty and endoscopic sinus surgery. The concurrent approach appears safe when patients with mild to moderate sinus disease are selected and acute bacterial or fungal infections have been excluded.

The placement of extensive nasal packing has become rare with atraumatic rhinoplasty techniques and infrequent with functional sinus surgery. Minimal resorbable packing of the middle meatus or sponges removed within a day of surgery typically provide excellent hemostasis and medialization of the middle turbinate. Nasal breathing is reinstituted quickly and patient comfort is enhanced. Additionally, middle turbinate medialization sutures or silicone stents extending lateral to the middle turbinates may be used to keep the middle turbinates from lateralizing during the healing phase.

Summary

A sound understanding of the physiological functions of the nose and their preservation is mandatory for excellent long-term outcomes after rhinoplasty. The functional residual capacity of the nose is unknown, and great reserve with regard to turbinate reduction, regardless of technique, is advised. Recognition of the nature and location of nasal valve pathologies allows for adequate correction and superb functional results in the majority of cases. Concurrent rhinoplasty and functional endoscopic sinus surgery can be performed safely. The evolution of atraumatic surgical techniques has resulted in substantially improved patient comfort and speedy recovery.

References

1. Tardy ME Jr. Surgical Anatomy of the Nose. New York: Raven Press; 1990:34
2. Griesman BL. Muscles and cartilages of the nose from the standpoint of typical rhinoplasty. Arch Otolaryngol Head Neck Surg 1944;39:334
3. Cole P. The four components of the nasal valve. Am J Rhinol 2003;17:107–110
4. Constantian MB. The incompetent external nasal valve: pathophysiology and treatment in primary and secondary rhinoplasty. Plast Reconstr Surg 1994;93:919–931
5. Drumheller GW. Topology of the lateral nasal cartilages: the anatomical relationship of the lateral nasal to the greater alar cartilage, lateral crus. Anat Rec 1973;176:321–327
6. Kienstra MA, Gassner HG, Sherris DA, Kern EB. A grading system for nasal dorsal deformities. Arch Facial Plast Surg 2003;5:138–143
7. Cauna N. Blood and nerve supply to the internal nasal lining. In: Proctor DF, Andersen I, eds. The Nose, Upper Airway Physiology, and the Atmospheric Environment. Amsterdam: Elsevier Biomedical Press; 1982:45–70
8. Stammberger HR, Kennedy DW. The Anatomic Terminology Group. Paranasal sinuses: anatomic terminology and nomenclature. Ann Otol Rhinol Laryngol Suppl 1995;167:7–16
9. Wigand ME. Endoscopic surgery of the paranasal sinuses and anterior skull base. Stuttgart: Theime Verlag; 1990
10. Stamm AC, Draf W. Microendoscopic Surgery of the Paranasal Sinuses and the Skull Base. Berlin: Springer; 2000
11. Orlandi RR, Kennedy DW. Surgical management of rhinosinusitis. Am J Med Sci 1998;316:29–38
12. Hasegawa M, Kern EB. The human nasal cycle. Mayo Clin Proc 1977; 52:28–34
13. Fry FA, Black A. Regional deposition and clearance of particles in the human nose. J Aerosol Sci 1973;4:113–124
14. Itoh H, Smaldone GC, Swift DL, Wagner HN. Mechanisms of aerosol deposition in a nasal model. J Aerosol Sci 1985;16:529–534
15. Jones N. The nose and paranasal sinuses physiology and anatomy. Adv Drug Deliv Rev 2001;51:5–19
16. Anderson SD, Togias AG. Dry air and hyperosmolar challenge in asthma and rhinitis. In: Busse WW, Holgate ST, eds. Asthma and Rhinitis. Boston: Blackwell Science; 1995:1178–1195
17. Cole P. Modification of inspired air. In: Proctor DF, Andersen I, eds. The Nose, Upper Airway Physiology, and the Atmospheric Environment. Amsterdam: Elsevier Biomedical Press; 1982:351–375
18. Kern EB. Surgery of the nasal valve. In: Sisson GA, Tardy ME Jr, eds. Plastic and Reconstructive Surgery of the Face and Neck: Proceedings of the Second International Symposium. Vol. 2. New York: Grune & Stratton; 1977:43–59
19. Gassner HG, Remington WJ, Sherris DA. Quantitative study of nasal tip support and the effect of reconstructive rhinoplasty. Arch Facial Plast Surg 2001;3:178–184
20. Kienstra MA, Gassner HG, Sherris DA, Kern EB. Effects of the nasal muscles on the nasal airway. Am J Rhinol 2005;19:375–381
21. Masing H. Rhinomanometry, different techniques, and results. Acta Otorhinolaryngol Belg 1979;33:566–571
22. Kern EB. Standardization of rhinomanometry. Rhinology 1977;15:115–119
23. Hilberg O, Jackson AC, Swift DL, Pedersen OF. Acoustic rhinometry: evaluation of nasal cavity geometry by acoustic reflection. J Appl Physiol 1989;66:295–303
24. Taverner D, Bickford L, Latte J. Validation by fluid volume of acoustic rhinometry before and after decongestant in normal subjects. Rhinology 2002;40:135–140
25. Beaty MM, Dyer WK II, Shawl MW. The quantificaiton of surgical changes in nasal tip support. Arch Facial Plast Surg 2002;4:82–91
26. Wolfensberger M, Schnieper I, Welge-Lessen A. Sniffin'Sticks: a new olfactory test battery. Acta Otolaryngol 2000;120:303–306
27. Kobal G, Hummel C. Cerebral chemosensory evoked potentials elicited by chemical stimulation of the human olfactory and respiratory nasal mucosa. Electroencephalogr Clin Neurophysiol 1988;71:241–250
28. Wei JL, Remington WJ, Sherris DA. Work-up and evaluation of patients with nasal obstruction. Facial Plast Surg Clin North Am 1999;7:263–278

29. Constantian MB. Differing characteristics in 100 consecutive secondary rhinoplasty patients following closed versus open surgical approaches. Plast Reconstr Surg 2002;109:2097–2111
30. Lanza DC, Kennedy DW. Adult rhinosinusitis defined. Otolaryngol Head Neck Surg 1997;117:S1–S7
31. Ponikau JU, Sherris DA, Kern EB, et al. The diagnosis and incidence of allergic fungal sinusitis. Mayo Clin Proc 1999;74:877–884
32. Braun H, Stammberger H, Buzina W, Freudenschuss K, Lackner A, Beham A. Incidence and detection of fungi and eosinophilic granulocytes in chronic rhinosinusitis [German]. Laryngorhinootologie 2003;82:330–340
33. Gosepath J, Brieger J, Vlaschtsis K, Mann WJ. Fungal DNA is present in tissue specimens of patients with chronic rhinosinusitis. Am J Rhinol 2004;18:9–13
34. Moore EJ, Kern EB. Atrophic rhinitis: a review of 242 cases. Am J Rhinol 2001;15:355–361
35. Dykewicz MS, Fineman S, Skoner DP, et al. American Academy of Allergy, Asthma and Immunology. Diagnosis and management of rhinitis: complete guidelines of the Joint Task Force on Practice Parameters in Allergy, Asthma, and Immunology. Ann Allergy Asthma Immunol 1998;81 (Pt 2):478–518
36. Ratner PH, Paull BR, Findlay SR, et al. Fluticasone propionate given once daily is as effective for seasonal allergic rhinitis as beclomethasone dipropionate given twice daily. J Allergy Clin Immunol 1992;90(Pt 1):285–291
37. Haye R, Gomez EG. A multicentre study to assess long-term use of fluticasone propionate aqueous nasal spray in comparison with beclomethasone dipropionate aqueous nasal spray in the treatment of perennial rhinitis. Rhinology 1993;31:169–174
38. Stern MA, Dahl R, Nielsen LP, Pedersen B, Schrewelius C. A comparison of aqueous suspensions of budesonide nasal spray (128 micrograms and 256 micrograms once daily) and fluticasone propionate nasal spray (200 micrograms once daily) in the treatment of adult patients with seasonal allergic rhinitis. Am J Rhinol 1997;11:323–330
39. Axelsson A, Lindholm B. The effect of triamcinolone acetonide on allergic and vasomotor rhinitis. Acta Otolaryngol 1972;73:64–67
40. Mygind N, Laursen LC, Dahl M. Systemic corticosteriod treatment for seasonal allergic rhinitis: a common but poorly documented therapy. Allergy 2000;55:11–15
41. Laursen LC, Faurschou P, Pals H, Svendsen UG, Weeke B. Intramuscular betamethasone dipropionate vs. oral prednisolone in hay fever patients. Allergy 1987;42:168–172
42. von Bechem FL, Knottnerus JA, Schrijnemaekers VJ, Peeters MF. Primarycare-based randomized placebo-controlled trial of antibiotic treatment in acute maxillary sinusitis. Lancet 1997;349:683–687
43. Savolainen S, Pietola M, Kiukaanniemi H, Lappalainen E, Salminen M, Mikkonen P. An ultrasound device in the diagnosis of acute maxillary sinusitis. Acta Otolaryngol Suppl 1997;529:148–152
44. Sinus and Allergy Health Partnership. Antimicrobial treatment guidelines for acute bacterial rhinosinusitis. Otolaryngol Head Neck Surg 2000;123(Pt 2):5–31
45. Ponikau JU, Sherris DA, Weaver A, Kita H. Treatment of chronic rhinosinusitis with intranasal amphotericin B: a randomized, placebo-controlled, double-blind pilot trial. J Allergy Clin Immunol 2005;115: 125–131
46. Sherris DA. Caudal and dorsal septal reconstruction: an algorithm for graft choices. Am J Rhinol 1997;11:457–466
47. Sherris DA, Kern EB. The versatile autogenous rib graft in septorhinoplasty. Am J Rhinol 1998;12:221–227
48. Schulte DL, Sherris DA, Kern EB. M-plasty correction of nasal valve obstruction. Fac Plast Surg Clin 1999;7:405–409
49. Alsarraf R, Murakami CS. The saddle nose deformity. Facial Plast Surg Clin North Am 1999;7:303–310
50. Paniello RC. Nasal valve suspension: an effective treatment for nasal valve collapse. Arch Otolaryngol Head Neck Surg 1996;122:1342–1346
51. Kienstra MA, Sherris DA, Kern EB. Osteotomy and pyramid modification in the Joseph and Cottle rhinoplasty. Facial Plast Surg Clin North Am 1999;7:279–294
52. Webster RC, Davidson TM, Smith RC. Curved lateral osteotomy for airway protection in rhinoplasty. Arch Otolaryngol Head Neck Surg 1977;103:454–458
53. Guyuron B. Nasal osteotomy and airway changes. Plast Reconstr Surg 1998;102:856–860
54. Byrne PJ, Walsh WE, Hilger PA. The use of "inside-out" lateral osteotomies to improve outcome in rhinoplasty. Arch Facial Plast Surg 2003; 5:251–255
55. Passali D, Passali FM, Damiani V, Passali GC, Bellussi L. Treatment of inferior turbinate hypertrophy: a randomized clinical trial. Ann Otol Rhinol Laryngol 2003;112:683–688
56. Moore GF, Freeman TJ, Ogren FP, Yonkers AJ. Extended follow-up of total inferior turbinate resection for relief of chronic nasal obstruction. Laryngoscope 1985;95(Pt 1):1095–1099
57. Lindemann J, Leiacker R, Sikora T, Rettinger G, Keck T. Impact of unilateral sinus surgery with resection of the turbinates by means of midfacial degloving on nasal air conditioning. Laryngoscope 2002;112: 2062–2066
58. Millman B, Smith R. The potential pitfalls of concurrent rhinoplasty and endoscopic sinus surgery. Laryngoscope 2002;112(Pt 1):1193–1196
59. Toffel PH. Simultaneous secure endoscopic sinus surgery and rhinoplasty. Ear Nose Throat J 1994;73:554–556, 558–560, 565
60. Rizk SS, Edelstein DR, Matarasso A. Concurrent functional endoscopic sinus surgery and rhinoplasty. Ann Plast Surg 1997;38:323–329
61. Lee JH, Sherris DA, Moore EJ. Combined open septorhinoplasty and functional endoscopic sinus surgery. Otolaryngol Head Neck Surg 2005;133:436–440

40 Philosophy and Principles of Rhinoplasty

M. Eugene Tardy Jr., Dean M. Toriumi, and David A. Hecht

Rhinoplasty is a continually evolving operation, but the fundamental philosophy and principles have not changed dramatically over recent years. Advances have been made in the refinement of rhinoplasty through a better understanding of nasal analysis, anatomy, function, and long-term postoperative healing. Novel surgical maneuvers and techniques have also been developed that improve the long-term results of rhinoplasty from both aesthetic and functional standpoints. Furthermore, technological advances in computer imaging and innovative surgical instrumentation have widened the armamentarium available to the surgeon performing rhinoplasty as well as other facial plastic procedures.

Aesthetic surgery of the nose is considered to be the most challenging, rewarding, and humbling of all facial plastic procedures. Every rhinoplasty operation presents the surgeon with a diversity of nasal anatomy, contours, and proportions, requiring a series of organized and interrelated surgical maneuvers tailored to each patient's anatomical and functional needs. The surgeon controls the operative event and must also become skilled at manipulating and controlling the dynamics of postoperative healing to attain optimal long-term aesthetic results. A necessary prerequisite is the skill to visualize the ultimate healed outcome while modifying nasal structures.

Such skills require many years of study and experience as the surgeon observes, analyzes, and modifies surgical results. With the improved methods of analysis and the increased popularity of open (external) rhinoplasty, young surgeons may be able to perform precise maneuvers under direct visualization. The key to self-education through experience is accurate diagrammatic record keeping coupled with long-term patient follow-up and evaluation (**Fig. 40.1**).[1,2]

The unique anatomy of the nose is the critical factor influencing the final result of each individual rhinoplasty procedure. Variability in anatomy demands refined diagnostic skills to identify the infinite variety of problems encountered. The aesthetic judgment of the surgeon, guided by patient expectation, determines the surgical changes planned. No single procedure or technique will suffice to reconstruct every nose in an aesthetically pleasing fashion. Therefore the surgeon must be skilled in many different approaches and maneuvers to handle the wide range of nasal anatomical combinations. The ability to identify correctable deformities and limitations inherent in each patient exists as the single most critical prerequisite to attainment of outstanding results on a consistent basis. Misguided attempts to create changes greater than the tissues will permit (overoperating) frequently results in aesthetic and functional complications resulting from overaggressive resection of supportive structures (**Fig. 40.2**).

Nasal Anatomy

The nose can be separated into several anatomical components, including the covering skin, the bony pyramid (nasal bones, bony septum, and ascending process of the maxilla), the cartilaginous pyramid (upper lateral cartilages and cartilaginous septum), and the nasal tip (lower lateral cartilages) (**Fig. 40.3A**).[3] The nasal tip can be further broken down into the domal region, infratip lobule, alar sidewalls, and columella (**Fig. 40.3B**).

The nose has a rich arterial blood supply derived mainly from branches of the facial and superior labial arteries.[4] These arterial branches are accompanied by corresponding veins and lymphatics that run together in a plane within the superficial musculoaponeurotic system (SMAS) layer of the nose. This relationship of the nasal blood supply to the SMAS layer of the nose bears clinical importance.[5] By elevating the skin–soft tissue envelope off the nasal skeleton *below* the SMAS layer during rhinoplasty, maximal blood supply and SMAS layer cushioning will be preserved in the overlying skin–soft tissue envelope.

Patient Evaluation

Throughout the entire evaluation process, ongoing analysis of the patient's motivations, expectations, and rapport with the surgeon is vital. This important information may help identify the problem patient with unrealistic expectations.[6] If the patient's anatomy suggests significant surgical limitations, surgical management should be planned only if outcome limitations are clearly understood and accepted by both patient and surgeon.

Careful examination of the nose and surrounding facial structures is critical before any decisions regarding the actual surgical plan can be made. The ideal nose differs for every patient and depends on facial features, the surgeon's sense of aesthetics, and the ability to surgically create the desired nasal shape.

Balance and harmony of proportionate facial features are critical in determining the ideal nose for a particular face. For example, the degree of nasal projection that is appropriate for an individual patient may be influenced by the projection and shape of the chin and mandible. An overprojected nose may not appear to be as unsightly in a patient with a strong chin and mandible. However, an adequately projected nose may appear overprojected in a patient with an underprojected chin or retrognathia. This relationship can be exploited in the case of an overprojected nose with an underprojected chin. In these cases, moderate retroprojection of the nose can be performed and supplemented by chin augmentation. Nasal projection will not have to be reduced to a point where the structure and balance of the nose are compromised, yet the increased chin projection will balance even a slightly overprojected nose.

The thickness of the skin overlying the nasal structure is perhaps the most critical factor in achieving ideal results in rhinoplastic surgery. Skin of moderate thickness is ideal because it usually conforms to the underlying cartilage and bone; therefore, surgical changes made in the nasal skeleton (cartilage and bone) translate the desired soft tissue changes. In addition, nasal skin of moderate thickness possesses enough subcutaneous fibrofatty tissue to provide a satisfactory cushion over the nasal skeleton to hide small irregularities of the nasal dorsum or asymmetries of the lower lateral cartilages.

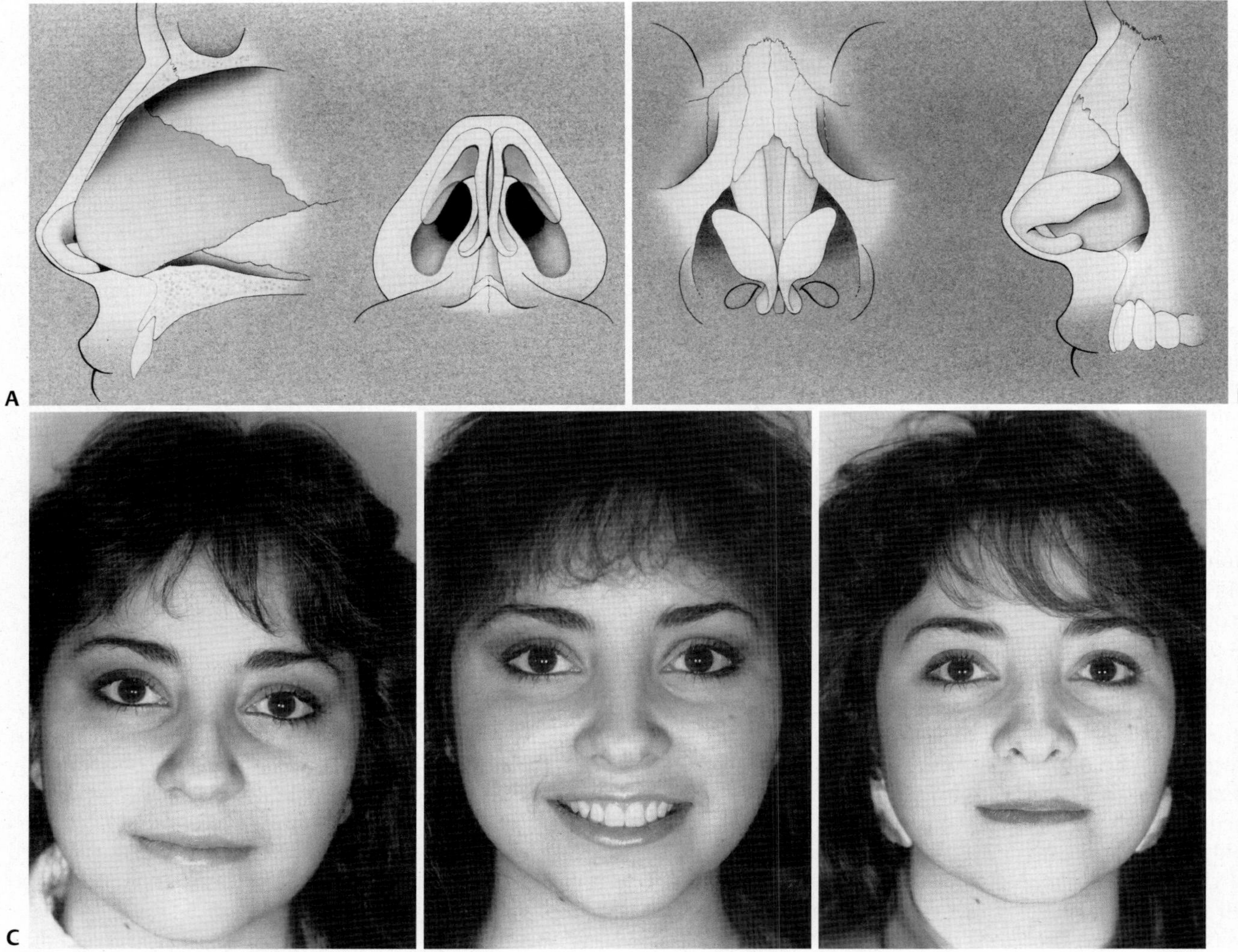

Fig. 40.1 **(A,B)** Graphic charts used in visual record keeping of the techniques and maneuvers performed during rhinoplasty. Comparison of this graphic record with the long-term outcome provides an instructive self-analysis of the usefulness of particular surgical techniques. Long-term follow-up of young girl who has undergone aesthetic septorhinoplasty (5 years). Column 1 illustrates the preoperative condition, column 2 the result at 1 year, and column 3 the final outcome at 5 years. Note the evolutionary progression of healing refinements over time.

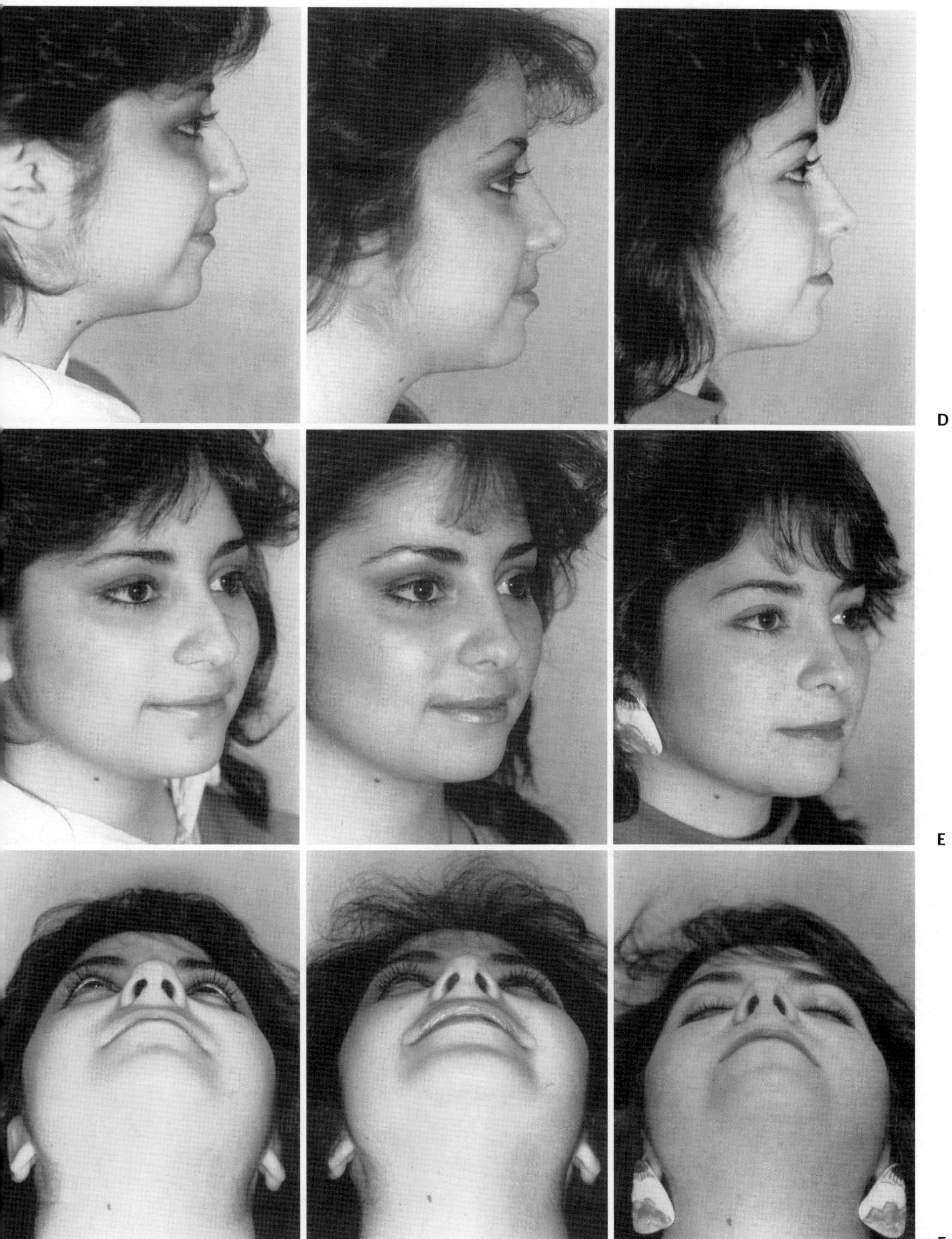

Fig. 40.1 (*Continued*)

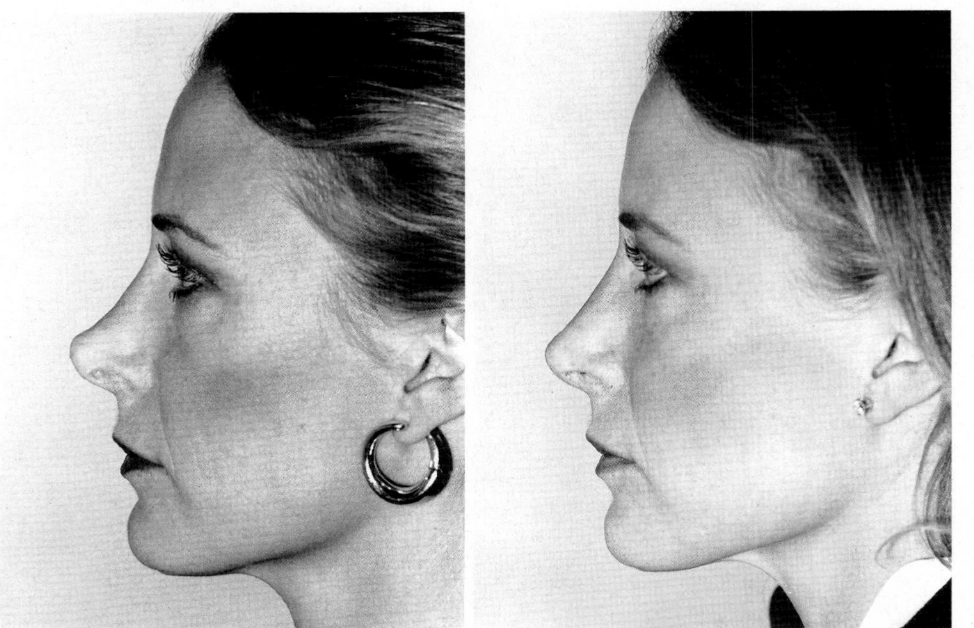

Fig. 40.2 Patient with iatrogenic overprojection of the tip several years following rhinoplasty surgery. (**A**) Inappropriate tip refinement technique was chosen, resulting in disproportion of the nose. Original operative record was unavailable. (**B**) Revision surgery consisted of exploration of the nasal tip with retropositioning of the overprojection phenomenon, intended to bring the nose into better balance.

Thick sebaceous skin tends to be inelastic, possessing a memory of its own. A nose with thick skin may suggest the temptation for aggressive changes in the shape of underlying cartilages to effect a change in soft tissue nasal contour. These aggressive maneuvers tend to weaken the support of the nasal skeleton, which may ultimately buckle and collapse under the forces of scar contracture. In some cases, the memory of the skin is so great that

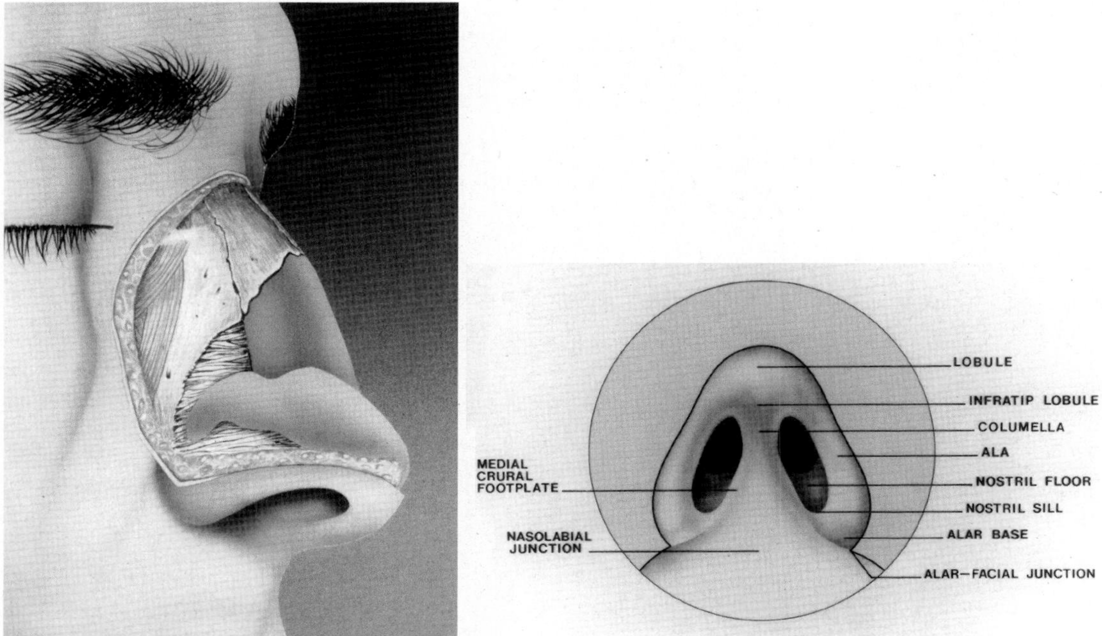

Fig. 40.3 (**A**) Artist's rendering of the anatomical components of the nose. (**B**) The anatomy and topographic designations of the nasal base.

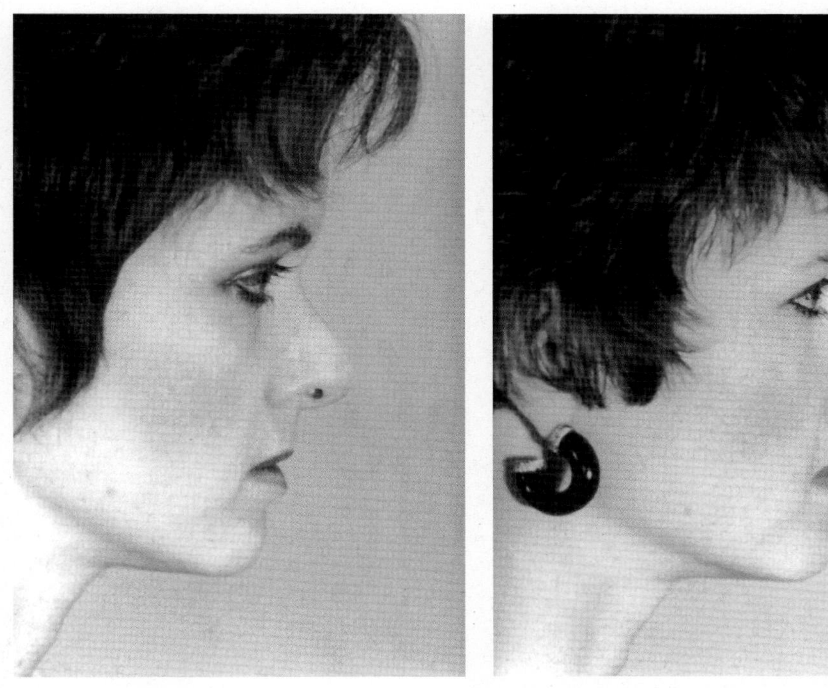

Fig. 40.4 (**A**) Patient requesting revision rhinoplasty following overaggressive procedure performed elsewhere. (**B**) Revision repair utilizing autogenous cartilage grafts to augment the overdeep bony dorsum and nasofrontal angle, with reduction of the soft tissue and cartilaginous pollybeak deformity.

no matter what is done to the nasal skeleton, the skin will not drape, leaving a dead-space void. This void may become occupied by scar tissue producing an amorphous nasal tip and soft tissue pollybeak (**Fig. 40.4**).[7]

Extremely thin skin is often pale and freckled and must be recognized and respected for its inherent limitations. Although ideal for obtaining critical definition, thin skin with limited subcutaneous tissue provides almost no cushion to hide even the smallest skeletal irregularities or contour imperfections. Working with thin skin requires near-perfect surgery to achieve the desired result. These patients also tend to demonstrate undesirable progressive skin retraction and shrinkage over several years, rendering the nose potentially unnatural and angular.

Evaluation of the skin is performed by close inspection and by palpation in the form of gentle pinching of the overlying skin to see how it glides over the nasal skeleton. In the non-Caucasian nose, the skin is commonly so thick and the cartilages so weak that at times it may be difficult to even appreciate the cartilages. In revision cases, skin thickness may be deceiving because of dense scar tissue, obliterating what once was a well-defined, subcutaneous fibrofatty tissue plane.[8]

When examining the patient, it is essential to evaluate the inherent strength and support of the lower third of the nose by using fingertip depression to test tip recoil.[9] The tip of the nose is firmly depressed toward the upper lip and then released, allowing the tip to recoil (**Fig. 40.5**). This is a reliable support test of the mobile lower third of the nose. A nose that lacks tip support probably has weak lower lateral cartilages that will not tolerate much loss

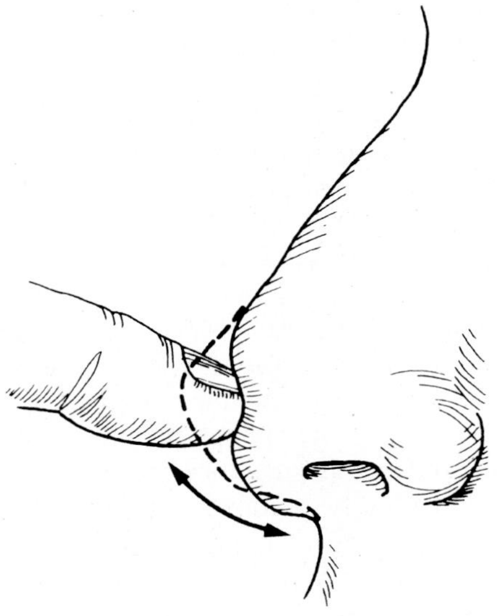

Fig. 40.5 Tip recoil phenomenon demonstrated on nasal tip. A degree of resilience of the nasal tip supportive structures provides a reliable guide to the ability of the nasal tip to retain satisfactory support and projection following tip refinement procedures.

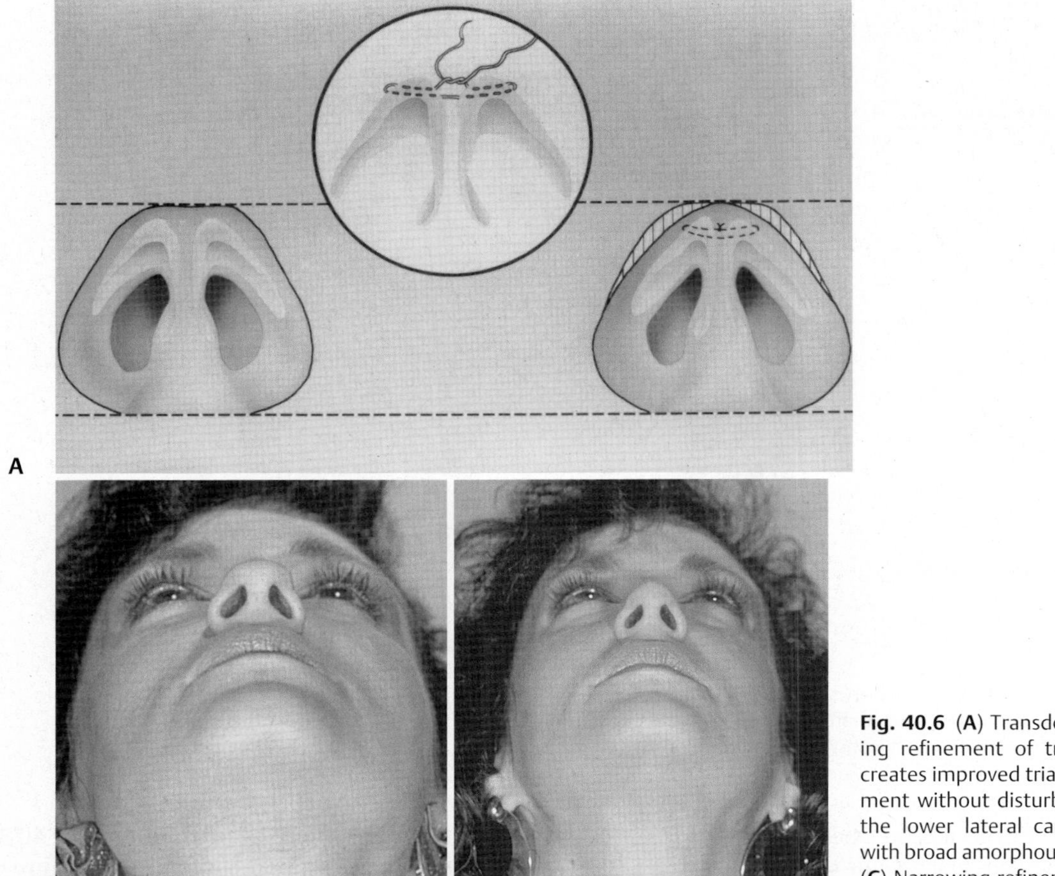

Fig. 40.6 (**A**) Transdomal suture narrowing refinement of trapezoidal nasal tip creates improved triangularity and refinement without disturbing the integrity of the lower lateral cartilages. (**B**) Patient with broad amorphous tip prior to surgery. (**C**) Narrowing refinement 2 years following transdomal suture refinement.

of support through aggressive tissue excision, suggesting the addition of supportive struts to prevent postoperative loss of tip projection. If tip recoil is vigorous and the tip cartilages resist the force exerted by fingertip depression, reasonable surgical manipulation of the lower lateral cartilages can usually be performed without a significant loss of tip support. Palpation or ballottement of the lateral crura between two fingers can provide important information about the size, shape, and strength of the alar cartilages. Buckles or asymmetry of the lower lateral cartilages should be identified before surgery, because these findings may influence the manner in which the cartilages are manipulated. The domal region should be examined to determine the distance between the domes. Significant tip bifidity requires narrowing the interdomal distance to achieve refinement (**Fig. 40.6**). The relationship between the anterior septal angle and domes should also be evaluated.

The length and strength of the upper lateral cartilages should be compared with the length of the nasal bones. Short nasal bones are usually associated with longer upper lateral cartilages. Patients with short nasal bones tend to possess less support in the region of the internal nasal valve because the long upper lateral cartilages can collapse inward on inspiration (negative pressure).[10,11] This is particularly true if a sizable dorsal hump is removed, leaving the caudal margin of the upper lateral cartilages with even less support. The internal nasal valve is composed of the angle defined by the caudal margin of the upper lateral cartilages, the nasal septum, and the floor of the nose. If the caudal margin of the upper lateral cartilages is weakened, allowing it to collapse inward, the dimensions of the internal nasal valve can decrease dramatically. To prevent such problems, when a large dorsal hump is removed leaving long-flail upper lateral cartilages, spreader grafts can be positioned between the dorsal edge of the septum and the upper lateral cartilages to prevent their collapse and prevent overnarrowing of the nasal middle third, characterized by an "inverted-V" deformity.[11]

The columella and caudal margins of the septum can be palpated between the thumb and index finger to supply information about the relationship between these two structures. On occasion, the caudal septum may be twisted or the quadrangular cartilage overdeveloped

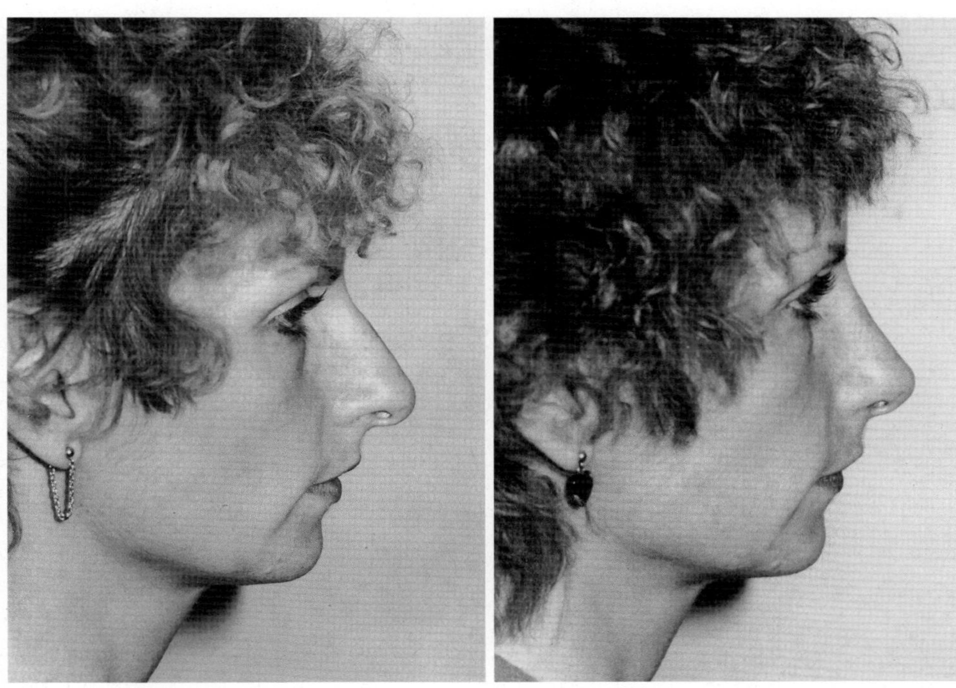

Fig. 40.7 (**A**) Patient with a large nose demonstrating overdevelopment and alar–columellar disproportion, as well as elongation of the caudal septum, creating a "hanging" infratip lobule phenomenon. (**B**) Correction involves reduction of the length of the quadrangular cartilage, excision of redundant vestibular skin, and shave-excision of the caudal margin of the medial and intermediate crura.

pushing the medial crura and columella inferiorly and creating a convex, overly prominent columella in relation to the alar rim (**Fig. 40.7**). Palpation in this region can also provide information about the anterior nasal spine and its relationship to the posterior septal angle.

The width and length of the columella and medial crura should be determined because of the support provided by this anatomical complex. Short medial crura usually require a cartilaginous strut to provide support and prevent postoperative loss of tip projection.[11] In the overprojecting nose, extremely long or flaring medial crura can be reduced in width and length to retroproject the lower third of the nose. Whether the tip–lip complex is tethered by an active musculus depressor septi nasi must also be determined.

A thorough intranasal examination before and after shrinkage of the mucosa of the septum and turbinates is an essential part of the initial examination. Shrinkage of the mucosa permits superior visualization of septal deviations and spurs along the floor of the nose. Identification of a deviated ethmoid plate is critical because it may be responsible for nasal obstruction after osteotomy and infracture of the bony sidewalls. Careful examination of the nasal valve region and turbinates is performed to determine if surgical reduction of the turbinates is required to improve overall nasal function. Finally, the surgeon must ensure that no septal perforations or synechiae exist.

The position and inclination of the nasofrontal and nasolabial angles must be carefully evaluated (**Fig. 40.8**). The nasofrontal angle can vary greatly from patient to patient. The deepest point of the nasofrontal angle is called *the sellion* and corresponds to the nasal starting point.[3] The nasal starting point in women should ideally be at or just below the level of the superior palpebral fold. In men, the nasal starting point should be at or just above the level of the superior palpebral fold. In some patients, the nasofrontal angle is blunted with a poorly defined nasal starting point. This can be due to a bony prominence in this region or a thick procerus muscle that tents across and blunts the nasofrontal angle. To correct this deformity, it may be necessary to excise bone or muscle to produce a well-defined nasal starting point. An overly acute or retracted nasolabial angle can be effaced by placing cartilage plumping grafts at the columellar–labial junction. In more severe cases, such as is seen in non-Caucasian noses, larger premaxillary grafts can be positioned on the premaxilla through a sublabial incision to help bring out the acute nasolabial angle.[12]

The size and shape of the alae and alar base should also be examined, with assessment regarding how this

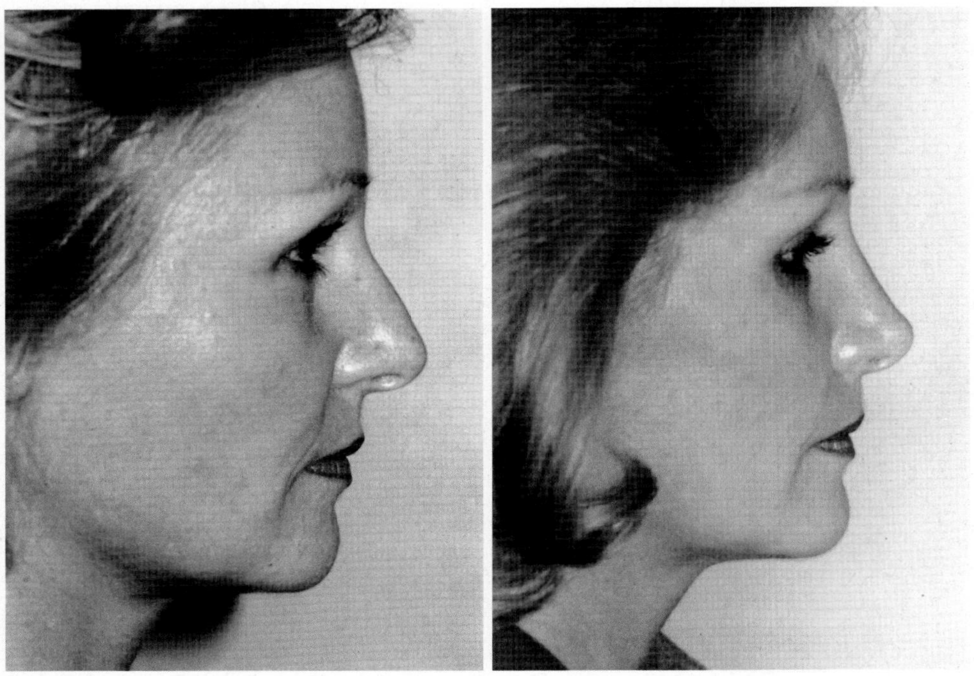

Fig. 40.8 (**A**) Patient requesting rhinoplasty. (**B**) Postoperative view shown 5 years following surgery, demonstrating near-ideal configuration of the nose, nasofrontal angle, and nasolabial angle.

shape may change with an increase or loss in nasal tip projection (**Fig. 40.9**). In some cases, alar base excisions may be necessary to provide harmony with the size and shape of the rest of the nose.

Finally, a functional assessment of the nose should be performed with an emphasis on dynamic forms of nasal airway obstruction, particularly the internal and external nasal valve regions. The internal nasal valve, as described previously, can be evaluated in two different ways. The Cottle maneuver is performed by retracting the cheek soft tissue and adjacent nasal wall laterally while the patient inspires through the nose. Alternatively, a blunt instrument (such as a nasal speculum or cerumen curette) can be inserted in the nose and used to directly displace the lateral nasal wall outward.[10] Both of these maneuvers result in decreased air flow resistance in the widened internal nasal valve region and are noted by the patient as conferring an improvement in nasal breathing. External nasal valve collapse is best evaluated from a basal view of the nose and manifests as collapse of the nostril margin (alar collapse) on nasal inspiration. It is important to evaluate and recognize nasal valve collapse because it is surgically correctable with the use of various grafting techniques.[10,11]

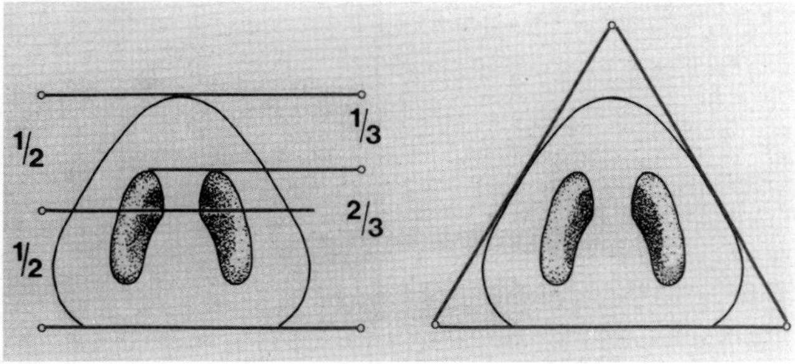

Fig. 40.9 Ideal proportionate configuration of the nasal base.

Photographic and Computer Imaging

Standard and uniform color photographs of the rhinoplasty patient, recorded before and after surgery, are important because they provide permanent records of the patient's deformity and how it has been corrected. The preoperative photographs are important guides to operative planning and execution. The entire set of preoperative and postoperative photographs provide a means of evaluating the progress of the patient, an invaluable teaching tool, and a vital medicolegal record.

Standard 35-mm color slides (Kodachrome or Ektachrome) in six standard head positions are preferred. Standard views in rhinoplasty photography include full frontal, right and left lateral, right and left oblique,

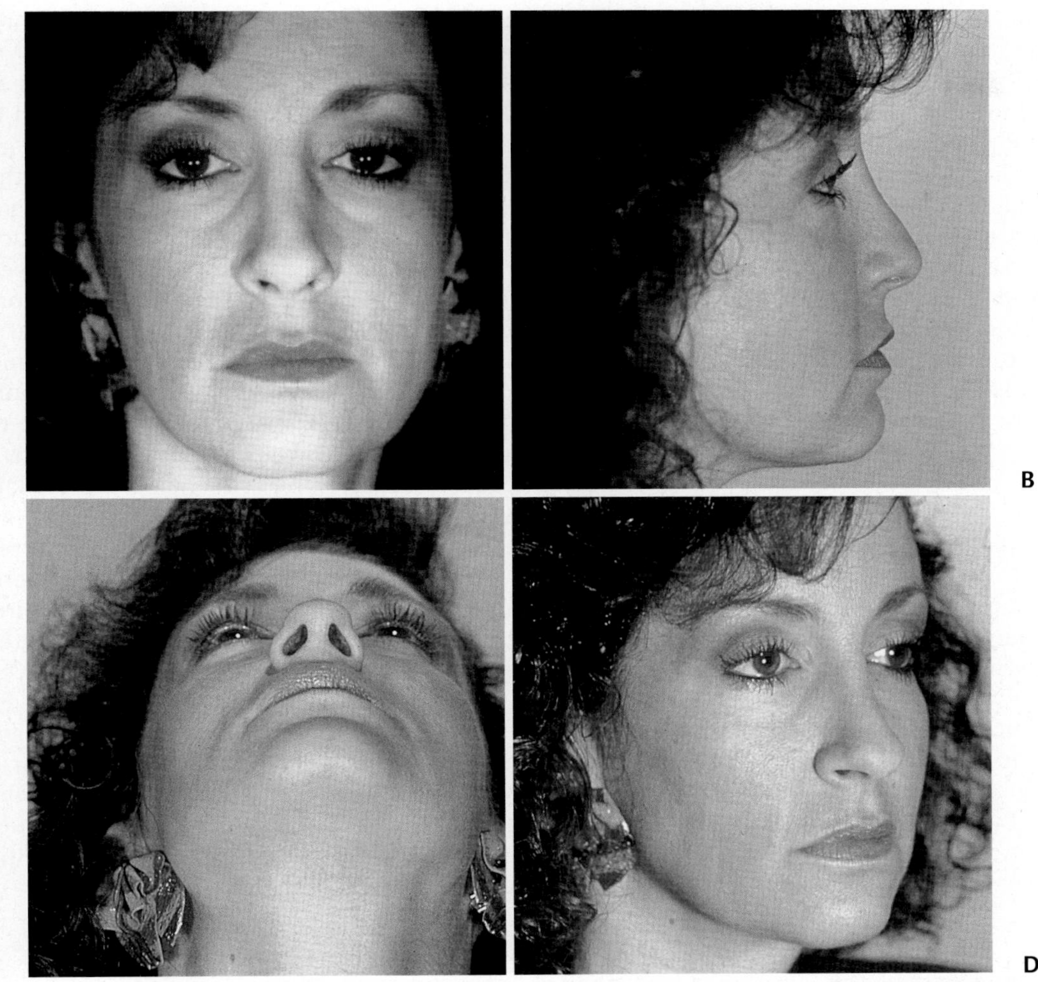

Fig. 40.10 (**A–D**) Typical preoperative photographic views obtained for rhinoplasty planning and documentation. Additional close-up views are recorded when required.

and basal views (**Fig. 40.10**). Use of a standard 105-mm portrait lens with dual-flash strobe units and an overhead slave key flash provides high-quality shadow-free representations of the nose and surrounding facial features.[13] A light blue background works well because this color complements skin tones. The photographic technique used should remain constant from sitting to sitting to produce standardized and uniform photographic records.

Computer imaging can be useful in facilitating communication between the surgeon and the patient.[14] Oftentimes, patients have difficulty describing the nasal deformities of concern and expressing the changes they desire. This also provides an opportunity for the surgeon to demonstrate to a patient what changes are realistic and surgically attainable. The nasal profile view lends itself well to computer imaging manipulation because the flesh-colored nasal contour is contrasted sharply against a selected colored background. Furthermore, profile changes can be made in the chin region to demonstrate to the patient the importance of balance between nasal and chin projection. The frontal view is more difficult to manipulate on the computer than the profile view because the nose is contrasted against the flesh-colored background of the face. However, by shifting shadows on frontal view it is possible to effect changes in nasal appearance. Finally, it must be emphasized to the patient that the images produced by the computer serve as a guideline of the proposed changes and hold no guarantee of the final results.

Anesthesia

Rhinoplasty can be performed under general anesthesia or local anesthesia with intravenous sedation.[15] No matter what mode is used, the key to anesthesia is comfort, safety, and good communication between the surgeon and the anesthesia provider. The patient must be made as comfortable as possible without compromising oxygenation. Proper use of the local anesthetic agents (1% lidocaine with 1:100,000 epinephrine, freshly mixed) provides good anesthesia and limited bleeding. The surgeon must dissect within the correct tissue planes during the operation to prevent unnecessary bleeding, violation of muscle, or thinning of skin flaps. Dissection in proper nonvascular areolar tissue planes prevents bleeding, decreases postoperative edema, and reduces scar tissue formation.

Choice of injection site depends on the particular approach to the nose that is used. The smallest amount of local anesthesia possible should be used to prevent distortion of tissues.

Principles in Shaping the Nasal Tip

Shaping of the nasal tip is the most exacting aspect of nasal plastic surgery. The surgeon must modify the lower lateral cartilages with a symmetric surgical technique, factoring in the dynamics of healing. Furthermore, no single surgical technique can be used on all noses because of the endless anatomical tip variations encountered. The surgeon must devise a surgical plan based on factors such as skin thickness, strength and shape of the alar cartilages, domal angle anatomy, dorsal contour, length and width of the nose, tip–lip angulation, requirements for tip projection and rotation, and, most importantly, patient expectations.

A fundamental principle of tip surgery is that normal or ideal anatomical features of the tip should be preserved and abnormal features analyzed, exposed and modified. Experienced nasal surgeons realize that radical excision of alar cartilages and other tip support mechanisms frequently leads to loss of tip support, buckling, and an unnatural appearance. What may appear satisfactory immediately after surgery may heal poorly because of overaggressive tissue excision. The goal of rhinoplasty is to achieve a more favorable appearance without compromising nasal support. The philosophy of a graduated, systematic anatomical approach to tip surgery is highly useful to achieve consistent long-term natural results.[13] Conservative reduction of the cephalic margin of the lateral crus, preserving at least 5 to 7 mm of complete strip of residual alar cartilage, is preferred. As the severity of the tip deformity becomes more profound, more aggressive techniques may be required (**Fig. 40.11**). These procedures may involve interruption of the lateral crural strip, resection of excess cartilage, followed by suture reconstitution of the divided edges. In cases where these more aggressive maneuvers are needed to produce a change, it is prudent to resect less cartilage and reconstitute all flail segments to control healing and use sutured-in-place columellar struts and sutured-in-place tip grafts to provide the desired shape.[16]

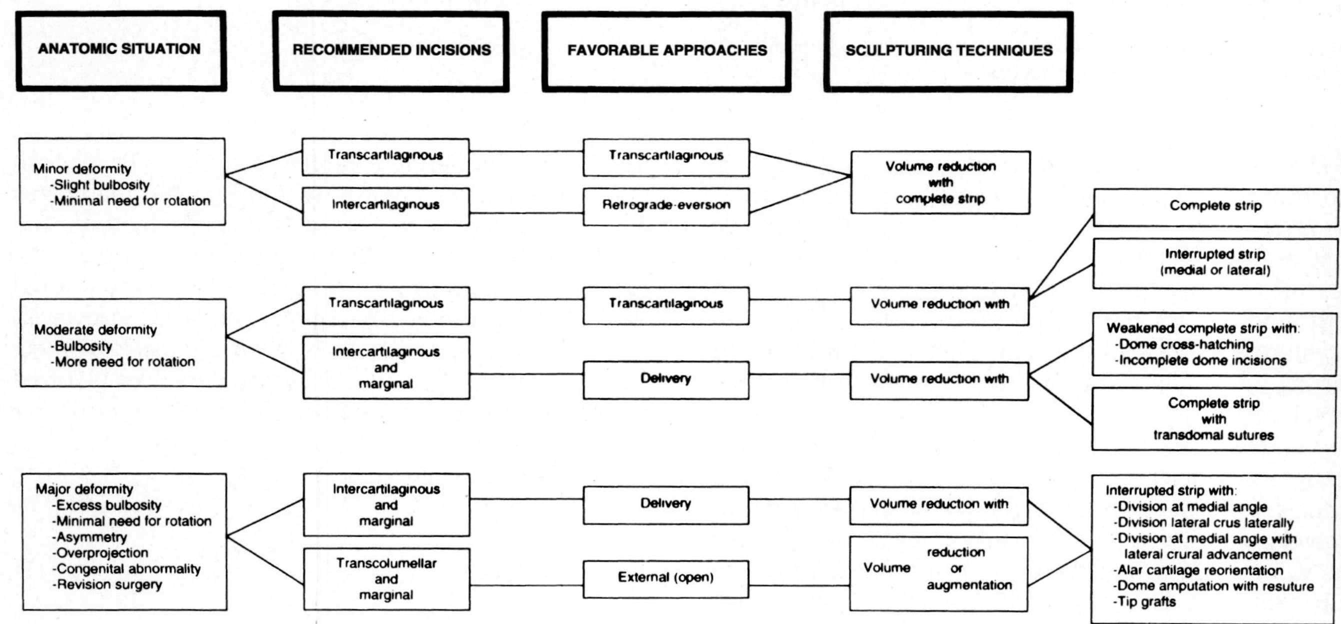

Fig. 40.11 An operative algorithm is useful in selecting the incisions, approaches, and techniques used in nasal tip surgery. In every case, the patient's anatomy dictates the selection.

Tip reshaping techniques cannot be performed with success until the major and minor tip support mechanisms are recognized, respected, and preserved or at least reconstructed.[17] Postoperative loss of tip support and projection is one of the most common iatrogenic consequences of rhinoplasty surgery. This loss of support is usually secondary to the sacrifice of one or more tip support mechanisms.

In most patients the major tip support mechanisms include (1) the size, shape, and resilience of the medial and lateral crura; (2) the wrap-around attachment of the medial crural footplates to the caudal margin of the quadrangular cartilage; and (3) the connective tissue attachment of the cephalic margin of the alar cartilage to the caudal margin of the upper lateral cartilage (scroll or recurvature). Whenever possible, an attempt should be made to reconstruct these major support mechanisms when they are divided.

The minor tip support mechanisms, which in certain anatomical configurations may assume major importance as a support mechanism, include (1) the interdomal ligament; (2) the dorsal cartilaginous septum; (3) the membranous septum; (4) the sesamoid complex; (5) the skin and subcutaneous fibrofatty tissues; and (6) the nasal spine. On occasion, because of extreme anatomical variability, a minor tip support may assume the importance of one of the more major supports. In light of the importance of these support mechanisms, tip incisions, approaches, and techniques should be planned to preserve as many tip supports as possible.

In Caucasian patients, nasal tip projection is usually adequate, and attempts should be made to preserve that degree of tip projection. Unfortunately, many of the maneuvers used to correct profound tip anomalies actually weaken tip support and result in a postoperative loss in tip projection. Thus columellar struts and tip grafts are recommended in selected patients to reestablish the preoperative level of tip projection.

The correct use of terminology is critical in communicating technical aspects of rhinoplasty procedures. The frequently misused terms *incision, approach,* and *technique* must be differentiated. An incision is a cut or the act of cutting to gain access to the underlying skeletal structures (in this case, bone and cartilage) of the nose. An approach is the specific anatomical dissection that provides surgical exposure of the skeletal structures, in this case consisting of procedures to deliver the tip cartilages or to avoid complete delivery, by operating on the alar cartilages without removing them from their anatomic beds. A technique is the specific method of procedure and the details of the surgical operation (i.e., excision, reorientation, or reconstruction of the alar cartilages to produce a predicted change in the projection, size, shape, and definition of the nasal tip).

Before making any changes in the tip, the surgeon must determine if the tip requires (1) a change in projection; (2) a reduction in the volume of the alar cartilages; (3) cephalic rotation with an increase in the columellar inclination; or (4) a change in the shape or orientation of the alar cartilages. In patients requiring *limited* refinement of the nasal tip, conservative reduction in the volume of the cephalic margin of the lateral crus can be executed, preserving the majority of the lateral crus and maintaining a complete (uninterrupted) strip of alar cartilage. When properly used, this technique provides the subtle tip refinement and minimal rotation while conferring little risk of postoperative deformity secondary to loss of tip support.

As the nasal tip deformity increases in size and complexity, more aggressive techniques must be considered. The philosophy of the graduated, incremental anatomical approach to the nasal tip is useful. This approach implies that no routine tip procedure is used; instead, the appropriate incisions, approaches, and tip sculpturing techniques are selected based entirely on the analysis of the varying anatomy encountered.

Surgical Approaches to the Tip

Nondelivery Approaches

In many patients the surgeon may encounter favorable nasal tip anatomy, composed of minimal tip bulbosity, medium skin thickness, and tip–cartilage symmetry. In such individuals, conservative tip refinement can be performed using nondelivery approaches. Less dissection and tissue manipulation is required, thereby reducing the possibilities of surgical error, tip support loss, asymmetries, and unfavorable healing. Properly executed, nondelivery approaches permit the surgeon to control healing to a greater extent than more radical approaches (delivery) and techniques (dome division).

The transcartilaginous approach (**Fig. 40.12**) is the preferred nondelivery approach because of its simplicity;

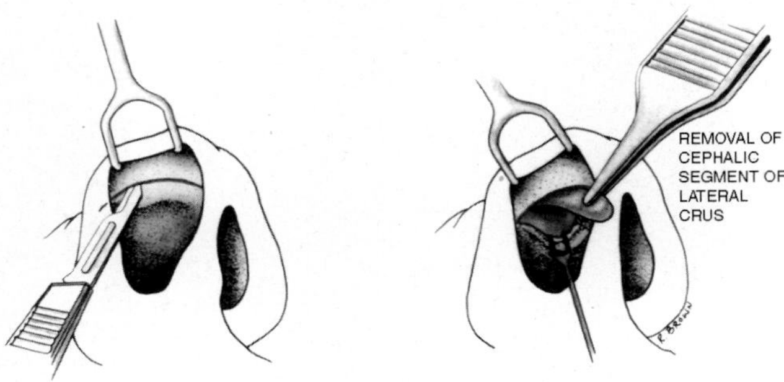

Fig. 40.12 Nondelivery approach to the nasal tip cartilages via the cartilage splitting (transcartilaginous) approach.

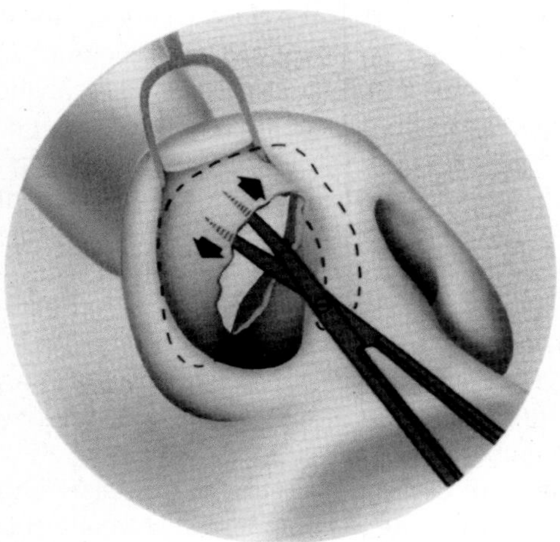

Fig. 40.13 Alternative nondelivery approach to the nasal tip cartilages via a retrograde approach.

similar tip modifications can be accomplished through the retrograde approach (**Fig. 40.13**). These approaches are most effective in patients with limited nasal tip bulbosity that only requires modest volume reduction of the cephalic margin of the alar cartilages. Such noses have a favorable triangularity of the tip, manifested as an equilateral triangle on the basal view (**Fig. 40.14**). In the case of widely arched, bifid, or bulbous lower lateral cartilages, the domal region requires aggressive alterations that cannot be accomplished through a nondelivery approach.

Delivery Approaches

In the case of more severe tip deformities requiring alteration of alar cartilage shape or orientation, the alar cartilages may be effectively delivered through intercartilaginous

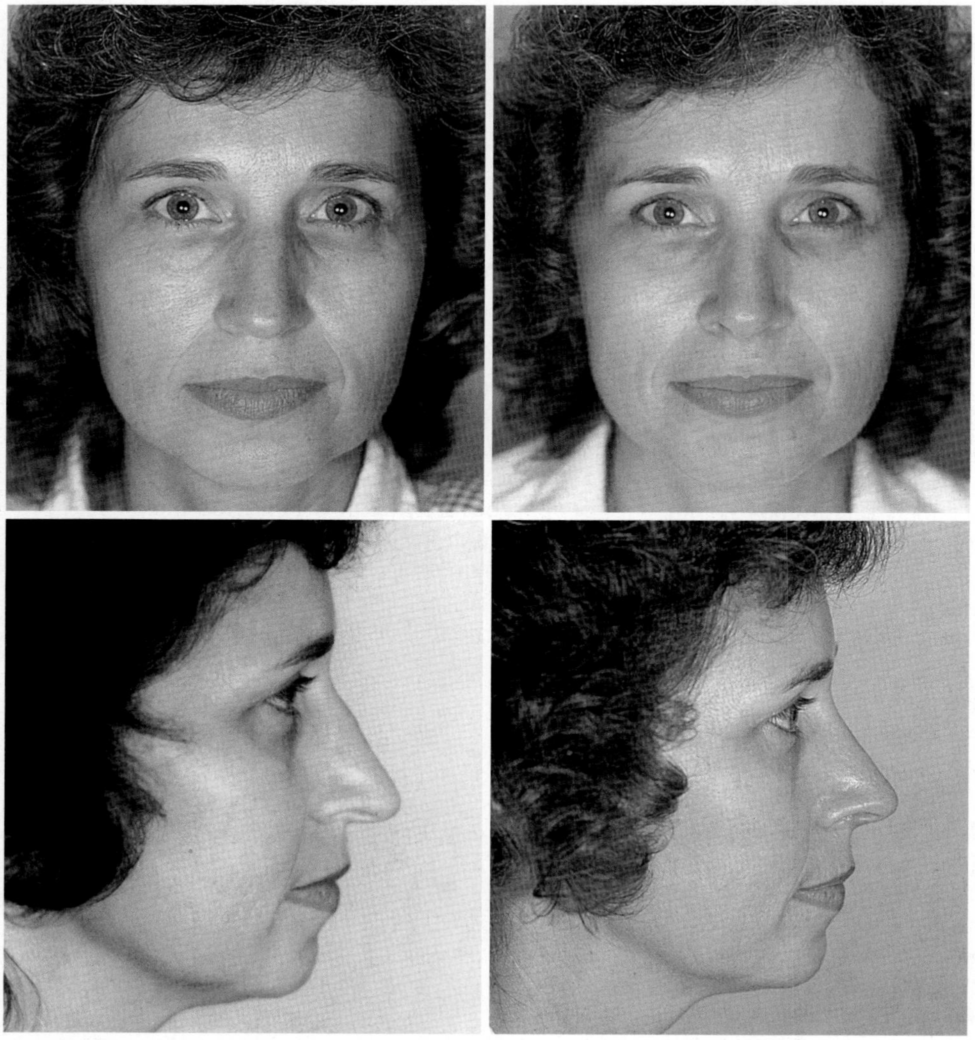

A B C D

Fig. 40.14 Two-year follow-up of patient operated utilizing a nondelivery cartilage splitting approach to the nose. Preoperative (column 1) and postoperative (column 2) condition.

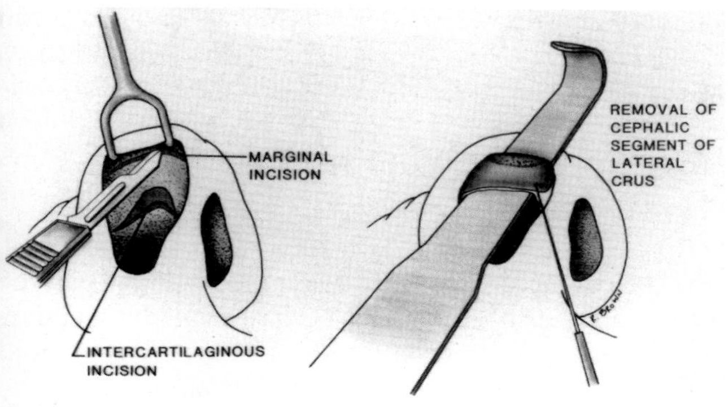

Fig. 40.15 Delivery of the nasal tip cartilages via intercartilaginous incisions combined with marginal incisions, utilized to deliver the cartilages as chondrocutaneous flap for evaluation and tip refinement surgery.

and marginal incisions as chondrocutaneous flaps (**Fig. 40.15**). The basal view can provide important information in the determination of triangularity of the nasal tip. If the alar cartilages are widely arched and bulbous with flared nostrils, tip triangularity is unsatisfactory and a delivery approach may be necessary to correct these deformities. A highly useful and effective technique involves transcartilaginous suture narrowing of broad, widely arched domes through the delivery approach (**Fig. 40.16**).[18] For more radical tip narrowing and cephalic rotation, interrupted-strip techniques can be performed, almost always by reconstituting the strip with fine sutures. The surgical exposure provided by the delivery approach is superior to that of nondelivery approaches but involves more disturbance of normal tissues. The open (external) approach provides maximal exposure.

External Rhinoplasty Approach

The open or external rhinoplasty approach requires bilateral marginal incisions connected by a transcolumellar incision at the level of the midcolumella (**Fig. 40.17**). The visualization provided by the open approach is unparalleled, affording the surgeon diagnostic and technical capabilities unavailable through traditional endonasal approaches (**Fig. 40.18**). This approach appears aggressive; however, the means of exposing the nasal skeleton does not in itself divide any major support mechanisms. The transcolumellar scar is of negligible importance if it is closed using proper techniques of skin eversion and early suture removal.[19] Disadvantages of the open approach include an enlarged region of dissection with possible scar formation, prolonged nasal tip edema, and increased operating time. None of these disadvantages can be considered major problems for experienced surgeons; however, the diagnostic and technical virtues must be weighed with the potential disadvantages. Indications for the open approach include a nasal tip that is asymmetrical, markedly bulbous, severely overprojected or underprojected, or anatomically complex (revision or cleft noses, infantile nostrils).[19,20] Relative indications include a nose with thick skin, poor tip support, or large perforations. One of the most valuable uses of the open approach is for teaching purposes. When subtle and conservative tip surgery is indicated

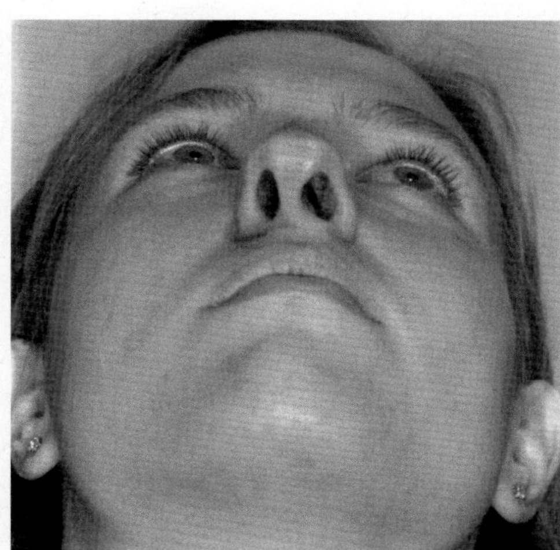

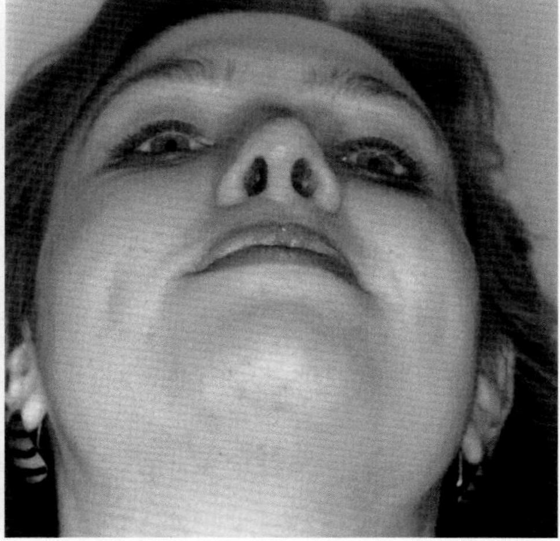

Fig. 40.16 Nine-year follow-up of patient with bifid, trapezoidal, twisted, and overprojected tip, approached through a delivery procedure. (**A**) Preoperative view. (**B**) Volume reduction and transdomal suture refinement of the nasal tip resulted in an improved triangular configuration to the nasal tip. Bilateral alar reduction procedures were necessary to improve the flaring of the alae secondary to retropositioning of the overprojected tip.

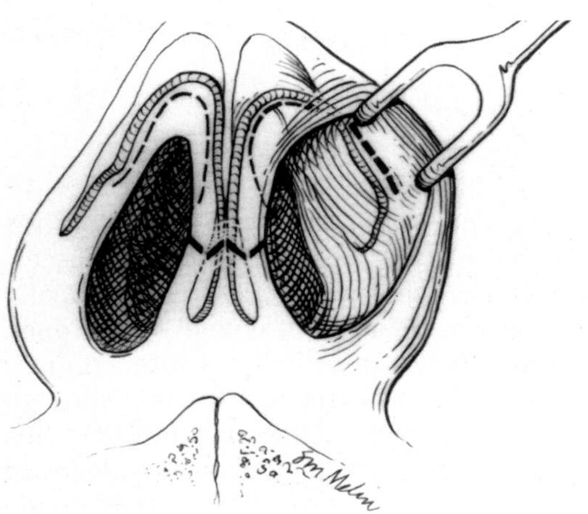

Fig. 40.17 Open rhinoplasty approach to the nasal tip cartilages.

by the patient's nasal contour, the open approach is unnecessary.

With the increased popularity of the open approach, techniques stressing a structurally sound nasal structure have been reemphasized. Open structure techniques may incorporate a sutured-in-place columellar strut, dome-binding sutures, and sutured-in-place tip graft. These basic maneuvers are more readily performed via the open approach to allow precise placement of struts and grafts, although in expert hands the closed approach can be preferable. The key to this technique is the precise control of tip shape, projection, and rotation, while preserving support and structure for long-term stability and control of healing.

Alar Cartilage–Shaping Techniques

The choice of technique used to alter the shape and position of the alar cartilages should be based on the anatomy encountered, the patient's wishes, and the predicted result defined by the dynamics of long-term healing.

Management of the alar cartilages can be divided essentially into four major categories. Although technical variations, such as the actual amount of cartilage to be resected, can vary, the four major categories are (1) volume reduction with residual complete strip; (2) volume reduction with transdomal suturing; (3) volume reduction with interrupted and resutured strip; and (4) tip refinement without volume reduction.

Whenever the presenting anatomy permits, preservation of the complete strip is preferred to prevent loss of support and projection. When the domes are divided, resuturing of the cut ends of the alar cartilage preserves structure and support.

In some cases, the complete residual strip is altered with a dome-binding suture to effect reorientation of the domes, narrowing, or changes in projection. In rare cases, stiff cartilages may need to be weakened by gentle crosshatching.

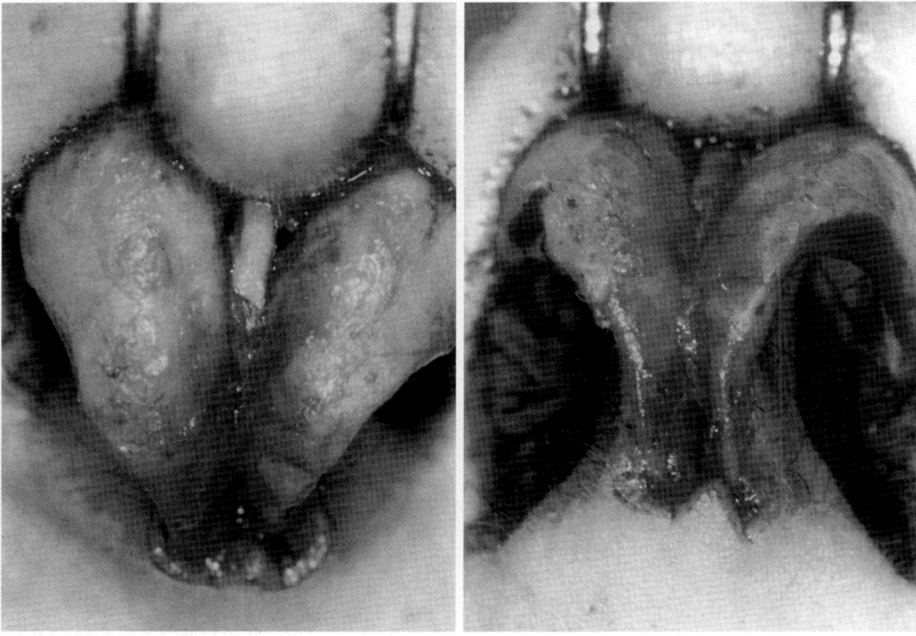

Fig. 40.18 Substantial exposure and visualization of the precise anatomy of the nasal tip cartilages is afforded through the open approach. (A) Frontal view. (B) Basal view.

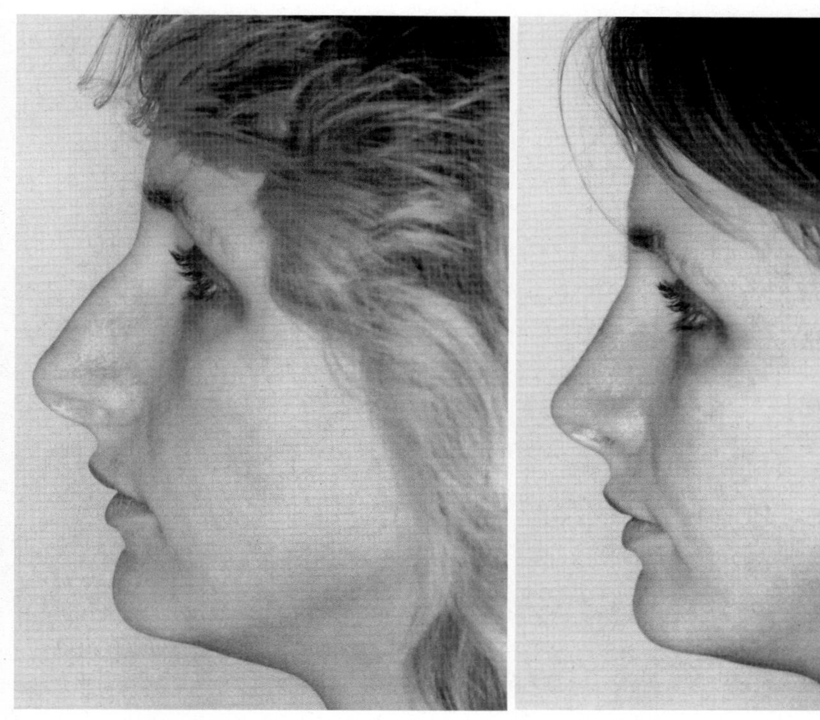

ig. 40.19 Patient (A) before and (B) after rhinoplasty in which a strong, high dorsum was maintained.

In more severe deformities, the alar cartilages may equire division to correct asymmetries or change proection. These maneuvers tend to produce healing in a ess controlled fashion, with a greater tendency to asymetry and deformity. In some cases, domal suturing is ombined with dome division in an effort to stabilize the ail segments. Despite such suturing, the risk of asymetric healing and loss of support is higher when the omes are divided and not reconstituted in a precise anner.

ip Projection

Modification of the alar cartilages may require division f one or more of the major support mechanisms of he nose, resulting in a potential loss of tip projection. ne of the keys to successful rhinoplasty is preservaion of existent nasal tip projection by preservation of s many support mechanisms of the nose as possible.[21] Many of the maneuvers performed to carry out other esthetic changes result in loss of tip projection. In he case of the overprojected nose, these changes are alculated and desirable. In other cases, nasal projecion is appropriate or deficient, requiring special surical techniques to increase tip projection. All involve eorientation of the alar cartilages or addition of carilaginous struts or tip grafts to support or increase the projection of the nasal tip and infratip lobule. The surgeon should avoid decreasing dorsal height to compensate for an inadequately projected nasal tip. Examples of techniques used to enhance tip projection include transdomal suturing, lateral crural steal, tip grafting, and the use of a columellar strut. Most of these techniques are covered in detail elsewhere in this book.

Tip Rotation

Some patients have a need for rotation of the nasal tip complex (alar cartilages, columella, and alar base), whereas in others rotation must be prevented. The dynamics of healing and scar contracture play a significant role in tip rotation. The upturned, short, overrotated nose of years past has fortunately given way to a more natural look, preserving a strong dorsum with sufficient length to impart character and suitable proportions to the rest of the face (**Fig. 40.19**). The degree of tip rotation depends on several factors, the most important being nasal length. To understand tip rotation, it must be distinguished from tip projection. Certain tip rotation techniques may result in increased tip projection because tip rotation and projection are complementary to each other and control of one variable is related to the other. The surgeon can imagine the alar cartilages acting as a tripod,

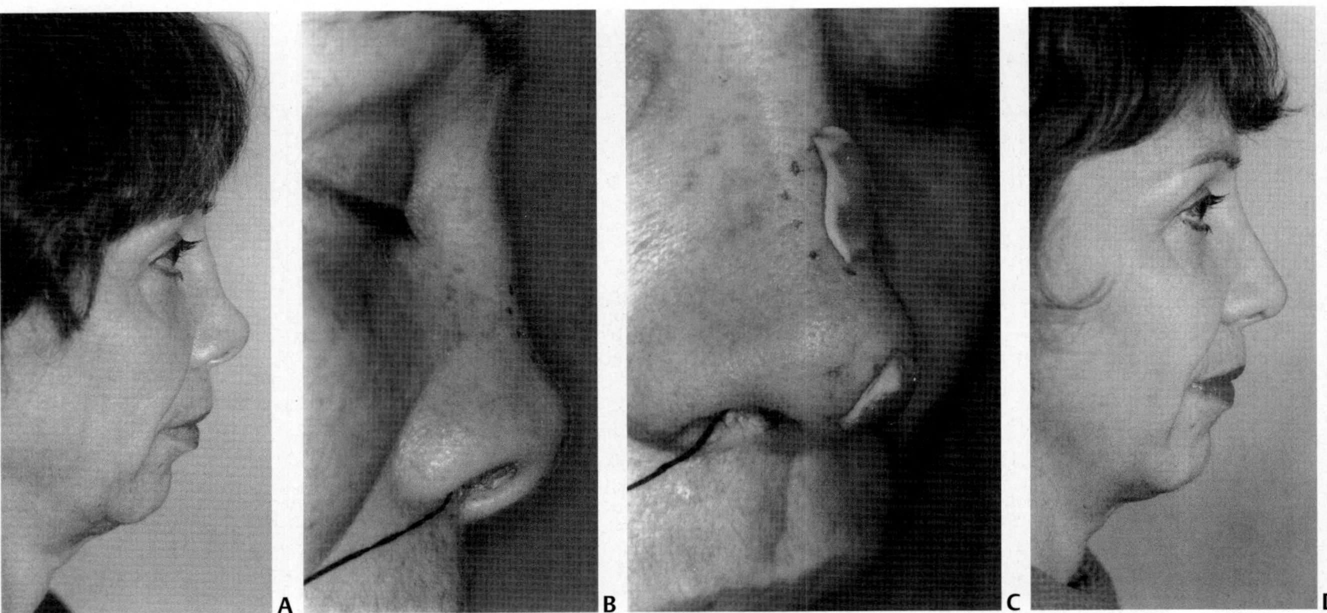

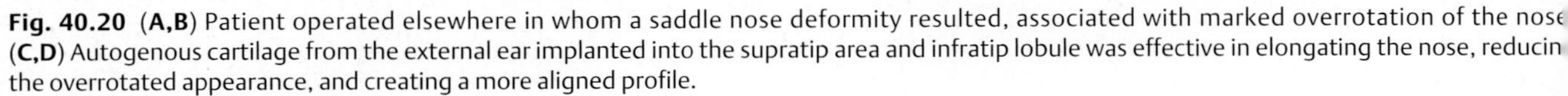
Fig. 40.20 (**A,B**) Patient operated elsewhere in whom a saddle nose deformity resulted, associated with marked overrotation of the nose (**C,D**) Autogenous cartilage from the external ear implanted into the supratip area and infratip lobule was effective in elongating the nose, reducin the overrotated appearance, and creating a more aligned profile.

with the conjoined medial crura making up one leg and the lateral crus making up the other two legs of the tripod. Using this simplified concept, the surgeon can conceptualize how tip rotation and projection are closely related.[13] The surgeon can produce the illusion of tip rotation by angulating the infratip lobule in a cephalic direction or by blunting the nasolabial angle. Placement of tip grafts along the caudal surface of the medial and intermediate crura can increase tip rotation. Use of double-layer tip grafts can give the illusion of increased nasal length by lengthening the dorsal line of the nose (**Fig. 40.20**). Modifications of the tip–lip complex profile with autogenous cartilage grafts can provide the illusion of tip rotation and preserve the length of the nose.

Fundamentally, nasal tip rotation results from planned surgical modification of the alar cartilages, such as conservative excision of the cephalic margin of the lateral crus. Tip rotation can also be obtained by shortening the caudal septum, shortening the septum with a high transfixion incision, setting back the medial crura on the caudal septum, and interrupting and overlapping the residual complete strip (**Figs. 40.21 and 40.22**).[22] Because tip rotation is only one of the objectives of rhinoplasty, the technique that is chosen must not interfere with the other aspects of the operation.

Volume reduction of the alar cartilage produces a tissue void along the cephalic margin of the lateral crus and results in limited tip rotation, with possible valve collapse and supraalar pinching in the long term. By interruptin the lower lateral cartilages at the domes, upward sca contracture will increase tip rotation, with possibl asymmetrical healing, loss of support, and overrotation. A reliable alternative involves resection of a segment of cartilage just lateral to the domes, followed b resuturing of the cut ends to reconstitute the intact stri (**Fig. 40.22B**). Lateral interruption of the lower lateral cartilages with a lateral crural overlay reconstitu tion technique also produces tip rotation, with less of chance of deformity in the domal region; however, th possibility of asymmetry and overrotation still exist if surgery is inexact. A columellar strut can be suture between the medial crura to stabilize and support. Alternatively, the medial crura can be stabilized by a “set-back fixation to the caudal septum. If necessary, a shield shaped tip graft can be sutured to the caudal margin c the medial crura at a designated angulation to provid precisely the tip projection and rotation that are desire (**Fig. 40.23**).

Profile Alignment

The structures responsible for the nasal profile are th nasal bones, the cartilaginous septum, and the alar cartilages. All three structures must be carefully realigned t create a well-balanced, natural profile. The nasal dorsur

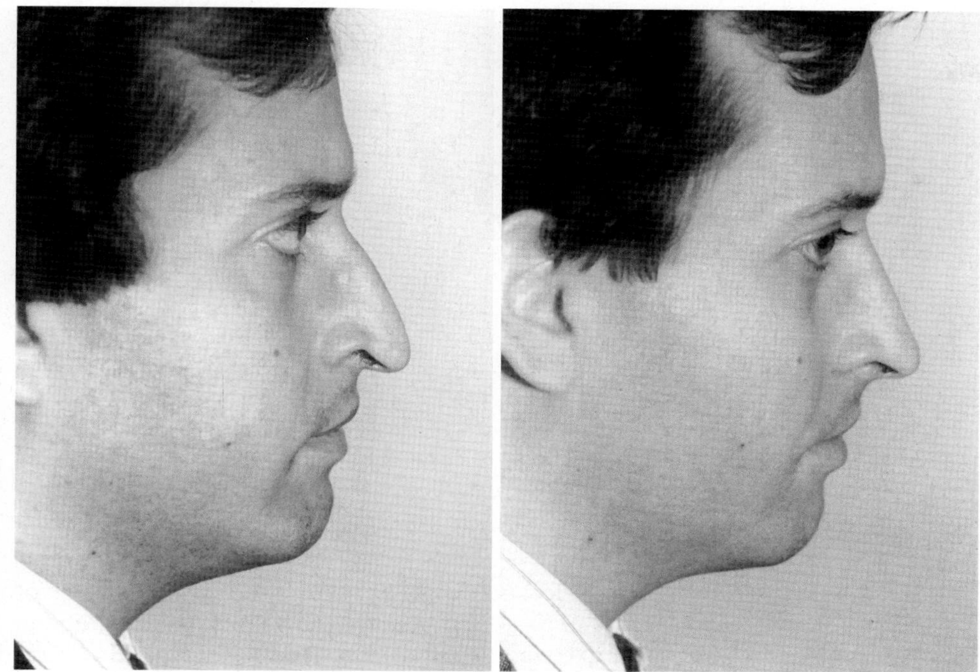

ig. 40.21 (**A**) Patient with elongated, dependent nose in need of a profile alignment and cephalic rotation of the asal tip. (**B**) Tip rotation was accomplished by shortening of the caudal septum, excision of redundant vestibular kin, and lateral interruption of the residual complete strip with suture reconstitution as shown in Fig. 40.22.

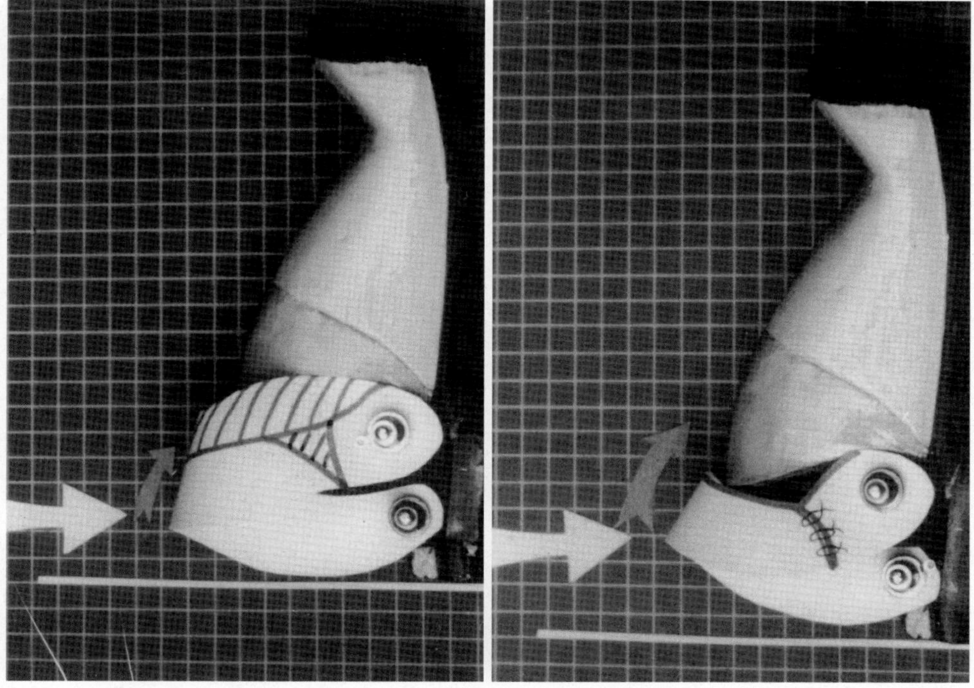

ig. 40.22 (**A**) Representation on teaching model of the extent of cephalic excision of lateral crus performed ith a representation of the interruption of the residual complete strip, demonstrating the triangular wedge xcision preparatory to cephalic rotation. (**B**) Cephalic rotation of alar cartilage (and therefore nasal tip) subsequent to suture reconstitution of the interrupted strip to yield a reconstituted complete strip.

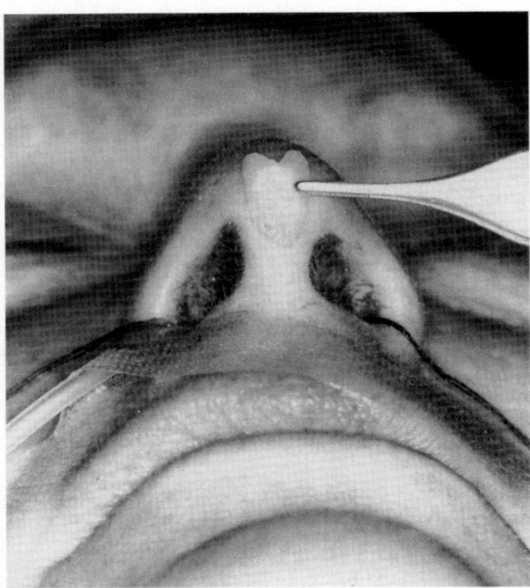

Fig. 40.23 Nasal tip grafts, either sutured in place or positioned in precise pockets in the infratip lobule, are effective in providing contour and projection to the nasal tip.

remains strong, with a well-defined nasal starting point at or just below the level of the superior palpebral fold (slightly higher in a man is acceptable). The nasal starting point is defined by the deepest point of the nasofrontal angle or sellion. The dorsal line of the nose extends from the sellion to the tip-defining points. In women, this line should be straight or have a slight concavity. The dorsal line in men should be straight or have a slight convexity.

The extent of reduction or augmentation of the profile depends on the final position of the nasal tip; setting the projection of the tip at the beginning of the operative procedure is therefore recommended. Overreduction of the dorsum should be avoided because it produces a washed-out, infantile appearance on the frontal view, separating the eyes inadequately and reflecting desired light reflexes poorly. A strong dorsum provides good shadowing along the nasal walls, giving the appearance of dorsal height. A slight supratip depression should exist at the junction between the tip and dorsum. Preservation of a supratip depression depends on strong support of the lower third of the nose.

Surgical access to the dorsum is gained through a transcartilaginous or intercartilaginous incision or an open approach. The plane of dissection over the dorsum should be just intimate to the perichondrium of the cartilaginous vault and just beneath the periosteum of the bony vault. The dorsal hump can be removed en bloc or incrementally, depending on the surgeon's

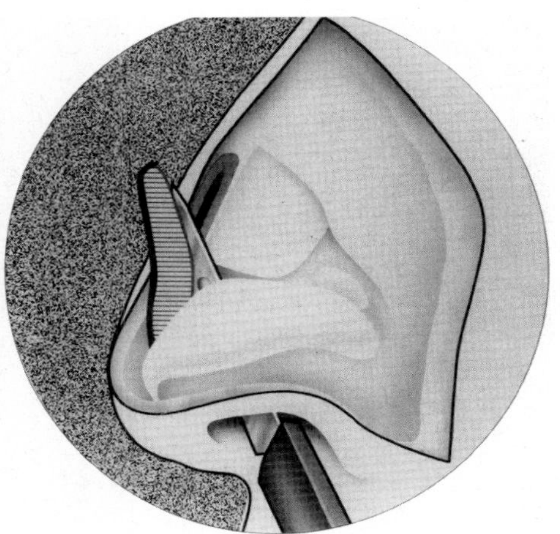

Fig. 40.24 Incremental sharp-knife reduction of the cartilaginous dorsum.

preference (**Fig. 40.24**).[12,23] A sharp Rubin osteotome can be used to remove the bony dorsum, extending the excision to the nasofrontal angle (**Fig. 40.25**). A common error is to overresect thinner nasal bone near the rhinion and underresect the thicker bone near the nasofrontal angle.

In patients with a poorly defined nasofrontal angle resulting from bony excess, special excision of the thick frontal bone may be necessary to deepen this angle. A 2-mm straight osteotome can be inserted transcutaneously to precisely define the upper margin of the resection (**Fig. 40.26**).[17] Then, a Rubin osteotome can be directed cephalically, completing hump removal at the point where the bone was scored with the 2-mm osteotome.

Any small irregularities can be corrected using traditional tungsten-carbide rasps or the newer powered

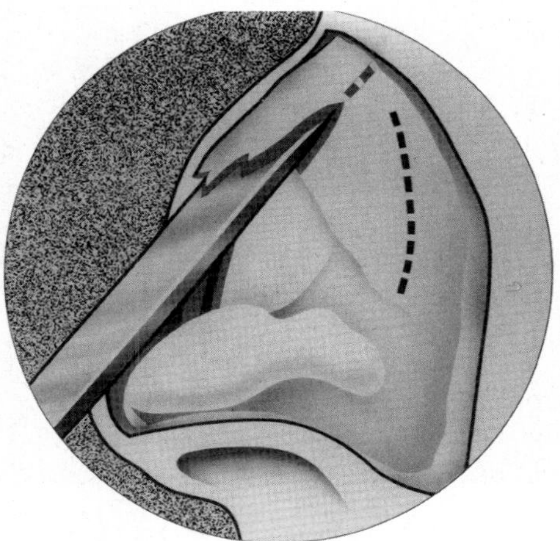

Fig. 40.25 Excision of the bony profile utilizing a thin, sharp, Rubin osteotome.

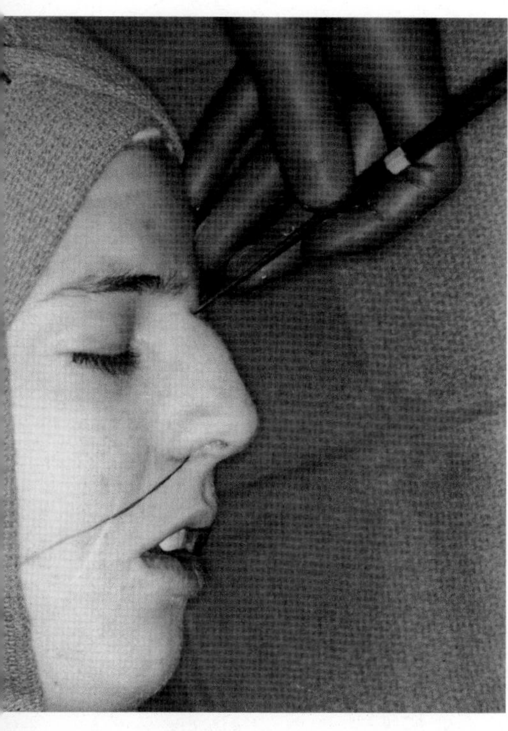

ig. 40.26 When deepening of the nasofrontal angle is indicated, the recise site of the angle break is created by driving a 2-mm osteotome ranscutaneously into the nasal bony root, scoring the bone with several erforations to ensure the exact site of its eventual cephalic removal.

nstrumentation (Rhinobur, Xomed, Jacksonville, FL).[24] The owered instrument consists of a bur partially encased y a sheath that provides protection and suction. This bur llows precise modification of limited areas of the nasal orsum while sparing unnecessary trauma to surrounding tissues. Fine-tuning of the profile can then be accomplished with small dorsal grafts, radix grafts, soft tissue esection in the supratip region, and plumping grafts or the nasolabial angle. A new method of camouflaging dorsal contour irregularities or raising dorsal nasal eight involves the use of a thin sheet of acellular dermal llograft, such as Allo-Derm (LifeCell Corp., The Woodlands, X). As healing occurs, this allograft is replaced by a layer of car tissue that maintains the desired contour alterations.

Narrowing the Bony Pyramid

After dorsal hump removal, the bony and cartilaginous yramids must be narrowed to restore the normal frontal ppearance to the operated nose. The bony lateral walls nust be completely mobilized and moved medially, avoiding greenstick fractures. To facilitate high-low-high lateral steotomies and control the exact site of fracture, medial blique osteotomies angled laterally at 15 to 20 degrees

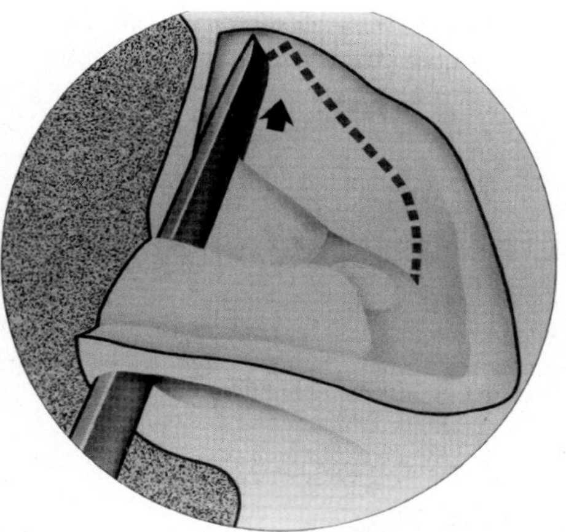

Fig. 40.27 In the majority of patients, medial oblique osteotomies, directed 15 to 20 degrees from midline, are useful in siting the exact position of the eventual back-fracture created by the low, curved, lateral osteotomy.

from the vertical midline are preferred (**Fig. 40.27**). This medial fracture provides control for the exact site of back-fracture in the lateral bony sidewall. A 2- to 3-mm sharp microosteotome is ideal for the medial oblique osteotomies.[17]

The low lateral curved osteotomy is started at the piriform aperture at or just above the inferior turbinate. A 2- to 3-mm microosteotome is recommended. The osteotome should be driven toward the base of the maxilla, curving up along the nasal maxillary junction to encounter the previously created small medial oblique osteotomy via a controlled back-fracture (**Fig. 40.28**). Immediate pressure is applied to prevent bleeding and ecchymosis.

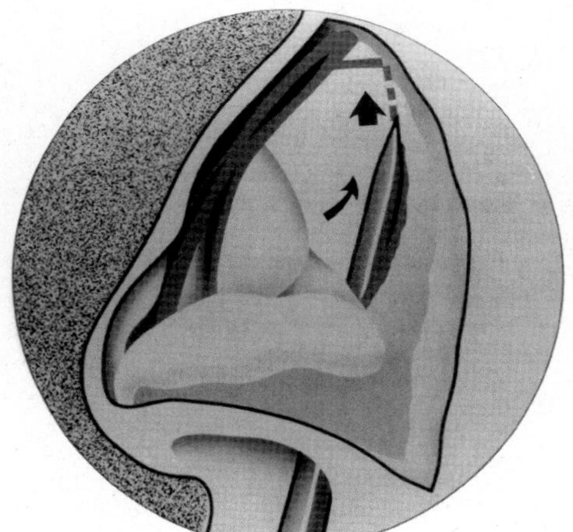

Fig. 40.28 The low, curved, lateral osteotomy is created with 2- or 3-mm microosteotomes. The osteotome is driven cephalically in a curvilinear direction to encounter the exact site of the back-fracture created when the lateral osteotomy meets the medial oblique osteotomy site.

If alar base reduction is indicated, the appropriate geometrical excision is performed as the final maneuver. All incisions are suture-repaired, the nose is taped and splinted, and the procedure is completed.

Postoperative Considerations

Patients should be given a postoperative instruction sheet, which guides their postoperative activities and care. Any nasal packing should be removed as soon as possible. If an open rhinoplasty approach was used, sutures from the columellar incision should be removed within 5 to 7 days. Care should be taken during cast removal at 5 to 7 days to present hematoma by avoiding elevating the skin off the underlying structures. Patients and their families must clearly understand that at least a year must pass before the near-final result of the surgery can be observed (**Fig. 40.29**). In many patients, changes will continue for a lifetime.

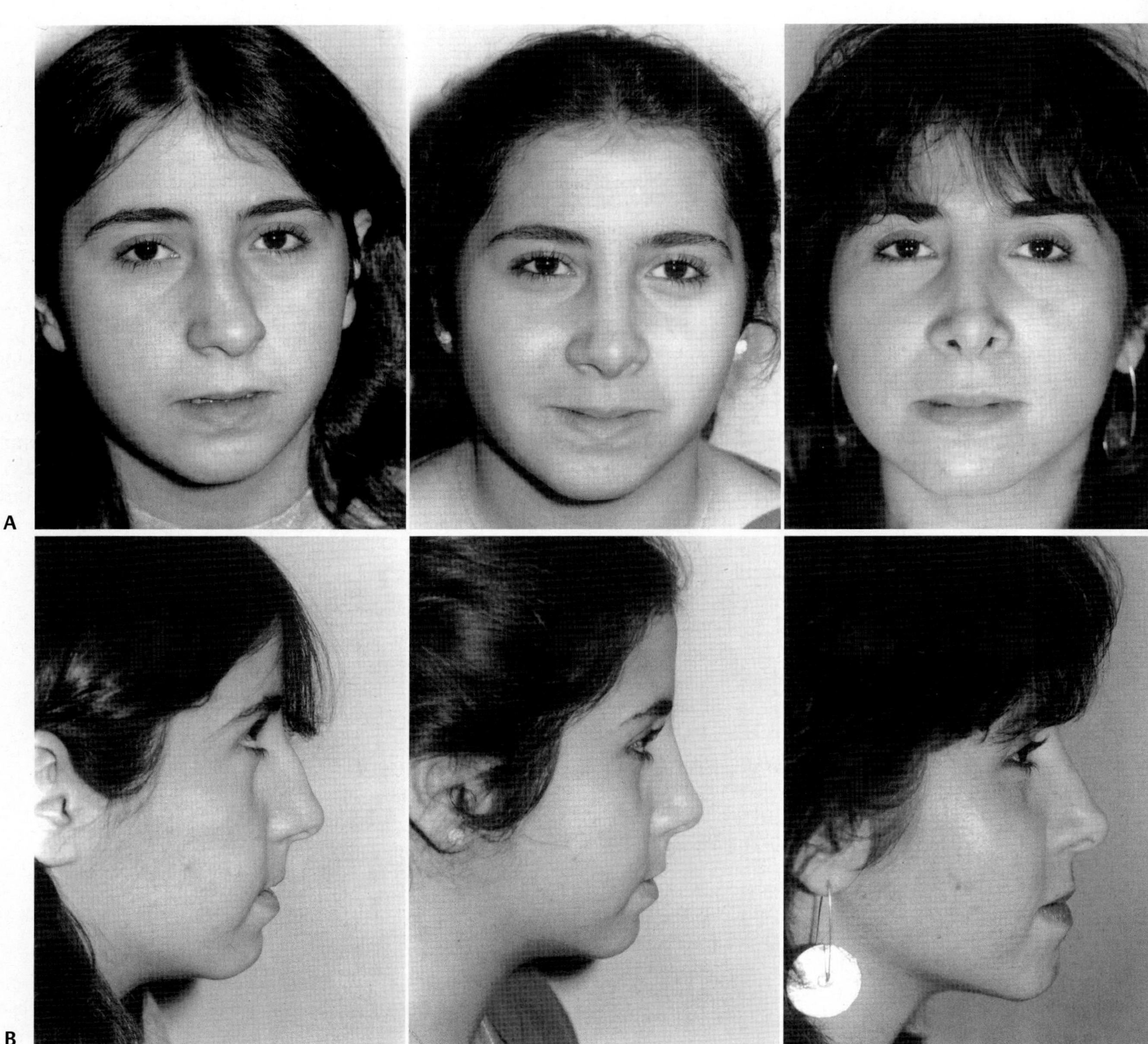

Fig. 40.29 Patient with severely twisted nose and nasal airway blockade. Postoperative result is shown 1 year and 7 years following surgery. Note the evolutionary healing changes that occur with the passage of time.

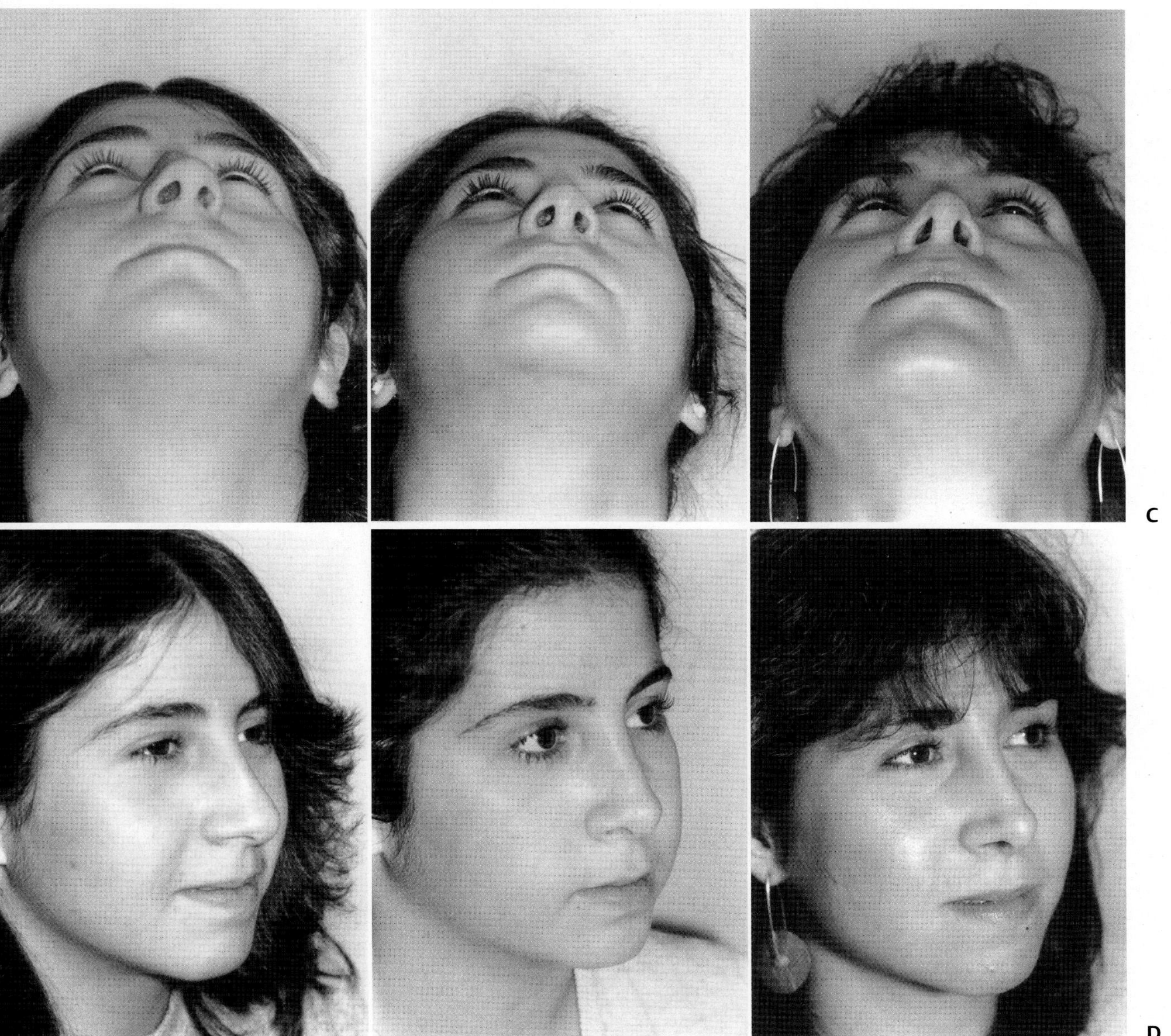

Fig. 40.29 *(Continued)*

References

1. Gunter JP. Anatomical observations of the lower lateral cartilages. Arch Otolaryngol 1969;89:61
2. Tardy ME, Broadway D. Graphic record-keeping in rhinoplasty: a valuable self-learning device. Facial Plast Surg 1989;6:2
3. Natvig P, Sether LA, Gingrass RP, Gardner WD. Anatomical details of the osseous-cartilaginous framework of the nose. Plast Reconstr Surg 1971;48:528
4. Toriumi DM, Meuller RA, Grosch T, et al. Vascular anatomy of the nose and the external rhinoplasty approach. Arch Otolaryngol Head Neck Surg 1996;122:24–34
5. Gilbert JG, Felt LJ. The nasal aponeurosis and its role in rhinoplasty. Arch Otolaryngol 1955;61:433
6. Wright MR, Wright WK. A psychological study of patients undergoing cosmetic surgery. Arch Otolaryngol 1975;101:145
7. Tardy ME, Kron TK, Younger R, et al. The cartilaginous pollybeak: etiology, prevention, and treatment. Facial Plast Surg 1989;6:2
8. Sheen JH. Secondary rhinoplasty. Plast Reconstr Surg 1975;56:137
9. Tardy ME. Rhinoplasty tip ptosis: etiology and prevention. Laryngoscope 1973;83:923
10. Toriumi DM, Josen J, Weinberger M, Tardy ME. Use of alar batten grafts for correction of nasal valve collapse. Arch Otolaryngol Head Neck Surg 1997;123:802–808
11. Toriumi DM. Management of the middle nasal vault in rhinoplasty. In: Operative Techniques in Plastic and Reconstructive Surgery. Vol 2. St. Louis: Mosby; 1995;16–30
12. Webster RC. Advances in surgery of the tip: intact rim cartilage techniques and the tip–columella–lip esthetic complex. Otolaryngol Clin North Am 1975;8:615
13. Tardy ME. Rhinoplasty: The Art and the Science. Philadelphia: WB Saunders; 1997
14. Schoenrock LD. Five-year facial plastic experience with computer imaging. Facial Plast Surg 1990;7:18–25
15. Tardy ME, Tom L. Anesthesia in rhinoplasty. Facial Plast Surg 1984;1(2):146

16. Ortiz-Monasterio F, Olmedo A, Oscoy LO. The use of cartilage grafts in primary aesthetic rhinoplasty. Plast Reconstr Surg 1981;67:597
17. Tardy ME, Denneny JC. Micro-osteotomies in rhinoplasty—a technical refinement. Facial Plast Surg 1984;1(2):137
18. Tardy ME. Transdomal suture refinement of the nasal tip. Facial Plast Surg 1987;4:4
19. Toriumi DM. External rhinoplasty approach. In: Bailey BJ,ed. Head and Neck Surgery—Otolaryngology. 2nd ed. Philadelphia: Lippincott-Raven Publishers; 1998:2599–2608
20. Patiovan IF. External approach in rhinoplasty. Surg ORL Lug 1966;3:354
21. Janeke JB, Wright WK. Studies on the support of the nasal tip. Arch Otolaryngol 1971;93:458
22. Parkes ML, Brennan HG. High septal transfixion to shorten the nose. Plast Reconstr Surg 1970;45:487
23. Webster RC, Smith RC. Rhinoplasty. In RM Goldwyn, ed. Long-term Results in Plastic and Reconstructive Surgery. Boston: Little, Brown and Company; 1980
24. Becker DG, Toriumi DM, Gross CW, Tardy ME. Powered instrumentation for dorsal reduction. Facial Plast Surg 1997;13:291-297

41 Open Rhinoplasty

Peter A. Adamson and Jason A. Litner

Open rhinoplasty is not a new operation. Around 600 BC, the Sushruta Ayurveda described external nasal surgery being performed in India.[1] Photos documenting Joseph's first published reduction rhinoplasty case are often shown in profile view. Sometimes overlooked, though, is the full-length nasal incision that was utilized for his approach.[1] In 1920, Gillies degloved the nasal tip using an "elephant trunk incision" placed in the inferior columella. The modern era of open rhinoplasty began in 1934 with Rethi's description of a high transcolumellar incision to expose the tip alone.[2] Sercer, in Zagreb, Yugoslavia, performed nasal decortication by extending the exposure to include the entire nasal pyramid in 1956.[3] Padovan, a student of Sercer, further utilized this external exposure to perform a septoplasty.[4] The era of open rhinoplasty in North America was ushered in by his presentation of this technique at the First International Symposium of the American Academy of Facial Plastic and Reconstructive Surgery in 1970. The technique has since stirred controversy, and until the last decade it was promoted mainly by a handful of advocates. Goodman, of Toronto,[5,6] is generally recognized as the first North American to embrace the technique, followed by Anderson,[7] Wright,[8] and others. Today, open rhinoplasty has achieved a respected position among rhinoplasty techniques and has become the one most commonly practiced by facial plastic surgeons.[9] Teaching of this technique in residency and postgraduate programs is ubiquitous. Now, almost 70 years since its modern day origins in Europe, renewed interest in the technique is being seen there as well.

Indications

It is recognized that each rhinoplasty surgeon has a varied surgical experience and therefore will have unique indications for the open technique. In years past, the approach was grudgingly supported for difficult or revision cases. However, indications have expanded commensurate with widespread increasing levels of comfort and familiarity with this technique. In our experience, open rhinoplasty is the technique of choice for all cases unless a comparable improvement for a definable deformity can be obtained with the closed approach. The open approach offers clear diagnostic and therapeutic advantages for many challenging functional and cosmetic nasal deformities, primarily resulting from the broad undistorted exposure it affords. This is especially true with respect to the premaxillary spine, caudal septum, dorsal and superior septum, lobule, and superior dorsum. An unparalleled diagnosis of the underlying anatomy resulting in the external deformity can be made via the open approach. Sutures can be placed, grafts exactly trimmed, and asymmetries corrected without distortion of surrounding tissues. Scar tissue and redundant subcutaneous tissue are more easily excised. The valve region can be well protected, and the absence of incisions in the intercartilaginous region diminishes subsequent obstructive phenomena by precluding scar formation and disruption of one of the tip support mechanisms. A majority of facial plastic surgeons in North America now relies on this technique to achieve consistently good and reproducible results for a wide variety of indications (**Figs. 41.1–41.6**).

Preoperative Evaluation

At the initial consultation, a complete history and examination is performed with specific emphasis placed on functional and aesthetic nasal diagnosis. The patient's wishes are determined and standard photos are reviewed to clarify the surgical goals. Patient education regarding realistic expectations and the possibility of minor postoperative asymmetries are underscored. Surgical protocols and risks are outlined. Referral for further investigations, including nasal airflow studies, imaging, and allergy testing, may be warranted, as mucosal disorders are optimally treated preoperatively. We routinely review details of the surgical plan with the patient at a second sitting along with any relevant test results. A rhinoplasty assessment sheet is completed, and a detailed written surgical plan is formulated for each patient.

Anesthesia

Most rhinoplasty patients are treated on an outpatient basis using general or neuroleptic anesthesia with an anesthesiologist in attendance. Clindamycin (300 mg) is given intravenously for bacterial prophylaxis. We do not routinely treat patients with postoperative antibiotics. Local infiltration anesthesia of the entire external and internal nose is performed with lidocaine 1% with 1:100,000 epinephrine, mixed in equal parts with bupivacaine (Marcaine) 0.5% with 1:200,000 epinephrine. This

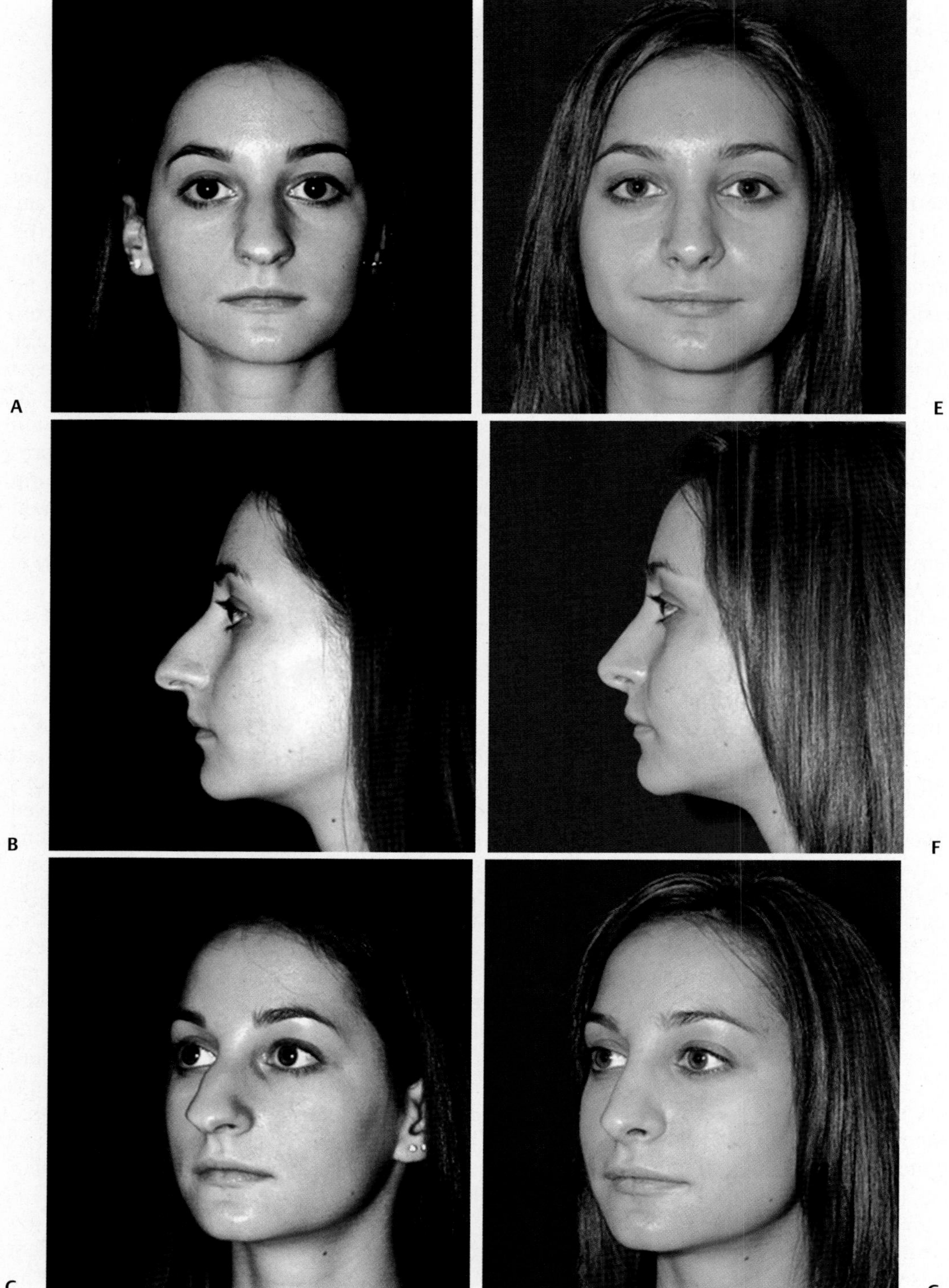

Fig. 41.1 (**A–D**) An 18-year-old female with large nose and dorsal hump. (**E–H**) Postoperative results showing M-Arch shortening with vertical lobule division, dorsal reduction, and osteotomies. (**I,J**) Dynamic diagrams.

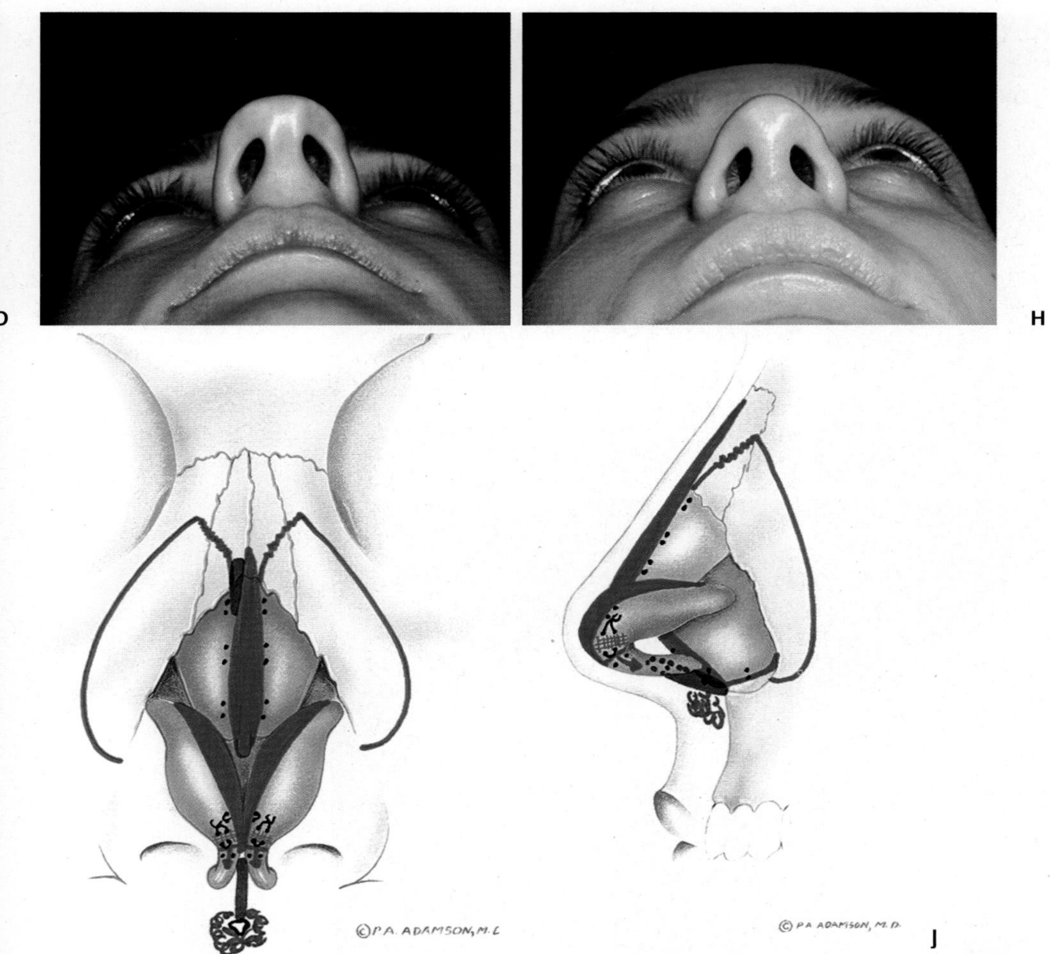

Fig. 41.1 (*Continued*)

provides long-acting anesthesia with a satisfactory vasoconstrictive effect. About 15 to 20 mL is required. We do not find added topical vasoconstriction to yield any additional benefit.

Surgical Technique

Incision Planning and Exposure

Some surgeons, primarily not in favor of the open technique, have cited the columellar scar as a major disadvantage of this procedure. However, if designed and closed judiciously, this is rarely, if ever, cause for revision. A retrospective study of patients who undewent cosmetic open rhinoplasty revealed a subjective dissatisfaction incidence of 1% and objective unsatisfactory scar incidence of 2%.[10] The first step in obtaining an ideal scar is incision planning. Our preferred open rhinoplasty incision involves a transverse midcolumellar inverted gull-wing approach (**Fig. 41.7**). The gull-wing incision heals better aesthetically than V-shaped, staircase, or straight transverse incisions. It should curve around the caudal margin of the medial crus to meet the marginal incision at right angles. The marginal incision is placed just behind the caudal margin of the medial crus as this allows for both a wider columellar flap and improved scar camouflage. Care is taken to place the incision above the feet of the medial crura, especially in blacks and Asians in whom these structures are often foreshortened, and who are at risk for postoperative columellar notching. The columellar flap should be handled delicately to avoid jeopardizing its vascularity. The junction of the transverse columellar and vertical marginal incisions is most at risk for an unfavorable scar as forces of contraction tend to cause a trapdoor effect in this location. This effect can be minimized through undermining of the inferior columellar skin prior to closure, and by placement of the angle suture

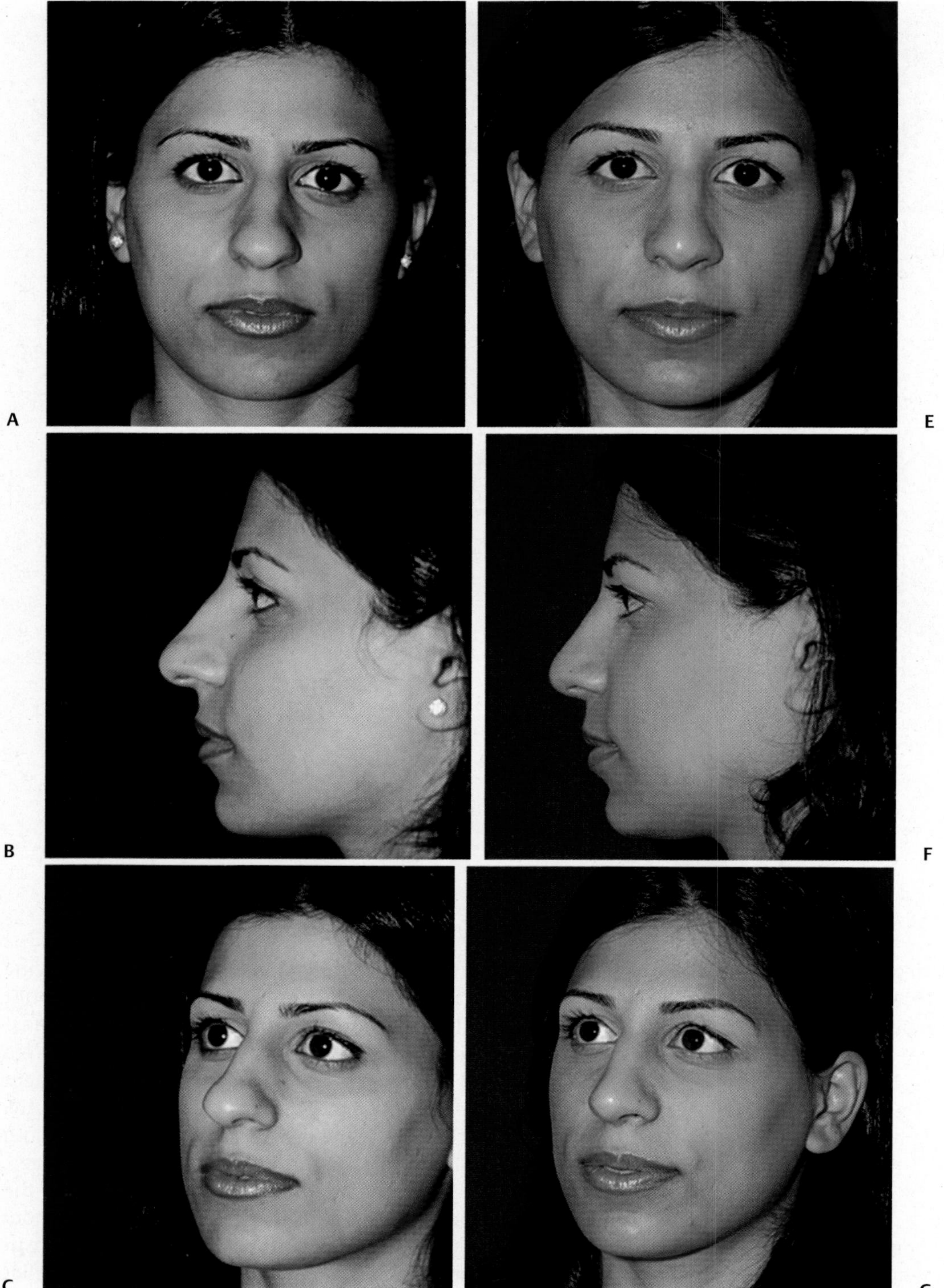

Fig. 41.2 (**A–D**) A 20-year-old female with large nose and bulbous tip. (**E–H**) Postoperative result following M-Arch shortening with vertical lobule division and lateral crural overlay. Also dorsal reduction, osteotomies, and alar base reduction. (**I,J**) Dynamic diagrams.

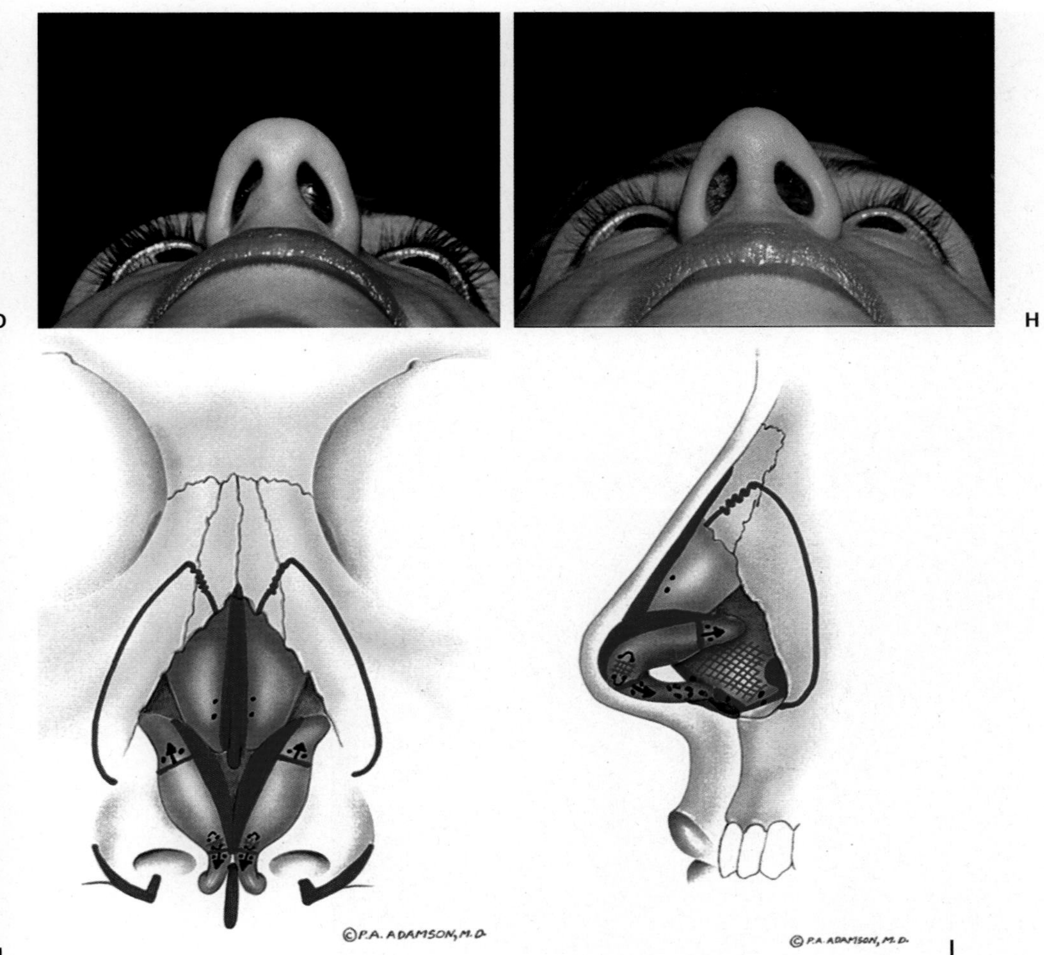

Fig. 41.2 (*Continued*)

full thickness inferiorly but only partial thickness superiorly, to "tuck in" the thicker superior flap edge. A single, simple inverted 6–0 polyglycolic acid suture may be placed intradermally in the central columella to decrease tension. We prefer simple 6–0 nylon everting skin sutures alone for columellar closure. In cases where significant deprojection of the tip has been performed, the columellar flap may be slightly long. Truncation of the flap by 1 or 2 mm will diminish the risk of a mild hanging columella effect in this instance. Conversely, when significant tip projection has been achieved, the columellar flap may appear relatively short on closure. Closing tension can be relieved by bilateral inferior extension of the vertical marginal incisions, allowing development of an inferior columellar advancement flap. If this potential problem is recognized preoperatively, a V-shaped columellar incision may be later closed in a V-to-Y fashion to achieve a similar columellar lengthening, although this tends to leave a slightly inferior scar.

The transverse columellar incision is made initially with a no. 11 blade. It is joined with a vertical marginal incision made superficially, so as not to incise the underlying crus, beginning at the soft tissue triangle. The columellar flap is freed up with scissors dissection up to the angle. We prefer to carry blunt and sharp scissors dissection superolaterally over the dome and along the lower lateral crus, allowing exposure of the tip cartilages under direct vision. However, it is occasionally necessary to first make the marginal incision with retrograde exposure in cases of severe scarring or unusual lobular configurations that render scissors dissection over the domes precarious. Elevation of dorsal skin may be performed blindly as in the closed technique. In cases of severe scarring, poorly defined deformities, or thin skin, exposure is performed under direct vision with scissors or knife dissection. Bleeding from the inferior columellar artery or from branches of the facial artery in the region of the pyriform aperture may be controlled with conservative bipolar cautery. The dorsal skin is elevated in a submucoperichondrial and submucoperiosteal plane to

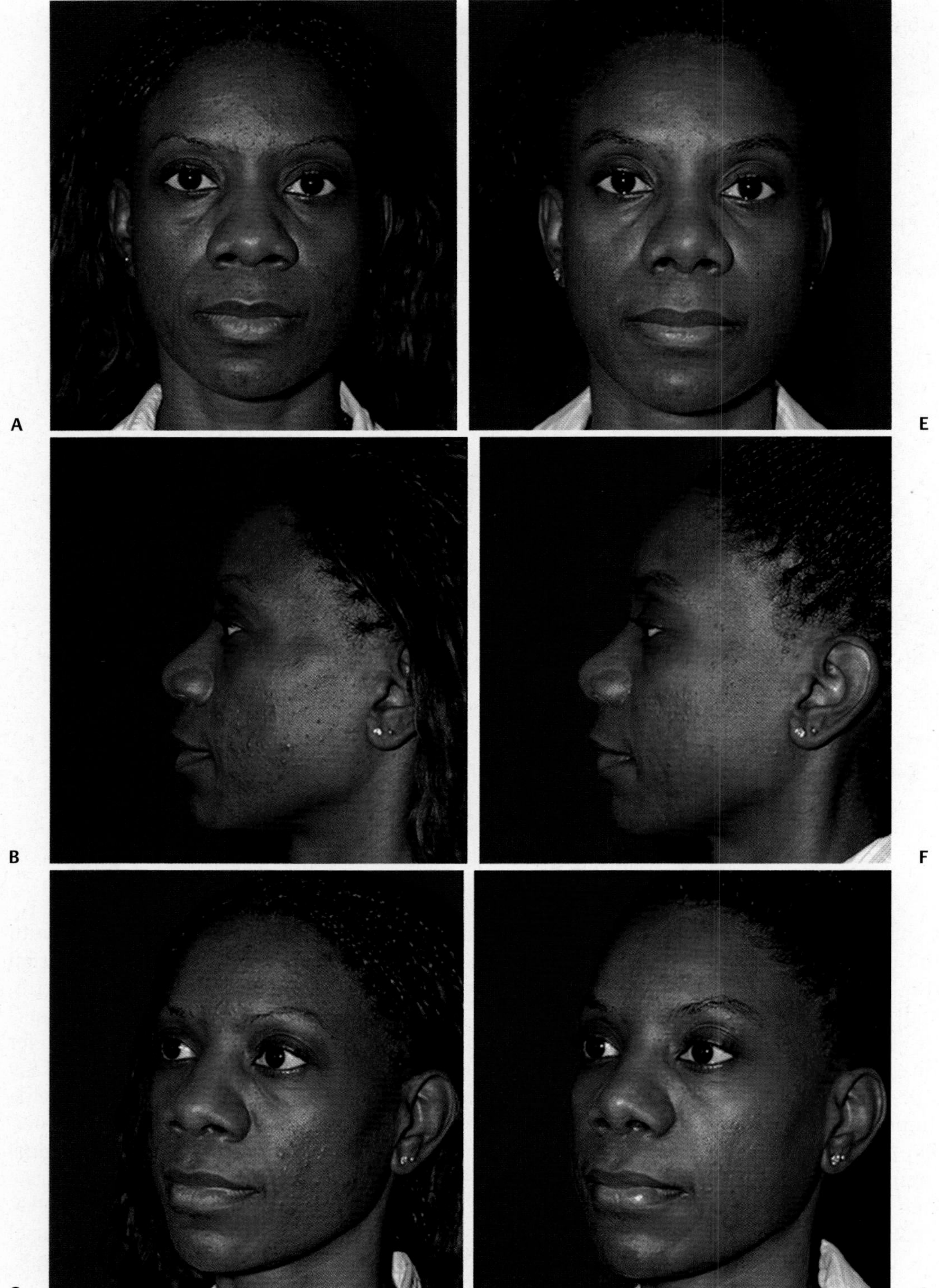

Fig. 41.3 (**A–D**) A 42-year-old female with bulbous tip, wide alar base, and thick skin. (**E–H**) Postoperative results showing lateral crural steal, columellar strut and batten, and two-layered infratip lobule graft. Also osteotomies and alar base reduction. (**I,J**) Dynamic diagrams.

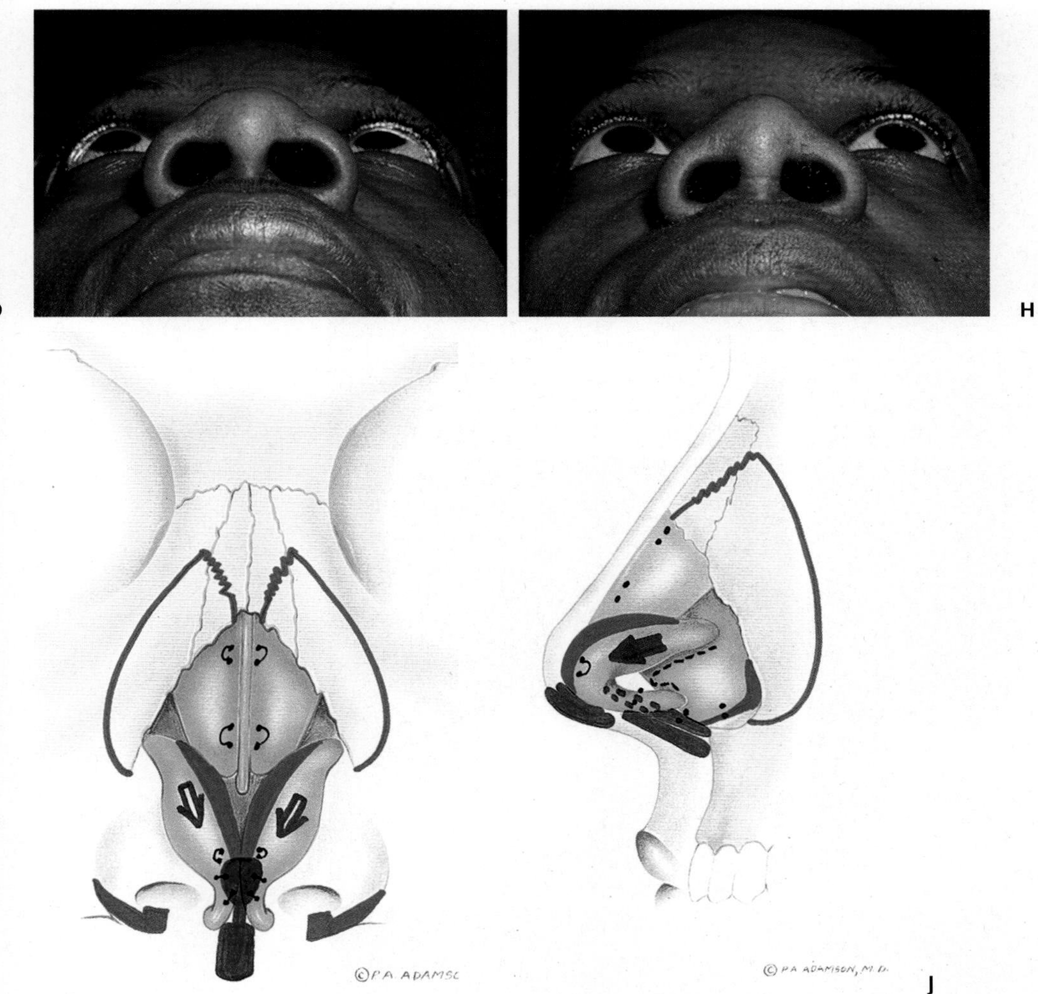

Fig. 41.3 *(Continued)*

diminish bleeding and tissue trauma. A balance is struck between maintenance of soft tissue support and skin elevation sufficient to allow appropriate surgical maneuvers and postoperative skin redrapage.

Septal Deformities

Septoplasty is usually performed first to correct functional problems and to obtain any cartilage that may be necessary for grafting. The superior septal angle is easily identified, and soft tissue is removed from between the medial crura down to the premaxilla. This provides excellent exposure of the caudal septum and allows the columella to be narrowed. This is especially helpful if a columellar strut is to be placed because struts widen the columella inferiorly. If nasolabial augmentation is required, this soft tissue may be retained as a flap based inferiorly and turned on itself to provide additional nasolabial angle augmentation.[11] It is secured with a through-and-through premaxillary transfixion suture. We often deepen or flatten the premaxilla at this juncture with a rongeur. The wide exposure offered by the open approach is much superior to closed techniques for this purpose. The nasal spine may be flattened to create an optimal platform for a columellar strut, but its excision is highly inadvisable. Beginning at the anterior septal angle, complete submucoperichondrial and submucoperiosteal septal flaps are elevated bilaterally. The upper lateral cartilages are separated from the septum such that the nasal dorsum and septum are "ouvert au ciel" or open to the sky. This affords a superb undistorted view unavailable with closed techniques, allowing any desired septoplasty technique to be executed (**Fig. 41.8**). Of note, the view is more anterosuperior than that seen in closed techniques and may require some adjustment of orientation in the mind's eye.

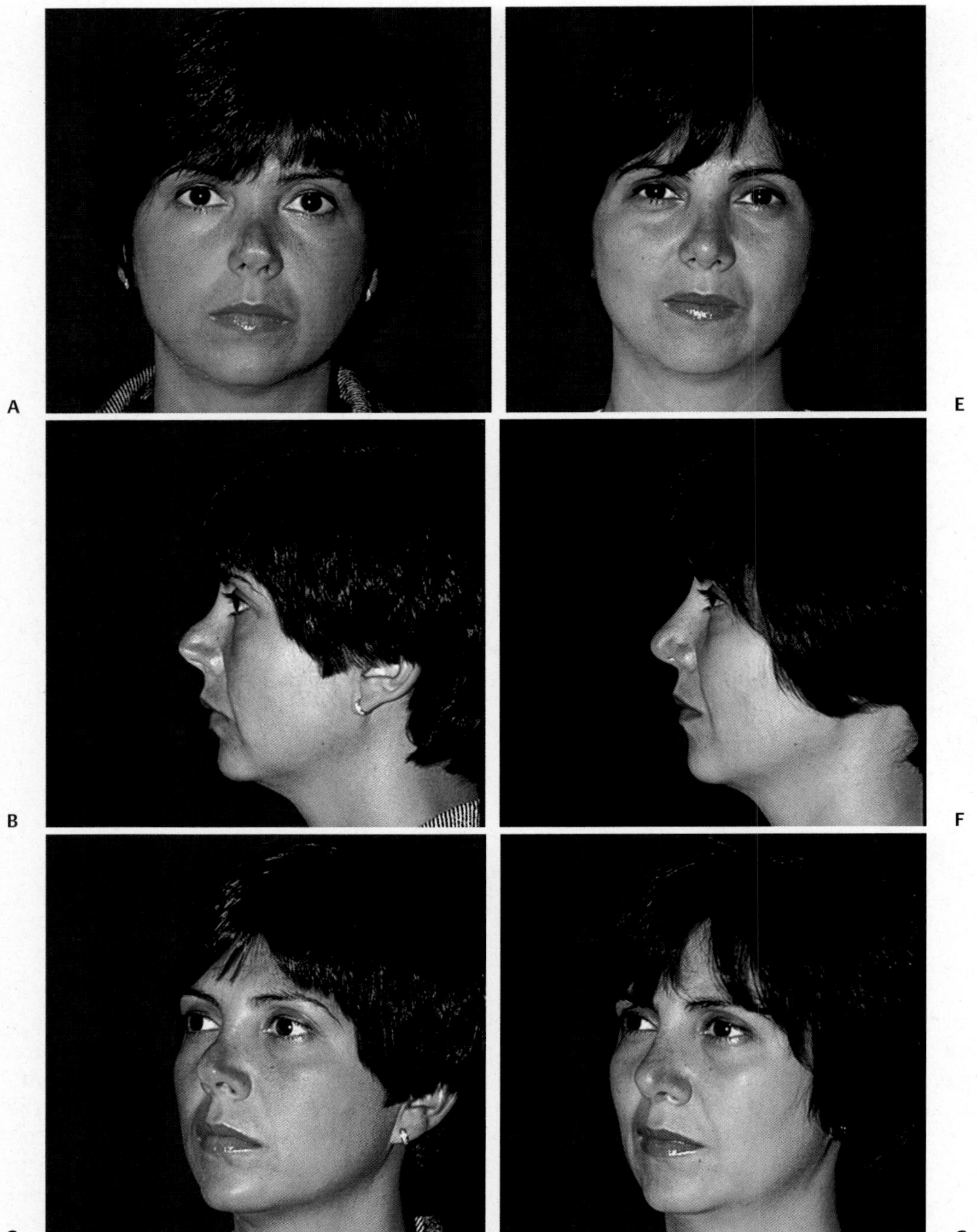

Fig. 41.4 (**A–D**) A 37-year-old female following previous closed septorhinoplasty with airway obstruction, cartilaginous pollybeak, radix over-resection, and tip asymmetry. (**E–H**) Postoperative results showing multiple septal and conchal cartilage grafts. These included columellar strut, infratip lobule, left supratip onlay, and radix and cephalic dorsum grafts. Cartilage pollybeak reduction. No osteotomies. (**I,J**) Dynamic diagrams.

Special Considerations in Septoplasty

Problematic areas of the septum may be managed with greater ease and assurance with the open approach. These include posterior septal spurs or deflections and high subradix deviations, along with dorsal or caudal curvatures. The high subradix deviation is important to identify, as it can be a cause of residual dorsal curvature if left uncorrected. This is treated by vertical shaving of the

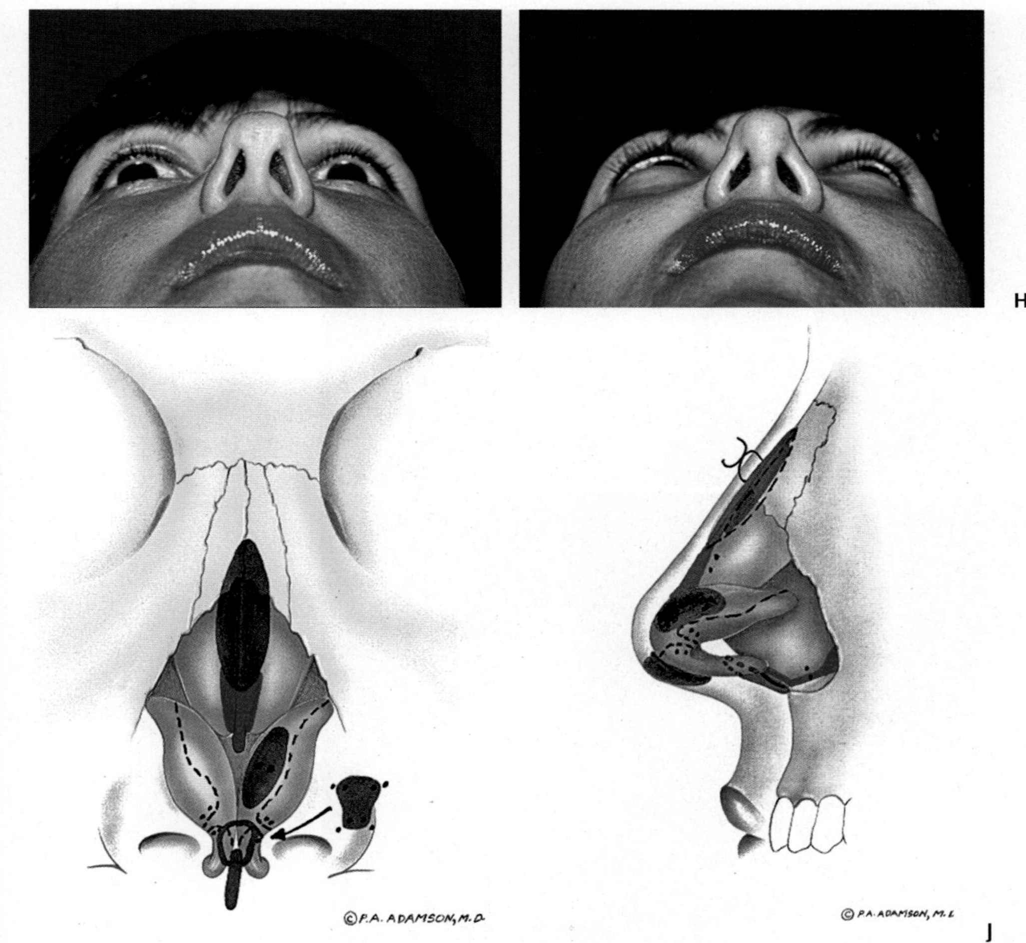

Fig. 41.4 (*Continued*)

dorsal septal cartilage, followed by careful mobilization of the ethmoid plate to the midline, taking care not to fracture the plate superiorly. Severe deflections may require complete disarticulation of the bony and cartilaginous dorsal strut with subsequent midline fixation to the upper lateral cartilages. Likewise, dorsal septal curvatures are frequently overlooked and difficult to assess, more so with the closed than with the open approach. Direct visualization of the dorsal septum without instrumentation distortion is valuable in spotting a subtle deviation. This may be treated by cartilage scoring or limited castellation and by asymmetric placement of septal to upper lateral cartilage transfixion sutures with or without cartilaginous spreader grafting. In this instance, the spreader may act as a spacer graft, camouflage graft, and to increase dorsal septal strength within the middle third.

The open approach also offers unparalleled exposure to the caudal septum, allowing enhanced diagnostic capability at this site. Postoperative curvatures of the caudal septum may result from alteration of the tensional forces within the cartilage following traditional septoplasty. For this reason, we almost routinely perform a "swinging door" technique to allow the inferior caudal septum to swing freely to the midline and come to rest in the maxillary groove. The cartilage may be scored on both the concave and convex surfaces to break its inherent spring. The effect of these maneuvers can be assessed immediately without distortion. In the rare instance of unyielding septal deviation, the septum may be removed in toto and replaced back to front following excision of the deviated portion. Iatrogenic or traumatic cartilaginous-bony disarticulations of the septum can be similarly secured to the upper lateral cartilages.

Septal Perforation

The open approach offers incomparable access to surgically repair septal perforations. Perforations that are asymptomatic need not mandate closure. Symptomatic

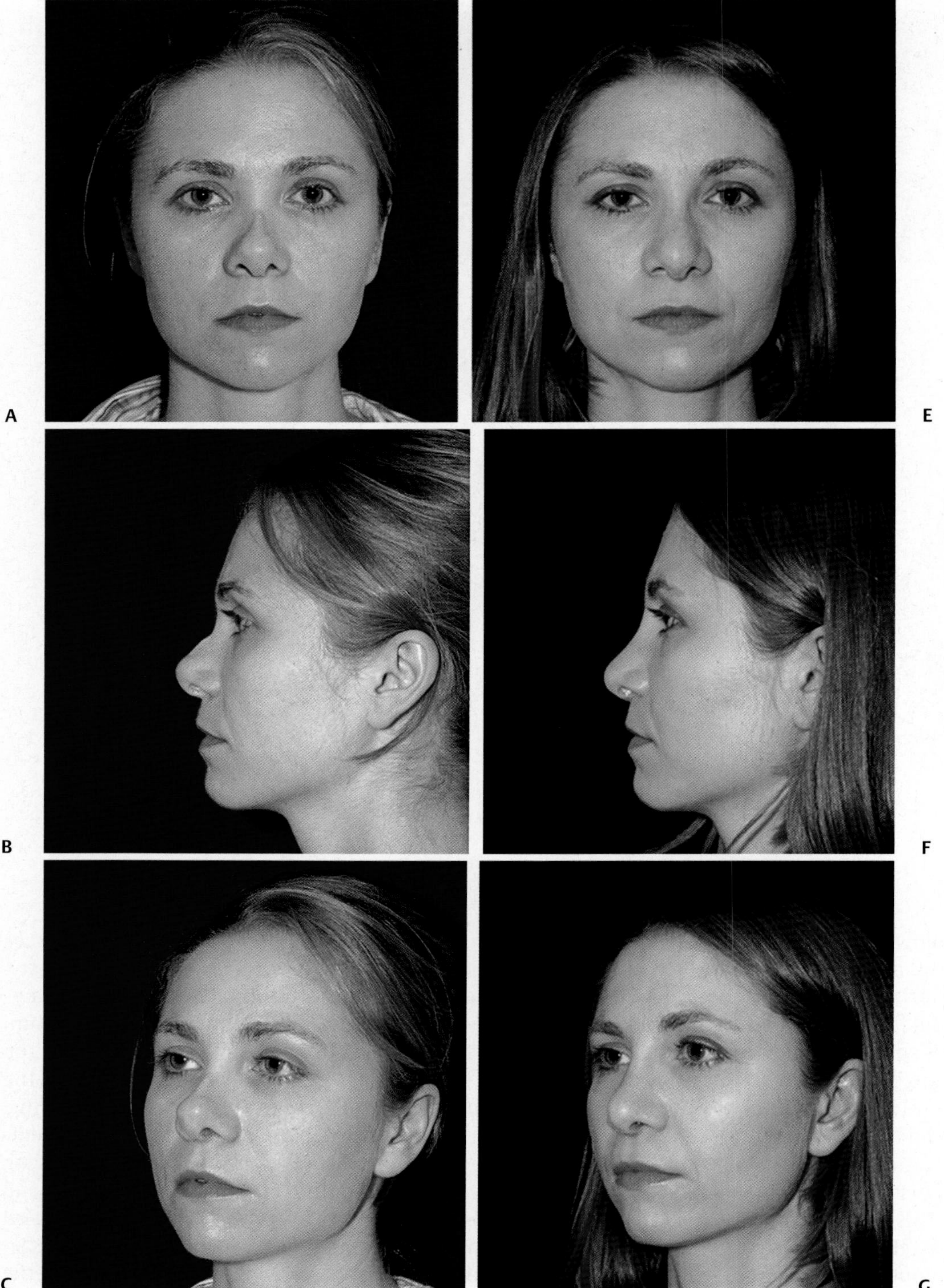

Fig. 41.5 (**A–D**) A 29-year-old female following previous open septorhinoplasty. Tip broad, hanging columella, dorsal hump, and deep radix. (**E–H**) Postoperative results following residual septoplasty and bilateral conchal cartilage donor grafts. These included caudal septal extension, bilateral spreader, radix, columellar strut, and nasolabial angle batten grafts. Vertical arch division of medial crura and single dome unit tip sutures. No osteotomies. (**I,J**) Dynamic diagrams.

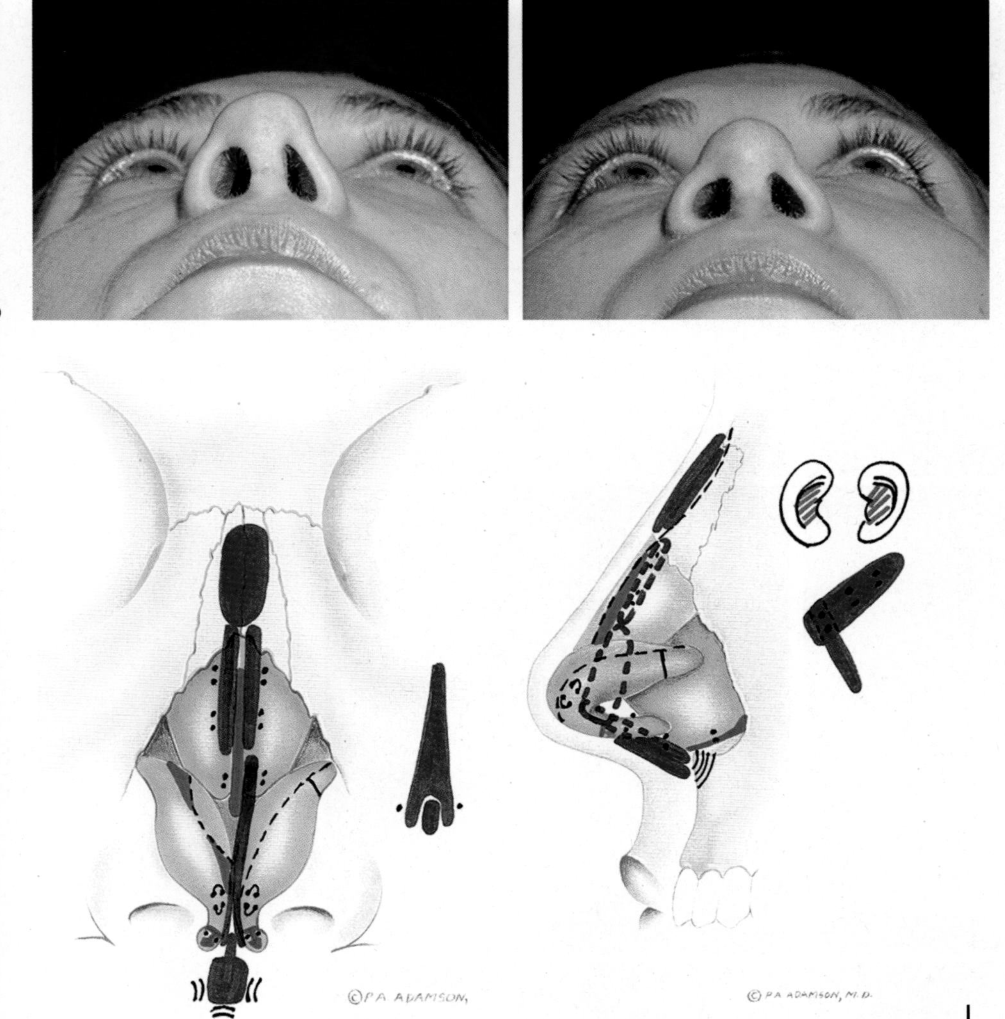

Fig. 41.5 (*Continued*)

perforations of up to 3 cm may be closed by the development of superior and inferior septal mucosal advancement flaps. Larger perforations require more aggressive techniques that are associated with a high risk of failure except in experienced hands.

Related Functional Conditions

Additional conditions contributing to nasal obstructive symptoms may be readily addressed via the open technique in a fashion similar to that using the closed approach. Synechiae, if present, may be incised and the airway maintained by placement of an allograft spacer such as Surgicel gauze or a Silastic stent. Likewise, vestibular stenosis can be addressed directly via an open approach. Of interest, symptomatic vestibular stenosis is more frequently observed following closed rhinoplasty owing to the greater number of vestibular or mucosal incisions, and their locations within the nasal valve area. In the open approach, by contrast, internal incisions are limited to the cartilage margins and, therefore, do not predispose to narrowing. A Z-plasty may be adequate to treat a minimal stenosis. However, we find this condition is best remedied by release of the scar band with interposition of a full-thickness skin graft, in combination with amputation of the head of the inferior turbinate and widening of the pyriform margin. Prolonged stenting with molded Silastic or alternative material is often required to prevent circumferential cicatrisation.

Completing the Septoplasty

The septoplasty is completed with plain gut transfixion sutures to appose the septal mucosal flaps and an inferior

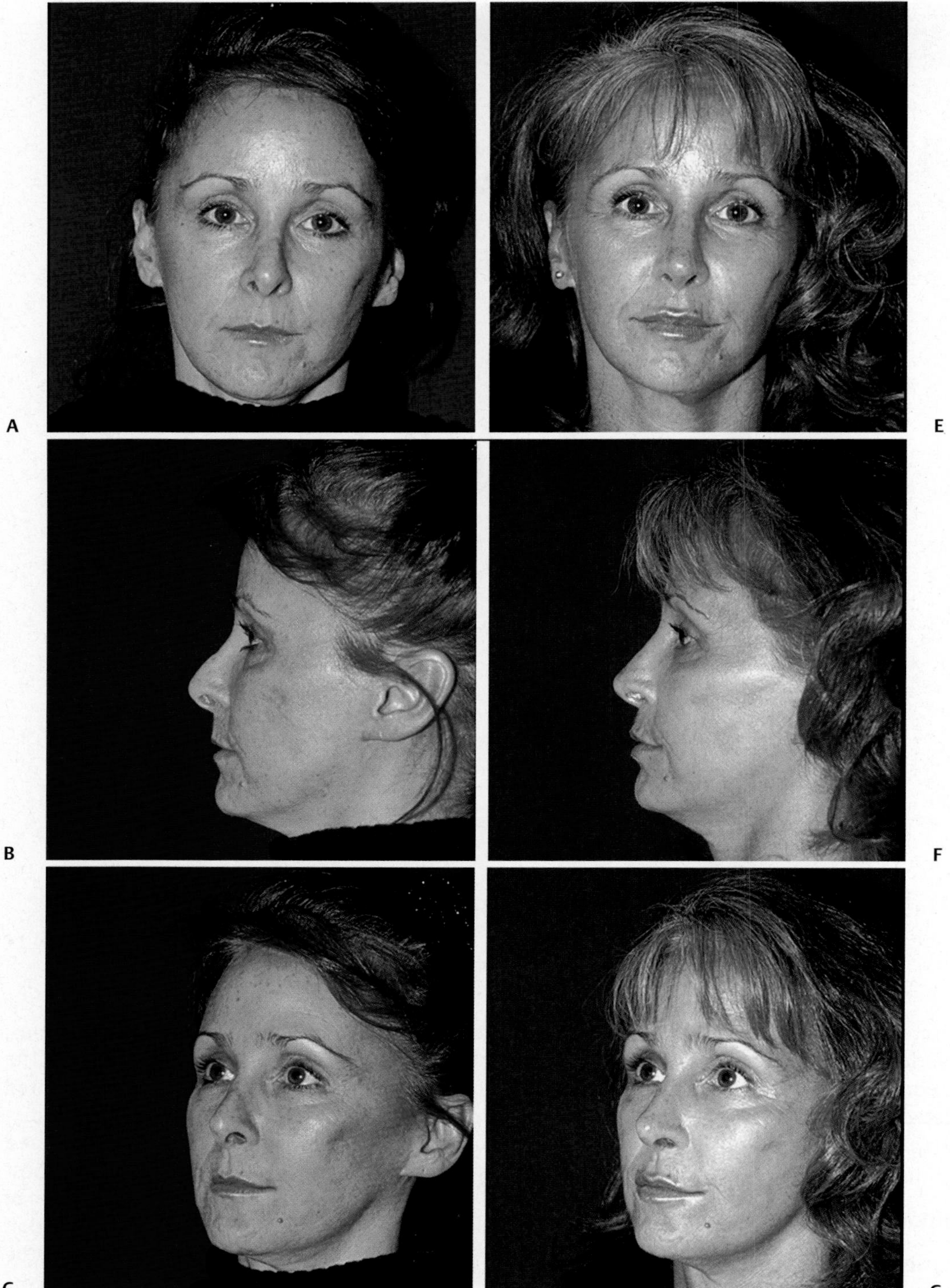

Fig. 41.6 (**A–D**) A 48-year-old female following previous open septorhinoplasty with nasal airway obstruction, crooked nose, tip irregularities, hanging columella, and cartilaginous pollybeak. (**E–H**) Postoperative septoplasty and bilateral conchal cartilage donor grafting. Grafts included columellar strut, infratip lobule, bilateral alar margin, right alar batten and alar strut, lobule spacer, left lobule cap, bilateral spreader, and left upper lateral cartilage onlay grafts. Dorsal reduction, no osteotomies. (**I,J**) Dynamic diagrams.

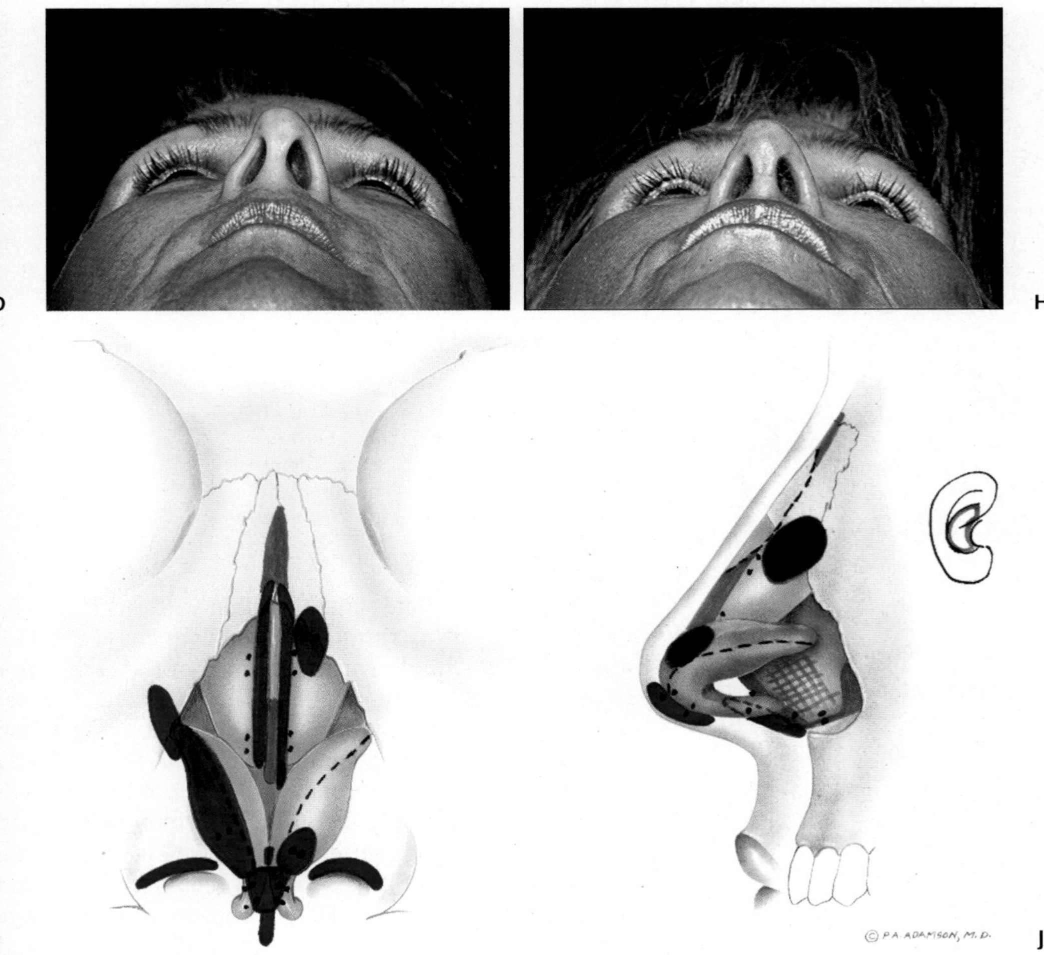

Fig. 41.6 (Continued)

horizontal flap drainage incision to prevent hematoma formation. If the caudal septal strut has been freed up inferiorly at the maxillary crest, it is resecured with transfixion sutures of 4–0 polyglycolic acid (Vicryl; Ethicon, Inc., Somerville, NJ). When minimal dorsal or septal work is required, some surgeons advocate performance of the open rhinoplasty technique in conjunction with a closed septoplasty, without division of the intervening soft tissues of the membranous septum.[12] This maneuver enhances tip stability by maintaining columellar integrity. We, rather, choose to reconstitute the normal septocolumellar relationship via careful suture placement and use of a columellar strut in most instances. The wider access of the open septoplasty permits unencumbered correction of all septocolumellar deformities. If a strut is to be used, it is often desirable to shorten the caudal septum marginally to avert a potential hanging columella effect.

At this juncture, we often treat the inferior turbinates as needed. Unless markedly prominent, simple out-fracture is generally sufficient to maximize the nasal airway. Submucosal electrocautery may be performed in those with a significant mucosal component. We do not routinely perform turbinate resection. However, this technique has been shown to objectively improve nasal airflow postoperatively in cases of documented anterior nasal obstruction.[13]

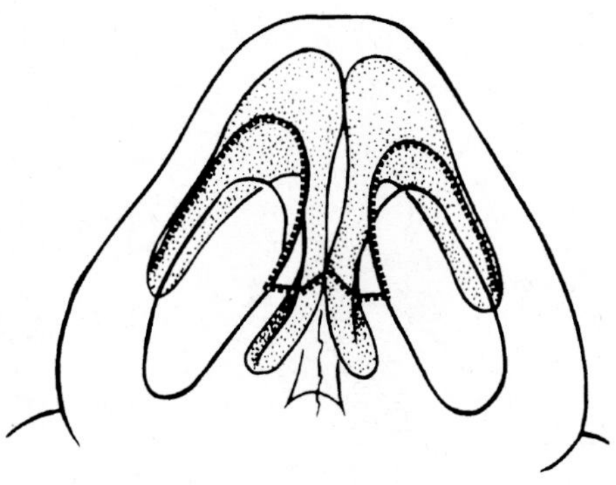

Fig. 41.7 Open rhinoplasty incision. The transverse midcolumellar incision should be placed above the medical crural feet and extend around to meet the vertical marginal incision at a right angle.

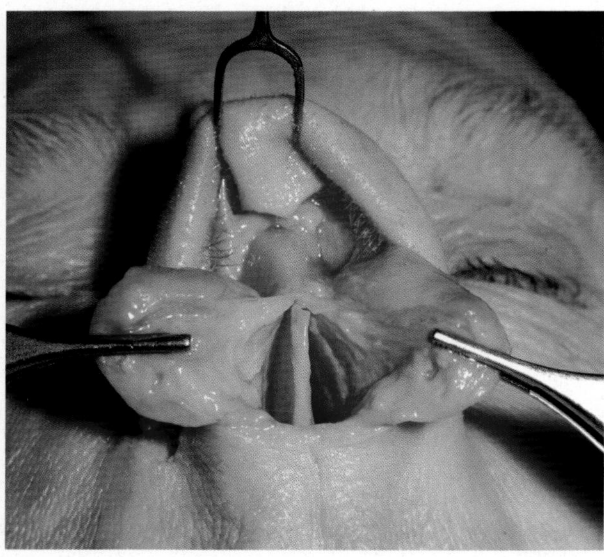

Fig. 41.8 Open rhinoplasty exposure. With elevation of the tip and dorsal skin, superb exposure of the entire nasal structure is obtained. Separation of upper lateral cartilages from the septum provides a direct and undistorted view of the entire septum.

Nasal Base Maneuvers

The nasal base is usually managed before the nasal dorsum. In this way, the major nasal parameters of length, projection, and rotation can be set, whereas the dorsum is adjusted accordingly. Occasionally, a tension tip deformity dictates preliminary dorsal reduction to resolve its distorting effect on the tip. The senior author (PAA) approaches tip alteration based on his contemporary model of tip dynamics, termed the M-Arch Model. This concept expands on Anderson's well-proven Tripod Arch Concept to consider the lower lateral cartilages as a set of M-shaped arches resembling the golden arches of the McDonald's Corporation. Through understanding the three-dimensional representations of these arches, the surgeon is able to influence the major nasal parameters by suitable modifications of the arches' shapes and spatial projections. The overall arch length and the site of the alteration are the most critical determinants of the resultant tip adjustment (**Figs. 41.9 and 41.10**). Shortening or lengthening of the arch closer to the vertex at the tip-defining point will have a greater impact on projection, whereas an identical modification further from the tip-defining point will more greatly influence rotation and, secondarily, length. Moreover, arch shortening lateral to the tip-defining point serves to deproject, rotate, and shorten the nose, whereas shortening medial to this point will deproject, counter-rotate, and lengthen the nose (**Fig. 41.11**). The degree of change correlates with the extent of the shortened segment, and the distance from the tip-defining point. We define division of the arch at any point along its length as a *vertical arch division* (VAD). Specifically, division within the domal or lobular segment of the arch, encompassing the intermediate crus and the anterior segment of the lateral crus, we

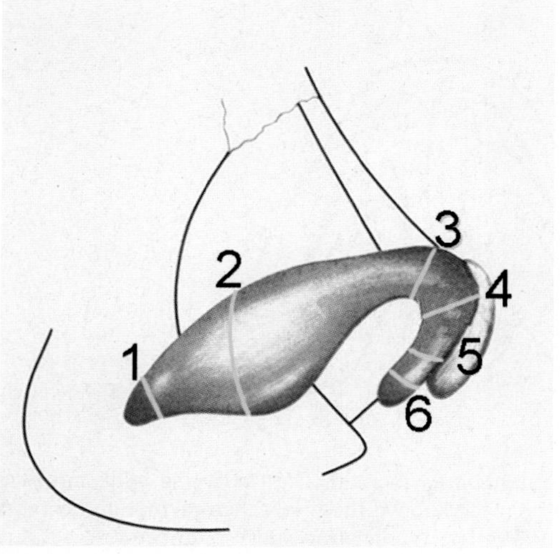

Fig. 41.9 Decreasing M-Arch length by vertical division. The M-Arch model states that a long tip arch can be shortened, and the appropriate tip projection, rotation, and lobule refinement achieved, by dividing the arch at an appropriately selected site. The Goldman division is the exception, in that it lengthens the arch.

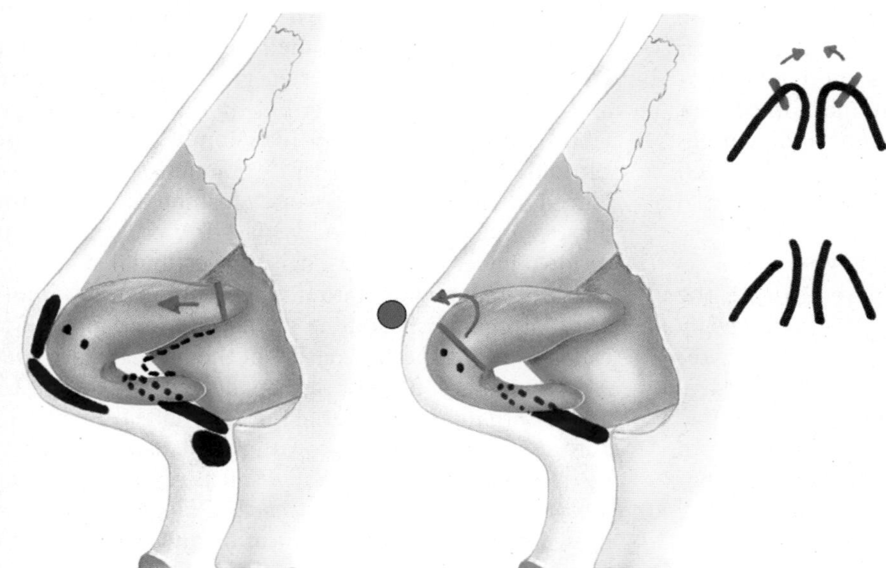

Fig. 41.10 Techniques to increase M-Arch length. (**A**) The M-Arch model states that a short tip arch can be lengthened and the appropriate tip projection, rotation, and lobule refinement achieved, by lateral crural steal, suturing, and cartilage grafting techniques. (**B**) The Goldman vertical arch division borrows cartilage from the lateral crus to become the intermediate crus to increase projection and lobule refinement.

term a *vertical lobule division* (VLD). These concepts apply equally well in closed or open approaches, but the superb exposure of the open approach enables more accurate diagnosis and definitive undistorted, bimanual correction of nasal base deformities.

Medial and Intermediate Crura

An advantage of the open approach is the degree of accuracy with which crural deformities can be distinguished and ameliorated. Not uncommonly, the open approach reveals marked asymmetry of the lower lateral cartilages despite a relatively symmetrical external appearance. Soft tissue excision between the medial crura produces a slight degree of columellar narrowing and gives wide and direct access to the premaxilla. The medial crural feet can be shortened to decrease projection or incised and bunched to decrease their inferior flare. Excision of prominent caudal margins of the medial crura is also facilitated by the open approach. Excessive crural curvature can be improved with scoring techniques. Most often a columellar strut is utilized to set the crural height, and to increase crural support. This is secured just above the premaxillary spine via two 4–0 Vicryl sutures placed through the strut–crural complex and the membranous septum. By varying the angle of its placement in the inferior columella, the strut can also be used to augment the nasolabial angle or increase columellar show. We prefer to set crural support and symmetry working from the base upward, which provides a scaffold for further grafting. Following adjustment of the medial crura, we find that prudent use of one or more vertically oriented intermediate crural horizontal mattress sutures of 5–0 nylon is especially effective in setting the contour and symmetry of the lobular arches. The precise location of this suture can be adjusted to effect changes in the intercrural and alar–columellar angles, to narrow the infratip columella, or to reduce a hanging infratip lobule.

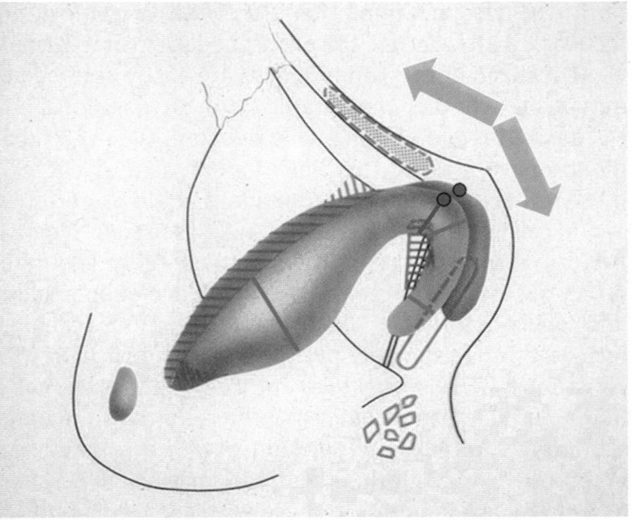

Fig. 41.11 M-Arch and rotation. The M-Arch model states that shortening the arch lateral to the tip-defining point serves to deproject, rotate, and shorten the nose, whereas shortening medial to this point would deproject, counter-rotate, and lengthen the nose.

Lateral Crura

The lateral crura are initially addressed to effect some degree of lobule refinement. Horizontal resection of the cephalic margin of the lower lateral cartilage can achieve some reduction in supratip fullness and may allow for rotation by other means, though it does not in itself produce substantial rotation. Considerably more important than the cartilage resected is the amount and symmetry of cartilage retained, a principle that is readily noted using the open technique. Reduction of the crural arch to less than 8 to 10 mm will serve only to heighten the risk of postoperative alar retraction and buckling.

As lobule reconstruction becomes more intricate, the value of the open approach increases. This is especially true if vertical arch division or lobule grafting is required.[14] Vertical arch division can be used at this stage to achieve adjustments in tip rotation and projection. Though warned against by some surgeons because of the propensity for tip irregularities, we find this maneuver, when employed thoughtfully, to be extraordinarily robust in its applications. In fact, when the cut cartilage edges are overlapped and stabilized, the M-Arch is actually strengthened as compared with its native state. Prior to arch division, the vestibular skin is widely undermined. The arch is incised vertically and overlapped cartilage edges are secured with two 6–0 nylon transfixion sutures to set the span and axis of the neo-arch. Alternatively, 4–0 Vicryl sutures can be used to stabilize the cartilages through the vestibular skin. This technique can be applied predictably to generate rotation, deprojection, or lobular refinement; to diminish a hanging infratip; to correct asymmetries; or to improve the nostril:columellar ratio.

The hinge area, or junction of the lower lateral crus with the sesamoid cartilage, can be observed especially well in the open approach. Accurate dissection and resection of the hinge can be performed to produce somewhat less tip rotation and deprojection than the lateral crural overlay (VAD within the lateral crus). By keeping such incisions well lateral in the more substantial tissues of the alae, the risk of vestibular and valve deformities can be minimized. Although surgeons might conceivably employ such maneuvers via a delivery approach, both visualization and bimanual dexterity are appreciably enhanced with the open approach.

Cartilage Grafting

The open approach is ideally suited for lobular and alar grafting, as these grafts can be easily secured and sculpted under direct vision. Autologous septal or conchal cartilage is preferred.[15] Infratip onlay grafts can be used to increase tip projection, improve definition, camouflage asymmetries, and to impart a degree of apparent counter rotation and lengthening. These are secured with peripherally placed 6–0 nylon sutures. Such grafts may be extended along the length of the columella or placed as a distinct columellar batten to enhance columellar contour or to increase columellar show. Similarly, lateral crural batten, strut, or margin grafts may be fashioned and used to increase structural support in cases of previous overresection or for inversion of alar concavities, contour irregularities, or rim retractions. These may be placed in an underlay or overlay fashion as the situation dicates and are transfixed with 4–0 Vicryl through the residual lower lateral cartilage and vestibular skin.

Nasolabial augmentation is most frequently required after iatrogenic shortening of the inferior aspect of the caudal septum and/or excision of the premaxillary spine. A premaxillary pocket can be developed easily from above with implant material inserted under direct vision. Care should be taken not to enter the labial sulcus and to restrict dissection to the bony–soft tissue plane to retain a substantial soft tissue pocket. Autologous cartilage is most satisfactory for this indication and may be secured in a layered fashion to achieve the desired correction. The columellar soft tissue flap already described may give an additional small degree of correction.

Dorsal Refinement

The open approach greatly enhances the performance of techniques for dorsal refinement. The experienced closed rhinoplasty surgeon may encounter frustration with the altered sense of feel in the assessment of the dorsum with the open technique. However, with time this can be exploited to achieve outstanding dorsal outcomes. Dorsal reduction and osteotomies are performed much the same as with closed techniques, only under improved visualization. This offers the surgeon direct feedback with regard to the effects of a particular maneuver. Localized dorsal prominences are easily assessed to determine whether they are bony or cartilaginous, and the desired mode of removal is selected. We prefer diamond rasps to lower the bony dorsum as they confer a more refined and natural reduction than do osteotomes. Septal cartilage is lowered with angled scissors. We next perform fading, abbreviated medial osteotomies under direct vision. This decreases the incidence of bone chips and rocker deformities. Low lateral osteotomies are performed through separate pyriform margin incisions after elevation of the periosteum internally and externally. Rarely, double osteotomies may be required to manage a broadly vaulted bony pyramid or a severe unilateral bony convexity. Caution is advised in patients with short or brittle nasal bones or in those with a low nasal bridge because of an increased risk of collapse or eggshelling of the bones exists. Should this occur, the bones are supported with Surgicel packing. The relative positions of the nasal bones and upper lateral cartilages with respect to the septum may be altered with osteotomies. Therefore, final refinement of the dorsum is deferred until the osteotomies are completed.

Open rhinoplasty offers specific advantages in achieving an ideal dorsal configuration. In particular, subtle irregularities of the septal or upper lateral cartilages can be readily identified and trimmed under direct vision, as can pollybeak deformities. Curved or collapsed upper lateral cartilages can be secured across the midline with 4–0 Vicryl transfixion sutures. Such suturing may remedy open roof deformities and provide added stability to the middle third of the nose. Spreader grafts can be interposed between the septum and upper lateral cartilages to achieve both functional and aesthetic widening of the middle vault. In addition, small cartilage wafers may be placed to fill areas of bone chips or open roof deformities. Dorsal augmentation grafts can also be easily tapered and layered as necessary beneath the dorsal flap. These and smaller camouflage onlay grafts can be precisely placed and fixed trancutaneously until ingrowth has commenced. Distinct advantages of the open technique include accurate graft placement, firm suture fixation, and protection from intranasal exposure. Proponents of closed techniques will note that the absence of a precise soft tissue pocket is offset by these advantages.

Final Lobule Refinement

Ultimate lobule refinement is best left to the conclusion of the case. This can be achieved by scoring of the domes to create a more defined tip-defining point or to eliminate cartilage convexity. We avoid aggressive cartilage morselization or crushing techniques as these only destabilize the tip. Suture techniques can be utilized such as single dome unit sutures to narrow the domal angle and double dome unit sutures to draw the domes medially. Supratip bunching sutures are useful if greater supratip narrowing is desired. Finally, excision of a prominent membranous septum may be accomplished to diminish a hanging columella effect. Although this can be undertaken concurrently with an open approach, it must be recognized that blood supply to the columella is disrupted both anteriorly and posteriorly via this course of action and caution should be exercised.

Soft Tissue Refinement

Skin is the most significant factor affecting the final aesthetic result for the experienced rhinoplasty surgeon. Patients having thick, sebaceous skin or older, less elastic skin may require a longer time for skin contraction, especially in the supratip. Judicious postoperative care is compulsory to minimize risk of a soft tissue pollybeak deformity in these patients. The soft tissue may be guardingly defatted and the skin lightly crosshatched to aid in redrapaging. Care must be taken not to compromise the subdermal vascular plexus. We find that postoperative supratip massage and nightly taping encourages redrapaging and obviates the need for routine use of steroid injections in such cases. Surgeons who regularly perform open rhinoplasty have not encountered difficulties with prolonged edema or increased risk of abnormalities with skin redrapage.

Columellar Scar

It is rarely necessary to refine the columellar scar of a previous open rhinoplasty.[10] The most likely deformity is a small irregularity at the junction of the horizontal and vertical components of the columellar incision. This is best treated with light dermabrasion or laser resurfacing. In revision open rhinoplasties, the original incision may be used without excising the initial scar.

Alar Base Narrowing

Alar narrowing is considered if the ala extends lateral to a perpendicular dropped from the medial canthus or if the nasal base is proportionately large for the nose owing to excessive alar width. Alar refinement is commonly performed when significant nasal tip deprojection results in undesirable flaring of the alae. A variety of nasal sill and alar excisions have been used.[16] The appropriate amount of resection from the internal and external nostril circumference and alar length is effected. We place the incision within the sill to retain the natural curvilinear contour of the nostril and to prevent notching. A generous back-cut placed just above the alar facial groove allows for advancement-rotation of the ala. A wedge may be excised from the alar wall at this time to decrease alar flare. The incision is closed meticulously with 6–0 nylon sutures, with special care taken to evert the sill incision. This technique narrows the nasal base, decreases nostril size, and alters the nostril axis.

Alar Hooding

Alar hooding repair is corrected after tip rotation and columella position is optimized. On lateral view, hooding appears as a curvilinear ptosis of the middle and posterior alar margin. The hooded skin is excised via a horizontal fusiform wedge excision at the caudal margin of the alar rim followed by a running 6–0 nylon closure.

Postoperative Care

Septal stents of exposed x-ray film are secured with 4–0 Vicryl transfixion sutures. Minimal packing placed at the osteotomy incision sites is removed the following day. Columellar and alar sutures are removed on day 4, with the exception of sutures at the transverse columellar-vertical marginal incision junction. These are removed at day 8 along with the septal stents and nasal cast. Light bimanual compression of the nasal bones is commenced for a period of 5 weeks. Patients are cautioned to avoid active exercise for 3 weeks and contact sports for 6 weeks.

Summary

Surgeons well versed in closed rhinoplasty techniques may find few indications for an open approach. Open rhinoplasty closure does consume greater time than a closed approach, and surgeons may find themselves spending more time correcting deformities that are more easily identified. Both intraoperative assessment and postoperative settling constitute a departure from the familiar healing experience with closed techniques; yet, they are no less effective. Recognition of the benefits of the open rhinoplasty approach continues to expand.[17] It is an educational approach in itself, with both novice and experienced rhinoplasty surgeons enhancing their diagnostic and therapeutic rhinoplasty skills. The improved exposure and technical advantages accrued using this technique ensure that it will continue to be held in high esteem for a long time to come.

References

1. Snell GE. A history of rhinoplasty. Can J Otolaryngol 1973;2(3): 224–230
2. Rethi A. Operation to shorten an excessively long nose. Rev Chir Plast 1934;2:85
3. Sercer A. Dekortication der Nose. Chirureie Maxillofac-Plast (Zagreb) 1958;1:49
4. Padovan T. External approach in rhinoplasty (decortication). Symp ORL 1966;4:354
5. Goodman WS. External approach to rhinoplasty. J Otolaryngol 1973; 2(3):207–210
6. Goodman WS, Charbonneau PA. External approach to rhinoplasty. Laryngoscope 1974;84(12):2195–2201
7. Anderson JR, Johnson CM Jr, Adamson P. Open rhinoplasty: an assessment. Otolaryngol Head Neck Surg 1982; 90(2):272–274
8. Wright WK, Kridel RW. External septorhinoplasty: a tool for teaching and for improved results. Laryngoscope 1981;91(6): 945–951
9. Adamson PA, Galli SK. Rhinoplasty approaches: current state of the art. Arch Facial Plast Surg 2005;7(1):32–37
10. Adamson PA, Smith O, Tropper GJ. Incision and scar analysis in open (external) rhinoplasty. Arch Otolaryngol Head Neck Surg 1990;116(6):671–675
11. Adamson PA, McGraw B. Soft tissue premaxillary augmentation flap. Laryngoscope 1991;101(1):86–88
12. Johnson CM, Toriumi D. Open Structure Rhinoplasty. Philadelphia: WB Saunders; 1990
13. Smith O, Adamson P, Tropper G, et al. The role of partial turbinectomy in aesthetic septorhinoplasty. In: Plastic and Reconstructive Surgery of the Head and Neck: Proceedings of the Fifth International Symposium. Philadelphia: B.C. Decker; 1991
14. Constantinides MS, Adamson PA. Vertical lobule division in open septorhinoplasty. Face 1997;5(2):63–72
15. Adamson PA. Nasal tip surgery in open rhinoplasty. Facial Plast Surg Clin North Am 1993;1:39–52
16. Adamson PA, Van Duyne JM. Alar base refinement. Aesthetic Plast Surg 2002;26(Suppl 1):20
17. Gunter JP. The merits of the open approach in rhinoplasty. Plast Reconstr Surg 1997;99(3):863–867

42 Surgery of the Bony Nasal Vault

Sam P. Most, Craig S. Murakami, and Wayne F. Larrabee Jr.

n important challenge to the surgeon wishing to master nodern rhinoplasty is the consideration of nasal function in ddition to traditional aesthetic concerns. The importance f nasal function is evidenced by the proposition that the istinguishing features of the human nose arose in *Homo rectus* in response to the need for more moisture conser-ation.[1] Recognition of nasal function is particularly impor-ant to the surgeon manipulating the bony skeleton of the ose. Although suboptimal aesthetic results may occur with ither inadequate or inappropriate mobilization of the asal bony–cartilaginous framework, significant reduction f the nasal airway may also occur. Several techniques are vailable to appropriately mobilize and reposition the bony asal vault. Herein we review our experience with a variety f techniques and consider some special situations.

natomy

xternal Landmarks and Soft issue Components

equisite to the use of the techniques described below is n understanding of the bony anatomy of the nose and its elation to the external nasal contour. The external contour f the upper third of the nose is defined by the two side-valls, the dorsum, and the nasofrontal angle.[2,3] The nasion s the bony junction between the frontal and nasal bones. he nasofrontal angle is the external landmark identifying he deepest or most posterior portion of the nasal dorsum nd may lie several millimeters inferior to the nasion. The hinion is the osseocartilaginous junction of the nasal bones o the superior edge of the upper lateral cartilages.

The external appearance of the nose is affected by oth the bony–cartilaginous framework and the shape nd consistency of components of the overlying soft tis-ue envelope. This soft tissue varies in thickness over the asal bones. As shown in **Fig. 42.1**, the nasal skin is thicker uperiorly and inferiorly and quite thin over the central asal rhinion.[2] Thus surgery on the nasal profile must ompensate for this to avoid a saddle nose appearance. For xample, a slight hump must be left at the bony rhinion if straight soft tissue profile is desired.

ony and Cartilaginous Framework

he nasal bones are paired structures that attach superi-rly to the frontal bone and laterally to the nasal process of the maxillary bones. These structures together form the bony nasal vault. The keystone area is the junction of the perpendicular plate of the ethmoid with the nasal bones at their inferior edge in the midline. This is an important area as destabilization here in the setting of aggressive septoplasty can lead to a saddle nose deformity. The side-walls are formed by the nasal bones themselves and the frontal process of the maxilla. The nasal bones are thin inferiorly and become thick superiorly.[2,4] This is demon-strated by transillumination of the skull (**Fig. 42.2**). The variable thickness of the bony structures of the nose has implications for osteotomy placement, as discussed later in the chapter.

The septum supports the nose below the inferior edge of the nasal bones. The septum and upper lateral cartilage complex provides the skeletal component of the lower na-sal dorsal profile. Preservation of adequate (>1 cm) dorsal and caudal struts of septum during septoplasty is para-mount in the preservation of this profile. In the setting of dorsal hump reduction, the amount of septum to be re-moved during hump reduction must be taken into account. For this reason, the authors regularly perform hump reduc-tion and medial osteotomies prior to removal of any septal cartilage, if septoplasty is being performed concurrently.

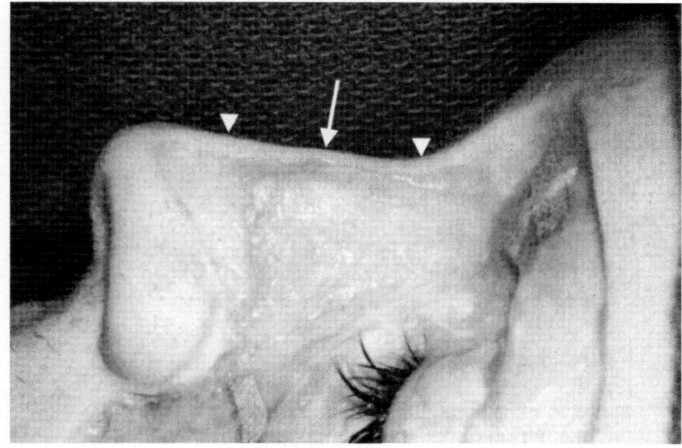

Fig. 42.1 Skin thickness of the nasal dorsum. The nasal thickness varies greatly from patient to patient but in general is thicker in the supratip and nasion areas (*arrowheads*). Reduction of the bony–cartilaginous framework in rhinoplasty must allow for variations in the thickness of the soft tissue–skin envelope. To maintain a straight soft tissue profile, the framework must maintain a slight hump at the rhinion (*arrow*). (Adapted from Larrabee WF Jr., Makielski KH. Surgical Anatomy of the Face. New York: Raven; 1993:164.)

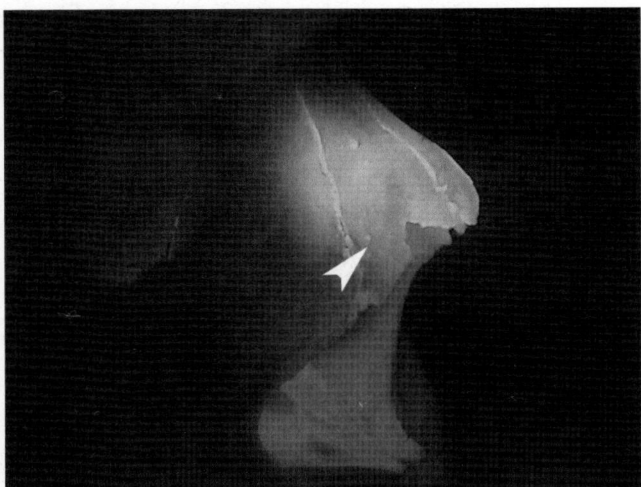

Fig. 42.2 Transillumination of the skull reveals the thinner aspect of the nasal bones, which are mobilized with osteotomies in rhinoplasty (*arrow*). Osteotomies that are carried into the thicker bone of the maxilla or frontal bone are ineffective or result in inappropriate fracture sites.

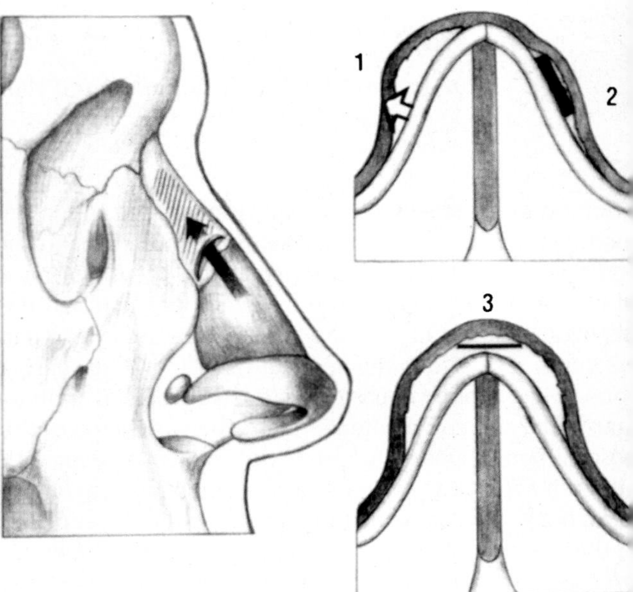

Fig. 42.3 Elevation of the periosteal flap begins with (1) sharp dissection a few millimeters above the caudal end of the nasal bones, followed by the development of pockets bilaterally (2) and the connection of these pockets in the midline with sharp dissection (3). (Adapted from Larrabee WF Jr. Open rhinoplasty and the upper third of the nose. Facial Plast Surg Clin North Am, Elsevier, 1993;1(1):26.)

Surgical Techniques

Hump Reduction

The soft tissue envelope is elevated from the bony–cartilaginous framework up to the level of the nasofrontal angle (via incisions described elsewhere in this text). Care is taken to undermine conservatively and yet widely enough to permit adequate hump reduction and subsequent skin redraping (**Fig. 42.3**). Although adequate exposure is obtained to perform the desired reduction or refinement of the profile, as much soft tissue support is preserved as possible. Either an osteotome or a rasp can be used to lower the dorsum, depending on the surgeon's experience and preference. In general, an osteotome may be used for larger humps and a rasp for smaller reductions and refinements. To remove larger humps, a conservative correction is performed with a double-guarded osteotome (**Fig. 42.4**). Refinements are then made with a tungsten carbide pull rasp. The rasp is angled slightly obliquely off the midline to avoid avulsing the upper lateral cartilages from the undersurface of the nasal bones. Removal of a dorsal hump creates a so-called open roof deformity, necessitating osteotomies for closure (**Fig. 42.5**).

Osteotomies

Jacques Joseph was one of the first surgeons to promote osteotomy.[5] The path of his osteotomy extended from the inferior piriform aperture up into the nasal process of the frontal bone. The mobilization of the nasal bones by Joseph and other early rhinoplastic surgeons resulted in a high rate of nasal airway compromise postoperatively. The recognition that preservation of the periosteum and lateral

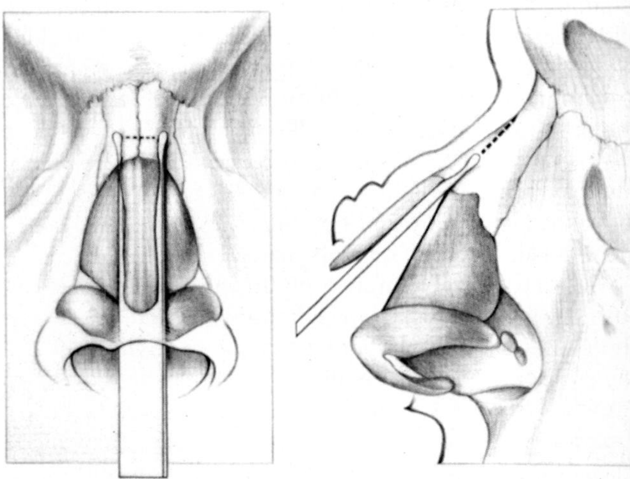

Fig. 42.4 The cartilaginous dorsum to be removed is incised sharply and left attached to the nasal bones. After elevating the periosteum, a double-guarded osteotome is then used to complete the hump removal. Care is used to follow the planned profile superiorly to the nasion and to avoid canting the osteotome to the right or left. The hump removal is done conservatively with fine adjustments made with the rasp. (Adapted from Larrabee, WF Jr. Open rhinoplasty and the upper third of the nose. Facial Plast Surg Clin North Am, Elsevier, 1993;1(1):28.)

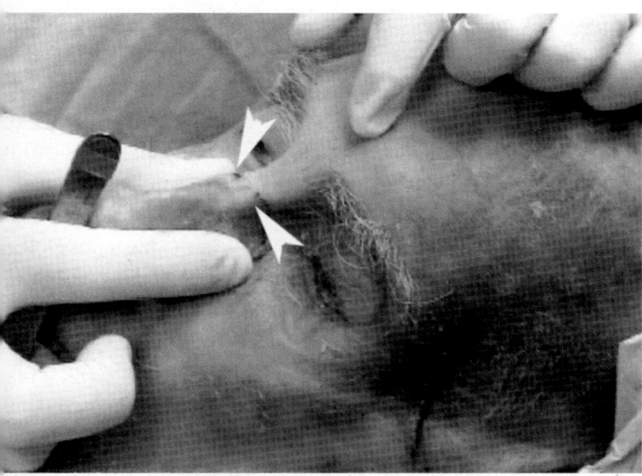

Fig. 42.5 An open roof deformity is created after removal of a bony and cartilaginous dorsal hump, as demonstrated in this cadaver dissection. The flattened nasal dorsum is the external manifestation of an open roof (*arrowheads*). Osteotomies are performed to close the open roof (see text).

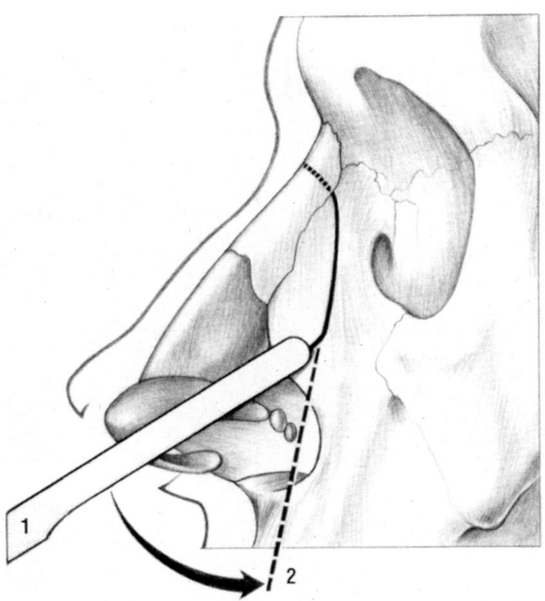

Fig. 42.6 The lateral osteotomy is begun at the anterior end of the inferior turbinate and is first made perpendicular to the face of the pyriform aperture (position 1). After this cut, the osteotomy is carried in a curved fashion toward the medial canthal area (position 2). (Adapted from Larrabee, WF Jr. Open rhinoplasty and the upper third of the nose. Facial Plast Surg Clin North Am, Elsevier, 1993;1(1):30.)

suspensory ligaments of the lower lateral cartilage helped to lower the incidence of postoperative airway compromise has been an important positive technical modification.[6–8] Thus modern techniques of osteotomy have evolved to take into account the effects of bony repositioning on functional as well as aesthetic outcome.

The indications for performing osteotomies are: (1) to close an open nasal vault (**see Fig. 42.5**); (2) to straighten a deviated nasal dorsum; or (3) to narrow the nasal sidewalls. From a functional standpoint, the surgeon must consider the possible effects of the osteotomy on the patient's nasal airway. Each patient's nasal architecture is unique. In general, an osteotomy should be limited to the thinner aspect of the nasal sidewall. The average thickness of the nasal sidewall along the osteotomy path is 2.5 mm.[9] Commonly used osteotomy techniques include the lateral osteotomy, performed either with a perforation or linear technique; the medial osteotomy; the superior osteotomy; and the intermediate osteotomy.

The Lateral Osteotomy

Lateral osteotomies are performed to close an open dorsum (open roof) and to narrow or straighten the nasal pyramid. There are two basic techniques: the linear (single-cut) technique and the perforating technique. With the linear technique, the osteotome is used to make a bony cut along the nasal facial groove (**Fig. 42.6**). The most widely accepted path of the osteotomy follows a high (anterior), low (posterior), high (anterior) pathway. The course of the lateral osteotomy begins just at or slightly above the level of the attachment of the inferior turbinate (**Fig. 42.7A**). A small triangle of bone at the pyriform aperture is left intact to preserve the lateral attachments of the suspensory ligaments. This helps to preserve the nasal airway. Next, the osteotomy is continued along the nasal facial groove until it curves superiorly and anteriorly into the thinner aspect of the nasal bone at the level of the inferior orbit (**Fig. 42.7B**). The cut is then terminated at the level of the medial canthus. If it is carried higher into the thicker bone of the nasofrontal suture a rocker deformity may result, in which in-fracture of the nasal bone results in protrusion at the superior fracture site.[10]

The superior back-fracture can be created by turning the osteotome, applying digital pressure, or using a percutaneous transverse superior osteotomy. In the latter technique, a small cutaneous puncture is created with a 2-mm osteotome midway between the nasal dorsum and the medial canthal region. Through this site, the same osteotome is used to create three or four small perforations, allowing mobilization of the nasal bone without disrupting the overlying periosteal support.

The perforating technique can also be used to create a lateral osteotomy. A small series of perforations are placed along the desired fracture site using a transnasal or transcutaneous approach (**Fig. 42.8**). The perforating intranasal osteotomy can also be used to "push out" the nasal bones

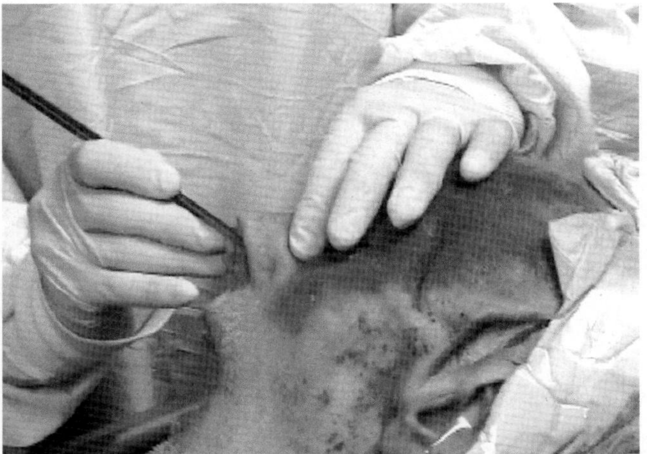

A

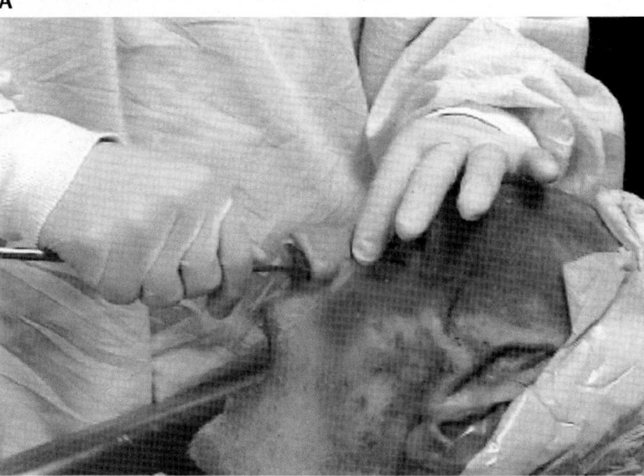

B

Fig. 42.7 Lateral osteotomy technique demonstration. (**A**) The osteotome is placed just above the level of attachment of the inferior turbinate, thus preserving lateral suspensory ligamentous attachments. (**B**) As the cut progesses superiorly, note the change in angle of the osteotome and the switch from an underhand to overhand grip on the instrument.

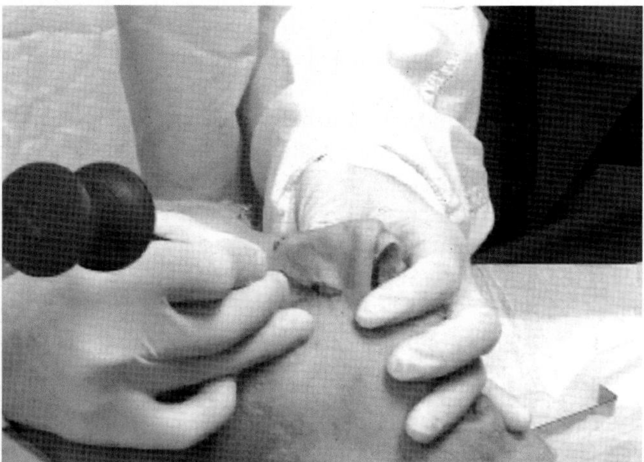

Fig. 42.8 External perforating lateral osteotomy technique. Using a sharp 2-mm straight osteotome, multiple postage-stamp osteotomies are made through one or two external incisions.

that have been medially displaced by previous trauma or surgery.[11] The objective is to move the nasal sidewall laterally. Although the perforating osteotomy is often preferred in difficult cases, such as revision rhinoplasty or posttraumatic nasal surgery, it is becoming more popular for performing osteotomies for the traditional indications. One reason for this is the ability to more directly visualize the path of the desired osteotomy, and another is the preservation of periosteal attachments to the nasal bones (**Fig. 42.9**). Cadaveric studies have demonstrated preservation of considerably more periosteal support with the perforating technique in comparison with the linear technique.[12,13] Noses that are extremely deviated or those that have thick nasal sidewalls are more appropriately treated with a linear osteotomy.[14]

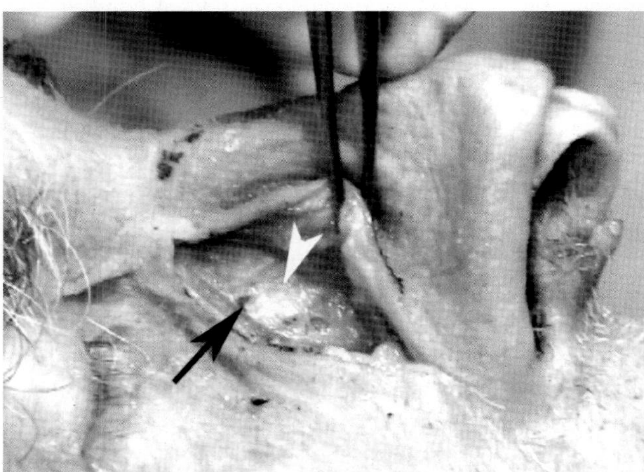

A

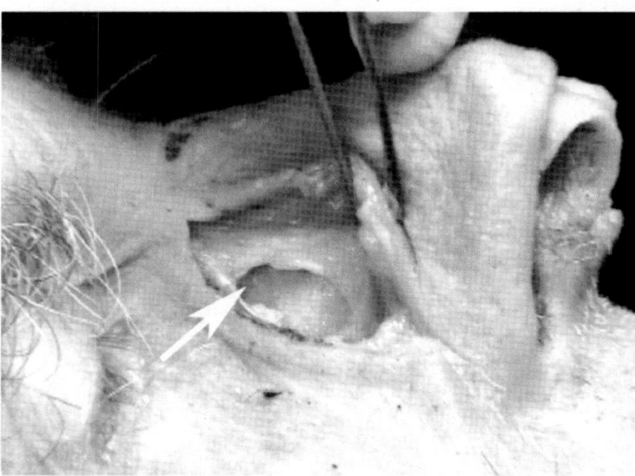

B

Fig. 42.9 Preservation of the periosteum using the perforating technique. (**A**) Dissection of periosteum after perforating osteotomy in this cadaver demonstrates an intact periosteum, still attached to the underlying (but mobilized) bone (*white arrowhead*). Black arrow indicates a postage-stamp periosteal and corresponding bony cut. (**B**) After incision of the periosteum, the bony sidewall falls into the nasal cavity (*white arrow*), demonstrating the importance of periosteal attachments in preventing flail segments during osteotomy.

The Medial Osteotomy

The indications for medial osteotomies are: (1) when mobilization of the entire nasal sidewall is required; (2) to help prevent uncontrolled or irregular back-fracture from the upper portion of a lateral osteotomy; and (3) to widen an overly narrowed bony nasal vault. The medial oblique osteomy technique is used for the former two indications, the medial vertical technique for the latter. The medial oblique osteotomy can be performed linearly or percutaneously. Linear medial osteotomies are performed in an angulated fashion between the nasal bone and septum and are carried superiorly to meet the superior osteotomy site or back-fractured site (**Fig. 42.10**). They are often used to correct the deviated nose or to narrow the wide nose without a hump. In the severely deviated or wide nose, medial osteotomies can be considered essential. However, in cases where less correction is required, they may actually cause bony irregularities and should be used judiciously.

The medial vertical osteotomy is performed to separate the septum from the bony nasal vault. It is often used alone (without lateral osteotomy) to widen the nasal vault that is natively or iatrogenically narrowed. After separation of the upper lateral cartilages from the septum, a straight osteotome is placed between the septum and inferior edge of the nasal bone. A vertical cut is performed, with care taken not to extend into the frontal bone. Care must also be taken during initiation of medial osteotomies in the keystone area, as destabilization of the septum can result, especially in the setting of prior septoplasty. A slight twisting motion at the end of the cut provides the 1 mm or so of space required for placement of a spreader graft.

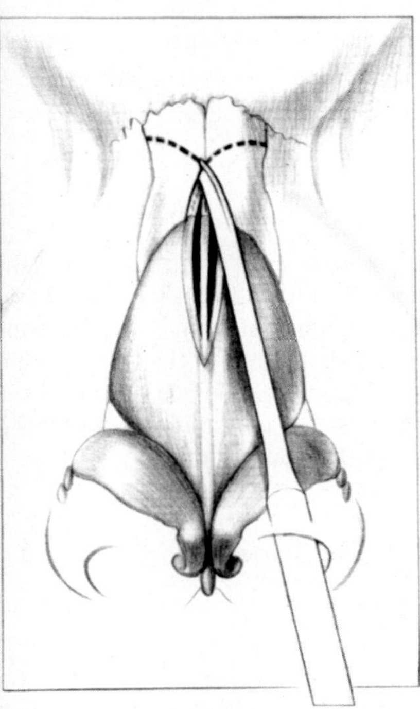

Fig. 42.10 Medial osteotomies are not done routinely but are performed when necessary, such as in the extremely wide or deviated nose. Either a straight or a curved osteotome creates a controlled cut at the transition to the thicker frontal bone. (Adapted from Larrabee WF Jr. Open rhinoplasty and the upper third of the nose. Facial Plast Surg Clin North Am, Elsevier, 1993;1(1):29.)

The Intermediate Osteotomy

The primary uses of the intermediate osteotomy are: (1) to narrow the extremely wide nose that has good height (bilateral osteotomy); (2) to correct the deviated nose with one sidewall much longer than the other; and (3) to straighten a markedly convex nasal bone.[14,15] The intermediate osteotomy is made parallel to the lateral osteotomy somewhere along the midportion of the nasal sidewall. The exact medial/lateral placement of the osteotomy along the lateral nasal wall may vary depending on the surgical goals. In a closed rhinoplasty, it is usually performed via an intercartilaginous incision with a small osteotome (e.g., 3 mm) and carried cephalad to the superior fracture site. Through the open rhinoplasty approach it can be performed with more precision. The intermediate osteotomy is performed before the lateral osteotomy, as the intermediate cut cannot be made easily after the bone is mobilized laterally. Soft tissue should be left attached to the nasal bone for added support.

Postoperative Care

Osteotomy causes mild to moderate soft tissue swelling and, in addition, may cause ecchymosis and periorbital edema. Postoperative edema can be greatly reduced by the application of cold compresses and by elevation of the head to 30 degrees during the first 24 hours after surgery. Perioperative antibiotics may be used. Nasal packing, if used, is removed in 24 hours, and nasal casts or surgical splints are removed after 1 week. Some surgeons encourage nasal exercises, in which the patient places a finger on either side ofthe nose and exerts moderate inward pressure to prevent displacement of the newly medialized osteotomized bony pyramid.

Special Considerations

The Extremely Deviated Nose

The previous osteotomies may be used in combination to correct any given anatomical deformity of the bony nasal pyramid. For example, in the posttraumatic or longstanding

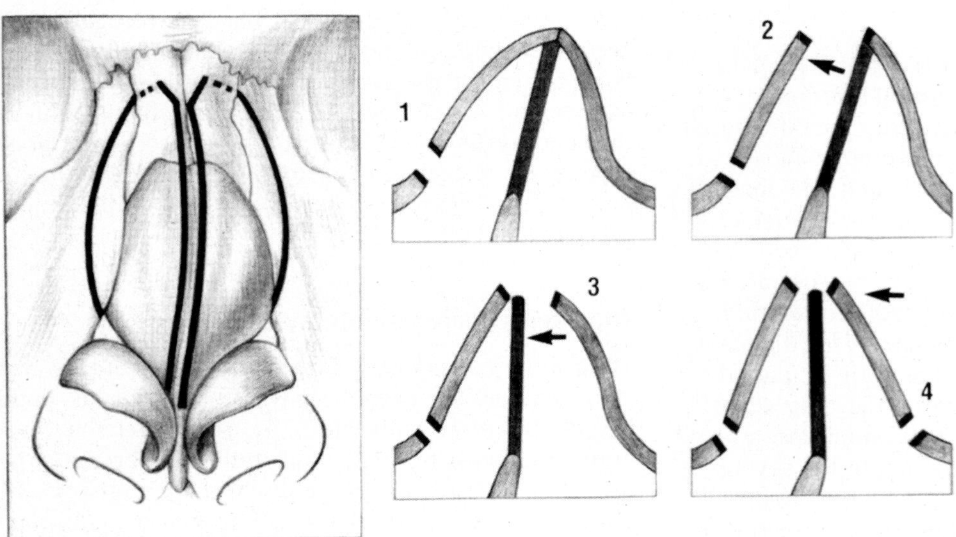

Fig. 42.11 To correct a deviated nose, sequential osteotomies are performed in a fashion similar to opening a book. (Adapted from Larrabee WF Jr. Open rhinoplasty and the upper third of the nose. Facial Plast Surg Clin North Am, Elsevier, 1993;1(1):33.)

severely crooked nose, it is important to completely mobilize the segments of the bony pyramid to avoid persistent postoperative deviations. In this situation, the osteotomies are performed sequentially beginning on the side opposite the deviation (e.g., for a pyramid displaced to the left, begin with the right lateral osteotomy). Note that this is similar to turning the pages of an open book, with the nasal walls and septum simulating the pages (**Fig. 42.11**). This allows creation of a space in which to realign the deviation.

Wide Nose

Removal of a significant hump from the wide nose may result in a wide open dorsum. Standard osteotomies may allow the nasal bones to be moved to close the open roof. Debris or residual wedges of bone or cartilage may persist at the junction of the nasal bone and septum. This must be removed prior to closure. In some cases, when nasal height is appropriate and the nasal bones are extremely wide or convex, bilateral intermediate osteotomies may be necessary to obtain adequate narrowing.[14]

Short Nasal Bones

Preoperative evaluation of the patient should include assessment of the length of the nasal bones and the composition of the nasal hump (bone versus cartilage). Patients with short nasal bones, as determined by palpation, often have a primarily cartilaginous hump. In this case, the surgeon must avoid both overmobilization o the nasal bones with osteotomies and over-resectio of the dorsal nasal bones with a rasp or osteotome. Th dorsal hump can sometimes be lowered without osteotomies. A perforating osteotomy may be used to preserv maximal soft tissue support. In these cases, a greenstic fracture superiorly is desirable as it also avoids overmobilization of the delicate, short nasal bones.

Summary

A systematic approach must be used when addressing th deviated nasal pyramid. This includes precise preoperative and intraoperative anatomical analysis of the bon deformity. A thorough understanding of the various techniques available to address these deformities allows th surgeon to address the deviated pyramid most appropriately and with optimal postoperative outcome.

References

1. Franciscus RG, Trinkaus E. Nasal morphology and the emergence o Homo erectus. Am J Phys Anthropol 1988; 75(4):517–527
2. Larrabee WF Jr, Cupp CC. Advanced nasal anatomy. Facial Plast Sur Clin North Am 1994;2(4):393–416
3. Most SP, Murakami CS. A modern approach to nasal osteotomies Facial Plast Surg Clin North Am 2005; 13(1):85–92
4. Harshbarger RJ, Sullivan PK. Lateral nasal osteotomies: implication of bony thickness on fracture patterns. Ann Plast Surg 1999;42(4 365–370, discussion 370–361
5. Aufricht G. Joseph's rhinoplasty with some modifications. Surg Cli North Am 1971;51(2):299–316
6. Farrior RT. The osteotomy in rhinoplasty. Laryngoscope 1978;88(9 Pt 1 1449–1459

7. Thomas JR, Griner NR, Remmler DJ. Steps for a safer method of osteotomies in rhinoplasty. Laryngoscope 1987;97(6):746–747
8. Webster RC, Davidson TM, Smith RC. Curved lateral osteotomy for airway protection in rhinoplasty. Arch Otolaryngol 1977;103(8):454–458
9. Larrabee WF Jr, Murakami CS. Osteotomy techniques to correct posttraumatic deviation of the nasal pyramid: a technical note. J Craniomaxillofac Trauma 2000; 6(1):43–47
10. Anderson JR. A new approach to rhinoplasty. Trans Am Acad Ophthalmol Otolaryngol 1966;70(2):183–192
11. Byrne PJ, Walsh WE, Hilger PA. The use of "inside-out" lateral osteotomies to improve outcome in rhinoplasty. Arch Facial Plast Surg 2003;5(3):251–255
12. Rohrich RJ, Minoli JJ, Adams WP, Hollier LH. The lateral nasal osteotomy in rhinoplasty: an anatomic endoscopic comparison of the external versus the internal approach. Plast Reconstr Surg 1997;99(5): 1309–1312, discussion 1313
13. Murakami CS, Larrabee WF. Comparison of osteotomy techniques in the treatment of nasal fractures. Facial Plast Surg 1992;8(4): 209–219
14. Larrabee WF Jr. Open rhinoplasty and the upper third of the nose. Facial Plast Surg Clin North Am 1993;1:23–38
15. Parkes ML, Kamer F, Morgan WR. Double lateral osteotomy in rhinoplasty. Arch Otolaryngol 1977;103(6): 344–348

43 Surgery of the Middle Vault

Ira D. Papel

Management of the middle vault in rhinoplasty was for many years considered little more than removal of a hump deformity. The traditional reduction rhinoplasty often included sharp resection of the middle vault apex (cartilage and mucosa) with little regard to nasal function or long-term sequelae. In the 1980s, surgeons began to describe long-term complications of this approach[1] and modified rhinoplasty techniques to avoid these problems. Reconstructive rhinoplasty techniques were also developed to repair damaged middle vaults. Nasal valve pathology is often overlooked as a source of nasal obstruction. Many surgeons concentrate on the septum, turbinates, and presence of mucosal abnormalities before considering the lateral nasal wall as a problem. Although it is important to rule out inflammatory, immunologic, septal, and other abnormalities in the nose, it is also important to consider the internal and external nasal valves in a differential diagnosis. In this chapter we will describe these techniques and identify patients who are at risk of middle vault pathology in rhinoplasty.

Anatomy

Beneath the nasal skin and soft tissue, the middle vault is composed of the paired upper lateral cartilages and attached mucosa. At the cephalic end the upper lateral cartilages are fused with the nasal bones, inserting just under the caudal end of the bones. Medially the cartilages fuse with the cartilaginous septum, the caudal end separating from the septum and lying fairly mobile. The caudal end of the upper lateral cartilages may have a recurvature or scroll that has attachments to the lower lateral cartilages. Laterally the upper lateral cartilages approach the pyriform apertures, fusing with dense fibrous tissue. Mucosa is tightly attached to the internal surface of the cartilages and is continuous with the lining of the septum and lateral nasal wall (**Fig. 43.1**).

The caudal margin of the upper lateral cartilage, the septum, the floor of the nose, and possibly the anterior head of the inferior turbinate define the internal nasal valve. This is generally regarded as the narrowest point of air flow through the nose. The angle between the septum and the upper lateral cartilage has a normal range of 10 to 20 degrees, and narrowing of this angle due to trauma, surgery, or disease can cause significant nasal obstructive symptoms. The nasal valve has a cross-sectional area of 55 to 83 mm^2 and represents the narrowest area of the nasal passage. The nasal valve is the site of greatest nasal resistance[2] (**Fig. 43.2**).

Significance of Middle Vault Anatomy in Rhinoplasty

Rhinoplastic surgeons must be able to evaluate and address the middle vault region to provide acceptable functional and cosmetic results. Many patients present with a wide middle vault and internal nasal valve where hump reduction and narrowing of the internal valve do not cause later problems. This is particularly true in the African American population. However, the surgeon must be able to identify patients in whom further narrowing is ill advised. In addition, repair of the incompetent internal nasal valve, with appropriate nasal width, must be part of the rhinoplastic surgeon's capabilities.

Hump reduction is probably the most common maneuver in rhinoplasty. In traditional hump reduction surgery, the cartilaginous hump is excised as a block with the underlying mucosa. This separates the upper lateral cartilages from the natural attachment to the septum and usually interrupts the continuity of the mucoperichondrium. This leads to inferomedial collapse of the upper lateral cartilages, which is worse if the mucosa is also severed.[3] This may not be apparent immediately after rhinoplasty but may present gradually over a period of years, with tell-tale deformities. The capacity of the middle vault to withstand the inward pressure of inspiration may be reduced. Chronic nasal obstruction due to valve narrowing may develop gradually or be apparent immediately. There are other conditions that may precipitate internal nasal valve obstruction. Facial paralysis can lead to ptosis of the lateral nasal soft tissues and narrowing of the valve, causing symptomatic obstruction. Cancer resection of the lower two thirds of the nose may lead to scar contraction and distortion of the valve. Senile tip ptosis can also cause significant narrowing and congestion (**Fig. 43.3**).

Risk Factors for Middle Vault Problems

Several risk factors have been identified as predisposing to middle vault problems in rhinoplasty.[4] Not recognizing these warning signs may inadvertently result in physical

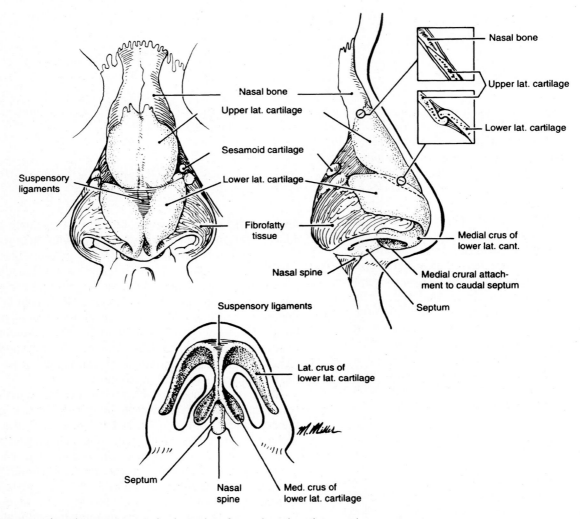

Fig. 43.1 Nasal cartilage anatomy, with relationship of upper lateral cartilage to other structures.

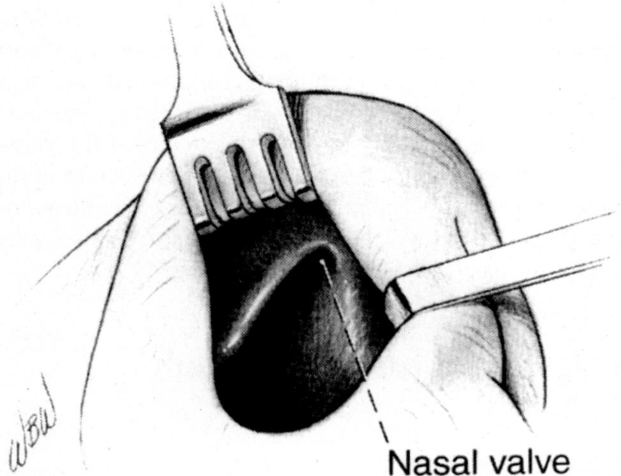

Fig. 43.2 Clinical appearance of internal nasal valve, which is the narrowest cross section of the nasal airway.

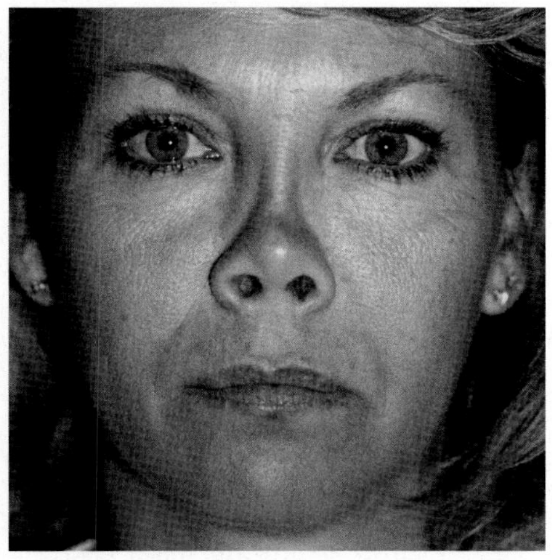

Fig. 43.3 Appearance of patient after rhinoplasty with narrowing of the middle vault causing nasal obstruction.

signs, such as inverted-V deformity, middle vault collapse on inspiration, overly narrow radix line, dorsal asymmetry, and eventual nasal obstruction.

The inverted-V deformity has been recognized as the classic sign of middle vault pathology following rhinoplasty. The cause seems to be posterior displacement of the nasal bones and upper lateral cartilages after osteotomies, combined with overresection or posterior displacement of the upper lateral cartilages. If dorsal reduction involves mucosal interruption or detachment of soft tissue over the nasal bones and upper lateral cartilages, these structures have little to support them after osteotomy.[5]

Specific risk factors associated with middle vault postoperative problems include short nasal bones, long and weak upper lateral cartilages, thin skin, tall and narrow noses, and previous trauma or surgery.[6]

Prevention of Middle Vault Problems

Proper preoperative evaluation and planning can prevent most middle vault complications. This allows preventive rhinoplastic techniques to be employed and improves functional and aesthetic results. These techniques include preservation of middle vault support structures, judicious use of spreader grafts, use of conservative osteotomies, and replacement of cartilage support in revision rhinoplasty cases. Every rhinoplasty patient deserves individual assessment and operative planning. Many middle vault characteristics may not be appreciated on the initial physical examination. Good quality photographs can be invaluable in preoperative evaluation and should be studied prior to surgery.

Toriumi and Johnson[4] have demonstrated that preservation of the middle vault mucosa helps to minimize posterior displacement of the upper lateral cartilages during hump removal. This mucosal bridge between the septum and upper lateral cartilages can be preserved by the creation of junction tunnels under the attachment area of the septum and upper lateral cartilage. Preserving this mucosa also helps to maintain a blood-free surgical field.

When performing dorsal reduction a conservative resection should be done. Maintenance of a strong dorsal line is usually desirable for both aesthetic and functional reasons. In a patient with dorsal convexity and a narrow vault, it may be necessary to reduce the dorsum minimally, widen the middle vault with spreader grafts, and increase tip projection to achieve nasal harmony.

A common postoperative problem is overnarrowing of the nose due to medial displacement of the nasal bones after aggressive complete osteotomies. Although many rhinoplasty patients desire a narrower nose, narrowing can be excessive and detrimental to both aesthetics and function. By maintaining the soft tissue attachments of the nasal bones and upper lateral cartilages, excessive medial and posterior displacement can be prevented. Internal splinting can also prevent excessive narrowing in the early postoperative period.

Correction of Middle Vault Pathology

Surgical correction of middle vault problems can be preventive or corrective. When the risk factors identified are present, preventive action may be required. In a revision

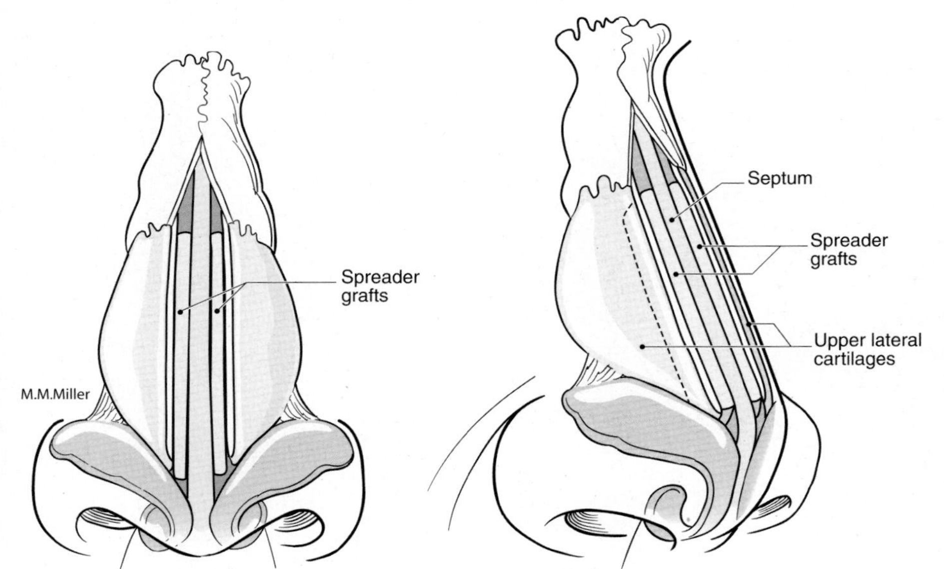

Fig. 43.4 Ideal placement of spreader grafts between septum and upper lateral cartilages. (A,B) Spreader grafts. Upper lateral cartilage.

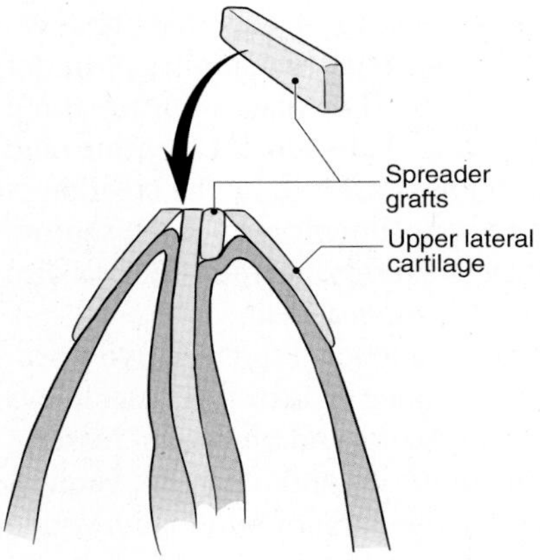

Fig. 43.5 Placement of spreader graft lateralizes and elevates the upper lateral cartilage widening the middle vault.

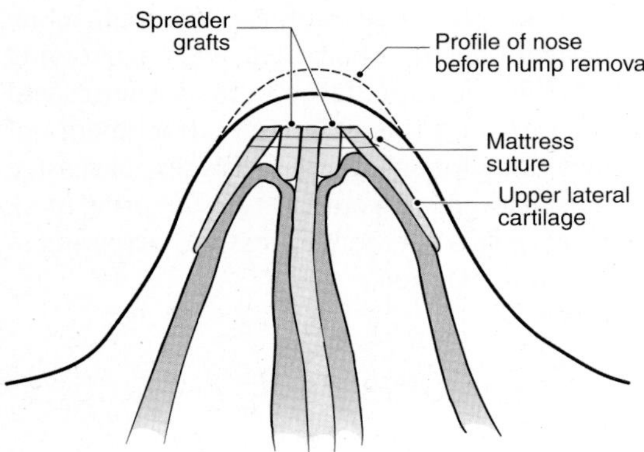

Fig. 43.6 Spreader grafts in place and fixed with mattress sutures. The original dorsal height is identified.

rhinoplasty multiple modalities may be utilized. These techniques may include cartilage grafts, precise structural realignment, and fixation of nasal valve structures.

Spreader grafts are probably the most common corrective modality used for middle vault rehabilitation. First described by Sheen and Sheen,[7] these are rectangular cartilage grafts placed between the junctions of the upper lateral cartilages and septum to widen the nasal valve. These cartilage grafts not only lateralize the upper lateral cartilages but add rigidity to the middle vault to resist inward motion on inspiration. They can be placed either through open or closed rhinoplasty techniques, but they are easier to stabilize with direct sutures via the open approach. Septal cartilage is the most frequently used grafting material, but auricular cartilage may be used if septum is not available. Spreader grafts can also be utilized for aesthetic purposes. For patients with unilateral middle vault depressions due to congenital, traumatic, or iatrogenic causes, a single spreader graft can elevate and lateralize the upper lateral cartilage and restore symmetry.

The surgical technique for placement of spreader grafts varies with the surgical approach. Sheen and Sheen[7] and Constantian and Clardy[8] describe placing the grafts in precise submucoperichondrial tunnels along the dorsal edge of the septum without separation of the existing upper lateral cartilages from the septum. This is accomplished through a closed rhinoplasty approach.

In many revision rhinoplasty cases involving middle vault pathology, separation of the septum and upper lateral cartilages has occurred due to hump removal. There is usually fibrous tissue instead of a fusion of

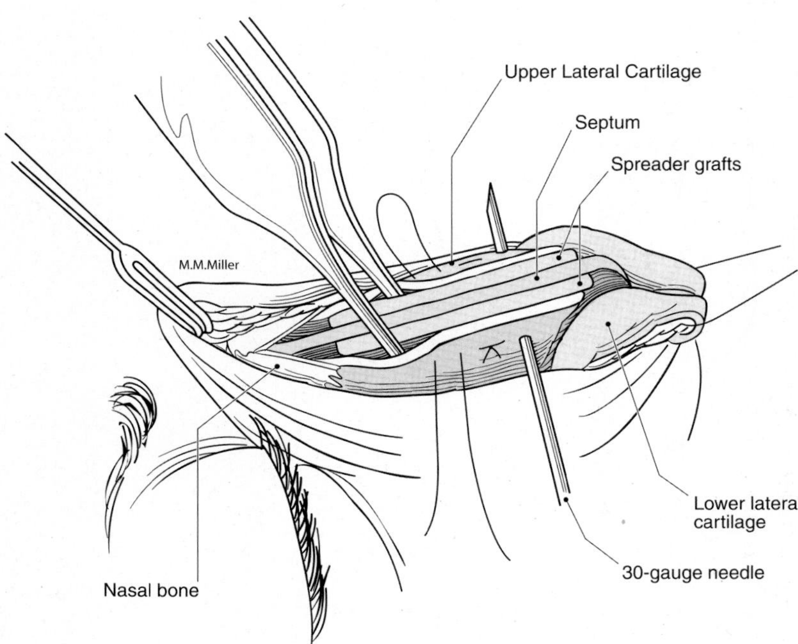

Fig. 43.7 Demonstration of mattress suture technique for fixation of spreader grafts.

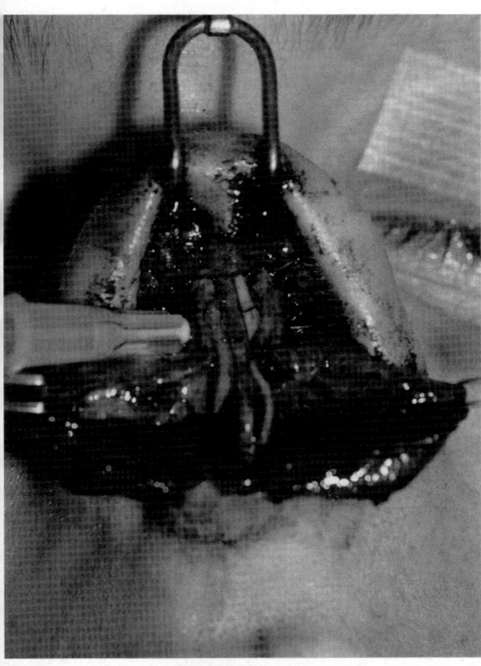

Fig. 43.8 Temporary placement of a 30-gauge needle fixes grafts and makes placement of mattress sutures technically easier.

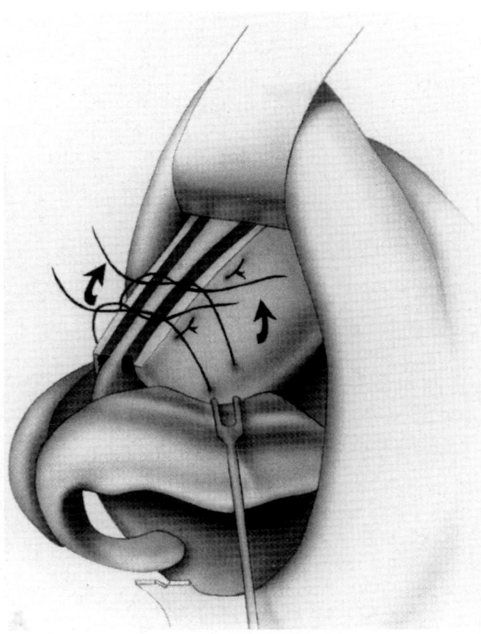

Fig. 43.9 Flaring suture can be used to cause further widening of the middle vault when combined with spreader grafts. (From Park SS. Treatment of the internal nasal valve. Facial Plast Clin North Am 1999;7:333–345. Reprinted by permission.)

cartilage at the internal nasal valve. Therefore, preservation of the mucoperichondrium and creation of a pocket for the graft placement through an open approach is usually preferred. If the upper lateral cartilages are fused with the septum, sharp dissection from the internal side with an elevator will preserve the mucoperichondrial flap attachments and preserve stability. At times the upper lateral cartilages may have been almost completely resected. In this situation, conchal cartilage grafts may be necessary to provide lateral support in addition to spreader grafts. The grafts are carved, aligned, and fixed in position with 5–0 PDS (polydiaxonone; Ethicon, Inc., Somerville, NJ) mattress sutures. Most spreader grafts are 1.5 to 2.5 cm in length and 1 to 3 mm in width. In general, the grafts should run along the dorsal septum from below the bony–cartilaginous junction to the anterior septal angle. In severe cases the grafts may be layered to provide additional bulk. Grafts of unequal width may be used to accommodate asymmetries in the middle vault. Spreader grafts may also be used as internal stents to help straighten a caudal septal deflection. The technique of spreader graft placement and fixation is demonstrated in **Figs. 43.4 to 43.7.** Placement of a 30-gauge needle through the cartilage complex makes placement of the sutures much easier (**Fig. 43.8**).

Grafts that are wide at the end may lateralize the caudal portion of the upper lateral cartilages, creating fullness in the lateral supratip area. Releasing the lateral crura from the scroll area allows for free motion, some overlap, and prevents distortion. In some cases it may be advisable to place a graft of crushed cartilage over the dorsum and spreader grafts to smooth the profile. AlloDerm (LifeCell Corp., Branchburg, NJ) may also be used for this purpose.

In an effort to further support the nasal valve, Schlosser and Park[9] described the use of flaring sutures to improve the cross-sectional area of the internal nasal valves. The additional treatment here is a 5–0 nylon clear mattress suture that spans the upper lateral cartilages

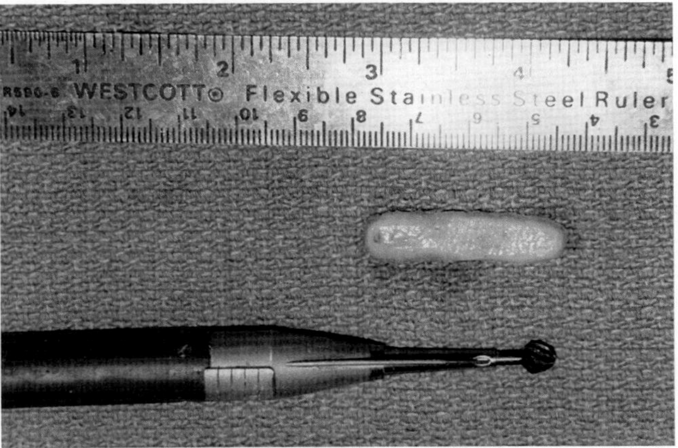

Fig. 43.10 Cranial bone grafts can be used for dorsal reconstruction and provision of middle + vault support.

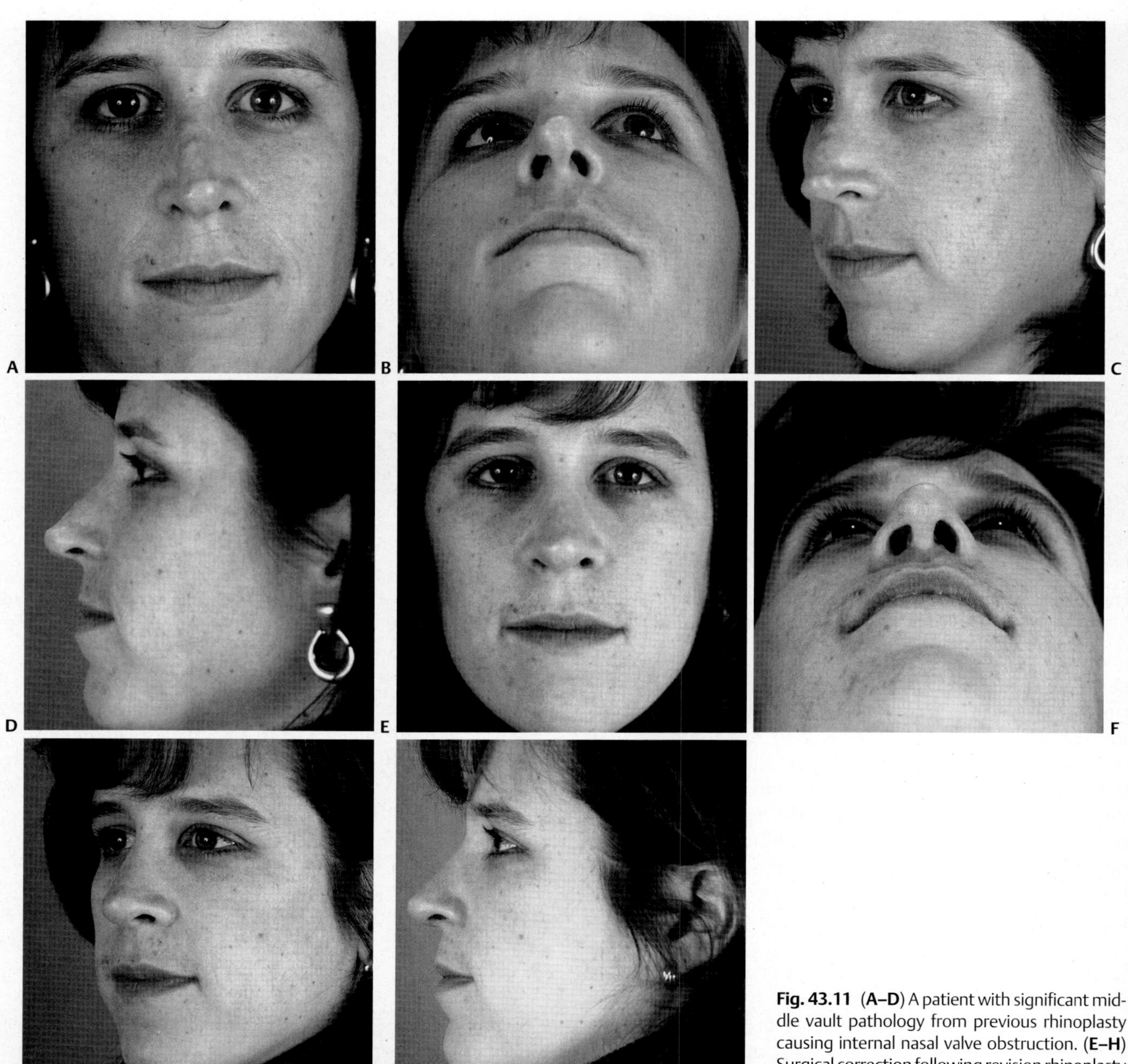

Fig. 43.11 **(A–D)** A patient with significant middle vault pathology from previous rhinoplasty causing internal nasal valve obstruction. **(E–H)** Surgical correction following revision rhinoplasty with spreader grafts and tip correction.

and the nasal dorsum horizontally. Tightening the suture increases the angle of the nasal valve, theoretically improving nasal function. Park's study indicated that flaring sutures used concomitantly with spreader grafts increase air flow more than spreader grafts alone[10] (**Fig. 43.9**).

Patients with saddle nose defects may have middle vault collapse with no support for the soft tissue. Fixated of a dorsal graft may help support the inferior soft tissues and stabilize the nasal valve. The use of cranial bone grafts combined with lag-screw fixation has been very helpful in these patients.[11] The cranial bone can serve as an anchor for reconstructive grafts and provide vertical height to the middle vault[12] (**Fig. 43.10**).

Nasal obstruction in rhinoplasty may have multiple causes. The middle vault may present with congenital, traumatic, or iatrogenic pathology that must be addressed during rhinoplasty. Specific physical signs and symptoms should alert the surgeon that middle vault intervention is necessary to prevent unwanted sequelae later. This will lead to better functional and aesthetic rhinoplasty results.

Case Example

The patient shown in **Fig. 43.11** presented with a history of previous rhinoplasty and increasing nasal obstruction for 10 years. The symptoms had gotten progressively worse and were not relieved by multiple medications. Examination revealed internal valve collapse bilaterally, with physical evidence of significant upper lateral cartilage resection. The residual middle vault cartilage was inferomedially displaced, causing narrowing of the middle vault. The cartilage edges and bone were also irregular and asymmetric. The lower lateral cartilages were also asymmetric with a bossa on the right. The preoperative condition is exhibited in **Fig. 43.11A–D.**

This patient underwent an open rhinoplasty procedure with use of spreader grafts, reduction of tip projection, interdomal sutures, columellar strut, and smoothing of the dorsal bone. The 2-year postoperative photographs are shown in **Fig. 43.11E–H**. The middle vault is more symmetrical and has appropriate width for function and cosmesis.

References

1. Sheen JH. Spreader graft: a method of reconstructing the roof of the middle nasal vault following rhinoplasty. Plast Reconstr Surg 1984; 73:230–237
2. Kasperbauer JL, Kern EB. Nasal valve physiology: implications in nasal surgery. Otolaryngol Clin North Am 1987;20:669–719
3. Toriumi DM. Management of the middle nasal vault in rhinoplasty. Facial Plast Surg Clin North Am 1995;3:77–91
4. Toriumi DM, Johnson CM. Open structure rhinoplasty: featured technical points and long-term follow-up. Facial Plast Surg Clin North Am 1993;1:1–22
5. Tebbetts JB. Primary Rhinoplasty: A New Approach to the Logic and Technique. St. Louis: CV Mosby; 1998
6. Robin JL. Extramucosal method in rhinoplasty. Aesthetic Plast Surg 1979;3:179–200
7. Sheen JH, Sheen AP. Aesthetic Rhinoplasty. St. Louis: CV Mosby; 1987
8. Constantian MB, Clardy RB. The relative importance of septal and nasal valvular surgery in correcting airway obstruction in primary and secondary rhinoplasty. Plast Reconstr Surg 1996;98:38–58
9. Schlosser RJ, Park SS. Surgery for the dysfunctional nasal valve. Arch Facial Plast Surg 1999;1:105–110
10. Park SS. The flaring suture to augment the repair of the dysfunctional nasal valve. Plast Reconstr Surg 1998;101:1120–1122
11. Frodel JL Jr, Marentette LJ, Quatela VC, Weinstein GS. Calvarial bone graft harvest. Techniques, considerations, and morbidity. Arch Otolaryngol Head Neck Surg 1993;119:17–23
12. Papel ID. Augmentation rhinoplasty utilizing cranial bone grafts. Md Med J 1991;40:479–483

44 Surgery of the Nasal Tip: Intranasal Approach

Gilbert J. Nolst Trenité

Nasal tip surgery is the most challenging part of rhinoplastic surgery. In the great variety of procedures for nasal tip surgery and individual differences in tip anatomy, a systematic rational approach as advocated by Tardy is obligatory (**Table 44.1**). Of the three basic approaches—nondelivery, delivery, and the external approach—the external approach is the most traumatic. Nevertheless, that approach has gained enormous popularity over the past decade. The possibility of accessing the anatomical deformities by direct inspection of the nasal cartilaginous and bony framework, and much easier bimanual sculpturing under direct vision, has stimulated, in particular, less experienced surgeons to choose this approach. One should keep in mind that the less the surgical trauma the more predictable will be the long-term outcome.

In modern rhinoplasty, the basic philosophy is to use the least traumatic approach that will enable us to apply the appropriate techniques to correct the specific deformities. In this chapter, the less traumatic approaches (nondelivery and delivery) will be emphasized.

Facial Analysis

Before analyzing the typical nasal deformity, the surgeon should consider other major aesthetic components in the facial complex—forehead, eyes, lips, and chin—so as to create harmony and balance between these components. Aesthetic parameters of the nasal tip are, in the frontal view (**Fig. 44.1**),

- tip-defining points
- width of the tip

in the lateral view (**Fig. 44.2**),

- tip projection
- nasolabial angle
- ratio between ala and lobule
- extension of the columella below the nares
- columella double break

and in the basal view (**Fig. 44.3**),

- equilateral triangle of the tip
- lobular, intermediate, and basal part of the columella
- nostril shape and lateral alar side walls
- columella base

With these aesthetic guidelines in mind, the surgeon should assess and document the tip deformities (shape, projection, and rotation) (**Fig. 44.4A**). Furthermore, standardized photographic documentation (at least six standard views) is obligatory. The quality of the skin (thickness, elasticity, and pathological conditions), evaluation of the tip support (tip recoil; **Fig. 44.5**), and shape, size, and thickness of the alar cartilage play an important role in assessment of the surgical possibilities. Taking into account the desires of the patient and the information obtained by examination (inspection and palpation), the physician should devise a well-documented operative plan (**Fig. 44.4B**) and discuss it with the patient during a second consultation.

Surgical Approaches and Incisions

There are two basic surgical approaches in intranasal tip surgery, the delivery and the nondelivery approach. Indications for each of these approaches depend on the

Table 44.1 Approaches to Nasal Tip Surgery

Approaches	Incisions	Indications	Techniques
Nondelivery	Transcartilaginous or intercartilaginous	Slight bulbosity; minimal tip rotation	Cephalic resection of lateral crus (complete strip)
Delivery	Intercartilaginous and marginal	Moderate bulbosity; extra tip rotation; bifidity; asymmetry	Cartilage resection; scoring and morselization; alar (domal) suturing (complete or interrupted strip)
External	Broken columellar and marginal	Congenital deformities; extensive revisions; severe nasal trauma; elaborate reduction and augmentation; shield graft; columella strut	Cartilage resections lateral/medial crura; alar cartilage modifications and reorientation (complete strip/interrupted strip)

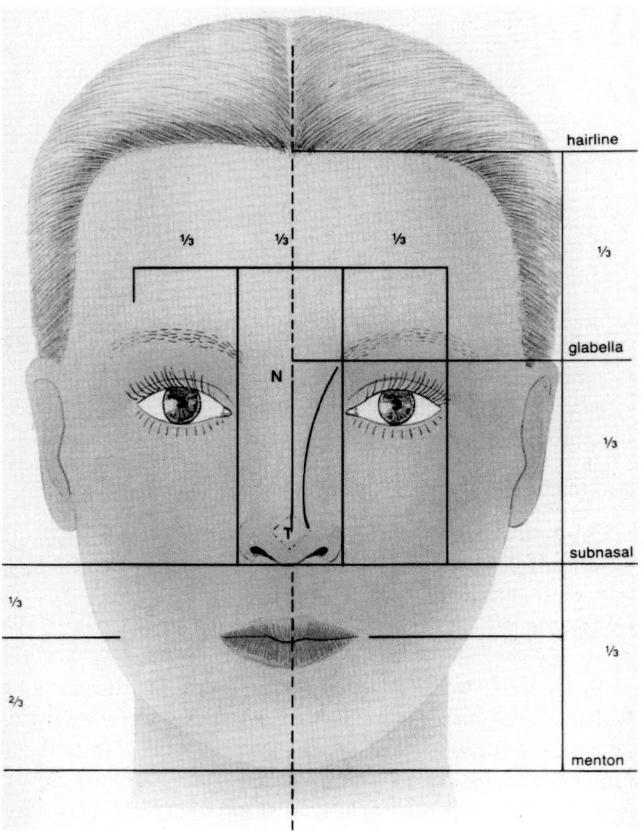

Fig. 44.1 Frontal view of the face divided into aesthetic proportions (equal thirds) with a gently curving unbroken line from the supraorbital ridge along the lateral border of the dorsum to the tip-defining point on the same side.

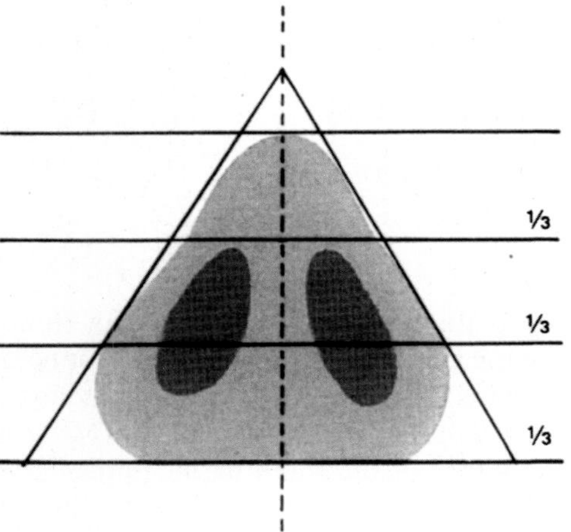

Fig. 44.3 Basal view of the nose, which should have approximatel the form of an equilateral triangle with the lobular, intermediate, and basal parts of the columella as three equal segments.

specific anatomy of the nose and what proposed changes (**Table 44.1**), including volume reduction, reconstruction, rotation, and change of projection, are planned.

The Nondelivery Approach

The nondelivery approach is very appropriate for (1) small volume reduction of the lateral crus and (2) slight cephalic rotation of the tip.

Volume reduction can be easily accomplished with a *transcartilaginous incision,* in which only slight surgical trauma occurs. The operative procedure of the cartilage-splitting nondelivery approach is as follows: after drawing

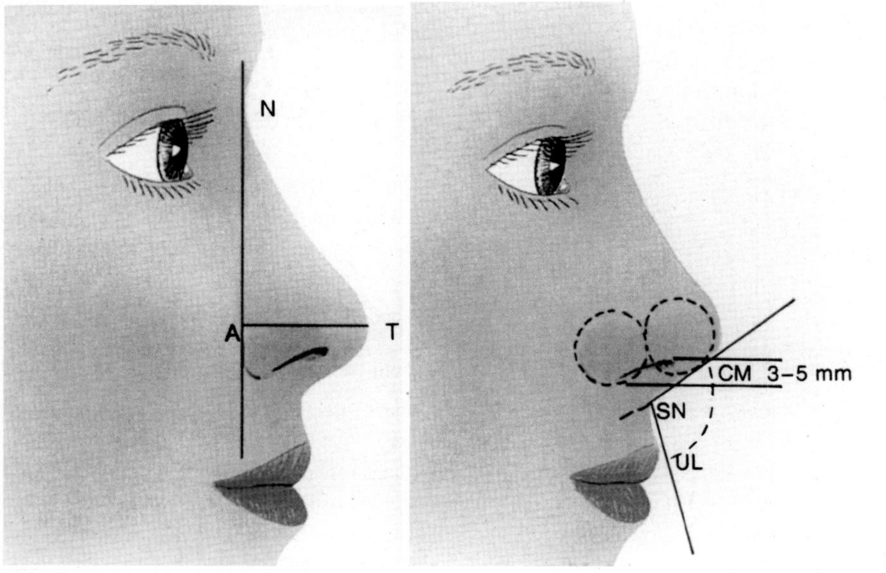

Fig. 44.2 (**A**) The ratio TA/TN as a measure for tip projection. (**B**) The nasolabial angle (CM-SN-UL), the ratio between ala and lobule and extension of the columella below the nares (3 to 5 mm).

SEPTO-RHINOPLASTY ASSESSMENT FORM

born ... ☐ male ☐ female

Septo-rhinoplasty: ☐ functional ☐ aesthetic ☐ both
Type: ☐ primary ☐ revision ☐ non-caucasion ☐ cleft lip

Septum, valve and turbinates

Septum pathol.
☐ deviation
area 1 2 3 4 5 L
area 1 2 3 4 5 R
☐ perforation
diam. ... cm.
☐ cartilage loss
area 1 2 3 4 5
☐ other

Turbinate pathol.

		atroph.	hypertr.	other
inf.	→	☐	☐	☐
med.	→	☐	☐	☐

Valve pathol.
☐ too narrow
☐ too wide
☐ other

Tip columella, vestibulum and ala

Tip pathol.
☐ bulbous
☐ bifid
☐ asym.
☐ overproj.
☐ underproj.

Tip recoil
weak →1→2→3→4→5 strong

Columella pathol.
☐ retracted
☐ deviated
☐ broadened
☐ other

Vestibulum pathol.
☐ stenosis
☐ other

Alar pathol.
☐ insuff. ☐ flaring ☐ other

Osseo-cartilaginous vault

Skin qual.
thin →1→2→3→4→5 thick

Vault pathol.
☐ deviated
☐ cartil. ☐ bony ☐ both
☐ irregular
☐ cartil. ☐ bony ☐ both
☐ saddle
☐ cartil. ☐ bony ☐ both
☐ hump
☐ tension nose

Rhinometry
☐ acoustic
☐ mano

Photography
☐ standard
☐ other

Anesthesia: ☐ local
☐ iv analgesia
☐ general

☐ day care
☐ hospitalization

☐ pre-assessment

Expected operation time ..... Operation date ......

Fig. 44.4 **(A)** Septorhinoplasty assessment form.

SEPTO-RHINOPLASTY OPERATION FORM

Name ... born ... □ male □ female
pat. reg. nr. .....
operating date .... anaesthesia: □ local □ i.v. □ general

Approach

□ endonasal
□ delivery
□ open

Incisions

□ hemitransf.
□ Killian
□ part. transf.
□ compl. transf.
□ marginal
□ rim
□ intercartil.
□ transcartil.
□ V-Y procedure
□ Z-plasty
□ broken columella

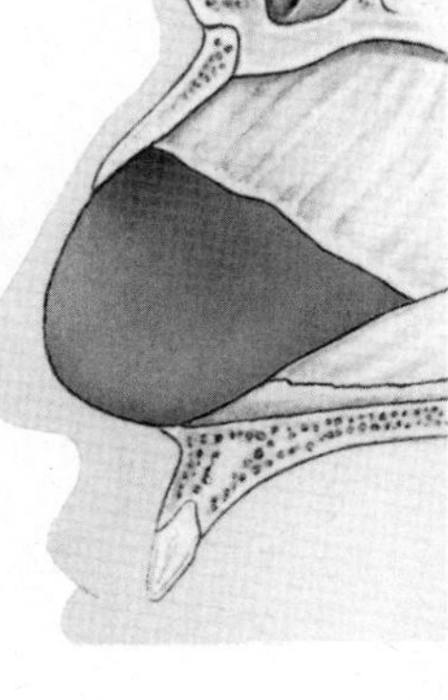

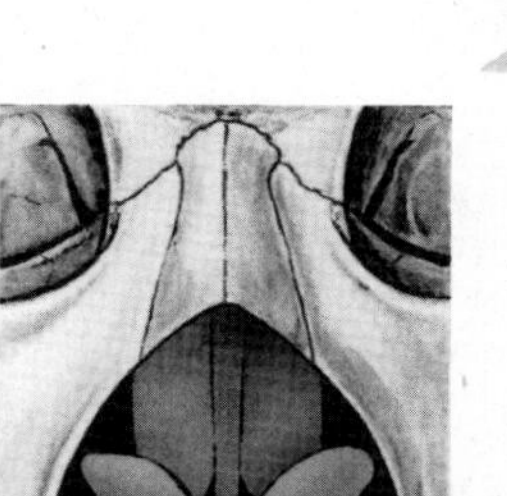

Type of grafts

□ autog. septal
□ autog. ear
□ autog. rib
□ composite ear
□ allogeneic
□ xenograft
□ alloplast
□ skin

Graft site

□ spreader
□ columella strut
□ shield
□ tip onlay
□ dorsal onlay
□ dorsal lat.
□ alar batton
□ maxillary
□ naso-front.
□ naso-lab.

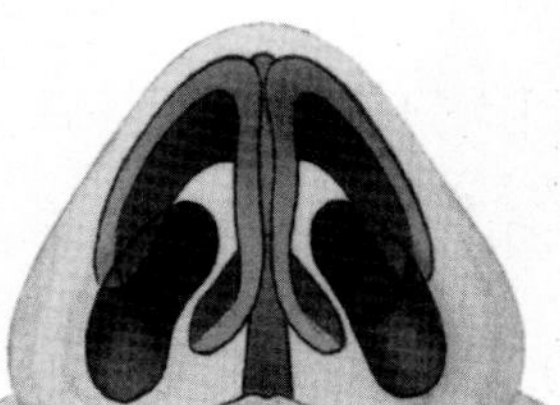
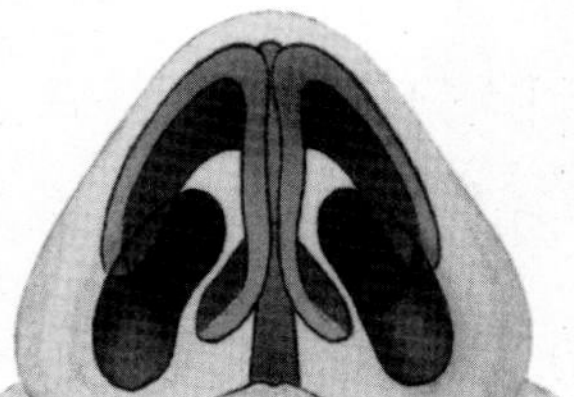
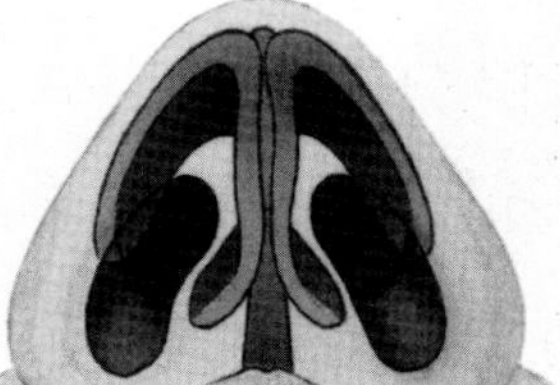
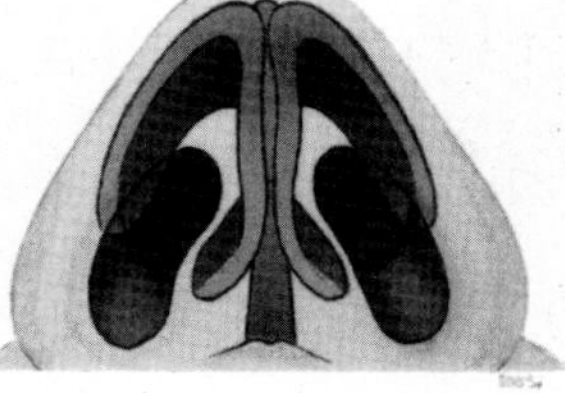
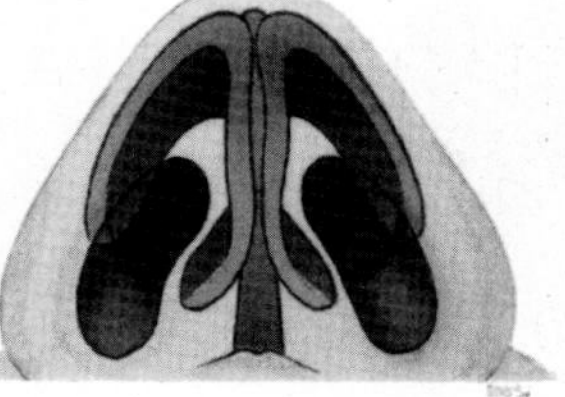
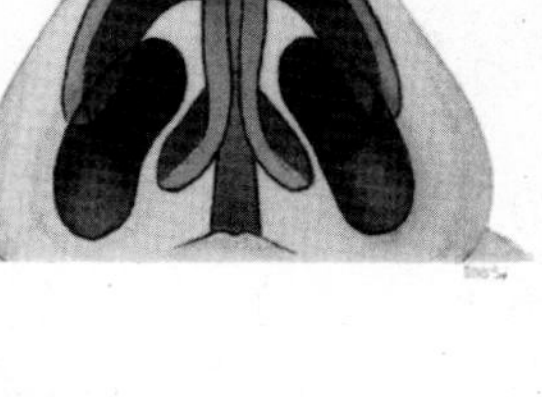

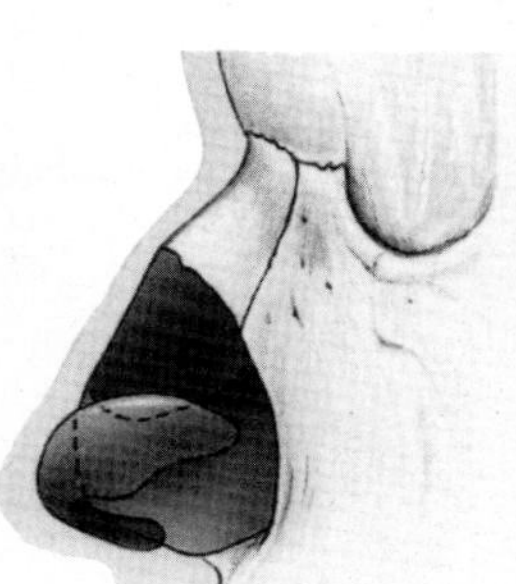

Technique

Septoplasty

Cart. septal work
□ basal strip
□ post. chondrotomy
□ scoring
□ splinting
□ resection

Bony septal work
□ ant. spine red.
□ ant. spine realignm.
□ perpend. plate
□ vomer
□ grafting

Turbinate reduct.
□ inf. □ L □ R
□ med. □ L □ R

Tip surgery

□ cephalic resection
□ complete strip
□ incomplete strip
□ suturing
□ interdomal
□ transdomal
□ lat. crural steal

Bony cart. vault surg.
□ hump resection
□ upper lateral
□ augmentation

Osteotomies
□ medial-oblique
□ intermediate
□ lateral (intranasal)
□ lateral (percutaneous)
□ infraction
□ outfraction
□ realignment

Alar base surgery

□ V-shape wedge
□ invert. V-shape wedge
□ rectang. shape wedge

Direct postoperative care

□ packing removal . . . days p.o. □ daycare
□ dressing removal . . . days p.o. □ hospitalization
□ sutures removal . . . days p.o. □ antibiotics
post op. consultation date . . . . . . □ other med.

Fig. 44.4 *Continued* (**B**) Septorhinoplasty operation form.

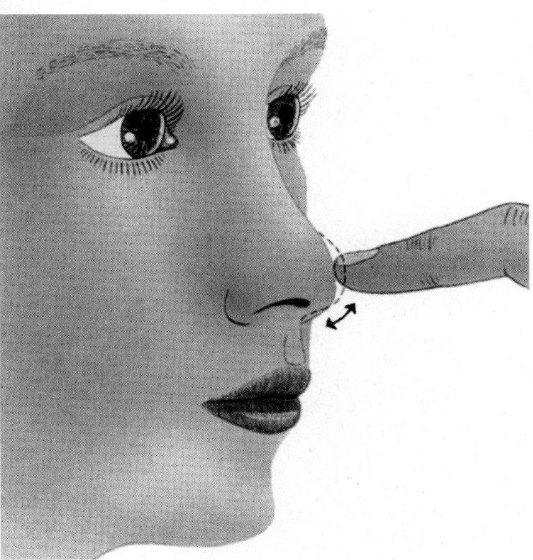

Fig. 44.5 Tip recoil.

the skeletal landmarks and boundaries on the skin of the nose, the most cephalic part of the lateral crus to be resected is outlined with a marking pen on the external skin (**Fig. 44.6**). It is helpful to indicate on the vestibular skin where the transcartilaginous incision should be made. This can be done either by a through-and-through needle from the outside or more elegantly by using the imprint of a surgical instrument on the vestibular skin. Care should be taken to preserve at least 8 to 10 mm of uninterrupted cartilage (in a vertical dimension) of the lateral crus. Although some surgeons make their incisions through the vestibular skin and cartilage concurrently, it facilitates the dissection of the vestibular skin to do this in two stages.

Hydraulic dissection with small depots of local anesthesia at the site of the vestibular incision facilitates dissection in the subperichondrial plane. A vestibular skin incision with a no. 15 blade (**Fig. 44.7**) is followed by dissecting the vestibular skin free from the proposed resection of the cephalic part of the lower lateral cartilage with a pair of sharp, pointed curved scissors, leaving the integrity of the lower lateral intact to ensure the best chance for an uncomplicated healing process (**Fig. 44.8**). Nowadays the retrograde-eversion approach is performed less often. Instead of a transcartilaginous incision, an intercartilaginous incision is made, followed by retrograde dissection over the lateral crus at the nonvestibular side, eversion of the lateral crus, and resection of the planned cephalic portion of the cartilage.

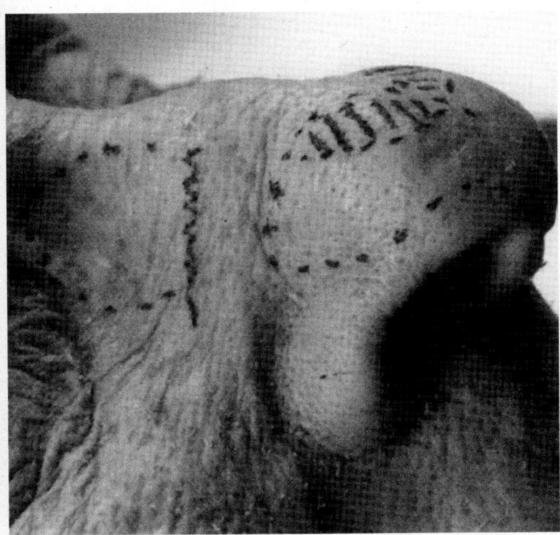

Fig. 44.6 Marking of the skeletal boundaries and the cephalic parts of the lateral crura to be resected.

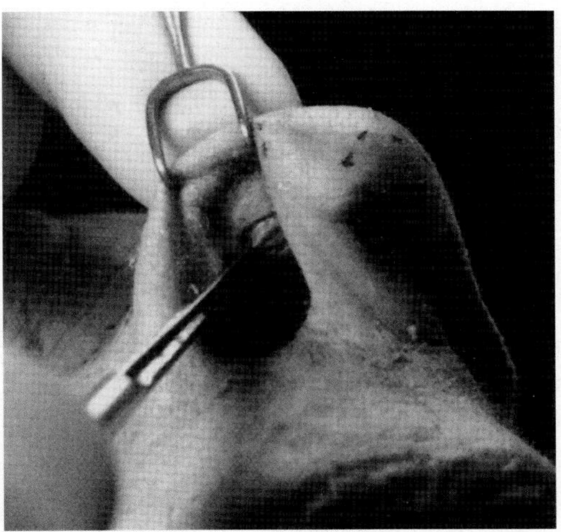

Fig. 44.7 Vestibular skin incision.

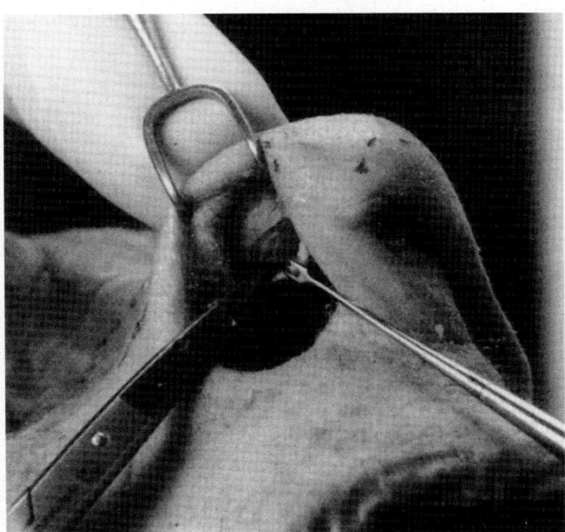

Fig. 44.8 Dissection of vestibular skin and perichondrium (subperichondrially).

The Delivery Approach (Bipedicle Chondrocutaneous Flap)

The delivery approach, though more traumatic, is indicated when the planned changes to the nasal tip constitute more

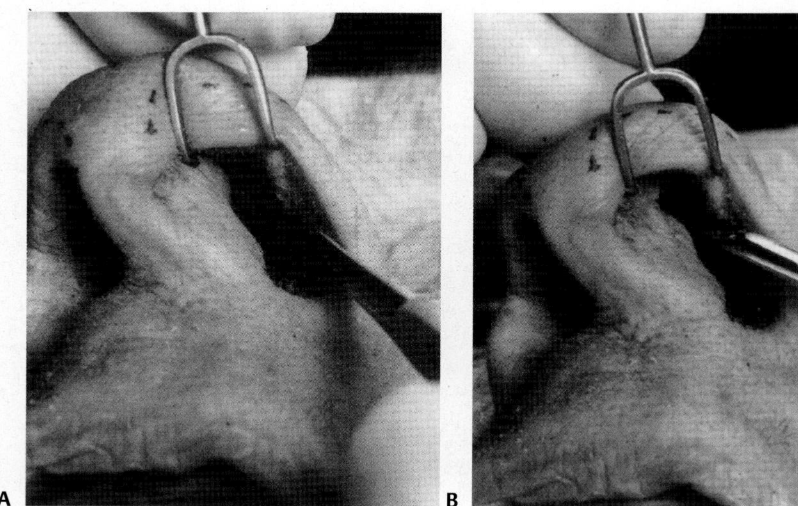
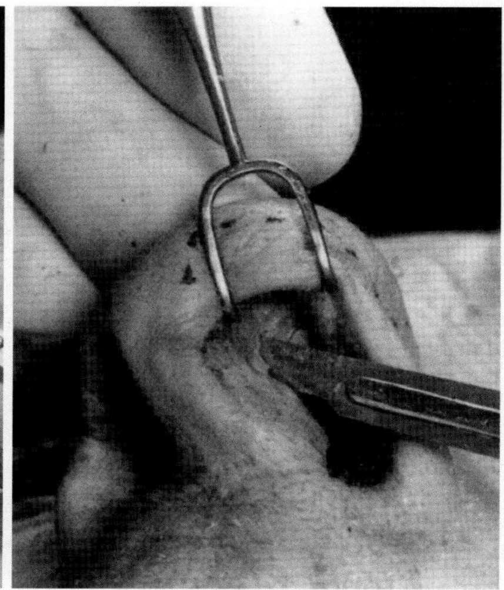

Fig. 44.9 Intercartilaginous incision starting (**A**) (1 to 2 mm) laterally to the internal valve, then (**B**) medially, and (**C**) caudally well around the anterior septal angle.

than a small-volume reduction. The indications for this approach are

- Asymmetry
- Bifidity
- Extracephalic tip rotation
- Alteration of the tip projection

With this approach, it is possible to modify the alar cartilage under direct vision up to the dome and interdomal area. Different operative techniques can be applied including

- Precise excision of cartilage to achieve good symmetry
- Remodeling of the alar cartilage by scoring and morselization
- Interdomal suturing to correct bifidity
- Interruption of the continuity of the alar cartilage to reduce an extremely overprojected tip ("Pinocchio" nose) or to enhance cephalic tip rotation
- Lateral crural steal to enhance tip projection

To ensure a dry operation field depots of local anesthesia are used along the caudal margin of the alar cartilages extending to the nonvestibular side. The infiltration procedure should be performed ~15 to 20 minutes before the dissection has started.

The surgical procedure to deliver the alar cartilages starts with an *intercartilaginous incision* with a no. 15 blade. It is important to make this incision caudally to the valve area to prevent unnecessary scarring in that area. This intercartilaginous incision should be carried well around the anterior septal angle (**Fig. 44.9**). If not, delivery could

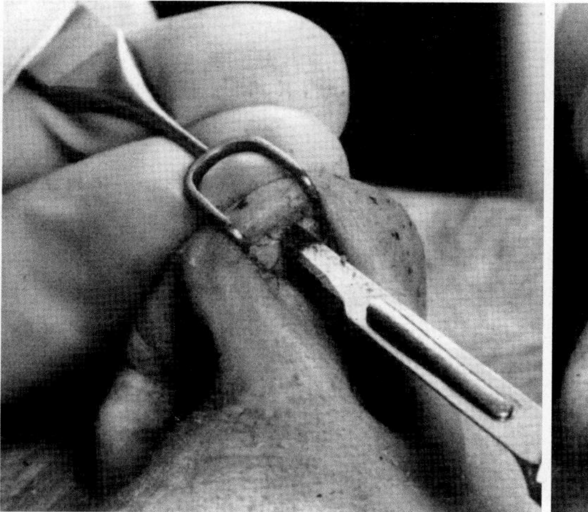
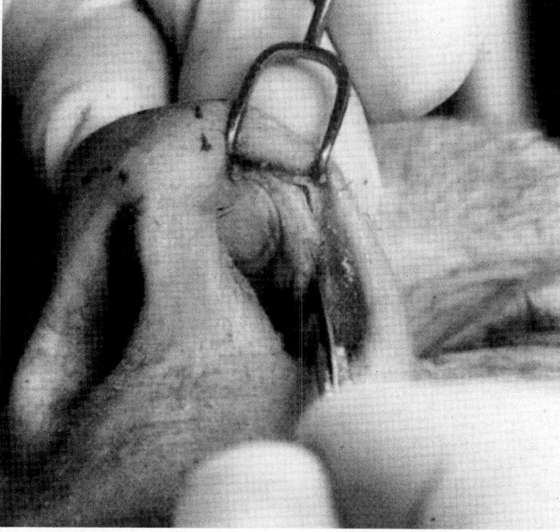

Fig. 44.10 (**A,B**) Marginal incision in a lateral to medial direction along the caudal rim of the lower lateral crus.

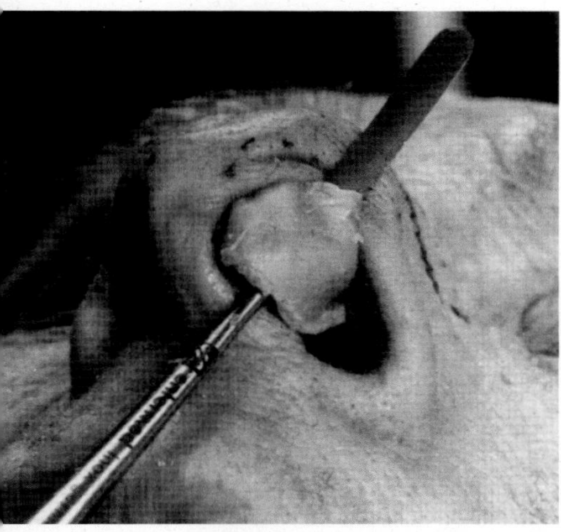

Fig. 44.11 The bipedicle chondrocutaneous flap is delivered.

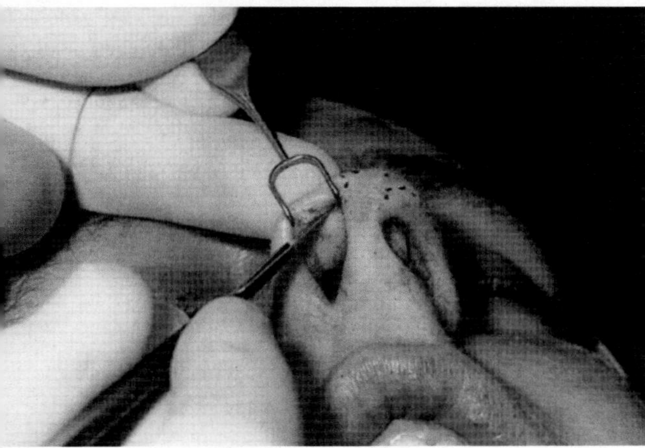

Fig. 44.12 Marginal incision along the caudal border of the lower lateral crus.

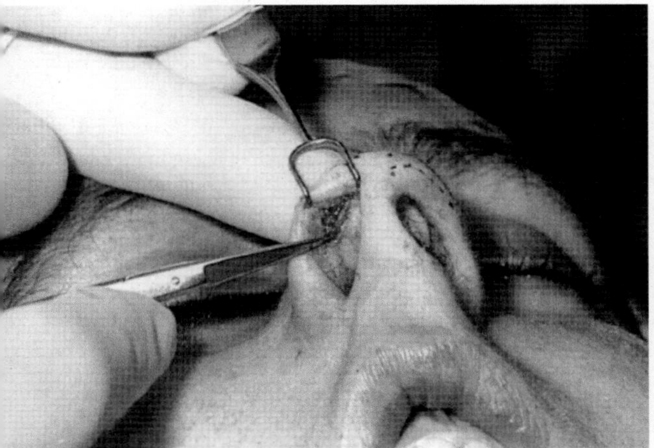

Fig. 44.13 Subperichondrial dissection at the vestibular side of the lateral crus with a pair of sharp curved scissors.

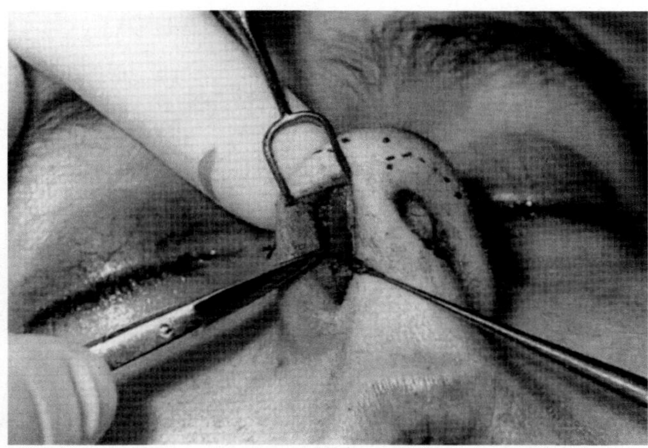

Fig. 44.14 Supraperichondrial dissection of the lateral crus at the nonvestibular side.

be difficult. The next step is to make a *marginal incision* (no. 15 blade), hugging the caudal edge of the lower lateral to prevent surgical damage to "the soft triangle."

To determine the caudal margin of the lower lateral, it is helpful to know that the skin overlying the cartilage does not consist of hair follicles. Palpation with a no. 15 blade helps to locate the caudal margin of the lateral crus.

The incision starts at the upper part of the caudal margin of the medial crus, goes around the dome, and follows the caudal margin of the lateral crus as far as necessary (**Fig. 44.10**). After these two incisions, the nonvestibular side of the lateral crus is freed from the soft tissue by dissection with a pair of sharp curved scissors. To deliver the bipedicle chondrocutaneous flaps, a small hemostat or a Joseph periost elevator is very handy (**Fig. 44.11**).

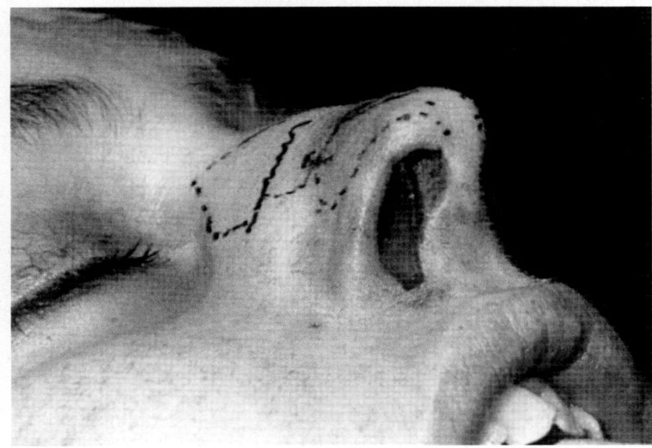

Fig. 44.15 Delivery of the lateral crus.

The Delivery Approach (Lateral Crus Delivery)

Local anesthesia depots, extending to both sides of the lateral crus, are used to ensure a dry operation field and to facilitate especially the subperichondrial dissection at the vestibular side of the lateral crus. A standard marginal incision (no. 15 blade) is made along the caudal border of the lower lateral crus, including the domal area (**Fig. 44.12**). With a pair of sharp curved scissors, the vestibular skin, including the underlying perichondrium,

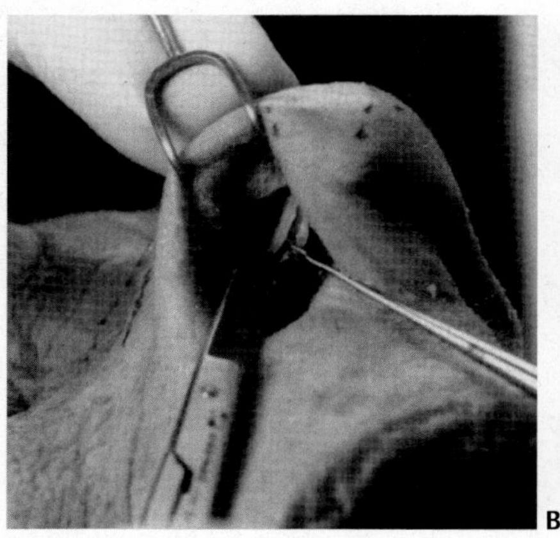

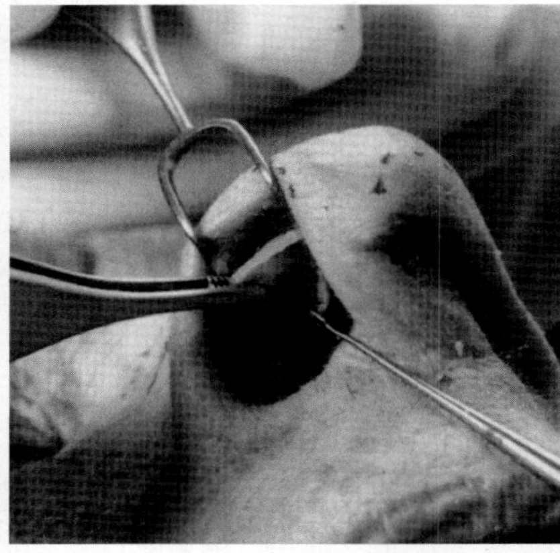

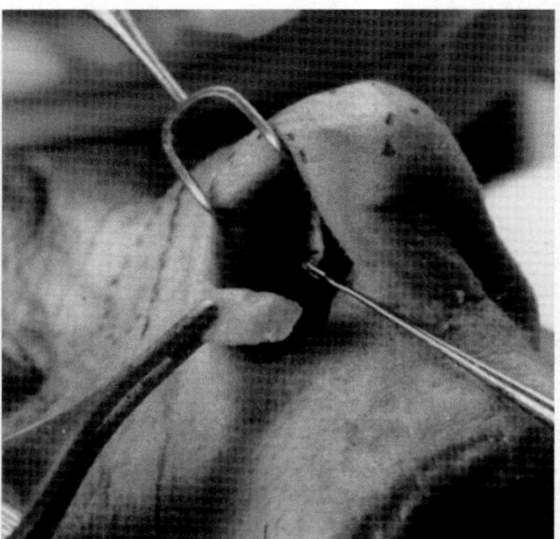

Fig. 44.16 (**A–C**) Resection of the chosen cephalic part of the lateral crus.

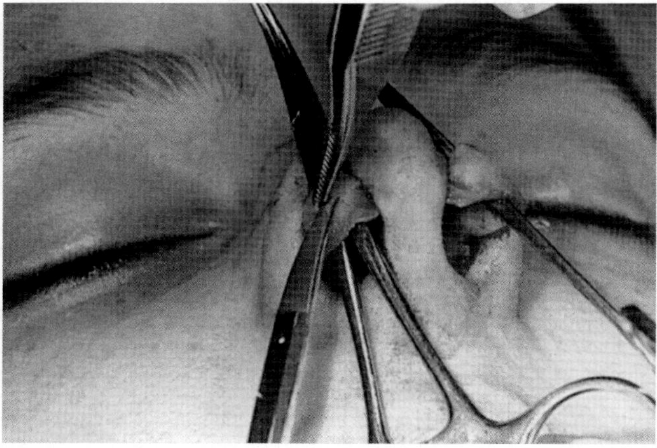

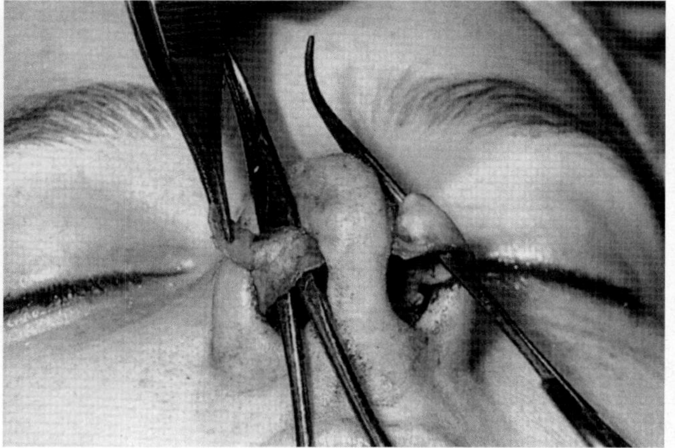

Fig. 44.17 (**A,B**) Precise dissection and excision of a cephalic portion of the lateral crus.

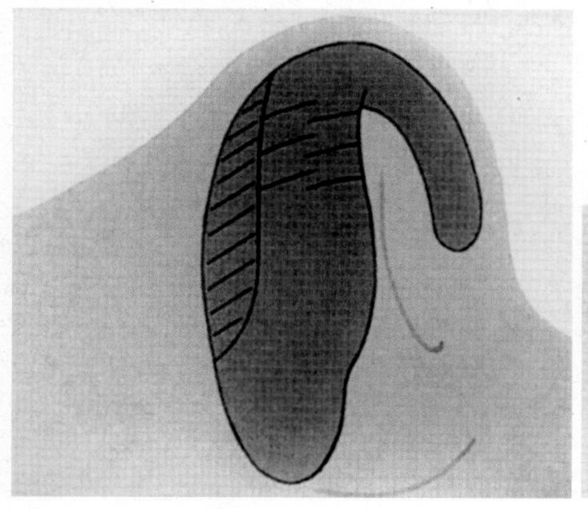

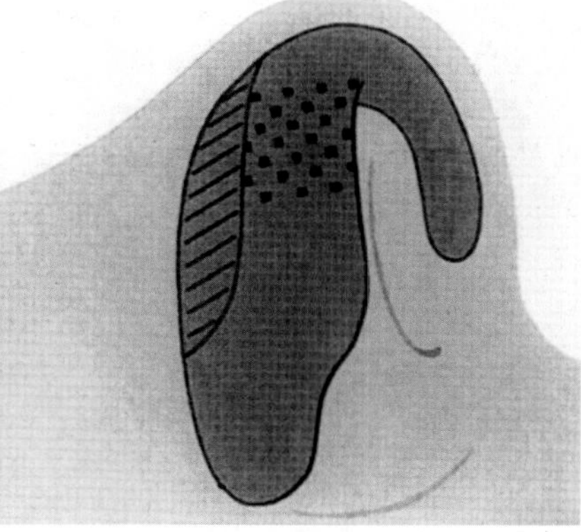

Fig. 44.18 Weakening procedure of the lateral crus: (**A**) scoring; (**B**) morselization.

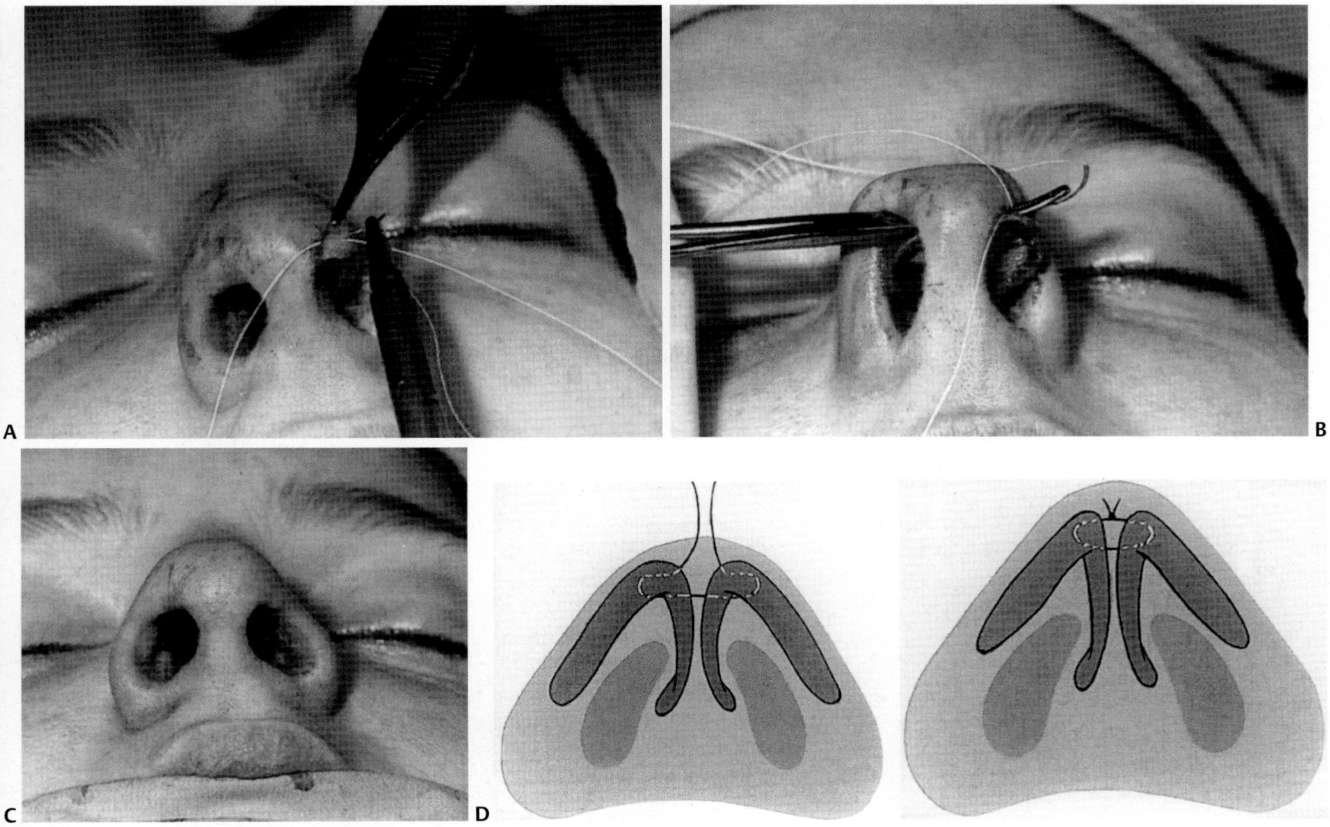

Fig. 44.19 (**A,D,E**) Horizontal-mattress suture technique to correct bifidity of the tip. (**B**) Mattress suture with 6–0 Gore-Tex of left lower lateral crus followed by transportation of the needle with a mosquito clamp to the right side for the same procedure. (**C**) Direct postoperative result after advancing the domes with horizontal mattress suture technique.

is freed from the lateral crus (**Fig. 44.13**). When starting the dissection, it is easier to begin just lateral of the dome, rather than far lateral where the right surgical plane is more difficult to find. After freeing the vestibular side of the lateral crus around the dome up to the medial crus, the nonvestibular side is dissected free from the overlying soft tissue in a supraperichondrial plane (**Fig. 44.14**). The lateral crus can easily be delivered now (**Fig. 44.15**).

The external approach, which is out of the scope of this chapter, although even more traumatic and time consuming, gives the best exposure of the three approaches. This approach enables the surgeon to perform bimanual surgery, and it makes judgment of the specific deformities much easier. Therefore, it is especially indicated in the case of

- Congenital deformities such as the cleft-lip nose
- Extensive revision surgery
- Severe nasal trauma
- Elaborate reduction and augmentation procedures
- Large septal perforations

Nevertheless, there is a tendency to use the external approach routinely, especially by less experienced nasal surgeons. This is justified as long as the surgeon weighs the surgical trauma of the chosen approach against the possibilities of a satisfying postoperative result in each case.

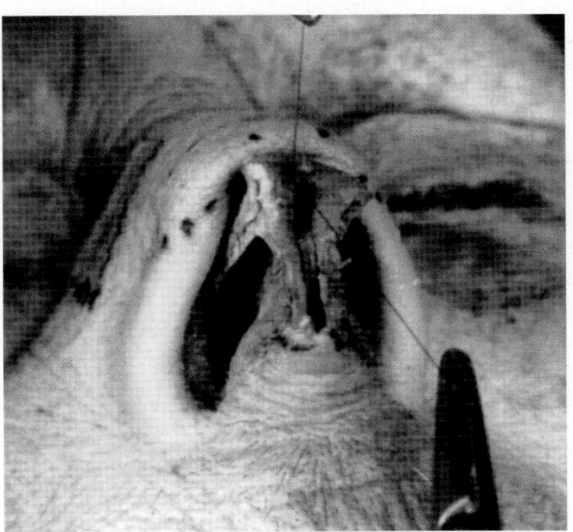

Fig. 44.20 Transdomal suture with lateral crural steal to enhance tip projection.

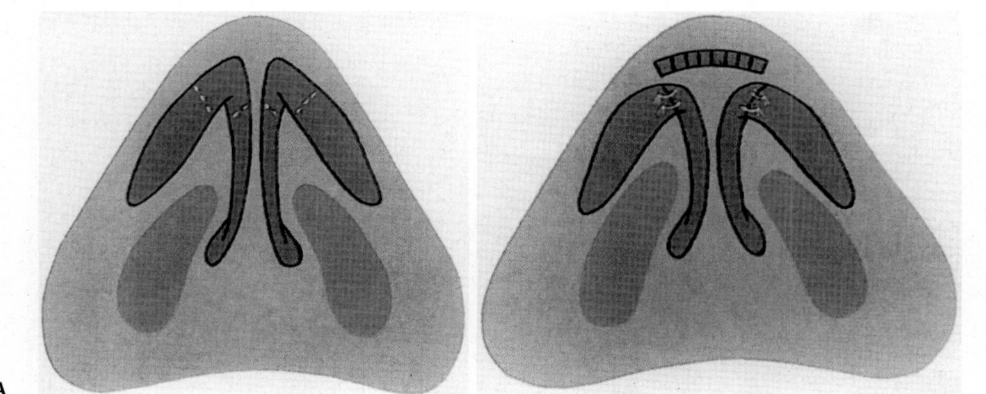

Fig. 44.21 (**A**) Dome amputation. (**B**) Sutured lower laterals with an onlay tip graft to hide possible postoperative irregularities.

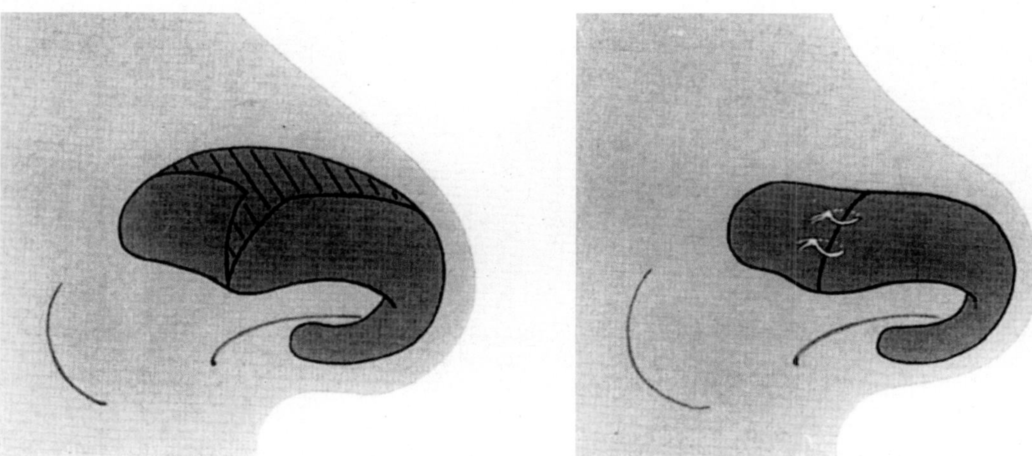

Fig. 44.22 Interrupted strip technique to obtain adequate cephalic tip rotation in case of a tension nose.

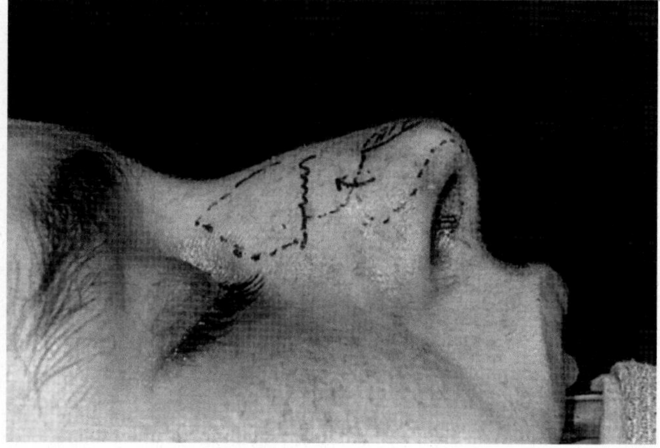

Fig. 44.23 Landmarks outlined on the nasal skin with marking of the new position of the lateral crus (*arrow*) and partial resection of the cephalic part of the lateral crus (*striped area*).

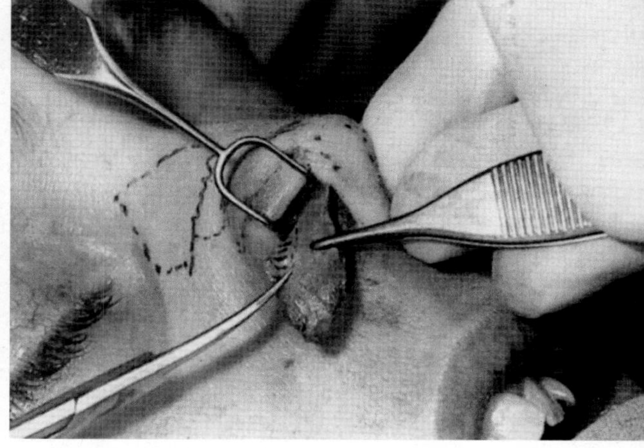

Fig. 44.24 Resection of the marked cephalic part of the lateral crus.

Surgical Techniques (Table 44.1)

With the *nondelivery approach,* the vestibular skin is freed from the proposed resection area of the cephalic part of the lateral crus. After splitting of the cartilage (no. 15 blade), the nonvestibular side of the cephalic part to be resected is dissected free from the overlying soft tissue and removed (**Fig. 44.16**). Pressure of the middle finger of the surgeon's hand (holding the double-hooked ala retractor) on the lateral crus will give excellent exposure and control during surgery. After sufficient and symmetrical volume reduction, the vestibular skin should be sutured carefully with 5–0 atraumatic absorbable suture material. This simple tip-refinement procedure gives minimal surgical trauma, leaving the integrity of the lower lateral crus intact and ensuring the best chance for an uncomplicated healing process.

The larger the portion of cartilage resection of the cephalic part of the lateral crus, the more upward rotation will be induced. A supplementary procedure to enhance tip rotation is resection of a caudal strip of the septal cartilage.

With the *delivery approach,* the alar cartilages are now delivered as bipedicle chondrocutaneous flaps. Precise excision of cartilage is now possible under direct vision (**Fig. 44.17**). In the case of bulging of the lateral crus, the weakening procedure (scoring or morselization) is performed, if indicated, in combination with resection of a cephalic portion of the lateral crus (**Fig. 44.18**).

The *delivery approach* is also appropriate in the case of bifidity of the nasal tip, in which the horizontal mattress-suture technique can be performed to advance the domes with a nonabsorbable (Gore-Tex; W. L. Gore & Associates, Inc., Flagstaff, AZ) or a slow absorbable (PDS [polydiaxonone], Ethicon, Inc., Somerville, NJ) atraumatic suture (**Fig. 44.19**). Another tip-suturing technique is the lateral crural steal in which the lateral crus is freed from the vestibular skin, after which the dissected area is advanced medially and fixed in the new position with a mattress suture (**Fig. 44.20**).

Interrupting the continuity of the alar cartilage (incomplete strip technique) can give some unpredictable scarring, especially visible in thin-skinned noses. In the case of dome amputation to reduce a Pinocchio nose, an onlay tip graft will hide possible irregularities in the healing process (**Fig. 44.21**).

To reduce tip projection and to obtain sufficient cephalic tip rotation, as is indicated in correction of a tension nose, the continuity of the alar cartilage is interrupted by transection of the lateral crus at the junction of its middle

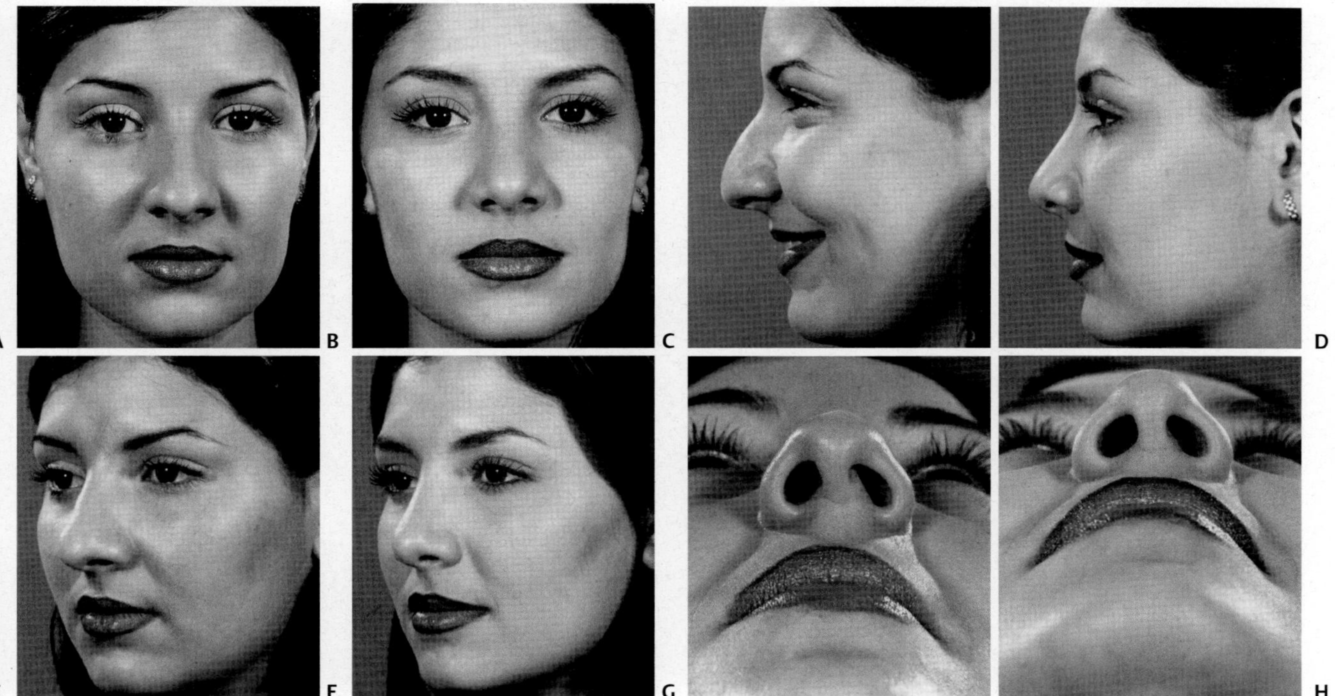

Fig. 44.25 (**A–H**) Pre- and postoperative views of a patient who underwent a rhinoplasty: first a septoplasty, followed by a cephalic resection of the lower laterals by a nondelivery approach and removal of a bony cartilaginous hump, micro-osteotomies, and infracture of the nasal bones.

and lateral third, followed by resection of the cartilage segment of the lateral third and cephalic part (**Fig. 44.22**).

With the *modified delivery approach,* whereby the lateral crus is freed from soft tissue at both sides, it is possible to deproject the tip as described by Peck or to correct alar insufficiency by rotating the lateral crus in a cephalic position (**Fig. 44.23**) as described by Rettinger and Masing. Upward rotation results in a slight bulbosity due to the new position of the lateral crus, which should be corrected by resection of a cephalic part of the lateral crus (**Fig. 44.24**).

The surgeon should be aware that with the delivery approach the healing process is less predictable than with the nondelivery approach, with a higher likelihood of postoperative asymmetries.

Pitfalls

Basic knowledge of surgical anatomy, tip-supporting mechanisms, tip dynamics, tripod theory and of the basic approaches and techniques in rhinoplasty are prerequisites to the prevention of serious sequelae in rhinoplasty. The impact of a disastrous surgical result on a patient's emotional and social life puts a heavy responsibility on the surgeon. Before starting surgical procedures on a patient, an intensive learning process, both theoretical and practical (with cadaver dissection), and including watching and assisting in live surgery, is obligatory.

Common pitfalls of the *nondelivery approach* and tips for their prevention are

- *Asymmetric resection* resulting in tip asymmetry. (To prevent asymmetry, the resected cephalic cartilage parts should be compared.)
- *Overresection* resulting in alar insufficiency (external valve collapse). (A caudal strip of 4 to 8 mm, depending on the strength of the alar cartilage, should be preserved.)
- A *wrong cartilage incision line* resulting in an incomplete strip can lead to weakening, asymmetry in shape, extra upward rotation, and bossa formation. (Knowledge

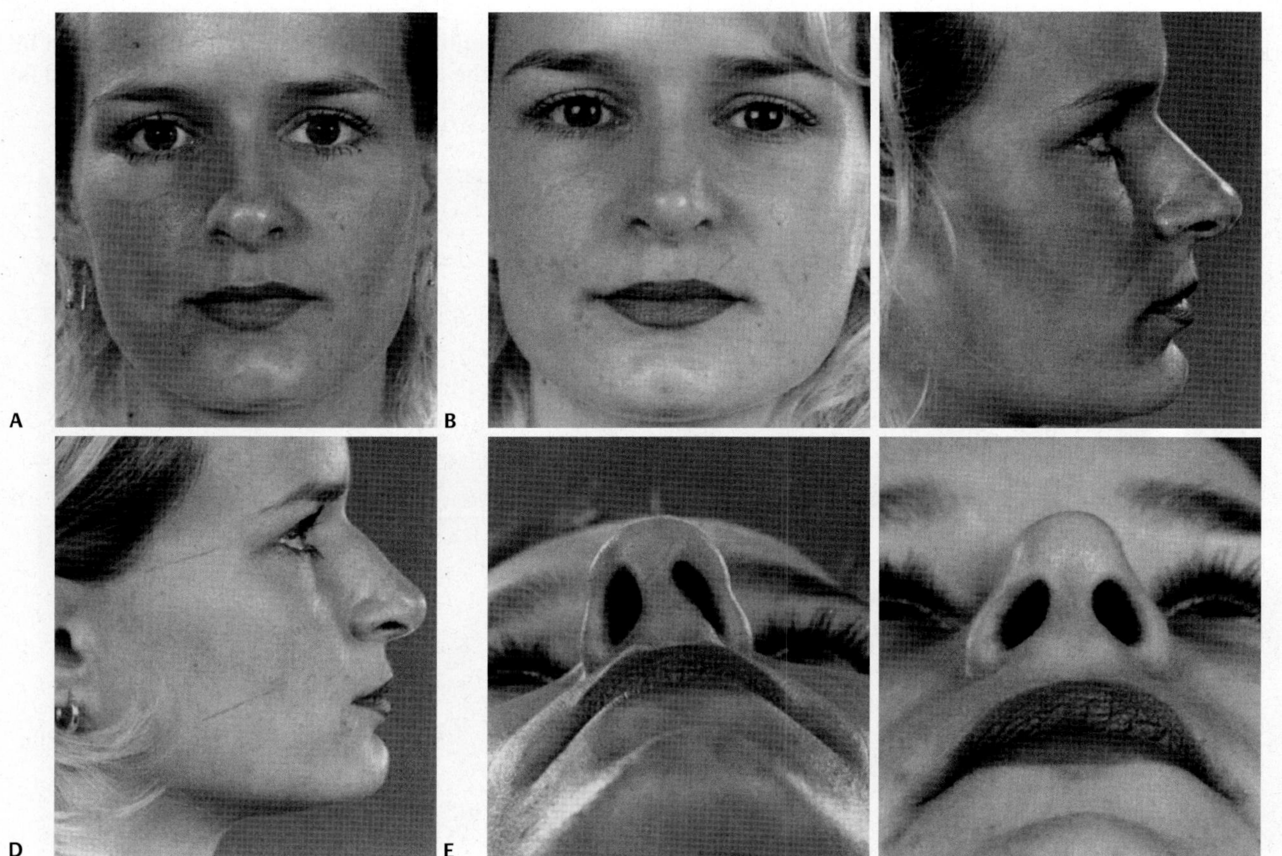

Fig. 44.26 (**A–F**) Pre- and postoperative views of a rhinoplasty by the delivery approach to narrow the broad trapezoid tip with transdomal and interdomal suturing, followed by a bilateral cephalic resection of the lower laterals and a small resection of the cartilaginous dorsum. The asymmetry of the nostrils due to a caudal septal deviation to the left was corrected by a septoplasty through a hemitransfixion incision.

of the pathway of the caudal margin of the alar cartilage can prevent such a sequela.)

Common pitfalls of the *delivery approach* (bipedicale chondrocutaneous flap) and tips for their prevention are

- *Incomplete delivery* due to insufficient extension, medially and laterally, of the intercartilaginous and marginal incisions. This can make the planned technical procedures difficult or even impossible.
- *Asymmetric delivery* due to a different extension of the incision lines at one side. (Helpful in preventing this is to determine the tip-defining point corresponding with the domal area by placing a one-prong at either side after which the flap should be delivered and the exact tip-defining point can be marked.)
- *Asymmetric resection* resulting in tip asymmetry. (Marking of the cephalic part with Bonney's blue dye or a marking pen will help to prevent this.)
- *Asymmetric inter- and transdomal suturing.* (This can be prevented by checking for smooth level of the domes in the horizontal plane and of the medial crura in the vertical plane.)
- *Overscoring and overmorselization,* which can result in asymmetry of the tip with typical bossa formation.
- *Compromising the tip support* by performing a complete transfixion (disturbing a major tip support mechanism, i.e., the medial crural footplate attachment to the septum) without the intention to diminish tip projection.

Common pitfalls of the *delivery approach* (lateral crus delivery) and tips for their prevention are

- Careless preparation resulting in *tearing the lateral crus* in the domal area. (Suturing and placing a small cartilage splint can restore the continuity.)
- *Wrong indication* for the rotation technique to treat alar insufficiency when there is no malposition of the lateral crus and protrusion in the vestibulum.
- *Overrotation* resulting in weakening of the alar support or supratip fullness. Keep in mind that the goal in modern rhinoplasty is to minimize surgical trauma to achieve a more predictable long-term outcome. The low-trauma approaches described in this chapter should be part of the armamentarium of all rhinoplastic surgeons (**Figs. 44.25–44.27**).

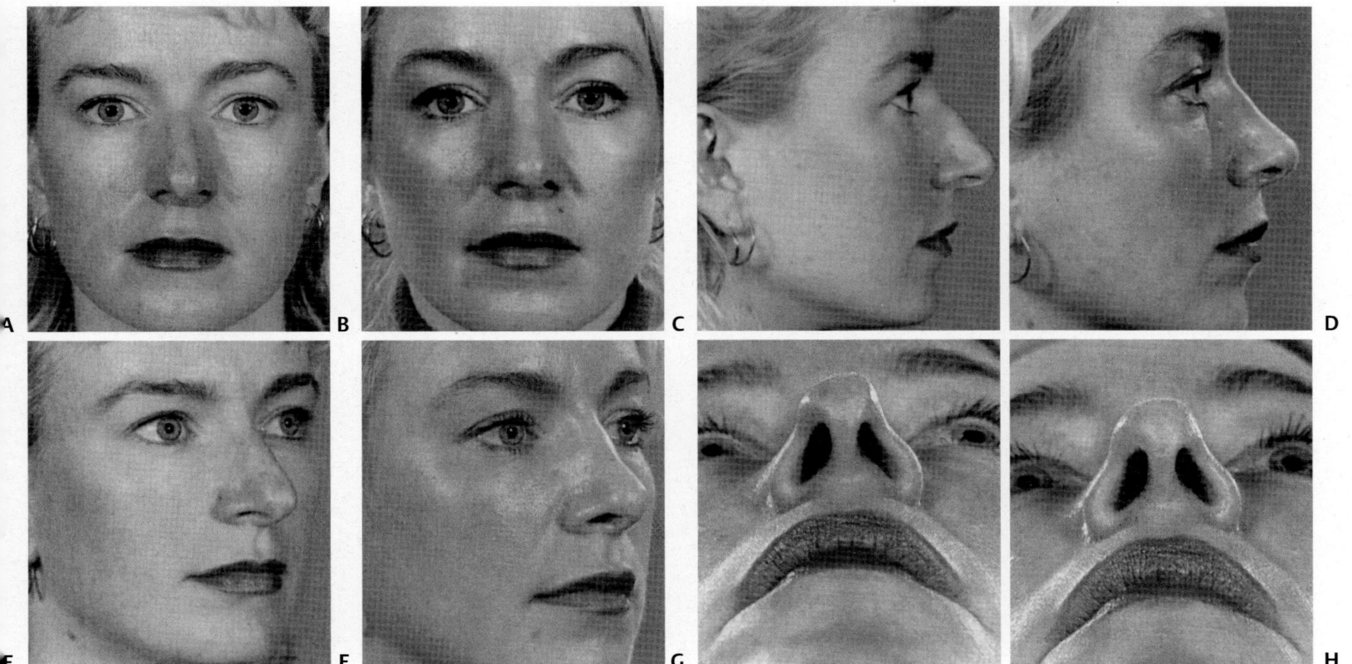

Fig. 44.27 **(A–H)** Pre- and postoperative views of a patient with alar collapse due to a malposition of the lateral crura. Furthermore, there is a bony cartilaginous hump with a slight deviation of the dorsum to the left and slight asymmetry of the nasal tip. Through marginal incisions the lateral crura were delivered (up to the dome), bilateral cephalic resection and at the left side a scoring procedure in the dome area to correct tip asymmetry were performed. Through the marginal incision the overlying soft tissue was dissected from the osseocartilaginous vault, followed by hump resection, medial oblique micro-osteotomies, and repositioning of the lateral crura with a guiding suture into a prepared pocket in a more cephalic position. Finally, lateral micro-osteotomies were performed, followed by realignment of an infraction of the dorsum.

Suggested Reading

Adamson PA. Refinement of the nasal tip. Facial Plast Surg 1988;5:115

Berman WE. Surgery of the nasal tip. Otolaryngol Clin North Am 1975;10:563

Bull TR. The tip. In: Rees TD, ed. Rhinoplasty: Problems and Controversies—A Discussion with the Experts. St. Louis: CV Mosby; 1988;5:35

Denecke HG, Meyer R. Plastische Operationen an Kopf und Hals. Vol 1. Nasenplastik Berlin: Springer-Verlag; 1964:82

Goodman WS. External approach to rhinoplasty. Can J Otolaryngol 1973;2:207

Kridel RWH, Konior RJ. The underprojected tip. In: Krause CHK, ed. Aesthetic Facial Surgery. Philadelphia: JB Lippincott Co; 1991:191

Mahe E, Gambling J. La voie transcartilagineuse dans la chirurgie de la pointe du nez. Ann Chir Plast 1982;27:147

Nolst Trenité GJ. The surgical approach to the nasal tip. Clin Otolaryngol 1991;16(1):109

Nolst Trenité GJ. Surgical correction of nasal tip deformities. In: Proceedings of the XVI World Congress of Otorhinolaryngology Head and Neck Surgery, Sydney. Bologna: Monduzzi Editore SpA; 1997:138–144

Nolst Trenité GJ, ed Rhinoplasty: A Practical Guide to Functional and Aesthetic Surgery of the Nose. 2nd ed. (with interactive CD-ROM). New York: Kugler Publications; 1998

Nolst Trenité GJ. Alar insufficiency surgery. In: Nolst Trenité GJ, ed. Rhinoplasty: A practical Guide to Functional and Aesthetic Surgery of the Nose. 2nd ed. New York: Kugler Publications; 1998;8:67

Nolst Trenité GJ. Guidelines to cadaver dissection. In: Nolst Trenité GJ, ed. Rhinoplasty: A Practical Guide to Functional and Aesthetic Surgery of the Nose. 2nd ed. New York: Kugler Publications; 1998;23:237

Parell GJ, Becker GD. The "tension nose." Facial Plast Surg 1984;1(2):81

Peck GC. Techniques in Aesthetic Rhinoplasty. New York: Gower Medical 1990

Ponti L. Aesthetic problems in surgical technique of the nasal tip. In: Plastic and Reconstructive Surgery of the Face and Neck. Proceedings of the 2nd International Symposium. Vol 1. New York: Grune & Stratton; 1977

Rettinger S, Masing H. Rotation of the Alar cartilage in collapsed Alar. 2nd ed. Rhinol 19:81,1981

Tardy ME, Hewell TS. Nasal tip refinement: reliable approaches and sculpture techniques. Facial Plast Surg 1984;1(2):87

Tardy ME, Younger R, Key M, et al. The overprojecting tip: anatomic variation and targeted solutions. Facial Plast Surg 1987;4:4

Tardy ME. Transdomal suture refinement of the nasal tip. Facial Plast Surg 1987;4:4

Tardy ME, Toriumi DM. Philosophy and principles of rhinoplasty. In: Papel ID, Nachlas NE, eds. Fac plast reconstr surg. Vol 31. St. Louis CV Mosby; 1991:278

Tardy ME. Rhinoplasty. The art and science. Vol 2. Philadelphia: WB Saunders; 1997

Webster RC. Advances in surgery of the tip: intact rim cartilage techniques and the tip–columella–lip esthetic complex. Otolaryngol Clin North Am 1975;8:615

45 Surgery of the Nasal Tip: Vertical Dome Division

Robert L. Simons and John S. Rhee

In recent years, three major trends have influenced the changes in nasal tip surgery. First, techniques have incorporated methods of greater medial stabilization and support of the nasal base. Second, more surgeons are relying on cartilage incisional and suture techniques of the alar cartilages rather than excisional ones to achieve desired changes. Finally, the use of the external approach for visualization of the alar cartilages has become commonplace, with the endonasal approach becoming an increasingly lost art form.

Philosophical Tenets of Vertical Dome Division

Ironically, the first two trends were longstanding philosophical tenets of Irving Goldman back in 1957.[1] Since his first published report on the importance of the medial crura and through subsequent articles on vertical dome division (VDD),[2–5] the message has been consistent: preserve and conserve rather than resect and regret. Yet the concept of incising the alar cartilage at the domal region has been labeled by many as dangerous, destructive, and radical rather than conservative and reasonable. It is vitally important not to combine excisional techniques and philosophy with an incisional procedure such as VDD. The complications of postoperative alar notching, collapse, unnatural tent-pole appearance, pinching, and bossae formation are caused more often by too much excision of the lateral crura than by dome division.[6]

In almost all primary cases and in most revision cases, our approach to tip surgery is an endonasal one, using the marginal incision delivery technique. Sufficient delivery of this bipedal flap requires vestibular incisions at the caudal border of the alar cartilages and medial extension along 50% of the anterior columellar border. Attention to these details will allow a wide and adequate exposure to irregularities and asymmetries in the lobular tissues. More importantly, it will allow symmetrical incisions and suturing of tissue without the need for a transcolumellar incision. Insertion of additional filler or onlay cartilage in the lobular or columellar area can be easily accomplished via the marginal incisions.

Preoperative Evaluation

As with all rhinoplasty, preoperative evaluation of the nasal tip is critical in choosing the correct tip procedure. Decisions about where and when to incise cartilage and how much to remove are made during the preoperative assessment. With adequate tip projection, two factors are generally seen. First, the lateral view evidences a 1:1 relationship between the length of the base of the nose and the upper lip (**Fig. 45.1**). Second, the base view shows a triangular orientation with an equilateral appearance, suggesting sufficient lateral battens of cartilage and strong medial support. The length and strength of the medial crura are evidenced in the ideal 2:1 relationship of the columella to the lobule (**Fig. 45.2**). The desired double break occurs naturally from the retroussé curve of the medial crus at the columellar–lobular junction (**Fig. 45.3**).

The cephalic movement of the nasal tip along the same radial arc from the facial plane defines tip rotation (**Fig. 45.4**). Rotation is accomplished through the interrelated steps in rhinoplasty involving lowering of the nasal dorsum, shortening of the caudal septum, plumping of an acute nasolabial angle, and resection

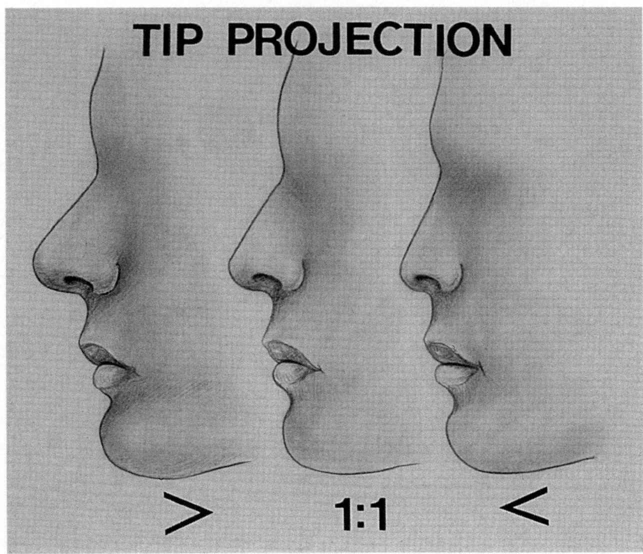

Fig. 45.1 Desired 1:1 ratio of length of nasal base to upper lip. Note that the change in lobular length directly affects tip projection.

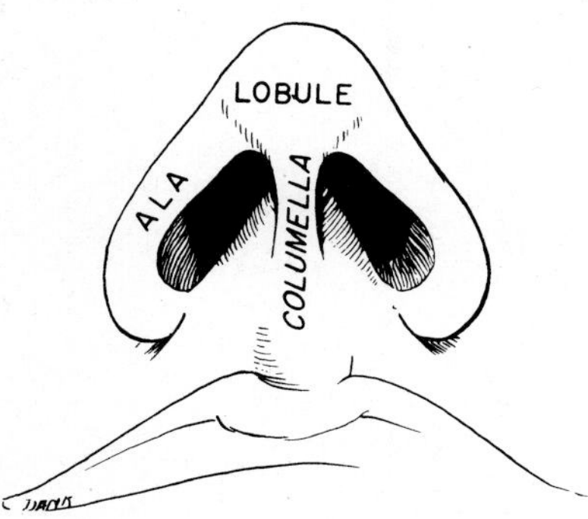

Fig. 45.2 Strong base view with desired 2:1 ratio of columella length to lobule.

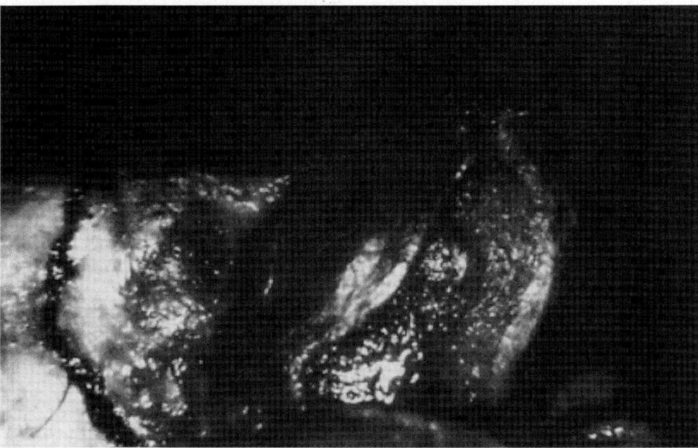

Fig. 45.3 Anatomical evidence of double break created by curvature of strong medial crura.

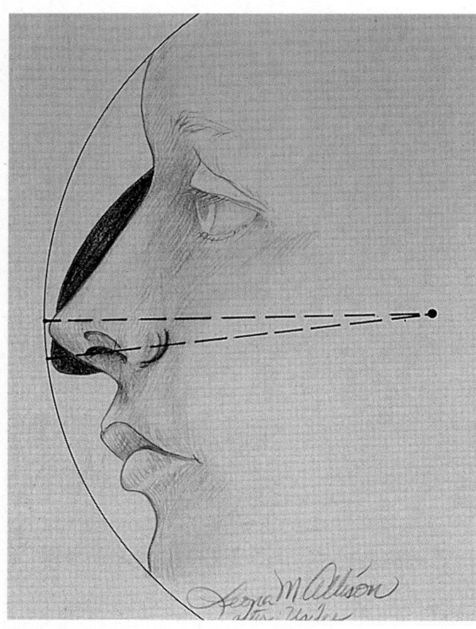

Fig. 45.4 Rotation of tip maintains same radial distance from facial plane.

of the cephalic portion of the lower lateral cartilage. A conservative cephalic resection of alar cartilage alone does little to effect tip rotation. Also, overzealous resection leads to postoperative sequelae of alar collapse and nasal bossae.

Surgical Technique

Over the past 30 years, we have used various forms of VDD in more than 1000 patients. The rationale behind VDD is the ability to change projection directly as well as to narrow and rotate the lobule with minimal cartilage excision. These desired effects can be accomplished without the use of additional struts or tip grafts because of the medial stabilization and strength provided by VDD techniques. Inherent in the philosophy is the preservation of surrounding tissues, such as the septal angle or caudal septum, further decreasing the risk of the postoperative appearance of an overrotated or "overoperated" nose.

There are three distinct VDD techniques that are effective in addressing the nasal tip: the classic Goldman prototype, the Simons modification, and the hockey-stick modification. The indications and surgical technique for each of these procedures will be discussed.

Goldman Technique

The prototype of VDD procedures is the classic Goldman technique, which calls for the creation of a chondrocutaneous strut by division of the alar cartilage along with the underlying vestibular skin. When employing the Goldman technique, the septal and dorsal alignment generally precedes the tip surgery. It is both crucial and advantageous that the initial lowering of the dorsum be minimal and that dorsal strength be maintained before the projection of the tip is changed.

The alar cartilages are delivered through marginal incisions. The high point of the lobular apex is marked on delivery by a right-angled hook. It is important to remember not to borrow more than 2 or 3 mm from the lateral crus (**Fig. 45.5**). The 3-mm borrowing boundary is measured along the caudal margin of the alar crus. The obliquity of the vertical cut at the dome allows more than 3 mm to be mobilized superiorly, thereby necessitating trimming of the posterior excess once the medial crura are brought together. The chondrocutaneous strut is sutured together with anterior, posterior, and superior horizontal mattress sutures of 4–0 chromic catgut (**Fig. 45.6**).

It is critical to preserve at least 8 to 10 mm of width of the lateral crura when trimming the cephalic border. It is worth reemphasizing that one should not borrow

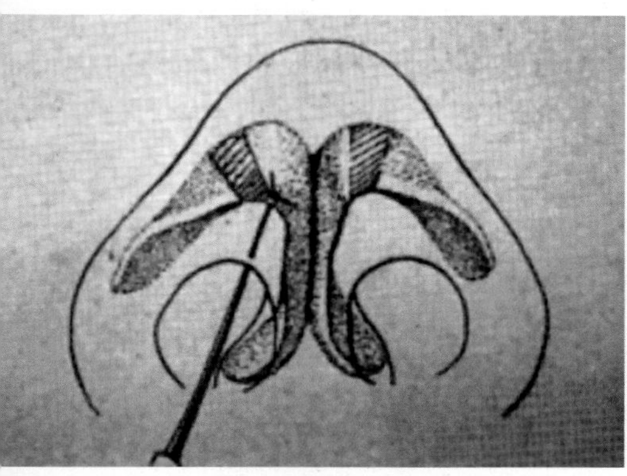

Fig. 45.5 Borrowing boundaries relate to distance from lobular apex marked with right-angled hook) to cut at caudal margin.

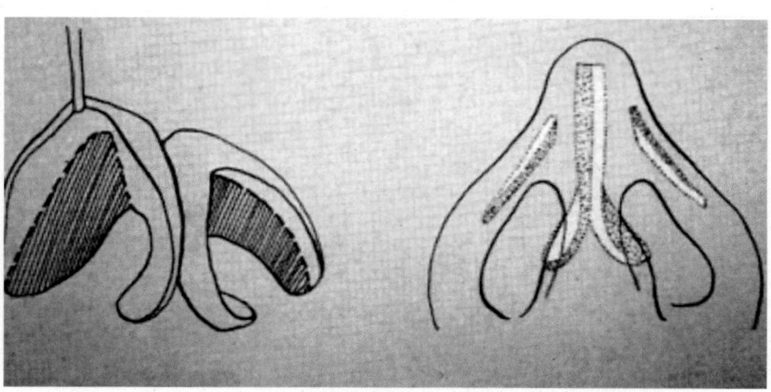

Fig. 45.7 Unnatural tent-pole appearance created by combining large excision of lateral crura with vertical dome division.

nore than 2 or 3 mm from the lateral crus when dividing the dome vertically. Remembering these admonitions will help one to avoid the outcome of an unnatural tent-pole appearance (**Fig. 45.7**).

Sharp edges of cartilage are trimmed and the sutured crura are repositioned in the lobule. A final, high, securing suture closes the space between the caudal septum and membranous septum. No effort is made to suture medial crura directly to septum. The marginal incisions are closed and no attempt is made to suture the medial to the lateral crura (**Fig. 45.8**).

The Goldman technique is preferred by the authors for the ptotic or aging situation whereby the vertically displaced alar complex requires direct redirection (**Figs. 45.9 and 45.10**).[7]

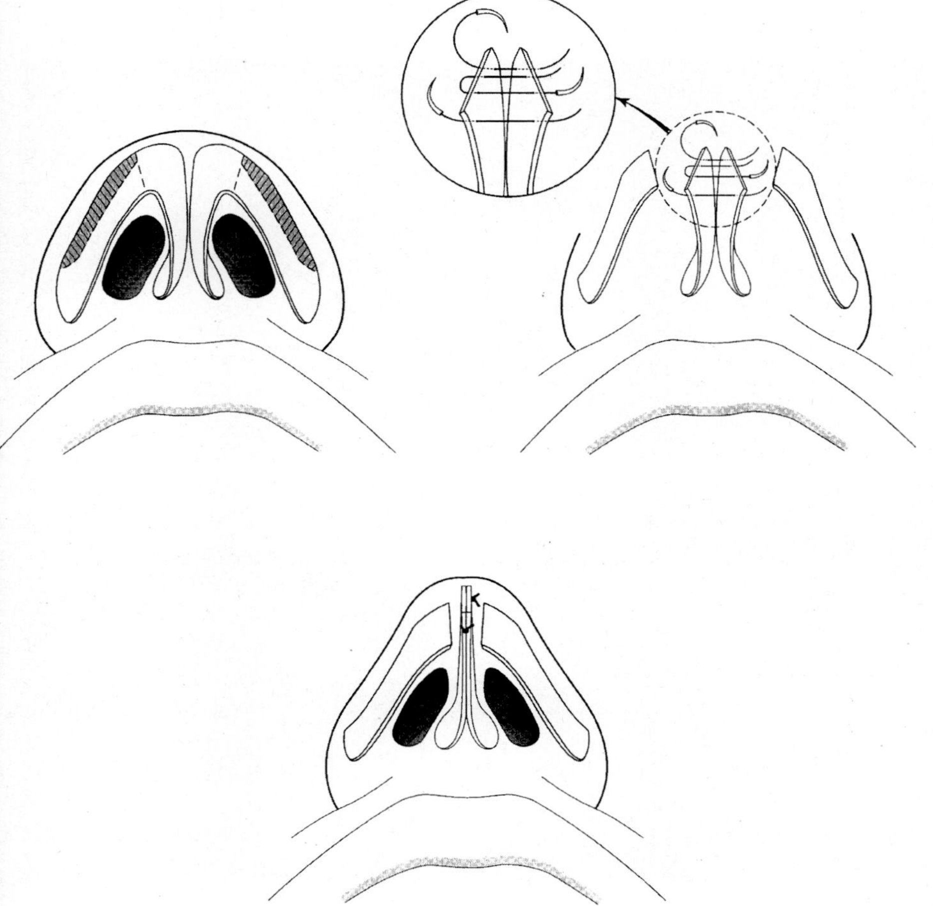

Fig. 45.6 Schematic representation of the Goldman technique.

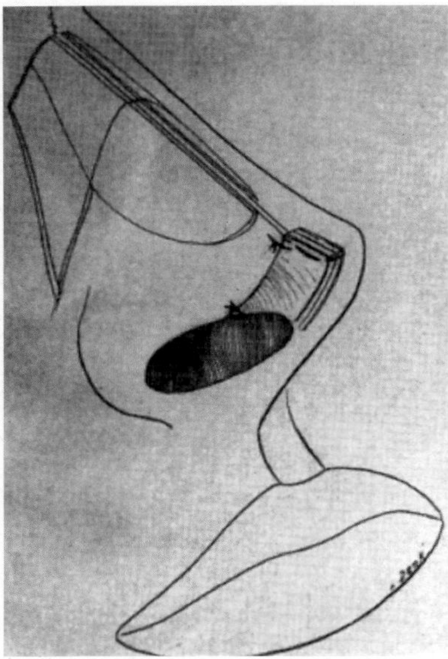

Fig. 45.8 Limited distance between cut medial strut and septal angle critical in classic Goldman technique.

If the nasolabial angle is particularly acute and the strength of the cartilage is suspect in regard to its ability to support the thick overlying skin, we often use a cartilaginous strut between the medial crura. Septal cartilage is generally used for the strut, which extends from the feet of the medial crura to the superior cut edges. This "sandwich" of chondrocutaneous leaves and cartilage is sutured together in the same manner as in the classic Goldman technique.

By rotating the medial crura together, the convex columella–lobular angle or so-called double break is at times created or accentuated. With a weaker, straight, or retracted columella, a cartilaginous batten or plumping grafts may further augment the tip procedure. Plumping grafts are small pieces of cartilage placed beneath the feet of the medial crura through a separate stab incision at the base of the columella. The cartilaginous batten is placed anterior to the medial crus via the medial aspect of the marginal incision (see section "Adjunctive Techniques").

Simons Modification

More common than the underprojected or ptotic tip is the lobule needing more subtle changes of increased medial strength and medial movement of the lobular domes. A widened or divergent lobule is defined as one in which the domal highlights are more than 4 mm apart. In these more frequent situations, we use our own modification of the VDD technique[3–5] (**Fig. 45.11**).

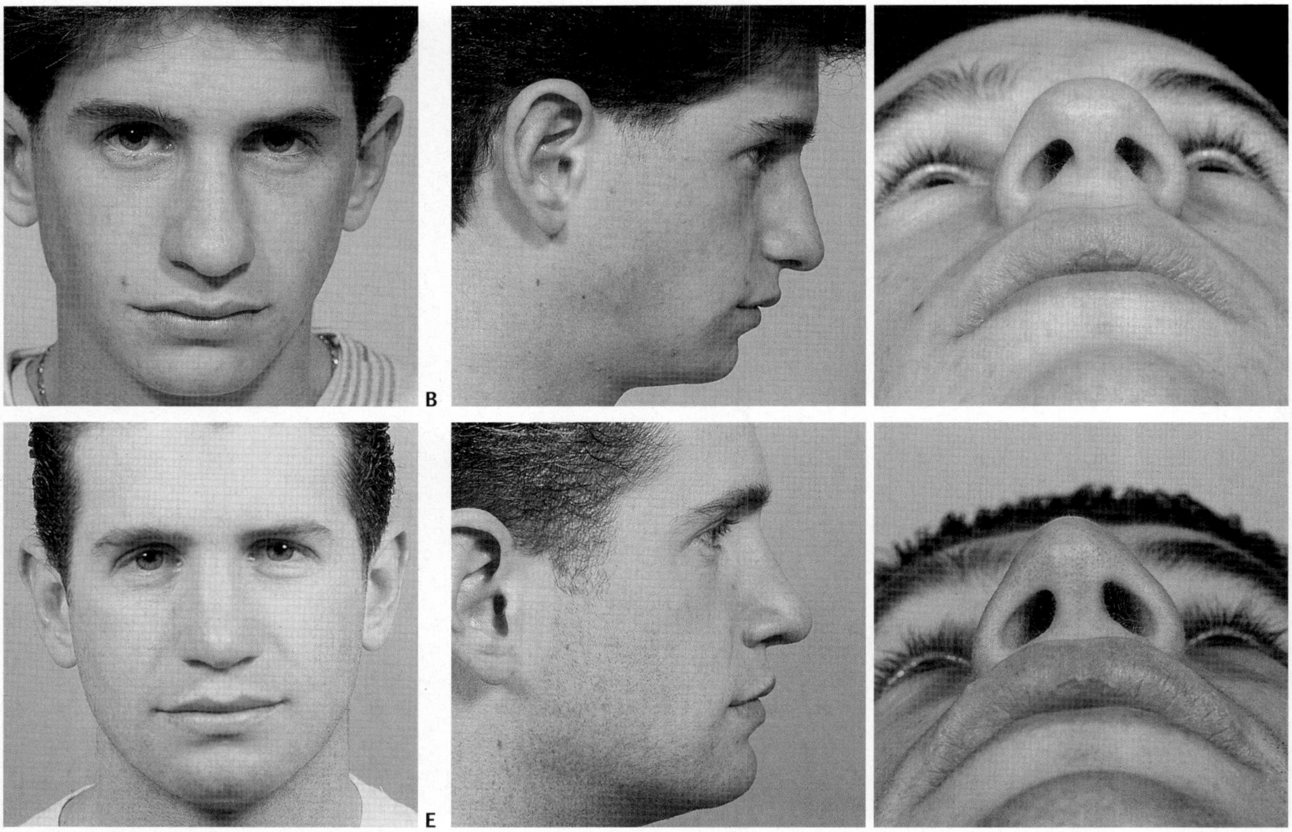

Fig. 45.9 (**A–C**) Preoperative views of patient with heavy ptotic tip. (**D–F**) Six-year postoperative views following Goldman technique.

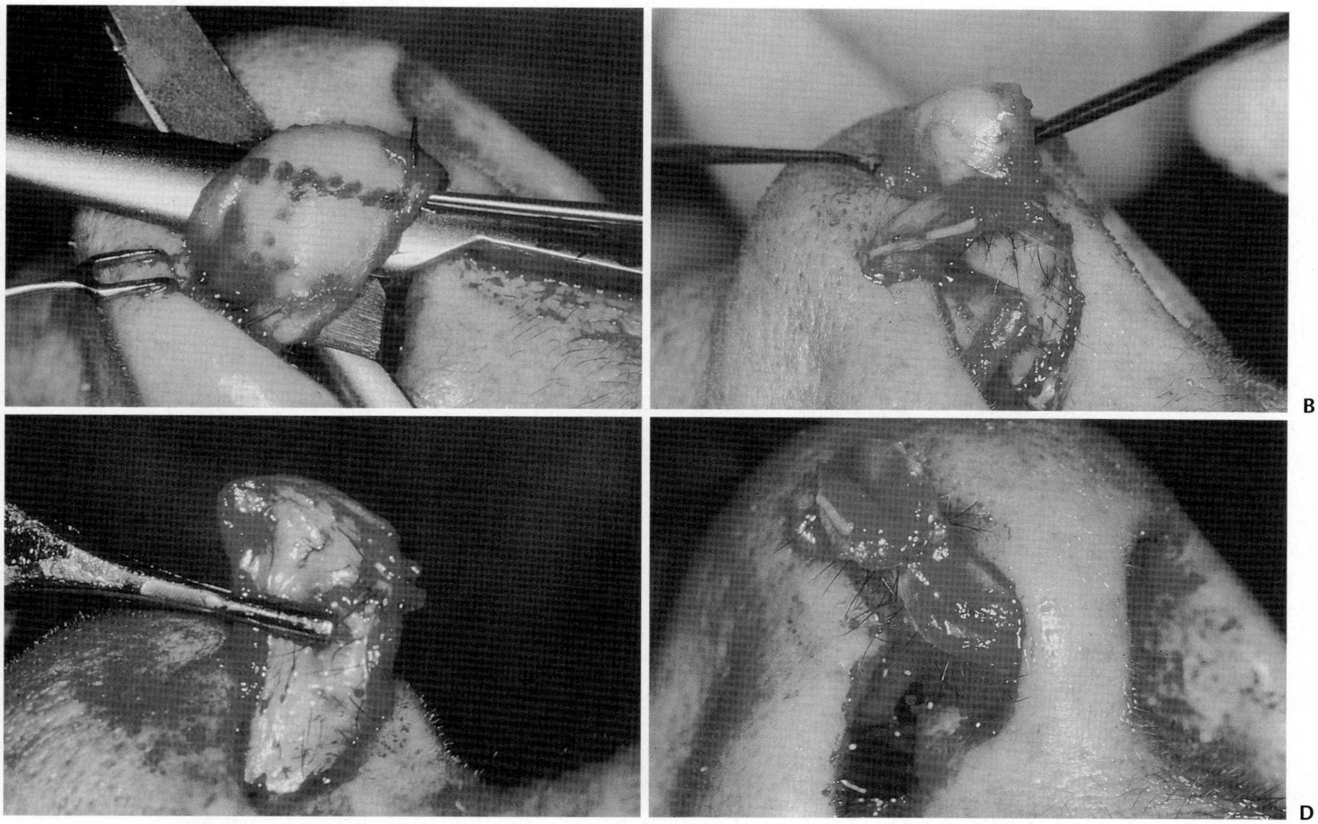

B

D

g. 45.10 (**A–D**) Intraoperative demonstration of Goldman technique.

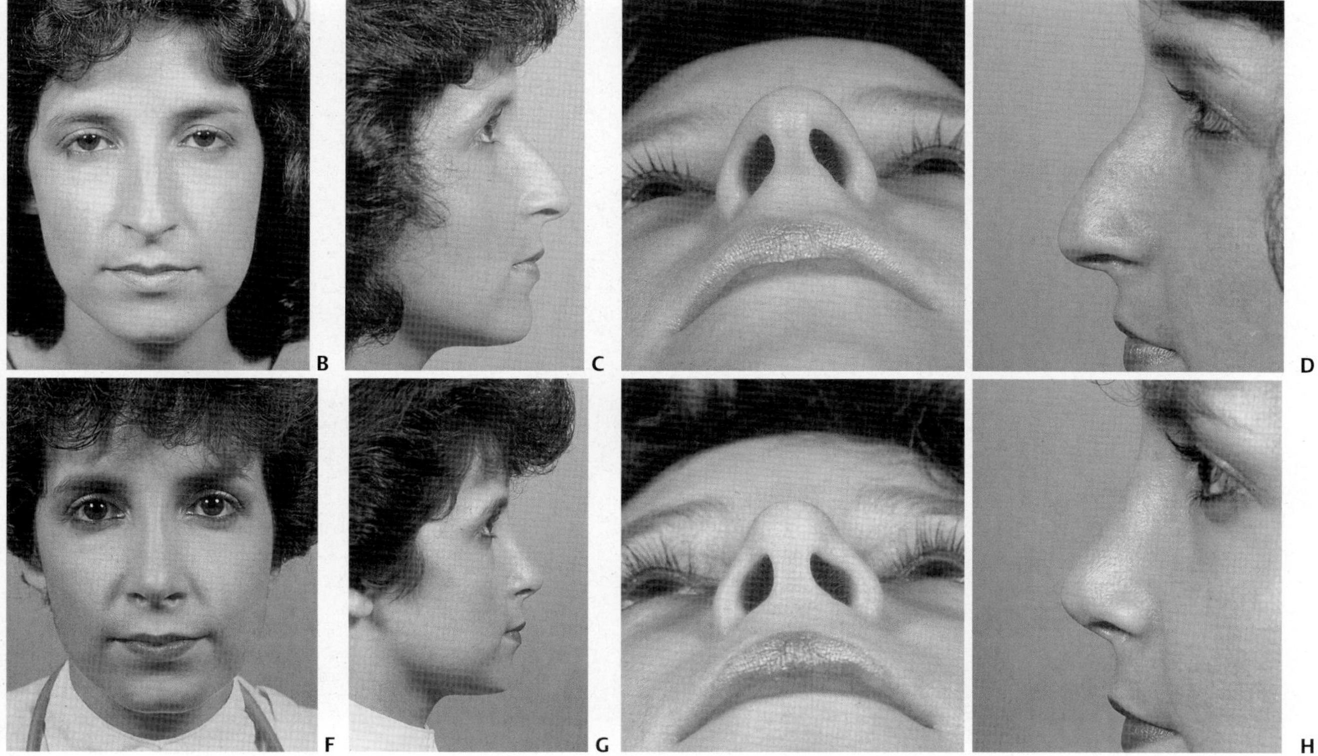

g. 45.11 (**A–D**) Preoperative views of patient with divergent and dependent lobule. (**E–H**) Two-year post-
ɔerative views after Simons modification of vertical dome division.

As outlined previously, the anatomical apex of the lobular dome is marked by a right-angled hook as the bipedal flap is delivered through marginal incision. The high point or anatomical apex of the dome is not synonymous with the junction of the medial crura and lateral crura or the cartilaginous isthmus between the inferior and superior genus. Rather, it represents the most anterior cartilaginous point of the nasal base, most easily punctured and identified by the right-angled hook.

Following delivery of both domes, soft tissue overlying the alar cartilage is removed. It is important to clear out the fatty fibrous tissue between the two domes, especially when there is intralobular weakness or frank bifidity. Even if intradomal sutures are not used, the postoperative scarification will aid intradomal stabilization.

The alar cartilages are vertically incised but, unlike the Goldman tip, the underlying vestibular skin is kept intact. Vertically cutting the dome allows direct inward and upward movement of the medial lobular portion. As with the classic Goldman maneuver, limiting the lateral distance of the cut to 3 mm from the lobular apex at the caudal margin prevents notching. Preserving at least 6 to 8 mm of the lateral crus after horizontal cephalic excision prevents alar collapse and helps to stabilize the pyramid base.

Maintenance of symmetry and further medial stabilization depends on proper placement of the intradomal suture. On presentation of both domes into the right nostril, a 5–0 clear nylon suture is used in a horizontal mattress fashion to bind the medial edges of the vertically divided alar cartilages. The first pass of the needle is closer to the left superior edge than the more medial inferior exit, with no attempt made to go beyond the interior perichondrium. A mirror image of that needle passage is performed on the right side with the knot buried between the medial crura superiorly (**Figs. 45.12 and 45.13**).

When the cut medial edge gently leads the lateral, nature does a wonderful job of reconstituting the dome. Our use of sutures in the tip is limited to stabilizing medial components. Attempting to reconstruct the dome by suturing the medial crus to the lateral crus is unnecessary and may lead to asymmetries. Moreover, suturing medial to lateral or lateral to lateral crural components defeats the purpose of VDD and may again result in an unnatural narrowing of the lobular apices.

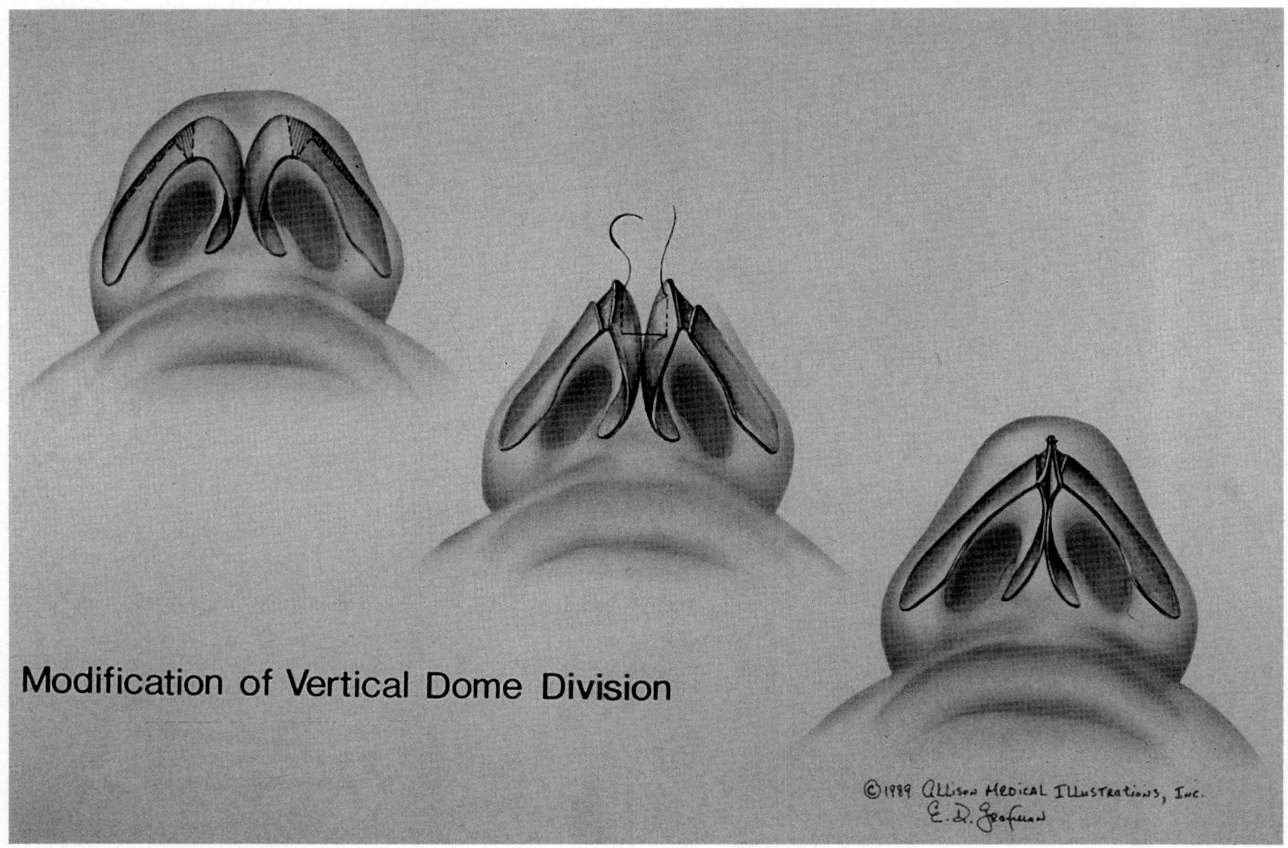

Fig. 45.12 Schematic representation of Simons modification of vertical dome division. Note the oblique placement of the intradomal horizontal mattress suture. Superior tie of intradomal suture helps to ensure the desired narrowing and symmetry of the newly defined tip.

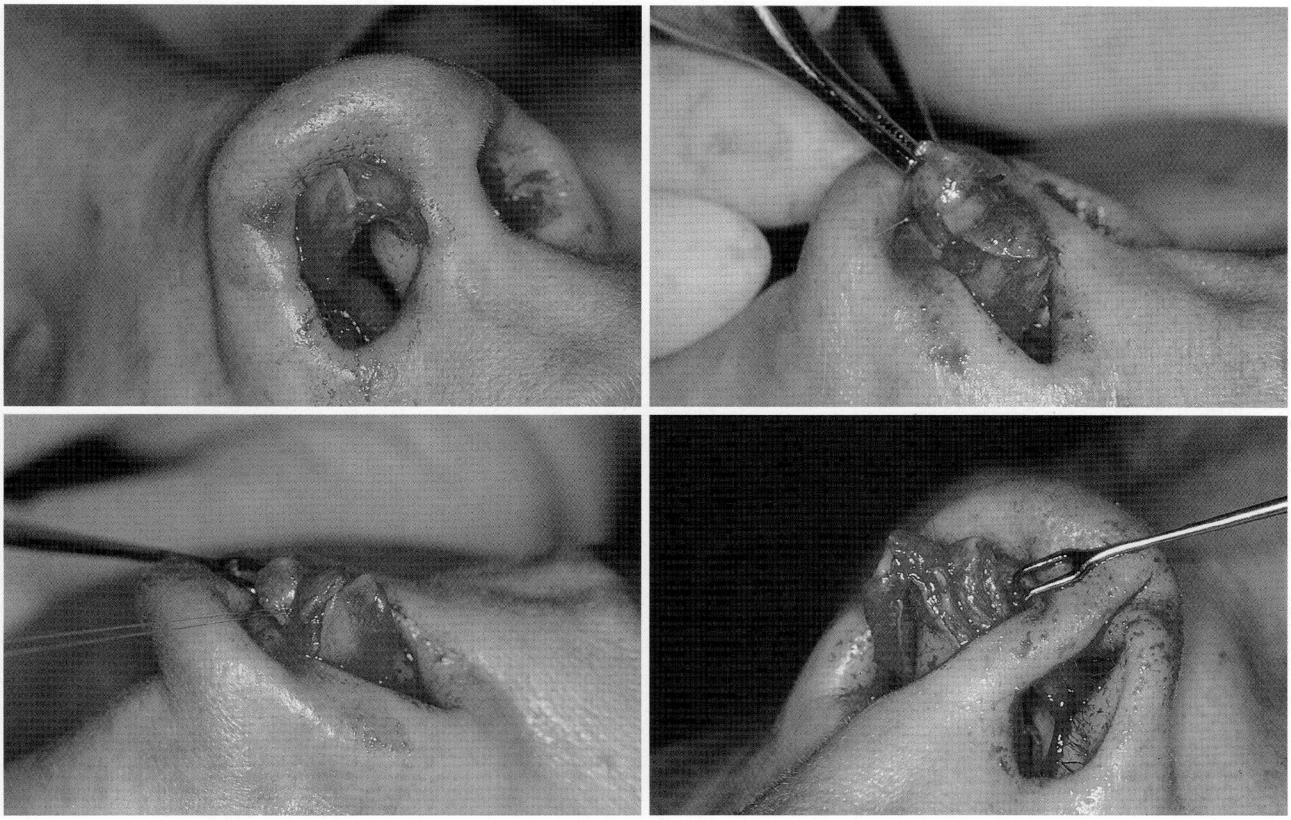

ig. 45.13 **(A–D)** Intraoperative views of the Simons modification of vertical dome division.

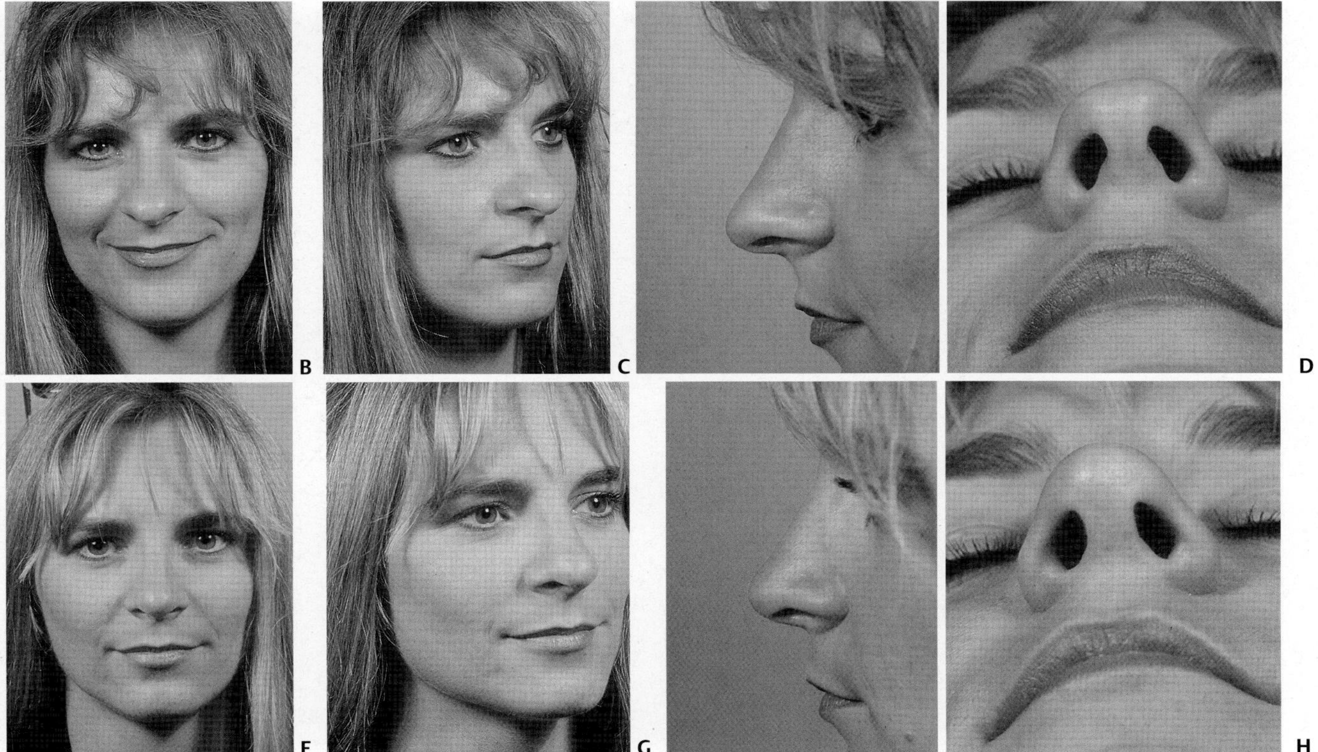

ig. 45.14 **(A–D)** Preoperative views of patient with boxy tip. **(E–H)** Two-year postoperative views after hockey-:ick modification of vertical dome division.

"Breaking the spring" or "relaxing the incision" is the conceptual precept of the VDD technique. In our experience, depending on sutures alone to produce medial strength has proven less effective than the combination of vertical domal incision and suture medial stabilization.

Hockey-Stick Modification

The boxy tip and overprojected tip present not infrequently with excessive cartilage both laterally and anteromedially (**Fig. 45.14**). Too much projection and excess width is an undesirable combination that is encountered frequently. This is the one situation in which a combination of incisional and excisional techniques is employed.

Reduction of volume is performed by the hockey-stick excision of cartilage.[3–5] As opposed to the previously described Goldman and Simons modification procedures, whereby the domal incision is made at or lateral to the lobular apex, the initial cuts in this case are made medial to the domal apex. Segmental sections of the dome (no more than 2 mm to either side of the apex) and a cephalic portion of the lower lateral cartilage are removed (**Fig. 45.15**).[8]

The intact underlying vestibular skin acts as a scaffold for reconstitution of the less projected dome. Again, the only suture advised is between the medial crura to narrow and obliterate intralobular width or bifidity. A 5–0 clear nylon suture is placed in a horizontal mattress fashion in the same manner as in the Simons modification procedure. The lateral crural batten, if not overly resected or undermined from the underlying tissues, will heal medially, achieving a more pyramidal appearance.

As with any tip procedure, the hockey-stick procedure is not the only technique to be considered in reducing the overly projected tip. In thinner-skinned individuals with long, angular lobular configurations, resection of cartilage lateral and inferior to the domal area will retrodisplace the tip by shortening the lateral and medial components of the tripod base.

If the quadrangular septal cartilage is excessive, creating a tension-like overprojection of the tip, resection of the dorsal and caudal elements of the septum is in order. Seldom in our experience has a full transfixion incision alone allowed an overly projected tip to retrodisplace. At times, excision of the feet of the elongated medial crura or reduction of a prominent anterior nasal spine helps to settle or reduce tip projection.

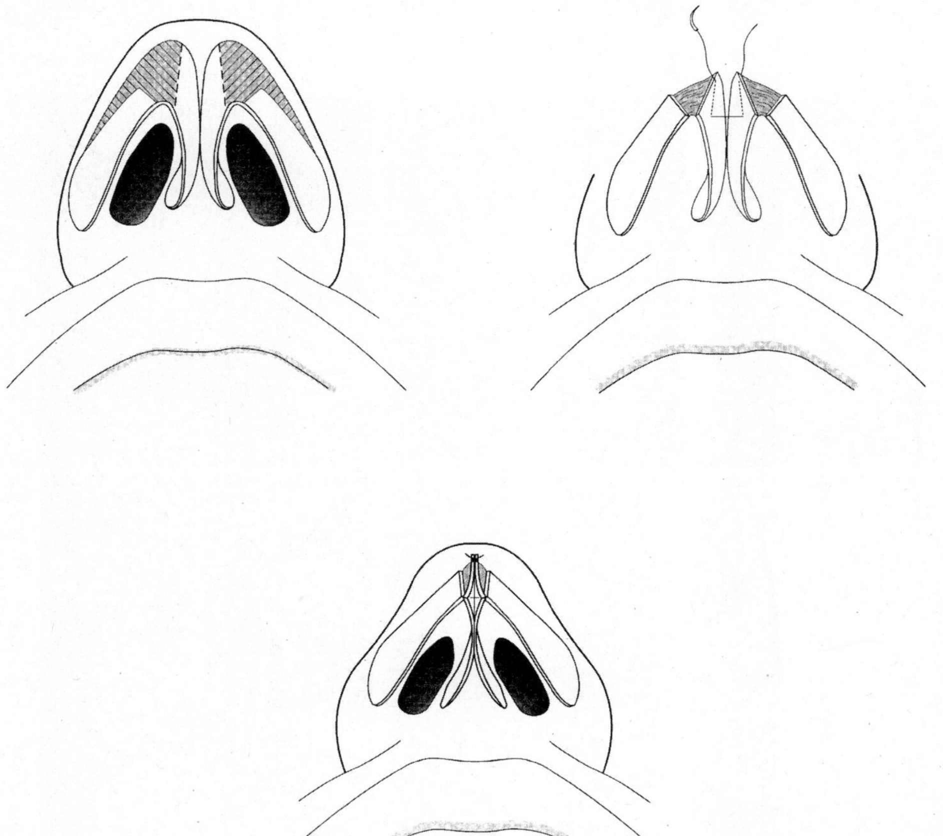

Fig. 45.15 Schematic representation of the hockey-stick modification, combining incisional and excisional techniques.

Adjunctive Techniques

We have increasingly employed the use of a soft onlay of crushed septal cartilage in the lobule. Using a Cottle crusher, septal cartilage can be crushed into a thin, lacy, malleable graft or lightly bruised to form a thicker, firmer, filler graft. This cartilage is placed into the infratip area through the medial aspect of the right marginal incision (**Fig. 45.16**). Depending on the needs of the tip, this onlay of crushed cartilage may serve as a delicate cover, camouflaging sharply incised alar cartilages, or as an augmentation lobular graft if a larger amount of bruised cartilage is introduced into the lobule.[9]

When the columella is somewhat retracted or inadequate, a batten contoured from septal cartilage may be positioned anterior to the medial crura through the marginal incision (**Fig. 45.17**). The batten is differentiated from a strut, which extends from below the feet of the medial

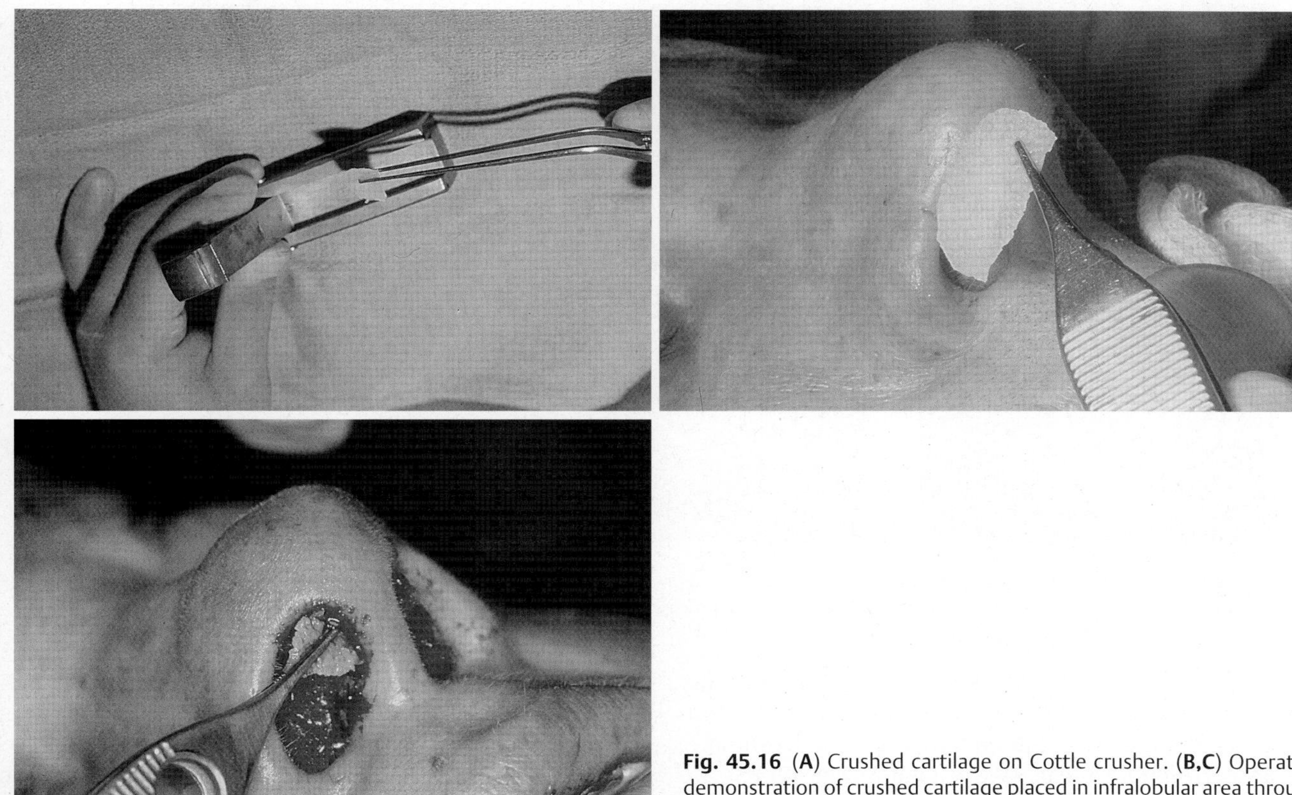

Fig. 45.16 (**A**) Crushed cartilage on Cottle crusher. (**B,C**) Operative demonstration of crushed cartilage placed in infralobular area through right marginal incision.

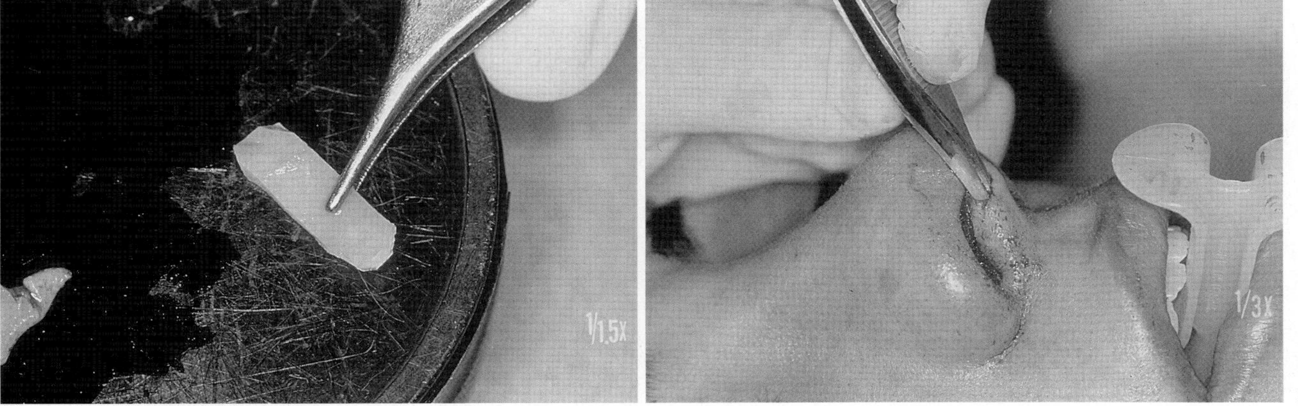

Fig. 45.17 (**A,B**) Batten contoured from septal cartilage being placed anterior to the medial crura via right marginal incision.

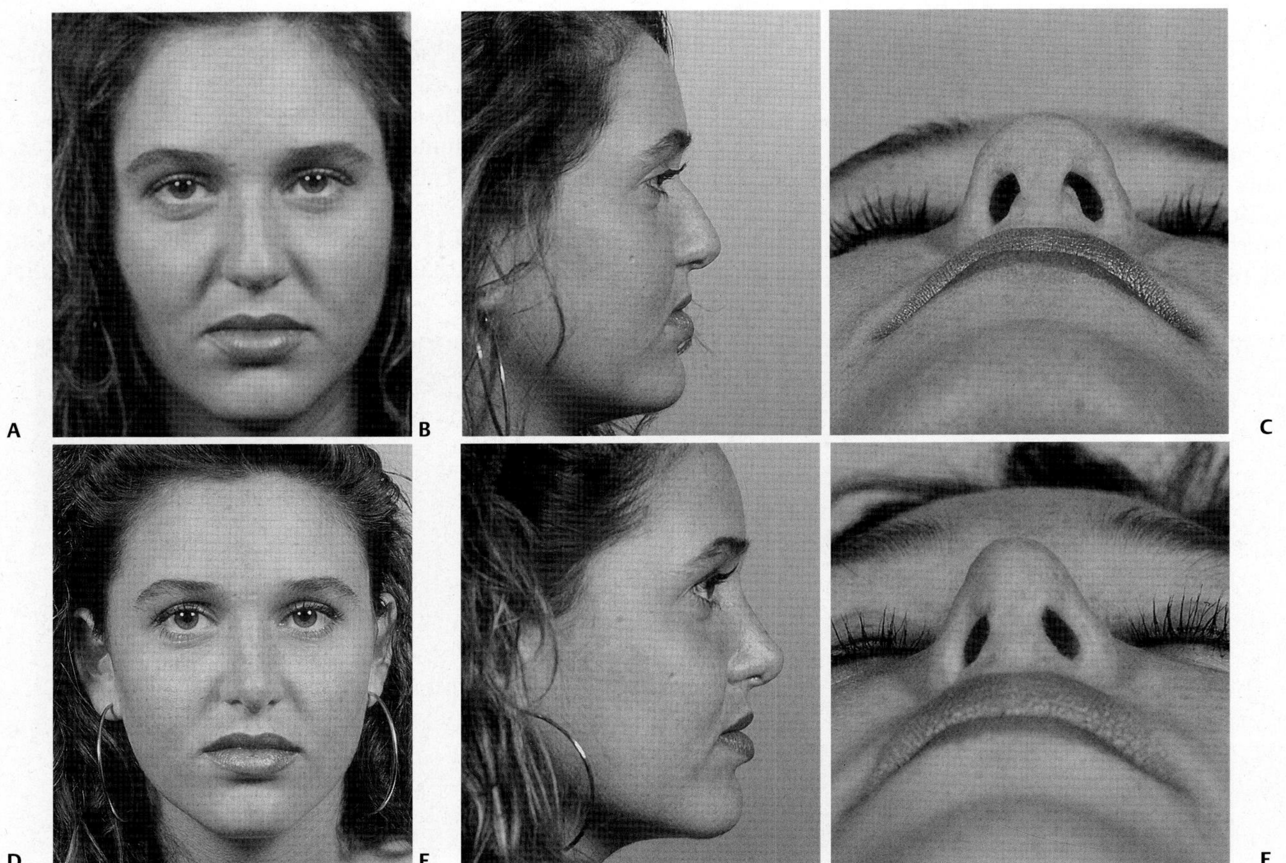

Fig. 45.18 (**A–C**) Preoperative views of patient with dependent tip and poor lobule definition. (**D–F**) Two-year postoperative views after Simons modification of vertical dome division, columellar batten, and infralobular crushed cartilage.

crura to the interdomal space and is placed between the medial crura before they are sutured together. In certain situations, the use of the batten may create or accentuate the desired double break of the lobule (**Fig. 45.18**). In addition, the batten can be used in conjunction with lobular crushed cartilage to lengthen the short nose.

Marginal incisions should be closed by placing two or three interrupted sutures of 4–0 chromic catgut in an oblique fashion. This maneuver encourages medial movement of the bipedal chondrocutaneous flap during the healing process. It is important not to create notching by placing the more medial exit of the suture too close to the alar rim. A lobular "cinch dressing" of clear tape is kept in place for 3 to 4 days with Telfa pads (Kendall, Mansfield, MA) used as internal splints. The tape and plaster cast external dressing is removed from the nose ~5 to 6 days postoperatively.

Summary

In summary, VDD is an excellent method for achieving long-lasting domal highlights, narrowing, and appropriate projection of the nasal tip. It creates medialization and stabilization of the alar cartilages, providing an alternative to tip grafts in primary and some revision cases. The use of extended marginal incisions to deliver the medial and lateral crura allows for accurate placement of incisions and excisions of cartilage and symmetrical suturing of the medial elements. When defining tip cartilages in primary cases, there is little need for the external approach. The classic Goldman technique is used on patients requiring a substantial increase in tip projection, support, or a change in lobular direction. The Simons modification allows for more frequently needed adjustments in tip position and narrowing when simple cephalic resection of the lateral crura is inadequate or when the divergence of the medial crura demands better medial stabilization. The hockey-stick procedure employs a combination of incisional and excisional techniques and is a reliable way to address the overprojected or boxy tip. Whatever the choice of tip procedures, the admonition to preserve and conserve rather than resect and regret rings true. Incisional techniques allow for strong, natural-looking, long-lasting results, often without the need of additional struts or grafts. A better understanding of the nuances of VDD procedures will only strengthen a surgeon's armamentarium of answers for the rhinoplasty patient.

References

1. Goldman IB. The importance of the medial crura in nasal tip reconstruction. Arch Otolaryngol 1957;65:143–147
2. Simons RL, Fine IB. Evaluation of the Goldman tip in rhinoplasty. In: Plastic and Reconstructive Surgery of the Face and Neck: Proceedings of the Second International Symposium. Vol 1. New York: Grune & Stratton; 1977:38–46
3. Simons RL. The difficult nasal tip. In: Current Therapy in Otolaryngology-head and neck surgery: 1982–83. Philadelphia: BC Decker; 1983:122–125
4. Simons RL. Vertical dome division in rhinoplasty. Otolaryngol Clin North Am 1987;20:785–796
5. Simons RL. Vertical dome division techniques. Facial Plast Surg Clin North Am 1994;2:435–458
6. Gillman GS, Simons RL, Lee DJ. Nasal tip bossae in rhinoplasty. Arch Facial Plast Surg 1999;1:83–89
7. Davis AM, Simons RL, Rhee JS. Evaluation of the Goldman tip procedure in modern-day rhinoplasty. Arch Facial Plast Surg 2004;6:301–307
8. Chang CW, Simons RL. Hockey-stick vertical dome division technique for overprojected and broad nasal tips. Arch Facial Plast Surg 2008;10:88–92
9. Simons RL. A personal report: emphasizing the endonasal approach. Facial Plast Surg Clin North Am 2004;12:15–34

46 Secondary Rhinoplasty

Ira D. Papel

Revision rhinoplasty has become a commonplace procedure. As the number of rhinoplastic surgeons has expanded, and the depth of experience has diminished, it is not unusual to see revision rate as high as 15 to 20% after primary procedures.[1] Factored into this rate is the phenomenon that patients expect near perfect results, a trend created by the media and optimistic advertisements by the surgeons themselves. This atmosphere of unrealistic expectations certainly adds to the demand for revision rhinoplasty.

Rhinoplasty as a procedure presents certain problems unique to facial surgery. The combination of skin and soft tissue, cartilage, bone, and mucosa brings together a mix

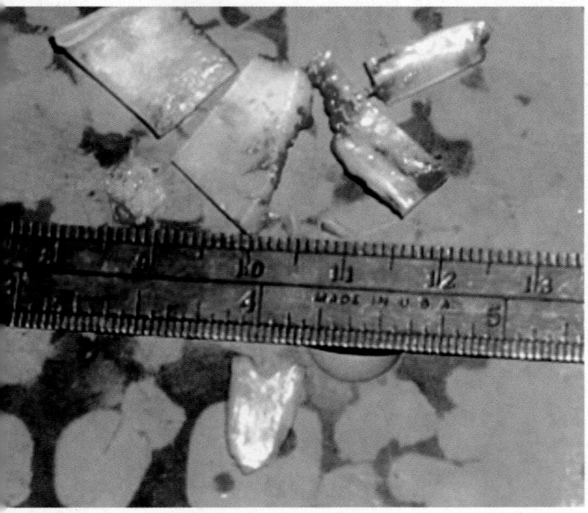

Fig. 46.1 Septal cartilage grafts.

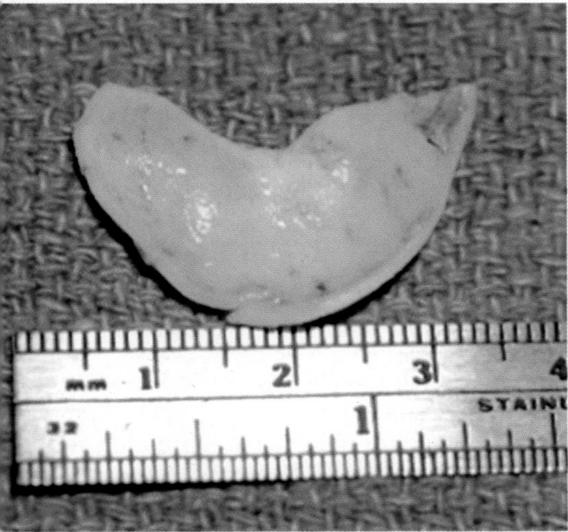

Fig. 46.2 Auricular cartilage grafts.

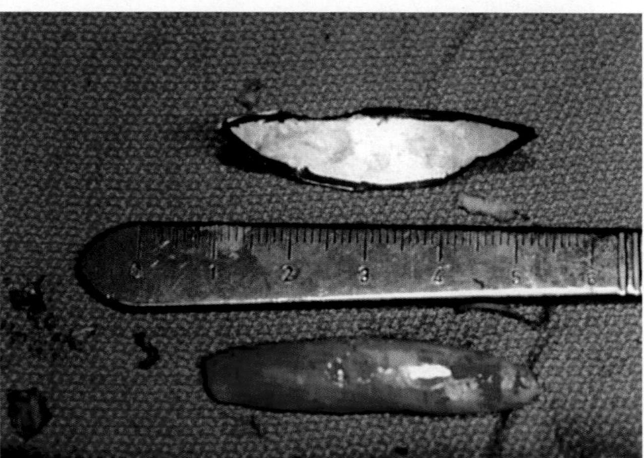

Fig. 46.3 Rib cartilage graft.

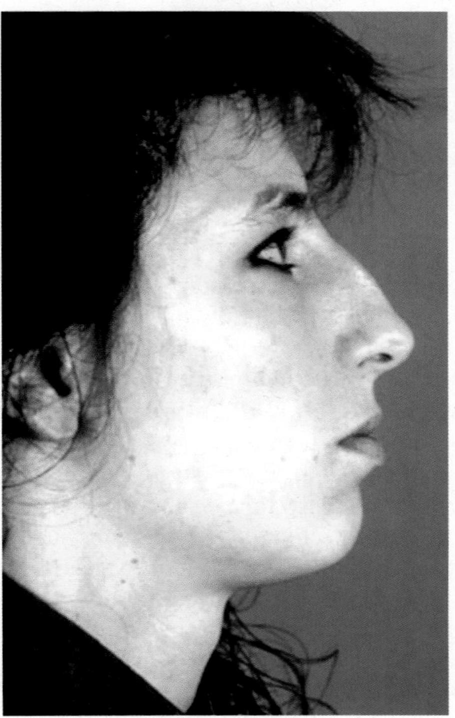

Fig. 46.4 Dorsal contour deformity.

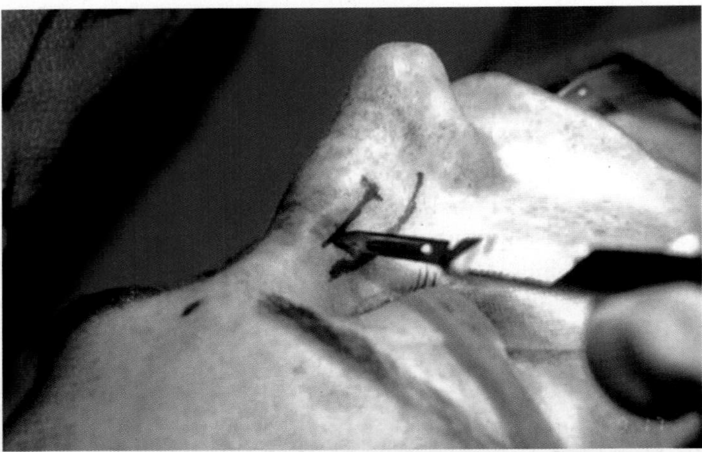

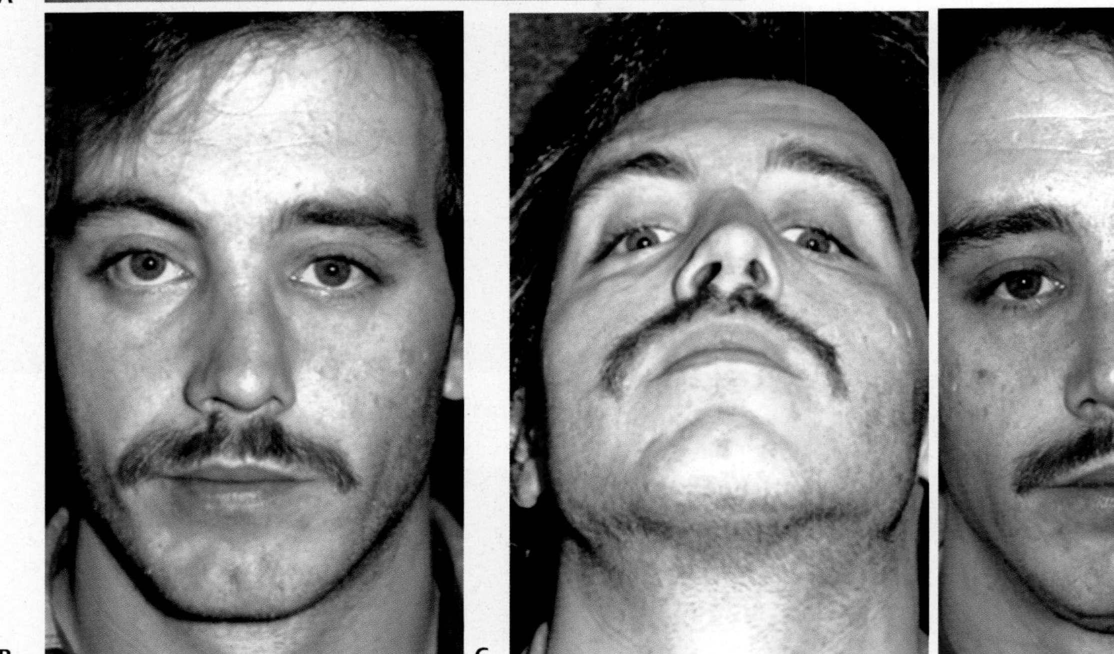

Fig. 46.5 Intermediate osteotomy (**A**); (**B**) and (**C**) show a patient with bony deformities after primary rhinoplasty. (**D**) and (**E**) show patient after intermediate and lateral osteotomies.

of tissue with varying healing characteristics. This puts the onus on the surgeon to predict how these tissues will heal in concert with each other. Although mostly predictable, even a well-performed rhinoplasty operation may result in an unfavorable result. With experience the rhinoplastic surgeon must learn to anticipate healing patterns, and thus minimize the need for revision surgery.

In the history of rhinoplasty, especially in the early twentieth century, most techniques were reductive in nature. The early works of Roe[2] and Joseph[3] specifically addressed altering the nose to reduce prominence in the dorsum and tip. Combined with an emphasis on intranasal incisions at all costs, these techniques often led to inaccurate and uneven resection of nasal structures. The results were often not apparent for years, due to the prolonged tissue edema and patients unfamiliar with expected results. Functional sequelae were often no reported for years, if at all, in the first two thirds of th twentieth century.

The latter part of the century brought a better under standing of the relation between nasal form and functio The rhinoplasty techniques are now less aggressive, wit an emphasis on preservation of key structures. Aestheti norms are now more widely recognized, which togethe with structural preservation helps prevent the notoriou ski-sloped, pinched tip results that were so common u into the 1970s. The reintroduction of the open rhinoplast technique has allowed for more accurate modifications i some cases. The open approach, however, has created som new problems as the surgeon tends to be more inclined t make more alterations. In general, the more alterations in nose, the more likely complications are to occur.

ʾreoperative Evaluation

ʾhe first order of business in evaluating a revision rhi-oplasty patient is to determine what surgery has been one in the past, and by what techniques. It is impor-ant to determine the number and timing of past proce-ures, and also how the patient feels about the current tatus. Questions should be asked about the original ose, function before and after the surgical interven-ions, and what the expectations of further surgery re. Operative notes may be helpful, and should be equested. If the previous surgery was more than 0 years before the consultation, it may be difficult to btain these records.

The patient interview is also vital to determine if the atient has realistic expectations. There is a subset of atients who will never be satisfied with any result, and hus keep seeking revision surgery for even small, insig-ificant physical traits. Patients with body dysmorhic isorder are not good candidates for surgery, and they nust be identified as early as possible to avoid further omplications.[4] The experienced surgeon learns how to pot these patients, and steers them to more appropriate sychological consultation.[5]

Physical diagnosis is the key to successful revision asal surgery. An accurate assessment of the aesthetic nd functional problems will help the surgeon determine he best course of action. Therefore a detailed inter-al and external nasal examination is essential during he initial, and subsequent, consultations. Specific areas o examine include the nasal septum, turbinates, and nternal valves. Externally, the upper, middle, and lower aults with their associated anatomical components must be individually assessed. The status of the skin–soft tissue envelope must be evaluated with regard to thickness and rigidity. Old scars should be documented. In revision rhinoplasty patients the stability of the nasal valves is often in question. The surgeon should determine if pathology exists in the internal valve, external valve, or both. This area is frequently overlooked by rhinoplasty surgeons. Not all patients with nasal obstruction have problems limited to the septum and turbinates.

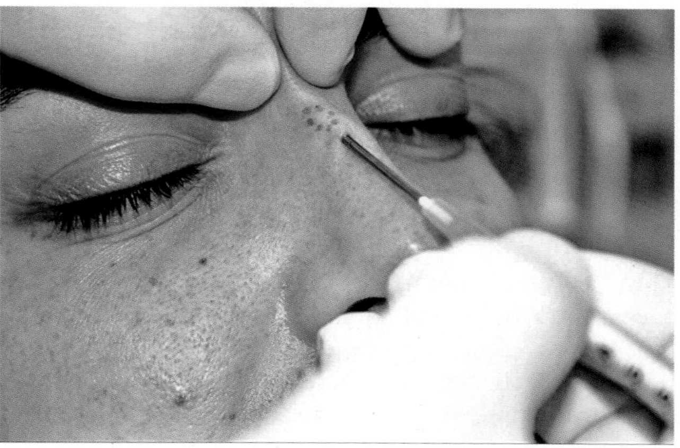

Fig. 46.7 Needle shave for minor dorsal deformity

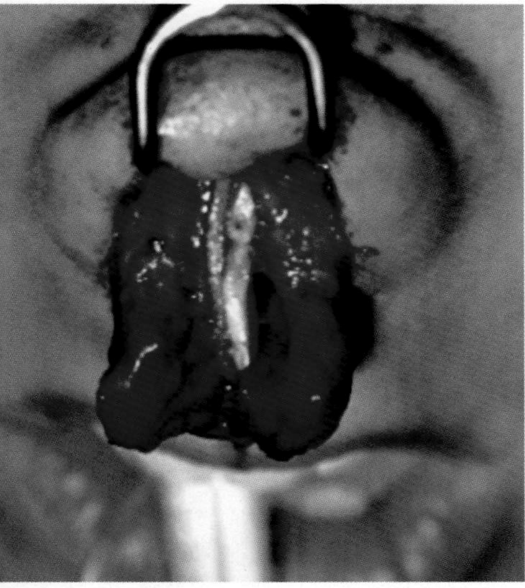

ig. 46.6 Intraoperative view of extended spreader graft used to traighten nose.

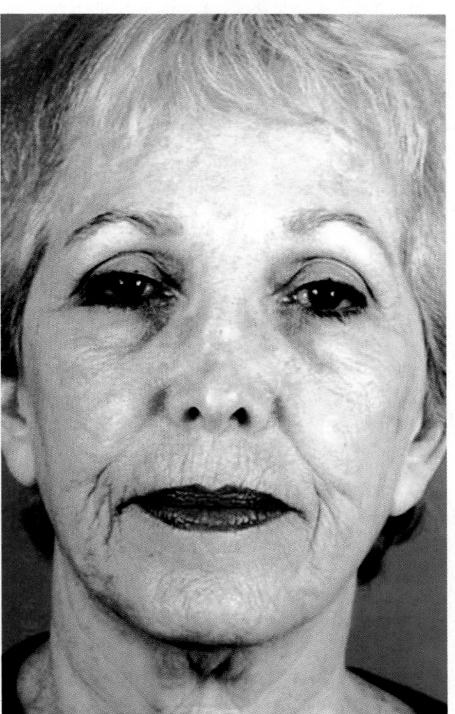

Fig. 46.8 Inverted-V deformity 40 years after primary rhinoplasty.

Therefore, a thorough aesthetic, functional, and psychological assessment must be obtained before deciding if a patient is a proper candidate for revision rhinoplasty surgery.

Timing of Revision Surgery

Most revision rhinoplasty patients present more than 1 year after the initial surgery. This occurs due to several factors. Most surgeons will accurately point out to patients that the soft tissue takes at least 1 year to mature, reassuring their patients that in time certain deformities will diminish. This is often true, but not universal. Many patients are satisfied for several years before deformities become more obvious, often associated with functional problems. This patient group demonstrates graphically that the final results of rhinoplasty may actually encompass 10 to 15 years or longer. Serial photographs taken over a 20- to 30-year period clearly show continuous soft tissue changes and movement of cartilaginous structures. This phenomenon of "shrink wrapping" of the skin–soft tissue envelope has been well described.[6]

When surgery has been in the recent past, it is usually wise to wait until 1 year to let the initial soft tissue edema resolve. In most circumstances this will be sufficient to

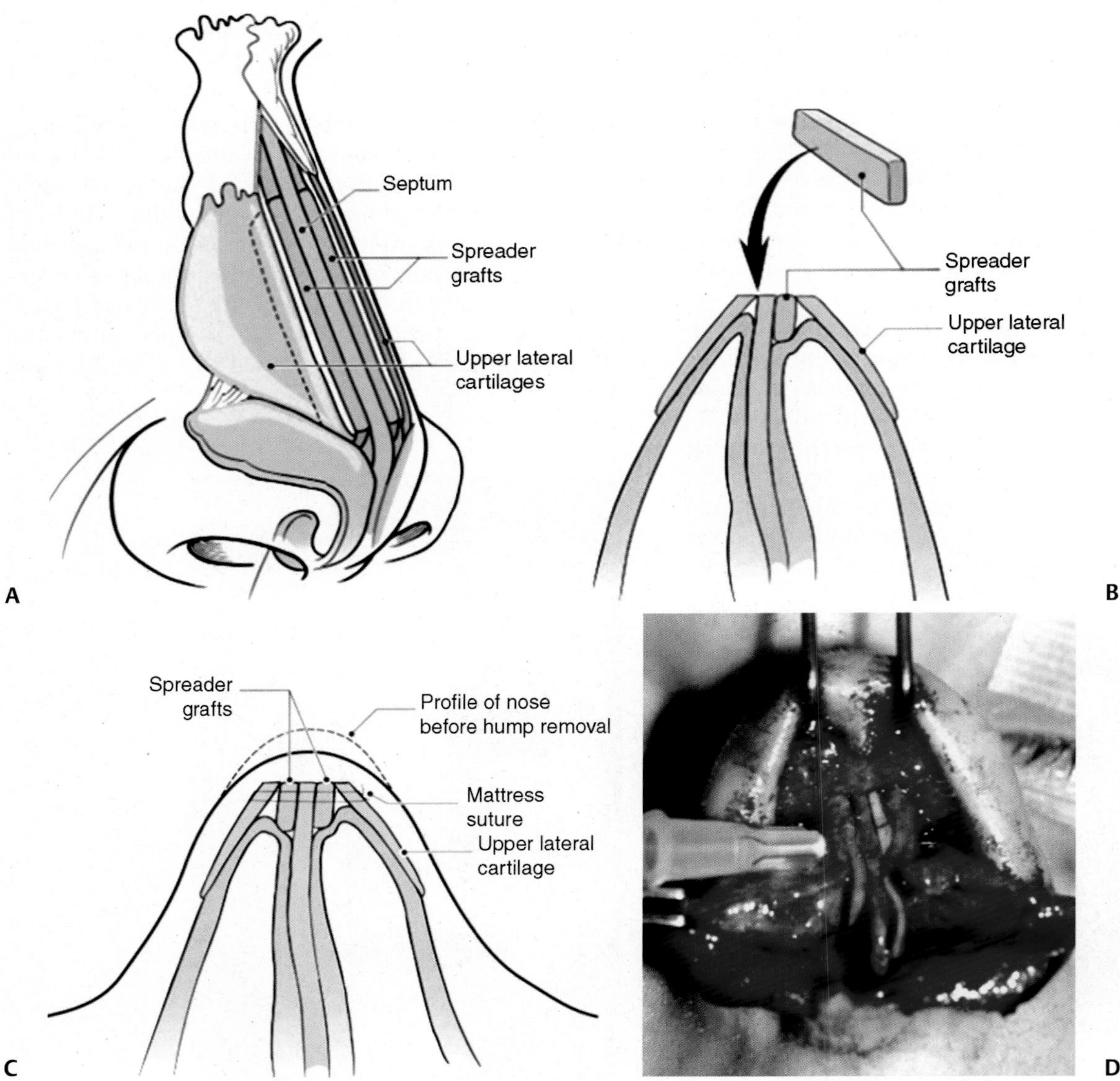

Fig. 46.9 Spreader grafts. (**A**) Classic positioning of spreader grafts. (**B**) Placement between septum and upper lateral cartilage. (**C**) Axial view of spreader grafts with widening of internal valve. (**D**) Operative view of spreader grafts.

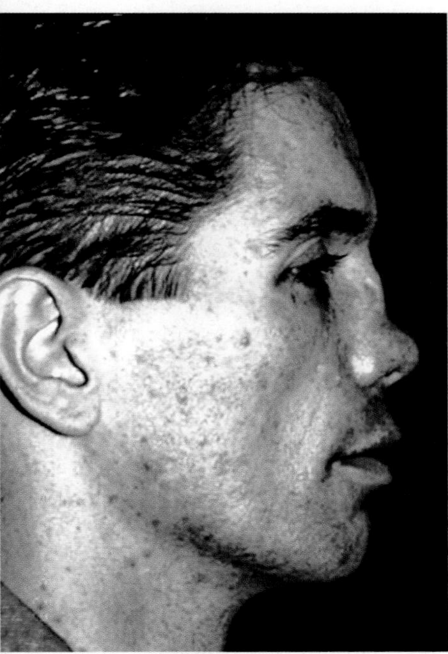

Fig. 46.10 Saddle nose deformity.

determine if deformities will continue to be a concern. One exception to this rule is if there is a gross deformity that has no chance to improve. A significant saddle nose, or severe loss of tip support, are examples of problems that will likely get worse while waiting a full year. The added factors of scar contraction and loss of tissue planes will only make the correction more difficult at a later date. Therefore for some deformities the correction should be undertaken as soon as the problem is recognized.

Surgical Technique

In recent years the open approach has become more popular for primary rhinoplasty. In revision rhinoplasty the choice of approach should be dictated by the deformity or problems being addressed. The surgeon should choose the exposure that provides the best chance to repair the problem, balanced with the least invasion/alteration required to get that result.

For example, a simple dorsal contour deformity is best addressed through an intranasal intracartilaginous incision. This will preserve the tip structures, which require no further alteration. Simple alar grafting may actually be easier to perform via a marginal incision than an open method. On the other hand, a patient with significant middle vault collapse needing structural grafts may require an open approach for proper placement and fixation of grafts. Significant tip asymmetry also lends itself to open procedures.

The choice of approach should be dictated by the individual needs of the patient. All rhinoplastic surgeons should have an array of techniques available to treat the wide range of deformities encountered.

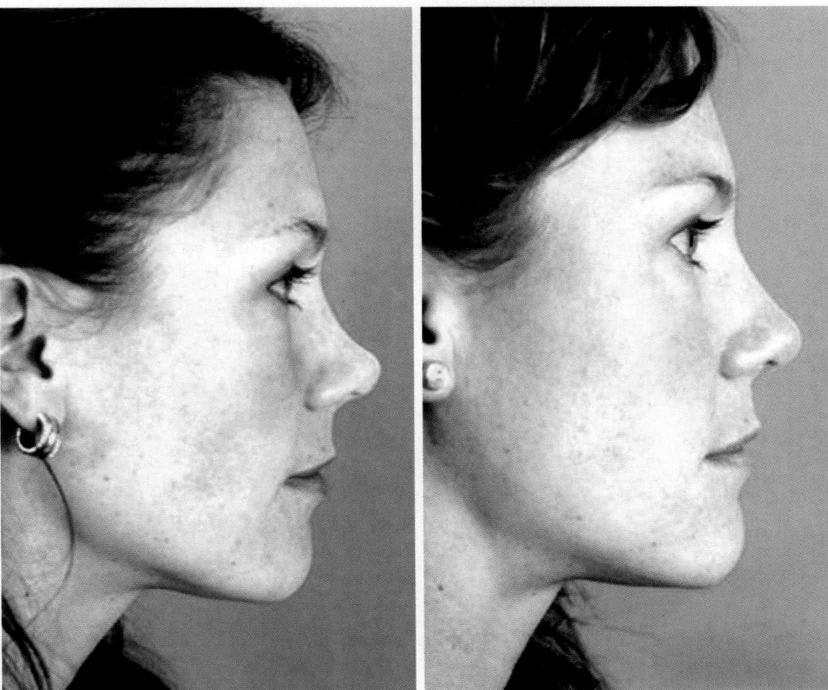

Fig. 46.11 (**A**) Patient with overresected dorsum after primary rhinoplasty. (**B**) After correction with septal cartilage grafts.

Grafting Materials

Revision rhinoplasty often requires replacement of structural anatomy. As a general principle of reconstruction the surgeon should replace anatomical structures with like materials. In the nose this implies autologous cartilage grafts to repair the lower two thirds of the nose. Cartilage is often used to repair the upper bony structures as well.

If septal cartilage is available, this is usually the easiest to obtain with minimal morbidity. Unfortunately, many revision rhinoplasty patients have already had resection of septal cartilage in previous procedures. The next choice is auricular cartilage, which is present in most patients. Auricular cartilage is obtained from the conchal bowl via either a lateral or medial incision. Composite grafts can also be obtained from the conchal area.

The auricular cartilage is especially helpful in alar reconstruction due to its inherent curvature and thickness.

Costal cartilage is a rich bank of cartilage for patients in need of more extensive reconstruction. This may be needed if septal and/or auricular grafts are not available. Harvesting of rib cartilage does require more time, and is associated with more donor site discomfort than septal or ear cartilage. Care should be taken to avoid pleural puncture, and the incision should be meticulously closed to minimize the scar.

Cranial bone has been utilized for dorsal nasal reconstruction with some success.[7] The bone is harvested from the outer table of the parietal skull, and is available in large amounts. Donor site morbidity is minimal with careful technique.[8] Fixation of the bone grafts is essential, and using a sunken lag screw into the preexisting nasal bones is a reliable method. Cranial bone grafts in the nose do tend to create an unnatural stiffness, often noted by patients.

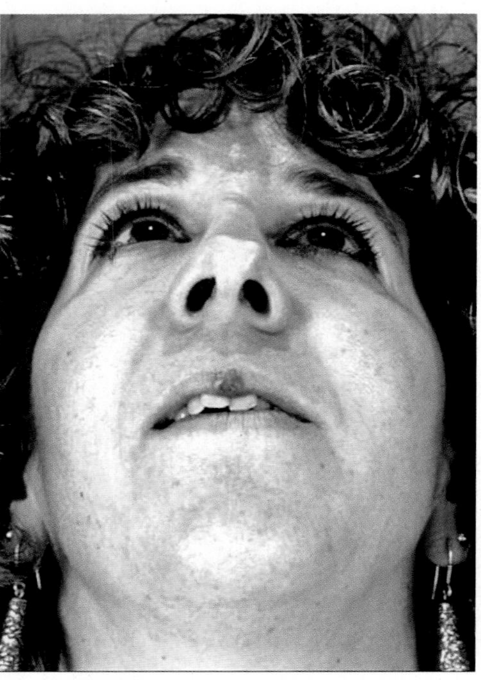

Fig. 46.13 Asymmetric tip.

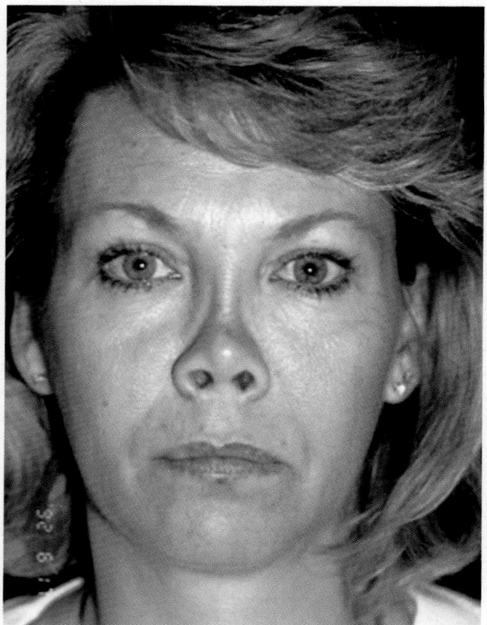

Fig. 46.12 Open roof deformity.

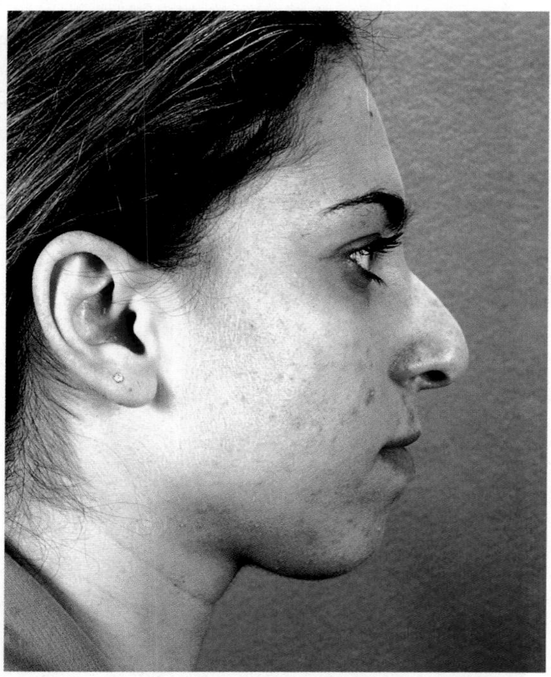

Fig. 46.14 Pollybeak deformity.

Synthetic materials have been utilized in primary and revision rhinoplastic surgery for many years. The rate of extrusion or infection of materials such as Gore-Tex (W. L. Gore & Associates, Inc., Flagstaff, AZ) or Medpor (Porex Surgical Inc., Newman, GA) in primary cases has been ~3%.[9] This complication rate in revision rhinoplasty patients is much higher. With longer studies the rate of extrusion seems to increase.[10] Therefore, many surgeons will utilize synthetic materials in revision rhinoplasty only if no other options are unavailable or the patient will not allow the use of autologous grafts (**Figs. 46.1–46.3**).

Bony Dorsal Deformities

The most common deformity of the bony dorsum after rhinoplasty is a visual contour deformity. This may be midline or lateral. These contour defects are due to uneven resection or augmentation of the upper one third of the nose. Due to thin skin coverage in this area the defect is usually apparent early, and does not improve with time. Treatment will usually require an intranasal approach, undermining of the skin–soft tissue envelope, and correcting the contour by rasping the bone edges or augmenting depressions with small cartilage grafts (**Fig. 46.4**).

Deviation of the nasal bones after rhinoplasty is also very common, especially if there was asymmetry beforehand. Correction may require a combination of revision osteotomies and/or onlay grafts to camouflage bony concavities. An intermediate osteotomy on bony convexities combined with lateral osteotomies may help even out the bony dorsum (**Fig. 46.5**).

Stair-step deformities of the upper lateral dorsum are the result of a lateral osteotomy being placed too high on the nasal process. This results in a visible and palpable deformity, often asymmetric. Treatment will require medial and lateral osteotomies to mobilize and properly place the lateral bony fragments.

Rocker deformities can result when the osteotomy produces a fracture that extends beyond the nasal bone and into the medial orbital wall. Pressing on the nasal bone causes the superior bones to lateralize, thus named a rocker deformity. Treatment will require splinting the bones in the original position and allowing healing for 8 to 12 weeks. After the bones are fully healed the proper osteotomy can be accomplished.

Middle Vault Deformities

Middle vault deformities are the result of asymmetry or malposition of the upper lateral cartilages. This pair of cartilages supports the airway and determines the external contour. The middle vault is important in hump reduction, and if certain anatomical relationships are not

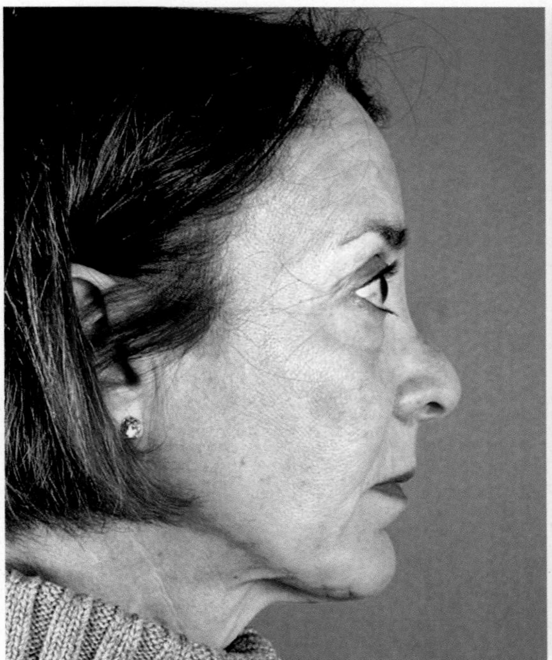

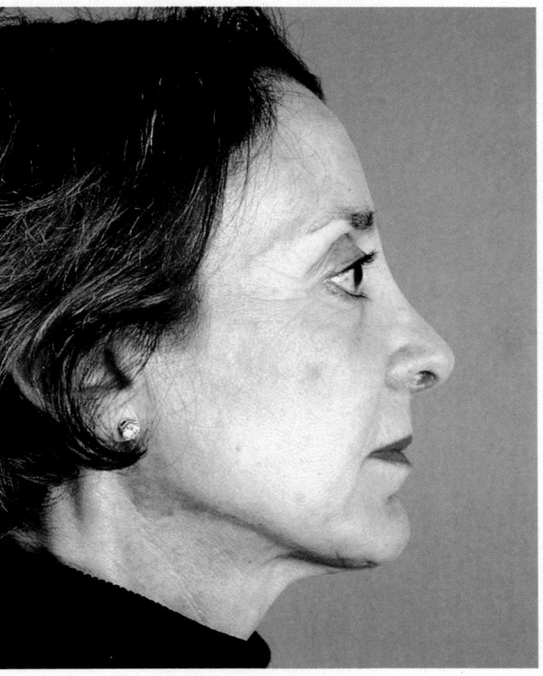

Fig. 46.15 (**A**) Lateral view of patient with pollybeak deformity after primary rhinoplasty. (**B**) After correction with columellar strut, tip sutures, reduction of supratip septum, and radix grafts.

preserved, both aesthetic and functional sequelae may occur.

Asymmetry is the most common middle vault deformity. Uneven lowering of the upper lateral cartilages may not be apparent for several months after surgery. Due to upward retraction during surgery asymmetries may be hidden. It is best to check the height of the upper lateral cartilages when minimal or no retraction is used. Palpation is a valuable tool to assess the dorsal contour during surgery to avoid this deformity.

Correction of asymmetry will require lowering the offending cartilage edge, or cartilage grafting when a depression is noted. Spreader grafts can be used to elevate and lateralize a depressed upper lateral cartilage for contour or function. Minor cartilage defects can be addressed by utilizing a transcutaneous needle to shave or soften the cartilage under local anesthesia (**Figs. 46.6 and 46.7**).

The inverted-V deformity occurs after rhinoplasty when the middle vault becomes displaced in a posterior and inferior direction. The mechanism appears to be lack of support for the middle vault after surgery. The typical signs

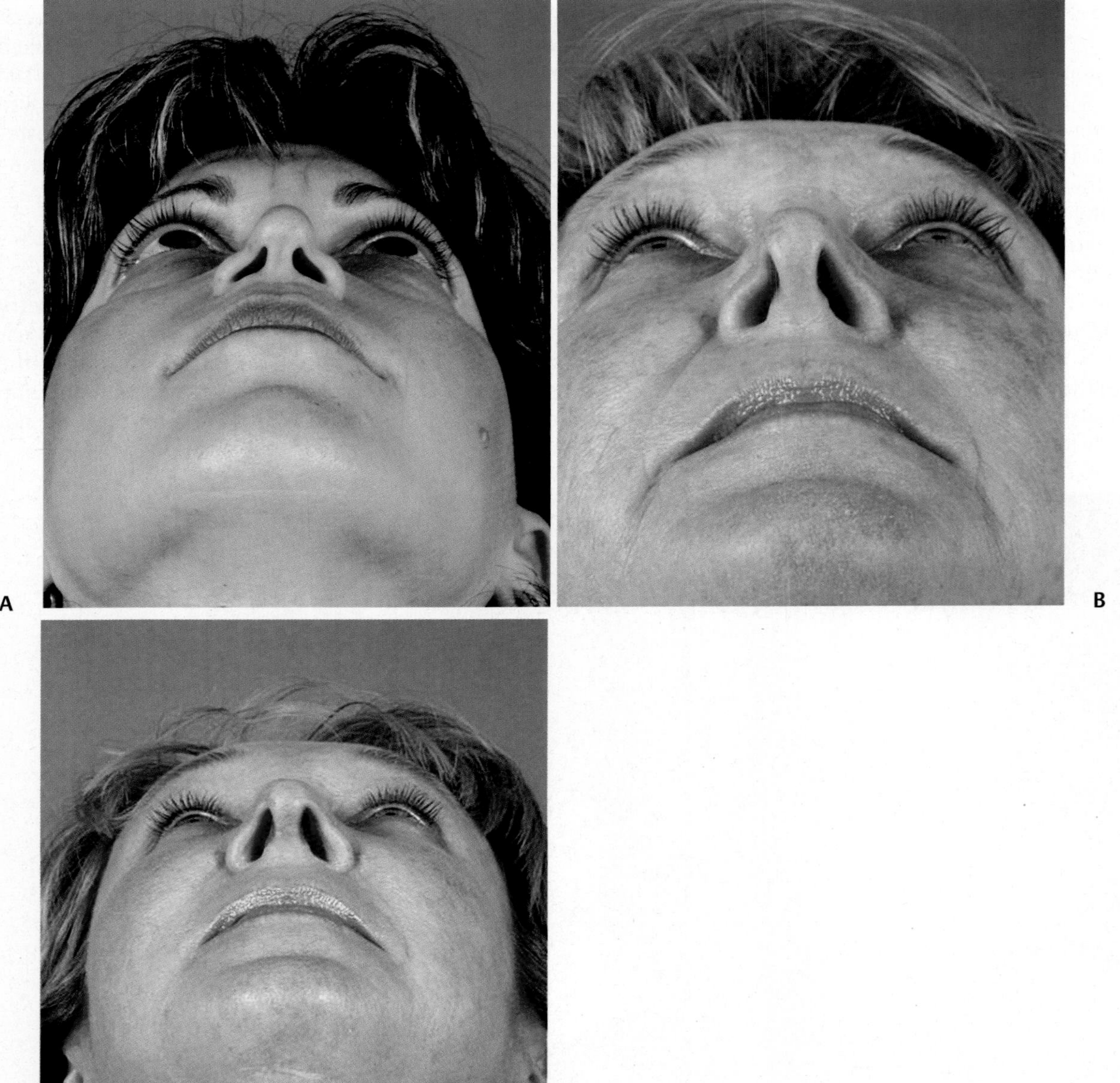

Fig. 46.16 (**A**) Patient with bilateral alar collapse. (**B**) Unilateral right alar collapse. (**C**) Correction of right alar collapse with batten graft.

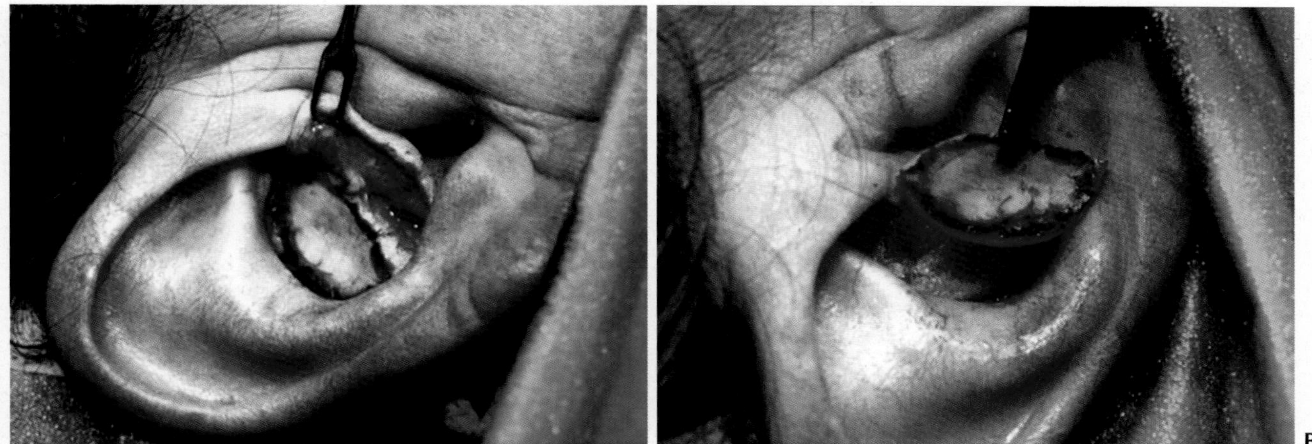

Fig. 46.17 (**A**) Obtaining cymba concha graft from right ear with skin flap raised. (**B**) Excised cartilage that can be divided into two equal batten grafts.

may not be apparent for years after the procedure. Reestablishing the natural relationship between the upper lateral cartilages and the septum at the initial procedure may prevent this problem. The placement of spreader grafts for position and stability may be utilized in both primary and secondary operations.[11] In some patients a permanent suture reestablishing the anatomical relationship of the septum and upper lateral cartilages may prevent these late sequelae (**Figs. 46.8 and 46.9**).

The most obvious middle vault deformity is the saddle nose. This may result from collapse of the cartilaginous dorsum, or it can be combined with a bony dorsal deficiency (**Fig. 46.10**).

Saddle nose defects can result from overresection of the skeleton, or from lack of support provided by the septum. Cocaine abusers and those who have had aggressive septal surgery are the most common patients to present with this disorder. There are patients with granulomatous disorders, such as sarcoid or syphilis, who can develop saddle noses without any previous surgery.

Correction will require replacement of the supporting skeleton with cartilage grafts. Smaller defects can be repaired with auricular cartilage, but significant saddle defects will require rib cartilage to reestablish proper dorsal strength and contour (**Fig. 46.11**).

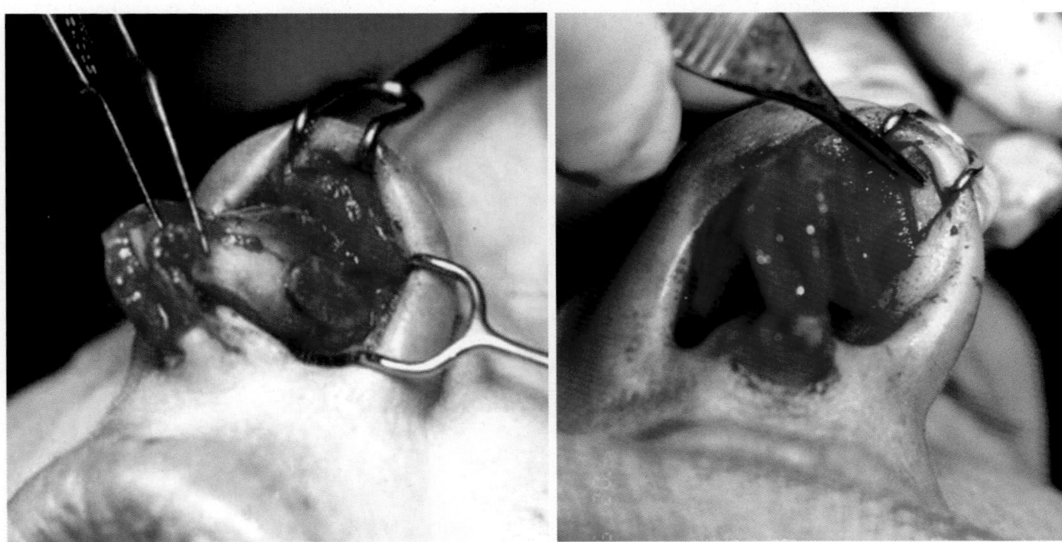

Fig. 46.18 (**A**) Alar batten graft in place. (**B**) Alar rim graft being placed.

Open Roof Deformity

After hump removal a gap may exist between the lateral nasal walls and the septum. This is typically closed by either osteotomies or the use of spreader grafts. If this gap remains open an obvious contour defect of the dorsum may develop. Revision will require completion of the lateral osteotomies, spreader grafts, or dorsal grafting to correct the contour deformity (**Fig. 46.12**).

Nasal Tip

The nasal tip presents unique problems in rhinoplasty. This portion of the nose contains the most variable anatomy among humans. In addition, the skin of the nasal tip is thicker than the rest of the nose, which contributes to the length of healing and camouflage of defects for months to years. The lower lateral cartilages are often asymmetric, with overlying soft tissues of varying thickness that may disguise the differences. Attempts to force the lower lateral cartilages into a symmetric formation may actually yield a more asymmetric result. Preoperative and intraoperative assessment is critical to obtaining predictable results. Therefore asymmetry of the nasal tip is probably the most common complication in the tip requiring revision.

Correction of the asymmetric tip often depends on the nature of the previous procedures. Cartilage-splitting techniques may require reconstitution of the domes with supporting grafts. Previous tip grafts may need to be carved or relocated. Resection of large portions of the lower lateral cartilages may demand alar batten or rim grafts. Composite grafts may be necessary to correct alar retraction and/or valve collapse. Suture techniques may help to bring the domes into better position relative to each other.[12] There are a myriad of techniques described to correct the asymmetric nasal tip (**Fig. 46.13**).

Supratip Fullness/Pollybeak

Supratip fullness after rhinoplasty, the so-called pollybeak deformity, can result from several technical errors or a combination of physical traits. If there is significant tip edema during a rhinoplasty procedure, it is often difficult to judge the proper height of the nasal dorsum. In an effort not to overresect the cartilaginous dorsum the area around the anterior septal angle may be left too high. This leads to supratip fullness, especially true during intranasal techniques (**Fig. 46.14**).

Tip projection and support are major factors in supratip fullness. If the tip does not have the strength to stand

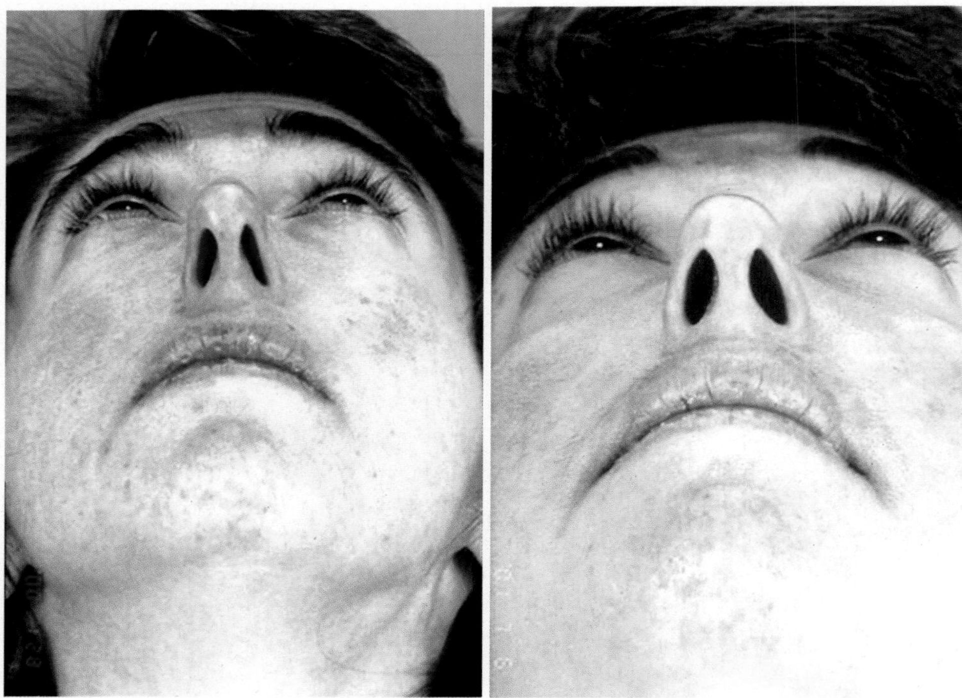

Fig. 46.19 (**A**) Patient with bilateral external valve insufficiency after primary rhinoplasty. (**B**) Base view after bilateral batten graft placement to strengthen nasal valve.

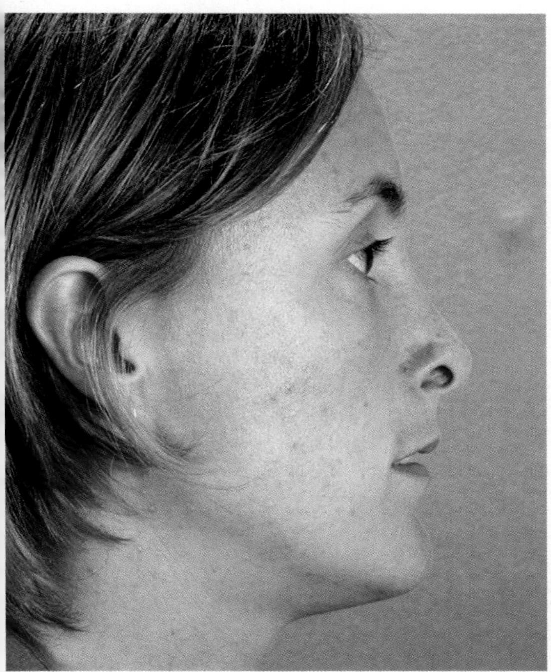

Fig. 46.20 Alar retraction.

up to postoperative tissue contraction, it will be pulled posterior and create a roundness in the profile. This has a major impact on profile aesthetics, and possibly on nasal function. It is critical that the surgeon understand the role of tip projection, and be familiar with ways to support the tip so that projection will be maintained in the healing process. Correction may include columellar advancement, columellar struts, tip grafts, or lateral crural steal procedures.[13]

Overresection of the bony dorsum can also give the impression of supratip fullness. Combined with inadequate tip projection the appearance may be the most extreme version of pollybeak deformity. In addition to improving tip projection, dorsal augmentation at the radix may be indicated (**Fig. 46.15**).

Alar Collapse

In an attempt to sculpt the tip many surgeons have overresected the lower lateral cartilages, leading to weakness of the lateral crura. The result may be external valve collapse, in addition to unsightly notching in the alar margin. In past

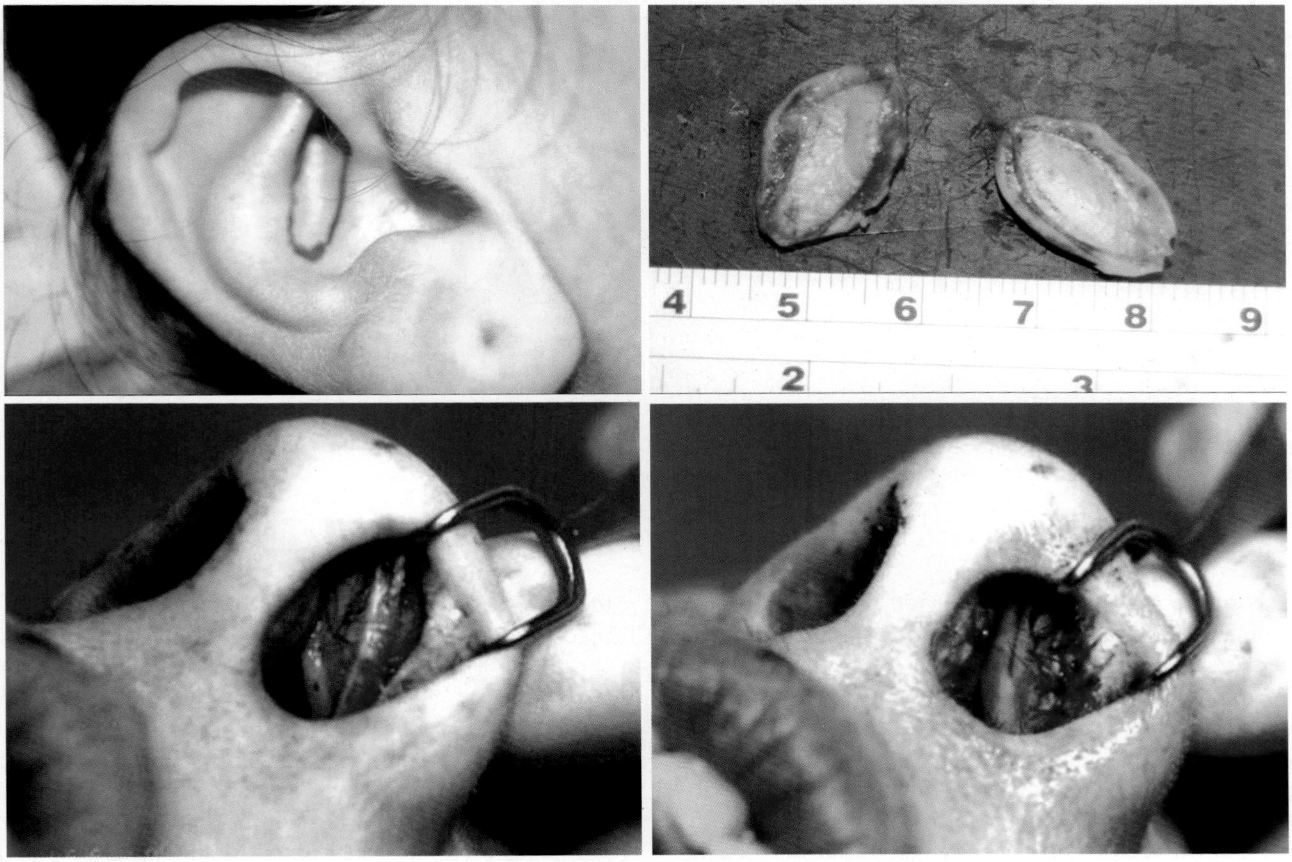

Fig. 46.21 (**A**) Donor site for auricular composite graft. (**B**) Bilateral grafts prior to placement. (**C**) Marginal incision prepared for composite graft placement. (**D**) Composite graft in place.

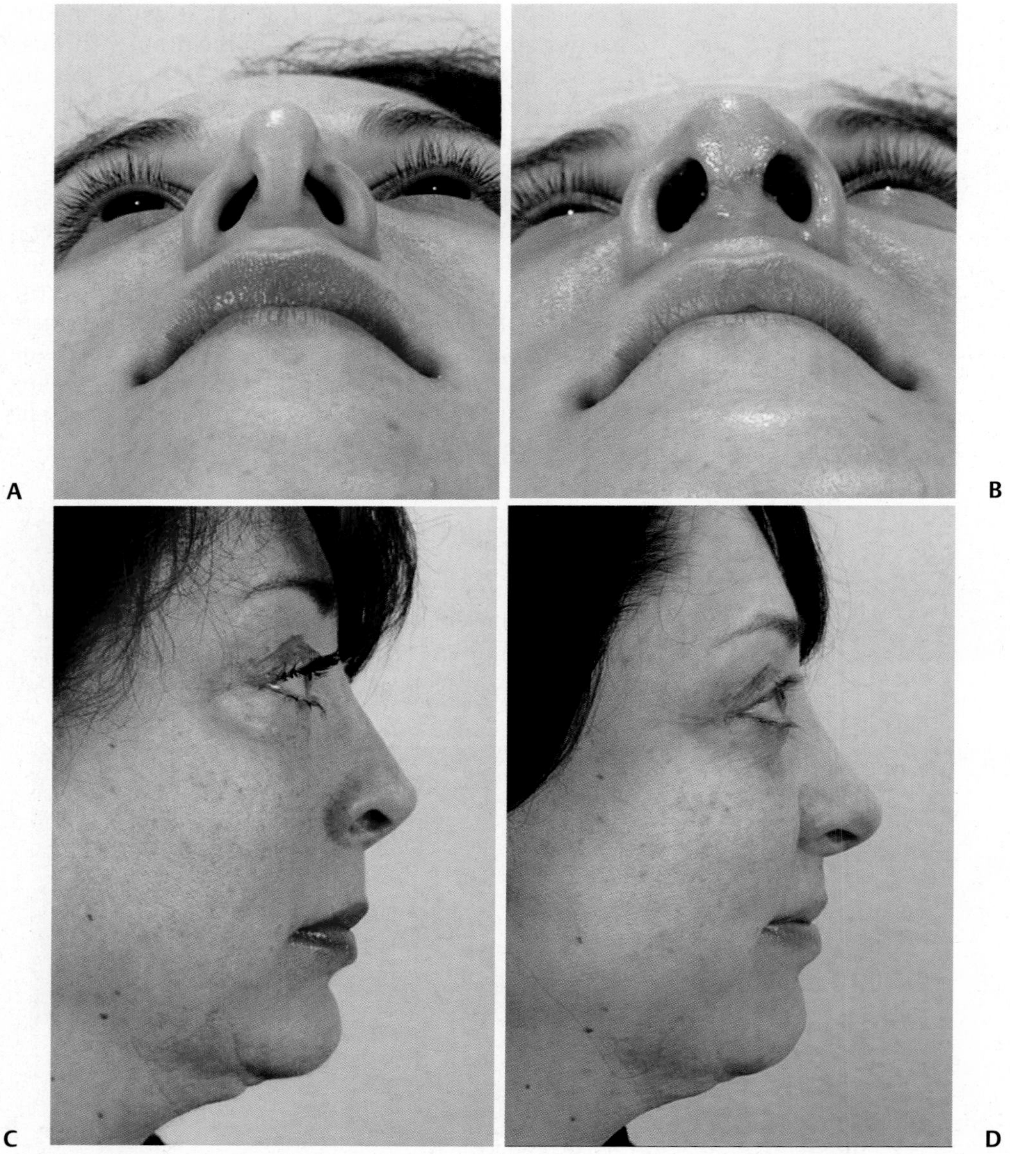

Fig. 46.22 (**A**) Base view of patient with alar retraction and collapse. (**B**) base view after placement of bilateral composite grafts. (**C**) Lateral view of patient with alar retraction. (**D**) Lateral view after composite grafts.

years many surgeons were instructed to leave only 2 to 4 mm of cartilage in the lateral crura. This often was adequate for several years, but resulted in a combination of deformities later. Alar retraction, collapse, and notching have been the most significant (**Fig. 46.16**).

Correction of these deformities will often include cartilage grafting. Septal cartilage may be used if available, but auricular cartilage often has a better natural shape to reconstruct the ala. The grafts are easily harvested from the cymba concha of the ear via either an anterior or posterior approach. It is helpful to avoid making the skin and cartilage incisions in one place to avoid a contour deformity. Mattress sutures should be placed to prevent a hematoma postsurgery (**Fig. 46.17**).

The grafts may be placed as an alar batten graft on the surface of the residual cartilage, or as an alar strut graft between the mucosa and the existing lower lateral cartilage. Direct suture fixation with long-term suture material is desirable. In either case an alar rim graft may be necessary to improve the contour of the alar margin[14] (**Fig. 46.18 and Fig. 46.19**).

Alar Retraction

Another complication of overresection of the lower lateral cartilages is alar rim retraction. Loss of support and extensive undermining will result in superior retraction of the alar margin, leading to excessive columellar show and cosmetic deformity. The usual appearance is very obvious, and is a tell-tale sign of an aggressive rhinoplasty. Alar retraction with excess columellar show must be distinguished from an overlong septum (**Fig. 46.20**).

Treatment of this deformity will usually include auricular composite grafts to force the alar margin to move caudally. The composite graft will concurrently provide support to correct external valve collapse. If the septum is too long a caudal resection can be performed to reduce excess columellar show (**Fig. 46.21 and Fig. 46.22**).

Bossae

Another complication of lower lateral cartilage resection is deformity of the dome areas due to scar contraction in the healing process. The combination of weak cartilage, thin skin, and overresection can lead to this obvious deformity. The usual sign is asymmetry of the domes, which becomes worse over time. Treatment may include shaving off the deformity via a marginal incision or cartilage grafting on top of the deformity[15] (**Fig. 46.23**).

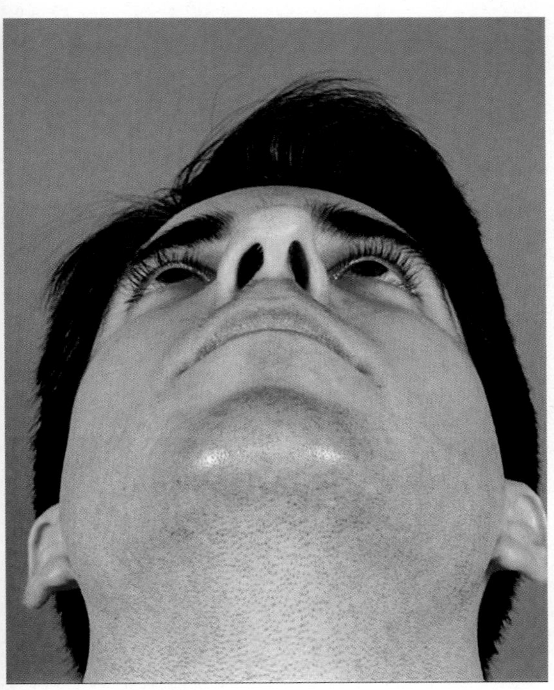

Fig. 46.23 Nasal tip bossae 10 years after primary rhinoplasty.

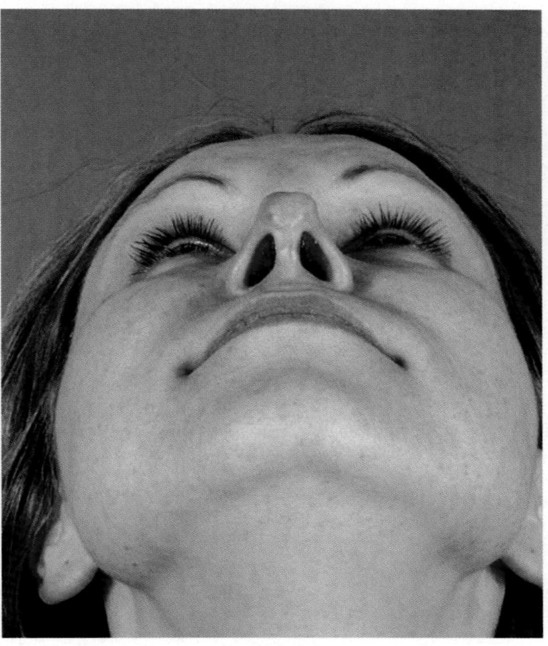

Fig. 46.24 Prominent tip graft in patient with thin skin 5 years after placement.

Prominent Tip Graft

In the era of open rhinoplasty tip grafts have been used much more frequently. Shield grafts to increase projection and shape the tip have become commonplace. In patients with thin skin these grafts can become very obvious over time as tissue contraction takes place (**Fig. 46.24**).

Correction of this deformity will require a revision open procedure with softening or trimming of the graft edges. Covering the graft with a layer of temporalis fascia or allograft dermis is helpful in preserving the support and contour of the area (**Fig. 46.25**).

Short Nose

The overshortened nose is one of the most difficult rhinoplasty sequela to repair. The result of overzealous resection of the caudal septum, overrotation will result as healing and scar contraction evolves. Correction will include caudal septal extension grafts and extended spreader grafts, in addition to grafting of the columella and ala[16–18] (**Fig. 46.26**).

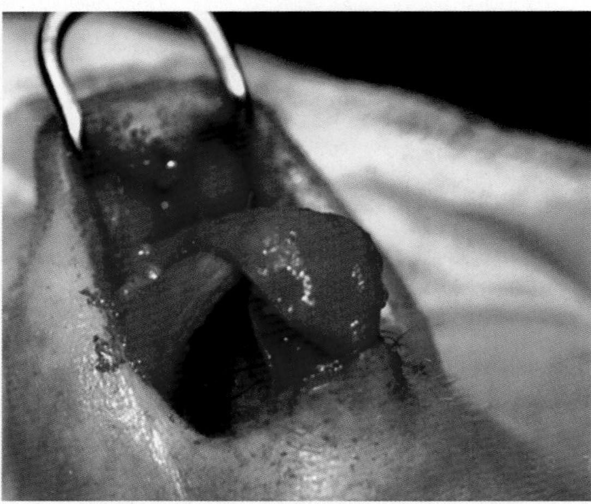
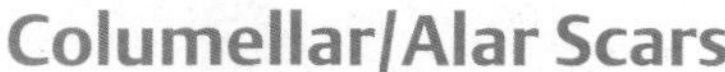

Fig. 46.25 Allograft dermis used to cushion tip graft in patient with thin skin during revision rhinoplasty.

Columellar/Alar Scars

The open rhinoplasty approach has made correction of many nasal deformities more predictable. The transcolumellar incision, however, does have the potential to heal poorly if the incision is not executed or closed carefully. Proper placement of the incision at the narrowest portion of the columella, over a part of the medial crura, will result in a well-healed barely visible scar. If the incision does not overlay the crura a contraction will take place, with an obvious contour deformity. The shape of the incision, either inverted-V or stair-step is not important, as long as the tissue is handled gently and closed appropriately. Scar revision in this area is difficult, and attempts at excising and reclosing old scars are rarely helpful.

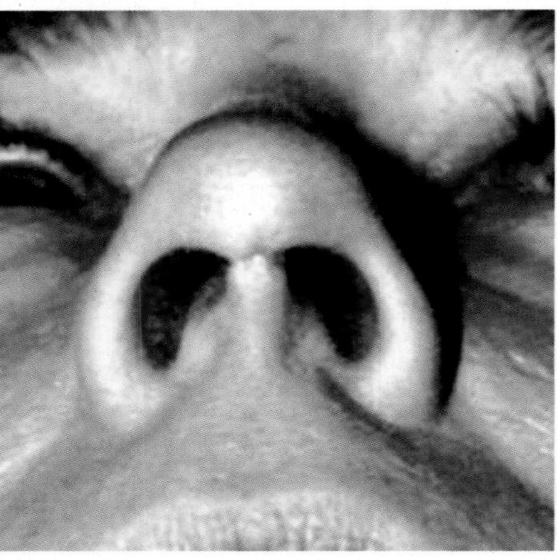

Fig. 46.27 Columellar scar after primary rhinoplasty.

Scars secondary to alar base resection are also difficult to revise. Prevention is possible by proper placement

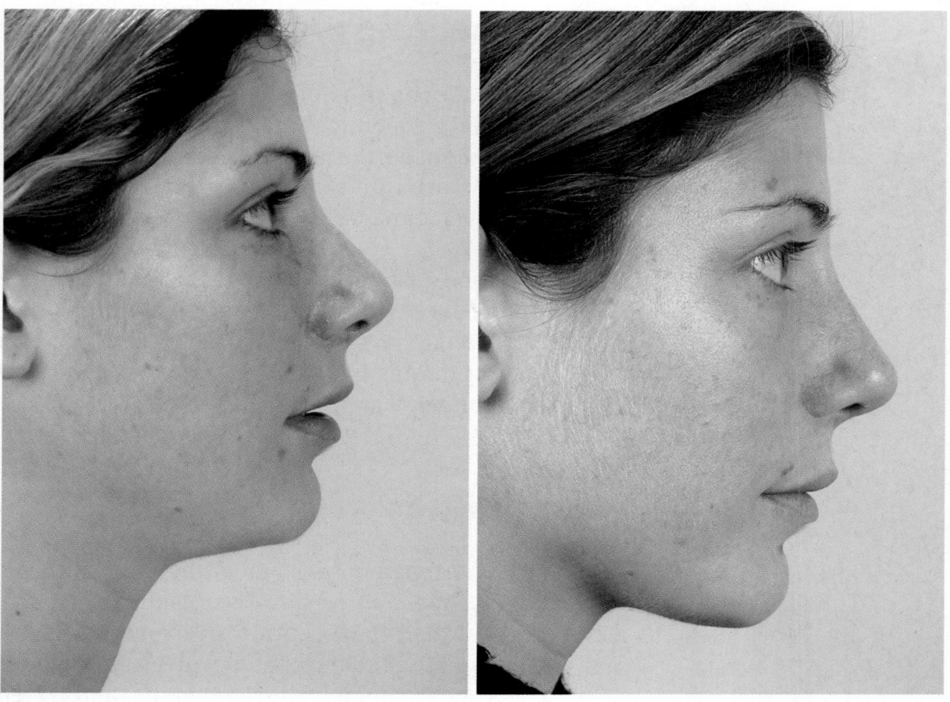

Fig. 46.26 (**A**) Overshortened nose after primary rhinoplasty. (**B**) After utilizing extension spreader grafts, septal extension graft, and infratip graft to lengthen nose.

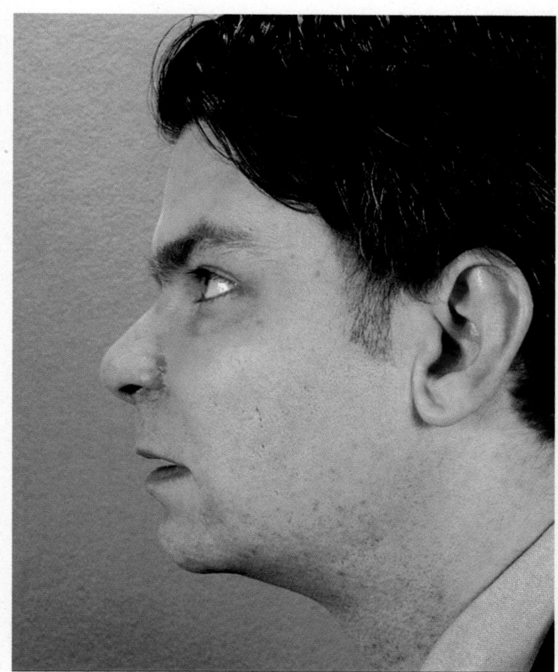
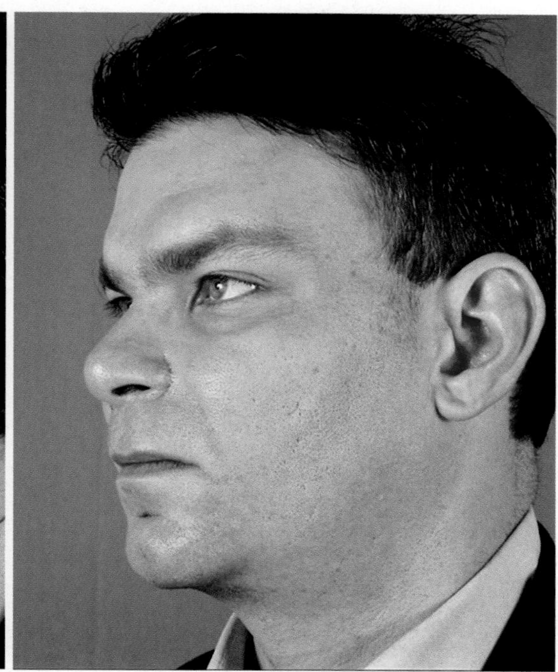

Fig. 46.28 (A,B) Alar base reduction scars.

and closure of alar incisions. In general, the base incision should be ~0.5 mm outside the natural crease, and should not extend so far lateral that the end is visible beyond the natural curve (**Figs. 46.27 and 46.28**).

In summary, revision rhinoplasty as a topic represents a wide range of clinical presentations. The rhinoplastic surgeon must be prepared to deal with the challenge of both physical and psychological factors. Experience with a multitude of techniques will help the surgeon obtain appropriate results in this difficult patient group.

References

1. Mazzola RF, Felisati G. Secondary rhinoplasty: analysis of the deformity and guidelines for management. Facial Plast Surg 1997;13(3):163–177
2. Roe JO. The deformity termed "pug nose" and its correction, by a simple operation. Arch Otolaryngol Head Neck Surg 1989;115:156–157
3. Joseph J. Rhinoplasty and Facial Plastic Surgery with a Supplement on Mammaplasty. Leipzig: Verlag von Curt Kabitzsch; 1931
4. Jerome L. Body dysmorphic disorder: symptom or syndrome. Am J Psychiatry 1994;151(3):460–461
5. Sarwer DB, Crerand CE, Didie ER. Body dysmorphic disorder in cosmetic surgery patients. Facial Plast Surg 2003;19:7–18
6. Tardy ME. Rhinoplasty: The Art and the Science. Philadelphia, WB Saunders; 1997
7. Papel ID. Augmentation rhinoplasty utilizing cranial bone grafts. Md Med J 1991;40(6):479–483
8. Frodel JL. Calvarial bone graft harvest in children. Otolaryngol Head Neck Surg 1999;121(1):78–81
9. Godin MS, Waldman SR, Johnson CM. Nasal augmentation using Gore-Tex. A 10-year experience. Arch Facial Plast Surg 1999; 1(2):118–121
10. Ahn J, Honrado C, Horn C. Combined silicone and cartilage implants: augmentation rhinoplasty in Asian patients. Arch Facial Plast Surg 2004;6(2):120–123
11. Sheen J. Spreader graft: a method of reconstructing the roof of the middle nasal vault following rhinoplasty. Plast Reconstr Surg 1984;73(2):230–239
12. Papel ID. Interlocked transdomal suture technique for the wide interdomal space in rhinoplasty. Arch Facial Plast Surg 2005;7(6): 414–417
13. Foda HM, Kridel RW. Lateral crural steal and lateral crural overlay: an objective evaluation. Arch Otolaryngol Head Neck Surg 1999;125(12): 1365–1370
14. Toriumi DM, Josen J, Weinberger M, Tardy ME Jr. Use of alar batten grafts for correction of nasal valve collapse. Arch Otolaryngol Head Neck Surg 1997;123(8):802–808
15. Gillman GS, Simons RL, Lee DJ. Nasal tip bossae in rhinoplasty. Etiology, predisposing factors, and management techniques. Arch Facial Plast Surg 1999;1(2):83–89
16. Gruber RP. Surgical correction of the short nose. Aesthetic Plast Surg 2002;26(Suppl 1):6
17. Lovice DB, Mingrone MD, Toriumi DM. Grafts and implants in rhinoplasty and nasal reconstruction. Otolaryngol Clin North Am 1999; 32(1):113–141
18. Beaty MM, Dyer WK, Shawl MW. The quantification of surgical changes in nasal tip support. Arch Facial Plast Surg 2002;4(2):82–91

47 Rhinoplasty in Children

Gilbert J. Nolst Trenité

Traditionally, septorhinoplasty in children has been postponed until after puberty, unless there is a severe impairment of the nasal airway or a severe external deformity with obvious psychological impact on the young patient. In addition, there are specific indications such as acute nasal trauma, septal abscess, dermoid cyst, and progressive distortion of the nose that demand early surgical intervention.

In septal surgery, the submucosal septal resection in the growing nose leads to saddle nose deformities and obvious growth disturbance of the nose and retroposition of the maxilla. These clinical observations[1,2] and experimental studies[3–10] confirm the importance of this clinical attitude.

The introduction of a more conservative submucosal septal correction (SSC) has led to a decline in the traditional restraint.[11–14]

Some authors have stated that conservative septal surgery does not interfere with nasal growth.[14,15] Clinical studies in favor of SSC in the growing nose have lacked information about previous surgical intervention and have had too short follow-up periods.[15–17] However, long-term follow-up until after the puberty growth spurt has shown evident growth inhibition of the nose and maxilla.[18,19]

Experimental studies in young, New Zealand, female white rabbits have shown comparable outcome with clinical observation with patients after nasal trauma and surgical intervention in childhood.[3,10,20] Not only septal surgery but also surgery of the cartilaginous vault will lead to growth inhibition and skeletal malformation.[21]

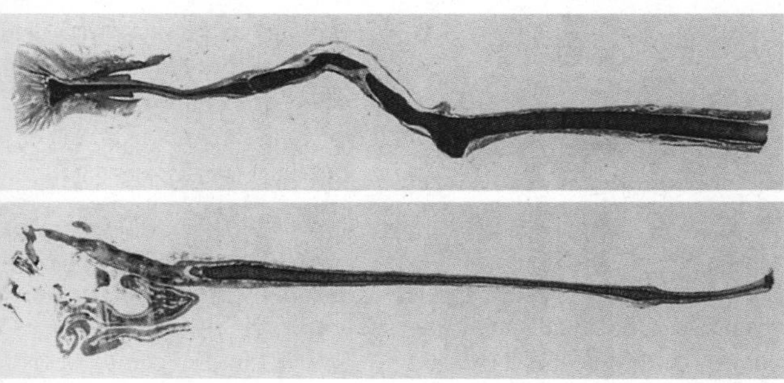

Fig. 47.1 (A) Resection of 1 cm of the cartilaginous septum followed by replacement of autogenous cartilage in a 4-week-old New Zealand white rabbit with septal deviation in the adult stage (24 weeks). (B) Same surgical procedure with a 0,15 mm PDS foil (polydioxanone) splint in the adult stage straight septum.

Anatomical studies in fetal and infant nasal skeleton[22] have helped in the understanding of the impact on outgrowth of surgical intervention in specific stages of development of the nose.[23]

The outcome of experimental surgery on the growing nose in rabbits, which is in concordance with clinical observations, gives scientific support to practical guidelines for rhinoplasty on the growing nose. There are distinct and relative indications for rhinoplasty in children. Especially in the latter, the surgeon has to weigh the possible growth inhibition against functional and/or aesthetic improvement.

In this chapter I discuss the theoretical background and experimental data of the morphogenetic function of the nasal septum for the outgrowth of the nose and maxilla, wound healing of the nasal cartilaginous skeleton, and new experimental developments to improve cartilaginous wound healing. Furthermore, the consequences of autogenous, homologous, and nonbiological implant material in the growing nose is discussed. These experimental studies and clinical observations are the pillars for practical guidelines for rhinoplasty (approaches and techniques) on the growing nose. Finally, timing of the operation and general guidelines for septorhinoplasty in the growing nose are discussed, with illustration of specific clinical cases.

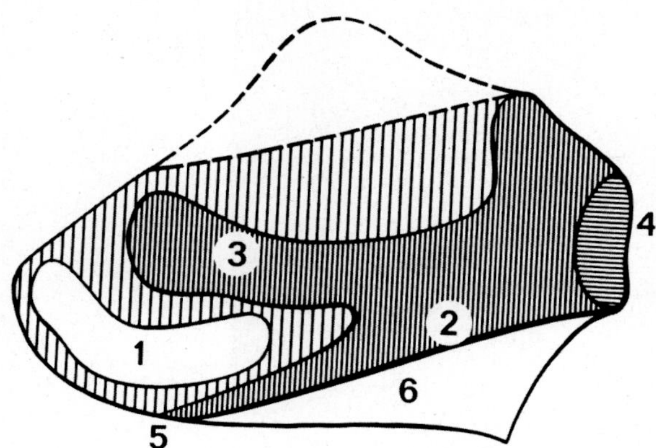

Fig. 47.2 Specific patterns of difference in thickness; (1) anterocentral area of the cartilage (0,75 mm thick); (2) sphenospinal zone from (4) sphenoid to (5) the anterior nasal spine (1.5–3 mm thick); (3) sphenodorsal zone (0,75–1,5 mm thick); and (6) vomer anlage between the basal rim of the cartilaginous septum and the palate. (From Verwoerd CDA, Verwoerd-Verhoef HL. In: Nolst Trenité GJ, ed. Rhinoplasty. 3rd ed. The Hague: Kugler Publications; 2005: ch 20. Reprinted by permission.)

Theoretical Background

Clinical observations of development of the midface after nasal surgery or trauma have shown typical anatomical findings that are in concordance with experimental work done by the interdisciplinary working group of skull development in Amsterdam and Rotterdam.[24–32]

Early experimental work by Urbanus and by Verwoerd-Verhoef on New Zealand female white rabbits in producing an artificial cleft lip and palate resulted in the same growth disturbances as in cleft palate patients. The morphogenetic function of the nasal septum for the development of the midface and specific surgical procedures such as SMR and SSC have shown obvious similarities between the experimental animals and human beings.[24,25]

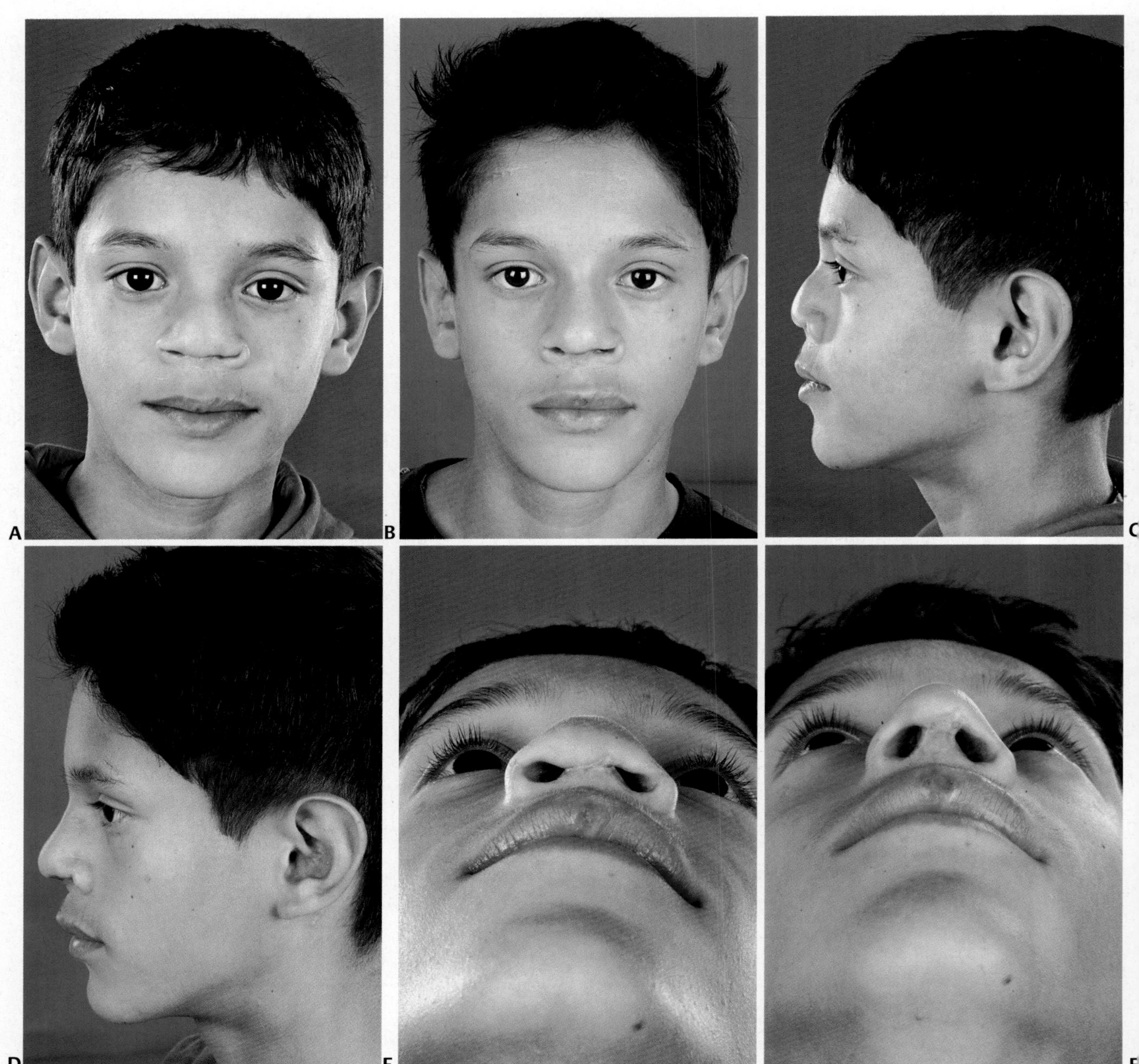

Fig. 47.3 Pre- (**A,C,E**) and postoperative (**B,D,F**) views of a 7-year-old patient with an earlier nasal trauma with lack of tip projection due to loss of caudal septal cartilage and short scarred columella. Due to psychological problems and disturbance in outgrowth a septorhinoplasty was done at the age of 11 before the final growth spurt. Septal reconstruction with autogenous conchal cartilage and columella reconstruction with an auricle composite graft.

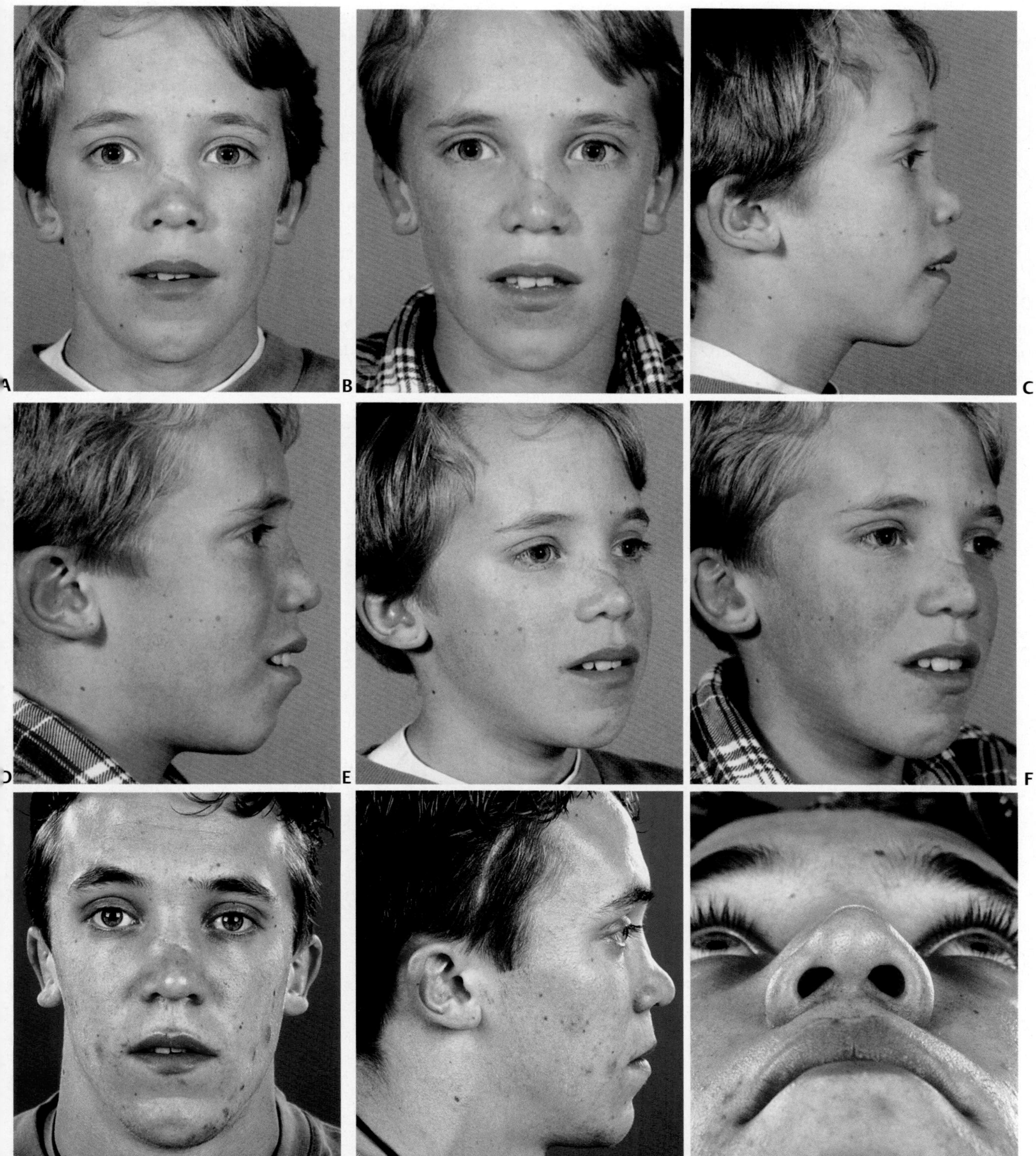

Fig. 47.4 Pre- (**A,C,E**) and postoperative (**B,D,F**) views of an 11-year-old boy with severe psychological problems with his facial appearance due to a severe nasal trauma resulting in a saddle nose deformity. He underwent an endonasal septorhinoplasty to straighten the deformed septum, to narrow the bony pyramid with micro-osteotomies, and to augment the nasal dorsum with a conchal cartilage onlay graft. Late postoperative views after the puberty growth spurt **(G,H,I)** at the age of 18 clearly show an underdeveloped short nose, retracted columella, underprojected tip, moderate saddling, and retroposition of maxilla and anterior nasal spine.

One of the major problems after surgery of the cartilaginous skeleton is wound healing. Instead of cartilaginous healing there is always a fibrous layer in between the surgically induced cartilaginous wound edges, which leads to distortion and or deviations of the cartilaginous structure based on the interrupted "interlocked stress."[33–37]

Experimental Data of Surgical Procedures in the Growing Nose

Basic procedures in surgery of the septum and bony pyramid are: resecting a basal strip, a vertical posterior chondrotomy, scoring, resection and reimplantation of autogenous material, and osteotomies. Analysis of the effect of these surgical intervention results in the following:

- Resection of a part of the cartilaginous septum, resulting in a discontinuity of the septum, disturbs the morphogenetic function resulting in an underdevelopment (shortening and saddling) of the nose and retroposition of the maxilla.[3,5,10]
- Vertical incision (complete height of the septum) leads to deviation of the septal cartilage and/or duplicature (overlap of cartilage) and consequently moderate growth inhibition[3,28,30,33]
- Removal of a basal strip results in lowering of the nasal dorsum with normal length and lowering of the cartilaginous dorsum and retroposition of the maxilla.[3,27]

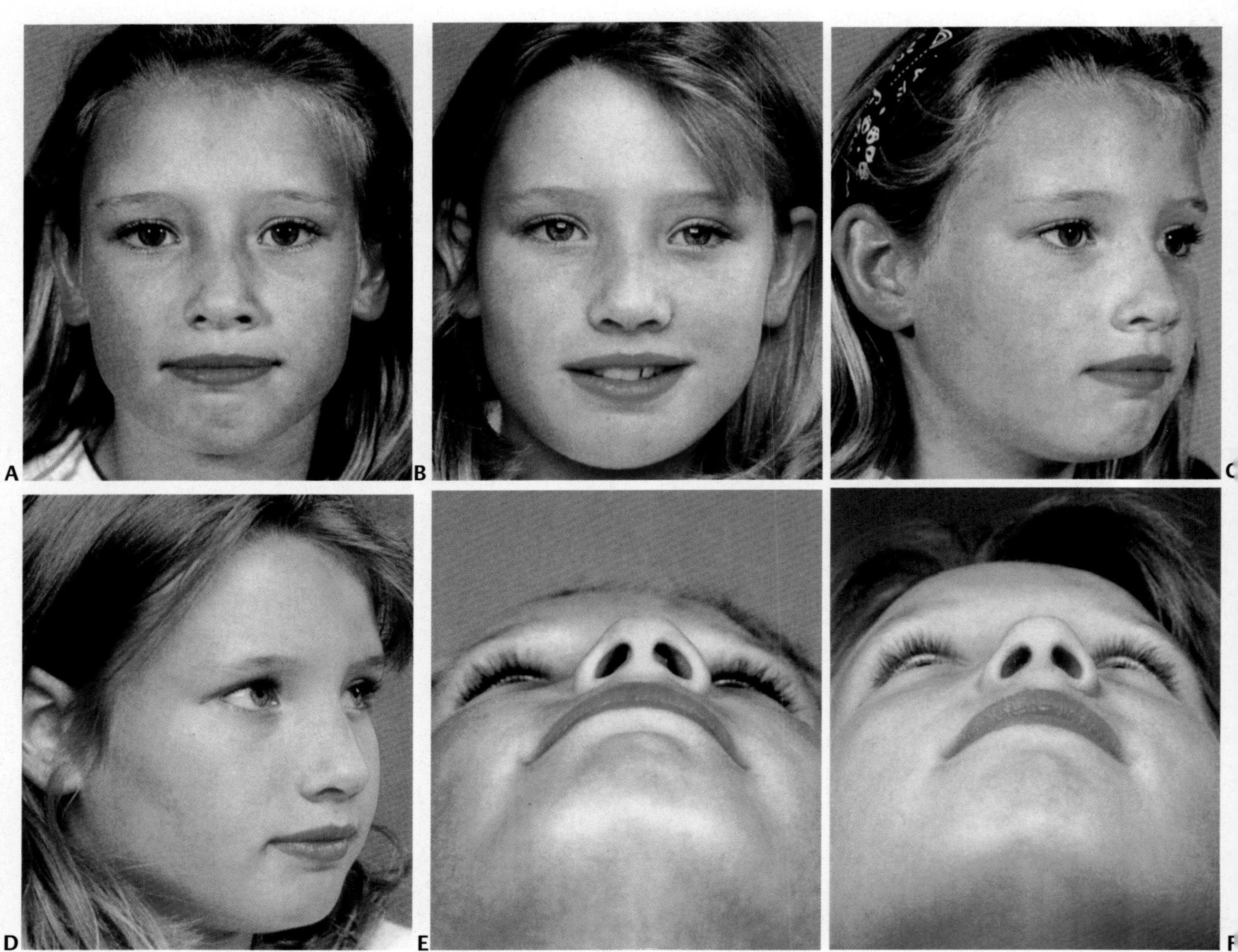

Fig. 47.5 Pre- (**A,C,E**) and postoperative (**B,D,F**) views of a 10-year-old girl who underwent a septorhinoplasty due to a posttraumatic septal deviation with nasal airway impairment and a gradually increasing deviation of the nasal dorsum. Realignment of the dorsum was performed with medial oblique and (endonasal) lateral osteotomies.

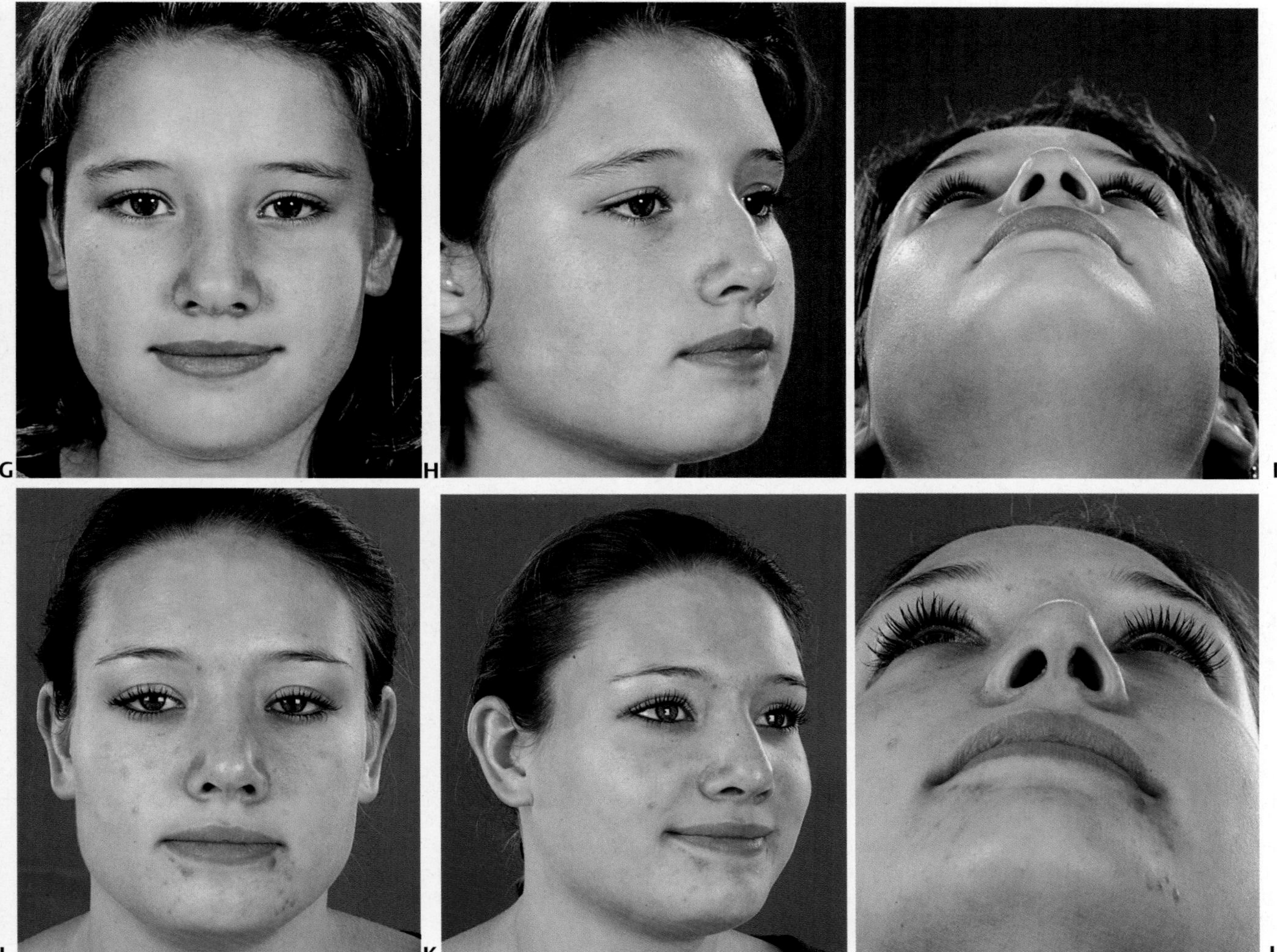

Fig. 47.5 (*Continued*) Late postoperative views (**G–I**) at the age of 17 (after her puberty growth spurt) showing normal outgrowth with a little "traumatic hump formation," which was corrected with a endonasal approach (**J–L**).

- Reinplantation of autogenous (septal cartilage) material leads to overlap, deviation, and moderate growth inhibition, whereas homologous implants and nonbiological material (Proplast) induce severe underdevelopment of the nose and retroposition of the maxilla.[10]
- The autogenous implant shows intrinsic growth.[10,30]
- The use of an intraseptal splint of PDS foil (polydioxanone) results in significantly fewer deviations of the septum[38] (**Fig. 47.1A,B**).
- Resection of a central part of the thin area of the septal cartilage (e.g., septal perforation) does not lead to underdevelopment of the nose.[39]
- Surgical intervention of the cartilaginous vault leads to malformation of the nasal dorsum.[29]
- Mobilization and/or partial resection of the nasal bones and/or vomer does not lead to growth disturbance of the nose.[10,29,30,39]

Development of the Anatomical Structures of the Nose during Childhood

There is a significant difference between the nose of a child and an adult regarding shape and underlying cartilaginous bony skeleton. Typical features of the child's nose are:

- less projection of dorsum and tip
- larger nasolabial angle
- shorter dorsum
- flat nasal tip
- round nares
- short columella

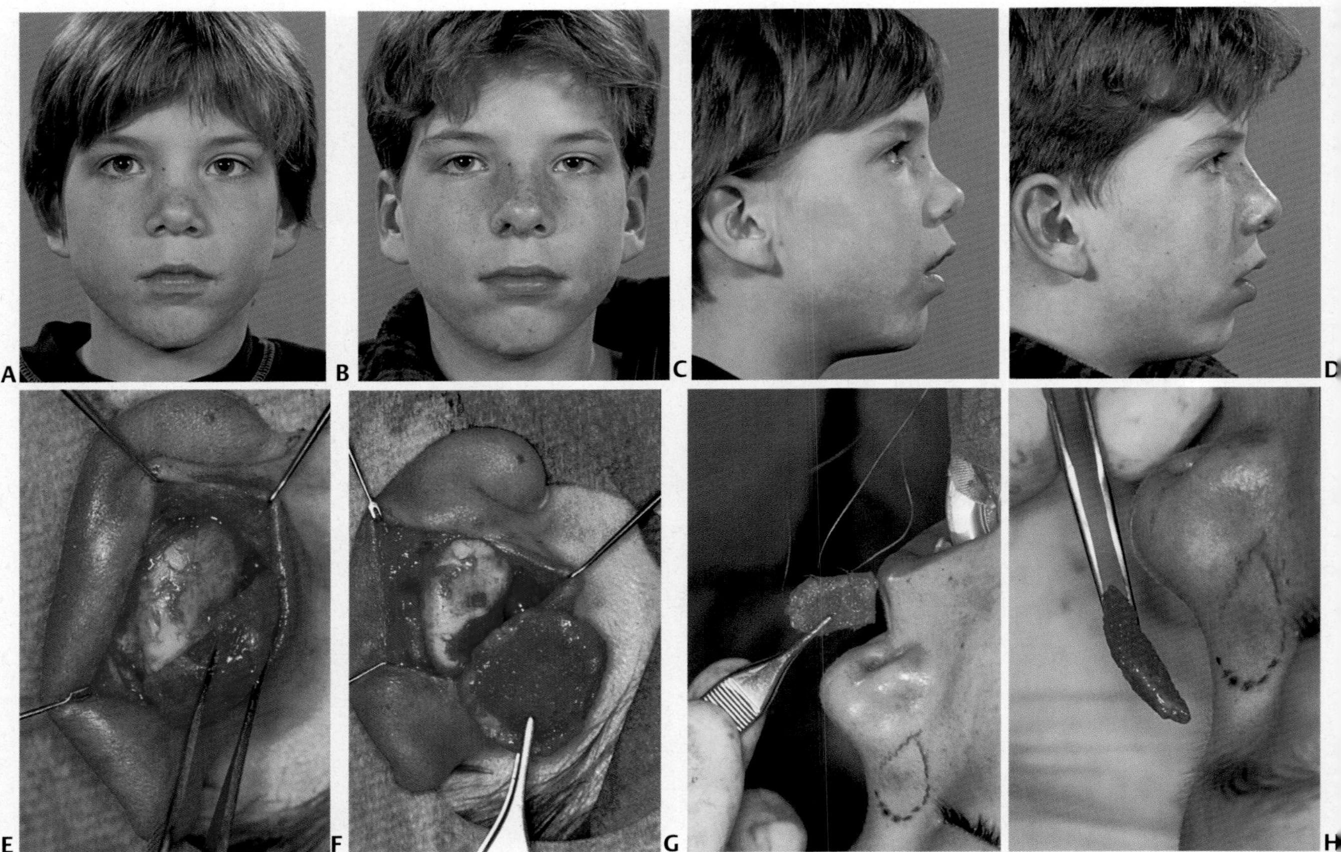

Fig. 47.6 (**A,C**) A 7-year-old patient with underdevelopment of the nose due to a septal abscess that was reconstructed with allogeneic (bank) cartilage (with no growth potential). Secondary surgery was done at the age of 10 years (**B,D**) with tissue engineered cartilage (bovine collagen matrix, wrapped in retroauricular perichondrium during 6 weeks) for septal reconstruction and dorsal onlay (**E–H**).

The nasal skeleton of the infant differs considerably with that of the adult nose.[29,31]

- The cartilaginous skeleton forms a larger part, which makes the nose more flexible and less vulnerable for trauma.
- The septal cartilage of the neonate reaches from the nasal tip to the interior skull base.
- The upper lateral cartilages extent under the nasal bones over their total length and merge with the cartilaginous structure of the interior cranial skull base.
- The perpendicular plate has not yet developed.
- The T-bar structure of septum and upper laterals is directly based on the sphenoid, supports the nasal bones, and determines largely the contour of the dorsum.
- The vomer is only rudimentarily developed.

During childhood the nasal skeleton changes through ossification of the cartilaginous septum with the formation of the perpendicular plate that finally merges with the vomer at the age of 6 to 8 years, and the extension of the upper laterals to the anterior cranial base regress, leaving only an extension of 3 to 15 mm under the nasal bones in the adult stage.

The specific pattern of difference in thickness of the cartilaginous septum especially the thicker zones, diverging in the sphenospinal and sphenodorsal zone play an important role in normal outgrowth of the nose and maxilla[22,23,39,40] (**Fig. 47.2**).

The two growth centers increase the length and height of the bone (sphenodorsal zone) and outgrowth of the maxilla (sphenospinal zone). Trauma or surgical loss of one these two growth centers cause growth inhibition in a specific pattern.[31,39]

Timing of the Operation

The adage to postpone septorhinoplasty after the puberty growth spurt to prevent growth inhibition and redeviation is still valid. However, severe functional and aesthetic sequelae ask for surgical intervention (**Fig. 47.3A–F**).

Distinct indications for immediate intervention are cute nasal trauma, septal abscess, and malignancies, vhereas severe septal deviations causing nasal airway bstruction, benign tumors such as dermoid cysts, highly rogressive distortion, and stigmatic deformities such as left-lip nose stigmata ask for surgery before the end of he puberty growth spurt.

With the more sophisticated modern techniques and reat demand by patients (and/or parents), there is a endency to perform septorhinoplasty before the final puberty) growth spurt.

Short follow-up has given rise to misleading statements n the literature that septorhinoplasty in children does not have consequences for the outgrowth of the nose and maxilla. There are two significant growth spurts: the first two postnatal years and during puberty when the nose grows faster then during the other periods of life. Consequently, surgery performed in the period between growth spurts can disguise a possible surgically induced growth disturbance until the final growth spurt (**Fig. 47.4A–I**).

The surgeon should be aware that even after the final growth spurt there can be some further growth of the septum up to the age of 25 that can lead to late postsurgical distortion. Therefore, parents and patients should be informed that late results cannot be predicted, and the possibility of revision surgery should be discussed.

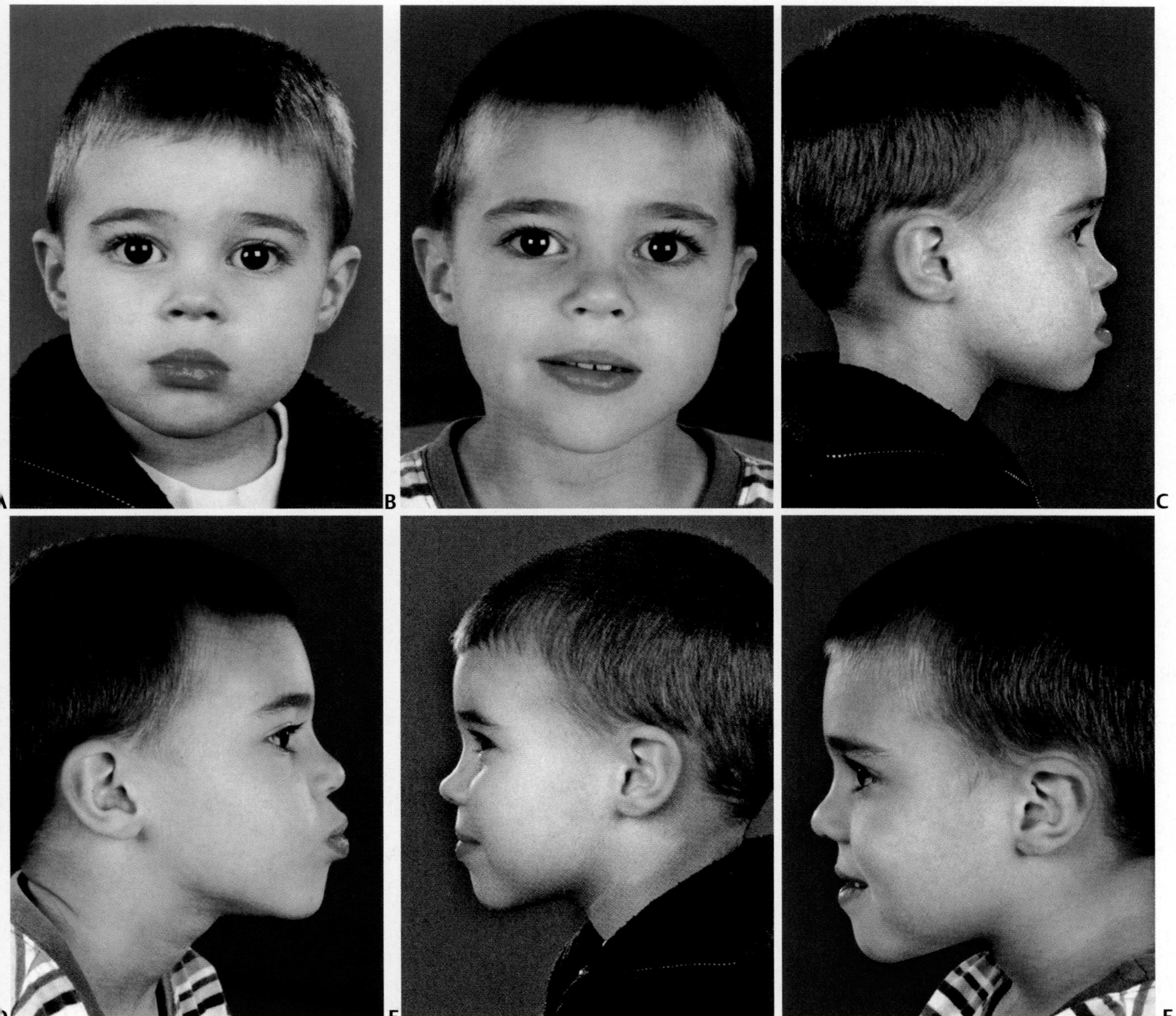

ig. 47.7 (**A,C,E**) Preoperative views of a 4-year-old child 1 week after a septal abscess with destruction of the cartilaginous septum. Postoperative views (**B,D,F**) nore then 2 years after septal reconstruction with PDS-conchal cartilage graft and, up until now, normal growth and septal support of the nasal dorsum.

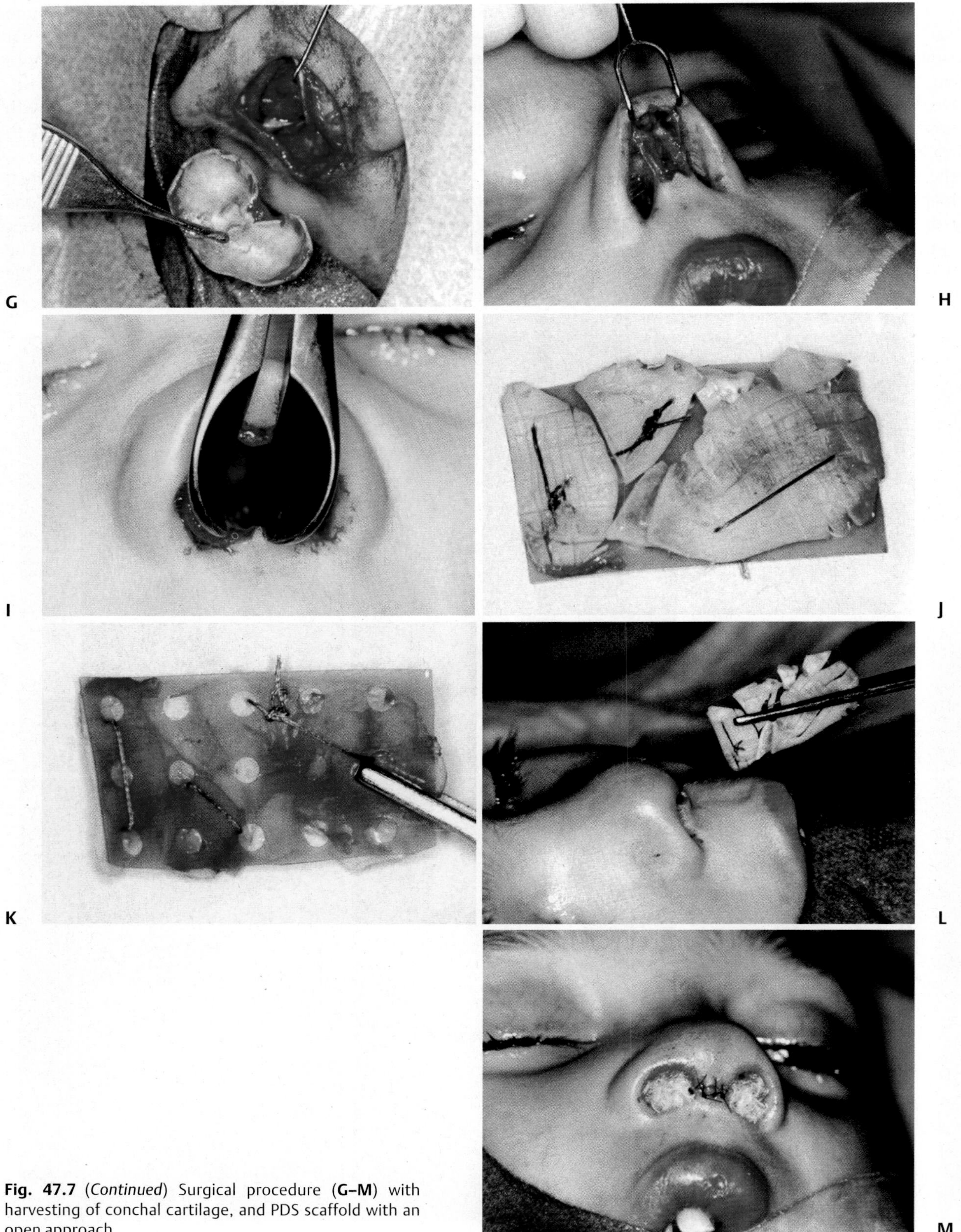

Fig. 47.7 (*Continued*) Surgical procedure (**G–M**) with harvesting of conchal cartilage, and PDS scaffold with an open approach.

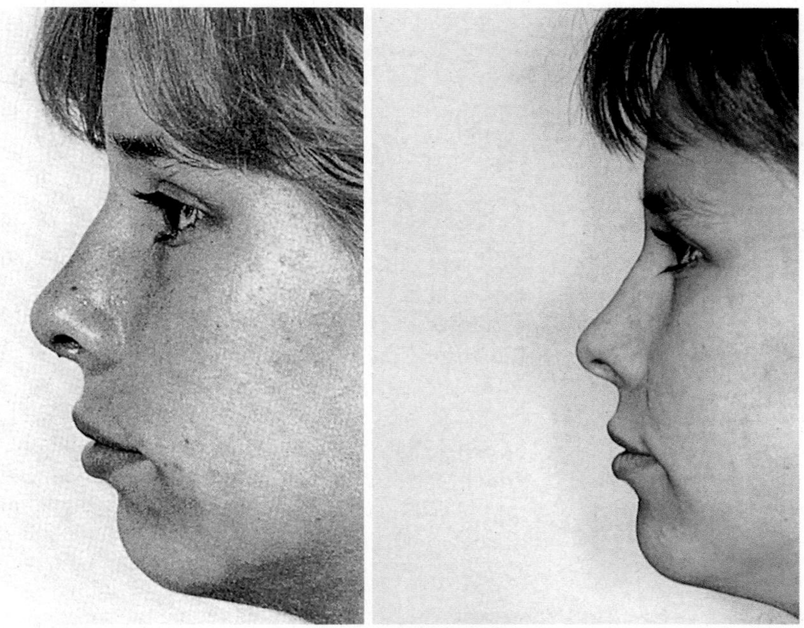

Fig. 47.8 (**A**) Lateral view of a 14-year-old girl 4 weeks after immediate reconstruction (with autogenous rib cartilage) of a completely destroyed cartilaginous nasal septum due to an abscess. (**B**) Lateral view of the same girl at the age of 19 years with adequate outgrowth of the nose and maxilla.

Guidelines for Septorhinoplasty in Children

Based on clinical observation, experimental data of surgical procedures, and knowledge of the anatomical development of the nose, "conservative" guidelines can be given:

- Elevation of the mucoperichondrium on one or both sides will not interfere with normal growth, and it is advisable to perform septal mattress sutures to ensure good approximation of the end of the septoplasty.
- The long-term result of scoring and incisions in the cartilage to realign the cartilaginous septum is not predictable.
- To stabilize the straightened septum, PDS foil (0,15 mm) at one side submucoperichondrially can improve long-term results.
- Vertical posterior chondrotomy or separation of the cartilaginous septum from the perpendicular plate should be avoided.
- If resection of the cartilaginous part of the septum is necessary for realignment or reconstruction, the thinner central part has the least chance of growth inhabitation.
- Resection of larger parts of the sphenodorsal "growth center" leads to disturbance in outgrowth of the nasal dorsum and of the sphenospinal growth center leads to retroposition of the anterior nasal spine and maxilla.
- Leftover crushed cartilage should be put back in the resected area to improve regeneration of cartilage and to prevent septal perforations.
- Resection of the bony deviation of premaxilla and the vomer (crista/vomeral spine) with mobilization and/or partial resection will not disturb the outgrowth of the nose.
- Hump resection in which the T-bone structure of the cartilaginous vault is disturbed can lead to outgrowth of the septum anterior of the upper laterals and subsequently irregularities of the dorsum.
- Osteotomies of the bony pyramid to realign the nasal dorsum do not create growth disturbances.
- Transcolumellar incision in an open approach (e.g., to remove a dermoid cyst), leaving the nasal skeleton in tact, will not disturb nasal growth.

Nevertheless, often, long follow-up after the puberty growth spurt shows obvious sequelae of early nose surgery. Still, more experimental data and clinical observations with long-term follow-up after the puberty growth spurt are essential to prevent unnecessary iatrogenic sequelae after surgery of the growing nose.

Nasal Trauma in Childhood

Fractures and dislocation of the nasal skeleton in children demand precise analysis to prevent sequelae that will express themselves more prominently during growth (**Fig. 47.5A–L**).

The following guidelines can be given:

- Inspection and palpation under general anesthesia (in most cases) is necessary to obtain the correct diagnosis and subsequently the appropriate treatment.
- Manual realignment with a speculum and elevator (closed reduction) is often possible.
- Elevation of the periosteum should be avoided and in case of surgical realignment a 2-mm osteotome is very useful. The still-attached periosteum will act like an internal splint.
- Inspection of the nasal cavity to diagnose mucosal tears and "fresh" cartilaginous deviations, is of utmost importance. Especially complex vertical fractures can lead to growth disturbances.
- Realignment and a supporting internal splint with PDS foil (0,15 mm) can be helpful to prevent early septal deviations.
- Septal mattress sutures and nasal packing will help to prevent hematoma and keep the realigned segment in place.
- In young children nasal packing is contraindicated as they are obligatory nose breathers.

Septal Abscess

A septal abscess in childhood often results in total destruction of the cartilaginous septum and consequently a saddle nose deformity and severe underdevelopment of the nose if inadequatedly treated.[41]

In the earlier literature[41,42] the standard therapy is drainage and packing. Some authors describe the use of immediate implantation with homologous cartilage, which can give a good short-term aesthetic result but finally will lead to midfacial growth inhibition (nose and maxilla)[43,44] (**Fig. 47.6A–H**).

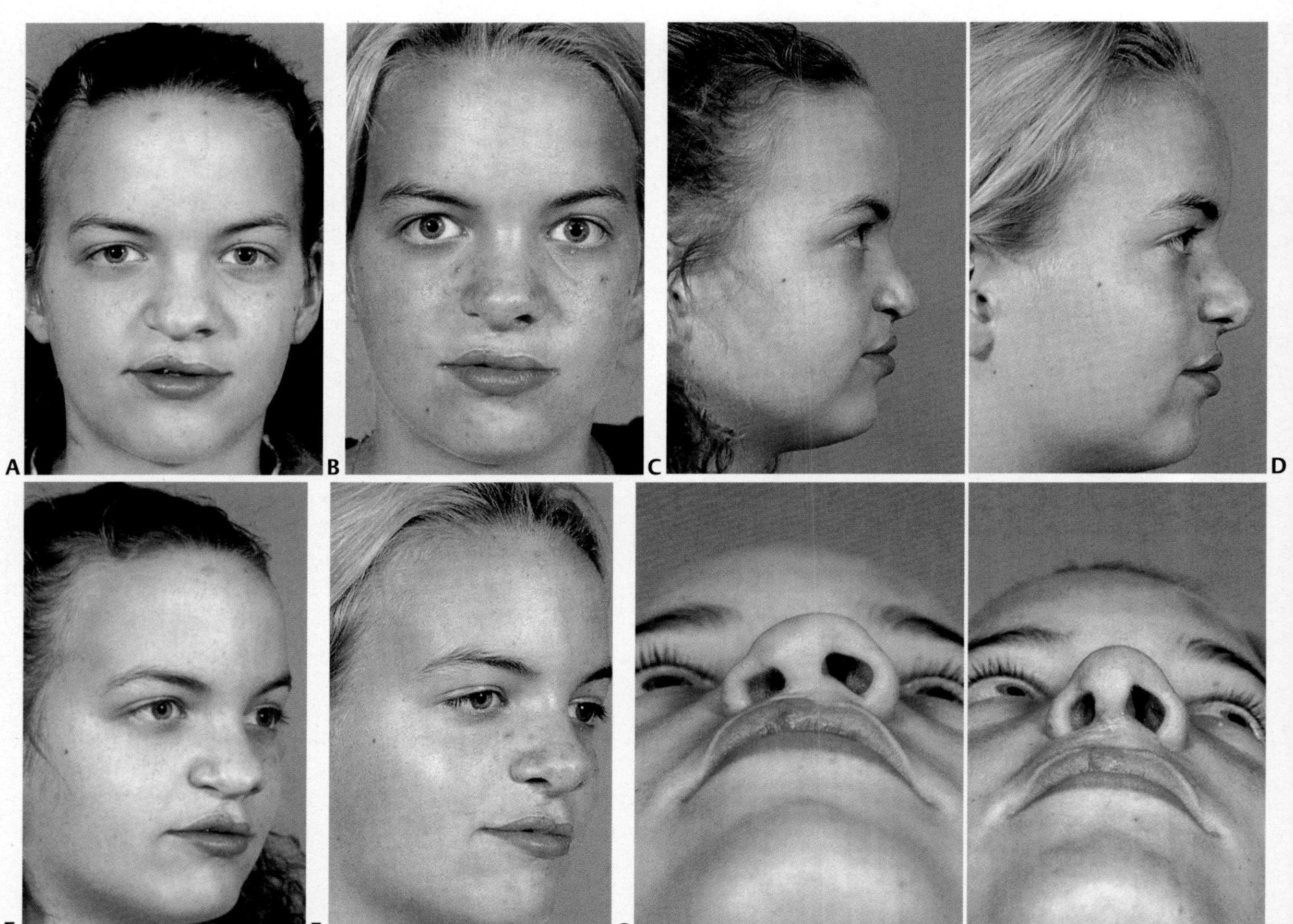

Fig. 47.9 Pre- (**A,C,E,G**) and postoperative (**B,D,F,H**) views of a 14-year-old girl with psychological and functional problems due to the typical unilateral cleft-lip nose deformity. Through an external approach, the septal deviation was corrected, followed by repositioning of the distorted lower lateral and the cleft side and endorotation of the alar base.

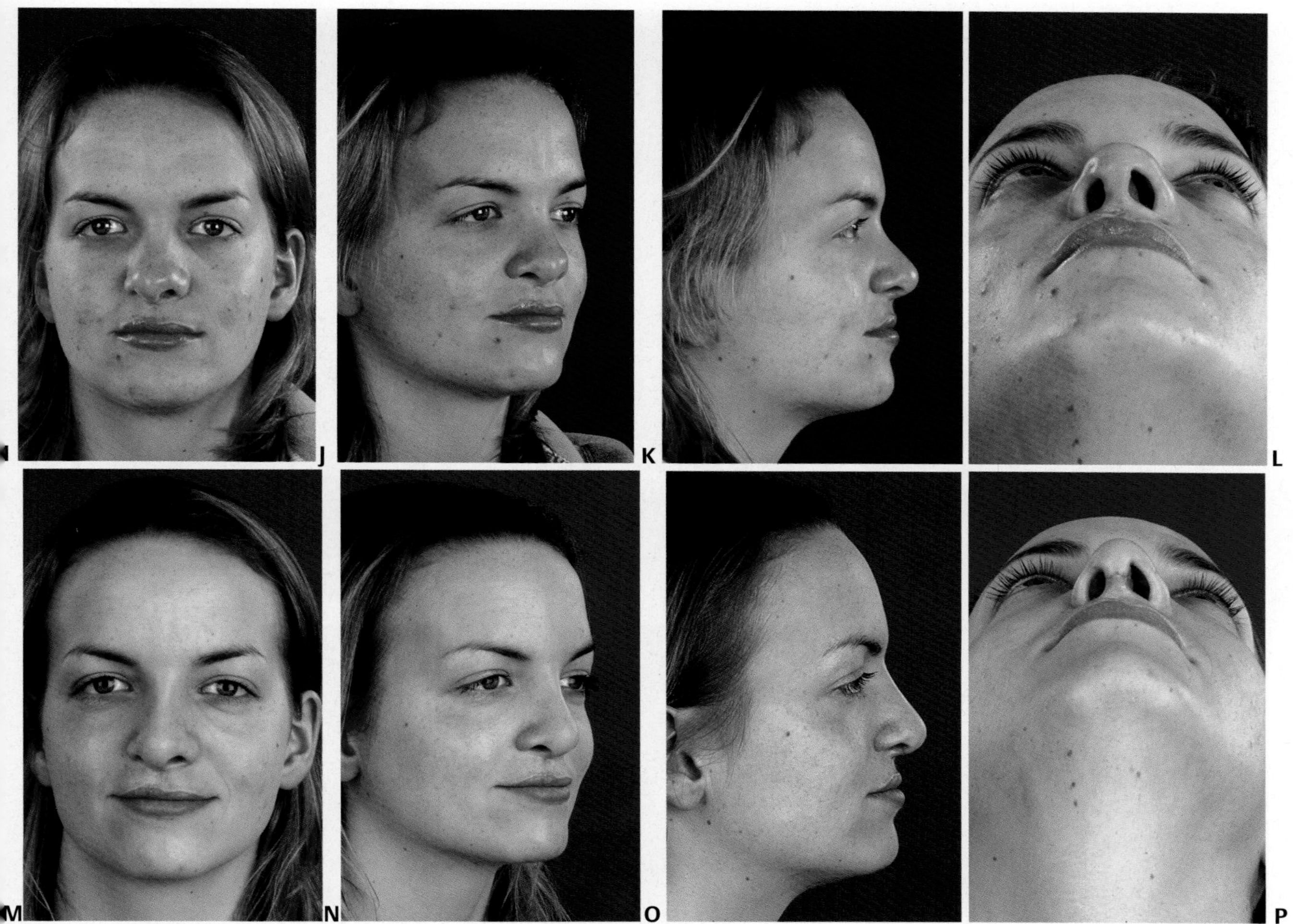

Fig. 47.9 (*Continued*) Tip projection was restored with a columella strut and a shield graft. Late postoperative views (**I–L**) at the age of 24, showing normal outgrowth of the nose, followed by (recent) minimal revision surgery (**M–P**).

Experimental and clinical observations show that immediate reconstruction of the destroyed septum with autogenous ear or rib cartilage shows better outgrowth of nose and maxilla, due to the fact that the implanted autogenous cartilage shows further growth[10,45–47] (**Figs. 47.7A–M and 47.8A,B**).

Approaches and Techniques

For septal work an endonasal approach, hemitransfixion incision, and elevation of the mucoperichondrium are suitable for children. Take care not to cause an injury of the incisival nerves. Conservative surgery (see guidelines) is mandatory to prevent discontinuity in anteroposterior direction.

Intercartilaginous incisions to approach the nasal dorsum in a growing nose should be avoided, which excludes the use of a delivery approach. The external approach, particularly in the growing nose, has the advantage that the cartilaginous nasal skeleton stays intact. This "open" approach enables the surgeon to excise dermoid cysts, to realign lower lateral cartilages (unilateral cleft), and to suture in place autogenous camouflage grafts, without disturbing the integrity of the cartilaginous skeleton (**Fig. 47.9A–P**). As discussed before, micro-osteotomies to mobilize and realign the nasal bone without elevating the periosteum are very suitable. Hump resection should be avoided in a growing nose to keep the T-bar structure of septum and upper laterals intact. Due to the delicate structures in children, the use of magnifying glasses is advisable. Meticulous closure of a broken columella incision with slight eversion of the wound edges will leave a more or less invisible scar (**Fig. 47.10A–F**).

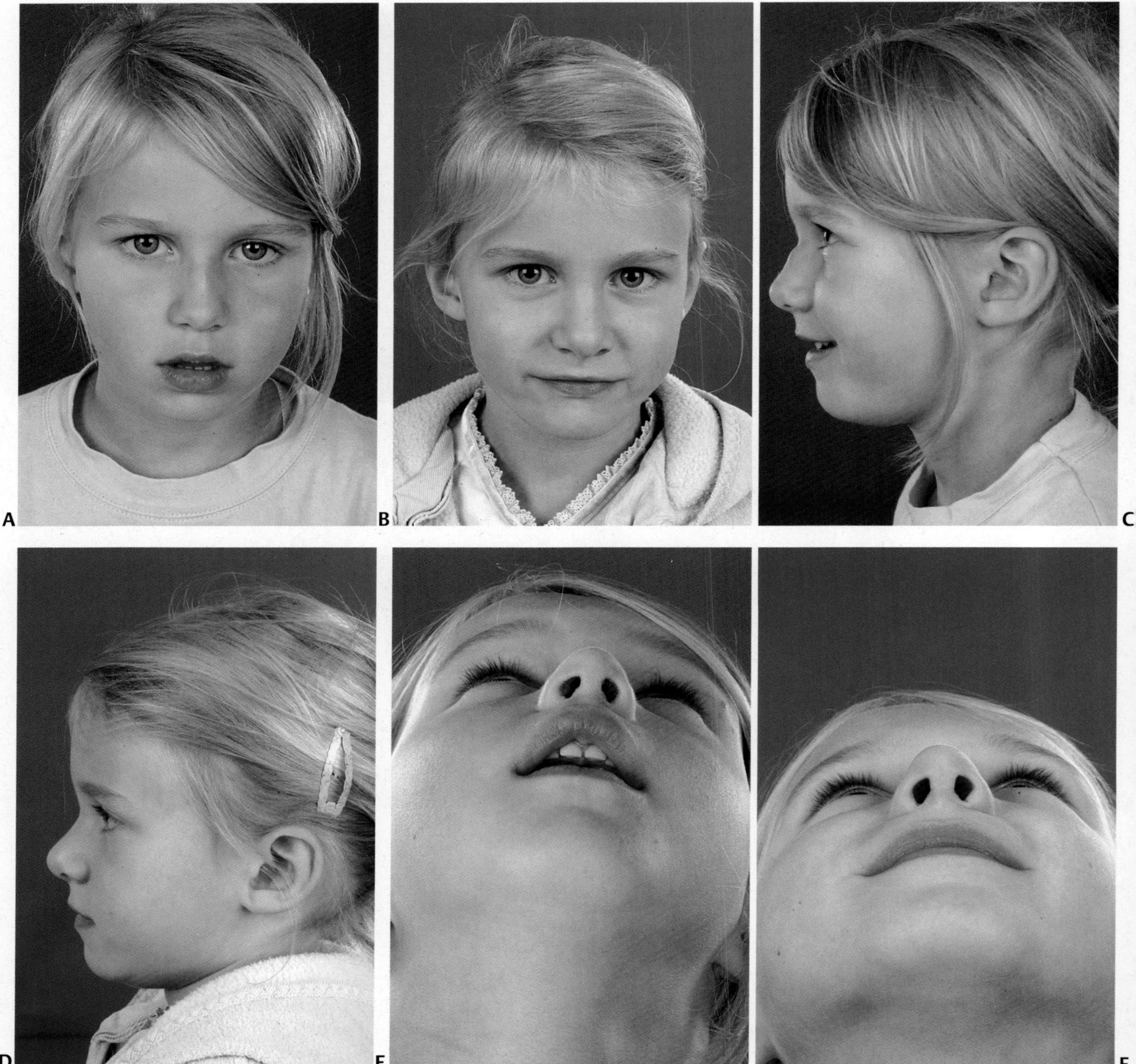

Fig. 47.10 Pre- (**A,C,E**) and postoperative (**B,D,F**) views of a 5-year-old girl with a dermoid cyst of the nasal dorsum that was excised through an open approach. The scar of the broken columellar incision (**F**) is nearly invisible. Due to the fact that the nasal skeleton was left intact, no growth inhibition of nose and maxilla can be expected.

Summary

When performing rhinoplasty in children, the surgeon should weigh the functional and aesthetic improvement against the possible growth disturbances. To avoid severe sequelae the integrity of the cartilaginous skeleton should be respected as much as possible.

The patient's parents should be informed about the chance of secondary surgery, which should be performed, if possible, after the last growth spurt.

Autogenous cartilage is the graft of choice, especially in children, due to the growth potential of the graft.

More experimental work and well-documented clinical studies with a follow-up until the puberty growth spurt is finished have to be done.

cknowledgment

Vith decennia long (1974–2005) experimental research in he growing nose, (now emeritus) Professor Carel Verwoerd nd his wife, Dr. Jetty Verwoerd, have made a major contri- ution to pediatric nose surgery with their research, from vhich guidelines have been developed for septorhinoplasty n children.

These preliminary guidelines will develop further with ew knowledge from experimental data and clinical stud- s. Nevertheless, the contemporary guidelines will help he surgeon to prevent severe sequelae after performing urgery in the growing nose.

eferences

1. Hayton CH. An investigation into the results of the submucous resection of the septum in children. J Laryng. 1916;31:132–138
2. Ombrédanne M. Les deviations traumatiques de la cloison chez l'enfant avec obstruction nasale. Traitement chiurgical et resultants eloignés. Arch Fr Pediatr 1942;1:20
3. Verwoerd CD, Urbanus NA, Nijdam DC. The effects of septal surgery on the growth of nose and maxilla. Rhinology 1979a;17:53–64
4. Sarnat BG, Wexler MR. The snout after resection of nasal spetum in adult rabbits. Arch Otolaryngol 1967b;63:467–478
5. Nordgaard JO, Kvinnsland S. Influence of submucous septal resection on facial growth in the rat. Plast Reconstr Surg 1979;64(1):84–88
6. Kremenak CR Jr, Searls JC. Experimental manipulation of midfacial growth: a synthesis of 5 years of research at the Iowa Maxilla Facial Laboratory. J Dent Res 1971;50:1488–1491
7. Kvinnsland S. Partial resection of the cartilaginous nasal septum in rats: its influence on growth. Angle Orthod 1974;44(2):135–140
8. Freer OT. The correction of deflections of the nasal septum with a minimum of traumatism. J Am Med Assoc 1902;38:636–642
9. Killian G. Beiträge zur sub submukösen Fensterresektion der Nasenscheidewand. Passow U Schaefer Reits. 1908;1:183–192
0. Nolst Trenité GJ, Verwoerd CD, Verwoerd-Verhoef HL. Reimplantation of autologous septal cartilage in the growing nasal septum, I: the influence of resecrtion and reimplantation of septal cartilage upon nasal growth: an experimental study in growing rabbits. Rhinology 1988;26:25
1. Conle MH, Loring RM. Surgery of the nasal septum: new operative procedures and indications. Ann Otol Rhinol Laryngol 1948;57:705–713
2. Cottle MH. Nasal surgery in children. Eye Ear Nose Throat Mon 1951;30:32–38
3. Goldman JB. New technique in surgery of the deviated nasal septum. Arch Otolaryngol 1956;64:183–189
4. Masing H. Eingriffe an der Nase. In: Kurze HNO-Operationslehre, bd. I, G. Theissing. Stuttgart: Thieme; 1971
5. Jennes ML. Corrective nasal surgery in children. Arch Otolaryngol 1964;79:145–151
6. Pirsig W, Knahl R. Rhinoplastische Operation bei Kindern: Erfahrungen an 92 Fällen. Z Laryngol Rhinol Otol 1974;53:250
7. Pirsig W. Septal plasty in children: influence on nasal growth. Rhinology 1977;15:193–204
8. Huizing EH. Septum surgery in children: indications. surgical technique, and long-term results. Rhinology 1979;17:91–100
9. Verwoerd CD, Verwoerd-Verhoef HL. Developmental aspects of the deviated nose. Facial Plast Surg 1989;6:95–100
0. Grymer LF, Bosch C. The nasal septum and development of the midface. A longitudinal study of a pair of monozygotic twins. Rhinology 1997; 35:6–10
1. Poublon RML, Verwoerd CDA, Verwoerd-Verhoef HL. Anatomy of the upper lateral cartilages in the human newborn. Rhinology 1990;28:41
2. van Loosen J, Verwoerd-Verhoef HL, Verwoerd CD. The nasal septal cartilage in the newborn. Rhinology 1988;26:161–165
23. Van Loosen J, Van Zanten GA, Howard CV, Verwoerd-Verhoef HL, Van Velzen D, Verwoerd CD. Growth characteristics of the human nasal septum. Rhinology 1996;34:78–82
24. Urbanus NAM. Schedelgroei na sluiting van lip-kaak-en gehemeltespleten. Experimentele toetsing van de beginselen van enige chirurgische methoden bij het konijn [thesis]. University of Amsterdam; 1974
25. Verwoerd-Verhoef HL. Schedelgroei onder invloed van aangezichtsspleten. Een experimentele studie bij het konijn [thesis]. University of Amsterdam; 1974
26. Mastenbroek GJ. De invloed van partiële resectie van het neustussenschot op de uitgroei van bovenkaak en neus [thesis]. University of Amsterdam; 1978
27. Nolst Trenité GJ. Implantaten in een groeiend neustussenschot [thesis]. Rotterdam: Erasmus University; 1984
28. Nijdam DC. Schedelgroei na partiële submukeuze resectie van het neustussenschot [thesis]. University of Amsterdam; 1985
29. Poublon RMC. The cartilaginous nasal dorsum and postnatal growth of the nose [thesis]. Rotterdam: Erasmus University; 1987
30. Meeuwis CA. Wondreacties in het kraakbenige neustussenschot [thesis]. Rotterdam: Erasmus University; 1988
31. Loosen J. Postnatal development of the human nasal septum and its related structures. Rotterdam: Erasmus University; 2000
32. ten Koppel PG. Woundhealing, distortion, and generation of cartilage [thesis]. Rotterdam: Erasmus University; 2005
33. Verwoerd CD, Verwoerd-Verhoef HL, Meeuwis CA, van der Heul RO. Wound healing of autologous implants in the nasal septal cartilage. ORL J Otorhinolaryngol Relat Spec 1991;53:310–314
34. Verwoerd-Verhoef HL, ten Koppel PG, van Osch GJ, Meeuwis CA, Verwoerd CD. Wound healing of cartilage structures in the head and neck region. Int J Pediatr Otorhinolaryngol 1998;43:241–251
35. ten Koppel PG, van der Veen JM, Hein D, et al. Controlling incision-induced distortion of nasal septal cartilage: a model to predict the effect of scoring of rabbit septa. Plast Reconstr Surg 2003;111(6):1948–1957
36. Fry H. Nasal skeletal trauma and the interlocked stresses of the nasal septal cartilage. Br J Plast Surg 1967;20:146–158
37. Fry HJH. The aetiology of so-called "septal deviations" and their experimental production in the growing rabbit. Br J Plast Surg 1968;21:419–422
38. Boenisch M, Hajas T, Nolst Trenité GJ. Influence of polydioxanone foil on growing septal cartilage after surgery in an animal model. Arch Facial Plast Surg 2003;5:316–319
39. Verwoerd CDA, Verwoerd-Verhoef HL. Rhinosurgery in children, developmental and surgical aspects. In: Nolst Trenité GJ, ed. Rhinoplasty. 3rd ed. The Hague: Kugler Publications; 2005
40. van Velzen D, van Loosen J, Verwoerd CDA, Verwoerd-Verhoef HL. Persistent pattern of variations in thickness of the human nasal septum: implications for stress and trauma as illustrated by a complex fracture in a 4-year-old boy. Otolaryngology in ASEAN countries. Adv Otorhinolaryngol 1997;51:46–50
41. Ambrus PS, Eavey RD, Baker AS, Wilson WR, Kelly JH. Management of nasal septal abscess. Laryngoscope 1981;91:575–582
42. Pirsig W. Historical notes and actual observations on the nasal septal abscess especially in children. Int J Pediatr Otorhinolaryngol 1984;8:43–54
43. Huizing EH. Long-term results of reconstruction of the septum in the acute phase of a septal abscess in children. Rhinology 1984;22:55–63
44. Dispenza C, Saraniti C, Dispenza F, Caramanna C, Salzano FA. Management of nasal septal abscess in childhood: our experience. Int J Pediatr Otorhinolaryngol 2004;68(11):1417–1421
45. Schrader M, Jahnek K. Tragal cartilage in the primary reconstruction of defects resulting from a nasal septal abscess. Clin Otolaryngol 1995;20:527–529
46. Nolst Trenité GJ. Postoperative care and complications. In: Nolst Trenité GJ, ed. Rhinoplasty. 3rd ed. The Hague: Kugler Publications; 2005:31–37
47. Bönisch M, Nolst Trenité GJ. New concepts in reconstructive septoplasty. In: Nolst Trenité GJ, ed. Rhinoplasty. 3rd ed. The Hague: Kugler Publications; 2005:285–296

48 Asian Rhinoplasty

Yong Ju Jang

Anatomical Characteristics

Asians include people living in East Asia, Southeast Asia, India, and the Middle East who have different ethnic origins and different aesthetic features. As a result of the diverse ethnicities in these populations, the anatomical characteristics of Asians vary greatly. Because the author has experience in performing rhinoplasties predominantly on Koreans, the following chapter should be understood as rhinoplasty for patients with an ethnic Mongoloid background (i.e., Chinese, Koreans, Japanese, and some Philippinos).

Although there are substantial variations, in the typical Asian nose, the nasal skin tends to be thicker than in the Caucasian nose, with abundant subcutaneous soft tissue. The tip of the nose is usually low and the lower lateral cartilages are small and weak. The nasal bones are poorly developed and thick, thus having a low radix (**Fig. 48.1**). The septal cartilage is thin and small. Altogether, when compared with the Caucasian nose, the typical Asian nose appears to be relatively small and flat, and has poor tip definition. In aesthetic analysis of the nasal profile, the nasolabial angles of Asians are typically more acute than those of Caucasians, but the nasofrontal angles do not differ greatly.[1]

Dorsal Augmentation

General Consideration

Dorsal augmentation is the most commonly addressed issue in Asian rhinoplasty and also the most common reason for revision surgery. When performing dorsal augmentation, it is unwise to determine the final shape of the patient's nose based soely on numerical factors without considering the overall harmony of the patient's face. When performing augmentation rhinoplasty on Asians, it is preferable or mandatory to first perform tip surgery using autologous cartilage, followed by dorsal augmentation using available implant material. The thickness of the patient's skin must be taken into consideration. If excessive dorsal augmentation is performed on a patient whose skin is too thin, there is a risk of implant visibility through the skin or an extrusion of the implant. Conversely, too thick skin can decrease the effect of nasal augmentation. Therefore, in patients with thin skin, it is preferable to use soft

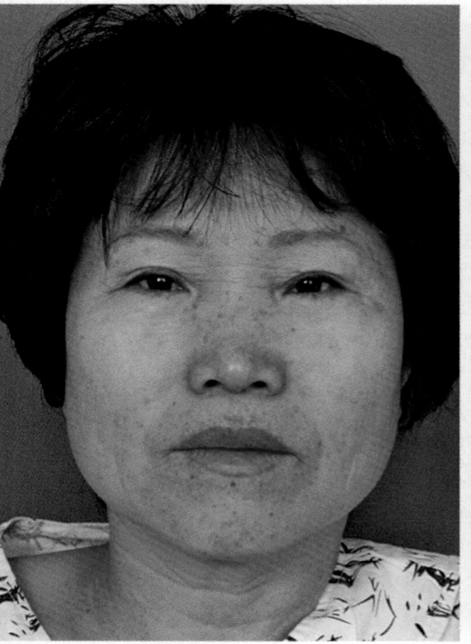

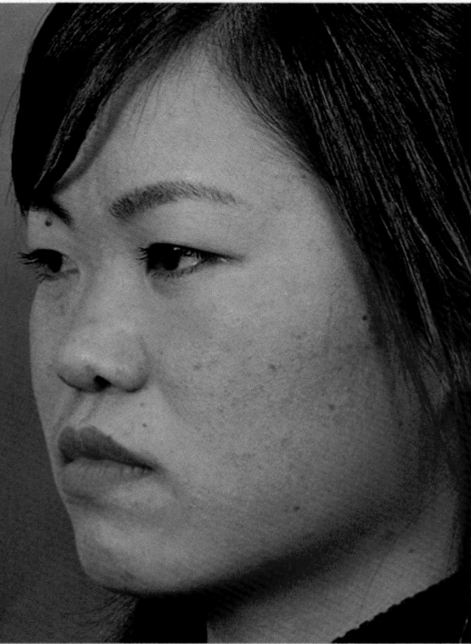

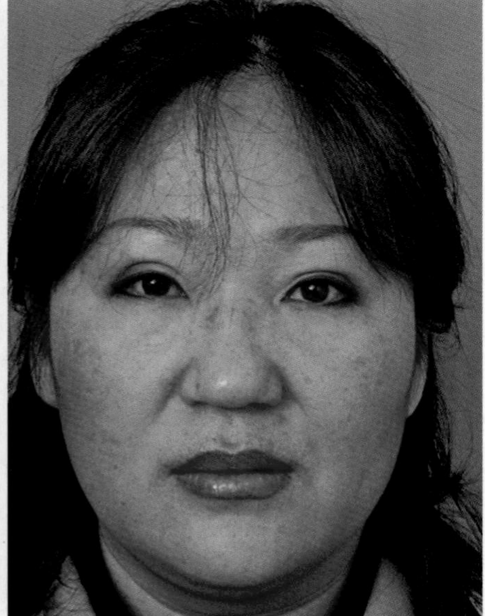

Fig. 48.1 Patients showing exaggerated features of noses with thick skin, low tip, low dorsum, and poor tip definition.

implants such as Gore-Tex (W. L. Gore & Associates Inc., Flagstaff, AZ) or autologous tissues such as morselized cartilage or fascia rather than silicone. In patients with thick skin, a relatively solid material such as silicone, reinforced Gore-Tex, or costal cartilage can be used without significant problems. In particular, when using implants with a certain level of hardness, such as silicone or costal cartilage, the base of the implant should be trimmed well so that it conforms to the contour of the nasal dorsum. Otherwise an up and down motion by palpation or deviation of the implant can occur, leading to implant visibility through the skin.

Implant Material

Various implant materials have been used for dorsal augmentation. Materials used in rhinoplasty can be divided largely between biologic tissues (autologous and homologous tissue) and the alloplastic materials.[2] In rhinoplasty for Caucasians, the use of an alloplastic implant, especially silicone, on the nasal dorsum has been condemned.[3] In Asian rhinoplasty, however, alloplastic implants still play a role due to the differing anatomical characteristics of Asians, such as thick skin and a poorly developed cartilaginous framework, compared with Caucasians. Alloplastic implants generally need to be biocompatible, nontoxic, chemically safe, and nonimmunogenic.[2] They must also not induce infection or cancer or produce toxic substances within the body. Additionally, during recovery, these implants should maintain their original size, shape, and hardness. At present, the most commonly used alloplastic implants that meet these conditions are silicone, Gore-Tex, and Medpor (Porex Surgical, Inc., Newman, GA).

Autologous Tissue

The advantage of autologous material for the dorsal augmentation of the nose cannot be questioned as these implants are well tolerated and carry the least risk of infection. However, if any autologous tissue other than septal cartilage is selected, the additional operative time required to harvest the graft and donor site morbidity become limiting factors. Common autologous tissues used for dorsal augmentation include septal cartilage, conchal cartilage, costal cartilage, fascia, and dermofat. As it is easy to harvest and shape the septal cartilage, it can be used to moderately elevate the nasal dorsum, to camouflage a partial concavity on the dorsum, and for nasal tip surgery. Because Asian patients have relatively small noses, it is practically difficult to harvest enough septal cartilage, leaving at least a 1-cm width of the L-strut, suitable for a full-length dorsal graft. Unlike septal cartilage, conchal cartilage has an intrinsic curvature that hampers its routine use in a dorsal augmentation in its original shape. Rather, in surgery on the Asian nose conchal cartilage is more frequently used for nasal tip surgery, to camouflage a partial concavity, or to cover the tip of the silicone implant to prevent extrusion. In addition, the conchal cartilage is frequently too small to yield a cartilage piece suitable for one-piece dorsal augmentation. To reduce the visibility and migration of the septal cartilage, and to overcome the limitation in size, the author prefers to place the septal cartilage onto the nasal dorsum after gentle crushing using a cartilage crusher. Also, when using conchal cartilage, it may be necessary to overlap pieces of cartilage in their opposite directions of curvature to neutralize their intrinsic curvature. Although costal cartilage is difficult to harvest and is associated with more serious donor site morbidity such as pneumothorax, as well as the problem of warping, it is the most useful autologous cartilage for substantial augmentation or in patients who have experienced complications with alloplastic implants.[4] Although strongly advocated by some surgeons for routine use in Asian rhinoplasty,[5] during the primary rhinoplasty, however, it is very difficult to persuade Asian women to use costal cartilage because the harvesting procedure leaves scars on the chest. One other critically important limitation of autologous tissue is that, except for only a few highly experienced surgeons, most rhinoplasty surgeons have difficulty using these implants to form an aesthetically pleasing nose, resulting in a high revision rate. Warping, graft visibility, and unnatural looking noses are common complications of augmentation using costal cartilage (**Fig. 48.2**). To avoid warping, it is best to soak the cartilage in saline solution to let the maximal warping occur, and to perform careful carving after a certain time elapsed (**Fig. 48.3A**). To reduce the risk of warping, the author prefers to use costal cartilage in a laminated form (**Fig. 48.3B**). Although autologous cartilage has the lowest risk of infection among graft materials, autologous cartilage including costal cartilage is associated with a significant risk of revision surgery, with rates as high as 15.5%.[6] The primary reasons for this high revision rate is that autologous tissue is usually used to treat more difficult cases and use of these implants is associated with unpredictable scarring, warping, and, at times, visible graft contours.

Autologous fascia, including temporalis fascia, can be used in rhinoplasty as radix graft or dorsal onlay grafts. However, harvesting autologous fascia requires an additional incision and hence is associated with additional morbidity. Furthermore, it is not always possible to harvest sufficient fascia of reasonable thickness because harvested fascia shrinks in volume as it dries, and, when wet, it is hard to manipulate. Compared with the temporalis fascia, fascia lata can provide a sufficient amount of connective tissue with significant thickness suitable for dorsal augmentation.

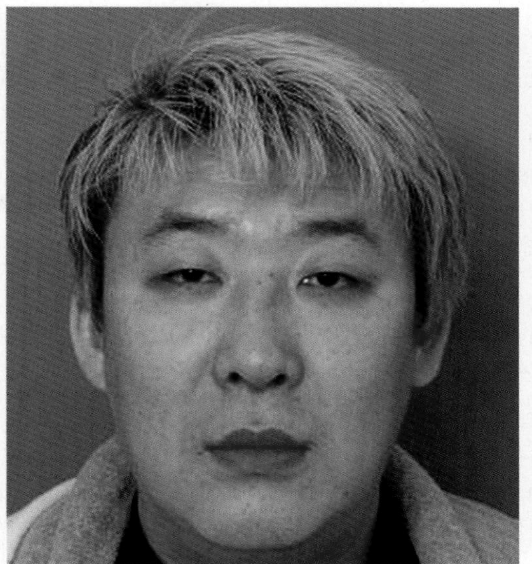

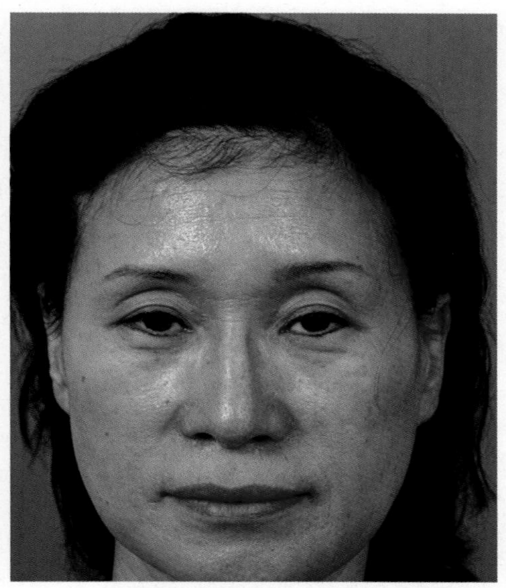

Fig. 48.2 Patients showing cartilage warping (**A**) and visible graft contour (**B**), years after dorsal augmentation using autologous costal cartilage.

However, harvesting this tissue also requires an additional incision distant from the main operative field. Nonetheless, in rhinoplasty, fascia lata could be used for dorsal augmentation, especially in secondary rhinoplasty for the correction of a failed alloplastic implant. One other advantage of fascia is that this material, placed right underneath the skin and over the crushed or morselized cartilage, or used after wrapping up the morselized cartilage, can nicely camouflage the irregular contour of diced cartilage or crushed cartilage, maximizing the full use of the small pieces of autologous tissues that remain after other procedures, and making it an alternate method of dorsal augmentation (**Fig. 48.4**). Studies have shown that diced cartilage-fascia–wrapped grafts survived and demonstrated normal

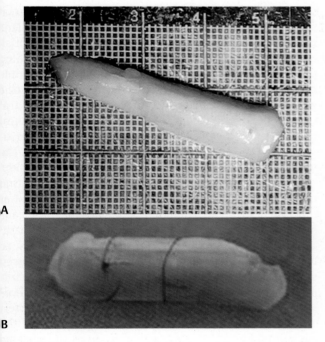

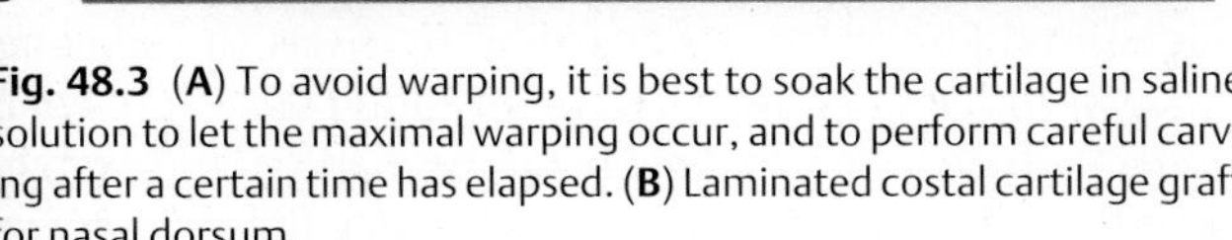

Fig. 48.3 (**A**) To avoid warping, it is best to soak the cartilage in saline solution to let the maximal warping occur, and to perform careful carving after a certain time has elapsed. (**B**) Laminated costal cartilage graft for nasal dorsum.

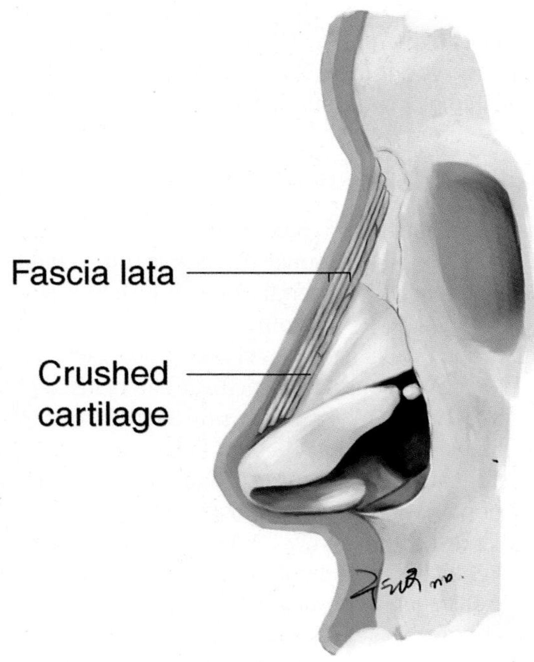

Fig. 48.4 Dorsal augmentation using fascia with crushed cartilage.

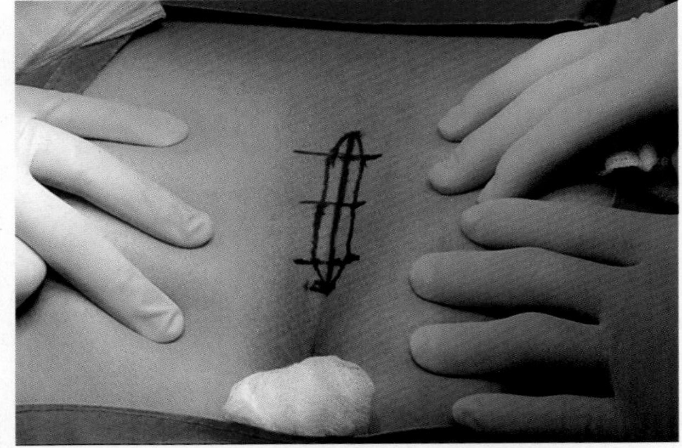

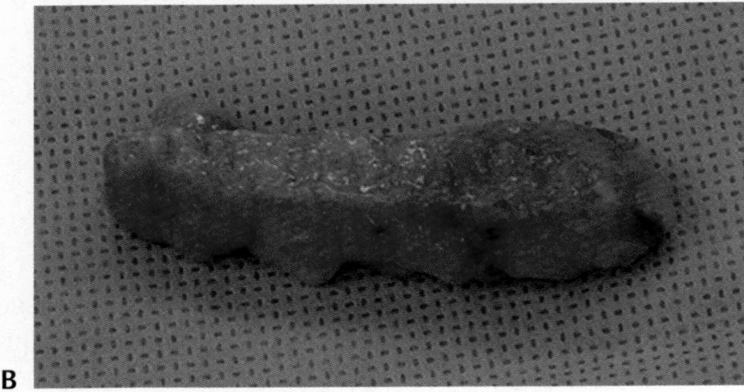

Fig. 48.5 Harvesting dermofat from coccygeal area (**A**) and harvested dermofat (**B**).

cartilage survival.[7] Dermofat, harvested from various locations, can also be used in dorsal augmentation. Although dermofat can be harvested in great quantities (**Fig. 48.5**), its absorption is difficult to predict, making it unsuitable for substantial dorsal augmentation. However, dermofat can be useful for patients with thin skin or contracture of the nose due to complicated primary rhinoplasty.[8]

Homologous Tissue or Tissue Allograft

Homologous costal cartilage, which is not associated with harvesting morbidity or additional operation time, could serve as an alternative graft material. For example, homologous costal cartilage harvested from cadaveric donors and processed in various ways has been shown to be useful in rhinoplasty.[9–11] Homologous costal cartilage can be used in revision rhinoplasties requiring structural reconstruction of the nasal framework in which patients resist harvesting their own costal cartilage. The use of homologous costal cartilage in rhinoplasty has shown conflicting results regarding the degree of resorption and warping.[9–11] In the author's experience, a significant number of patients had unpredictable complications such as resorption, warping, and graft visibility when this cartilage was used as a full-length dorsal graft. The high complication rate associated with homologous cartilage may limit its utility for dorsal augmentation.

Tutoplast processed fascia lata (TPFL) (IOP Inc., Costa Mesa, CA) is commercially available homograft fascia that has been successfully used as human tissue grafts for physical support procedures such as slings for stress incontinence, filler material, facial paralysis, or congenital ptosis.[12,13] The author has used TPFL in rhinoplasty for dorsal and radix onlay grafts. TPFL can be used for smoothening grafts for dorsal irregularity following correction of a deviated nose, as additional graft material when an inadequate amount of septal or conchal cartilage is available for dorsal augmentation, in patients who dislike the use of alloplastic material for dorsal augmentation, and for complicated revision surgery in which silicone has been used on the dorsum (**Fig. 48.6**). The soft contour of TPFL means that it can be nicely blended with the overlying skin–soft tissue envelope. Although TPFL has very low risks of infection, displacement, and extrusion, an unpredictable degree of resorption could be a problem.[13]

Silicone

Nasal dorsal augmentation with silicone rubber is the most popular rhinoplasty procedure in East Asia. Due to its stable chemical structure, silicone has several advantages including its lack of tissue reaction and ease of handling. Moreover, the availability of ready-made products makes application convenient and the relative hardness of silicone makes it suitable for fashioning the desired nasal shape for Asians with thick skin.[3,14,15] The skin of Asians is thicker than that of Caucasians, so there is a lower risk of an implant extrusion after surgery. The prefabricated products can be divided largely into L- and I-shaped implants (**Fig. 48.7**). Some surgeons favor an L-shaped or a variation of an I-shaped silicone (covering the nasal tip) capable of covering from the radix all the way down to the nasal tip. However, because the nasal tip area is an area that is always exposed to exterior stimulation, the use of L-shaped silicone carries a higher risk of extrusion, regardless of the thickness of nasal subcutaneous tissue in Asians. Thus the placement of an I-shaped implant at the nasal dorsum area and tip plasty using an autologous material (septal cartilage, conchal cartilage) at the nasal tip area is a preferable surgical method. In addition to using prefabricated silicone implants, the author has used silicone sheeting for nasal dorsal augmentation, which is more versatile but without an increased risk of complications[16] (**Fig. 48.8**). In trimming the silicone, it should preferably be ~3.5 to 4.0 cm long and ~8 mm wide and the edge should be as thin as possible. To insert the silicone, an open rhinoplasty approach or an endonasal approach is used. The size of the pocket should be made slightly larger than the implant, with just enough space for insertion of

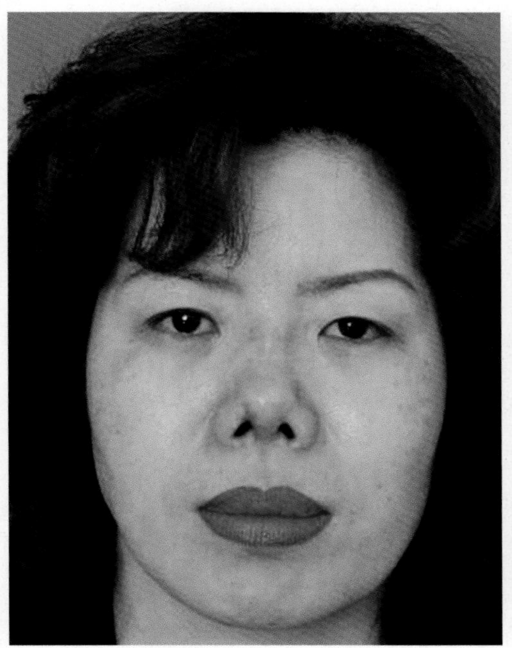
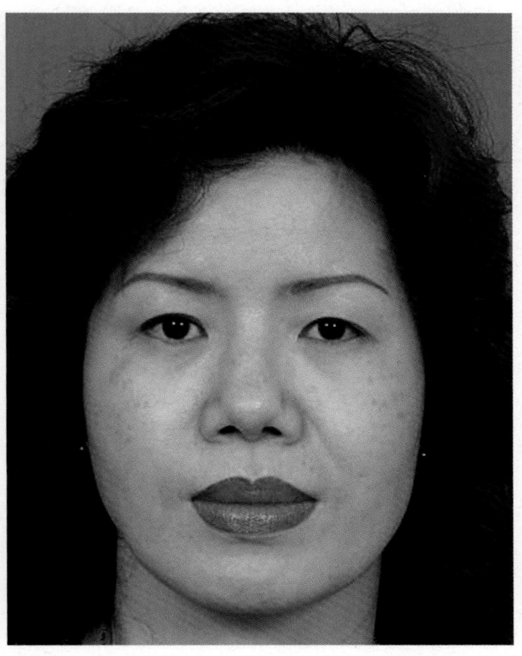

Fig. 48.6 Patient before (**A**) and after (**B**) undergoing rhinoplasty using Tutoplast processed fascia lata for management of contracted nose caused by infection due to silicone implant.

the implant held by a surgical tool. Revision rhinoplasty after silicone implants may be needed for implant deviation, floating, displacement, extrusion, impending extrusion, and infection[14] (**Fig. 48.9**). Although infection is one of the most dreadful complications of silicone implants, early infections can be prevented by the use of aseptic techniques and prophylactic antibiotics. Infection can also be treated by implant removal, antibiotic administration, and delayed reinsertion. Extrusion of the implant can occur through the nasal skin or mucosa, with tension over the implant being the most common cause of extrusion. The most likely cause of implant displacement is supraperiosteal placement of implants. Thus implant displacement can be reduced by placing it immediately below the periosteum.

Fig. 48.7 Various shapes of prefabricated silicone implants.

Gore-Tex

Gore-Tex enjoys a long history of use in vascular surgery and millions of grafts have been implanted with remarkably good biocompatibility.[17] Gore-Tex (expanded polytetrafluoroethylene [ePTFE]), next to silicone, is the most widely used alloplastic implant in the Asian nose, and currently its use is on the increase. Gore-Tex implants are porous, inducing the surrounding tissue to grow inward through the pore, and have the advantages of increased stability and lower incidence of capsule formation. In addition, the risk of extrusion is lower with Gore-Tex than with silicone. The soft texture of Gore-Tex reduces patient discomfort and the occurrence of unnatural visible implant contours through the skin. One important disadvantage of Gore-Tex is that it decreases in volume after insertion. In addition, it is more difficult to remove a Gore-Tex implant than a silicone implant. Reports of a

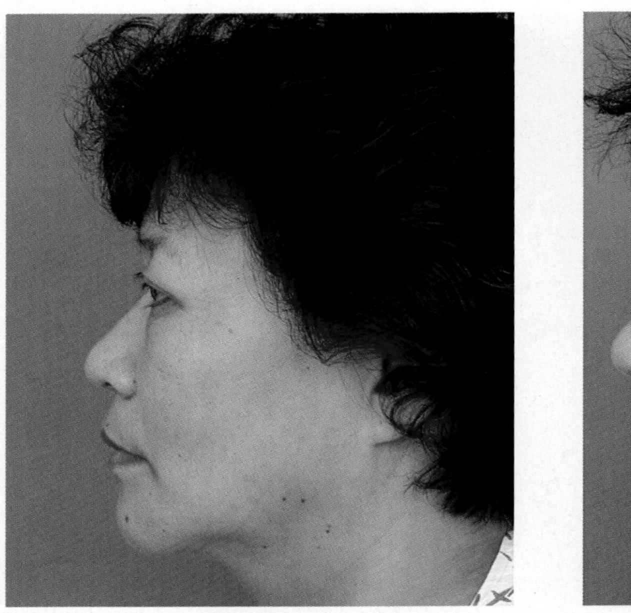
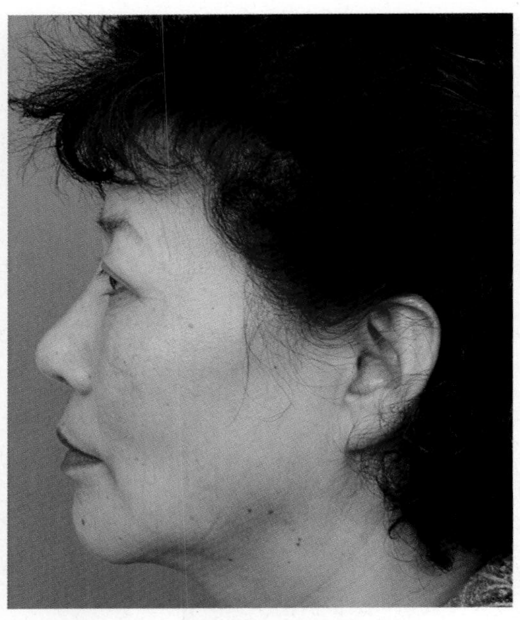

Fig. 48.8 Patient before (**A**) and after (**B**) undergoing dorsal augmentation using silicone sheeting.

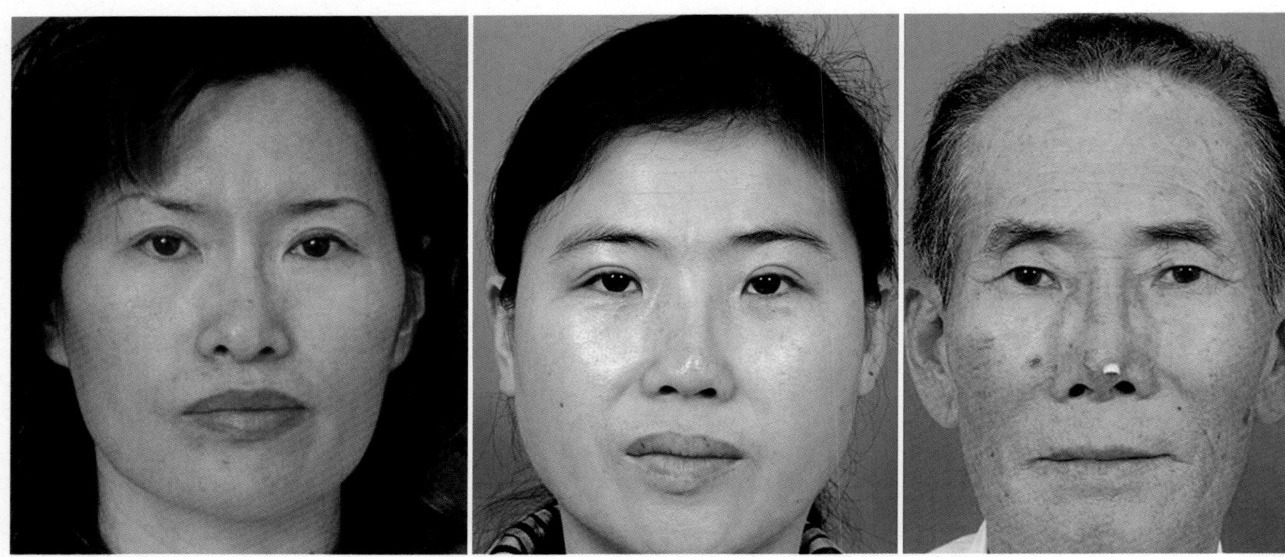

Fig. 48.9 Complication of rhinoplasty using silicone. Implant deviation (**A**), impending extrusion (**B**), and extrusion (**C**) are the most common complications.

delayed inflammation (**Fig. 48.10**) are increasing, and outcome data are not adequately accumulated to date. One must be cautious when using Gore-Tex in the presence of inflammation within the nasal cavity (sinusitis, vestibulitis, and active acne). Moreover, when performing operations that may create microcommunication with the nasal cavity (e.g., osteotomy or septal reconstruction), there is an increased risk of infection. It has been recommended that patients be treated with antibiotics prior to inserting the Gore-Tex as well as after surgery, and it is essential to soak the Gore-Tex in saline solution containing Betadine (povidone-iodine) or antibiotics before use. Also, before handling the Gore-Tex, surgical personnel should wash their gloves to remove powder or other foreign substances. It has been reported that infection rate in primary surgery is 1.2%, whereas infection rate in secondary surgery is 5.4%.[18]

Radix Augmentation

The ability to display adequate nasofrontal and nasofacial angles is an important requirement for an attractive

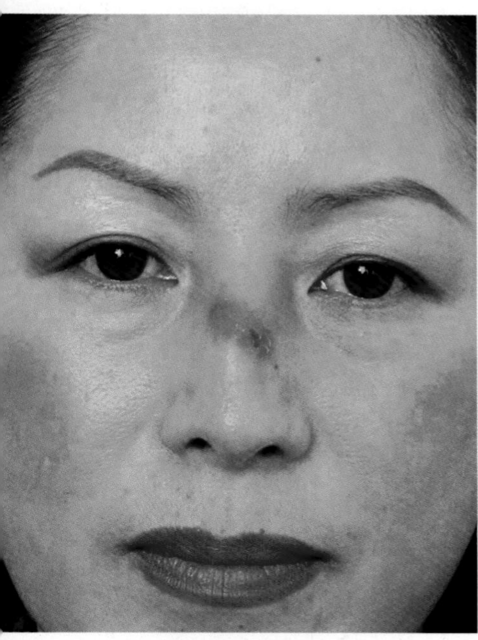

Fig. 48.10 Delayed inflammation two years after rhinoplasty using Gore-Tex.

nose.[19] In Asians, the height of radix is sometimes very low, and a significant proportion of patients have a low, flat forehead, making the nasal starting point blunt. In general, Asian women are highly concerned about the location of the nasal starting point after dorsal augmentation. Thus properly addressing the radix area is a very important aspect of Asian rhinoplasty. Furthermore, because many patients complain of a short nose, these patients require proper radix augmentation to make their noses look longer. Among Asians, the nasion is located at various levels, but the general consensus is that the nasion is best located around the horizontal midpupillary line or just above for women, and between the upper eyelash and eyelid crease for men (**Fig. 48.11**).

Surgical manipulation of the radix can alter the nasion level. If a patient desires a softer-looking nose, the new nasion can be created at about the midpupil level, whereas, if a patient wants a nose with a stronger appearance, the nasion can be relocated closer to the glabella. If the nasofacial angle becomes broader as a result of an excessively deep radix, the nose can appear short; whereas, if the nsaofacial angle becomes narrower, the nose can appear elongated as a result of shallow radix (**Fig. 48.12**). In a frontal photograph, the radix must appear to form a soft line that connects naturally with the supraorbital curve.

Osteotomy

Osteotomy is an important technique for correction of a deviated nose, hump reduction, and modification of brow-tip aesthetic line. Although osteotomy can be used as frequently for rhinoplasty in Asians as in Caucasians, osteotomy for Asian noses carries a special challenge

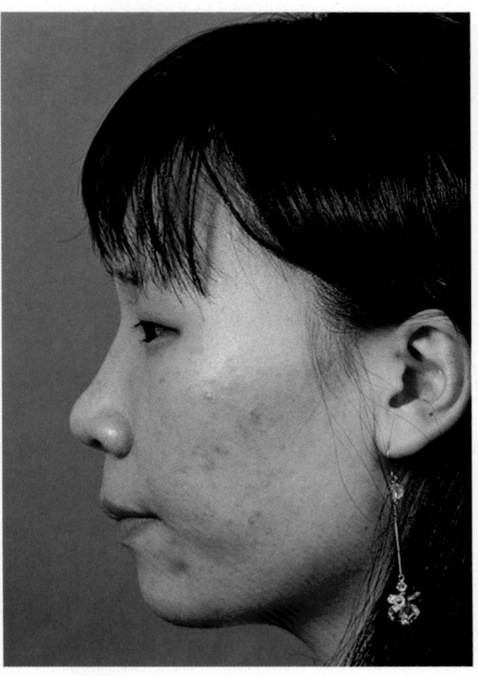

A

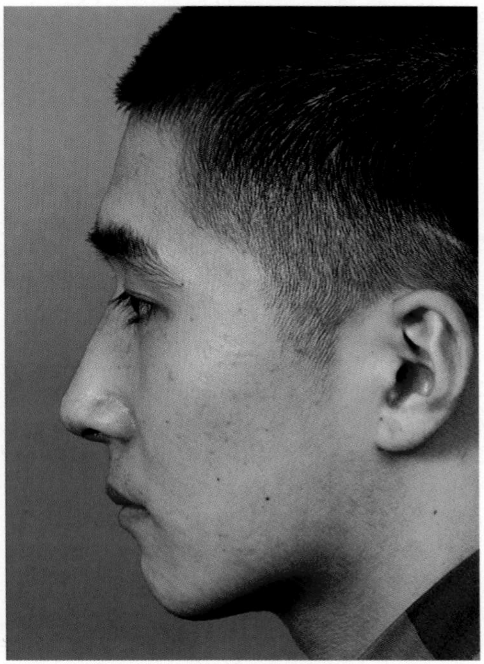

B

Fig. 48.11 Nasal starting point favored by Asian female (**A**) and male (**B**) patients.

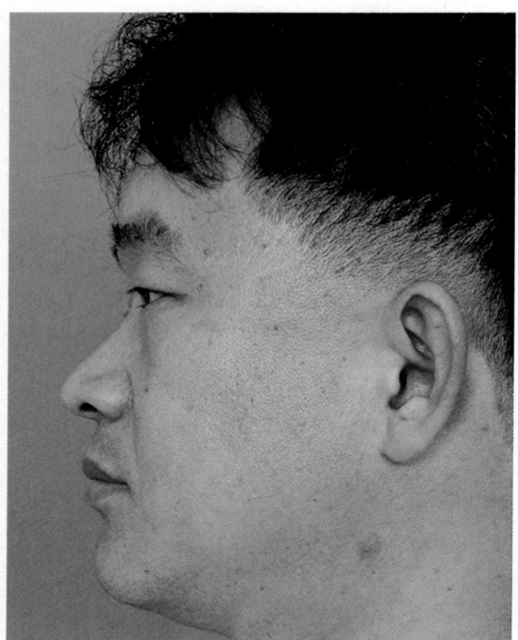

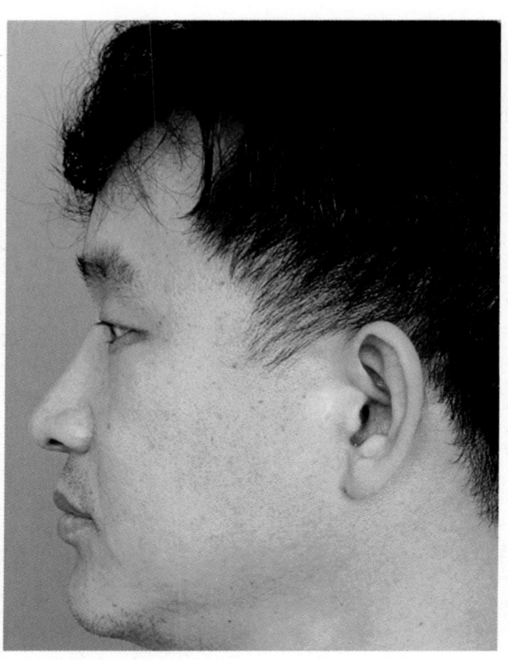

Fig. 48.12 Before (**A**) and after (**B**) radix augmentation. Following surgery the nasofacial angle became narrower and the nose appears elongated.

due to the size and thickness of the bone. In Asians, the nasal bones are generally small and thick, thus increasing the risk of shattering the bone and fracturing it into small pieces (**Fig. 48.13**). In these patients, alternative procedures, such as onlay grafts, are recommended in place of an osteotomy. In addition, percutaneous lateral osteotomy, which is widely performed during rhinoplasty in Caucasians,[20] is not suitable for patients with thick and small nasal bones. It is difficult to make several holes in thick nasal bone, and to connect the holes using digital pressure. Thus the author recommends that medial and lateral osteotomy be performed using the internal continuous method, not the percutaneous route. Also, among patients with excessively thick skin, a common trait in Asian populations, the changes induced by an osteotomy frequently do not appear externally, making the effect of osteotomy less prominent.

Correction of a deviated nose is not possible if the direction of the midline bony septum left over from medial and lateral osteotomy is not straight. The midline bony septum should therefore be fractured to completely mobilize the midline structure. However, when the central bony structure is so thick as to resist fracturing by digital compression, a percutaneous root osteotomy can be performed to fracture the bony septum and relocate it in the desired direction.[21] Percutaneous root osteotomy is performed at the eyebrow level using a 2-mm osteotome (**Fig. 48.14**). As a prerequisite, the dorsal part of the cartilaginous septum must be separated from the upper lateral cartilages. At times, however, the severed bony segment can collapse toward the nasal cavity following a root osteotomy. In such cases, it is recommended that an onlay graft be performed using a bony fragment or cartilage.

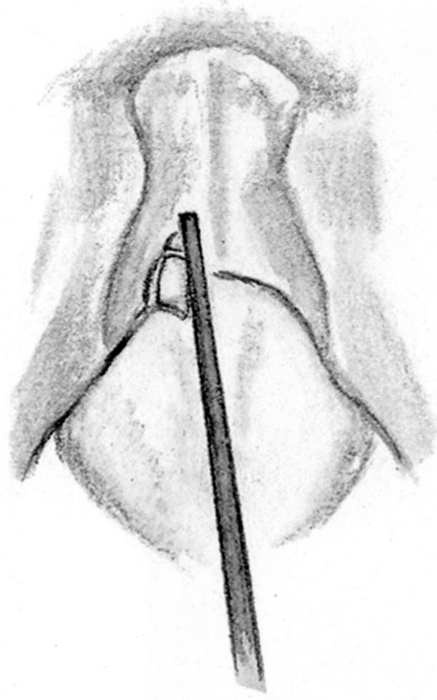

Fig. 48.13 Osteotomy performed on small but thick nasal bones have a high risk of inducing comminuted fracture of the nasal bone.

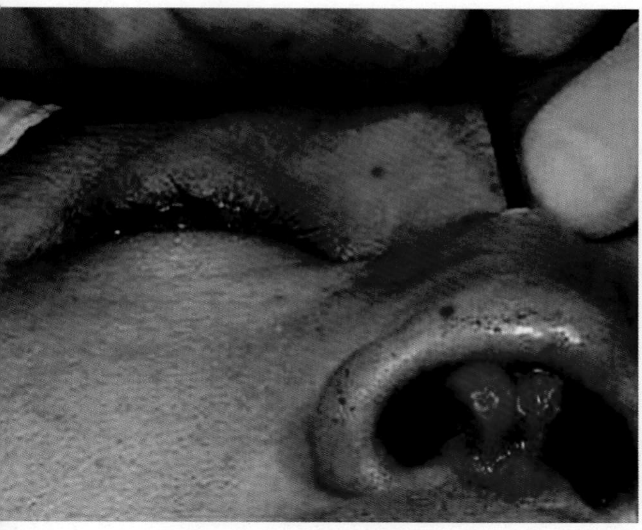

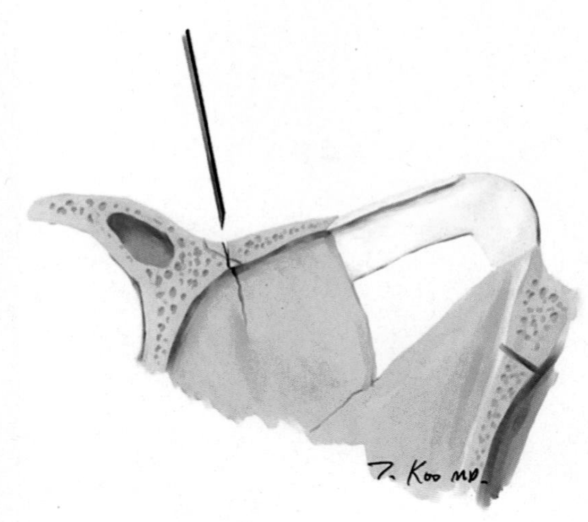

Fig. 48.14 Percutaneous root osteotomy, which can be performed to make a controlled fracture line of the bony septum and relocate it in the desired direction.

Dorsal Hump Reduction

Reduction rhinoplasty for dorsal hump is one of the most common rhinoplasty procedures performed on Caucasian noses, from which a variety of rhinoplasty techniques evolved. In contrast to the well-developed and prominent noses of Caucasians, noses of Asians are generally small and less prominent. Accordingly, the prevalence of a hump nose among Asians is relatively low. Rhinoplasties for Asian noses have traditionally been oversimplified and overrepresented as augmentation rhinoplasty using alloplastic material such as prefabricated silicone. However, this simple approach is not a universal remedy for various aesthetic features in Asian noses, particularly for the correction of a dorsal hump. Dorsal hump reduction in Caucasian noses frequently consists of humpectomy followed by osteotomy and tip surgery. However, in treating dorsal humps in underdeveloped and underprojected noses, a different treatment strategy, such as reduction in combination with dorsal augmentation, may be required. Certainly, dorsal humps are present in Asians, with the degree and type of deformity varying greatly among patients seeking treatment for a dorsal hump. Furthermore, in examining a patient's nose, a typical hump as well as a hump-like deformity can be identified. Dorsal hump nasal deformities of Asian noses can be classified into three types: generalized hump, isolated hump, and relative hump due to low tip. Generalized hump represents the typical hump commonly seen in Caucasian populations, in which the curvature of the hump begins from the bony vault and extends to the cartilaginous dorsum in a gentle curve (**Fig. 48.15**). Isolated hump represents instances of abrupt protrusion of a small hump in a triangular or round shape at the dorsal line. The total length of the hump is short, with most of it located around the rhinion (**Fig. 48.16**). Relative hump with low tip represents patients in which the height of the nasal dorsum is not so prominent but the nasal tip is underdeveloped, giving a false impression of a nasal dorsal hump (**Fig. 48.17**).

For treating the generalized hump type of deformity, an open approach is preferred. Excessive septal cartilage in the dorsal aspect is resected using a blade, the bony hump is reduced using a osteotome, and a judicious removal of the dorsal aspect of the upper lateral cartilages then follows.[22] Open roof deformities in the bony dorsum are closed mostly by medial and lateral osteotomies. Placement of a spreader graft is the preferred way of reconstructing the cartilaginous dorsum. In most cases, tip surgery techniques are required to project the nasal tip and improve the tip support. When a patient presents with a low radix, the latter can be augmented using crushed cartilage, resected hump, or fascia. Some patients, even those with generalized hump, want dorsal augmentation, in which case, the level of which was adjusted by the newly created tip height can be augmented to make an ideal dorsal profile. In treatment of isolated hump, either open approach or closed approach is selected depending on the degree of associated deformity. Hump reduction is usually performed by en bloc removal, and osteotomy is performed depending on the width of the open roof deformity. Osteotomies are not performed when the removed hump is small and the remaining dorsal flatness is not so prominent. Placement of spreader grafts is also performed in selected patients. Tip surgery and dorsal augmentation is performed as described for generalized hump. In some

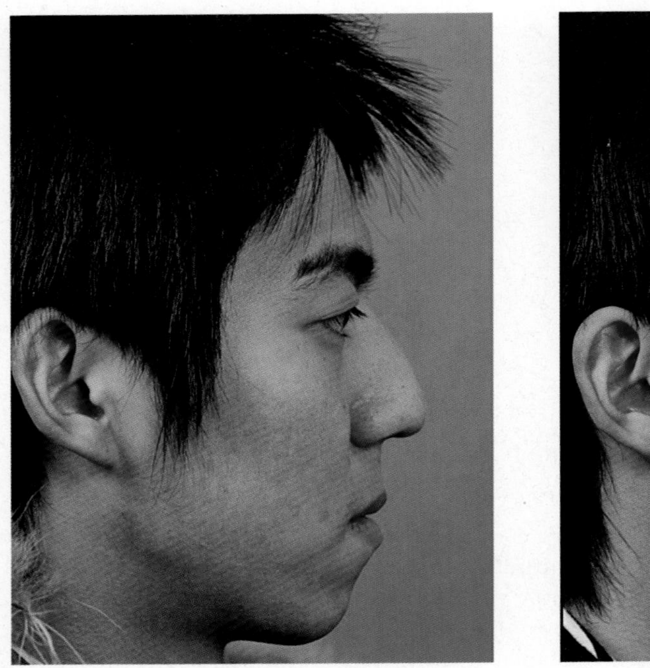

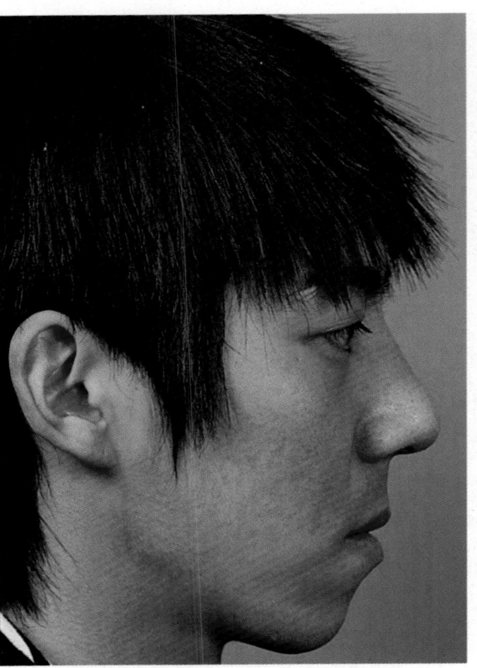

Fig. 48.15 Typical features of a generalized hump, preoperative (**A**) and postoperative (**B**).

patients with a convex nasal dorsum, there are instances of accompanying severely underprojected tip giving the false impression of a hump nose. In this type of patient, surgery to improve the tip projection and support is the mainstay of the treatment. Various surgical techniques are used, including caudal septal extension graft, columellar strut, shield graft, and suture techniques. These patients also require dorsal augmentation. The dorsum, particularly the cartilaginous dorsum, should be elevated in correspondence with the newly elevated nasal tip. The rationale for

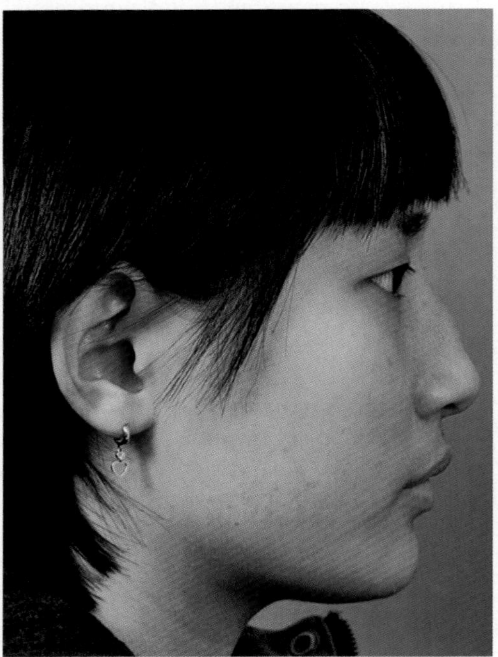

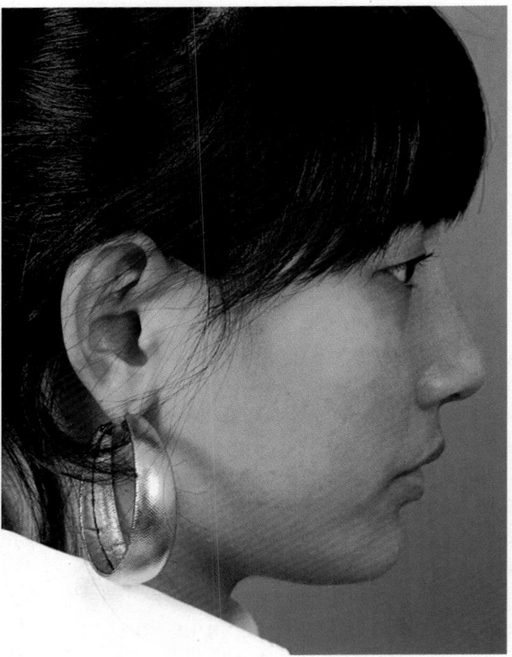

Fig. 48.16 Typical features of a isolated hump, preoperative (**A**) and postoperative (**B**).

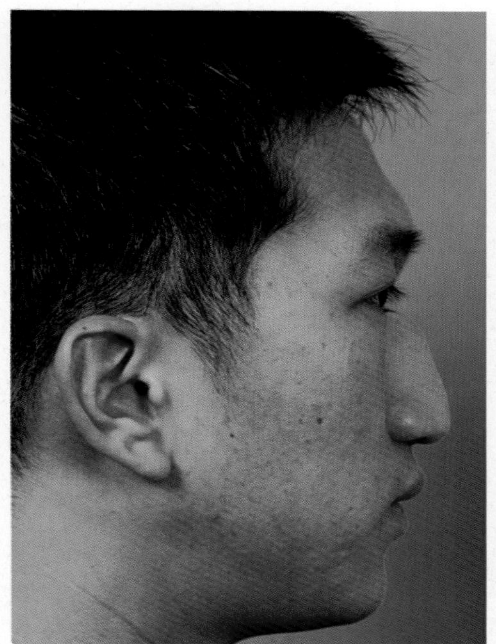

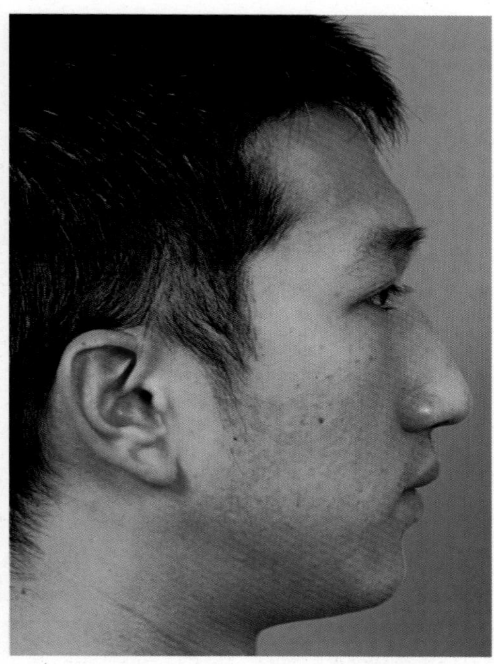

Fig. 48.17 Typical features of a relative hump with low tip, preoperative (**A**) and postoperative (**B**).

dorsal augmentation in hump management is that many patients need correction of minor contour irregularities, and hence require a smoothening graft. Second, many patients want augmentation together with reduction. Thus, the correction of a dorsal hump in Asian patients is closer to redistribution surgery than to simple reduction.

Correction of Deviated Nose

The surgical principles applicable to the management of the bony vault, middle vault, and lower third of the Caucasian nose are also applicable to the correction of deviated noses in Asians.[23] But the difficulty in the management of this problem is that many patients lack a sufficient amount of septal cartilage for simultaneous use in reconstructing the septal framework, tip surgery, and dorsal augmentation. Thus the surgeon frequently must harvest costal cartilage for complete correction of the deviated nose. In addition, many patients undergoing correction of a deviated nose also want dorsal augmentation as a result of surgery (**Fig. 48.18**). Thus dorsal augmentation may be regarded as an important part in the correction of the deviated Asian nose. Dorsal augmentation is performed during the last stage in the correction of a deviated nose. Through this procedure, the surgeon reestablishes the harmony between the bone and the skin–soft tissue envelope as well as the balance between the function and the aesthetics of the nose. The sutures used to secure the osteotomy or spreader graft performed during the correction of a deviated nose may lead to postsurgical irregularity of the dorsum, particularly among patients with thin skin. In addition, unexpected events, such as a saddle nose deformity caused by the destruction of the keystone area, may occur during surgery, emphasizing the need for dorsal augmentation. Some patients with deviated noses manifest contracture of the skin and soft tissues in the severely deviated area. Proper dorsal augmentation can help overcome the deformity of the soft tissue that contributes to the formation of the deviation. In addition, dorsal augmentation in itself helps the nose look longer and narrower. The supporting structure of the new dorsum created during surgery, by osteotomy or septal reconstruction, is weaker than the original dorsum. Therefore, if hard implant materials such as silicone or costal cartilage are positioned at sites without sufficient room between the skin and the dorsum, these implants will exert excessive force downward with the result being that the dorsum will be pressed down toward the nasal cavity and become flat or cause a relapse of the deviation (**Fig. 48.19**). Thus, if possible, a less bulky implant, made of soft material, should be selected. In addition, reconstruction of the dorsum can create a microcommunication between the nasal cavity and the dorsum, increasing the risk of infection, when alloplastic implants such as Gore-Tex or silicone are used. Thus choosing the ideal implant material becomes difficult. During the correction of a deviated nose, the author prefers to use material such as crushed cartilage or fascia because of its relative softness and its easy blending with the skin.

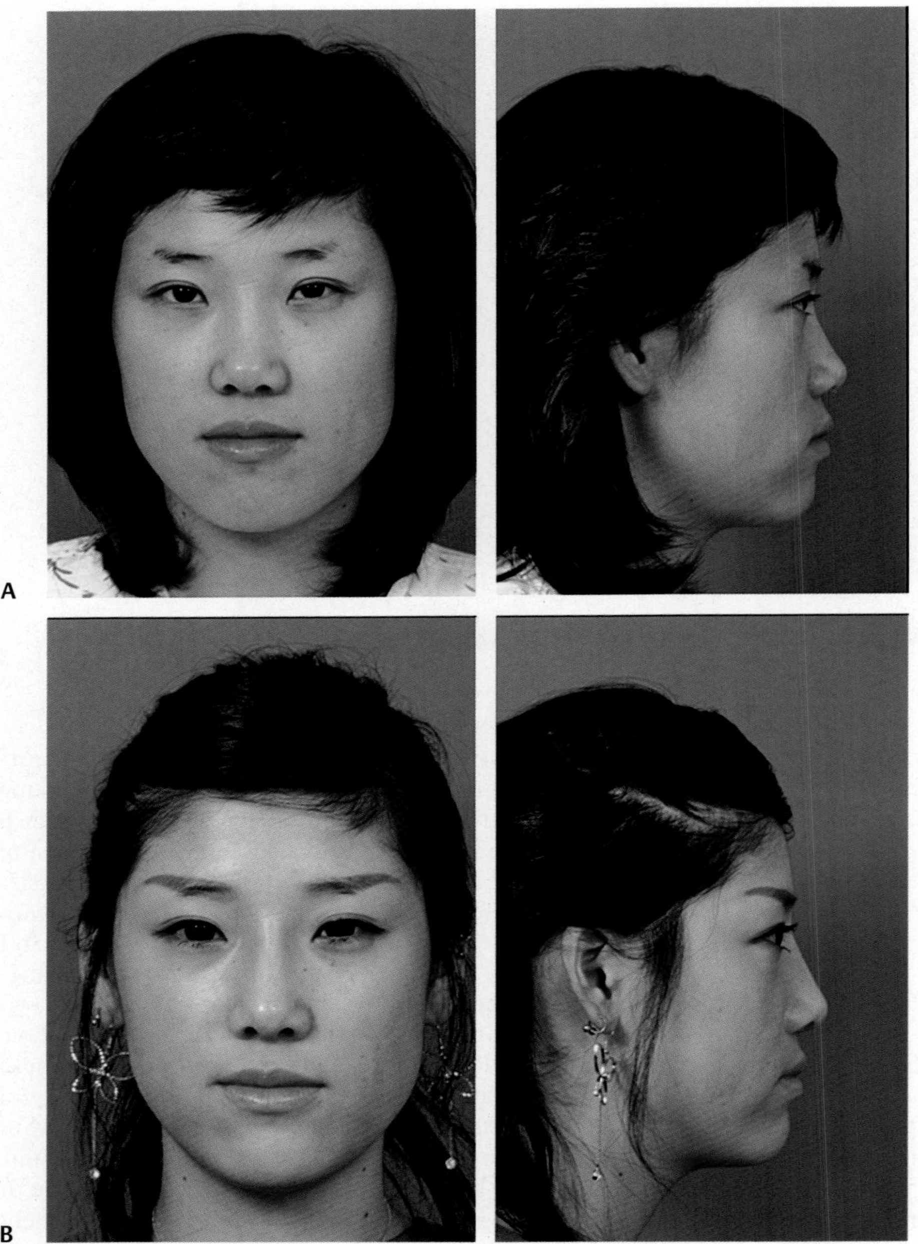

Fig. 48.18 Patient before (**A**) and after (**B**) undergoing correction of deviated nose in association with dorsal augmentation.

Surgery of the Nasal Tip

Traditionally, tip surgery has been a point of emphasis in rhinoplasty among Caucasians, but its importance has been generally underestimated among Asians. A careful observation of the Asian nose reveals a surprising diversity in the shape of the nasal tip. Thus it is incorrect to conclude outright that the Asian nose as a whole is unsuitable for a conventional tip surgery technique. Rather, various tip surgery techniques once thought to be applicable only to Caucasians are also largely applicable to Asians. It is important to emphasize that such tip surgery techniques are essential for managing Asian noses.

The typical endonasal approach for Caucasian noses involve cephalic resection through a delivery or nondelivery approach, and placement of transdomal and interdomal sutures and a columellar strut. This approach can also be used for the placement of shield or onlay graft.

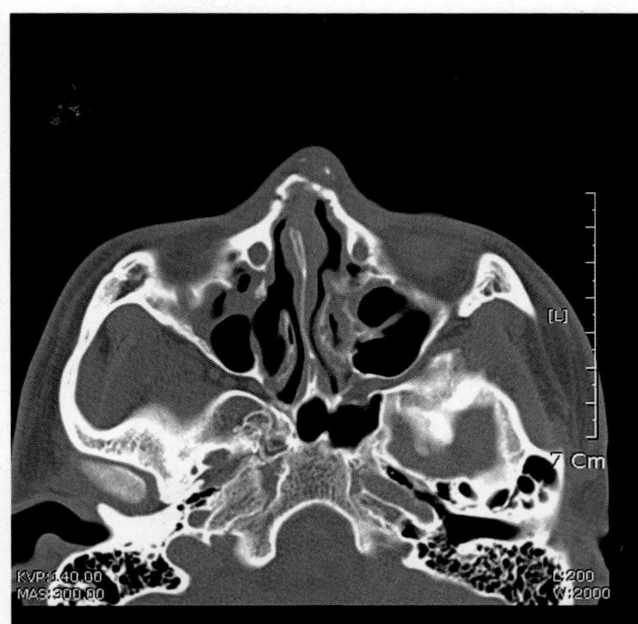

A

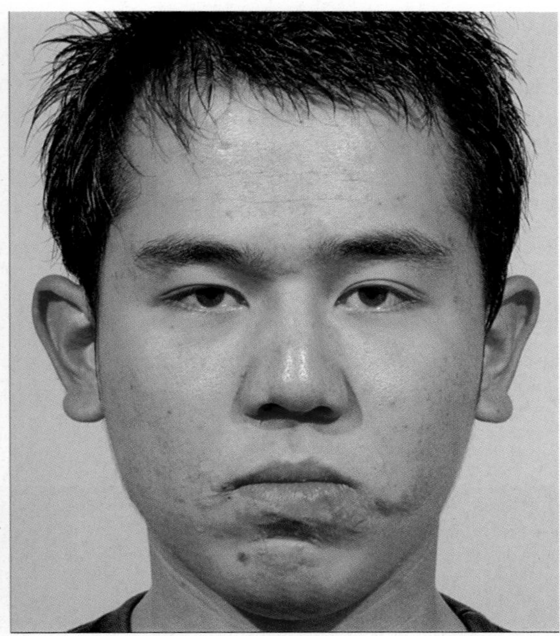
B

Fig. 48.19 Collapsed bony dorsum (*thin arrow*) after placement of costal cartilage (*thick arrow*) dorsal onlay grafting (**A**), and resultant recurrence of bony deviation (**B**).

Cephalic resection using the nondelivery approach is impractical for Asian patients because tip surgery requiring only a cephalic resection is very rare in Asian patients. Meanwhile, a certain level of tip projection and rotation can be achieved through the incision on the skin from the middle crus of the lower lateral cartilage to the vestibule side.[24] Using this limited marginal incision and subsequent dissection of the caudal area of the lower lateral cartilage can enable a surgeon to place the onlay graft at the tip area (**Fig. 48.20**). The external rhinoplasty approach is a versatile approach that enables the surgeon to precisely diagnose nasal tip deformity and to tailor treatment using various tip surgery techniques.[25] The most common of these tip surgery techniques include

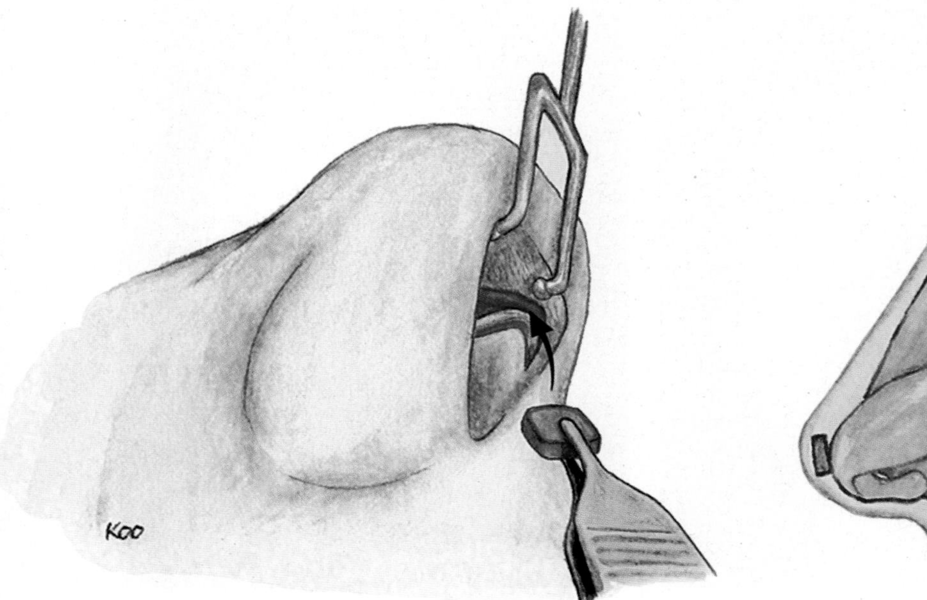

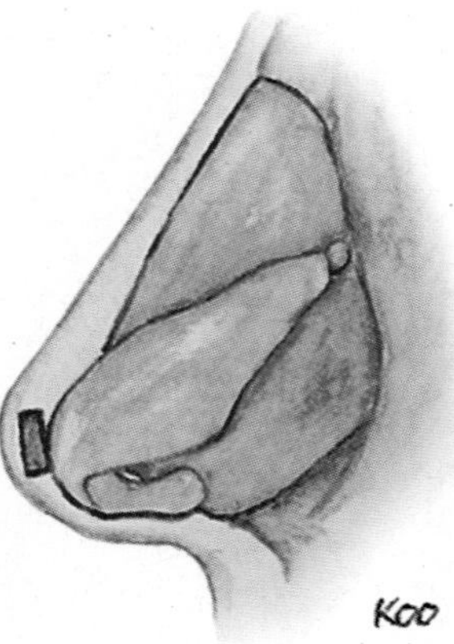

Fig. 48.20 An onlay graft can be placed on a dorsum using the closed approach.

columellar struts; shield, onlay, and septal extension grafts; and transdomal, interdomal, suture, and septocolumellar sutures.[26–29] Selection of the specific maneuver is dependent on the shape of the patient's deformity, the availability of grafting material, and the surgeon's preference. Among the multitude of tip surgery techniques, the following have important roles and should be emphasized for the Asian tip.

Defatting

When the skin–soft tissue envelope of the nasal tip is too thick, it is almost impossible to create an ideal tip with a distinct definition. Nevertheless, cosmetic improvement is possible, even in such patients. For patients with excessively thick soft tissue at the tip, the author uses an external approach to expose the tip. During the process of dissecting the skin flap, a method that elevates the flap with the yellowish fibro-fatty tissue left attached to the surface of the lower lateral cartilage is preferred, rather than the more common supraperichondrial dissection method. If the supraperichondrial dissection of the lower lateral cartilage is performed after the flap is elevated in this manner, the fibro-fatty tissue can be removed safely and the removed tissue can be used as a filler for other areas during surgery (**Fig. 48.21**). At times, the soft tissue

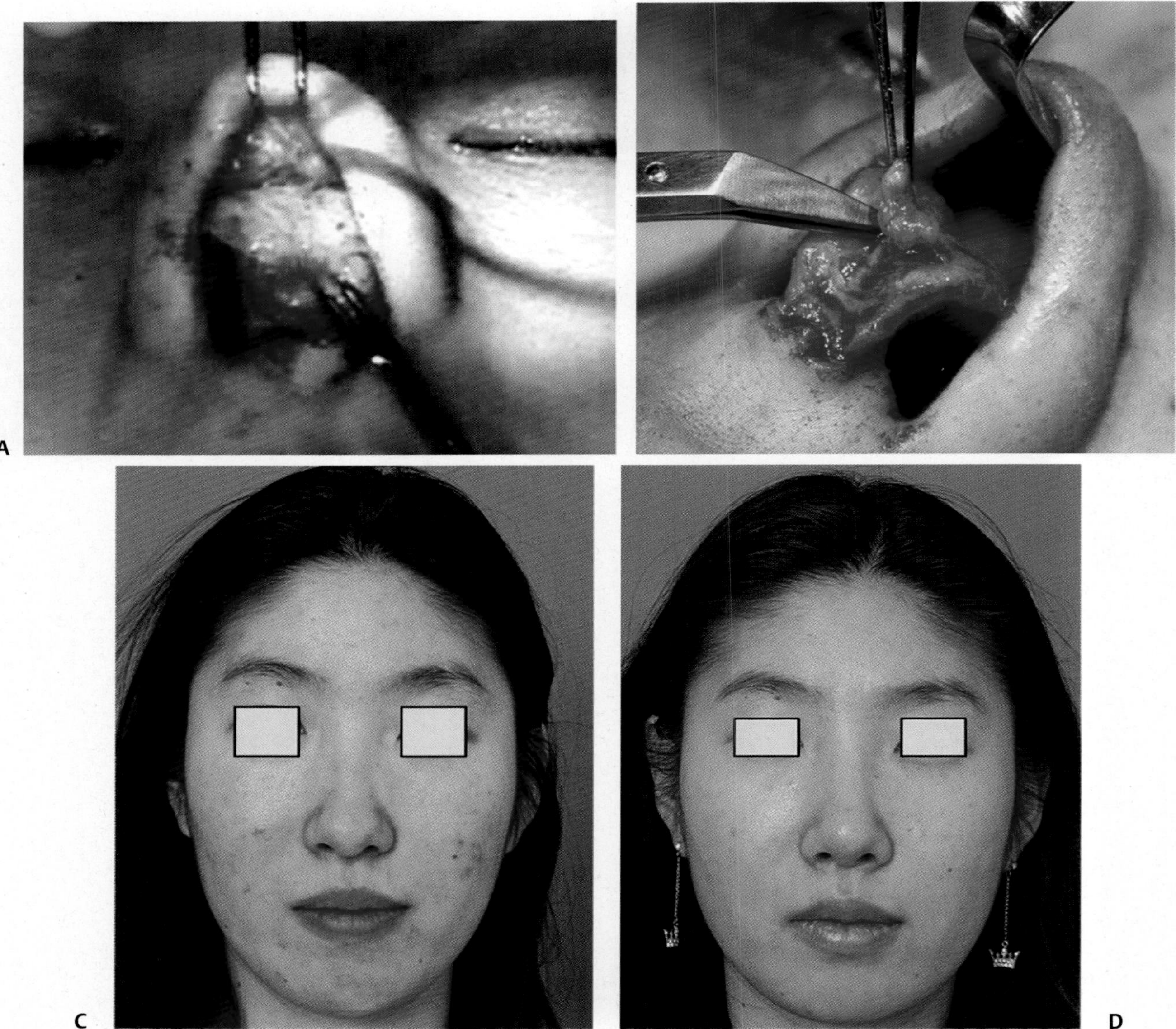

Fig. 48.21 A certain level of defatting becomes possible if the fibro-fatty tissue left on the lower lateral cartilage after elevation of the skin flap (**A**) is dissected and removed in the manner shown (**B**). Before (**C**) and after (**D**) the operation.

attached to the elevated skin flap can also be additionally removed, but this procedure requires extreme caution as it may cause irreversible damage to the skin. Most patients with a bulbous nose, which necessitates this technique, also have extremely poorly developed lower lateral cartilages. Therefore, the tip projection must be enhanced through transdomal or interdomal sutures, columellar struts, or onlay grafting.

Columellar Plumping Graft and Premaxillary Graft

These grafts are used to correct an acuteness of the columellar–labial angle, which can easily be seen in Asian noses. These grafts, usually consisting of crushed, morselized cartilage, are placed near the anterior nasal spine[28] (**Fig. 48.22**). When significant augmentation of the premaxillar is required, prefabricated silicone implants or large cartilage pieces of costal cartilage can be used (**Fig. 48.23**).

Septal Extension Graft

Although the underprojection of the tip among Asians frequently results from an inadequately developed lower lateral cartilage, it may also be caused by poor caudal septal support. If an adequate quantity of septal cartilage can be obtained after preserving its L-strut, this cartilage can be used as a septal extension graft to elevate the anterior septal angle of the septal cartilage as well as to strengthen the support.[30,31] As a result, the tip support can be strengthened along with the creation of a significant projection. One of the advantages of this technique is that, besides the projection/rotation of the tip, it can be useful in correction of the short nose deformity, which can be commonly found in the Asian population (**Fig. 48.24**). In particular, in patients with a retracted columella, a caudal extension of the graft can be particularly effective in improving the columellar retraction, as well as in correcting the caudal septal deflection. Septal extension grafts can be classified into three types, depending on the graft[28] (**Fig. 48.25**). Type I takes the form of a spreader graft that extends over the area between the front of the anterior septal angle to the interdomal space. Type II takes on the form of a pair of batten grafts that extending to the tip-lobule complex in a slightly slanting manner from the caudal and dorsal septal L-strut. Type III is a graft that involves the enlargement of the septal batten graft, is fixed to the anterior nasal spine or the nasal floor posteriorly, and is placed in a protruding manner toward the caudal and dorsal directions of the anterior septal angle. Because type III graft is the most effective in supporting the caudal septum, this type is preferred by the author. Grafts of this type should be made of septal or costal cartilage. This method is easy to perform during an open rhinoplasty when both sides of the crura are already separated at the middle and both sides of the septal mucosa and upper

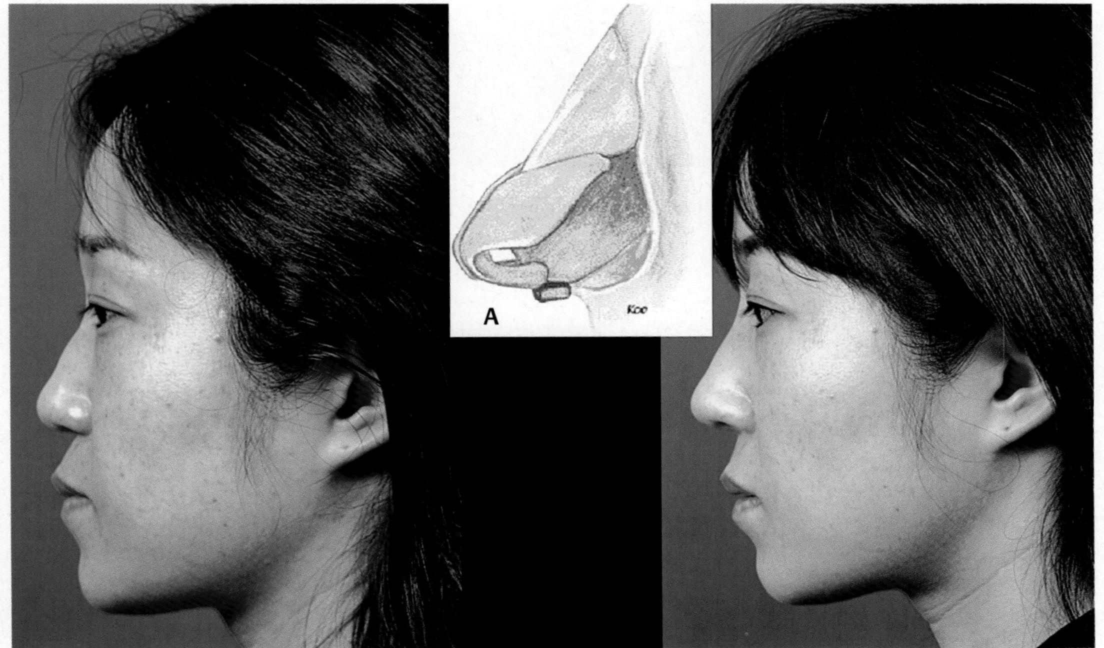

Fig. 48.22 (**A**) Pluming graft. It can be used for the purpose of widening the columellar–labial angle. Before (**B**) and after (**C**) plumping graft.

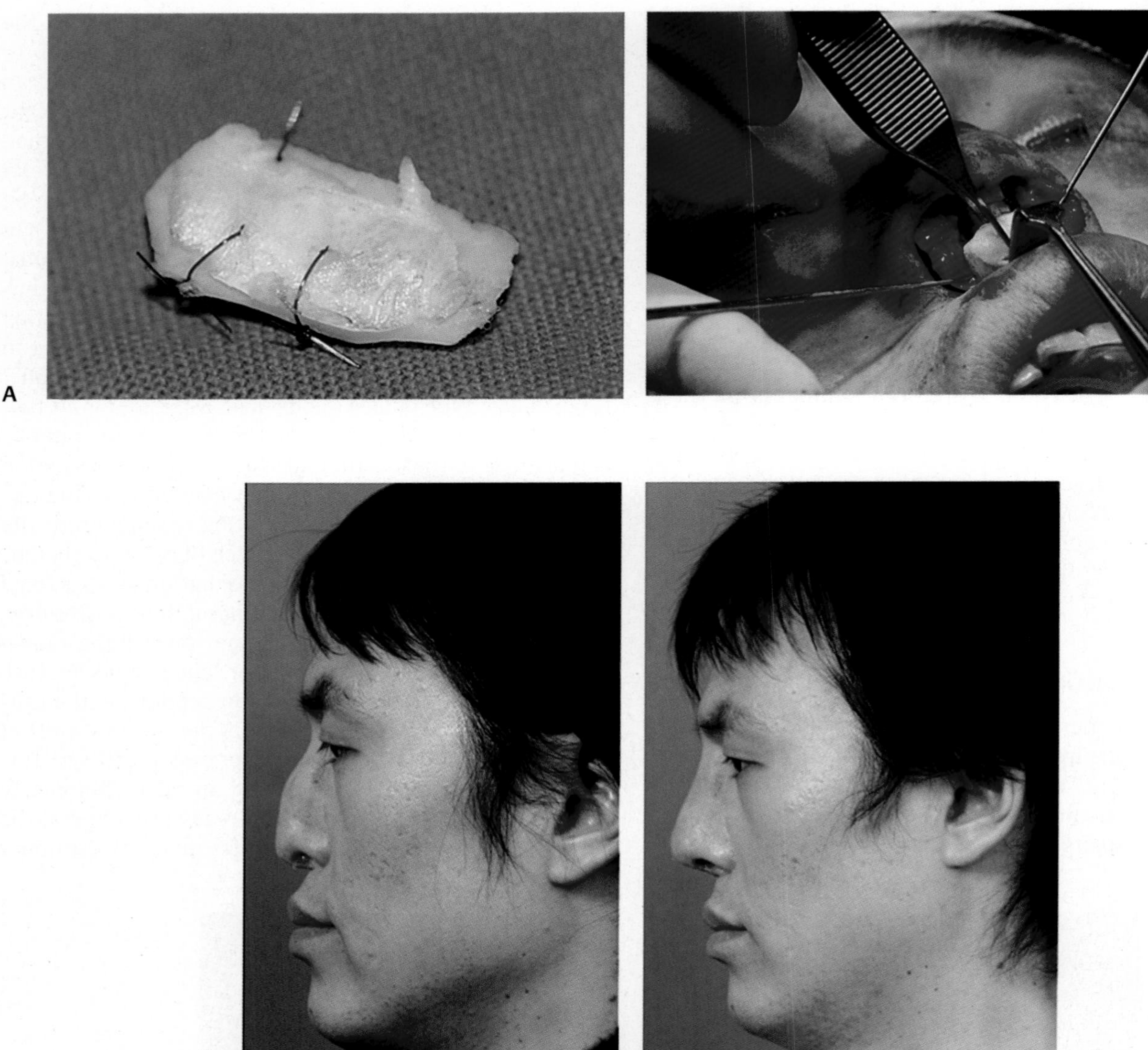

Fig. 48.23 (**A**) Placement of premaxillary graft. Before (**B**) and after (**C**) the premaxillary grafting using costal cartilage.

lateral cartilage are also in a dissected state. If the cartilage fragment is sufficiently large, it can be extended to the anterior nasal spine area. However, when the usable cartilage fragment is small, it should be made to protrude above the anterior septal angle in a type II form and be fixed to the septal cartilage using suture. In performing septal extension graft surgery, it is preferable to position the graft at both sides of the caudal septal cartilage due to the reduced risk of causing nostril asymmetry, as well as the stronger nature of the grafting. In reality, however, it is difficult to obtain sufficient cartilage to place the graft on both side,s and hence the procedure is generally performed only on one side. The graft can later be secured by applying a columellar-septal suture to the bilateral middle crura in a tongue-in-groove fashion and a through-and-through suture to the newly created anterior septal angle.

Alar Base Surgery

Because many Asian patients tend to have a broad alar base, alar base surgery is a very important supplementary surgical technique in Asian rhinoplasty that is used to construct a cosmetically balanced nasal base. Most alar base surgeries are performed to reduce the width of the nose and are known by an assortment of names, including as alar base reduction, alar base resection, and alar wedge resection.[32]

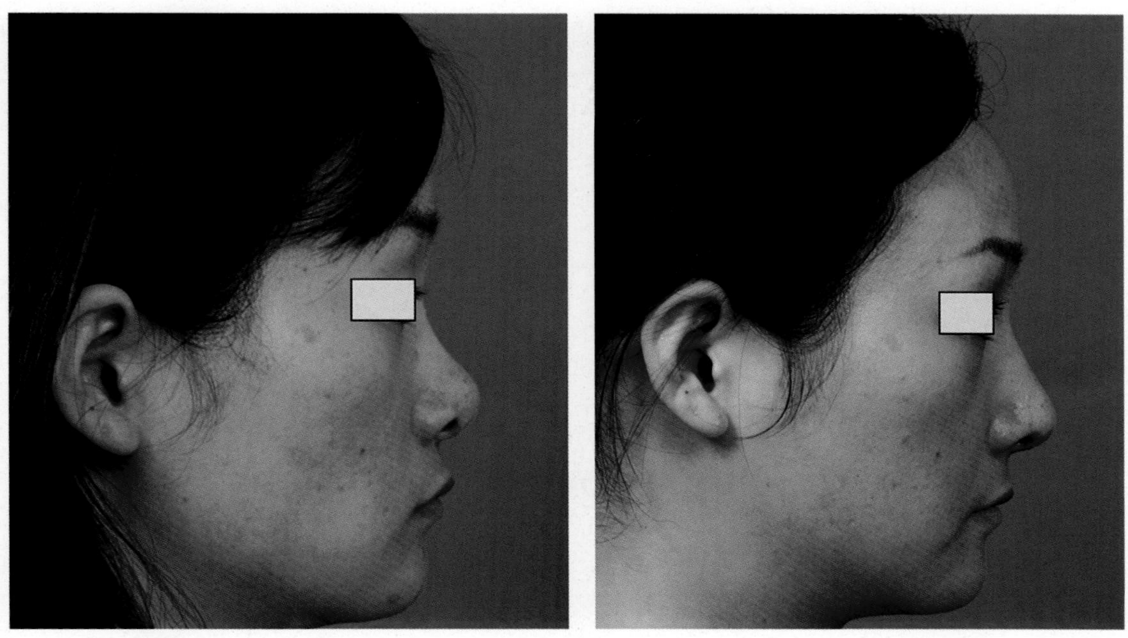

Fig. 48.24 Patient with a short nose, before (**A**) and after (**B**) undergoing lengthening procedure using septal extension graft.

Surgical Technique

Alar Flair Reduction (Alar Wedge Excision)

Nostrils close to normal in size but with an alar flair are treated using an inverted V-shaped or elliptical wedge. When performing an inverted V-shaped resection, the apex of the wedge must be located at the nostril groove, with only the skin of the ala included in the resection. During an oval resection, a wedge resection should be performed 2 to 5 mm in thickness and 1 mm above the alar crease. This type of surgery can also be represented as an alar wedge excision.

Nostril Size Reduction (Nostril Sill Excision)

In the case in which the nostril is wide and the alar flair is not severe, a V-shaped wedge resection can be performed, such that the apex of the wedge reaches the alar groove. This type of resection must include both the ala and vestibular skin.

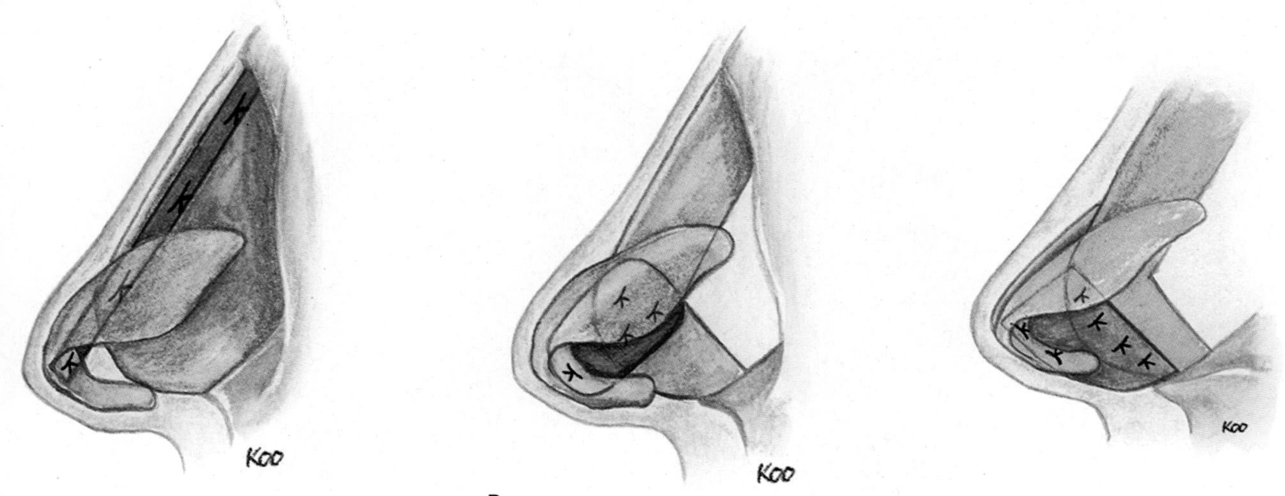

Fig. 48.25 Illustration depicting caudal septal extension graft.

Combination of Alar Flair Reduction and Nostril Size Reduction (Combined Sill/Alar Excision)

Wide nostrils with alar flair should be treated with an oblong-shaped resection. The resection can also be performed using a shape that combines the oval and wedge shapes. Such a method is also called the combined sill/alar excision (**Fig. 48.26 and 48.27**).

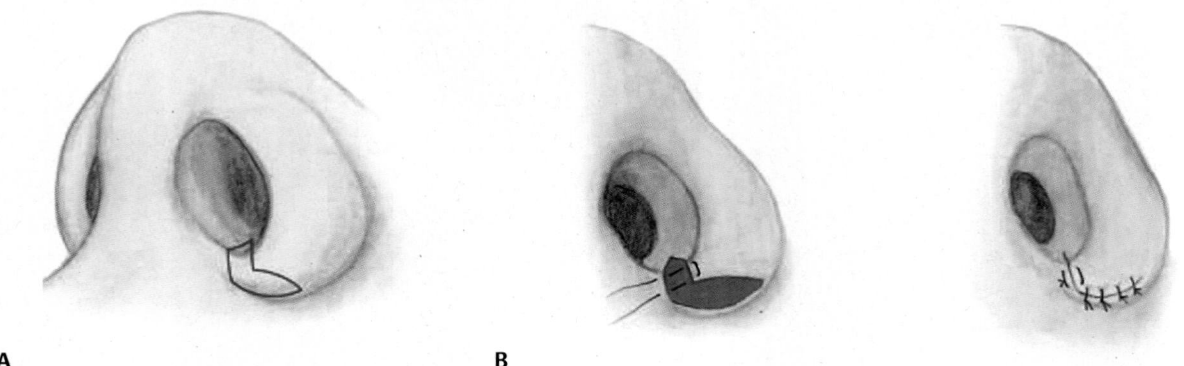

Fig. 48.26 Combined sill/alar excision. When the nostril is wide and there is a case of alar flair, a resection that combines the oval and wedge can be performed.

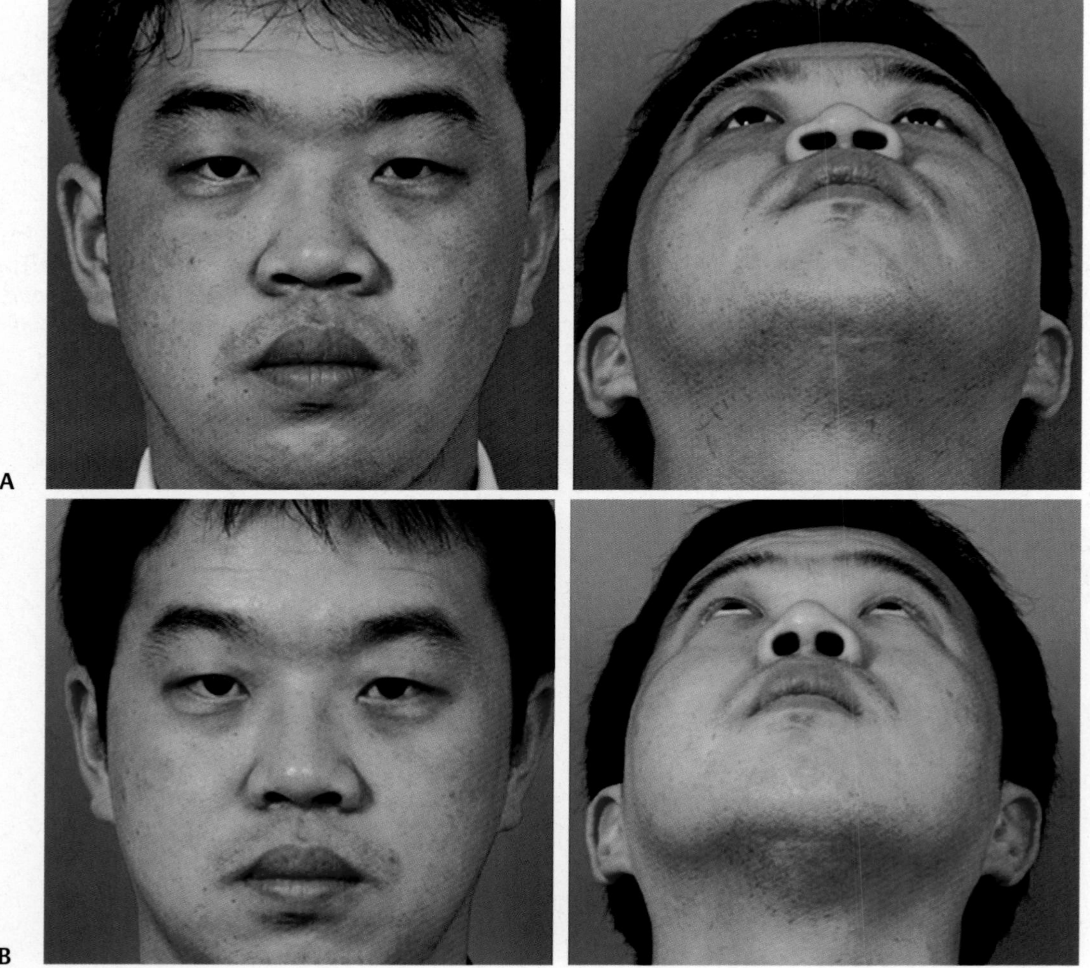

Fig. 48.27 Preoperative (**A**) and postoperative (**B**) photos of patient who underwent alar base surgery.

References

1. Leong SCL, White PS. A comparison of aesthetic proportions between the Oriental and Caucasian nose. Clin Otolaryngol 2004;29:672–676
2. Stucker FJ, Shaw G, Ephrat M. Biologic tissue implants. In: Papel ID, ed. Facial Plastic and Reconstructive Surgery. 2nd ed. New York: Thieme; 2002:73–78
3. McCurdy JA. The Asian nose: augmentation rhinoplasty with L-shaped silicone implants. Facial Plast Surg 2002;18:245–252
4. Guerrerosantos J. Nose and paranasal augmentation: autogenous fascia and cartilage. Clin Plast Surg 1991;18:65–86
5. Toriumi DM, Swartout B. Asian rhinoplasty. Facial Plast Surg Clin North Am 2007;15:293–307
6. Bateman N, Jones NS. Retrospective review of augmentation rhinoplasties using autologous cartilage grafts. J Laryngol Otol 2000;14:514–518
7. Calvert JW, Brenner K, DaCosta-Iyer M, et al. Histological analysis of human diced cartilage grafts. Plast Reconstr Surg 2006;118:230–206
8. Yang SJ, Kim BS, Kim JH. Secondary augmentation rhinoplasty with dermofat graft. J Korean Soc Plast Reconstr Surg 1998;25:152–160
9. Welling DB, Maves MD, Schuller DE, et al. Irradiated homologous cartilage grafts. Long-term results. Arch Otolaryngol Head Neck Surg 1988;114:291–295
10. Strauch B, Wallach SG. Reconstruction with irradiated homograft costal cartilage. Plast Reconstr Surg 2003;111:2405–2013
11. Lefkovits G. Nasal reconstruction with irradiated homograft costal cartilage. Plast Reconstr Surg 2004;113:1291–1292
12. Ghoniem GM. Allograft sling material: is it the state of the art? Int Urogynecol J Pelvic Floor Dysfunct 2000;11:69–70
13. Jang YJ, Wang JH, Sinha V, et al. Tutoplast-processed fascia lata for dorsal augmentation in rhinoplasty. Otolaryngol Head Neck Surg 2007;137:88–92
14. Tham C, Lai YL, Weng CJ, et al. Silicone augmentation rhinoplasty in an oriental population. Ann Plast Surg 2005;54:1–5
15. Erlich M, Parhiscar A. Nasal dorsal augmentation with silicone implants. Facial Plast Surg 2003;19:325–330
16. Wang JH, Lee BJ, Jang YJ. Use of silicone sheets for dorsal augmentation in rhinoplasty for Asian noses. Acta Otolaryngol 2007;127(Suppl 558):115–120
17. Maas CS, Gnepp DR, Bumpous J. Expanded polytetrafluoroethylene (Gore-Tex soft-tissue patch) in facial augmentation. Arch Otolaryngol Head Neck Surg 1993;119:1008–1014
18. Godin MS, Waldman SR, Johnson CM. Nasal augmentation using Gore-Tex: a 10-year experience. Arch Facial Plast Surg 1999;1:118–121
19. Becker DG, Pastorek NJ. The radix graft in cosmetic rhinoplasty. Arch Facial Plast Surg 2001;3:115–119
20. Bull TR. Percutaneous osteotomy in rhinoplasty. Plast Reconstr Surg 2001;107:1624–1625
21. Jang YJ, Wang JH, Sinha V, et al. Percutaneous root osteotomy for correction of the deviated nose. Am J Rhinol 2007;21:515–519
22. Rohrich RJ, Muzaffar AR, Janis JE. Component dorsal hump reduction: the importance of maintaining dorsal aesthetic lines in rhinoplasty. Plast Reconstr Surg 2004;114:1298–1308
23. Gunter JP, Rohrich RJ. Management of the deviated nose: the importance of septal reconstruction. Clin Plast Surg 1988;15:43–55
24. Sheen JH. Tip graft: a 20-year retrospective. Plast Reconstr Surg 1993;91:48–63
25. Adamson PA. Open rhinoplasty. Otolaryngol Clin North Am 1987;20:837–852
26. Behmand RA, Ghavami A, Guyuron B. Nasal tip sutures, part I: the evolution. Plast Reconstr Surg 2003;112:1125–1129
27. Gruber RP, Friedman GD. Suture algorithm for the broad or bulbous nasal tip. Plast Reconstr Surg 2002;110:1752–1764
28. Gunter JP, Landecker A, Cochran CS. Frequently used grafts in rhinoplasty: nomenclature and analysis. Plast Reconstr Surg 2006;118:14–29
29. Vuyk HD. Suture tip plasty. Rhinology 1995;33:30–38
30. Byrd HS, Andochick S, Copit S, et al. Septal extension grafts: a method of controlling tip projection shape. Plast Reconstr Surg 1997;100:999–1010
31. Hubbard TJ. Exploiting the septum for maximal tip control. Ann Plast Surg 2000;44:173–180
32. Anderson JR. A reasoned approach to the nasal base. Arch Otolaryngol Head Neck Surg 1984;110:349–358

49 Complications in Rhinoplasty

Daniel G. Becker

The nose plays a functional role in nasal breathing, and also an aesthetic role as it represents the most prominent and central facial feature. That the nose has enormous psychological, emotional, social, and symbolic importance is indisputable.[1] Most studies suggest that the great majority of rhinoplasty patients benefit psychologically from the operation.[1] Although rhinoplasty can be a satisfying procedure for both patient and surgeon, the literature reports an incidence of postoperative rhinoplasty complications ranging from 8 to 15%.[2–4] The rhinoplasty surgeon must take great care to minimize the incidence of both functional and cosmetic complications.

How is a "complication" defined? In most cases with an unacceptable result, the patient and surgeon recognize an unacceptable result, and a corrective plan is agreed upon. At times, the surgeon may notice a relatively subtle abnormality that is amenable to correction, but the patient is not concerned by it. It should be a rare situation that the surgeon is proud of the outcome whereas the patient is displeased.[5]

A candid discussion with the patient regarding the goals and expectations of surgery is an essential aspect of preoperative planning. A discussion of the potential complications is critical, so that the patient understands the risks. Although most complications are relatively minor and correctable, more serious and debilitating complications do occur. All complications must be addressed with forthright recognition, close attention to the patient, and appropriately timed corrective measures.

Careful preoperative anatomical diagnosis and a conservative approach guided by an understanding of the postoperative changes that occur during healing are critical in minimizing or avoiding complications. Failure to recognize the precise anatomical cause of a nasal feature is a common reason for failure to effect the desired change. Failure in execution (e.g., greenstick osteotomies, dorsal irregularities) is another cause. Despite careful preoperative analysis and meticulous attention to surgical detail, complications will occur.

Complications in rhinoplasty may be categorized as functional or aesthetic in nature; often, there are elements of both. In considering this subject, it may also be helpful to organize aesthetic complications by the specific nasal subunit affected.

Problems after rhinoplasty commonly relate to issues of underresection, overresection, and/or asymmetry. In general, it is easier to address a problem relating to underresection because the surgeon needs only to "take a little more." Problems relating to overresection can be difficult, and are often complicated by scarring, need for graft material, and other issues.[2]

Anatomical diagnosis is helpful in the prevention of complications, and it is also critical in the proper evaluation and treatment of complications when they occur. In this chapter we will address many of the more commonly described surgical complications with special attention to their cause and treatment. Emphasis is placed on the anatomical basis of each complication, as this approach provides a guide to correction. Although complications have been generally arranged by anatomical location, there are naturally some topics that cross categories.

Nasal tip

General Considerations

In the nasal tip, overreduction may violate critical tip-support mechanisms (**Table 49.1**),[5,6] which can lead to complications including tip ptosis and inadequate tip projection. Alternatively, overresection of the caudal septum can result in overrotation of the nasal tip with excessive shortening of the nose. Overresection may also contribute to other complications such as bossae, alar retraction, and alar collapse.[2,7–9]

Underreduction may be simply due to overcaution but is commonly due to a failure to correctly assess preoperatively the anatomical situation. For example, failure to recognize an overprojected nose, or to diagnose the steps required based on the patient's anatomy to adequately address this, can lead to a persistent overprojected state.[7,10] Failure to adequately resect cartilaginous dorsum may result in a pollybeak deformity.[2,7–9,11]

Asymmetries of the nasal tip may be due to unequal reduction of the lower lateral cartilages or to asymmetric application of dome-binding sutures.[7] It may also be caused by unequal scarring that can occur during the natural healing process and may not be evident for months or even years after surgery. Also, asymmetry is often present preoperatively and should be recognized and pointed out to the patient prior to surgery.

Specific Complications

Ptotic Tip

A critical principle in avoiding undesired changes of the nasolabial angle is assessment of tip anatomy and tip support, followed by maneuvers that maintain or augment

Table 49.1 Tip-Support Mechanisms

Major tip-support mechanisms
1. Size, shape, and strength of lower lateral cartilages
2. Medial crural footplate attachment to caudal septum
3. Attachment of caudal border of upper lateral cartilages to cephalic border of lower lateral cartilages
[The nasal septum is also considered a major support mechanism of the nose.]
Minor tip-support mechanisms
1. Ligamentous sling spanning the domes of the lower lateral cartilages (i.e., interdomal ligament)
2. Cartilaginous dorsal septum
3. Sesamoid complex of lower lateral cartilages
4. Attachment of lower lateral cartilages to overlying skin–soft tissue envelope
5. Nasal spine
6. Membranous septum

tip support and restore the nose to a more natural appearance. As mentioned above, however, maneuvers that result in loss of tip support may lead to a droopy tip (tip ptosis with an overly acute nasolabial angle). The normal nasolabial angle (angle defined by columellar point to subnasale line intercepting with subnasale to labrale superius line) is 90 to 120 degrees.[12] Within this range, a more obtuse angle is more favorable in females, a more acute angle in males. Loss of tip support can lead to a ptotic, underprojected drooping nose.

Treatment of complications relating to a ptotic nose rely on restoration of tip support and tip projection. When faced with an operative complication such as a droopy, ptotic tip, appropriate diagnosis will guide correction.[7] There are numerous rhinoplasty maneuvers to increase tip support, reproject the nose, and rotate the nose (**Table 49.2**).[6]

Overrotated Tip

Conversely, one may face a patient with a nose that has been overrotated, with an overly obtuse angle. Overresection of the caudal septum is a common cause of overrotation of the tip. Overrotation of the nose creates an unsightly, overshortened appearance.

Careful preoperative assessment can identify those patients in whom operative rotation should be avoided. Treatment of complications relating to a short, overrotated nose rely on maneuvers that lengthen and counterrotate the nose.[7] There are specific rhinoplasty maneuvers to lengthen and counterrotate the nose (**Table 49.2**).[6]

Bossae[2,7–9]

A bossae is a knuckling of the lower lateral cartilage at the nasal tip due to contractural healing forces acting on weakened cartilages. Patients with thin skin, strong cartilages, and nasal-tip bifidity are especially at risk. Excessive resection of lateral crus and failure to eliminate excessive interdomal width may play some role in bossae formation. Bossae are felt to be the result of scar contracture on an overly narrowed complete rim strip, causing a bulging during postoperative healing. Some have described an association between cartilage splitting techniques and bossae formation.[2] Others, however, maintain that vertical dome division techniques are reliable when performed correctly and do not contribute to these difficulties.[9,13]

As an isolated deformity, bossae are typically treated through a small marginal incision with minimal undermining over the offending site followed by trimming or excising the offending cartilage. In some cases, the area is covered with a thin wafer of cartilage, fascia, or other material to further smooth and mask the area

Alar retraction

Cephalic resection of the lateral crus of the lower lateral cartilages is commonly undertaken to effect refinement of the nasal tip. If inadequate cartilage is left, then the contractile forces of healing over time will cause the ala to retract (**Fig. 49.1**).[2,7–9,14] This is a commonly seen sequelae of overresection of the lateral crus. The surgical rule of thumb is to preserve at least 6 to 9 mm of complete strip. Nevertheless, an anatomical study of the alar base recognized that in a normal patient population, 20% of patients had a thin alar rim. This anatomical variation must be recognized, as these patients may require even more conservative approaches to avoid the risk of alar retraction and/or external nasal valve collapse.[15] Also, vestibular mucosa should be preserved, as excision of vestibular mucosa contributes to scar contracture with alar retraction.

Table 49.2 Operative Maneuvers

Increase Rotation
Lateral crural steal
Transdomal suture that recruits lateral crura medially
Base-up resection of caudal septum (variable effect)
Cephalic resection (variable effect)
Lateral crural overlay
Columellar strut (variable effect)
Plumping grafts (variable effect)
Illusions of rotation: increased double break, plumping grafts (blunting nasolabial angle)
Decrease Rotation (Counter-rotate)
Full-transfixion incision
Double-layer tip graft
Shorten medial crura
Caudal extension graft
Reconstruct L-strut, as in rib graft reconstruction (integrated dorsal graft/columellar strut) of saddle nose
Increase Projection
Lateral crural steal (increased projection, increased rotation)
Tip graft
Plumping grafts
Premaxillary graft
Septocolumellar sutures (buried)
Columellar strut (variable effect)
Caudal extension graft
Decrease Projection
High-partial, or full-transfixion incision
Lateral crural overlay (decreased projection, increased rotation)
Nasal spine reduction
Vertical dome division with excision of excess medial crura, with suture reattachment
Increase Length
Caudal extension graft
Radix graft
Double-layer tip graft
Reconstruct L-strut
Decrease Length
See "Increase Rotation"
Deepen nasofrontal angle

Alar retraction may be treated by cartilage grafts in more minor cases (1–2 mm).[2] The area of retraction is marked prior to injection, and a small marginal incision allows dissection of a precise pocket. A contoured cartilage graft (commonly of auricular or septal cartilage) may be inserted into the precise pocket that should extend inferiorly to the sesamoids and should be wide enough to simulate the normal shape of the lateral crus at the dome.

Auricular composite grafts are commonly used in more severe cases. The cymba concha of the opposite ear (example, left ala, right ear) provides the best contour. An incision several millimeters from the nostril rim is followed by careful dissection with freeing of adhesions, creating a defect and displacing the alar rim inferiorly. The fashioned composite graft is carefully sutured into place.[2,16]

Alar–Columellar Disproportions (protruding or hanging columella)

These can be areas of significant patient concern.[17,18] The range of normal columellar show is generally considered to be 2 to 4 mm. The complexities of the alar–columellar relationship have been categorized by Gunter,[18] who describes the position of the ala and the columella in relationship to a line drawn through the long axis of the nostril.[18] All patients have a hanging, normal, or retracted ala and a hanging, normal, or retracted columella . Thus there are nine possible anatomical combinations making up the alar–columellar relationship (**Fig. 49.2**).

Alar–columellar disproportion may exist in the unoperated nose; also, it may be caused by surgical misadventure (**Fig. 49.1**). A protruding or hanging columella may be due to a persisting uncorrected deformity, such as overly wide medial crura or overlong caudal septum.[7] The deformity may be increased columellar show secondary to retraction of the alar margins, rather than an actual protrusion of columella. A deficient or retracted columella may be due to a preexisting uncorrected deformity, or it may be due to excessive resection of soft tissue, cartilage, or nasal spine. The surgeon should avoid excessive resection of the caudal septum, and should avoid resection of the nasal spine.[2,7,17]

Treatment of a protruding or hanging columella may include resecting full-thickness tissue from the membranous columella, including skin, soft tissue, and perhaps a portion of the caudal end of the septum itself. If the medial crura is excessively wide, excision may include a conservative excision of the caudal margin of the medial crura.[7,17]

Retracted columella may be improved with plumping grafts inserted at the base of the columella to address an acute nasolabial angle; columellar struts may also be helpful for minor deformities. A cartilage graft may be used to lengthen the overshortened nose. The use of composite grafts have also been described.[2,7]

Pollybeak[2,7,9,11]

A pollybeak refers to postoperative fullness of the supratip region, with an abnormal tip–supratip relationship

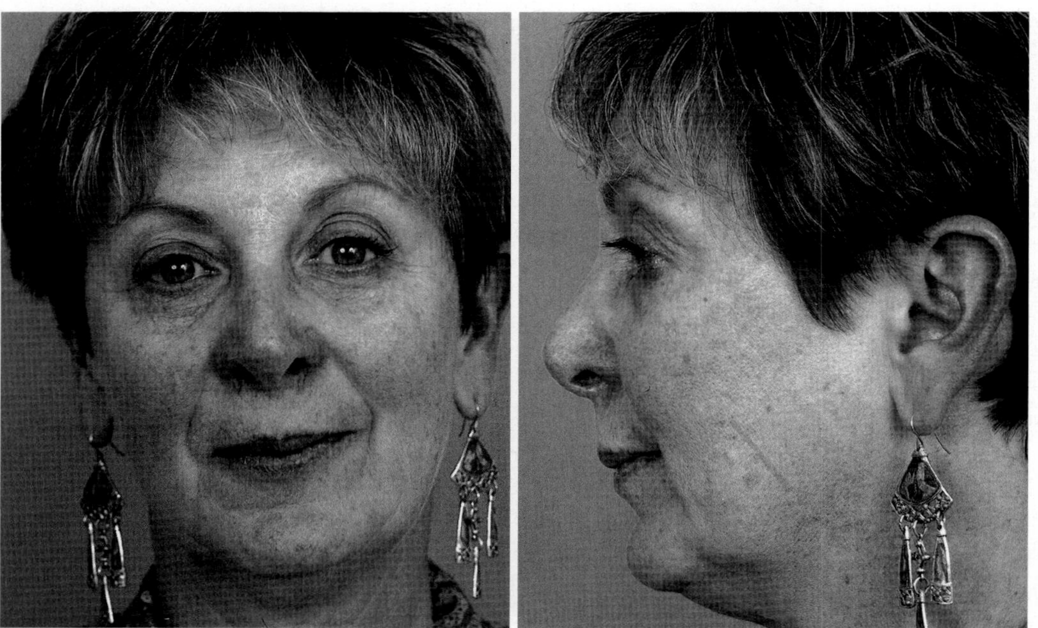

Fig. 49.1 (**A,B**) Patient many years after rhinoplasty, with alar–columellar disproportion due to alar retraction.

(**Fig. 49.3**). This may have several etiologies, including failure to maintain adequate tip support (postoperative loss of tip projection), inadequate cartilaginous hump (anterior septal angle) removal, and/or supratip dead space/scar formation.

Treatment of the pollybeak deformity depends upon the anatomical cause. If the cartilaginous hump was underresected, then the surgeon should resect additional dorsal septum. Adequate tip support must be ensured; maneuvers such as placement of a columellar strut may be of benefit. If the bony hump was overresected, a graft to augment the bony dorsum may be beneficial. If a pollybeak is from excessive scar formation, Kenalog (triamcinolone) injection or skin taping in the early postoperative period should be undertaken prior to any consideration of surgical revision.

Columellar Incision

The external rhinoplasty approach includes a columellar incision.[19] Great care must be taken when making this incision not to bevel it but rather to carefully ensure that the incision is perpendicular to the skin, thereby avoiding the complication of a trapdoor deformity. Great care must be taken in closing the incision to avoid notching at the margins or other deformity (**Fig. 49.4**).

A single, subcutaneous 6–0 PDS suture (polydiaxonone) can be positioned in the dermal tissues to enhance skin edge eversion and take tension off of the closure. This suture should provide skin-edge alignment and slight eversion. Excessive eversion will create a deformity that may require many months to resolve. The level of the skin edges must be precisely aligned with this suture; otherwise an unsightly scar may result. If there is no tension on the closure, a subcutaneous suture may not be necessary.

To close the skin, a minimum of five sutures should be used. The first suture lines up the apex of the inverted V. The next two sutures are angled from medial on the lower flap to lateral on the upper flap to properly align the closure. A 6–0 chromic suture is used to line up the vestibular skin at the corner of the columellar flap. This corner suture is important because aberrant healing of this corner can result in a visible notch defect.

The Nasal Vault (Middle and Upper Nasal Thirds)

General Considerations

The aesthetic importance of the nasal profile and the tip–supratip relationship make profile reduction a critical step in rhinoplasty. Overreduction of the bony component may lead to a flattened appearance that simulates pseudohypertelorism. Overreduction of the bony and cartilaginous nasal vault results in an overly concave, operated appearance. Overreduction may lead to iatrogenic saddle nose deformity. When undertaking profile reduction, great care must be taken to preserve support of the middle nasal vault—failure to do so can lead to complications such as nasal valve collapse and inverted-V deformity.[2,7,9]

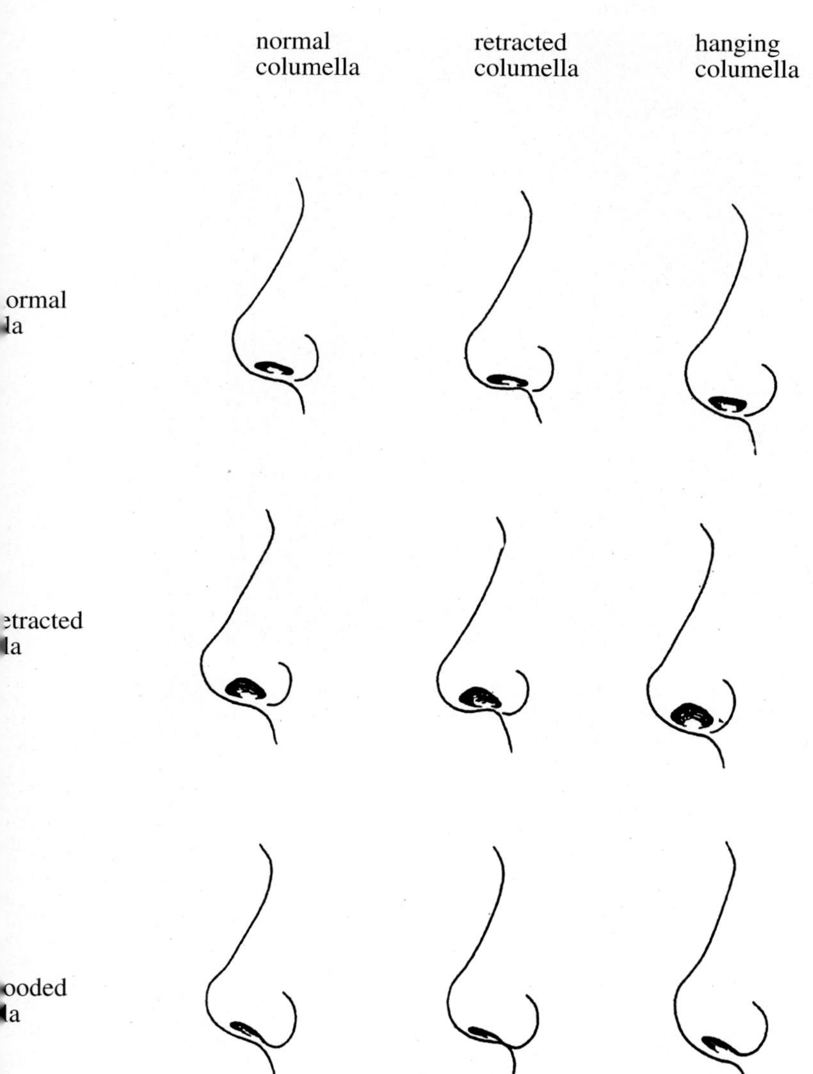

Fig. 49.2 The alar–columellar relationship can be described with nine possible anatomical combinations.

Prevention of over- or underresection requires knowl-dge of skin thickness and the anatomical contributions f bone and cartilage to the nasal dorsum. The bony con-ibution of the nasal dorsum is less than the cartilaginous ructures; great care must be taken in the resection of ach component. The skin–soft tissue envelope is thicker ver the nasofrontal angle and the supratip region and inest over the rhinion. Relatively less hump is taken at e rhinion to accommodate this.

Underreduction leads to a persistent deformity. nderreduction may not only leave a persistent dorsal ump but may also create a supratip prominence or ollybeak, or alternatively an unsightly prominence at the pper nasal third. Nevertheless, this deformity is prefer-ble to overreduction because it is easier to correct the nderreduction secondarily when indicated.

Asymmetric resection may lead to unsightly appearance. orrection of this deformity is challenging. This may be treated with onlay grafts, either through a precise pocket placement or via an external rhinoplasty approach.

Specific Complications of the Nasal Vault

Saddle Nose

Saddle nose refers to the appearance of the nose after loss of support of the nasal vault with subsequent collapse (**Fig. 49.5**). This deformity has been described after overresection of the septum, with failure to preserve an adequate L-strut. A minimum of 15 mm of cartilage is recommended as a rule of thumb; if a dorsal hump resection is also planned, this must be accounted for in planning adequate L-strut for nasal support. Other causes of saddle nose deformity include septal hematoma, septal abscess, and severe nasal trauma. Excessive dorsal hump resection also leads to saddle nose deformity.

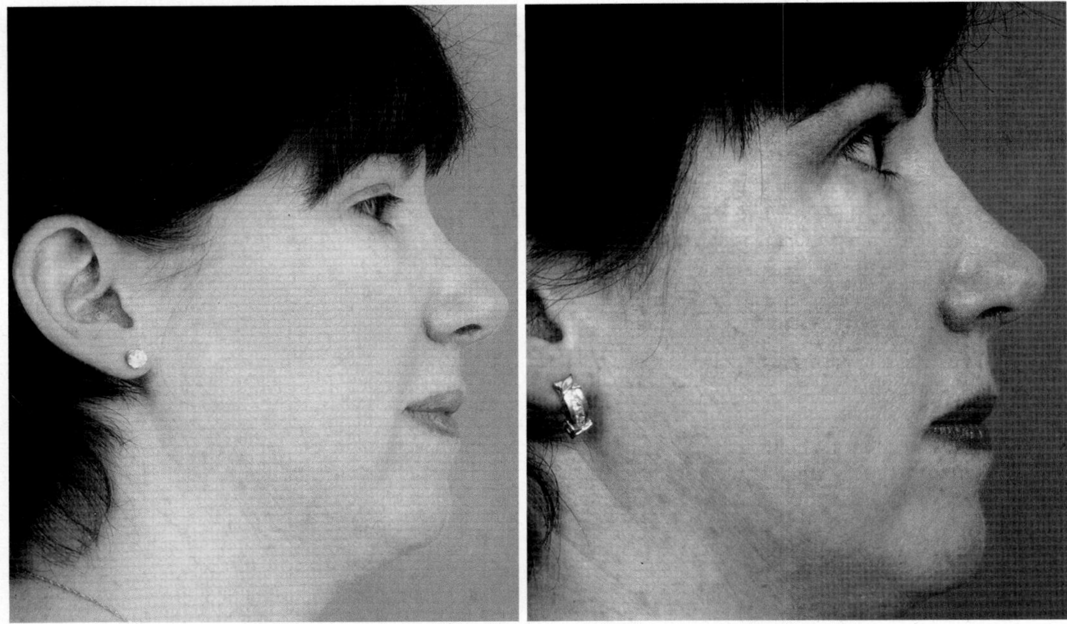

Fig. 49.3 (**A,B**) Patient with overresected bony dorsum and underresected cartilaginous dorsum. Her pollybeak deformity was due to persistent cartilaginous dorsum and was therefore corrected by additional excision of cartilaginous dorsum. Her overresected upper nasal third was augmented to create a more balanced profile.

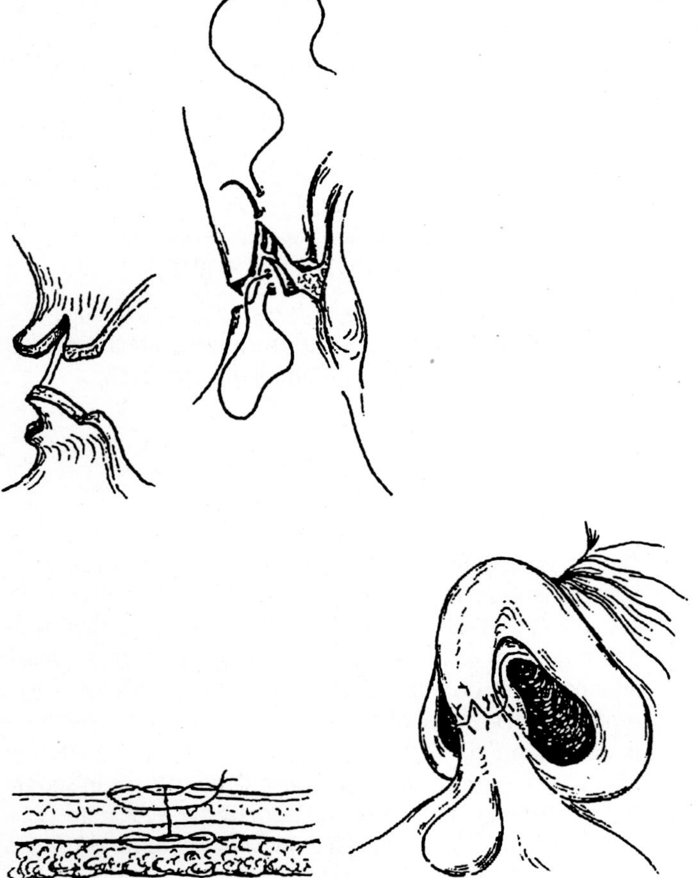

Fig. 49.4 Special attention should be given to the columellar incision, and to its closure, when undertaking external rhinoplasty. Great care should be taken to perform these maneuvers properly (see text) to avoid a visible deformity.

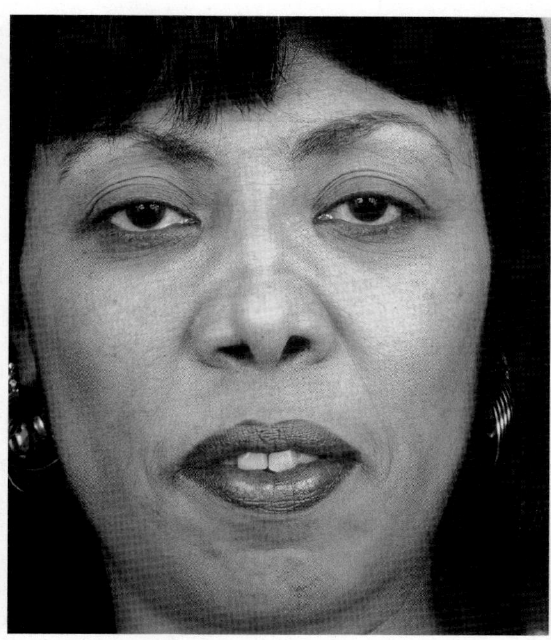
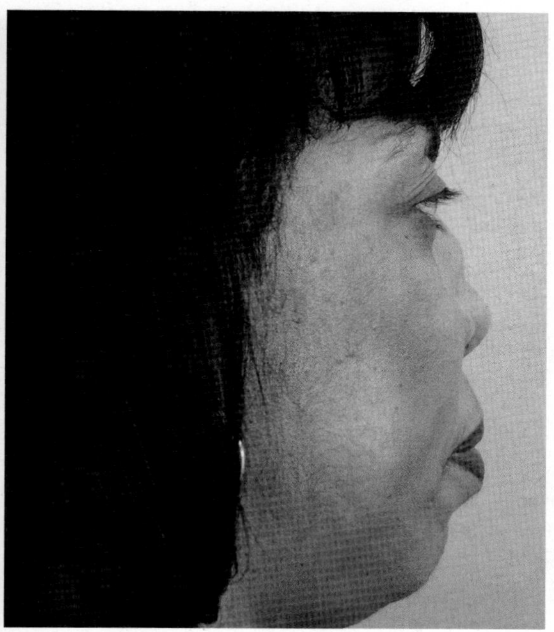

B

ig. 49.5 (**A,B**) Patient with large septal perforation, loss of cartilaginous nasal support, and subsequent severe saddle ose deformity. On frontal view the caudal aspect of the patient's nasal bones are visible in broad relief, demonstrating ne inverted-V deformity.

Onlay grafting can effectively camouflage and correct nild and moderate saddle deformities. Single or multiple ayers of septal cartilage or auricular cartilage are comnonly used effectively.[20,21] Severe saddle nose deformity nay require major reconstruction with cantilevered cartiage or bone grafts.[22–24]

nverted-V Deformity

n this deformity, the caudal edge of the nasal bones is isible in broad relief (**Fig. 49.5**). Inadequate support of ne upper lateral cartilages after dorsal hump removal an lead to inferomedial collapse of the upper lateral artilages and an inverted-V deformity.[25] Inadequate nfracture of the nasal bones is another significant cause f inverted-V deformity.

When executing hump excision, it is helpful to preserve ne underlying nasal mucoperichondrium (extramucosal issection), which provides significant support to the upper teral cartilages and helps decrease the risk of inferomedial ollapse of the upper lateral cartilages after hump excision. Vhen undertaking osteotomies after hump excision, approriate infracture and narrowing of the bony vault must be chieved.

asal Valve Collapse

he internal nasal valve is bounded by the caudal margin f the upper lateral cartilage and the septum.[25–30] The external nasal valve refers to the area delineated by the cutaneous and skeletal support of the mobile alar wall, anterior to the internal nasal valve.[30] Excessive narrowness or flaccidity in either of these locations may cause nasal obstruction. Weakness at either of these locations may result in collapse with the negative pressure of inspiration, resulting in nasal airway obstruction. Nasal valve collapse is seen most often as a sequelae of overresection of lateral crura or middle vault collapse. Overaggressive resection of the lateral crura and the subsequent postoperative soft tissue contraction frequently leads to nasal valve compromise. Failure to maintain proper middle vault support may lead to inferomedial collapse of the upper lateral cartilages, with internal nasal valve compromise.

Treatment of internal nasal valve collapse may include the use of spreader grafts. Spreader grafts act as a spacer between the upper lateral cartilage and septum, correcting an overnarrow middle vault and internal nasal valve, or preventing excessive narrowing when undertaking a rhinoplasty in the high-risk patient.[25–30]

Careful preoperative analysis should determine the need for other supportive and reconstructive maneuvers, such as conchal cartilage grafts to restore support to a collapsed lateral nasal wall. Alar batten grafts, typically of curved septal or auricular cartilage, placed to support the alar rim can correct internal or external nasal valve collapse (**Fig. 49.6**).[25–30]

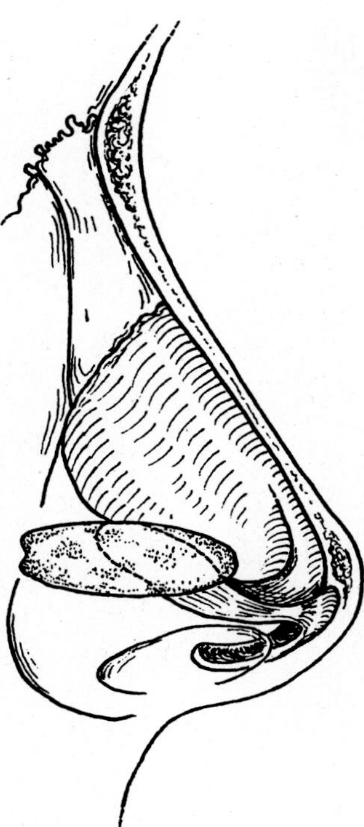

Fig. 49.6 Alar batten grafts may be used to treat nasal valve collapse.

Deviated Nose

Persisting deviation after rhinoplasty may occur at the upper third, middle third, or tip of the nose, or it may occur postoperatively in a previously straight nose. Preoperative anatomical diagnosis is a critical component of successful treatment. Persisting deviation of the nasal bones may occur due to greenstick fractures or other problems with osteotomies.[31,32] Inherent deviations in the cartilage of the middle nasal vault may prove especially challenging.[33] Also, hump removal may uncover asymmetries that result in postoperative deviation where none existed previously. Tip asymmetry may be overlooked preoperatively, or it may due to asymmetric excision of lateral crura, asymmetric placement of a columellar strut, or placement of an overlong columellar strut, as well as other causes. Several surgical maneuvers are available to address the deviated nose.[25,31–33]

The Upper Third of the Nose

Specific Complications

Rocker Deformity

If osteotomies are taken too high, into the thick frontal bone, the superior aspect of the osteotomized nasal bone may project or "rock" laterally when the bone is infractured. This is a rocker deformity. A 2-mm osteotome may be employed percutaneously to create a more appropriate superior fracture line and correct the rocker deformity.[31]

Dorsal Irregularities

After creation of an "open roof" by hump removal, the bony margins should be smoothed with a rasp. Any bony fragments should be removed, making sure that all obvious particles are removed from under the skin–soft tissue envelope. Failure to remove all fragments may lead to a visible and/or palpable dorsal irregularity.

Bony dorsal irregularities are a well-recognized complication of rhinoplasty. In the search for an approach that could reliably assure a smoother contour without sharp edges, irregularities, or asymmetries, surgeons have reported on the use of various onlay grafts, including homograft sclera,[34] gelatin film,[35] temporoparietal fascia,[36] and superficial musculoaponeurotic system (SMAS).[37] Becker et al[38] have described the use of a powered drill or rasp, which they felt may decrease the incidence of dorsal irregularities. The multiple proposals in the literature on this subject may suggest the lack of a completely satisfactory solution.

Open Roof Deformity

After hump removal, the free edges of the nasal bones are palpable beneath the skin–soft tissue envelope. Failure to perform lateral osteotomy, or inadequate osteotomy results in an open roof deformity. Lateral osteotomies are typically undertaken to "close" the open roof.

Greenstick Fracture

This incomplete fracture of the nasal bones after osteotomy may lead to the recurrence of a deformity (such as nasal deviation) due to "memory" and "spring" in the nasal bone. Although they may be acceptable in certain circumstances, such as the elderly rhinoplasty patient with thin, brittle bones, greenstick fractures commonly lead to a recurrence of a preoperative nasal bony deformity.

Skin–Soft Tissue Envelope

The skin–soft tissue envelope has well-defined tissue planes in which avascular dissection may be undertaken. Operating in more superficial planes not only leads to a bloody surgical field but also risks damage to the vascular supply with potential damage to the skin. Once the skin–soft tissue envelope is damaged, it can never be fully restored. The damaged skin creates an aesthetically displeasing appearance.[39]

Vascular supply and lymphatics are found superficial o the nasal musculature.[40] The soft tissue layers in the ıose are epidermis, dermis, subcutaneous (this plane conains blood vessels and lymphatics, and also a [typically] hin layer of fat), muscle, and fascia (musculoaponeurotic) ›lane, areolar tissue plane, and perichondrium/perioseum. Dissection during rhinoplasty in the proper tissue ›lanes (areolar tissue plane, i.e., submusculoaponeurotic) ›reserves nasal blood supply and minimizes postoperaive edema.

Alloplastic implants risk skin complications. The nose ulfills few of the requirements for use of alloplastic naterials. If the alloplast extrudes through the skin, the kin–soft tissue envelope is permanently and irreparably lamaged.

Infection of the skin–soft tissue envelope is a rare omplication of septorhinoplasty. Nevertheless, cellulitis haracterized by erythema, edema, and pain is a potential isk that must be identified and treated promptly. If oral ntibiotics are not quickly effective, intravenous antibiotics nust be used to quickly control this rare but potentially erious complication. Nasal culture may guide therapy in lifficult cases.[39]

Functional Complications

he list of possible functional complications can be xhaustive. Note must be made of possibly serious com›lications.[41,42] Intracranial complications may occur in ssociation with septal surgery, as the perpendicular plate of he ethmoid has an attachment superiorly in the floor of he cranial cavity. Great care must be taken, particularly n the elderly, to avoid avulsing ethmoid bone and creatng a fracture with cerebrospinal fluid leak. Other funcional complications of septoplasty and septorhinoplasty nclude septal perforation, toxic shock syndrome, septal ematoma or abscess.

Airway complications merit a chapter in itself. In brief, he surgeon must take a careful history to recognize nedical causes of obstruction such as allergy, sinusitis, or nedication misuse (rhinitis medicamentosa).

It is critical that rhinoplasty maintain or improve the ıasal airway. Failure to preserve nasal airway function an be crippling. The causes of nasal airway obstrucion must be identified and addressed. Conservatism nust be emphasized. For example, overresection of urbinates can lead to atrophic rhinitis, which can be rippling. Overnarrowing of the bony pyramid, with ailure to preserve the airway at the nasal valve, can ılso lead to nasal obstruction.[43] Overresection of the ateral crus can lead to aesthetic complications that are ›ften accompanied by nasal valve collapse and breathing omplications.

Summary

An overview of rhinoplasty complications addresses the avoidance, diagnosis, and management of common complications of rhinoplasty. Careful preoperative diagnosis and a conservative approach guided by an understanding of the postoperative changes that occur during healing are critical in minimizing and avoiding complications. These principles are also essential in the treatment of complications when they occur.

References

1. Goin JM, Goin MK. Changing the Body—Psychological Effects of Plastic Surgery. Baltimore: Williams & Wilkins; 1981
2. Kamer FM, Pieper PG. Revision rhinoplasty. In: Head and Neck Surgery Otolaryngology, ed. Byron Bailey. Lippincott: Philadelphia; 1998
3. Rees TD. Postoperative considerations and complications. In: Rees TD, ed. Aesthetic Plastic Surgery. Philadelphia: W.B. Saunders; 1980
4. McKinney P, Cook JQ. A critical evaluation of 200 rhinoplasties. Ann Plast Surg 1981;7:357
5. Tardy ME. Rhinoplasty: The Art and the Science. W.B. Saunders: Philadelphia 1997
6. Tardy ME, Toriumi DM. Philosophy and principles of rhinoplasty. In: Cummings CW, ed. Otolaryngology-Head & Neck Surgery. 2nd ed. St. Louis: Mosby Year Book; 1993:278–294
7. Thomas JR, Tardy ME. Complications of rhinoplasty. Ear Nose Throat J 1986;65:19–34
8. Tardy ME Jr, Cheng EY, Jernstrom V. Misadventures in nasal tip surgery. Analysis and repair. Otolaryngol Clin North Am 1987;20(4): 797–823
9. Simons RL, Gallo JF. Rhinoplasty complications. Facial Plast Surg Clin North Am 1994;2(4):521–529
10. Tardy ME, Walter MA, Patt BS. The Overprojecting nose: anatomic component analysis and repair. Facial Plast Surg 1993;9(4): 306–316
11. Tardy ME, Kron TK, Younger RY, Key M. The cartilaginous pollybeak: etiology, prevention, and treatment. Facial Plast Surg 1989;6(2): 113–120
12. Ridley MB. Aesthetic facial proportions. In: Papel ID, Nachlas NE, eds. Facial Plastic & Reconstructive Surgery. Philadelphia: Mosby-Year Book; 1992:99–109
13. Simons RL. Vertical dome division techniques. Facial Plast Surg Clin North Am 1994;2(4):435–458
14. Tardy ME, Patt BS, Walter MA. Alar reduction and sculpture: anatomic concepts. Facial Plast Surg 1993;9(4):295–305
15. Becker DG, Weinberger MS, Greene BA, Tardy ME Jr. Clinical study of alar anatomy and surgery of the alar base. Arch Otolaryngol Head Neck Surg 1997;123(8):789–795
16. Tardy ME, Toriumi DM. Alar retraction: composite graft correction. Facial Plast Surg 1989;6(2):101–107
17. Tardy ME, Genack SH, Murrell GL. Aesthetic correction of alar–columellar disproportion. Facial Plast Surg Clin North Am 1995;3(4):395–406
18. Gunter JP, Rohrich RJ, Friedman RM. Classification and correction of alar–columellar discrepancies in rhinoplasty. Plast Reconstr Surg 1996;97(3):643–648
19. Johnson CM, Toriumi DM. Considerations in open rhinoplasty. Facial Plast Surg Clin North Am 1993;1(1):1–23
20. Tardy ME, Schwartz M, Parras G. Saddle nose deformity: autogenous graft repair. Facial Plast Surg 1989;6(2):121–134
21. Gunter JP, Rohrich RJ. Augmentation rhinoplasty:dorsal onlay grafting using shaped autogenous septal cartilage. Plast Reconstr Surg 1990;86(1):39–45
22. Wang TD. Aesthetic structural nasal augmentation. Oper Tech Otolaryngol Head Neck Surg 1990;1:116

23. Daniel RK. Rhinoplasty and rib grafts: evolving a flexible operative technique. Plast Reconstr Surg 1994;94(5):597–611
24. Murakami CS, Cook TA, Guida RA. Nasal reconstruction with articulated irradiated rib cartilage. Arch Otolaryngol Head Neck Surg 1991;117:327–330
25. Toriumi DM. Management of the middle nasal vault. Plast Reconstr Surg 1995;2(1):16–30
26. Toriumi DM, Josen J, Weinberger MS, Tardy ME Jr. Use of alar batten grafts for correction of nasal valve collapse. Arch Otolaryngol Head Neck Surg 1997;123:802–808
27. Constantian MB, Clardy RB. The relative importance of septal and nasal valvular surgery in correcting airway obstruction in primary and secondary rhinoplasty. Plast Reconstr Surg 1996;98(1):38–54
28. Goode RL. Surgery of the Incompetent Nasal Valve. Laryngoscope 1985;95:546–555
29. Sheen JH. Spreader graft: a method of reconstructing the roof of the middle nasal vault following rhinoplasty. Plast Reconstr Surg 1984;73(2):230–237
30. Constantian MB. The incompetent external nasal valve: pathophysiology and treatment in primary and secondary rhinoplasty. Plast Reconstr Surg 1994;93(5):919–933
31. Larrabee WF Jr. Open rhinoplasty and the upper third of the nose. Facial Plast Surg Clin North Am 1993;1(1):23–38
32. Thomas JR. Steps for a safer method of osteotomies in rhinoplasty. Laryngoscope 1987;97(6):746–747
33. Toriumi DM, Ries WR. Innovative surgical management of the crooke nose. Facial Plast Surg Clin North Am 1993;1(1):63–78
34. Michel RG, Patterson CN. Evaluation of sclera as a homograft i facial plastic and reconstructive surgery. Otolaryngology 1978;86 ORL206–ORL214
35. Kamer FM, Parkes ML. Gelatin film: a useful adjunct in rhinoplasti surgery. Arch Otolaryngol 1977;103:667
36. Guerrerosantos J. Temporoparietal free fascia grafts in rhinoplasty Plast Reconstr Surg 1984;74(4):465
37. Leaf N. SMAS autografts for the nasal dorsum. Plast Reconstr Sur 1996;97(6):1249
38. Becker DG, Toriumi DM, Gross CW, Tardy ME. Powered Instrumen tation for dorsal nasal reduction. Facial Plast Surg 1997;13(4):291 297
39. Rettinger G, Zenkel M. Skin and soft tissue complications. Facial Plas Surg 1997;13(1):51–59
40. Toriumi DM, Mueller RA, Grosch T, Bhattacharyya TK, Larrabee WF J Vascular anatomy of the nose and the external rhinoplasty approacl Arch Otolaryngol Head Neck Surg 1996;122:24–34
41. Schwab JA, Pirsig W. Complications of septal surgery. Facial Plast Sur 1997;13(1):3–14
42. Thumfart WF, Völklein C. Systemic and other complications. Faci Plast Surg 1997;13(1):61–69
43. van Olphen A. Complications of pyramid surgery. Facial Plast Sur 1997;13(1):15–23

50 Reconstructive Surgery of the Nasal Septum

Jan L. Kasperbauer, George W. Facer, and Eugene B. Kern

he deviated nasal septum has been addressed in multiple fashion in the past and currently. Prominent 9th-century rhinologists, including Bosworth, Roe, Vatson, Gleason, Asch, and Douglas, utilized a variety of techniques to address nasal septal deformities.[1] he most common approach was that of Bosworth,[2] which employed a saw to remove the deformity and preserved one side of the septal mucosa. Septal perfoation was a common complication. Watson[3] described n early septoplasty technique with preservation of mucosa, and Asch[4] introduced cartilage modification techiques. The twentieth century in rhinology opened with he development of the submucous resection technique. reer[5] and Killian[6] introduced the concept of submucous esection, which allowed relief from a septal obstruction vithout sacrifice of mucosa. Briefly, an incision is made n the respiratory mucosa 1.5 to 2 cm behind the olumella. The incision is carried through the cartilage, nd subsequent elevation of mucoperichondrium in a posterior direction on each side of the septum allows emoval of obstructive septal structures (**Fig. 50.1**). Closure s accomplished by mattress stitch approximating mucoperichondrium. Precepts associated with the submucous esection dictate preservation of a dorsal caudal strut f ~1 cm of cartilaginous septum. Although the submuous resection was a significant advancement, several shortcomings were noted (**Table 50.1**), with a significant problem involving the inability to address caudal end deformities. Metzenbaum[7] and others[8–12] proposed alternative methods for addressing management of caudal end deformities.

Modern reconstruction surgery of the nasal septum is based on principles forwarded by Maurice Cottle[13] and provides a method to address the nasal septum in a comprehensive fashion. When compared with the submucous resection, the incision is placed through skin (i.e., stratified squamous epithelium rather than respiratory mucosa) and is located at the distal end of the quadrangular cartilage. This subsequently allows access to all borders of the bony and cartilaginous septum (**Fig. 50.2**). Cottle termed this the *maxilla–premaxilla*

Table 50.1 Limitations of the Submucous Resection

- Caudal end deformities are not addressed.
- Access to the premaxilla and nasal spine is limited.
- Convexities of the nasal valve area are not addressed.
- Submucous resection is not applicable to children.
- Revision surgery is more difficult due to lack of cartilage or bone.

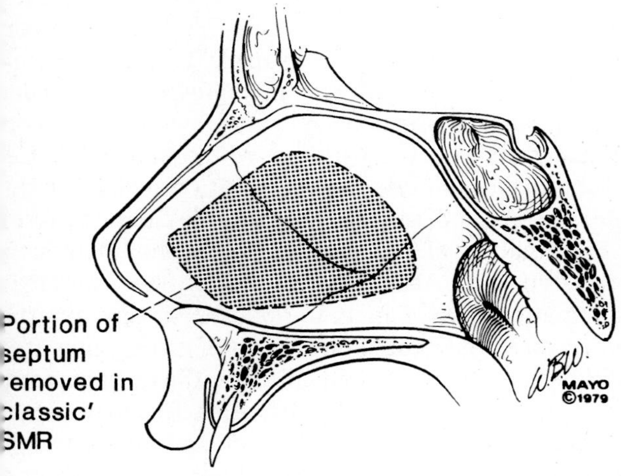

ig. 50.1 Shaded area represents the portions of the nasal septum at can be approached by submucous resection (SMR).

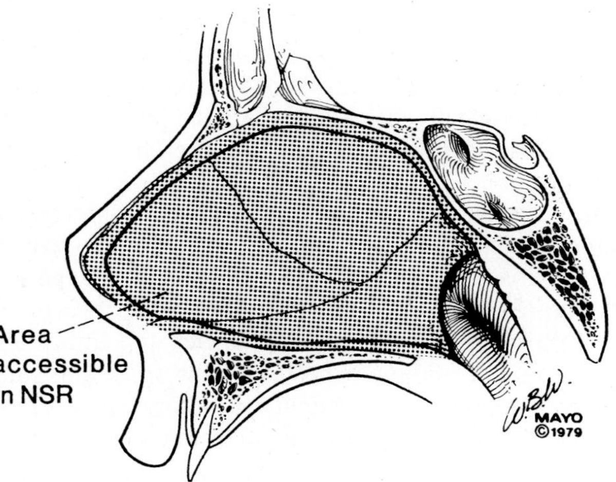

Fig. 50.2 Structures of the nasal septum and upper lateral cartilage that can be approached by the nasal septal reconstruction (NSR) concept using the maxillar–premaxilla approach. The shaded area represents the portions of the entire septum that can be exposed by this method.

approach.[14] Basic principles formulated with this approach include preservation of mucosa, repair of mucosal tears experienced during the dissection, avoidance of circumferential incisions, and replacement of bony and cartilaginous fragments to reconstruct the septum. This is the approach favored by the authors and described in some detail subsequently. The major advantages are significant and include mobilization of the entire septum when necessary and preservation or replacement of the caudal septum. Realistically, practicing rhinologists use their knowledge of both procedures when operating on nasal septal deformities. Rhinologic innovation in the late twentieth century included endoscopic approaches to paranasal sinus disease and, subsequently, endoscopic septoplasty.[15] In this situation, endoscopic equipment in use for paranasal sinus surgery is utilized to complete a submucous resection of limited septal deformities. This technique promotes teaching when video monitors are used, avoids the use of a headlight, and minimizes mucoperichondrial flap dissection.

Nasal septal surgery has evolved as knowledge of the anatomy, physiology, and pathophysiology of the nose has become better understood. Rhinomanometry has significantly advanced the understanding of nasal physiology and pathophysiology while providing objective pre- and posttherapy data.[16] This information has led to a confirmation of the importance of the anterior septum, nasal valve area, and mucosa (turbinates) in nasal respiration,[17,18] regulating air flow, and mass transfer.[19] The structures in the nasal valve area (valve angle, septum, anterior inferior turbinate, and anterior floor of nose) require careful investigation. This dynamic area requires a straight, stable septum and an appropriately flexible upper lateral cartilage that provides variable resistance, such as a Starling resistor.[20] Thus, combined with the maxilla–premaxilla approach, rhinomanometry and an understanding of nasal physiology allow the rhinologic surgeon to selectively address septal, mucosal (turbinates), and nasal valve pathologies, thereby improving patient care.

The most common application of the maxilla–premaxilla approach is in addressing caudal septal deformities, which result in airway obstruction. The true flexibility and potential wide exposure of this approach enable incorporation with open and closed rhinoplasties and utilization as a method of midline exposure of the sphenoid sinus (e.g., transseptal transsphenoidal pituitary surgery). In addition, this approach allows mobilization of the septum to allow adequate exposure of the lateral wall of the nose when septal deviations limit exposure to the ethmoids. The least common application of the maxilla–premaxilla approach is to reduce septal deformities associated with facial pain.

Preoperative Evaluation

Patients with disturbed nasal physiology require a complete history, a careful clinical examination, laboratory tests, and a frank discussion prior to surgical intervention. The nose plays a key role in active breathing and ultimately in oxygen and carbon dioxide exchange at the alveoli (respiration). Disturbances of respiration can have far-reaching somatic and psychological effects. A major diagnostic goal is to determine whether the patient's disturbed physiology is related primarily to a mucosal disturbance, a structural abnormality, or both. If the history suggests a mucosal component to the patient's complaints, then appropriate medical therapy should be initiated and improvement evaluated following an adequate therapeutic trial prior to addressing structural abnormalities. The key elements sought in the history are the symptoms of allergic and nonallergic rhinitis, chronic and acute sinusitis, topical nasal decongestant abuse, use of hypertensive medications, and a history of hypothyroidism or pregnancy. These are but a few of the causes of mucosal abnormalities that can produce disturbed nasal physiology and nasal symptoms.

In addressing structural abnormalities that may be associated with disturbed air flow or abnormalities of mass transfer, it is important to assess the location of the septum and its upper lateral cartilaginous extensions as well as the structure and position of the lower lateral cartilage, the nasal valve area, and the lateral nasal wall (especially the head of the inferior turbinate) (**Fig. 50.3**). Historical points that may be significant include a history of congenital abnormalities predisposing to structural defects, such as a cleft lip or cleft palate deformity, Binder's syndrome, or septal trauma with dislocation. Inflammatory diseases, which may produce structural abnormalities, include Wegener granulomatosis, sarcoidosis, and syphilis. A history of trauma is common but important to note, as is a prior history of rhinologic surgery. Certainly, the history suggestive of any neoplastic process is important to note preoperatively, as is a history of sleep apnea. Keep in mind that patients with atrophic rhinitis may present with a complaint of nasal obstruction, and patients with overzealous turbinate surgery seem to present with complaints related to abnormalities in mass transfer (dry, crusted, congested nose; bleeding and pain may be part of the clinical picture).

Examination of the patient's nose should then be correlated with the historical facts. The rhinologic examination should include notation of any external deformities. The caudal end, including the valve area, must be carefully evaluated, as this is the most common site of symptomatic septal deformities. This may require trimming of the vibrissae and utilization of either a pediatric nasal speculum or a four-pronged retractor to allow visualization of the vestibule and nasal valve area with minimal distortion. The position of the septum

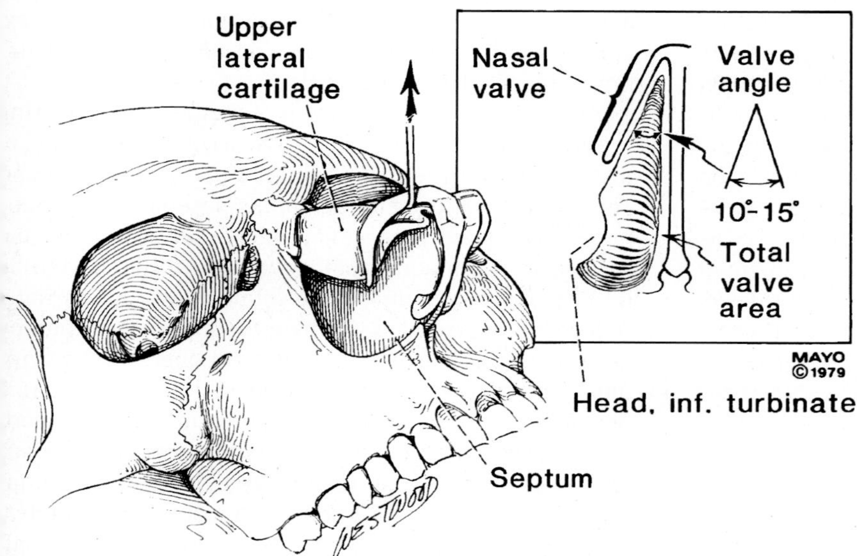

Fig. 50.3 The nasal valve area is bounded by the nasal septum, the caudal end of upper lateral cartilage, soft fibrofatty tissue overlying pyriform aperture and floor of the nose, and posteriorly by the head of the inferior turbinate. This area is shaped like an inverted cone or teardrop, the slit-like apex of which is the nasal valve angle and normally subtends an angle of 10 to 15 degrees.

should be evaluated in relationship to the lower lateral cartilage, the nasal spine, the premaxilla, and the remainder of the nasal valve area. As depicted in **Fig. 50.3**, the normal valve angle is 10 to 15 degrees. This examination should be done prior to and following decongestion. After a thorough visualization of the nasal cavity, it is often beneficial to use a rigid or a flexible endoscope to further assess the mid and posterior portions of the nasal cavity. This can be easily done following topical application of 1% phenylephrine hydrochloride (Neo-Synephrine). Midseptal deformities can frequently be noted and generally are asymptomatic from an obstructive standpoint. However, they may present with a history of facial pain or a predisposition to recurrent sinusitis.

Sensitive, specific, cost-effective, and reliable tests of nasal function would ideally quantify abnormal nasal physiology and confirm response to treatments. Today the documentation of many nasal functions remains elusive or impractical for most facial plastic or rhinologic surgeons. Pertinent to nasal septal surgery, measures of respiratory and olfactory function are available but problematical. The tools readily available for the measurement of olfaction include the University of Pennsylvania Smell Identification Test (UPSIT) and commercially available odorants used in an individualized fashion. Threshold detection testing is complex, time consuming, not readily available, and not considered further in this review. The UPSIT is an easily administered forced-choice test based on microfragrance samples from the 3M Company (St. Paul, Minnesota). The test consists of scratch-and-sniff methods of odorant presentation and interpretation based on data from a large number of individuals with "normal" olfactory function. Results from the UPSIT are scored from 0 to 40, with higher scores representing greater olfactory function. Tables are provided that allow scoring of an individual's result as a percentile of the normal population. Scores can also be categorized into normosmia, microsmia (decreased but not anosmic), total anosmia, and probable malingering. It is difficult to interpret results at age extremes in part due to the sample size and score variability in the normal population studied. Currently this kit called UPSIT is available from Sensonics, Inc. (Haddonfield, NJ).

The utility of olfactory testing is easily recognized when a patient who has had nasal surgery presents with the complaint of decreased olfactory function. Mechanisms responsible for olfactory injury from nasal surgery include direct trauma to the olfactory epithelium, traction on the olfactory nerve due to cribriform plate motion, vascular compromise of the olfactory neuroepithelium during surgery, drug effects, atrophic rhinitis due to excessive removal of intranasal tissue, mucosal edema due to or exacerbated by surgical trauma preventing odorant access to the neuroepithelium, and idiopathic development of anosmia in the postoperative period. Kimmelman[21] utilized the UPSIT to study 93 patients before and after nasal surgery to identify the risk to olfaction. Thirty-four percent of patients scored lower on the UPSIT postoperatively, with a mean decline of 2.25 correct responses resulting in a decline in percentile rank of 25 percentile points. In the group of patients studied, 1.1% developed total anosmia postoperatively and 66% either improved or were unchanged.

Olfactory testing is not routinely performed for patients undergoing nasal and paranasal sinus surgery because it adds time and cost. However, the utility of routine olfactory testing becomes clear when the surgeon is faced with a disturbed patient who reports altered olfaction following nasal surgery.

Rhinomanometry provides objective information regarding the respiratory function of the nasal airway. Rhinomanometry quantifies nasal air flow and pressure, allowing calculation of airway resistance. Three methods exist to measure air flow based on the location of the pressure catheter. Anterior rhinomanometry relies on a catheter placed in a sealed nasal vestibule to measure pressure changes in the opposite side of the nose. Posterior rhinomanometry involves peroral placement of a catheter in the oropharynx, which allows both sides of the nose to be measured simultaneously. Pernasal rhinomanometry requires passing a pressure catheter transnasally to the nasopharynx. This is similar to posterior rhinomanometry, which provides simultaneous measurement of flow and pressure from both sides of the nose. In each method, the patient either wears a mask or is in a chamber that allows measurement of pressure and air flow changes related to breathing. Posterior rhinomanometry requires the greatest degree of patient education and has the highest rate of test failure. Pernasal rhinomanometry causes some irritation with the catheter placement but provides the most consistent results.[22] Anterior mask rhinomanometry is the most common method because it requires the least patient cooperation and has the least complicated equipment.

Data gained from rhinomanometry include the simultaneous pressure and flow of nasal respiration, which are nonlinear during the respiratory cycle. Although a variety of results can be computed, nasal resistance (pressure/flow) is most commonly reported. However, resistance varies at different points on the pressure–flow curve due to the nonlinear relationship. A consistent point on the pressure–flow curve must be selected to allow comparison between tests in the same patient as well as among patient groups. It is important to report the nasal resistance at a given pressure (150 Pa)[23] and at a given radius.[24] Additional parameters that can be reported include maximal nasal resistance[25] and mean resistance.[26] Both maximal and mean resistance can be calculated for all patients, which is advantageous over measuring resistance at set points along the pressure–flow curve because some patients require a voluntary increase in ventilation to reach these points. The challenge for any data gathered from rhinomanometry is variability as well as correlation with clinical symptoms. Some variability is due to nasal sources and includes variable mucosal congestion from exercise, postural changes, pressure applied to certain body areas, nasal secretions, and the nasal cycle. Medications, height, anthropological type, and age may also induce variability. Methodological sources of variability include mask leakage, equipment repositioning, and inadequate equipment warm-up. Factors that minimize variability include symmetrical patient sitting position, avoiding exercise 30 minutes prior to testing, consistent temperature and humidity, avoidance of medications prior to testing and alleviation of patient anxiety by appropriate explanation of the testing procedure.[27]

Acoustic rhinomanometry is a method of measuring the cross-sectional area of the nasal cavity as a function of distance from the nostril. This technique requires a sound generator, wave tube, microphone, nosepiece, and computer. The sound generator produces an acoustic signal (pulsed or continuous) that travels down the wave tube into the measured object. The sound waves are partially reflected by narrowings in the measured object, thereby representing a change in the cross-sectional area. A microphone measures the transmitted and reflected sound which is digitized with reconstruction of the impedance and area profile plotted as a function of area versus distance. These calculations are based on several assumptions. First, the measured object is a series of cylinders of the same length. Second, there is an infinite signal-to-noise ratio. And third, significant wall inertia exists. All of the above assumptions can contribute to inaccuracies in the measurement of cross-sectional areas. Despite these limitations, accurate measurements can be obtained and have been confirmed by a variety of models.[28] A critical portion of the apparatus to measure acoustic rhinomanometry is the nosepiece. The nosepiece must form an acoustic seal with the wave tube and nose yet not distort the nasal tip/valve region. Nosepieces of different shapes and materials yield different data values when the same object is measured. It is best to use nosepieces that are composed of the same material and that are anatomically conformed to obtain accurate measurements.

The results from acoustic rhinomanometry represent the cross-sectional area (cm^2) of the nasal cavity as a function of distance (cm) from the end of the nosepiece. The data from acoustic rhinomanometry in normal individuals can vary with race, craniofacial development, mucosal variations, environmental conditions, and skeletal variations. Data from acoustic rhinomanometry reveals an initial decrease in cross-sectional area related to the narrowing in the region of the nasal valve followed by a subsequent narrowing due to the anterior head of the inferior turbinate. These constrictions are typically noted at ~1.3 and 3.6 cm from the nosepiece. The cross-sectional area distal to the head of the inferior turbinate gradually increases to the region of the nasopharynx. Acoustic rhinomanometry should be performed with the patient in a comfortable, symmetrical sitting position before and after decongestion. Several studies have reported the results on normal individuals and patients with allergic rhinitis, vasomotor rhinitis, and patients before and after septal surgery.[29–31]

Although acoustic rhinomanometry provides data on the cross-sectional area of the nasal cavity, it does not detail the shape of the airway. Therefore, acoustic rhinomanometry annot provide information on nasal airway resistance. Rhinomanometry determines overall nasal patency but annot provide information about the geometry of the irway. One can conclude that these are complementary methods of investigating key elements of the nasal airway. The utility of rhinomanometry and acoustic rhinomanometry is limited by the potential need for both studies, equipment-related expense, lack of reimbursement, and est variability. Routine use cannot be mandated, but the benefits are realized in the context of complex procedures or potentially litigious patients.

The final aspect of the preoperative assessment consists of discussing the findings of the history, physical examination, and laboratory studies, including the etiology of the disturbed nasal physiology and the planned therapeutic approach. This includes a frank discussion regarding alternative therapies, potential complications, an estimate of the likelihood of success, and, if surgery s required, postoperative recovery time and possible reoperation.

Surgical Technique

The outlined approach to reconstructive surgery of the nasal septum is based on the following precepts and concepts. First, the goal of surgery is to remove pathology and reconstruct the abnormal septal parts into normal position so that normal physiological airway function can take place. Second, the aim of the incisions and subsequent dissection is to completely expose the pathological septal tructures. Third, the mucosal lining is the valuable organ of the nose where the defense and biochemical reactions occur and incisions should be in the skin to preserve the integrity of the mucosa. Fourth, the goal of surgery is to help relieve the patient of symptoms that distort his or her well-being.

Positioning on the operating table for nasal surgery hould provide comfort for both the patient and the surgeon. The patient should be placed on a well-padded table or chair (dental flexible chair) as close to the right side of the table as possible to minimize the distance the surgeon must reach to address the nose. A semi-Fowler's position s frequently used to aid in patient comfort. Two power surgical loops are very helpful in the performance of this delicate surgery.

Nasal septal surgery can be performed under either general anesthesia or local anesthesia with intravenous sedation. Premedication should include analgesics and sedatives. In either situation the nose is infiltrated with solution containing epinephrine. The concentration of pinephrine varies; in general, a concentration of 1:100,000 s safe. The solution should be injected in the areas to be pproached surgically and additionally focused in areas of incisions and vascular areas. Therefore, areas that are generally infiltrated include that of the hemitransfixion incision between the medial crura, the region of the incisive foramen, the heads of the inferior and middle turbinate (to allow decongestion and increased visualization of the nose), and the region between the upper and lateral cartilage and lower lateral cartilage near the intercartilaginous incision. The external cartilaginous and bony pyramid of the nose is also anesthetized at a similar time. Frequently, 5 cm^3 is adequate to accomplish this. It is often advisable, especially under local anesthesia with intravenous sedation, to first spray the nose and vasoconstrict with 1% phenylephrine hydrochloride and then topically anesthetize the nose by spraying two or three puffs of 4% lidocaine. Subsequent application of ~100 to 150 mg of cocaine flakes on cotton carriers directly to the region of the anterior ethmoid nerves and sphenopalatine ganglion provides excellent anesthesia. Halothane, enflurane, and isoflurane are commonly used inhalation anesthetics. These agents and cocaine sensitize the myocardium to the actions of the sympathomimetics.[27] Therefore, the combination of these agents with the infiltration of an epinephrine-containing solution requires careful cardiac monitoring and minimal dosages of cocaine and epinephrine.[32]

The opening incision for septal surgery is the right hemitransfixion incision (**Fig. 50.4**). The hemitransfixion incision extends from the anterior part of the caudal end of the septum to the area just anterior to the nasal spine. This incision parallels the caudal end of the septum in the skin. Instruments used to expose the caudal septum and identify the caudal end of the septum include a Cottle clamp and an alar protector. For a more advanced surgeon, a nasal speculum may be all that is required. After the caudal end of the cartilaginous septum is isolated, the elevation of the mucoperiosteum from the left side of the

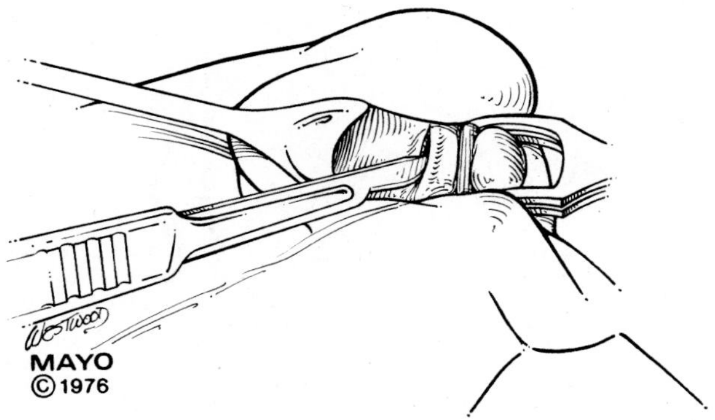

Fig. 50.4 A right-handed surgeon holds a Cottle columellar clamp in the left hand and the assistant holds an alar protector. After a columellar clamp has been applied to identify the caudal end of the septum, a right hemitransfixion incision is made ~1 to 2 mm behind the caudal end of the nasal septum with a no. 15 blade.

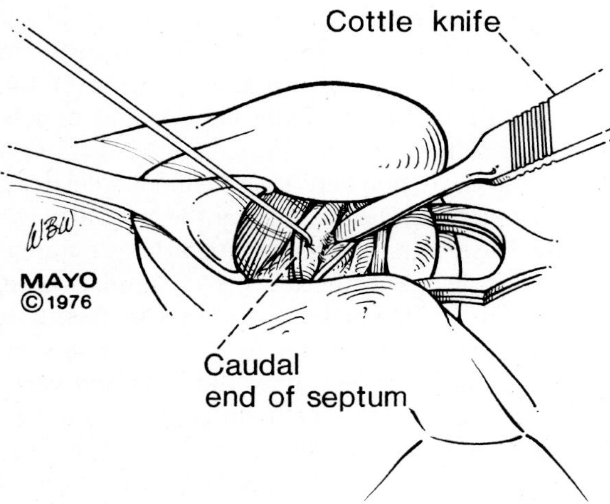

Fig. 50.5 Through the right hemitransfixion incision, the quadrangular septal cartilage is retracted to the right with a hook, and the Cottle knife is used to begin the dissection beneath the mucoperichondrium of the septal cartilage.

septum or left anterior tunnel is begun (**Fig. 50.5**). It is important to obtain a dissection plane between the cartilage and perichondrium to maintain the vascular supply to the perichondrium. Several instruments are helpful in this dissection. Selection varies on the history of previous surgery and the particular deformity encountered. When the plane is clearly identified elevation of the mucoperichondrium proceeds quickly, with an appropriate length nasal speculum providing retraction onto the mucoperichondrium as well as visualization of the area where the mucoperichondrium is still attached to the septum (**Fig. 50.6**). With adequate vasoconstriction, anesthesia, hypotension, and dissection in the correct plane below the perichondrium, bleeding is usually not a significant

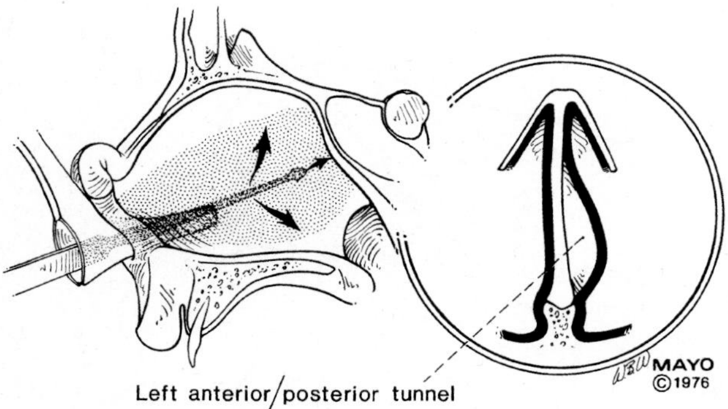

Fig. 50.6 As the dissection continues, the left anterior tunnel becomes a left anterior/posterior tunnel, with elevation of the mucoperiosteum of the perpendicular plate of the ethmoid bone and the vomer in the posterior portion of the nose. Following placement of a nasal speculum through the hemitransfixion incision into the left anterior tunnel, a Cottle elevator is used to continue mucoperichondrial and mucoperiosteal elevation back to the face of the sphenoid.

problem and blood loss is minimal. A Cottle dissector is an excellent instrument to effect elevation of the perichondrial flap away from the septal skeleton. This technique works for the majority of the anterior septum as well as the posterior septum after the bony cartilaginous junction has been passed. The ligamentous attachments of the inferior septum to the spine and premaxilla are somewhat thick and the mucosa tenuous because it is frequently here that a deviation is present requiring careful dissection to maintain continuity of the mucoperichondrial flap.

Specific Problems

Transverse Anterior Septum

A nose that has had significant trauma may have a deformity of the anterior septum being nearly transverse with a fracture line in the cartilage extending from the spine superiorly to the "K" area formed by the junction of the upper lateral cartilage and nasal bones. This results in a particularly unstable caudal end of the septum when the subsequent deflections are removed or reduced. In situations where this results in lack of adequate support for the tip or a concern about maintenance of a correct position for airway patency, the anterior septum may require removal and subsequent reconstruction with an autogenous (cartilage or bone) material. In this situation it is helpful if the posterior bony septum is intact to allow harvesting of a large piece of septal skeleton that can subsequently be shaped to replace the anterior cartilaginous septum. It is frequently helpful in this situation to use the caudal end as a template to size the height of the graft which will be placed in the caudal end. The bony segment is subsequently shaped to resemble the cartilaginous caudal end and a small pocket created anterior to the hemitransfixion incision between the medial crura with the implant subsequently placed using 4–0 chromic guide sutures on a Keith needle (**Fig. 50.7**).

Broad Deviated Premaxillary Crest

A common finding in septal deformities is that the deformity includes a broad and frequently asymmetric premaxillary wing or crest. As in other areas of septal surgery exposing the underlying structures while maintaining mucoperichondrial integrity is helpful. Two approaches to this problem may be applicable. If the deformity is located anteriorly, a plane of dissection adjacent to bone can often be found posteriorly; subsequently, careful dissection anteriorly with concomitant dislocation of the cartilaginous septum to the opposite side is frequently successful in exposing this region. This allows removal of the deviated

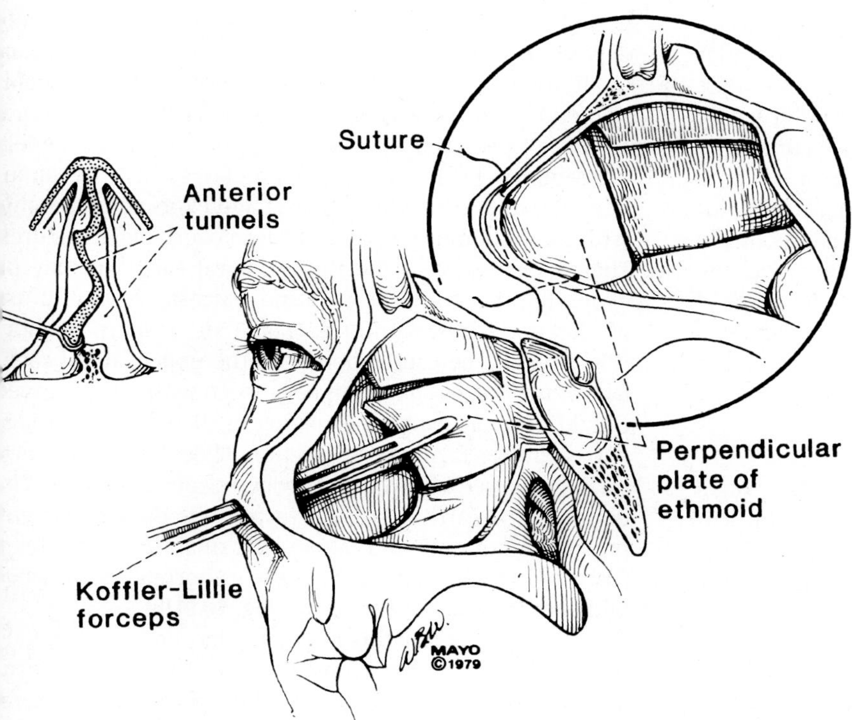

Fig. 50.7 Bilateral anterior and posterior tunnels have been created to allow removal and replacement of deformed caudal end of the septum with autogenous bone graft from the perpendicular plate of ethmoid.

premaxillary crest by using a chisel, heavy scissors, or a rongeur. A second approach to this problem involves identifying the nasal spine and pyriform aperture with subsequent elevation of the mucoperiosteum from the floor of the nose and onto the premaxillary crest. This inferior tunnel is connected to the anterior tunnel adjacent to the septum, allowing direct visualization and removal of the bony deformity (**Fig. 50.8**).

Large Posterior Septal Spur

Frequently, patients with septal deformities have as part of their abnormality a large, sharp septal deformity in the mid- or posterior-septal region. This may be associated with intermittent facial pain and possibly recurrent sinusitis. The approach favored by the authors is extension of the submucoperichondrial dissection on each

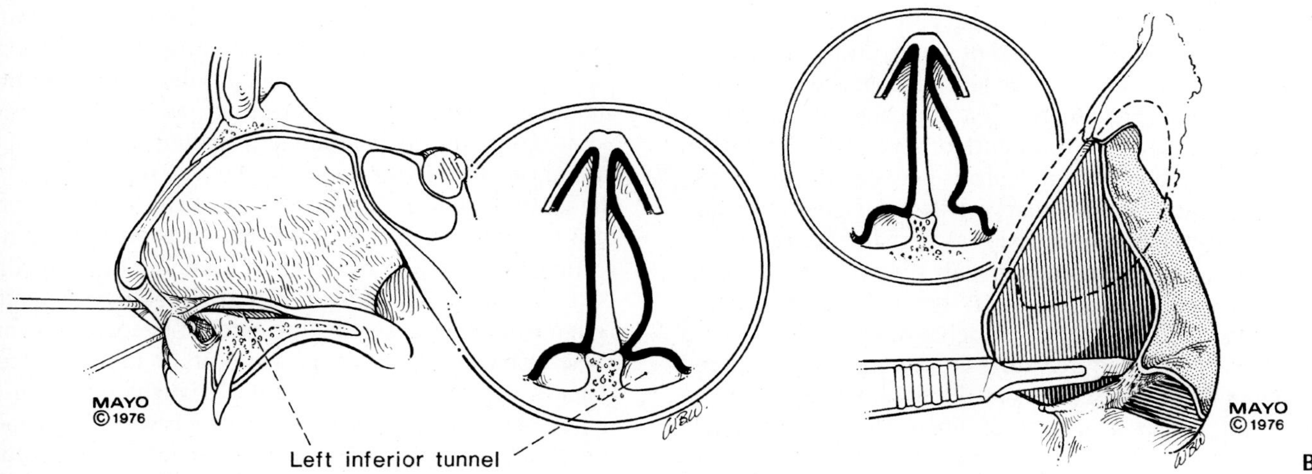

Fig. 50.8 Development of a left inferior tunnel. (**A**) The crest of the pyriform aperture is identified, and a curved Cottle elevator is used to elevate mucosa along the floor of the nose on the left. Three tunnels have now been developed; a left anterior/posterior, a right inferior, and a left inferior. (**B**) The joining of the left anterior and left inferior tunnels by sharp dissection of the fibrous tissue that binds the mucosa in this area to the crest of the premaxilla. Care is taken not to perforate the mucosa.

side of the septum to the anterior margin of the spur and beyond the spur on the side opposite the spur. A similar dissection is performed inferior to the spur, if possible. The bony margins above and below the spur are freed by a bone scissors or an ostetome, and the spur is dissected from the mucosa. In the unusual situation in which a sharp posterior septal spur is the only deformity for which one is performing septal surgery, such as in the case of unilateral facial pain or sinusitis, then an incision just anterior to the spur with subsequent elevation of the mucosa in the region of the spur will allow removal with an osteotome.

Upper Lateral Cartilage Surgery

Surgery on the upper lateral cartilage is best performed early in the operation, when the field is dry. Hemostasis and precision exposure are the keys to surgery of the upper lateral cartilage. This is probably best done after the septal surgery and before surgery on the tip and pyramid. The intercartilaginous incision is the most commonly used approach to the dorsum of the nose; yet, as pointed out by Anderson,[33] the cartilage-splitting incision (cutting through the lower lateral, i.e., alar or lobular, cartilage) can be used to modify both the dorsum of the nose and the lower lateral cartilages without violating the skin or mucosa of the nasal valve.

Because of the need for accurate surgical technique in this region, the details of technique will be described. Gray[34] deserves credit for first developing this exacting technique. The authors of this chapter favor the intercartilaginous incision in most instances because it affords the most direct approach to the upper lateral cartilage. This incision is made along the caudal end of the upper lateral cartilage from lateral to medial aspects, preferably with a no. 15 blade and with the aid of a four-pronged retractor and the middle finger of the left hand (if the operator is right-handed) (**Fig. 50.9A**). First, the skin is incised. Then the incision is carried to a depth of several millimeters to the intercartilaginous aponeurosis between the upper and lower lateral (alar or lobular) cartilages. If a hemitransfixion or full-transfixion incision was made for the septal surgery, care is taken not to join the intercartilaginous incision with these incisions; however, should these incisions be inadvertently or deliberately joined (for tip rotation), then accurate suture approximation is required to avoid excessive scarring at the nasal valve angle. The assistant places a weighted, single Joseph skin hook, 16 cm, into the upper lateral cartilage and retracts it downward, while the operator holds either a four-pronged retractor or another retractor to expose upper lateral cartilage in his left hand and holds cotton swabs or suction in his right hand for removal of blood from the field. A no. 66 Beaver knife blade is used to reach the perichondrium of the upper lateral cartilage. This technique not only exposes the upper lateral cartilage but prevents injury to the overlying canopy of neuromuscular and vascular structures (**Fig. 50.9B**). By this method, the upper lateral cartilage up to and over the nasal bones can be widely undermined in a relatively avascular plane. The upper lateral cartilage may be explored and exposed bilaterally with minimal injury to any of these overlying structures. The undersurface of the upper lateral cartilage may be exposed, preserving the skin and mucosa, by careful use of the no. 66 Beaver knife blade or a sharp scissors (**Fig. 50.9C**). The caudal border of the upper lateral cartilage or the mucosa itself can be grasped with a 7 in., curved Gerald dressing forceps. Grasping of the skin or cartilage with a forceps facilitates dissection. Thus the upper lateral cartilage is freed from the mucocutaneous coverings. The upper lateral cartilage may be evaluated after it has been precisely exposed and after abnormalities have been corrected in an attempt to restore a "normal" nasal valve with a normal nasal valve angle (**Fig. 50.9D–F**).

Thickening or twisting in this region can be adequately managed by resection. Gray[34] believes that some returning (also termed *curling* or *scrolling*) of the upper lateral cartilage may be a normal finding. Yet other workers, including Cottle (cited by Hinderer[35]) believe that returning is almost always a pathological finding. "Physiological" returning of the upper lateral cartilage affords some stiffness to resist collapse, whereas "pathological" and "excessive" returning may interfere with the flexible valve action of the upper lateral cartilage. In attempting to achieve a normal nasal valve angle and avoid either increased rigidity or increased collapsibility, the surgeon can use his or her resourcefulness in reconstructing a normal nasal valve. Resection of the upper lateral cartilage (and lower lateral cartilage as part of tip surgery) should be conservative so as to avoid mobile inspiratory collapse. The amount of caudal end of upper lateral cartilage that should be removed is determined, as Hinderer[35] has pointed out, so as to maintain the relationship of the upper lateral cartilage to the caudal end of the septum. Thus, if the septum is being shortened by 2 to 4 mm, then resection of 2 to 4 mm from the caudal end of the upper lateral cartilage should be considered. The amount of the medial portion of upper lateral cartilage that should be removed is determined by resecting the amount needed to reconstruct a normal nasal valve angle of 10 to 15 degrees. Usually the removal of a medial triangular section of upper lateral cartilage (base of triangle is caudal and apex is cephalic) can open the nasal valve angle when the upper lateral cartilage is thickened, deflected, or twisted. In addition, when the valve angle is narrow it may be advantageous to trim the caudal end of the upper lateral cartilage and then to remove a medial triangle of the upper lateral cartilage.

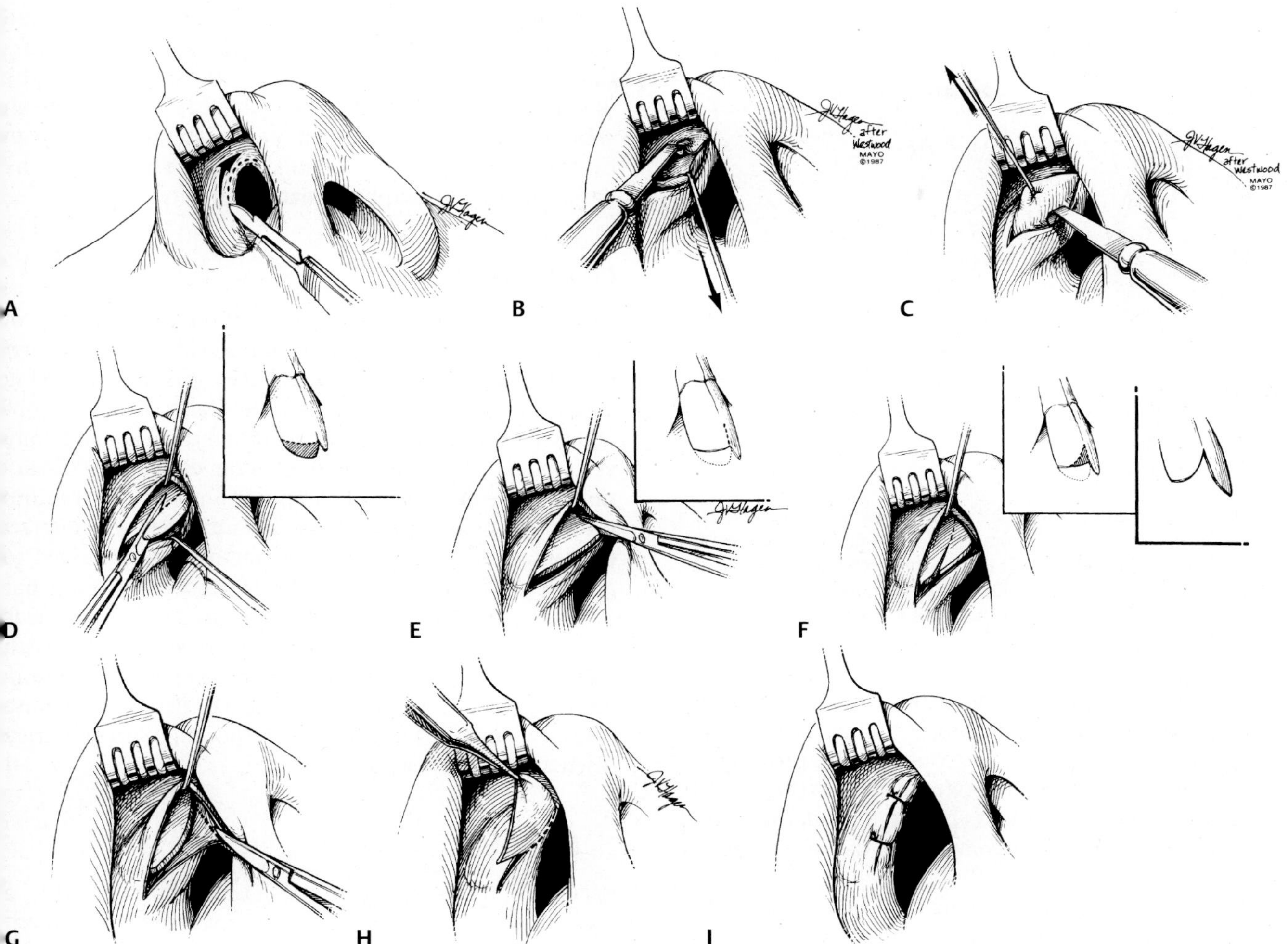

Fig. 50.9 (**A**) Intercartilaginous incision with no. 15 blade carried just beneath the skin. (**B**) A weighted hook is applied to upper lateral cartilage for countertraction, and dissection with a no. 66 Beaver knife blade is made down to perichondrium. (**C**) Undersurface of upper lateral cartilage may be exposed, preserving skin. (**D**) Resection of caudal end of upper lateral cartilage may be performed directly, and mucocutaneous tissue can be preserved. (**E**) Upper lateral cartilage can be completely separated from nasal septum medially, and submucosa can be preserved if desired. (**F**) Medial triangle of upper lateral cartilage can be removed submucosally from its attachment to septum. (**G**) After caudal end and medial triangle of upper lateral cartilage have been removed, mucocutaneous tissue is separated from septum. (**H**) Excess tissue is trimmed, and intercartilaginous incision is closed (**I**) thereby opening and widening the apex of the valve angle. (Courtesy of Mayo Foundation.)

After the medial triangle of upper lateral cartilage adjacent to the septum has been removed and the valve angle opened, several millimeters of the mucocutaneous tissue is separated from the septum (**Fig. 50.9G**), and a mucosal relaxing incision is created that extends cephalad from the intercartilaginous incision in the valve apex. The tissue from the cephalic margin of the intercartilaginous incision can be flapped back and trimmed (**Fig. 50.9H**) and the intercartilaginous incision closed with 4–0 chromic catgut on a curved cutting needle (Ethicon no. 744; Ethicon, Inc., Somerville, NJ) **(Fig. 50.9I),** thereby opening and widening the valve angle. The upper lateral cartilage is supported in a more dorsal position. Subsequent scar formation aids in maintaining a greater valve angle. We term this flap the *Lopez-Infante flap* because we learned about it from Dr. Fausto Lopez-Infante of Mexico City.

After surgery on the upper lateral cartilage, there are times when widening of the nasal valve angle cannot be satisfactorily accomplished by resection of a triangular portion of the upper lateral cartilage or by creation of the Lopez-Infante flap because of a congenitally narrowed nose or a previous rhinoplasty in which the upper lateral cartilage was scarred close to the septum after hump removal and in-fracture were accomplished. When the upper lateral cartilage is displaced against the septum, two procedures can be used to reopen the nasal valve

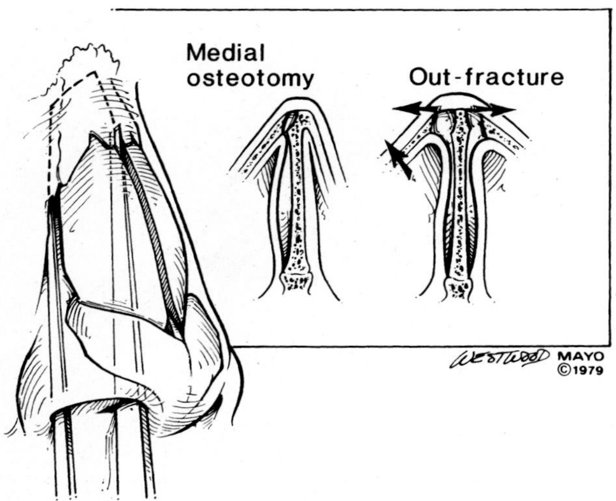

Fig. 50.10 Upper lateral cartilage can be completely separated from nasal septum submucosally (intraseptal separation). These medial, lateral, transverse osteotomies, with out-fracture on one or both sides as indicated, can be performed to carry the upper lateral cartilage away from the septum to open the nasal valve angle. (Courtesy of Mayo Foundation.)

angle. When a significant mobilization of the upper lateral cartilage is required, medial, lateral, and transverse osteotomies may be necessary, with out-fracture carrying the upper lateral cartilage away from the septum (**Fig. 50.10**). If a dorsal hump deformity has been removed, then a roof repair is required in which available tissue is used for grafting.

Special situations or problems may arise that test the surgeon's ingenuity. For example, during nasal septal reconstruction with modification of the external nasal pyramid or during rhinoplasty, modification of the upper lateral cartilage may be required before or after the osteotomies and in-fracture to prevent permanent narrowing of the nasal valve area and closing of the nasal valve angle. Thus a medial triangle of upper lateral cartilage can be removed for prophylaxis, that is, to maintain a normal nasal valve angle and prevent a fixed collapse of the nasal valve angle. In the situation of mobile collapse of the nasal valve caused by either a nonresilient upper lateral cartilage or previous trauma (surgical or nonsurgical), with partial or complete absence of the upper lateral cartilage, either a conchal (ear) cartilage or septal cartilage autograft, or even rotation of the lower lateral (alar) cartilage over the remnant of the upper lateral cartilage, may be attempted to prevent or lessen an increase in collapsibility of the nasal valve. This subject has been reported on by Goode.[36] He believes that missing cartilage that produces valve collapse is best replaced by a cartilage graft. Scar contraction is repaired by skin graft, and composite loss (skin and cartilage) is probably best reconstructed by composite graft.

During treatment of the severely twisted or smashed nose, if "ballooning" or flaring of the upper lateral cartilage is present, with widening of the valve angle, the upper lateral cartilage may be separated from the septum submucosally, and a section of upper lateral cartilage can be removed to reconstruct and, in this case, narrow the nasal valve angle to approximate normality.

Prior Surgery

Patients with nasal airway obstruction and a history of previous rhinologic surgery present a challenge for several reasons. First, prior surgery produces scar tissue, making surgical dissection difficult. Second, there is a high probability that a significant portion of the cartilage and bony skeleton may be absent, increasing the difficulty of dissection and the likelihood of complications that may require the use of an autograft from a distant site or an allograft for septal reconstruction. These factors not only lead to a more difficult dissection of the mucoperiosteum but increase the risk of tearing of the mucosal flap. Thus one is operating in a technically more difficult environment with fewer resources available for reconstruction. In addition, both physiological and psychological difficulties are more complex, and a thoughtful and thorough preoperative discussion is mandatory.

Reconstruction

Reconstructive surgery of the nasal septum is truly a reconstruction, with the final steps involving replacement and fixation of the appropriately trimmed cartilage and bone in the septal mucosal envelope. Bone is replaced where bone existed and cartilage is replaced where cartilage existed (**Fig. 50.11**). Lack of adequate septal cartilage (dorsal or caudal support) will lead to various degrees of saddle deformity, with columellar retraction and even inadequate tip support. Inadequate tip support can be overcome with a caudal cartilaginous strut placed between the medial crura and sutured in place. This strut should span the distance from the spine to the intradomal tip region. If a saddle deformity results, then replacement of the cartilaginous septum, either with autogenous septal structures or with autograft rib, may be required. For the cosmetic defect a dorsal onlay cartilage graft through either the hemitransfixion or an intercartilaginous incision can be considered.

Closure and Dressing

Completion of reconstructive septal surgery includes closure of the hemitransfixion incision and repair of any significant tears (greater than 1 cm) in the mucosa. Absorbable

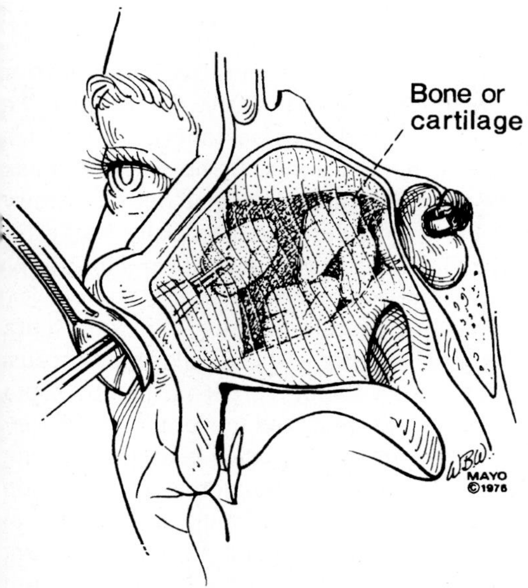

ig. 50.11 Crushed cartilage and bone replaced within septal space.

utures are satisfactory in both situations to close and epair the septal envelope. Mucosal tears are approximated with 4–0 chromic on a G-2 needle (Ethicon no. 798) and a Castroviejo needle holder. If mucosal tears are present at pposing sites, cartilage and Gelfilm (Pharmacia & Upjohn Co., Kalamazoo, MI) are placed in the septal space in the ope of providing a surface for mucosal healing.

Closure also includes a mechanism to retain the reconstructed septum in the midline and prevent hematoma ormation. Two options are available to accomplish this. Most commonly, the authors utilize plastic nasal stents utured to the septum with subsequently placed antibiotic-impregnated petroleum jelly gauze nasal packing Fig. 50.12). An alternative method is to mattress suture the mucoperichondrial flaps with an absorbable suture, thus obviating the need for nasal packing. However, if significant reconstructive efforts have been undertaken or if bone has been transplanted anteriorly in the septal space due to the cartilaginous deformity, mattress suturing would not be advisable. Finally, an external tape dressing is applied. A firm, external nasal stent is applied to support and protect the dorsal septal dissection.

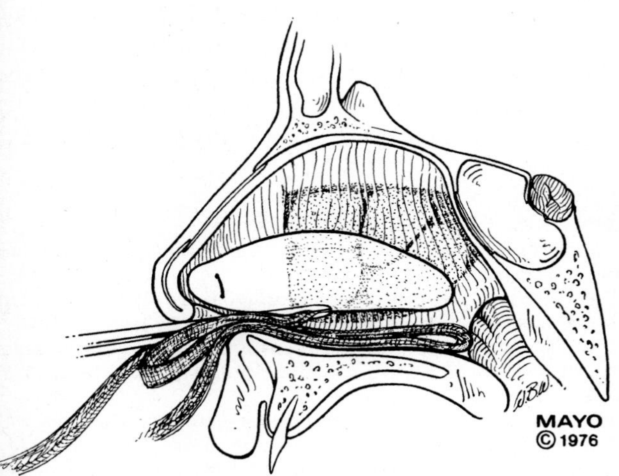

ig. 50.12 Nasal stents are secured on either side of the septum, and asal packing is introduced to complete the closure of the procedure.

Postoperative Care

Reconstructive surgery of the septum frequently is performed on an outpatient basis. The patient is discharged from the hospital with a small amount of pain medication, antibiotics, and sedatives. Patients are instructed to avoid lifting anything over 20 pounds for 10 days. Lozenges and added humidification to prevent symptomatic drying of the upper airway can be helpful. If packing is placed in the nose to aid in maintaining the septum in its reconstructed position, the timing of the pack removal is variable. Certainly, if there is any history of cardiac disease, significant pulmonary dysfunction, or sleep apnea, then administering oxygen and monitoring arterial oxygen saturation while the packs are in place may be warranted. The timing of pack removal is individualized, with individual surgeons preferring the following day to 4 to 7 days following surgery. Plastic stents are usually removed 7 to 10 days following surgery, depending on the need to protect the mucosa and prevent adhesions.

Complications

Intraoperative Complications

The use of local anesthetics either singly or associated with general anesthesia carries an inherent risk of toxicity of the local anesthetics, additives, or a potential interaction of these agents with a general anesthetic. Established safe doses should not be exceeded, and arterial oxygen saturation as well as mental status should be monitored during the procedure. Monitoring the mental status of the patient allows one to be aware of early signs of central nervous system toxicity, whereas monitoring arterial oxygen saturation prompts one to maintain a high PaO^2, which is key in preventing local anesthetic–induced seizures.

Excessive intraoperative bleeding is not common. However, during the course of elevation of the mucoperichondrial and mucoperiosteal flaps, the incisive artery may be encountered and torn. This can be easily handled with electrocautery using steps to protect the integrity of the mucoperichondrial flaps. In addition, a very light electrocautery may be applied to focal sites of hemorrhage that are particularly bothersome. Temporary packs soaked in solutions containing 1:100,000 epinephrine may be helpful.

Broadening of the alar base may be noted following hemitransfixion incision and dissection of the soft tissues near the region of the nasal spine. The preoperative soft tissue relationships can be restored by inserting a base stitch prior to the closure of the hemitransfixion incision utilizing a medium-sized Keith needle and a chromic suture. The Keith needle is placed via the inferior extent of the hemitransfixion incision through the subcutaneous tissues and brought out through the left alar facial groove, and it is subsequently reinserted adjacent to the exit site and passed in the subcutaneous tissues just inferior to the nasal spine and again exiting the alar facial groove on the right. Finally, the Keith needle is again passed through the subcutaneous tissues, entering adjacent to the exit site on the right alar facial groove, and is brought out through the hemitransfixion incision. A nasal speculum placed in the hemitransfixion incision forms a firm back-stop by which the Keith needle can be directed from the hemitransifixion incision atraumatically. The free ends of the suture are then tied, with the tension adjusted so that the preoperative appearance is restored.

It is possible during a hemitransfixion incision for inadvertent lacerations of the alar rim to occur. These should be approximated using 6–0 Prolene (Ethicon, Inc.), with meticulous technique to prevent any notching or residual scarring.

Early Postoperative Complications

Hemorrhage following reconstructive surgery of the nasal septum is rare but requires prompt treatment. If the hemorrhage is minimal, local measures, such as mild pressure, may suffice. If the bleeding is subsequent to removal of the packing, application of a topical vasoconstrictor may be useful. If other measures fail, repacking may be required.

Normally, reconstructive surgery of the nasal septum produces minimal discomfort. Pain in the nose warrants immediate reevaluation due to the possibility of a septal hematoma or abscess. The presence of fever or toxic symptoms requires pack removal and consideration of drainage and intravenous antibiotic therapy, with coverage for *Staphylococcus aureus* due to reported cases of toxic shock syndrome.[36–38] Although not proven to be preventative against toxic shock syndrome, patients are routinely administered an oral antistaphylococcal antibiotic, and nasal packing is impregnanted with antibiotic ointment to prevent bacterial overgrowth.

Late Postoperative Complications

The most frustrating late postoperative complication is recurrence of the septal deformity, although this is uncommon. It can occur due to postoperative scar tissue contracture or nasal trauma. If the patient's nasal breathing is disturbed because of a recurrent deformity then reoperation is considered. It is usually suggested that 12 months elapse prior to reoperation. This allows scar tissue to contract and mature.

Septal perforations are not common following septal surgery, yet surgical trauma is the most common cause of septal perforation.[39] Factors predisposing to septal perforation include devascularized mucosal flaps (dissection performed in the incorrect plane), bilateral opposing mucoperichondrial flap tears, hematoma, and infection. To minimize the possibility of developing perforations, an appropriate plane of dissection should be maintained and tears repaired with absorbable suture. Careful attention during closure and packing placement should minimize hematoma formation.

Occasionally, patients may note transient palatal and dental anesthesia. This is most likely due to injury to branches of the nasopalatine nerve, which pass through the incisive foramen. Anosmia is an unusual complication following septal surgery and potentially results if the dissection is carried high in the region of the perpendicular plate of the ethmoid.[40] More significant disruption of structures in this region may lead to cerebrospinal fluid leakage.[41]

Summary

Surgery involving the nasal septum is both challenging and rewarding. The rhinologic surgeon requires extensive knowledge of nasal anatomy, physiology, and pathophysiology to effectively plan therapy that will relieve the patient's often wide-ranging symptoms. Use of nasal septal reconstruction techniques and principles should provide a means to consistently achieve success.

References

1. Bailey BJ. Nasal septal surgery 1896–1899: transition and controversy. Laryngoscope 1997;107:10–16
2. Bosworth FH. Treatment of nasal stenosis due to deflective septa, with or without thickening of convex side. Laryngoscope 1899;7:337–339
3. Watson AW. Treatment of nasal stenosis due to the deflective septa with or without thickening of convex side. Laryngoscope 1899;7:348–351
4. Asch MJ. Treatment of nasal stenosis due to the deflective septa, with or without thickening of convex side. Laryngoscope 1899;7:340–343
5. Freer OT. The correction of deflections of the nasal septum with a minimum of traumatism. JAMA 1902;38:636–642
6. Killian G. The submucous window resection of the nasal septum Ann Otol Rhinol Laryngol 1905;14:363–393

7. Metzenbaum M. Replacement of the lower end of the dislocated septal cartilage versus submucous resection of the dislocated end of the septal cartilage. Arch Otolaryngol 1929;9:282–296
8. Peer LA. An operation to repair lateral displacement of the lower border of the septal cartilage. Arch Otolaryngol 1937;25:475–477
9. Salinger S. Deviation of the septum in relation to the twisted nose. Arch Otolaryngol 1939;29:520–532
10. Seltzer AP. The nasal septum: plastic repair of the deviated septum associated with a deflected tip. Arch Otolaryngol 1944;40:433–444
11. Fomon S, Gilbert JC, Silver AG, et al. Plastic repair of the obstructing nasal septum. Arch Otolaryngol 1948;47:7–20
12. Fomon S, Bell JW, Berger EL, et al. New approach to ventral deflections of the nasal septum. Arch Otolaryngol 1951;54:356–366
13. Cottle MH, Loring RM. Surgery of the nasal septum: new operative procedures and indications. Ann Otol Rhinol Laryngol 1948;57:705–713
14. Cottle MH, Loring RM, Fischer GG, et al. The "maxillapremaxilla" approach to extensive septum surgery. Arch Otolaryngol 1958;68:301–313
15. Hwang PH, McLaughlin RB, Lanza DC, Kennedy DW. Endoscopic septoplasty: indications, technique, and results. Otolaryngol Head Neck Surg 1999;120:678–682
16. Gordon AS, McCaffrey TV, Kern EB, et al. Rhinomanometry for preoperative and postoperative assessment of nasal obstruction. Otolaryngol Head Neck Surg 1989;101:20–26
17. Mertz JS, McCaffrey TV, Kern EB. Objective evaluation of anterior septal surgical reconstruction. Otolaryngol Head Neck Surg 1984;92: 308–311
18. Pallanch JF, McCaffrey TV, Kern EB. Normal nasal resistance. Otolaryngol Head Neck Surg 1985;93:778–785
19. Scherer PW, Hahn II, Mozell MM. The biophysics of nasal airflow. Otolaryngol Clin North Am 1989;22:265–278
20. Kasperbauer JL, Kern EB. Nasal valve physiology. Otolaryngol Clin North Am 1987;20:669–719
21. Kimmelman CP. The risk to olfaction from nasal surgery. Laryngoscope 1994;104:981–988
22. Cole P, Ayiomanimitis A, Ohki M. Anterior and posterior rhinomanometry. Rhinology 1989;27:257–262
23. Clement PA. Committee report on standardization of rhinomanometry. Rhinology 1984;22(3):151–155
24. Broms P, Jonson B, Lamm CJ. Rhinomanometry. Acta Otolaryngol 1982;94:157–168
25. McCaffrey TV, Kern EB. Clinical evaluation of nasal obstruction. Arch Otolaryngol 1979;105:542–545
26. Cole P, Fastag O, Niinimaa V. Computer-aided rhinometry: a research rhinometer for clinical trial. Acta Otolaryngol 1980;90:139–142
27. Pallanch JF. Rhinometry: the application of objective airway testing in the clinical evaluation of nasal obstruction. In: McCaffrey TV, ed. Rhinology and Sinusology. New York: Thieme; 1997:125–154
28. Lenders HG. Acoustic rhinometry. In: McCaffrey TV, ed. Rhinology and Sinusology. New York: Thieme; 1997:125–154
29. Grymer LF, Hilberg O, Pedersen OF, Rasmussen TR. Acoustic rhinometry: values from adults with subjective normal controls. Rhinology 1991;29:35–47
30. Lenders H, Pirsig W. Diagnostic value of acoustic rhinometry: patients with allergic and vasomotor rhinitis compared with normal controls. Rhinology 1990;28:5–16
31. Grymer LF, Hilberh O, Elbrond O, Pederson OF. Acoustic rhinometry: evaluation of the nasal cavity with septal deviations, before and after septoplasty. Laryngoscope 1989;99:1180–1187
32. Verlander JM, Johns ME. The clinical use of cocaine. Otolaryngol Clin North Am 1981;14:521–531
33. Anderson JR. A new approach to rhinoplasty. Trans Am Acad Ophthalmol Otolaryngol 1966;70:183–192
34. Gray VD. Physiologic returning of the upper lateral cartilage. Int Rhinology 1970;8:56–59
35. Hinderer KH. Fundamentals of Anatomy and Surgery of the Nose. Birmingham, AL: Aesculapius Publishing Co.; 1971
36. Goode RL. Surgery of the incompetent nasal valve. Laryngoscope 1985;95:546–555
37. Hull HF, Mann JM, Sands CJ, et al. Toxic shock syndrome related to nasal packing. Arch Otolaryngol 1983;109:624–626
38. Barbour SD, Shalaes DM, Guertin SR. Toxic shock syndrome associated with nasal packing: analogy to tampon-associated illness. Pediatrics 1984;73:163–165
39. Jacobson JA, Kasworm EM, Crass BA, et al. Nasal carriage to toxigenic *Staphylococcus aureus* and prevalence of serum antibody to toxic shock syndrome toxin 1 in Utah. J Infect Dis 1986;153:356–359
40. Fairbanks DN, Fairbanks GR. Nasal septal perforation: prevention and management. Ann Plast Surg 1980;5:452–459
41. Hinderer KH. Fundamentals of Anatomy and Surgery of the Nose. Birmingham, AL: Aesculapius Publishing Co.; 1971

51 Prevention, Management, and Repair of Nasal Septal Perforation

Russell W. H. Kridel and Hossam M. T. Foda

Perforation of the nasal septum presents a difficult surgical challenge to the otolaryngologist/head and neck surgeon. Although the most common causes are self-inflicted or iatrogenic, a clear-cut etiology must be established from a long list of potential causes, some of which can be life threatening. Septal perforation repair is technically difficult because the perforation represents a hole in three distinct tissue layers, constituting the right and left septal mucoperichondrial flaps, and the intervening cartilage, all three of which must be distinctly separated and repaired individually. Many procedures have been described to repair septal perforations. Those that are based on an attempt to stretch the septal mucosa through an advancement flap without adequate mobilization generally fail because the septal membrane is relatively inelastic. Those techniques that have the best physiological result, highest success rate, and best patient acceptance generally require the use of extensively mobilized bilateral intranasal mucosal advancement flaps with the interposition and anchoring of a connective tissue type of graft.

Patient Evaluation

Patient Presentation

Patients who are symptomatic with their septal perforation usually present with complaints about crusting, bleeding, whistling if the perforation is small, nasal obstruction if the perforation is large, pain, and/or rhinorrhea. The more anterior the perforation is on the septum, the more commonly the patient will be symptomatic because this area of the nose is drier than the more posterior portions. Sometimes if the perforation is small and especially if it is posterior, the patient will not have any symptoms and the perforation will be found simply on examination by a physician. Large perforations generally cause more symptoms of nasal obstruction because they disrupt the normal separate lamellar flow.[1,2] The symptom of pain is often more ominous because it suggests the possibility of chondritis, which can occur around the edges of the exposed cartilage at the circumference of the perforation. When normal air flow is not restored by surgical repair or the interposition of a button, the turbulent air flow can change normal respiratory epithelium to dry mucosa, which is often noted by crusting on the mucosa, not at the perforation site, in patients with long-term perforation.

Crusting and bleeding usually occur with septal perforations at the edge of the perforation because of the difficulty for the mucosa to heal over any exposed cartilage. Significant bleeding can occur and must be treated appropriately. In patients with large amounts of crusting and inflammation, one needs to consider a chronic inflammatory process and must rule out cocaine abuse or a granulomatous process.

On examination, the septum should be palpated to ascertain if there is any residual cartilage between the mucosal flaps around the perforation site. In perforations after septoplasty, there is usually very little cartilage left around the perforation, and this makes dissection of the adherent flaps much more difficult (**Fig. 51.1**). Self-inflicted trauma and previous cocaine use often leave large amounts of intervening septal cartilage and bone, thus making the repair easier. In patients with granulomatous processes or vasculitis, the intervening septal cartilage is usually of poor quality.

Patients often have no understanding of the complexity of a septal perforation or the difficulty of its repair. A great deal of education is important in helping patients understand that the operative repair is not always successful but is often necessary to restore normal physiology. Showing the patient an endoscopic view of the

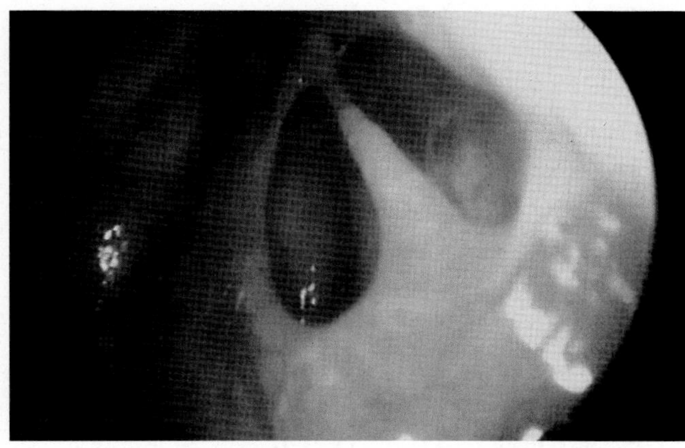

Fig. 51.1 An endoscopic view of a septal perforation in a patient who had previous septoplasty with removal of almost all of the septal cartilage and bone. Note the paper-thin adherent flaps with a small bridge of tissue within the perforation.

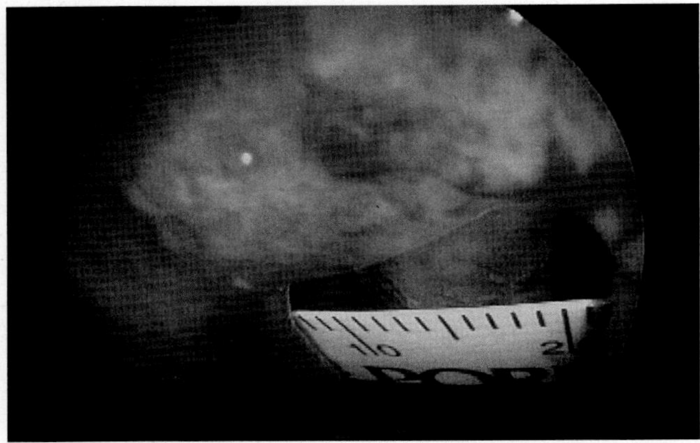

Fig. 51.2 A paper ruler is placed in the nose and an endoscopic picture taken to show the patient the size and shape of the perforation.

perforation on a monitor is often helpful in this educational process (**Fig. 51.2**).[3]

History and Etiologic Factors

Once iatrogenic or traumatic causes for the perforation have been ruled out, a very thorough history and examination are necessary in all patients. The septal perforation may be the first sign of a potentially life-threatening generalized systemic process. **Table 51.1** clearly identifies the multiple causes of septal perforation, and the reader of this chapter is directed to a previous paper by the author (RWHK) that delineates these etiologies in detail.[4]

Table 51.1 Causes of Septal Perforation

Causes of Septal Perforation
Trauma
External
Fracture
Septal hematoma
Piercing injuries
Self-inflicted
Nose picking
Foreign bodies
Iatrogenic
Nasal Surgery
Septoplasty
Sinus surgery
Turbinate surgery
Rhinoplasty
Septal cauterization
Septal packing
Septal splinting
Cryosurgery
Transsphenoidal hypophysectomy
Postoperative suctioning
Nasotracheal intubation
Drugs—Legal and Otherwise
Vasoconstrictive nasal sprays
Steroid nasal sprays
Cocaine
Smoking
Chemical Irritants
Chromic, sulfuric, and hydrochloric acids
Chlorines and bromines
Agricultural aerosolized dust
Rice and grain elevator dust
Chemical and industrial dusts
Lime
Cement
Glass
Salt
Dust
Heavy metal
Cyanide, arsenicals
Neoplastic Causes
Adenocarcinoma
Squamous cell carcinoma
Metastatic carcinoma
Midline destructive granuloma
Inflammatory Causes
Vasculitides
Collagen vascular diseases
Sarcoidosis
Wegener granulomatosis
Renal failure/renal disease
Infections
Tuberculosis
Syphilis
Rhinoscleroma
Lepromatous leprosy
Rhinosporidiosis
Multiple fungal species infection
Mucor infection
Typhoid
Diphtheria

Iatrogenic Causes

Unfortunately, the most common cause of a septal perforation stems from previous nasal surgery, especially septoplasty, and from treatment for epistaxis. During septoplasty, there may have been tears in both septal membranes in a contiguous area where the intervening septal cartilage or bone has been removed. If these are not repaired immediately at the time of surgery, the contraction of healing itself will enlarge the perforation. It is unwise to believe that a perforation will heal on its own; in fact, it is more likely that the perforation will enlarge postoperatively with the contraction of healing. Not only should the membrane tears be repaired but the insertion of intervening cartilage or connective tissue graft as a barrier to perforation is prudent.[5] The author (RWHK) when performing a septoplasty, always places crushed cartilage between the septal flaps and the area where the cartilage has been removed, whether or not there have been tears in the septal membranes. Often the obstructing cartilage that is removed during septoplasty is discarded or sent to pathology. Placing it back between the flaps, after it has been straightened or crushed, makes it act as a barrier against perforation and also, even if it does not survive, against fibrosis between the septal flaps, and may strengthen areas that have been weakened by the removal of cartilage (**Fig. 51.3**).

The secret to preventing corresponding tears in both mucoperichondrial flaps during septoplasty is to ensure that one has undermined broadly and elevated the mucoperichondrium away from the deviated cartilage or septal spur areas prior to attempting to remove the spur or the deviation. Even when there is a large spur, where penetrating the overlying membrane is common, the opposite mucoperichondrium usually can easily be elevated and maintained intact. If only one membrane is torn, the chance of a through-and-through perforation is markedly decreased. When a large posterior bony spur is encountered, the cartilage is separated from the bony septum and then the mucoperichondrium is elevated over the bony portion of the spur on the opposite side of the spur prior to removal. Becker scissors are used to cut above and below the bony spur, and then the tip of the nasal speculum is used to push the intervening spur closer to the midline as one teases the mucoperichondrium off the protruding portion of the spur prior to its removal.

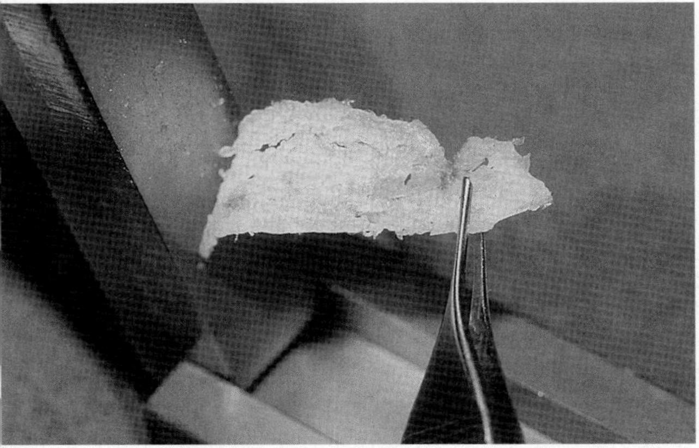

Fig. 51.3 A piece of septal cartilage is crushed in a cartilage crusher and then placed back between the mucoperichondral flaps to reskeletonize the septum and help prevent a perforation.

Bilateral corresponding tears in septal membranes can still cause septal perforation, even if there is intervening cartilage left; therefore these tears should be repaired. The blood supply to the cartilage comes from the overlying mucoperichondrium, and if this is disrupted bilaterally the intervening cartilage may necrose and ultimately perforate.

Nasal Sprays and Cocaine Usage

Some steroid nasal sprays can be very irritating to the septal mucosa when used on a long-term basis and can lead to perforation.[6] It is the obligation of the physician who places patients on such sprays to periodically examine the nasal mucosa for any untoward effect of the medication.

Cocaine use has increased dramatically as a major cause of septal perforations. The drug itself causes intense vasoconstriction compromising blood supply to the flaps. As most street cocaine is adulterated with filler substances that can be quite irritating, such as borax or talc, the insult to the septal membrane can be even worse, and even one-time usage of intranasal street cocaine has been known to cause a septal perforation.[7] Chronic cocaine use can totally destroy the inside of the nose because quite often infection complicates the inflammation, irritation, and lack of blood supply. The necrosis can proceed not only to perforation but also to total nasal collapse, dorsal saddling, intranasal stenosis, and scarring. Because cocaine is so addictive, patients often need to be screened for continued use despite their denial of continued use. It would be useless to attempt to repair a septal perforation in a patient who is still using cocaine.

Disease Processes

Septal perforations can be the sequelae of serious systemic diseases, whether they be neoplastic, inflammatory, or infectious. When no obvious cause has been determined, the physician must rule out potential serious medical illnesses. Renal failure and renal disease, vasculitides, and collagen vascular disorders such as lupus, rheumatoid arthritis, and polychondritis can predispose to septal perforation.

Unfortunately, some of these latter conditions may recur following remission. Therefore, prior to repairing such perforations, it is important to consult with the primary physician who is treating the patient. Patients must be told that even though repair may be successful, recurrence is possible if the disease flares up again at a later date.

One of the authors has noted this in several patients with renal and small-vessel disease.[8] Wegener granulomatosus, sarcoidosis, and other granulomatous diseases are less common causes, but computed tomography (CT) of the nose and paranasal sinuses helps to rule out these conditions. The workup of individuals with no known cause and a negative head and neck examination, and negative CT scans, should include laboratory evaluation for collagen vascular and renal disease. It should also include fluorescent treponemal antibody, absorbed (FTA-ABS), Venereal Disease Research Laboratory (VDRL), cytoplasmic antineutrophilic cytoplasmic antibody (C-ANCA), and Epstein-Barr virus titers. Nasal cultures for fungi and bacteria are helpful in the presence of any inflammatory process. Skin testing for anergy, tuberculosis, and fungal infections may also be helpful. If all of these tests come up negative and no clear cause has been elicited, then a biopsy of the perforation may be indicated prior to any surgery. Such a biopsy should be taken from the posterior edge of the perforation and should be large enough to include tissue away from the perforation so that the pathologist can get a definitive diagnosis and just not render a report of chronic inflammation. It is important not to biopsy at the superior or inferior edge of the perforation where one would increase the vertical perforation height, which is the dimension of the perforation that is most critical in one's ability to close a perforation. In addition, biopsies at the anterior portion of the perforation should be avoided because that area must be closed preferentially to decrease symptoms.

Medical Treatment

Asymptomatic patients with perforations rarely require treatment. Such patients should be advised to keep the nose moist when in dry climates with the use of petrolatum-based ointment. For patients with a great deal of crusting, frequent therapy with a nasal irrigant as well as ointments and emollients is indicated. David Fairbanks recommends an antiseptic wash of 1 teaspoon of table salt dissolved in 1 quart of warm water as a nasal irrigant delivered via a Water Pik–type device with a nasal adapter.[7] Corn syrup or glycerin can be added to the saline mixture as a moisturizing and coating substance, which further reduces nasal crusting. A teaspoon of vinegar or 1 to 3 tablespoons of boric acid powder helps decrease *Staphylococcus aureus* and *Pseudomonas aeruginosa* growth. If there is a chronic infection, antibacterial ointments such as bacitracin or Bactroban (mupirocin) may be applied.

Patients often are bothered by such laborious treatment regimens and often opt for other solutions. A silicone grommet prosthesis does not fix the perforation but helps to restore better nasal air flow and keeps the edges of the perforation more moist. The commercially available buttons are not always of proper size to fit larger perforations, in which case a custom silicone button can be fabricated by the local prosthetist once given the proper dimensions. The standard or the custom-made septal buttons usually can be inserted in the office under local and/or topical anesthesia. When these buttons are in place, occasional nasal irrigants may still be needed to keep the obturator clean, and they may have to be removed for more adequate cleaning and integrity check on a yearly or more frequent basis. Such buttons are ideal for patients who are not good surgical candidates for medical reasons and should also be considered for patients with chronic or recurrent disease as well as patients with continued cocaine usage.

Surgical Treatment

Goals and Options

Surgery should not only repair the perforation but should also restore normal nasal function and physiology. The literature is replete with different techniques described for closure, but only those that use intranasal advancement flaps successfully achieve normal nasal physiology because nasal respiratory epithelium is utilized for closure. Methods that use skin grafts or oral buccal mucosal grafts may be successful in closing the perforation but leave the patient with a dry nose that continues to crust as these grafts either shed or dry because normal respiratory epithelium is not present. The normal flow of air through the nose exacerbates the problem as it dries out these grafts.

The surgical method chosen should also facilitate a tension-free closure so that the repair will not break down postoperatively as healing causes contraction. Because there is no elastic tissue in septal mucosa, methods that rely on septal advancement without adequate mobilization usually fail because the graft will not stretch. The open external rhinoplasty approach provides the necessary access and exposure for adequate mobilization and development of mucosal flaps, which are advanced into place without an attempt to stretch the flaps. By using sliding bipedicle or unipedicle flaps, usually from the floor of the nose and under the inferior turbinates, the surgeon can close the mucosal portion of the perforation with normal nasal respiratory mucosa. Because these flaps have a blood supply, their success rate is much higher than that of any composite graft that may not vascularize. In addition to

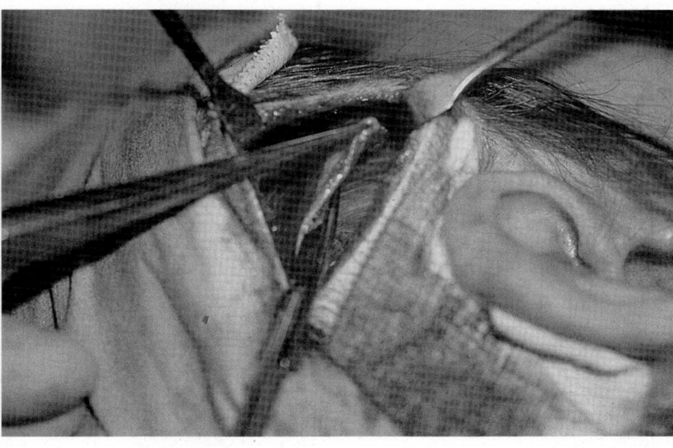
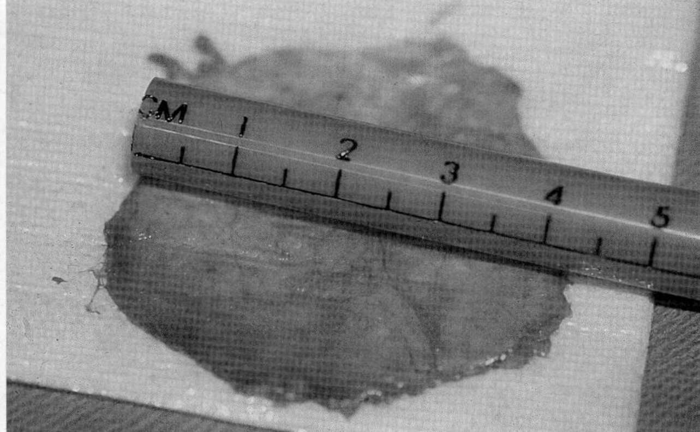

Fig. 51.4 (**A**) The temporalis fascia as it is being harvested. (**B**) A 4 × 4 cm piece of temporalis fascia spread out to dry prior to insertion between the mucoperichondral flaps.

closing the perforation in each mucoperichondrial flap, it is absolutely critical that a connective tissue interposition graft be placed between the flaps at the perforation repair site to prevent recommunication and reperforation, and to act as a continuous surface in which the edges of the sewn perforation can migrate and mucosalize closed. This method of mucosalized flaps with an interposition graft has been described with more than a 90% success rate in perforations of 2 to 3 cm by several authors, including Fairbanks,[9] Gollom,[10] Wright and Kridel,[11] and Goodman and Strelzow.[12] As perforations increase in size, the chances for their successful closure decrease proportionately and patients need to be so informed. Romo et al[13] described a method of tissue expansion by which to create larger advancement flaps for closure of these more difficult large perforations. Murrell[14] even described a repair utilizing a forearm free flap that was anastomosed with the facial artery.

The anterior to posterior size of the perforation is not very important in closure because the tension of the closure is from the floor of the nose to the dorsum, which is perpendicular to this dimension. Therefore, the height of the perforation is the most helpful determinant for the possibility and success of repair. Furthermore, the absolute size of the perforation is not as important as the proportion of septal membrane remaining. Perforations that extend all the way up to the nasal dorsum or all the way back to the sphenoid are almost impossible to repair unless there is some small cuff of membrane to which the inferior advance flap can be sewn. A previous septoplasty may make the dissection of the adherent mucosal flaps more difficult if a large amount of septal cartilage has been removed, and such dissection can lead to further worsening of the perforation during envelope separation. Adhesions between the remaining septal membranes and the lateral nasal wall or turbinates may need to be lysed during a separate preceding procedure with the placement of Silastic sheeting (Dow Corning, Midland, MI) on the septum for several weeks to prevent reformation prior to the attempt at perforation repair.

Graft Selection

Many types of connective tissue grafts have been used to interpose between the repaired septal flaps; these include mastoid periosteum, temporalis fascia, pericranium, septal bone or cartilage, fascia lata, and, most recently, acellular dermal allografts.[15] Interposing such a connective tissue graft between the repaired septal flaps helps to strengthen the repair and acts as a scaffold for the mucosa to creep on during the healing phase; this is especially important in cases where complete closure of the mucosal defect was not possible. Currently, the most commonly used grafts are the temporalis fascia and the dermal allografts (**Figs. 51.4 and 51.5**). The temporalis

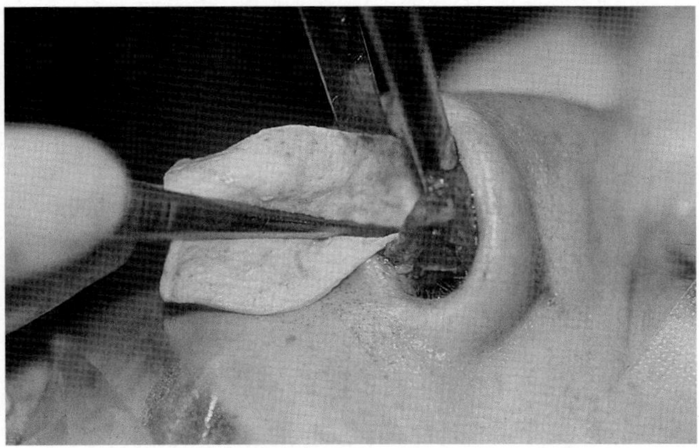

Fig. 51.5 AlloDerm (LifeCell Corp., Branchburg, NJ) is shown being inserted between the mucoperichondral flaps as an interposition acellular dermal graft.

fascia is harvested through a horizontal temporal incision, and the incision is beveled to parallel the hair shafts to avoid injury to the hair follicles. Dissection is taken down to the deep temporal fascia. Injection of saline under the deep temporal fascia helps to elevate it off the temporalis muscle. A curved scissor is used to harvest the graft, which should be considerably larger than the septal perforation as the perforation itself may get enlarged during the process of flap dissection. After complete hemostasis is achieved, the temporal incision is closed in two layers and a mastoid-type pressure dressing is applied.

Surgical Approaches

The endonasal approach to perforation repair has been popularized by David Fairbanks.[7] This method is associated with a high success rate but is extremely difficult, especially in large perforations or in patients with small nostril apertures. When more exposure is needed, Fairbanks does a lateral alotomy, which has the potential for a visible incision. The external rhinoplasty approach is quite advantageous in that it provides access to not only the anterior but also the superior and posterior aspects of the perforation. This provides increased surgical exposure and visualization and avoids distortion that normal intranasal retraction can cause. Furthermore, as no transfixion incision is made, the anterior septal blood and lymphatic supply is preserved, which may improve nasal advancement flap viability. With the external technique, one approaches the caudal end of the septum by totally separating the medial crura from themselves and from the septum. This process cuts the normal fibrous connections between the medial crura, the septum, and the overlying skin, which normally help to support and preserve tip projection. The careful surgeon must reconstitute tip-support mechanisms after the perforation is repaired not only by sewing the medial crura back together with interrupted sutures but also at times by placing a columellar strut.

Surgical Technique

The patient is placed in the supine position. After an adequate level of general oral endotracheal anesthesia is obtained, an oral pharyngeal throat pack is placed to prevent any blood from trickling down into the esophagus and stomach, thus reducing the chance of any postoperative nausea. The nose and septum are then infiltrated with 1% xylocaine with 1:100,000 units of epinephrine. Time is allowed to elapse for the vasoconstrictive and anesthetic effect of the infiltrated solution while the patient is prepped and draped in the usual sterile fashion. Careful intranasal examination is done, and any intranasal synechia or hypertrophied turbinates are dealt with at this stage.

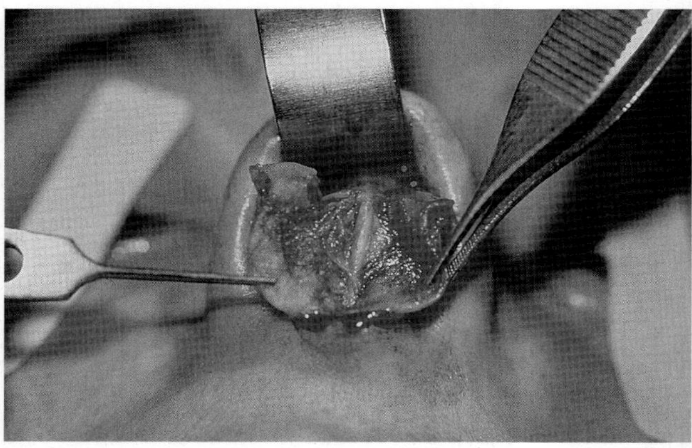

Fig. 51.6 Intraoperative photograph showing the dissection and spreading apart of the medial crura to gain access to the caudal part of the septal cartilage.

A classic external rhinoplasty approach is performed whereby bilateral alar marginal incisions are started laterally along the caudal edge of the lateral crus, and dissection is continued medially down the length of the columella where the incisions are connected via an inverted V-shaped transcolumellar incision. The columellar skin is elevated off the medial crura and skin dissection is continued upward, with care taken to stay in the supraperichondrial avascular plane until reaching the nasal bones where the periosteum is elevated using a Joseph-type periosteal elevator. Dissection is performed between the medial crura to gain access to the caudal septal cartilage followed by bilateral caudal septal membrane elevation in a strict submucoperichondrial plane (**Fig. 51.6**). Septal flap elevation is continued upward until reaching the cartilaginous edge of the perforation where an increased resistance is met during the dissection due to the adherence of the septal flaps to each other with no intervening cartilage. At this stage the dissection is taken downward to elevate the mucosa off the maxillary crest, nasal floor, and laterally until reaching the root of the inferior turbinate. Any bleeding encountered from the penetrating vessels at the maxillary crest should be cauterized using an insulated-tip suction cautery. After completing the nasal-floor flap elevation a posterior-to-anterior backcut incision is made using a no. 15 blade at the root of the inferior turbinate, thus creating a bipedicled mucosal flap that is attached both anteriorly and posteriorly to preserve its vascular supply (**Fig. 51.7**). This flap could be mobilized medially and upward on both sides of the nasal septum to facilitate checking the amount of mucosal redundancy provided by the created flaps. In larger perforations, the inferior advancement floor flaps alone cannot provide enough mucosa for closure, and a superiorly based flap may also be needed. In these cases, the septal flap elevation is continued dorsally between the superior edge of the perforation and the upper lateral cartilages. The upper

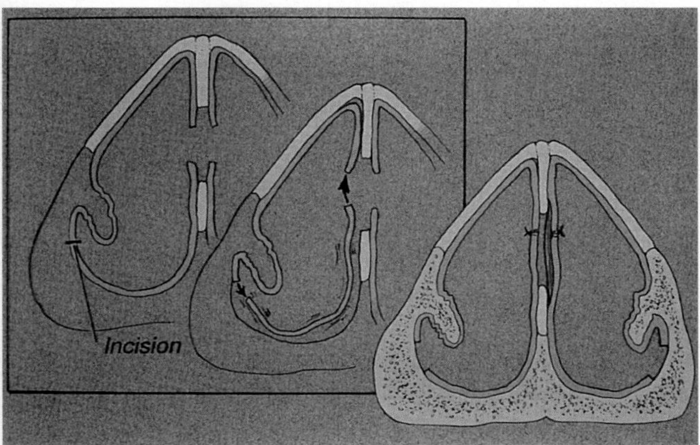

Fig. 51.7 The effect of making a floor/inferior turbinate flap with advancement of the mucosal floor flap toward the septum to close the perforation. (From Kridel R. The open approach for repair of septal perforations. In: Daniel RK, ed. Aesthetic Plastic Surgery: Rhinoplasty. Boston: Little Brown & Company; 1993:555–556. Reprinted by permission.)

lateral cartilages are then sharply separated from the septum extramucosally (**Fig. 51.8**). The roof flap that now bridges between the superior edge of the perforation and the undersurface of the upper lateral cartilage could be dropped downward to help in closing the mucosal perforation on each side.

In cases involving large perforations, more length could be added to the roof flap by extending the dissection to include the mucoperichondrium of the undersurface of the upper lateral cartilage. In exceptionally large perforations, a back-cut could be made in the mucosa under the upper lateral cartilage, thus transforming the roof flap into a bipedicled flap allowing more downward advancement. This can only be performed on one side for fear that the dorsal cartilaginous septum would be exposed bilaterally.

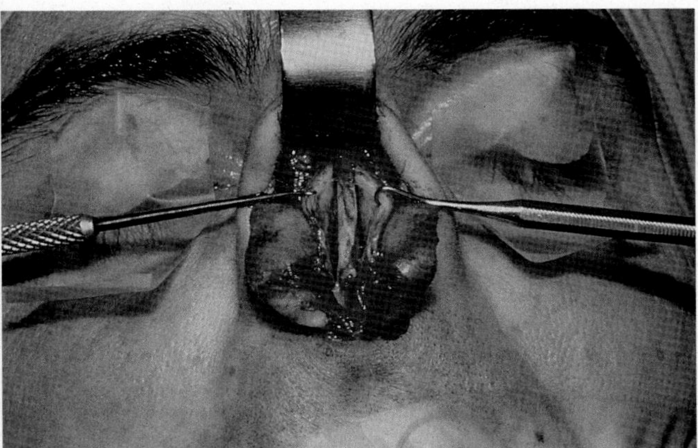

Fig. 51.8 The upper lateral cartilages are sharply cut away from the septum to provide improved access to the perforation. The mucoperichondrium is left intact and attached to the undersurface of the upper lateral cartilage.

Loss of cartilaginous viability in the cartilaginous dorsal area may result in dorsal saddling or a high perforation.

Only after completion of the roof and floor flaps can the mucosal perforation be opened from the front, using a broad exposure technique and careful dissection to avoid enlargement of the existing perforation. Dissection must proceed posteriorly for at least 1 cm back behind the perforation, and any residual bony cartilaginous deviations can be corrected at this time.

Once enough mucosal laxity has been provided by these advancement flaps, the perforation in each mucoperichondrial flap is closed, under no tension, using interrupted sutures of either 4–0 or 5–0 chromic or plain gut sutures (**Fig. 51.9**). Any granulation tissue or scarring that is present at the periphery of the perforation should be removed prior to suturing to provide fresh edges that would be more likely to heal. At this point, the temporalis fascia graft, the pericranium, or the human acellular dermal graft is utilized. The interposition graft is then placed between the mucoperichondrial flaps and brought back posteriorly at least 1 cm beyond the closed perforation. The graft should then be stabilized to prevent postoperative movement by utilizing a few individual sutures to affix it directly to the septal cartilage remnant. After fixation, the grafting site should be inspected to

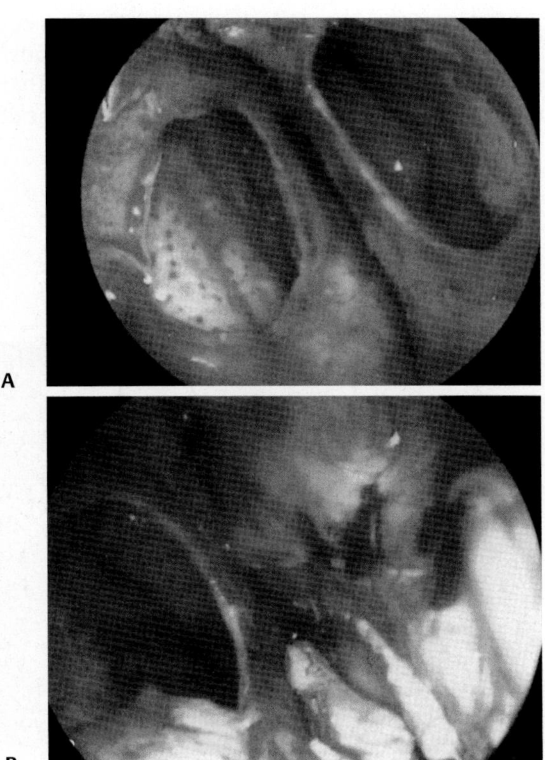

Fig. 51.9 (**A**) The mucoperichondral flaps, separated with the perforation in each flap, are readily seen. (**B**) The perforation sutured closed on one side with dark marks identifying the interrupted sutures.

ensure that the center of the closed perforation is well covered by the graft.

The upper lateral cartilages must then be resutured to the septum. If the perforation was large and required superior advancement flaps, it may be difficult to reattach the upper lateral cartilages to the septum at their original height and at the same time avoid tension on the newly closed perforation site. The surgeon may be forced to resecure the upper lateral cartilages to the septum at a lower level, with the potential cosmetic outcome being a pinched appearance to the nasal dorsum. The pinched appearance results from the upper laterals being lower than the central septal dorsum. Recognition of this potential problem would necessitate placing cartilaginous onlay grafts over the reset upper lateral cartilages to provide better dorsal symmetry. If a reduction rhinoplasty was performed at the same time, this problem would be less of an issue.

The intranasal septal flaps must then be mattressed together reapproximating both flaps and sandwiching the interposition graft. Mattressing the septum aids in the healing of the perforation and speeds the revascularization of the graft. It furthermore helps to prevent the occurrence of a postoperative hematoma. The mattress stitch is usually a 4–0 chromic suture and a continuous suture technique is utilized (**Fig. 51.10**). The needle must be extremely sharp so that it passes freely through not only the flaps, but also the graft and causes little displacement of the interposition graft. Mattress sutures must be used above and below the repaired perforation so that the sutures are placed in a perpendicular plane to that of the perforation repair. This suture technique strengthens and reinforces closure.

As noted previously, resupport of the nasal tip support mechanisms is crucial.[4] The medial crura must be resewn together with or without a columellar strut. The nose should also be evaluated at this time to see if there has been any unwanted rotation of the tip due to tension of the closure, or continuity of the septal flaps with the mucosa of the medial crura. If unwanted rotation and shortening of the nose have occurred, the surgeon may use a caudal septal replacement graft to lengthen the nose or place a large cartilaginous batten in front of the medial crura to camouflage such rotation. A tip graft can also be added that does not extend above the dorsum and so provides extra length to the tip without increased rotation or projection. The dome cartilages must then be sewn together with permanent sutures, reconstructing the dome complex and preventing postoperative bossae. At completion of the rhinoplasty part of the procedure, the nasal skin is redraped to its normal anatomical position and the external rhinoplasty incisions are closed. The transcolumellar incision is closed using a deep 6–0 polydioxanone suture to take the tension off the skin edges, which are then approximated using a combination of interrupted 6–0 polypropylene sutures and 6–0 fast-absorbing plain gut in a running locking fashion. The marginal incision is closed on each side using a 5–0 plain suture.

To protect the repaired septal flaps during their healing phase, 0.020-in.-thick polymeric silicone sheeting (Silastic) is placed on both sides of the septal flaps, covering almost

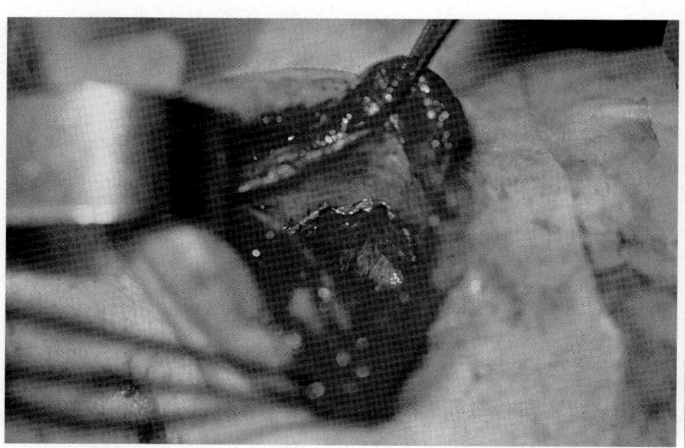

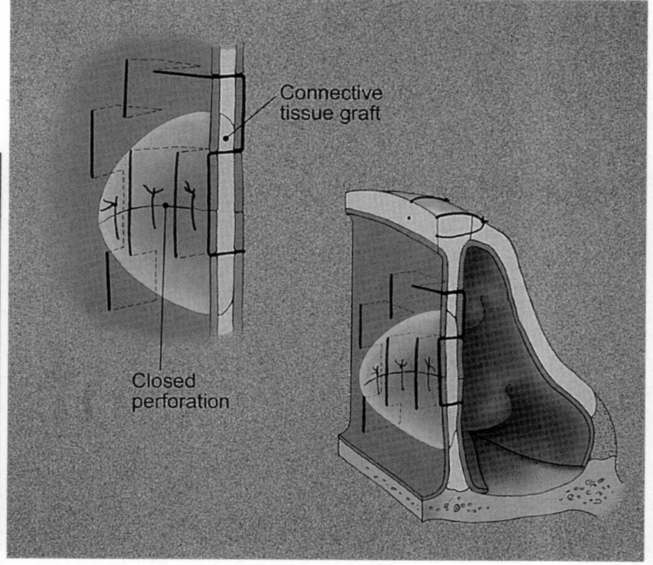

Fig. 51.10 (**A**) In this case, the temporalis fascia graft is shown covering the cartilage perforation and has been sewn to the surrounding septal cartilage to prevent migration. (**B**) The interposition graft is centered under the closed perforation. Mattress sutures go through both mucosal flaps and the graft to prevent migration of the graft, to hold the graft in apposition to the flaps as an aid in healing, and to prevent postoperative bleeding or hematoma formation.

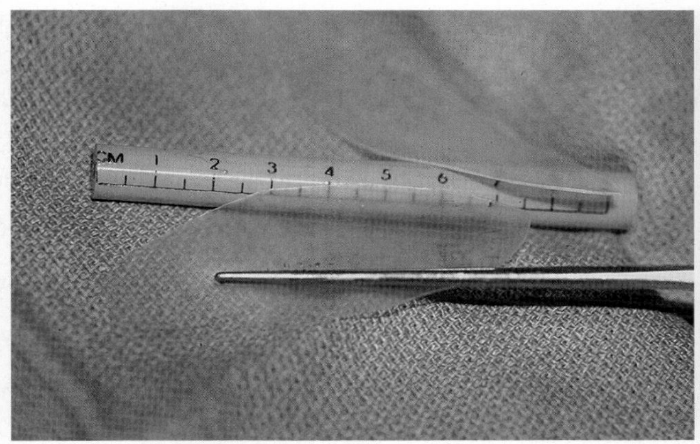

A

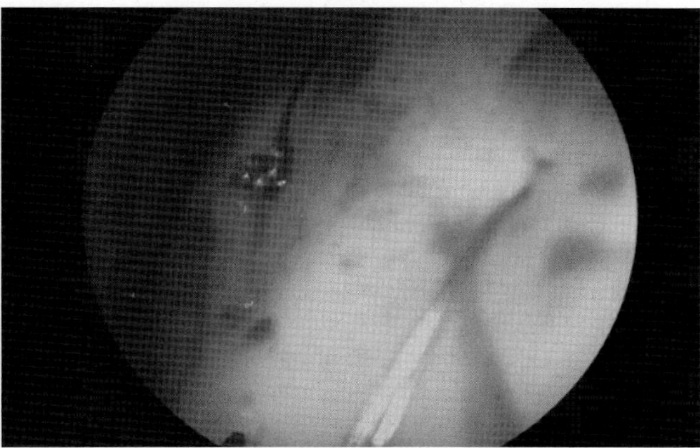

B

Fig. 51.11 (**A**) Clear 0.02-in.-thick silicone soft sheeting that is shaped to cover the perforation repair on each side of the septum. (**B**) The silicone sheeting sewn into place with three through-and-through mattress sutures of 5–0 Prolene. Care was taken not to constrict the flaps and compromise the blood supply. One can easily monitor the healing of the septal perforation repair through these transparent sheets.

all of the septum on each side, and is secured into place by approximately three 5–0 nonabsorbable sutures (**Fig. 51.11**). These sutures should not be overly tight so as not to constrict the blood supply to the septum. Because the polymeric silicone sheets are transparent, the repair site can be visualized postoperatively with monitoring of the healing mucosa. Monitoring of the protected repaired site is especially helpful if the surgeon is unable to close the perforation fully. The sheeting protects the graft site from air flow drying and keeps the area moist to accelerate the healing process. The nose is then very lightly packed with Gelfoam (Pfizer Inc., New York, NY) strips underneath the inferior turbinates, followed by a small Telfa pack (Kendall, Mansfield, MA) impregnated with antibiotic cream. If too much packing is placed, vascular compromise of the repair site could ensue as nasal swelling develops. The Gelfoam is additionally helpful because it absorbs any bleeding as the result of the development of the bipedicled flaps. The nose is then externally taped and splinted, whether or not any dorsal modifications, osteotomies, or grafts have been used. Elevation of the open rhinoplasty flap creates a potential space for blood accumulation and fibrosis postoperatively, and a standard external splint must be placed for prevention. A drip pad is placed, and the patient is then extugated by anesthesia.

Postoperative Care

All patients are told that there will probably be some bloody discharge postoperatively because of the raw areas underneath the inferior turbinates. This nasal discharge often subsides after the first 24 hours.

On the first postoperative day, the Telfa packs are removed and the Gelfoam is usually left in place. No attempt is made to remove all of the Gelfoam on the first postoperative day.

The patient is instructed to use saline nose drops three to four times per day. This helps to keep the Gelfoam moist and allows easier suctioning over the next 7 to 10 days. Using cotton-tipped applicators, the patient is encouraged to place antibacterial ointment in the nose to prevent postoperative crusting. The external nasal splint is usually removed ~5 to 7 days later, and then the nose is usually retaped for another 5 days. The nonabsorbable columellar sutures are removed on about the fifth day.

Careful examination of the site of the previous perforation is performed through the clear Silastic sheeting at each visit. In most cases, we leave the sheeting in place for 3 weeks, but we will prolong that time if the perforation does not appear to be fully healed. If upon removal of the Silastic sheeting we discover a small area that is unhealed, the patient is instructed to keep this area moist, using antibacterial ointment three to four times per day in addition to a saline mist.

The patient is instructed not to use any vasoconstrictive sprays, to refrain from smoking, and to avoid noxious fumes during the postoperative phase. Blowing of the nose is also to be avoided for the first month postoperatively.

If the patient had a temporalis fascia graft harvested, the drain is removed on the first day, the pressure dressing is maintained for 2 or 3 additional days, and the sutures are removed in ~7 to 10 days.

Outcomes

The successful outcome of this operation is dependent on many factors, including the cause of the perforation, size and location of the perforation, surgical skill of the operating physician, and cooperation of the patient postoperatively. If one has not been successful in totally closing the perforation, it is usually made smaller with this surgery. If complete closure is not likely, all perforations should be closed from an anterior-to-posterior direction, moving the perforation more posteriorly, thus decreasing the patient's symptoms. A repeat operation can be attempted in ~6 months, if necessary.

After the perforation has healed completely, the patient can experience the same satisfaction as the physician in the successful closure. Photographic documentation once again can assist the patient in understanding this difficult and complex problem and in seeing the successful outcome. It is remarkable to observe how well the septum heals with little or no evidence of previous perforation.

References

1. Belmont JR. An approach to large nasoseptal perforations and attendant deformity. Arch Otolaryngol Head Neck Surg 1985;3:450–455
2. Kuriloff DB. Nasal septal perforations and nasal obstructions. Otolaryngol Clin North Am 1989;22:333–350
3. Kridel RWH. Combined septal perforation repair with revision rhinoplasty. Facial Plast Surg Clin North Am 1995;3:459–472
4. Kridel RWH. Septal perforation repair. Otolaryngol Clin North Am 1999;32(4):695–724
5. Trenite GJN, Verwoerd CDA, Verhoef V. Reimplantation of autologous septal cartilage in the growing nasal septum. Rhinology 1987;25:225–236
6. Schoelzel EP, Menzel ML. Nasal sprays and perforation of the nasal septum. JAMA 1985;253:2046
7. Fairbanks DN. Nasal septal perforation repair: twenty-five-year experience with the flap and graft technique. Am J Cosmet Surg 1994;11:189–194
8. Adler D, Ritz E. Perforation of the nasal septum in patients with renal failure. Laryngoscope 1980;90:317–321
9. Fairbanks DN. Closure of nasal septal perforations. Arch Otolaryngol Head Neck Surg 1980;106:509–513
10. Gollom J. Perforation of the nasal septum, the reverse flap technique. Arch Otolaryngol Head Neck Surg 1968;888:518–522
11. Kridel RWH, Appling D, Wright W. Closure of septal perforations: a simplified method via the external septorhinoplasty approach. In: Ward P, Berman W, eds. Plastic and Reconstructive Surgery of the Head and Neck: Proceedings of the Fourth International Symposium, Los Angeles, 1983. Vol 1. St. Louis: CV Mosby; 1984:183–188
12. Goodman WS, Strelzow VV. The surgical closure of nasoseptal perforations. Laryngoscope 1982;92:121–124
13. Romo T III, Jablonski RD, Shapiro AJ, McCormick SA. Long-term nasal mucosal tissue expansion using repair of large nasoseptal perforations. Arch Otolaryngol Head Neck Surg 1995;121:327
14. Murrell GL, Karakla DW, Messa A. Free flap repair of septal perforation. Plast Reconstr Surg 1988;818–821
15. Kridel RWH, Foda H, Lunde K. Septal perforation repair with acellular human dermal allograft. Arch Otolaryngol Head Neck Surg 1998;124:73–78

IV

Reconstructive Surgery of the Face and Neck

52 Diagnosis and Treatment of Cutaneous Malignancies

John D. Hendrix Jr. and Craig L. Slingluff

Cutaneous malignancies, which are the most common cancers in the world, include melanoma and nonmelanoma skin cancers, principally squamous cell carcinoma (SCC) and basal cell carcinoma (BCC). These tumors originate from the upper layer of the skin, called the epidermis. Many factors can play a role in the development of skin cancer, but exposure of the epidermis to ultraviolet (UV) radiation—principally from sunlight—is the most important factor. Less common cutaneous malignancies can arise from the deeper layers—the dermis and subcutaneous fat—or from other structures, such as hair follicles, sebaceous glands, eccrine glands, blood vessels, and nerves. Sometimes skin cancers are misdiagnosed because they mimic benign growths that arise from these structures in the skin.

The incidence of skin cancer in the United States is approaching epidemic proportions. Currently, one in five Americans will develop a skin cancer during his or her lifetime.[1] There are now over one million cases of nonmelanoma skin cancer in the United States annually.[2] It is predicted that one in 75 individuals in the United States will develop melanoma by the year 2000.[1] It is postulated that the increase in incidence of skin cancer may be explained by changes in lifestyle or depletion of the ozone layer, which filters out the carcinogenic UV radiation from sunlight.[3] Epidemiological studies suggest that an individual who develops a skin cancer is more likely to develop not only additional skin cancers but other internal malignancies, such as lung cancer.[4–6] An individual who develops one nonmelanoma skin cancer has an estimated risk of developing one or more additional skin cancers of 35% at 3 years and 50% at 5 years.[7]

In this chapter, we will focus on the diagnosis and treatment of skin cancer, particularly SCC and BCC. The biology and histology of these neoplasms will be included when relevant to management. Other unusual cutaneous malignancies will also be reviewed.

Squamous Cell Carcinoma

Epidemiological and Etiologic Factors

Cutaneous SCC, a malignant tumor of keratinizing epidermal cells, is the second leading cause of skin cancer death after melanoma and the second most common type of skin cancer after BCC.[8] The incidence of SCC, and all skin cancer, is increasing. SCC has been found to occur on all cutaneous surfaces but most often occurs on the sun-exposed areas of the head and neck. In the United States, one study estimated a fourfold increase in SCC incidence in men and a 15-fold increase in women from 1977 to 1994.[9]

The cause of SCC is multifactorial. Exposure to sunlight, fair skin, and reduced immunity are major risk factors. Certain environmental exposures and medical conditions are associated with an increased risk of SCC. When many predisposing elements are present in a patient, such as high cumulative sun exposure, fair skin, and immunosuppression (which many organ transplant patients have), the likelihood of developing SCC is extremely high.

The principal cause of SCC is ultraviolet (UV) radiation from sunlight. The majority of SCCs occur in elderly, fair-complexioned Caucasians who have had years of sun exposure.[10] Pigmentation plays an important role in protecting the skin from UV radiation; therefore, skin cancer is uncommon in individuals with dark pigmentation. Clinical signs of chronic sun exposure that can be used to identify those at risk for SCC and skin cancer in general include freckling, telangiectasia, atrophy, rhytides, and precancerous lesions.[11,12] People who are engaged in an outdoor occupation or recreation, live close to the equator (where the sun is more intense), or are elderly (with more cumulative exposure to UV radiation) are at higher risk for the development of SCC.[13] Both epidemiological and experimental evidence points to UV-B as the major component in sunlight responsible for causing cutaneous SCC.[14–16] UV-A may also play a role in the development of SCC, particularly when a photosensitizer is used.[14]

Chemical exposure to organic hydrocarbons, pesticides, and arsenic (most commonly in contaminated well water) can be associated with the development of SCC.[17–19] Ionizing radiation can be associated with SCC.[20] Cigarette smoking has also been shown to be a risk factor for development of SCC.[21] Certain genetic disorders and syndromes (such as xeroderma pigmentosum and albinism) are also associated with the development of SCC.[22–24] Chronic skin conditions, such as draining sinuses, burn scars,[25] ulceration, and infection, can also be associated with the development of SCC.[18]

Impaired cell-mediated immunity (either drug- or disease-induced) is linked with the development of cutaneous SCC. Organ transplant patients requiring chronic immunosuppressant medications, such as cyclosporine, azathioprine, and prednisone, are at increased risk for SCC. T-cell depletion (particularly CD4± T cells) is associated with increased risk of skin cancer in long-term renal transplant recipients.[26] The incidence of malignancy increases with time after transplantation. One study showed the overall risk for a transplant patient to develop a first skin cancer increased from 10% after 10 years to 40% after 20 years of graft survival.[27] In one study of heart transplant patients, SCC was the predominant skin malignancy, constituting 90% of the lesions. Another study showed the mean number of skin malignancies per transplant patient to be greater than four, with some patients having more than 100 cutaneous cancers.[28,29] Development of SCC is also more common in diseases with impaired cell-mediated immunity, such as lymphoma or leukemia,[30,31] autoimmune disease,[32] and epidermodysplasia verruciformis (a rare hereditary immune deficiency in which human papillomavirus is associated with SCC).[33]

Clinical Characteristics and Precursors

The most common precursor to SCC is the actinic keratosis (AK). AKs, also called solar keratoses, are sun-induced precancerous lesions. These scaly, circumscribed, rough, erythematous lesions are often better recognized by palpation than inspection. They are typically found on the head and neck of many middle-aged and elderly individuals (**Fig. 52.1**). They are usually asymptomatic, but the patient may occasionally complain of itching or tenderness. Size varies from pinpoint size to large plaques, but they usually are 3 to 6 mm in diameter. AKs are clinical markers of long-term sun exposure, a major risk factor for nonmelanoma skin cancer, and may be the most significant predictor for a person's developing cutaneous SCC.[34] Although AKs are biologically considered to be premalignant, histologically they appear to represent early SCC in situ.[35] About 20% of AKs will spontaneously involute.[36] An AK can evolve into SCC with the potential for metastases when there is active growth with invasion into the dermis. Malignant conversion has been estimated to be on the order of a 1 in 1000 chance per year and may involve p53 mutations.[37,38] Hyperkeratotic AKs may have a higher rate of malignant transformation.[39]

Another less common precursor to invasive SCC often associated with AKs is Bowen's disease (SCC in situ). Histologically, one sees malignant cells filling the epidermis but not invading the dermis. Clinically, Bowen's disease most often appears as a single erythematous, slightly scaly, minimally indurated patch that can be mistaken for eczema, fungus, or psoriasis (**Fig. 52.2**). There can sometimes be multiple areas on a background of sun damage and AKs. The lesions measure from millimeters to centimeters. Bowen's disease is most commonly found on the trunk. Any induration or hyperkeratotic thickening should alert the clinician to the possibility of invasive SCC in that area and a biopsy should be done.

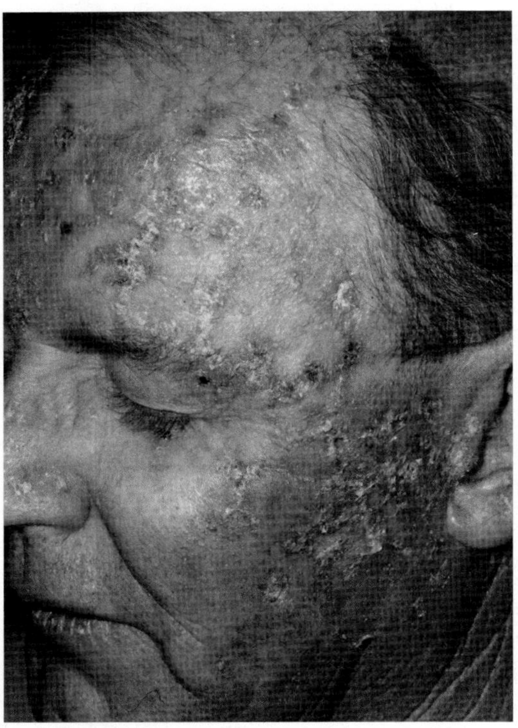

Fig. 52.1 Severely sun-damaged skin and multiple actinic keratoses on the left side of the face.

Invasive SCC typically presents on the sun-exposed areas of the head, neck, and arms. They can arise de novo or from preexisting AKs. Clinically, SCC most often presents as a hyperkeratotic growth or a crusted, indurated papule

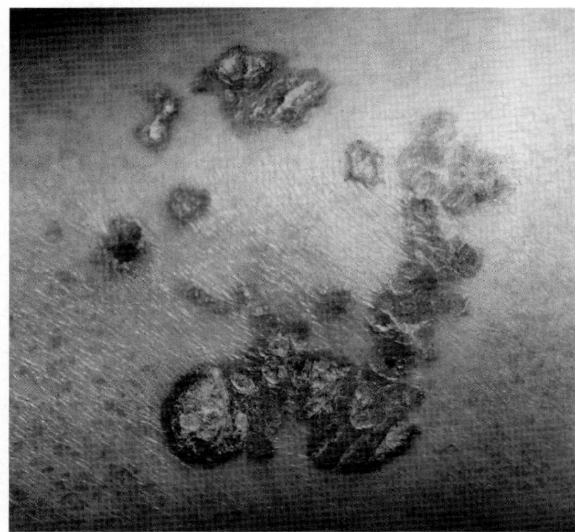

Fig. 52.2 Bowen's disease (squamous cell carcinoma in situ) on the trunk. These lesions could be mistaken for psoriasis, eczema, or fungus.

carcinoma syndrome. UV radiation–induced mutations in the human *PATCHED* gene have also been implicated in sporadic cases of BCC as well as nevoid basal cell carcinoma syndrome.[57]

Clinical Characteristics and Precursors

There is no common clinical precursor to BCC as there is with SCC. BCC typically occurs on sun-exposed areas, especially the head and neck, in particular the nose. Patients often present with a nonhealing "sore" of varying duration. Bleeding on slight injury is a common sign. Some BCCs heal spontaneously and form scar tissue as they extend. The lesions are sometimes itchy but often asymptomatic. There is gradual enlargement, with the tumor roughly doubling its 6-month volume at 1 year and quadrupling it at the end of 2 years.[58]

BCC can have a variety of clinical appearances, such as nodular, pigmented, cystic, or superficial. Nodular BCC is the most common variety and is usually composed of one or a few small, waxy, semitranslucent "pearly" papules or nodules that sometimes form around a central depression (**Fig. 52.6**). The tumor may be eroded, ulcerated, crusted, or bleeding. The trauma necessary for ulceration is usually slight, and patients frequently insist that the lesion is a scratch or razor nick. The edges of larger lesions have a characteristic rolled or raised border and are well circumscribed. Telangiectasias are visible coursing through the lesion. BCC may also be pigmented with brown or black pigmentation. Pigmented BCCs are seen more commonly in dark-skinned individuals and can mimic a mole or even a melanoma (**Fig. 52.7**). Cystic BCCs (**Fig. 52.8**) are filled with fluid that makes them look translucent blue-gray. These cystic nodules may mimic benign cystic lesions, especially around the eye where they may be confused with hidrocystomas. Superficial BCCs (**Fig. 52.9**) usually are pink to reddish brown scaly macules or plaques, seen occasionally with central clearing. Ulceration is less common than in nodular BCC. Superficial BCCs are more common on the trunk where they can be multiple. There is little tendency to become invasive. Superficial BCC may mimic psoriasis, fungus, or eczema. Occurrence of numerous superficial BCCs may be a clue to arsenic exposure.

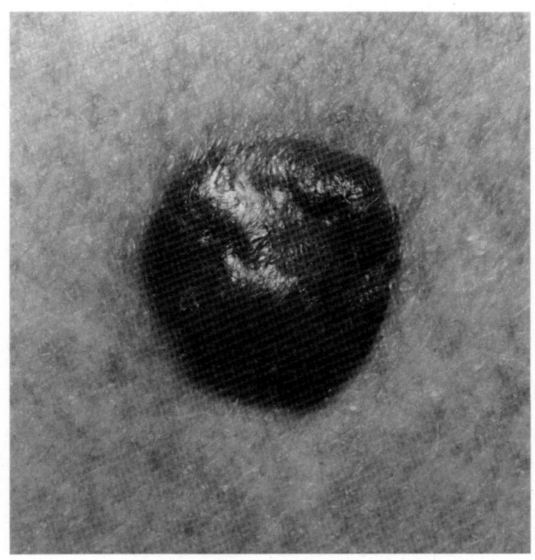

Fig. 52.7 Pigmented basal cell carcinoma on the trunk. One might mistake this growth for a melanoma.

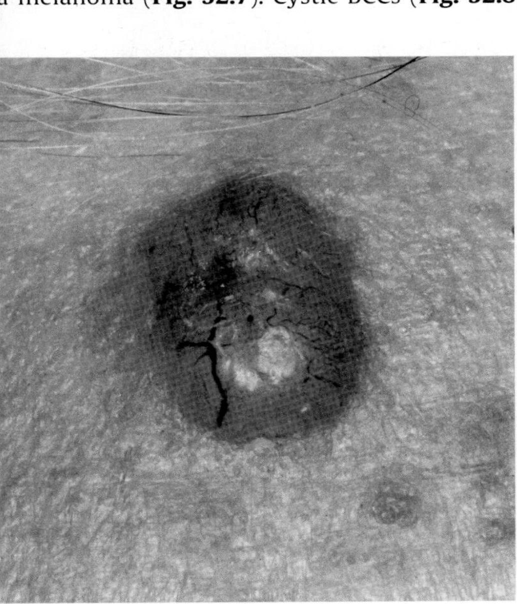

Fig. 52.6 Nodular basal cell carcinoma on the left forehead. Note the pearliness, well-circumscribed border, and telangiectasia.

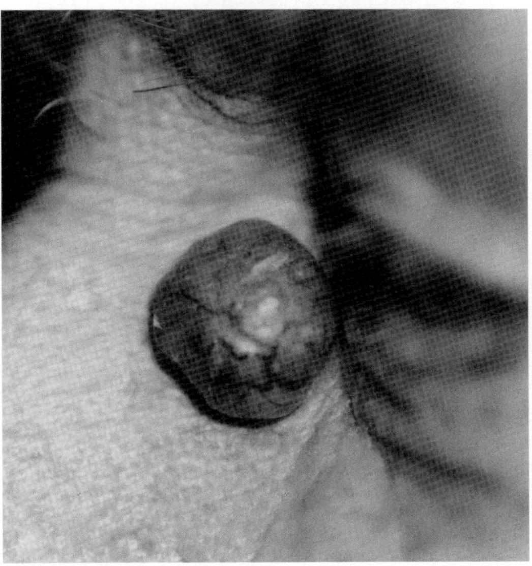

Fig. 52.8 Cystic basal cell carcinoma on the left medial canthus/nose.

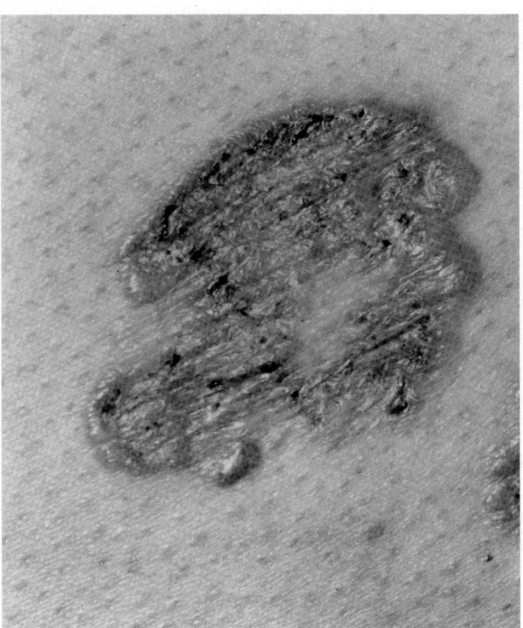

Fig. 52.9 Superficial basal cell carcinoma on the trunk, which could be mistaken for a patch of eczema, fungus, or psoriasis. Note the scaly crusted surface, pearliness, and well-defined borders.

BCCs can also have the appearance of pale, flat, smooth-surfaced plaques or macules that are typically ill defined (**Fig. 52.10**). They are usually referred to as "aggressive" BCCs because they have ill-defined borders with deeper extension of tumor that cannot be detected clinically. They are also called "sclerosing" BCCs because they can masquerade as a scar. Telangiectasia, ulceration, erosion, scaling, and crusting are often absent. Clinically this tumor appears as a yellowish white, indurated plaque with ill-defined borders. This is in contrast to nodular BCCs, which usually have well-defined borders. Oftentimes this deeper growth of aggressive BCC goes undetected for a long period and there is enormous destruction of normal tissue by the time the tumor is discovered. This hidden growth is referred to as subclinical extension. Subclinical extension refers to the portion of a tumor that is present histologically but cannot be detected clinically. Even if the border is seemingly well defined, a tumor can invisibly extend far beyond clinically apparent margins. BCCs with subclinical extension may appear yellowish white when the skin is stretched and be firm to the touch (**Fig. 52.11**). Significant subclinical extension is most commonly seen with the morpheaform, infiltrating, and micronodular histological subtypes, to be discussed under "Biological Behavior and Risk Factors."

When examining possible skin cancers, it is best to use good lighting and magnification. The affected skin should be stretched, squeezed, and palpated to better estimate the tumor size and depth (**Figs. 52.10 and 52.11**). Oblique illumination of the tumor can highlight surface changes

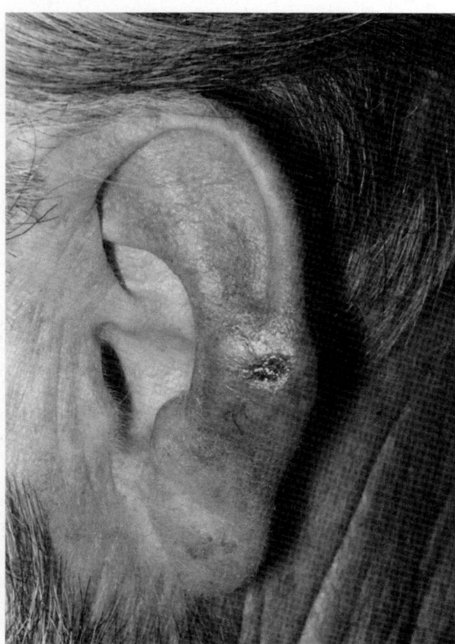

Fig. 52.10 "Aggressive" basal cell carcinoma (infiltrative histology) on the left helix. Note the ill-defined border and white, scar-like appearance.

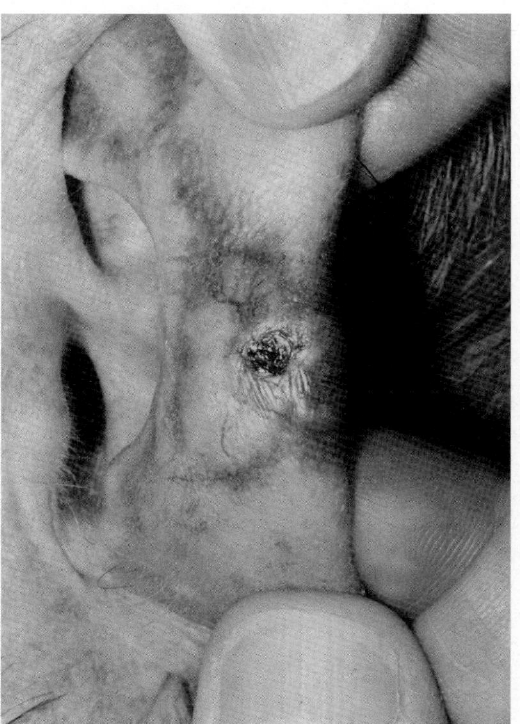

Fig. 52.11 The same basal cell carcinoma as shown in Fig. 52.10. Note that the clinical extent of tumor becomes more evident when the skin is stretched.

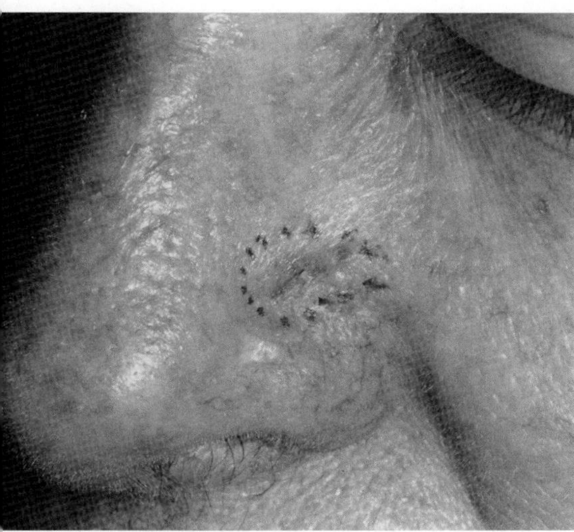

ig. 52.12 A basal cell carcinoma (nodular-infiltrative histology) on he left ala (before Mohs micrographic excision). Gentian violet dots utline the extent of tumor that could be detected clinically.

uch as a "rolled" border. A gentian violet pen can be sed to mark the clinical margin of the tumor. Occasion- lly, the true extent of the tumor can be grossly under- stimated because of subclinical extension (**Figs. 52.12 nd 52.13**).

iological Behavior and Risk Factors

ike SCC, BCC is a locally growing neoplasm that is usu- lly easily diagnosed and treated. In some cases, BCC may nfiltrate the surrounding skin and adjacent structures. lthough the clinical appearance of the BCC can alert the clinician to the possibility of subclinical extension, the histological appearance of the BCC obtained from a generous skin biopsy (see "Biopsy Techniques" discussed under "Melanoma") can more accurately predict which BCC will have a greater chance of incomplete surgical removal (and subsequent recurrence).[59] The micronodular, infiltrative, and morpheaform histological subtypes of BCC can be more difficult to detect clinically and to eradicate than the nodular histological subtype of BCC because of the patterns of growth within the skin. Micronodular, infiltrative, and morpheaform BCCs grow in a dispersed pattern, enlarging beneath the epidermis by small, diffuse finger-like extensions that can permeate through tissue without much displacement of normal tissue. Extension from the epidermis is minimal so that there is little surface change to reveal the tumor during skin examination. In contrast, nodular BCCs have an aggregated pattern that enlarges in a circumscribed expansile manner, displacing more tissue and becoming more raised and clinically evident with time. BCC of any histological subtype can have malignant extension that is invisible to the eye, but micronodular, infiltrative, and morpheaform types are consistently deceptive and actually much larger than they appear clinically in comparison with nodular BCC.[60–63] Micronodular, infiltrative, and morpheaform BCCs often need larger excision margins to effect complete removal of these subtypes.[64] The invisible portion of tumor may invade deeply into subcutaneous tissue, bone, and cartilage, causing extensive local destruction and mutilation.[65,66] Death from BCC is uncommon. Metastatic BCC is rare but more cases are being reported.[67,68] In a study of skin cancer mortality in Rhode Island from 1979 to 1987, there were 51 deaths from nonmelanoma skin cancer. Of these deaths, 20% were due to BCC, the mean age was 85 years, and refusal of surgical intervention was documented in 40%. BCCs that metastasize have almost always been subjected to repeated incomplete excisions or represent lesions that have been so neglected as to reach extremely large size without the benefit of treatment.[44] A BCC that metastasizes has an extremely poor prognosis; according to the English literature, the median survival of patients with metastatic basal cell carcinoma is 10 months.[68]

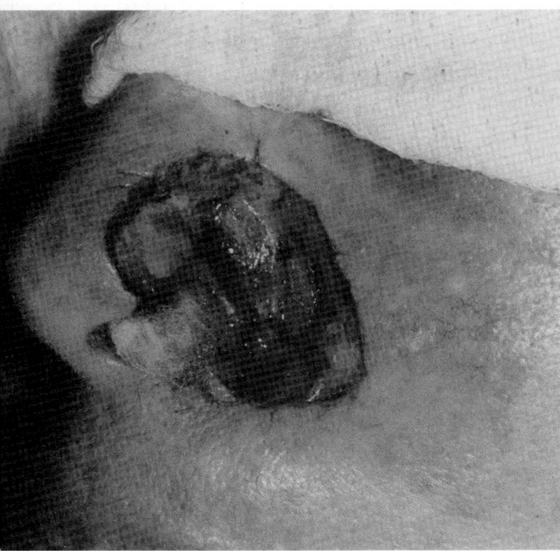

ig. 52.13 The same basal cell carcinoma in Fig. 52.12 but after Mohs nicrographic excision. Note the great quantity of tumor that could not e detected clinically (subclinical extension).

Treatment Options for SCC and BCC

Superficially destructive measures provide adequate treatment for AKs. Cryotherapy or the application of liquid nitrogen (with a temperature of –195°C) to the skin is most commonly used to destroy AKs. Other treatments include topical 5-fluorouracil cream, electrodesiccation and curettage, CO2 laser, dermabrasion, and chemical peel. If the AK is markedly hyperkeratotic and raised, then a shave or punch biopsy should be done to rule out the

Table 52.2 Treatment Options for Basal Cell Carcinoma and Squamous Cell Carcinoma

If one or more of these factors are present, then consider
Mohs micrographic excision:
Recurrent tumor
Tumor size 72 cm in diameter
Tumors with an aggressive histology (such as morpheaform, infiltrative, micronodular BCC, or poorly differentiated SCC)
Tumors with ill-defined margins
Tumors that are incompletely excised
Tumors with perineural invasion
Tumor location where maximal conservation of normal tissue is important (such as eyelid, nose, ear, lip, digit, genitalia)
Otherwise consider **standard excision** and use at least:
*4- to 6-mm margins to a depth of mid- to deep-subcutaneous tissue if small (62 cm) primary BCC/SCC with clinically well-defined borders and nonaggressive histology **OR** 7-mm margins to a depth that includes all of the subcutaneous tissue if factor(s) are present for consideration of Mohs but Mohs is unavailable or patient refuses Mohs.*
Radiation therapy should be considered if patient is a poor surgical candidate or refuses surgery. If Mohs or standard excision shows perineural invasion or positive margins, then radiation therapy should be considered as postoperative treatment.
Consider therapies other than radiation therapy if the patient has connective tissue disease (i.e., lupus, scleroderma) or patient is younger than 50 years.
Less commonly used modalities to consider if none of the above factors are present (these modalities are primarily used for superficial BCC and SCC on the trunk and extremities):
Cryosurgery
Curettage and electrodesiccation
Laser
Photodynamic therapy

Abbreviations: BCC, basal cell carcinoma; SCC, squamous cell carcinoma.

possibility of SCC. Those patients who develop AKs have had sufficient chronic photodamage to produce skin cancer, and regular skin cancer checks are recommended. Use of sunscreen has been shown to prevent the development of actinic keratoses and, possibly, future skin cancer.[69] Interestingly, a low-fat diet has been shown to reduce the incidence of AK.[70]

The choice of therapeutic modalities is the same for SCC and BCC (**Table 52.2**). Selection of the most appropriate therapy depends on many factors, including size of the tumor, location, whether the tumor is primary or recurrent (or incompletely treated), histology, and individual patient factors. Careful consideration of the options should be undertaken—especially with SCC, given the greater potential for morbidity and mortality. Standard treatment can be divided into excision and field therapy.

Excision of the tumor is followed by permanent or frozen sectioning of the specimen to check the margins. Field therapies destroy tissue in an area within and around the tumor, and the tissue is not evaluated histologically for margins. Commonly used field therapies include radiation therapy, cryosurgery, and curettage and electrodesiccation. Excision is the treatment of choice for most SCCs and BCCs. A standard excision is usually done under local anesthetic, and the tumor is removed with a margin of clinically normal-appearing skin. Selected vertical sections (either frozen or permanent) from the specimen are then examined microscopically to determine if margins are free of tumor. Unfortunately, this method samples less than 1% of the true surgical margin, leaving the possibility that the examined sections may not include areas in the specimen where there are tumor extensions. Despite this disadvantage, cure rates greater than 90% can be obtained in many cases with standard excision for SCC and BCC.[43,71] Although it is potentially dangerous to assign a "standard" margin, current surgical recommendations call for margins of 4 mm of healthy tissue in excision of nodular BCC and more than 7 mm in aggressive BCC.[60–62,72] For SCC, one study proposed minimal margins of excision of 4 to 6 mm around the clinical borders.[73]

Mohs micrographic excision (MME) uses horizontal frozen sections and intraoperative tumor mapping to provide a higher cure rate for SCC and BCC than standard excision while leaving a smaller wound. When compared with other modalities, MME obtains higher cure rates—as high as 99% for primary BCC and SCC[43,74] (**Table 52.3**). The reason for the high cure rate is that 100% of the surgical margin (deep and peripheral) is examined microscopically

able 52.3 Long-Term (5-Year) Recurrence Rates for Treatment of Primary and Recurrent Basal Cell Carcinoma (BCC)

	Recurrence Rate (%)	
	Primary BCC	**Recurrent BCC**
Treatment modality		
Surgical excision	10.1	17.4
Curettage and electrodesiccation	7.7	40.0
Radiation therapy	8.7	9.8
Cryotherapy	7.5	None reported
All non-Mohs modalities	8.7	19.9
Mohs micrographic surgery	1.0	5.6

Source: From Rowe DE, Carroll RJ, Day CL. Long-term recurrence rates in previously untreated (primary) basal cell carcinoma: implications for patient follow-up. J Dermatol Surg Oncol 1989;15:315–328, and Rowe DE, Carroll RJ, Day CL. Mohs surgery is the treatment of choice for recurrent (previously treated) basal cell carcinoma. J Dermatol Surg Oncol 1989;15:424–431. Reprinted by permission of Blackwell Science, Inc.

n combination with precise mapping of the surgical site nd histological specimen.

At the beginning of Mohs excision (**Fig. 52.14**) the skin s anesthetized and the tumor is excised just beyond the linical margin. The tissue is frozen and very thin sections re mounted on microscope slides. The tissue is oriented o that the sections are made horizontally across the deep and lateral margins of the specimen instead of vertically (the usual method). The pathologist then reads these sections, looking for remaining tumor cells by examining the entire periphery. By mapping the tumor site, the surgeon can pinpoint the location of residual disease and remove only the area that contains cancerous tissue. One or more layers may need to be excised and inspected before all residual cancer cells are found. A more detailed description can be found elsewhere.[75]

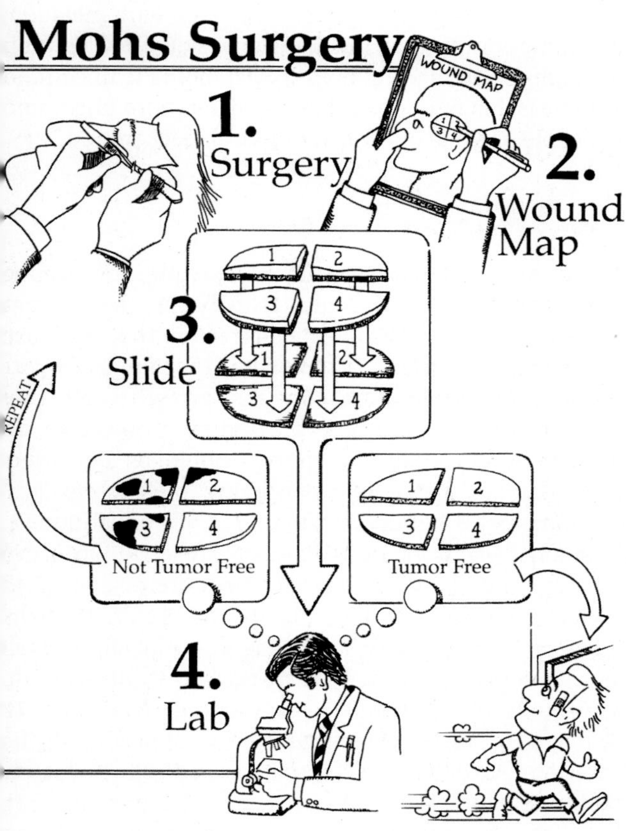

g. 52.14 Steps in Mohs micrographic surgery.

MME should be very seriously considered for SCCs or BCCs that are recurrent, large (greater than 1 cm), or that have indistinct margins or are in critical locations. A critical location may be defined as one where tissue sparing is paramount (e.g., nasal tip, eyelid, concha) or recurrence is common (e.g., nose, ear, periocular). MME should also be considered for the more difficult histological patterns, such as poorly differentiated SCC or BCC with morpheaform, infiltrative, micronodular, or mixed morphology or tumors with perineural involvement. If positive margins are reported after standard excision with no obvious clinical tumor, then MME should be considered. The need for MME increases when several these factors are present (i.e., recurrence, infiltrative histology, perineural invasion, etc.).

Cryosurgery, a field therapy, destroys tissue by freezing (usually with liquid nitrogen) to a tumoricidal temperature. In most cases, cryosurgery is best limited to small, superficial SCCs and BCCs. In skilled hands, cryosurgery will give a cure rate in excess of 95% on selected SCCs and BCCs.[76] Wounds heal with secondary intention and leave hypopigmented, soft, sometimes depressed scars. The technique for freezing skin cancers is distinctly different from the light freeze for AKs.[77]

Curettage followed by electrosurgery is indicated only for the smallest, most superficial, and well-circumscribed SCCs and BCCs. The curette has a sharp edge that scrapes away soft tumor tissue followed by electrodesiccation of the wound base. The cosmetic appearance is usually minimally satisfactory. In one study, for sites at low risk for recurrence (neck, trunk, and extremities), BCCs of all diameters responded well to curettage and electrodesiccation, with an overall 5-year recurrence rate of 3.3%.[78]

Radiation therapy, another field therapy, can be used as a primary therapeutic alternative to surgery if the case dictates, or as an adjunctive therapy to surgery.[79] The latter approach should receive consideration when dealing with high-risk cutaneous SCCs and BCCs (e.g., an SCC that is poorly differentiated, large, recurrent, deeply penetrating, or perineural). In high-risk SCCs, radiation therapy is sometimes employed to treat the nodal basin prophylactically after the primary tumor has been excised.[80–82] Radiation therapy is a proven field therapy that achieves cure rates in excess of 90% for appropriately selected patients with SCC and BCC. It is an excellent choice for patients who are not good surgical candidates or who do not wish to have surgery.[83]

In summary, SCCs and BCCs are the most commonly encountered skin cancers in the world. Clinicians should be familiar with their clinical appearance so that diagnosis and treatment can be initiated early. When treatment is delayed significant morbidity and mortality can ensue. Many therapies obtain reasonable cure rates, but Mohs micrographic excision remains the gold standard.

Melanoma

Epidemiological and Etiologic Factors

Melanoma is a malignancy arising from melanocytes, the pigment-producing cells of the skin. It accounts for ~4% of skin cancers, with more than 41,000 new invasive melanomas, 21,000 new melanomas in situ, and ~7300 melanoma deaths annually in the United States.[2] Usually, it arises in sun-exposed areas. Commonly, melanomas in women arise on the lower extremities. In men, they commonly arise on the trunk and the head and neck region (**Fig. 52.15**). The primary cause of melanoma is believed to be exposure to UV radiation from the sun.[84] Experimental data from a possum model suggest that exposure of animals to UV light early in life can lead to metastatic melanoma in later life.[85] Other studies suggest that UV-B irradiation of human skin engrafted on mice leads to the development of nevi and melanomas.[86] However, the exact etiologic role of UV light is not entirely understood, and there are melanomas that arise in areas not exposed to the sun. The association between melanoma and sun exposure is based on several observations, including studies showing that people with severe burns in childhood seem to be at higher risk for developing melanoma later in

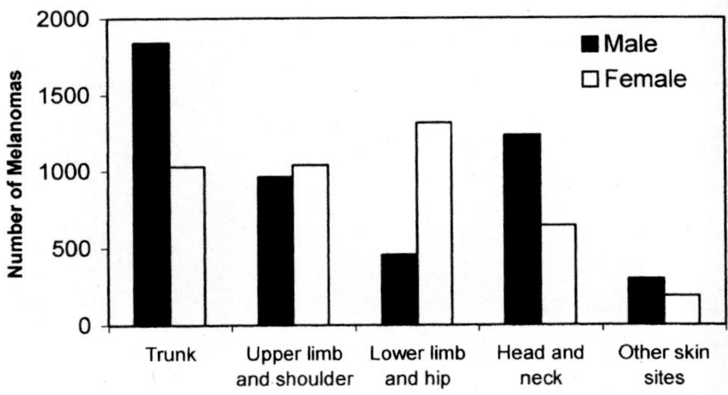

Fig. 52.15 In a population-based registry, there is association b[illegible] tween patient gender and body site of primary melanoma. Wome[illegible] are much more likely to develop melanomas of the lower extremit[illegible] whereas men are more likely to develop melanomas of the trunk an[illegible] of the head and neck. (Adapted from data in Norris SLW. Melanoma [illegible] Virginia 1970–1996. In: Pugh AM, Slingluff CL Jr, and Woolard D, ed[illegible] Virginia Cancer Registry, Virginia Department of Health, 1999.)

life.[84] It is of interest that people who have been expose[illegible] to the sun on a regular basis appear not to be at increase[illegible] risk of melanoma. Chronic sun exposure in people wh[illegible] tan well does not appear to be associated with increase[illegible] risk and may even be protective.[87] Persons at highest ris[illegible] for melanoma are those with fair complexions who hav[illegible] had intermittent sun exposure and severe sunburns. I[illegible] particular, the skin type most associated with melanom[illegible] is a Celtic complexion, including pale skin, freckles, blon[illegible] or reddish hair, and light eyes. Melanoma is uncommo[illegible] in Caucasians with dark skin and even more uncommo[illegible] in people of Asian or African American background.

Clinical Characteristics

Many melanomas arise from preexisting nevi, thoug[illegible] most probably arise de novo. Usually they have irreg[illegible] lar borders and variations in color. Often they are raise[illegible] above the skin surface. Occasionally, they are black wit[illegible] out any other coloration. Any skin growths with thes[illegible] characteristics should be evaluated by a physician, an[illegible] if there is any doubt, a biopsy should be performe[illegible] A mnemonic useful for identifying melanomas is: [illegible] (asymmetry), B (border irregularity), C (color variation), [illegible] (diameter >6 mm). Lesions that are also elevated are of eve[illegible] greater concern. All of these features are evident in th[illegible] melanoma shown in **Figs. 52.16 and 52.17**. Realizin[illegible] however, that the goal is to diagnose melanoma earl[illegible] small and flat lesions that satisfy the A-B-C criteria or th[illegible] are totally black should be considered suspicious. Th[illegible] lesion in **Fig. 52.18** is extensive but was almost totally fla[illegible] Excision revealed the lesion to be a dysplastic nevus co[illegible] taining a 3 mm wide melanoma, only 0.8 mm thick. Th[illegible] patient's prognosis is good and can be attributed to ear[illegible] diagnosis. If a melanoma is diagnosed and removed whe[illegible]

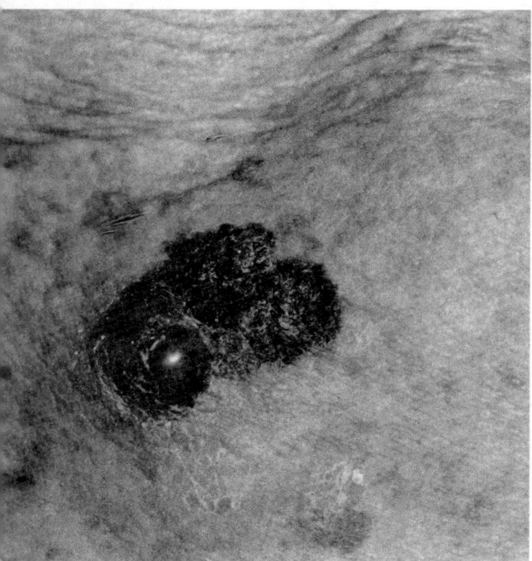

ig. 52.16 A thick melanoma on the upper chest that is characterized by symmetry, border irregularity, color variations, diameter greater than mm, and marked elevation. The black, flatter portion measured 11 × 4 mm across. The raised reddish nodule was 1 cm across and 4 mm high. he Breslow thickness was 4.3 mm. (From Slingluff CL Jr. Pigmented skin esions. In: Schirmer B, Rattner DW, eds. Ambulatory Surgery. Philadel-hia: WB Saunders, 1998:386–392. Reprinted by permission.)

ery thin, cure is likely. If it is diagnosed when thick, netastasis may have occurred and cure is less likely. Signs hat are particularly worrisome in a primary lesion would e itching, bleeding, ulceration, and the presence of satel-ite lesions.

Unfortunately, some melanomas do not have brown or lack pigment and look very much like normal skin. These an be very difficult to diagnose, even by an experienced hysician. Among these amelanotic melanomas, there are

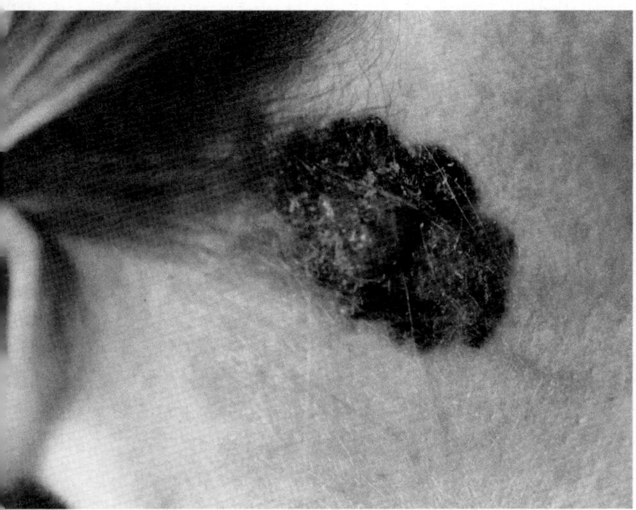

ig. 52.17 An intermediate-thickness melanoma was diagnosed on he right temple on a woman in her mid-30s with fair skin and red hair. t was Breslow thickness 2.9 mm, with a raised nodule in the center.

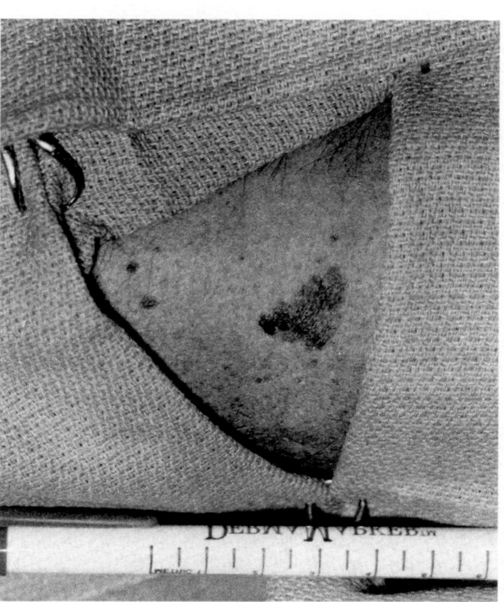

Fig. 52.18 The melanoma arising in this large dysplastic nevus was in the more darkly pigmented portion and was only 3 mm across and 0.8 mm deep. The remainder of the lesion was benign. The entire lesion was excised with a 1 cm margin. (From Slingluff CL Jr. Pigmented skin lesions. In: Schirmer B, Rattner DW, eds. Ambulatory Surgery. Philadelphia: WB Saunders, 1998:386–392. Reprinted by permission.)

a disproportionate number that fit into an uncommon histological group: the desmoplastic melanomas.[88] Given the variable presentations of melanoma, any pigmented skin lesion that has changed should be evaluated for possible biopsy.

Though melanoma arises in defined cutaneous sites in ~90% of cases, it can also arise from mucous membranes, from the eye, from unknown sites, or, rarely, from viscera. These presentations are uncommon but well described, and familiarity with each is important in the management of patients with melanoma.

Approximately 1 to 2% of melanomas arise from mucous membrane sites, and these are distributed equally among three different body areas: the mucous membranes of the head and neck (oropharynx, nasopharynx, and sinuses), the anorectal region, and the female genital tract.[89] These lesions are usually large when diagnosed because they are in areas not readily visible to the patient or to family. They are usually associated with a very poor prognosis.[90] Though up to 10 to 20% of patients may be alive at 5 years, the vast majority of patients will ultimately succumb to the disease. Radical resection does not appear to improve patient survival, compared with wide excision, but it may improve local-regional control.[91]

Ocular melanomas account for 2 to 5% of melanomas, and they may arise from the retina, the iris, the ciliary body, or other sites in the eye. These melanomas are often identified as small lesions as they may be visible or may affect vision. Often they can be treated by radiation, but advanced lesions require enucleation. Though these tumors share many phenotypic features with cutaneous melanomas, they behave in a distinct pattern. Nodal metastases are rarely seen, presumably because of the lack of ocular lymphatics.[92] Instead, the first site of metastasis is almost always the liver. In many cases, it is the only site of metastasis and the liver metastases are the cause of death.

Very rarely, melanomas arise primarily in viscera, such as esophagus and lung. The esophagus contains normal melanocytes in 3% of normal individuals, and these can transform into melanoma.[93] These, like mucosal melanomas, are usually diagnosed when they have become large.

In 5 to 10% of patients who present with metastatic melanoma, no primary melanoma can be identified. These most commonly present as melanoma in a lymph node or in cutaneous sites.[94] In some cases, a history of a pigmented lesion that spontaneously regressed can be elicited. In some cases, it is believed that the immune system may have destroyed the primary melanoma. Another hypothesis for melanoma in a lymph node without a known primary is that the melanoma may have arisen there primarily, as isolated nests of nevus cells can be found incidentally in some lymph nodes. However, most cases remain unexplained.

Biological Behavior

Although wide excision of melanoma is curative in some cases, all invasive melanomas have some risk of metastasis; the risk correlates well with the maximal thickness (Breslow thickness) of the primary melanoma.[95] Melanomas typically metastasize through lymphatic channels, usually to the regional nodes draining the primary melanoma. If a melanoma arises on an extremity, the most common place for metastases to be found is in the axillary or inguinal nodes, respectively. However, when a melanoma arises on the trunk or on the head and neck, lymphatic drainage patterns can be less predictable.

A total of 80 to 90% of first metastases of melanoma can be found on physical examination, either in the skin or in lymph nodes. Metastases in the skin typically appear as nodules that are either black or dark blue, but they may appear without any color. When melanoma metastasizes to lymph nodes, the nodes usually appear round and hard, resembling marbles. Usually there is no tenderness or pain associated with them. Surgery often permits complete removal of cutaneous and isolated nodal metastases, and some patients treated surgically for nodal or cutaneous metastases survive for years without distant disease.

Unfortunately, however, melanoma is also prone to metastasize to visceral sites through hematogenous dissemination. Often little can be done to effect cure in those cases, but some treatments may be helpful, including chemotherapy and cytokine therapy. There are novel experimental immunotherapy approaches available in certain circumstances, including several melanoma vaccine approaches. In rare cases, durable complete responses occur after systemic therapy with chemotherapy or with immunotherapy, including administration of interleukin-2.

Biopsy Techniques

The diagnosis of a skin lesion can be made easily with a simple biopsy. It is important to realize that there can be a difference between removing a skin lesion and making a diagnosis. Shave biopsies are often performed for the easy removal of benign skin lesions, such as keratoses, but significant diagnostic and prognostic information can be lost if a shave biopsy is performed for a lesion suspected to be melanoma. In particular, there are difficult diagnostic dilemmas for pathologists that can be made more difficult without complete tissue excision. One of these is distinguishing a melanoma from a Spitz nevus.[96,97] Spitz nevi are much more common in children but can be found in adults. Because some of the distinction is based on the architecture of the entire lesion, a shave biopsy that does not encompass the entire lesion may result in an inaccurate diagnosis or a delayed diagnosis. A more common problem is that a shave biopsy may not include the base of the lesion, thus preventing an accurate assessment of the tumor thickness. This limits the prognostic information available to patients and may affect the extent of subsequent surgery and the candidacy for adjuvant therapy. The goals, if melanoma is suspected, should be to (1) make a diagnosis; (2) collect the most prognostic information possible; and (3) facilitate subsequent therapy.

The principles that will ensure fulfillment of these goals are as follows: (1) always take full-thickness biopsies; (2) include a rim of normal skin in the biopsy; and (3) on extremities, orient the incision longitudinally. A full-thickness biopsy should, by definition, include all layers of the skin, so that the subcutis is entered during the biopsy. Excision of a small ellipse of skin with a scalpel is usually done for a full-thickness biopsy. Normal skin included in the biopsy need not be extensive. A 1 to 2 mm margin of normal skin permits the pathologist to examine the junctional changes that are critical to identifying melanoma and to determine if it is a primary or a metastatic lesion.

These biopsies are easily performed in the outpatient or ambulatory setting. No preoperative laboratory studies are needed. Under local anesthesia, the lesion is then excised with a 1- to 2-mm margin, lifting the skin up with an Adson forcep. Hemostasis can usually be achieved without electrocautery by a combination of gentle pressure and suture losure. The incision is closed, in many cases, with a sub-uticular 4–0 absorbable suture and sterile strips. If there s significant tension, a few interrupted nonabsorbable 4–0 sutures will suffice. The wound can be covered with a sterile dry dressing for 2 to 3 days.

In some cases, the lesion of concern is large enough hat even simple excision would leave a large wound, with concern for functional and cosmetic implications. In hose cases, excision of the portion of the lesion of great-est concern may be adequate for a diagnosis. Again, some normal skin should be included at a margin. It is impor-ant that the full thickness of the lesion be evaluated in he biopsy. Because wide reexcision is always performed after the biopsy, partial excision of a melanoma is not generally thought to compromise subsequent therapy; however, the possibility of effects on prognosis has not been ruled out.[98] Thus, it is wise to perform complete excisional biopsy when feasible.

In some cases, a punch biopsy technique may be use-ul, such as with small nevi. A punch biopsy instrument is a disposable circular blade on a handle that can be used to excise a small circle of full-thickness skin. Punch biopsy instruments for excisions 4, 5, or 6 mm in diameter are use-ul for quick excisions of small nevi. It is important when using a punch to be certain the lesion can be completely excised with a 1- to 2-mm margin and also to be careful not to crush the lesion when excising it. After punching out he skin, the circle of skin containing the lesion must be excised with scissors just below the dermis. A fine forcep can be used to elevate the skin circle while cutting underneath t. After excision, the lesion should be placed in formalin and sent for histological evaluation. Lesions larger than 2 to 4 mm should not be excised with a punch biopsy because evaluation of the junctional zone at the edge of the lesion an be very important for a definitive diagnosis.

At least as important as the instructions listed previ-ously is the choice of skin incision. Especially on extremi-ies, the orientation of the initial skin biopsy is a critical determinant of the subsequent therapy. If the pigmented esion is melanoma, a wide excision will be needed, the orientation of which is determined largely by the orienta-ion of the initial excision. It is difficult to close a trans-verse incision on an extremity primarily; thus, a transverse incision is more likely to require a skin graft. Also, because he innervation to skin surfaces runs longitudinally, a ransversely oriented excision will interrupt more of the innervation to skin distal to the lesion. On the other hand, an incision that crosses a joint may lead to a contracture hat limits range of motion; so extremity excisions near a oint may need to be oriented transversely or closed with Z-plasty across the joint. On the head and neck region, he orientation of a biopsy incision should be selected with consideration of how it may affect subsequent reex-ision or node dissection incisions.

Prognosis and Staging

The pathologist looks for several characteristics when a primary melanoma is diagnosed in a skin biopsy. The most important of these is thickness (Breslow thickness), which is measured in millimeters. Melanomas thinner than 0.76 mm have classically been considered thin melanomas and are unlikely to recur once removed.[99,100] Currently, thin melanomas include lesions up to 1 mm thick. Melanomas thicker than 4 mm are considered thick melanomas and have a greater than 50% chance of recurring or metastasizing to other organs.[101] Melanomas that are intermediate in thickness have a likelihood of recurrence that averages roughly 30 to 40%. As examples, the patients with the melanomas pictured in **Figs. 52.16 and 52.18** developed axillary nodal metastases and systemic metastases, respectively, within 3 years of diagnosis.

Several additional histological features of melanomas can be important in considering the overall prognosis. These include the Clark level, growth phase, ulceration, mitotic rate, lymphovascular invasion, satellite lesions, and the presence or absence of tumor-infiltrating lymphocytes. Clark level refers to the depth of invasion of the lesion, relative to the anatomical layers of the skin.[102] A Clark level I lesion is a melanoma in situ, confined to the epidermis, with no significant metastatic potential. A Clark level II lesion involves the superficial (papillary) dermis and is usually associated with a good prognosis. A Clark level III lesion fills the papillary dermis, and a Clark level IV lesion invades the reticular dermis and is associated with a poor prognosis. A Clark level V lesion invades full thickness into the subcutaneous fat and is generally associated with a very high mortality risk. Although these measures are useful, distinction between levels III and IV is not always reproducible among good pathologists, and the Breslow thickness is a more reproducible prognostic factor. Also, in multivariate analyses, Clark level adds little to Breslow thickness in determining prognosis.

Most melanomas go through two growth phases, the first being a radial growth phase (RGP), when the tumor cells proliferate at the dermal–epidermal junction and the tumor expands radially. This may include lesions confined to the epidermis and those with superficial dermal involvement. Subsequently, the lesion begins to invade more deeply into the dermis, with expansile nests of cells growing vertically. This is often associated with the development of a palpable nodule in the lesion, and this is considered the vertical growth phase (VGP). A common presentation of melanoma in the head and neck region is Hutchinson's melanotic freckle (lentigo maligna), which is a form of melanoma in situ commonly arising on the face, more commonly in women. A VGP is that portion of the tumor associated with metastatic risk. In some cases, a desmoplastic melanoma may arise from a lentigo maligna.

Similar patterns of radial and vertical growth also occur with superficial spreading melanomas and acral lentiginous melanomas. The exception to this sequence of growth phases involves the nodular type of melanoma, which only has a VGP. Some lesions are excised early, while still in the RGP, and there are data to suggest that these lesions have no metastatic potential.[103–105] Usually, patients with thin melanomas have an excellent prognosis, but a small percentage go on to develop metastatic disease, and it appears that part of the explanation for this may be attributed to thin VGP lesions that do have metastatic potential. Most of the thicker melanomas are in VGP.

Ulceration is a poor prognostic sign and is more common in thicker lesions.[101,106] A high mitotic rate is also associated with a poor prognosis, with lesions containing more than 6 mitoses/mm^2 being at higher risk than those with fewer mitoses. Similarly, lesions with microscopic satellites or lymphovascular invasion appear to be at higher risk. A protective feature may be the presence of a cellular immune response to the tumor, as evidenced by lymphocytes infiltrating into the tumor mass itself.

When tumor-infiltrating lymphocyte response is brisk, there is a significantly improved prognosis.[105,107] When a patient presents for definitive therapy following initial diagnosis, it is important to make an initial assessment of the stage of disease. The vast majority of melanomas present with clinically localized disease, but occasionally patients have clinically evident nodal or visceral metastases. The first step in evaluation includes a history and review of systems, looking for evidence of bone pain, mental status changes, cough, headaches, weight loss, or other new systemic symptoms that may suggest metastases to bone, lung, liver, or brain. A careful physical examination should focus on evaluation of the regional nodal basins for lymphadenopathy, as the first site of metastasis is usually to those nodes. The examination should also include a detailed evaluation of the skin and subcutis between the primary site and the regional nodes, as in-transit metastases are also common. In addition, distant skin metastases should be sought, as they are fairly common metastatic sites and are best identified by physical examination. A chest x-ray and a serum lactate dehydrogenase are reasonable screening studies to identify patients who may have metastases to lung and liver, though the yield is low in patients without clinical evidence of metastases.[108–110] Routine computed tomography (CT) scans or bone scans are not indicated if these evaluations are all negative. However, specific studies to evaluate worrisome symptoms or physical findings may be indicated.

If a patient has evidence of distant metastases, then aggressive management of local and regional disease is not indicated. Instead, systemic therapy must be considered. Fortunately, this is uncommon, and most patients will present without evidence of metastasis. In these patients, the focus of definitive therapy will be on wide excision of the primary lesion and consideration of surgical staging of the regional nodes.

American Joint Council on Cancer (AJCC) staging for melanoma is based on the TNM (tumor, node, metastasis) system. The T stage is based on the tumor thickness (T1: <0.76 mm or Clark II; T2: 0.76–1.5 mm or Clark III; T3: 1.6–4 mm or Clark IV; T4: >4 mm or Clark V). Stage I includes T1 N0 M0 and T2 N0 M0. Stage II includes T3 N0 M0 and T4 N0 M0. Nodal metastases or intransit metastases qualify for N1 status. Bulky nodes are graded as N2. Stage III includes T any N1 M0 and T any N2 M0, and stage IV includes T any N any M1. Recommendations in 1999 for changing the AJCC staging criteria are being formally considered, and they likely will be adopted. With these changes, ulceration will be included as a part of staging the primary lesion, and the N staging will also take into account the number of positive nodes, which is well documented as the single most important prognostic factor in patients with nodal metastases.[106]

Treatment

The definitive treatment of melanoma of the skin includes wide excision of the initial biopsy site. The goal is to remove an area of normal skin around the primary melanoma to remove dermal or subcutaneous micrometastases that often occur as a result of lymphatic spread. By doing so, we reduce the chance of the melanoma recurring locally. For melanomas in situ (Clark level I, confined to the epidermis and epidermal–dermal junction), a 5-mm margin is adequate. Thin melanomas, up to 1 mm in thickness, should be excised with a 1-cm margin.[111] Thicker melanomas are usually managed with a 2-cm margin. In many locations on the body, this can be accomplished with an elliptical skin incision and the wound can be closed primarily. In some locations, a skin graft may be required. This is particularly true on the face, hands, and feet but may be true on other parts of the body as well. In some of these locations, concern for appearance or function may require taking smaller margins to permit primary closure.

The basis for the current recommendations for wide excision margins is clinical experience with 2-cm margins showing good local control in thick lesions. Also, randomized clinical trial data from the Intergroup trial show that 2-cm margin provide the same local control and survival as 4-cm margin for melanomas 1 to 4 mm thick.[101,112,11] Furthermore, 1-cm margin provide the same local and distant control as 2-cm margin for melanomas up to 1 mm in thickness.[114] For melanomas 1 to 2 mm thick, a slight increase in local recurrence (<5% of patients) was observed without impact on survival.[114] Thus for some lesions up to 2 mm in thickness it is reasonable to perform excisions with a 1-cm margin.[115] It is common in the head and neck region for cosmetic concerns and anatomical constraints to prevent excisions larger than 1 cm in some cases, and these data justify use of narrower margins in certain cases.

Wide excisions can generally be performed easily in the outpatient or ambulatory setting but require more time than a simple skin biopsy. The goals of the wide excision are to (1) obtain an adequate margin of normal tissue radially; (2) resect full-thickness skin and subcutaneous tissue in the area of concern; and (3) minimize morbidity. This is usually best performed in an operating room using local anesthetic (lidocaine 1%, with epinephrine 1:100,000 to slow systemic distribution and sodium bicarbonate 0.084% to decrease patient discomfort) and intravenous sedation. In most cases, a complete excision has been performed prior to the wide excision; however, in cases where residual melanoma is present, it may be wise to cover the lesion with an adherent plastic barrier to prevent possible transfer of melanoma cells to the wound edges. An incision is planned, first by measuring the appropriate margin of excision around the initial scar or residual melanoma, then by extending the ellipse in the direction that will best permit primary closure under the least tension. After the planned ellipse of skin has been marked out, a field block can be performed with the lidocaine, being careful to anesthetize deeply through the full thickness of the subcutaneous tissue. The incision is then made with a scalpel and deepened through full thickness of subcutis, down to the muscle fascia with electrocautery in all directions. The attachments to the fascia are divided with electrocautery as the specimen is lifted from the wound. An Allis clamp is useful for grasping one end of the skin as the dissection progresses. When large cutaneous nerves are encountered deep to the subcutis along the surface of the deep fascia, they can be preserved. When they run through the superficial subcutaneous tissue or innervate the excised skin, they should be sacrificed. Closure of the wide excision can usually be accomplished, under some tension, in two layers, using interrupted 3–0 absorbable sutures to reapproximate the subcutaneous fascia, followed by 3–0 nonabsorbable monofilament sutures in a full-thickness vertical mattress pattern to reapproximate the skin and to reinforce the subcutaneous closure. Where the subcutaneous tissue is not substantial, vertical mattress sutures in the skin will suffice. The closure will usually heal well, and the skin and scar will stretch with time, much as is observed with tissue expanders; so the tension will resolve over a few weeks to months. When there is significant tension, the sutures generally should be left in place for 2 weeks.

Where the wide excision wound does not close easily, some limited undermining of the skin can permit closure. If this fails or is not feasible, a skin graft may be needed. Large myocutaneous flaps are not usually recommended because of the difficulty of evaluating for early local recurrences in that setting. However, split-thickness skin grafts, harvested from areas distant from or contralateral to the primary site, can be used to cover a defect. In body sites where cosmesis is a major concern, a full-thickness skin graft may be harvested from the inguinal area, neck, abdomen, or inferior gluteal region and used in a fashion similar to that of a split-thickness graft. A graft placed near a joint will heal better if the limb is immobilized in a splint. The dressing and splint may be removed after 5 days and the surgical site cared for in a routine fashion. With 1- to 2-cm margins of excision, skin grafts are rarely required on the back or proximal extremities. However, wide excisions are often difficult to close on the distal extremities and on the face and scalp; therefore, these areas are more likely to require skin grafts.

Melanomas of the head and neck can arise in many different locations, and for many of them there are special considerations related to the wide excision (**Fig. 52.19**). For these melanomas, the deep margin of excision often is not muscle; the extent of resection must be individualized depending on the location and the extent of the lesion. Melanomas of the external ear, unless very superficial, often require wedge resection of the cartilage and primary closure. In patients who wear glasses, preservation of the upper portion of the external ear is particularly important. Amputation and reconstruction of the external ear is generally reserved for patients with very extensive local disease. For melanomas of the nose, the perichondrium often can be spared unless there is gross involvement of the subcutaneous tissue with tumor. Scalp melanomas tend to have

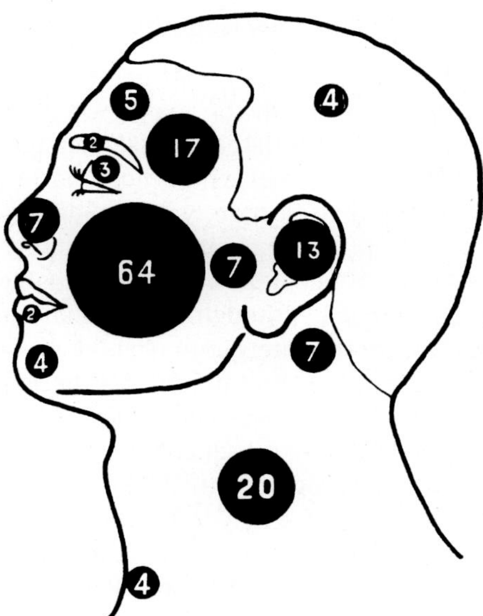

Fig. 52.19 The number of melanomas arising in each area of the head and neck, based on experience in Queensland. (From Harris TJ, Hinckley DM. Melanoma of the head and neck in Queensland. Head Neck Surg, Elsevier, 1983;5:197–203. Reprinted by permission.)

a particularly poor prognosis, and they should be excised with the underlying fascia but not with periosteum. Melanomas overlying the parotid gland should be excised down to the parotid fascia. In cases where the deep or lateral margins are expected to be close to important anatomical structures, it is reasonable to perform the excision and to leave the wound open until the final pathology report is available. At that point, reexcision or coverage can be performed as a separate procedure. This approach can permit sparing of critical structures while ensuring adequate margins before any local flaps or grafts are applied.[116]

For melanomas of the scalp, appropriate methods of closure include local advancement flaps, pinwheel flaps, or split-thickness skin grafts. The hair will usually cover these areas well. On the face and neck, the cosmetic concerns are more substantial. Alternatives to free skin grafts include simple advancement flaps or rotational or free vascularized flaps. Free flaps or large rotational flaps are generally discouraged for closure of melanoma wide-excision wounds because of the difficulty in following these areas in the event of local recurrence and because some patients will have unsuspected satellite lesions at or near the margins. Creation of a large complex wound puts the patient at risk for a local recurrence that extends over a large area and that may be very difficult to manage. However, small rotation flaps and simple advancement flaps can be used with good cosmesis. It is critical to ensure adequate margins of excision prior to any major reconstructive effort, especially where local recurrence may threaten adjacent structures.

Surgical Management of Clinically Negative Regional Nodal Basins

One of the most debated issues in the management of melanoma has been the appropriate surgical management of clinically negative regional lymph node basins. Evidence is accumulating that elective lymph node dissections (ELND) do not provide a survival advantage over selective dissections of nodal basins when palpable nodal metastases are evident. Although subset analysis of the published data from the Intergroup trial has been interpreted to show that for a subset of patients there is a survival advantage to ELND, when reasonable statistical principles are applied to these subset analyses the differences are not statistically significant.[117] More recent follow-up data suggest that there may in fact be a small improvement in survival for melanomas 1 to 2 mm thick when elective node dissection is performed (Balch CM, abstract presented at Society of Surgical Oncology meeting, March 1999). However, an earlier World Health Organization study and a Mayo Clinic study found no evidence for a survival advantage with ELND when compared with delayed, selective lymphadenectomy in patients with isolated nodal metastases.[118–120] Even the Intergroup data, when considering the entire population of patients with melanomas 1 to 4 mm thick, show no difference in survival with ELND. The only studies that show a significant improvement in survival after ELND were retrospective nonrandomized studies.[121,122] More recent reviews from the same institutions, with longer follow-up, found that patients with ELND had the same likelihood of survival as patients managed with wide excision only.[123,124]

Independent of the potential effects of ELND on patient survival, there is strong prognostic value in knowing the status of the regional nodes in patients with melanoma. Also, knowing the status of regional nodes can affect therapeutic decisions. Interferon-α is FDA-approved for the adjuvant therapy of melanoma patients with thick melanomas or with positive nodes, and there are numerous experimental trials of melanoma vaccines for which the status of the regional nodes is required for entry in those trials. Unfortunately, the morbidity of lymphadenectomy can be significant, especially for inguinal nodes. An approach that permits accurate staging of the regional nodes without complete lymphadenectomy is sentinel lymph node biopsy. The technique for sentinel lymph node biopsy was first described by Dr. Donald Morton and colleagues in the early 1990s[125] and has been widely adopted since for the management of melanoma. It has been demonstrated that the node (or nodes) draining a primary tumor site can, in the vast majority of cases, be identified either by lymphatic mapping using a vital blue dye or a technetium-labeled sulfur colloid injected into the skin. Current estimates are that the sentinel node reflects the status of the entire nodal basin in 98 to 99% of cases.[126] Thus, if 20% of patients with intermediate-thickness melanomas have nodal metastases, 1 to 2% of these metastases may not be detected by sentinel node biopsy. This represents ~5 to 10% of persons with positive nodes. On the other hand, the application of serial sectioning and immunohistochemistry on the sentinel nodes may identify nodal metastases that would have been missed on routine evaluation of one face of each node using hematoxylin and eosin (H&E) stains. In one large series, 26% of nodal metastases detected in the sentinel nodes were found by serial sectioning and immunohistochemistry only.[127] Thus the net sensitivity of sentinel node biopsy may exceed that of standard complete node dissections because the pathologist can examine the sentinel nodes more carefully than is practical for an entire node dissection (i.e., by serial sectioning and immunohistochemistry).

After a negative sentinel node biopsy, 4.1% of patients may develop palpable nodal metastases in that basin.[128] This compares favorably with the 4% rate of nodal recurrences following a negative elective complete node dissection.[123]

The attractiveness of sentinel node biopsies is that reliable staging information can be obtained with minimal morbidity, using a technique that requires only local anesthesia and that can be performed at the time of wide local excision. This procedure can generally be performed on an outpatient basis, and it often requires only a local anesthetic. If metastatic melanoma is found in the nodal basin, then a complete node dissection can be scheduled electively. The finding of a positive sentinel node upstages a patient to stage III, making him or her eligible for adjuvant therapy with high-dose interferon-α or for inclusion in experimental tumor vaccine protocols. It is reasonable to consider sentinel node biopsy in patients with melanomas thicker than 1 to 1.5 mm. Some patients may be offered sentinel node biopsy in the setting of more minimal disease. It can be argued that the risk of metastatic disease is so low in patients with melanomas in situ or with radial growth phase melanomas that sentinel node biopsy is not indicated in those cases.

Most surgeons use technetium-99-labeled sulfur colloid to identify the draining nodal basin and to localize the sentinel nodes preoperatively. A handheld gamma camera can then be used intraoperatively to localize the sentinel nodes definitively prior to and after excision. Simultaneous injection of vital blue dye can further confirm the identity of radiolabeled nodes as sentinel; some surgeons use both techniques together. The use of technetium-99-labeled sulfur colloid for intraoperative localization has been found to be effective without blue dye[129] and can improve the accuracy of intraoperative mapping better than blue dye alone.[130]

Routine use of lymphoscintigraphy has permitted a detailed understanding of the variability of lymphatic patterns among individuals. In 34 to 84% of patients with head and neck melanomas, the draining nodes are in basins that would not have been predicted clinically.[131,132] The impact of sentinel node biopsy techniques on patients with head and neck melanoma is that it permits accurate staging without performance of a complete neck dissection and without parotidectomy in the majority of cases. This may spare many patients the substantial morbidity of that surgery while still permitting detailed staging.

Surgical Management of Palpable Nodal Metastases

When melanoma recurs in a regional nodal basin, complete resection of the nodal basin is associated with regional control in the vast majority of cases and with long-term survival in a significant minority (**Fig. 52.20**). For patients with a single nodal metastasis, 10-year survival is ~40% after complete node dissection, and for patients with more nodes, there still is a significant chance of long-term survival.[133] Thus resection of nodal metastases is pursued

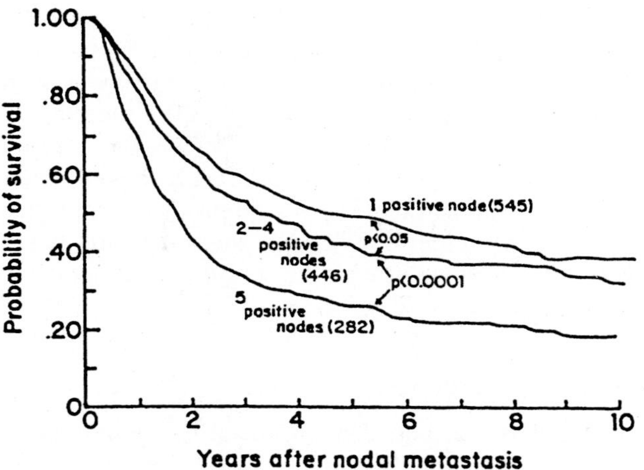

Fig. 52.20 The 10-year survival of patients treated with lymphadenectomy for regional nodal metastases of melanoma is demonstrated for patients with one positive node and for groups of patients with a larger number of positive nodes. (From Slingluff CL, Vollmer R, Seigler HF. Stage II malignant melanoma: presentation of a prognostic model and an assessment of specific active immunotherapy—1273 patients. J Surg Oncol 1988;39:139–147. Reprinted by permission.)

aggressively in the absence of detectable systemic disease. It is recommended that CT scans of the chest, abdomen, and pelvis be obtained prior to node dissection.[134] In patients with nodal metastases from an unknown primary, survival after surgical resection is as good as or better than survival of similar patients with a known primary.[133,135]

In the case of cervical metastases, the extent of the neck dissection does not appear to affect recurrence or survival; thus preservation of function with a modified neck dissection is advocated.[136] There has been some experience with adjuvant radiotherapy to the surgical site after neck dissection for nodal metastases of melanoma. Although there has been some suggestion of increased regional control, the differences are not significant and there is no evidence that survival is affected.[137] Randomized prospective trials are under way to determine if any significant differences in patient outcome can be detected with radiation therapy after therapeutic lymphadenectomy. Patients with many positive nodes or with extracapsular extension are at higher risk of regional recurrence, so that radiation therapy, if beneficial, may have the greatest impact in these patients.

Adjuvant Systemic Therapy for Melanoma

In patients with thick melanomas (T4 N0 M0) or nodal metastases (Tany N1 M0), the risk of systemic recurrence is greater than 50%. Interferon-α is FDA-approved for the adjuvant therapy of melanoma in these patients, based on a randomized trial (ECOG 1684), which showed a modest improvement in survival in patients treated with high-dose interferon.[138] The toxicity has been high with this therapy, limiting its acceptability to patients and to physicians. A repeat trial (ECOG 1690) has also been completed, but no difference in survival was seen in this larger trial (presentation at ECOG meeting in November 1998). Interferon-α does have some activity in melanoma, but these conflicting results have further diminished the willingness of patients to accept this therapy. Experimental adjuvant therapies are being investigated in this same patient group, primarily using melanoma vaccines.

Therapy for Systemic Disease

Only ~20% of patients diagnosed with melanoma are expected to die of their disease. However, the progression of melanoma can be relentless and can be associated with great morbidity. Melanoma can metastasize to any site, but common visceral sites include the lung, liver, bone, and brain. It may also metastasize to the gastrointestinal tract, to adrenal glands, and to soft tissue sites. Cytotoxic chemotherapy is associated with a modest response rate of 20 to 40%, with the single most active agent being dacarbazine (DTIC). However, durable complete responses occur in only 1 to 2% of patients at most. High-dose interleukin-2 therapy has been associated with response rates of 15 to 20% but with 5 to 10% durable complete responses.[139,140] Combination therapy with cytotoxic chemotherapy and biologic therapy (interleukin-2 and interferon-α) has been associated with higher response rates (60 to 70%), but to date has not been associated with improved survival compared with dacarbazine alone.[141] Similarly, the addition of chemotherapy to interleukin-2 and interferon appears to increase response rates but also does not improve long-term survival.[142,143]

An area of active clinical investigation is immunotherapy. Melanoma expresses numerous antigens recognized by cytotoxic T cells and numerous antigens recognized by antibodies. Attempts to treat melanoma with immunotherapy are not new and date back to the work of W. B. Coley at the end of the nineteenth century, and even earlier. However, these approaches are being revolutionized by new knowledge about the molecular nature of melanoma antigens, about the role of cytokines in modulating immune responses, and about the critical role of antigen-presenting cells called dendritic cells.[144] Many clinical trials of tumor vaccines for melanoma are now under way; these include peptide-based vaccines, DNA vaccines, carbohydrate-based vaccines, adoptive cellular therapy, and cytokine therapy.[145,146]

Monitoring of Patients after Treatment or Therapy

Follow-up of patients with melanoma focuses on detection of treatable recurrences. Primarily this includes local recurrences, in-transit metastases, and nodal recurrences. The vast majority of these are evident on physical exam; therefore, physical examination should be the primary focus of follow-up visits. Various schedules of follow-up are used in different treatment centers, depending in part on the level of risk for individual patients. A reasonable schedule for follow-up exams is every 3 to 4 months for 2 years, then every 6 months for the next 3 years, and then annually after 5 years.

Follow-up should also include a history focused on identifying any signs or symptoms of systemic disease. Any suspicious symptoms should be evaluated in detail. In the absence of clinical evidence of recurrence, it is reasonable to perform screening chest x-rays and a serum lactate dehydrogenase and complete blood count annually.

In summary, the surgical management of early melanoma can usually be handled on an ambulatory basis for most procedures, from initial diagnosis by biopsy of a suspicious lesion to wide excision and sentinel node biopsy. Keys to optimal management include early diagnosis, aggressive resection of the primary lesion with attention to the orientation of the incision, and complete staging of patients with intermediate and thick melanomas by sentinel node biopsy where appropriate. Aggressive surgical therapy for nodal metastases is the standard of care and can lead to long-term survival or cure in many patients. Unfortunately, visceral disease or distant metastatic disease is difficult to manage and can only rarely be cured with existing therapy. New hope for advances in this field include ongoing studies of novel therapy directed at modulating the immune response to melanoma.

Unusual Cutaneous Malignancies

Angiosarcoma

Cutaneous angiosarcoma (AS), a highly malignant soft tissue sarcoma of vascular origin, accounts for less than 0.1% of all head and neck cancers. Half of all ASs occur on the scalp and face, most often in elderly Caucasian men. Sun exposure does not appear to play a role in development of AS.[147] Chronic lymphedema, usually on the edematous arm of women with a radical mastectomy and axillary node dissection for carcinoma of the breast, can be associated with AS (Stewart-Treves syndrome).[148] Rarely, AS can develop following radiation therapy for breast or cervical cancer.[149]

AS typically presents as painless enlarging purple-blue macules, plaques, or nodules and can be mistaken for infection or bruising (**Fig. 52.21**). They can range in size from a quarter to a softball. Lesions often have ill-defined borders and may be solitary or multiple. Ulceration and bleeding can occur in advanced cases.

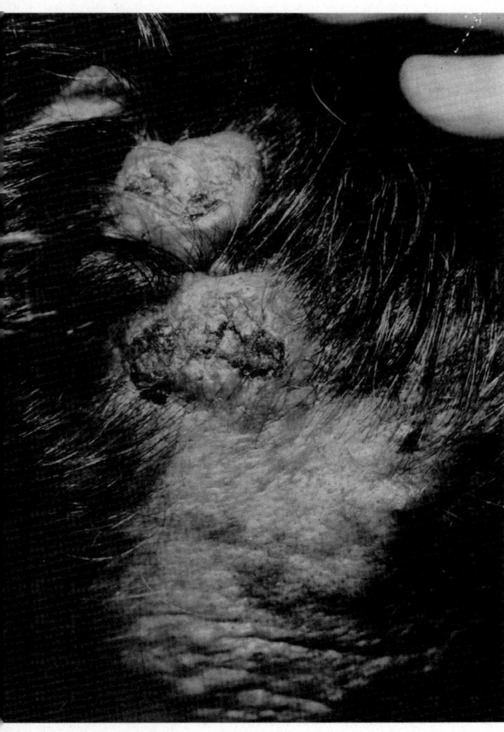

ig. 52.21 Angiosarcoma on the anterior scalp with noduloulcerative ppearance.

AS frequently presents with multifocal disease. There s a propensity for both local recurrence and distant netastasis. The rate of lymph node metastases is 13% for \S—the highest of all soft tissue sarcomas of the head and ıeck.[150] Elective lymph node dissection is not routinely lone. Distant metastases occur in up to 50% of patients vith AS—most commonly involving lung and liver.[151,152]

The prognosis of patients with AS is poor. A recent study reported an overall survival rate of 33%.[147] If an extremity is involved, amputation probably offers the best chance for survival.[152] Mohs micrographic excision may offer some treatment benefit with improved margin conrol in the treatment of AS.[153] The literature suggests that ıggressive combined modality therapy with surgery, radiıtion, and chemotherapy offers the best chance for longerm control in patients with AS.[151] Unfortunately, the areness of this tumor is why no large controlled studies o evaluate treatment have been done.

Atypical Fibroxanthoma

Atypical fibroxanthoma (AFX) is an uncommon spindle cell neoplasm that usually presents as an innocuousıppearing skin growth on the head or neck of elderly men (**Fig. 52.22**). UV radiation appears to play a role in the development of AFX because it appears most often on ıctinically damaged skin, such as the ear and nose.[154]

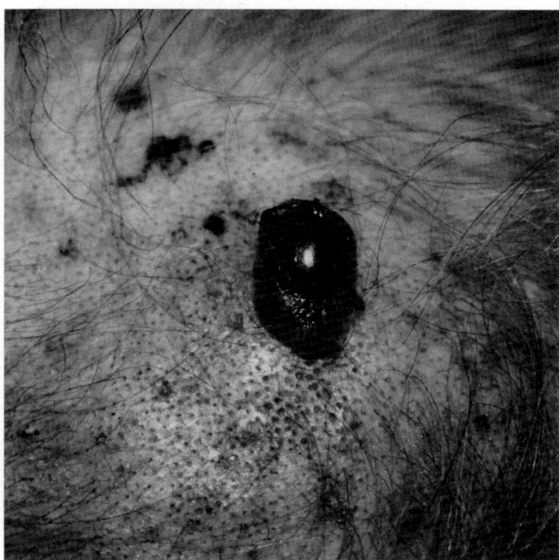

Fig. 52.22 Atypical fibroxanthoma on the vertex scalp. Note typical nodular appearance with an eroded glistening surface.

AFX most commonly appears as a solitary, nickel-sized erythematous nodule. It is often mistaken clinically for BCC, SCC, or amelanotic melanoma. The nodule can enlarge quickly over a period of weeks. Quite often the lesion is friable and there is ulceration with bleeding and pain. The term *atypical* refers to the bizarre, malignant-looking giant cells sometimes seen histologically in AFX. AFX is usually only locally aggressive, sometimes recurring after excision but rarely metastasizing.[155,156] Management of AFX should be similar to that of cutaneous SCC with wide local excision. In advanced cases, radiation has been combined with surgery to manage AFX.[156] Mohs micrographic excision has been associated with a lower recurrence rate than wide local excision.[157] Because of its histological appearance, AFX is felt by some to be a superficial form of malignant fibrous histiocytoma (which carries a poor prognosis).

Dermatofibrosarcoma Protuberans

Dermatofibrosarcoma protuberans (DFSP) is an intermediate-grade sarcoma thought to arise from fibroblasts in the dermis.[158] DFSP usually occurs in early to middle adult life. Occasionally, there is a history of antecedent trauma.[159] There is no racial predisposition, although there is a slight male predominance. Rarely, DFSP occurs in childhood.[160]

DFSP initially presents as a solitary, asymptomatic, firm, half-dollar–sized plaque that is usually violaceous to reddish brown in color. DFSPs arise most often on the trunk or proximal extremities and occasionally on the head and neck. The tumor enlarges slowly over months

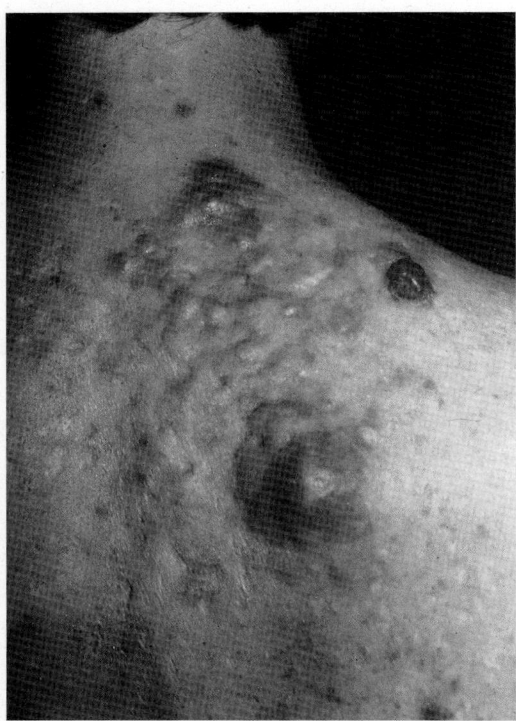

Fig. 52.23 Dermatofibrosarcoma protuberans on the right upper back. Elevated firm papules and nodules could be mistaken for cystic acne and scarring.

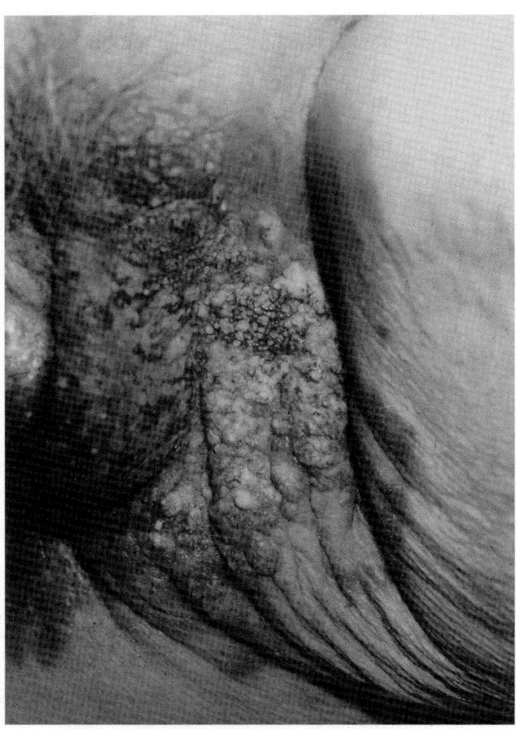

Fig. 52.24 Extensive extramammary Paget's disease of the left labium majora and inguinal crease that could be mistaken for a yeast infection of the skin.

to years and gradually develops small raised nodules within the plaque (**Fig. 52.23**). The growth is usually fixed to overlying skin but not underlying structures. The initial lesion can sometimes be confused with a scar, lipoma, cyst, or neurofibroma. The patient becomes aware of the lesion when there is a sudden change in size or it becomes tender.

Although DFSP is known to be locally aggressive, it metastasizes only rarely. Clinically DFSP may appear to be well circumscribed, but beneath the skin the tumor diffusely infiltrates the dermis and subcutaneous tissue with root-like projections. In the past, this large subclinical spread caused physicians to underestimate the extent of the tumor and use narrower margins for removal than required. In part, this underestimation explains the high rate of recurrence after excision, as much as 60%, in one study.[161] After multiple recurrences, invasion into fascia, muscle, bone, and even brain has occurred.[162] Metastases are usually preceded by two or more local recurrences. One recent review of 913 cases of DFSP reported that only 1% of patients had regional lymph node metastases, and ~4% had suspected distant metastases, principally in the lung. Most patients with metastases died within 2 years.[163]

DFSP is best treated by wide surgical excision. A minimal margin of 3 cm of surrounding skin, including the underlying fascia, is recommended.[163] Radiotherapy has been useful in selected cases.[164,165] Treatment of primary and recurrent DFSP by Mohs micrographic excision has been shown to result in a lower recurrence rate than wide local excision.[166,167]

Extramammary Paget's Disease

Paget's disease is an adenocarcinoma that can develop not only around the breast but also at other apocrine gland-bearing extramammary sites, such as vulva, scrotum, and perianal area (**Fig. 52.24**). Extramammary Paget's disease (EP) occurs primarily in elderly Caucasians and is seen more frequently in women than in men. EP occasionally is associated with an underlying adenocarcinoma or internal malignancy, in contrast to mammary Paget's disease which almost always is associated with an underlying intraductal carcinoma of the breast.[168]

EP presents most often as an ill-defined erythematous patch or plaque in the anogenital area. In women the site most often affected is the labium majora and in men the scrotum.[169] Size can range from a few millimeters to the entire anogenital area. Itching and burning are common symptoms. Scaling and crusting can occur, as can ulceration. EP can easily be mistaken for psoriasis, eczema, seborrheic dermatitis, or fungal infection, delaying diagnosis.

Most cases of EP are superficial, confined to the epidermis without invasion. However, one study found that 24% of patients with EP have an associated underlying cutaneous adnexal adenocarcinoma. The mortality rate of EP with an underlying carcinoma was 46% and dropped to 18% without an underlying carcinoma. Concurrent internal malignancy, such as bladder carcinoma or prostate cancer, was found in 12% of patients with EP.[170] The location of the underlying internal malignancy appears to be closely related to the location of the EP, so that a finding of perianal EP should trigger a search for carcinoma of the digestive system and genital EP an investigation of the genitourinary system.[171,172] The risk of an underlying neoplasm is highest with perianal EP (especially rectal carcinoma), resulting in the poorest prognosis of any location.[173,174] Of patients with EP disease, 26% will ultimately die of it or of associated internal malignancy.[170]

Therapy consists of wide local excision with frozen section margin control, preferably followed by permanent section margin control.[175] Excision may be very difficult or even impossible if the disease is widespread or located in a critical anatomical site. Recurrences after excision are notoriously common—probably because the tumor almost always extends beyond clinically apparent margins and can be multifocal.[176,177] Mohs micrographic excision of EP can provide tissue sparing of critical anatomical structures.[178] Field-destructive modalities, such as radiotherapy, laser, and 5-fluorouracil cream, have been used as adjuvant or primary therapy with varying success.[179–182]

Kaposi's Sarcoma

Kaposi's sarcoma (KS) is a relatively indolent vascular neoplasm that is most often seen in AIDS patients, sometimes as the presenting sign of HIV infection (epidemic KS).[183] Less commonly, KS is seen in HIV-negative individuals—usually on the lower extremities in elderly men of eastern European or Mediterranean descent (endemic KS). There is also an African variant. KS can also be observed in immunosuppressed patients, such as organ transplant recipients. Recently, human herpesvirus type 8 has been shown to be involved in the pathogenesis of AIDS-related KS.[184,185]

KS most often appears as bilaterally symmetrical, bruise-like, violaceous to brown macules, plaques, and nodules on the lower extremities. Involvement of the ears, lips, nose, mucous membranes, and trunk can also be observed. Most cases are asymptomatic. The lesions can be solitary or multiple (**Fig. 52.25**), and multiple lesions can coalesce. Gradually, the lesions of KS darken and become thickened and raised. Advanced lesions can become painful, ulcerated, and edematous, especially on the extremities.

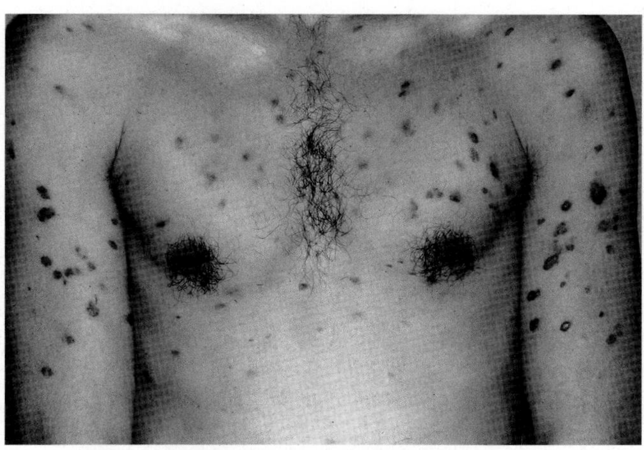

Fig. 52.25 Extensive Kaposi's sarcoma on the chest and arms of an HIV-positive young man.

Immunosuppression, brought on either by drug therapy (e.g., cyclosporin in organ transplant patients) or by infection (e.g., HIV), appears to play a role in the development of KS. Cessation of immunosuppressive therapy in organ transplant patients or improvement of CD4± cell counts in AIDS patients may result in regression of the KS.[186,187] Quite often KS remains indolent and is not a threat to a patient's general health. Internal organ involvement in patients with KS is common but without consequence unless gastrointestinal or pulmonary bleeding or obstruction occurs.[188]

Asymptomatic KS may not require treatment. Cosmetic improvement can be accomplished with cryotherapy, radiation therapy, or intralesional injection of a substance such as vinblastine sulfate.[189–191] Systemic chemotherapy, with a cytotoxic agent such as etoposide or an antiviral agent such as cidofovir, can be administered if KS becomes life threatening.[192,193]

Merkel Cell Carcinoma

Merkel cell carcinoma (MCC) is a highly malignant neoplasm derived from neuroendocrine cells thought to function as touch receptors.[194] Most MCCs occur in elderly Caucasian men and women on the head and neck. MCC is often associated with other skin neoplasms, the most common of which is SCC. This suggests that UV radiation may have an etiologic role in the development of MCC.[195]

MCC appears as a rapidly growing purple to red nodule with telangiectasia. The nodule is usually painless, firm, raised, and red, pink, or occasionally blue (**Fig. 52.26**). Advanced lesions may be ulcerated. The tumors range in size from a few millimeters to many centimeters; they average 2 cm.

The recurrence and metastatic rate for MCC is high. One review reported a 40% local recurrence rate, 55% nodal

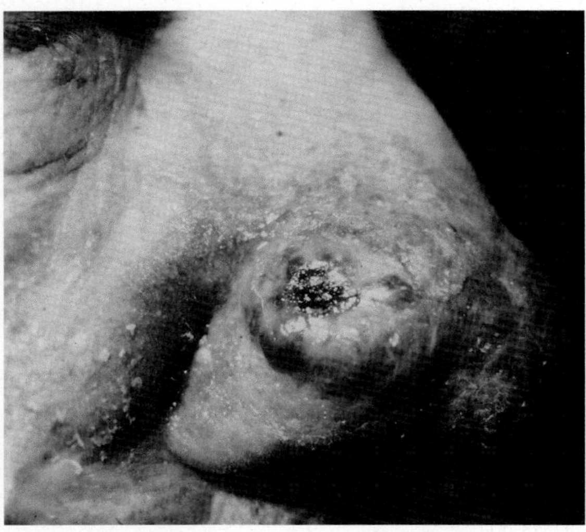

Fig. 52.26 Merkel cell carcinoma on the right ala.

recurrence rate, and a 36% incidence of distant metastases.[196] One study found an overall median survival of 24 months, with 65% of patients succumbing to metastatic disease.[197] There are no reliable microscopic features that differentiate MCC from metastatic oat cell carcinoma; therefore, it is always necessary to rule out oat cell carcinoma metastatic from the lung to the skin by radiological studies.

There is currently no standardized treatment for MCC due to the rarity of this neoplasm.[198] Most authors recommend wide local excision.[199] Prophylactic lymphadenectomy is controversial.[200] MCC is chemosensitive, and a wide variety of chemotherapeutic agents have been used for palliation.[201,202] MCC is also a radiosensitive tumor, and postoperative radiation therapy has been recommended for all patients.[203,204]

Microcystic Adnexal Carcinoma

Microcystic adnexal carcinoma (MAC) most likely originates from sweat ducts.[205] It usually occurs on the head and neck in middle-aged to older Caucasian men and women. The tumor is sometimes associated with a history of previous radiation therapy.[206] Diagnosis of MAC is often delayed because of its slow growth, innocuous clinical appearance, and lack of symptoms. A patient's report of sensory changes, such as pain, numbness, or paresthesias, should alert the physician to the perineural involvement that can be seen with MAC. The incidence of perineural invasion has been reported to be as high as 80%.[207] Clinically, MAC presents as an indurated white to yellow smooth-surfaced plaque or nodule, most often on the upper lip, eyebrow, or, occasionally, the scalp

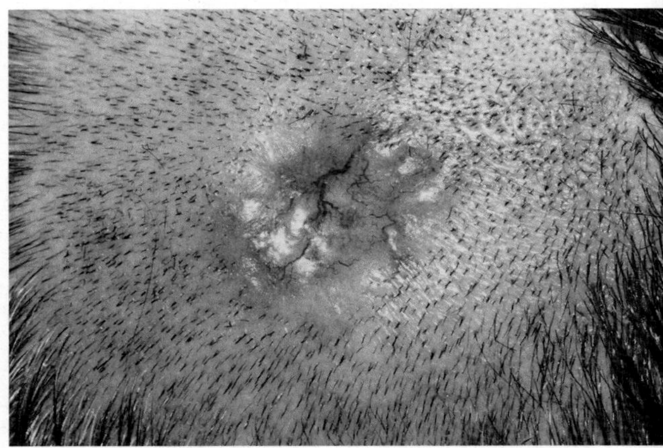

Fig. 52.27 Microcystic adnexal carcinoma of the scalp. Note typical ill-defined whitish plaque with central depression and telangiectasia.

(**Fig. 52.27**).[208,209] MAC is a locally destructive tumor with a high rate of local recurrence (as high as 47% after conventional surgical excision).[205] Frequently MAC is deeply infiltrating, invading muscle and bone, and the tumor often extends far beyond clinically apparent margins.[210,21] MAC has rarely been reported to metastasize.[212] The clinically inapparent extension and perineural involvement of MAC make Mohs micrographic excision the treatment of choice.[213] MAC has been reported to be radioresistant in many cases.[207,208,210]

Sebaceous Gland Carcinoma

Sebaceous gland carcinoma (SGC) may arise from any sebaceous gland in the body but most commonly arises from the sebaceous glands of the eyelid [usually the meibomian glands (51% of cases) or, less commonly, the glands of Zeis (10% of cases)].[214] Extraocular SGC most often occurs on the head and neck.[215] SGC has been associated with ionizing radiation.[216] Mutational inactivation of p53 may be involved in the progression of sebaceous carcinoma.[217]

SGC most commonly arises in elderly women as a slowly growing, indurated, painless, yellow to red nodule on the conjunctival surface of the upper eyelid. The upper eyelid is involved more often than the lower eyelid (**Fig. 52.28**).[21] SGC is often mistaken for a benign inflammatory condition of the eyelids (such as chalazion), and delay in diagnosis is common.[218]

SGC has a propensity for recurrence and metastasis. Both ocular and extraocular SGCs often recur after treatment with approximately one third of all patients having local recurrences.[219] Metastasis occurs in 14 to 25% of cases and is most often to the regional lymph nodes.[215] Orbital invasion occurs in 6 to 17% of cases.[220] Delay in diagnosis and increased tumor size of ocular SGC correlate with increased

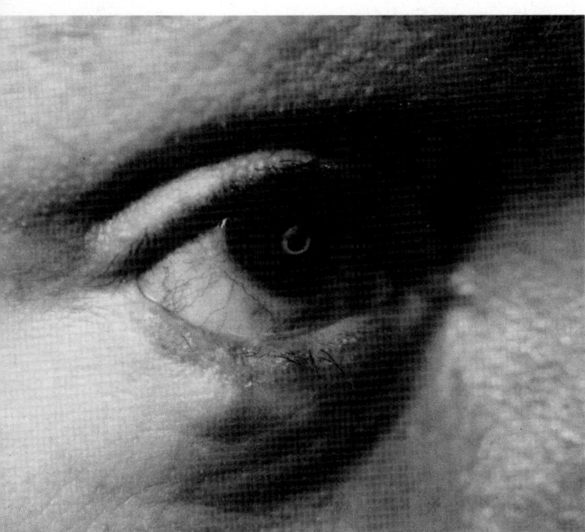

Fig. 52.28 Sebaceous gland carcinoma on the right lower eyelid. Note the margin irregularity, subcutaneous nodule, and eyelash loss.

mortality.[214] SGC of the lower eyelid reportedly has a better prognosis; however, prognosis is poor if both eyelids are involved, with a mortality of 83%.[214,215] Extraocular SGC has a better prognosis than ocular involvement. A patient with an SGC occurring in association with a gastrointestinal malignancy should alert the physician to the possibility of Muir-Torre syndrome, an autosomal dominant genodermatosis.[221]

Wide surgical excision with 6-mm surgical margins controlled by frozen section or permanent section is the primary management for SGC.[215] Orbital exenteration for ocular SGC has been recommended for orbital disease, extensive intraepithelial neoplasia, tumors greater than 2 cm in diameter, or lesions present for more than 6 months.[220] Better margin control and tissue sparing have been obtained with Mohs micrographic excision, but the multicentricity and pagetoid spread of SGC may still allow tumor to be missed and thereby lower the cure rate.[222,223] Cryosurgery for conjunctival pagetoid spread of SGC may have a role in treatment and may preclude exenteration.[224] Although radiotherapy has been used with some success for treatment of SGC, it is usually reserved for treatment of patients who cannot undergo surgery, for palliation, or as adjuvant therapy after surgery.[223,225]

Summary

Unusual cutaneous malignancies often have unusual clinical presentations. For many, the prognosis is usually poor because of failure to discern the true diagnosis. Unusual cutaneous malignancies should always be included in the differential of a suspicious skin growth. If in doubt, a generous biopsy should always be performed. Unfortunately, treatment of many of these unusual cutaneous malignancies is suboptimal, not only because the diagnosis is delayed but also because their rarity precludes any standardized approach to examination.

References

1. Rigel DS, Friedman RJ, Kopf AW. Lifetime risk for development of skin cancer in the U.S. population: current estimate is now 1 in 5 [editorial]. J Am Acad Dermatol 1996;35:1012–1013
2. Landis SH, Murray T, Bolden S, et al. Cancer statistics, 1998 [published erratum appears in CA Cancer J Clin 1998;48(3):192]. CA Cancer J Clin 1998;48(3):6–29
3. Urbach F. Ultraviolet radiation and skin cancer of humans. J Photochem Photobiol B 1997;40:3–7
4. Karagas MR, Greenberg ER, Mott LA, et al. Occurrence of other cancers among patients with prior basal cell and squamous cell skin cancer. Cancer Epidemiol Biomarkers Prev 1998;7:157–161
5. Marghoob AA, Slade J, Salopek TG, et al. Basal cell and squamous cell carcinomas are important risk factors for cutaneous malignant melanoma: screening implications. Cancer 1995;75:707–714
6. Levi F, La Vecchia C, Te VC, et al. Incidence of invasive cancers following basal cell skin cancer. Am J Epidemiol 1998;147:722–726
7. Karagas MR. Occurrence of cutaneous basal cell and squamous cell malignancies among those with a prior history of skin cancer. The Skin Cancer Prevention Study Group. J Invest Dermatol 1994;102:10S–13S
8. Weinstock MA. Epidemiologic investigation of nonmelanoma skin cancer mortality: the Rhode Island Follow-Back Study. J Invest Dermatol 1994;102:6S–9S
9. Miller DL, Weinstock MA. Nonmelanoma skin cancer in the United States: incidence. J Am Acad Dermatol 1994;30:774–778
10. Gloster HM Jr, Brodland DG. The epidemiology of skin cancer. Dermatol Surg 1996;22:217–226
11. English DR, Armstrong BK, Kricker A, et al. Demographic characteristics, pigmentary and cutaneous risk factors for squamous cell carcinoma of the skin: a case-control study. Int J Cancer 1998;76:628–634
12. Harvey I, Frankel S, Marks R, et al. Nonmelanoma skin cancer and solar keratoses, II: analytical results of the South Wales Skin Cancer Study. Br J Cancer 1996;74:1308–1312
13. Strom SS, Yamamura Y. Epidemiology of nonmelanoma skin cancer. Clin Plast Surg 1997;24:627–636
14. Stern RS, Liebman EJ, Vakeva L. Oral psoralen and ultraviolet-A light (PUVA) treatment of psoriasis and persistent risk of nonmelanoma skin cancer: PUVA follow-up study. J Natl Cancer Inst 1998;90:1278–1284
15. Nomura T, Nakajima H, Hongyo T, et al. Induction of cancer, actinic keratosis, and specific p53 mutations by UVB light in human skin maintained in severe combined immunodeficient mice. Cancer Res 1997;57:2081–2084
16. English DR, Armstrong BK, Kricker A, et al. Case-control study of sun exposure and squamous cell carcinoma of the skin. Int J Cancer 1998;77:347–353
17. Gallagher RP, Bajdik CD, Fincham S, et al. Chemical exposures, medical history, and risk of squamous and basal cell carcinoma of the skin. Cancer Epidemiol Biomarkers Prev 1996;5:419–424
18. Preston DS, Stern RS. Nonmelanoma cancers of the skin [see comments]. N Engl J Med 1992;327:1649–1662
19. Markey AC. Etiology and pathogenesis of squamous cell carcinoma. Clin Dermatol 1995;13:537–543
20. van der Laan BF, Baris G, Gregor RT, et al. Radiation-induced tumors of the head and neck. J Laryngol Otol 1995;109:346–349
21. Grodstein F, Speizer FE, Hunter DJ. A prospective study of incident squamous cell carcinoma of the skin in the nurses' health study [see comments]. J Natl Cancer Inst 1995;87:1061–1066
22. Copeland NE, Hanke CW, Michalak JA. The molecular basis of xeroderma pigmentosum. Dermatol Surg 1997;23:447–455

23. Halder RM, Bridgeman-Shah S. Skin cancer in African Americans. Cancer 1995;75:667–673
24. Hendrix JD Jr, Patterson JW, Greer KE. Skin cancer associated with ichthyosis: the MAUIE syndrome. J Am Acad Dermatol 1997;37:1000–1002
25. Phillips TJ, Salman SM, Bhawan J, et al. Burn scar carcinoma: diagnosis and management. Dermatol Surg 1998;24:561–565
26. Ducloux D, Carron PL, Rebibou JM, et al. CD4 lymphocytopenia as a risk factor for skin cancers in renal transplant recipients. Transplantation 1998;65:1270–1272
27. Hartevelt MM, Bavinck JN, Kootte AM, et al. Incidence of skin cancer after renal transplantation in the Netherlands. Transplantation 1990;49:506–509
28. Lampros TD, Cobanoglu A, Parker F, et al. Squamous and basal cell carcinoma in heart transplant recipients. J Heart Lung Transplant 1998;17:586–591
29. Christiansen TN, Freije JE, Neuburg M, et al. Cutaneous squamous cell carcinoma metastatic to the parotid gland in a transplant patient. Clin Transplant 1996;10:561–563
30. Hartley BE, Searle AE, Breach NM, et al. Aggressive cutaneous squamous cell carcinoma of the head and neck in patients with chronic lymphocytic leukaemia. J Laryngol Otol 1996;110:694–695
31. Frierson HF Jr, Deutsch BD, Levine PA. Clinicopathologic features of cutaneous squamous cell carcinomas of the head and neck in patients with chronic lymphocytic leukemia/small lymphocytic lymphoma. Hum Pathol 1988;19:1397–1402
32. Rosenthal AK, McLaughlin JK, Gridley G, et al. Incidence of cancer among patients with systemic sclerosis. Cancer 1995;76:910–914
33. Drolet BA, Neuburg M, Sanger J. Role of human papillomavirus in cutaneous oncogenesis. Ann Plast Surg 1994;33:339–347
34. Marks R, Rennie G, Selwood T. The relationship of basal cell carcinomas and squamous cell carcinomas to solar keratoses. Arch Dermatol 1988;124:1039–1042
35. Cohn BA. Squamous cell carcinoma: could it be the most common skin cancer? [letter]. J Am Acad Dermatol 1998;39:134–136
36. Marks R, Foley P, Goodman G, et al. Spontaneous remission of solar keratoses: the case for conservative management. Br J Dermatol 1986;115:649–655
37. Sober AJ, Burstein JM. Precursors to skin cancer. Cancer 1995;75: 645–650
38. Einspahr J, Alberts DS, Aickin M, et al. Expression of p53 protein in actinic keratosis, adjacent, normal-appearing, and non-sun-exposed human skin. Cancer Epidemiol Biomarkers Prev 1997;6:583–587
39. Suchniak JM, Baer S, Goldberg LH. High rate of malignant transformation in hyperkeratotic actinic keratoses. J Am Acad Dermatol 1997;37:392–394
40. Hodak E, Jones RE, Ackerman AB. Solitary keratoacanthoma is a squamous-cell carcinoma: three examples with metastases [see comments]. Am J Dermatopathol 1993;15:332–342 ,discussion 343–352
41. Schwartz RA. Keratoacanthoma. J Am Acad Dermatol 1994;30:1–19, quiz 20–12
42. Manstein CH, Frauenhoffer CJ, Besden JE. Keratoacanthoma: is it a real entity? Ann Plast Surg 1998;40:469–472
43. Rowe DE, Carroll RJ, Day CL Jr. Prognostic factors for local recurrence, metastasis, and survival rates in squamous cell carcinoma of the skin, ear, and lip: implications for treatment modality selection [see comments]. J Am Acad Dermatol 1992;26:976–990
44. Weinstock MA, Bogaars HA, Ashley M, et al. Nonmelanoma skin cancer mortality: a population-based study. Arch Dermatol 1991;127:1194–1197
45. Immerman SC, Scanlon EF, Christ M, et al. Recurrent squamous cell carcinoma of the skin. Cancer 1983;51:1537–1540
46. Friedman HI, Cooper PH, Wanebo HJ. Prognostic and therapeutic use of microstaging of cutaneous squamous cell carcinoma of the trunk and extremities. Cancer 1985;56:1099–1105
47. Breuninger H, Black B, Rassner G. Microstaging of squamous cell carcinomas. Am J Clin Pathol 1990;94:624–627
48. Dinehart SM, Nelson-Adesokan P, Cockerell C, et al. Metastatic cutaneous squamous cell carcinoma derived from actinic keratosis. Cancer 1997;79:920–923
49. Frierson HF Jr, Cooper PH. Prognostic factors in squamous cell carcinoma of the lower lip. Hum Pathol 1986;17:346–354
50. Clouston PD, Sharpe DM, Corbett AJ, et al. Perineural spread of cutaneous head and neck cancer: its orbital and central neurologic complications. Arch Neurol 1990;47:73–77
51. Hayat G, Ehsan T, Selhorst JB, et al. Magnetic resonance evidence of perineural metastasis. J Neuroimaging 1995;5:122–125
52. Dinehart SM, Pollack SV. Metastases from squamous cell carcinoma of the skin and lip: an analysis of 27 cases [see comments]. J Am Acad Dermatol 1989;21:241–248
53. Dinehart SM, Chu DZ, Maners AW, et al. Immunosuppression in patients with metastatic squamous cell carcinoma from the skin. J Dermatol Surg Oncol 1990;16:271–274
54. Miller SJ. Biology of basal cell carcinoma (Part I). J Am Acad Dermatol 1991;24:1–13
55. Kricker A, Armstrong BK, English DR, et al. Does intermittent sun exposure cause basal cell carcinoma? A case control study in Western Australia. Int J Cancer 1995;60:489–494
56. Xie J, Murone M, Luoh SM, et al. Activating smoothened mutations in sporadic basal-cell carcinoma. Nature 1998;391:90–92
57. Brash DE, Ziegler A, Jonason AS, et al. Sunlight and sunburn in human skin cancer: p53, apoptosis, and tumor promotion. J Investig Dermatol Symp Proc 1996;1:136–142
58. Salasche SJ. Status of curettage and desiccation in the treatment of primary basal cell carcinoma [editorial]. J Am Acad Dermatol 1984;10:285–287
59. Rippey JJ. Why classify basal cell carcinomas? Histopathology 1998;32:393–398
60. Hendrix JD Jr, Parlette HL. Micronodular basal cell carcinoma: a deceptive histologic subtype with frequent clinically undetected tumor extension. Arch Dermatol 1996;132:295–298
61. Hendrix JD Jr, Parlette HL. Duplicitous growth of infiltrative basal cell carcinoma: analysis of clinically undetected tumor extent in a paired case-control study. Dermatol Surg 1996;22:535–539
62. Salasche SJ, Amonette RA. Morpheaform basal-cell epitheliomas: a study of subclinical extensions in a series of 51 cases. J Dermatol Surg Oncol 1981;7:387–394
63. Orengo IF, Salasche SJ, Fewkes J, et al. Correlation of histologic subtypes of primary basal cell carcinoma and number of Mohs stages required to achieve a tumor-free plane. J Am Acad Dermatol 1997;37:395–397
64. Sexton M, Jones DB, Maloney ME. Histologic pattern analysis of basal cell carcinoma: study of a series of 1039 consecutive neoplasms. J Am Acad Dermatol 1990;23:1118–1126
65. Mohs F, Larson P, Iriondo M. Micrographic surgery for the microscopically controlled excision of carcinoma of the external ear. J Am Acad Dermatol 1988;19:729–737
66. Morselli P, Tosti A, Guerra L, et al. Recurrent basal cell carcinoma of the back infiltrating the spine: recurrent basal cell carcinoma. J Dermatol Surg Oncol 1993;19:917–922
67. Tavin E, Persky MS, Jacobs J. Metastatic basal cell carcinoma of the head and neck. Laryngoscope 1995;105:814–817
68. Mall J, Ostertag H, Mall W, et al. Pulmonary metastasis from a basal-cell carcinoma of the retroauricular region. Thorac Cardiovasc Surg 1997;45:258–260
69. Thompson SC, Jolley D, Marks R. Reduction of solar keratoses by regular sunscreen use [see comments]. N Engl J Med 1993;329: 1147–1151
70. Black HS, Herd JA, Goldberg LH, et al. Effect of a low-fat diet on the incidence of actinic keratosis. N Engl J Med 1994;330:1272–1275
71. Silverman MK, Kopf AW, Bart RS, et al. Recurrence rates of treated basal cell carcinomas, III: surgical excision [see comments]. J Dermatol Surg Oncol 1992;18:471–476
72. Wolf DJ, Zitelli JA. Surgical margins for basal cell carcinoma. Arch Dermatol 1987;123:340–344

73. Brodland DG, Zitelli JA. Surgical margins for excision of primary cutaneous squamous cell carcinoma. J Am Acad Dermatol 1992;27: 241–248
74. Rowe DE, Carroll RJ, Day CL Jr. Mohs surgery is the treatment of choice for recurrent (previously treated) basal cell carcinoma. J Dermatol Surg Oncol 1989;15:424–431
75. Swanson NA, Grekin RC, Baker SR. Mohs surgery: techniques, indications, and applications in head and neck surgery. Head Neck Surg 1983;6:683–692
76. Kuflik EG. Cryosurgery for cutaneous malignancy: an update. Dermatol Surg 1997;23:1081–1087
77. Graham GF. Cryosurgery. Clin Plast Surg 1993;20:131–147
78. Silverman MK, Kopf AW, Grin CM, et al. Recurrence rates of treated basal cell carcinomas, II: curettage-electrodesiccation [see comments]. J Dermatol Surg Oncol 1991;17:720–726
79. Geohas J, Roholt NS, Robinson JK. Adjuvant radiotherapy after excision of cutaneous squamous cell carcinoma. J Am Acad Dermatol 1994;30:633–636
80. Cottel WI. Perineural invasion by squamous-cell carcinoma. J Dermatol Surg Oncol 1982;8:589–600
81. Goepfert H, Dichtel WJ, Medina JE, et al. Perineural invasion in squamous cell skin carcinoma of the head and neck. Am J Surg 1984;148:542–547
82. McCord MW, Mendenhall WM, Parsons JT, et al. Skin cancer of the head and neck with incidental microscopic perineural invasion. Int J Radiat Oncol Biol Phys 1999;43:591–595
83. Zablow AI, Eanelli TR, Sanfilippo LJ. Electron beam therapy for skin cancer of the head and neck. Head Neck 1992;14:188–195
84. Elwood JM. Melanoma and sun exposure. Semin Oncol 1996;23: 650–666
85. Robinson ES, Hubbard GB, Colon G, et al. Low-dose ultraviolet exposure early in development can lead to widespread melanoma in the opossum model. Int J Exp Pathol 1998;79:235–244
86. Atillasoy ES, Seykora JT, Soballe PW, et al. UVB induces atypical melanocytic lesions and melanoma in human skin. Am J Pathol 1998;152:1179–1186
87. White E, Kirkpatrick CS, Lee JA. Case-control study of malignant melanoma in Washington State, I: constitutional factors and sun exposure. Am J Epidemiol 1994;139:857–868
88. Quinn MJ, Crotty KA, Thompson JF, et al. Desmoplastic and desmoplastic neurotropic melanoma: experience with 280 patients. Cancer 1998;83:1128–1135
89. DeMatos P, Tyler DS, Seigler HF. Malignant melanoma of the mucous membranes: a review of 119 cases. Ann Surg Oncol 1998;5:733–742
90. Welkoborsky HJ, Sorger K, Knuth A, et al. Maligne Melanome der Schleimhaute des oberen Aerodigestivtraktes: klinische, histologische, und immunhistochemische Charakteristika. Laryngorhinootologie 1991;70:302–306
91. Slingluff CL Jr, Vollmer RT, Seigler HF. Anorectal melanoma: clinical characteristics and results of surgical management in 24 patients. Surgery 1990;107:1–9
92. Tojo D, Wenig BL, Resnick KI. Incidence of cervical metastasis from uveal melanoma: implications for treatment. Head Neck 1995;17:137–139
93. Kanavaros P, Galian A, Periac P, et al. Melanome malin primitif de l'oesophage developpe sur une melanose: etude histologique, immunohistochimique, et ultrastructurale d'un cas. Ann Pathol 1989;9:57–61
94. Norman J, Cruse CW, Wells KE, et al. Metastatic melanoma with an unknown primary. Ann Plast Surg 1992;28:81–84
95. Balch CM, Murad TM, Soong SJ, et al. Tumor thickness as a guide to surgical management of clinical stage I melanoma patients. Cancer 1979;43:883–888
96. Walsh N, Crotty K, Palmer A, et al. Spitz nevus versus spitzoid malignant melanoma: an evaluation of the current distinguishing histopathologic criteria. Hum Pathol 1998;29:1105–1112
97. Paredes B, Hardmeier T. Naevus Spitz und Naevus Reed: bei Erwachsenen ein Melanomsimulator. Pathologe 1998;19:403–411
98. Austin JR, Byers RM, Brown WD, et al. Influence of biopsy on the prognosis of cutaneous melanoma of the head and neck. Head Neck 1996;18:107–117
99. Breslow A. Thickness, cross-sectional areas, and depth of invasion in the prognosis of cutaneous melanoma. Ann Surg 1970;172:902–908
100. Slingluff CL Jr, Vollmer RT, Reintgen DS, et al. Lethal "thin" malignant melanoma: identifying patients at risk. Ann Surg 1988;208:150–161
101. Heaton KM, Sussman JJ, Gershenwald JE, et al. Surgical margins and prognostic factors in patients with thick (74-mm) primary melanoma. Ann Surg Oncol 1998;5:322–328
102. Clark WH Jr, From L, Bernardino EA, et al. The histogenesis and biologic behavior of primary human malignant melanomas of the skin. Cancer Res 1969;29:705–727
103. Elder DE, Van Belle P, Elenitsas R, et al. Neoplastic progression and prognosis in melanoma. Semin Cutan Med Surg 1996;15:336–348
104. Guerry DT, Synnestvedt M, Elder DE, et al. Lessons from tumor progression: the invasive radial growth phase of melanoma is common, incapable of metastasis, and indolent. J Invest Dermatol 1993;100: 342S–345S
105. Clark WH Jr, Elder DE, Guerry DT, et al. Model predicting survival in stage I melanoma based on tumor progression [see comments]. J Natl Cancer Inst 1989;81:1893–1904
106. Buzaid AC, Ross MI, Balch CM, et al. Critical analysis of the current American Joint Committee on Cancer staging system for cutaneous melanoma and proposal of a new staging system [see comments]. J Clin Oncol 1997;15:1039–1051
107. Clemente CG, Mihm MC Jr, Bufalino R, et al. Prognostic value of tumor infiltrating lymphocytes in the vertical growth phase of primary cutaneous melanoma. Cancer 1996;77:1303–1310
108. Terhune MH, Swanson N, Johnson TM. Use of chest radiography in the initial evaluation of patients with localized melanoma [see comments]. Arch Dermatol 1998;134:569–572
109. Provost N, Marghoob AA, Kopf AW, et al. Laboratory tests and imaging studies in patients with cutaneous malignant melanomas: a survey of experienced physicians. J Am Acad Dermatol 1997;36: 711–720
110. Khansur T, Sanders J, Das SK. Evaluation of staging workup in malignant melanoma. Arch Surg 1989;124:847–849
111. Anonymous. NIH Consensus conference: diagnosis and treatment of early melanoma [see comments]. JAMA 1992;268:1314–1319
112. Cascinelli N. Margin of resection in the management of primary melanoma. Semin Surg Oncol 1998;14:272–275
113. Balch CM, Urist MM, Karakousis CP, et al. Efficacy of 2-cm surgical margins for intermediate-thickness melanomas (1- to 4-mm): results of a multi-institutional randomized surgical trial [see comments]. Ann Surg 1993;218:262–267, discussion 267–269
114. Veronesi U, Cascinelli N. Narrow excision (1-cm margin): a safe procedure for thin cutaneous melanoma. Arch Surg 1991;126:438–441
115. Cascinelli N, Santinami M. Excision of primary melanoma should allow primary closure of the wound. Recent Results Cancer Res 1995;139:317–321
116. Harris TJ, Hinckley DM. Melanoma of the head and neck in Queensland. Head Neck Surg 1983;5:197–203
117. Balch CM, Soong SJ, Bartolucci AA, et al. Efficacy of an elective regional lymph node dissection of 1- to 4-mm-thick melanomas for patients 60 years of age and younger. Ann Surg 1996;224:255–263, discussion 263–266
118. Veronesi U, Adamus J, Bandiera DC, et al. Stage I melanoma of the limbs. Immediate versus delayed node dissection. Tumori 1980;66:373–396
119. Veronesi U, Adamus J, Bandiera DC, et al. Delayed regional lymph node dissection in stage I melanoma of the skin of the lower extremities. Cancer 1982;49:2420–2430
120. Sim FH, Taylor WF, Pritchard DJ, et al. Lymphadenectomy in the management of stage I malignant melanoma: a prospective randomized study. Mayo Clin Proc 1986;61:697–705
121. Balch CM, Soong SJ, Milton GW, et al. A comparison of prognostic factors and surgical results in 1786 patients with localized (stage I)

melanoma treated in Alabama, USA, and New South Wales, Australia. Ann Surg 1982;196:677–684
122. Reintgen DS, Cox EB, McCarty KS Jr, et al. Efficacy of elective lymph node dissection in patients with intermediate-thickness primary melanoma. Ann Surg 1983;198:379–385
123. Slingluff CL Jr, Stidham KR, Ricci WM, et al. Surgical management of regional lymph nodes in patients with melanoma: experience with 4682 patients [see comments]. Ann Surg 1994;219:120–130
124. Coates AS, Ingvar CI, Petersen-Schaefer K, et al. Elective lymph node dissection in patients with primary melanoma of the trunk and limbs treated at the Sydney melanoma unit from 1960 to 1991 [see comments]. J Am Coll Surg 1995;180:402–409
125. Morton DL, Wen DR, Wong JH, et al. Technical details of intraoperative lymphatic mapping for early-stage melanoma. Arch Surg 1992;127:392–399
126. Kelley MC, Ollila DW, Morton DL. Lymphatic mapping and sentinel lymphadenectomy for melanoma. Semin Surg Oncol 1998;14: 283–290
127. Joseph E, Messina J, Glass FL, et al. Radioguided surgery for the ultrastaging of the patient with melanoma [see comments]. Cancer J Sci Am 1997;3:341–345
128. Gershenwald JE, Colome MI, Lee JE, et al. Patterns of recurrence following a negative sentinel lymph node biopsy in 243 patients with stage I or II melanoma. J Clin Oncol 1998;16:2253–2260
129. Gogel BM, Kuhn JA, Ferry KM, et al. Sentinel lymph node biopsy for melanoma. Am J Surg 1998;176:544–547
130. Gershenwald JE, Tseng CH, Thompson W, et al. Improved sentinel lymph node localization in patients with primary melanoma with the use of radiolabeled colloid. Surgery 1998;124:203–210
131. Wells KE, Cruse CW, Daniels S, et al. The use of lymphoscintigraphy in melanoma of the head and neck. Plast Reconstr Surg 1994;93: 757–761
132. O'Brien CJ, Uren RF, Thompson JF, et al. Prediction of potential metastatic sites in cutaneous head and neck melanoma using lymphoscintigraphy. Am J Surg 1995;170:461–466
133. Slingluff CL Jr, Vollmer R, Seigler HF. Stage II malignant melanoma: presentation of a prognostic model and an assessment of specific active immunotherapy in 1273 patients. J Surg Oncol 1988;39: 139–147
134. Buzaid AC, Tinoco L, Ross MI, et al. Role of computed tomography in the staging of patients with local regional metastases of melanoma. J Clin Oncol 1995;13:2104–2108
135. Anbari KK, Schuchter LM, Bucky LP, et al. Melanoma of unknown primary site: presentation, treatment, and prognosis: a single institution study. University of Pennsylvania Pigmented Lesion Study Group. Cancer 1997;79:1816–1821
136. Van de Vrie W, Eggermont AM, Van Putten WL, et al. Therapeutic lymphadenectomy in melanomas of the head and neck. Head Neck 1993;15:377–381
137. O'Brien CJ, Petersen-Schaefer K, Ruark D, et al. Radical, modified, and selective neck dissection for cutaneous malignant melanoma. Head Neck 1995;17:232–241
138. Kirkwood JM, Strawderman MH, Ernstoff MS, et al. Interferon alfa-2b adjuvant therapy of high-risk resected cutaneous melanoma: the Eastern Cooperative Oncology Group Trial EST 1684 [see comments]. J Clin Oncol 1996;14:7–17
139. Rosenberg SA, Yang JC, White DE, et al. Durability of complete responses in patients with metastatic cancer treated with high-dose interleukin-2: identification of the antigens mediating response. Ann Surg 1998;228:307–319
140. Keilholz U, Conradt C, Legha SS, et al. Results of interleukin-2-based treatment in advanced melanoma: a case record–based analysis of 631 patients. J Clin Oncol 1998;16:2921–2929
141. Falkson CI, Ibrahim J, Kirkwood JM, et al. Phase III trial of dacarbazine versus dacarbazine with interferon alpha-2b versus dacarbazine with tamoxifen versus dacarbazine with interferon alpha-2b and tamoxifen in patients with metastatic malignant melanoma: an Eastern Cooperative Oncology Group study. J Clin Oncol 1998;16:1743–1751
142. Keilholz U, Goey SH, Punt CJ, et al. Interferon alfa-2a and interleukin-2 with or without cisplatin in metastatic melanoma: a randomized trial of the European Organization for Research and Treatment of Cancer Melanoma Cooperative Group. J Clin Oncol 1997;15:2579–2588
143. Rosenberg SA, Yang JC, Schwartzentruber DJ, et al. Prospective randomized trial of the treatment of patients with metastatic melanoma using chemotherapy with cisplatin, dacarbazine, and tamoxifen alone or in combination with interleukin-2 and interferon alfa-2b. J Clin Oncol 1999;17:968–975
144. Fernandez N, Duffour MT, Perricaudet M, et al. Active specific T-cell-based immunotherapy for cancer: nucleic acids, peptides, whole native proteins, recombinant viruses, with dendritic cell adjuvants or whole tumor cell–based vaccines: principles and future prospects. Cytokines Cell Mol Ther 1998;4:53–65
145. Maeurer MJ, Storkus WJ, Kirkwood JM, et al. New treatment options for patients with melanoma: review of melanoma-derived T-cell epitope-based peptide vaccines. Melanoma Res 1996;6:11–24
146. Slingluff CL Jr. Tumor antigens and tumor vaccines: peptides as immunogens. Semin Surg Oncol 1996;12:446–453
147. Lydiatt WM, Shaha AR, Shah JP. Angiosarcoma of the head and neck. Am J Surg 1994;168:451–454
148. Woodward AH, Ivins JC, Soule EH. Lymphangiosarcoma arising in chronic lymphedematous extremities. Cancer 1972;30:562–572
149. Robinson E, Neugut AI, Wylie P. Clinical aspects of postirradiation sarcomas. J Natl Cancer Inst 1988;80:233–240
150. Fong Y, Coit DG, Woodruff JM, et al. Lymph node metastasis from soft tissue sarcoma in adults: analysis of data from a prospective database of 1772 sarcoma patients. Ann Surg 1993;217:72–77
151. Mark RJ, Tran LM, Sercarz J, et al. Angiosarcoma of the head and neck: the UCLA experience 1955 through 1990. Arch Otolaryngol Head Neck Surg 1993;119:973–978
152. Sordillo PP, Chapman R, Hajdu SI, et al. Lymphangiosarcoma. Cancer 1981;48:1674–1679
153. Goldberg DJ, Kim YA. Angiosarcoma of the scalp treated with Mohs micrographic surgery [see comments]. J Dermatol Surg Oncol 1993;19:156–158
154. Dei Tos AP, Maestro R, Doglioni C, et al. Ultravioletinduced p53 mutations in atypical fibroxanthoma. Am J Pathol 1994;145:11–17
155. Fretzin DF, Helwig EB. Atypical fibroxanthoma of the skin: a clinicopathologic study of 140 cases. Cancer 1973;31:1541–1552
156. Helwig EB, May D. Atypical fibroxanthoma of the skin with metastasis. Cancer 1986;57:368–376
157. Davis JL, Randle HW, Zalla MJ, et al. A comparison of Mohs micrographic surgery and wide excision for the treatment of atypical fibroxanthoma [see comments]. Dermatol Surg 1997;23:105–110
158. Allan AE, Tsou HC, Harrington A, et al. Clonal origin of dermatofibrosarcoma protuberans. J Invest Dermatol 1993;100:99–102
159. Mbonde MP, Amir H, Kitinya JN. Dermatofibrosarcoma protuberans: a clinicopathological study in an African population. East Afr Med J 1996;73:410–413
160. Pappo AS, Rao BN, Cain A, et al. Dermatofibrosarcoma protuberans: the pediatric experience at St. Jude Children's Research Hospital. Pediatr Hematol Oncol 1997;14:563–568
161. Mark RJ, Bailet JW, Tran LM, et al. Dermatofibrosarcoma protuberans of the head and neck: a report of 16 cases. Arch Otolaryngol Head Neck Surg 1993;119:891–896
162. Rockley PF, Robinson JK, Magid M, et al. Dermatofibrosarcoma protuberans of the scalp: a series of cases. J Am Acad Dermatol 1989;21:278–283
163. Rutgers EJ, Kroon BB, Albus-Lutter CE, et al. Dermatofibrosarcoma protuberans: treatment and prognosis. Eur J Surg Oncol 1992;18:241–248
164. Marks LB, Suit HD, Rosenberg AE, et al. Dermatofibrosarcoma protuberans treated with radiation therapy. Int J Radiat Oncol Biol Phys 1989;17:379–384
165. Haas RL, Keus RB, Loftus BM, et al. The role of radiotherapy in the local management of dermatofibrosarcoma protuberans. Soft Tissue Tumours Working Group. Eur J Cancer 1997;33:1055–1060

166. Gloster HM Jr, Harris KR, Roenigk RK. A comparison between Mohs micrographic surgery and wide surgical excision for the treatment of dermatofibrosarcoma protuberans. J Am Acad Dermatol 1996;35: 82–87
167. Ratner D, Thomas CO, Johnson TM, et al. Mohs micrographic surgery for the treatment of dermatofibrosarcoma protuberans: results of a multiinstitutional series with an analysis of the extent of microscopic spread. J Am Acad Dermatol 1997;37:600–613
168. Heymann WR. Extramammary Paget's disease. Clin Dermatol 1993; 11:83–87
169. Perez MA, LaRossa DD, Tomaszewski JE. Paget's disease primarily involving the scrotum. Cancer 1989;63:970–975
170. Chanda JJ. Extramammary Paget's disease: prognosis and relationship to internal malignancy. J Am Acad Dermatol 1985;13:1009–1014
171. Feuer GA, Shevchuk M, Calanog A. Vulvar Paget's disease: the need to exclude an invasive lesion. Gynecol Oncol 1990;38:81–89
172. Allan SJ, McLaren K, Aldridge RD. Paget's disease of the scrotum: a case exhibiting positive prostate-specific antigen staining and associated prostatic adenocarcinoma. Br J Dermatol 1998;138:689–691
173. Beck DE, Fazio VW. Perianal Paget's disease. Dis Colon Rectum 1987;30:263–266
174. Merot Y, Mazoujian G, Pinkus G, et al. Extramammary Paget's disease of the perianal and perineal regions: evidence of apocrine derivation. Arch Dermatol 1985;121:750–752
175. Barlow RJ, Ramnarain N, Smith N, et al. Excision of selected skin tumours using Mohs' micrographic surgery with horizontal paraffin-embedded sections. Br J Dermatol 1996;135:911–917
176. Gunn RA, Gallager HS. Vulvar Paget's disease: a topographic study. Cancer 1980;46:590–594
177. Wagner RF Jr, Cottel WI. Treatment of extensive extramammary Paget disease of male genitalia with Mohs micrographic surgery. Urology 1988;31:415–418
178. Coldiron BM, Goldsmith BA, Robinson JK. Surgical treatment of extramammary Paget's disease: a report of six cases and a re-examination of Mohs micrographic surgery compared with conventional surgical excision. Cancer 1991;67:933–938
179. Besa P, Rich TA, Delclos L, et al. Extramammary Paget's disease of the perineal skin: role of radiotherapy. Int J Radiat Oncol Biol Phys 1992;24:73–78
180. Burrows NP, Jones DH, Hudson PM, et al. Treatment of extramammary Paget's disease by radiotherapy [see comments]. Br J Dermatol 1995;132:970–972
181. Arensmeier M, Theuring U, Franke I, et al. Topische Therapie des extramammaren Morbus Paget. Hautarzt 1994;45:780–782
182. Eliezri YD, Silvers DN, Horan DB. Role of preoperative topical 5-fluorouracil in preparation for Mohs micrographic surgery of extramammary Paget's disease. J Am Acad Dermatol 1987;17: 497–505
183. Rabkin CS. Epidemiology of AIDS-related malignancies. Curr Opin Oncol 1994;6:492–496
184. Moore PS, Chang Y. Detection of herpesvirus-like DNA sequences in Kaposi's sarcoma in patients with and without HIV infection [see comments]. N Engl J Med 1995;332:1181–1185
185. Kennedy MM, Cooper K, Howells DD, et al. Identification of HHV8 in early Kaposi's sarcoma: implications for Kaposi's sarcoma pathogenesis. Mol Pathol 1998;51:14–20
186. Montagnino G, Bencini PL, Tarantino A, et al. Clinical features and course of Kaposi's sarcoma in kidney transplant patients: report of 13 cases. Am J Nephrol 1994;14:121–126
187. Aboulafia DM. Regression of acquired immunodeficiency syndrome-related pulmonary Kaposi's sarcoma after highly active antiretroviral therapy. Mayo Clin Proc 1998;73:439–443
188. Requena L, Sangueza OP. Cutaneous vascular proliferations, III: malignant neoplasms, other cutaneous neoplasms with significant vascular component, and disorders erroneously considered as vascular neoplasms. J Am Acad Dermatol 1998;38:143–175, quiz 176–178
189. Tappero JW, Berger TG, Kaplan LD, et al. Cryotherapy for cutaneous Kaposi's sarcoma (KS) associated with acquired immune deficiency syndrome (AIDS): a phase II trial. J Acquir Immune Defic Syndr 1991;4:839–846
190. Kirova YM, Belembaogo E, Frikha H, et al. Radiotherapy in the management of epidemic Kaposi's sarcoma: a retrospective study of 643 cases. Radiother Oncol 1998;46:19–22
191. Gascón P, Schwartz RA. Treatment of Kaposi's sarcoma. Dermatol Clin 1994;12:451–456
192. Schwartsmann G, Sprinz E, Kromfield M, et al. Clinical and pharmacokinetic study of oral etoposide in patients with AIDS-related Kaposi's sarcoma with no prior exposure to cytotoxic therapy. J Clin Oncol 1997;15:2118–2124
193. Hammoud Z, Parenti DM, Simon GL. Abatement of cutaneous Kaposi's sarcoma associated with cidofovir treatment. Clin Infect Dis 1998;26:1233
194. Ratner D, Nelson BR, Brown MD, et al. Merkel cell carcinoma. J Am Acad Dermatol 1993;29:143–156
195. Pitale M, Sessions RB, Husain S. An analysis of prognostic factors in cutaneous neuroendocrine carcinoma. Laryngoscope 1992;102:244–249
196. Hitchcock CL, Bland KI, Laney RG, et al. Neuroendocrine (Merkel cell) carcinoma of the skin: its natural history, diagnosis, and treatment. Ann Surg 1988;207:201–207
197. Boyle F, Pendlebury S, Bell D. Further insights into the natural history and management of primary cutaneous neuroendocrine (Merkel cell) carcinoma. Int J Radiat Oncol Biol Phys 1995;31: 315–323
198. Queirolo P, Gipponi M, Peressini A, et al. Merkel cell carcinoma of the skin: treatment of primary, recurrent and metastatic disease: review of clinical cases. Anticancer Res 1997;17:2339–2342
199. O'Connor WJ, Roenigk RK, Brodland DG. Merkel cell carcinoma: comparison of Mohs micrographic surgery and wide excision in eighty-six patients [published erratum appears in Dermatol Surg 1998;24(2):299]. Dermatol Surg 1997;23:929–933
200. Kokoska ER, Kokoska MS, Collins BT, et al. Early aggressive treatment for Merkel cell carcinoma improves outcome. Am J Surg 1997;174:688–693
201. Wynne CJ, Kearsley JH. Merkel cell tumor: a chemosensitive skin cancer. Cancer 1988;62:28–31
202. Krasagakis K, Almond-Roesler B, Zouboulis CC, et al. Merkel cell carcinoma: report of ten cases with emphasis on clinical course, treatment, and in vitro drug sensitivity. J Am Acad Dermatol 1997;36:727–732
203. Morrison WH, Peters LJ, Silva EG, et al. The essential role of radiation therapy in securing locoregional control of Merkel cell carcinoma. Int J Radiat Oncol Biol Phys 1990;19:583–591
204. Fenig E, Brenner B, Katz A, et al. The role of radiation therapy and chemotherapy in the treatment of Merkel cell carcinoma. Cancer 1997;80:881–885
205. Cooper PH. Sclerosing carcinomas of sweat ducts (microcystic adnexal carcinoma). Arch Dermatol 1986;122:261–264
206. Borenstein A, Seidman DS, Trau H, et al. Microcystic adnexal carcinoma following radiotherapy in childhood. Am J Med Sci 1991;301:259–261
207. Cooper PH, Mills SE, Leonard DD, et al. Sclerosing sweat duct (syringomatous) carcinoma. Am J Surg Pathol 1985;9:422–433
208. Sebastien TS, Nelson BR, Lowe L, et al. Microcystic adnexal carcinoma. J Am Acad Dermatol 1993;29:840–845
209. Chow WC, Cockerell CJ, Geronemus RG. Microcystic adnexal carcinoma of the scalp. J Dermatol Surg Oncol 1989;15:768–771
210. Billingsley EM, Fedok F, Maloney ME. Microcystic adnexal carcinoma: case report and review of the literature. Arch Otolaryngol Head Neck Surg 1996;122:179–182
211. Yuh WT, Engelken JD, Whitaker DC, et al. Bone marrow invasion of microcystic adnexal carcinoma. Ann Otol Rhinol Laryngol 1991;100:601–603
212. Bier-Lansing CM, Hom DB, Gapany M, et al. Microcystic adnexal carcinoma: management options based on long-term follow-up. Laryngoscope 1995;105:1197–1201

213. Burns MK, Chen SP, Goldberg LH. Microcystic adnexal carcinoma: ten cases treated by Mohs micrographic surgery. J Dermatol Surg Oncol 1994;20:429–434
214. Rao NA, Hidayat AA, McLean IW, et al. Sebaceous carcinomas of the ocular adnexa: a clinicopathologic study of 104 cases, with five-year follow-up data. Hum Pathol 1982;13:113–122
215. Nelson BR, Hamlet KR, Gillard M, et al. Sebaceous carcinoma. J Am Acad Dermatol 1995;33:1–15, quiz 16–18
216. Lemos LB, Santa Cruz DJ, Baba N. Sebaceous carcinoma of the eyelid following radiation therapy. Am J Surg Pathol 1978;2:305–311
217. Gonzalez-Fernandez F, Kaltreider SA, Patnaik BD, et al. Sebaceous carcinoma: tumor progression through mutational inactivation of p53. Ophthalmology 1998;105:497–506
218. Margo CE, Lessner A, Stern GA. Intraepithelial sebaceous carcinoma of the conjunctiva and skin of the eyelid. Ophthalmology 1992;99:227–231
219. Doxanas MT, Green WR. Sebaceous gland carcinoma: review of 40 cases. Arch Ophthalmol 1984;102:245–249
220. Kass LG, Hornblass A. Sebaceous carcinoma of the ocular adnexa. Surv Ophthalmol 1989;33:477–490
221. Schwartz RA, Torre DP. The Muir-Torre syndrome: a 25-year retrospect [see comments]. J Am Acad Dermatol 1995;33:90–104
222. Yount AB, Bylund D, Pratt SG, et al. Mohs micrographic excision of sebaceous carcinoma of the eyelids. J Dermatol Surg Oncol 1994;20:523–529
223. Folberg R, Whitaker DC, Tse DT, et al. Recurrent and residual sebaceous carcinoma after Mohs' excision of the primary lesion. Am J Ophthalmol 1987;103:817–823
224. Lisman RD, Jakobiec FA, Small P. Sebaceous carcinoma of the eyelids: the role of adjunctive cryotherapy in the management of conjunctival pagetoid spread [see comments]. Ophthalmology 1989;96:1021–1026
225. Nunery WR, Welsh MG, McCord CD Jr. Recurrence of sebaceous carcinoma of the eyelid after radiation therapy. Am J Ophthalmol 1983;96:10–15

53 Minimally Invasive Options and Skin Grafts for Cutaneous Reconstruction

David B. Hom and Whitney D. Tope

Conservative options for cutaneous facial reconstruction comprise of healing by second intention, primary closure, the use of skin grafts, and skin flaps. Quite often, minimally invasive techniques for facial reconstruction are the best choice in reconstructing facial defects. This chapter focuses on these minimally invasive reconstructive options for facial repair. In treating patients requiring facial reconstruction, the major objectives and time course for healing should be carefully discussed with the patient and family so that a mutual agreement is made regarding the reconstructive goals.

Patient Evaluation

Assessment of the Facial Defect

To determine the optimal method for reconstruction, one must fully define the given defect. The complexity of the defect is defined by the tissue layers that are missing: location, surface area of involvement, and its relationship to the aesthetic subunits.

The initial wound assessment involves determining the size, location, and depth of the facial defect while being cognizant of the possibility that underlying neurovascular or glandular structures might also be missing. Evaluating the depth of the defect (subcutaneous space, facial musculature, cartilage, and bone) is crucial for planning the appropriate repair. By palpating the wound and its surrounding structures, the structural support of the area is determined. If structural support is missing, computed tomography (CT) might be helpful in determining if additional underlying support is required. The extent of the tissue loss and orientation of the wound in proximity to surrounding mobile facial structures (eyelids, nasal alae, nasal tip, auricle, vermilion, commissures, and philtral ridges) should also be evaluated.

The major reconstructive goal is to reestablish functional structural support and soft tissue coverage, maintaining the most aesthetic appearance with minimal distortion. Ideally, the absent tissue should be repaired with like tissue that is similar in color, texture, and thickness. Absent supporting structures (bone and cartilage) should be replaced to obtain appropriate projection and contour. Wound healing should be optimized to avoid infection, excessive contraction and scarring.

Planning Guidelines and Facial Subunits

The extent of the missing facial subunits should be evaluated. If the contralateral face is normal, it can be used as a visual template for guidance. Dividing the face into six major facial aesthetic units (forehead, eye/eyebrow, nose, lips, chin, and cheek) is helpful in reconstructive planning (**Fig. 53.1**). Aesthetic units of the face represent anatomical boundaries, and scars lying on these boundaries appear more concealed. This is because the borders of the aesthetic units are defined by light reflections and shadows of the facial contours. Within some aesthetic units, additional anatomical boundaries can be divided into subunits. This boundary division is applicable to the nose, which can be divided into the subunits—nasal dorsum, nasal tip, columella, nasal alae, soft tissue triangles, and nasal sidewalls.[1]

Scars are concealed maximally by adhering to techniques of tensionless wound closure, wound edge eversion, and planning to have the wound lie within the relaxed skin tension line (RSTL) of the face (**Fig. 53.2**) or at the border of facial aesthetic units.

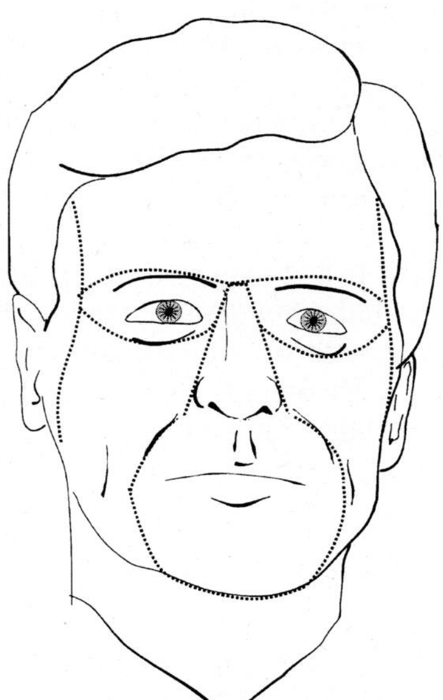

Fig. 53.1 Aesthetic units on the face (forehead, eye/eyebrow, nose, cheek, mouth, and chin). (From Hom DB, Odland RM. Prognosis for facial scarring. In: Harahap M, ed. Surgical Techniques for Cutaneous Scars Revision. New York: Marcel Dekker; 2000:25–37.)

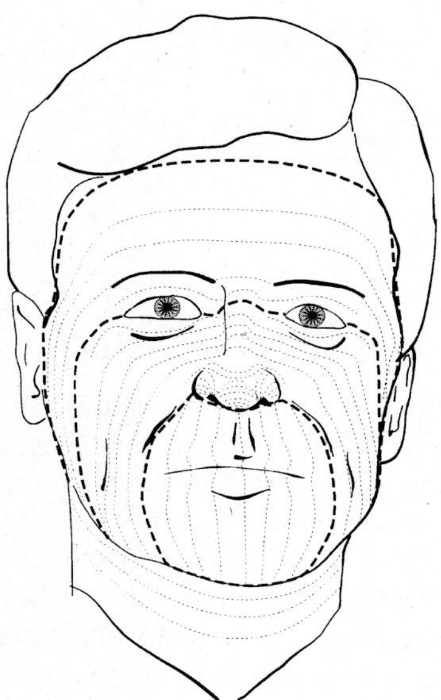

Fig. 53.2 Facial relaxed skin tension lines. The long axis of fusiform excisions should lie parallel to the relaxed skin tension lines. (From Hom DB, Odland RM. Prognosis for facial scarring. In: Harahap M, ed. Surgical Techniques for Cutaneous Scars Revision. New York: Marcel Dekker; 2000:25–37.)

With any wound, the proximity of the tissue loss with respect to nearby mobile facial structures (eyelids, nasal alae, nasal tip, auricle, vermilion, commissures, and philtrum) should be recognized. This is to avoid distortion of these neighboring structures during closing of the wound, which can make the scar much more noticeable.

When a wound from tissue loss cannot be adequately closed primarily without undue tension or vital structure deformity, planning for reconstruction is required. Reconstructive options include healing by second tension, local skin flaps, skin grafts, regional flaps, or free flaps. For wound sites having the majority of a facial aesthetic unit missing, considerations can be made for removal of the remaining aesthetic skin unit followed by local skin flaps or skin grafting. This technique can maintain uniformity of skin color and contour of the facial unit and make scars less visible by having them lie on the aesthetic unit boundaries. For defects encompassing more than one facial aesthetic unit, the units can be reconstructed independent of one another.

Primary Closure

Tensionless closure of each layer (mucosa, muscle, subcutaneous tissue, and skin) should be achieved. To avoid distortion of nearby structures, differential undermining of the wound edges in the subcutaneous plane may be necessary. Differential undermining signifies dissecting in the subcutaneous plane only on one side of the wound. This is performed only to advance the undermined side of the wound edge to avoid distorting the nonundermined side of the wound. The deeper layers can be closed individually with buried absorbable suture to avoid transmitting tension to the skin surface. With dermal closure, eversion of the skin edges can then be performed. To minimize a "trap door" deformity with a beveled wound edge, excessive dermal tissue can be conservatively excised in a tangential fashion to the wound surface to create a more vertical skin edge. When a defect cannot be adequately closed primarily, other conservative options include healing by second intention, local flaps, skin grafts, or skin flaps.

Healing by Second Intention

History and Background

It is easy to overlook the fact that the healthy human body possesses the capability to repair damaged or lost tissue without surgical intervention. This phenomenon of complete tissue restoration[2] of soft tissue defects occurs through processes of replacement of lost tissue volume (granulation), reestablishment of defect surface integrity (reepithelialization), and reduction of wound volume (wound contraction). However, the healing of full-thickness dermal wounds does not transform into an intact layered integument complete with adnexal structures. Hence second-intention healing results in an appearance and scar texture different from that of normal adjacent skin.

It is interesting that even in the preantiseptic, preantibiotic, and preanesthetic eras, healing of wounds by surgical reconstruction was judged to be the surgeon's first intention. In first-intention healing, surgical apposition of the wound's edges allows healing without the intervention of exposed granulation tissue. Advances in surgical technique have expanded the scope of first-intention healing beyond linear closures to include use of local, regional, and free flaps, and skin grafting.

These improvements led to a mindset that surgeons could create results superior to those afforded by "natural" healing. Thus healing achieved through the natural processes of granulation, reepithelialization, and wound contraction was judged to be the surgeon's second intention. Fortunately, observant physicians who felt compelled to allow second-intention healing in a variety of clinical situations rediscovered the positive attributes of this approach, it being the most conservative form of wound management.

Perhaps foremost among the early observers of second-intention wound healing was Dr. Frederic E. Mohs. While a University of Wisconsin medical student, Mohs created a surgical technique combining in situ tissue fixation and complete microscopic margin examination for the treatment of skin cancer. Similar to wounds created by cryosurgery and electrosurgery, residual devitalized tissue present in the postoperative wound bed fixed by Mohs' zinc chloride paste precluded immediate wound closure. Thus most wounds created through the original Mohs micrographic technique, known as the fixed-tissue technique, were allowed to heal by second intention. Any reconstruction performed typically awaited slough of the devitalized fixed wound tissue, usually within a week on facial skin. By 1948, Mohs was able to report 5-year follow-up of 577 cases of primary and recurrent basal cell carcinoma (BCC) and squamous cell carcinoma (SCC), largely managed by second-intention healing.[3] Over the next 3 decades, several authors reported the adequacy of second-intention healing, particularly after surgical treatment of lower eyelid and medial canthal BCC[4] and in large traumatic or surgical defects of the central face.[5]

In 1978, Mohs reported his 30 years of experience in treating cutaneous malignancies by his micrographic technique.[6] Well over 10,000 cutaneous BCCs and SCCs had been followed through wound healing with a final 5-year follow-up. Mohs noted that "healing by granulation yields surprisingly good cosmetic and functional results. In some areas the results are superior to those obtained by standard surgical or radiation procedures. Prime examples are the forehead, temples, scalp, eyelid margins, canthi, nasal root and alae, ears, fingers, hands and plantar surfaces of the feet. The good results partly are attributable to the saving of maximal amounts of normal tissues as a consequence of microscopic control, but much is also attributable to the surprisingly good healing that can occur by granulation."[6] Again, other authors also advocated second-intention healing to prevent hypertrophic scar formation[7] to produce smaller, more manageable facial defects for delayed flap or graft reconstruction[8] and to manage medial canthal and lower eyelid margin defects.[9,10]

In the 1970s, Mohs' fixed-tissue technique was supplanted by the fresh-tissue technique. Whereas Mohs reported use of tumor excision using frozen tissue sections and without application of zinc chloride fixative for eyelid tumors,[6,11] it was later advocated for virtually all cutaneous tumors using Mohs technique. Today widely practiced by surgeons trained in Mohs technique the fresh-tissue technique avoids the pain and tissue slough associated with in situ tissue fixation and allows immediate reconstruction. Despite the wound's readiness for reconstruction and their confidence in tumor-free margins, Mohs surgeons commonly employ second-intention healing of selected, clean surgical wounds. Certainly, wounds with clear margins as assessed by "frozen section control" or those confirmed by permanent sections may be allowed to heal by second intention as well.

General Considerations

In addition to tumor-free wound margins, other factors suggest that second-intention healing may or should be considered. Clinical factors include the shape and contour of the wound, potential for compromised healing of flaps or grafts, patient at high risk for local tumor recurrence, patients ill suited to undergo surgical reconstruction, and a wound requiring a granulation tissue bed for receiving grafts. In addition, a desire to decrease the initial size of large facial wounds prior to reconstruction may give an early option for second-intention healing. Finally, the expected function and cosmesis resulting from second-intention healing may be superior to that expected from first-intention healing.

Mohs surgery involves creation of a beveled wound edge. Microscopic margin examination allows the surgeon to track out subclinical tumor extensions. Mohs defects typically are gently rounded and concave. Such beveled curvilinear wounds lend themselves to second-intention healing with less contraction than that seen with angulate wounds.[12,13]

Second-intention healing is an excellent option to manage compromised wound healing. Compromised vasculature increases the risk of graft or flap failure. Compromised wound beds occur in persons with previously irradiated skin, in diabetics, in users of tobacco, and in persons with contaminated wounds. Hemorrhagic diatheses may cause hematoma and failure of flaps or grafts while not greatly interfering with second-intention healing. In particular, aspirin, nonsteroidal anti-inflammatory agents, ticlopidine, heparins, coumarins, a-tocopherol, garlic, and ethanol should be avoided preoperatively. Still, many patients may be unable to or fail to discontinue these agents, making immediate reconstruction more difficult.

Despite careful performance of Mohs micrographic surgery, some patients remain at high risk for local tumor recurrence. Such tumors may manifest perineural, perivascular, muscular, cartilaginous, or osseous invasion, or may possess an inherently aggressive histopathological growth pattern. This is especially true of sclerosing, morpheaform, and keratinizing (metatypical) BCC, poorly differentiated SCC, microcystic adnexal carcinoma, extramammary Paget's disease, and sebaceous carcinoma. In fact, some authors advocate against immediate reconstruction of recurrent basal cell cancers.[5,14] Reconstruction in such patients may obscure and delay diagnosis of clinical tumor recurrence. Also, photodamaged, field-cancerized skin imported for reconstruction may harbor a subclinical tumor, leading to pseudorecurrence.

Certain patients are ill suited to surgical reconstruction. They may be unable to cooperate with appropriate local anesthesia, may be at significant medical risk for general anesthesia, or may not want more surgery.

Second-intention healing may effectively aid rather than supplant reconstruction. Deep wounds amenable to full-thickness skin grafting may benefit from filling of the defect with granulation tissue prior to grafting. This approach can reduce graft depression and poor post-operative tissue contour. Large facial wounds healing by second intention may contract sufficiently to make possible delayed reconstruction[5,8] or create smaller scars than the original. Finally, second-intention healing can be used concurrently with flap or graft reconstruction. Especially in a setting of complex facial wounds involving two or more facial cosmetic subunits, one can select second-intention healing for one appropriate subunit while reconstructing the adjacent one (**Fig. 53.3**). Use of certain flaps may allow a defect to shift to an area more likely to heal better by second intention. Upper forehead

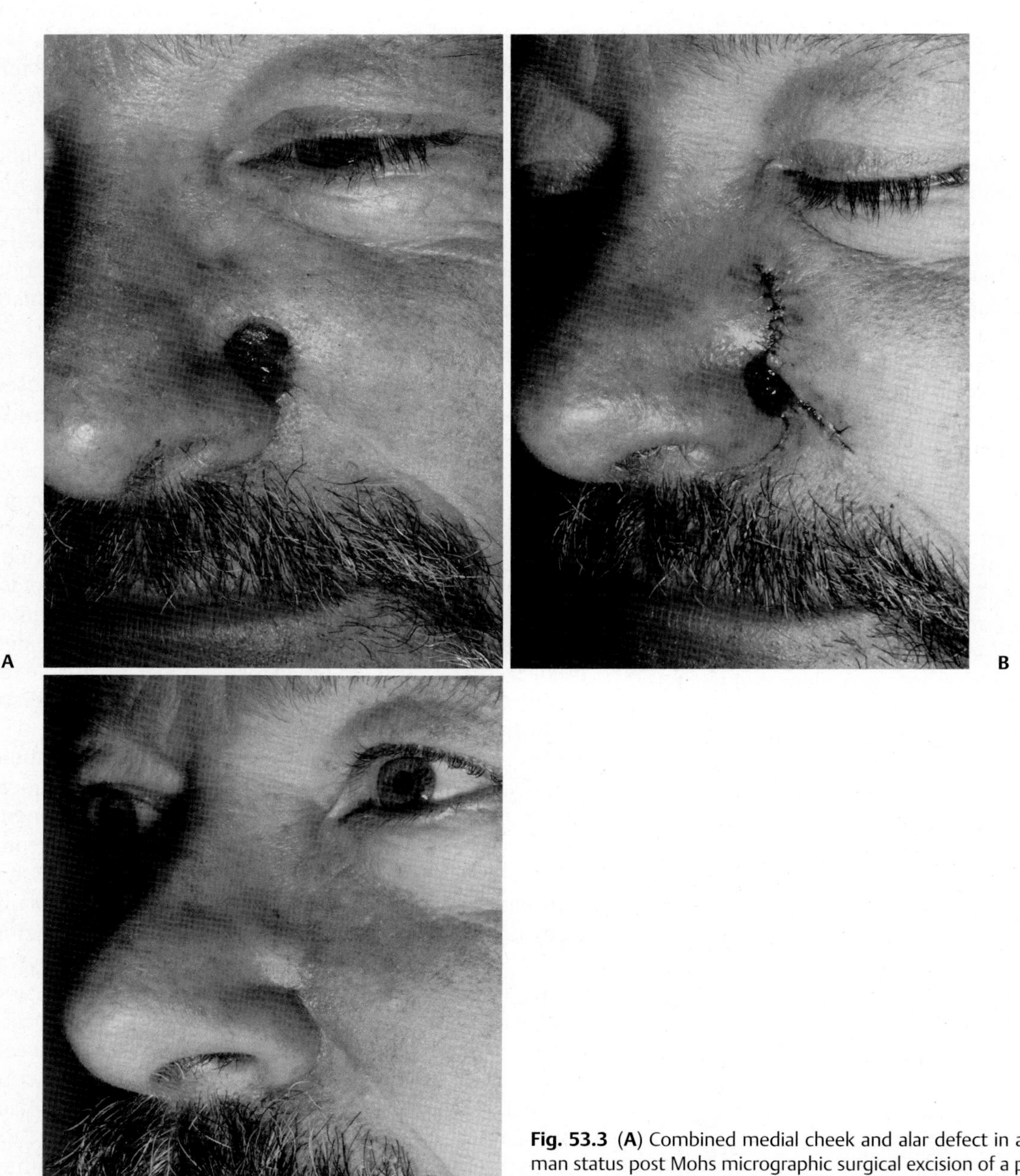

Fig. 53.3 (**A**) Combined medial cheek and alar defect in a 50-year-old man status post Mohs micrographic surgical excision of a primary basal cell carcinoma. (**B**) Immediate postoperative view after cheek advancement flap reconstruction of the medial cheek portion of the surgical defect. Based on the superficial nature of the alar portion of the defect, it was allowed to heal by second intention. (**C**) Postoperative view with complete healing 5 weeks later. No alar retraction or elevation resulted from second-intention healing.

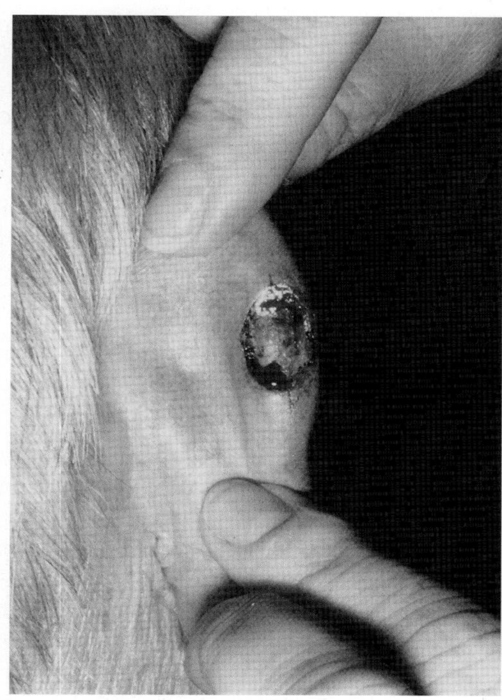
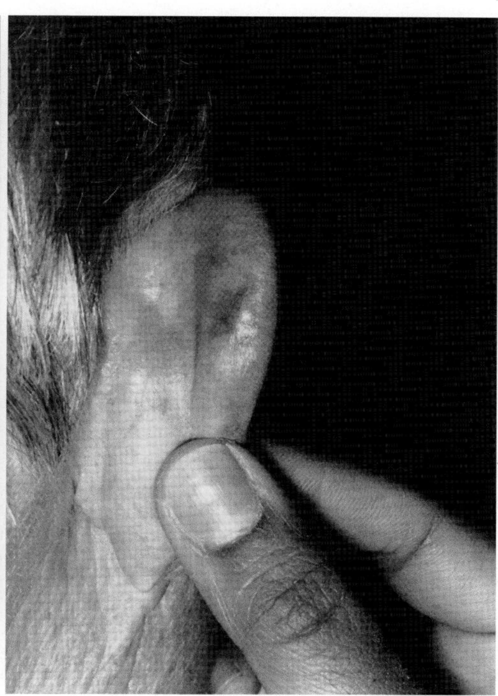

ig. 53.4 (A) Posterior view of a helical rim defect n an 87-year-old man status post Mohs micrographic surgical excision of a recurrent invasive quamous cell carcinoma. Second-intention healing was selected based on the defect size, location, and the tumor's recurrent nature. (B) Healing of helical defect from second intention 2 months later.

vounds resulting from donor site defects of paramedian orehead flaps used in nasal reconstruction often heal y second intention with very satisfactory cosmesis. Full-thickness skin defects at the posterior auricular sulcus and midhelical rim usually heal with minimal scarring by second intention (**Figs. 53.4 and 53.5**).[15]

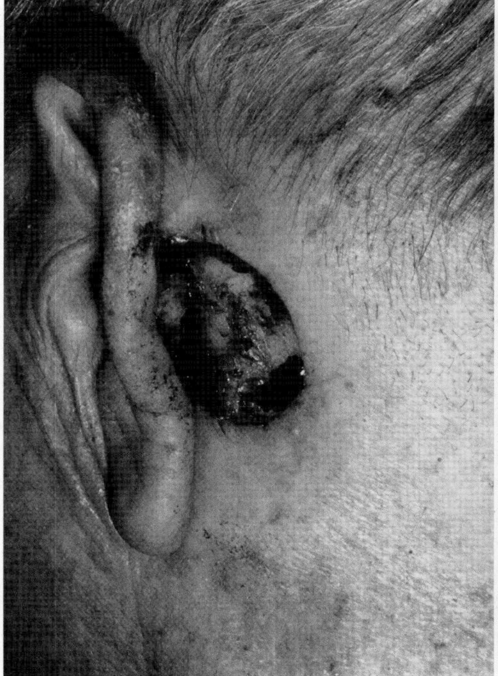
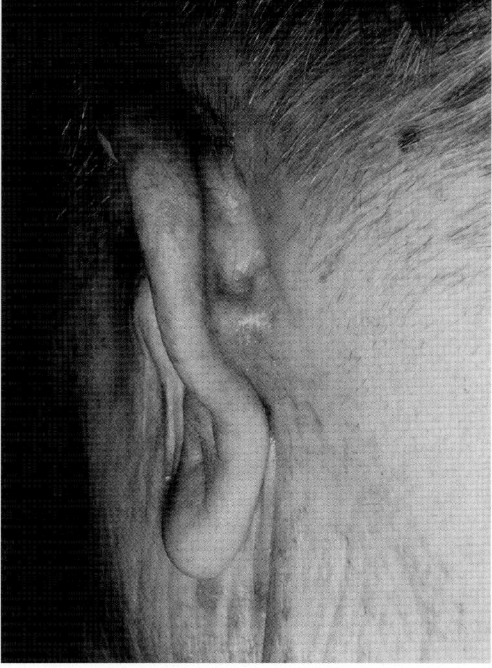

ig. 53.5 (A) Posterior auricular sulcus defect in an 82-year-old man following Mohs micrographic surgical xcision of a squamous cell carcinoma in situ. (B) Healing by second intention 8 weeks later.

Linear closures with dehiscence or necrotic areas on flaps or grafts should be allowed to heal by second intention before corrective techniques are considered.[5]

Second-intention healing should be given serious consideration for anatomical locations in which excellence in both function and cosmesis are expected. Second-intention healing most frequently leads to poor function when wounds are large or deep and involve or lie in proximity to anatomical free margins, lip, ala, eyelid, and, occasionally, the external ear canal. The process of wound contraction literally pulls on free margins distorting position and creating dysfunction. Tension on the lip, eyelid, and nasal ala will cause distortion. Defects involving a significant portion of the circumference of the auditory meatus may cause meatal stenosis. Except for these situations, which are prevented by appropriate reconstruction, second-intention healing usually does not result in anatomical dysfunction. Dr. John Zitelli first classified expected cosmesis of second intention healing by facial regions[16,17] based on his observation of several thousand patients. He observed that healing in anatomical sites characterized by concave surfaces (on the nose, eye, ear, and temple—or NEET—areas) produced superior cosmetic results. Convex surface defects (on the nose, oral lip, cheeks, chin, and helix—NOCH—areas) healed with obvious scars. And flat surface defects (on the forehead, antihelix, eyelids ["I"], and remainder of the nose, lips, and cheeks—FAIR—areas) healed with satisfactory cosmetic results (**Fig. 53.6**). Several other factors contribute to the expected cosmetic result of second-intention healing. The pallor of mature scars stands out more in patients with darker pigmentation (Fitzpatrick phototypes III to VI). In a given anatomical subunit, smaller and more superficial wounds leave less noticeable scars particularly when the defect retains appendages that recreate the pore pattern of normal skin. Skin with large and numerous sebaceous glands (distal nose, medial cheeks, or in early rhinophyma) are more prone to have visible scarring (**Fig. 53.7**).[16,17]

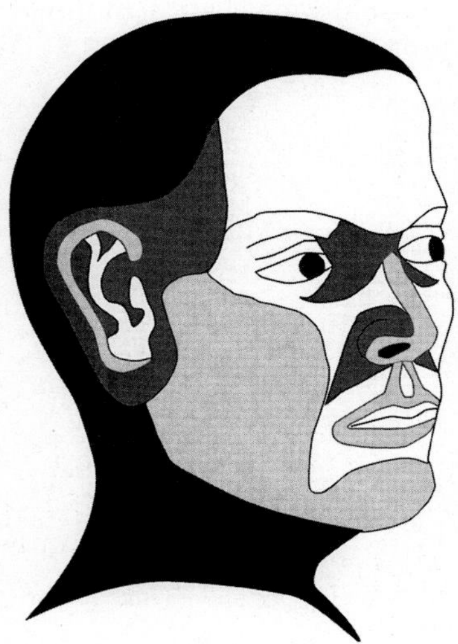

Fig. 53.6 Aesthetic result of facial areas healing by second intention. Dark gray (NEET area, concave surfaces of the nose, eye, ear, and temple) —excellent results. White (FAIR area, forehead, antihelix, eyelids ["I"], and rest of the nose, lips and cheeks)—satisfactory results, could result in hypopigmented scars. Light gray (NOCH area, convex surfaces of the nose, oral lips, cheeks, chin and helix)—variable results, superficial wounds acceptable to some patients but deeper wounds heal with depression or potential for hypertrophic scars. (From Zitelli JA. Wound healing by secondary intention: a cosmetic appraisal. J Am Acad Dermatol 1983;9:407–415.)

Comparison of First-Intention and Second-Intention Healing

Second-intention healing possesses distinct advantages over first-intention reconstruction. Tissue defects reconstructed with flaps have greater skin tension, which contributes to postoperative pain. Second-intention healing also obviates the possibility of nerve injury during reconstruction and the creation of a second wound at graft donor sites. Contrary to popular and "informed" opinion, open healing wounds are universally not painful. Whereas desiccated wounds can be uncomfortable, second-intention healing within a moist healing environment typically is not painful,[18] rarely requiring analgesia stronger than acetaminophen. Significant pain may suggest the presence of infection. Even irradiated wound beds heal well, though more slowly. Postoperative hemorrhage easily drains away from the wound, avoiding hematoma and seroma formation. The wounds of patients at risk for hemorrhage are easily treated with topical hemostatic agents, such as oxidized cellulose (OxyCel, Becton Dickinson, Franklin Lakes, NJ). Devitalized tissue from electrocautery readily sloughs from the wound, and no suture is present to incite a foreign-body reaction. Wounds healing by second intention are no more likely to develop infection than reconstructed wounds if kept clean.[6]

Selection of Wounds for Second-Intention Healing

When does the surgeon select second-intention healing for a patient? First, the final decision of repair should be based on an agreement between the surgeon and the patient. For education purposes, the patient should view the wound to be aware of the amount of tissue removed to eradicate the tumor. The expected appearance of the scar, time for wound healing, and the patient's (family's or home nurse's) role in wound care are discussed. If the patient is willing to consider second-intention healing, the surgeon must assess the whole patient as well as the specific wound characteristics. During second-intention healing, one must rely on published criteria, such as Zitelli's guide, for advice on appropriate wound management.[16,17]

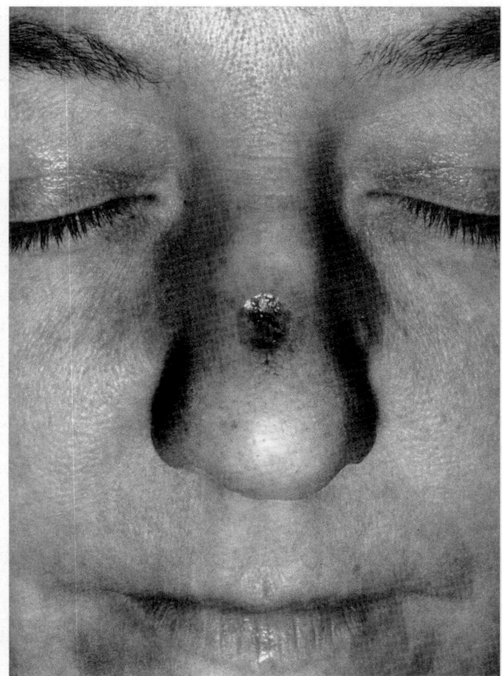

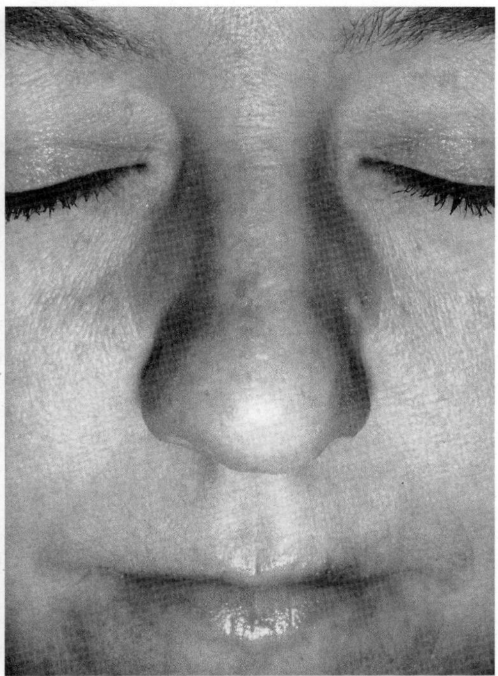

A B

ig. 53.7 (A) Full-thickness nasal dorsal defect in a 8-year-old woman following Mohs micrographic surgi-al excision of a primary nodular basal cell carcinoma. Second-intention healing was selected. (B) The wound reepithelialized over 6 weeks, and at 3 months some residual scar telangiectasia is evident.

Wound Preparation and Care

We practice the following routine in managing wounds selected to heal by second intention. To optimize wound healing, the tenets listed in **Table 53.1** are followed. The patient or caregivers, if available, are involved in initial dressing application. If a significant amount of periosteum is removed, decortication of bone to expose the diploic layer is required for adequate granulation tissue formation.[19] This may be achieved using a rotating bone bur, rongeur, CO_2 laser,[20] or an erbium:yttrium-aluminum-garnet (Er:YAG) laser.[21] Bone decortication should create exposed bone segments smaller than 1 cm or be performed to the soft tissue periphery. Bone exposed in this manner, if not kept moist, may become devitalized and impede wound healing. Hydrogen peroxide should not be consistently applied to exposed cartilage or bone due to its desiccating effects.[19] Wounds with exposed bone should be reviewed regularly to remove devitalized tissue until a complete granulation tissue bed has formed.[19] The presence of significant infection (chondritis or osteomyelitis) in either of these settings is unusual.[19]

Table 53.1 Major Tenets for Optimal Local Wound Care Management

Debride necrotic tissue.	Removal of necrotic tissue minimizes bacterial growth.
Identify and treat infection.	Infection inhibits all stages of wound healing.
Pack dead spaces lightly.	Tightly packed spaces hinder wound cavity contraction.
Divert any salivary drainage away from the wound.	Salivary seepage increases bacteria wound load.
Drain any excess fluid collection.	A fluid collection becomes a reservoir for infection.
Absorb excess exudates.	Excess wound exudate macerates surrounding skin.
Maintain a moist wound surface.	Moist surfaces enhance granulation tissue formation and epithelial cell migration.
Maintain open fresh wound edges.	Closed, well-epithelialized wound edges prevent epithelial migration across the wound surface.
Protect the wound from trauma and infection.	Trauma and infection cause damage to new tissue.
Insulate the wound.	Warmth maximizes blood flow and cell function, thus optimizing wound healing.

Source: From R. Bryant. Science and reality of wound healing—wound healing: state of the science, 1997. Program of the Wound Healing Society and the Wound, Ostomy, and Continence Nurses Society. Nashville, TN: The Wound, Ostomy, and Continence Nurses Society; 1997; June 12.

Residual clot or cautery debris is removed and adequate hemostasis achieved in the wound bed. Sufficient antibiotic ointment (bacitracin zinc) is applied to prevent tissue desiccation. If the patient has known contact allergy to bacitracin, then another antibiotic agent or white petrolatum may be used. Next, a pressure dressing (composed of a layer of nonadherent gauze dressing; packing of cotton gauze, dental rolls, or cotton balls to overfill the wound; and paper tape) is applied. Adherent (Medipore, 3M Health Care, St. Paul, MN) or nonadherent elasticized materials (Coban, 3M Health Care) can be used for additional pressure, if required. Three-dimensionally complex areas, such as external ear sites, may require a mold such as heat-sensitive plastic (Aquaplast, WFR Aquaplast Corp., Wyckoff, NJ) and suture to achieve a rigid, well-conformed dressing. If contact allergy to tape components exists, Aquaplast or Coban avoids irritation or allergy. The patient is sent home with written wound care instructions and contact telephone numbers.

Patients are instructed to remove pressure dressings after 24 or 48 hours. Wounds are cleansed with tap water, normal saline, or H_2O_2 soaks or cotton-tipped applicators to remove crust and debris from the wound and surrounding skin. We encourage patients to attempt to remove soft fibrinous material from the wound bed, but not so vigorously as to cause more than pinpoint bleeding. The wound is blotted dry. Antibacterial ointment and a lighter dressing of nonadherent gauze (Telfa, Kendall Healthcare Products, Mansfield, MA) and paper tape (Micropore, 3M Health Care) are applied. Patients are specifically cautioned to ensure a moist environment and not to allow dry scabs to form because dry eschars dramatically slow wound healing[22] and contribute to postoperative pain. Wound cleansing is performed and new dressings applied twice daily for the first week, then decreased to once daily until complete healing has occurred. To help determine the kind of dressing to use, **Tables 53.2 and 53.3** describe the types of dressings available and their reasons for use.

Wounds are reexamined within a week to judge the adequacy of wound care, provide coaching technique, and perform surveillance for adverse events. Wound examinations then occur monthly until the wound has healed completely. Once healing has taken place, patients are seen annually, or as dictated by changes in status, for surveillance of recurrence or development of new suspicious lesions. Wounds managed by second intention often heal initially with an indurated, red or violaceous central papule or ridge. This resolves with time or its resolution may be accelerated by twice-daily digital massage with lotion or ointment. Massage enhances blood flow and speeds scar tissue remodeling. Oral antibacterial agents are used only in patients judged to have a clinically significant propensity for infection, a strong history of prior wound infections or a need for antibiotic prophylaxis to protect artificial valves, prosthetic joints, and so forth. In our experience the occurrence of wound infection in second-intention healing is a rarity, even in immunosuppressed individuals. We do find that an occlusive hydrocolloid dressing (DuoDerm, ConvaTec, Princeton, NJ) may adhere well, retain drainage, require less frequent dressing changes, and provide an excellent environment for second-intention wound healing. Use of hydrocolloid dressings allows serum enzymes to perform painless autolytic debridement of fibrinous eschar. Some patients prefer this wound dressing to those described previously, especially for wounds on an alopecic scalp or difficult-to-reach areas of the trunk.

Steps in Second-Intention Wound Healing

Wound healing is dependent on the following physiological steps: hemostasis (occurring over minutes), inflammation (occurring over 3 days after injury), proliferation (occurring from the third to 12th day after injury), and remodeling (occurring over months after injury). In open wounds healing by secondary intention, contraction plays a critical role. All of these components must be present in a coordinated sequence for optimal healing to occur.

When one healing step is delayed, all subsequent healing steps are affected. When one or more of these steps is impaired, delayed healing becomes apparent, resulting in more scarring. Wound remodeling is the last and longest phase of soft tissue wound healing. During this period, granulation tissue recedes, collagen remodels, and a mature scar forms. Scar maturation takes place over years, with gradually increasing tensile strength. However, the strength of healed tissue never reaches that of uninjured skin.

As long as a wound remains open, inflammation persists. This is because in an exposed wound, continual exposure to microorganisms and foreign material acts as an inflammatory stimulus. For inflammation to resolve, this stimulus must be eliminated. The epithelium is the key barrier that protects the wound from the external environment. After a wound becomes reepithelialized, the underlying tissue is further protected and inflammation is curtailed.

It is believed that something in the epithelium suppresses inflammation. Clinically, this is supported by observing that closing a wound primarily or covering a wound with a graft reduces the inflammation. If an open wound fails to reepithelialize within 2 to 3 weeks, the likelihood of a hypertrophic scar developing increases.[23]

Table 53.2 Dressing Purpose and Product Classifications

Purpose of Product	Wound Product Classifications
Cleanse topically	Normal saline
	Commercial wound cleaners
Absorb exudate	Absorption beads, pastes, and powders
	Alginates
	Composite dressings
	Foams
	Gauze
	Hydrocolloids
	Hydrogels
Cover a wound to allow autolytic enzymes of the wound fluid to self-digest eschar and fibrinous slough	Absorption beads, pastes and powders
	Alginates
	Composite dressings
	Foams
	Gauze
	Hydrocolloids
	Hydrogels
	Transparent film
Topically debride devitalized tissue chemically	Enzymatic debridement agents
Mechanically debride devitalized tissue	Wound cleansers
	Gauze (wet to dry)
Add moisture to the wound	Gauze (impregnated or with saline)
	Hydrogels
	Wound care systems (two-part)
Maintain a moist wound environment	Ointments
	Foams
	Gauze (impregnated or with saline)
	Hydrocolloids
	Hydrogels
	Transparent films
	Wound care systems (two-part)
Fill dead space	Absorption beads, pastes, and powders
	Alginates
	Hydrocolloid pastes, powders
	Foam
	Gauze
Cover and protect wound	Composites
	Compression bandages/wraps
	Foams
	Gauze dressings (covers/wraps)
	Hydrocolloids
	Hydrogels (with covers/borders)
	Transparent film dressings
Protect surrounding skin from moisture and trauma	Moisture barrier ointments
	Foams
	Hydrocolloids
	Securement devices
	Skin sealants
	Transparent film dressings

Source: From Krasner, D. Dressing decisions for the 21st century. In: Krasner D, Kane D. Chronic Wound Care. 2nd ed. Wayne, PA: Health Management Publications; 1997:139–151 and Hom DB, Adams G, Koreis M, Maisel R. Choices of wound care management for irradiated soft tissue wounds. Otolaryngol Head Neck Surg 1999;121(5):591–598.

Table 53.3 Tailoring Wound Dressings to the Particular Characteristics of the Wound

Type	Wound Description	Dressings to Consider	Objective
Necrotic	Wound cavity with excessive yellow exudate, slough, dark eschar (black to tan)	Calcium alginate rope, hypertonic saline gauze, hypertonic gel, enzymatic debriding ointment	To absorb exudate and promote debridement
Granular	Granulating wound, minimal or moderate exudate	Hydrogel gauze, calcium alginate	To provide a moist environment
Requiring reepithelialization	Pink, shallow	Hydrogel sheet, hydrocolloid, foam when wound is moist	To maintain moisture, promote resurfacing, and protect new epithelium

Source: Adapted from Krasner, D. Dressing decisions for the 21st century. In: Krasner D, Kane D. Chronic Wound Care. 2nd ed. Wayne, PA: Health Management Publications; 1997:139–151 and Hom DB, Adams G, Koreis M, Maisel R. Choices of wound care management for irradiated soft tissue wounds. Otolaryngol Head Neck Surg 1999;121(5):591–598.

Complications

Significant hemorrhage following Mohs surgery may rarely occur, typically in the first 24 hours. Most commonly, diffuse oozing occurs in patients with an organic or iatrogenic bleeding diathesis. This may be sufficient to soak through the initial pressure dressing but should be controllable through direct pressure, application of new dry dressings, rest, and wound elevation. Occasionally, arteriolar bleeding manifests within several hours of surgery when the epinephrine effect wanes. The presence of exposed large vessels dictates management by tissue coverage. Slow wound healing may be expected to occur in previously irradiated skin (**Fig. 53.8**) or may develop concurrently with bacterial colonization or wound infection. Wounds suspected of microbial colonization or infection should be cultured, any dry eschar removed (often revealing purulent foci), appropriately aggressive wound care reemphasized, and gram-positive antibacterial coverage begun. If necessary, antibiotic coverage is later adjusted

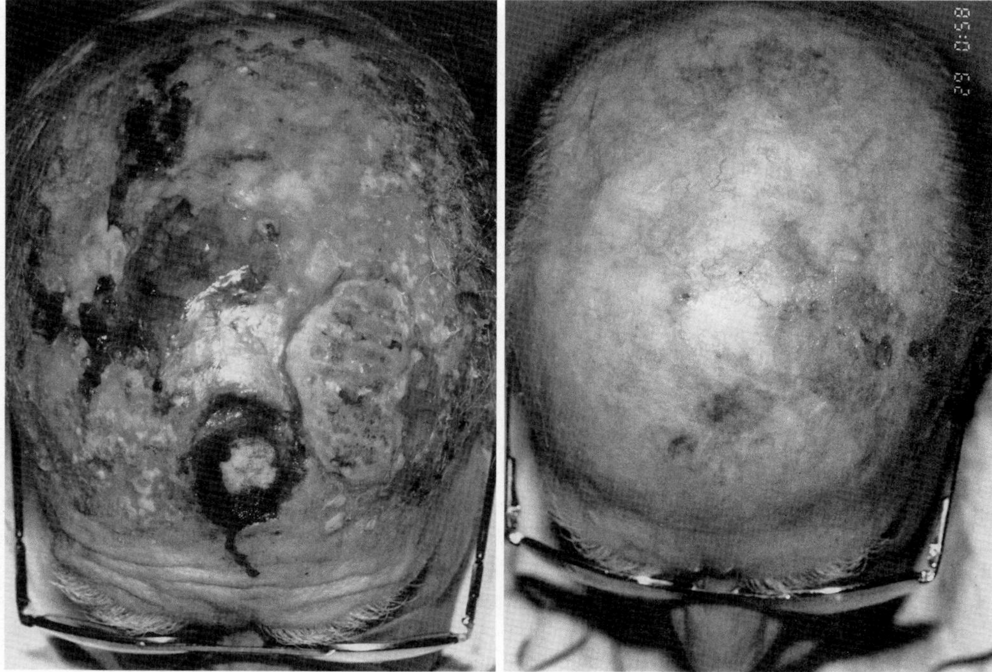

Fig. 53.8 An 82-year-old man who presented with a persistent, chronic, nonhealing full-thickness wound on his scalp of 2 years' duration following excision of a squamous cell cancer 2 years previously. Ten years previously he had received radiation to his scalp. He had no evidence of tumor recurrence by multiple biopsies. (**A**) Inadequate granulation tissue and bare calvarial bone exposed. (**B**) After the outer table of skull was burred down and the scalp kept moist with antibiotic ointment, new granulation tissue formed to allow for later coverage with a split-thickness skin graft.

based on culture results. Rarely, even in healthy-appearing wounds, nonhealing may be observed. In this instance, one observes granulation tissue formation followed by only partial reepithelialization. Such wounds should be cultured to rule out colonization by yeast or bacteria and antibiotics employed as necessary. A recent clinical report[24] suggests that wound healing arrest may be reversed by topical or oral corticosteroids or oral ibuprofen in combination. Provided that sufficient granulation tissue has developed, grafts may be placed or flaps constructed to cover the wound. Development of proud flesh, an exuberant growth of granulation tissue, that overfills the wound bed, may impede wound healing. Proud flesh has been associated with the presence of foreign bodies, such as hair shafts on hair-bearing skin, which should be removed to allow regression of abundant granulation tissue. Regression may be induced by application of chemical cautery (silver nitrate sticks), electrocautery, topical steroids,[25] pulsed laser irradiation targeting oxyhemoglobin (532 nm, 577 to 600 nm), or CO_2 laser targeting tissue H_2O. Alternatively, proud flesh may be sharply debrided, particularly if pedunculated or overgrowing the wound edges.[16,17] Ironically, the moist wound environment, which promotes wound healing in some cases, may contribute to the formation of proud flesh. If other treatment modalities fail, use of less occlusion (less ointment, more gas-permeable dressings) or astringent wound care (acetic acid wet-to-dry dressings) can bring about regression of proud flesh. In a wound created by removal of a skin malignancy, failure of proud flesh to respond to common measures should prompt a biopsy to rule out recurrence.

Once reepithelialized, second-intention wounds may still not achieve complete healing. Inadequate filling of the wound to a level that recreates the normal tissue contour commonly occurs on convex surfaces, making scars more noticeable and less cosmetically appealing. In addition, some scars may heal with a shelf-like drop-off at the periphery. This contour abnormality readily casts a shadow and brings attention to the scar. Hypertrophic scarring is unusual but may follow second-intention healing. Hypertrophic scar tissue is marked by significant red or violaceous erythema, induration, pruritus or pain, and progressive growth. Common facial sites include the cutaneous and vermilion lip, upper medial canthi, and central cheeks. Hypertrophic scarring diagnosed early may be treated with topical or intralesional corticosteroids, intralesional 5-fluorouracil, intralesional interferon-α, topical silicone gel sheeting, or pulsed dye laser irradiation (585 nm). Tissue contraction associated with second-intention healing may distort surrounding normal anatomical structures. Appropriately placed guiding sutures can alter contraction force vectors to minimize or prevent distortion of adjacent structures.[26] Finally, second-intention healing of wounds deep to the pilosebaceous units can leave alopecic scars on hair-bearing skin. This can make second-intention healing a relatively poor choice on the male beard area or on hair-bearing scalp.

A successful approach to wound management is based on an appreciation for the expected outcome of wounds managed by both first and second intention. One should consider that the choice of second-intention healing need not produce inferior results and therefore should not be a secondary consideration.

Skin Grafts

A skin graft consists of a segment of dermis and epidermis that has been completely separated from its blood supply and donor site and transferred to a recipient location. Skin grafts are classified as split-thickness skin grafts (STSGs) and full-thickness skin grafts (FTSGs) (**Fig. 53.9**).

Skin grafts are often considered when local skin flaps are not feasible. Compared with skin flaps, skin grafts give less optimal color match and texture on the face. STSGs (0.010 to 0.018 in.) can provide temporary coverage of soft tissue defects if adjacent soft tissue viability is uncertain or if a large amount of soft tissue coverage is required. However, they give poorer color and texture match than FTSGs, giving a lighter, more atrophic, and glistening appearance. They also have less skin durability to infection and to future trauma with increased wound contracture. FTSGs give more acceptable facial color and texture match in comparison with STSGs if they are taken from the preauricular, postauricular, upper eyelid, nasolabial, or supraclavicular donor areas.

When obtaining skin grafts, one should be aware that skin thickness varies with age, sex, and region of the body. Skin is 3.5 times thinner in newborns than in adults. By 5 years of age, the skin thickness in children is close to that of adults. Females have thinner skin than males. By body region, skin is thinnest at the eyelids (0.017 in.) and thickest over the soles of the feet and palms (0.150 in.).[27]

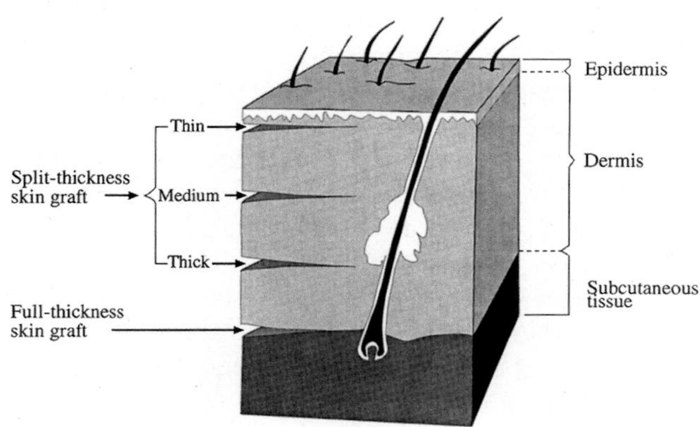

Fig. 53.9 Various skin graft thicknesses taken from the skin.

STSGs can be used to cover any wound that has a blood supply sufficient to support its survival. Areas that cannot furnish enough blood supply to a graft are on cortical bone without periosteum, cartilage without perichondrium, tendon without paratenon, nerve with perineurium, and any surface with stratified squamous epithelium intact. In addition, a previously irradiated recipient site has a lower blood supply and results in a decreased "take rate" than a nonirradiated site.

Wound Healing of Skin Grafts

Immediately after a skin graft is brought in contact with its recipient bed, it begins to absorb the plasma wound fluid like a sponge by capillary action (plasmatic imbibition) during the first 48 hours. In addition, over the first 24 hours, a fibrin layer forms underneath the graft, keeping the graft adhered to the wound bed to allow for vascular budding to occur. Within 4 to 7 days after transplantation, the skin becomes revascularized by three major mechanisms. One mechanism is the direct connection of vascular buds from the bed with preexisting vessels in the graft (inosculation). The second method is ingrowth of the host vessels through preexisting endothelial channels of the graft. The third method is random ingrowth of vascular buds into the graft, thus forming a new vascular network.[28] Thin STSGs (<0.014 in.) are thought to revascularize faster than thicker skin grafts. This is because penetrating blood vessels travel shorter distances through the dermis in thinner skin grafts. In addition, thin STSGs have a lower metabolic rate; thus, plasma imbibition is able to maintain the graft survival longer, before revascularization occurs.[28]

Split-Thickness Skin Grafts

STSGs contain epidermis and a portion of the dermis. They can be further defined by their thickness: thin (0.008 to 0.010 in.), medium (0.011 to 0.015 in.), and thick (0.016 to 0.018 in.). Thin STSGs contract more than thick STSGs. Thin STSGs do not grow hair at the recipient site. The advantages of using STSGs for reconstruction of facial defects are as follows: (1) they can be an expedient technique for covering soft tissue defects if adjacent soft tissue viability is uncertain and (2) they can cover large defects when close surveillance is required of the site for tumor recurrence. Disadvantages of partial thickness skin grafts are as follows: (1) they have poor color and texture-match with the surrounding skin, giving a lighter, more atrophic, and glistening appearance; (2) they result in decreased skin durability to future trauma; (3) there is increased wound contracture; and (4) there is a donor site scar.

Donor Sites

Common donor sites include thigh, abdominal wall, and buttock. If a larger amount of STSG is required, the scalp can be used repeatedly in 7-day intervals because its dermis is so thick with dense hair follicles and a robust blood supply. Up to five or six harvestings can be taken from the same site.[29]

Surgical Technique

Common instruments used in obtaining a STSG are the Brown electrical or air-driven dermatome, the Padgett-Hood dermatome, or the Humby knife. The choice of instrument is based on the surgeon's preference. To obtain the preferred STSG thickness using the electrical dermatome, adjust the pitch of the blade in the instrument by closing the knobs down completely and use this reading as the zero point on each side. After the preferred thickness and width have been set, it is recommended that the space between the blade and the instrument be double-checked to ensure that a consistent and proper thickness is obtained. The skin is cleaned with bactericidal solution and dried, then treated with sterile mineral oil. The dermatome is set between 0.008 and 0.018 in. with the desired STSG thickness. The dermatome is operated so that its flat surface lies against the skin with even pressure.

After the graft has been placed at the recipient site, it is immobilized for 5 to 7 days to prevent hematoma formation and shearing. A pressure dressing using a bolster or stent with tie-over sutures is helpful. Cotton balls, dental rolls, fluffed gauze, or sponges are effective as bolus materials to secure even pressure over the graft site. A heat-sensitive mold splint (Aquaplast) is used to conform and secure the bolus material in place for 5 to 7 days. The skin graft donor site can be covered with an occlusive dressing (such as Opsite [Smith & Nephew Healthcare, UK]) for several days and changed when needed until adequate reepithelialization has occurred. A moist donor area will heal more rapidly than a dry area (**Fig. 53.10**).

Full-Thickness Skin Grafts

FTSGs consist of the entire epidermal and dermal layers of the skin. After transfer, they do not change in color or texture. As hair follicles are transferred with these grafts, hair growth is preserved. Because they are thicker than STSGs, they are more slowly revascularized. Intrinsically, they do not contract; however, their recipient bed does contract with healing. Facial areas for which FTSGs are very useful are at the nasal tip, eyelids, and auricle (**Figs. 53.11 and 53.12**).

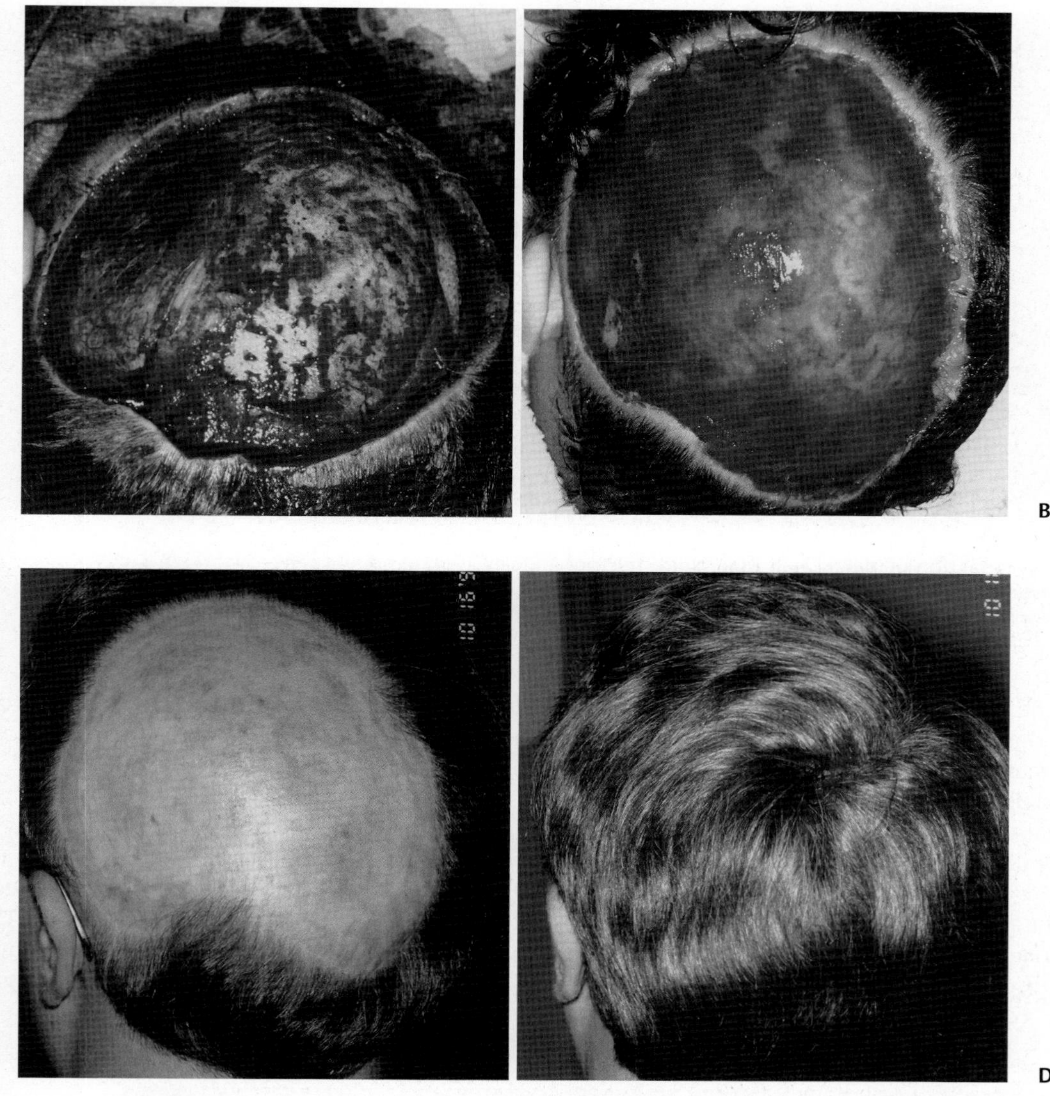

ig. 53.10 (A) A 27-year-old man who required full-ıickness scalp excision and burring down of outer alvarial bone to remove dermatofibrosarcoma rotuberans. (B) Scalp was allowed to granulate. (C) Split-thickness skin graft placed over well-granulated bed. (D) After healing, the patient wears a hairpiece to cover site.

Advantages in using FTSGs are as follows: (1) they ive a more acceptable facial color and texture match ıan STSGs if taken from the preauricular, postauricu-ır, upper eyelid, or supraclavicular donor sites, and 2) they are a single-stage procedure. Disadvantages of TSGs are as follows: (1) they have a decreased "take ate" in comparison with STSGs; (2) deep defects may equire adequate granulation tissue before grafting; 3) there is decreased durability to trauma in compari-ɔn with skin flaps; and (4) there is increased donor te morbidity.

Donor Sites

Skin on different regions of the body differs in color, texture, thickness, vascularity, and hair-bearing nature. The closer in proximity the donor site is to the recipient site, the more likely the skin match. Thus skin grafts taken above the clavicles tend to retain their natural blush state, in contrast to skin taken below the clavicle, which has a yellowish or brownish hue.[30] The most common donor sites used are the postauricular, preauricular, supraclavicular, and upper eyelid skin areas. Postauricular skin

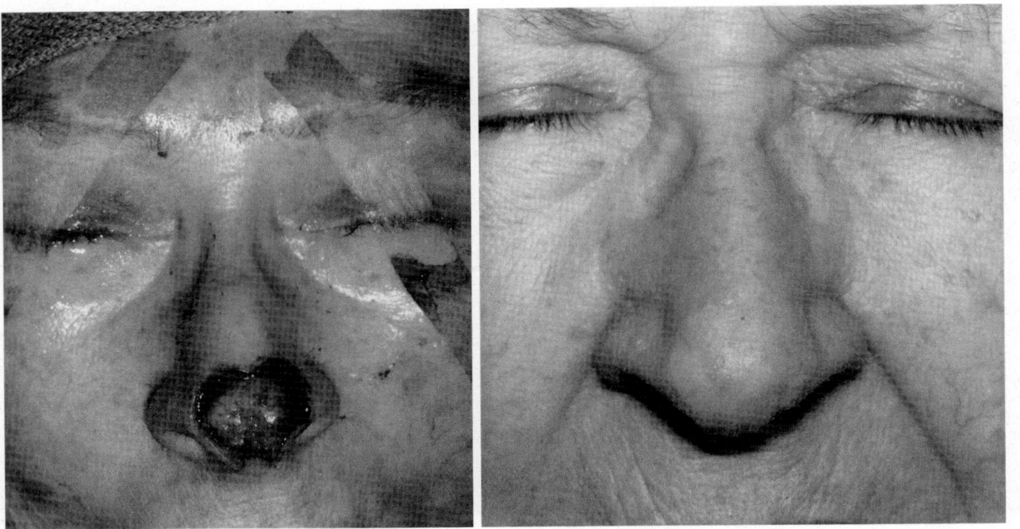

Fig. 53.11 (**A**) Full-thickness nasal tip skin defect following Mohs' micrographic excision of a basal cell carcinoma in 70-year-old women. A posterior auricular full-thickness skin graft was used to cover the defect. (**B**) Appearance 1 year later.

grafts 3 × 5 cm can be taken from the postauricular sulcus, encompassing the area from the helical rim to the hairline over the mastoid region. If necessary, this donor site can be closed primarily or with an STSG. At the supraclavicular and preauricular sites, the color match and texture are also good, with the skin being thicker. Upper eyelid skin can be used as a donor site when a small, thin FTSG is required for another eyelid site. Other donor sites are at the flexor crease of the antecubital or inguinal regions. When obtaining an FTSG, the subcutaneous fat should be removed because the adipose layer will act as barrier to reduce revascularization of the dermis.

Storage of Skin Grafts

When it is anticipated that the skin graft may be neede in the future, it can be stored by two methods. STSC can be placed back on the donor site and removed up t 14 days later. Another method is to wrap the skin gra

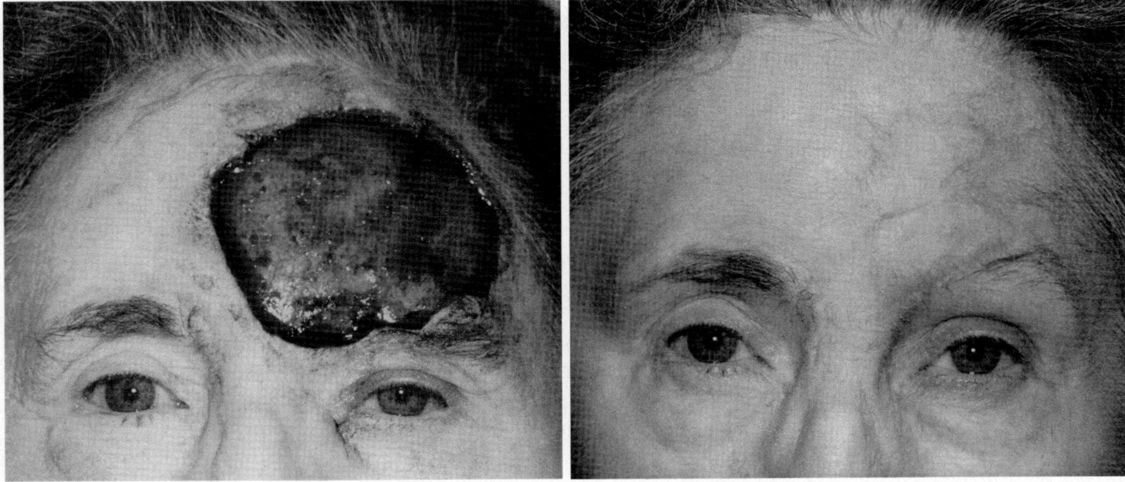

Fig. 53.12 (**A**) Full-thickness forehead skin defect following Mohs micrographic excision of a basal cell carcinoma in a 65-year-old women. A preauricular full-thickness skin graft was used to cover the defect. (**B**) Appearance 1 year later.

in saline- or Ringer's lactate–soaked gauze and place it in a sterile jar in a refrigerator at 4°C. By this method, STSG can be refrigerated up to 21 days and still be used for grafting. It appears that using an STSG taken for the second time from its donor site gives a higher take rate than grafts stored in saline at 4°C.[31]

Dermis Grafts

A dermis graft consists of an FTSG without the epidermis. By removing the epidermal surface, vascularization can occur on both surfaces of the graft. After a dermis graft is transplanted, an intense granulation reaction occurs within the graft mesoderm, which fibroses and contracts over several months.

Dermis grafts should be placed in areas where soft tissue contraction will not distort neighboring structures. They can be stacked in several layers before transplantation to give additional bulk for augmentation. Dermis grafts are useful in augmenting facial regions where bulk is required, but not for support.

Composite Skin–Cartilage Grafts

Composite skin–cartilage grafts can give both covering and contour to a facial defect. To optimize perfusion of a composite skin–cartilage graft, all points of the graft should be within 5 mm of the edge.[32] Larger composite grafts up to 3.0 cm have been reported; however, beyond 1.0 cm diameter, the predictability of composite graft survival decreases.[33] Transferring more skin than cartilage can enhance neovascularization of larger composite grafts, thus converting the graft to more of a full-thickness type. Skin cartilage grafts are useful for closing defects of the nasal alar rim, columella, and eyelid when adequate vascularity of the surrounding tissue bed exists. Advantages of composite skin–cartilage grafts are that (1) it is a one-stage procedure, and (2) structural and epithelial coverage are transferred.

The disadvantages of composite grafts are that (1) once the size of the grafts is beyond 1.0 cm diameter, the predictability of composite skin–cartilage graft survival decreases, and (2) composite graft contraction occurs gradually, which can compromise the final cosmetic result.

In some instances, the revascularization of composite grafts can be improved by increasing the host bed surface area. This can be done by rotating an adjacent turnover flap to increase graft–host surface contact, rather than depending solely on edge-to-edge contact (**Fig. 53.13**).

Wound Healing of Skin–Cartilage Composite Grafts

The healing of composite skin–cartilage grafts is similar to that of skin grafts in that revascularization of grafted skin is essential for its long-term survival. During the revascularization process of composite skin–cartilage grafts, host vessels cannot penetrate cartilage. Hence, the host vessels spread along the underside of the cartilage until they reach the dermis of the graft. After 48 hours, vascularization begins at the host–dermis interphase of the composite graft, followed by vascularization toward the dermal center of the graft.[33]

Wound Care

For wound cleaning, skin cleansers (Betadine [povidone-iodine] and Hibiclens [Mölnlycke Health Care US, LLC, Norcross, GA) should not be repetitively used in a wound to avoid cell damage. Wound cleaning can be performed using normal saline or commercial wound cleansers. Moisture-retentive dressings or ointments should be used until reepithelization of the wound is complete.

Local factors that impede wound healing, such as infection, hematoma, and seroma, will increase the likelihood of scarring. Another factor that increases scarring potential is excessive tension at the incisions. With careful preoperative planning and meticulous surgical technique, these risks can be minimized.

New Products for Improving Wound Healing

Several new products over the last decade signify the beginning of a new era for actively improving wound healing for the surgeon. In 1998, the first FDA growth factor product, recombinant human platelet derived growth factor, (PDGF) becaplermin (Regranex, Ortho-McNeil, Inc., Titusville, NJ) was approved to actively improve wound healing. Specifically, it is used to induce granulation tissue formation in diabetic, neuropathic, nonischemic ulcers. The becaplermin gel is applied topically to the wound site every 24 hours. Recently, the off-label use of becaplermin has been reported by clinicians to help transform a chronic problem wound into an acute healing state.[34,35] However, at the present time, becaplermin should not be used at sites of active neoplasia because of the possible risk of propagating the malignancy. Thus, in facial plastic surgery, becaplermin should not be used in patients with active head and neck cancer until further studies can clarify this issue.

Another FDA-approved growth factor product is allogeneic living epidermal and dermal skin derived from cultured neonatal foreskin (Apligraf, Organogenesis Canton, MA). This product is a living bilayer graft having cellular and growth factor components. Its dermal layer consists of living fibroblasts within a bovine collagen matrix. On its surface, it has living keratinocytes in the epithelium. The

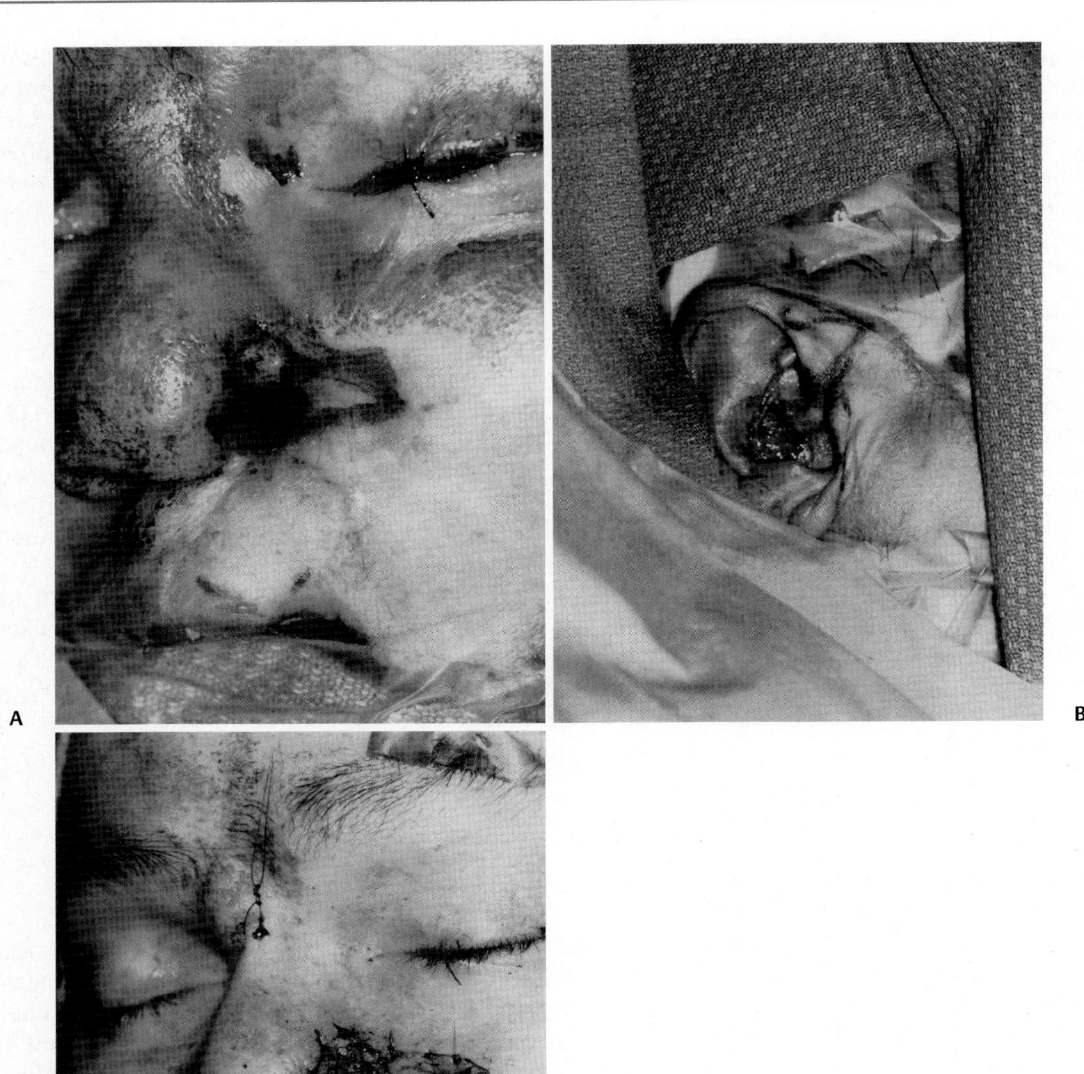

Fig. 53.13 (**A**) Composite skin–cartilage graft for nasal ala defect. To increase composite graft–recipient surface contact for revascularization, an adjacent turnover flap was used, instead of solely depending on edge-to-edge contact. (**B**) Donor site of composite skin cartilage graft. (**C**) Placement of composite skin–cartilage graft at nasal alar rim and full-thickness skin graft over donor site.

Langerhans cells have been removed to remove the immunogenicity of the graft. Currently, it is approved for use in venous ulcers and diabetic foot ulcers. For facial plastic surgeons, it would especially be helpful in patients who are unable or unwilling to have an autogenous partial-thickness skin graft. These newer products such as becaplermin and Apligraf have the potential to help the facial plastic surgeon to more actively improve chronic wounds of the skin to heal.

References

1. Burget G, Menick F. The subunit principle in nasal reconstruction. Plast Reconstr Surg 1985;76:239
2. Carrel A. The treatment of wounds. JAMA 1919;68:2148–2150
3. Mohs FE. Chemosurgical treatment of cancer of the skin. JAMA 1948;138:564–569
4. Brown JB, Fryer MP. Carcinoma of eyelids and canthal region. Geriatrics 1957;12:181–184
5. Goldwyn RM, Rueckert F. The value of healing by secondary intention for sizeable defects of the face. Arch Surg 1977;122:285–292

6. Mohs FE. Chemosurgery, Microscopically Controlled Surgery for Skin Cancer. Springfield, IL: Charles C. Thomas; 1978:3–337
7. Goldwyn RM. Value of healing by secondary intention seconded. Ann Plast Surg 1980;4:435
8. Panje WR, Bumsted RM, Ceilley RI. Secondary intention healing as an adjunct to the reconstruction of midfacial defects. Laryngoscope 1980;90:1148–1153
9. Mehta HK. Spontaneous reformation of lower eyelid. Br J Ophthalmol 1981;65:202–208
10. Moscona R, Pnini A, Hirshowitz B. In favor of healing by secondary intention after excision of medial canthal basal cell carcinoma. Plast Reconstr Surg 1983;71:189–195
11. Tromovitch TA, Stegman SJ. Microscopically controlled excision of skin tumors—chemosurgery (Mohs): fresh tissue technique. Arch Dermatol 1974;110:231–232
12. Billingham RE, Russell PS. Studies on wound healing with special reference to the phenomenon of contracture in experimental wounds in rabbits' skin. Ann Surg 1956;144:961–981
13. Kopke LFF, Konz B. Mikrographische chirurgie: eine methodische bestandsaufnahme. Hautarzt 1995;46:607–614
14. Albom MJ. The management of recurrent basal cell carcinomas: please no grafts or flaps at once. J Dermatol Surg Oncol 1977;3:382–384
15. Clark DP, Hanke CW. Neoplasms of the conchal bowl: treatment with Mohs micrographic surgery. J Dermatol Surg Oncol 1988;14:1223–1228
16. Zitelli JA. Wound healing by secondary intention. J Am Acad Dermatol 1983;9:407–415
17. Zitelli JA. Secondary intention healing: an alternative to surgical repair. Clin Dermatol 1984;2:92–106
18. James JH, Watson ACH. The use of Opsite, a vapor permeable dressing, on skin graft donor sites. Br J Plast Surg 1975;28:107–110
19. Baillin PL, Wheeland RG. Carbon dioxide (CO2) laser perforation of exposed cranial bone to stimulate granulation tissue. Plast Reconstr Surg 1985;75:898–902
20. Walsh JT, Flotte TJ, Deutsche TF. Er:YAG laser ablation of tissue: effect of pulse duration and tissue type on thermal damage. Lasers Surg Med 1989;9:314–326
21. Snow SN, Staff MA, Bullen R, et al. Second-intention healing of exposed facial scalp bone after Mohs surgery for skin cancer: review of 91 cases. J Am Acad Dermatol 1994;31:450–454
22. Hinman CD, Maibach H. Effect of air exposure and occlusion on experimental human skin wounds. Nature 1963;200:377–378
23. Deitch E, Wheelahan TM, Rose MP, Clothier J, Cotter J. Hypertrophic burn scars: analysis of variables. J Trauma 1983;23:895–898
24. Jaffe AT. Second-intention healing arrest: four case reports [abstract]. Presented at: American College of Mohs Micrographic Surgery and Cutaneous Oncology, 31st Annual Meeting; May 17, 1999;; Miami
25. Mandrea E. Topical diflorasone ointment for treatment of recalcitrant, excessive granulation tissue. Dermatol Surg 1998;24: 1409–1410
26. Albright SD. Placement of "guiding sutures" to counteract undesirable retraction of tissues in and around functionally and cosmetically important structures. J Dermatol Surg Oncol 1981; 7:446–449
27. Southwood W. The thickness of skin. Plast Reconstr Surg 1955;15:423
28. Gibson T. Physical properties of skin. In: McCarthy J, ed. Plastic Surgery. Philadelphia: WB Saunders; 1990:249
29. Crawford B. An unusual skin donor site. Br J Plast Surg 1964;17:311
30. Edgerton M, Hansen F. Matching facial color with split-thickness skin grafts from adjacent areas. Plast Reconstr Surg 1960;25:455
31. Shepard G. The storage of split-skin grafts and their donor sites. Plast Reconstr Surg 1972;49:115
32. Barton F, Byrd H. Acquired deformities of the nose. In: McCarthy J, ed. Plastic Surgery. Philadelphia: WB Saunders, 1990:1932
33. Rees T. Composite grafts. In: Transactions of the Third International Congress of Plastic and Reconstructive Surgery. Washington, DC: Excerpta Medica; 1963
34. Hom DB, Manivel JC. Promoting healing with recombinant human platelet-derived growth factor–BB in a previously irradiated problem wound. Laryngoscope 2003;113(9):1566–1571
35. Jakubowicz DM, Smith RV. Use of becaplermin in the closure of pharyngocutaneous fistulas. Head Neck 2005;27(5):433–438

54 Local and Regional Cutaneous Flaps

Stephen S. Park

Reconstruction of facial defects with local and regional cutaneous flaps is a challenging and rewarding part of facial plastic surgery. Over the years, the standard of care has risen significantly, and today's expectations are an inconspicuous aesthetic result with preservation of normal function. Many contemporary principles have allowed us to achieve these goals in a great number of patients.

Cutaneous lesions can be treated in a variety of ways, but Mohs micrographic surgery represents the gold standard for complex malignancies of the face and neck. Frederick Mohs first described this technique in the 1940s while a medical student at the University of Wisconsin.[1] This original fixation technique occurred in situ and required a postoperative slough of tissue, forcing a majority of these defects to heal by second intention. The development of immediate, fresh-tissue fixation allowed the definitive excision to be completed much more quickly and permitted immediate repair, thus catalyzing the interest in cutaneous reconstruction through local and regional flaps.

It is recognized that the primary risk for cutaneous malignancies is a series of high-intensity, short bursts of sun exposure at an early age, such as children with sunburns. Many adults today, however, grew up in an era when the importance of sun protection was less appreciated; consequently the incidence of cutaneous malignancies continues to rise. Ultraviolet-B (UV-B) rays are absorbed at the dermal–epidermal junction and are most responsible for malignant degeneration of epidermal cells. UV-C rays are the shortest wavelength and are absorbed by the ozone layer in their entirety. UV-A rays penetrate to the deeper dermal layer and are more associated with tanning and causing photoaging of skin.

Anatomy and Physiology

Vascular Supply

The cutaneous vascular network is a unique system with an abundant dermal and subdermal plexus that allows for dependable and versatile random donor flaps. This dermal plexus is regulated by arteriovenous shunts that are controlled by the adrenergic neural supply and function as one of the primary thermal regulators of our body. Skin may also have its arterial supply through an axial pattern based on a dominant artery in the subcutaneous layer. Muscular perforating arteries are also a dependable source to the cutaneous vascular bed. Local perfusion pressure is the driving force for random cutaneous flaps. Critical closing pressure is the pressure whereby capillary vessels collapse and all vascular flow ceases. This is thought to occur between 5 and 10 mm Hg.[2] The concepts of perfusion pressure and closing pressure have challenged the old dogma that random donor flaps require a length to width ratio of 3:1. Studies have now shown this to be a fallacy and that the essential variable for flap viability is the perfusion pressure and vascularity at the pedicle base.[3] This understanding has strongly supported the birth of pedicle flaps and microvascular free flaps.

Skin Lines

Langer's lines were defined by the way a circular wound takes on an elliptical shape as rigor mortis develops. Langer's assumption was that skin excisions oriented along the long axis of these wounds resulted in more favorable healing. Clinical experience has shown that this is not always accurate and they appear to conflict with other described skin lines. Today Langer's lines are of historical interest only. Relaxed skin tension lines (RSTL) are derived from vectors within facial skin that reflect the intrinsic tension of skin at rest.[4] These properties of skin are defined by the microarchitecture, such as the alignment of elastic and collagen fibers, and to a lesser degree, by the influence of underlying bone and soft tissue bulk. RSTLs are the lines of intrinsic skin tension that appear when the skin is in repose and represent the directional pull on wounds. They have the greatest cumulative effect on wound tension and final healing. The RSTLs are generally parallel to external skin wrinkles but represent a distinct entity from them and occasionally conflict (**Fig. 54.1**).

Lines of minimal tension that are also known as natural skin creases or wrinkles are the lines that are externally visible and result from repeated bending of skin from muscular contraction until a permanent cutaneous crease has formed with adhesions between the dermis and deeper tissues. These natural skin creases run perpendicular to muscular fibers and can guide wound orientation for favorable healing. The glabella, nose, and lateral canthal areas have conflicting RSTLs and lines of minimal tension where repeated muscular pull creates permanent skin creases that override the intrinsic tension lines of the skin. In these regions, it is usually best to orient wounds and scars within skin creases rather than the RSTLs for best camouflage.

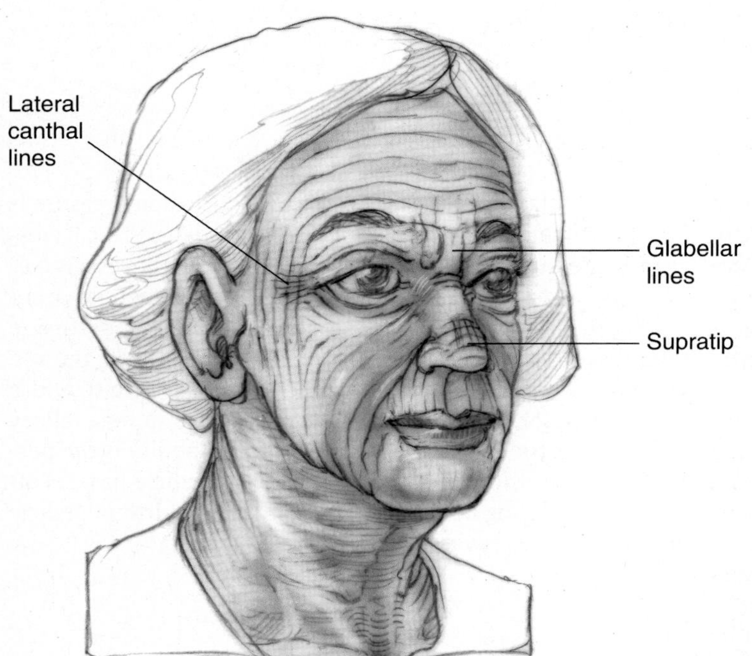

Fig. 54.1 Relaxed skin tension lines (RSTLs) and natural skin creases of the face. Generally these coincide, but three areas of conflict are lateral canthus, nasal supra tip, and glabella.

Sleep lines represent the skin creases that result from the patient's habitual positioning while asleep, where the skin is unnaturally folded and remains independent of the intrinsic skin forces as well as muscular contraction.

Lines of maximum extensibility are important when recruiting tissue from adjacent areas. The tension on the flap is an essential consideration and can be minimized by studying the lines of maximum extensibility (LME). These lines typically run perpendicular to the RSTLs and parallel to muscular fibers. Extensibility must be distinguished from elasticity, the latter being the property of recoil as skin returns to its original shape.

Timing of Wound Repair

There is a general surgery dictum that soft tissue wounds that are not closed within 6 hours be left open to heal by second intention. The rationale for this is the concern with contamination and subsequent soft tissue infection. Although this is a significant concern with lower extremity wounds, it is not as applicable to the soft tissues of the face and neck. The robust vasculature of the face affords a very low incidence of soft tissue infections, and there is essentially no limit to the delay for facial wound closure. There are occasions where the repair of soft tissue wounds is best delayed for a couple weeks, such as when the accumulation of granulation tissue will improve the contour of the wound bed. Prior to closure of a delayed wound, it should be aggressively debrided with removal of the thin layer of fibrinous exudate that forms on the bed. Wound margins are "freshened" as peripheral epithelialization has often occurred. An important consideration with regard to delayed wound repair is soft tissue contracture, which may be favorable as the overall dimensions of the soft tissue deficit decrease. However, once this contracture distorts surrounding structures, such as eyelids, lips, or the alar rim, its surgical correction can be far more challenging than the original defect.

Wound Care

Closed incisions are cleansed with dilute hydrogen peroxide followed by a thick moisturizing ointment. The purpose of the peroxide is to remove any small blood clots and crusts within the skin incision itself. Left alone, these small scabs may contribute to a slightly wider scar as epithelialization occurs beneath it. Sufficient hemostasis has usually occurred after a few days, and peroxide is no longer needed. Continued moist wound coverage is essential and simple petrolatum gel is sufficient. All open wounds and skin grafts are managed with mild soap and water followed by ointment. Hydrogen peroxide is strictly avoided due to its cellular toxicity and the potentially delayed healing that may occur. Diligent sun protection is critical for at least 6 months following reconstructive surgery and is continually reiterated to the patients. All undermined skin as well as incisions are more sensitive to actinic injury and prone to early tanning and burning.

Premature sun exposure may result in a permanent discoloration or a "tattooing" effect on the cutaneous scars.

Flap Nomenclature

Different disciplines participate in cutaneous flap surgery, and it remains important to use consistent nomenclature. Four systems are utilized, as follows, to characterize flaps.

1. *Blood supply*. Skin flaps may be characterized by their arterial blood supply as either *random donor*, *axial pattern*, or *pedicled*. The dermal and subdermal plexus alone nourishes random pattern flaps. Axial pattern flaps have more dominant superficial vessels that are oriented longitudinally along the flap axis. Pedicled flaps have large, named vessels that directly supply the skin paddle, often through muscular or fascial perforators (**Fig. 54.2**).
2. *Location*. The region from which tissue is mobilized is another means of classification. Local flaps generally imply utilizing adjacent tissue. Regional flaps are from different areas of the same part of the body (e.g., forehead flaps for nasal reconstruction). Distal flaps are from different parts of the body, such as a pectoralis myocutaneous flap for the head and neck.
3. *Tissue content*. The embryologic layers of tissue contained within the flap are another means of classification. *Cutaneous flaps* are limited to the skin. As deeper layers are incorporated into the flap they are classified accordingly (e.g., *myocutaneous*, *fasciocutaneous*, and *composite*).
4. *Method of transfer*. Method of transfer is probably the most frequently utilized system of nomenclature but often inaccurately defined. *Advancement flaps* are mobilized in a unilinear fashion toward the defect. *Rotational flaps* pivot around a specific point and maintain that radius. Therefore, pure rotational flaps are rarely utilized. Most local flaps combine advancement and rotational elements. *Transposition* refers to a flap that is elevated and mobilized toward an adjacent defect and transposed over an incomplete bridge of skin. A rhombic flap is an example of a transposition flap in that the flap is elevated and transposed over a small triangle of undisturbed adjacent skin. *Interposition flaps* are similar to transposition flaps; however, the incomplete bridge of adjacent skin is also elevated and mobilized, usually in the opposite direction to fill the secondary defect. A Z-plasty is an example of an interposition flap. Interpositioned flaps differ from transposition flaps in that the skin flap is elevated and transferred over a complete bridge of intact skin. By definition, this creates

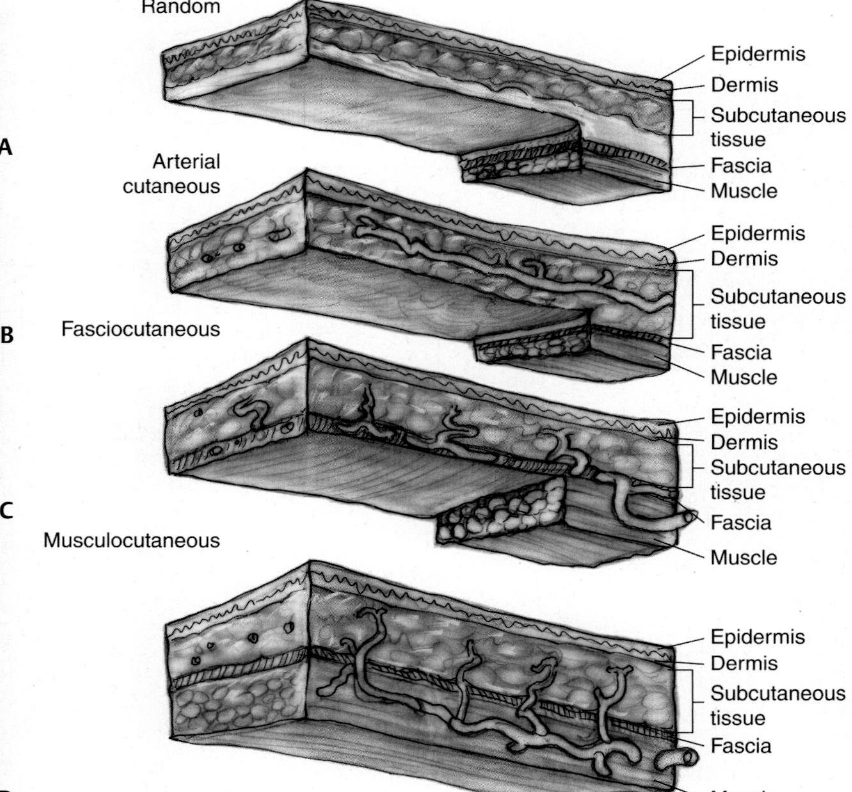

Fig. 54.2 Vascular anatomy of cutaneous flaps. (**A**) Random pattern flap based on subdermal plexus. (**B**) Axial pattern flap. (**C**) Fasciocutaneous flap with named vessel. (**D**) Musculocutaneous flap with named vessel.

a cutaneous pedicle and mandates a second stage for pedicle division. The forehead flap is an *interpolated flap* wherein the glabella represents the undisturbed bridge of skin. The island flap is a variation of an interpolated flap where the pedicle is deepithelialized and contains subcutaneous tissue alone. This pedicle can then be buried beneath the intact bridge of skin, thus obviating the second stage. *Free microvascular flaps* are based on a detached vascular pedicle and transferred to a different region for reanastomosis.

Patient Evaluation: Defect Analysis

During the initial evaluation of a cutaneous defect, the optimal method of reconstruction is not always immediately obvious and an algorithmic method of analysis can assist with flap selection and design. By reviewing four specific areas, one may lay out the most aesthetic cutaneous flap while avoiding gross facial asymmetry or distortion.

1. *Immobile structures.* What are the specific structures relevant to this facial defect that must not be distorted or come under any tension? These include such landmarks as the hairline, eyelid, melolabial fold, and so forth.
2. *Area of recruitment.* Which of the areas surrounding the defect is most readily accessible and has sufficient laxity to allow mobilization toward the defect?
3. *Relaxed skin tension lines and aesthetic units.* How are the RSTLs, skin creases, and LMEs oriented in that region to best accommodate additional skin incisions while minimizing wound tension? In addition, the borders of the aesthetic units represent imaginary lines that can accept skin incisions and their subsequent scars in an inconspicuous manner. The principle of the aesthetic unit is based on the fact that our eyes tend to see objects and faces as a series of block images that are spatially organized. For example, the face is characterized by several distinct aesthetic units, each seen by the casual observer as a single block image. The nose has been further divided into aesthetic subunits and has served as one of the major advances in contemporary nasal reconstruction[5] (**Fig. 54.3**). These aesthetic units of the face and nose are defined by subtle changes in topography, reflections of light, preexisting creases, and transition zones of skin texture. They do not necessarily correlate with the underlying bony and cartilaginous framework. Scars that lie at the junction of two adjacent aesthetic units tend to be inconspicuous because one expects delineation between these facial areas.

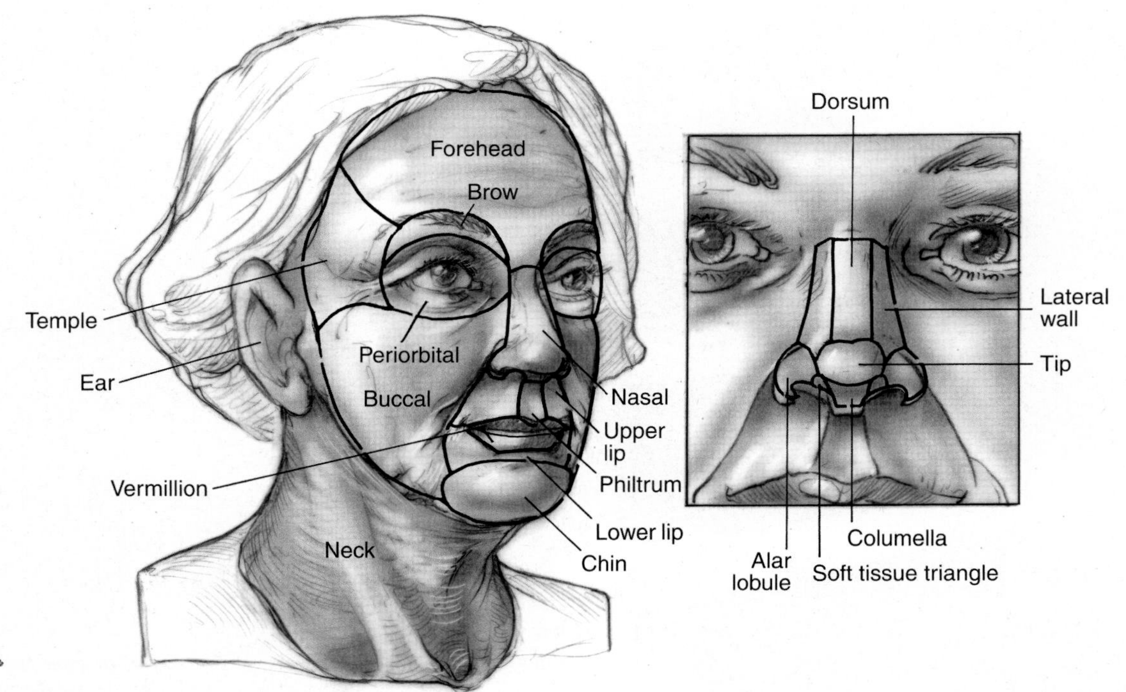

Fig. 54.3 Facial aesthetic units. (**A**) The face is perceived as a series of block images and incisions/scars along unit borders tend to be less conspicuous. (**B**) The nose is further broken down to aesthetic subunits.

4. *Resultant scar.* One must always anticipate the final resultant scar of any local and regional flap. Oftentimes these flaps can be oriented in such a way as to comply with the preexisting variables discussed previously, for example, relaxed skin tension lines and aesthetic unit borders.

This algorithm for defect analysis will often lead to the optimal reconstructive flap with the least functional problems and inadvertent distortion.

Case 1 (Fig. 54.4A)

An 82-year-old woman is referred for repair of a nasal Mohs defect. **(B–D)** The nasal aesthetic subunits are outlined and illustrate a majority of the tip unit to be missing along with 40% of the dorsal unit and 20% of the left lateral sidewall. A small superficial defect of the right ala is repaired independently with a full-thickness skin graft. **(E)** The aesthetic units are excised and resurfaced with a single flap. **(F–I)** The 18-month postoperative view demonstrates the camouflage that can be achieved by designing wound edges, flap borders, and subsequent scars consistent with principles of aesthetic subunits.

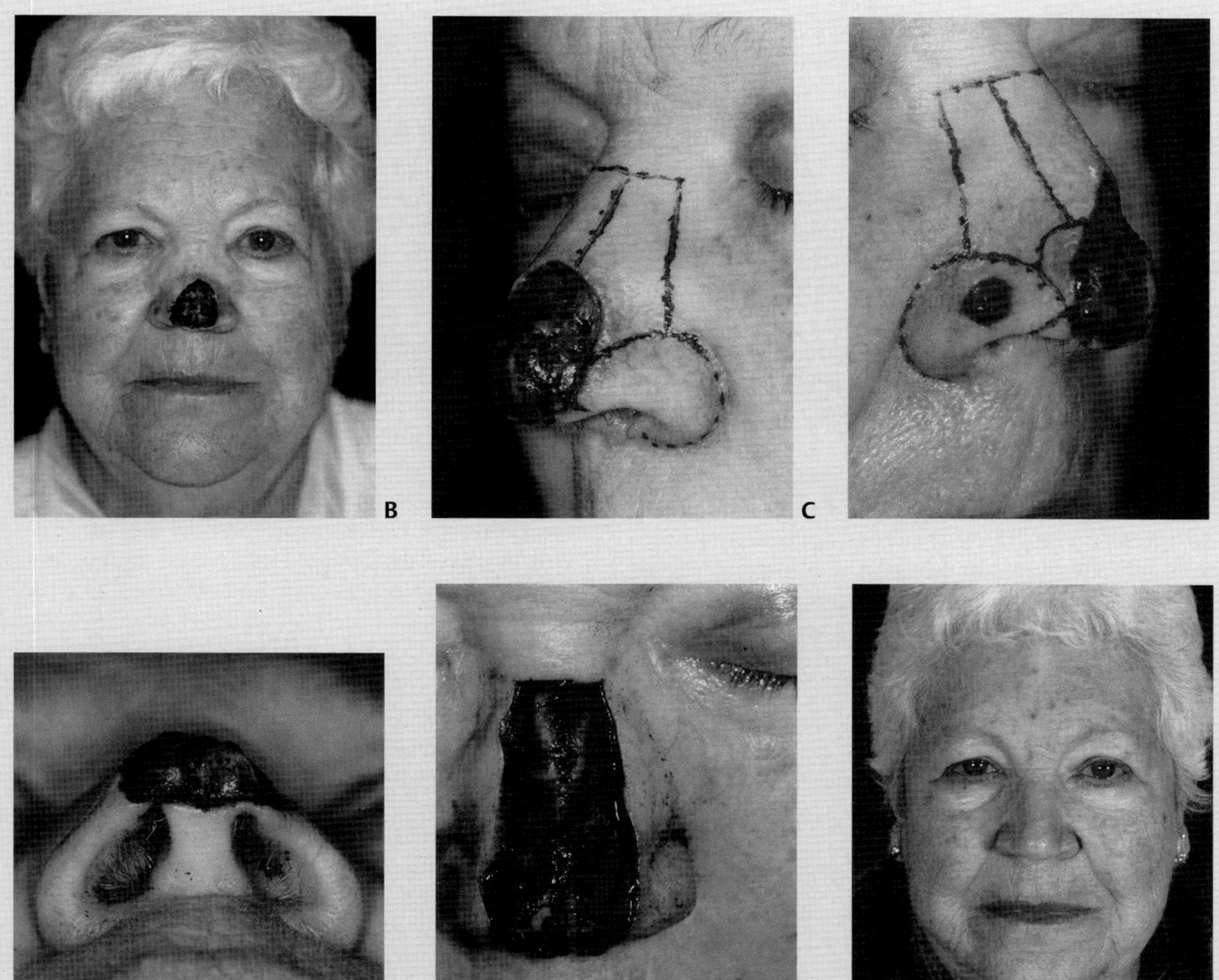

Fig. 54.4 **(A–I)** Case 1. The nasal aesthetic subunits.

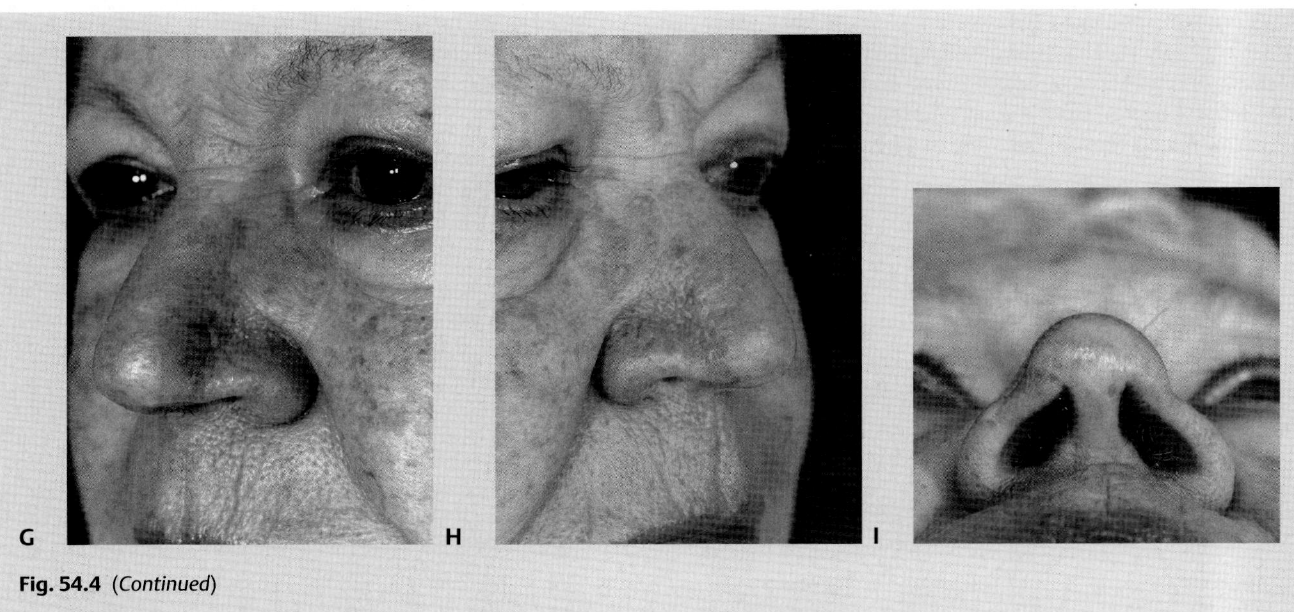

Fig. 54.4 *(Continued)*

Second-Intention Healing

Second-intention healing is often overlooked by facial plastic surgeons but is often employed by dermatologic surgeons and has several advantages. On occasion, second-intention healing may be the method of choice for obtaining the best aesthetic and functional outcome. Wounds that lend themselves to second-intention healing are superficial, concave, and not in close proximity to mobile structures that might be distorted during normal wound contracture. Patients who are exceptionally high surgical risks are also good candidates for this method of repair. A disadvantage of second-intention healing is the length of time required for complete healing; an average 1-cm defect may take close to 4 weeks for total reepithelialization. The inconveniences of continued wound care often exceed that of a surgical repair. If wound contracture occurs and causes significant distortion to adjacent structures, the secondary repair can represent a formidable challenge. Soft tissue contracture usually involves deeper tissues, and a multilayer reconstruction may be needed for correction.

Surgical Treatment

Advancement Flap

Wound edges from a Mohs defect must be "freshened" prior to definitive closure. The technique of Mohs surgery leaves wound edges beveled toward the center of the wound to analyze the entire specimen margin. When closing cutaneous wounds, it is preferable for the edges to bevel away from the center to allow maximal skin eversion during subcuticular closure.

Primary closure is the simplest form of an advancement flap. An advancement flap refers to mobilizing tissue in a unilinear dimension without a rotational element. Circular defects closed primarily must be modified to an elliptical shape to avoid standing cutaneous deformities. The terminal angles of a defect should be roughly 30 degrees or less to avoid this "dog ear" deformity. This 30-degree angle serves as a reference to dictate how far one must extend the ellipse and how much normal tissue will be discarded. When this tissue cannot be readily sacrificed, the ellipse can be converted to a W-plasty with the apices of the "W" 30 degrees or less (**Fig. 54.5**). This preserves some surrounding tissue and also avoids extension of the resultant scar. AW-plasty can be very useful for cutaneous defects in close proximity to facial landmarks, such as a lip defect repaired primarily using an inferior W-plasty to avoid a scar that traverses the mental crease.

Pure advancement flaps have the feature of limiting wound tension to a single vector with minimal perpendicular tension (**Fig. 54.6A**). Advancement flaps are often utilized in the forehead and eyebrow areas to capitalize on the natural forehead furrows while causing no vertical distortion of the hairline superiorly or the brow margin inferiorly. The skin edges from the flap and nonflap sides are of different lengths, and their

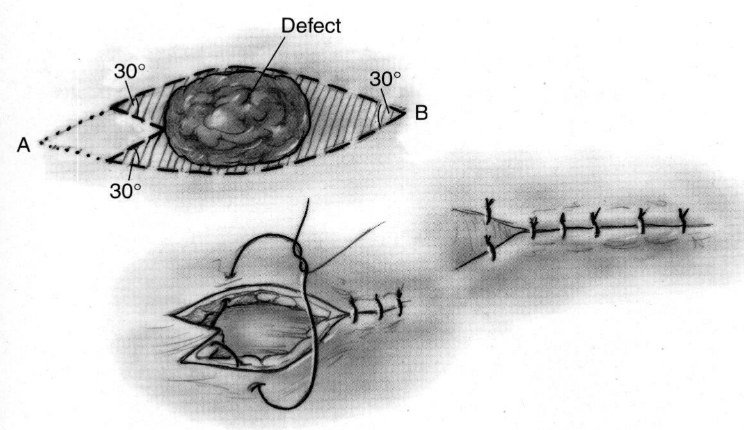

Fig. 54.5 Primary closure with W-plasty. The terminal angles for any primary closure with advancement flaps must be 30 degrees or less to avoid the standing cutaneous deformity.

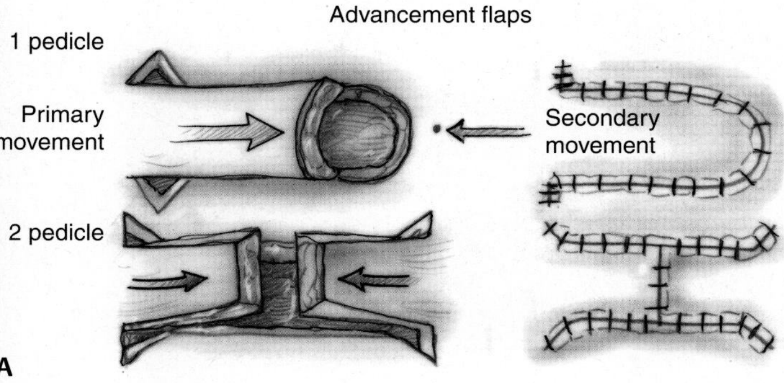

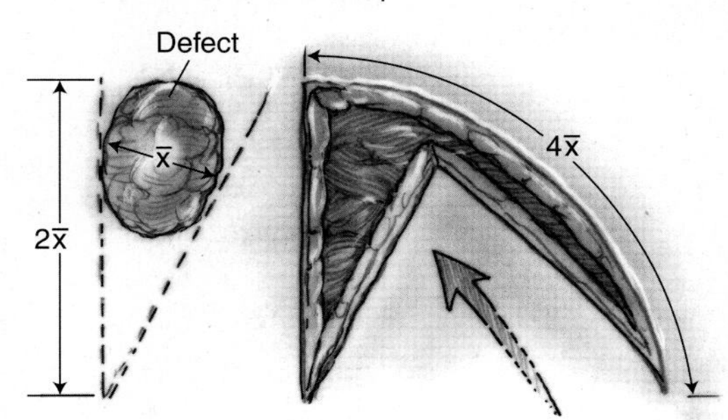

Fig. 54.6 Unilateral and bilateral advancement flaps. (**A**) The primary tension vector is along a single axis with very little surrounding distortion. (**B**) Rotation flap around a given pivot point with an arc that is roughly four times the diameter of the defect.

closure may create one or several standing cutaneous deformities that may require direct excision (Burrow's triangles). These excisions create scars perpendicular to the flap margin, which are generally undesirable and should be positioned as inconspicuously as possible. When smaller discrepancies exist, the flap borders may be closed primarily through serial halving sutures; that is, each sequential suture is placed midway along the incision such that the length discrepancy becomes evenly distributed along the length of the wound.

V-Y flaps are also advancement flaps in that they are mobilized in a linear direction. They are based on a subcutaneous pedicle, which may limit the amount of advancement the flap can achieve. The secondary defect is closed primarily and the resultant scar resembles the letter "Y." Cheek defects along the alar facial groove are amenable to a V-Y flap repair, recruited from the melolabial fold. This minimizes distortion to the nose and upper lip while preserving the general orientation of the melolabial fold.

Case 2 (Fig. 54.7A)

A 74-year-old woman presents with a Mohs defect of the left cheek and lip that crosses the melolabial fold and is up to the alar facial groove. A preexisting scar is noted in the left cheek. (**B**) This is repaired with a V-Y advancement flap, with primary closure of the donor site leaving a scar within the melolabial fold. (**C**) The advancement flap is based on a subcutaneous pedicle and mobilized up to the alar facial groove. (**D**) The resultant scar is in the configuration of the letter "Y." (**E**) A 6-month postoperative view.

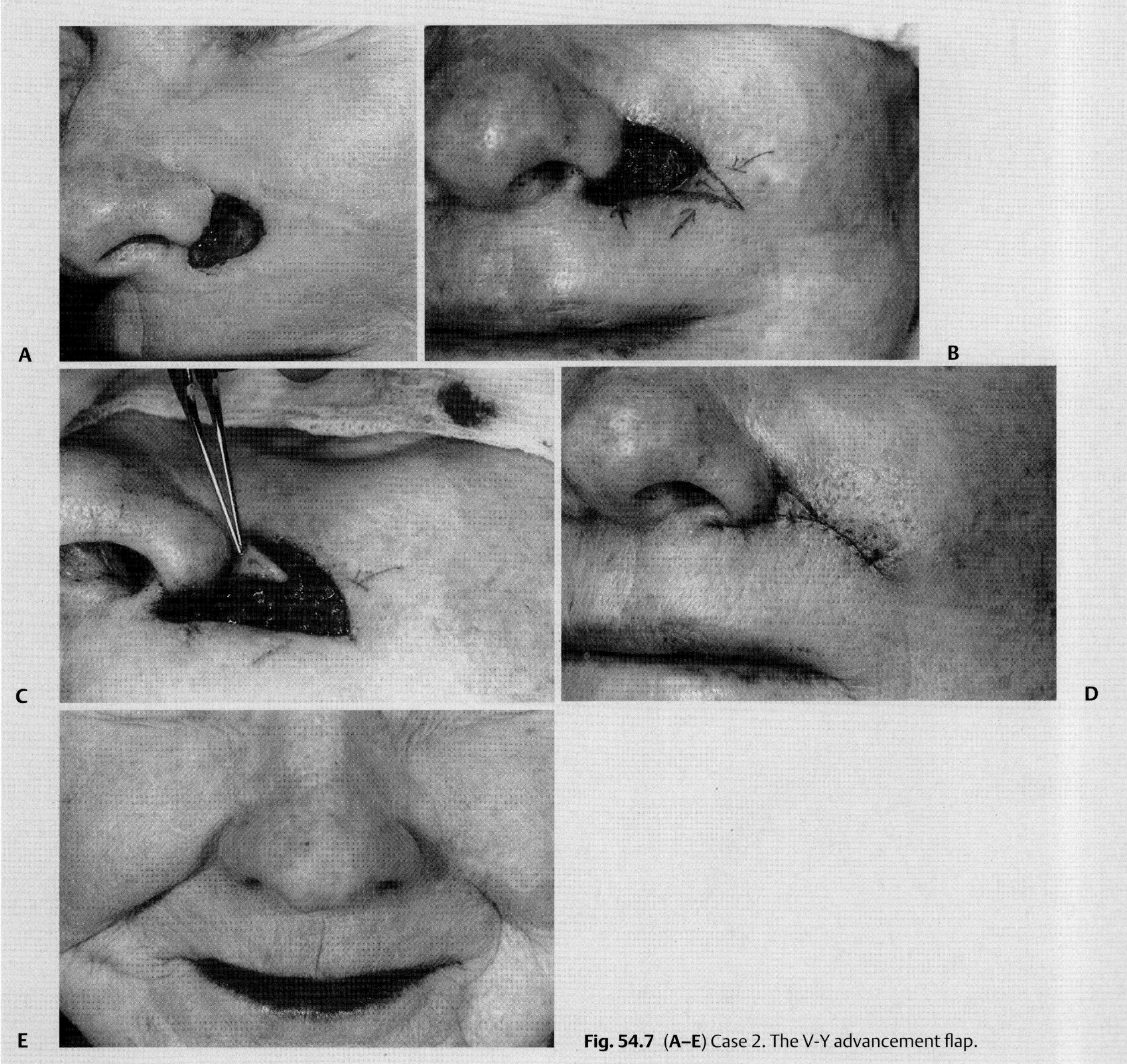

Fig. 54.7 **(A–E)** Case 2. The V-Y advancement flap.

Scalp Flap

The scalp flap is a unique example of a pure rotation flap due to the extreme inextensibility of the galea in and around the flap. Many facial defects can be closed with a rotation flap designed with an arc four times the diameter of the defect (**Fig. 54.6B**). On the scalp, however, the arc must be roughly six times the wound diameter to allow primary defect coverage. Galeal incisions, galeatomies, can improve the extensibility of these tissues and are best performed parallel to the arterial flow and perpendicular to lines of tension. Multiple rotation flaps can be designed around the primary defect in a spiral fashion.[6] Scalp defects occasionally require preoperative tissue expansion to create adequate coverage.[7] The advantage of using a scalp flap for defects of the head is coverage with like tissue (i.e., adjacent hair-bearing tissue). A reasonable alternative is to allow second-intention healing or skin graft coverage followed by serial excisions every 2 months.

Cheek Flap (Cervical Facial Flap)

The cheek flap is a common example of a combination rotation and advancement flap that is ideally suited for moderate to large cutaneous defects of the medial cheek area. It utilizes the usually abundant tissue laxity in the adjacent cheek and jowl areas. Although it requires a moderate amount of undermining and skin elevation, the strategic placement of incisions makes the resulting scar relatively inconspicuous and is a dependable and aesthetic flap for many cheek defects. The disadvantage of a cheek flap relates to the amount of skin mobilization needed for adequate coverage. In addition, some patients are left with cheek asymmetry wherein one side has notably fewer wrinkles and smaller jowls. When improperly done, the cheek flap may cause distortion to important landmarks, such as the lower eyelid and nasal ala.

The superior incision for a cheek flap typically extends along a subciliary crease and out the lateral canthal and temporal area. There is a tendency to allow the incision to drift inferiorly as one extends beyond the lateral canthus, and this should be deliberately avoided. It is more useful to extend this lateral extension in a superior direction prior to turning inferiorly toward a standard facelift or parotidectomy incision. This superior extension allows a more rotational element to the cheek flap with less advancement. The inferior extension can be similar to a parotidectomy incision with a horizontal limb in the upper neck. When necessary, this flap can be enlarged inferiorly to incorporate a deltopectoral flap. More skin recruitment can be achieved by extending the incision to the postauricular, non–hair-bearing area and transposing this over the ear in a bilobe fashion. The medial incision should be along the nasal facial groove and continued into the melolabial fold; it does not extend to the upper lip. There is usually some flap redundancy or standing cutaneous deformity around the melolabial fold that requires direct excision, which should be performed liberally. The plane of elevation is in the subcutaneous layer, superficial to the facial nerve. It is critical that the flap be suspended in a superior medial direction via direct anchoring to the periosteum of the zygoma, infraorbital rim, or nasal facial groove. There should be no tension on the lower eyelid, nasal ala, or upper lip during closure. The suspending sutures can be done with long-lasting resorbable material such as 4–0 polydioxanone (PDS, Ethicon, Inc., Somerville, NJ). Small cutaneous “dimples” may arise from the suspension sutures, but these are temporary and can be massaged out over time. The superomedial tip of the flap should maintain an acute angle and fit precisely in the borders of the cheek, eye, and nasal aesthetic units. There is a tendency to round this corner of the flap, which leaves a more conspicuous resultant scar that is more likely to pull the lower lid during contracture. The portion of the flap that is repositioned over the lower eyelid should be aggressively thinned to mimic the thickness of skin native to this area.

Case 3 (Fig. 54.8A)

A 77-year-old woman presents with a Mohs defect of the left medial cheek down to the subcutaneous fat. She has reasonable tone to the left lower eyelid. **(B)** The borders of the facial units extend along the subciliary crease, vertically along the nasal facial groove and into the melolabial fold. Although closure along the long axis of the defect would require less skin mobilization, the resultant scar would be more unfavorable because it would lie within the cheek unit. **(C)** The cheek flap is advanced medially, with the resultant scar along the borders of the facial aesthetic units. A small dimple can be seen in the medial aspect of the cheek flap that represents a suspension suture between the dermis and the periosteum along the pyriform aperature. The lower lid is not shortened, although this can be done when significant laxity exists. There is no inferior tension to the lid margin. **(D, E)** Nine-month postoperative views with scars less conspicuous due to their placement. The lower eyelid margin is maintained, although there is some asymmetry to the fullness of the lower eyelids and cheek.

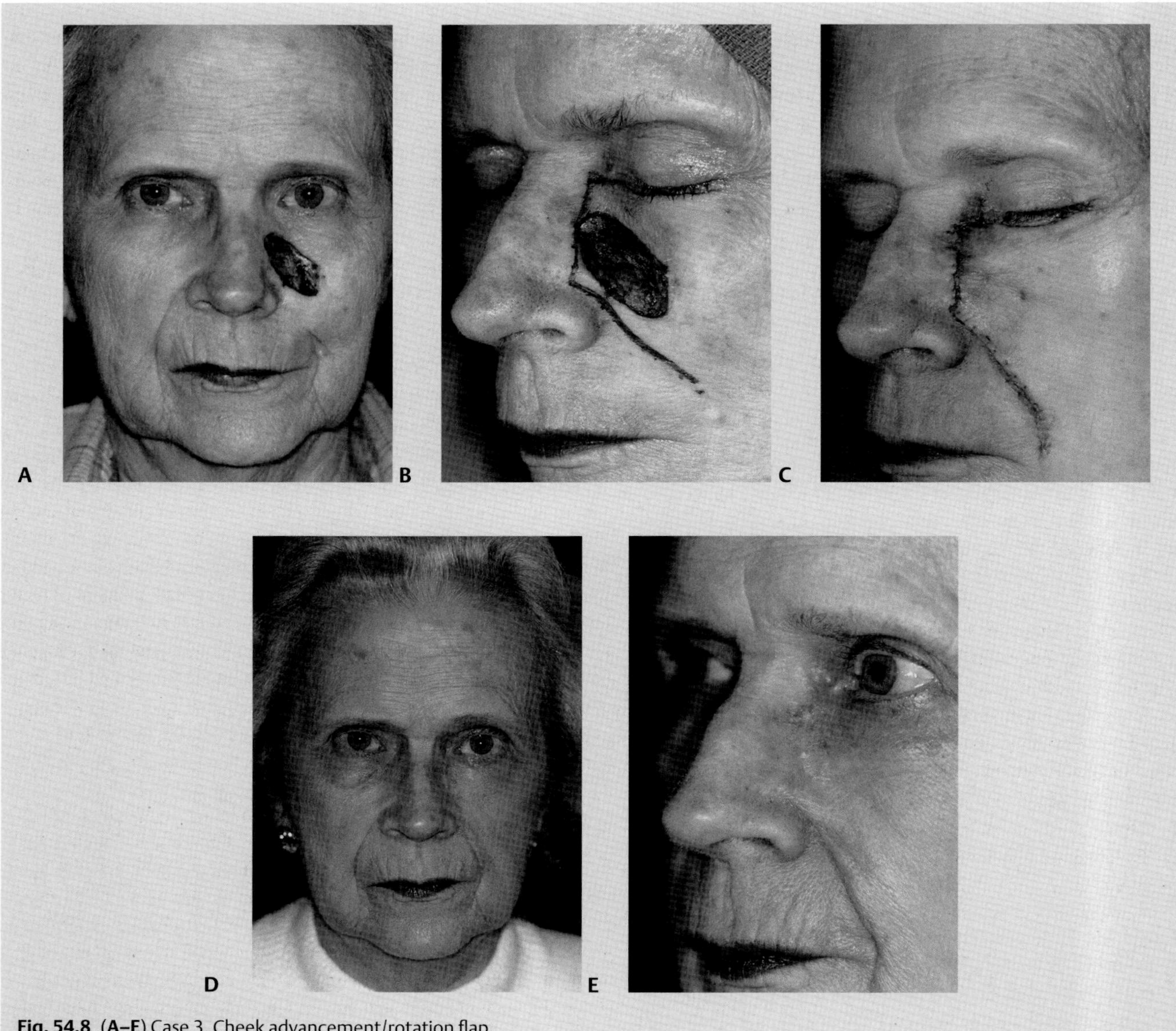

Fig. 54.8 **(A–E)** Case 3. Cheek advancement/rotation flap.

O-T Flap

This flap converts a circular defect to a T-shaped scar. It incorporates advancement and rotational vectors with the distinct feature of recruiting adjacent tissue from a specific area around the defect while leaving one border undisturbed. This design is well suited for defects juxtaposed to important aesthetic landmarks on which the closure must not exert tension or distortion. For example, a cutaneous defect along the hairline is easily repaired with the O-T flap because it avoids mobilization of hair-bearing skin onto the face. Other areas in which O-T flaps are frequently utilized include forehead, temple, and lips. These flaps have the disadvantage of leaving an unfavorable scar containing two perpendicular limbs, one usually opposing natural skin creases. In addition, the central limb from the circular defect must be extended to avoid the standing cutaneous deformity, requiring the excision of some normal tissue.

Case 4 (Fig. 54.9A)

A 62-year-old woman has a defect of the left temple. The regional immobile structures include the hairline, eyebrow, and lateral canthus. The greatest area of recruitment can come from the left cheek and, to a lesser extent, from the forehead. (**B**) An O-T advancement/rotation flap is designed leaving the hairline and brow undisturbed. Both flaps are mobilized in the subcutaneous plane, superficial to the facial nerve. (**C**) Flap closure is complete, with one horizontal limb running perpendicular to the RSTLs of the temple area. This is accepted as a tradeoff for maintaining eyebrow and hairline position. Scar resembles the letter "T." (**D**) One-year postoperative view showing the oblique limb of the defect closure. Regional facial landmarks remain undisturbed.

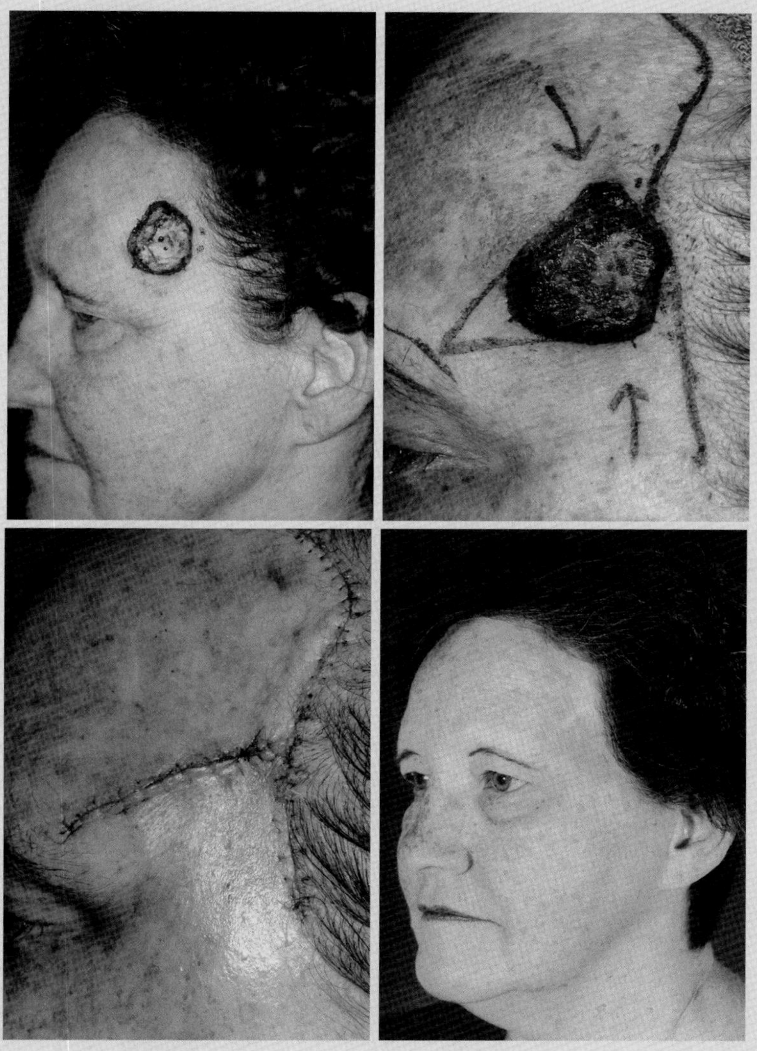

A B C D

Fig. 54.9 (**A–D**) Case 4. The O-T advancement/rotation flap for the temple.

O-Z Flap

The O-Z flap is an advancement/rotation flap similar to the O-T flap, except that the adjacent flaps are based on opposing sides of the defect and the final incision resembles the letter "Z." The unique characteristic of this design is the resultant scar; rather than two perpendicular limbs, the O-Z flap creates scars that run oblique to one another and can be more closely aligned with skin creases. This flap can be useful in the temple and cheek regions where scar alignment has a significant impact on the cosmetic outcome.

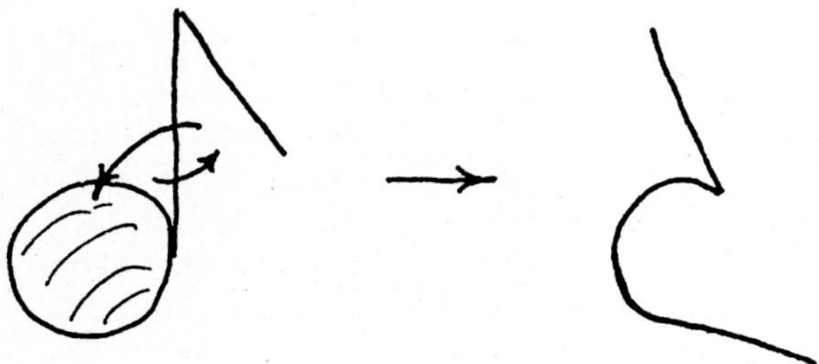

Fig. 54.10 Note flap. The triangular flap can fill the circular defect as either a transposition or interposition flap. The circular defect can be converted to a triangle to maintain sharp angles.

Note Flap

The note flap is a simple transposition flap whereby a circular defect is repaired with an adjacent triangular flap and the donor site closed primarily.[8] The flap design resembles the musical eighth note and is transposed over a small incomplete bridge of adjacent skin. A Burrow's triangle is excised from the defect margin, along the base of the flap. The resultant scar has a circular and straight component. The incomplete bridge of adjacent skin can also be mobilized to fill the donor site as an interposition flap (**Fig. 54.10**).

Rhombic Flap

The rhombic flap is a precise, geometric modification of the note flap and is a classic flap that remains the workhorse for many small cutaneous defects of the face. It is a transposition flap in that the mobilized tissue is elevated over an incomplete and undisturbed bridge of skin. The rhombic flap recruits and mobilizes tissue from a specific area and results in a predictable scar with well-defined vectors of tension.

The Limberg rhombic flap is the traditional design whereby the defect has 60 and 120 degree angles and the limbs are of equal length.[9] The flap begins by extending an incision along the short axis of the defect, equal in length to one side of the rhombic defect. The second incision is 60 degrees from the first and equal in length. A disproportionate amount of tension (58%) can be found at a single point of the flap corresponding to the closure of the secondary defect. More importantly, the vector of this tension is predictable and runs roughly parallel to the adjacent limb of the original defect[10] (**Figs. 54.11 and 54.12A,B**). The resultant scars run in multiple directions and it is not possible to align them all parallel to RSTLs. This vector of maximum tension, therefore, dictates flap orientation such that it runs parallel to the existing LMEs. One of the disadvantages of the classic Limberg flap is the significant tension at the closure point as well as the amount of discarded tissue needed to convert circular defects to a geometrical rhombus. Dufourmentel modified the Limberg flap to accommodate defects that are more square and to minimize discarded normal tissues[11] (**Fig. 54.12C,D**). The transposed flap is proportionally wider than the Limberg one and still creates a vector of tension that dictates the orientation for flap design.

The Webster 30-degree rhombic transposes a narrower flap with more acute angles, facilitating donor site closure without dog ears and creating a more even distribution of tension around the defect.[12] This distribution of tension may translate to small amounts of distortion to neighboring structures, which must be anticipated. A W-plasty is often incorporated into the defect to preserve more tissue but at the expense of an additional limb of scar (**Fig. 54.12E,F**).

Most defects that are repaired with a rhombic-type transposition flap utilize a combination of these modifications. Very rarely is the cutaneous defect converted to an exact rhombus; more often, the transposed flap is slightly narrower and oriented more along the long axis of the defect, both of which facilitate donor site closure and create an even distribution of tension around the defect. Multiple rhombic flaps can be designed around larger cutaneous defects of rectangular or circular shapes.

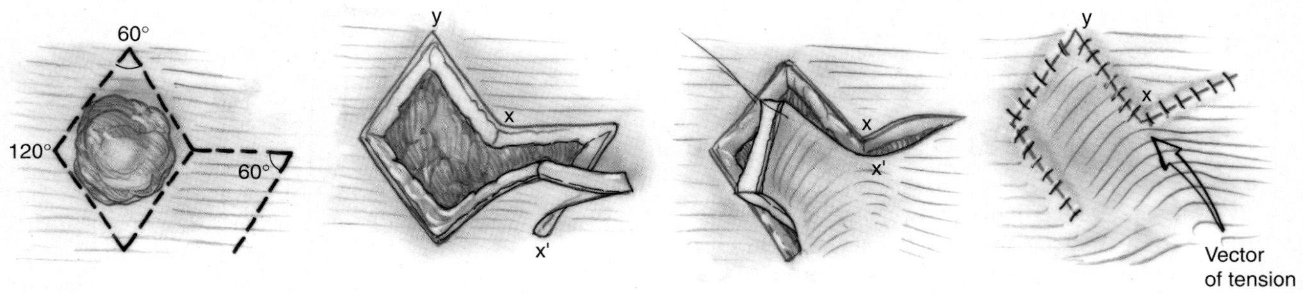

Fig. 54.11 Rhombic flap. Limberg flap design and transposition. Note the primary vector of tension being parallel to an adjacent limb of the primary cutaneous defect.

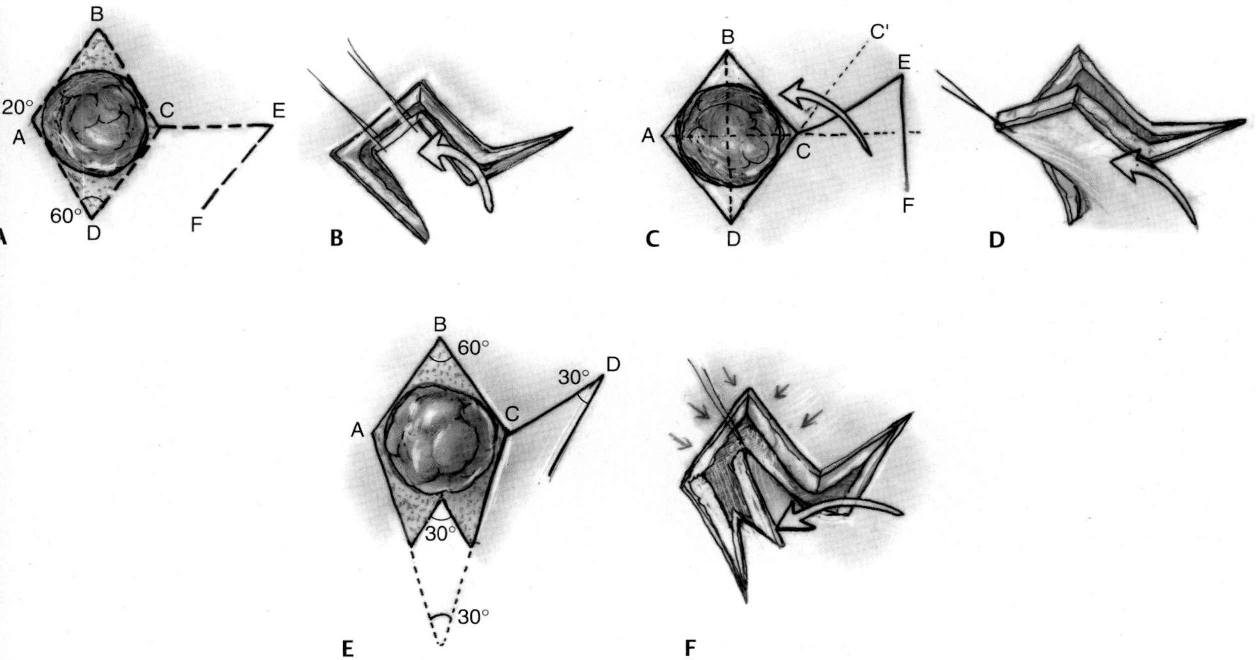

Fig. 54.12 (**A,B**) Classic Limberg flap. (**C,D**) Dufourmentel modification for closure of square defects. (**E,F**) Webster 30 degree modification with inferior W-plasty.

Case 5 (Fig. 54.13A)

A circular defect of the left cheek area measures 23 mm in diameter and extends to the subcutaneous tissues. (**B**) A modified rhombic flap is designed with components from both the Dufourmentel and Webster modifications. Less normal tissue is discarded from the apices of the defect. The flap is recruited from the lower cheek area and oriented such that the vector of maximum tension during flap mobilization runs parallel to the LME. (**C**) The flap is closed with a predictable resultant scar that crosses many natural skin creases and RSTLs; however, it is under the least possible tension and causes no distortion to the lower eyelid. (**D**) A 12-month postoperative view demonstrates acceptable healing due to closure under minimal tension.

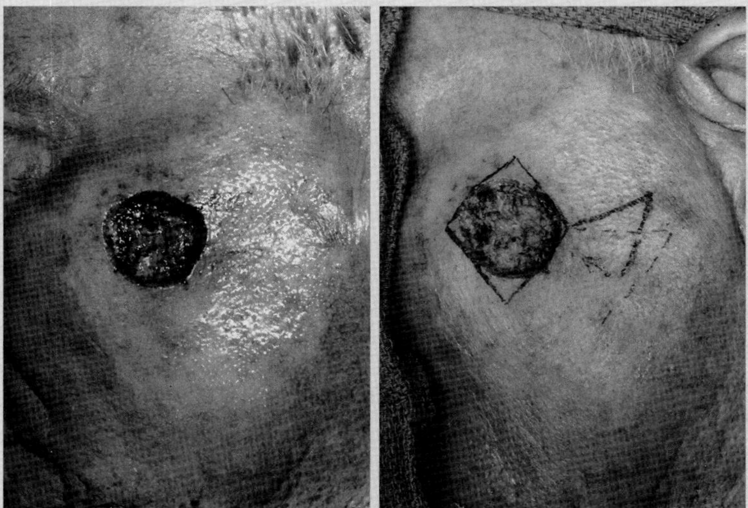

Fig. 54.13 (**A–D**) Case 5. Rhombic flap for a cheek defect.

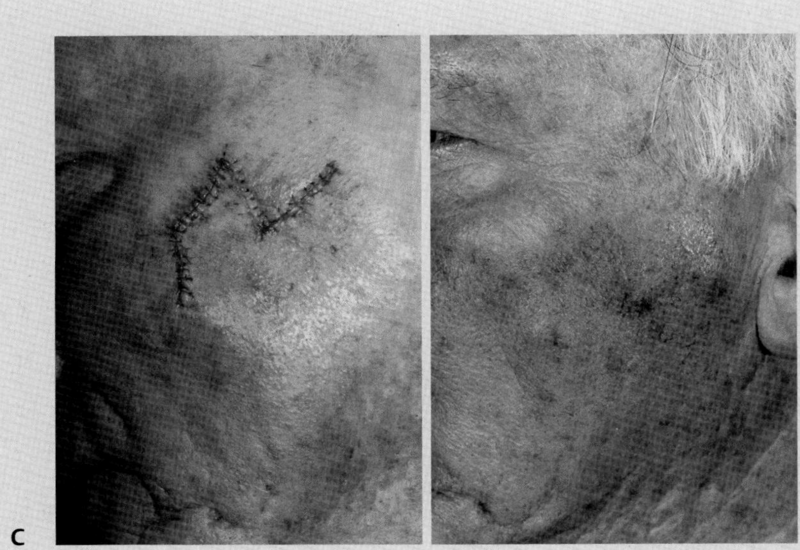

Fig. 54.13 *(Continued)*

Bilobe Flap

The bilobe flap is a transposition flap with two circular skin paddles based on a common cutaneous base, transposed over an in complete bridge of skin. It is primarily a rotational flap around a pivot point, but it incorporates small degrees of advancement. These bilobe flaps have the distinct advantage of moving the areas of recruitment, and therefore tension, further from the primary defect. This second lobe allows the transfer of tension from donor site closure further from the primary defect, which is especially useful for small defects of the lower nose and temple areas. Earlier designs oriented the skin paddles 90 degrees to each other. The secondary flap, therefore, had its axis 180 degrees away from the original defect and created a large arc of rotation with more standing cutaneous deformities. The bilobe design has been modified to rotate around a smaller arc, usually 90 to 100 degrees, thus reducing the amount of dog ear[13] (**Fig. 54.14**).

The disadvantages of bilobe flaps are that they leave circular scars that will not blend easily with existing creases or RSTLs. Moreover, bilobes frequently develop some "pin cushioning" of the skin paddle for several reasons: (1) the flap is typically based on a narrow pedicle and prone to congestion, especially when superiorly based; (2) a wide bed of scar develops beneath the flap and impedes lymphatic drainage; and (3) most importantly, the cutaneous scars are curvilinear: they contract and tend to bunch the flap up as the incision shortens. This pin cushioning typically resolves over the course of a year and is facilitated by steroid injections.

The design for a bilobe flap begins with identifying the area of recruitment and a pivot point. This pivot point is roughly a radius of the defect away from the wound margin. The first lobe of the flap can be the exact size of the primary defect and the second lobe slightly smaller, with a triangular apex to allow primary closure. The axis of the second flap is ~100 degrees from the primary defect, with the plane of elevation for the nose immediately above the

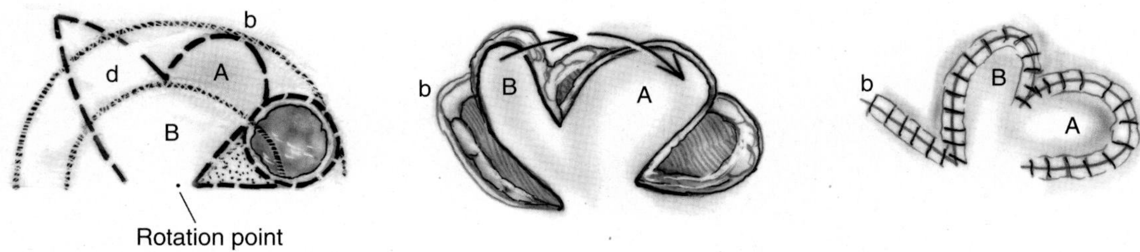

Fig. 54.14 Bilobe closure for nasal tip defect oriented such that the resultant scar from the secondary lobe is along the aesthetic subunit border. The Burrow's triangle off the primary defect is positioned along the supraalar crease. This flap receives its random pattern blood supply off the angular artery.

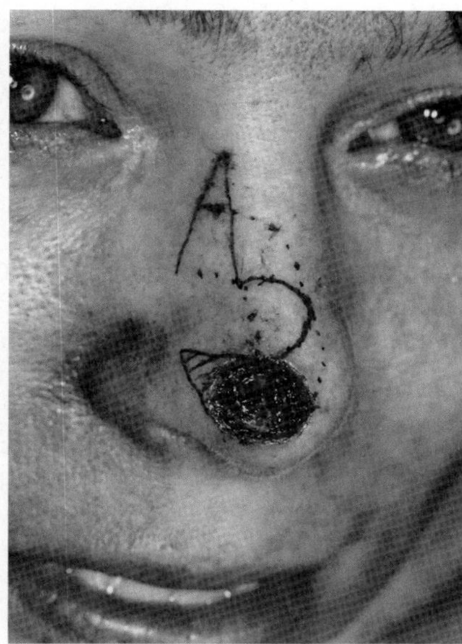

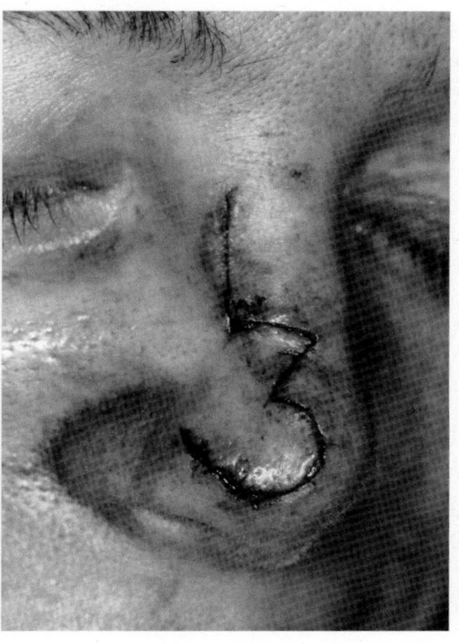

A B

Fig. 54.15 Bilobe flap. The axis of the second flap is roughly 100 degrees from the axis along the primary defect, thus decreasing the arc of rotation and standing cutaneous deformity.

perichondrium/periosteum. Elsewhere, the flap is elevated in the standard subcutaneous layer. Wide undermining best distributes tension. Whereas the primary and secondary defects result in curvilinear scars, the tertiary defect is linear. One can take advantage of this and orient the flap such that this linear scar comes to lie at the border of aesthetic subunits or at least parallel to skin creases (**Fig. 54.15A,B**). This primarily rotational flap tends to exert some tension along the border of the primary defect, and this should be kept in mind for defects along the nasal tip and ala. Paradoxically, the tension to the border of the defect is often in an inferior direction due to the rotation of the flap.

Forehead Flap

The forehead flap is a workhorse flap for large nasal defects and can be traced back to antiquity.[14] Historically, several forehead flaps have been described as being based on a variety of vessels, including the anterior branch of the superficial temporal artery, supraorbital artery, and others on both supratrochlear vessels.[15–17] The contemporary forehead flap is primarily based on a single supratrochlear vessel with a relatively narrow pedicle (1.0 to 1.5 cm) and utilizes a skin paddle from the midforehead area.[18] This flap is transposed as an interpolated flap over the intact glabellar skin and mandates a second-stage procedure for pedicle division.

The forehead flap is the flap of choice for larger cutaneous nasal defects because it is characterized by many of the virtues of a regional cutaneous flap: (1) there is abundant tissue allowing resurfacing of the entire nasal unit with a single flap; (2) it follows the principle of replacing tissue with like tissue in that there is an excellent match of skin color and texture to the native nose; (3) there is acceptable donor sight morbidity; and (4) the flap has proven to be extremely robust and dependable, even in individuals with small-vessel disease. The primary disadvantage is the need for additional stages and the fact that the pedicle is cumbersome and requires continued wound care for a longer postoperative period.

The technique for elevating and transferring a forehead flap has been described.[19,20] A template of the nasal defect is useful for defining the outline of the skin paddle on the forehead. This accounts for the three-dimensional contours of the nose that may be lost if one simply uses a ruler to measure defect dimensions. Forehead flaps can be designed as either a paramedian or a midline flap. The distinction between these flaps refers to the precise location of the skin paddle, not the pedicle base. The paramedian is centered on the supratrochlear artery, whereas the midline is located in the precise anatomical center of the forehead. However, both flaps utilize a narrow pedicle (61.5 cm) centered on a unilateral supratrochlear artery and can easily extend below the level of the brows. There is a rich anastomosis in this region between the supratrochlear and angular arteries, allowing for a robust perfusion pressure at the base of the pedicle.[21] The advantage of the paramedian flap is that it is centered on the supratrochlear artery, incorporating more of the main trunk and its dermal branches within the pedicle and skin paddle. Improved clinical viability with this design has not been shown over the midline flap. The advantage of a *midline* flap is that the resultant scar is located in the exact center of the forehead and tends to be less conspicuous than a paramedian one. In spite of the fact that both flaps leave a vertical forehead scar running perpendicular to RSTLs, they tend to heal quite well. However, the midline scar is consistent with aesthetic units in that the casual observer tends to see the face as two halves. The midline design also gives greater length to the flap than the paramedian one, an important consideration in individuals with a low anterior hairline.

The skin paddle is elevated in either the subgaleal or the subcuticular plane, but in either case, additional debulking in selective areas is needed prior to inset. It is imperative to maintain crisp corners at the edge of the flap to inset precisely with the borders of the aesthetic subunits of the nose. The pedicle portion of the flap is always elevated in the subgaleal plane, incorporating the frontalis muscle with the pedicle. On occasion, one can elevate subperiosteally around the base of the pedicle to achieve greater length and rigidity around the supratrochlear vessel. The width of the pedicle need not be greater than 1.5 cm and is more often closer to 1.0 cm, allowing for easier rotation and less kinking of the pedicle. During dissection at the base of the pedicle, the corrugator muscle must be divided; this is done carefully under direct vision to preserve all major feeding vessels. The pedicle can easily extend beneath the level of the eyebrow, providing additional length as needed. Immediately prior to flap inset the skin paddle can be selectively thinned again to match the native skin thickness that is variable for different areas of the nose. The pedicle is typically divided 3 weeks later and aggressively thinned in a cephalad to caudad direction, particularly because the native skin in that area is thin. The base of the pedicle is usually amputated with a small inset into the glabellar area to reestablish brow symmetry.

Case 6 (Fig. 54.16A,B)

A 73-year-old man presents with a cutaneous nasal defect following Mohs excision of a recurrent basal cell carcinoma. **(C)** The aesthetic units of the nose are defined and modified slightly. **(D)** A template is formed of the modified nasal defect. **(E)** The template is transferred to the midline forehead. **(F)** The midline forehead flap is elevated, based on the unilateral supratrochlear area. The pedicle is no wider than 1.5 cm to facilitate rotation. The arterial supply in this area is through rich collaterals between the supratrochlear and angular arteries. **(G)** The skin paddle of the forehead flap is aggressively thinned to resemble the native nasal skin. A characteristic cobblestone appearance is seen on the undersurface of the flap. The frontalis muscle and galea are not included in the skin paddle. **(H)** The periosteum at the base of the pedicle can be included to further facilitate the rotation and pedicle stability. **(I)** The forehead flap is transferred and a small bolster suture is left in the left supraalar crease to accentuate that area. **(J)** Three weeks postoperatively, the patient is ready for pedicle division. **(K, L)** Twelve-month postoperative view demonstrating acceptable donor site scar and full viability of all corners of the midline forehead flap.

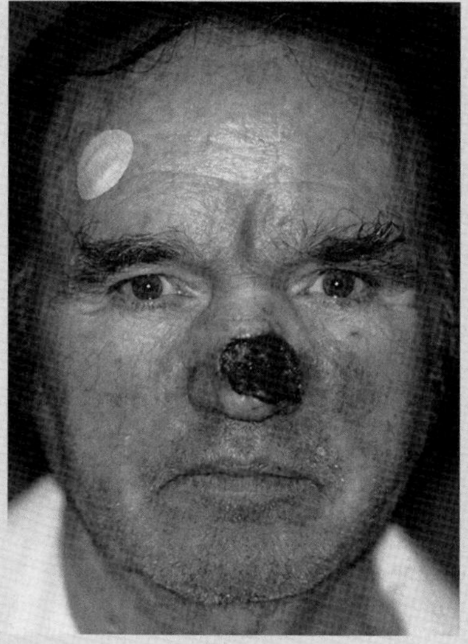
A

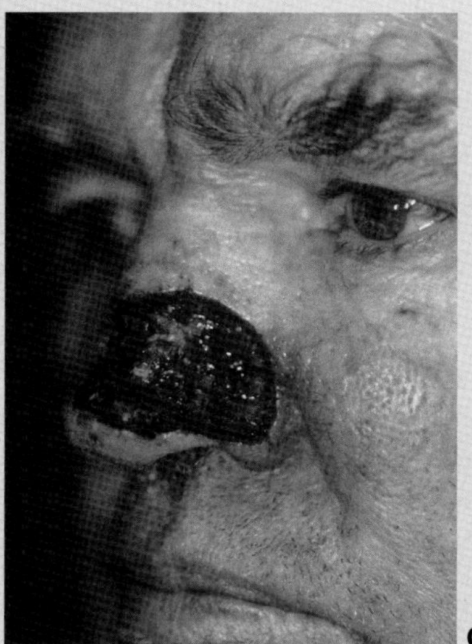
B

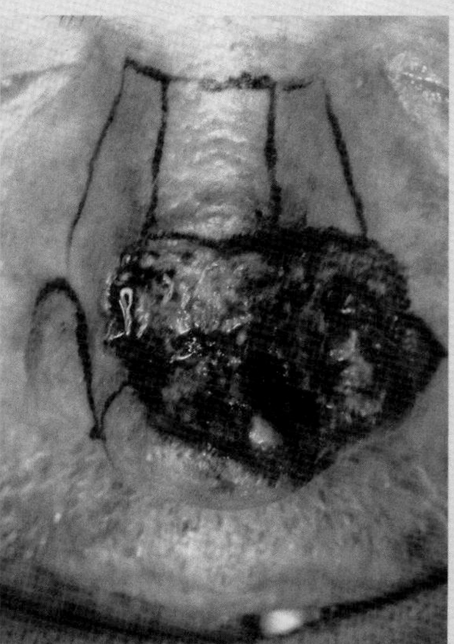
C

Fig. 54.16 **(A–L)** Case 6. Midline forehead flap for a nasal defect.

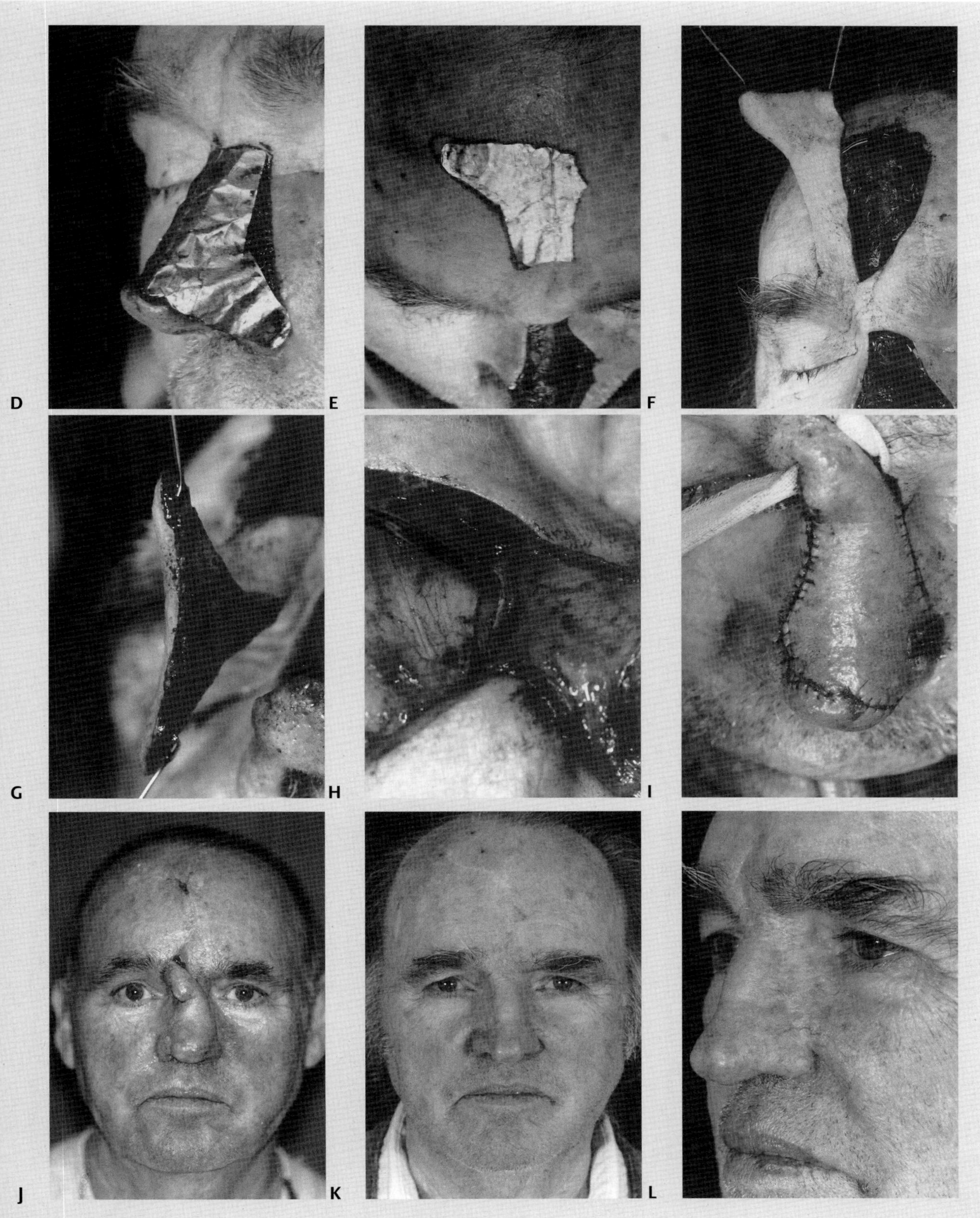

Fig. 54.16 (*Continued*)

High-risk individuals, such as those with known small-vessel disease, can have the entire flap elevated and transferred in the subgaleal plane. This requires an intermediate stage at 3 weeks at which the flap is elevated and debulked from the lateral aspect while remaining perfused in a bipedicle fashion through the pedicle and columella.[20] Three weeks following this intermediate stage, the pedicle is divided in the standard fashion. The advantage of this method is that it further ensures flap viability while neovascularization occurs. This comes at the expense of an additional stage and requires the patient to endure the pedicle for 6 weeks rather than 3.

The other extreme allows a forehead flap to be transferred as a single-stage flap and is reserved for those individuals free of small-vessel disease. The pedicle of the flap is deepithelialized and transferred under intact glabellar skin, thus converting the interpolated forehead flap to an island flap and obviating the need for a second-stage pedicle division. The procerus muscle is usually resected to minimize bulk in that region. For elderly individuals with any systemic vascular disease and for smokers, the procedure is contraindicated. The advantage of this "single-stage forehead flap" is that it completes the reconstruction in one operation, although it does leave some fullness to the glabellar area that tends to recede with time. On occasion, patients will desire a debulking procedure for that region, which can be done at any time.

Case 7 (Fig. 54.17A)

A 52-year-old woman presents with a nasal and cheek defect following Mohs surgery. (**B**) The cheek portion is repaired with a cheek advancement/rotation flap, up to the nasal facial groove. The nasal aesthetic units are outlined. (**C**) The defect is modified to resemble the borders of the nasal aesthetic subunits. (**D**) A template of the modified nasal defect is transferred to the precise midline. (**E**) The forehead flap is based on a subcutaneous pedicle. (**F**) The forehead flap is transferred under the intact glabellar skin as a single-stage procedure. The procerus muscle has been resected to better accommodate the subcutaneous pedicle. (**G**) The forehead flap is approximated to the local cheek flap. (**H**) Twelve months postoperatively, the forehead flap is viable but some discoloration is evident, reflective of the patient's forehead skin.

A
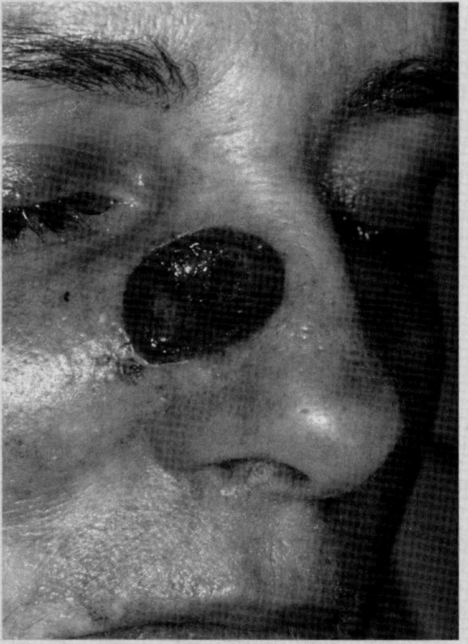

B
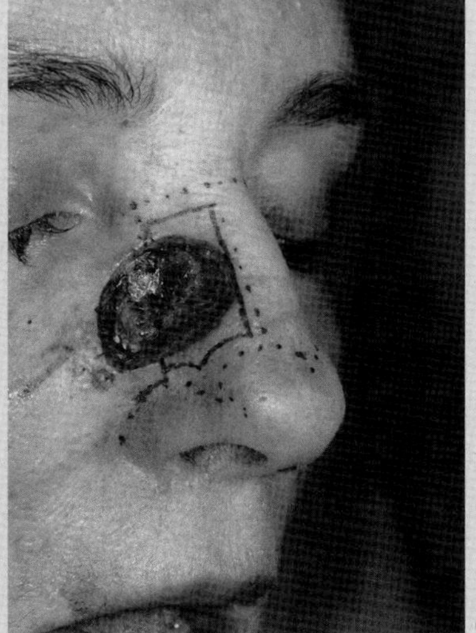

C
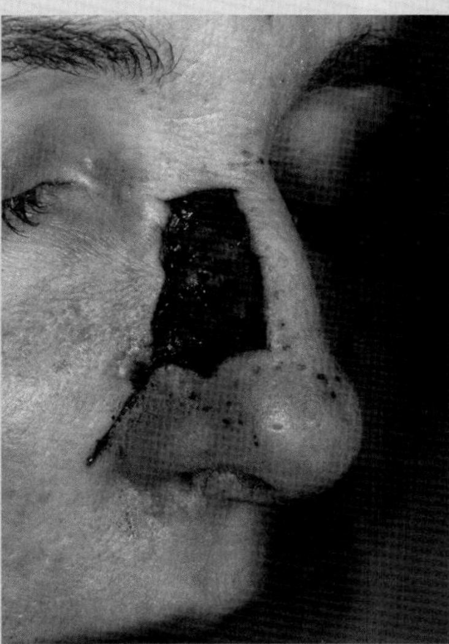

Fig. 54.17 (A–H) Case 7. Single-stage forehead flap.

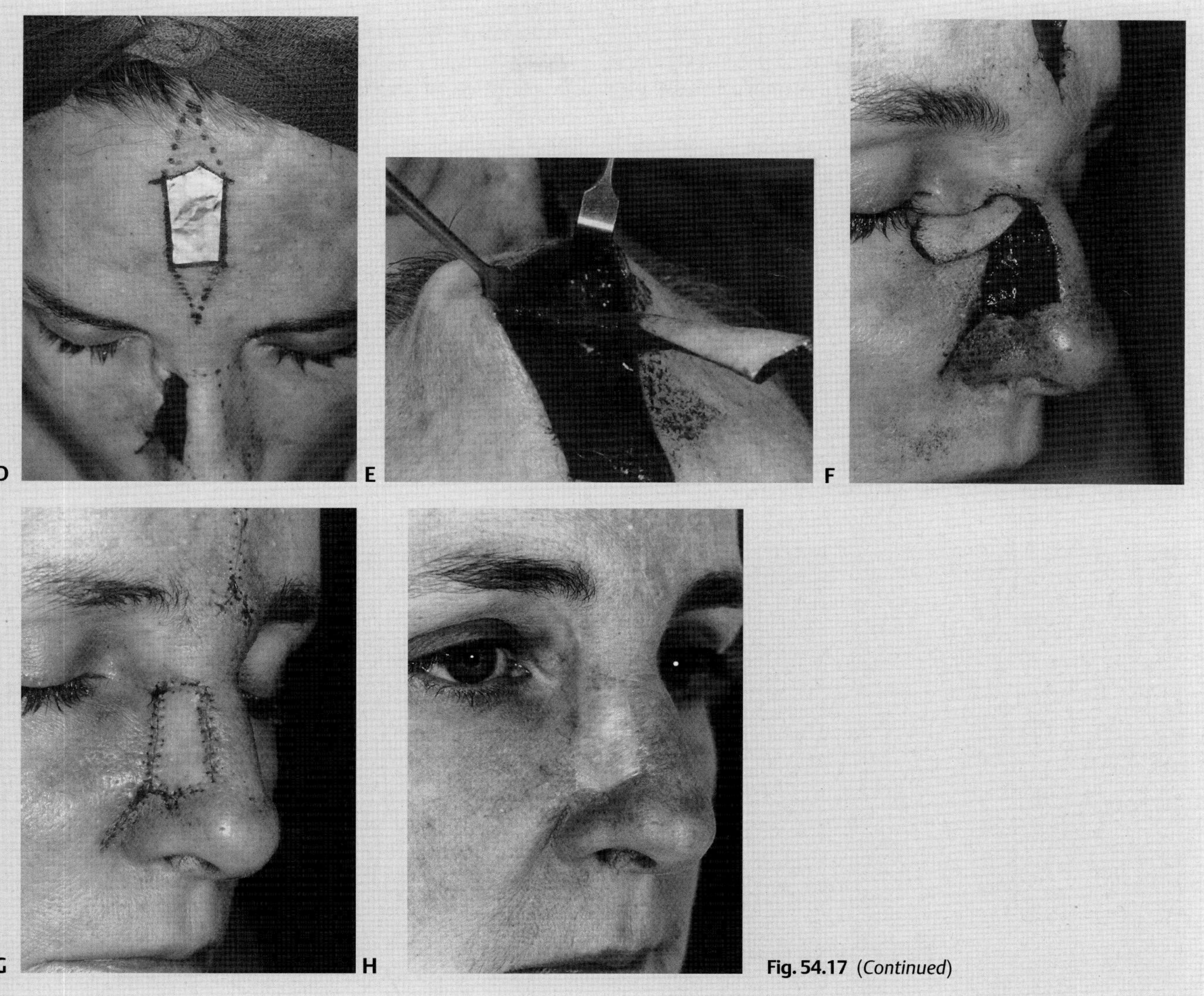

Fig. 54.17 *(Continued)*

Melolabial Flap

The melolabial flap is a useful flap for reconstructing defects of the lower third of the nose, especially the alar lobule or columella.[22] It can be transposed as either an interpolated flap requiring subsequent pedicle division or a single-stage transposition flap. The flap is primarily based on the angular artery off the facial artery. When based inferiorly, the pedicle may capture the artery itself, but when based superiorly, as is more frequently done, the pedicle contains only perforators from this main artery and is converted to an axial pattern arterial flap. The skin paddle is thinned aggressively to minimize bulk to the nose.

For nasal reconstruction, a melolabial flap has the advantage over a forehead flap that the area of recruitment is in closer proximity to the primary defect. This results in less translocation of tissue and a shorter pedicle that does not traverse between the eyes, which is often a significant complaint. The disadvantage of the melolabial flap is limited donor tissue availability for resurfacing. In addition, there may be more problems with the donor site than the forehead flap; noticeable facial asymmetry can occur along the melolabial folds.

When designing the melolabial flap, it is useful to use a precise template of the primary defect to ensure sufficient width of the flap. A "pivot point" is identified to ensure sufficient length to the flap; often the skin paddle is harvested more inferiorly than first impression. The pedicle base can be designed with a wide skin paddle to capture subdermal vascularity, but this not only creates problems with the donor site scar but also impedes mobilization of the flap. The melolabial flap is better designed with a wide subcutaneous pedicle centered on the angular artery and an elliptical, shallow skin incision. This serves to improve the rotational movement of the flap and extends its reach. Furthermore, it lends itself to primary closure of the secondary donor site during pedicle division.

During pedicle division, the defect can be closed primarily with a resultant scar situated along the nasal facial junction and melolabial fold. This requires undermining and advancement of the cheek, which may lead to some facial asymmetry. Alternatively, the entire skin pedicle can be returned to the cheek. The latter method will maintain symmetry to the melolabial folds but will result in two vertical scars, the lateral one being located within the cheek aesthetic unit and running obliquely across natural RSTLs.

Case 8 (Fig. 54.18A)

A 68-year-old man presents with a left nasal defect that includes small portions of left lower lateral cartilage but has not violated the intranasal mucosa. **(B)** The defect's shape is modified to mimic the natural aesthetic alar unit. Although it is superior to the contralateral supraalar crease, this modification tends to be more accepting to the casual observer. Conchal cartilage is placed as a batten graft along the caudal border of the left ala. Note the nonanatomical position of this support graft, which reinforces the lobule and prevents collapse. **(C)** A left melolabial flap is designed, based on perforators from the angular artery. The skin portion of the pedicle tapers to a point to allow easy rotation and inset. The subcutaneous pedicle, however, remains at least 1.5 cm wide. **(D)** After 3 weeks, the pedicle is ready for division and closure. **(E, F)** A 6-month postoperative view demonstrating the reconstructed alar lobule and the donor site scar within the melolabial fold.

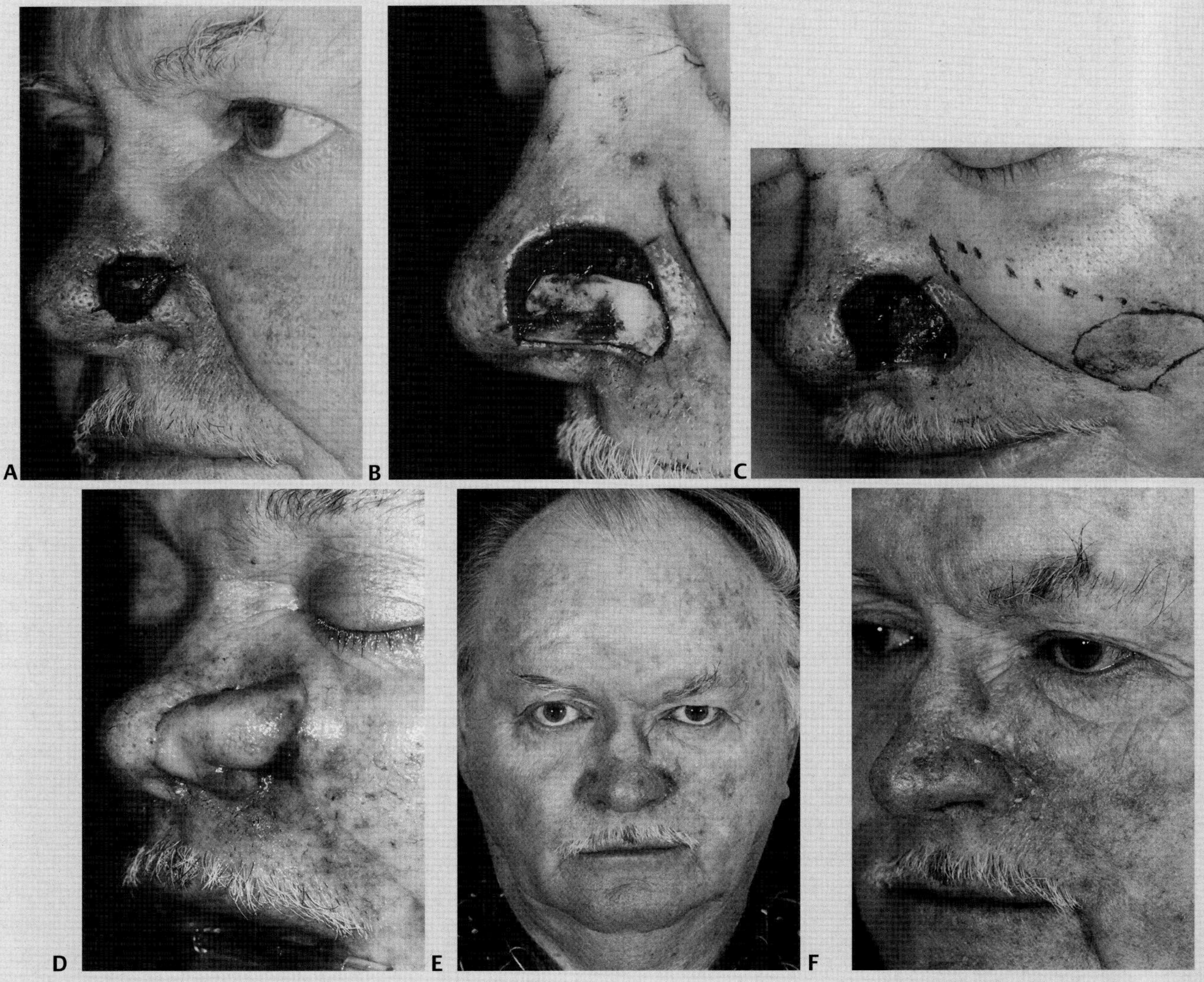

Fig. 54.18 **(A–F)** Case 8. Melolabial flap for alar reconstruction.

Single-stage melolabial flaps are transposition flaps with primary closure of the donor sight. These flaps are useful for small, lateral nasal defects but have the disadvantage of creating nasal asymmetry. When mobilizing cheek skin across the aesthetic border onto the nose, the nasal facial junction is often blunted and leaves fullness to the side of the nose.

Complications

A detailed history can identify those individuals with various risk factors involving small vessels. They include any systemic collagen vascular disorder, hypertension, diabetes, previous irradiation, preexisting scars, and tobacco use. It is important to keep in mind that replacement of smoking with nicotine patches is not a beneficial alternative. It is possible to minimize postoperative complications through early recognition, careful flap design, and enhancement of soft tissue viability.

Flap Delay

Flap delay has been consistently shown to enhance flap length and viability by as much as 100%.[23] The method of delaying the flap involves incising the borders of the flap with or without partial subcutaneous elevation but leaving it in situ for 2 weeks. Following this, the flap is fully elevated and transposed. The mechanism of action for this process remains unclear but several hypotheses exist:

1. *Metabolic adaption*. One of the early assumptions was that a biochemical adaptation occurring at the cellular level allows this tissue to better tolerate relative ischemia.[24] This has been disproved because it is now known that delaying the base of the flap or pedicle is more important than delaying the tip or skin paddle itself. In fact, delayed tissue appears to tolerate degrees of ischemia more poorly than nondelayed tissue.[25]
2. *Adrenergic spasm*. On cutting nerve endings, there is a sudden release of norepinephrine and subsequent vasoconstriction, thus exacerbating flap ischemia and diminishing flap viability. The delayed procedure could sympathectomize the flap by depleting the surrounding nerve endings of norepinephrine and preventing the adrenergic spasm to occur during definitive flap elevation and transposition.[26] If this were the only mechanism of action, however, only a single day of delay would be necessary because norepinephrine is rapidly depleted from neural endings following transection and is cleared from local tissues. A 1-day delay has been shown to be ineffective for flap enhancement.[27]
3. *Arteriovenus shunt*. The neural sympathectomy should close arteriovenous (AV) shunts along the flap borders and increase perfusion pressure and nutrient supply via capillary levels. However, tests with radiolabeled microspheres have shown that AV shunts are not closed during the delayed process.[28]
4. *Vascular collateral*. The density of capillary flow within the flap appears enhanced during the delayed period, and the border of capillary perfusion is similarly extended.[29] Some angiographic studies, however, do not support this concept, although the sensitivity of these tests may not be sufficient.[30] Although animal studies have reproduced the beneficial effects of a delayed process, its mechanism is probably multifactorial and its understanding limited by biotechnical studies available today.

Hyperbaric Oxygen

Hyperbaric oxygen has a proven beneficial effect on the vascularity of marginal tissues.[31] Whereas normal tissues are not significantly affected, relatively ischemic tissues have a greatly amplified ischemic gradient, which serves as an angiogenic stimulus for new-vessel ingrowth. This occurs in all areas where marginal oxygenation exists, such as diabetic foot wounds, irradiated mandibles prior to dental extraction, and cutaneous flap enhancement. The primary role for prophylactic hyperbaric oxygen therapy in cutaneous flap surgery is with the irradiated tissue bed, characterized by vascular sclerosis, hypoxia, and hypocellularity. A course of hyperbaric oxygen treatments pre- and postoperatively can enhance flap dependability. This involves a significant patient commitment and should be used only selectively on individuals with known preexisting hypoxic tissues (e.g., prior irradiation to the head and neck).

Congestion

Early recognition of the compromised flap is essential to maximize salvage. Most vascular problems with facial flaps involve congestion and, less frequently, arterial ischemia. It is possible for different areas of a single flap to be suffering from both venous congestion and arterial ischemia. Typical signs of a congested flap are warmth, edema, and a purplish blue color that blanches with pressure but promptly refills (**Fig. 54.19**). A pinprick demonstrates dark venous blood. Arterial ischemia, on the other hand, is characterized by a cool, pale, and flat skin paddle and does not blanch with gentle pressure. A pinprick will often not bleed.

When venous congestion is significant, it can lead to arterial compromise and flap necrosis. This can be managed

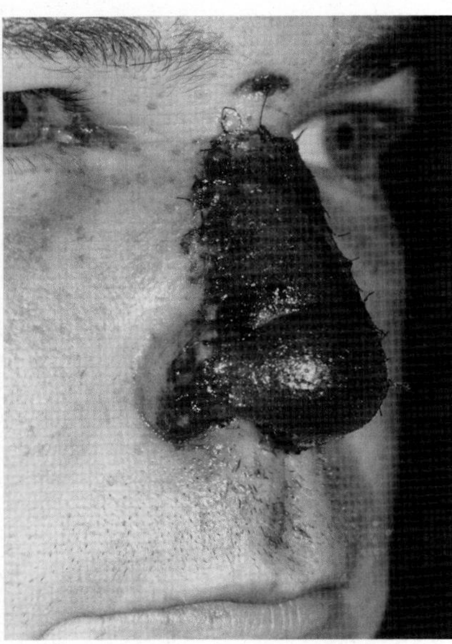

Fig. 54.19 Congested flap. A reimplantation of an amputated nose demonstrating signs of congestion. This flap did not survive and required a midline forehead flap for definitive repair.

in several ways. Sutures can be temporarily released to allow the flap edges to decompress. Tight bandages or closure around the flap pedicle may also be released. Medicinal leeches (*Hirudo medicinalis*) are effective in decompressing venous blood in a congested flap through a transcutaneous route. Leeches should only be used in flaps that are congested with venous blood and are not beneficial when arterial ischemia exists. Fortunately, they generally do not adhere to flaps that are not already engorged. Saliva from a leech contains an anticoagulant and a vasodilator that facilitate continued oozing from the bite site for 6 hours after they detach, decompressing the flap of roughly 50 mL of blood. Usually, several leeches are utilized simultaneously and therapy continues for several days until revascularization is under way. Most medical centers maintain an inventory of leeches, but they may also be purchased from private companies and delivered via overnight service.

Hyperbaric oxygen is beneficial to congested flaps by creating a local arterial vasoconstriction through the dramatic rise in tissue oxygen content, thus reducing the volume of inflow. In spite of this vasoconstriction and reduction in vascular perfusion, tissue oxygen levels in the flap continue to rise due to improved diffusion and net oxygen delivery.

Ischemia

Arterial ischemia to a cutaneous flap is less common than congestion and more challenging to rectify. The most significant and direct means of enhancing viability is through administration of hyperbaric oxygen. This ca maintain flap viability while continued neovasculariza tion occurs and a more definitive arterial supply is estab lished. Heparin and dipyridamole have been shown t increase the survival of an ischemic flap, presumably b preventing clot formation in small vessels that wer injured during ischemia.[32,33] After tissue necrosis ha been established, it is better to debride the dry eschar an maintain a clean, moist wound bed, which will allow fo more rapid healing and epithelialization.

Summary

Local and regional cutaneous flaps continue to be a important tool for the facial plastic surgeon. Despite th many years that such techniques have been employed the art and science of local flaps continue to evolve an improve. Our understanding of wound healing, loca tension vectors, aesthetic units, and flap enhancemen techniques has allowed us to repair most cutaneous facia defects with a dependable, acceptable, and functiona outcome.

References

1. Mohs FE. Chemosurgery, a microscopically controlled method of cance excision. Arch Surg 1941;42:279
2. Cutting CA. Critical closing and perfusion pressure in flap surviva Ann Plast Surg 1982;9:524
3. Milton S. Fallacy of the length–width ratio. Br J Plast Surg 197 57:502
4. Borges AF. Relaxed skin tension lines (RSTL) versus other skin line Plast Reconstr Surg 1984;73:144–149
5. Burget GC, Menick FJ. The subunit principle in nasal reconstructio Plast Reconstr Surg 1985;76:239–247
6. Orticochea M. Four flap–scalp reconstruction technique. Br J Plast Su 1967;20(2):159–171
7. Wang TD, Park SS. Tissue expansion in head and neck reconstructio In: Reonigk RK, Reonigk HH, eds. Cosmetic Dermatologic Surger 2nd ed. London: Martin Dunitz 1996:897–909
8. Walike JW, Larrabee WF. The note flap. Arch Otolaryngol 198 111:430
9. Limberg AA. The Planning of Local Plastic Operations on the Bod Surface: Theory and Practice. Toronto: Cullamore Press; 1984
10. Larrabee WF Jr, Trachy R, Sutton D. Rhomboid flap dynamics. Arc Otolaryngol 1981;107:755–757
11. Lister GD, Gibson T. Closure of the rhomboid skin defects: the flaps c Limberg and Dufourmentel. Br J Plast Surg 1972;25:300
12. Webster RF, Davidson TM, Smith RC. The 30-degree transposition fla Laryngoscope 1978;88:85
13. Zitelli JA. The bilobed flap for nasal reconstruction. Arch Dermat 1989;145:957
14. "BL," Letter to the Editor. Gentleman's Magazine, London, October 179 p. 891; reprinted in Plast Reconstr Surg 1969;44:67–69
15. New GB. Sickle flaps for nasal reconstruction. Surg Gynecol Obst 1945;80:497
16. Kazanjian VH. The repair of nasal defects with the median forehea flap: primary closure of the forehead wound. Surg Gynecol Obst 1946;37:83–87
17. Converse JM. New forehead flap for nasal reconstruction. Proc R So Med 1942;35:811

8. Shumrick KA, Smith TL. The anatomic basis for the design of forehead flaps in nasal reconstruction. Arch Otolaryngol Head Neck Surg 1992;118:373–379
9. Quatela VC, Sherris DA, Rounds MF. Esthetic refinements in forehead flap nasal reconstruction. Arch Otolaryngol Head Neck Surg 1995;121(10):1106–1113
0. Burget GC, Menick FJ. The paramedian forehead flap. In: Aesthetic Reconstruction of the Nose. St. Louis: Mosby; 1994:57–92
1. McCarthy JG, Lorenc ZP, Cutting C, Rachesky M. The median forehead flap revisited: the blood supply. Plast Reconstr Surg 1985;76: 866–869
2. Younger RA. The versatile melolabial flap. Otolaryngol Head Neck Surg 1992;107:721–726
3. Myers M, Cherry G. Differences in the delay phenomenon in the rabbit, rat, and pig. Plast Reconstr Surg 1971;47:73
4. McFarlane R, Heagy FC, Radin S, Aust JC, Wermuth RE. et al. A study of the delay phenomenon in experimental pedicle flaps. Plast Reconstr Surg 1965;35:245
5. Cutting C, Bardach J, Rosewall D. Skin–flap delay procedures: proximal delay versus distal delay. Ann Plast Surg 1980;14:293
26. Norberg K, Palmer B. Improvement of blood circulation in experimental skin flaps by phentolamine. Eur J Pharmacol 1969;8:36
27. Cutting C, Robson M, Koss N. Denervation supersensitivity and the delay phenomenon. Plast Reconstr Surg 1978;61:881
28. Guba A. Arteriovenous shunting in the pig. Plast Reconstr Surg 1980;65:323
29. Cutting C, Bardach J, Tinseth F. Hemodynamics of the delayed skin flap: a total blood flow study. Br J Plast Surg 1981;34:133
30. Myers M. Attempts to augment survival in skin flaps: mechanism of the delay phenomenon. In: Graff W, Myers MB, eds. Skin Flaps. Boston: Little, Brown and Company; 1975
31. Zamboni WA, Roth AC, Russell RC, Smoot EC. The effect of hyperbaric oxygen on reperfusion of ischemic axial skin flaps: a laser Doppler analysis. Ann Plast Surg 1992;28:339–341
32. Myers M, Cherry G. Enhancement of survival in devascularized pedicles by the use of phenoxybenasmine. Plast Reconstr Surg 1968; 42:254
33. Kinkead L, Zook E, Card E. Vasoactive drugs and skin flap survival in the pig. In: Abstracts of Plastic Surgery Research Council meeting, Springfield, IL, May 22, 1981.

55 Tissue Expansion in Reconstruction of the Head and Neck

John F. Hoffmann

Large and complex defects of the head and neck pose difficult challenges for the reconstructive surgeon. Whenever feasible, traditional local and regional skin flaps should always be the first choice as they offer optimal aesthetic results. In selected circumstances, skin grafts may be employed but routinely offer distinctly inferior cosmetic results and have unique problems. Microvascular free tissue transfer, which can transfer large volumes of tissue reliably, has become the standard for extensive and complex defects of the head and neck. However, as free flaps come from distant areas in the body, the tissue match and ultimate aesthetic result is often poor. In addition, it may be difficult to provide sensate or functional tissues in a free flap. When adequate local or regional tissue is not available, and if microvascular transfer is a less optimal option, then adjunctive techniques such as tissue expansion may be necessary or beneficial. Tissue expansion may allow a surgeon to develop large local flaps, which have optimal tissue characteristics. Tissue expansion may also enhance regional or microvascular flaps prior to transfer. The decision to employ tissue expansion should be made carefully as complications from this technique are not unusual and the patient will need to endure certain hardships during the tissue expansion process. This chapter will summarize the physiology, surgical techniques, applications, and complications of tissue expansion in the realm of reconstructive surgery of the head and neck.

History

Surgical tissue expansion is simply an application of a natural physiological process. The classic example of tissue expansion in nature is pregnancy where the uterus and abdominal tissues undergo dramatic and gradual expansion. Many cultures have employed forms of tissue expansion for decoration, enhancement, and occasionally mutilation of facial and body structures such as the ear lobes and nostrils. During the 1970s extensive experimental and clinical experience with tissue expansion was reported. Neumann[1] reported the first use of tissue expansion with a subcutaneous balloon in 1957, but it was not until the works of Austed[2] and Radovan[3] were published separately in the 1970s and '80s that tissue expansion became a widely accepted technique. These authors' works established the foundation for the basic understanding of the physiology of tissue expansion as well as the clinical applications of the techniques. In the following decades, numerous reports of clinical[4–12] and experimental[13–18] experience with tissue expansion have demonstrated the safety and efficacy of the techniques.

Tissue Responses to Expansion

Human tissues exhibit dynamic effects when exposed to sustained pressure and expansion. The histological and biochemical changes that occur during tissue expansion have been studied extensively in both animal models and in humans. Different tissues respond variably to the forces of expansion, and the rate and duration of expansion have a significant impact on the tissue response. Not surprisingly, many tissues do not tolerate rapid or extreme expansion as well as controlled, gradual expansion.

A distinction must be made between the similarly named but physiologically distinct techniques of conventional, long-term tissue expansion and rapid intraoperative expansion (ITE). Sustained and progressive tissue expansion results in significant physiological and histological changes in the skin and subcutaneous tissues. In contrast, ITE most likely induces principally mechanical changes within the skin or it may represent an enhanced undermining and recruitment of surrounding tissues.[19–21] The differences between these techniques will be discussed further in this chapter.

Long-Term Tissue Expansion

Extensive biological and morphological changes occur in tissues that are subjected to prolonged and progressive tissue expansion. Even though the surface area of the expanded skin is ever increasing during expansion, the overlying epidermis does not thin and has even been found to slightly thicken.[13,14,22] Studies have shown that the mitotic activity of the expanded skin is increased,[23] and this enhanced mitotic rate helps to maintain and enhance the epidermal height while the normal stratified epithelial appearance is preserved. These changes within the epidermis appear to be temporary and the microscopic appearance of the skin returns to normal within a year or two after the conclusion of the expansion. Clinically, the most common noticeable skin changes are increased dryness, erythema, and occasionally hyperpigmentation.

The dermis, meanwhile, does not respond as favorably to chronic expansion. Typically the dermis thins dramatically (30 to 50%), particularly when expansion is accelerated.[14,24] Increased metabolic activity has been observed in many of the cell populations that reside within the dermis. Fibroblast activity is increased and collagen synthesis is enhanced while the physical arrangement of the collagen fibers is altered and elastic fibers become fragmented. Increased pigmentation may occur during expansion resulting from temporarily enhanced melanin production. Hair follicles become less dense due to the increased surface area of the epidermis as the actual number of hair follicles remains the same. The thickness of the basal layer has been seen to increase and additional myofibroblasts are found within the expanded tissues. The enhanced myofibroblast population is largely responsible for the contracture that may occur in expanded flaps after removal of the tissue expander. The histological changes seen within the dermis and associated appendages account for the clinical characteristics of stiffness, striae, erythroderma, alopecia, and diminished sensation commonly seen in expanded tissues.[25]

The expansion process also affects the associated structures located within the subcutaneous tissues. Adipose tissue is very intolerant of expansion and thins dramatically losing up to 50% of its initial thickness. The fat cells become flattened, lose their fat content, and may be replaced with fibrous tissue. However, some of this adipose loss may be regained following expansion. Vascular changes during expansion are quite dramatic as chronic tissue expansion is a strong stimulus for vascular proliferation.[26] This enhanced vascularity is one of the benefits of expansion as the enhanced blood supply of the tissue allows for the elevation of the vigorous, extensive local flaps, which are more resistant to infection.[27] This can be particularly helpful in instances where the vascularity of the tissue is already compromised. During expansion there is a proliferation of capillaries and, ultimately, the venules and arterials, and lengthening of vascular structures occurs.[28] Clinical experience has shown that expanded flaps do have an enhanced survival rate similar to delayed flaps.[29] A dense fibrous capsule forms around the expander balloon, which contains not only high concentrations of fibroblasts but is also highly vascular (**Fig. 55.1**). The capsule is lined with macrophages surrounded by fibroblasts that are actively producing collagen. The capsule may contribute some to the enhanced vascularity of expanded flaps, but it also contributes to the contracture and shrinkage of the flap after the expander has been removed and the flap inset. This subsequent contracture may cause the flap to become thickened and aesthetically undesirable for certain reconstructions that require thin and pliable flaps as in the case of forehead flaps for nasal reconstruction[30] (**Fig. 55.2**). If needed, this capsule may be excised cautiously, and in most instances this will not significantly compromise the vascularity of the flap.[31]

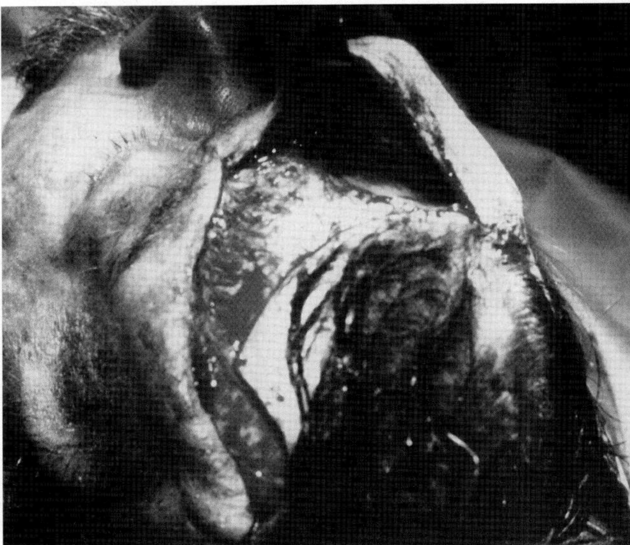

Fig. 55.1 Flaps raised after long-term expansion of the forehead. Note thickness of the flaps and the capsule on their undersurface.

Muscular tissue does not tolerate expansion nearly as well as vascular tissue. Muscle thinning, necrosis

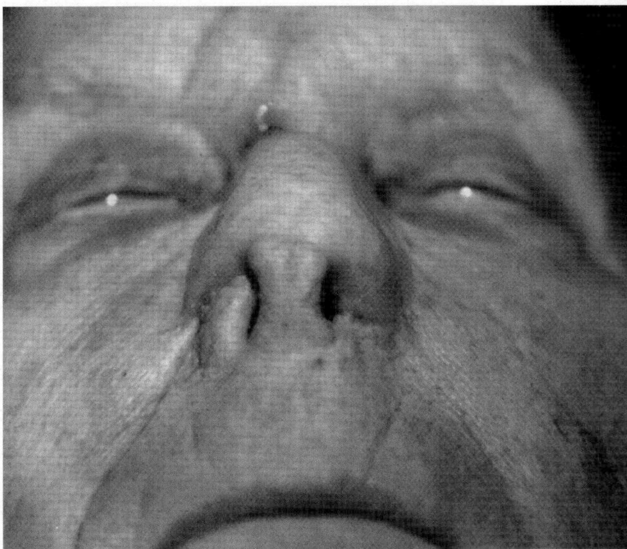

Fig. 55.2 Thickened and contracted paramedian forehead flap that was expanded prior to elevation and transfer to the nose. Excision of the capsule may have avoided this.

atrophy and clinical weakness have all been observed.[32] n the head and neck, this would be most concerning if it were to affect the frontalis or muscles of facial expression. Neural tissue is rather tolerant of expansion and gradual lengthening of nerves can be accomplished without necrosis. Experimental studies have hown that peripheral nerves can be lengthened up to 32% with long-term expansion but perhaps with some diminished function.[33] The facial nerve has been studied during rapid expansion by Martini et al,[34] who found the acial nerve of a cat to be significantly lengthened with intraoperative expansion. However, 40% of the expanded nerves failed to regenerate, likely due to mechanical axonal disruption or from compromised vascularity. herefore, it is probably prudent to place expanders n the face and neck superficial to the facial nerve and uperficial musculoaponeurotic system (SMAS) in the heek or platysma in the neck to minimize potential njury to the facial nerve.

Rapid Intraoperative Expansion

Rapid ITE is a technique that has been championed by asaki as an extension of his experiences with conventional, long-term tissue expansion.[35] In essence, TE involves a rapid, cyclical stretching of the skin performed during the same operative session in which ne elevates and mobilizes tissue flaps. Early on, it was ecognized that one could temporarily overinflate a ong-term tissue expander balloon immediately prior o its removal, thereby gaining some apparent additional flap length. This concept was then applied on its wn without any preceding chronic expansion. Sasaki as reported his experience with almost 300 cases in which he felt that an additional 1 to 3 cm of flap length s gained with this technique. The rapid nature of ITE bviously does not allow the physiological or metabolic hanges seen in long-term tissue expansion to occur. ather, the increase in skin flap length is thought to rise principally from mechanical "creep" and maximization of the skin's natural extensibility. Mechanical creep involves the displacement of interstitial luid and ground substance, fragmentation of elastin, ollagen fiber realignment, and adjacent tissue dislacement into the expanded field.[24] Recent studies ave also suggested that ITE may result in the induction f several genes that may be involved in cell growth egulation.[36] Rapid ITE remains a controversial technique and debate has largely centered on whether there re true expansion effects or whether ITE represents rincipally enhanced undermining, tissue recruitment, nd redraping.[19,37–40] Recent reports in the literature, owever, have continued to support ITE as a viable echnique.[36,41,42]

Indications for Tissue Expansion

Tissue expansion is theoretically possible anywhere within the head and neck. Clinical experience, however, has shown that some areas are better suited to expansion because of thick overlying skin and a robust blood supply. Tissue expansion works best in locations where there is a solid bony support under the expander balloon device. For example, the scalp[43,44] and forehead[45] (**Fig. 55.3**) are optimal locations for long-term expansion. Staged repair of extensive scalp defects (**Fig. 55.4**) and hair replacement[46,47] are excellent opportunities to employ tissue expansion. Some surgeons have also advocated tissue expanders in auricular or microtia reconstruction.[48–50] However, as mentioned previously, the potential for contracture of an expanded flap as well as thickening of the tissue from the expander capsule may limit the application of expansion of flaps used for ear and nose reconstruction as at these are instances in which a thin and pliable soft tissue coverage is essential to allow the underlying cartilaginous framework to show through. Expansion may also be used for large defects in the cheek secondary to skin cancer (**Fig. 55.5**) or congenital lesions such as hairy nevi.[51–53] The surgeon should remember however, that the cheek skin may not tolerate expansion well because the skin is relatively thin and there is potential for damage to the facial nerve and musculature. When an expander is employed in the cheek, it may be necessary to inflate the expander with smaller volumes of fluid over an extended period of time to minimize complications. Similarly, tissue expansion in the neck may be limited by the thin skin and underlying neurovascular structures. Tissue expansion may be particularly helpful in previously irradiated areas because of the enhancement of the vascularity, which is provided by the expansion.[54] However, one should be particularly cautious in these patients as their tissues will be more fragile and are potentially more prone to breakdown leading to exposure or extrusion of the expander. Romo and colleagues[55] have described a series of patients in whom a small tissue expander was placed intranasally to provide additional tissue for the successful repair of large septal perforations. Several reports have appeared in the literature describing the application of tissue expansion in regional or distant free flaps prior to their elevation and transfer to head and neck defects.[56–60] Preexpansion of flaps may lessen donor site morbidity as well as provide more tissue for transfer that has an enhanced blood supply. Whenever possible, the reconstructive surgeon should try to anticipate the size of the defect prior to its resection and plan the expansion accordingly. If one is faced with a large defect that will optimally be repaired with an expanded flap, consideration could be given to a temporary coverage with a skin graft while

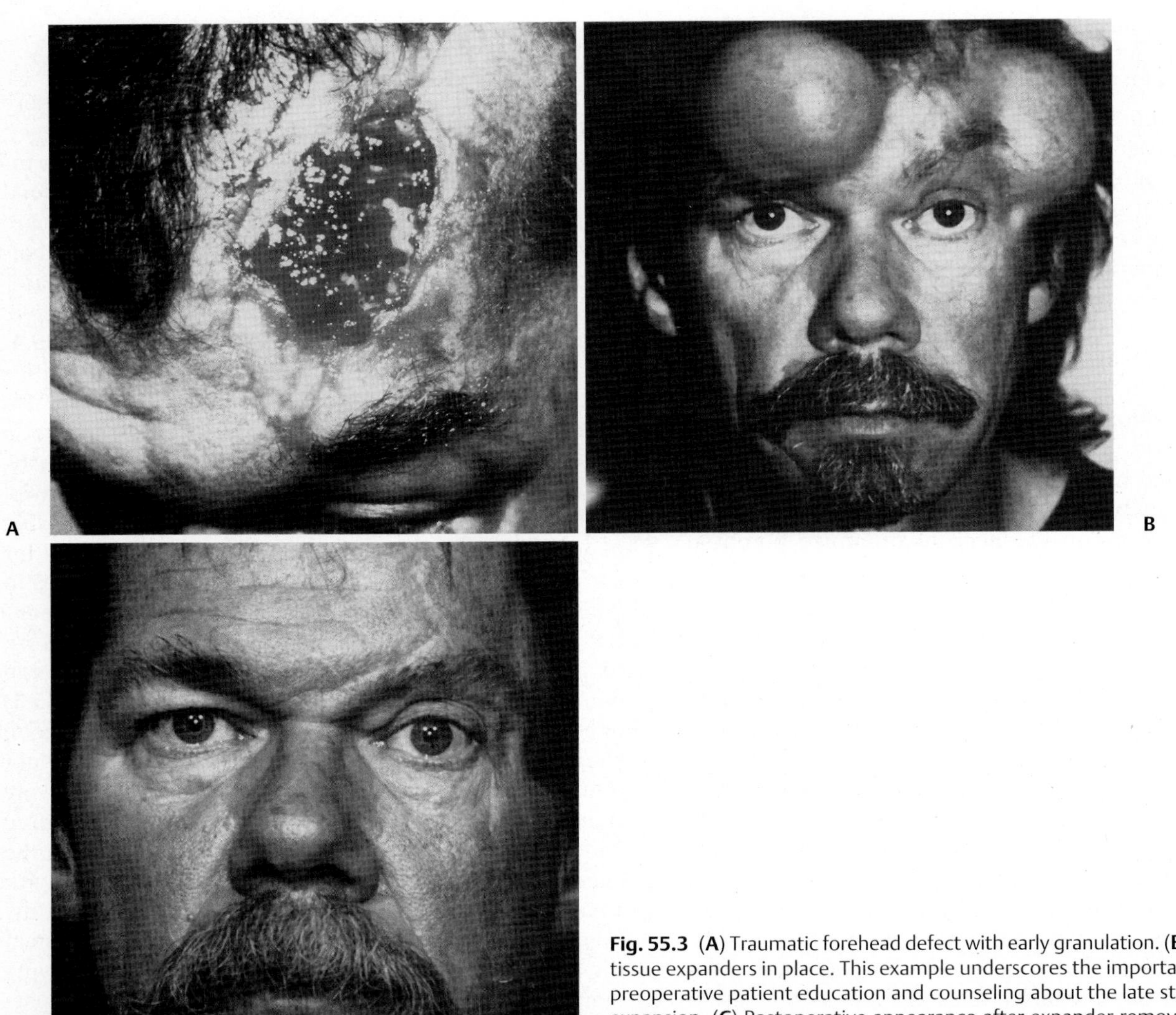

Fig. 55.3 (**A**) Traumatic forehead defect with early granulation. (**B**) Two tissue expanders in place. This example underscores the importance of preoperative patient education and counseling about the late stage of expansion. (**C**) Postoperative appearance after expander removal and repair with two advancement flaps.

the expansion is underway. Once the expansion is completed, the skin graft can be excised and replaced with the expanded flap.

Surgical Technique

Conventional Tissue Expansion

A wide variety of shapes and sizes of tissue expanders are available for clinical use (**Fig. 55.6**). Most often, an expander with a remote injection port is utilized in head and neck reconstruction. The remote port allows the surgeon to place the port away from critical structures and in areas that are less sensitive and painful during the inflation process. In children, it is important to place the injection port in an area that is less sensitive and out of their field of view and therefore less frightening. Common places for placement of the injection port are the poste rior scalp or neck. Templates of the various expanders ar available from the manufacturers, and these can be ver useful in selecting the appropriate size and shape of th expander required (**Fig. 55.7**). Templates are models o the expanders that can be helpful in patient educatio by allowing the patient to visualize the deformity th expander will create when fully inflated. Patient prepara tion and education is essential to help minimize the anxi ety and emotional duress that many patients experienc during the tissue expansion process. Multiple surgerie are required not only to place the expander but also t create the flaps and patients need to visit the surgeon' office numerous times to inflate the expander and t monitor the expansion process. In some instances, it ma be helpful to educate the patient's family to perform th expansion at home, particularly if they live some distanc away. During the final phases of the expansion, patient

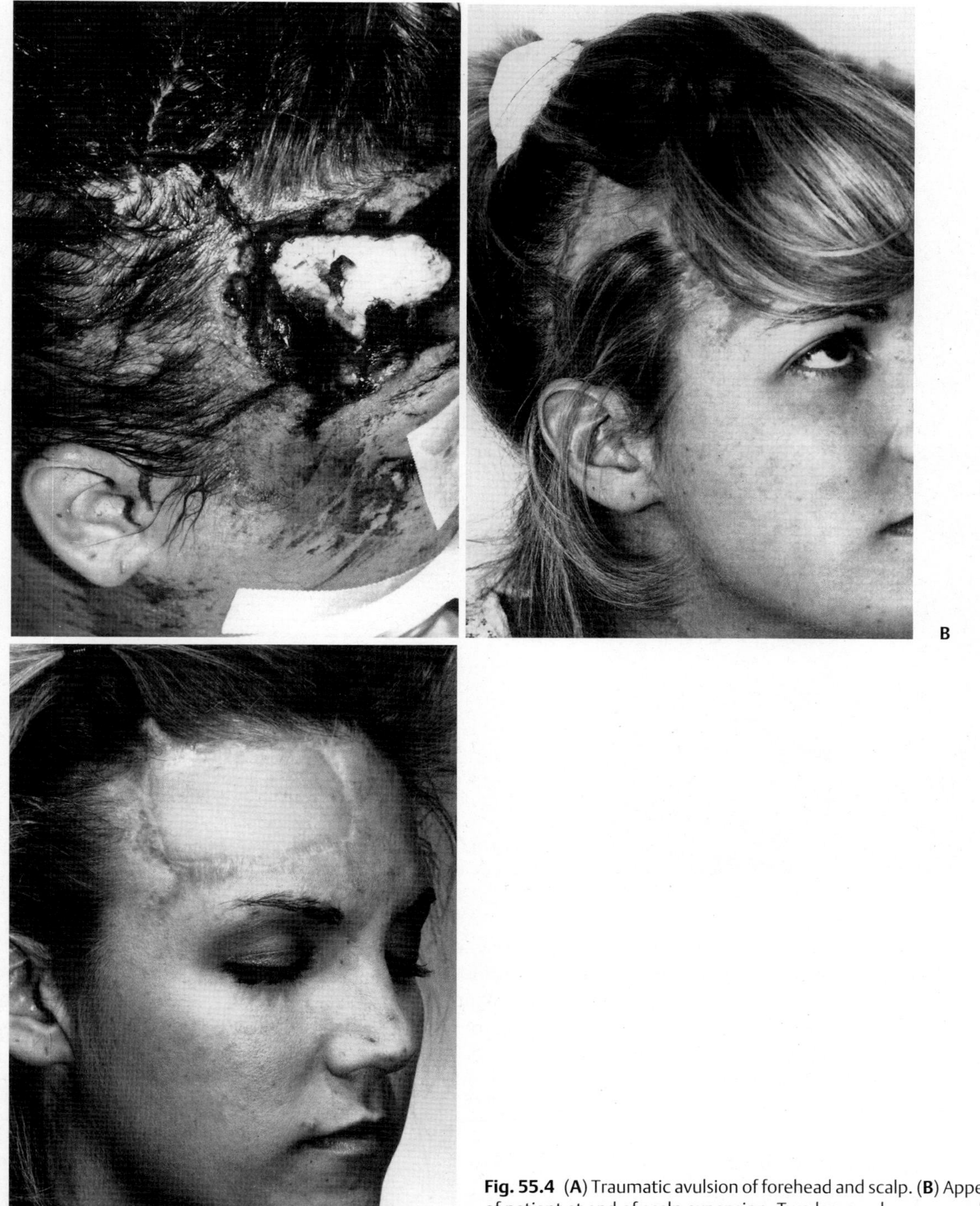

Fig. 55.4 (**A**) Traumatic avulsion of forehead and scalp. (**B**) Appearance of patient at end of scalp expansion. Two large-volume expanders are in place superior and posterior to the scalp scar. The forehead has been repaired with a radial forearm free flap. (**C**) Postoperative appearance after repair with expanded scalp flaps.

will have very conspicuous and embarrassing bulges that can make social interactions difficult (**Fig. 55.3**). The better educated the patients and their families are, the easier it will be for them to accept this. As tissue expansion commonly leads to complications, a thorough discussion of all of these preoperatively is essential.

Selection of the proper size and shape of the expander remains somewhat of an art that is guided by experience;

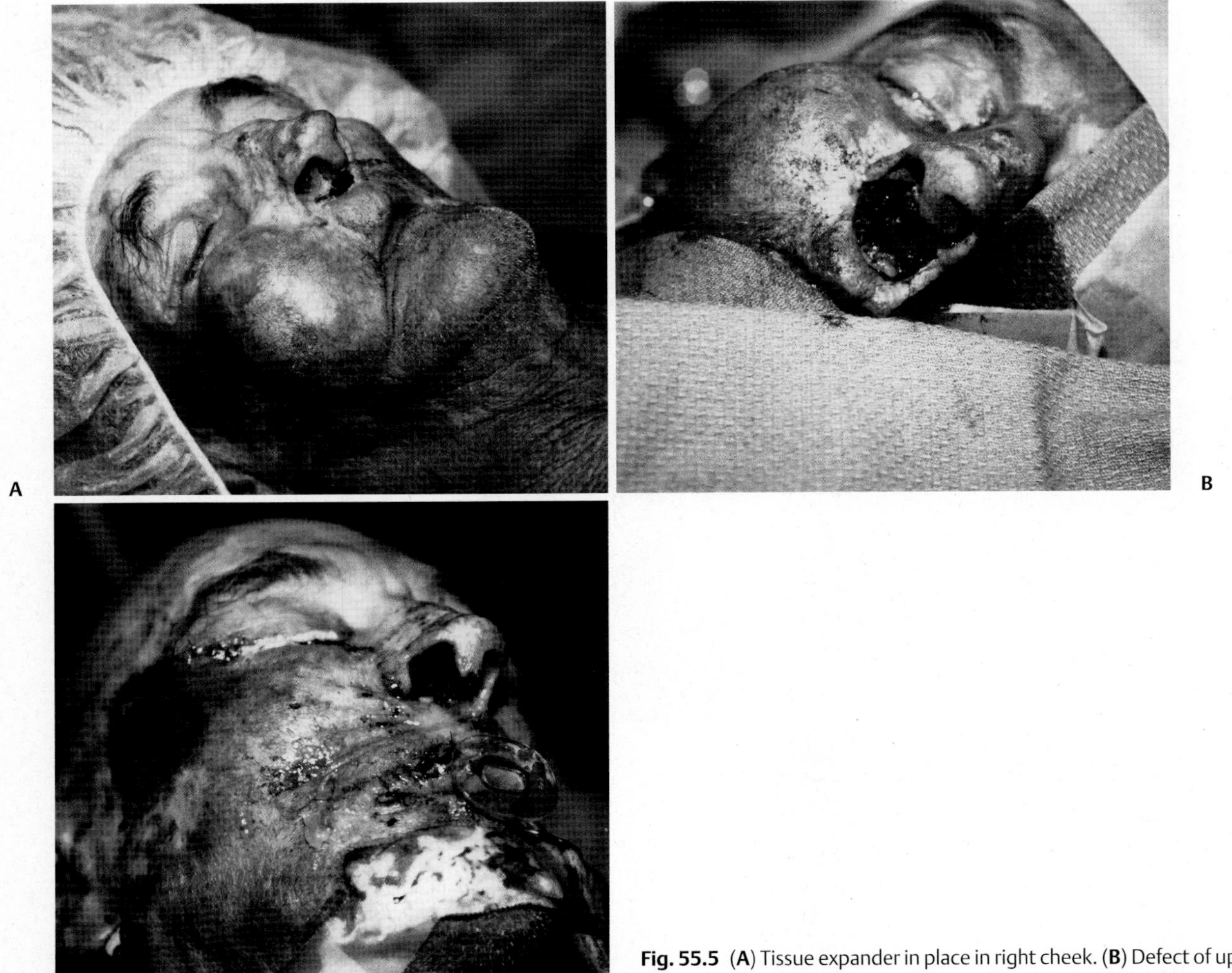

Fig. 55.5 (**A**) Tissue expander in place in right cheek. (**B**) Defect of upper lip and cheek following tumor removal. (**C**) Expanded flap in place.

however, there are guidelines to follow. The most commonly used shapes in head and neck reconstruction are the rectangle, crescent, and oval. Often, the type and shape of a flap that is planned will dictate the shape of the expander. For example, an advancement of flap planned for the forehead may be best expanded with a rectangular expander. In contrast, a large curved rotation scalp flap may be best expanded with either a crescentic or circular expander. Selection of the proper expander should take into account the size of the defect and the availability and location of the donor flap skin. One should always assume that less skin will be available for reconstruction after expansion than one expects preoperatively and choose a somewhat larger expander. A general guideline for the selection of an expander base size is 2.5 to 3 times the area to be reconstructed.[61] Sasaki,[62] in his excellent text on tissue expansion, proposed the following general guidelines for expander selection and inflation: Fill the expander to a width of 2.0 to 2.5 times the width of the defect for flat areas and 2.5 to 3.0 times the width over curved area (**Table 55.1**). For some defects, this would mean that th expander required would be larger than the availabl surrounding tissues. In that case, it would be necessary t

Table 55.1 Guidelines for Expander Selection and Inflation

Site	Expanded Flap Width (cm)	Expected Flap Advancement (cm)
Scalp	12–16	Up to 8
Forehead	8–14	Up to 7
Midface	10–14	Up to 7
Ear	4–8	Up to 4
Neck	12–16	Up to 8

Source: Adapted from Saski GH. Tissue expanders and general guidelines for tissue expansion technique. In: Tissue Expansion in Reconstructive and Aesthetic Surgery. St. Louis: CV Mosby; 1998. Reprinted by permission.

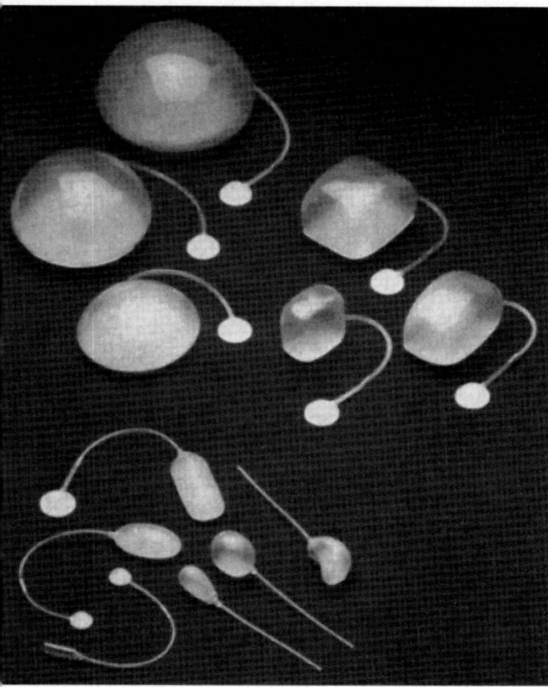

Fig. 55.6 Examples of available Silastic expanders with remote injection ports. (From Swenson RW. Tissue expansion. In: Papel ID, Nacklas NE, eds. Facial Plastic and Reconstructive Surgery. St. Louis: Mosby; 1992:60. Reprinted by permission.)

place two or more expanders around the defect and have multiple expanded flaps available to advance into the defect (**Figs. 55.3 and 55.4**).

When an appropriate expander size and shape has been selected, the first stage of reconstruction is performed to implant the expander. The surgeon should carefully outline the flaps intended end of the location of the expander and the injection port. The surgeon should bear in mind where the final incisions will be required for the ultimate flap. One should also carefully identify nearby neural and vascular structures that may be important for the flap so that they will not be damaged by placement of the expander or elevation of the flap. The incision should be as unobtrusive as possible and is far from the expander as is feasible to minimize the risk of wound dehiscence and expander exposure. The depth of placement and expander varies depending on area to be expanded. In the scalp, the most common location is between the galea and pericranium. Too superficial a placement in the subcutaneous tissues could injure the hair follicles and lead to alopecia. In the forehead, the expander is also placed deep to the frontalis and atop the periosteum. In the cheek and neck, the expander is usually placed in the subcutaneous plane to avoid injury to the facial nerve, although a sub-SMAS (subplatysmal) placement could be considered particularly in patients in whom the overlying skin has a questionable vascularity as a sub-SMAS flap is inherently more robust. Standard facelift and cervical incisions can be employed for access.

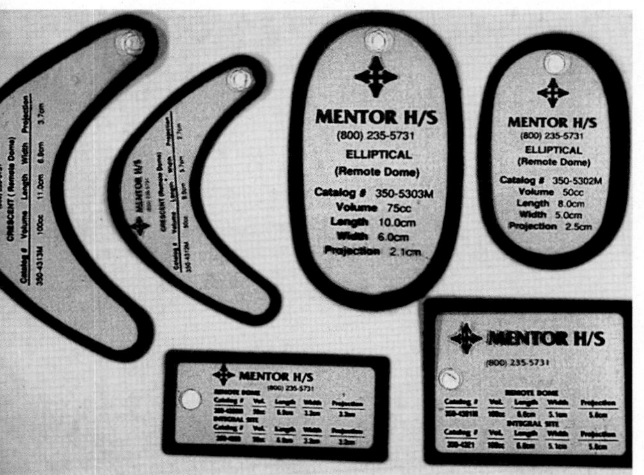

Fig. 55.7 Examples of various tissue expander templates for preoperative planning.

Wide undermining of the pocket into which the expander is placed is necessary. The pocket for the balloon must be large enough to allow the expander to lie completely flat with no folding or buckling and an appropriate location for the injection port should also be selected. Most commercially available tissue expanders come with a preattached port at a given length from the balloon, but the tubing can be shortened by the surgeon as needed. Many surgeons employ permanent sutures even in the deeper layers of tissue closure to minimize the risk of early wound dehiscence during the initial phases of inflation. Slight inflation of the balloon can be done at the time of insertion to obliterate any dead space and to aid hemostasis around the expander pocket. However, there should not be any tension on the wound at closure. Typically, ~2 weeks are allowed to lapse before the sequential inflation is begun.

Inflation of the expander balloon via the injection port is done using a sterile technique. The expander is inflated with sterile saline solution typically once and occasionally twice a week. The volume injected varies depending on the expander size, where in the stage of the expansion you are, the comfort of the patient, and the tolerance of the tissue being expanded. Expansion should proceed more slowly in those areas where the skin is more sensitive and painful and in those areas where the skin is thin and more at risk for breakdown and expander exposure. A small butterfly needle (23 to 25 guage) is convenient for injection. Most injection ports have a raised, palpable ring on top that facilitates palpation through even the thick tissues such as the scalp. If saline is inadvertently injected into the surrounding tissues rather than into the expander, one should simply allow the saline solution to gradually reabsorb while carefully observing that no infection has occurred. In general, each inflation session continues until the overlying skin becomes quite firm or the patient becomes uncomfortable. If pallor or blanching occurs in the overlying skin, then some saline should be withdrawn until the tissue is reperfused. In most cases, 4 to 6 weeks are required to reach full inflation. It is essential that these patients be followed closely and that one tailor the inflation schedule to the individual patient and his or her tissue. Patients will often benefit from the administration of a mild analgesic shortly prior to their scheduled expansion session. When an adequate area of tissue has been expanded, then one can proceed with the definitive flap elevation and inset.

During flap elevation it may be beneficial to briefly overinflate the balloon immediately prior to its removal. This can provide some rapid expansion of the flap, aid the elevation of the flap itself, and perhaps help disrupt some of the capsular fibers around the expander. Some authors have advocated the excision of some or all of the capsule at the time the flap elevation even though this may deprive the flap of some of its blood supply. The advantage of capsular removal is that the bulk of the flap will be reduced and subsequent flap contracture will be lessened. This may be especially critical during auricular or nasal reconstructions where any contracture seriously affects the final results. Because of these concerns, Burget and Menick[63] advise that one never use expansion in paramedian forehead flaps used for nasal reconstruction. Instead, they advocate

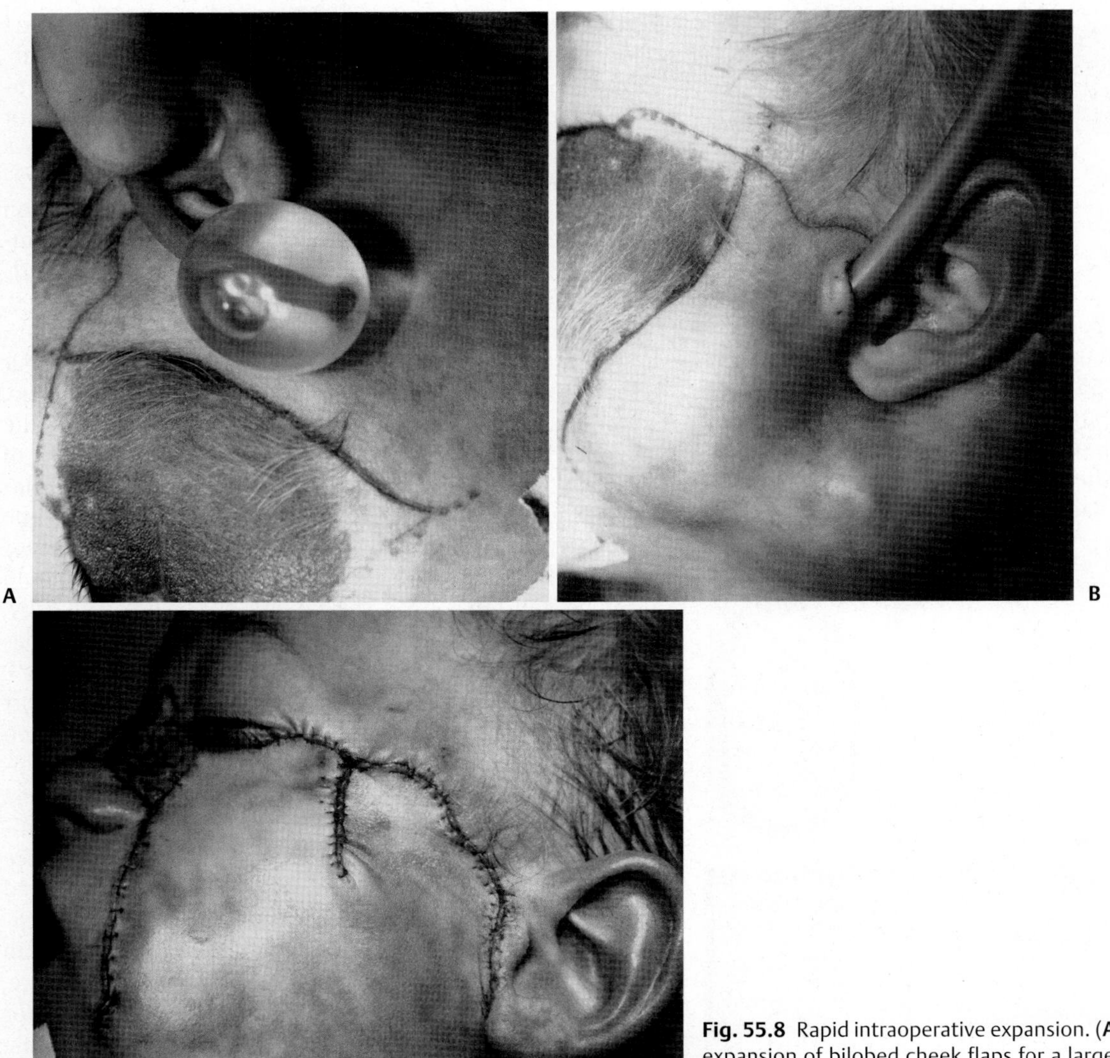

Fig. 55.8 Rapid intraoperative expansion. (**A**) Foley catheter used for expansion of bilobed cheek flaps for a large congenital hairy nevus (**B**) Two catheters in place under each lobe of the flap. (**C**) Flaps in place after excision of the nevus.

raising a thin unexpanded flap even for total nasal reconstructions and then allow the forehead defect to heal by secondary intention.

Rapid Intraoperative Expansion

In rapid ITE, the flap is elevated and expanded simultaneously. One can utilize either a large Foley catheter balloon or a commercially designed intraoperative expander. Sasaki[64] has provided guidelines for how much lengthening one can expect with intraoperative expansion (**Table 55.2**). After the flap has been designed, cyclic expansion is performed (**Fig. 55.8**). The balloon is filled until tissue pallor and firmness are reached. Inflation is typically maintained for 3 minutes, then the saline is withdrawn and the tissue is allowed to rest for several minutes. The cycle is then repeated twice more at which time the flap is transferred and the donor site closed. Surgeons who wish to employ intraoperative expansion must have realistic expectations as to how much additional tissue will be made available with this technique. Some authors believe that there is a lot of immediate stretch-back of the rapidly expanded tissue, which may limit the usefulness of this technique.[19] Occasionally, this technique may be helpful in the closure of donor sites adjacent to the flap rather than for expansion of the flap itself (**Fig. 55.9**).

Table 55.2 Lengthening Provided by Intraoperative Expansion

Site	Average Tissue Gain per Expander (cm)
Scalp	1.0–1.5
Forehead	1.0–2.5
Upper half of nose	1.0–1.5
Nasal tip	0.5–0.75
Midface	1.0–2.5
Neck	1.0–2.5

Source: Adapted from Saski GH. Intraoperative tissue expansion as immediate reconstructive technique. In: Tissue Expansion in Reconstructive and Aesthetic Surgery. St. Louis: CV Mosby; 1998. Reprinted by permission.

Complications

Tissue expansion may subject facial tissues to significant mechanical and biological stresses. As such, these techniques should be used with caution and close clinical observation. One may expect complications

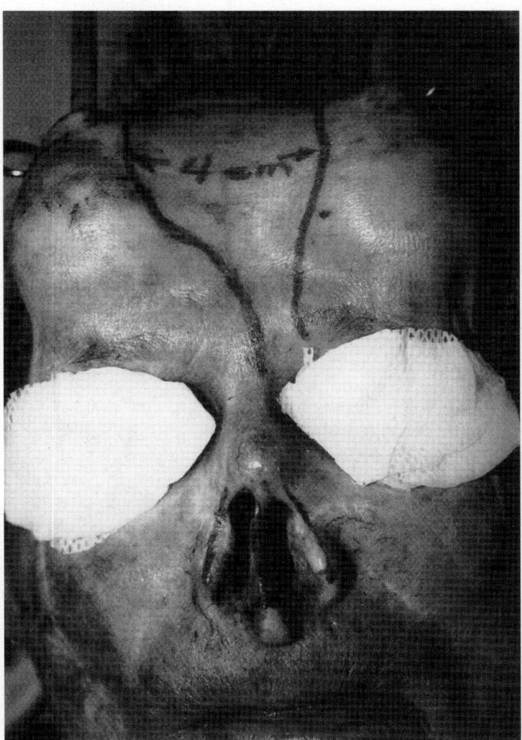
A

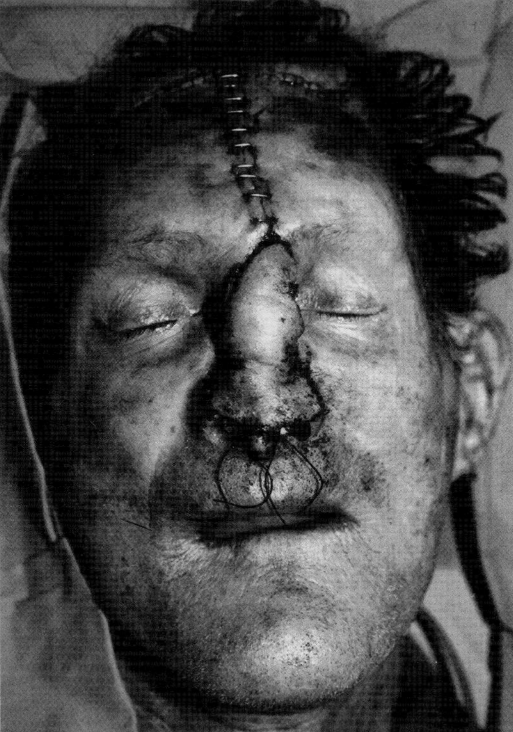
B

Fig. 55.9 (**A**) Intraoperative expansion utilized to aid closure of the forehead after elevation of a large paramedian forehead flap for total nasal reconstruction. (**B**) Forehead closed primarily and flap in place.

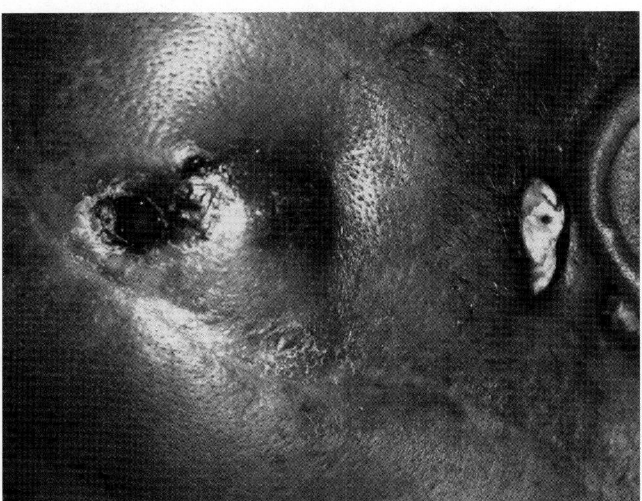

Fig. 55.10 Exposed expander in a previously operated and irradiated scalp.

in ~10% of patients; however, most of the time the expansion and reconstruction can proceed even when problems occur. The most common complication is exposure or extrusion of the expander balloon (**Fig. 55.10**). Typically, this occurs through an incision line but may occur through thin intact skin particularly in those cases that are compromised as with previous irradiation. If exposure occurs early in the course of the expansion, the procedure may well need to be aborted. If, however, it occurs near the completion of expansion—as is most common—then the inflation may be completed or perhaps abbreviated. Exposure occurs most commonly in thin-skinned areas such as over the mastoid, in the midface, or in the neck. Slow, cautious inflation may reduce this risk and careful clinical judgment is essential.

Infection around expanders in the head and neck is unusual and is most commonly seen around the ear or in the scalp. Again, if infection occurs early, then removal of the expander may be required. If appropriate antibiotic therapy controls the infection adequately then the expansion process may proceed to completion although with some delay. Careful sterile technique during the inflation process should minimize the risk of infection. Ischemia and necrosis of flaps in the head and neck during expansion is rare and is most likely the result of too rapid or overzealous inflation techniques. Risk factors for this disastrous complication include a history of smoking, diabetes, extensive scarring, and previous irradiation. Actual failure of the expander device is quite rare and again is more likely to be the result of poor inflation technique. Most inflation ports are quite durable and immune to leakage, but the main balloon itself is susceptible to injury from needle punctures or other penetrating injuries. Neuropraxias during expansion are unusual and typically temporary. The nerves most at risk in the face are the mandibular or frontotemporal branches of the facial nerve and the greater auricular nerve in the neck. As during facelift and other facial surgeries, the location of these nerves should be carefully identified and avoided.

Future Directions

The basic techniques of and indications for tissue expansion are well accepted. Recent research has been devoted to further elucidating the physiology of expansion and to enhance the techniques. Minimally invasive endoscopic techniques have been described for expander placement.[65] Various authors have described attempts to enhance and facilitate the expansion process pharmaceutically.[66,67] Self-inflating osmotic expanders have also recently been described that do not require painful injections for inflation.[68] These and other developments to come will likely only expand the applications and usefulness of tissue expansion.

Summary

Tissue expansion has become a widely accepted and valuable adjunctive technique in head and neck reconstruction. Expansion should be considered when one cannot close a defect primarily or if conventional facial flaps are inadequate. With careful planning, surgical technique, and appropriate inflation, chronic tissue expansion is a safe and reliable technique. Tissue expansion can optimize conventional local, regional, and free flaps and provide robust and appropriate tissue for extensive defects of the head and neck.

References

1. Neumann CG. The expansion of an area of skin by progressive distention of a subcutaneous balloon. Plast Reconstr Surg 1957;19:124
2. Austed ED, Rose GL. A self-inflating tissue expander. Plast Reconstr Surg 1982;70:588
3. Radovan C. Adjacent flap development using expandable silastic implants Paper presented at: Annual Meeting of the American Society of Plastic and Reconstructive Surgery; September 1976; Boston
4. Radovan C. Tissue expansion in soft tissue reconstruction. Plast Reconstr Surg 1984;74:482
5. Austed ED. Evolution of the concept of tissue expansion. Facial Plast Surg 1988;5:277
6. Malata CM, Williams NW, Sharpe DJ. Tissue expansion: clinical applications. J Wound Care 1995;4:37
7. Cunha MS, Nakamoto HA, Herson MR, Faes JC, Gemperli R, Ferreira MC. Tissue-expander complications in plastic surgery: a 10-year experience. Rev Hosp Clin Fac Med Sao Paulo 2002;57:93

8. Bauer BS, Few JW, Chavez CD, Galiano RD. The role of tissue expansion in the management of the large congenital pigmented nevi of the forehead in the pediatric patient. Plast Reconstr Surg 2001;107:668
9. Hoffmann JF. Tissue expansion in the head and neck. Facial Plast Surg Clin North Am 2005;13:315
10. Hudson DA, Grob M. Optimizing results with tissue expansion: 10 simple rules for successful tissue expander insertion. Burns 2005;31:1
11. Rivera R, LoGiudice J, Gosain AK. Tissue expansion in pediatric patients. Clin Plast Surg 2005;32:35
12. LoGiudice J, Gosain AK. Pediatric tissue expansion: indications and complications. J Craniofac Surg 2003;14:866
13. Austed ED, Pasyk KA, McClatchey KD, et al. Histomorphologic evaluation of the guinea pig skin and soft tissue after controlled expansion. Plast Reconstr Surg 1982;70:704
14. Pasyk KA, Argenta LC, Hassett C. Quantitative analysis of the thickness of human skin and subcutaneous tissue following controlled expansion with a silicone implant. Plast Reconstr Surg 1988;81:516
15. Belkoff SM, Naylor EC, Walshau R, et al. Effects of subcutaneous expansion on the mechanical properties of porcine skin. J Surg Res 1995;58:117
16. Guida RA, Cohen JI, Cook TA, et al. Assessment of survival and microscopic changes in porcine skin flaps undergoing immediate intraoperative tissue expansion. Otolaryngol Head Neck Surg 1993;109:926
17. Preyer S. Skin expansion and skin growth: molecular proof of collagen synthesis in long-term expansion. HNO 1996;44:117
18. DeFilippo RE, Atala A. Stretch and growth: the molecular and physiologic influences of tissue expansion. Plast Reconstr Surg 2002;109:2450
19. Machida BK, Liu-Shindo M, Sasaki GH, et al. Immediate versus chronic tissue expansion. Ann Plast Surg 1991;26:227
20. Suegert R, Weerda H, Hoffman S, Mohadjer C. Clinical and experimental evaluation of intermittent intraoperative short-term expansion. Plast Reconstr Surg 1993;92:248
21. Wee SS, Logan SE, Mustoe TA. Continuous versus intraoperative expansion in a pig model. Plast Reconstr Surg 1992;90:808
22. Johnson TM, Lowe L, Brown MD, et al. Histology and physiology of tissue expansion. J Dermatol Surg Oncol 1993;19:1074
23. Austed ED, Thomas SB, Pasyk KA. Tissue expansion: dividend or loan? Plast Reconstr Surg 1986;78:63
24. Pasyk KA, Argenta LC, Austed LC. Histology of human expanded tissue. Clin Plast Surg 1987;14:435
25. Sasaki GH. Reactive patterns and dysfunctional changes in expanded tissue. In: Tissue Expansion in Reconstructive and Aesthetic Surgery. St. Louis: Mosby; 1998:40
26. Cherry GW, Austed ED, Pasyk KA. Increased survival in the vascularity of random pattern skin flaps elevated in controlled, expanded skin. Plast Reconstr Surg 1983;72:68
27. Baker DE, Dedrick DK, Burney RE, et al. Resistance of rapidly expanded random skin flaps to bacterial infection. J Trauma 1987;27:1061
28. Hong C, Stark GB, Futrell W. Elongation of axial blood vessels with a tissue expander. Clin Plast Surg 1987;14:465
29. Saxby PJ. Survival of island flaps after tissue expansion in a pig model. Plast Reconstr Surg 1988;81:30
30. Burget GC, Menick FJ. Subtotal and total nasal reconstruction. In: Aesthetic Reconstruction of the Nose. St. Louis: Mosby; 1994
31. Morris SF, Pang CY, Mahoney J, et al. Effect of capsulectomy on the hemodynamics and viability of a random pattern skin flaps raised on expanded skin in the pig. Plast Reconstr Surg 1989;84:323
32. Sasaki GH. Reaction patterns and dysfunctional changes in expanded tissue. In: Tissue Expansion in Reconstructive and Aesthetic Surgery. St. Louis: Mosby; 1998:35–37
33. Milner RH, Wilkins PR. The recovery of peripheral nerves following tissue expansion. J Hand Surg [Br] 1992;17:78
34. Martini DV, Har-El G, McKee J, et al. Rapid intraoperative facial nerve expansion. Otolaryngol Head Neck Surg 1996;114:605
35. Sasaki GH. Intraoperative sustained limited expansion as an immediate reconstructive technique. Clin Plast Surg 1987;14:563
36. Zhu Y, Luo J, Barker J, Hochberg J, Cilento E, Reilly F. Identification of genes induced by rapid intraoperative tissue expansion in mouse skin. Arch Dermatol Res 2002;293:560
37. Shapiro AL, Hochman M, Thomas JR, Braham G. Effects of intraoperative tissue expansion and skin flaps on wound closing tension. Arch Otolaryngol Head Neck Surg 1996;122:1107
38. Mackay DR, Saggers GC, Kotval W, et al. Stretching skin: undermining is a more important than intraoperative tissue expansion. Plast Reconstr Surg 1990;86:722
39. Siegert R, Weerda H, Hoffman S, et al. Clinical and experimental evaluation of intermittent intraoperative short-term expansion. Plast Reconstr Surg 1993;92:248
40. Wee SS, Logan SE, Mustoe TA. Continuous versus intraoperative tissue expansion in the pig model. Plast Reconstr Surg 1992;90:808
41. Chandawarkar RY, Cervino AL, Pennington GA. Intraoperative acute tissue expansion revisited: a valuable tool for challenging skin defects. Dermatol Surg 2003;29:834
42. Zeng YJ, Xu CQ, Yang J, Sun GC, Xu XH. Biomechanical comparison between conventional and rapid expansion of skin. Br J Plast Surg 2003;56:660
43. Manders EK, Graham WP, Scheiden MJ, et al. Skin expansion to eliminate large scalp defects. Ann Plast Surg 1984;12:305
44. Earnest LM, Byrne PJ. Scalp reconstruction. Facial Plast Surg Clin North Am 2005;13:345
45. Azzolini A, Riberti C, Cavalca D. Skin expansion in head and neck reconstruction. Plast Reconstr Surg 1992;90:799
46. Konior RJ, Kridel RWH. Tissue expansion in scalp surgery. Facial Plast Surg Clin North Am 1994;2:203
47. Kolasinski J, Kolenda M. Algorithm of hair restoration surgery in children. Plast Reconstr Surg 2003;112:412
48. Bauer BS. The role of tissue expansion and reconstruction of the ear. Clin Plast Surg 1990;17:3129
49. Brent B. Auricular repair with autogenous rib cartilage grafts: 2 decades of experience with 600 cases. Plast Reconstr Surg 1992; 90:355
50. Zim SA. Microtia reconstruction: an update. Curr Opin Otolaryngol Head Neck Surg 2003;11:275
51. Baker SR, Swanson NA. Reconstruction of major facial defects following surgical management of skin cancer: the role of tissue expansion. J Dermatol Surg Oncol 1994;20:133
52. Bauer BS, Vicari F. Approach to excisions of congenital giant pigmented nevi in infancy and early childhood. Plast Reconstr Surg 1988;82:1012
53. Bauer BS, Corcoran J. Treatment of large and giant nevi. Clin Plast Surg 2005;32:11
54. Goodman CM, Miller R, Patrick CW, et al. Radiotherapy: effects on expanded skin. Plast Reconstr Surg 2002;110:1080
55. Romo T, Jablonski RD, Shapiro AJ, McCormick SA. Long-term nasal mucosal tissue expansion use in repair of large nasoseptal perforations. Arch Otolaryngol Head Neck Surg 1995;121:327
56. Forte V, Middleton WG, Briant TD. Expansion of myocutaneous flaps. Arch Otolaryngol Head Neck Surg 1985;111:371
57. Masser WR. Pre-expanded radial free flap. Plast Reconstr Surg 1990; 86:295
58. Russell RC, Khouri RK, Upton J, et al. The expanded scapular flap. Plast Reconstr Surg 1996;96:884
59. Acarturk TO, Glaser DP, Newton ED. Reconstruction of difficult wounds with tissue expanded free flaps. Ann Plast Surg 2004;52:493
60. Ninlovic M, Moser-Rumer A, Spanio S, Rainer C, Gurunluoglu R. Anterior neck reconstruction with pre-expanded free groin and scapular flaps. Plast Reconstr Surg 2004;113:61
61. Swenson RW. Tissue expansion. In: Papel ID, Nacklas ND, eds. Facial Plastic and Reconstructive Surgery. St. Louis: Mosby-Year Book; 1991:61
62. Sasaki GH. Tissue expanders and general guidelines for tissue expansion technique. In: Tissue Expansion in Reconstructive and Aesthetic Surgery. St. Louis: Mosby; 1998:11–14

63. Burget GC, Menick FJ. The paramedian forehead flap. In: Aesthetic Reconstruction of the Nose. St. Louis: Mosby; 1994:65
64. Sasaki GH. Intraoperative expansion as an immediate reconstructive technique. In: Tissue Expansion and Reconstructive and Aesthetic Surgery. St. Louis: Mosby; 1998:248
65. Shabaro VI, Moroz VY, Starkov YG, Strekalovsky VP. First experience of endoscopic implantation of tissue expanders and plastic and reconstructive surgery. Surg Endosc 2004;18:513
66. Tang Y, Luan J, Zhang X. Acceleration of tissue expansion by application of topical papaverine and cream. Plast Reconstr Surg 2004;114:1166
67. Copcu E, Sivrioglu N, Sisman N, Aktas A, Oztan Y. Enhancement of tissue expansion by calcium channel blocker: a preliminary study. World J Surg Oncol 2003;9:19
68. Ronert MA, Hofheinz H, Manassa E, Asgarouladi H, Olbrisch RR. The beginning of an era in tissue expansion: self-filling osmotic tissue expander—4-year clinical experience. Plast Reconstr Surg 2004;114:1025

56 Musculocutaneous Flaps

Donald J. Annino Jr., Russell S. Shu, and Daniel R. Gold

The development of the pedicled musculocutaneous flap in the 1970s heralded a new era of surgical advancement in head and neck reconstruction. These defined areas of muscle, centered around perpendicularly oriented myocutaneous perforating vessels, are an ideal source of reliable transplantable muscle and skin. These flaps provide well-vascularized, reliable, and versatile tissue to reconstruct a variety of head and neck soft tissue defects (**Table 56.1**).

The first reported use of a pedicled myocutaneous flap was by Tansini in 1896 with the use of a pedicled latissimus dorsi flap for breast reconstruction.[1] These flaps, however, were not utilized in the head and neck until Owens in 1955.[2] Instead, reconstruction was performed with fasciocutaneous flaps or skin grafts. This was ultimately overturned in 1979 when Ayrian described the use of the pectoralis major musculocutaneous flap for reconstruction of the head and neck.[3] These reports demonstrated that musculocutaneous pedicled flaps improved reliability, offered one-stage reconstruction, and provided more bulk than fasciocutaneous flaps. The myocutaneous flap rapidly rose to become the workhorse for head and neck reconstruction and still remains an important and integral tool in the field.

Pectoralis Major Musculocutaneous Flap

The pectoralis major musculocutaneous flap was first described in 1968 in the resurfacing of an anterior chest wall defect.[4,5] Its first use in head and neck reconstruction was not until 1979.[3] Since then it has become one of the most popular flaps for head and neck reconstruction. It can be used to reconstruct defects of the oral cavity, the oropharynx, the face, and the neck.

The pectoralis major musculocutaneous flap has the advantages of being easy to raise, reliable, and requiring only a single stage. It also offers the advantage of providing good carotid coverage and protection in patients who have undergone a neck dissection. The primary limitation of the flap is the bulkiness of the subcutaneous adipose tissue between the skin and the muscle. This can be reduced by stripping the skin and adipose and applying a skin graft to resurface the muscle.

Anatomy

The pectoralis major is a flat, fan-shaped muscle. It arises from the medial half of the anterior surface of the clavicle, the sternum, the costochondral cartilages of the first six ribs, and the aponeurosis of the external oblique muscle. The muscle inserts into the biceps groove of the humerus. On its deep surface, it lies superficial to the pectoralis minor.

The pedicle blood supply is from the pectoral branch of thoracicoacromial artery, which enters the muscle after piercing through the clavicopectoral fascia. The lateral thoracic artery also supplies the lateral portion of the pectoralis major, but frequently it must be sacrificed for adequate arc of rotation (**Fig. 56.1**).

Surgical Technique

The thoracicoacromial artery leaves the axillary artery at a right angle from below the medial third of the clavicle. The path of the pectoral branch can therefore be marked by

Table 56.1 Characteristics of Musculocutaneous Flaps

Myocutaneous Flap	Major Arterial Blood Supply	Innervation	Common Uses
Pectoralis major	Pectoral branch of thoracicoacromial artery	Lateral and medial pectoral nerves	Oral cavity, oropharynx, face and neck defects
Trapezius	Paraspinous perforators/occipital/TCA/DSA	Spinal accessory nerve	Lower two thirds of face, neck, temporal fossa defects
Sternocleidomastoid	Occipital/superior thyroid/thyrocervical trunk	Spinal accessory nerve	Resurfacing oral cavity, lining/protecting pharyngeal reconstruction, protecting great vessels
Platysma	Submental branch of facial artery/many anastamosis	Cervical branch of facial nerve	Intraoral, oropharyngeal, hypopharyngeal defects
Latissimus dorsi	Thoracodorsal artery	Thoracodorsal nerve	Oral cavity, oropharynx, face and neck defects. Protecting great vessels
Temporalis	Anterior and deep temporal artery	Trigeminal nerve	Dynamic facial rehabilitation, facial augmentation. Cheek and orbit defects

Abbreviations: DSA, dorsal scapular artery; TCA, transverse cervical artery.

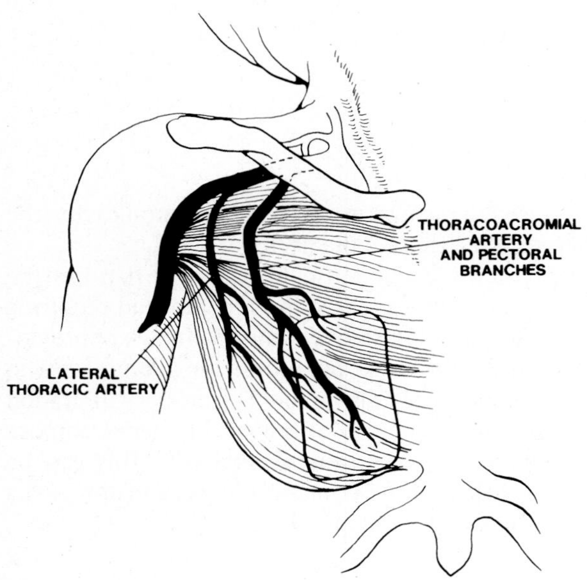

Fig. 56.1 Vascular anatomy of pectoralis major musculocutaneous flap.

drawing a line on the upper chest wall from the acromion process (medial third) to the xiphoid process. The skin paddle is designed between the nipple and the sternum along this line. Ideally, the skin paddle should not violate the territory of a deltopectoral flap, and the parasternal perforators of the second and third intercostal spaces are left intact. An incision is made from the upper lateral edge of the paddle to the axilla. In the female patient, the skin paddle is placed to give minimal distortion to the breast and the incision to the axilla placed in the inframammary crease.[6]

The lateral border of the pectoralis major muscle is then identified by wide undermining of medial and lateral skin flaps. The incision around the skin paddle is completed once it has been determined that the paddle is primarily located over the muscle with as small a random component as possible. When performing the incision around the skin paddle and elevating the flap, care must be taken to limit any shearing forces on the skin paddle. Tacking sutures may also be utilized to keep the skin paddle securely attached to the muscle.

Once the skin paddle has been raised, the inferior portion of the pectoralis major is sharply freed from the chest wall and dissected superiorly. The medial aspect of the muscle must also be freed from the sternum and any parasternal perforators ligated. Superiorly, the vascular pedicle is identified medially on the deep surface of the muscle and protected. The plane is carried laterally between the pectoralis minor and major with blunt dissection along the fascial plane. Along the lateral edge of the pectoralis minor, the lateral thoracic pedicle is encountered and usually needs to be sacrificed to allow for adequate mobilization and flap rotation. The arc of rotation is also improved by narrowing the segment of muscle overlying the vascular pedicle.

A subcutaneous tunnel is formed superficial to the clavicle connecting the neck and chest sites. A minimum of three fingers should fit comfortably through the tunnel to ensure that the pedicle will not be constricted. The flap is then passed over the clavicle effectively rotating it 180 degrees around the pedicle. It is important to ensure that the pedicle does not become twisted or kinked as it passes through the tunnel. The flap is then secured to the recipient site with care taken to preserve the integrity of the pedicle.

The donor site is closed primarily, with wide undermining of the surrounding skin. A perforating towel clamp can be helpful to keep tension off the incision during the closure and may be released after sufficient deep sutures are in place. A suction drain is placed in the donor site postoperatively to prevent seroma or hematoma.

Trapezius Musculocutaneous Flap

Three flaps can be created using the trapezius musculocutaneous unit: the lateral island, the superior-based and the anterior-based flaps. The first report of a trapezius flap came in 1842 when Mutter described use of a mastoid-occiput–based shoulder cutaneous flap to fill a defect of the anterior neck created by release of scar contracture.[7] Zovickian in 1957 used delaying procedures to extend the length of the flap farther onto the shoulder to repair pharyngocutaneous fistulas.[8] In 1979, McGraw et al described an undelayed Mutter-Zovickian flap by including underlying trapezius muscle to improve circulation.[9] This became known as the superior or upper trapezius musculocutaneous flap. The lateral island trapezius musculocutaneous flap was described by Demergasso and Piazza in 1977.[10] The lower trapezius island musculocutaneous flap was not described until 1980 by Baek et al.[11]

The ideal areas for reconstruction with these flaps are the lower two thirds of the face, neck, and temporal fossa. The trapezius muscle has the advantages of being thin, located outside the usual field for head and neck irradiation, and having a long arc of rotation and a long pedicle to help it reach most areas in the head and neck.

Its disadvantages are that it must be harvested in the lateral decubitus position, that there is a frequent need for skin grafting to resurface the donor site, and that the spinal accessory nerve must be sacrificed. The limitations on shoulder mobility following a neck dissection are exacerbated with the harvest of this flap.

Anatomy

The trapezius is a flat triangular muscle arising from the occiput, the superior nuchal line, the nuchal ligament, and the spinous processes of C-7 to T-12. The muscle inserts on the lateral third of the clavicle, the scapular spine, and the acromion. It helps to elevate and rotate the shoulder.

The blood supply to the trapezius is from four sources. The paraspinous perforators supply the muscle along its entire course. The superior portion of the muscle receives its blood supply from the occipital artery. The transverse cervical (TCA) and dorsal scapular (DSA) arteries supply the inferior part of the muscle.[12]

The TCA most commonly originates from the thyrocervical trunk but in 20% of individuals it originates directly from the subclavian artery.[13] This variation limits the use of the lateral island flap as the TCA may run deep to or through the brachial plexus exposing it to injury. The TCA usually travels in a superolateral direction superficial to the anterior scalene muscle, phrenic nerve, and brachial plexus, and deep to the omohyoid muscle. It enters the midpoint of the trapezius muscle, along with the spinal accessory nerve. The TCA then divides into a deep and superficial branch. The deep branch passes along the undersurface of the minor rhomboid muscle, emerges from between the minor and major rhomboids, and supplies the lower portion of the trapezius. This deep branch, also known as the dorsal scapular artery (DSA), may also originate directly from the subclavian artery. The superficial branch of the TCA passes over the levator scapulae divides into an ascending and descending branch as it runs along the undersurface of the trapezius.[14] The ascending branch supplies the superior portion of the muscle, whereas the descending branch supplies the lower portion of the muscle.

The concept of cutaneous angiosomes is helpful when designing the trapezius island flap.[12] The skin overlying the trapezius muscle can be divided into three vertical angiosomes: the superior supplied by the TCA, the middle supplied by the DSA, and the lower (overlying the latissimus dorsi) supplied by the intercostals. According to the concept of angiosomes, the skin of an angiosome may be removed from its supply vessel and be reliably perfused by an intact adjacent angiosome. Thus one can reliably include the lower trapezius angiosome if the DSA (middle angiosome) is preserved.

The nerve supply to the trapezius is from the spinal accessory cranial nerve.

Lower Trapezius Island Musculocutaneous Flap

The lower trapezius island musculocutaneous flap is the most versatile of the trapezius flaps due to its great arc of rotation. It is possible to reach anywhere from the midline of the neck, to the lateral skull base or the cheek. When using this flap shoulder restriction may be minimized by preserving the superior portion of the trapezius and utilizing only the portion of the muscle inferior to the skin paddle.

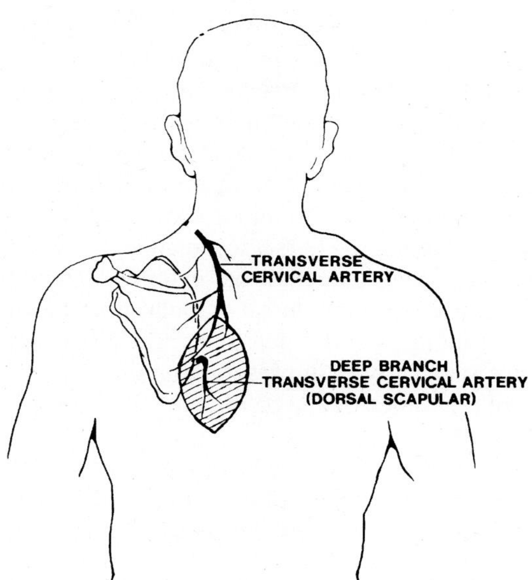

Fig. 56.2 Vascular anatomy of lower trapezius island musculocutaneous flap.

The blood supply for this flap is the TCA and DCA and veins. However, the flap can be harvested on the TCA and vein alone, as long as the inferior end of the flap does not extend beyond the rhomboids. Elevation of the flap with sacrifice of the dorsal scapular pedicle improves the arc of rotation. Inclusion of both TCA and DSA allows the inferior end of the flap to extend 10 to 15 cm beyond the inferior end of the scapula. Therefore, when utilizing this flap it is critical that the TCA and vein are intact and have not have been sacrificed during a previous neck dissection (**Fig. 56.2**).

Surgical Technique

The flap is elevated with the patient in the lateral decubitus position. Adduction and internal rotation of the arm helps to increase the working area available between the medial surface of the scapula and the spine. The skin paddle is marked on the skin between the medial border of the scapula and the midline of the back. It should not extend more than 5 cm beyond the inferior border of the scapula to ensure a dependable skin paddle. The course of the TCA is exposed by incising a line superior and medially from the skin paddle toward the posterior triangle of the neck. Skin flaps are raised and the trapezius muscle is exposed along its entire length leaving the skin paddle attached. Starting laterally, the trapezius is dissected from the rhomboids. Medially the trapezius is separated from the vertebrae and the paraspinous perforators are ligated. The DSA and vein are identified as they enter the trapezius medially from between the rhomboids. If the dorsal scapular vessels are to be saved, the rhomboid minor must be transected. Care should be taken though not to divide both rhomboid major and minor, which will result in a free-floating scapula. The dorsal scapular vessels must also remain intact if the skin paddle has extended beyond the scapula tip; otherwise the dorsal scapular vessels are ligated and the rhomboid muscle left intact. The dissection then continues superiorly with preservation of the anterior segment of the trapezius and passing the flap beneath the eleventh nerve.

Donor site closure is performed primarily with wide undermining of the margins. A suction drain is placed to decrease the risk of a seroma, which may occur following this flap.

Superior Trapezius Flap

The superiorly based trapezius flap is based on the paraspinous perforators and the occipital artery (**Fig. 56.3**). The blood supply is, therefore, not compromised by a previous neck dissection. The flap provides excellent coverage for defects in the neck that do not extend across the midline. It is oriented with its base superiorly so gravity will not be pull the flap from the recipient site as occurs with many other flaps . It is the most reliable of the three trapezius flaps.[13,14]

Surgical Technique

The superiorly based trapezius flap is harvested in the lateral decubitus position. The flap is outlined over the superior portion of the trapezius with the superior incision overlying the anterior edge of the muscle. A parallel inferior incision is made to yield sufficient donor skin paddle and to include at least two paraspinous perforators. The flap usually incorporates the skin paddle along the entire length of the muscle, but it can also be designed as an island flap. The incision can be extended laterally up to 10 cm over the deltoid muscle as long as the fascia from the deltoid is included with the flap. The limitation to the rotation of this flap is the inferior incision at the midline. Panje introduced the modification of extending the incision beyond the midline and turning it superiorly, which improves the reach of the flap.[14]

The plane of dissection is deep to the trapezius muscle and above the supraspinatus, levator scapulae, rhomboid major, and deltoid. The transverse cervical pedicle is encountered medially and is ligated to allow adequate mobilization of the flap. Ideally, the pedicle should be saved, but this is not routinely done. A skin graft is used to close the donor defect.

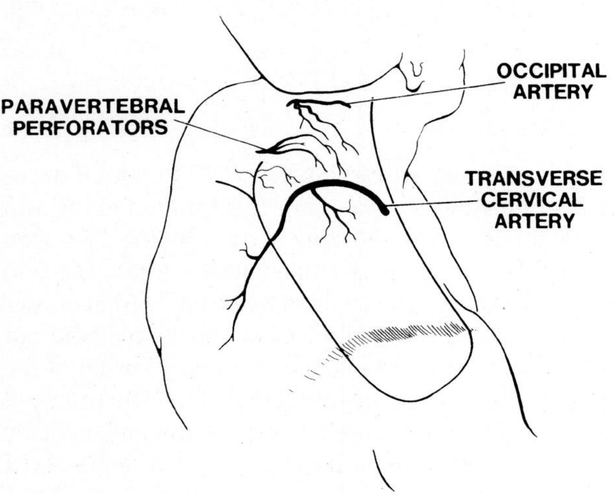

Fig. 56.3 Vascular anatomy of superiorly based trapezius musculocutaneous flap.

Lateral Trapezius Island Myocutaneous Flap

The Lateral trapezius island myocutaneous flap is based on the TCA and vein (**Fig. 56.4**) and is reported to be the least reliable of the trapezius flaps.[13,15] Caution must therefore be taken before elevating this flap if a neck dissection has been performed. One must either be certain that the transverse cervical vessels are intact or explore the neck prior to elevating the flap. The flap is used to reconstruct external defects of the neck or mucosal loss in the oral cavity and pharynx.

Surgical Technique

The lateral trapezius island flap is designed with a skin paddle overlying the superior lateral aspect of the trapezius

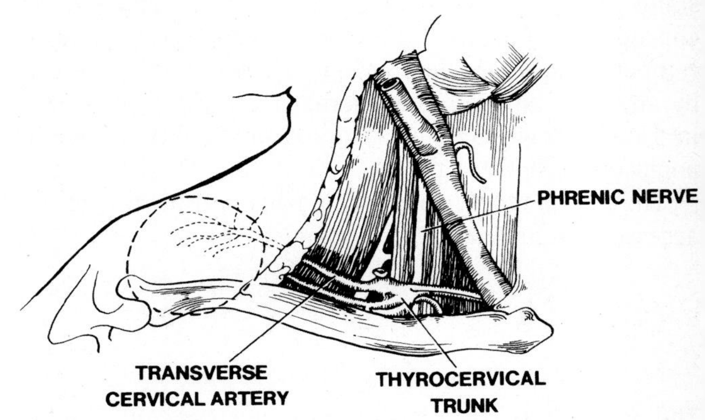

Fig. 56.4 Vascular anatomy of lateral trapezius island musculocutaneous flap.

muscle. The first step is to identify the TCA and vein in the posterior neck to ensure that use of the flap is viable. The skin paddle is then centered over the transverse cervical pedicle. The anterior border of the trapezius is identified and the skin edges are incised. The incisions are then continued through the subcutaneous tissue and muscle. Frequently, the DSA has to be ligated with the distal portion of the TCA to completely mobilize the flap. The skin paddle may also be extended distally to include random-pattern skin. In elevating this flap, care must be taken around the TCA, which may be intertwined with the roots of the brachial plexus. This is especially a risk when the TCA arises directly from the subclavian artery.

Sternocleidomastoid Musculocutaneous Flap

The use of the sternocleidomastoid musculocutaneous flap was first reported in 1955.[2] It was not, however, until 1980 that the arterial supply was properly understood.[16] It is supplied in three sections: the occipital artery supplies the superior third, the superior thyroid artery supplies the middle third, and the thyrocervical trunk supplies the inferior third of the muscle. This allows the flap to be designed as superiorly or inferiorly based depending on the area of reconstruction. Ideally, all flaps should include at least two vessels (the superior thyroid artery contribution is always included), otherwise it becomes a less reliable random-pattern flap rather than an axial-patterned flap. This flap can be used for resurfacing of the oral cavity or lining a pharyngeal reconstruction.[17–19] It is important when using this flap not to forget oncologic principles. It should not be used when neck disease would normally dictate resection of the muscle.

Anatomy

The sternocleidomastoid muscle arises from two sources: the sternum and the medial head of the clavicle. The two heads fuse to insert in the mastoid process. The muscle is innervated by the spinal accessory nerve.

Surgical Technique

The skin paddle is outlined over the bulk of the sternocleidomastoid muscle. Inferiorly, the skin may extend over the clavicle. The skin incision is carried down through the skin, the subcutaneous tissue, and the platysma. A vertical incision is than made to the mastoid process. In elevating the superiorly based flap the branches from the thyrocervical trunk are sacrificed. Ideally, the blood supply from the superior thyroid artery is preserved; however, this may limit the arc of the superiorly based flap. The harvesting of the inferiorly based flap is similar, except that the skin paddle is centered over the mastoid tip. In this case, the blood supply from the occipital artery is ligated. With both the inferiorly and superiorly based flaps, local skin undermining and advancement can usually close the donor defect. A suction drain is placed at the time of closure.

Platysma Musculocutaneous Flap

The platysma musculocutaneous flap was first described by Gersuny in 1887 for the reconstruction of a full-thickness cheek defect.[20] The flap was rotated inward to provide a new lining for the buccal mucosa. In 1978, Futrell et al reported the first large series involving use of the platysma flap for head and neck reconstruction.[21]

This flap has been most frequently used in reconstruction of intraoral defects, such as those of buccal mucosa and floor of mouth.[21–26] In addition, oropharyngeal and hypopharyngeal defects have been reconstructed with this flap.[23] Outer skin of the midface and lip region are other reported sites of reconstruction.[25]

The accessibility of this flap in the surgical field, lack of bulk, pliable nature, one-stage reconstruction capability, and primary closure with minimal donor site deformity have made this flap a very attractive option for head and neck reconstruction.[26]

Anatomy

The platysma muscle lies within the superficial fascial layer of the neck. The muscle originates from the subcutaneous tissue of the upper thorax, drapes the anterior neck extending the border of the mandible, to insert in the facial skin at the lateral angles of the oral commissure. It is innervated by the cervical branch of the facial nerve. The platysma's main blood supply is from the submental branch of the facial artery.[22] It also is supplied inferiorly by the superficial branch of the TCA, medially from the thyroid vessels, and laterally from the occipital and posterior auricular vessels.

Early reports questioned the reliability of this flap after the facial artery has been ligated during neck dissection. McGuirt et al showed, however, that among 19 of 20 patients whose facial artery was ligated and divided (bilaterally in two) the flap was only compromised when both facial arteries were ligated.[23] Numerous anastomoses exist between the anterior facial artery system and both ipsilateral internal and external carotid systems. These ipsilateral and contralateral contributions allow retrograde filling of a proximally ligated facial artery. All that is absolutely requires is an intact submental artery distal to the submandibular gland. Venous drainage of the flap is in a vertical orientation. Tension and kinking should be limited with adequate length and back-cuts to ensure good venous outflow.

There has also been concern over preoperative irradiation resulting in vascular changes that would compromise flap viability[27]; however, this flap can be successfully used in previously irradiated patients.[28] Use of the flap in patients with prior radical neck dissection should be based on the previous neck incisions. A transverse neck incision may divide the pedicle and compromise viability. If flap loss does occur, there are reports of successfully using the nonviable flap as a biologic dressing, managed conservatively with debridement without a secondary reconstruction.[24]

Surgical Technique

The outline of the platysma flap is initially made as an ellipse with the inferior margin low in the neck. Typically, the dimensions of the skin ellipse are 5 × 10 cm to 7 × 14 cm.[21] When an apron flap is used for the neck dissection, the inferior margin of that flap will become the inferior margin of the platysma flap. The inferior skin incision will pass through the platysma, whereas the superior skin incision will pass only through skin. A skin-only flap is then raised superior to the skin paddle up to the mandible, leaving the platysma down. At this point, the distal skin island with its supporting platysma is elevated superiorly in a subplatysmal plane, typical for standard exposure for neck dissection. After the tumor ablation and neck dissection, the platysma musculocutaneous flap is rotated superiorly and 180 degrees into the defect and sutured in position. The donor site is closed primarily with undermining of the upper chest wall skin.

Latissimus Dorsi Musculocutaneous Flap

The latissimus dorsi flap was the first musculocutaneous flap described.[1,29] It offers the advantages of substantial bulk, a site distant from the usual head and neck irradiation fields, and provides protection to the carotid artery following a neck dissection. It is also the largest volume of transplantable regional soft tissue for reconstruction of the head and neck. It is relatively hairless, and the donor site can be more aesthetically acceptable to some patients than the pectoralis major.

The latissimus dorsi flap has the following disadvantages: bulkiness of the flap, necessity to position the patient in the lateral decubitus position, and increased shoulder weakness and loss of range of motion, particularly in conjunction with sacrifice of the accessory nerve. Special care must be taken to position the ipsilateral arm so that brachial plexus injury does not occur while harvesting the flap.[30]

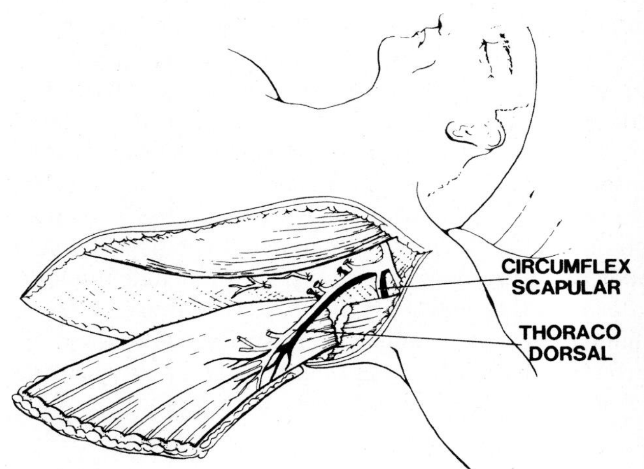

Fig. 56.5 Vascular anatomy of latissimus dorsi musculocutaneous flap.

Anatomy

The latissimus dorsi muscle is a flat muscle that arises from the thoracic, lumbar, and sacral vertebrae, the thoracolumbar fascia, the external oblique fascia, and the iliac crest. It inserts on the intertubercular groove of the humerus. It has an axial blood supply from the thoracodorsal artery, an end artery of the subscapular artery, which arises from the axillary artery (**Fig. 56.5**).

The thoracodorsal nerve innervates the latissimus dorsi muscle.

Surgical Technique

The patient is placed in the lateral decubitus position. The skin paddle is drawn over the muscle based on the size of the defect. The incision is made from the superior margin of the skin paddle to the axilla. Skin flaps are elevated to expose the muscle and the muscle is released inferiorly and anteriorly. The vascular pedicle is identified just medial to the anterior border of the muscle as the dissection proceeds superiorly. Superior dissection separates the latissimus from the serratus anterior, and the branch of the thoracodorsal to the serratus anterior is identified and ligated. When the dissection has reached the circumflex scapular vessels the flap will be of sufficient mobility to reach most areas in the head and neck. If extra length is needed, the circumflex vessels can be sacrificed as well. The muscle is separated from the humerus and the posterior border from the vertebrae. The flap is then passed into the neck through a subcutaneous tunnel from the axilla. To prevent constriction of the pedicle the arm should be elevated for the first few days. The wound can be closed primarily if the width of the skin paddle is 10 cm or less. Defects greater than this require a skin graft to assist with closure. A suction drain is routinely placed into the donor site.

Temporalis Muscle Flap

The temporalis muscle flap was first described in 1898 in the reconstruction of an orbital defect.[31] The temporalis muscle flap is most commonly used today for dynamic facial rehabilitation and facial augmentation. It was first used for rehabilitation of facial nerve paralysis in the 1930s.[32] It can be useful for reconstruction of the orbit and cheek; however, a short arc of rotation and the lack of transplantable overlying skin coverage limit the use of this flap. It can be used and then easily covered with a skin graft. An additional disadvantage is the resulting depression in the temporal region following rotation of this flap. This can be improved with augmentation of the area with various alloplastic materials as well as the use of folded temporoparietal fascia.

Anatomy

The temporalis muscle is a broad, thin muscle. It arises from the pericranium and passes obliquely forward and inferiorly to the coronoid process of the mandible. The blood supply is from the anterior and deep temporal arteries off the internal maxillary artery. It is innervated by the mandibular division of the trigeminal nerve along with the other muscles of mastication.

Surgical Technique

The incision is Y-shaped, extending from the superior temporal line to the helix of the ipsilateral ear. A sinusoid incision is made to best camouflage the scar postoperatively. The incision is continued inferiorly preauricularly, usually not beyond the level of the tragus. The depth of the incision should be through the temporoparietal fascia to the level of the deep temporal fascia. Reflection of the scalp flaps exposes the deep muscular fascia. Care must be taken anteriorly to avoid injuring the frontal branch of the facial nerve, which runs anterior to the temporal hairline. The nerve runs in the superficial temporal fascia, also known as the temporoparietal fascia.

A section of the temporalis is elevated from superiorly starting at the superior temporal line. Once the junction of the deep fascia and the periosteum is divided, the muscle is dissected bluntly from the skull with a periosteal elevator. The dissection proceeds inferiorly toward the zygomatic arch and the insertion onto the coronoid process. Care must be taken as the dissection approaches the zygomatic arch to avoid injury to the vessels entering the deep surface of the muscle. It is helpful either to section the zygomatic arch or, if the flap is to obliterate the orbit, to create a lateral orbitotomy to improve the arc of rotation and reach of the flap. When elevating this flap it is possible to tailor its size as needed; either the entire muscle or a strip can be used.

Caution should be exercised when using this flap in conjunction with a temporoparietal fascial flap in patients who have received radiation. The skin flaps will likely not survive following mobilization of the temporoparietal fascia with its supplying superficial temporal artery and vein.

Summary

The primary goals of surgical treatment and reconstruction of head and neck cancer are tumor-free survival, preservation, restoration of function, and normalization of appearance. The ideal procedure is a single-stage resection followed by immediate reconstruction. For this purpose, musculocutaneous flaps offer the advantage of dependability, bulk, and single-stage reconstruction. Each regional musculocutaneous flap has its own characteristics, making it suitable for specific defects. These include the total area of the defect, the thickness of the flap, its pliability, length of the vascular pedicle, ease of harvest, and donor site morbidity.

The most common etiology for musculocutaneous flap failure is technical error during the preparation and insetting of the flap. Complications can range from total or partial loss, suture line dehiscence, fistulas, wound infection, and hematoma and seroma formation. These complications can occur either at the donor site, the recipient site, or both. Limiting any trauma during elevation, transposition, and insetting of the flap is extremely helpful in preventing complications. In addition, utmost care must be taken to ensure that the pedicle is not constricted or kinked. Whenever possible, the flap should be designed to avoid excess bulk and tension.

Microvascular free flaps have helped to increase the spectrum of reconstructive options available but have not eliminated the myocutaneous pedicled flaps from daily practice. The pedicled musculocutaneous flap remains a reliable and technically easier reconstruction option when compared with a microvascular free tissue transfer.

References

1. Tansini I. Nouvo processo per l'amputazione della mammella per cancro. Riforma Med 1896;12:3
2. Owens N. Compound neck pedicle designed for repair of massive facial defects. Plast Reconstr Surg 1955;15:369
3. Ayrian S. The pectoralis major myocutaneous flap: a versatile flap for reconstruction in the head and neck. Plast Reconstr Surg 1979;63:73
4. Hueston JT, McConchie IH. A compound pectoral flap. Aust N Z J Surg 1968;38:61
5. Pickerel KL, Baker HM, Collins JP. Reconstructive surgery of the chest wall. Surg Gynecol Obstet 1947;84:465
6. Colman MF, Zemplenyi J. Design of incisions for pectoralis myocutaneous flaps in women. Laryngoscope 1986;96:695

7. Mutter TD. Cases of deformity relieved by operation. Am J Med Sci. 1842;4:66
8. Zovickian A. Pharyngeal fistulas: repair and prevention using mastoid-occiput based shoulder flaps. Plast Reconstr Surg 1957;19:355
9. McGraw JB, Magee WP, Kalwaic H. Uses of the trapezius and sternomastoid myocutaneous flaps in head and neck reconstruction. Plast Reconstr Surg 1979;63:49
10. Demergasso F, Piazza MV. Trapezius myocutaneous flap in reconstructive surgery for head and neck cancer: an original technique. Am J Surg 1977;138:533
11. Baek SM, Biller HP, Krespi YP, et al. The lower trapezius myocutaneous flap. Ann Plast Surg 1980;5:108
12. Urken ML, Naidu RK, Lawson W, et al. The lower trapezius island musculocutaneous flap revisited. Arch Otolaryngol Head Neck Surg 1991;117:502
13. Netterville JL, Panje WR, Maves MD. The trapezius myocutaneous flap. Arch Otolaryngol Head Neck Surg 1987;113:271
14. Panje WR. Myocutaneous trapezius flap. Head Neck Surg 1980;2:206
15. Netterville JL, Wood DE. The lower trapezius flap. Arch Otolaryngol Head Neck Surg 1991;117:73
16. Ayrian S. The strenocleidomastoid myocutaneous flap. Laryngoscope 1980;90:676
17. Conley J, Gullane PJ. The sternocleidomastoid muscle flap. Head Neck Surg 1990;2:308
18. Littlewood M. Compound skin and sternocleidomastoid flap for repair in extensive carcinoma of the head and neck. Br J Plast Surg 1967;20:403
19. Bakamajian VY. A technique for primary reconstruction of the palate after radical maxillectomy for cancer. Plast Reconstr Surg 1963; 31:103
20. Gersuny R. Plastischer Ersatz der Wangenscheimhaut. Zentralbl Hi 1887;14:706
21. Futrell JW, Johns ME, Edgerton MT, et al. Platysma myocutaneous flap for intraoral reconstruction. Am J Surg 1978;136:504
22. Coleman JJ, Nahai F, Mathes SJ. The platysma musculocutaneous flap clinical and anatomic considerations in head and neck reconstruction Am J Surg 1982;144:477
23. McGuirt WF, Matthews BL, Brody JA, et al. Platysma myocutaneous flap: caveats reexamined. Laryngoscope 1991;101:1238
24. Conley JJ, Lanier DM, Tinsley P. Platysma myocutaneous flap revisited Arch Otolaryngol Head Neck Surg 1986;112:711
25. Coleman JJ, Jurkiewicz MJ, Nahai F, et al. The platysma musculocutaneous flap: experience with 24 cases. Plast Reconstr Surg 1983;72:31
26. Ozcelik T, Aksoy S, Gokler A. Platysma myocutaneous flap: use fo intraoral reconstruction. Otolaryngol Head Neck Surg 1997;116:493
27. Persky MS, Kaufman D, Cohen NL. Platysma myocutaneous flap fo intraoral defects. Arch Otolaryngol Head Neck Surg 1983;109:463
28. Cannon CR, Johns ME, Atkins JP, et al. Reconstruction of the oral cavity using the platysma myocutaneous flap. Arch Otolaryngol Head Neck Sur 1982;108:491
29. Quillen CG, Shearin JC Jr, Georgiade NG. Use of the latissimus dors myocutaneous island flap for reconstruction of the head and neck area Plast Reconstr Surg 1978;62:113
30. Quillen CG. Latissimus dorsi myocutaneous flaps in head and nec reconstruction. Plast Reconstr Surg 1979;63:664
31. Golovine SS. Precede de cloture plastique de 1'orbite après 1'exenteration J Fr Ophtalmol 1898;18:679
32. Gillies HD. Experience with fascia lata grafts in the operative treatmen of facial paralysis. Proc R Soc Med 1934;27:1372

57 Microvascular Flaps

Brian B. Burkey, Cecelia E. Schmalbach, and John R. Coleman Jr.

With the current advances in surgical technique, titanium plating, and vascular physiology, microvascular free tissue transfer has become the reconstructive choice for many complex three-dimensional head and neck defects. Although these defects can arise in the setting of trauma and congenital malformations, the vast majority of patients suffer from head and neck cancer. This patient population poses several unique challenges in that patients are often heavy smokers, in poor health, and suffering from malnutrition. In addition, the head and neck region carries the potential risks of fistula, salivary contamination, and compromised vasculature secondary to irradiation. Unlike regional flaps and nonvascularized bone grafts, microvascular free tissue transfer enables reconstruction with nonirradiated, well-vascularized, and reliable tissue.

The purpose of this chapter is to provide the reader with an overview of head and neck microvascular free tissue transfer. We will discuss surgical technique, flap monitoring, and the management of flap failures. Ten commonly used donor sites will be highlighted, including the anatomy, surgical technique, advantages, and disadvantages of each site. The chapter will conclude with a review of the reconstruction of site-specific head and neck defects, with an emphasis on speech and swallowing.

Preoperative Evaluation and Patient Selection

The first step to successful transfer begins in the office with appropriate patient selection. A thorough history and physical examination is required. Poor cardiopulmonary status may preclude the patient from undergoing the long general anesthetic often required for free tissue transfer. In such cases, a regional flap or secondary reconstruction may be a better choice. In addition, patients with a history of diabetes mellitus often have significant peripheral vascular disease. For this reason, we prefer to reconstruct bony defects in diabetics using either the iliac crest–internal oblique or scapula free tissue rather than the fibula donor site. It is important to inquire about prior trauma, femoral bypass surgery, axillary nodal dissection, and inguinal hernia repair, all of which can lead to vascular pedicle injury. Ultimately, the decision to utilize free tissue transfer for head and neck reconstruction depends upon the surgeon's experience and the specific defect, as well as the patient's overall health, personal wishes, and social support system.

Surgical Technique

Successful transfer of free tissue necessitates the use of meticulous surgical technique during flap harvest, vessel preparation, microvascular anastomosis, and insetting of the flap, with specific attention to vessel geometry.

Flap Harvest

Successful and efficient flap harvest requires a detailed knowledge of the donor site anatomy and elevation planes. The surgeon must respect the location of the vascular pedicle and make every effort to protect it during harvest. It is imperative to avoid separating the pedicle from the tissue to be transferred. All branches and perforators not included with the flap should be separated from the pedicle at the greatest distance possible using surgical clips, bipolar electrocautery, or surgical ties depending upon vessel size. The use of unipolar cautery in close proximity to the pedicle is discouraged. After the pedicle has been dissected a sufficient distance to create adequate pedicle length, it can be divided and the flap taken to a back table for vessel preparation.

Vessel Preparation

The back table allows the microvascular surgeon the opportunity to prepare the flap and its vessels for transfer. Jeweler's forceps; sharp, straight, and curved microscissors; a vessel dilator; and curved needle holder are required to ensure gentle handling of the vessels (**Fig. 57.1**). The interior of the vessels should never be handled directly because intimal tears lead to exposed subendothelium, which is highly thrombogenic.[1] Traditionally, an operating microscope is used for illumination and magnification (4 to 16 times). Some surgeons use high-powered loupe magnification with equal success.[2] Preparation begins by flushing the vessels with heparinized saline to remove blood and thrombogenic precursors. The loose layers of adventitia are removed from the distal 2 to 3 cm of the vessels to allow for anastomosis. This dissection is easily accomplished with the surgeon and the assistant grasping the vessel at 180-degree opposite points to create traction and open space for tissue dissection. Although it is important to remove adventitia, which could potentially prevent intima contact

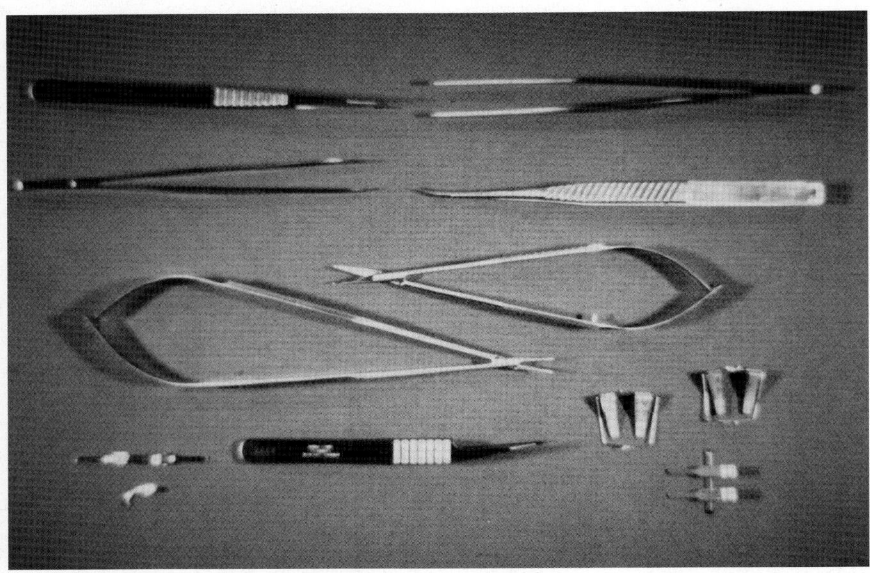

Fig. 57.1 The basic microvascular equipment tray, including straight and curved scissors, jeweler's forceps, right-angled forceps, vessel dilator, and vessel clamps with clamp holder.

between the donor and recipient vessels during the anastomosis, it is important to keep in mind that overzealous cleaning leads to devascularization of the intima and subsequent tissue death. The artery and veins should be separated from one another to allow for optimal vessel geometry and tension-free spacing during anastomosis. Vessel dilators and heparinized saline are used to gently dilate the artery and veins.

Anastomosis

After analogous cleaning of the recipient neck vessel adventitia, microvascular anastomosis is performed. Typically, the arterial anastomosis is performed in an end-to-end fashion, whereas the venous anastomosis is accomplished either end-to-end or end-to-side. It is important to choose appropriate recipient vessels when multiple ones are available. The vessels should share similar caliber and demonstrate brisk bleeding. Unfortunately, this luxury is not always available. If a lumen size mismatch beyond 2:1 exists, the surgeon can fish-mouth the smaller vessel and take unequal bites to achieve adequate approximation.[3] An alternative means for addressing large vessel mismatch is to perform an end-to-side anastomosis (**Fig. 57.2**). Most microvascular surgeons prefer to use an end-to-side anastomosis between the donor vein and the internal jugular vein. A statistical difference in vessel thrombosis has not been demonstrated when comparing end-to-side anastomosis versus end-to-end venous anastomosis.[4] However, increased thrombosis has been demonstrated with anastomosis into the external jugular system compared with the internal jugular system.[5] For this reason, we favor the latter recipient vessel whenever available.

The traditional technique for the anastomosis involves the use of interrupted 9–0 or smaller nylon stitches. An equivalent rate of vessel patency has been reported with the use of continuous compared with interrupted suture technique.[6] Running a continuous suture allows for faster anastomosis, leading to decrease ischemia time, and it is particularly helpful with vessel size mismatch. However, these advantages come at the expense of potential narrowing of the vessel lumen at the anastomotic site

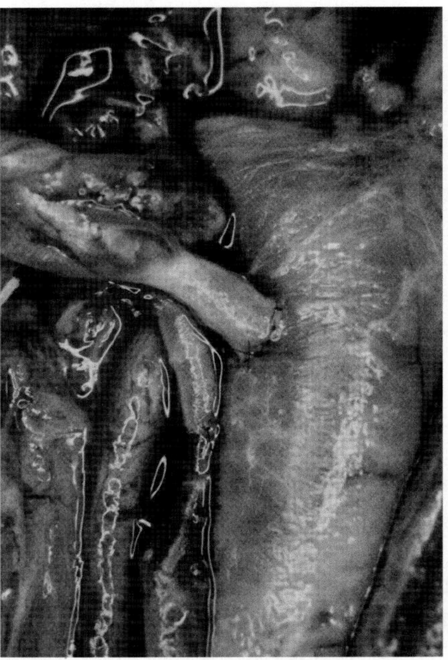

Fig. 57.2 Anastomoses for a lateral arm free flap showing an arterial end-to-end anastomosis and a venous end-to-side anastomosis into the internal jugular vein.

Framed artery and vein clamps are commonly used for end-to-end anastomosis, whereas end-to-side anastomosis is generally done freehand following the placement of vessel loops. Other authors report the use of anastomotic devices with similar safety, efficacy, and thrombosis rates as traditional anastomoses.[7,8] The advantage of the device is decreased operative time and the ability to perform the anastomosis even when exposure is less than ideal. Shindo reported a series in which the only failure occurred with the arterial anastomosis; therefore, her group recommends use of the ring anastomotic device for venous anastomosis only.[7]

Vessel Geometry

Vessel geometry refers to the orientation of the anastomotic vessels. Although this appears to be a simple concept, ultimate success of the flap hinges on the orientation of the pedicle.[9] It is essential that the vessels rest in a tension-free environment, allowing sufficient length to create gentle curves rather than tight turns that can potentially kink and lead to anastomotic thrombosis. Resection of the posterior belly of the digastric muscle, generous 360-degree dissection around the internal jugular vein, back-cutting the sternocleidomastoid muscle, and mobilization of the recipient vessels such as the facial artery or external carotid artery beneath a carefully dissected hypoglossal nerve may help to remove undue tension. It is preferable for the anastomosis to sit down in the neck rather than ride up immediately under the skin. With bone flaps, the surgeon must decide whether to take the pedicle over or under the bone segment, keeping in mind that pressure can be placed on the pedicle by a tight tunnel under the bone or external compression over the bone. At each step in the reconstruction, the surgeon should check the orientation of the vessels as well as the overlying external forces. Often times, a simple tacking suture or strategically placed piece of Gelfoam (Pfizer, Inc., New York, NY) can help to maintain ideal vessel geometry.

Flap Monitoring

Early detection of ischemia through reliable flap monitoring is critical to the success of microvascular free tissue transfer. Monitoring of perfusion begins in the operating room, immediately following anastomosis. In this setting, most surgeons rely on direct examination of the flap to assess perfusion. This examination includes observation of bleeding from the cut edges of the flap, capillary refill of the skin paddle when available, flap warmth, and ultrasonic Doppler signal directly over the vessels.

Once the flap has been inset and the case completed, the choice of postoperative flap monitoring is surgeon-dependent, and varies in part on the type and location of the flap itself. An ideal monitoring technique would be safe, cost-effective, 100% sensitive and specific, continuous, reproducible, noninvasive, and easily interpreted by nursing and physicians alike.[10] The vast number of monitoring devices reported in the literature lends credence to the fact that an ideal technique has yet to emerge. The techniques range from assessment of a monitoring segment for buried flaps,[11] monitoring vascular perfusion via Doppler ultrasonography or laser Doppler flow,[12] as well as measuring tissue perfusion using oxygen tension,[13,14] photoplethysmography,[15] and tissue metabolism (hydrogen clearance).[16]

Despite all of the above noted techniques, the vast majority of microvascular surgeons employ clinical assessment as their primary monitoring modality. At our institution we rely upon capillary refill, cutaneous flap temperature, and if applicable, bleeding of the skin paddle following gentle pinprick with a 20-guage needle. Doppler ultrasonographic signals over the flap and presumed path of the pedicle are also used to evaluate both arterial and venous flow. The nursing staff monitors the flap every hour during the first 72 hours, followed by every 4 hours during the subsequent 48 hours, and finally every 8 hours until hospital discharge. If changes occur, the surgeon is notified and the examination is immediately repeated.

Normal flap examination includes a pink skin paddle that is warm to touch, 3-second capillary refill, and production of bright red blood within seconds of pinprick. Arterial insufficiency presents as a cool, pale skin paddle, with prolonged capillary refill beyond 5 seconds, loss of the Doppler signal, and a prolonged bleeding time following needlestick. Conversely, the hallmarks of venous insufficiency include a congested, hyperemic skin paddle with brisk capillary refill, brisk, dark bleeding that returns immediately when the 20-guage needle is withdrawn, and a pistol shot quality on Doppler exam. Patients with the above noted changes on exam warrant immediate flap exploration under general anesthesia. In the event of a postoperative hematoma, the patient should return to the operating room in a timely fashion. In the interim, the wound should be opened at the bedside to immediately alleviate pressure from the pedicle. It has been our experience that the setting of an infected surgical bed carries an increased risk of venous thrombosis. For this reason, we also return immediately to the operating room to perform a surgical wash-out on all patients who develop purulent drainage from their wound or suction drains.

The majority of postoperative flap monitoring focuses upon the free tissue that was transferred. However, it is important to examine the donor site to ensure that a wound infection or hematoma does not develop. Radial forearm and fibular free flaps usually require casting. In this setting, neurovascular integrity of the donor extremity should be monitored on a routine basis to ensure that undue pressure beneath the cast does not develop.

Flap Failure

The current success rate of free tissue transfer ranges from 95 to 98%. Vessel thrombosis accounts for the majority of failures during the immediate postoperative period. Specifically, arterial thrombosis accounts for ~20% of failures and tends to occur within the first 24 hours of anastomoses.[16] Venous thrombosis is much more common, accounting for more than 50% of failures, and presents later. Flap failure can be related to inappropriate preoperative planning. Ideally, the type of free tissue transfer should optimize vessel geometry and avoid vein grafts. Other important factors impacting flap survival include detailed attention to flap harvest, appropriate vessel geometry, vessel anastomosis, and thorough postoperative flap monitoring.[17–19]

Salvage of a failing flap ultimately depends on timely identification of the problem and swift intervention. The goal is to limit ischemia time to avoid the "no-reflow phenomenon" in which prolonged ischemia leads to irreversible endothelial damage.[20] Once this damage occurs, the vessels can only exist in a thrombosed state. Despite reperfusion of the larger vessels, the injury cannot be overcome, and thrombosis is permanent. The amount of ischemia time leading to the no-reflow phenomenon remains unknown. Therefore, it is imperative that flap ischemia be promptly identified and rapidly corrected. Salvage rates in this setting range from 70 to 100%.[19,20]

Many surgeons use anticoagulation during the perioperative period to decrease the likelihood of vessel thrombosis. Anticoagulation has a proven benefit in the setting of traumatic amputation and reimplantation; however, its role in microvascular reconstruction remains to be determined.[21,2] Common agents used to prevent platelet deposition and clot formation include aspirin, low-molecular-weight dextran, heparin, and prednisone. Currently, we use dextran-40 intravenously at a rate of 25 mL per hour during the first 36 hours following surgery. Dextran is a volume expander that can cause pulmonary edema and anemia. For this reason, we follow hematocrit levels closely and avoid its use in patients with poor cardiac and/or pulmonary function. In addition, aspirin (325 mg/day) is started on postoperative day 1 and continued until 3 weeks following the free tissue transfer.

Microvascular Flaps Used in Head and Neck Reconstruction

A detailed description of the major free flaps utilized in head and neck reconstruction is provided below. Emphasis is placed on both anatomy and surgical technique in flap harvest. Please refer to **Table 57.1** for a summary of the flaps and their associated neurovascular components.

Fascial and Fasciocutaneous Flaps

Radial Forearm Free Flap

The radial forearm free flap has gained tremendous popularity since its introduction in 1978. In fact, it is now

Table 57.1 Summary of Head and Neck Free Flap Neurovascular Components

Flap	Artery	Vein	Nerve
Superficial temporoparietal fascial	Superficial temporal	Superficial temporal	N/A
Radial forearm	Radial	Cephalic	Lateral antebrachial cutaneous
Lateral arm	Posterior radial collateral	Venae comitantes	Posterior cutaneous nerve of the arm
Lateral thigh	Profunda femoris perforators	Venae comitantes	Lateral femoral cutaneous
Anterior lateral thigh	Lateral circumflex femoral artery	Venae comitantes	Lateral femoral cutaneous
Latissimus dorsi	Thoracodorsal	Thoracodorsal	Thoracodorsal (m.) Intercostal (s.)
Rectus	Deep inferior epigastric	Deep inferior epigastric	N/A
Jejunum	Superior mesenteric arterial arcade	Superior mesenteric venous arcade	N/A
Fibula	Peroneal	Peroneal	Lateral sural cutaneous
Scapula	Circumflex scapula	Circumflex scapula	N/A
Iliac crest—internal oblique	Deep circumflex	Deep circumflex	N/A

Abbreviations: m., motor innervation; N/A, not applicable; s., sensory innervation.

regarded as the workhorse flap for head and neck reconstruction. The relative ease in harvest, reliable anatomy, and thin, soft tissue with the potential for innervation allow for a variety of reconstructive applications. The radial forearm free flap is commonly used to reconstruct defects of the oral cavity/oropharynx, hypopharynx, total pharyngoesophagus, skull base, external skin and scalp.[23]

Anatomy

The radial forearm free flap can be harvested as a fascial flap, fasciocutaneous flap, or osteocutaneous flap, with or without sensory innervation. The classic design includes a variable skin paddle usually averaging 9 × 6 cm in size; however, nearly the entire skin of the forearm can be transferred if necessary. The skin paddle is centered over the vascular pedicle, which consists of the radial artery and two venae comitantes and/or cephalic vein. Distally, the pedicle travels within the intermuscular fascial septum, which separates the flexor carpi radialis and the brachioradialis muscles. Within the proximal forearm, the pedicle courses deep to the brachioradialis muscle. Multiple perforators are given off from the pedicle to the skin, muscles, and lateral surface of the distal radius bone. The superficial drainage of the flap is usually incorporated into the harvest by recruiting branches of the cephalic vein. The deep and superficial venous systems often unite in the region of the antecubital fossa to form one common vein. Thus tracing the venous drainage system proximately will allow for one, as opposed to two, venous anastomoses. Clinical work has demonstrated that flap survival is not dependent on both systems, and adequate venous drainage can be achieved with either the deep or superficial system alone.[24] The medial and lateral antebrachial nerves are encountered during flap elevation. If a sensate skin paddle is desired, the nerves can be incorporated into the harvest and anastomosed to a local sensory nerve.

If composite reconstruction is required, 10 to 12 cm of bone can be harvested from the distal radius. Long-term immobilization of the donor site is required in the postoperative period. Despite limiting the harvest to only 40% of the radius circumference, pathological fractures occur in up to 23% of cases.[25–27] Therefore, the transfer of bone in the setting of a radial forearm free flap is discouraged by many microvascular surgeons.

Lastly, the palmaris longus muscle can be incorporated into the radial forearm free tissue transfer to support complex reconstructions such as total lip[28] and hemilarynx.[29] This muscle originates from the deep fascia near the medial epicondyle. The tendon inserts into the palmar aponeurosis. Removal of this muscle–tendon complex for reconstructive purposes is associated with little morbidity.

Surgical Technique

In preparation for sacrifice of the radial artery, all patients must undergo preoperative assessment of collateral blood flow to the hand. Most surgeons rely upon an Allen's test performed in the clinic setting to assure a patent deep palmer arch. It is the preference at our institution to verify adequate flow using a Doppler-aided Allen's test because this test provides additional information about the patency of the radial artery itself.

Intraoperatively, the patient is positioned supine with the operative arm resting on two arm boards. The outline of the skin paddle is centered over the pedicle. Proximally, an S-shaped incision is extended up to the antecubital fossa (**Fig. 57.3**). If tourniquet control is desired to provide bloodless dissection, care should be taken to exsanguinate the forearm using an elastic Esmarch bandage prior to inflating the tourniquet to 250 mm Hg.

Dissection begins from either the ulnar or radial side of the flap. Elevation proceeds from each side in a subfascial plane until the pedicle is reached in the intermuscular septum between the brachioradialis and the flexor carpi radialis. Radial dissection requires attention to the superficial venous drainage system and the branches of the superficial radial nerve that provide sensation to the thumb and dorsal surface of the first two fingers. During ulnar dissection, the ulnar artery and paratenon overlying the muscular tendons must be identified and preserved. The paratenon provides the necessary vascular supply to the split-thickness skin graft used in closing the donor site (**Fig. 57.4**). Once the pedicle has been approached from both sides, it can be elevated from its deep muscular and bony attachments. Dissection proceeds proximally toward the antecubital fossa until sufficient pedicle length is obtained. Typically the pedicle is traced back to the junction of the radial, ulnar, and brachial arteries. The takeoff of the recurrent radial artery tends to be the proximal limit of the pedicle. Before the distal pedicle is ligated, an intraoperative Allen's test can be performed by placing a microvascular clamp on the

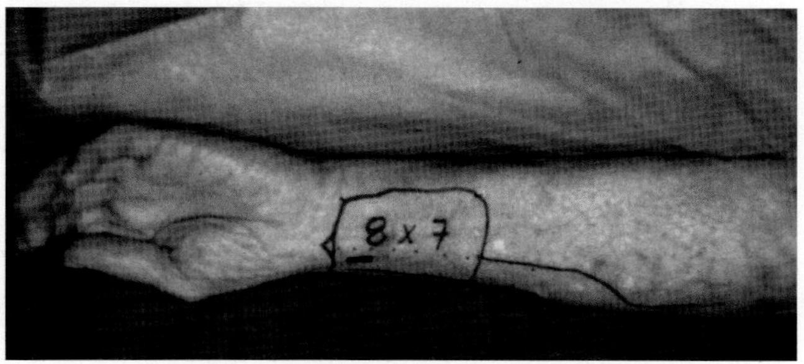

Fig. 57.3 Proposed incisions for a radial forearm free flap, with dots indicating the course of the radial artery and a curvilinear incision from the skin paddle to the antecubital fossa.

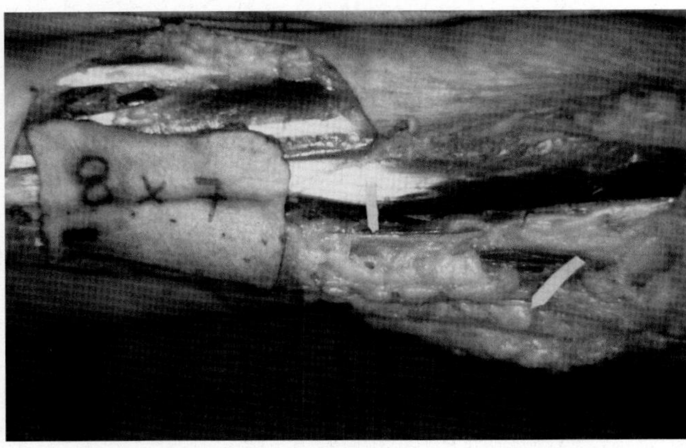

Fig. 57.4 The radial forearm skin paddle elevated from the underlying paratenon. The distal arrow denotes the pedicle and the proximal arrow points to the lateral antebrachial cutaneous nerve.

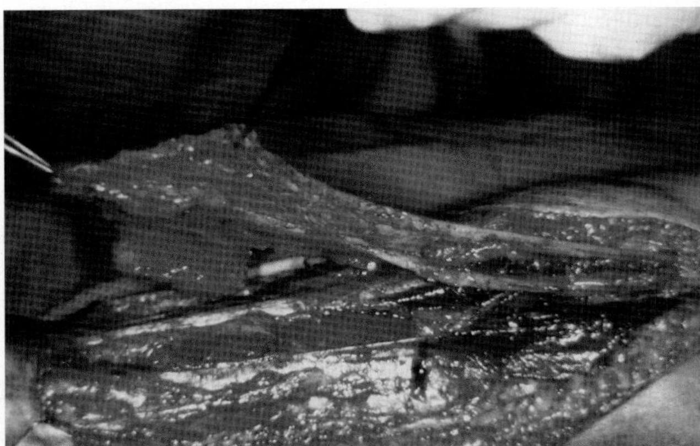

Fig. 57.6 A radial forearm flap raised on its pedicle after the tourniquet has been released. Note the thinness and vascularity of the flap as well as the long vascular pedicle.

radial artery, deflating the tourniquet, and confirming capillary reperfusion of the hand. Closure of the donor site usually requires placement of a split-thickness skin graft from the anterior thigh (**Fig. 57.5**). A dorsal splint is placed for 6 days to immobilize the forearm and enhance graft success.

Advantages and Disadvantages

The radial forearm free flap is considered the workhorse of microvascular reconstruction because the thin, pliable tissue can be adapted to meet the needs of multiple reconstructions (**Fig. 57.6**). The skin has little hair, the pedicle has adequate vessel size as well as length, and the anatomy is highly reliable. The flap can be sensate, and the harvest can incorporate bone and/or tendon to enhance reconstruction.

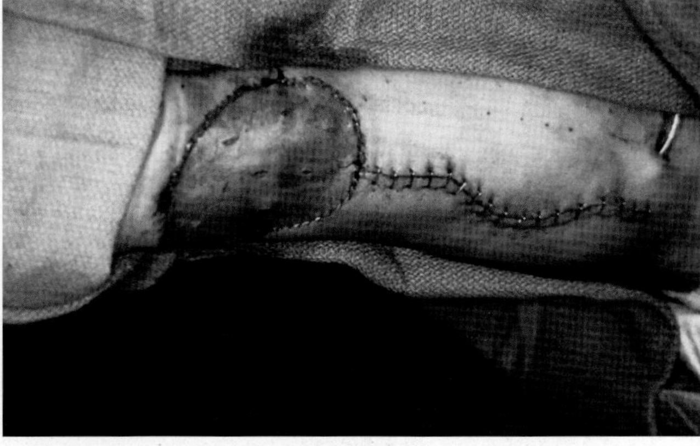

Fig. 57.5 The donor site closed with a split-thickness skin graft covering the original location of the skin paddle. Note the closed suction drain. A pressure dressing and dorsal splint fashioned with the hand in extension is placed at the end of closure to promote success of this graft.

The disadvantages of the flap are related to donor site morbidity. The most devastating complication is hand ischemia following sacrifice of the radial artery. Fortunately, it is exceptionally rare in the setting of a normal Allen's test.[30] The appearance of the harvest site after skin graft closure is less than cosmetically appealing. Local flap and tissue expanders have been used, but the overall benefit is limited.[31,32] Exposure of the forearm tendons and decreased hand function have been reported.[33] However overall wrist range of motion, grip strength, and sensation over the radial, ulnar, and median distribution mirror that of patients who have not undergone radial forearm free tissue transfer. Finally, the risk of pathological fracture after harvest of radial bone is significant, with reported rates as high as 43%.[34]

Lateral Arm Free Flap

Song et al introduced the lateral arm free flap in 1982.[35] This versatile flap can be harvested in either a fascial or fasciocutaneous manner. A segment of humeral bone (1 × 10 cm) two cutaneous nerves, and a portion of the triceps muscle can be included in the harvest to enhance reconstruction The unique feature of the lateral arm free flap is the variability of skin thickness within a single paddle. This variability allows for tongue base reconstruction with the thicker proximal skin, and lateral pharyngeal wall reconstruction with the thinner, distal skin.[36]

Anatomy

The lateral arm flap is based on the posterior radial collateral artery, which arises as a terminal branch from the deep brachial artery. The posterior radial collateral artery is found in the lateral intermuscular septum between the brachioradialis and the triceps muscle. The septum can be

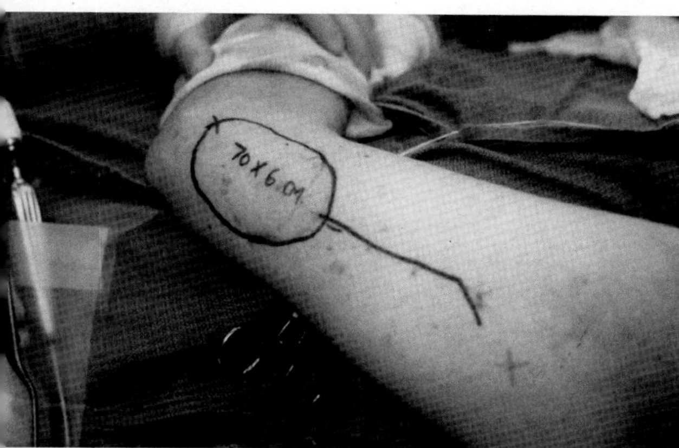

ig. 57.7 Proposed incisions for a lateral arm free flap. The incision rom the flap superiorly to the deltoid insertion is shown. The back-cut s used to facilitate pedicle exposure.

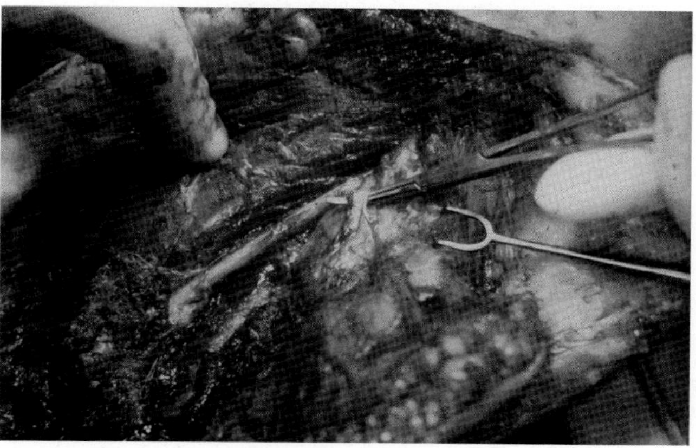

Fig. 57.8 Neural dissection during lateral arm flap elevation. The radial nerve is easily identified. The clamp is located under the posterior cutaneous nerve of the arm, which branches from the radial nerve and provides sensory innervation to the flap.

pproximated by a line drawn from the deltoid insertion o the lateral epicondyle. The skin paddle for the flap is entered over the lateral intermuscular septum in the disal third of the arm (**Fig. 57.7**). Many authors recommend imiting the cutaneous paddle to one third the width of he circumference of the arm (~6 cm). However, the vasular territory extends into the upper forearm, and, subtantially, larger paddles can be safely harvested.[37] This xtension is necessary if variability in skin thickness is reuired for reconstruction. Perforators from the artery give lood supply to the triceps and the periosteum overlying he humerus. This allows for composite transfer with he triceps, providing additional bulk, and the humerus roviding bone stock.

Similar to the radial forearm free flap, the lateral arm as a dual venous drainage. The deep venous system onsists of paired venae comitantes which typically join n the proximal arm to form one common deep system. he superficial venous system consists of branches of the ephalic vein. Although either venous system can be used or free transfer, the deep system alone is utilized with reater frequency.[38]

Three nerves should be identified during the lateral rm harvest. The radial nerve is the largest and travls with the profunda brachii in the spiral groove of the umerus. It then pierces the lateral intermuscular septum o run the length of the arm. The radial nerve provides two ranches that can be used in reconstruction. The posterior utaneous nerve of the arm supplies cutaneous sensation o the skin paddle and surrounding tissue, whereas the osterior cutaneous nerve to the forearm accompanies he pedicle and provides more distal sensation to the orearm (**Fig. 57.8**). Because of the close proximity of the osterior cutaneous nerve of the forearm to the vascular edicle, this nerve can be harvested as a vascularized erve graft.

Surgical Technique

The lateral arm flap can be harvested simultaneously during the head and neck extirpation. A tourniquet can be used but is rarely necessary. Elevation proceeds from either the anterior or posterior limb of the incision. Below the epicondyle, the plane of dissection is superficial to the fascia. Above the epicondyle, dissection proceeds in the subfascial plane over the brachioradialis and brachialis muscles until the intermuscular septum is encountered. Fibers of the brachioradialis originate from the septum itself and must be separated to facilitate identification of the radial nerve, posterior cutaneous nerves, and the vascular pedicle. The approach from the posterior incision is in the subfascial plane overlying the triceps muscle until the intermuscular septum is once again identified. Unlike the brachioradialis, the triceps muscle does not originate from the septum. For this reason we prefer to complete the posterior dissection first because these tissues are less adherent to the septum and underlying vasculature. The pedicle is identified adjacent to the humerus. To maximize vessel caliber and length, the pedicle is traced with the accompanying radial nerve in the spiral groove to its junction with the deep brachial artery and vein (**Fig. 57.9**). Usually the two venae comitantes will join to form a single venous system prior to joining the brachial vein. The lateral head of the triceps is released from its humeral attachment to facilitate this portion of the dissection. The harvest is completed by mobilizing the radial nerve away from the pedicle and transecting the posterior cutaneous nerves.

It is advisable to close the donor site by approximating the brachioradialis and triceps muscles to cover and protect the radial nerve. A closed suction drain is place. After wide undermining, the defect can usually be closed primarily. On rare occasion, a split-thickness skin graft may be required.

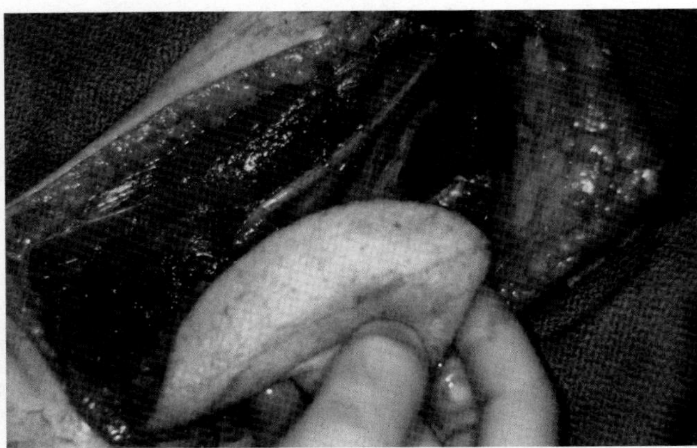

Fig. 57.9 The lateral arm flap elevated, showing its thinness. The vascular pedicle lies in the spiral groove.

Advantages and Disadvantages

The lateral arm free flap represents a supple, fasciocutaneous flap with the potential for reinnervation. The overall skin thickness is greater than a radial forearm, but not as bulky as scapular or parascapular skin. The two major advantages of the lateral arm flap are (1) variable skin thickness of the paddle for reconstructing tongue and pharyngeal wall defects simultaneously and (2) a nonessential vascular pedicle that is a terminal branch of the brachial artery. Therefore, sacrifice of the posterior radial collateral artery during flap harvest has no effect on upper extremity or hand viability. Graham et al reviewed their series of 123 lateral arm free flaps.[39] Principle disadvantages included hair growth at the recipient site (78%), lateral arm numbness (59%), donor site appearance (27%), and elbow pain (19%).

Lateral Thigh Free Flap

The lateral thigh free flap is a fasciocutaneous flap originally introduced by Baek in 1983,[40] and subsequently popularized by Hayden.[41] This flap is similar to both the radial forearm and lateral arm free flaps in that there are a multitude of reconstructive applications. The thickness of the flap is directly related to patient habitus and must be taken into consideration during flap selection. Thin flaps are used in situations analogous to those fitting for a radial forearm free flap, and they can even be used in a tubed fashion to reconstruct long pharyngoesophageal defects. Thicker flaps can be used for total glossectomy reconstruction.

Anatomy

The lateral thigh free flap is a fasciocutaneous flap based on a cutaneous perforator of the profunda femoris. The profunda femoris artery, also termed the *deep femoral artery*, originates from the femoral artery several centimeters inferior to the inguinal ligament. As the profunda femoris courses through the posterior compartment it gives rise to anywhere between two to six perforators. Most often there are four perforators, with the dominant blood supply to the lateral thigh being the third perforator. Each perforator provides muscular branches, a fasciocutaneous branch, as well as branches that anastomose with the adjacent perforators. The first perforator gives off a large muscular branch that serves as the primary blood supply to the adductor musculature. The second perforator provides the critical nutrient artery to the femur. As mentioned above, the third perforator is most frequently the dominant blood supply to the flap. The fourth perforator is commonly the terminal branch of the profunda femoris. In 15% of cases, the third perforator will not be the dominant vessel. For this reason, Hayden advised inclusion of the fourth perforator in all harvests.[4] In the rare event that the second perforator is found to be the dominant blood supply, it is imperative to terminate pedicle dissection at the takeoff of the muscular branches to preserve the vascular supply of the femur.

The fasciocutaneous branches from these perforators travel through the intermuscular septum between the vastus lateralis and biceps femoris en route to the skin. This septum can be approximated by drawing a line from the greater trochanter to the lateral femoral epicondyle. In thin individuals, the location is palpable. Miller et al demonstrated that the third perforator exits 14.5 ± 3.5 cm superior to the lateral epicondyle.[42] This site typically corresponds to the halfway point between the greater trochanter and the lateral epicondyle. The venous drainage of the lateral thigh free flap is via paired venae comitantes that travel adjacent to the arteries. The venae comitantes usually form a common vein prior to joining the profunda femoris vein.

The skin paddle is based around the midpoint of the intermuscular septum, with the long axis paralleling the septum. Skin flaps up to 27 × 14 cm have been described.[43] The thickness of the flap will vary with body habitus. Sensory innervation of the paddle is provided by the lateral femoral cutaneous nerve. To harvest a sensate flap, an additional incision over the sartorius muscle is made to allow for identification of the main nerve trunk prior to arborization over the lateral thigh.

Surgical Technique

The lateral thigh free flap is harvested with the patient supine, knee flexed, and lower extremity rotated medially for adequate exposure of the lateral thigh. This position allows simultaneous flap harvest and tumor extirpation. The greater trochanter and lateral femoral epicondyle are marked. A fusiform skin paddle is centered along a line lrawn between these two landmarks. This line represents he anticipated course of the intermuscular septum and he midpoint approximates the location of the third asciocutaneous perforator.

The anterior incision is brought down to the level of he iliotibial tract and fascia overlying the vastus lateralis. Dissection proceeds toward the intermuscular septum in his suprafascial plane. Upon identification of a perforaor, it is traced proximally through the short head of the biceps femoris. Significant branches to the muscle must be identified, and a small portion of the muscle itself can be ncluded in the flap if composite tissue is required. The pedicle is traced to the adductor fascia where the third perforator will travel through the semilunar hiatus of he adductor magnus muscle. To obtain adequate pedicle ength and larger caliber vessels, the adductor attachnents are released from the linea aspera of the femur, and the profunda is traced proximally to the origin of the econd perforator. The pedicle is ligated just distal to this point to preserve the femoral vasculature. Upon compleion of the pedicle dissection, the posterior aspect of the lap is elevated. This dissection remains superficial to the biceps femoris fascia. The posterior dissection is reserved as the last step to minimize vascular shearing during dissection and to provide oxygen to the skin paddle during he majority of the harvest.[43]

The donor site is closed by reapproximating the biceps emoris and iliotibial tract. A closed suction drain is placed. Wide undermining usually allows for primary closure; f necessary, a split-thickness skin graft can be used.

Advantages and Disadvantages

The principle advantage of the lateral thigh flap is the mount of tissue available from a single donor site. The arge surface area, bulk, and pliability of tissue allow for variety of reconstructive applications. The flap provides long pedicle. When primary closure of the defect is posible, donor site morbidity is quite low, with a linear scar occurring along the lateral leg.

The disadvantages of this flap are primarily related to he harvest. There is anatomical variability with respect o the perforators that can make the harvest considerably hallenging. The blood supply to the femur can be at risk f the second perforator is the dominant vessel harvested with the free flap.

Anterolateral Thigh Flap

The anterolateral thigh flap was first reported in 1984 by Song et al[44] as a septocutaneous perforator flap. More ecent clinical applications describe its use as a subcutaneous, fasciocutaneous, myocutaneous, and adipofascial lap depending upon the individual thickness of the soft tissue defect.[44–50] For this reason, the anterolateral thigh is considered a versatile flap for head and neck reconstruction, often being utilized for tongue, laryngopharyngeal, oropharyngeal, maxillary, and external soft tissue defects.

Anatomy

The anterolateral thigh flap is most often supplied by perforating vessels arising from the descending branch of the lateral circumflex femoral artery.[44,46] This branch travels inferiorly within the intermuscular space bound by the rectus femoris and the vastus lateralis muscles. During its descent in the midportion of the lateral thigh, the descending branch provides several perforators to the overlying skin. These perforators travel one of two possible routes. They follow a course between the rectus femoris and vastus lateralis to traverse the fascia lata as septocutaneous perforators supplying the skin of the lateral thigh. Alternatively, the vessels traverse the vastus lateralis muscle and the deep fascia as musculocutaneous perforators to supply the skin.[50] In this latter setting, there are two variations from which the musculocutaneous perforators may arise. The first variation is the vertical musculocutaneous perforators. Similar to the septocutaneous perforators, these vessels arise from the descending branch of the lateral circumflex femoral artery. They then pass through the vastus lateralis perpendicularly and into the fascia lata before supplying the subdermal tissue and skin. The second variation is the horizontal musculocutaneous perforators that pass through the vastus lateralis muscle in a horizontal fashion, after arising from the transverse branch of the lateral circumflex artery. In a series of 28 anterolateral thigh flaps by Yildirim et al, the blood supply to the anterior lateral thigh flap was via septocutaneous perforators in 10% of cases, musculocutaneous perforators from the descending branch in 89% of cases, and musculocutaneous perforators from the transverse branch in only 4% of cases.[51] Ultimately, the exit point of the septocutaneous and musculocutaneous perforators is located ~2 cm lateral and 2 cm inferior to the midpoint of a line joining the anterior superior iliac spine and the lateral border of the patella.[47] The venous drainage system to the anterolateral thigh flap parallels that of the arterial supply.

The lateral femoral cutaneous nerve is the dominant sensory nerve for this flap. It is a direct branch of the lumbar plexus and enters the thigh deep to the lateral aspect of the inguinal ligament, near the anterior superior iliac spine. It follows the path of the deep circumflex iliac artery and vein, running anterior, posterior, or through the sartorius muscle and continuing through the fascia lata, where it divides to emerge on the anterolateral thigh as multiple small branches.[47]

The maximum size of the anterolateral thigh flap originally described by Song et al extended from a horizontal line at the level of the greater trochanter down to a parallel line 3 cm above the patella, spanning the anterior and lateral aspect of the thigh.[44] More recent descriptions reported skin paddles measuring up to 20 × 26 cm.[51]

Surgical Technique

The anterolateral thigh free flap is harvested in the supine position, allowing for a two-team surgical approach. The intermuscular septum between the rectus femoris and vastus lateralis muscles is estimated by drawing a line between the anterior superior iliac spine and lateral border of the patella. Using the midpoint of this line as a landmark, the skin perforators are identified with a Doppler. Dissection begins along the medial aspect of the skin paddle. If a thicker, fasciocutaneous flap is planned, dissection is brought down through the fascia of the rectus femoris and subfascial dissection proceeds laterally until the major perforators to the skin are identified. Conversely, if a thinner, cutaneous flap is desired, the skin incision is brought down through the underlying subcutaneous tissue and dissection proceeds in the suprafascial plane toward the intermuscular septum. The cutaneous flap can be elevated as thin as 5 mm, although excessive thinning should be avoided to prevent marginal necrosis.[48] In both harvests, the remaining skin incisions are then completed, and subfascial dissection proceeds toward the intermuscular septum. The rectus femoris muscle is retracted medially to allow exploration of the intermuscular space and identification of either septocutaneous or musculocutaneous perforators. The pedicle is carefully dissected in a retrograde fashion either to the descending branch in the case of septocutaneous perforators or through the vastus lateralis muscle in patients with myocutaneous perforators. In the later setting, a small cuff of muscle should be left surrounding the pedicle. The lateral femoral cutaneous nerve to the thigh can be incorporated into this harvest if sensory reinnervation is desired. Lastly, if an adipofascial flap is desired, the methods of harvest are similar to the conventional subfascial method outline above, except that only the adipofascial layer, without the cutaneous portion, is elevated.[52,53] If the skin-paddle width measures less the 8 cm, the donor site can be closed primarily. Otherwise, a split-thickness skin graft is recommended.

Advantages and Disadvantages

The anterolateral thigh flap provides great versatility in terms of it potential size as well as its use as a subcutaneous, fasciocutaneous, myocutaneous, or adipofascial flap. The flap provides a long vascular pedicle measuring more than 16 cm in length, large caliber vessels, and a large, reliable skin paddle. An additional advantage is the ability to harvest this flap simultaneously during tumor extirpation. With respect to disadvantages, the donor site morbidity is minimal. Kimata et al demonstrated that the morbidity is dependent on the extent of vastus lateralis injury and the need for a split-thickness skin graft closure.[54] The vascular anatomy of the anterolateral thigh free flap is variable, and dissection of the perforators can be technically challenging. In addition, the flap can be bulky in a patient with excessive subcutaneous fat secondary to obesity. In this setting, an alternative flap should be used because a large body habitus leads to a technically challenging harvest, as well as a high risk of postoperative dysphagia. Lastly, patients who have undergone previous upper thigh surgery, including major vascular bypass procedures, are not candidates for this flap.[55]

Superficial Temporal Parietal Fascia Flap

The superficial temporal parietal fascia flap (STPFF) is a thin pliable flap used in head and neck reconstruction. Although the fascia flap is usually utilized as a pedicled flap, it can be transferred as free tissue to reconstruct sites such as the oral cavity, skull base, and auricle. This flap is exceptionally versatile, with the ability to transfer overlying hair-bearing tissue from the scalp, split-thickness calvarial bone grafts, and cartilage from the helical root.[56] It also provides a vascularized bed for the use of split-thickness skin grafts.

Anatomy

The superficial temporal parietal fascia (STPF) is located immediately beneath the skin and subcutaneous tissues. It is an extension of the superficial musculoaponeurotic system. Above the superior temporal line it is contiguous with the galea aponeurosis. A loose layer of areolar tissue separates the STPF from the underlying deep temporal fascia (DTF) (**Fig. 57.10**). The DTF splits into a deep and superficial layer to envelop the temporalis muscle, both of which attach inferiorly to the zygomatic arch.

The superficial temporal artery and vein supply the SPTF. The artery is the terminal branch of the external carotid artery, which takes a tortuous path through the parotid gland before arborizing over the lateral scalp. The artery has three main branches. The first branch is the middle temporal artery, which is located approximately at the level of the zygomatic arch and provides blood to the DTF. More superiorly, at the level of the helical root, the superficial temporal artery branches into an anterior frontal branch and a posterior parietal branch. Safe dissection can precede ~3 to 4 cm along the frontal branch before there is significant risk to the temporal branch of the facial nerve, which courses 1 to 1.5 cm posterior to the lateral orbital

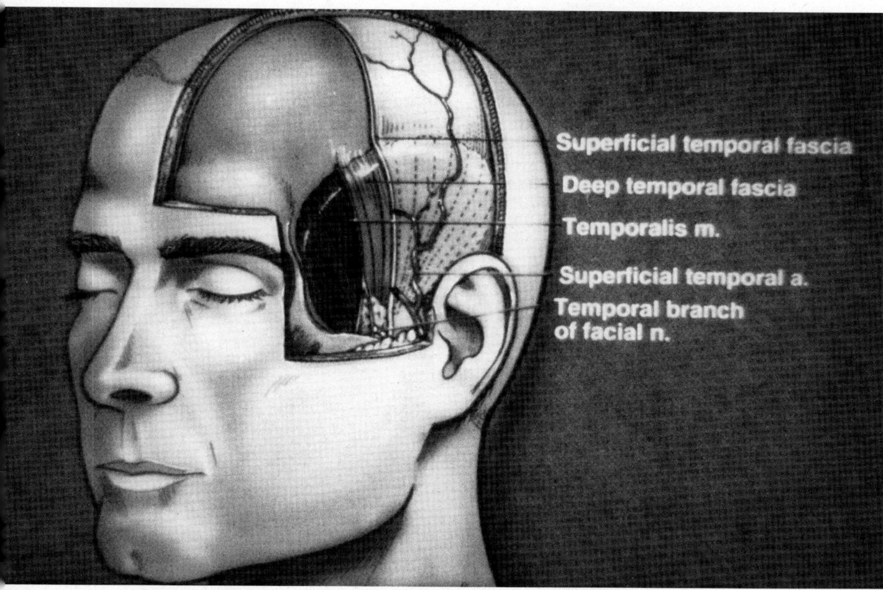

Fig. 57.10 Layers of the scalp and infratemporal fossa. Understanding this relationship is vital to the successful elevation of the superficial temporal parietal fascia flap.

im. The parietal branch provides the major blood supply f this flap. The artery runs within the fascia, whereas the ccompanying veins lie superficial to the fascia. Successful issection can yield a flap measuring up to 14 × 17 cm in urface area, and a thickness ranging from 2 to 4 mm.[57]

urgical Technique

he STPFF is harvested with the patient in the supine poition. A preauricular incision extends superiorly into the calp. The skin is elevated in a plane just beneath the hair ollicles and subcutaneous tissue to prevent injury to the nderlying venous drainage system. Electrocautery is disouraged because of the potential for alopecia. After skin levation, the pedicle is identified proximally and protected. he fascia flap is incised according to the desired size and levated off of the DTF (**Fig. 57.11**). Primary closure of the onor site is almost always possible. Closed suction drains nd a pressure dressing help to prevent seroma formation.

dvantages and Disadvantages

he STPFF is a thin, pliable, yet durable flap that can be harested solely as a fascia flap or as a composite flap. Disadantages include the potential for donor site alopecia.[58] The emporal branch of the facial nerve is at risk during harvest. astly, the superficial temporal vein travels along a superfiial course, making it vulnerable to damage during harvest.

lyocutaneous and Enteric Flaps

ectus Myocutaneous Free Flap

ennington and Pelly are responsible for first introducing he rectus myocutaneous free flap transferred on the deep inferior epigastric vessels.[59] This free flap can be transferred as a myocutaneous, myofascial, myogenous, or myosubcutaneous flap. Within the head and neck region, it is commonly used to reconstruct the skull base, oral cavity, and cutaneous/soft tissue defects.

Anatomy

The rectus free flap is supplied by two dominant vascular pedicles: the deep inferior and deep superior epigastric

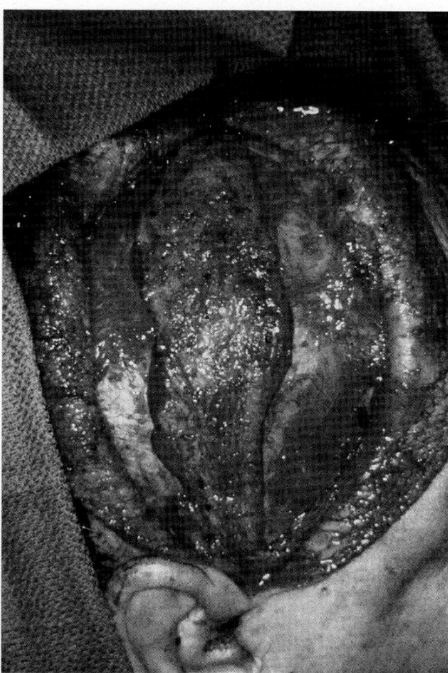

Fig. 57.11 The superficial temporal parietal fascia flap raised. Note the thinness of the flap and the length from the root of the helix to the vertex.

arteries that anastomose through a series of choke vessels surrounding the umbilicus. The deep inferior epigastric vessels are utilized more often due in part to larger vessel caliber and the tendency to supply a wider distribution of subcutaneous tissue.[60] The deep inferior epigastric artery is a branch of the external iliac artery. It travels cephalad, penetrating the transversalis fascia 3 to 4 cm caudal to the arcuate line, where it then crosses the rectus muscle transversely, giving off perforators to the muscle itself and overlying skin. In the region of the umbilicus, the deep inferior epigastric arteries anastomose with the deep superior epigastric vessels, intercostals, lumbar and deep groin vessels bilaterally. This vascular rich area contains a significant number of musculocutaneous perforators. The venous drainage usually consists of two venae comitantes, which parallel the arterial inflow and join to form a single vein before reaching the external iliac vein.

The numerous periumbilical perforators allow the skin paddle to be oriented in several ways over the rectus muscle. Ultimately, the anatomical defect dictates the design of the flap. Vascular studies demonstrated that the skin overlying both the ipsilateral rectus muscle, as well as skin lateral to the linea semilunaris can safely be harvested on the deep inferior epigastric artery.[60] Because of the rich, watershed area surrounding the umbilicus, the contralateral skin can also reliably be used.

Both sensory and motor function is provided to this region by segmental intercostal nerves. To date, a reliable technique for reinnervation of the rectus myocutaneous flap has not been described.[61]

Surgical Technique

This flap is harvested with the patient in the supine position, allowing for a two-team approach. The desired skin paddle is outlined over the rectus muscle. As mentioned above, there are a variety of possible designs depending on the amount of tissue required for reconstruction as well as the patient's habitus. To achieve a thinner flap, the skin paddle should be designed in an oblique fashion, at a 45-degree angle toward the scapula tip (**Fig. 57.12**).[62,63] Alternatively, a transverse skin paddle can be fashioned above or below the umbilicus, an extended flap can incorporate the contralateral periumbilical region, or a longitudinal skin paddle can be designed along the entire course of the rectus muscle. Regardless of exact orientation, the paddle should be centered at the level of the umbilicus to incorporate the dominant periumbilical perforators of this region. The arcuate line runs at approximately the level of the anterior superior iliac spine. Below this line, the aponeurotic layers of the external oblique, internal oblique, and transversus abdominis muscles all converge to form the anterior

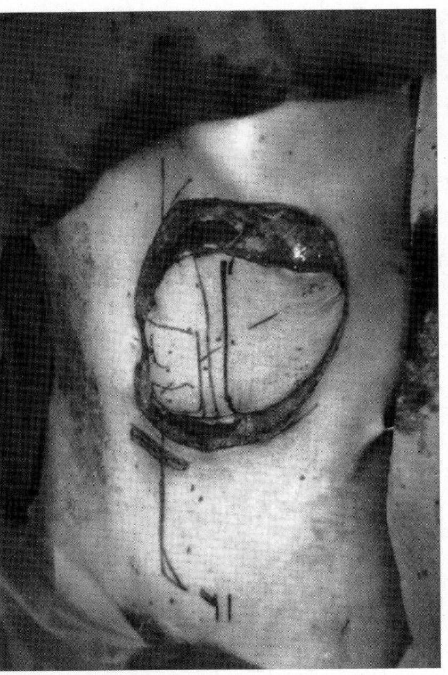

Fig. 57.12 Incisions for the rectus myocutaneous free flap. The fla is based on the paraumbilical perforators and extends at a 45-degre angle toward the tip of the scapula.

rectus sheath. This leaves a thin posterior rectus sheat consisting only of the transversalis fascia. For this reaso the anterior rectus sheath should not be harvested cauda to the arcuate line.[62]

Elevation begins along the lateral aspect of the ski paddle, in a plane just superficial to the fascia of th external oblique muscle. Dissection proceeds mediall with care. At approximately the level of the linea semilunaris, musculocutaneous perforators can be identifie To preserve these vessels, the fascia is incised lateral t these perforators. Dissection continues along the superior border of the skin paddle where the desired cuff c rectus muscle is incorporated (**Fig. 57.13**). The medi dissection is once again performed in the suprafasci plane above the anterior rectus sheath. The fascia an underlying muscle is then incised, usually lateral to th linea alba. In doing so, a small remnant of fascia is le to facilitate closure. During the ensuing elevation of th rectus muscle off of the posterior sheath, it is critical t maintain the integrity of the posterior fascia to preven disruption of the abdominal wall and postoperative herni formation. At the level of the arcuate line, the dee inferior epigastric vessels are identified and traced to th external iliac vessels to obtain adequate pedicle lengt To obtain adequate exposure for pedicle dissectio the anterior rectus fascia below the level of the arcuat line is incised vertically. The insertion of the rectus musc onto the pubic bone is then divided, and the flap is read for transfer (**Fig. 57.14**).

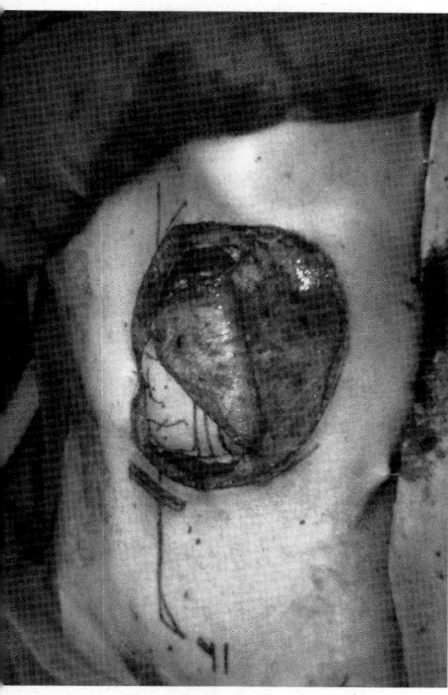

Fig. 57.13 The rectus flap is raised laterally to medially off of the external oblique muscle until the rectus fascia is encountered, at which point the fascia is divided and the muscle is elevated.

Wide undermining is required to close the donor site. It is critical that the anterior rectus fascia is carefully closed below the arcuate line to prevent postoperative hernia. If possible, the anterior rectus fascia is closed

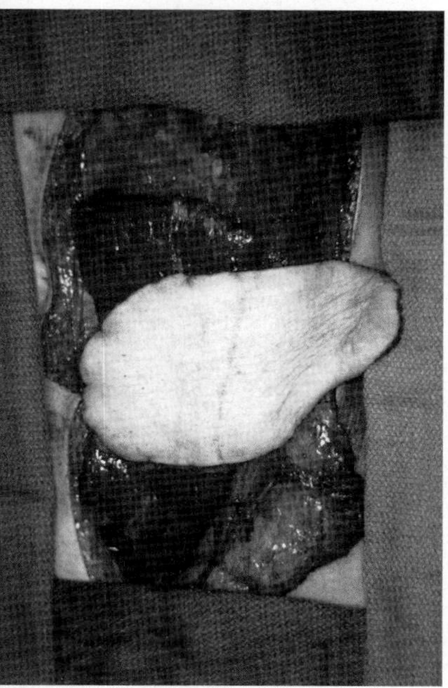

Fig. 57.14 The rectus muscle is divided superiorly and elevated inferiorly to the pubis. The muscle is divided at the pubic attachment, and the pedicle is dissected proximately. Note the large skin paddle.

above the arcuate line. Closed suction drains are place, and the skin is closed primarily with the aid of wide undermining.

Advantages and Disadvantages

The advantages of the rectus myocutaneous free flap include a long pedicle, the variety of composite tissue types that can be transferred, and the two-team surgical approach. Unfortunately, the tissue bulk in most patients relegates use of the rectus flap to large defects, where mobility of the surrounding tissue is not critical to the reconstruction. The most common complications are abdominal wall hernia, wound dehiscence, and infection. These complications can be minimized with attention to detail during flap design and donor site closure.

Latissimus Dorsi Free Flap

The latissimus dorsi free flap was introduced by Baudet in 1976, nearly 80 years after the first description of the pedicled latissimus flap.[64] The flap provides a large source of skin and soft tissue for head and neck reconstruction. The principal use of the flap is skull base and large soft tissue defects. Motor reinnervation has made this flap useful in the repair of total glossectomy reconstruction. The latissimus flap can also be incorporated with the subscapular system to produce the megaflap, which is useful in the setting of large defects.

Anatomy

The latissimus dorsi muscle is large, fan-shaped, and occupies the majority of the lower back. The muscular origin is broadly across the back, including the external oblique, serratus anterior and teres major musculature, the lower six thoracic vertebrae, the lower four ribs, and the fascia attaching to the lumbar and sacral vertebrae and the iliac crest. The muscle converges laterally over the scapular tip to insert onto the medial surface of the humerus. In the process of doing so, the tendon of the latissimus dorsi and the teres major muscle form the posterior axillary fold. The skin paddle can be placed in a variety of locations across the large muscle. The size of the paddle is usually limited by the ability to obtain primary closure.

Two vascular pedicles are associated with the flap. The primary pedicle is the thoracodorsal artery and vein; the secondary pedicle consists of perforators from the intercostal vessels. Free transfer of the musculocutaneous flap is based on the thoracodorsal artery and vein. The thoracodorsal artery is a branch of the subscapular artery, which in turn branches from the third portion of the axillary artery. The pedicle can be traced to the origin of the subscapular system to obtain a larger diameter artery (3 to 4 mm) and vein (3.5 to 4.5 mm), as well as additional pedicle length. In doing so, the circumflex scapular artery (CSA) is sacrificed unless a megaflap is planned, in which case the CSA is incorporated into the harvest as a means to supply the scapular free tissue. In 85% of cases, the thoracodorsal artery terminates into the latissimus dorsi by dividing into a medial and superior branch, which allows for separate skin paddles.[65] Venous outflow parallels the course of the thoracodorsal artery.

Both motor and sensory reinnervation of the latissimus dorsi muscle have successfully been performed.[66,67] The thoracodorsal nerve provides motor innervation of this flap. This nerve is a branch from the posterior cord of the brachial plexus. The nerve parallels the course of the vascular pedicle. The sensory innervation is via the segmental, cutaneous branches of the intercostal nerves.

Surgical Technique

Important landmarks for harvesting the latissimus dorsi free flap include the midpoint of the axilla, the anterior superior iliac spine, the posterior superior iliac spine, and the tip of the scapula. The anterior border of the latissimus muscle is estimated by a vertical line dropped from the midpoint of the axilla through the midpoint of a line joining the anterior and posterior superior iliac spines. The pedicle usually enters the undersurface of the muscle 8 to 10 cm below the level of the midaxilla. The skin paddle is centered vertically over the midportion of the muscle because the distal aspect of the muscle is less reliable (**Fig. 57.15**).[68]

The posterior incision is first brought down to the level of the muscle. The volume of muscle harvested is ultimately dependent on reconstructive needs and can include the entire muscle as well as a portion of the thoracolumbar fascia. The muscle is released from its origin and elevated using a combination of sharp and blunt dissection. The anterior incision is made in a similar fashion. As the dissection proceeds superiorly along the anterior boarder, the pedicle must be identified entering the muscle. This dissection can be accomplished by gently spreading the axillary fat along the border of the muscle. Frequently, the first vessels identified are branches to the serratus anterior muscle, which can be traced proximately to their origin from the thoracodorsal artery. Ultimately, these branches are ligated to mobilize the flap. With the pedicle identified and protected, the humeral insertion of the latissimus dorsi can safely be released. The final aspect of flap harvest requires defining the pedicle proximately toward the axillary system until adequate length and vessel caliber is achieved. Wide undermining is used to primary close the donor site.

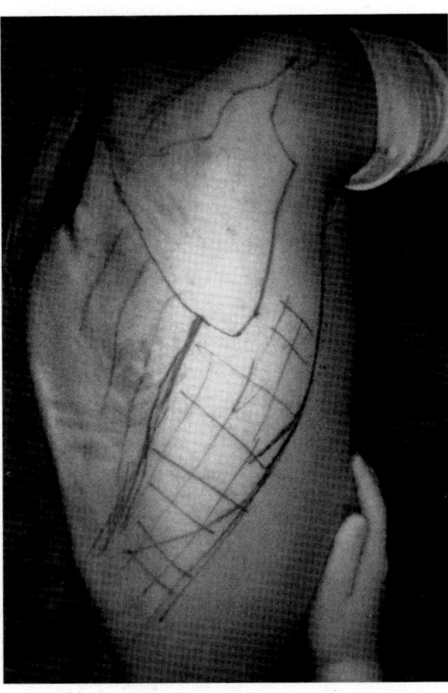

Fig. 57.15 The marked area represents the most common location of the skin paddle for the latissimus dorsi free flap. Note the scapula outlined as a reference.

Advantages and Disadvantages

The latissimus dorsi muscle provides a large amount of musculocutaneous tissue for reconstruction. Advantages include long pedicle length as well as larger vessel caliber. The primary disadvantage is muscle location, which requires lateral decubitus positioning. For this reason, it is extremely difficult to simultaneously complete both the tumor extirpation and flap harvest. Other disadvantages include decreased arm function following muscle sacrifice, possible injury to the long thoracic nerve, and the potential for brachial plexus injury.

Free Jejunal Flap

Seidenberg and colleagues introduced the free jejunal flap in 1958.[69] Subsequently, the flap has become a standard option for hypopharyngeal reconstruction. The flap is ideal for circumferential defects of the hypopharynx and cervical esophagus, as well as incomplete defects requiring a patch graft.

Anatomy

The jejunum is a portion of the small intestine bound by the duodenum and the ligament of Treitz. The blood supply is via segmental jejunal arterial arcades from the superior mesenteric artery. Typically, the second loop of jejunum provides an adequate 15- to 25-cm segment ased on a single artery. The artery ranges from 1 to 5 mm n diameter, whereas the vein ranges from 2 to 4 mm in liameter. The nervous supply to the bowel is intrinsic, nd contraction of the bowel resumes upon revasculari-ation of the flap.

urgical Technique

he jejunal free flap can be harvested with a two-team pproach. At our institution the general surgery depart-nent is in charge of the flap harvest. Traditionally the flap s harvested through a midline incision. Recently there as been increased interest in laparoscopic flap harvest,[70] vhich can decrease abdominal pain, recovery time, and norbidity associated with the harvest. Transillumina-ion of the bowel aids in identification of the vascular rcades. A gastrostomy and jejunostomy tube is often laced by the general surgeons to facilitate postoperative ehabilitation.

There are several key principles to the surgical tech-ique for jejunal free transfer. Once the jejunal free flap s disconnected, it is imperative to minimize bowel isch-mia. It is also critical that the harvesting surgeon marks he proximal end of the bowel to ensure isoperistaltic rientation within the head and neck. Although the size f the jejunum is a good match for that of the esophagus, lock-and-key configuration of the jejunoesophageal nastomosis should be used to minimize postoperative tricture. Finally, the flap must be fish-mouthed along he proximal antimesenteric border to allow for adequate pproximation with the pharynx while maintaining vas-ular integrity to the bowel.

Following revascularization, the flap becomes pink, eristaltic contractions begin, and mucus is released from ntestinal glands. Monitoring of the flap can easily be ccomplished by isolating a small segment of bowel utside the neck closure for direct visualization (**Fig. 57.16**).

dvantages and Disadvantages

he advantages of the jejunal free flap over more tradi-onal methods of total pharyngeal reconstruction include horter hospitalization, shorter time period to success-ıl oral alimentation, and lower incidence of fistula.[71] isadvantages include the morbidity associated with a ıparotomy, postoperative dysphagia secondary to bowel eristalsis, and poor vocal quality with tracheoesopha-eal puncture.[72] The most common abdominal compli-ations are dehiscence and gastrointestinal bleeding. he dysphagia can be improved by orienting the flap in an soperistaltic fashion, but a component will still exist due ɔ the lack of coordination between contractions of the ative tissue and the transferred bowel segment. The risk of a istal stricture can be minimized by using the lock-and-key

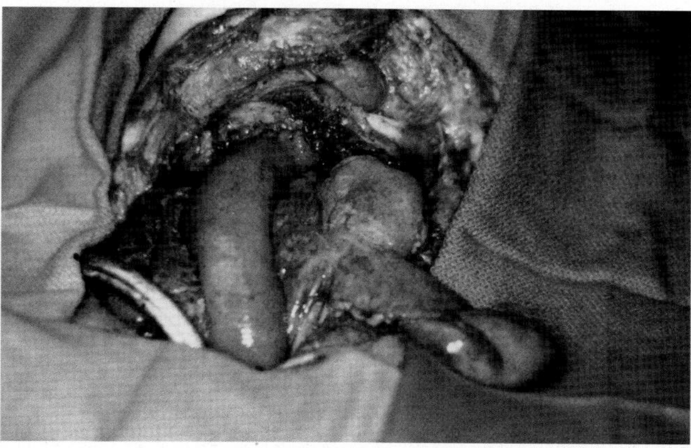

Fig. 57.16 The jejunal flap in place during reconstruction of a total laryngopharyngectomy defect. Note the segment of the jejunum to the right, which remains based on its mesentery, and is brought out to the neck for postoperative flap monitoring.

approach noted above. The poor voice quality is unavoid-able due to the jejunal mucosal folds and intrinsic mucus production. These features are responsible for the resulting "wet voice."

Bone Flaps Used in Head and Neck Reconstruction

Fibular Osteocutaneous Free Flap

The free transfer of the fibula was first proposed by Taylor et al.[73] Since its introduction in 1975, this flap has gained tremendous popularity and is now regarded as the workhorse for oromandibular reconstruction. The fibula provides a long bone segment (25 cm), long pedicle, and potential for skin flap sensation. With the use of ostecto-mies, the bone is readily contoured for use in mandible, palate, or midface reconstruction.

Anatomy

The fibula is the smaller of the two lower extremity bones and is non–weight bearing. It is necessary to preserve 6 to 8 cm of bone superiorly and inferiorly to protect the knee and ankle joints. In doing so, up to 25 cm of bone is still available for harvest. The average cross-sectional area is 90 mm^2.[74] This volume of bone is usually adequate for osseointegrated dental implants; however, a height discrepancy with the native mandibular bone will be present.[75]

The fibula free flap is based on the peroneal artery and accompanying venae comitantes that travel the length of the fibula between the flexor hallicus longus and poste-rior tibialis muscles. This artery arises from the posterior tibial artery, ~2 to 3 cm distal to the bifurcation of the popliteal artery. It provides a nutrient medullary branch to the fibula bone and segmental blood supply to the periosteum of the bone. This dual segmental and central blood supply allows for safe placement of multiple ostectomies (up to every 2 cm) when contouring bone.[76] On rare occasion, the peroneal artery will be the major vessel perfusing the foot or it can be completely absent.[77] For this reason we obtain preoperative lower extremity computed tomography arteriograms on all patients undergoing fibular free tissue transfer to ensure adequate three-vessel runoff to the foot. Other institutions utilize magnetic resonance angiography and color flow Doppler as alternatives to arteriography.[78]

The skin paddle is centered over the lateral intermuscular septum. This area is supplied by peroneal septocutaneous and musculocutaneous perforators, which tend to concentrate between the middle and distal thirds of the septum. If multiple perforators exist, the skin paddle can be divided to simultaneously resurface adjacent sites within the head and neck. Although the fibula skin paddle is deemed the least dependable of the osteocutaneous flaps, recent studies report a reliable skin paddle in 95% of all cases.[79] In addition to supplying the fibula and overlying skin, the peroneal artery also gives off muscular perforators that allow for the incorporation of a cuff of soleus and flexor hallicus longus into the harvest if bulk is needed in the reconstruction. The sensory input to the fibular flap is from the lateral sural cutaneous nerve, which is a branch of the common peroneal nerve.[80,81]

Surgical Technique

The harvest of the fibula free flap is performed with the patient in the supine position, with a slight bump under the hip to allow for internal rotation of the lower extremity. A two-team approach is quite feasible in this setting. Use of a tourniquet (350 mm Hg) during the harvest allows for bloodless dissection. The course of the lateral intermuscular septum is estimated by connecting a line from the posterior aspect of the lateral malleolus inferiorly to the posterior aspect of the fibular head superiorly (**Fig. 57.17**). A fusiform skin paddle is then centered over this septum, taking care to preserve 6 to 8 cm of bone inferiorly and superiorly to prevent injury to the ankle and knee joints respectively. A large skin paddle is recommended to capture the major septocutaneous perforators necessary for reliable transfer of the skin with the fibula.

First the posterior skin incision is brought down through the subcutaneous tissue and fascia of the gastrocnemius and soleus muscles. Elevation continues in the subfascial plane until the lateral border of the fibula and intermuscular septum are identified. Muscular perforators to the gastrocnemius are ligated in the process, and a small cuff of soleus should be preserved along the lateral

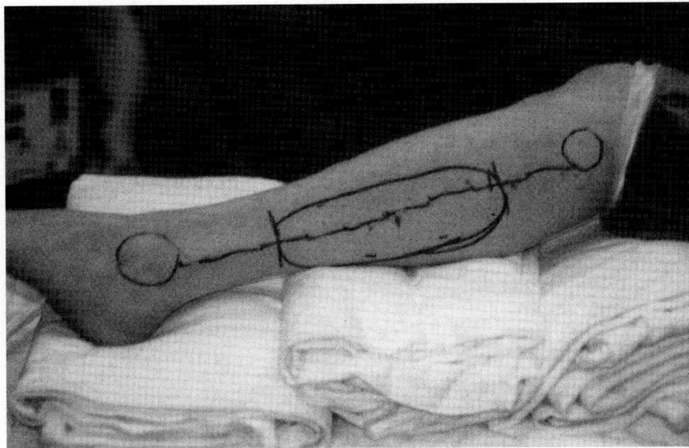

Fig. 57.17 Proposed incisions for a fibula osteocutaneous flap. Th flap is centered on a line connecting the posterior aspect of th lateral malleolus and the posterior aspect of the fibular head. A lon fusiform skin paddle is fashioned to include all possible perforators

border of the fibula. Septocutaneous perforators are care fully identified as they course through the septum t supply the overlying skin (**Fig. 57.18**). The approximat area of the perforators is marked on the overlying ski paddle for future reference. If necessary, the location o the skin paddle can be altered once these perforators a identified.

The anterior skin incision is then brought down throug skin, subcutaneous tissue, and the fascia of the peroneu longus and brevis muscles. Dissection proceeds fro anterior to posterior in the subfascial plane toward th intermuscular septum. Medial retraction of the pero-neu longus, peroneus brevis, and extensor hallicus longu reveals the contents of the anterior compartment, whic includes the anterior tibial artery, anterior tibial vein, an

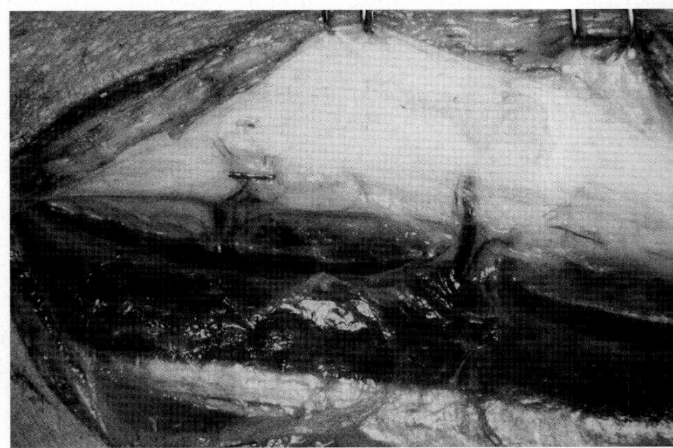

Fig. 57.18 Septocutaneous and myocutaneous perforators to the fi ula skin paddle that has been elevated over the soleus muscle towa the intermuscular septum. The left perforator is running in the septu alone as a fasciocutaneous perforator, whereas the right perforator coursing through the soleus as a musculocutaneous perforator.

deep peroneal nerve. As dissection continues along the medial fibular border, the interosseous septum is encountered and divided.

At the planned site of the proximal and distal osteotomies, gentle dissection is used to free the fibula bone completely from surrounding tissues. The fibula bone cuts are performed to allow distraction of the bone, which is necessary for safe pedicle dissection. The interosseous septum and underlying tibialis posterior muscle fibers are divided to allow identification of the peroneal artery and vein. The pedicle is ligated distally and traced superiorly to its origin at the posterior tibial artery. In the process of doing so, the flexor hallicus longus and soleus are released from the fibula with the pedicle under direct visualization. A cuff of each muscle can be harvested if additional bulk is required for the reconstruction. If the overlying skin paddle is supplied by musculocutaneous branches of the peroneal artery, it is imperative to harvest the associated muscle.

To increase pedicle length, a piece of fibula bone longer than the actual surgical defect is usually harvested. Once the free flap is disconnected, the surrounding soft tissue and associated pedicle is carefully stripped from the proximal portion of the harvested bone, which is not required for reconstruction. After completing an additional ostectomy, the surgeon is left with a distal portion of the fibula free flap matching the surgical defect and long pedicle.

The donor site can be closed primary if only a small skin paddle is harvested. In the majority of cases, a split-thickness skin graft will be required. Closed suction drainage is used, and a posterior splint is placed to immobilize the leg during the immediate postoperative period (6 days).

Advantages and Disadvantages

The fibula free flap provides the reconstructive surgeon with sufficient bone to address any defect (**Fig. 57.19**). It is unique in that it is only osteocutaneous flap that provides enough bone length to address subtotal and total mandibular defects. The bone stock is adequate to accept

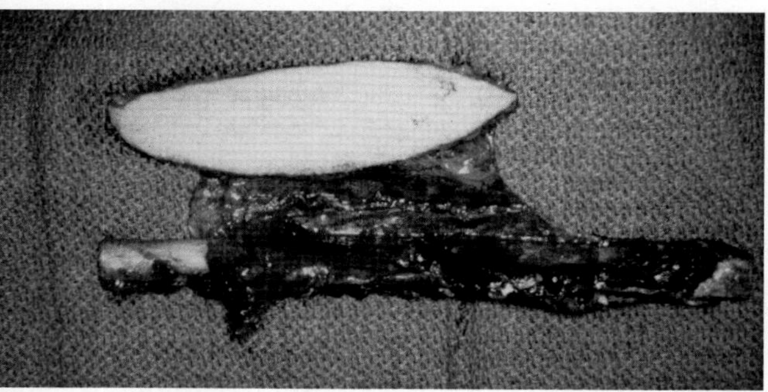

Fig. 57.19 The fibula osteocutaneous flap with its long sock of bone and attached skin paddle via the intermuscular septum.

osseointegrated implants. The skin paddle is reliable, with the ability for sensory reinnervation. An additional advantage is that the harvest can take place simultaneously during the extirpation. Disadvantages of the fibula free flap include postoperative weakness of great toe flexion, potential instability to the ankle, ankle pain and stiffness, the need for split-thickness skin graft closure of the donor site, the risk of foot ischemia due to peroneal artery sacrifice, and limited height of the fibula bone.

Scapula Free Flap

The scapula free flap was introduced for mandibular reconstruction by Swartz and colleagues in 1986[82] and remains the most versatile bone stock flap. The reconstructive surgeon has the ability to transfer up to three different skin paddles (scapular, parascapular, and latissimus), two muscles (latissimus dorsi and serratus anterior), and two bone segments (lateral scapular border and scapular tip), all on a single pedicle. This versatility allows for complex three-dimensional insetting of both bone and soft tissue. In addition, the scapula free flap provides large caliber vessels, a long pedicle, and a large skin surface area.

Anatomy

The lateral border of the scapula provides 10 cm of bone for transfer, and incorporation of the adjacent scapular tip provides an additional 4 cm. The cephalad extent of the harvest is limited by the glenohumeral joint. The lateral border is bicortical and thins toward the midline of the blade. Although vertical height is limited, up to 75% of cadaveric scapular bone samples supported osseointegrated implants.[79] The tip of the scapula provides an additional 4 cm of bone and is often used for reconstruction of the mandibular angle.

The CSA and vein compose the scapular free flap pedicle. The CSA is a branch of the subscapular artery, which originates along the distal third segment of the axillary artery. The CSA sends periosteal perforators to the lateral aspect of the scapular bone and terminates in two distinct cutaneous branches: the transverse branch supplying the scapular skin paddle and the descending branch supplying the parascapular skin paddle (**Fig. 57.20**). Conversely, the tip of the scapula is supplied by the angular artery, which is a branch of the thoracodorsal artery. The venous drainage parallels the arterial inflow.

As noted above, two separate skin paddles can be harvested based on the terminal, cutaneous, CSA branches. This skin is thicker than a radial forearm but thinner than rectus myocutaneous flap. The subcutaneous tissue can be harvested by itself as a vascularized fat graft. The segmental, intercostals cutaneous nerves, cervical plexus, and circumflex branch of the brachial plexus provide innervation to the skin.[83] However, the absence of a single,

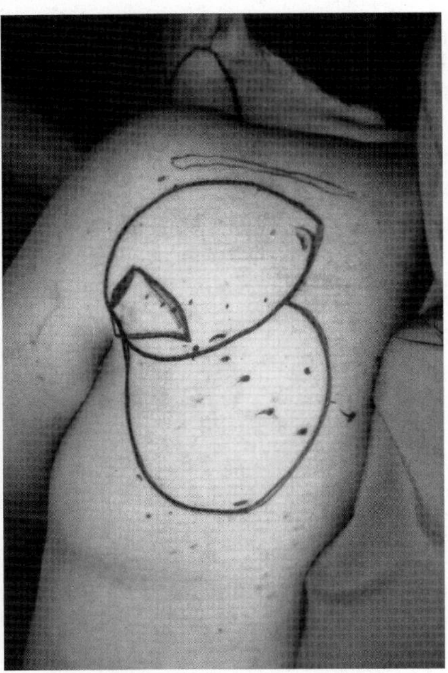

Fig. 57.20 The scapula skin paddle design for an osteocutaneous flap. Both the transverse scapular and longitudinal parascapular paddles are outlined around the triangular space.

dominant sensory nerve precludes reliable reinnervation of the scapular skin.

Surgical Technique

The scapula flap is harvested with the patient in the lateral decubitus position. To prevent injury to the brachial plexus, an axillary roll is carefully positioned such that a fist can fit superior to the roll, within the axilla itself. The arm of the donor side is prepped into the field for ease of manipulation during dissection. The triangular space, bound by the teres minor, teres major, and long head of the triceps, is the key body surface landmark. The circumflex scapular pedicle exits the triangle just prior to the takeoff of the terminal, cutaneous branches that supply the scapular skin (**Fig. 57.20**). Specifically, the transverse branch parallels the scapular spine, running ~2 cm inferiorly. The descending branch runs perpendicular to the spine, 2 cm medially to the lateral border of the scapula.[84] The two skin paddles can be harvested as two separate paddles, or as a large bilobed flap.

The harvest proceeds medial to lateral to avoid undue stress on the pedicle. The plane of dissection is superficial to the fascia of the infraspinatus musculature. The skin flap is elevated to the borders of the teres major and teres minor, where cutaneous branches of the CSA are found exiting the triangular space. The teres major muscle is divided along the lateral border of the scapula to expose the underlying bone. Care is taken to avoid exposing the underlying periosteum because perforators from the CSA enter in this region. The pedicle is traced proximally through the triangular space into the axilla. To incorporate the scapular tip into the harvest, care must be taken to preserve the thoracodorsal artery; otherwise, the vessel can be sacrificed to gain additional pedicle length. Upon completion of the pedicle dissection, a cutting saw is used to harvest the bone. An adequate superior bony margin must be preserved to avoid damage to the glenohumeral joint. Injury is avoided by placing the superior osteotomy below the long head of the triceps brachii muscle. The longitudinal bony cut that parallels the lateral scapula border must be made medial to the bony ridge to prevent injury to the pedicle. Prior to inset, ostectomies, with minimal periosteal elevation, are performed to contour the shape.

Closure of the donor site includes reapproximation of the teres major to the scapula. This goal can be accomplished by drilling holes through the remaining lateral bone and passing nonabsorbable sutures. With wide undermining, the skin can be closed primarily. Defects wider than 12 to 14 cm may require a split-thickness skin graft.[85] Normal restoration of preoperative arm and shoulder function requires intensive physical therapy, which we recommend beginning 3 days following surgery.

Advantages and Disadvantages

Advantages of the scapula free flap include diversity of flap design, abundant skin and soft tissue based on a single pedicle, as well as three-dimensional maneuverability of bone, skin, and muscle. The main disadvantage is surgical positioning, which makes a simultaneous, two-team surgical approach exceeding difficult. The bone stock is thin, especially in the central region of the scapula. Donor site morbidity is also a disadvantage but can be minimized with early, aggressive physical therapy.[86]

Iliac Crest–Internal Oblique Osteomyocutaneous Flap

The iliac crest osteocutaneous flap was first described by Taylor et al in 1979.[87] Ramasastry et al modified the harvest to include the internal oblique musculature,[88] and Urken et al popularized this modification for oromandibular reconstruction.[89] The iliac crest–internal oblique osteomyocutaneous flap plays a versatile role in head and neck reconstruction because it provides a large segment of naturally curved bone, a long pedicle, and both a muscle and skin paddle.

Anatomy

The iliac crest composes the superior aspect of the lateral pelvic girdle and provides a source of cancellous bone with a rich blood supply. Up to 16 cm of bone can be

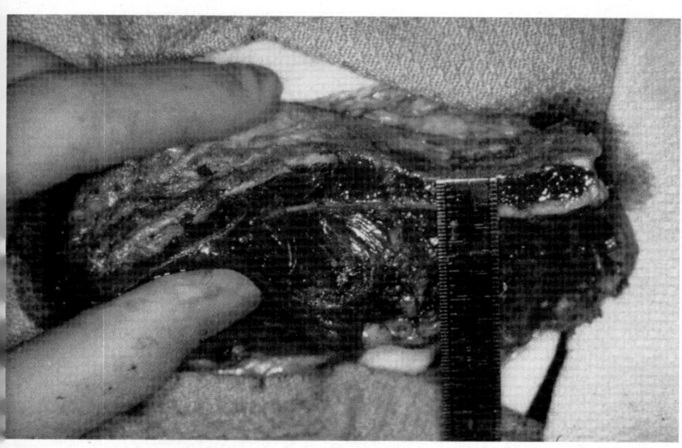

Fig. 57.21 The iliac crest–internal oblique osteocutaneous flap provides a thick bone segment that approximates the mandibular contour and height.

harvested from the anterior superior iliac spine to the posterior superior iliac spine. The natural curve of this bone allows mandibular reconstruction up to a hemimandibulectomy without the need for an ostectomy[90] (**Fig. 57.21**). In the setting of longer mandibular defects, ostectomies can be safely performed. Unlike the fibula free flap, the iliac crest can be harvested to match the height of the native mandible. Osseointegrated implants are accepted without difficulty.[91]

The vascular pedicle of the iliac crest–internal oblique flap is based on the deep circumflex iliac artery (DCIA) and vein (DCIV). These vessels join the external iliac system just cephalad to the inguinal ligament. From this point, the pedicle courses through a fibrous tunnel created by the decussation of the transversalis and iliacus fasciae. In the majority of cases, the DCIA gives off a large ascending branch at approximately the level of the anterior superior iliac spine. This ascending branch provides the dominant vascular supply to the internal oblique muscle. The artery continues along the medial aspect of the iliac crest, giving rise to numerous musculocutaneous perforators. These perforators penetrate the three layers of the abdominal musculature (transversus abdominis, internal oblique, and external oblique) to supply the skin above the iliac crest. The DCIA also provides the blood supply to the iliac bone via both periosteal perforators and a nutrient artery. Finally, the venous drainage parallels the arterial inflow as dual venae comitantes, which form a single vein (DCIV) prior to joining the external iliac vein.

Two separate paddles can be transferred with this harvest. The skin paddle is located over the iliac crest and can vary significantly in thickness depending on the patient's habitus. Flaps measuring as large as 20 × 10 cm have been successfully transferred.[90] The skin paddled has a limited arc of rotation with relation to the bone secondary to the perforators. The second paddle is composed of the internal oblique muscle, which is a broad, flat muscle that forms the middle layer of the abdominal musculature. The entire muscle can be transferred on the large ascending branch, providing a paddle up to 8 × 15 cm in size.[92] In contrast to the skin paddle, the muscle has a significant arc of rotation that can be wrapped around the harvested bone.[89] The lateral cutaneous branch of the 12th thoracic nerve provides the dominant sensory innervation to the skin paddle. Reinnervation based on this nerve has been described, but a large series has yet to be reported.[93]

Surgical Technique

The iliac crest–internal oblique free flap is harvested with the patient in the supine position and the hip bumped. The skin paddle is outlined along the iliac crest, centered along a line drawn from the anterior superior iliac spine to the tip of the scapula. To incorporate the maximum number of musculocutaneous perforators, the paddle should measure at least 8 cm from the anterior superior iliac spine along this line. First, the medial skin incision is brought down through the subcutaneous tissue, to the fascia of the external oblique muscle. Elevation proceeds from medial to lateral in the suprafascial plane. To preserve the musculocutaneous perforators, dissection ends 3 cm from the iliac crest. The external oblique is divided at this point to expose the underlying internal oblique musculature. After the internal oblique is exposed, it is released laterally, medially, and superiorly. Beginning at the superior–lateral margin, a plane is then developed between the internal oblique and underlying transversus abdominis muscle. The ascending branch of the DCIA can be identified on the undersurface of the internal oblique. Once the DCIA and DCIV are traced back to the external iliac system, the transversus abdominis muscle is divided. Again, care is taken to preserve approximately a 3-cm cuff of muscle to avoid inadvertent damage to the musculocutaneous perforators. Similarly, the underlying iliacus is transected. The lateral skin incision is then brought down through the subcutaneous tissue to the tensor fascia lata and gluteus medius. Elevation continues in a suprafascial plane toward the iliac crest. Transection of these muscles, along with the sartorius and iliopsoas, allows exposure of the iliac crest. Bone cuts are then made with the abdominal contents safely retracted and the pedicle protected.

Meticulous closure of the donor site is required to prevent the development of a hernia. Drill holes are place along the cut edge of the iliac crest so that the transversus abdominis and iliacus can be reliably approximated with permanent suture. Care should be taken to avoid injury of the femoral artery and nerve. The second layer of closure reapproximates the external oblique musculature and tensor fascia lata. A closed suction drain is placed, and the overlying skin can usually be closed primarily.

Advantages and Disadvantages

The iliac crest–internal oblique osteomyocutaneous flap provides a dependable source of well-vascularized bone for reconstruction. The primary advantage of this flap is the large, curved, bony segment that matches the native mandibular height, and often the nature contour of the hemimandible, thus avoiding multiple ostectomies. The flap provides both a muscle and skin paddle, allowing for simultaneous reconstruction of multiple surfaces. The skin paddle is often used in reconstructing chin and cutaneous neck defects, whereas the muscle provides excellent intraoral coverage. Finally, the donor site incisions are hidden by standard clothing.

Disadvantages of this flap include a limited arc of rotation for the skin paddle. For this reason, the skin should not be used to reconstruct defects superior to the lateral oral commissure. In addition, the flap tends to be quite thick because a cuff of the abdominal muscles must be harvested to adequately capture the musculocutaneous perforators. Donor site morbidity is of particular concern. In one large series, complications included sensory changes (27%), contour deformity (20%), hernia formation (9.7%), and gait disturbance (11%).[94]

Functional Review of Flap Options for Head and Neck Reconstruction

The final section of this chapter focuses on a functional and anatomical approach to head and neck reconstruction using the free flaps described above. Soft tissue and oral defects, hypopharyngeal reconstruction with an emphasis on swallowing, skull base defects, and mandibular reconstruction are addressed. A summary of common flap reconstructive applications is outlined in **Table 57.2**.

Soft Tissue and Oral Defects

Reconstruction of soft tissue and oral defects involve similar flaps, albeit for different reasons. The amount of skin required, native tissue bulk, and skin color match should all be taken into account when selecting a donor site. Oral cavity reconstructions require pliable, thin, potentially sensate tissue that can easily contour in three dimensions to prevent tethering of mobile tissue such as the tongue.[95] Options include the STPPF with overlying skin graft, radial forearm, lateral arm, anterior lateral thigh, lateral thigh, scapula, latissimus dorsi, and rectus free flaps. Although it will vary somewhat with patient habitus, these flaps are listed in increasing order of thickness. The flaps do not provide an ideal color match for facial and cervical skin; however, the upper extremity tends to be a better match relative to the abdomen, lower extremity, and back.

The STFF is used only on rare occasion, usually in the setting of floor of mouth reconstructions. When bulk is not required, the radial forearm remains the workhorse of oral cavity reconstruction. It provides ample flap size for nearly all oral cavity defects, a long and reliable vascular pedicle, limited donor site morbidity if collateral ulnar flow is sufficient to supply the hand, and reliable sensory innervation that facilitates swallowing rehabilitation (**Fig. 57.22**). In comparison, the lateral arm free flap can provide a combination of both thick and thin tissue within a single skin paddle, and the vascular pedicle has no impact on hand or arm viability. However, a much smaller skin paddle is provided by the lateral arm compared with the radial forearm, and the harvest is technically more difficult. The lateral arm is particularly useful for tongue base reconstruction where a thicker, sensate flap is advantageous. It is also useful for midface soft tissue defects that require bulk (**Fig. 57.23**).

The lateral thigh and anterior lateral thigh free flap can also be technically challenging to harvest due to the anatomical variability in blood supply. Both provide a large skin paddle and excellent bulk for large soft tissue defects. However, this bulk makes the thigh free flaps less then ideal for oral cavity reconstruction. Similarly, the scapular flap is usually too thick for oral cavity reconstruction. However, the availability of two skin paddles is ideal for reconstructing through-and-through defects in which both facial skin and oral cavity mucosa require reconstruction. Tissue bulk of the scapula, lateral thigh, and anterior lateral thigh flaps is also ideal in reconstructing total parotid defects. In such cases, almost the entire flap is deepithelialized prior to placement under the native skin.

The latissimus dorsi flap is the cornerstone for large soft tissue defects because it provides an extremely large, long, and reliable skin paddle. To achieve acceptable tissue contouring, long-term atrophy of the muscle secondary to denervation can be used to the surgeon's advantage. This flap is particularly useful for combined skull base and scalp defects (**Fig. 57.24**). The relatively thin nature of this flap allows it to be folded to reconstruct combined maxillectomy and orbital exenteration defects. Finally, the muscle alone with overlying skin grafts can be used for near total scalp defects with reasonable color and thickness match (**Fig. 57.25**).

The rectus flap provides a large skin paddle but is frequently too thick for application in the oral cavity. It is important to realize that the denervated muscle will eventually atrophy and that the reconstructive bulk is actually achieved with the vascularized fat. This flap is only used when bulk is acceptable such as cases involving maxillectomy and orbital exenteration (**Fig. 57.26**).

Lastly, if the oral cavity defect is secondary to a maxillectomy in the setting of residual dentition, a fibular free tissue transfer is favored. This donor site provides adequate bone stock for future osseointegrated implants, as well as

Table 57.2 Summary of Flap Donor Sites and Reconstructive Applications in the Head and Neck Region

Donor Site	Defect
Superficial temporoparietal fascial	Lateral skull base
	Oral cavity: floor of mouth
Radial forearm	Oral cavity/oropharynx
	Cutaneous soft tissue
	Pharynx (<10 cm length; above thoracic inlet)
	Lateral edentulous mandible
Lateral arm	Tongue base
	Cutaneous soft tissue
Lateral thigh	Pharynx (>10 cm length; above thoracic inlet)
	Maxillectomy with orbital exenteration
	Cutaneous soft tissue
	Total parotid defect
Anterior lateral thigh	Pharynx (>10 cm length; above thoracic inlet)
	Total glossectomy
	Maxillectomy with orbital exenteration
	Cutaneous soft tissue
	Total parotid defect
Latissimus dorsi	Maxillectomy with orbital exenteration
	Near-total scalp defect
	Anterior skull base
	Lateral skull base
	Combined skull base and scalp
	Total glossectomy
Rectus	Maxillectomy with orbital exenteration
	Anterior skull base
Jejunum	Pharynx (>10 cm length; above thoracic inlet)
Fibula	Mandible (up to 25 cm)
	Midface: maxilla and hard palate
Iliac crest–internal oblique	Mandible (up to 16 cm; cutaneous defect inferior to oral commissure)
Scapula	Through-and-through cheek
	Total parotid
	Anterior skull base requiring bone
	Mandible (up to 10 cm)

thin skin paddle for lining the palatal defect (**Fig. 57.27**). Other bony flaps such as the scapula and iliac crest–internal oblique transfer significant tissue bulk, which can lead to dysphagia during the oral phase of swallowing.

Hypopharynx Reconstruction

The choice of reconstructive option of the hypopharynx is primarily dependent on the defect size with respect to both circumference and length, the availability of donor sites, and patient characteristics including body habitus and wishes for vocal rehabilitation. For defects above the thoracic inlet measuring less than 270 degrees in circumference, we principally use pedicled regional flaps such as the pectoralis major or latissimus dorsi muscle. However, large, bulky, myocutaneous flaps tend to form poor tubes, leading to significant postoperative dysphagia. In such cases, we prefer free tissue transfer. Patch grafting can be successfully achieved with cutaneous free flaps (radial forearm, lateral or anterior lateral thigh) or a jejunal flap

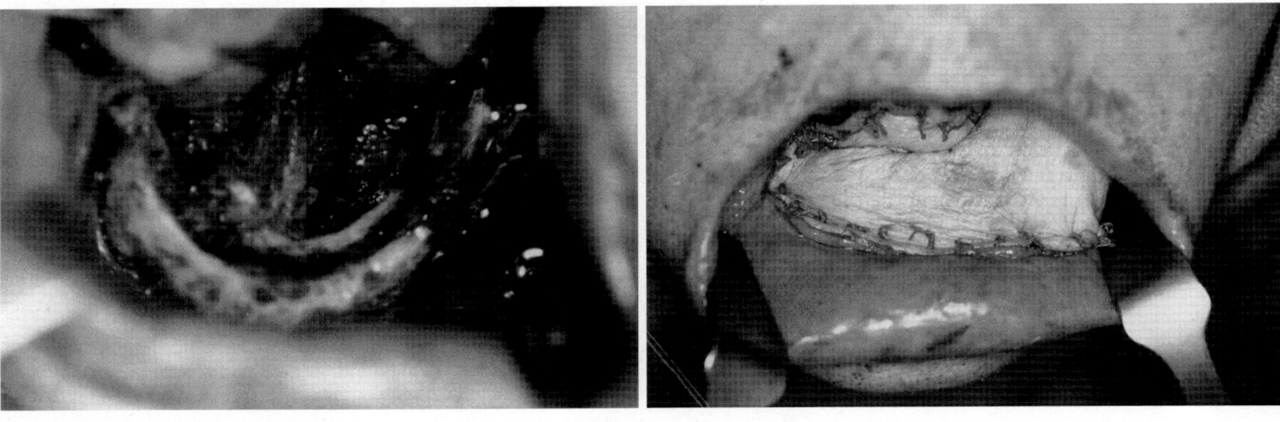

Fig. 57.22 (**A**) A composite resection that included a partial mandibulectomy and mucosa of the floor of mouth bilaterally. The genioglossus muscle is now visible. (**B**) The same view with a radial forearm flap inset.

opened completely along the antimesenteric border. Regardless of the donor site, it is important to avoid post-operative stenosis and associated dysphagia by utilizing a lock-and-key configuration during distal anastomosis with the native esophagus.

For defects greater than 270-degree circumference and above the thoracic inlet, we use free tissue transfer with either a cutaneous flap or jejunal flap. The cutaneous flaps provide a soft, supple conduit with a thickness that parallels the native pharynx and esophagus.[96] There are several differences between the radial forearm, lateral thigh, and anterior lateral thigh free flaps worth noting. The radial forearm provides less tissue compared with the thigh, but the skin paddle is thin and supple (**Fig. 57.28**). The thickness of the thigh flaps vary on an individual basis. A thicker flap will be more difficult to tube and carries a higher risk of postoperative dysphagia. Overall, a flap width of 9 cm, which is then tubed, provides an adequate neopharynx to prevent dysphagia. This width can be achieved from ei-ther the radial forearm or thigh. During the harvest of th radial forearm, the integrity of the skin over the ulnar sur face should be preserved. The available flap length is muc greater with the lateral and anterior lateral thigh compare with the radial forearm. For this reason, defects that spa from the nasopharynx to the thoracic inlet (greater tha 15 cm) should be reconstructed with either thigh free fla or a jejunal flap. Lastly, the radial forearm free flap is easie to harvest, provides a longer pedicle, and has been shown i long-term studies to be effective with vocal rehabilitation.[9

For hypopharyngeal defects above the thoracic inle but longer than 10 cm, or in patients with thick cutaneou flaps, we prefer the jejunal free flap because the dry epi thelial lining of a long, tubed cutaneous flap can promot stasis and dysphagia. The lining of the jejunal flap is mucou secreting, and the flap matches longer defects above th thoracic inlet well. However, disadvantages include dono

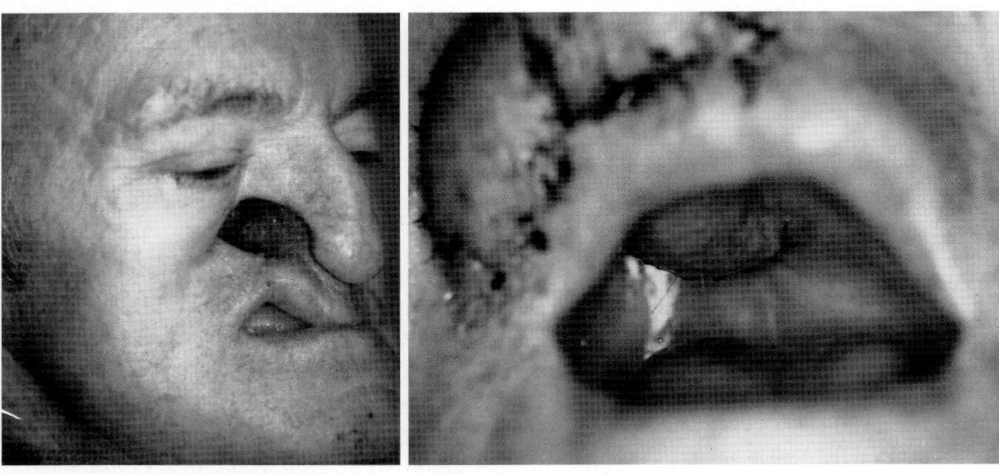

Fig. 57.23 (**A**) A combined fascial and palatal defect after partial maxillectomy and postoperative radiation therapy for cancer. (**B**) The same defect after reconstruction with a lateral arm flap. A portion of the flap was deepithelialized to allow both defects to be closed with a single skin paddle.

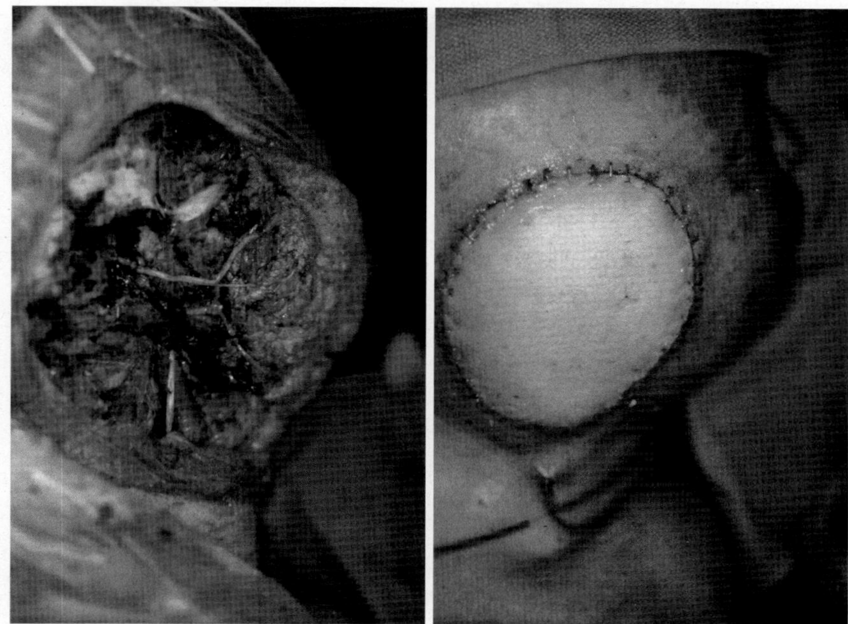

Fig. 57.24 (**A**) A combined skin and skull base defect after resection of a substantially invasive skin cancer. Note the facial nerve graft in the depth of the surgical bed. (**B**) The same view with a latissimus dorsi myocutaneous flap filling the defect.

site morbidity, dysphagia cause by mucosal folds and incoordination between muscle contraction and flap peristalsis, as well as a wet voice with tracheoesophageal speech.[98]

Hypopharyngeal defects extending below the thoracic inlet are traditionally reconstructed with a gastric pull-up. In doing so, a distal anastomosis within the thorax is avoided. Avoiding this anastomosis is important because leakage in this region carries a significant rate of mediastinitis and associated death. Unfortunately, the gastric pull-up is not without morbidity (32%) and mortality (5%).[98]

Skull Base Reconstruction

Skull base defects can be divided into anterior reconstructions involving the midface, sinuses, and orbit, and

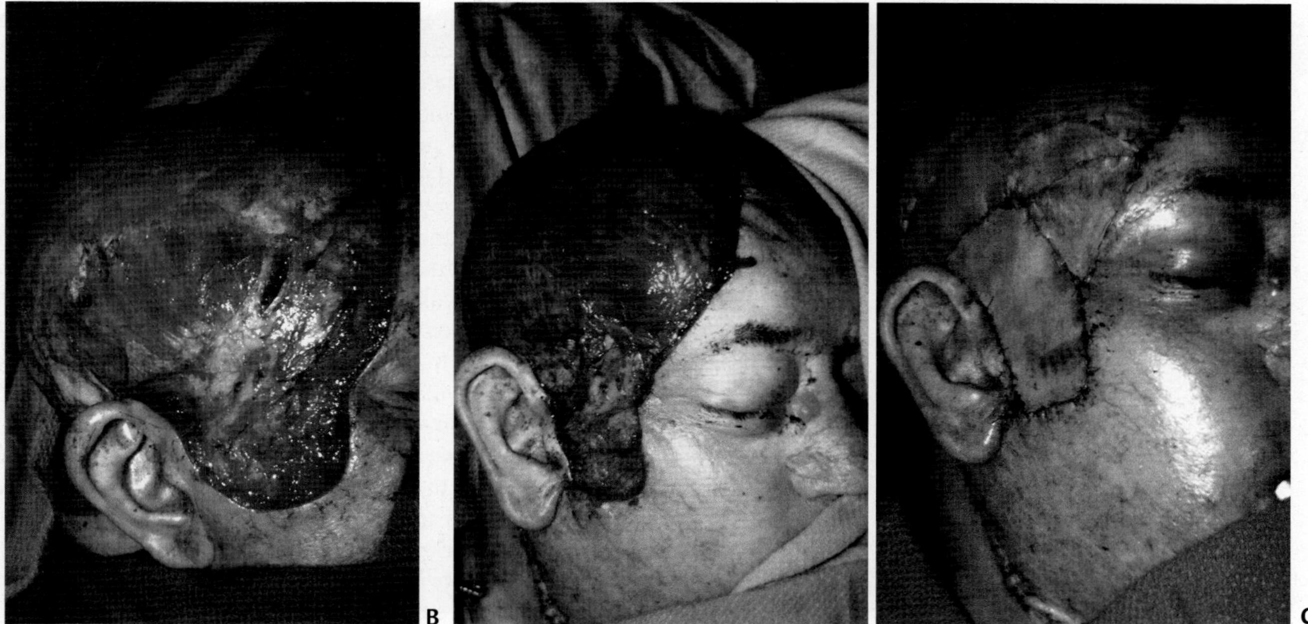

Fig. 57.25 (**A**) A massive resection of a scalp angiosarcoma. (**B**) The same defect reconstructed with a latissimus dorsi myogenous free flap. (**C**) The same view after split-thickness skin grafting of this muscle.

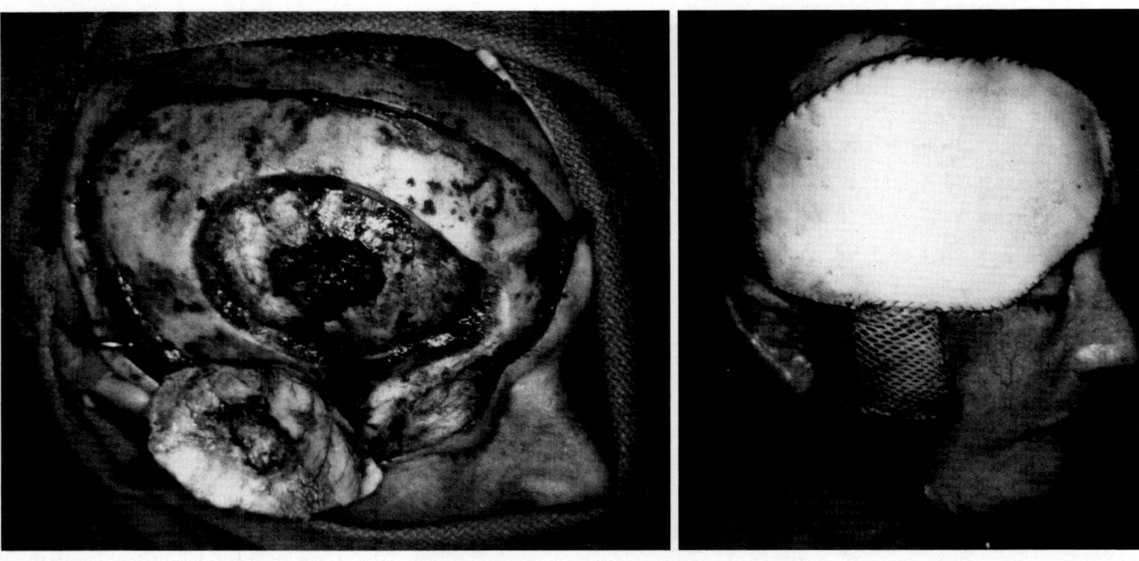

Fig. 57.26 (**A**) Another massive scalp and skull base defect after resection of skin cancer. Note the tumor still adherent to the dura, prior to dural resection. (**B**) The same defect with a rectus myocutaneous flap in place. The muscle reconstructing the lateral face/neck was skin grafted to avoid unnecessary tension over the pedicle.

posterior reconstructions that include the ear and temporal bone.

The central principle in anterior skull base reconstruction is the separation of brain and dura from contamination by sinus, oral cavity, and pharyngeal contents.[99] Secondary considerations include the obliteration of dead space, restoration of bone and soft tissue, and external cosmesis.[100]

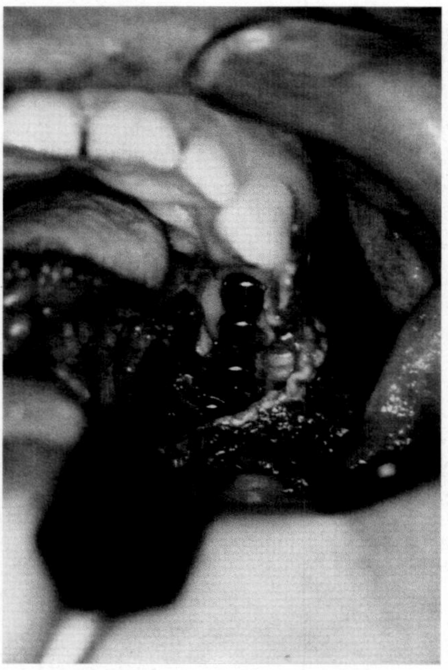

Fig. 57.27 Osseointegrated implants visible in a fibula free flap, used for reconstruction after near-total maxillectomy.

For anterior skull base defects involving the orbit or sinuses but not requiring significant tissue bulk, we prefer the radial forearm free flap or the superficial temporoparietal fascial flap.[101] As the need for tissue bulk increases, musculocutaneous flaps such as the rectus and latissimus dorsi are extremely useful. Both flaps provide large skin paddles that can be divided to resurface different surfaces in a three-dimensional configuration. They also provide a long vascular pedicle, which is necessary to reach the recipient vessels of the neck, as well as sufficient tissue bulk to obliterate dead space and enhance cosmesis. The key differences between the rectus and latissimus dorsi flaps are the harvest position and component of tissue bulk. The rectus muscle is harvested in the supine position with a two-team approach. In contrast, the latissimus dorsi harvest requires a lateral decubitus position, which often precludes the ability to perform simultaneous tissue harvest and tumor ablation. The majority of the tissue bulk supplied by the rectus free flap is from vascularized fat. Therefore, this tissue can reliably be contoured because it will not atrophy over time.[99] Conversely, the majority of the latissimus dorsi free flap is muscle, which will indeed atrophy with denervation. It is this latter point that makes the rectus free flap the workhorse for anterior skull base reconstruction.[102] When bony reconstruction is required, the scapula free flap is the preferred choice. This bone is thin and multiple bone flaps can be transferred on a single pedicle. As noted earlier in the chapter, this flap provides a variety of skin and muscle paddle configurations for complex three-dimensional reconstructions.

Posterior skull base defects also require separation of the brain and dura from contamination by the external

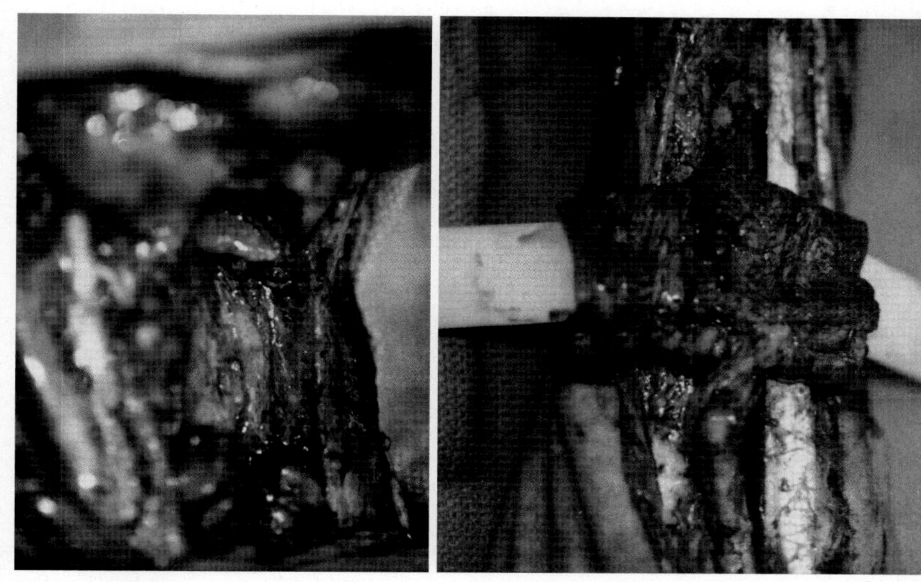

Fig. 57.28 (**A**) A total laryngopharyngectomy defect with the residual tongue base visible superiorly. (**B**) A radial forearm free flap with a penrose drain through the lumen of the tubed radial forearm. This portion of the reconstruction is done with the pedicle intact at the donor site to limit ischemia time.

and middle ear spaces. The majority of the defects can be reconstructed with either the STPPF or the latissimus dorsi flap. These flaps can be transferred as free tissue or as pedicled, regional flaps. Both flaps are readily available with the patient positioned in the lateral decubitus position, which is also a convenient position for resection. The STPPF is preferred when reconstruction calls for sealing cavities, whereas the latissimus dorsi flap is used when skin and tissue bulk are required. If these flaps are not available, we choose one of the anterior skull base flaps described above.

Oromandibular Reconstruction

The introduction of free tissue transfer has dramatically changed mandibular reconstruction. The 95% success rate and ability to restore function with osseointegrated implants revolutionized this reconstruction.[103] We achieve the majority of oromandibular reconstructions using an osteomyocutaneous flap such as the fibula, scapula, or iliac crest–internal oblique. Some surgeons utilize a composite radial forearm free flap for limited mandibular defects, but we do not harvest the radius due to the increased risk of pathological fractures. However, the radial forearm free flap is useful in reconstructing a lateral mandibular defect in an edentulous patient who does not desire dental restoration. In this setting, the vascularized tissue is draped over a mandibular reconstruction bar. This reconstructive option can also be considered in an ill patient with advanced disease and a poor prognosis. However, the reconstruction bar and radial forearm free flap is not an ideal option for patients who desire osseointegrated implants, for anterior mandibular defects that tend to lead to bar exposure over time, or for dentate patients because they have the ability to generate enough force over time to fracture the bar.

The fibula free flap is considered the workhorse flap for oromandibular reconstruction. It provides a long, well-vascularized bone segment as well as a potentially sensate skin paddle. The bone can be readily contoured because of the dual central and periosteal blood supply, and the skin paddle can be rotated to replace either the oral mucosa or cutaneous surface (**Fig. 57.29**). Although the height of the fibula bone may not match that of the native mandible, the bone stock is excellent and easily accepts osseointegrated implants (**Fig. 57.27**). The fibula provides up to 25 cm of bone length, making it the only bony flap for near total mandibular reconstruction. Soft tissue coverage provided by this flap is limited. Therefore, we do not utilize it in the setting of through-and-through mandibular defects. We also avoid utilizing this flap in the setting of diabetes mellitus, peripheral vascular disease, or prior lower extremity trauma because of increase donor site morbidity.

The scapula is our free flap of choice for reconstruction of oromandibular reconstruction in three specific situations: (1) a through-and-through cheek defect of the oromandibular complex superior to the oral commissure; (2) a patient with severe atherosclerotic disease precluding the use of a fibula free flap and; (3) very large soft tissue defects requiring bone as well as significant tissue bulk for adequate reconstruction.[104] The latter scenario is addressed

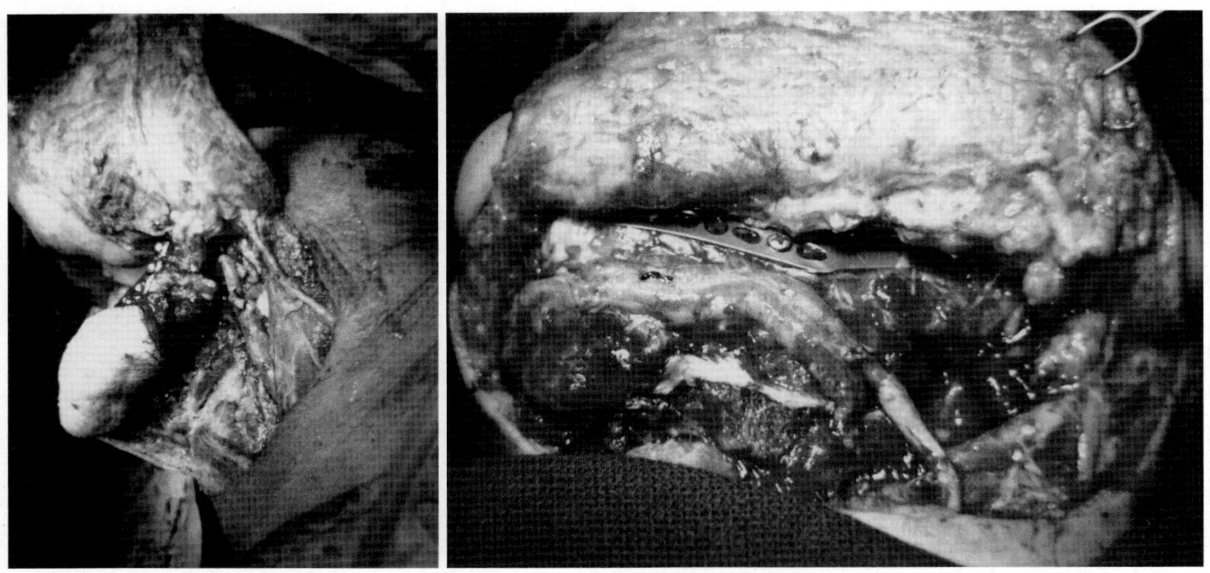

Fig. 57.29 (**A**) A fibula osteocutaneous flap in place, viewed from the posterior neck. Note the skin paddle, which can be rotated internally for mucosal coverage or left externally for skin reconstruction. (**B**) A fibula flap in place, attached to the mandibular reconstruction plate.

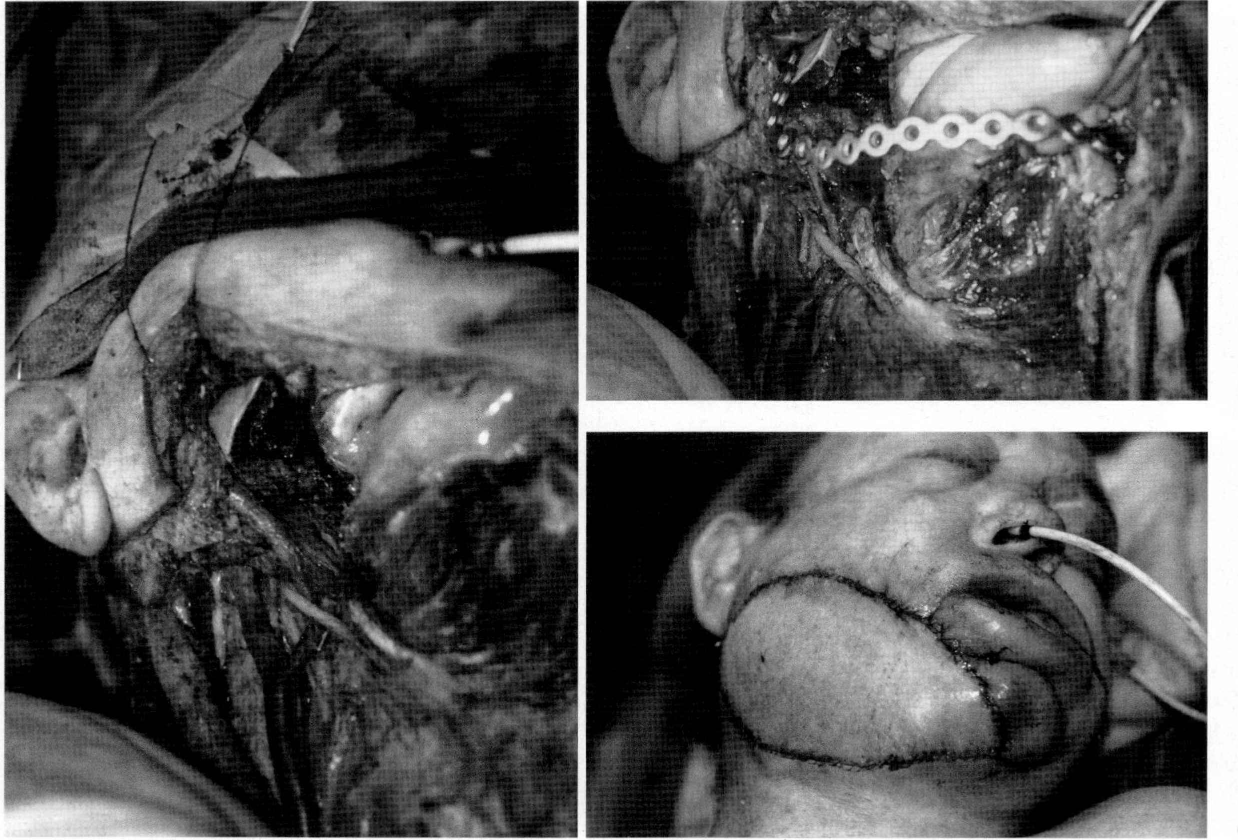

Fig. 57.30 (**A**) A view of the right neck after composite resection of the skin, mandible, and mucosa for a right oromandibular tumor. The native mandibular condyle remains present superiorly. (**B**) The same view with a mandibular reconstruction plate placed prior to inset of the scapula osteocutaneous flap. (**C**) The immediate postoperative result with one skin paddle achieving both internal mucosal and external skin closure.

by creating a megaflap base on the single pedicle of the scapula free flap. The ability to transfer a variety of bone, muscle, and skin paddles based on one pedicle allows this flap to be used for a variety of complex three-dimensional closures without shearing or tension (**Fig. 57.30**). This versatility is in marked contrast to the iliac crest–internal oblique skin paddle. Up to 10 cm of bone can successfully be transferred using the scapula; however, this bone tends to be thin and lacks vertical height. An additional disadvantage is increase operative time due to lateral decubitus positioning.

The iliac crest–internal oblique is most useful for through-and-through defects below the oral commissure and for cases involving massive tissue loss secondary to trauma. The limited arc of rotation of the skin paddle relative to the bone makes this flap ideal for cutaneous reconstruction of the chin, neck, and jowl. If necessary, the internal oblique musculature can then be used with or without a split-thickness skin graft to line the floor of mouth. The bone stock of the iliac crest provides up to 16 cm of thick bone with excellent height to match the native mandible and to accept osseointegrated implants (**Fig. 57.31**). A two-team approach is easily accomplished. The main disadvantages include risk of postoperative hernia, contour irregularity, gait disturbance, and donor site pain.[94] Finally, the bulk of this flap can be prohibitive for small composite oromandibular defects.

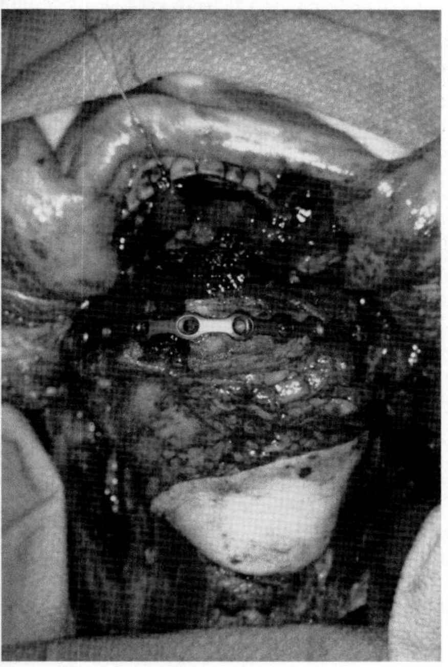

Fig. 57.31 The iliac crest–internal oblique osteocutaneous flap used for reconstruction of an angle-to-angle oromandibular defect. The bone is plated to a mandibular reconstruction plate, the skin paddle is used for a submental cutaneous defect, and the internal oblique muscle (marked with a suture) is rotated intraorally to line the floor of mouth.

We use the same surgical technique for reconstructing oromandibular defects, irrespective of donor site. The patient is placed in occlusion, which is maintained with standard mandibular-maxillary fixation. A 2.4-mm mandibular reconstructive locking plate (Synthes; Paoli, PA) is fashioned to span the defect. The bone is then carefully contoured using ostectomies to create a tight bone–plate interface. The bone is secured to the lingual aspect of the plate using monocortical screws. The vascular anastomoses are completed, and the soft tissue is positioned and sutured. If applicable, osseointegrated implants can be placed primarily (**Fig. 57.29**). Our experience has been that the flap tends to remucosalize over the implants during the immediate postoperative period. For this reason we prefer secondary osseointegrated implants at approximately 3 months following surgery unless postoperative radiation is required, in which case we advise patients to wait a minimum of 6 months.

Summary

Advances in surgical technique, titanium plating, and vascular physiology throughout the past 2 decades have enabled microvascular free tissue transfer to emerge as the reconstructive choice for complex three-dimensional head and neck defects. The ability to reliably and safely transfer healthy skin, muscle, and bone provides the microvascular surgeon with the necessary flexibility to reconstruct what were once deemed severely debilitating cancer defects, tissue loss secondary to trauma, as well as congenital abnormalities. Each defect must be closely analyzed on an individual basis to determine if free tissue transfer is truly advantageous, and to determine which donor site will yield the best result both from a functional, as well as a cosmetic standpoint. Exciting research in areas such as distraction osteogenesis and tissue engineering will further enhance the role of microvascular free tissue transfer in head and neck reconstruction.

References

1. Davie EW. Biochemical and molecular aspects of the coagulation cascade. Thromb Haemost 1995;74:1–6
2. Shenaq SM, Klebuc MJA, Vargo D. Free tissue transfer with the aid of loupe magnification: experience with 251 procedures. Plast Reconstr Surg 1995;95:261–269
3. Shindo ML, Nalbone VP. Clinical vessel anastomosis in head and neck free tissue transfer. Facial Plast Surg 1996;12:9–12
4. Ueda K, Harii K, Nakatsuka T, et al. Comparison of end-to-end and end-to-side venous anastomosis in free tissue transfer following resection of head and neck tumors. Microsurgery 1996;17:146–149
5. Chalian AA, Anderson TD, Weinstein GS, Weber RS. Internal jugular vein versus external jugular vein anastomosis: implications for successful free tissue transfer. Head Neck 2001;23:475–478

6. Cordeiro PG, Santamaria E. Experience with the continuous suture microvascular anastomosis in 200 consecutive free flaps. Ann Plast Surg 1998;40:1–6
7. Shindo ML, Costantino PD, Nalbone VP, et al. Use of a mechanical microvascular anastomotic device in head and neck free issue transfer. Arch Otolaryngol Head Neck Surg 1996;122:529–532
8. DeLacure MD, Wong RS, Markowitz BL, et al. Clinical experience with a microvascular anastomotic device in head and neck reconstruction. Am J Surg 1995;170:521–523
9. Moscoso JF, Urken ML. Why free flaps fail. Oper Techn Otolaryngol Head Neck Surg 1993;93:169–171
10. Stepnick DW, Hayden RE. Postoperative monitoring and salvage of microvascular free flaps. Otolaryngol Clin North Am 1994;27: 1201–1207
11. Cho BC, Shin DP, Byun JS, Park JW, Baik BS. Monitoring flap for buried free tissue transfer: its importance and reliability. Plast Reconstr Surg 2002;110:1249–1258
12. Yoshino K, Nara S, Endo M, Kamata N. Intraoral free flap monitoring with a laser Doppler flowmeter. Microsurgery 1996;17:337–340
13. Hirigoyen MB, Blackwell KE, Zhang WX, et al. Continuous tissue oxygen tension as a monitor of free-flap viability. Plast Reconstr Surg 1997;99:763–773
14. Wechselberger G, Rumer A, Schoeller T, et al. Free-flap monitoring with tissue-oxygen measurement. J Reconstr Microsurg 1997;13: 125–130
15. Futran ND, Stack BC, Hollenbeak C, Scharf JE. Green light photoplethysmography monitoring of free flaps. Arch Otolaryngol Head Neck Surg 2000;126:659–662
16. Kroll SS, Schusterman MA, Reece GP, et al. Timing of pedicle thrombosis and flap loss after free tissue transfer. Plast Reconstr Surg 1996;98:1230–1233
17. Khouri RE, Cooley BC, Kunselman AR, et al. A prospective study of microvascular surgery and outcome. Plast Reconstr Surg 1998;102: 711–721
18. Kroll SS, Schusterman MA, Reece GP, et al. Choice of flap and incidence of free flap success. Plast Reconstr Surg 1996;98:459–463
19. Hidalgo DA, Disa JJ, Cordeirp PG, Hu QY. A review of 716 consecutive free flaps for oncologic surgical defects: refinement on donor-site selection and technique. Plast Reconstr Surg 1998;102:722–732
20. Gapany M. Failing flap. Facial Plast Surg 1996;12:23–27
21. Walton RL, Beahm EK, Brown RE, et al. Microvascular replantation of the lip: a multi-institutional experience. Plast Reconstr Surg 1998;102:358–368
22. Pomerance J, Truppa K, Bilos ZJ, et al. Replantation and revascularization of the digits in a community microsurgical practice. Br J Plast Surg 1993;36:1–8
23. Moscoso JF, Urken ML. Radial forearm flaps. Otolaryngol Clin North Am 1994;27:1119–1140
24. Futran ND, Stack BC. Single versus dual venous drainage of the radial forearm free flap. Am J Otolaryngol 1996;17:112–117
25. Urken ML. Composite free flaps in oromandibular reconstruction; review of the literature. Arch Otolaryngol Head Neck Surg 1991;117:724–732
26. Calhoun KH. Radial forearm free flap for head and neck reconstruction. Facial Plast Surg 1996;12:29–33
27. Martin IC, Brown AE. Free vascularized fascial flap in oral cavity reconstruction. Head Neck 1994;16:45–50
28. Sadove RC, Luce EA, McGrath PC. Reconstruction of the lower lip and chin with the composite radial forearm–palmaris longus free flap. Plast Reconstr Surg 1991;88:209–214
29. Urken ML, Blackwell K, Biller HF. Reconstruction of the laryngopharynx after hemicricoid/hemithyroid cartilage resection. Arch Otolaryngol Head Neck Surg 1997;123:1213–1222
30. Jones B, O'Brien C. Acute ischemia of the hand resulting from elevation of the radial forearm flap. Br J Plast Surg 1985;38:396–397
31. Elliot D, Bardsley AF, Batchelor AG, Soutar DS. Direct closure of the radial forearm flap defect. Br J Plast Surg 1988;41:358–360
32. Hallock GG. Refinement of the radial forearm flap donor site using skin expansion. Plast Reconstr Surg 1988;81:21–25
33. Brown MT, Cheney ML, Gliklich RL, et al. Assessment of functional morbidity in the radial forearm free flap donor site. Arch Otolaryngol Head Neck Surg 1996;122:991–994
34. Timmons MJ, Missotten FEM, Poole MD, Davies DM. Complications of radial forearm donor sites. Br J Plast Surg 1986;39:176–178
35. Song R, Song Y, Yu U, Son Y. The upper arm free flap. Clin Plast Surg 1982;9:27–35
36. Civantos FJ, Burkey BB, Lu F, Armstrong W. Lateral arm microvascular flap in head and neck reconstruction. Arch Otolaryngol Head Neck Surg 1997;123:830–836
37. Sullivan MJ, Carroll WR, Kuriloff DB. Lateral arm free flap in head and neck reconstruction. Arch Otolaryngol Head Neck Surg 1992;118:1095–1101
38. Scheker LR, Kleinert HE, Handel DP. Lateral arm composite tissue transfer to ipsilateral hand defects. J Hand Surg [Am] 1987;12:665–672
39. Graham B, Adkins P, Scheker LR. Complications and morbidity of the donor and recipient sites in 123 lateral arm flaps. J Hand Surg [Br] 1992;17:189–192
40. Baek SM. Two new cutaneous free flaps: the medial and lateral thigh flap. Plast Reconstr Surg 1983;71(71):354–363
41. Hayden RE. Lateral cutaneous thigh flap. In: Baker S, ed. Microsurgical Reconstruction of the Head and Neck. New York: Churchill Livingstone; 1989:211
42. Miller MJ, Reece GP, Marchi M, Baldwin BJ. Lateral thigh free flap in head and neck reconstruction. Plast Reconstr Surg 1995;96: 334–340
43. Deschler DG, Hayden RE. Lateral thigh free flap. Facial Plast Surg 1996;12:75–79
44. Song YG, Chen GZ, Song YL. The free thigh flap: a new free flap concept based on the septocutaneous artery. Br J Plast Surg 1984;37:149–159
45. Koshima I, Fukuda H, Yamamato H, et al. Free anterolateral thigh flaps for reconstruction of head and neck defects. Plast Reconstr Surg 1993;92:421–428
46. Malhostra K, Lian TS, Chakradeo V. Vascular anatomy of the anterolateral thigh flap. Laryngoscope 2008;118:589–592
47. Zhou G, Qiao Q, Chen CY, et al. Clinical experience and surgical anatomy of 32 free anterolateral thigh flap transplantations. Br J Plast Surg 1991;44:91–96
48. Wei FC, Jain V, Ortho MC, et al. Have you found an ideal soft tissue flap? An experience with 672 anterolateral thigh flaps. Plast Reconstr Surg 2002;109:2219–2226
49. Makitie AA, Beasley NJP, Neligan PC, et al. Head and neck reconstruction with anterolateral thigh flap. Otolaryngol Head Neck Surg 2003;129:547–555
50. Koshima I, Fukuda H, Utunomiya R, et al. The anterolateral thigh flap: variations in its vascular pedicle. Br J Plast Surg 1989;42:260–262
51. Yildirim S, Avci G, Akov T. Soft tissue reconstruction using free anterolateral thigh flap: experience with 28 patients. Ann Plast Surg 2003;51:37–44
52. Hsieh CH, Yang CC, Kuo YR, et al. Free anterolateral thigh adipofascial perforator flap. Plast Reconstr Surg 2003;112:976–982
53. Agostini V, Dini M, Mori A, et al. Adipofascial anterolateral thigh free flap for tongue repair. Br J Plast Surg 2003;56:614–618
54. Kimata Y, Uchiyama K, Ebihara S, et al. Anatomic variations and technical problems of the anterolateral thigh flap: a report of 74 cases. Plast Reconstr Surg 1998;102:1517–1523
55. Lin DT, Coppit GL, Burkey BB. Use of the anterolateral thigh flap for reconstruction of the head and neck. Curr Opin Otolaryngol Head Neck Surg 2004;12:300–304
56. Cheney ML. Temporoparietal fascia. In: Urken ML, Cheney ML, Sullivan MJ, Biller HF, eds. Atlas of Regional and Free Flaps for Head and Neck Reconstruction. New York: Raven Press; 1995:197
57. Clymer MA, Burkey BB. Other flaps for head and neck use: temporoparietal fascial free flap, lateral arm free flap, omental free flap. Facial Plast Surg 1996;12:81–89

58. Cheney ML, Varvares MA, Nadol JB Jr. The temporoparietal fascial flap in head and neck reconstruction. Arch Otolaryngol Head Neck Surg 1993;119:618–623
59. Pennington DLM, Pelly A. The rectus abdominis free muscle transfer. Br J Plast Surg 1980;33:277–282
60. Boyd JB, Taylor GI, Corlett RJ. The versatile deep inferior epigastric (inferior rectus abdominis) flap. Br J Plast Surg 1984;37:330–350
61. Urken ML, Turk JB, Weinberg H, et al. The rectus abdominis free flap in head and neck reconstruction. Arch Otolaryngol Head Neck Surg 1991;117:857–866
62. Wanamaker JR, Burkey BB. Overview of the rectus abdominis myocutaneous flap in head and neck reconstruction. Facial Plast Surg 1996;12:45–50
63. Kosima I, Moriguchi T, Fukuda H, Yoshikawa YSS. Free thinned periumbilical perforator-based flaps. J Reconstr Microsurg 1991;7:313–316
64. Baudet J, Guimberteau J, Nascimento E. Successful clinical transfer of two free thoracodorsal axillary flaps. Plast Reconstr Surg 1976;58:680–688
65. Civantos FJ. Latissimus dorsi microvascular flap. Facial Plast Surg 1996;12:65–68
66. Haughey B. Tongue reconstruction: concepts and practice. Laryngoscope 1993;103:1132–1141
67. Schultes G, Karcher J, Gaggl A. Sensate myocutaneous latissimus dorsi flap. J Reconstr Microsurg 1998;14:541–543
68. Russell RC, Pribaz J, Zook E, et al. Functional evaluation of the latissimus donor site. Plast Reconstr Surg 1978;78:336–344
69. Seidenberg B, Rosenak S, Hurwitt ES, Som ML. Immediate reconstruction of the cervical esophagus by a revascularized isolated jejunal segment. Ann Surg 1959;142:162–171
70. Gherardini G, Gurlek A, Staley CA, et al. Laparoscopic harvesting of jejunal free flaps for esophageal reconstruction. Plast Reconstr Surg 1998;102:473–477
71. Alford EL. Free jejunal transfer. Facial Plast Surg 1996;12:69–73
72. Reece GP, Bengtson BP, Schusterman MA. Reconstruction of the pharynx and cervical esophagus using jejunal transfer. Clin Plast Surg 1994;21:125–136
73. Taylor GI, Miller GDG, Ham FJ. The free vascularized bone graft: a clinical extension of microvascular techniques. Plast Reconstr Surg 1975;55:533–544
74. Moscoso JF, Keller J, Genden EM, et al. Vascularized bone flaps in oromandibular reconstruction: a comparative anatomic study of bone stock from various donor sites to assess suitability of enosseous dental implants. Arch Otolaryngol Head Neck Surg 1994;120: 36–43
75. Roumanas ED, Markowitz BL, Lorant JA, et al. Reconstructed mandibular defects: fibula free flaps and osseointegrated implants. Plast Reconstr Surg 1997;99:356–365
76. Hidalgo DA. Fibula free flap: a new method of mandibular reconstruction. Plast Reconstr Surg 1989;84:71–79
77. Young DM, Trabulsy PP, Anthony JP. The need for preoperative arteriogram in fibula free flap. J Reconstr Microsurg 1994;10:283–287
78. Futran ND, Stack BC Jr, Payne LP. Use of color Doppler flow imaging for preoperative assessment in fibular osteoseptocutaneous free tissue transfer. Otolaryngol Head Neck Surg 1997;117:660–663
79. Day TA, Resser JR. Mandibular reconstruction. Cur Opin Otolaryngol 1998;6:255–262
80. O'Leary MJ, Martin PJ, Hayden RE. The neurocutaneous free fibula flap in mandibular reconstruction. Otolaryngol Clin North Am 1994;47: 544–547
81. Wei FC, Chuang SS, Yim KK. The sensate fibula osteoseptocutaneous flap: a preliminary report. Br J Plast Surg 1994;47:544–547
82. Swartz WM, Banis JC, Newton ED, et al. The cutaneous scapular flap for mandibular and maxillary reconstruction. Plast Reconstr Surg 1986;77:530–545
83. Funk GF. Scapular and parascapular free flaps. Facial Plast Surg 1996;12:57–63
84. Baker SR, Sullivan MJ. Osteocutaneous free scapular flap for one-stage mandibular reconstruction. Arch Otolaryngol Head Neck Surg 1988;114:267–277
85. Robb GL. Free scapular flap reconstruction of the head and neck. Clin Plast Surg 1994;21:45–58
86. Sullivan MJ, Baker SR, Smith-Wheelock M. Free scapular osteocutaneous flap for mandibular reconstruction. Arch Otolaryngol Head Neck Surg 1988;114:267–277
87. Taylor GI, Townsend P, Corlett R. Superiority of the deep circumflex iliac vessels as the supply for free groin flaps: experimental work. Plast Reconstr Surg 1979;64:595–604
88. Ramasastry SS, Tucker JB, Swartz WM, Hurwitz DJ. The internal oblique muscle flap: an anatomic and clinical study. Plast Reconstr Surg 1984;73:721–730
89. Urken ML, Vickery C, Weinberg H, et al. The internal oblique–iliac crest osseomyocutaneous microvascular free flap in head and neck reconstruction. J Reconstr Microsurg 1989;5:203–214
90. Boyd JB. The place of iliac crest in vascularized oromandibular reconstruction. Microsurgery 1994;15:250–256
91. Frodel JL, Funk GF, Capper DT, et al. Osseointegrated implants: a comparative study of bone thickness for four vascularized bone flaps. Plast Reconstr Surg 1993;92:449–458
92. Ramasastry SS, Granick MS, Futrell JW. Clinical anatomy of the internal oblique muscle. J Reconstr Microsurg 1986;2:117–122
93. Blackwell KE, Urken ML. Iliac crest free flap. Facial Plast Surg 1996;12:35–43
94. Forrest C, Boyd B, Manktelow R, et al. The free vascularized iliac crest tissue transfer: donor site complications associated with 82 cases. Br J Plast Surg 1992;45:89–93
95. Wax MK. Soft tissue reconstruction of the oral cavity. Curr Opin Otolaryngol Head Neck Surg 1998;6:251–254
96. Burkey BB. Pharyngoesophageal reconstruction. Curr Opin Otolaryngol Head Neck Surg 1995;3:267–271
97. Stepnick DW, Hayden RE. Options for the reconstruction of the pharyngoesophageal defect. Otolaryngol Clin North Am 1994;27:1151–1158
98. Cahow C, Sasaki C. Gastric pull-up reconstruction for pharyngolaryngoesophogectomy. Arch Surg 1994;129:425–430
99. Wax MK, Burkey BB, Bascom D, Rosenthal EL. The role of free tissue transfer in the management of massive neglected skin cancers of the head and neck. Arch Facial Plast Surg 2003;5:479–482
100. Neligan PC, Boyd JB. Reconstruction of the cranial base defect. Clin Plast Surg 1995;22:71–77
101. Burkey BB, Gerek M. Repair of the persistent cerebrospinal fluid leak. Curr Opin Otolaryngol Head Neck Surg 1998;6:263–267
102. Nakatsuku T, Harii IK, Yamada A, Asotoh S. Versatility of a free inferior rectus abdominis flap for head and neck reconstruction: analysis of 200 cases. Plast Reconstr Surg 1994;93:762–769
103. Urken ML, Buchbinder D, Costantino PD, et al. Oromandibular reconstruction using microvascular composite flaps. Arch Otolaryngol Head Neck Surg 1998;124:46–55
104. Burkey BB, Coleman JR. Current concepts in oromandibular reconstruction. Otolaryngol Clin North Am 1997;30:607–628

58 Mandibular Reconstruction and Osseointegrated Implants

Eric M. Genden, Daniel Buchbinder, and Mark L. Urken

Since Crile introduced the concept of en bloc resection to head and neck surgery almost a century ago,[1] cure rates for head and neck cancer have improved significantly. However, as a result of this approach, extensive postablative defects were not uncommon. In the early nineteenth century, these defects were either closed primarily or left to heal by secondary intention, often resulting in debilitating oral dysfunction. Contraction of the surrounding soft tissues following composite resection resulted in mandibular drift, malocclusion, and often a compromise in speech, mastication, and swallowing. Gradually it became evident that the morbidity associated with a mandibulectomy defect varied depending on the location of the defect. Anterior defects of the mandible resulted in a structural disruption leading to collapse of the airway and a profound disturbance in oral function and facial appearance. In contrast, extensive lateral defects led to shifting of the mandible, resulting in pain and malocclusion. In spite of these repercussions, the clear curative advantage of wide-field ablation was evident. The profound cosmetic and functional disturbances associated with composite ablation provided the impetus for numerous attempts to ameliorate the impact of the segmental mandibulectomy defect through a variety of reconstructive methods.

The primary purpose of mandibular reconstruction is to restore the patient's oromandibular function to the predisease state. Aside from anchoring dentition and supporting mastication, the mandible also plays a crucial role in supporting the tongue and larynx, thus providing for a patent airway. Alloplastic implants, autogenous nonvascularized bone grafts, reconstruction plates, and free tissue transfer all have a role in contemporary mandibular reconstruction; however, each case must be evaluated critically, taking into consideration not only the size and position of the defect but the pathology of the disease process and the comorbid status of the patient. This chapter reviews the options for mandibular reconstruction with an emphasis on free tissue transfer, followed by a discussion regarding special considerations in contemporary mandibular reconstruction.

Materials for Mandible Reconstruction

Alloplasts

Alloplasts can be grouped into spacers, gap-bridging appliances, and reconstruction plates, all of which have been used to reconstruct the mandibulectomy defect. Temporary spacers, such as Kirschner wires and Steinmann pins, prevent collapse of the overlying tissues, which would otherwise occur. They are inserted into the intramedullary space of both the proximal and distal segments of bone. Retention bolts and contouring techniques have been employed to increase the stability of spacers, but the results have been disappointing. This method of reconstruction has largely been abandoned because of lack of stability, external extrusion, and an unacceptably high rate of infection.

Alternatively, gap-bridging devices, such as mesh cribs, can be used to bridge continuity defects in the mandible (**Fig. 58.1**). A metallic or polyurethane tray is tailored and contoured in situ to reconstruct the exact dimensions of the defect. The tray is fixed in place using wire or screws, and particulate bone grafts can then be placed in the tray and wrapped in vascularized tissue (pedicled myocutaneous flap). The trays are fenestrated, allowing for revascularization; however, salivary contamination can inhibit integration and lead to resorption of the graft.

Currently, reconstruction plates are the most commonly used form of alloplastic materials. Either alone or in combination with a bone graft, the titanium reconstruction plates and screws offer a reliable method of short-term

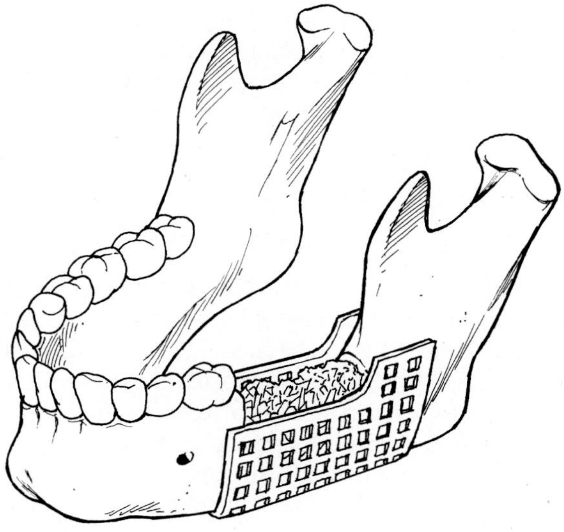

Fig. 58.1 Mesh tray for reconstruction of a lateral mandibular defect. The titanium mesh crib is filled with particulate bone graft.

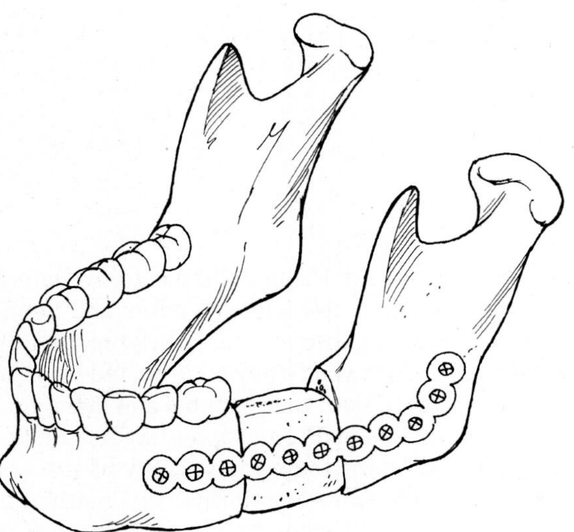

Fig. 58.2 Reconstruction plate and a nonvascularized bone graft for reconstruction of a lateral mandibular defect.

fixation (**Fig. 58.2**). These plates can be conformed to recreate a variety of mandibular defects and provide a rapid method of reconstruction; however, problems such as extrusion and plate fracture occur when these plates are placed in an irradiated field or when they are left in place for a prolonged period. This is particularly problematical in a functional mandible where the plate is subject to the forces of mastication. Although enveloping the reconstruction plate in vascularized muscle may delay plate exposure, extrusion rates remain as high as 45%.[2]

Finally, the insertion of osseointegrated dental implants is not possible with metal plate reconstruction; therefore, this type of reconstruction will not support dental rehabilitation, which is necessary for optimal oral rehabilitation.[3] As a group, alloplasts serve as a simple and temporary tool for the rapid bridging of small to medium-size lateral mandibular defects. However, larger and more complex defects of the anterior mandible require a more definitive method of reconstruction.[4]

Bone Grafts

Throughout the reconstructive era, bone grafting has been the most reliable method to achieve long-term mandibular reconstruction. Bone grafts can be classified as vascularized or nonvascularized. This section will focus on nonvascularized bone grafts, which can be categorized as autogenous, homologous, and xenogenic. Currently, autogenous bone grafts are most commonly used. The host–graft immunologic response characteristic of homologous and xenogenic grafts inhibits their osteoconductive properties and, as a result, has limited their application in contemporary mandibular reconstruction.

Autogenous Bone Grafts

Autogenous bone is recognized as the most osteoconductive material and the least likely to extrude. As a result, it has been considered the gold standard of treatment for limited mandibular defects. Autografts are harvested from one of several donor sites (**Table 58.1**). Three forms of autogenous bone grafts can be harvested: cancellous, cortical, and corticocancellous. The location of the defect commonly dictates the type of graft required for the reconstruction.

Cancellous bone grafts consist of both bone marrow and medullary bone matrix. They contain the highest concentration of viable cells and, as a result, have the highest potential for osteoconductivity. The large surface area associated with the cancellous matrix permits rapid revascularization, leading to a better chance of graft survival. However, because these grafts lack a cortical component, they have no source of structural rigidity and therefore must rely on a concomitantly placed scaffold, such as a mesh crib.

In contrast, cortical grafts are composed of lamellar bone, which is largely composed of osteocytes. The compact nature of this graft does not facilitate revascularization; hence, osteocytes rarely tolerate transplantation. Corticocancellous grafts are composed of a cortical segment combined with a cancellous portion (**Fig. 58.3**). These grafts possess the ideal composition of structurally sound cortical bone and viable osteoblastic cancellous bone. However, the cortical segment of bone can inhibit rapid revascularization, essential to graft integration, and as a result lead to decreased graft survival.

Each of the three forms of autogenous bone grafts haas advantages and disadvantages. Cortical bone grafts offer the dense structural bone necessary to reconstruct load-bearing areas; however, they do not permit revascularization and hence tend to undergo resorption. Conversely, cancellous bone grafts offer porous bone with a greater surface area, ideal for revascularization and hence new bone formation, but these grafts offer no structural component. In what appears to be an ideal balance, the

Table 58.1 Donor Sites for Autogenous Bone

Calvaria
Rib
Ilium
Tibia
Fibula
Scapula
Humerus
Radius
Metatrsus

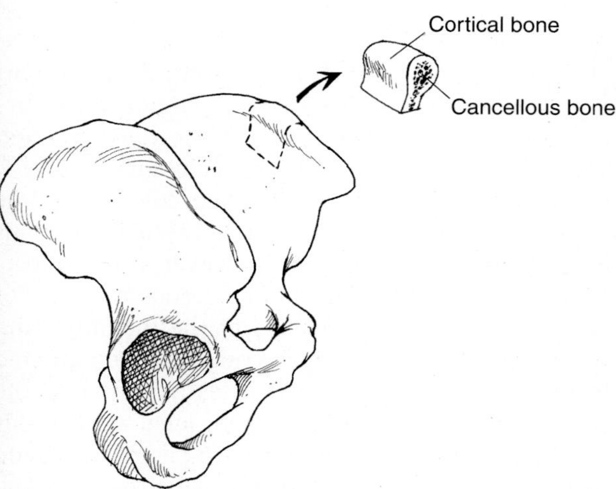

Fig. 58.3 Nonvascularized iliac bone graft. The corticocancellous block is composed of an external cortical graft and an internal cancellous graft.

autogenous corticocancellous bone graft may inhibit revascularization and undergo resorption, particularly in a previously irradiated field or a field exposed to salivary contamination. Although each of these grafts has a place in facial skeletal reconstruction, none is ideal for mandibular reconstruction.

Homologous Bone Grafts

Homologous bone grafts are harvested from individuals of the same species. Because of the major histocompatibility complex mismatch, these grafts are allogeneic. Lyophilization, irradiation, and cold pretreatment are methods used to reduce the antigenicity of the grafts; however, unlike autogenous bone, these grafts do not possess viable osteoblasts. It is theorized that these grafts harbor osteoconductive elements that induce the host's pluripotential cells to differentiate into osteoprogenitor cells. Homologous bone grafts are usually placed in a bioresorbable crib when autologous bone is unavailable.

Xenogenic Bone Grafts

Xenogenic bovine grafts were popular in the 1950s. However, they are no longer used because of host–graft antigenicity.

Bone Graft Incorporation

Two-Phase Theory

Graft incorporation occurs in two phases.[5] Phase I occurs during the first 4 weeks as new osteoid is formed by osteoblastic cells in transplanted bone. This phase determines the ultimate volume of bone because new-bone formation does not occur in the second phase. In the second phase, osteogenesis occurs as a result of the transformation of pluripotential stem cells into osteoblastic and osteoclastic cells—a process mediated by bone morphogenic protein. Phase II peaks at 6 weeks and is complete by 6 months. Failure to transfer living bone cells within the graft results in a nonvital sequestrum that will eventually be resorbed. As discussed earlier, the combination of particulate cortical bone and cancellous marrow offers the best long-term results because it offers the most reliable osteogenic potential and maintains the highest concentration of viable endosteal osteoblasts as well as mesenchymal cells to support both phase I and phase II osteogenesis. Unfortunately, the particulate nature of this bone graft is such that it lacks the structural integrity to support the stresses of mastication and must be placed in an alloplastic or allogeneic crib. This form of reconstruction has inherent shortcomings and requires an extended period before the newly formed bone is fully integrated and capable of withstanding the forces of mastication.

The Recipient Bed

The success of a free bone graft is dependent on the number of viable osteoblastic cells in the transplanted bone and the vascularity of the recipient bed. Osteoblastic cells provide mediators necessary for new-bone formation and the vascular supply within the recipient bed provides the nutrients essential to the survival of the osteoblasts. Radiotherapy has a negative impact on bone graft survival by causing a hypocellular, hypovascular reaction in the recipient bed.[6,7] In this circumstance, hyperbaric oxygen can be used to improve the quality of the recipient tissue bed by improving local oxygen tension and increasing neovascularity, which can aid in the incorporation of nonvascularized bone graft.[8,9] In the absence of a well-vascularized tissue bed, the nonvascularized bone will become a sequestrum and resorb.

Flaps for Mandible Reconstruction

Pedicled Osteomyocutaneous Flaps

In the early 1960s, it became apparent that bone grafts exposed to salivary contamination commonly became infected, resulting in resorption. As a result, the application of nonvascularized bone grafts in the contaminated recipient bed was limited. These shortcomings led to a series of animal experiments in the 1970s that defined the advantages of vascularized bone grafts.[10] Investigators found that pedicled vascularized rib resisted infection and extrusion, and maintained the osteogenic capacity, integrating with the adjacent mandible. Further investigation revealed that vascularized bone healed in an irradiated bed without a significant risk of infection or extrusion.[11,12] Combined, these studies demonstrated the unique advantages of vascularized bone over nonvascularized bone and subsequently led to a cascade of reports on mandibular reconstruction using pedicled vascularized bone.

In an effort to establish a form of definitive mandibular reconstruction, a variety of pedicled flaps incorporating an attached segment of bone were attempted in the early twentieth century. Rydygier first reported the use of a vascularized clavicular segment based on the sternocleidomastoid muscle for mandibular reconstruction in 1908.[13] Soon after, Blair described the use of composite flaps containing both clavicle and rib.[14] However, it was not until the 1970s that this concept was reapplied by Snyder et al[15] and Siemssen et al.[16] Conley reported the first large series of 50 cases of bone containing pedicled flaps for mandibulofacial reconstruction.[17] In this report, he applied a host of newly described techniques, including a deltopectoral acromion flap, a trapezius–scapular flap, and a temporalis–calvarial flap. Although novel in technique, the attendant donor site morbidity and poor bone volume limited the popularity of these flaps. The widespread use of the pectoralis major myocutaneous flap in the mid 1970s led Cuono and Ariyan to use muscle to carry a segment of the fifth rib. However, reports by Biller et al[18] and Bell and Barron[19] reflected poor results as a result of bone exposure and bone necrosis, highlighting the limited vascular supply to these bone segments as well as the lack of mobility of the soft tissue relative to the bone.

Panje and Cutting reported on the use of the lateral trapezius osteomyocutaneous flap for mandibular reconstruction in 1980.[20] This technique was originally described by Demergasso and Piazza.[21] Bone is harvested from the medial portion of the scapular spine, pedicled on the trapezius muscle. This composite flap is supplied by the transverse cervical vascular pedicle as well as contributions from the occipital artery and the paraspinous perforators. Unreliable vascular anatomy and sacrifice of this artery during a radical neck dissection prevented the routine use of this flap in head and neck reconstruction.

In summary, the limitations of pedicled osteomyocutaneous reconstruction are self-evident. However, the insights gained during these trials have led to a better understanding of the importance of vascularized bone and the role of periosteal blood supply. Consequently, these concepts have given rise to the development of bony free tissue transfer, presently considered the gold standard for definitive reconstruction of significant composite defects of the mandibulofacial complex.

Free Tissue Transfer

In 1974, Ostrup and Fredrickson were the first to report on experimental mandibular reconstruction using revascularized rib in the canine model.[12] Shortly thereafter, McKee[22] and Daniel[23] applied this technique clinically, reporting the first vascularized bone containing free flap for mandibular reconstruction. Revascularized rib is no longer used in this capacity; however, this pioneering work revolutionized mandibular reconstruction. For the first time, composite defects of the mandible and adjacent soft tissue could now be reliably reconstructed with vascularized bone as well as skin, obviating the need for a second soft tissue flap. Additional work in this area demonstrated that contouring osteotomies could be performed safely without jeopardizing the vascularity of the bone.[24] Baker and Sullivan later demonstrated that transferred bone healed within 8 weeks, forming a strong union with the adjacent native mandible, even in irradiated patients.[25] As the advantages of transplanted vascularized bone for mandibular reconstruction became evident and the techniques to perform this procedure were refined, several new donor sites were described (**Table 58.2**). However, this review will cover only those most commonly used in contemporary mandibular reconstruction, such as fibular, iliac crest, and scapular donor sites.

Fibula

In 1975, Taylor et al introduced revascularized fibular bone for the repair of an open fracture of the lower extremity.[26] Chen and Yan[27] subsequently examined and reported on the vascular supply to the fibula. It was not until 1989 that Hildalgo reported on the use of the fibular free flap as a method of mandibular reconstruction.[28] Soon thereafter, Hayden and O'Leary expanded the utility of the fibular free flap for oromandibular reconstruction by introducing a sensate flap innervated by the lateral sural cutaneous nerve.[29] The straightforward anatomy and the accessibility of the fibula have been responsible for the popularity of this flap in mandibular reconstruction.

Table 58.2 Donor Sites for Vascularized Bone Containing Free Flaps

Rib
Scapula
Fibula
Ilium
Radius
Ulna
Humerus
Metatarsus

The peroneal artery provides the primary blood supply to the overlying skin of the lateral aspect of the calf and the fibular bone by giving rise to an endosteal vascular supply via a nutrient medullary artery as well as numerous periosteal feeders. The vascular pedicle is limited in length by its bifurcation from the posterior tibial artery. The pedicle can be lengthened by the harvesting of more bone from the distal aspect of the fibula and the discarding of unneeded bone from the proximal aspect. By performing a subperiosteal dissection of the proximal bone, the blood supply to the distal flap can be maintained while pedicle length is gained proximally. Because it is a non–weight-bearing structure, up to 25 cm of dense cortical bone can be harvested with minimal donor site morbidity. The maximum length of bone harvested is predicated on preserving 6 to 7 cm of bone both proximally and distally to preserve normal function of the knee and ankle joints. The ability to harvest such a large portion of bone makes the fibula ideal for reconstruction of subtotal or total defects of the mandible.[30] Aside from supplying the fibula periosteum, the peroneal artery also gives rise to fasciocutaneous perforators located in the posterior cural septum, which supply the overlying skin.

Early reports of skin paddle necrosis were discouraging[28]; however, this was in part due to a poor understanding of the nature of the blood supply to the skin paddle, prompting numerous studies to better define this issue. Yoshimura et al[31] and others[32,33] have performed exhaustive investigations to better define the arterial anatomy as it relates to harvesting a skin paddle. The skin of the lateral aspect of the lower leg is supplied by either musculocutaneous or septocutaneous perforators that derive from the peroneal artery and vein (**Fig. 58.4**). Most surgeons use the approach described by Flemming et al, which favors an anterior subfascial dissection, creating a long flap that allows for variations in the location of the septocutaneous perforators.[34] Wei et al have since demonstrated the reliability of the skin paddle in reconstruction of composite defects, reporting 100% success rate in a total of 80 cases.[35]

The dense cortical bone is ideal for mandibular reconstruction as it effectively withstands the forces of mastication and easily accommodates osseointegrated implants.[36] Curvature of the neomandible can be achieved by the performance of multiple osteotomies without compromising vascularity to the distal bone. In pediatric patients or patients with unusually narrow fibula, the bone can be osteotomized and "double barreled," increasing the height of the bone stock.[37] We have found the fibula to be particularly useful in reconstruction of mandibular defects that involve the condyle. As discussed previously, a subperiosteal dissection of the proximal bone can be performed and the proximal bone may be discarded. The remaining fibula and proximal periosteal sheath can then be used to recreate a protective barrier over the cut end of the bone to prevent the risk of skull base erosion. The narrow fibula can easily be passed through a small tunnel up into the condylar fossa and secured to the glenoid fossa with a nonabsorbable suture. The suture is placed through the periosteal cuff, which serves to anchor the fibula as well as protect the glenoid fossa and prevent ankylosis.

The advantages of the fibular free flap include its uniquely dense cortical bone, which affords excellent primary stability when placing osseointegrated implants. With the vascular pedicle oriented on the lingual surface, multiple osteotomies can be safely performed to contour the bone, and the skin paddle can be transposed over the buccal surface, delivering the skin intraorally. Shortcomings include the limited pedicle length and restricted mobility of the skin paddle relative to the bone, which inhibits the reconstruction of complex composite defects. Finally, because of the high prevalence of peripheral vascular disease

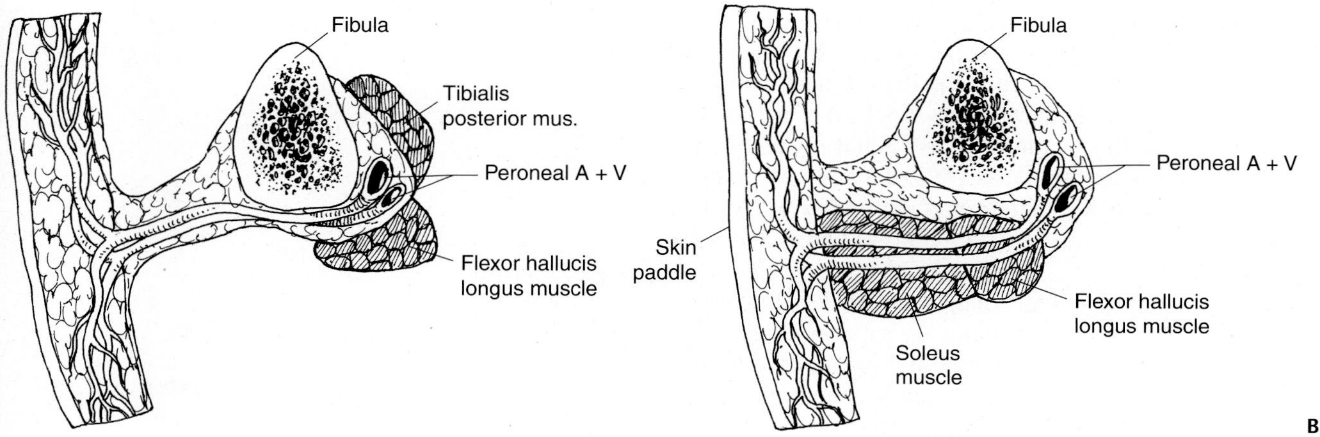

Fig. 58.4 (**A,B**) Vascular supply to the fibula skin paddle. (**A**) Septocutaneous perforators. (**B**) Musculocutaneous perforators. A cuff of soleus and flexor hallucis longus muscle is harvested to protect the perforators.

in head and neck cancer patients and the risk of vascular anomaly, we perform preoperative angiograms on all candidates for fibular free flap reconstruction. In 10 to 20% of patients, either the anterior or posterior tibial artery may become attenuated distally.[38] Although a communicating branch from the peroneal artery supplies the region of the diminutive vessel, if this anomaly is unrecognized, harvest of the fibula may result in ischemia of the foot. In cases where vascular compromise prohibits harvest of a fibula, we review the nature of the anticipated postablative defect and prepare for an alternative donor site.

Scapula

Although Saijo[39] was the first to recognize the potential for transferring free vascularized scapular skin, Swartz[40] popularized the scapular composite free flap for head and neck reconstruction. In contrast to the fibular free flap, the scapular free flap possesses several unique advantages, such as a long vascular pedicle with a large-vessel caliber, the potential for multiple soft tissue options, and mobility between the soft tissue and the bone flap. The independent nature of the vascular supply to the bone, skin paddle, and associated muscles provides an opportunity to reconstruct complex three-dimensional defects and the ability to combine the latissimus dorsi and/or serratus anterior muscles with an overlying skin paddle.[41] It is because of the wide range of hard and soft tissue options that this donor site is best referred to as the subscapular system of flaps.

The vascular pedicle, which is quite constant, is based on the subscapular artery. The subscapular vessels arise from the third part of the axillary artery and give rise to the circumflex scapular vessels (CSVs) and the thoracodorsal vessels (TDVs). The CSVs run through a triangular space formed by teres major, teres minor, and the long head of the triceps brachii muscles. They then divide into and terminate as a cutaneous horizontal branch and a vertical branch, allowing for the harvest of a scapular or parascapular skin paddle, respectively.[42,43] Up to 14 cm of pedicle length can be harvested when the subscapular vessels are included. When the circumflex scapular artery is harvested at its takeoff from the subscapular vessels, the pedicle ranges from 7 to 10 cm with a diameter of 4 mm.[43] The diameter of the subscapular pedicle averages 6 mm, with a range of 4 to 8 mm.[42]

The unique ability to freely maneuver the skin flaps relative to the bone segment facilitates the capacity to restore complex three-dimensional defects that would otherwise require two separate flaps. The skin can be manipulated to resurface large intraoral defects and external skin defects, or it can be deepithelialized and used for soft tissue augmentation. Furthermore, the fact that the lateral scapular border can be harvested separately from the scapular tip adds versatility to this flap. The scapular tip is supplied by the angular artery, a branch of the thoracodorsal artery or the serratus artery (**Fig. 58.5**). The medial half of the scapular tip is characteristically a thin area of bone that is ideal for palatal and orbital reconstruction. We have found that the harvesting of bone from the scapular tip and lateral scapula together is an excellent method for reconstructing combination defects of the palate, retromolar trigone, and mandible. The scapular tip is separated and secured to the remaining palate or adjacent maxilla. The bone from the lateral scapular border is used to reconstruct the lateral mandibular defect. A bilobed scapular–parascapular skin paddle design serves to reline the palate and buccal–gingival sulcus.

In comparison with the medial aspect of the scapular bone, the lateral scapular border provides a more substantial segment of bone measuring up to 10 to 14 cm, which will comfortably accommodate the placement of osseointegrated implants.[36] As with the fibula, the periosteal blood supply of the scapular bone permits the performance of osteotomies for bone contouring. For particularly large orofacial defects, the latissimus dorsi can be harvested on the thoracodorsal artery, in combination with the scapular flap, and used either for intraoral lining or to protect exposed vessels in the neck.

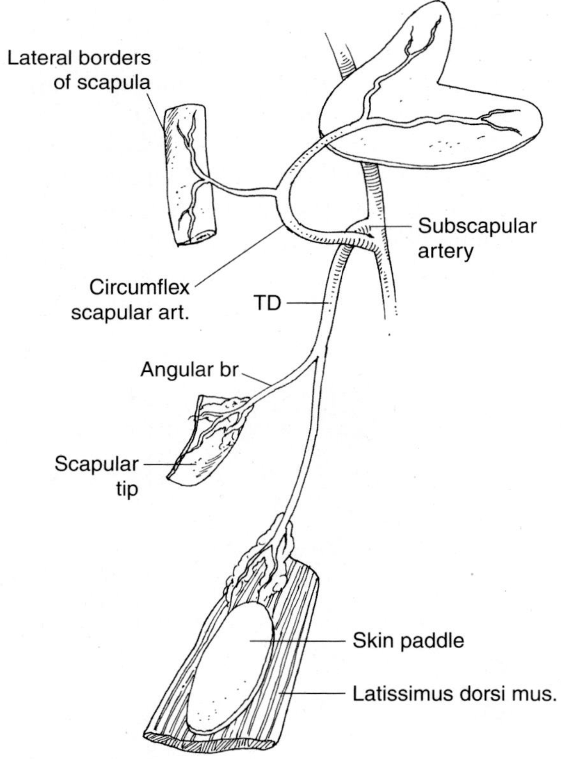

Fig. 58.5 The subscapular system of flaps.

One of the major drawbacks of the subscapular system of flaps is the intraoperative position required for harvest. Aside from precluding a two-team approach, patient positioning can be cumbersome and make an extensive surgery more tedious. As discussed earlier, the scapular bone will accommodate osseointegrated implants; however, pediatric patients may have insufficient bone stock for mandibular reconstruction. For this patient population, a donor site is advisable.

Iliac Crest

The groin and pelvis represent an area that has been the subject of much interest with regard to microvascular transfer. The four distinct vascular suppliers of the ilium—the superficial circumflex iliac artery (SCIA), deep circumflex iliac artery (DCIA), superior deep branch of the gluteal artery, and ascending branch of the lateral circumflex artery—have been responsible for several soft tissue and bone-containing free flaps. In 1980, Salibian reported one of the first free flaps, the groin flap, based on the SCIA.[44] He later found that the SCIA, which provides a rich vascular supply to the skin overlying the ilium, did not reliably supply the periosteum of the ilium.[45] In 1979, Sanders and Mayou[46] determined that the DCIA and DCIV reliably supplied the bone of the ilium as well as the skin overlying the ilium. Subsequent work by Ramasastry identified the ascending branch of the DCIA as the supply to the internal oblique muscle, setting the stage for the introduction of the iliac crest osteomusculocutaneous free flap for reconstruction of the lower extremity.[47] Subsequently, Urken et al applied the iliac crest–internal oblique composite flap to oromandibular reconstruction.[48]

The DCIA and the DCIV, which supply the iliac crest osteomyocutaneous flap,[49] originate from the lateral aspect of the external iliac artery and vein, cephalad to the inguinal ligament. From there, they course toward the anterior superior iliac spine where they enter a tunnel formed by the attachment of the transverse fascia and the iliac fascia to the inner table of the iliac crest. As the DCIA and DCIV course along the inner aspect of the iliac bone, they give rise to several branches, including those that supply the iliac bone, the muscular abdominal wall, and the overlying skin. These branches perforate all three layers of the abdominal wall; hence, a cuff of iliacus, transversus abdominis, internal oblique, and external oblique must be included in the harvest to preserve the deep circumflex iliac vessels and the vascular supply to both the internal oblique muscle and the overlying skin (**Fig. 58.6**). Through injection studies, Ramasastry et al defined a single dominant ascending branch of the DCIA in 80% of cases. However, in 20% of cases, there were several smaller branches supplying the muscle.[47] This independent axial blood supply affords

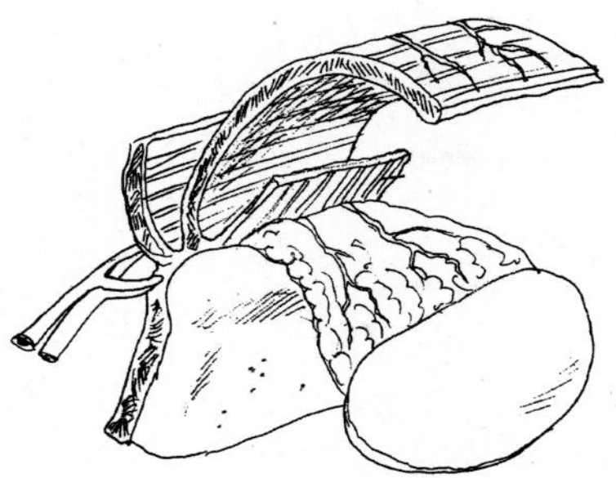

Fig. 58.6 The iliac crest free flap. A tripartate flap composed of a skin paddle, the internal oblique muscle, and the iliac crest.

mobility to the muscle relative to the bone such that it may be wrapped around the neomandible or transposed intraorally.

Over the past decade, the iliac crest has become commonly applied for reconstruction of complex composite defects that would otherwise require multiple flaps. A maximum of 14 to 16 cm of corticocancellous bone can be harvested, which is ideal for the placement of osseointegrated implants.[36] The nature of the donor bone is such that a ramus and condyle can be sculpted according to the principles described by Manchester.[50] The vast periosteal blood supply permits contouring osteotomies, making the iliac crest ideal for lateral and anterior mandibular arch reconstruction. Reconstruction of the mandible is usually achieved by harvesting from the ipsilateral hip. This configuration allows the anterior superior iliac spine to serve as the angle of the neomandible while the iliac crest forms the inferior border. The vascular pedicle remains on the lingual aspect of the neomandible so that the microvascular anastomosis is easily accessible. Urken and colleagues have demonstrated that whereas the bulky nature of the skin paddle often precludes its use for intraoral reconstruction, the thin pliable characteristics of the internal oblique muscle make it ideal for reconstituting intraoral defects.[48,51] In contrast to the scapular flap, the iliac crest skin paddle is often bulky and has poor mobility relative to the bone. Closure of the donor site must be meticulous to prevent a ventral hernia. Careful attention must be paid to the position of the femoral nerve to prevent incidental injury. We have been liberal in our use of synthetic mesh in obese patients or in patients whose closure is compromised by a thin transversus abdominis muscle, which limits the integrity of the abdominal wall.

The advantages of the iliac crest free flap include its unique tripartite design, ideal for complex three-dimensional reconstruction of composite defects of the mandible and oral cavity. In contrast to the scapula, it facilitates a two-team approach, which shortens operative time. Its most significant shortcoming is the bulky nature of the skin paddle, particularly in heavyset patients; however, this problem is circumvented by using the internal oblique muscle for intraoral reconstruction.

Reconstruction of the Temporomandibular Joint

One of the most important considerations related to evaluating and reconstructing the mandible is the presence of the temporomandibular joint (TMJ). Tumors involving the tonsillar fossa or the retromolar trigone often require resection of a portion of the ascending ramus, and extensive disease may necessitate resection of both the condyle and the coronoid process. In cases where a subcondylar ostectomy is appropriate, unless the mandible is primary reconstructed, the coronoid process should not be left intact because contraction of the pterygoid and temporalis muscles will draw the remaining bone superior and medial. Over time, progressive fibrosis leads to pain—a process that may be accentuated by external-beam radiation therapy. The optimal situation arises when an oblique subcondylar ostectomy can be performed. In this situation, the condyle and the posterior border of the ascending ramus are preserved, whereas the coronoid process and its attachments to the temporalis muscle are resected. The neomandible can be secured to the residual ascending ramus, and the coronoid process and its adverse muscular attachments have been eliminated.

If the primary disease process necessitates complete ablation of the ascending ramus, there are several reconstructive options available. Alloplastic joint replacement systems are available,[52] although our experience with these systems has been disappointing. However, autogenous bone or a costochondral graft integrates quite naturally with minimal resorption. As discussed earlier, the fibula can be fashioned with a periosteal cuff, which can then be secured to the glenoid fossa with nonabsorbable suture.

Primary versus Secondary Mandibular Reconstruction

There has been a great deal of debate regarding the timing of mandibular reconstruction. In the past, delayed management of the mandibular defect was considered standard for two reasons. First, prior to the implementation of free vascularized mandibular reconstruction, nonvascularized bone grafts were exposed to salivary contamination during primary reconstruction, which often resulted in an unacceptably high rate of graft infection and resorption. Second, because of the high recurrence rates associated with oral cavity carcinoma, some surgeons required a disease-free interval before embarking on a complex reconstruction.

Although there is merit to this logic, advocates of primary reconstruction contend that patients should not be forced to live with the cosmetic and functional consequences that commonly result from ablative surgery. The goal of primary oromandibular reconstruction is to restore both function and appearance in a manner that will allow the patient to assume as normal a lifestyle as possible. Furthermore, contraction and fibrosis of the operated field often complicate secondary reconstruction, increasing the risk of facial nerve paralysis and, in some cases, increasing the risk of postoperative morbidity.

Dental Rehabilitation

Despite advances in free tissue transfer and the capability of restoring continuity defects as well as soft tissue lining, the ultimate goal of occlusal and masticatory function restoration had remained elusive.[53] The quality of the soft tissue transplant or native mucosa, often irradiated, did not provide for a good environment for the retention of a conventional, removable dental appliance. The use of osseointegrated fixtures, popularized by the work of Branemark et al,[54] provided the solution to this problem. Endosteal titanium fixtures, strategically placed in the bone flap and allowed to osseointegrate, could provide for anchorage and allow for load sharing of the dental prosthesis, minimizing the risk of injury to the radiated native mucosa as well as the possibility of radiation-induced osteomyelitis of the underlying bone.

Over the past decade, several reports have described the importance and efficacy of this type of functional masticatory restoration.[55–57] However, one of the controversies in the use of this technique relates to the timing of the fixture placement and the effect of radiation on the process of integration of the endosteal fixtures. Whereas we have long advocated for the primary placement of the fixtures at the time of the reconstructive procedure,[58] others prefer to place the implants in a secondary procedure.[59] In theory, delayed placement of the fixtures allows one to position them in a more ideal location and inclination in terms of the opposing arch. The reality is that the buccolingual positioning of the fixtures is essentially dictated by the initial contouring of the bone flap. Furthermore, primary placement affords the best surgical access for assessment of the interarch relationship. Finally, primary placement of the fixtures takes advantage of a "window of opportunity" before the damaging effect of radiation affects the bone.[60] Implant placement in irradiated bone would require preoperative hyperbaric oxygen therapy,[61] thus adding to the cost and inconveniencing the patient.

Donor Site Selection

Donor site selection for oromandibular reconstruction is predicated on several factors, including:

1. The nature of the soft tissue defect
2. The relationship of the composite defect to the tongue and oropharynx
3. The nature of the bone defect
4. Donor site availability

The scapular, iliac, and fibular donor sites may all be used to successfully reconstruct composite defects involving the mandible; however, the nature of the soft tissue defect often dictates the donor site. As mentioned earlier, the mobility of the skin paddle relative to the bone segment plays an integral role in determining the optimal donor site. The immobile skin paddle, characteristic of the fibular free flap, often precludes its use in complex three-dimensional reconstructions. If the fibular skin paddle is used to reconstruct composite defects involving the tongue base, the restricted mobility of the skin relative to the bone flap may tether the tongue during deglutition, thus preventing optimal functional rehabilitation. However, this skin paddle is best suited for anterior and lateral floor-of-mouth defects as well as external defects of the neck.

In contrast, the iliac and scapular free flaps can be manipulated to resurface complex defects of the oral cavity, oropharynx, and the neck. The scapular donor site possesses the added advantage of allowing for harvest of the latissimus dorsi or serratus anterior muscle, which can be used to reline the oral cavity or insulate the great vessels. The iliac tripartite design allows for the internal oblique muscle to be used for relining the oral cavity, whereas the skin paddle can be employed to reconstruct the lateral tongue or external neck.

The nature of the bone stock associated with each donor site seldom dictates donor site selection. An exception is during the reconstruction of a total or near-total mandibular defect, which requires a long segment of bone that will tolerate multiple contouring osteotomies as well as sustain the forces of mastication. The fibula is the only donor site that will accommodate a total mandibular reconstruction because it offers the appropriate length as well as the ability to safely reconstruct both condyles. Another consideration is that total mandibular reconstruction and condylar replacement can place the facial nerve at risk. The characteristically narrow dimensions of the fibular bone are ideal for this purpose. The fibular bone can be drawn cephalad into the condylar fossa through a small tunnel and secured into the glenoid fossa with little risk of neural injury.

Finally, contraindications to using a donor site are rare, but they do occur. We recommend preoperative lower extremity angiography for all patients who are candidates for a fibular free flap. The role of preoperative angiography has been assessed in several recent studies, and angiographic findings preventing the use of the fibula have ranged from 10 to 25%.[62–64] Congenital vascular anomalies, vascular disease, and prior lower extremity injury are the most common contraindications to the use of this flap. However, the iliac crest can be evaluated by physical examination. Prior surgery to the hip, groin, or lower abdomen makes up the majority of contraindications to use of this donor site. Similarly, use of the scapular donor site has few contraindications; prior injury or surgery to this area should be evaluated.

Summary

Although there are a host of options for mandibular reconstruction, vascularized bone flaps are unique in that they permit reconstruction of the oromandibular complex even though the recipient bed is often compromised by salivary contamination and prior irradiation. In contrast to nonvascularized bone grafts, vascularized bone grafts remain capable of healing to the adjacent native mandible and eventually withstand the loading forces associated with mastication.[65,66] The fibular, iliac, and scapular donor sites all provide bone stock sufficient for dental implants in the majority of patients,[36] which has been demonstrated as an essential factor for full oral rehabilitation.[3] Furthermore, the soft tissue components harvested with each of these three composite flap donor sites provide a source of tissue for either intraoral lining or extraoral coverage.[67] Inherent differences with regard to bone stock, soft tissue quality, potential for sensory reinnervation, and pedicle geometry dictate which of the available donor sites will provide the optimal source for reconstruction.

References

1. Crile G. Excision of cancer of the head and neck. JAMA 1906;47:1780
2. Papel ID, Price JC, Kashima HK, Johns ME. Compression plates in the treatment of advanced anterior floor of mouth carcinoma. Laryngoscope 1986;96(7):722–725
3. Urken ML, Buchbinder D, Weinberg H, et al. Functional evaluation following microvascular oromandibular reconstruction of the oral cancer patient: a comparative study of reconstructed and nonreconstructed patients [see comments]. Laryngoscope 1991;101(9):935–950
4. Steckler RM, Edgerton MT, Gogel W. Andy Gump. Am J Surg 1974;128(4): 545–547
5. Axhausen W. The osteogenic phases of regeneration of bone: a historical and experimental study. J Bone Joint Surg 1956;38:593
6. Adamo AK, Szal RL. Timing, results, and complications of mandibular reconstructive surgery: report of 32 cases. J Oral Surg 1979;37(10): 755–763
7. Lawson W, Loscalzo LJ, Back SM, et al. Experience with immediate and delayed mandibular reconstruction. Laryngoscope 1982;92(1):5–10
8. Marx RE. Osteoradionecrosis: a new concept of its pathophysiology. J Oral Maxillofac Surg 1983;41(5):283–288

9. Marx RE. A new concept in the treatment of osteoradionecrosis. J Oral Maxillofac Surg 1983;41(6):351–357
10. McCullough D, Fredrickson J. Neovascularized rib grafts to reconstruct mandibular defects. Can J Otolaryngol 1973;2:96
11. Ostrup LT, Tam CS. Bone formation in a free, living bone graft transferred by microvascular anastomoses:_ a quantitative microscopic study using fluorochrome markers. Scand J Plast Reconstr Surg 1975;9(2):101–106
12. Ostrup LT, Fredrickson JM. Reconstruction of mandibular defects after radiation, using a free, living bone graft transferred by microvascular anastomose: an experimental study. Plast Reconstr Surg 1975;55(5):563–572
13. Rydygier L. Zum osteoplastischen Ersatz nach Unterkieferresektion. Zentralbl Chir 1908;36:1321
14. Blair V. Surgery and Diseases of the Mouth and Jaw. St. Louis: CV Mosby; 1918
15. Snyder CC, Bateman JM, Davis CW, Warden GD. Mandibulofacial restoration with live osteocutaneous flaps. Plast Reconstr Surg 1970;45(1):14–19
16. Siemssen SO, Kirkby B, O'Connor TP. Immediate reconstruction of a resected segment of the lower jaw, using a compound flap of clavicle and sternomastoid muscle. Plast Reconstr Surg 1978;61(5):724–735
17. Conley J. Use of composite flaps containing bone for major repairs in the head and neck. Plast Reconstr Surg 1972;49(5):522–526
18. Biller HF, Back SM, Lawson W, et al. Pectoralis major myocutaneous island flap in head and neck surgery: analysis of complications in 42 cases. Arch Otolaryngol 1981;107(1):23–26
19. Bell M, Baron PT. Reconstruction of floor of mouth defects with pectoralis major rib flaps. In: Williams HB, ed. Transactions of the Eighth International Congress of Plastic and Reconstructive Surgery. Montreal, 1983
20. Panje W, Cutting C. Trapezius osteomyocutaneous island flap for reconstruction of the anterior floor of the mouth and the mandible. Head Neck Surg 1980;3(1):66–71
21. Demergasso F, Piazza MV. Trapezius myocutaneous flap in reconstructive surgery for head and neck cancer: an original technique. Am J Surg 1979;138(4):533–536
22. McKee DM. Microvascular bone transplatation. Clin Plast Surg 1978;5(2):283–292
23. Daniel RK. Reconstruction of mandibular defects with revascularized free rib grafts [letter]. Plast Reconstr Surg 1978;62(5):775–776
24. Ariyan S. The viability of rib grafts transplanted with the periosteal blood supply. Plast Reconstr Surg 1980;65(2):140–151
25. Baker SR, Sullivan MJ. Osteocutaneous free scapular flap for one-stage mandibular reconstruction. Arch Otolaryngol Head Neck Surg 1988;114(3):267–277
26. Taylor GI, Miller GD, Ham FJ. The free vascularized bone graft: a clinical extension of microvascular techniques. Plast Reconstr Surg 1975;55(5):533–544
27. Chen Z, Yan W. The study and clinincal application of the osteocutaneous flap of fibula. J Microsurg 1983;4:11–16
28. Hidalgo DA. Fibula free flap: a new method of mandible reconstruction. Plast Reconstr Surg 1989;84(1):71–79
29. Hayden R, O'Leary MA. A neurosensory fibula flap: anatomical description and clinical applications. In: 94th Annual Meeting of the American Laryngological, Rhinological, and Otological Society. Waikoloa, Hawaii, 1991
30. Gilbert R, Dovion D. Near total mandibular reconstruction: the free vascularized fibula transfer. Oper Tech Otolaryngol Head Neck Surg 1993;4:145
31. Yoshimura M, Shimamura K, Iwai Y, et al. Free vascularized fibular transplant:_ a new method for monitoring circulation of the grafted fibula. J Bone Joint Surg Am 1983;65(9):1295–1301
32. Beppu M, Hanel DP, Johnston GH, et al. The osteocutaneous fibula flap: an anatomic study. J Reconstr Microsurg 1992;8(3):215–223
33. Carriquiry C, Aparecida Costa M, Vasconez LO. An anatomic study of the septocutaneous vessels of the leg. Plast Reconstr Surg 1985;76(3):354–363
34. Flemming AF, Brough MD, Evans ND, et al. Mandibular reconstruction using vascularised fibula. Br J Plast Surg 1990;43(4):403–409
35. Wei F, Seah C, Tsai Y, et al. Fibula osteoseptocutaneous flap reconstruction of the composite mandibular defect. Plast Reconstr Surg 1994;93:294
36. Moscoso JF, Keller J, Genden E, et al. Vascularized bone flaps in oromandibular reconstruction:_ a comparative anatomic study of bone stock from various donor sites to assess suitability for enosseous dental implants. Arch Otolaryngol Head Neck Surg 1994;120(1):36–43
37. Jones NF, Swartz WM, Mears DC, et al. The "double-barrel" free vascularized fibular bone graft. Plast Reconstr Surg 1988;81(3):378–385
38. Senior HD. An interpretation of the recorded arterial anomoloies in the human leg and foot. J Anat 1919;53:130
39. Saijo M. The vascular territories of the dorsal trunk: a reappraisal for potential flap donor sites. Br J Plast Surg 1978;31(3):200–204
40. Swartz WM, Banis JC, Newton ED, et al. The osteocutaneous scapular flap for mandibular and maxillary reconstruction. Plast Reconstr Surg 1986;77(4):530–545
41. Harii K, Yamada A, Ishihara K, et al. A free transfer of both latissimus dorsi and serratus anterior flaps with thoracodorsal vessel anastomoses. Plast Reconstr Surg 1982;70(5):620–629
42. Dos Santos L. The vascular anatomy and dissection of the free scapular flap. Plast Reconstr Surg 1984;73:599
43. Nassif TM, Vidal L, Bovet JL, Baudet J. The parascapular flap: a new cutaneous microsurgical free flap. Plast Reconstr Surg 1982;69(4):591–600
44. Salibian AH, Rappaport I, Furnas DW, Achaver BM. Microvascular reconstruction of the mandible. Am J Surg 1980;140(4):499–502
45. Salibian AH, Rappaport I, Allison G. Functional oromandibular reconstruction with the microvascular composite groin flap. Plast Reconstr Surg 1985;76(6):819–828
46. Sanders R, Mayou BJ. A new vascularized bone graft transferred by microvascular anastomosis as a free flap. Br J Surg 1979;66(11):787–788
47. Ramasastry SS, Tucker JB, Swartz WM, Hurwitz DJ. The internal oblique muscle flap: an anatomic and clinical study. Plast Reconstr Surg 1984;73(5):721–733
48. Urken ML, Vickery C, Weinberg H, et al. The internal oblique–iliac crest osseomyocutaneous free flap in oromandibular reconstruction: report of 20 cases. Arch Otolaryngol Head Neck Surg 1989;115(3):339–349
49. Taylor GI. Reconstruction of the mandible with free composite iliac bone grafts. Ann Plast Surg 1982;9(5):361–376
50. Manchester W. Immediate reconstruction of the mandible and the temoromandibular joint. Br J Plast Surg 1965;18:291
51. Urken ML, Weinberg H, Vickery C, et al. Oromandibular reconstruction using microvascular composite free flaps: report of 71 cases and a new classification scheme for bony, soft-tissue, and neurologic defects. Arch Otolaryngol Head Neck Surg 1991;117(7):733–744
52. Wolford LM. Temporomandibular joint devices: treatment factors and outcomes. Oral Surg Oral Med Oral Pathol Oral Radiol Endod 1997;83(1):143–149
53. Komisar A. The functional result of mandibular reconstruction. Laryngoscope 1990;100(4):364–374
54. Brånemark PI, Hansson BO, Adell R, et al. Osseointegrated implants in the treatment of the edentulous jaw. Experience from a 10-year period. Scand J Plast Reconstr Surg Suppl 1977;16:1–132
55. Schmelzeisen R, Hausamen JE, Neukam FW, et al. Combination of microsurgical tissue reconstruction with osteointegrated dental implants:_ presentation of a technique. Int J Oral Maxillofac Surg 1990;19(4):209–211
56. Reideger D. Restoration of masticatory function by microsurgically revascularized iliac crest bone grafts using endosseous implants. Plast Reconstr Surg 1988;81:861
57. Neukam F, Schmelzeisen R, Schliephake H. Oromandibular reconstruction with vascularized bone grafts in combination with implants. In: Davis W, Sailer F, ed. Preprosthetic Surgery: Oral Maxillofacial Surgery. Philadelphia: WB Saunders; 1990

58. Urken M, Buchbinder D, Weinberg H, et al. Primary placement of osseointegrated implants in mandibular reconstruction. Otolaryngol Head Neck Surg 1989;101:56
59. Reychler H, Iriarte Ortabe J, Pecheur A, Brogniez V. Mandibular reconstruction with a free vascularized fibula flap and osseointegrated implants: a report of four cases. J Oral Maxillofac Surg 1996;54(12):1464–1469
60. Jacobsson M, Telljström A, Albrektsson T, Thomsen P, Turesson I. Integration of titanium implants into irradiated bone. Ann Otorhinolaryngol 1988;97:337–340
61. Larsen PE, Stronczek MJ, Beck FM, Rohrer M. Osteointegration of implants in radiated bone with and without adjunctive hyperbaric oxygen. J Oral Maxillofac Surg 1993;51(3):280–287
62. Disa JJ, Cordeiro PG. The current role of preoperative arteriography in free fibula flaps. Plast Reconstr Surg 1998;102(4):1083–1088
63. Young DM, Trabulsy PP, Anthony JP. The need for preoperative leg angiography in fibula free flaps. J Reconstr Microsurg 1994;10(5):283–287; discussion 287–289
64. Blackwell KE. Donor site evaluation for fibula free flap transfer. Am J Otolaryngol 1998;19(2):89–95
65. Urken ML. Composite free flaps in oromandibular reconstruction: review of the literature. Arch Otolaryngol Head Neck Surg 1991;117(7):724–732
66. Duncan MJ, Manktelow RT, Zuker RM, Rosen IB. Mandibular reconstruction in the radiated patient: the role of osteocutaneous free tissue transfers. Plast Reconstr Surg 1985;76(6):829–840
67. Wilson KM, Rizk NM, Armstrong SL, Gluckman JL. Effects of hemimandibulectomy on quality of life. Laryngoscope 1998;108(10):1574–1577

59 Major Nasal Reconstruction

Shan R. Baker

)ver the last decade, reconstruction of the nose has eached a high level of sophistication, with enhancement ›f aesthetic results.[1–3] This has been achieved by empha-izing the necessity of replacing surgically ablated tissue vith like tissue. Skin is replaced with skin that matches t in color and texture as closely as possible. Cartilage and one are replaced, and mucosa is used to replace any loss f the nasal lining. The concept of nasal aesthetic units has merged with an emphasis on reconstructing an entire nit, if the majority of the unit is missing. Another impor-ant concept that has led to enhancement in the results of estorative surgery has been the emphasis on the place-nent of incisions for local flaps along borders of aesthetic egions or units to maximize camouflage of scars. When-ver possible, local flaps are designed so that they are not ransferred across the borders of aesthetic regions, partic-larly if the border has a concave topography. An example f such a border is the alar facial sulcus, which represents concave border between three aesthetic facial regions: he nose, the cheek, and the upper lip.[4,5]

·acial Aesthetic Regions

'he face can be divided into topographic regions, each vith its individual intrinsic characteristics of skin color, exture, contour, and hair growth.[5] Each has an individ-al shape created by the underlying facial skeleton. The ose is one of the aesthetic regions of the face and can be ivided into several aesthetic units (**Fig. 59.1**). Each unit may be proportionally over- or underdeveloped relative to other noses, but there is a consistent general configu-ration from nose to nose. There are nine aesthetic units of the nose identified by distinctive convex or concave surfaces, including the lobule, dorsum, paired sidewalls, paired alae, paired soft tissue facets, and the columella. The shape of the lobule is determined, in general, by the size and contour of the alar cartilages, and specifically by the domal portion of the nasal cartilages. The lobule is covered by relatively thick sebaceous skin. Each dome causes a point of reflected light. Above the lobule is a supratip depression, which separates the lobule from the dorsum. The skin of the dorsum tends to be less thick and sebaceous than that of the lobule, becoming progressively thinner as it ascends to the rhinion and thicker again as it approaches the glabella. The nasal bones together with the upper lateral cartilages and cartilaginous septum provide skeletal support for the dorsum. The lateral bor-ders of the dorsum are defined by the lateral shoulders of the upper lateral cartilages and the junction of the nasal bones with the frontal processes of the maxillae. These structures separate the dorsum from the sidewalls and create a line of reflected light and shadows separating the lateral walls from the dorsum. The nasal sidewalls are most often a combination of convex and concave elements extending laterally from the dorsum to the junction of the nose and cheek. Structurally, the sidewalls are supported by the lateral extensions of the nasal bones and upper lateral cartilages and the medial extension of the frontal processes of the maxillae. The skin of the

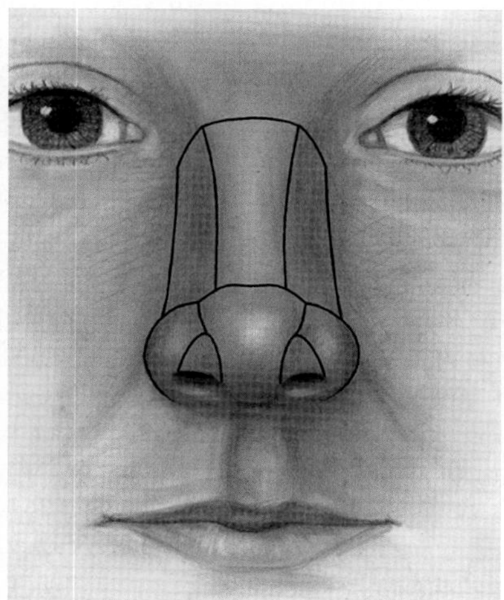

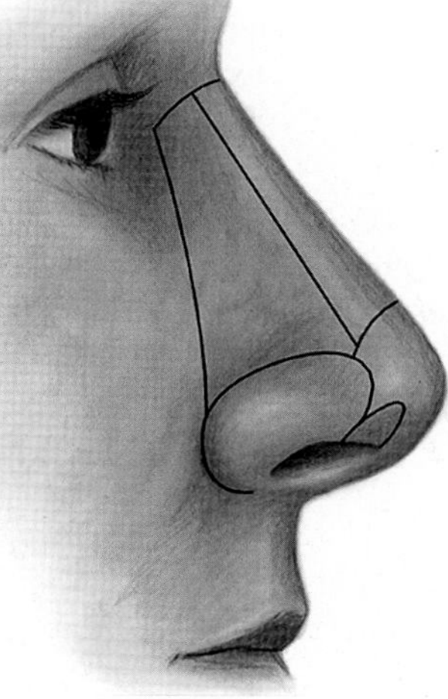

B

Fig. 59.1 (**A,B**) Topographic aesthetic nasal units.

sidewalls is thin and less sebaceous than that of the dorsum and lobule, and they are separated from the alae by the alar nasal crease, which is the deepest contour line of the nose. This crease is continuous laterally with the alar facial sulcus, and together they circle the alae, delineating them from the lobule, sidewalls, and cheeks. The alar unit itself is a smooth bulge reflecting a single spot of light and is covered with thick sebaceous skin similar in texture and porosity to that of the lobule. The structural support of the ala is provided by thick fibrofatty tissue that does not contain cartilage.

The soft tissue facets contribute to a portion of the nostril margin and span the notch between intermediate and lateral crura of each lower lateral cartilage. They are covered by thin, nonsebaceous skin and have only a small amount of fibrous connective tissue for structural support. They may be separated as distinct units by the shadow of the lobule. The columella, like the lobule and dorsum, is a nonpaired aesthetic unit extending from the caudal aspect of the lobule to the upper lip. It is covered by the thinnest of nasal skin and is supported structurally by the medial crura. The lining for each of the nine aesthetic units of the nose is also distinctive. Thin non–hair-bearing skin lines the lobule, whereas the nasal facets and alae are lined by thicker skin, the caudal aspect of which is hair bearing. The columella is backed by the membranous septum, which is skin-lined. At the piriform aperture, the lining transitions to mucosa that lines the dorsum and sidewall units.

Menick has stressed that the goal of restorative nasal surgery is not simply to fill a defect.[2] Depending on the extent of the defect, wounds should be altered in size, configuration, and depth to allow reconstruction of an entire unit. If the majority of the surface area of a unit is lost, resurfacing of the entire unit is usually preferable. This is accomplished by discarding the remaining skin of the unit and designing the surface flap so that it will compensate for the discarded skin. This arrangement places the scars in the junction between units where they will lie in depressions or along shadow lines, maximizing scar camouflage. By placing the scars in these junctions, they will blend with the normal contour lines of the nose and will not distract the viewing eye. Resurfacing the entire unit also takes advantage of the mild trap-door scar contraction phenomenon, which causes the entire unit to bulge slightly, simulating the normal convexity of the lobule, dorsum, and ala.[2] More important than resurfacing of an entire nasal unit, however, is the creation of the proper contour of the flaps so that it exactly duplicates the normal topography of the unit.

The surface area and pattern of each unit should be replaced so as to achieve exact duplication whenever possible. Because a fresh wound is always enlarged by retraction of the margins, the contralateral units should be used for the design of covering flaps. If the contralateral counterpart is missing or a unit does not have a matching pair, a template recreating the ideal unit size for that specific patient is used. Because the nose is a three-dimensional structure, each unit must duplicate the normal contour. This is accomplished by concomitantly integrating structural support in each step of the repair. Reconstructed skeletal elements must be attached to a stable foundation, such as remaining nasal cartilages or the bone of the maxilla, to prevent collapse or distortion during the healing process.[2] The reconstructed skeletal structures must span the entire defect. This is accomplished prior to wound healing to prevent distortion from scar contraction during the healing process.

Application of the aesthetic unit principles provides a logical cognitive approach to nasal reconstruction. Missing tissue must be replaced with like tissue at a quantity and quality that exactly replicates the pattern, surface area, and contour of the absent unit.

Flaps for Nasal Reconstruction

Lining Flaps

Burget and Menick have studied the vascularity of the nasal septal mucosa and discovered that the entire ipsilateral septal mucoperichondrium can be transferred with a narrow pedicle containing the septal branch of the superior labial artery.[1] Likewise, the entire contralateral mucoperichondrium can be turned laterally as a dorsally based hinge flap to line the sidewall of the nose based on the anterior and posterior ethmoid arteries (**Fig. 59.2**).[1] Burget and Menick have also shown that if both right and left septal branches are included in the pedicle, the entire septum can be rotated out of the nasal passage as a composite flap containing a sandwich of cartilage between the two mucoperichondrial leaves (**Fig. 59.3**).[1] Such flaps, whether composite or simple mucoperichondrial hinge flaps, can be designed to extend from the floor of the nose to within 1 cm of the junction of the upper lateral cartilage and cartilaginous septum. The flaps may extend posteriorly well beyond the bony–cartilaginous junction of the septum, producing a hinged mucosal flap as wide as 3 cm and as long as 5 cm.[1] Burget and Menick advocate a back-cut of the mucoperichondrium in the area of the anterior septal angle to facilitate flap transfer.[3] I prefer leaving the flap hinged on the entire length of caudal septum to maintain a wider pedicle and enhance the vascularity of the flap (**Fig. 59.3B**). These authors have also described a bipedicle flap of vestibular skin and mucosa based medially on the septum and laterally on the floor of the nasal vestibule. Such a flap is elevated from the undersurface of the lateral crus and mobilized inferiorly to reline alar defects (**Fig. 59.4**). All of these lining flaps have a reliable vascularity

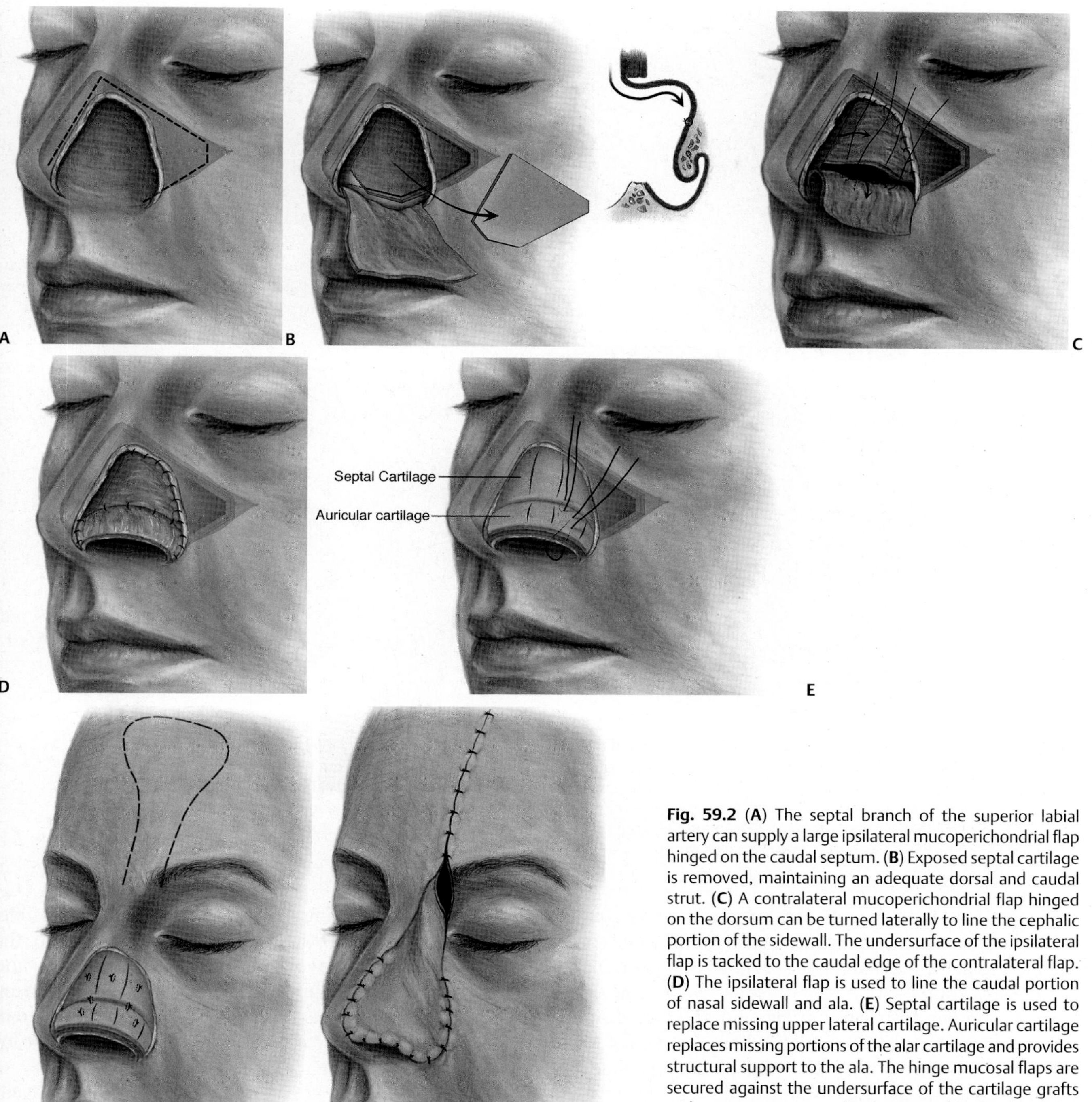

Fig. 59.2 (**A**) The septal branch of the superior labial artery can supply a large ipsilateral mucoperichondrial flap hinged on the caudal septum. (**B**) Exposed septal cartilage is removed, maintaining an adequate dorsal and caudal strut. (**C**) A contralateral mucoperichondrial flap hinged on the dorsum can be turned laterally to line the cephalic portion of the sidewall. The undersurface of the ipsilateral flap is tacked to the caudal edge of the contralateral flap. (**D**) The ipsilateral flap is used to line the caudal portion of nasal sidewall and ala. (**E**) Septal cartilage is used to replace missing upper lateral cartilage. Auricular cartilage replaces missing portions of the alar cartilage and provides structural support to the ala. The hinge mucosal flaps are secured against the undersurface of the cartilage grafts with mattress sutures. (**F,G**) Paramedian forehead flap is used to cover exposed cartilage grafts.

and are thin and supple, providing natural physiological material for the interior of the nasal passage. They do not distort the external shape of the nose, nor do they compromise the airway. Importantly, these well-vascularized lining flaps allow the primary placement of cartilage grafts for framework, which when properly fashioned prevents nasal distortion resulting from scar contraction.

Framework Grafts

The dorsum of the nose is supported by the nasal bones and cartilaginous septum: the sidewalls by the frontal processes of the maxillae and upper lateral cartilages, the lobule by the intermediate and lateral crura of the alar cartilages, the columella by the medial crura, and the ala

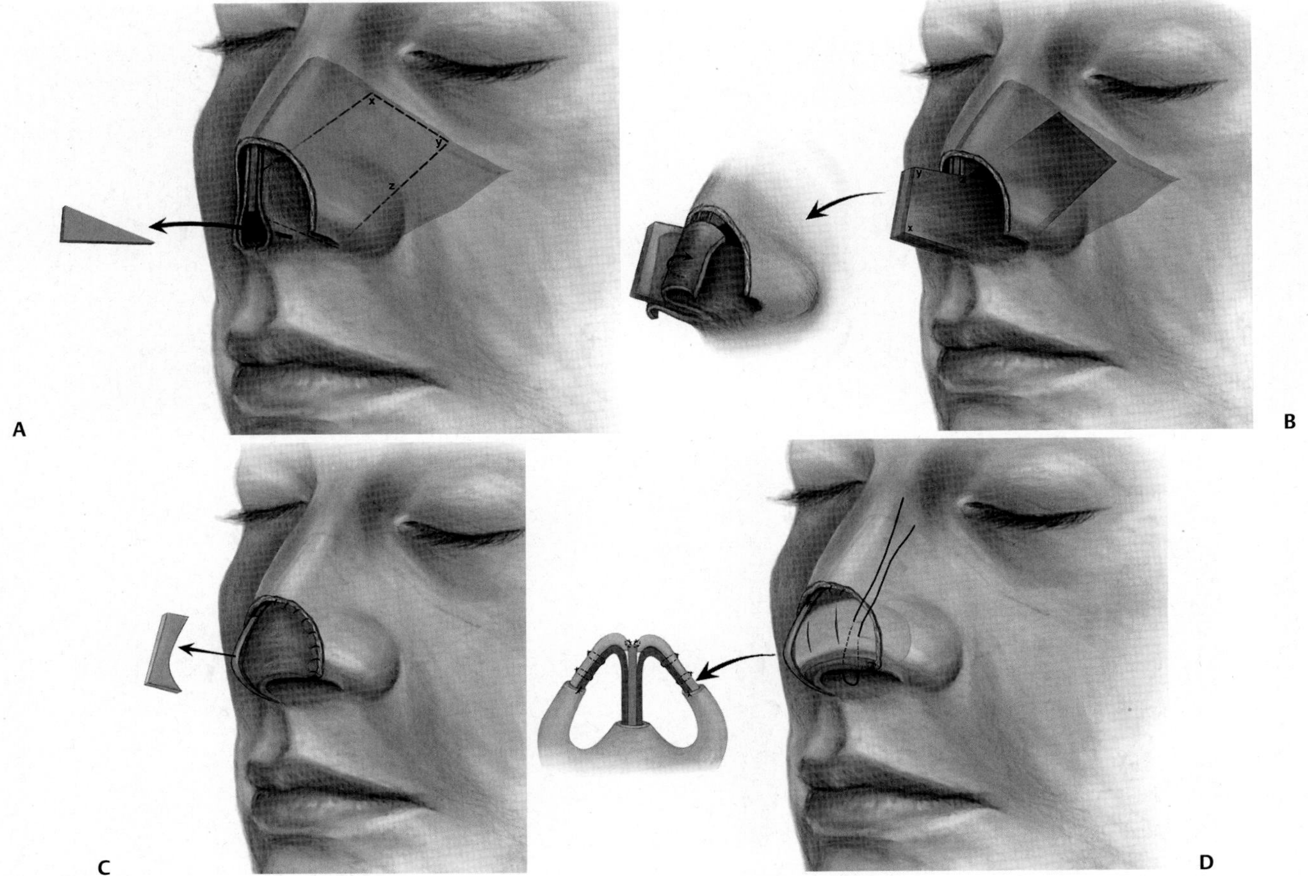

Fig. 59.3 (**A**) Composite flap based on the dual blood supply of the septal branches of the superior labial artery. A wedge of cartilage is removed to allow the flap to be turned outward. (**B**) Bilateral hinged mucoperichondrial flaps are turned downward to provide lining for the reconstructed nasal vestibule. (**C**) Excess septal cartilage is trimmed, and flaps are sutured to the lateral and superior borders of the vestibule. (**D**) Auricular cartilage grafts are used to replace missing portions of alar cartilages. Hinged mucoperichondrial flaps are secured against the undersurface of the cartilage grafts with mattress sutures.

and soft tissue facet by stiff fibrofatty connective tissue. If missing, the nasal framework of each unit must be completely replaced. Cartilage grafts can be used to replace the missing framework of the dorsum, lobule, and sidewalls. In addition, a strip of cartilage must be placed along the reconstructed nostril margin whenever the connective tissue framework is missing (**Fig. 59.4C**). In instances of alar reconstruction, this usually means placing a cartilaginous strip that spans the distance from the junction of the ala with the cheek to the region of the soft tissue facet, even though these areas do not normally contain cartilage. This is required to support the nostril rim and prevent upward migration of the nostril margin during wound healing.

The function of the framework is to provide contour and maintain a patent airway. Framework grafts must be placed at the time of initial reconstruction and should consist of grafts that replicate the exact size, shape, and contour of the missing framework as closely as possible When covered by a thin, conforming cutaneous flap, the contour of the framework is distinctively manifested and produces a normal appearing restoration of the missing part. Framework grafts fix in place the soft tissues used in nasal repair by virtue of providing a skeletal support for both lining and cover.

Bone and cartilage are the tissue-grafting materials available to the surgeon for replacing the framework of the nose. The framework of the nasal dorsum may be replaced with bone or cartilage. Cranial bone grafts are the preferred material for more cephalic skeletal defects and are anchored to the frontal bone with miniplates. Limited caudal dorsal skeletal defects are best replaced with septal or auricular cartilage when available. The dorsal framework prevents cephalic contraction and subsequent shortening of the nose. It also provides shape and projection to the bridge The framework of the sidewall can be replaced with septal

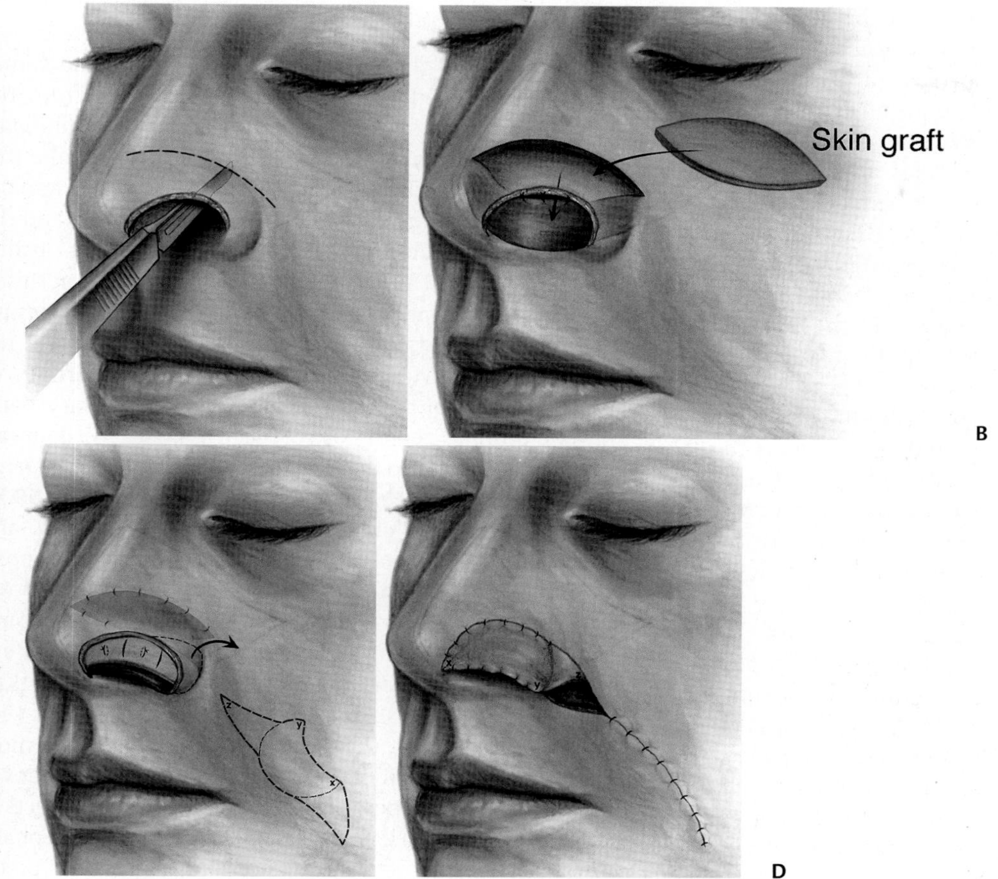

ig. 59.4 (**A**) Full-thickness defects of the ala that do not extend cephalad more than 1.5 cm may be lined by bipedicle advancement vestibular skin flap based medially on the septum and laterally on the floor of the asal vestibule. An extended intercartilaginous incision is needed to develop the flap. (**B**) The bipedicle flap is dvanced caudally and the donor site is covered with a thin full-thickness skin graft. (**C**) Any remaining skin of he ala is discarded (*arrow*). Auricular cartilage provides structural support to the nostril margin. A superiorly ased subcutaneous pedicled interpolated cheek flap is designed to cover the cartilage graft. (**D**) Interpolated heek flap sutured in place. The caudal border of the cheek flap is sutured to the caudal border of the bipedicle dvancement flap.

one and cartilage or cranial bone contoured into a trape-oid shape and fixed to the dorsum and maxilla. It supports he middle vault and prevents collapse. It also serves as a oundation for attaching the lower framework of the nose, pecifically the alar cartilages or their replacements.

The lobule is shaped by the alar cartilages, and the pre-erred replacement framework is conchal cartilage grafts. y coincidence, when turned upside down, the contralat-ral concha cymba often closely resembles the shape of he dome cartilage (intermediate crus) and the concha avum resembles the shape of the lateral crus. Grafts to 8 mm wide from the auricle can be scored and bent o replace the entire lower lateral cartilages. These grafts an be used bilaterally or unilaterally as needed and are ixed to any residual stumps of the medial and lateral rura. They support the dome and recreate the contour of the nasal lobule. Additional projection and shaping of the tip can be accomplished with Peck-type septal cartilage grafts anchored atop the reconstructed alar cartilages[2] or the fabrication of shield-shaped septal cartilage tip grafts placed caudad to the auricular cartilages.

Structural support for the columella can be provided by auricular cartilage grafts described for the lobule, but placed in such a way as to span the gap in the medial crus or extend all the way to the nasal spine if the entire medial crus is absent. Septal cartilage grafts are very effective for this purpose as well but must be thinned, scored, and bent so as to replicate the diverging angle that naturally occurs at the junction of the medial and intermediate crura.

An alar batten of septal or auricular cartilage 5 mm wide can be used for the framework of the ala and soft tissue facet. The natural curvature of the concha cartilage makes this material preferable to septal cartilage when available. When all or portions of the lateral crus are missing in addition to the ala, the auricular cartilage graft can be designed as a wider graft (0.75 to 1.0 cm) to concomitantly replace the lateral crus and provide support to the ala. The graft should be placed along the proposed margin of the missing nostril from the alar base to the nostril apex (see **Fig. 59.6D**). It is inserted into a deep-tissue pocket in the alar facial sulcus and attached medially to the framework of the dome. The tissue pocket serves to stabilize the graft laterally. Similar to the grafts used to replace missing alar cartilage, grafts must be thinned, scored, and bent to replicate the bulging contour of the ala. If the nasal defect extends to the soft tissue facet, the batten should extend beneath the diverging angles of the intermediate and lateral crura to span any gap present. The batten fixes the reconstructed alar rim in position, preventing upward migration and notching of the rim.

In summary, the surgeon must determine what part of the nasal framework is missing and replace it completely. Each replaced element must be carefully shaped, thinned, scored, bent, and fixed with regard to nasal projection, contour, alar rim position, and symmetry, so that it exactly replicates the contralateral counterpart or the ideal if both components of the framework are missing. The better the surgeon can achieve this goal, the better the aesthetic and functional results.

Covering Flaps

Small defects of the nasal skin (2 cm or less) can sometimes be repaired with local flaps harvested from the remaining nasal skin if there is sufficient redundancy of skin. Most notable of the local flaps is the bilobe flap as modified by Zitelli.[6] The bilobe flap was originally designed for repair of nasal tip defects. Each lobe and the defect were separated by 90 degrees for a total transposition over a 180-degree arc. Although this recruited tissue for repair at some distance from the defect, it also maximized the standing cutaneous deformities and the likelihood of development of a trap-door deformity or pincushioning of both the primary and secondary flaps. Zittelli[6] emphasized the use of narrow angles (45 degrees) between the lobes so that the total arc of tissue transferred occurs over no more than 90 to 100 degrees (**Fig. 59.5**). This reduces the standing cutaneous deformity and pincushioning effects. Bilobe flaps are double transposition flaps that transfer the wound closure tension from the initial defect through a 90-degree arc to the donor site areas. A major disadvantage of this flap is the extensive amount of linear scar that does not fall along nasal topographic borders. Postoperative dermabrasion is very helpful in obscuring the scar. The bilobe flap is the most commonly used local flap harvested within the confines of the nose itself. It is best limited to repair of skin defects of the lower third of the nose. It is not well suited for cephalic dorsal defects because the donor site for the secondary

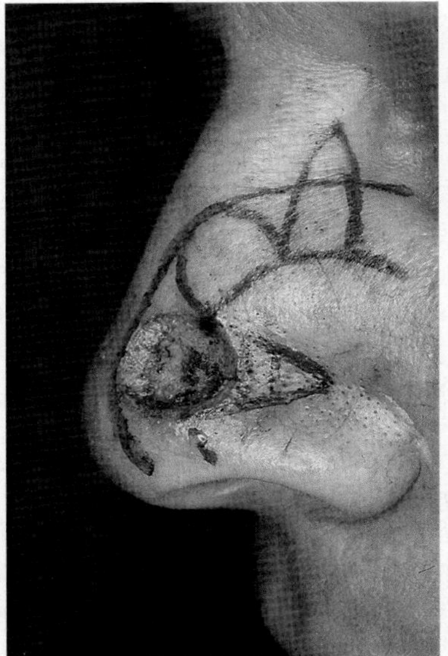
A

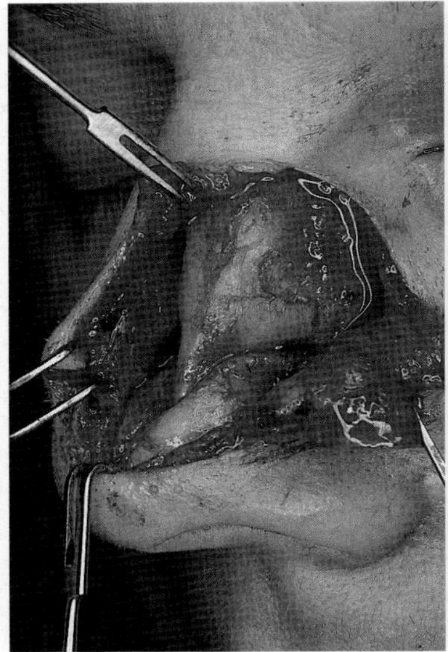
B

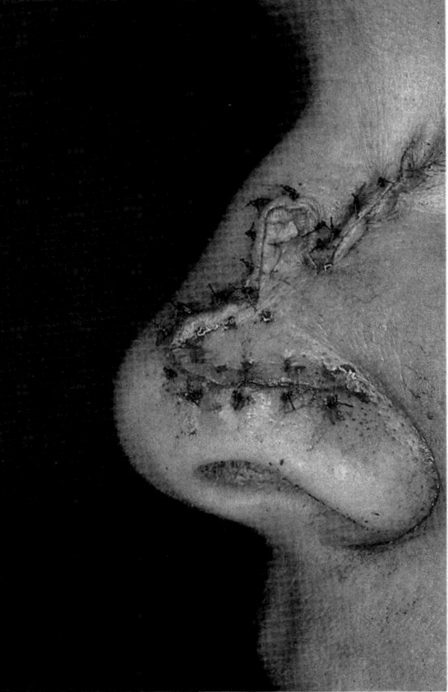
C

Fig. 59.5 (**A**) Bilobe flap designed so that each lobe has a linear axis 45 degrees from the other. Each lobe is designed around one arc through the center of the defect and another through the peripheral border of the defect. The center of each arc is at the apex of the standing cutaneous deformity that will form on flap transfer. The pivotal point for designing the arcs is set at a distance equal to the radius of the defect. (**B**) The flap and entire adjacent nasal skin are undermined. (**C**) Flap in position and standing cutaneous deformity excised.

flap must lie in the area of the medial canthus where the skin is immobile, making wound closure difficult.

As designed by Zitelli,[6] skin adjacent to the defect is used as the primary lobe of the flap, thus allowing for an excellent color and skin texture match. This lobe is designed nearly as large as the defect so that little wound closure tension is exerted at the recipient site. The second lobe is recruited from the lax skin of the upper dorsum and sidewall. The donor site for the second lobe is closed primarily. The base of the bilobe flap is usually positioned laterally, and the transverse nasalis muscle is included in the substance of the flap to enhance vascularity.

The ideal nasal defect for a bilobe flap is a small (less than 1.5 cm) defect at least 5 mm from the margin of the nostril located on the lobule or sidewall. The flap is preferably based laterally and is designed so that the standing cutaneous deformity or cone resulting from pivoting of the flap is removed parallel to or in the nasal alar crease. When designed as a laterally based flap, the base of the cone develops at the lateral border of the defect with its apex pointing laterally. The base of the cone is approximately one half to two thirds of the diameter of the defect. The apex of the cone-shaped excision serves as the pivot point for the flap. Each donor lobe is designed around one arc through the center of the defect and another through the peripheral border of the defect (**Fig. 59.5**).

The linear axis of each lobe is positioned ~45 degrees from the other, with the primary lobe axis positioned 45 degrees from the axis of the defect. The flap is elevated just above the perichondrium and periosteum of the underlying nasal framework. If the thickness of the primary lobe is greater than the recipient area, the distal portion of the lobe may require thinning even to the level of the dermis to match the thickness of the skin at the recipient site. Following incision of the flap, wide peripheral undermining of essentially all skin of the nose is important to reduce wound closure tension, facilitate flap transfer, and minimize trap-door deformity. The primary lobe of the flap is transposed to the defect and secured with sutures. Next, the donor site of the secondary lobe is closed primarily. Last, the secondary lobe is transposed and trimmed appropriately to fit, without redundancy, the donor defect of the primary lobe.

The bilobe flap is most useful in patients with thin nasal skin and laxity of skin along the nasal sidewall. The surgeon can estimate the laxity by pinching the lateral nasal skin between the thumb and index finger. Patients with thick sebaceous skin have a higher risk of flap necrosis and development of trap-door deformity. Dermabrasion, 6 weeks following flap transfer, is recommended for most patients reconstructed with a bilobe flap. Although local nasal flaps can be used to repair defects 2 cm or less on the nose, the majority of surface defects are best repaired with skin from the forehead or cheek.

Melolabial Interpolation Flap

The ala is best resurfaced with cheek skin from the area of the melolabial fold. The sebaceous quality of the skin of the fold closely resembles that of the ala. Menik noted that as melolabial flaps contract they become rounded, resembling the contour of the normal ala.[2] Skin of the melolabial fold is limited, and its use can flatten the fold causing marked asymmetry of the face. Nor can it easily be transferred to the nasal lobule or dorsum. Skin from this fold should be transferred to the ala as an interpolated flap, the pedicle of which crosses over, but not through, the alar facial sulcus (**Fig. 59.4**). The pedicle is superiorly based and may consist of skin and subcutaneous fat or subcutaneous fat only. It is detached from the cheek 3 weeks after the initial transfer to the nose. Although 3 weeks is a lengthy period for the patient to endure the deformity caused by the flap, this interval allows the surgeon to aggressively defat and sculpture the flap both at the time of the flap transfer and at the time of pedicle detachment and flap inset.

For resurfacing the ala, the remaining skin of the ala is usually removed, preserving a 1-mm-wide cuff of alar skin at the base, rather than extending the excision into the alar facial sulcus. A template is fashioned to exactly represent the shape and surface area of the ala. The contralateral ala can be used for the template when present. The template is used to design a flap that is positioned so that the center of the flap is on a horizontal plane with the lateral commissure of the lip. The medial border of the flap should lie in the melolabial sulcus. The flap is designed as an interpolation flap in which the donor site scar will lie precisely in the melolabial sulcus. The flap is based on perforating vessels from the facial artery that penetrate just superior and inferior to the zygomatic major muscle. Incorporation of these perforators gives the flap an axial nature with an excellent blood supply and allows elevation of the flap on a subcutaneous pedicle. Designing it as an island flap on a subcutaneous pedicle enables the base to be tapered superiorly to facilitate transposition (**Fig. 59.4**). This also reduces skin loss from the upper portion of the melolabial fold where the fold is more prominently manifested. A standing cutaneous deformity resulting from closure of the donor site is marked distally so that the scar resulting from its excision will follow the line of the melolabial sulcus. The flap is pivoted toward the midline to reach the nose, crossing over the alar facial sulcus. Fat on the distal one third of the flap is excised, leaving 1 to 2 mm of subcutaneous fat in place. The donor site is closed primarily through advancement and necessitates the excision of a standing cutaneous deformity. The pedicle is divided 3 weeks later at which time the attached flap is partially elevated to allow removal of additional subcutaneous fat from the more proximal portion of the covering flap.[4] The flap is then trimmed of its tail of skin (carried with it from the superior melolabial fold at the time of the initial transfer) and inset into the ala by joining it to the preserved cuff of alar skin adjacent to the alar facial sulcus and to the nasal sil.

Paramedian Forehead Flaps

Several studies of the vascular anatomy of the forehead have been reviewed by Baker and Alford.[7] These studies confirm that the supratrochlear artery is the primary axial blood supply of midforehead flaps, which include the median and paramedian vertically oriented flaps. In addition, the studies have shown that in the medial canthal region a rich anastomotic network exists between the supratrochlear, supraorbital, and angular arteries. Identification of this vascular network and the surgical techniques of flap harvest that preserve this regional blood flow have allowed surgeons to harvest paramedian forehead flaps based on pedicles narrower than those used for median forehead flaps. The narrower pedicle gives the flap more freedom to rotate about its pivot point and therefore provides more effective flap length. At the same time, this design reduces the donor site deformity in the glabellar area that results from transposition of the flap. Based on the supratrochlear artery and its anastomoses to surrounding vessels, the paramedian forehead flap is an axial pivotal interpolation flap with an abundant blood supply that allows transfer without delay.

Paramedian forehead flaps are the preferred local flap for resurfacing most large nasal defects. The flap is usually dissected under local anesthesia. The base of the pedicle is placed in the glabellar region centered over the supratrochlear artery on the same side as the majority of the nasal defect (**Fig. 59.6**). The origin of the supratrochlear artery is consistently found to be 1.7 to 2.2 cm lateral to the midline and usually corresponds to the vertical tangent of the medial border of the brow.[8] The artery exits the orbit by piercing the orbital septum and passing under the orbicularis oculi and over the corrugator supercilii muscle. At the level of the brow, the artery passes through orbicularis and frontalis muscles and continues in a vertical direction upward in a subcutaneous plane. Because of this, the portion of the flap extending from the level of the brow to the hairline can be trimmed of its frontalis muscle and much of the subcutaneous fat without harming the blood supply to the overlying skin. The axial nature of the flap, based on a single supratrochlear artery, enables the pedicle to be as narrow as 1.2 cm.[8] The narrow pedicle minimizes the standing cutaneous deformity as the flap pivots (**Fig. 59.7**). An exact template of the defect is used to design the paramedian forehead flap, which is centered over the vertical axis of the supratrochlear artery. The length of the flap is determined by measurement. If an adequate length necessitates extending the flap into the hair-bearing scalp, the author prefers turning the flap obliquely along the hairline to prevent transfer of hair-bearing skin to the nose. However, this design may not be prudent if the flap must be more than 3 cm wide. Oblique forehead flaps wider than 3 cm remove excessive skin from the lateral portion of the forehead, sometimes causing unsightly scars or upward distortion of the central portion of the brow. Thus, flaps wider than 3 cm should be extended into the hair-bearing scalp rather than designed in an oblique fashion. The flap is elevated in a subfascial plane just superficial to the periosteum of the frontal bone. To avoid injury to the arterial pedicle, blunt dissection is used near the brow to separate the corrugator muscle from the flap and facilitate mobility. Incisions can be extended below the brow if necessary to enhance the length of the flap. Adequate flap mobilization usually requires complete sectioning of the corrugator supercilii muscle to achieve free movement. Prior to inset, the flap is sculptured and contoured to fit the depth of the defect perfectly by removal of all or some of the muscle and subcutaneous tissue from the distal portion of the flap. When necessary, all but 1 mm of fat beneath the dermis may be removed. It is sometimes even necessary to resect a portion of the dermis along the edge of the flap so that the thickness of the skin of the flap matches the adjacent nasal skin in instances where the adjoining nasal skin is thin. Only the distal three fourths of the flap required for reconstruction is sculptured; the proximal one fourth is left thick and is debulked at the time of pedicle detachment 3 weeks later. Prudence in thinning the flap is advised in patients who smoke. Donor site closure is accomplished by undermining the forehead skin in the subfascial plane from the anterior border of one temporalis muscle to the other. Several parallel vertical fasciotomies 2 to 3 cm apart may be helpful to achieve primary wound closure. However, one must take care not to injure the supraorbital nerves when initiating this maneuver. Any portion of the donor site that cannot be closed primarily should be left to heal by second intention, keeping the open wound moist at all times. Healing by second intention usually results in an acceptable scar but may take 6 weeks for completion.

Three weeks after the initial flap transfer, the pedicle is divided under local anesthesia. The nasal skin surrounding the defect superiorly is undermined for a distance of ~1 cm. The portion of the flap not thinned at the time of transposition is now thinned appropriately. In the case of reconstruction of skin-only nasal defects that extend to the rhinion, the flap must be aggressively thinned to the level of the dermis to duplicate the thin skin that is normally found in this area. Deep-layer closure is not necessary because the wound should not be subjected to any closure tension. The base of the pedicle is returned to the donor site in such a way as to restore the normal anatomical and spatial relationship of the two eyebrows (**Fig. 59.7**). Care should be taken to maintain the muscular component of the proximal pedicle that is returned so that a depression between the brows does not occur. Any excess pedicle should be discarded rather than returned to the forehead above the level of the brow.

Local Flaps and Skin Grafts

The skin of the cephalic two thirds of the nose, columella, and soft tissue facets is thin, nonsebaceous, and mobile. In contrast, the lobule and ala are covered with immobile, thick sebaceous skin. Single-lobe transposition flaps may be satisfactory for smaller defects of the cephalic nose because of the redundancy and mobility of the skin covering the sidewall of the nose where the donor site is located. They work less well for the nasal tip and poorly for the ala because of secondary movement of adjacent free margins from wound contraction. Full-thickness skin grafts harvested from the preauricular area or forehead along the hairline match the thickness and texture of the cephalic nose and, if dermabraded postoperatively, often produce a satisfactory result. A skin graft is also useful for limited defects of the columella and soft tissue facets. Skin grafts are less favorable for the lobule and ala where they may appear as an island or patch rather than blend with adjacent nasal skin. If the depth of a nasal defect extends through the supporting framework, it must

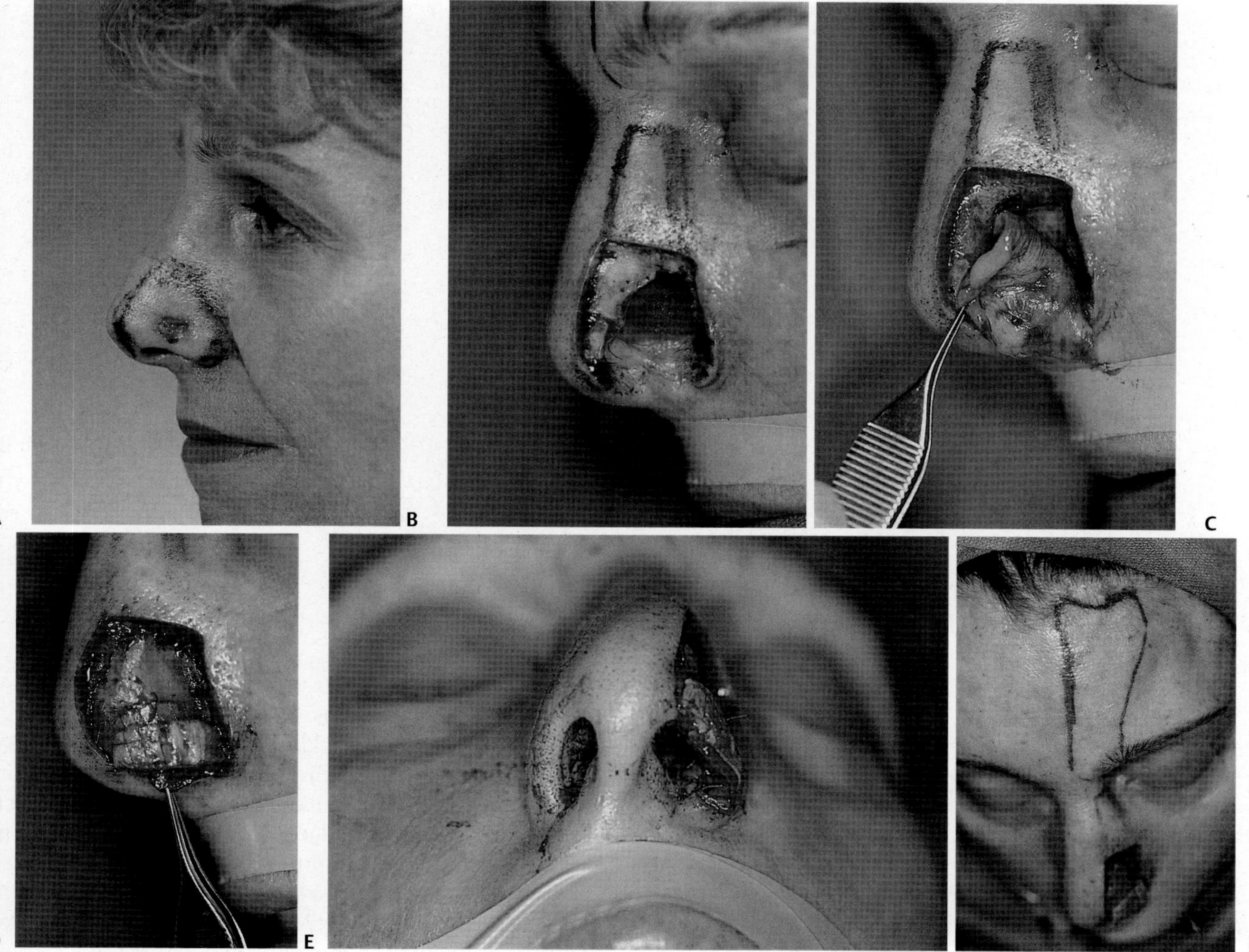

Fig. 59.6 (**A**) Preoperative photograph outlining resection borders for removal of a melanoma. (**B**) Following resection, a full-thickness defect of ala and lower sidewall is observed. (**C**) Ipsilateral septal mucoperichondrial flap hinged on the caudal septum will provide internal lining for the reconstruction. (**D**) Septal cartilage graft replaces caudal portion of the upper lateral cartilage. Auricular cartilage graft replaces missing lateral crus in addition to providing structural support to the ala. It is positioned caudad and lateral to septal cartilage graft. Forcep holds caudal border of hinge flap. (**E**) Curvature of auricular cartilage graft provides contour to the reconstructed ala and nostril. (**F**) Paramedian flap designed as cover for cartilage grafts. (*Continued*)

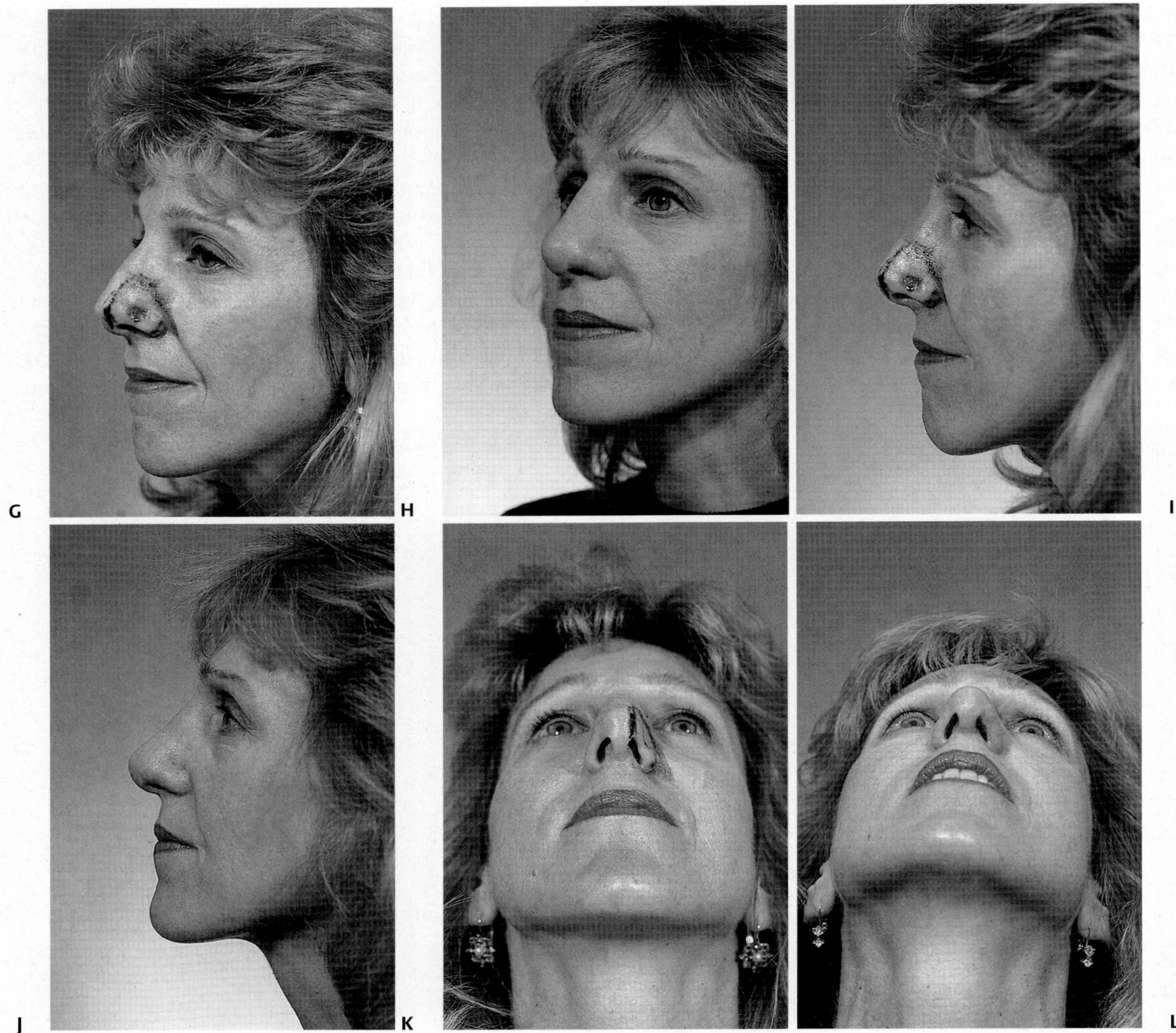

Fig. 59.6 (*Continued*) (**G,H**) Oblique view: preoperative and 1 year postoperative. (**I,J**) Lateral view: preoperative and 1 year postoperative. (**K,L**) Baseview: preoperative and 1 year postoperative.

be restored with primary cartilage grafts. In such instances, a skin graft or covering flap harvested from the nose itself is no longer advisable because contraction of such grafts and flaps often obscures the delicate topography of the replacement framework; a cheek or a forehead flap is the preferred covering flap. This approach replaces the missing skin rather than borrowing it from another area of the nose, keeping contracting forces of healing to a minimum.

Defect Classification

Defects of the nose may be classified according to location, depth, and size. Skin-only defects can be replaced with full-thickness skin grafts, local flaps (if the defect is small), or preferably, skin transferred from the cheek or forehead. Defects involving loss of skeletal structure require replacement with like tissue. Full-thickness defects of the nose require replacement of the missing lining with flaps harvested from the interior of the nose when possible. These defects always require replacement of the missing skeletal framework and thus should be resurfaced with a paramedian forehead or melolabial interpolation flap.

The size of the nasal defect determines the source of the covering flap. In the case of defects greater than 2 cm in greatest dimension, there is rarely sufficient residual nasal skin for closure by a local flap without creating undue wound closure tension. Thus the forehead or cheek should be used as a donor site.

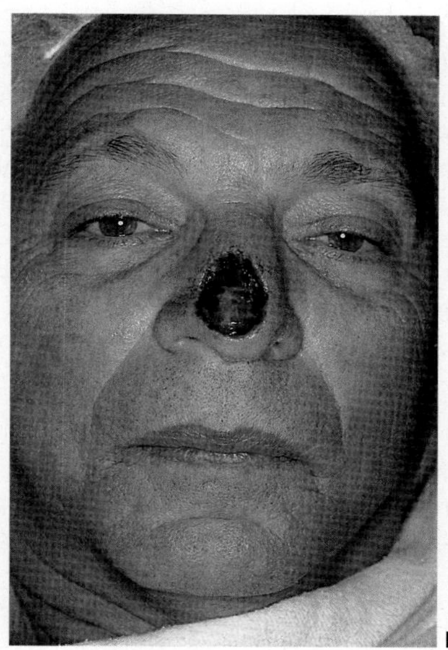
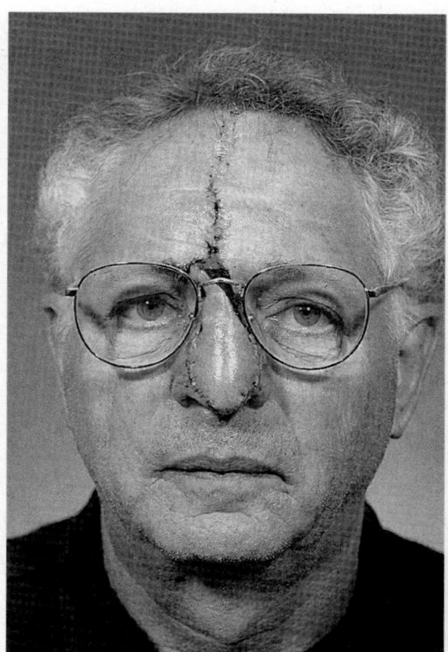
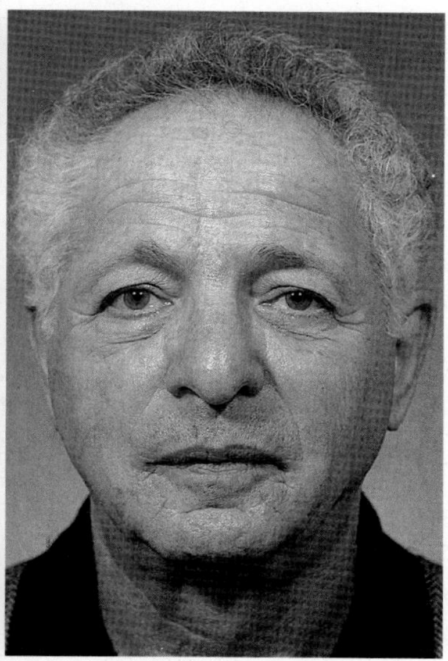

Fig. 59.7 (**A**) Skin defect of lobule. (**B**) The narrow pedicle of the paramedian forehead flap minimizes the standing cutaneous deformity resulting from pivoting of the flap. This has allowed the patient to position eyeglasses comfortably over the flap. (**C**) Six months following detachment of flap pedicle. No revision surgery was necessary. Note restored relationship of the medial aspect of eyebrows.

Surgical Technique

Reconstruction of the Columella

The columella is the most difficult region of the nose to reconstruct. Small defects limited to 1.5 cm in greatest dimension can occasionally be repaired with composite grafts from the auricle in nonsmokers. The grafts should be chilled for 3 days following transfer, and systemic steroids should be administered for 1 week. It is preferable to allow the initial defect to heal by second intention and then perform the composite graft after preparing a fresh recipient site by removing all scar tissue and new epithelium. The graft should be oversized by 2 mm to accommodate wound contraction.

Depending on extent of the tissue loss, larger defects of the columella are best repaired with unilateral or bilateral superiorly based interpolated melolabial flaps. Septal cartilage grafts should be utilized for the framework. The initial flap transfer will produce a thick columella that will require secondary thinning. Defects that extend into the lobule from the columella require structural support with cartilage grafts and a paramedian forehead flap for cover. By extending the incision for the forehead flap into or below the brow, the flap can be made to reach the upper lip without excessive wound closure tension.

Full-thickness defects of the columella and lobule are best reconstructed with a tilt-out, hinged, composite nasal septal flap (**Fig. 59.3**). Mucosa of the flap is peeled downward bilaterally to provide internal lining. Auricular cartilage grafts are attached to the composite flap to provide structural support laterally. A paramedian forehead flap is best for exterior covering.

Reconstruction of the Lobule

Small, skin-only superficial defects of the nasal tip may be covered with a local bilobe flap, as described in detail earlier, or a full-thickness skin graft. However, a paramedian forehead flap will usually give a more natural result because the entire aesthetic unit can be covered by the flap, placing scars in borders of aesthetic units. Cartilage grafts should be used routinely along the margin of the nostril when the defect extends from the lobule to the soft tissue facet. This is in addition to any missing lower lateral cartilage, which must be replaced as well.

Bilateral full-thickness defects of the lobule should be repaired with a tilt-out, hinged, composite septal flap as discussed (**Fig. 59.3**). However, unilateral full-thickness defects can be nicely reconstructed with an ipsilateral septal hinge mucosal flap for internal lining and a paramedian forehead flap for cover. The lining flap spans the nasal passage on the affected side. Following restoration of the absent cartilaginous framework, a paramedian forehead flap provides surface replacement. In instances of a hemitip defect, I usually only resurface the hemilobule rather than the entire lobule. Concomitant with detachment of the forehead flap 3 weeks after transfer, the hinge mucosal flap is released from the septum, thus restoring patency of the nasal airway.

Reconstruction of the Ala

Defects confined to the ala with or without limited extension to the lobule or sidewall are best resurfaced with an interpolated superiorly based melolabial flap. I routinely resurface the entire ala regardless of the size of the alar defect.[4] The melolabial flap based on a subcutaneous pedicle is preferred because this design minimizes the amount of skin that is disturbed in the upper melolabial fold. Preserving the upper fold is paramount in maintaining symmetry of the cheeks following reconstruction of the ala with a cheek flap. Cartilage grafts are used in the majority of alar defects. This is because most lesions involving resection of alar skin also require removal of the underlying firm fibrofatty subdermal tissue, which gives the ala form and structural support. This must be replaced by cartilage to prevent upward migration of the ala and notching of the margin of the nostril.

Internal lining for full-thickness alar defects is provided by bipedicle vestibular skin flaps or unilateral hinge septal mucosal flaps (**Fig. 59.6**). Occasionally, an additional contralateral hinge mucosal flap, as discussed in the earlier portion of this chapter, may be necessary if the vertical height of the defect is such that a single hinged mucosal flap will not provide sufficient tissue to replace the entire missing lining.

Reconstruction of the Nasal Dorsum

The nasal dorsum is perhaps the least complex portion of the nose to reconstruct. Forehead skin in the form of a paramedian flap is usually preferred for resurfacing skin-only

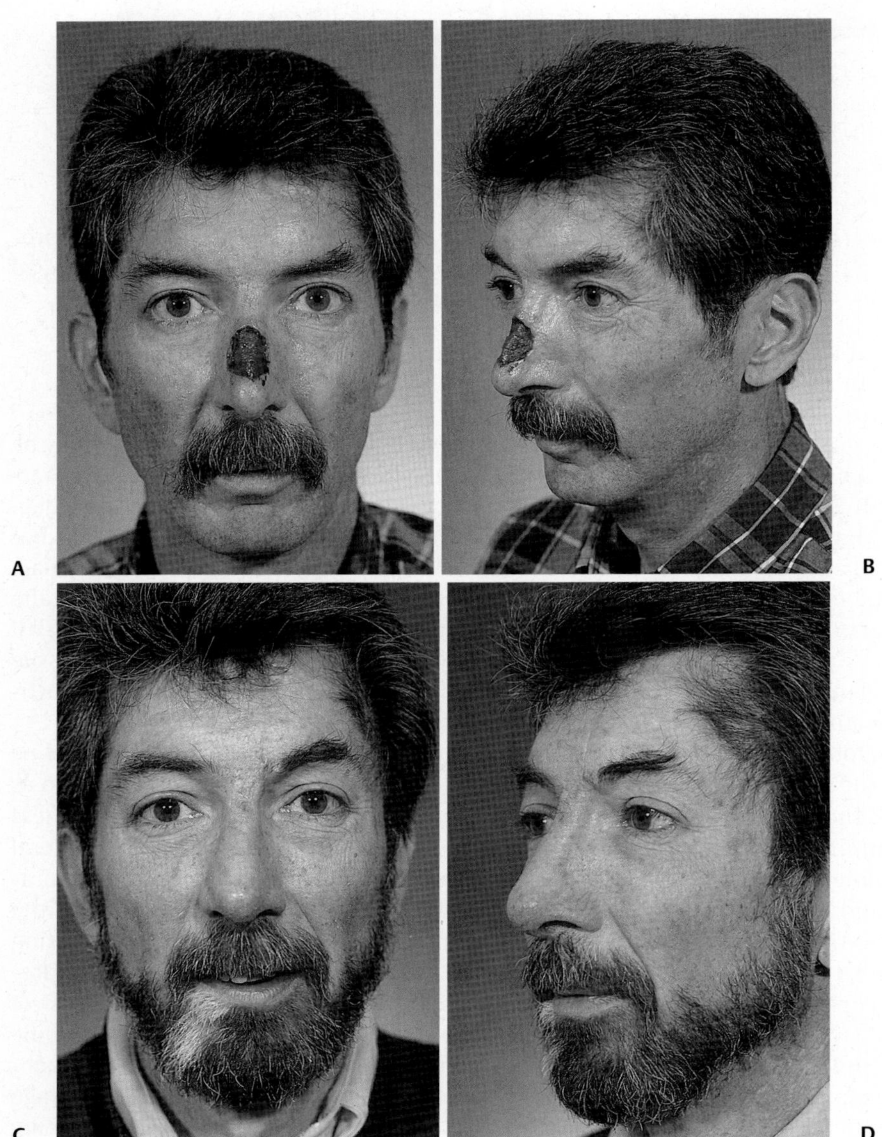

Fig. 59.8 (**A,B**) Skin defect of nasal dorsum. (**C,D**) Six months following reconstruction with a paramedian forehead flap. No intermediate surgical stage or revision surgery's necessary.

defects of the caudal dorsum. However, bilobe flaps or full-thickness skin grafts may also be used. Likewise, skin defects of the cephalic dorsum can be repaired with glabellar flaps, such as the dorsal nasal flap, or full-thickness skin grafts, but paramedian forehead flaps are preferred (**Fig. 59.8**). Small defects of the dorsal framework can be replaced with septal cartilage grafts. More extensive defects of the nasal skeleton extending from the frontal bone to the lobule are best replaced with calverial bone grafts secured to the frontal bone or remaining nasal bony root with plate-and-screw fixation. To prevent medialization of the nasal sidewall following wound healing, structural defects that extend into the nasal sidewall require replacement concurrent with replacement of the dorsal framework. Septal cartilage or additional cranial bone grafts plated to the dorsal graft work well for this purpose. Internal lining for full-thickness dorsal defects can usually be provided by mucosal hinge flaps reflected laterally from the exposed dorsum as long as there is sufficient height to the remaining septum. Unilateral or bilateral hinge septal mucosal flaps based on the caudal septum and including the septal branch of the labial artery can also sometimes be used for lining when there is considerable loss of dorsal septal height. A tilt-out composite septal flap, as discussed earlier in this chapter, should be used to provide lining and structural support for the dorsum in extensive bilateral full-thickness dorsal nasal defects (**Fig. 59.9**). In instances where this approach will not provide sufficient tissue, bilateral paramedian forehead flaps are recommended. One flap provides internal lining and the other provides external coverage. A cranial bone graft is placed between the flaps for structural support.

Reconstruction of the Nasal Sidewall

Reconstruction of the sidewall of the nose is relatively uncomplicated. Small skin-only defects may be repaired with a bilobe flap harvested from the remaining nasal sidewall skin. Full-thickness skin grafts harvested from the preauricular area of the cheek also provide a reasonable option for covering defects located in the superior portion of the sidewall because of the thinness of the skin at this location. Larger surface defects are best covered with a paramedian forehead flap. When structural support is absent from the upper third of the nasal sidewall, it should be replaced with a calverial bone graft, whereas the lower two thirds of the sidewall skeleton is best replaced with septal cartilage grafts. Full thickness unilateral sidewall

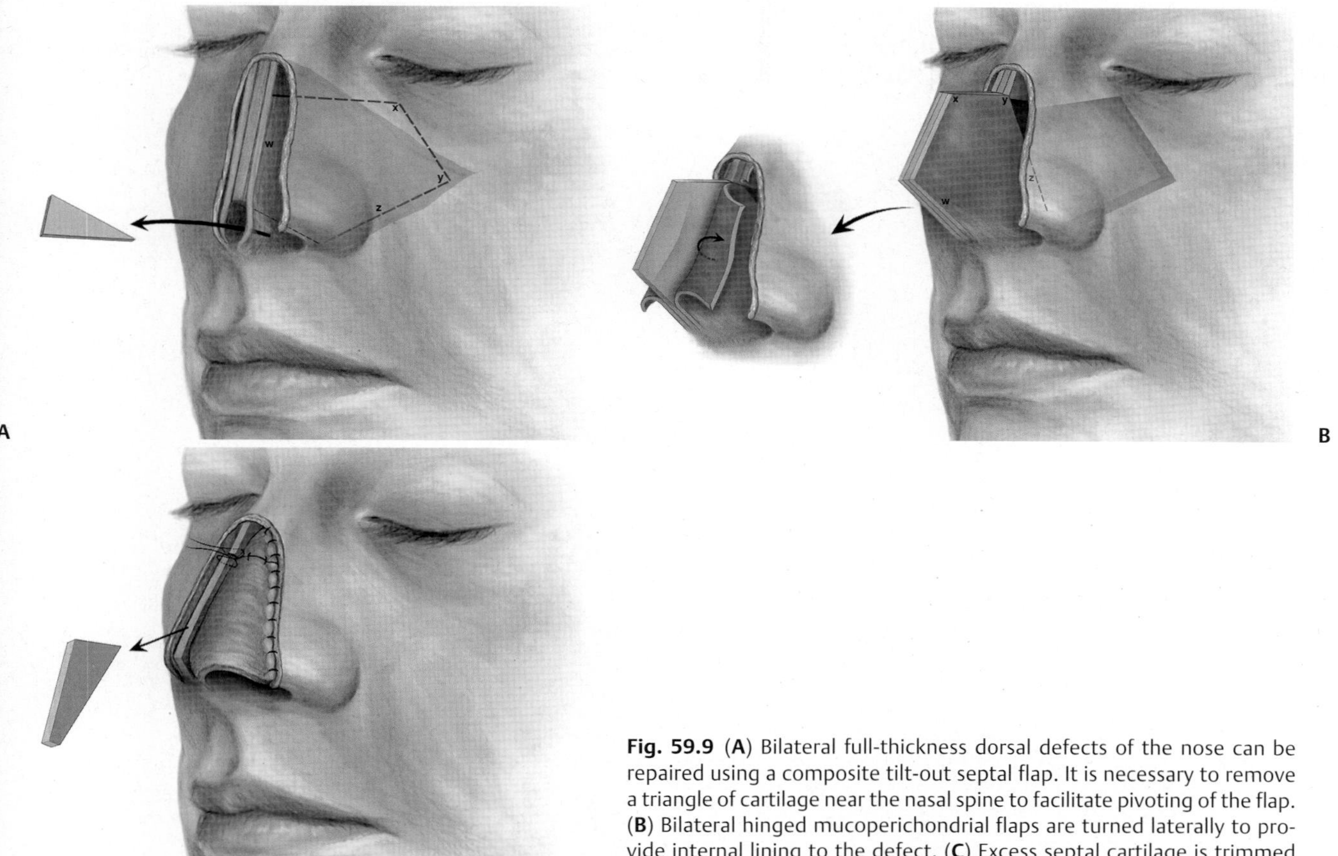

Fig. 59.9 (**A**) Bilateral full-thickness dorsal defects of the nose can be repaired using a composite tilt-out septal flap. It is necessary to remove a triangle of cartilage near the nasal spine to facilitate pivoting of the flap. (**B**) Bilateral hinged mucoperichondrial flaps are turned laterally to provide internal lining to the defect. (**C**) Excess septal cartilage is trimmed from the flap and used for grafting purposes.

defects can be lined using contralateral hinged septal mucoperichondrial flaps based on the nasal dorsum and delivered through a superiorly positioned nasal septal fenestrum. For more caudally located sidewall defects, an ipsilateral mucosal flap hinged on the caudal septum may provide sufficient lining (**Fig. 59.6**). However, this arrangement requires subsequent detachment of the pedicle. It is usually necessary to use both the contralateral dorsally based flap and the ipsilateral caudally based septal hinge mucoperichondrial flap to provide lining for full-thickness defects that involve the ala and extend the entire length of the nasal sidewall (**Fig. 59.2**).

Summary

During the last decade, reconstruction of the nose has progressed to a new level of finesse that allows the surgeon to restore near-normal form and function to all but the most extensive nasal defects. These advances are based on the contemporary concept of respecting the borders of aesthetic units of the nose. The nose is reconstructed separately from any extension of a nasal defect into the cheek or lip, which in turn is repaired by tissue within the respective aesthetic region. The other concept that has contributed to this higher level of surgical achievement is that of replacing missing tissue with like tissue. Internal lining is replaced with nasal mucosal flaps, which because of their nature provide adequate vascularity to nourish and sustain the cartilage and bone grafts used in skeletal replacement. Missing bone and cartilage are replaced with similar tissue, which is carefully crafted to replicate the exact size, configuration, and contour of the missing nasal skeleton. Surface defects are covered with cheek or forehead skin transferred by interpolation so as not to violate the aesthetic boundary between nose and the other regions of the face. This surgical approach provides natural building material precisely fitted to reconstruct nasal deficits to a condition as near normal as possible.

References

1. Burget GC, Menick FJ. Nasal support and lining: the marriage of beauty and blood supply. Plast Reconstr Surg 1989;84:189–202
2. Menick FJ. Reconstruction of the nose. In: Baker SR, Swanson NA, eds. Local Flaps in Facial Reconstruction. St. Louis: CV Mosby; 1995:305–337
3. Burget GC, Menick FJ. Aesthetic Reconstruction of the Nose. St. Louis: CV Mosby; 1993
4. Baker SR, Johnston TM, Nelson BR. The importance of maintaining the alar–facial sulcus in nasal reconstruction. Arch Otolaryngol Head Neck Surg 1995;121:617–622
5. Baker SR. Contemporary aspects of nasal reconstruction. In: Myer E, Krause CJ, eds. Advances in Otolaryngology: Head and Neck Surgery. Vol 12. St. Louis: CV Mosby; 1998:235–261
6. Zitelli JA. Bilobe flaps. In: Baker SR, Swanson NA, eds. Local Flaps in Facial Reconstruction. St. Louis: CV Mosby; 1995:165–180
7. Baker SR, Alford EL. Midforehead flaps: operative techniques. Otolaryngol Head Neck Surg 1993;4:24–30
8. Menick FJ. Aesthetic refinements in use of the forehead flap for nasal reconstruction: the paramedian forehead flap. Clin Plast Surg 1990;17:607–622

60 Auricular Reconstruction

Tom D. Wang

Auricular reconstruction poses one of the most difficult challenges in reconstruction surgery of the head and neck. This is due to the unique architectural topography of the external ear. The multiple concavities and convexities of the cartilage framework are enveloped by a very thin, tightly adherent skin envelope. This entire skin and cartilaginous framework exists as a protuberant three-dimensional structure standing alone and projecting away from the side of the head. The vascular supply for this unique structure, although well defined, can be tenuous and is often less robust than that of other regions of the face, such as nose and lips. In addition, this entire freestanding framework exhibits great delicacy in its various topographic convolutions, as well as a smooth, flowing curvature representing the outer helical rim. Finally, within the framework itself, there is variation of tissue type, blending varying amounts of cartilage with overlying skin and intervening soft tissue to create the components that make up the normal external ear.

Reconstructive Philosophy

The ultimate goal in any reconstruction is the precise duplication of the absent anatomical portions. This is certainly the intended goal in auricular reconstructions as well. Although this goal might be more achievable with smaller defects, it becomes much more challenging with the loss of significant portions of the ear. As important to the duplication of the precise anatomical landmarks, however, is the recognition and reproduction of normal auricular characteristics. A successful outcome, especially in the reconstruction of large auricular defects, depends more on respecting the characteristics of the normal ear than exact duplication of normal anatomical landmarks. The characteristics of the normal ear that need to be preserved in all reconstructive endeavors include the size, location, orientation, and finally, anatomical landmarks. A reconstructed ear will appear instantly recognizable as such only if these characteristics are observed. Conversely, if one or more of these

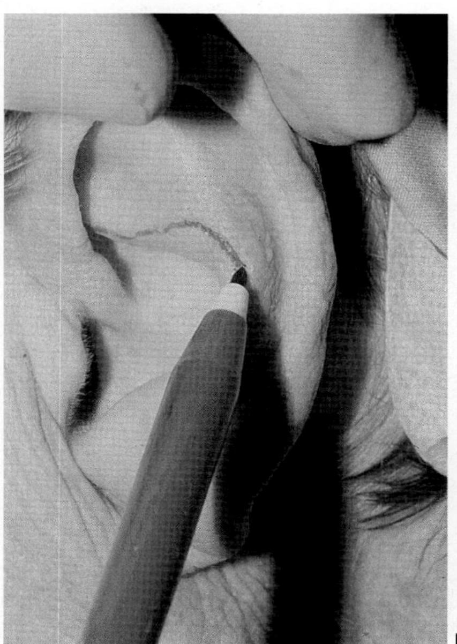
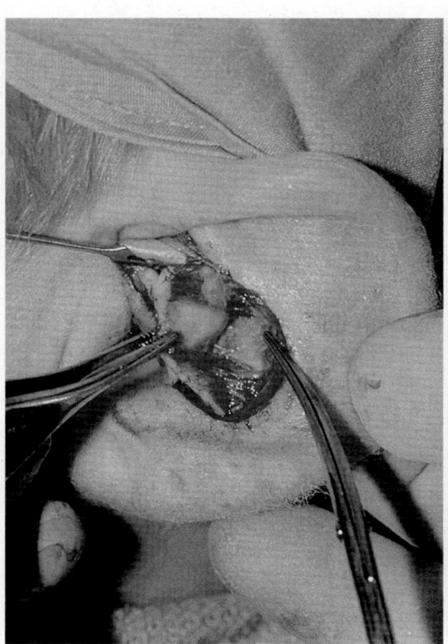
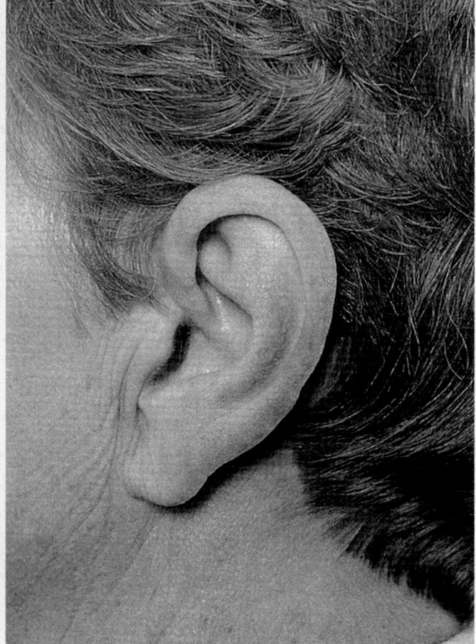

Fig. 60.1 (**A**) Access incision used for obtaining conchal cartilage for grafting purposes. The incision itself is placed along the antihelical ridge for camouflage. (**B**) Harvest of conchal cartilage via the anterior approach. (**C**) Postoperative appearance of donor ear with no distortion or morbidity.

characteristics is absent—for instance, if the ear is significantly deviant in size, location, or orientation—then despite the most accurate reproduction of anatomical detail that ear will appear to be abnormal.

One of the most useful ways to approach auricular reconstruction is via accurate classification of the auricular defect. In this respect, the classification of defects of the ear is not unlike the classification of defects elsewhere on the face. Because different portions of the ear constitute different tissue compositions—that is, the varying ratio of cartilage to overlying skin and intervening soft tissue—the reconstructive demands will similarly vary. As with nasal reconstruction, different aspects of the ear can be thought of as representing different "aesthetic subunits" requiring

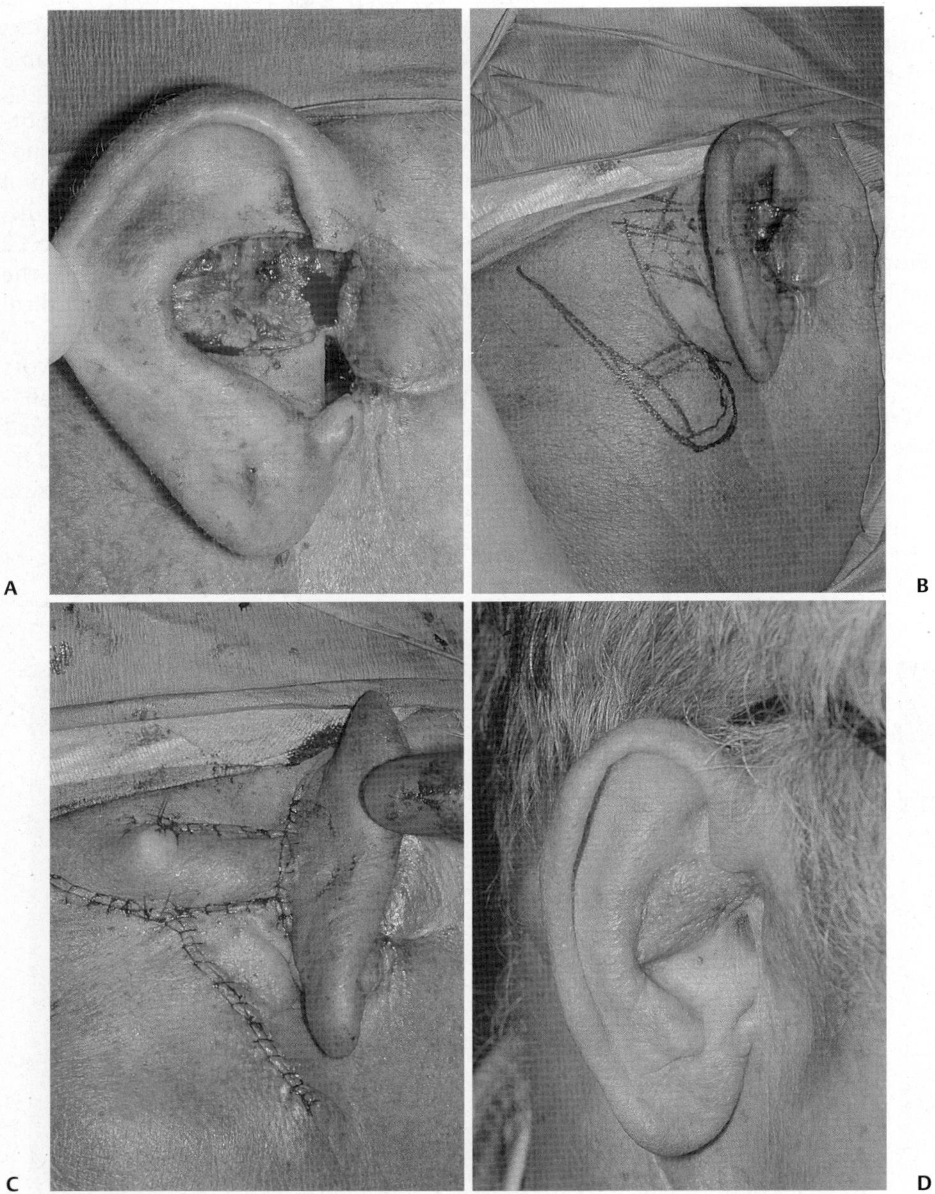

Fig. 60.2 (**A**) Defect of the helical root and conchal bowl involving skin and cartilage tissue loss. (**B**) Pedicle flap reconstruction of defect with superiorly based mastoid flap. (**C**) Donor site closed and flap transposed in position. (**D**) Long-term result with uneventful healing and maintenance of auricular contour.

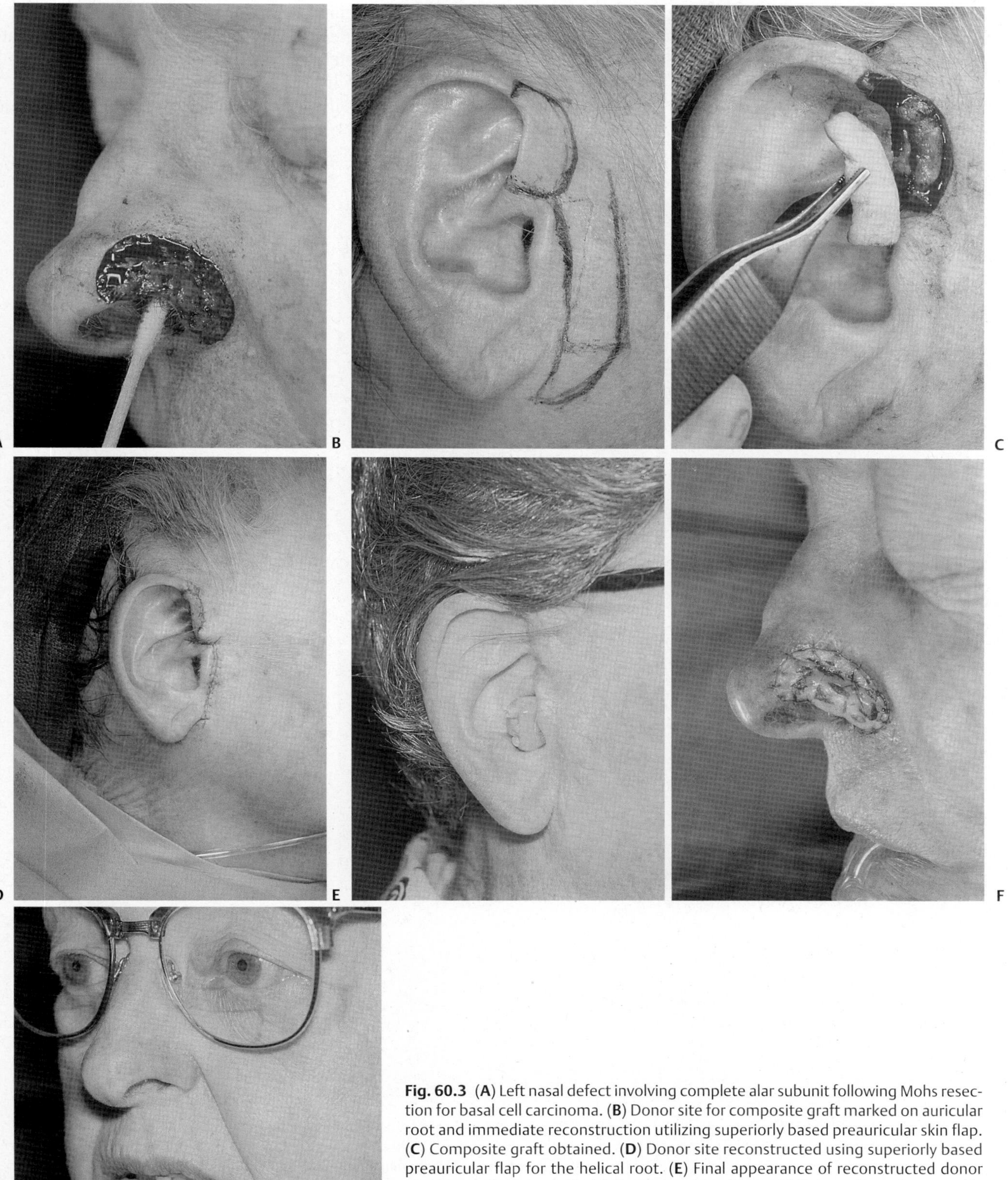

Fig. 60.3 (**A**) Left nasal defect involving complete alar subunit following Mohs resection for basal cell carcinoma. (**B**) Donor site for composite graft marked on auricular root and immediate reconstruction utilizing superiorly based preauricular skin flap. (**C**) Composite graft obtained. (**D**) Donor site reconstructed using superiorly based preauricular flap for the helical root. (**E**) Final appearance of reconstructed donor site demonstrating minimal deformity and morbidity. (**F**) Composite graft sutured in place in recipient bed. (**G**) Long-term result of composite grafting.

attention to the specific topographic contours and demands within that specific missing unit. From this perspective, auricular defects can be categorized as follows:

1. Central defects involving the conchal bowl and helical root
2. Peripheral defects involving the upper third of the ear
3. Peripheral defects involving the middle third of the ear
4. Peripheral defects involving the lower third of the ear
5. Defects involving the periauricular tissues
6. Large defects involving both the central and peripheral portions of the ear

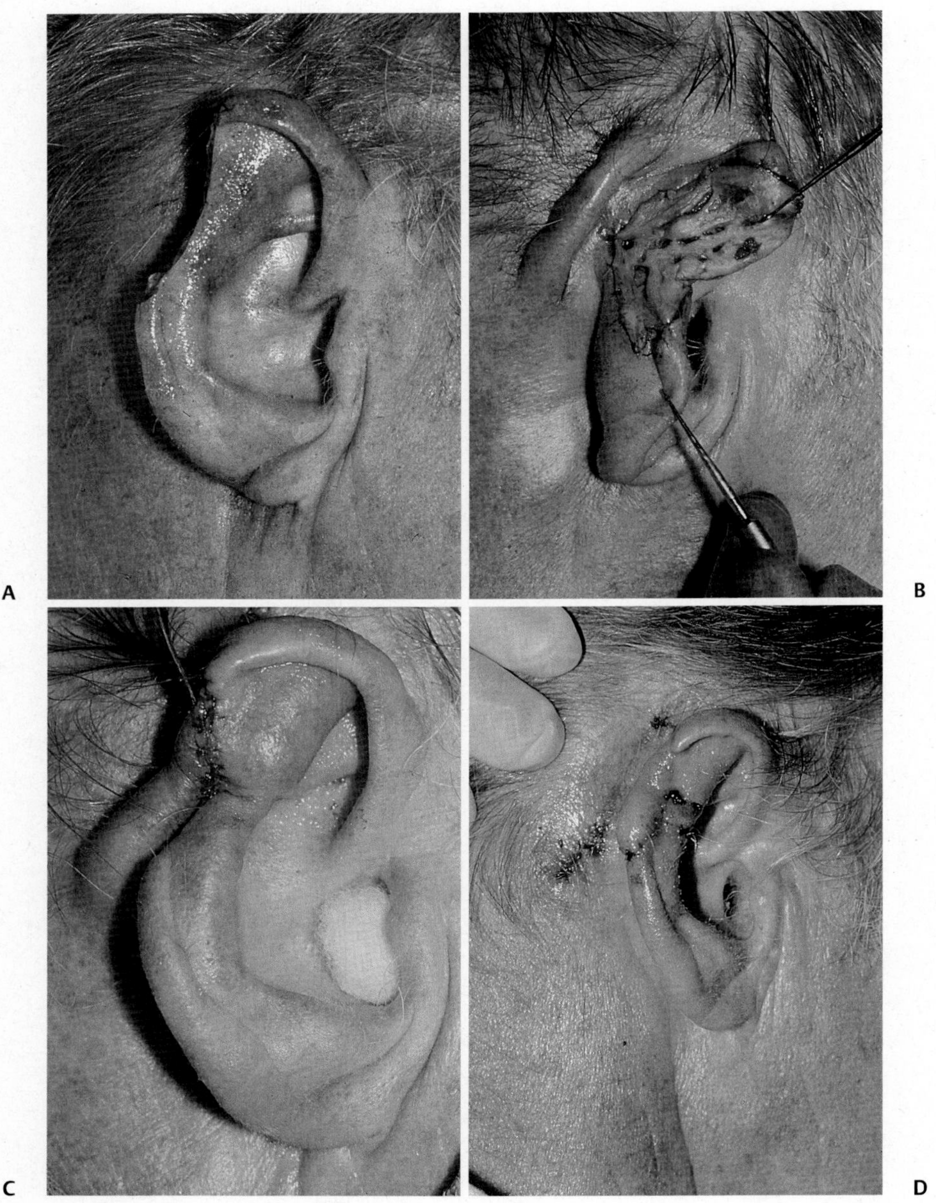

Fig. 60.4 (**A**) Full-thickness defect status post Mohs excision for squamous cell carcinoma involving helical rim and scapha of upper third of ear. (**B**) Staged reconstruction utilizing tube mastoid tissue and full-thickness skin grafting to postauricular defect. (**C**) First-stage attachment of superior portion of tube flap to superior aspect of defect. (**D**) Second-stage completion of reconstruction with attachment of inferior portion of tube flap to inferior portion of auricular defect to recreate auricular helical contour.

Central Auricular Defects Involving the Conchal Bowl and Helical Root

Central auricular defects can typically be successfully reconstructed by providing adequate skin coverage alone. We know this to be true from experience harvesting auricular cartilage for reconstruction elsewhere, leaving minimal—if any—residual donor site deformity (**Fig. 60.1**). As long as the remainder of the peripheral auricular cartilage framework is intact, an absence of conchal bowl cartilage is relatively inconsequential. In this respect, full-thickness skin grafting can work well in resurfacing defects in this region. If a more substantial amount of tissue is required, donor sites from the postauricular and retromastoid regions can be easily harvested for bulk and resurfacing requirements (**Fig. 60.2**).

The root of the helix is a preferred donor site for composite grafts for nasal reconstruction. The resulting donor defect can be easily reconstructed with a superiorly based preauricular flap with or without the introduction of cartilage to replace the missing tissue (**Fig. 60.3**).

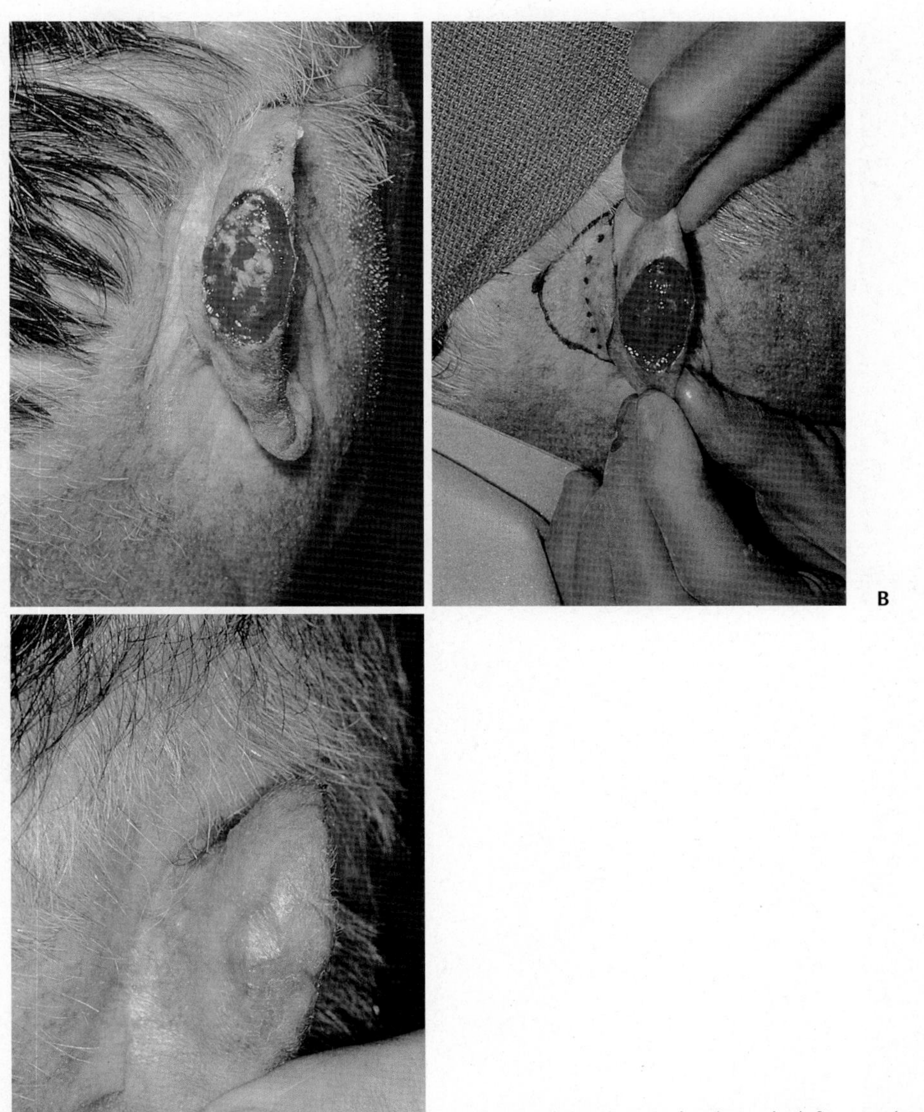

Fig. 60.5 (**A**) Postauricular skin only defect involving the middle-third portion of the helical rim. (**B**) Full-thickness skin graft planned from postauricular sulcus. (**C**) Final result with satisfactory healing of both donor and recipient sites.

Peripheral Defects Involving the Upper Third of the Ear

The primary consideration for defects involving the upper third of the rim is recreation of the normal anatomical curvature present here. When there is full-thickness loss, the postauricular and mastoid skin become convenient and suitable donor sites for reconstruction in this region (**Fig. 60.4**). These reconstructions can often be performed in a staged fashion with the use of skin grafts from the contralateral postauricular skin. In addition, excisions of lesions in this region require a stellate configuration to minimize pinching or notching of the helical rim contour. This approach allows appropriate apposition of the antihelix along with advancement of the helical rim to effect anatomical closure.

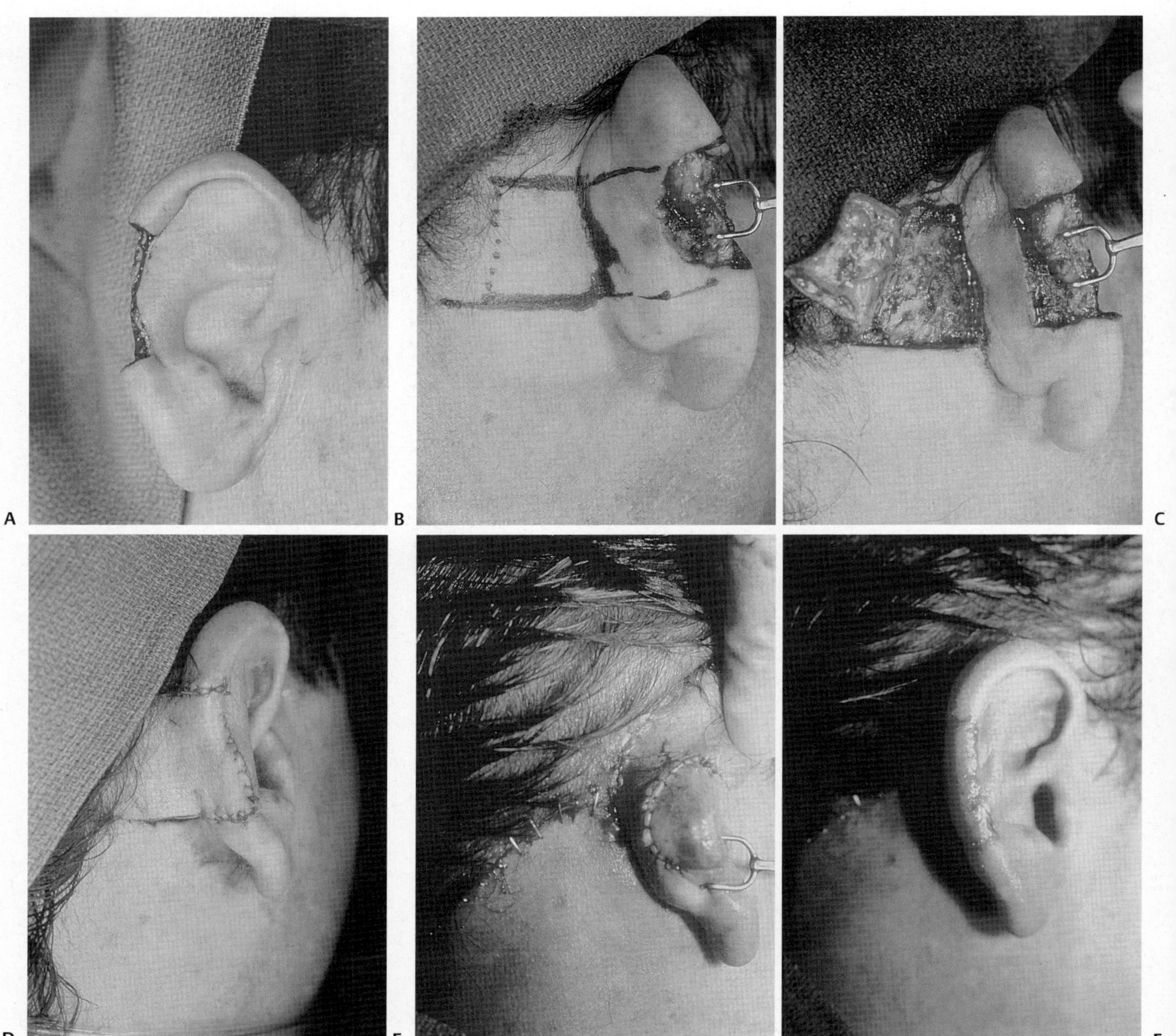

Fig. 60.6 (**A**) Defect involving middle third of the auricle with full-thickness loss of the helical rim. (**B**) Postauricular mastoid flap planned for coverage of defect. (**C**) Elevation of flap prior to closure with view of intervening skin bridge. (**D**) Flap sewn into position. (**E**) Second-stage transsection of flap pedicle with repair of donor site. (**F**) Final outcome with satisfactory recreation of auricular helical contour.

Peripheral Defects Involving the Middle Third of the Ear

The predominant consideration in reconstruction of this portion of the auricular subunit once again is concerned with reestablishing the appropriate auricular contour. However, in contrast to the upper third of the ear, which is quite curved, the auricular contour in the middle third is relatively straight. The use of postauricular and mastoid tissue advancement flaps has proved to be extremely helpful in reconstructing the full-thickness defects involving this region (**Figs. 60.5 and Fig. 60.6**). Interpositioned cartilaginous grafts may be required in larger defects involving this region of the ear. An additional source of

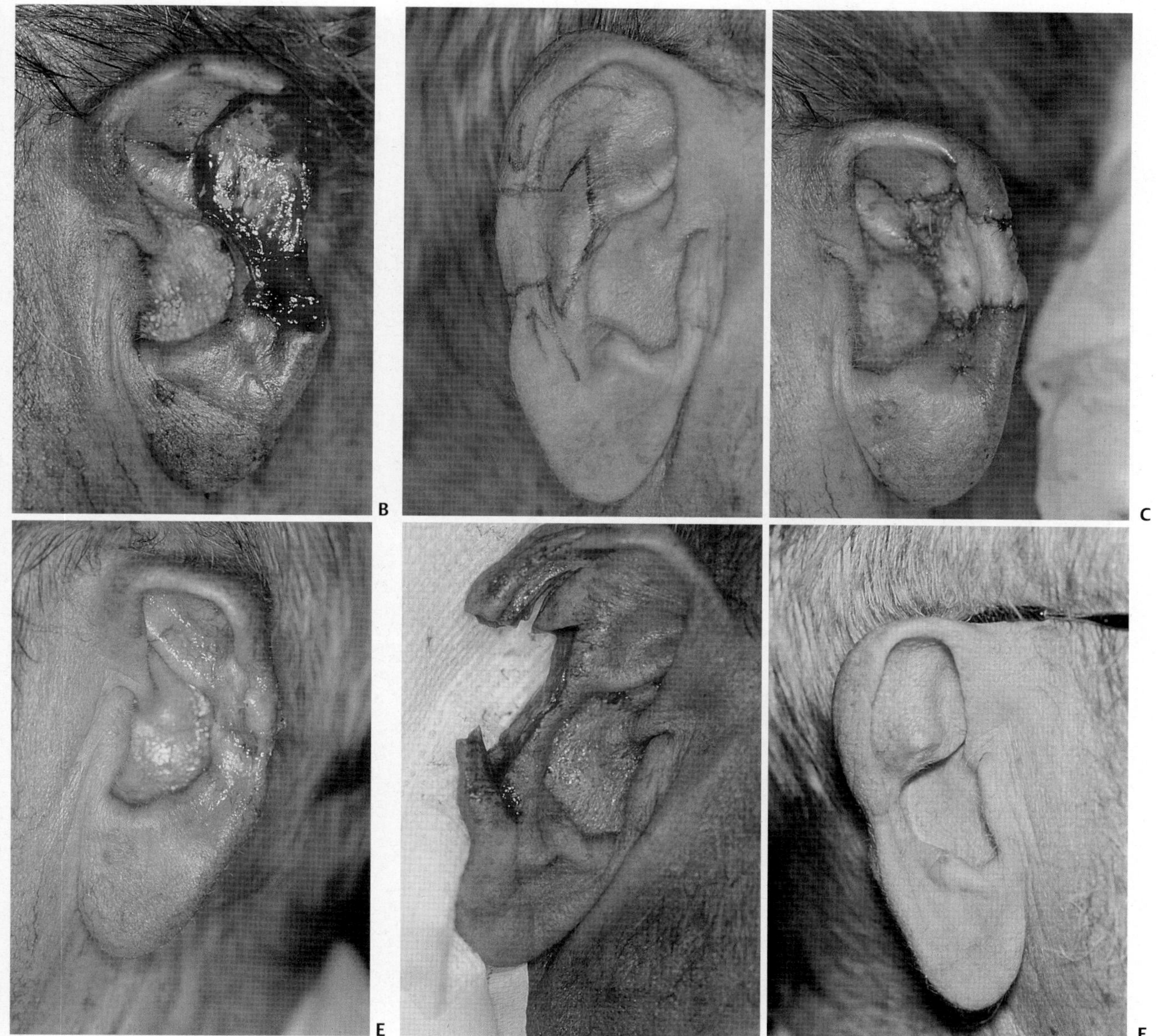

Fig. 60.7 (**A**) Central-third defect of left auricle following Mohs resection for basal cell carcinoma. Defect involved skin and cartilage. This is an elderly patient with elongated ears. (**B**) Contralateral normal ear marked for full-thickness composite graft for reconstruction. Note a stellate pattern of excision, which will minimize notching deformities. Also note the helical rim advancements to reconstruct the donor site deformity. (**C**) Composite graft in position at recipient site. (**D**) Complete take of composite graft. (**E**) Donor defect following stellate excision and preparation of helical rim advancement. (**F**) Satisfactory healing of donor site with minimal morbidity and anatomical deformity.

potential donor tissue is the contralateral normal ear, especially in the older patient who has experienced elongation of the soft tissue structures of the ear (**Fig. 60.7**). A full-thickness composite graft with replacement of both skin layers, as well as the intervening cartilage structure, can be used to restore appropriate helical architecture and contour. In addition, stellate excision and rim advancement of the donor site help achieve satisfactory closure and minimize donor site morbidity.

Peripheral Defects Involving the Lower Third of the Ear

In the area of the lower third of the ear, the predominant tissue is skin and subcutaneous fatty tissue with a minimal amount of intervening cartilage. For this reason, defects involving the earlobe can be simply and adequately reconstructed, again utilizing local soft tissue (**Fig. 60.8**).

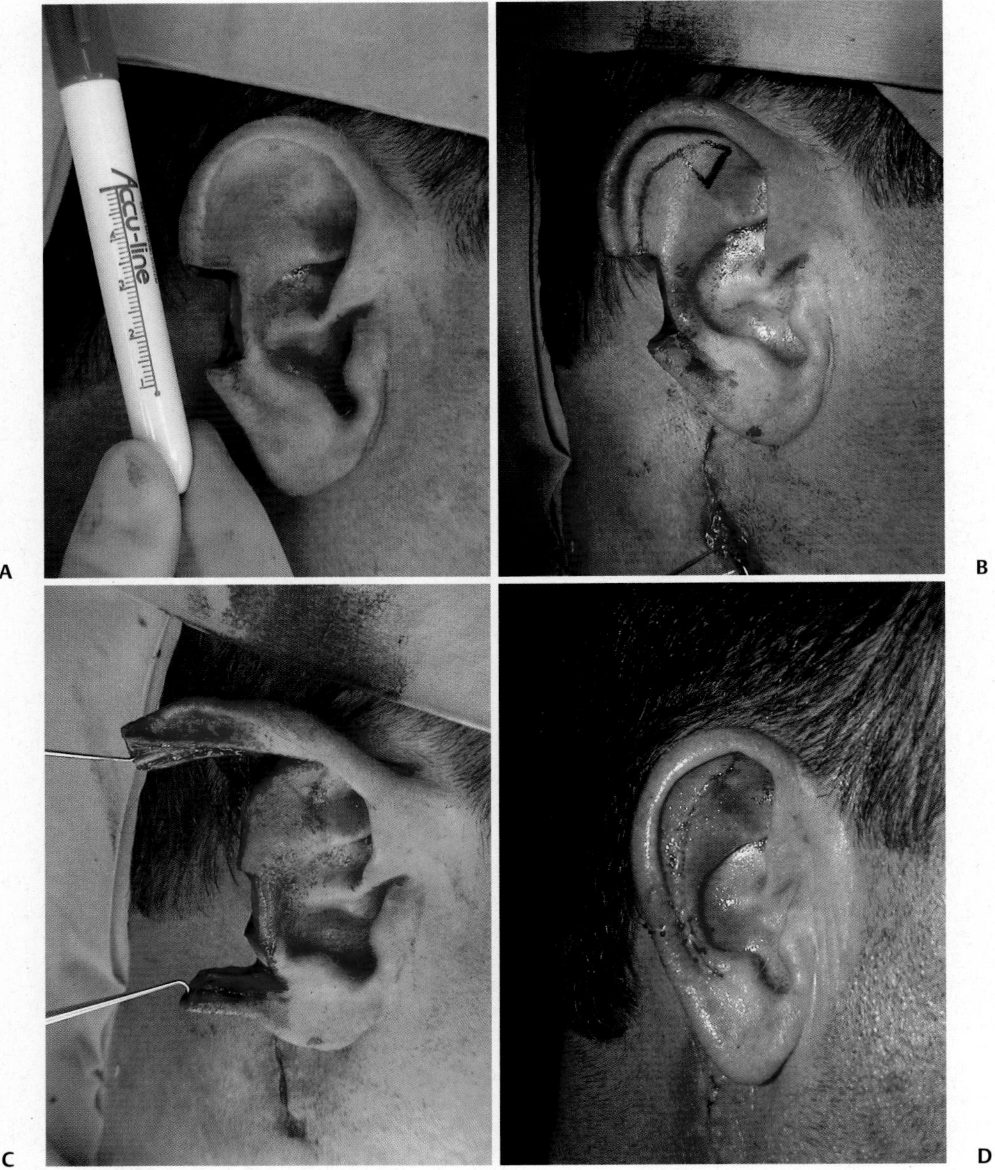

Fig. 60.8 (**A**) Full-thickness loss of left earlobe. (**B**) Bilobed flap reconstruction of earlobe. (**C**) Flap sutured into position to reconstruct earlobe with closure of donor site. (**D**) Satisfactory recreation of earlobe.

When a more significant portion of the lower third of the ear is absent, local tissue is recruited along with contralateral auricular cartilage to recreate the normal auricular architecture (**Fig. 60.9**). Auricular lobule elongation occurs as part of the aging-face syndrome. This can result in a pendulous lobule that patients find objectionable. This is a condition that can be easily corrected via simple wedge excisions to recreate a more youthful lobule contour (**Fig. 60.10**).

Defects Involving Periauricular Tissues

Significant tissue loss in the periauricular region can usually be reconstructed with recruitment and mobilization of cervical facial skin to resurface the defect (**Fig. 60.11**). When the defect involves the preauricular temporal hair tuft, reconstruction can be performed

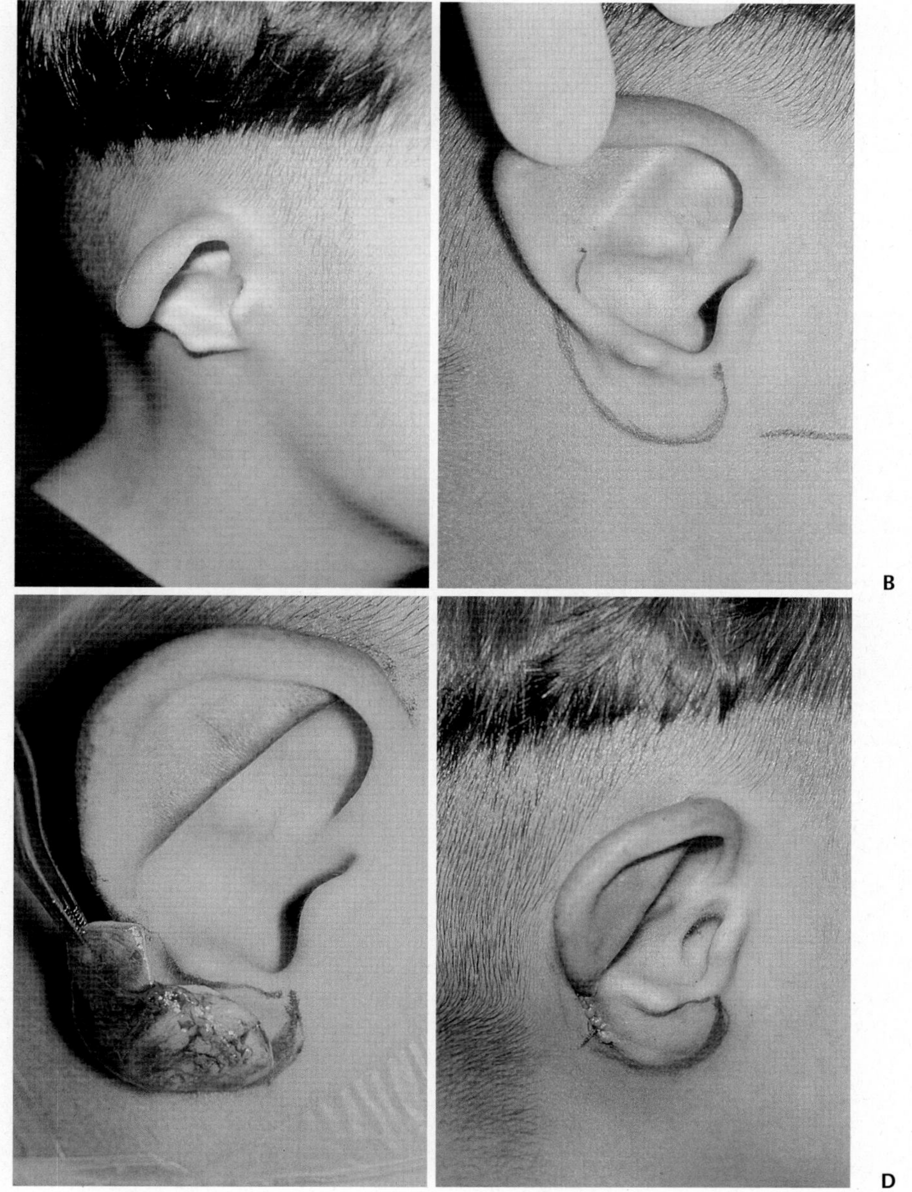

Fig. 60.9 (**A**) Child with cup-ear deformity and congenital complete absence of lower third of right ear. (**B**) Absent portion of ear marked based on contralateral auricular contour. (**C**) Conchal cartilage graft from contralateral normal ear to be used as cartilage graft to help define lower third of ear. Note also creation of antihelical ridge for correction of cup-ear deformity. (**D**) Completion of first stage with implantation of cartilage.

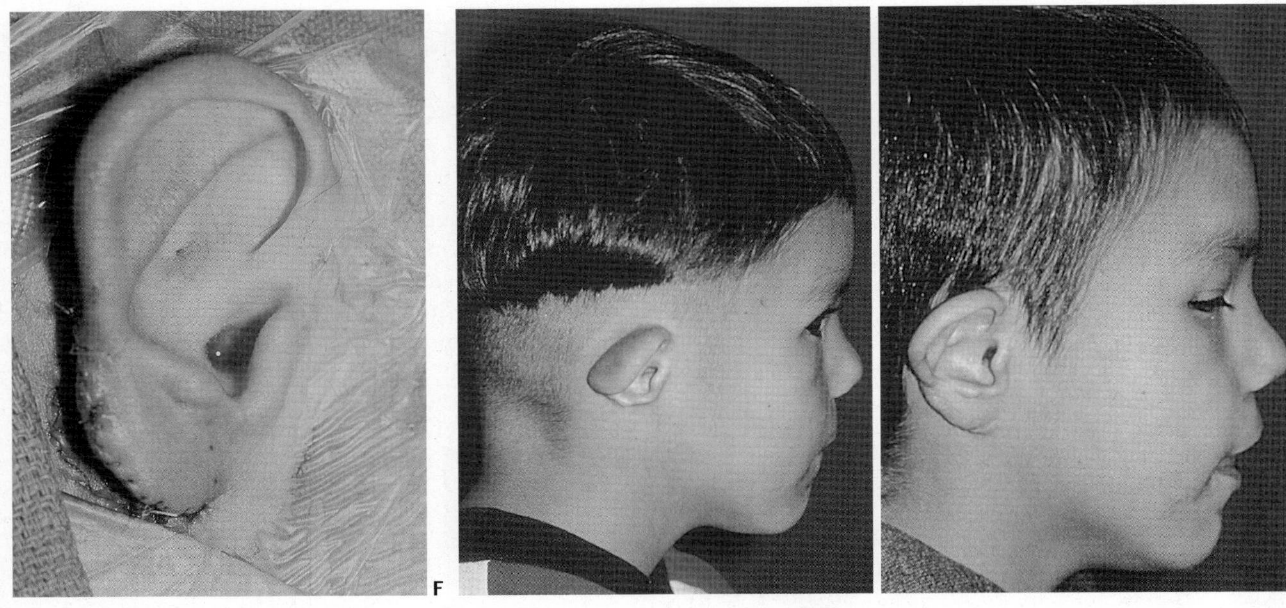

Fig. 60.9 (*Continued*) (**E**) Completion of second stage with elevation of cartilage graft and postauricular skin grafting. (**F**) Preoperative appearance with cup-ear deformity and congenital absence of inferior aspect of ear. (**G**) Complete postoperative result with improvement of cup-ear deformity and reconstruction of inferior aspect of ear.

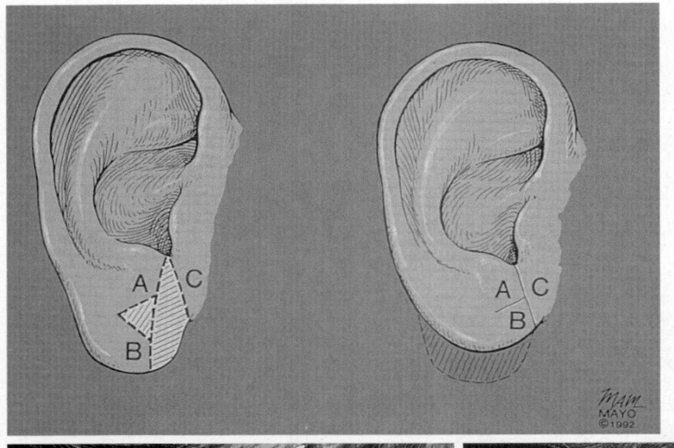

Fig. 60.10 (**A**) Reduction of the aging elongated earlobe via two triangular excisions. (**B**) Excisions marked intraoperatively on patient. (**C**) Completion of earlobe reduction. Note correction of pendulous earlobe. This procedure is routinely performed in conjunction with aging-face surgery.

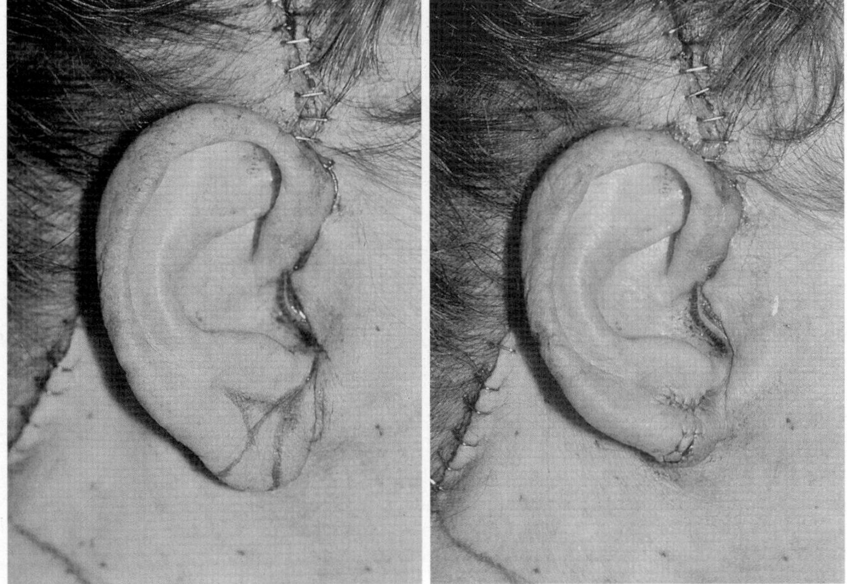

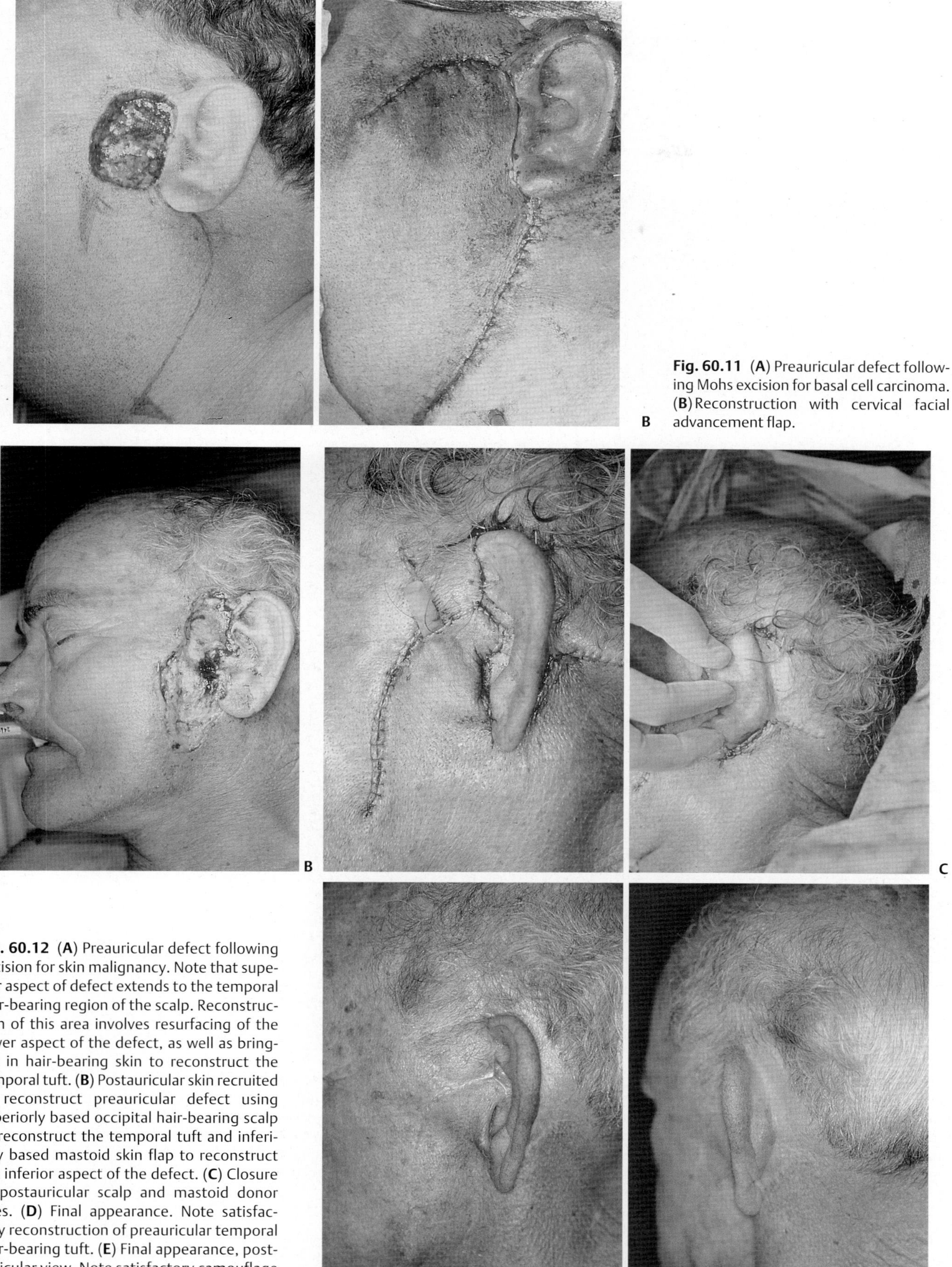

Fig. 60.11 (**A**) Preauricular defect following Mohs excision for basal cell carcinoma. (**B**) Reconstruction with cervical facial advancement flap.

Fig. 60.12 (**A**) Preauricular defect following excision for skin malignancy. Note that superior aspect of defect extends to the temporal hair-bearing region of the scalp. Reconstruction of this area involves resurfacing of the lower aspect of the defect, as well as bringing in hair-bearing skin to reconstruct the temporal tuft. (**B**) Postauricular skin recruited to reconstruct preauricular defect using superiorly based occipital hair-bearing scalp to reconstruct the temporal tuft and inferiorly based mastoid skin flap to reconstruct the inferior aspect of the defect. (**C**) Closure of postauricular scalp and mastoid donor sites. (**D**) Final appearance. Note satisfactory reconstruction of preauricular temporal hair-bearing tuft. (**E**) Final appearance, postauricular view. Note satisfactory camouflage of donor site scars and recreation of natural occipital hairline.

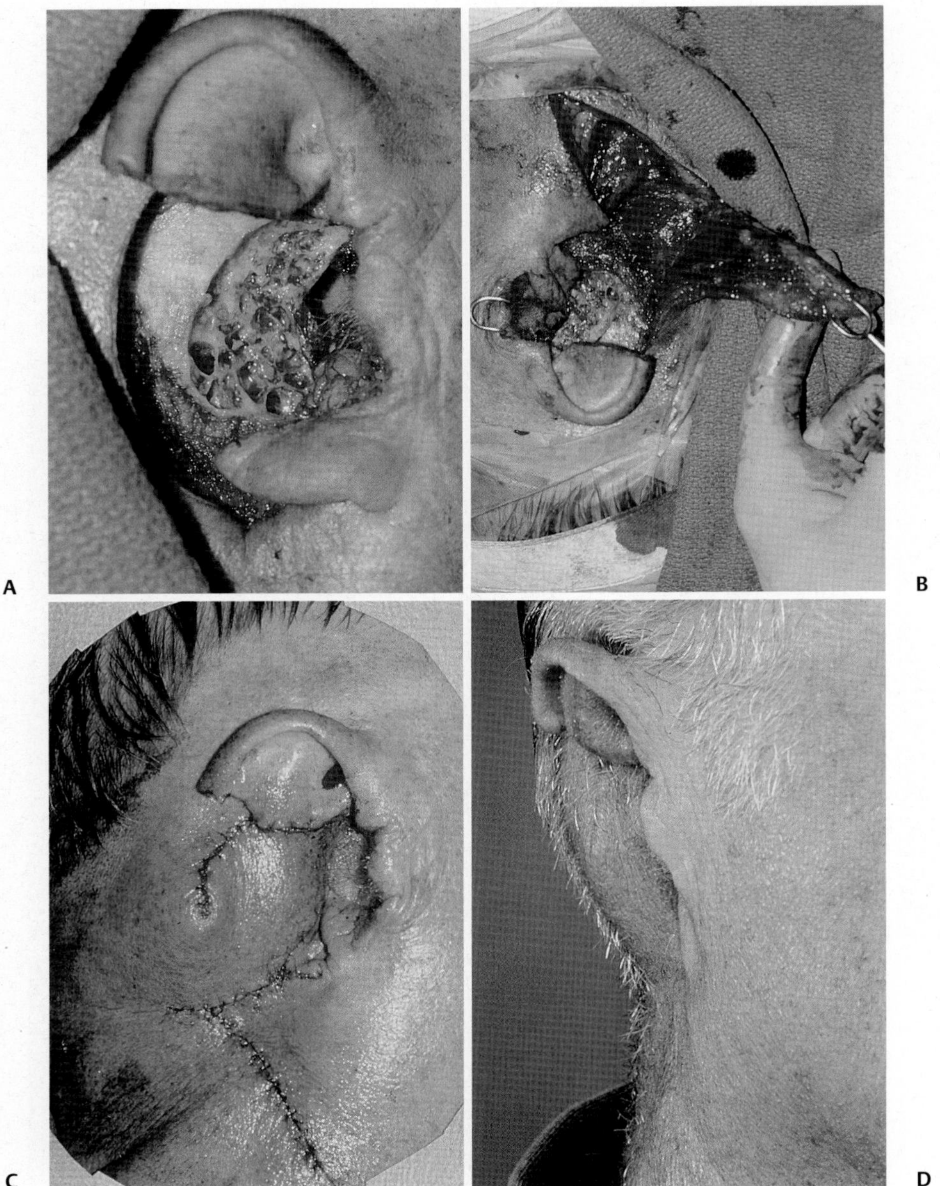

Fig. 60.13 (**A**) Auricular mastoid defect following removal for malignancy. Patient is only interested in having the superiormost portion of his ear intact to allow him to wear eyeglasses. He was not interested in further extensive reconstruction. (**B**) Myocutaneous flap elevated for reconstruction of exposed bony defect, as well as recreation of ear contour. (**C**) Flap swung into position and all raw surfaces satisfactorily covered. Note that no attempt was made at reconstructing the auricular defect other than simple closure of edge of excision. (**D**) Long-term follow-up showing satisfactory healing with superior auricular portion intact to allow patient to wear eyeglasses.

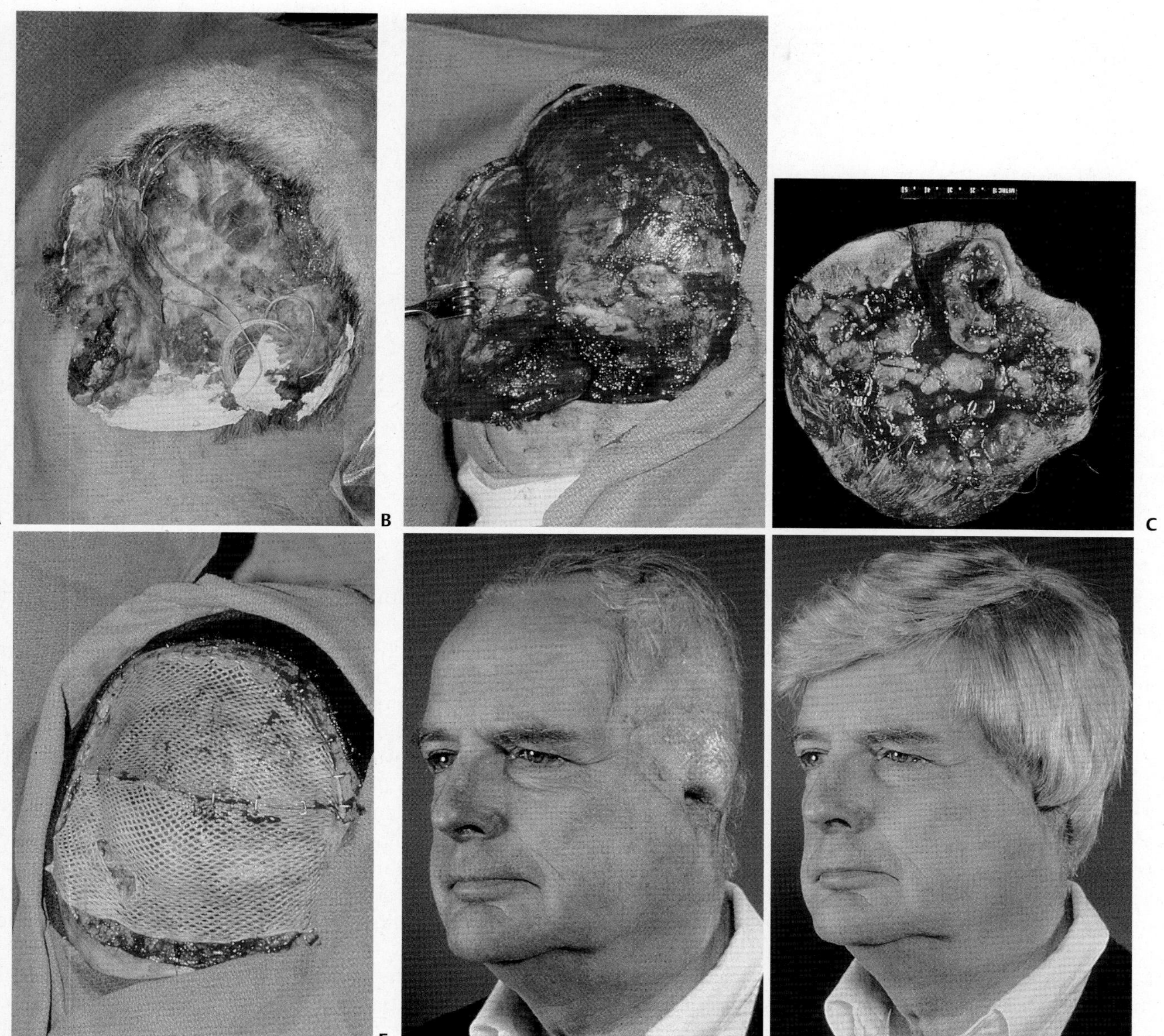

ig. 60.14 (A) Giant neglected basal cell carcinoma involving the ear, mastoid, and temporal region. Patient as been ignoring this lesion for years and has been dressing it with tissue paper. (B) Intraoperative excision f tumor down to temporalis muscle and mastoid bone. (C) Specimen with complete auriculectomy. (D) Due o the need for ongoing tumor surveillance and the history of patient's neglect, a full-thickness skin graft was sed to resurface the entire region. (E) Final postoperative appearance. (F) Patient camouflages the temporal nd auricular defect with wig.

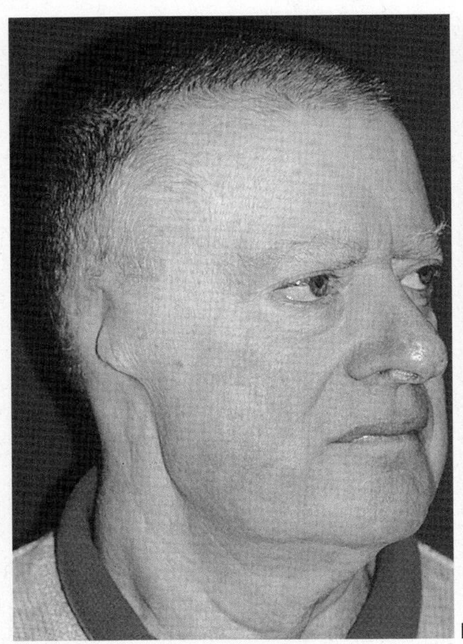

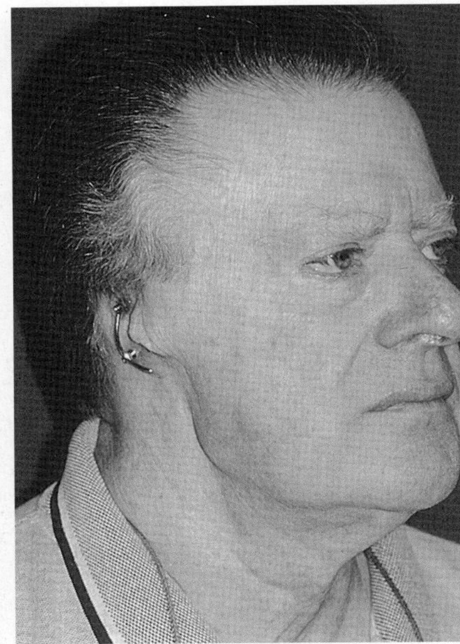

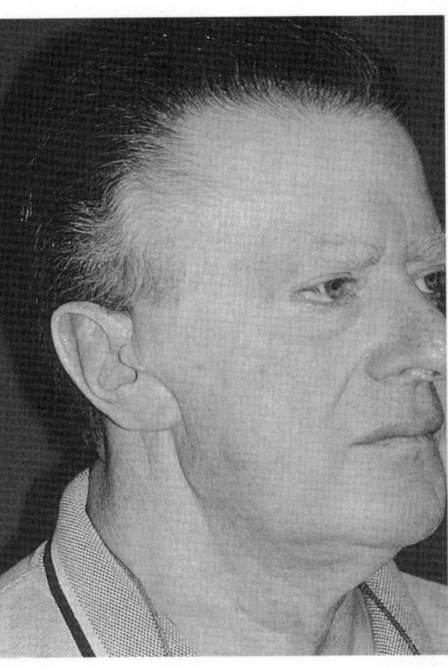

Fig. 60.15 (**A**) Patient status post total auriculectomy for recurrent malignant melanoma. (**B**) Patient with titanium osteointegrated implant in place with abutment attached to wire. (**C**) Prosthetic ear is easily attached to the wire framework.

using a hair-bearing scalp flap recruited from the postauricular region to recreate the preauricular temporal tuft. The postauricular donor region is closed with local advancement flaps (**Fig. 60.12**).

Large Defects Involving Both the Central and Peripheral Portions of the Ear

Large defects of the ear present the greatest challenge for the reconstructive surgeon. Several reconstructive options exist in these circumstances. The patient's wishes are critical in this decision-making process. Not all patients want to have their defects reconstructed. For some, the primary concern is retaining the helical root and superior helical rim portion of the ear, which will allow them to wear their glasses securely. In those instances, simple closure of the remainder of the defect would suffice to meet the patient's desires (**Fig. 60.13**). Other patients may not be candidates for total auricular reconstruction. For patients in whom neglect was a significant factor in the initial disease process, as well as patients in whom secondary tumor surveillance is critical, reconstruction should be deferred until a more appropriate time. In that circumstance, simply resurfacing the region and subsequent camouflage with a wig would fulfill the patient's onco logic requirements (**Fig. 60.14**).

For patients with total auricular loss who desir reconstruction but for whom continued tumor surveil lance is required, the use of an auricular prosthesi is a viable option. The prosthesis is anchored by clip to titanium osteointegrated implants placed in th mastoid bone. Placement of these implants involves simple outpatient procedure that is done in two stages The anaplastologist fabricates the prosthesis, whic is based on a mirror image of the patient's normal ea These reconstructions recreate an excellent fascimile o an ear while allowing simultaneous tumor surveillanc (**Fig. 60.15**).

In cases where the patient desires autogenous tis sue reconstruction of large auricular defects, the princi ple used in microtia reconstruction is incorporated. Thi involves the creation of a freestanding costal cartilag sculptural framework that is implanted in vascularize tissue (**Fig. 60.16**). This process is done in a staged fash ion to recreate a freestanding auricular contour. Whe additional vascularity is required, the temporoparietofas cial flap (**Fig. 60.17**) has been used in conjunction wit autogenous costal cartilage framework and primary ski grafting to recreate the appropriate auricular contou (**Fig. 60.18**). The advantage of this technique lies in the fac that complete reconstruction can take place essentiall

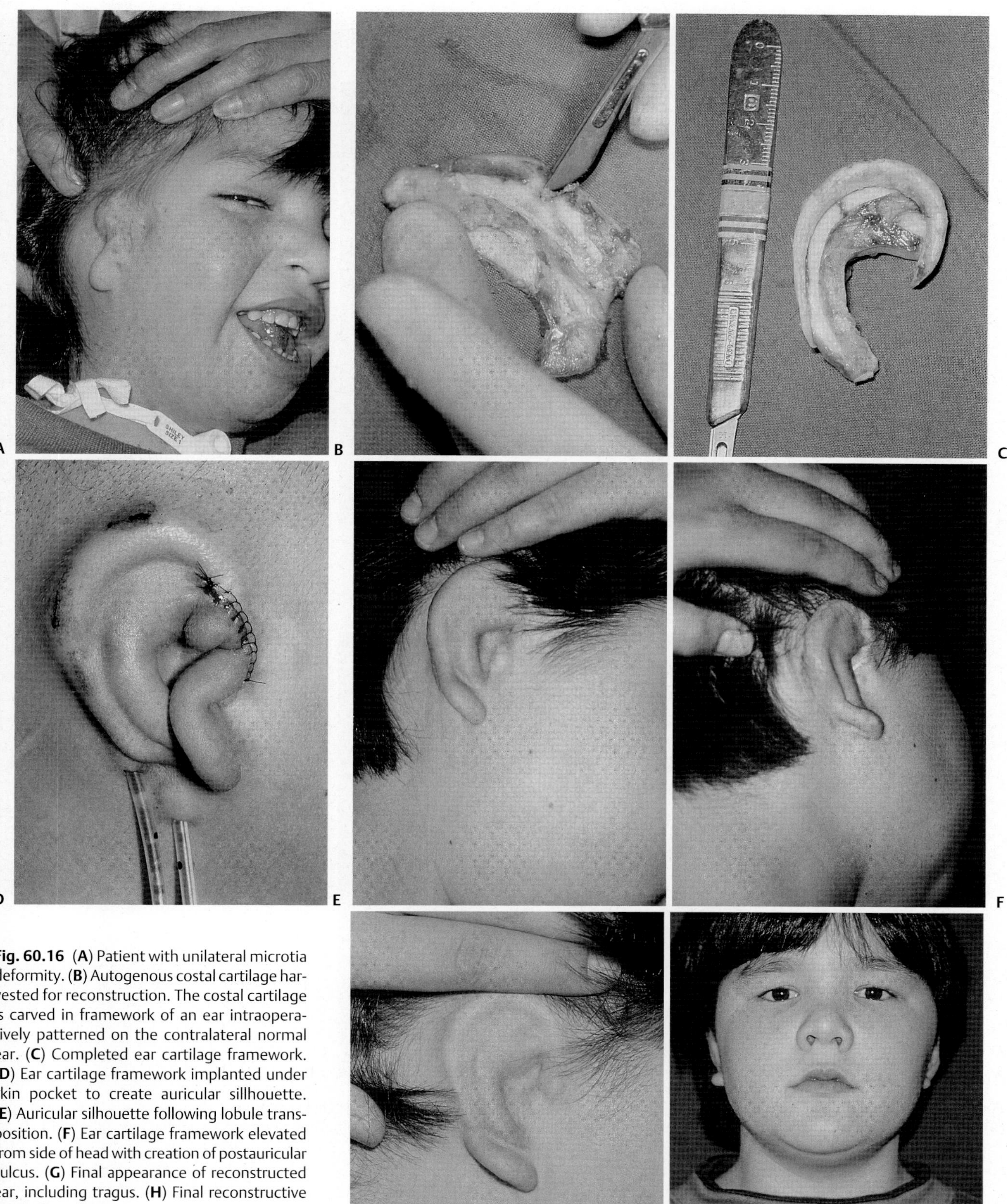

Fig. 60.16 (**A**) Patient with unilateral microtia deformity. (**B**) Autogenous costal cartilage harvested for reconstruction. The costal cartilage is carved in framework of an ear intraoperatively patterned on the contralateral normal ear. (**C**) Completed ear cartilage framework. (**D**) Ear cartilage framework implanted under skin pocket to create auricular sillhouette. (**E**) Auricular silhouette following lobule transposition. (**F**) Ear cartilage framework elevated from side of head with creation of postauricular sulcus. (**G**) Final appearance of reconstructed ear, including tragus. (**H**) Final reconstructive result, frontal view.

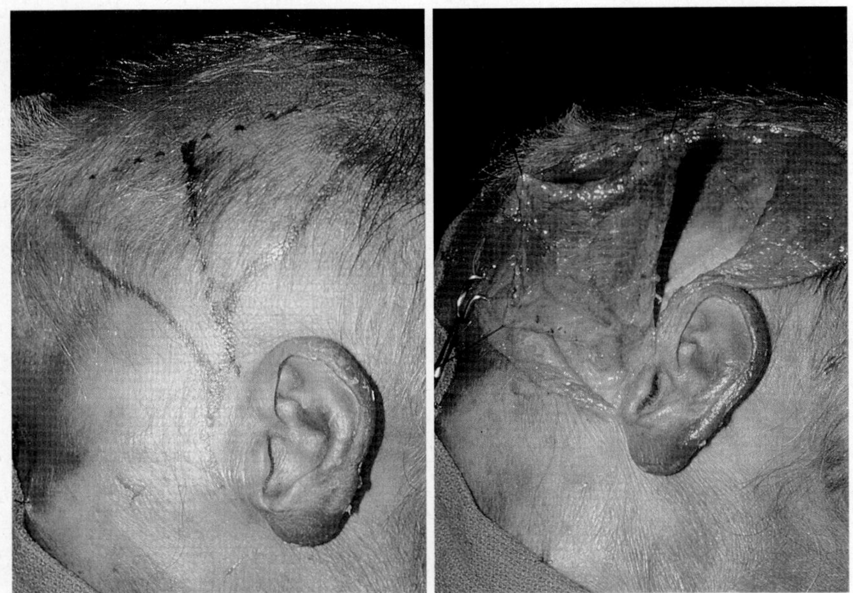

Fig. 60.17 (**A**) "T" incision used to harvest temporoparietofascial flap. Anterior and posterior superficial temporal vessels are also marked. (**B**) Anatomy of temporoparietofascial flap elevated based on superficial temporal vessels. Note the dense, white, conjoint temporal fascia found deep to the superficial temporoparietal fascia.

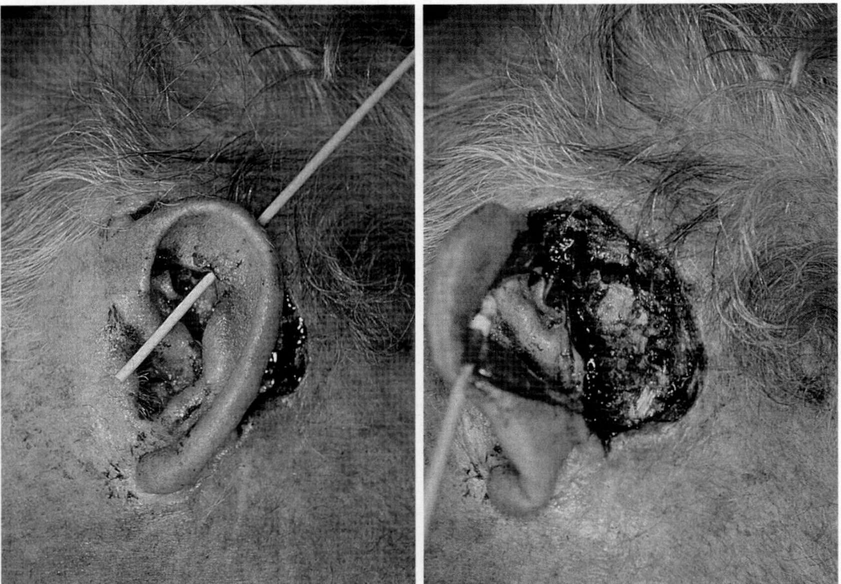

Fig. 60.18 (**A**) Large auricular defect involving full-thickness loss of midportion of ear following cancer excision. (**B**) Ear reflected forward to reveal the full-thickness loss, as well as postauricular defect down to mastoid bone.

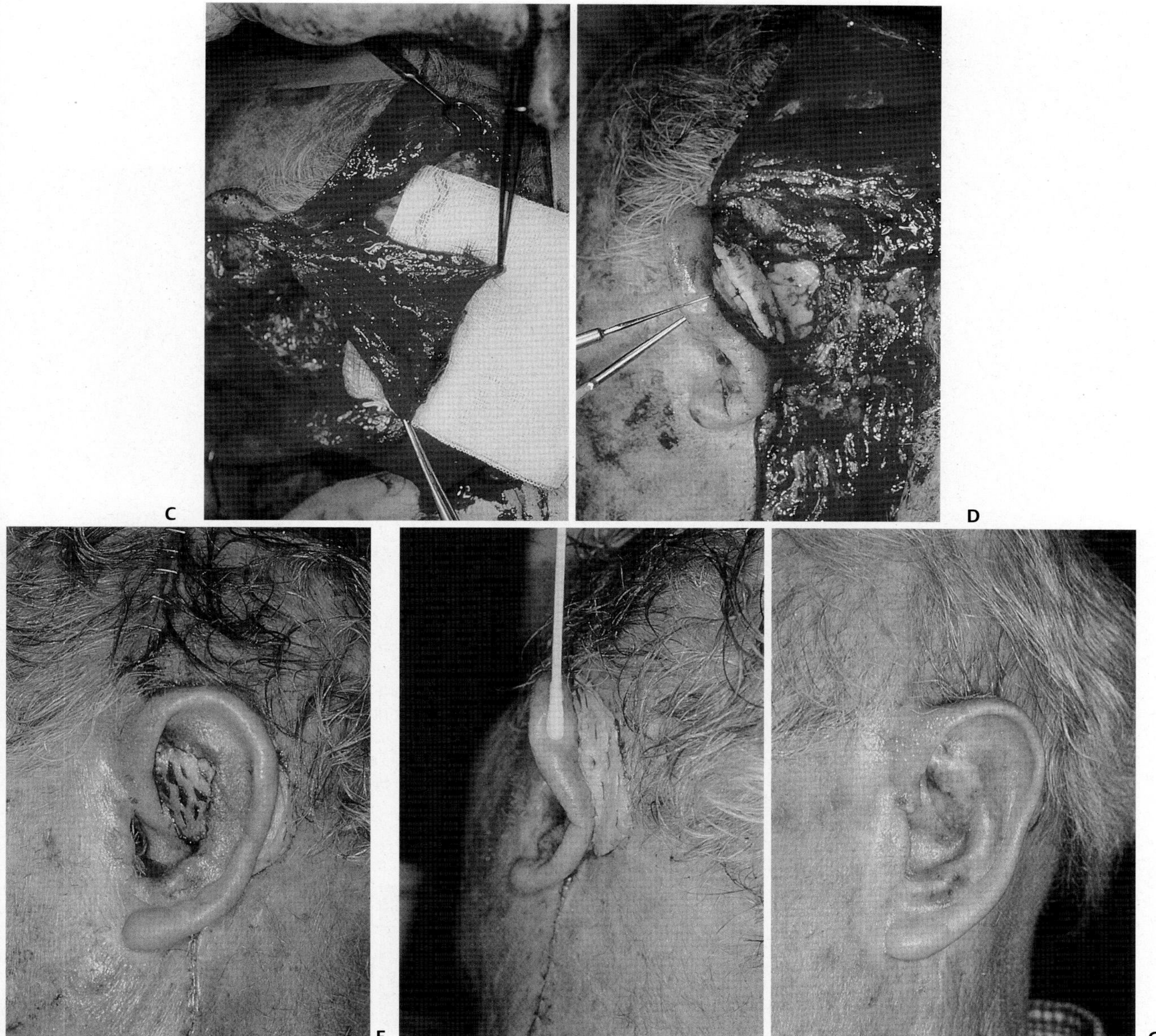

Fig. 60.18 (*Continued*) (**C**) Well-vascularized temporoparietofascial flap harvested to provide vascularity. (**D**) Autogenous costal cartilage shaped to recreate cartilaginous portion of defect and provide auricular structural framework. This will be wrapped with the vascular temporoparietofascial flap and covered with skin graft for reconstruction. (**E**) Completion of initial reconstruction. (**F**) Postauricular view of completed reconstruction. (**G**) Long-term follow-up with excellent maintenance of auricular contour and satisfactory healing of temporoparietal donor site.

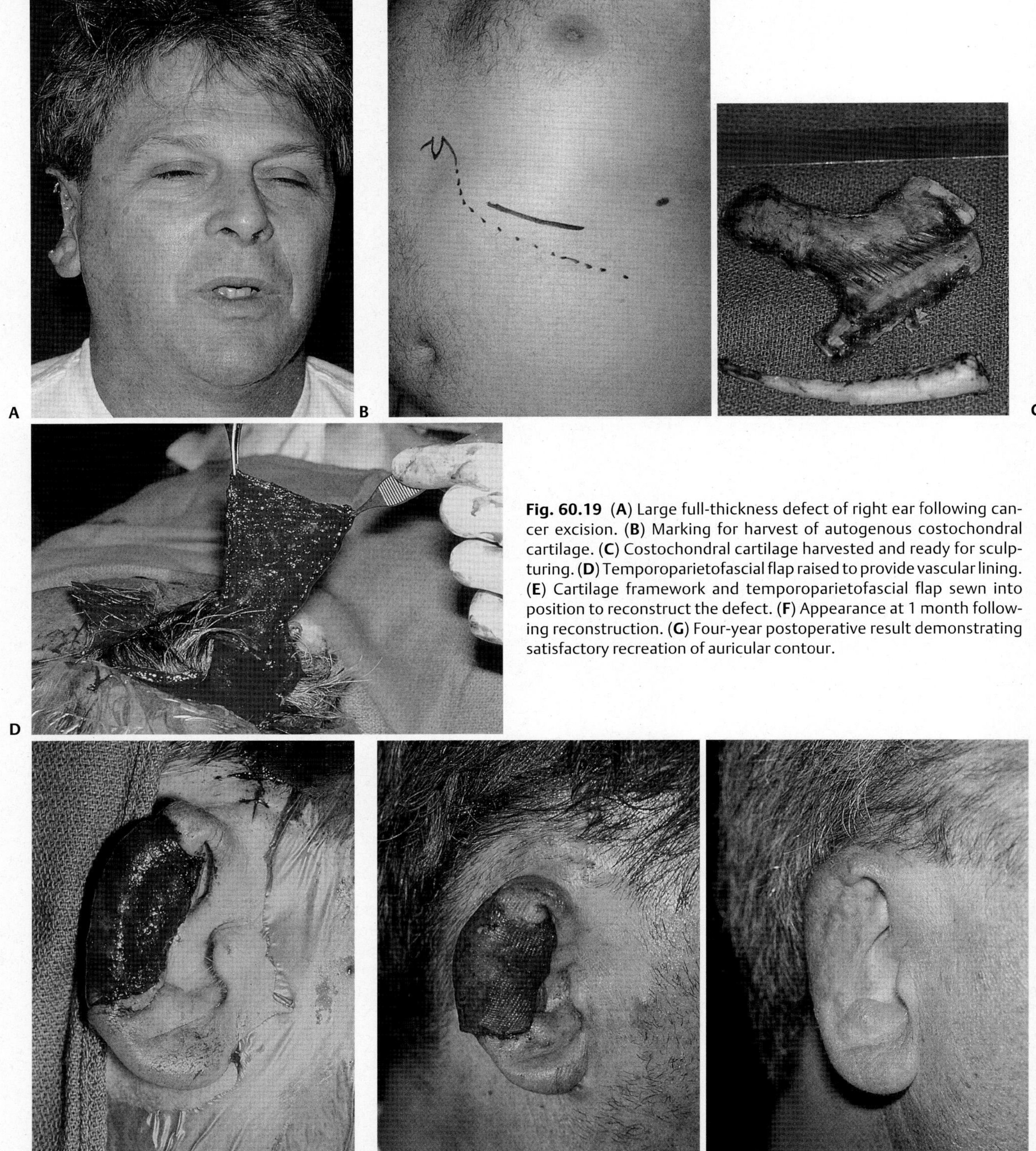

Fig. 60.19 (**A**) Large full-thickness defect of right ear following cancer excision. (**B**) Marking for harvest of autogenous costochondral cartilage. (**C**) Costochondral cartilage harvested and ready for sculpturing. (**D**) Temporoparietofascial flap raised to provide vascular lining. (**E**) Cartilage framework and temporoparietofascial flap sewn into position to reconstruct the defect. (**F**) Appearance at 1 month following reconstruction. (**G**) Four-year postoperative result demonstrating satisfactory recreation of auricular contour.

in a one-stage setting, allowing very satisfactory reconstruction of large defects of the ear (**Fig. 60.19**).

Summary

Auricular reconstruction can present myriad challenges for the reconstructive surgeon. As in reconstruction elsewhere in the head and neck, it is useful to approach defects in the ear from the standpoint of aesthetic subunits that will help guide the reconstructive effort. Appropriate reproduction of the missing anatomic region conforming to the appropriate subunit principle will yield a satisfactory reconstructive outcome.

Suggested Readings

Antia NH, Buch VI. Chondrocutaneous advancement flap for the marginal defect of the ear. Plast Reconstr Surg 1967;39:472

Brent B. Auricular repair with autogenous rib cartilage grafts: 2 decades of experience with 600 cases. Plast Reconstr Surg 1992;90:355

Brent B. Reconstruction of traumatic ear deformities. Clin Plast Surg 1978;5:437

Brent B, Byrd HS. Secondary ear reconstruction with cartilage grafts covered by axial, random, and free flaps of temporoparietal fascia. Plast Reconstr Surg 1983;72:141

Larrabee WF, Makielski KH. Surgical Anatomy of the Face. Philadelphia: Lippincott-Raven Publishers; 1992

Park SS, Wang TD. Temporoparietal facial flap in auricular reconstruction. Facial Plast Surg 1996;11(4):330–337

Tolleth H. Artistic anatomy: dimensions and proportions of the external ear. Clin Plast Surg 1978;36:466

Wazen JJ, Wright R, Hatfield RB, Asher ES. Auricular rehabilitation with bone-anchored titanium implants. Laryngoscope 1999;109(4):532–537

61 Lip Reconstruction

Robert J. DeFatta and Edwin F. Williams III

Historical Overview

Lip reconstruction for large defects of the lower and upper lip continues to be a formidable challenge. The first written description of lip reconstruction was by Susruta in 1000 BC, but an ancient Hindu description of facial, lip, and nasal reconstruction with a forehead flap is reported as early as 3000 BC.[1] Sabatini first described lip reconstruction using a cross-lip flap in 1837,[2] but a subsequent modification of this technique by Abbe and Estlander resulted in their names being ascribed to this method of reconstruction. Bernard and Burow later described a method of lip reconstruction for total and subtotal defects using bilateral full-thickness advancement flaps to the cheeks that were brought to the midline to fashion a new lip.[3,4] Full-thickness triangles were excised in the location of the nasal alar fold to alleviate puckering that resulted from tissue excess in that location. In the 1920s, Gillies described a classic fan flap using a full-thickness pedicle that allows redistribution of the remaining lip during the reconstructive effort and emphasized the use of a similar or like tissue.[5] This concept was further modified by Karapandzic in 1974, who made incisions through the skin and mucosa at a distance equal to the depth of the defect, but with primary emphasis on preservation of the underlying musculature and neurovascular structures.[6] More contemporary refinements for reconstruction of large lip defects by Burget and Menick include the importance of the subunit principle as it applies to the upper lip for an optimal aesthetic result.[7] Microvascular reconstruction using radial forearm free flap and temporal scalp free flap have been used for large and total defects of the lip, and their use may become more popular as more surgeons are trained in microvascular techniques and refinement procedures to maximize the functional and aesthetic outcomes.[8]

Evaluation of the patient in need of lip reconstruction requires a clear understanding of the lip anatomy, aesthetics, and function. In this chapter, a systematic approach will be emphasized based on the anticipated or presenting size and location of the lip defect for a given patient.

Anatomical Considerations

The primary objective of a reconstructive effort is an aesthetic result that approaches a normal appearance. Functional considerations, including oral competence, articulation, speech, and the role of the lips in mastication, must be kept in mind during reconstruction of large lip defects.

Anatomically, the lips extend vertically from the subnasale to the chin and horizontally from the oral commissure to oral commissure. Both upper and lower lips consist of a separate red lip and white lip component separated by a vermilion border.

The upper lip is a curved M-shaped structure with the highest points of the vermilion border just located at the philtral ridges. The philtral ridge extends bilaterally from the highest point of the vermilion border to the base of the columella, and between the lines is a central depression in the upper lip. The complexity of the surface topography, its lines and shadows, results in two medial and lateral subunits of the upper lip, first described by Ulloa-Gonzales and subsequently emphasized by Burget and Menick[7] as illustrated in **Fig. 61.1**. A reconstructive effort of the upper lip in which the surgical defect is simply filled without regard to the subunit principle is perceived by the observer as a patch. Aesthetically, for the lip to look normal, the observer's eye should perceive it as normal. The perception of normal is more accurately described as the absence of abnormal because the "mind's eye" of the observer ignores the defect it would see and focuses on the absence of aberrance. During lip

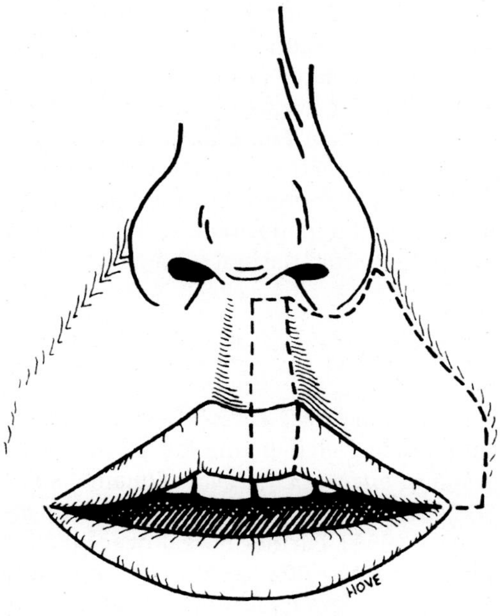

Fig. 61.1 Medial and lateral upper lip subunit.

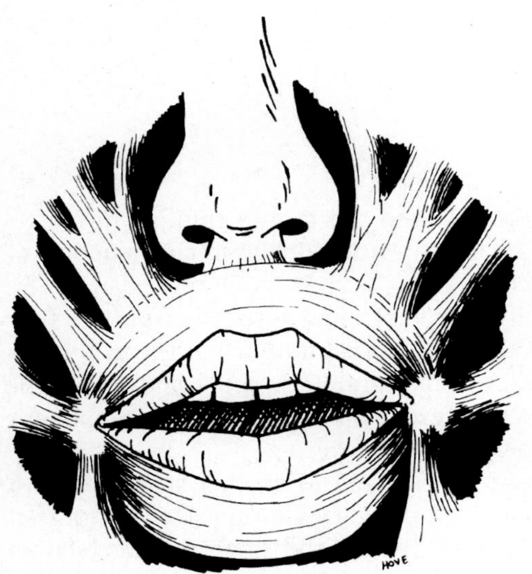

Fig. 61.2 Periorbital musculature and muscular modiolus.

reconstruction, one should attempt to duplicate appropriate height, projection, and the relationship of white to red lip. In addition, because regional or distant tissue is a different color, the use of local tissue with local flaps generally provides a superior result. The lower lip anatomy is considerably less complex and more forgiving of reconstructive effort. However, the same general principles apply for an optimal aesthetic result.

Functionally, the lips act as a sphincter to assist in phonation, mastication, and speech. Anatomical structures that are important to the function of the lips and oral sphincter include the perioral facial musculature, the neurovascular anatomy, and the muscular modiolus, all of which are located between the mucosal surface and the cutaneous surface of the lips. The muscular modiolus is a fibrous structure located at the oral commissure bilaterally and is a site of insertion of the oral sphincter musculature as illustrated in **Fig. 61.2**. The most successful functional reconstruction will address not only the integrity of the muscular oral sphincter, but also the importance of the orientation, position, and function of the muscular modiolus within the oral sphincter.

Lip Reconstruction Techniques

Although traumatic defects are routinely encountered, the most common defect challenging the facial plastic surgeon is a result of oncologic excision. Squamous cell carcinomas (SCCs) are the most common malignant neoplasm of the red lip (95%). Furthermore, lower lip SCCs outnumber upper lip SCCs (90% versus 10%), probably related to a more direct sun exposure encountered by the lower lip. However, in the authorss experience, most basal cell carcinomas of the upper lip arise from the cutaneous white upper lip.

Reconstructive procedures can be classified as:

1. *Minor reconstruction*
   a. Vermillion defects
   b. Small full-thickness defects (< 30% horizontal lip)
      i. Lower lip
      ii. Upper lip
   c. Combination of previous

2. *Major reconstruction*
   a. Medium-size defects (30–60% horizontal lip)
      i. Upper lip
      ii. Lower lip

3. *Subtotal/total lip reconstruction*
   a. Large defects (> 60% horizontal lip)
      i. Lower lip
      ii. Upper lip

4. *Microvascular reconstruction*

Minor Reconstruction

Vermilionectomy

Vermilionectomy is indicated in the patient with chronic actinic cheilitis or microinvasive SCC. Actinic cheilitis is almost exclusively seen in the lower lip and can persist for several months or years before progressing to SCC. A positive diagnosis is considered an indication for surgical treatment because of the long-term risk for invasive carcinoma. In the compliant patient where there is no concern regarding appropriate follow-up, the authors advocate an ablation procedure with the CO_2 laser. Local anesthetic is infiltrated, and a laser resurfacing mode is used at the same parameters one would utilize to treat eyelid skin. Two or three passes are performed, and the appropriate short- and long-term follow-up recommended. In the authors' experience with a compliant patient, this approach is very successful, and it is more cosmetically acceptable than the traditional vermilionectomy and lip advancement procedure.

Technique

A vermilionectomy procedure is the time-honored and traditional procedure for actinic cheilitis or carcinoma in situ especially in the patient for whom reliable follow-up might be a concern. A surgical marking pen is used to delineate the vermilion border from oral commissure to oral commissure. A fusiform-type excision of the vermilion is planned and a posterior incision is placed parallel to the anterior vermilion border incision. The lip is infiltrated with the appropriate amount to lidocaine with 1:100,000 epinephrine. Incisions are made and the vermilion is excised in a submucosal plane as illustrated in **Fig. 61.3**. A submucosal dissection is carried from the posterior incision toward the gingival–buccal sulcus approximately two times the width of the fusiform excision from anterior to posterior. Posterior red lip is advanced in a meticulous repair that is performed along the vermilion with a 5–0 chromic suture. Two back-cuts from each oral commissure toward the sulcus may be necessary to facilitate advancement. It is important that the vermilion border is repaired without tension on the incision line.

Wedge Excision and Primary Repair

A wedge or full-thickness excision is indicated with invasive SCC of the lower lip. A full-thickness wedge excision and repair can be utilized for surgical defects measuring up to one third the size of the horizontal lip. The length of the lower lip generally measures 7 to 7.5 cm, allowing a surgical defect of ~2.5 cm. However, one should exercise judgment in the patient at the upper limit of an acceptable excision for primary repair. In a patient with less tissue elasticity or one in whom repair will result in a significant and noticeable discrepancy of the upper

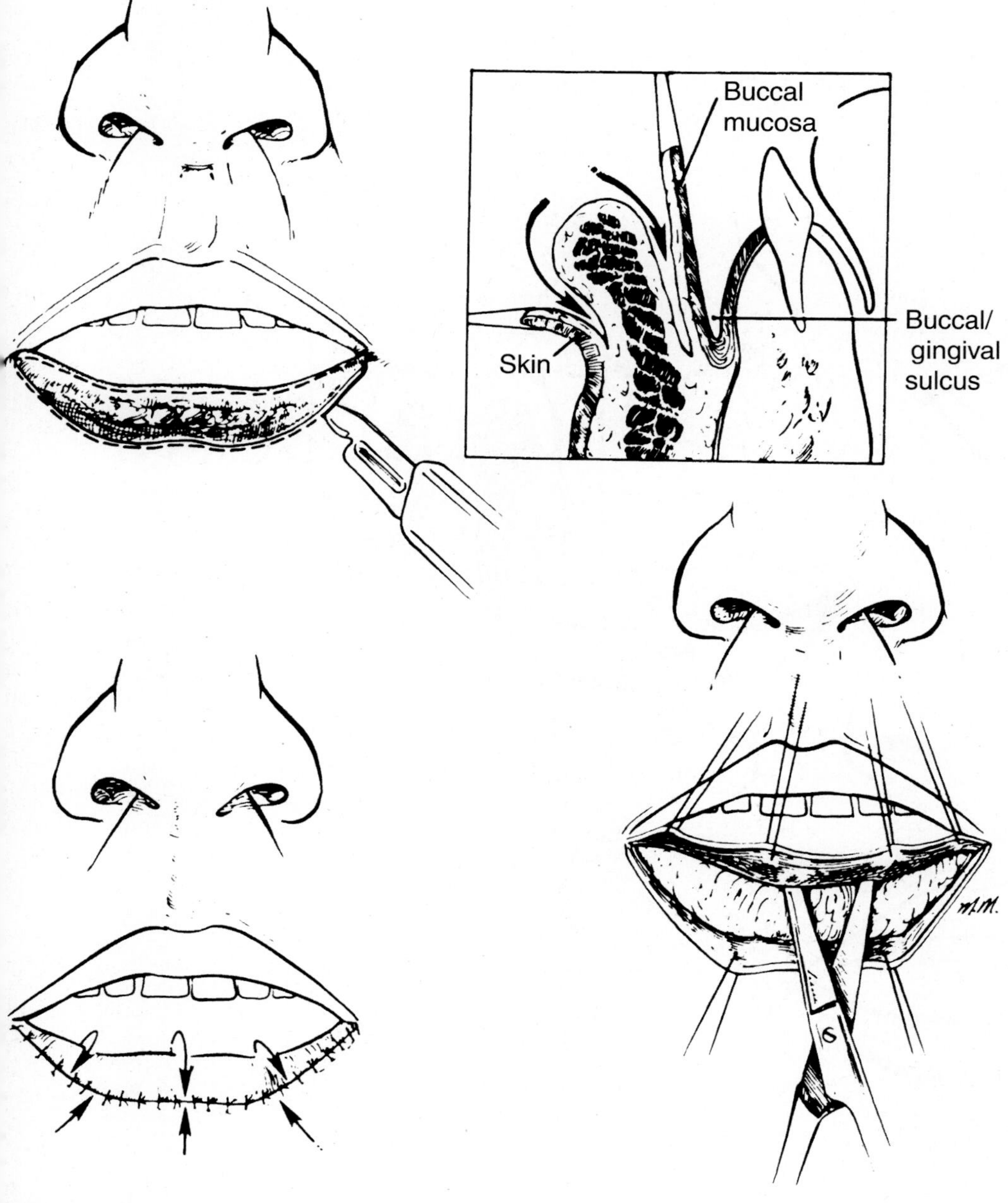

Fig. 61.3 Vermilionectomy technique.

and lower lip, it may be advisable to reconstruct using a cross-lip flap.

Technique

A surgical marking pen is used to plan for the reconstruction. It is generally recommended that the vermilion border be marked adjacent to the line of resection as local anesthetic, edema, and the blanching effect of epinephrine often make a precise repair at the vermilion border difficult. The line of resection through the red lip should be perpendicular to the long axis of the red lip and allowed to converge beginning on the white lip as illustrated in **Fig. 61.4**. The apex of the wedge should not extend beyond the mental crease or melolabial crease. Incorporation of an M-plasty in the repair is advised for larger wedge resections as it prevents the incision from crossing the lip–chin junction and assists in irregularizing a longer incision. The repair is begun by placing a 6–0 nonabsorbable, monofilament suture at the vermilion border (Prolene, nylon). Two or three interrupted sutures should then be placed in the orbicularis muscle with a longer lasting absorbable, monofilament polyglycolic suture (4–0 PDS, macron). A 4–0 chromic suture

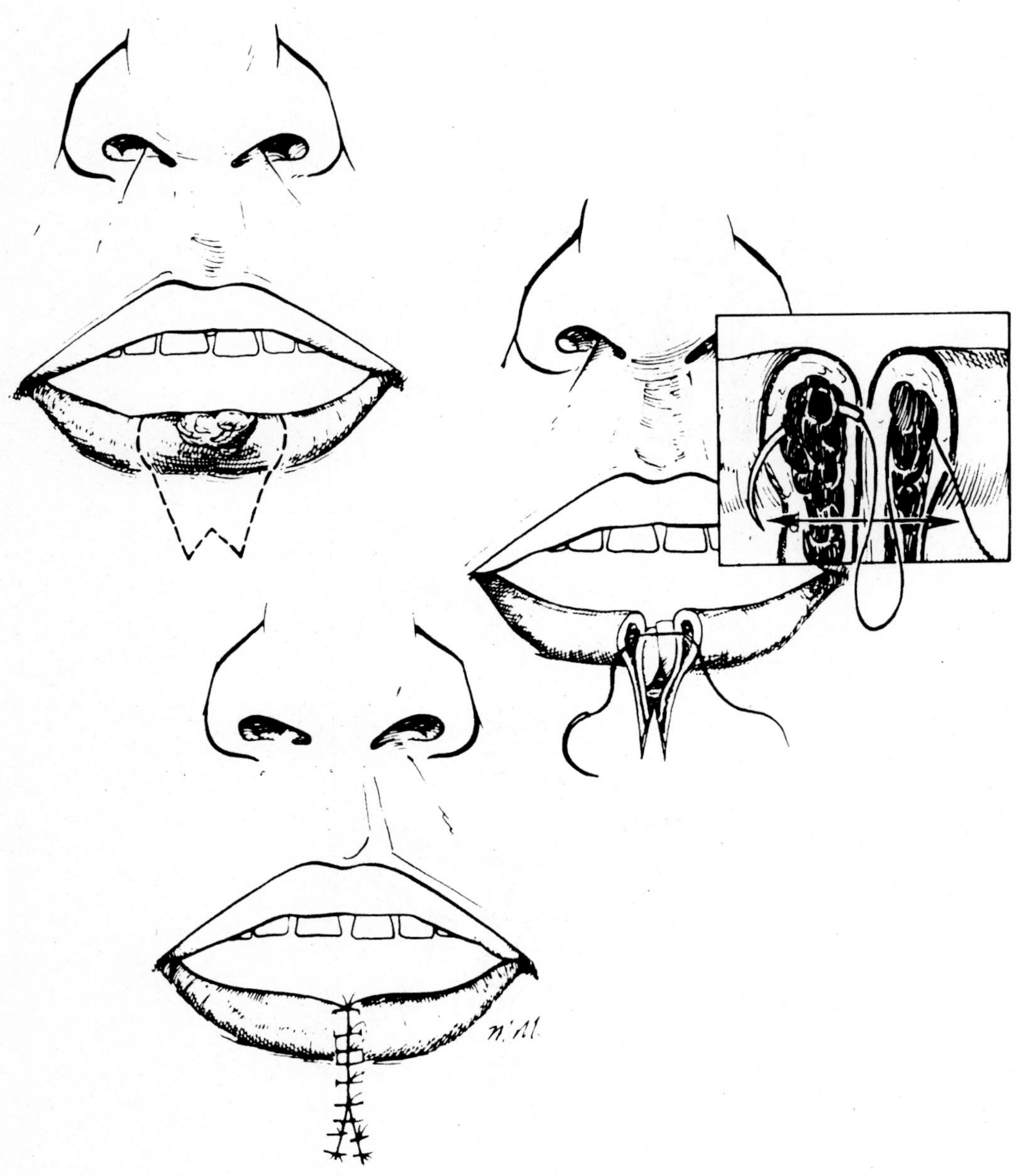

Fig. 61.4 Wedge excision and primary full-thickness repair.

is used for the intraoral red lip, and the author prefers a 5–0 chromic suture for the exposed red lip repair. The skin should be closed with a 6–0 nonabsorbable, monofilament suture (Prolene [Ethicon, Inc., Somerville, NJ], nylon).

Combined Defects

Occasionally, a patient presents with a discrete lower-lip lesion amenable to excision with a full-thickness repair. However, on inspection the remaining red lip has the clinical appearance of a severe actinic cheilitis, placing the patient at high risk for subsequent carcinoma of the lip. In this patient population, a full-thickness excision and repair should be performed in conjunction with vermilionectomy and lip advancement for the remaining red lip.

Major Reconstruction of Medium-Sized Defects: Cross-Lip Flap

Surgical defects measuring between 30 and 60% of the horizontal lip are best reconstructed with a staged cross-lip flap, as first described by Sabatini[2] and further modified by Abbe and Estlander. In general, this corresponds to a surgical defect between 2.5 and 4.5 cm. The cross-flap reconstruction has the benefit of reconstructing a relatively large full-thickness lip defect with tissue of similar texture, complexion, thickness, and muscular activity. Electromyography studies at 1 year following reconstruction have confirmed the ability of the transferred orbicularis muscle to reinnervate successfully and function as an animated segment.[7] Sensory function may also return after several months. In addition, the cross-lip reconstruction successfully redistributes the remaining upper and lower lip discrepancy to the deficient lip with a minimal effect on the

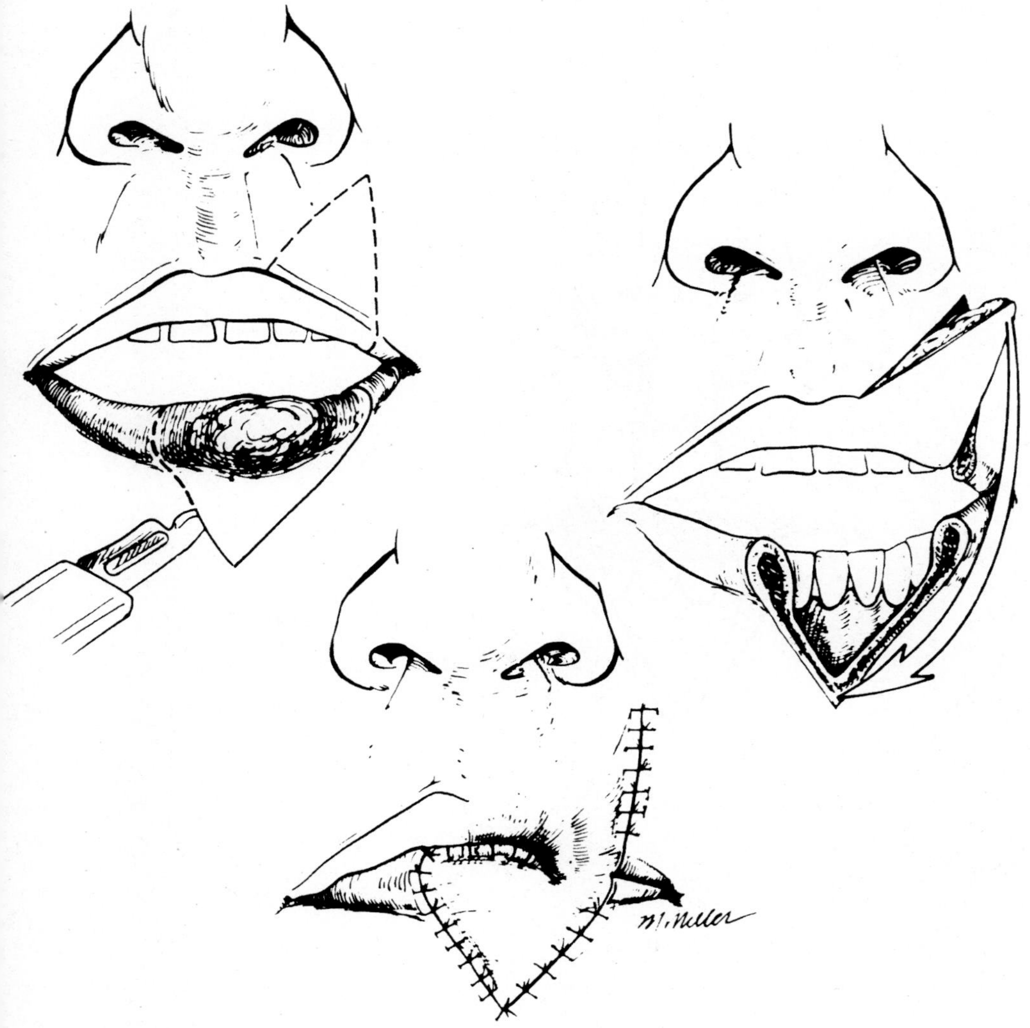

Fig. 61.5 Cross-lip flap technique.

muscular modiolus in orientation of the remaining musculature of the oral sphincter. Because of the complexity of the upper lip anatomy as compared with the lower lip anatomy, the primary consideration of a cross-lip flap reconstruction is generally the effect the reconstruction will have on the upper lip anatomy.

Lower Lip

The approach to lower lip defects of 30 to 60% with a cross-lip flap is fairly straightforward, with primary emphasis placed on how taking the upper lip donor flap will affect the upper lip aesthetically.

Technique

After a wedge resection of the lower lip has been performed, a triangular full-thickness flap is designed on the upper lip. Traditionally, a cross-lip flap is designed at a width of one half to two thirds of the horizontal lip surgical defect, as illustrated in **Fig. 61.5**. A full-thickness incision is carried ~2 to 3 mm to the vermilion border, and a meticulous dissection through the orbicularis muscle allows preservation of the labial artery. Burget emphasizes the importance of the blood supply provided by the vermilion mucosa and stresses the importance of preserving ~5 mm of mucosa in addition to the labial artery, which is included in the pedicle.[7] Division and inset of the flap should occur

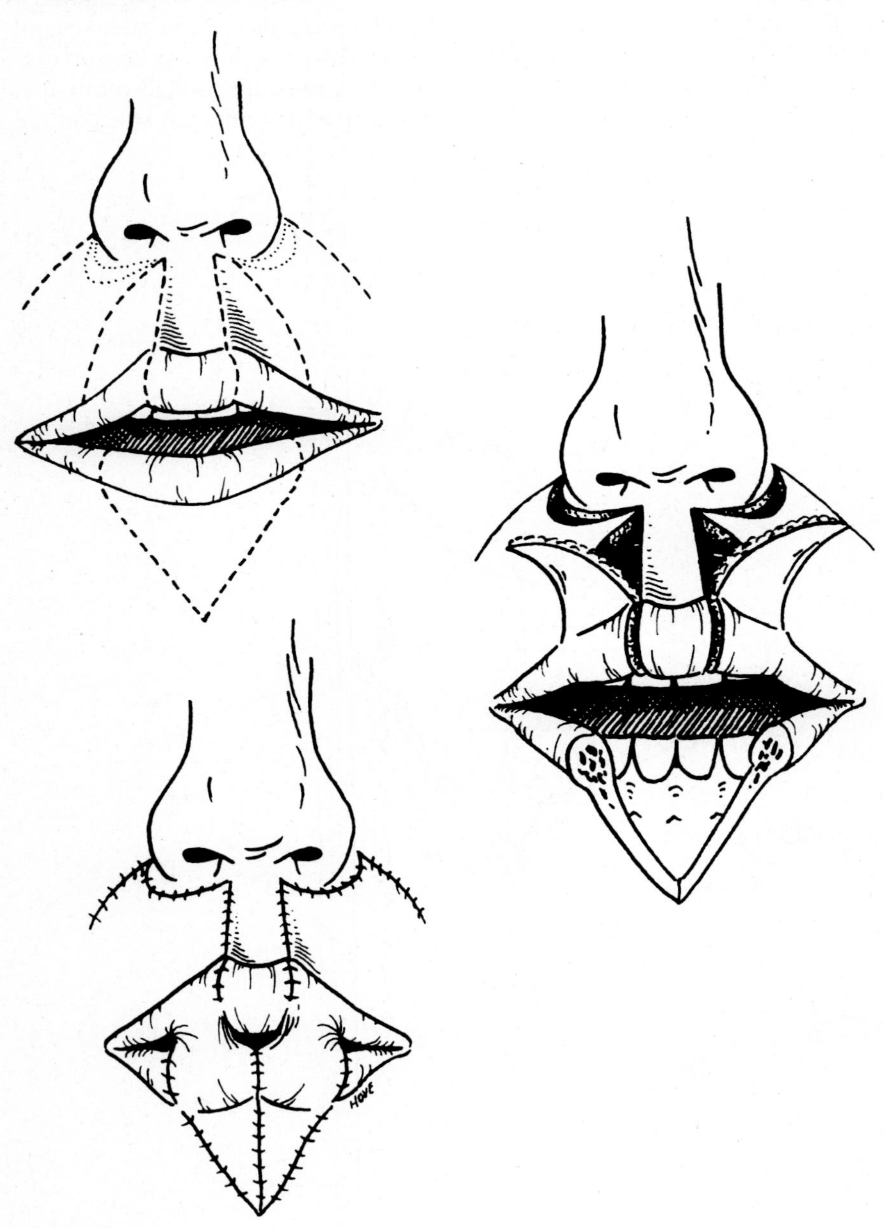

Fig. 61.6 Modified bilateral cross-lip flap for the lower lip.

at 14 to 21 days, and no attempt is made to test the flap with a tourniquet as suggested by some authors.

In the fastidious patient with a larger defect (60 to 70% lower lip), one should consider bilateral cross-lip flaps to fill the lower lip defect as shown in **Fig. 61.6**. This approach not only keeps the incision lines at the junction of the aesthetic subunits of the upper lip, but it also distributes the loss between the upper lip lateral subunits rather than recruiting all tissue from one side and causing a noticeable upper lip asymmetry.

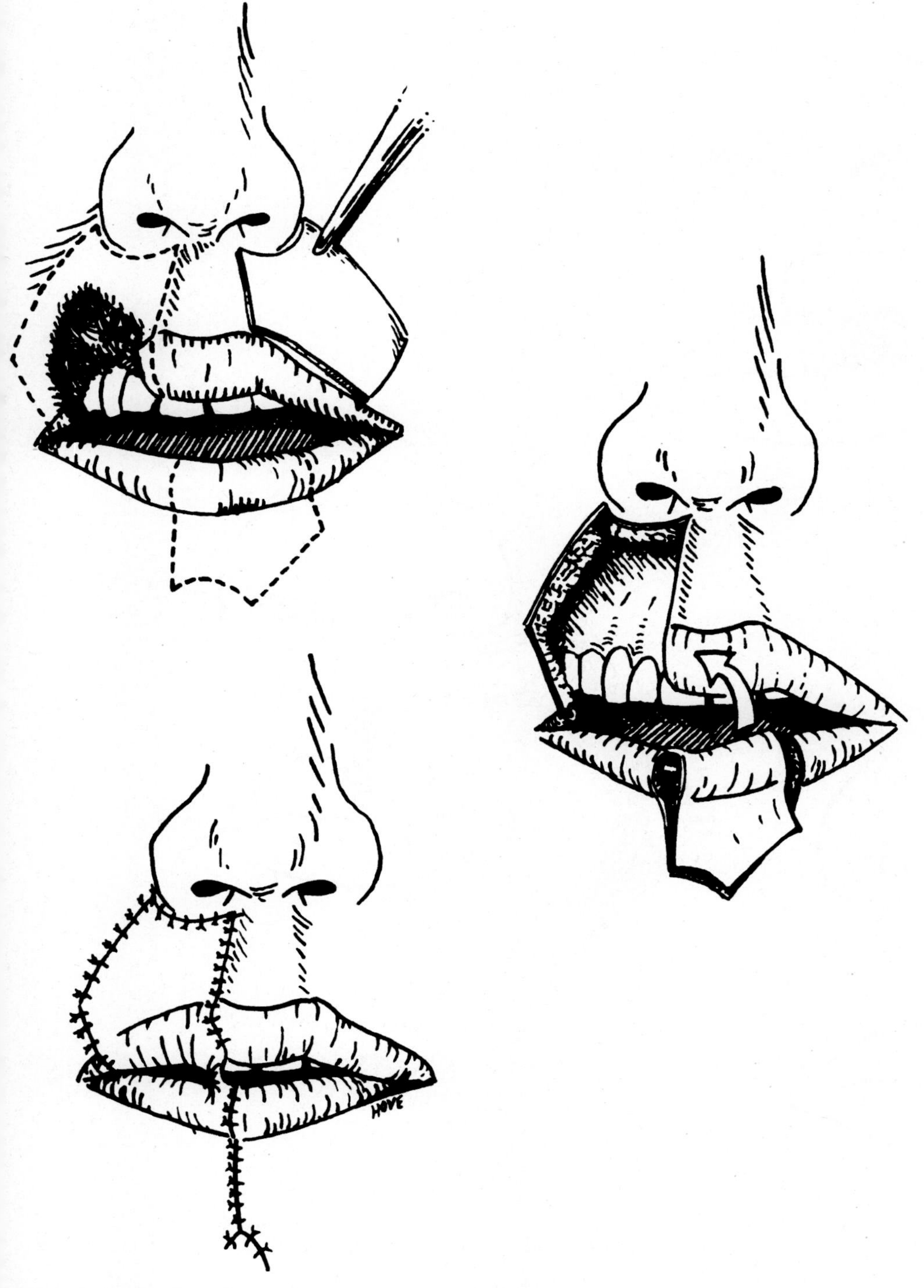

Fig. 61.7 Modified cross-lip flap for the upper lip with emphasis on the subunit principle.

Upper Lip

Upper lip defects pose a greater challenge for an optimal reconstruction because of the surface topography, complexity of the anatomy, and potential for distorting the upper lip subunits, thus creating a noticeable asymmetry.

Technique

In defects that result in more than 50% loss of the subunit, the reconstructive surgeon should excise the remaining normal tissue and replace the entire subunit from the lower lip, as shown in **Fig. 61.7**. The template from the contralateral normal subunit is outlined on the upper lip, and a

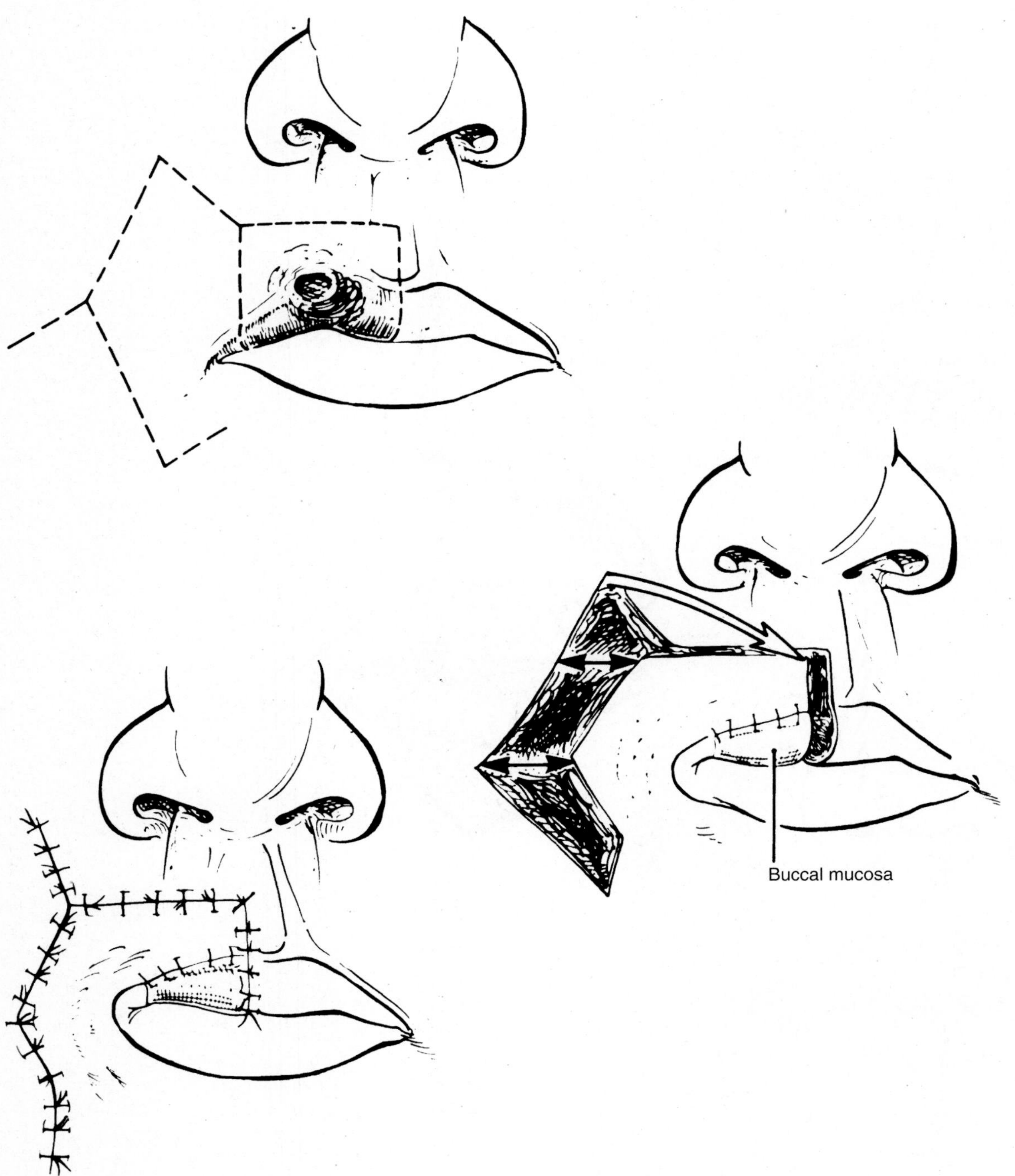

Fig. 61.8 Gillies fan flap technique.

similar technique is used for developing, transposing, and resecting the cross-lip flap. The contralateral normal lip is utilized for developing a template because the presence of local anesthetic, tumor, and edema will result in a less accurate template if one uses the involved lip and subunit.

Subtotal/Total Lip Reconstruction of Large Defects

Surgical defects measuring greater than 70 to 80% of the lip continue to be a formidable challenge. In the 1920s, Gillies[5] first described the classic fan flap using a full-thickness pedicle that allows redistribution of the remaining lip as illustrated in **Fig. 61.8**. Karapandzic[6] further modified this concept with an incision through both the skin and mucosa, with emphasis placed on preservation of the underlying musculature, as shown in **Fig. 61.9**. Both techniques are important for historical purposes but have shortcomings with regard to an optimal aesthetic and functional reconstruction as previously discussed. In a more recent report, Kroll described a similarly staged pro-

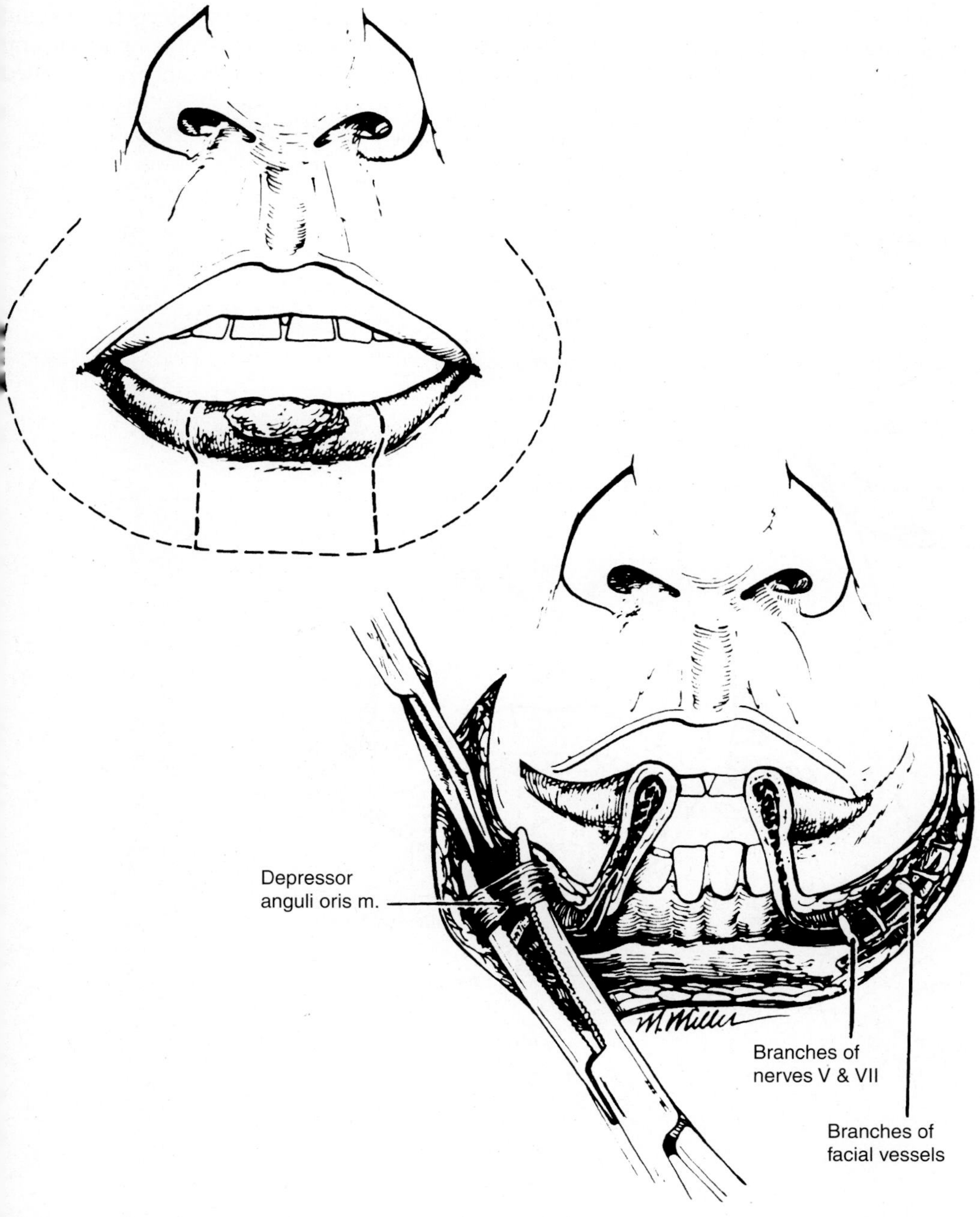

Fig. 61.9 Karapandzic flap technique.

cedure that uses the Bernard-Burow modification of the Karapandzic fan flap (**Fig. 61.10**) followed by a cross-lip flap at a different operative setting.[9–11] In principle, this accomplishes the same goal of reconstructing the missing lip with like tissue. This approach addresses the problem of lip tissue discrepancy between the lip that is reconstructed and the remaining lip by redistributing lip tissue in an area where it is needed. Williams et al further described the simultaneous use of a modified Bernard-Burow cheek advancement flap and a cross-lip flap for total lower or upper lip defects.[12] We believe that the modified cheek flap offers several advantages over sequential reconstruction described by Kroll. The extended intraoral incisions described allow for considerable advancement of the cheek into the surgical defect while preserving the neurovascular structures of the remaining lip. Furthermore, the procedure offers a theoretical advantage of less postoperative microstomia because it recruits new lip tissue into the perioral area rather than rearranging or sharing the remaining lip.

Subtotal/Total Lower Lip Defects

Technique

Total lower defects are full-thickness defects that extend from oral commissure to oral commissure or past the oral commissure to include a portion of the cheek, as detailed

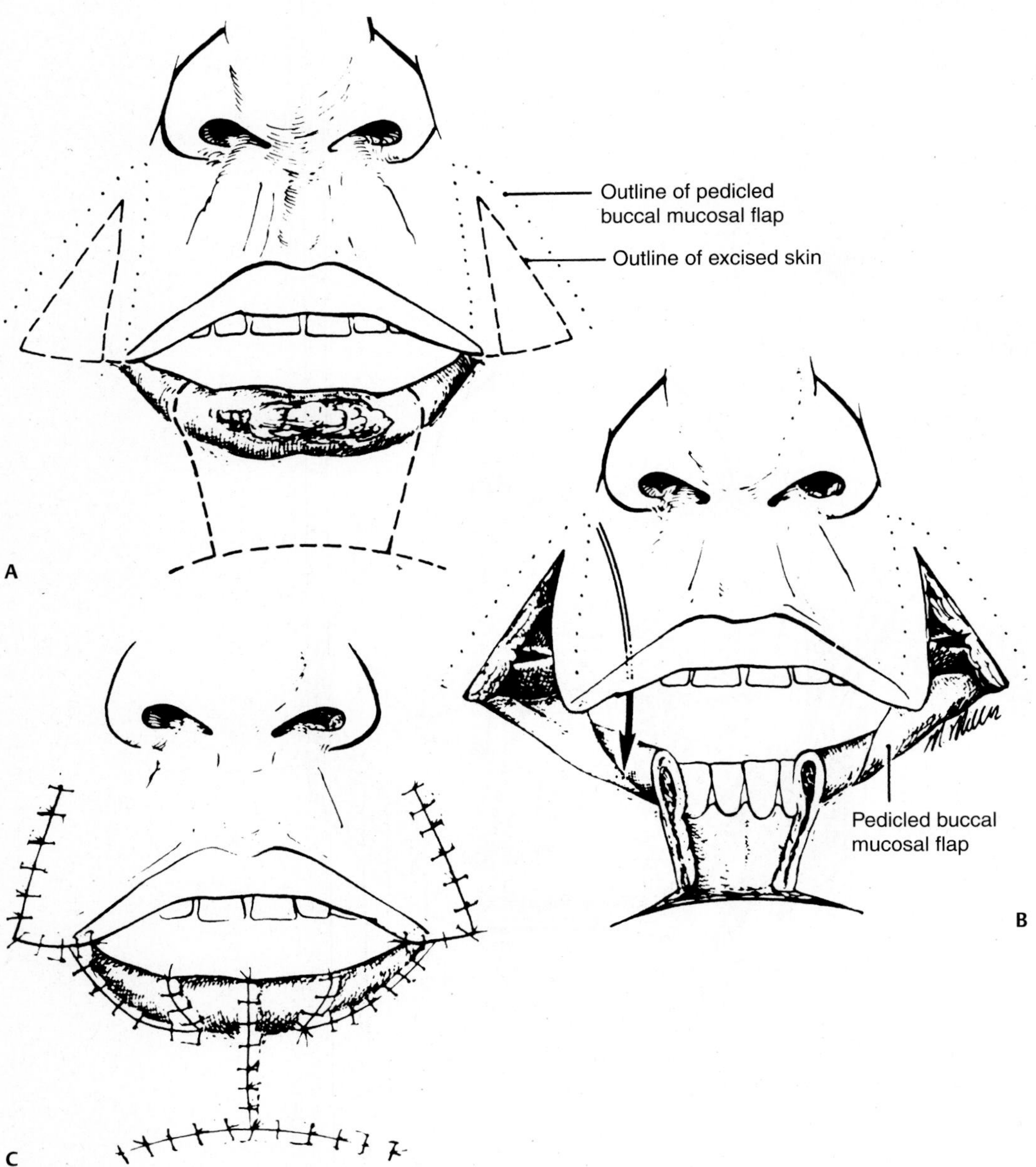

Fig. 61.10 Bernard-Burow flap technique.

n **Fig. 61.11**. During the first stage of reconstruction, the ateral aspect of the lip is reconstructed using a modifi-cation of the Bernard-Burow flap. Incisions only through the mucosa are created in the gingival–buccal sulcus from the surgical defect posterior to the angle of the mandible. Next, a horizontally oriented parallel incision s made through the mucosa only from the oral com-missure posteriorly so that it is at least 1 cm from the opening of Stenson's duct. An inferiorly based mucosal flap is created at the anterior aspect of this incision o be used for creation of the lateral oral commissure n red lip. Finally, a Burow's triangle full-thickness skin flap is excised from the most lateral aspect, allowing advancement.

These surgical maneuvers allow mobilization of the cheek for recruitment in the lower lip reconstruction. At this time, a midline cross-flap is developed and rotated into the central aspect of this large central defect. A three-layered, full-thickness defect closure is now per-formed between the laterally advanced lower lip and the transposed central cross-lip flap. A new oral com-missure is created by rotation and inset of the mucosal flap. At 2 weeks, a delayed section of the cross-lip flap is performed (**Fig. 61.12**).

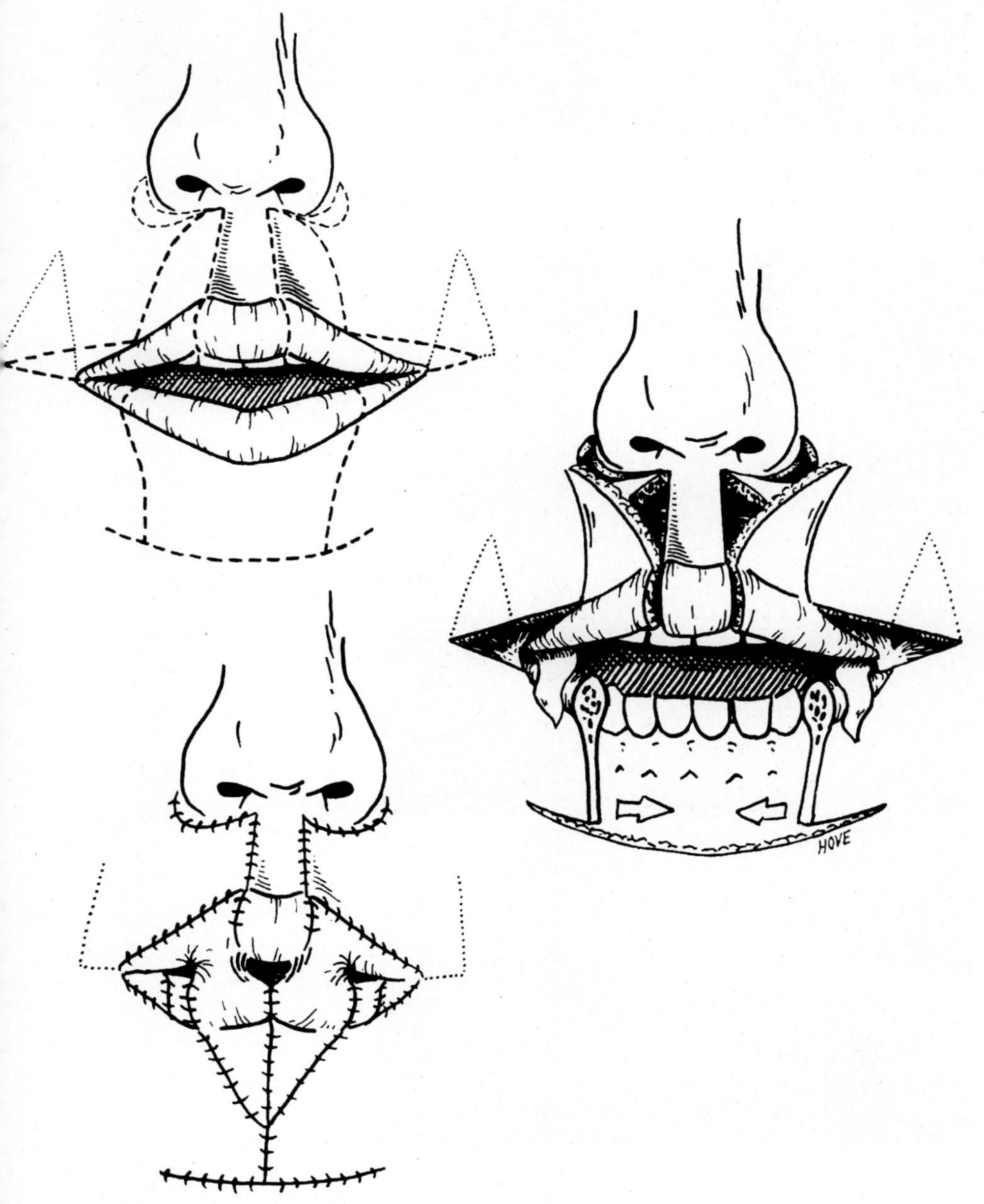

g. 61.11 Modified Bernard-Burow cheek advancement with simultaneous cross-lip flap.

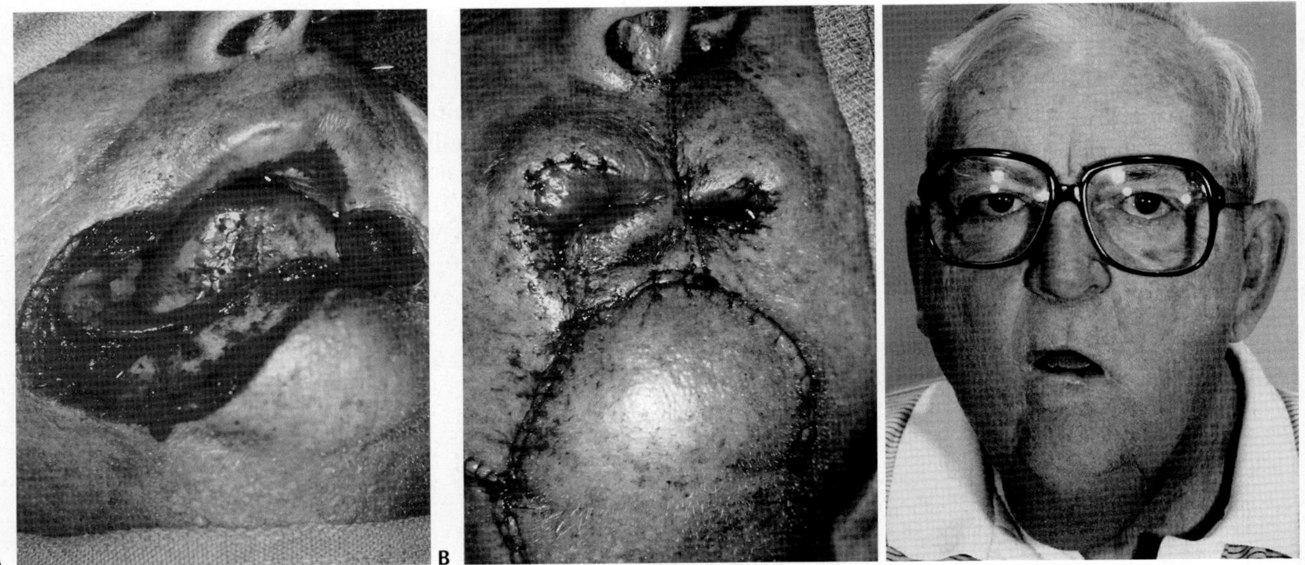

Fig. 61.12 Intraoperative (**A**), immediate postoperative (**B**), and 1-year (**C**) result of a surgical defect extending from left commissure to include entire lower lip, right oral commissure, and right cheek repaired with a modified Bernard-Burow cheek advancement with a simultaneous cross-lip flap.

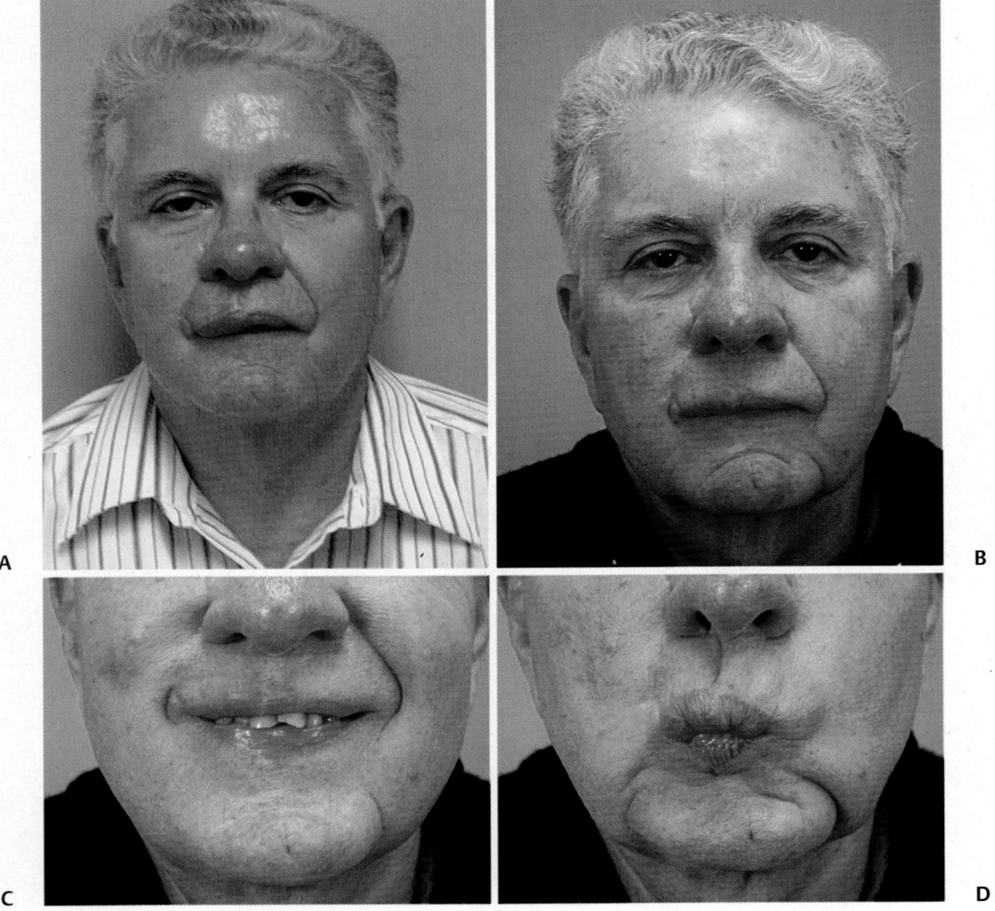

Fig. 61.13 This patient underwent lip reconstruction with right cross-lip and cheek advancement flaps. Three-month postoperative result (**A**), demonstrating significant upper lip edema. Twenty-three-month postoperative result (**B**) with vast improvement in edema as well as a good functional result (**C,D**).

Subtotal/Upper Lip Defects

Technique

For upper lip defects, the modified Bernard-Burow cheek advancement is performed in a similar fashion. In addition, it may be necessary to excise a perialar crescent of skin bilaterally. When used in conjunction with bilateral cheek advancement, the suture lines will be placed where the eye expects to see a shadow and will thus look more normal. In contrast to reconstruction of the lower lip, it is more important to emphasize and employ the subunit principle as previously described.

Microvascular Reconstruction

When the defect involves greater than 80% of the lower lip and cheek, the reconstruction is significantly more challenging. Not only does internal and external lining have to be replaced, but oral competence also has to be restored. Although one-stage reconstruction of these defects is possible with free flaps the functional result, such as maintaining oral competency is often lacking. It is important to note that this is one variable that does not come into play when reconstructing the upper lip with a free flap.

In 1989, Sakai used a composite radial forearm-palmaris longus flap for total lower lip reconstruction. The folded forearm skin provided both external and mucosal resurfacing, and both ends of the tendon were sutured to either cheek or modiolus to support the lip.[13] Although such a technique provides static suspension of the lower lip, it is not able to maintain adequate oral competence while the patients are speaking or eating.[14]

Hence, modifications of this reconstruction effort needed to focus on returning functionality to the lower lip. The first attempt to achieve this was undertaken by Shawney, where he sutured to the tendon to the transferred masseter muscle to achieve dynamic suspension of the lower lip.[15] In another attempt, Jeng passed both ends of the palmaris longus tendon intramuscularly through the bilateral modiolus at the angle of the mouth and anchored them to the remaining orbicularis muscle of the upper lip near the phitral columns in order to obtain dynamic function. This refinement allows the free flap to mimic the function of the horizontal fibers of the orbicularis oris, and hence, restore complete circumference of the oral sphincter.[16]

Recently, Cinar passed the free edges of the palmaris longus tendon through the modiolus bilaterally from the subcutaneous plan superficially to the malar eminence deeply while following the direction of the zygomaticus major muscle. This modification allowed the palmaris longus to be anchored to the proper point of the malar eminences while preserving the anatomic integrity of the modiolus. This malar-to-malar sling of the palmaris longus tendon was felt to add significant dynamic property to the reconstruction by transferring the force of the elevator muscles of the lips and even the orbicularis muscle of the upper lip to the tendon.[17]

Finally, the anterolateral thigh free flap with vascularized fascia has been recently introduced as a alternative to the radial forearm as a total reconstruction of the lower lip.[18] This flap is felt to have certain advantages over the radial forearm flap. These include less donor site morbidity since perforator vessels feed this flap versus the sacrifice of a major artery in the hand, no numbness which can be a significant morbidity with the radial forearm flap, and the donor-site scar is less conspicuous.

Postoperative Considerations

Postoperative edema is an unavoidable aspect of lip reconstruction that should be discussed with the patient prior to the procedure. Based on the authors' experience, the edema gradually resolves by between 12 and 18 months (**Fig. 61.13**). The patient should be counseled on performing oral exercise as much as possible in the postoperative period. These exercises help to reestablish neuronal connections and lymphatic channels that can improve the functional result and help decrease edema, respectively.

Asymmetry of the oral commissure or microstomia can result from surgical defects of the lips and present an aesthetic and functional dilemma.[19] Cross-lip flaps involving the commissure can result in blunting at the commissure. These problems can be addressed with a commissuroplasty, involving excision of a triangular piece of cutaneous skin at both commissures with mucosal advancement to the apex. Care must be taken to have precise alignment of the commissure at the appropriate level. This can be done as an office procedure under local anesthetic. Commissuroplasty is considered no sooner than 9 months after the lip reconstruction procedure.

References

1. Hessler F. Commentarii et Annotationes in Susrutae Ayurvedam Enlager. Enke 1855;12
2. Sabatini P. Cennestorico dell'origine e progressi della rhinoplastica e cheiloplastica. Bologna, Italy: Belle Arti; 838
3. Abbe RA. A new plastic operation for the relief of deformity due to double hairlip. Med Rec 1889;53:447
4. Estlander JA. Eine Methods ans der einen Lippe Substanzverluste der anderen zu ersetzen. Arch Klin Chir 1872;14:622
5. Gilles HD. Plastic Surgery of the Face. London: Hodder & Stoughton Ltd; 1920
6. Karapandzic M. Reconstruction of lip defects by local arterial flap. Br J Plast Surg 1974;27:93–97
7. Burget GC, Menick FJ. The subunit principle in nasal reconstruction. Plast Reconstr Surg 1985;76:239–247
8. Coppit GL, Lin DT, Burkey BB. Current concepts in lip reconstruction. Curr Opin Otolaryngol Head Neck Surg 2004;12:281–287
9. Bernard C. Cancer de la levre inferieure: resauration a laide de deux lambeaux gwaadrilatere. Querison Bull Mem Svc Chir Paris 1853;3:357

10. Burow CA. Beschreibung einer neunen Transplantations-Method (Method der seitlichen Dreiecke) zum Wiedersatz verlorengegangener Teile des Gesichts. Berlin: Nauck; 1855
11. Kroll SS. Staged sequential flap reconstruction for large lower-lip defects. Plast Reconstr Surg 1990;88:620–625
12. Williams EF, Setzen G, Mulraney MJ. Modified Bernard–Burow advancement and cross-lip flap for total lip reconstruction. Arch Otolaryngol Head Neck Surg 1996;122:1253–1258
13. Sakai S, Soeda S, Endo T, Ishii M, Uchiumi E. A compound radial artery forearm flap for the reconstruction of lip and chin defect. Br J Plast Surg 1989;42:337–338
14. Behmand RA, Rees RR. Reconstructive lip surgery. In: Coleman JJ, ed. Plastic Surgery Indications, Operations, and Outcomes. St. Louis: Mosby, Inc., 2000:1193–1210
15. Sawhney CP. Reanimation of lower lip reconstructed by flaps. Br J Plast Surg 1986;39:114–117
16. Jeng SF, Kuo YR, Wei FC, et al. Total lower lip reconstruction with a composite radial forearm-palmaris longus tendon flap: a clinical series. Plast Reconstr Surg 2004;113:19–23
17. Cinar C, Arslan H, Ogur S. Reconstruction of massive lower lip defect with the composite radial forearm-palmaris longus free flap: empowered static and partial dynamic reconstruction. J Craniofac Surg 2007;18: 237–241
18. Kuo Yr, Jeng SF, Wei FC, Su CY, Chien CY. Functional reconstruction of complex lip and cheek defect with free composite anterolateral thigh flap and vascularized fascia. Head Neck 2008;30:1001–1006
19. Gaylon SW, Frodel JL. Lip and perioral defects. Otolaryngol Clin North Am 2001;34(3):647–666

62 Periocular Reconstruction

Sara A. Kaltreider

Reconstruction of the periocular area is unique because of the specialized protective function of the periocular tissues in preserving vision. Specific functions of the eyelids include protection of the ocular surface from trauma, preservation of the tear film (which is crucial for clarity of vision), and tear excretion (which is dependent on the pumping action of the lids and the presence of an intact tear excretory apparatus). The principles of surgical reconstruction in the periocular area are generally the same whether the defect arises from excision of tumor, trauma, previous surgical procedures, or a pathological cicatrizing process.

The foremost goal of reconstruction is restoration of the three-dimensional anatomy of the eyelid as close to normal as possible. Attention to the microscopic anatomy and meticulous surgical technique are crucial to the success of the reconstruction. The details of the surgical anatomy are described and illustrated in other sources.[1–3] Areas deserving special attention during soft tissue reconstruction are the retractors of the eyelids, the lateral canthal tendon, the medial canthal tendon, the canalicular system, and the lacrimal sac. In addition to the complex microanatomy, the concavity of the medial canthal area presents particular challenges. Attention to postoperative care and splinting of the medial canthus after reconstruction will impact the outcome. As with reconstruction of any type, there is a potential need for secondary surgical revision.

Apposition of the eyelid conjunctiva to the ocular surface is important for a normal tear film and corneal clarity. If cicatricial forces disturb the delicate balance of the eyelid margin, then keratinized tissue and cilia may destroy the corneal epithelium and cause loss of vision. Therefore, reconstructive procedures must replace the anterior lamella of the eyelid with skin and the posterior lamella with mucous membrane while maintaining horizontal muscle tone, preserving the tear excretory microanatomy, and allowing the lids to open and close completely. The soft tissue reconstructive techniques described herein depend on the location, depth, and extent of the defect, and the potential sources for any tissue that may be missing or insufficient. Salient references are important for those who plan to become adept at eyelid reconstruction as details of each and every technique cannot be reproduced in a single chapter.

Anterior Lamellar Defects

Anterior lamellar defects involving skin or skin and the underlying orbicularis oculi muscle may be repaired using several techniques. Small defects may be left to granulate spontaneously, but judgment and experience must dictate those defects at risk for distorting the eyelid position or causing lagophthalmos.[4] Even large defects (>15 mm) in the medial canthal area may be allowed to heal by secondary intention as seen in **Fig. 62.1**.

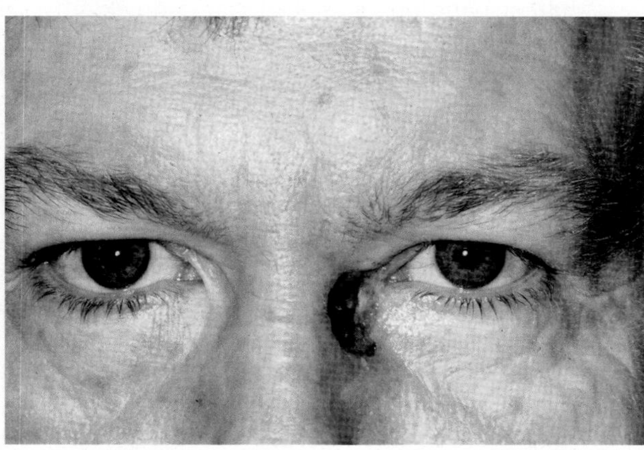

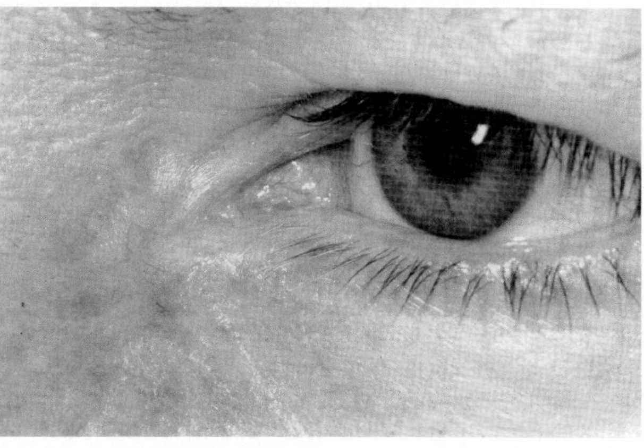

Fig. 62.1 This patient underwent Mohs excision of a basal cell carcinoma of the left medial canthus. The defect did not involve the canalicular system and was centered over the medial canthal area (**A**). Two months after excision and healing by granulation, the area is well covered, with no distraction of the eyelids from the ocular surface (**B**).

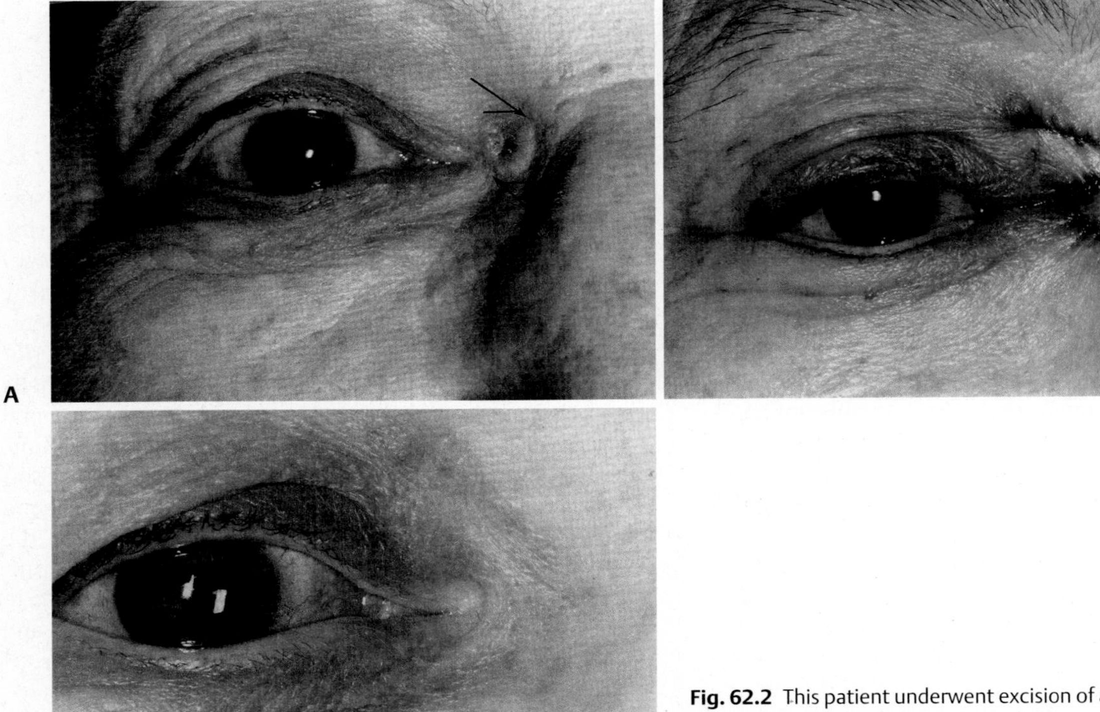

Fig. 62.2 This patient underwent excision of a basal cell carcinoma of the medial canthal area (**A**). The defect was reconstructed using an O- to Z-plasty, with mobilization of the flaps from the horizontal direction (**B**). No distortion of the medial canthal angle or web formation occurred (**C**).

The advantages of healing by secondary intention are preservation of tissue relationships and expediency for patients who may not wish to have additional surgery to cover the defect. Disadvantages are the presence of an open wound with serosanguinous discharge and crusting until epithelialization occurs, and the potential for ectropion and tearing if scarring distracts the eyelid margin from the ocular surface.

Alternatively, direct closure or local flaps such as an O- to Z-plasty, rotational flap, transpositional flap, rectangular advancement flap, V to Y advancement flap, Y to V advancement flap, or rhomboid flap may be used.[5,6] **Figure 62.2** demonstrates a nodular basal cell carcinoma that was removed and the defect closed using an O- to Z-plasty. The Z-plasty flaps are mobilized from the lateral and medial direction to avoid webbing in the medial canthus. Likewise, closure of defects in the upper or lower eyelid must be carefully planned to avoid vertical shortening of the eyelids and consequent lagophthalmos.

Myocutaneous flaps consisting of skin and orbicularis muscle may be transposed from the upper eyelid, where an excess of skin may be found in some patients, to a lower eyelid anterior lamellar defect. The lower incision of the flap is placed in the eyelid crease, and the upper incision is placed 10 to 12 mm below the brow cilia. The flap is carefully dissected to avoid damage to the underlying levator aponeurosis. The base of the pedicle is left intact medially or laterally. This procedure may produce some asymmetry of the upper lid fold with less redundancy on the side of the reconstruction, but it provides skin of matching color and texture. **Figure 62.3** shows a patient whose defect was repaired with a transpositional flap from the upper eyelid to the lower eyelid.

Multiple noncontiguous defects are closed with a variety of flaps. Often the bridging tissue is useful in forming one of the flaps, as in the patients shown in **Figs. 62.4 and 62.5**. The patient in **Fig. 62.4** has basal cell nevus syndrome and underwent Mohs excision of three defects in the temple area.

The bridge of tissue between the upper two defects was severed just above the brow cilia, and the tissue was advanced and lifted upward into the defect above the brow. The projection of tissue adjacent to the lower eyelid was lifted upward and laterally, and the cheek tissue was mobilized by pulling the skin edges together from the horizontal direction to create a vertical closure.

The patient in **Fig. 62.5** has two defects: one on the nose and one in the left medial canthus. The bridge of tissue was severed laterally and rotated clockwise into the lower defect. The longest line of closure was deliberately placed along the side of the nose rather than on

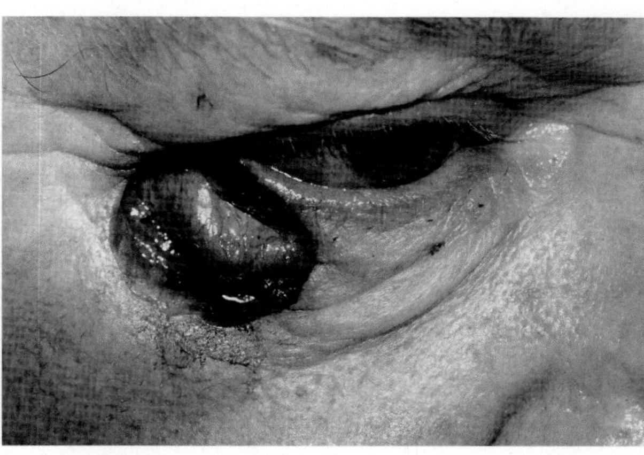

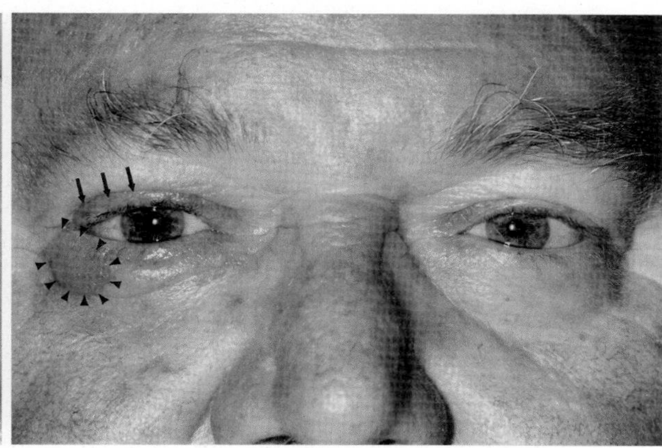

A B

Fig. 62.3 This patient underwent Mohs excision of a basal cell carcinoma in the lateral canthal area and lower eyelid (**A**). Reconstruction consisted of transposing a myocutaneous flap from the upper eyelid to the defect (**B**). The lower edge of the flap was placed in the eyelid crease, and the upper incision was placed 10 to 12 mm below the brow cilia. The flap was transposed, sutured into position, and splinted with a dressing. A postoperative photograph at 1 month shows good eyelid contour and symmetry (**B**). The arrowheads show the extent of the transposition flap, and the arrows show the closed donor site well hidden in the eyelid crease.

the dorsum. The remaining defect in the medial canthus was covered with a small flap from the redundant upper eyelid skin.

Large anterior lamellar defects may require repair with full-thickness skin grafts from the retroauricular area. Skin grafts from the neck and below have a sallow appearance when grafted to the eyelids, whereas retroauricular skin has a pink hue matching that of the eyelids.[7] Although split-thickness grafts may also be used, rarely does the deficiency of eyelid skin require a large enough surface area to warrant split-thickness grafting. **Figure 62.6** shows a defect too large to be repaired with local flaps alone. The area above the medial canthal tendon was covered with a flap from the upper eyelid, and the large defect in the lower eyelid and medial canthus was covered with a full-thickness skin graft from the retroauricular area. The component of the defect over the bridge of the nose was closed with adjacent skin, undermined, and closed in a horizontal fashion.

Posterior Lamellar Defects

Posterior lamellar defects are usually accompanied by anterior lamellar defects unless a cicatrizing conjunctival process is present. Those defects that are purely posterior

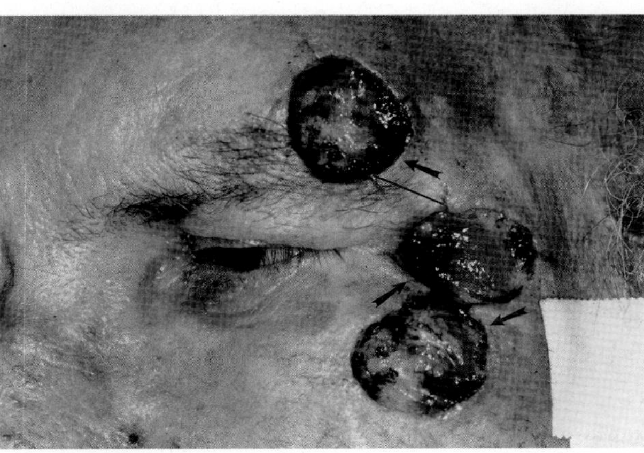

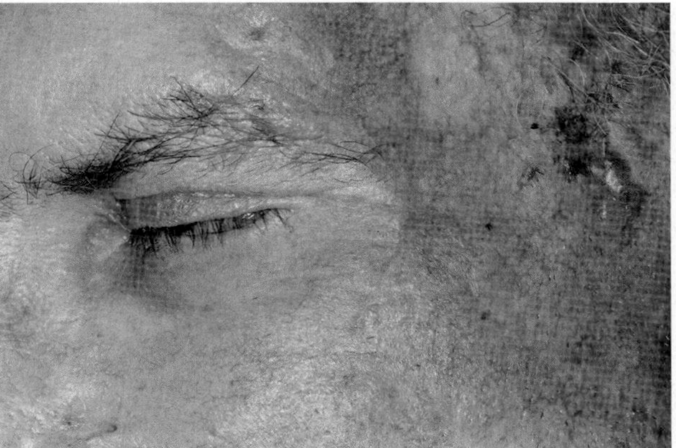

A B

Fig. 62.4 This patient with basal cell nevus syndrome had a bridge of tissue between the upper and middle skin defects that was severed (*line*) and mobilized (*arrows*) into the upper defect (**A**). The lower skin defects were repaired by undermining and advancing the adjacent tissue (*arrows*). Two months postoperatively, the area is well healed (**B**).

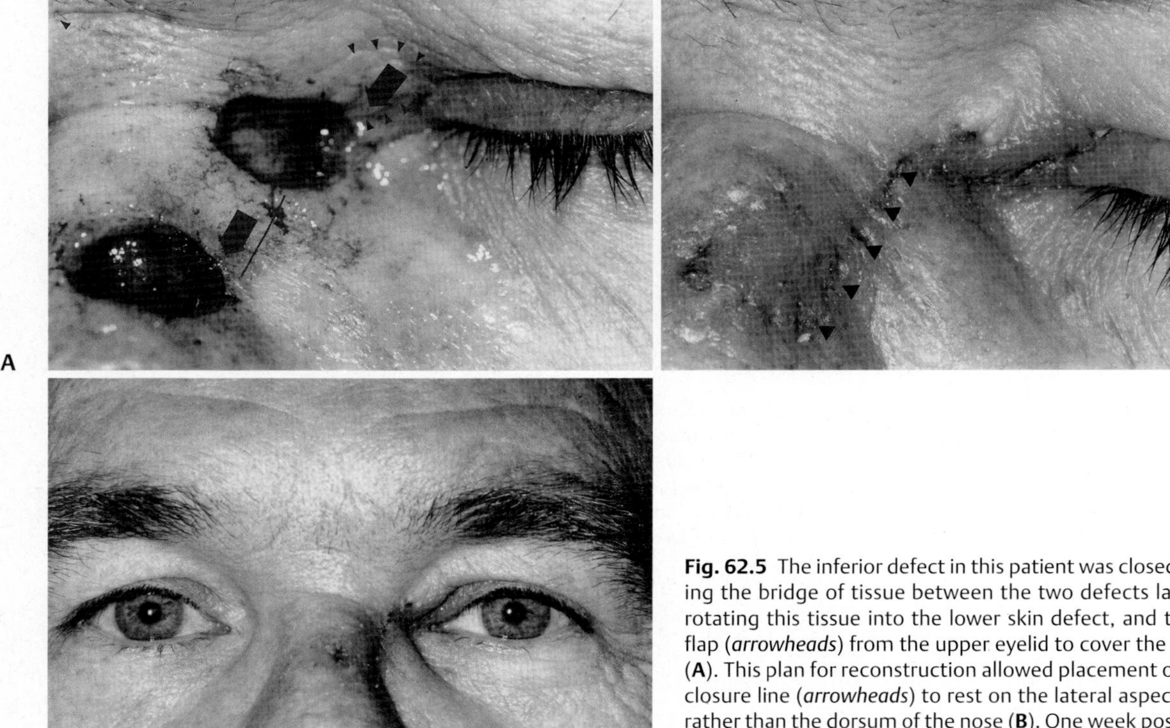

Fig. 62.5 The inferior defect in this patient was closed by transecting the bridge of tissue between the two defects laterally (*line*), rotating this tissue into the lower skin defect, and transposing a flap (*arrowheads*) from the upper eyelid to cover the upper defect (**A**). This plan for reconstruction allowed placement of the longest closure line (*arrowheads*) to rest on the lateral aspect of the nose rather than the dorsum of the nose (**B**). One week postoperatively, the contour of the reconstructed area is smooth and the eyelids and medial canthal angle are in a good position (**C**).

in nature and extensive require mucous membrane grafting from the buccal mucosa, lip mucosa, tarsoconjunctival graft, or hard palate.[7–10] Cicatricial entropion, which is caused by deficiency or scarring of the conjunctiva, may be repaired by the Wies procedure or a variation of an eyelid-splitting procedure. The Wies procedure is a transverse blepharotomy and rotation of the eyelid margin outward.[11] A bipedicle tarsoconjunctival flap, with or without mucous membrane grafting, is another means of rotating the eyelid margin outward.[12] The latter procedure is particularly useful in anophthalmic patients and when combined with a mucous membrane graft addresses the

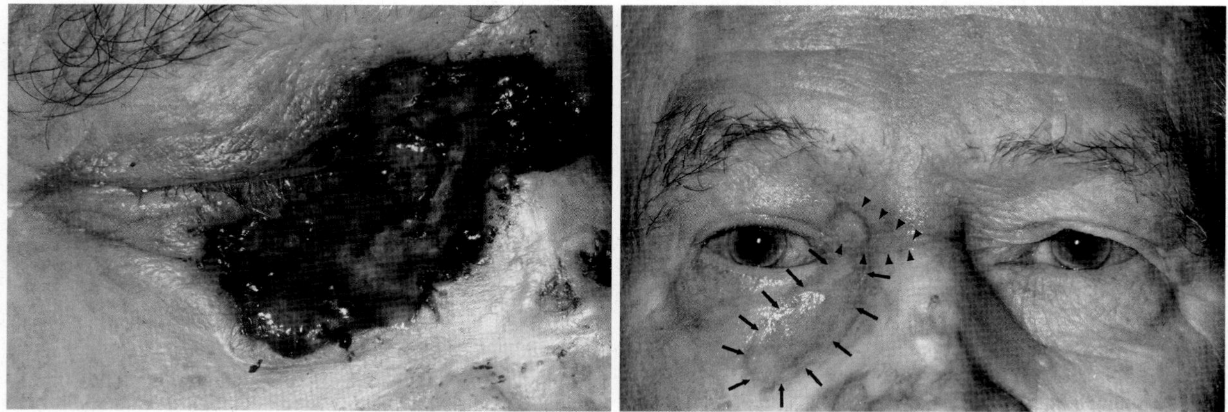

Fig. 62.6 This defect (**A**), too large to be covered by flaps alone, was reconstructed using a transposition flap from the upper eyelid to the upper part of the defect (*arrowheads*, **B**) and a full-thickness skin graft from the retroauricular area to the lower eyelid defect (*arrows*). Postoperatively, the eyelids are in an excellent position, and the skin graft matches the color of the lower eyelid nicely.

issue of the eyelid margin position and the deficiency of surface area of the socket.

Full-Thickness Defects

Some full-thickness defects may be closed primarily depending on the size, age of patient, and degree of horizontal laxity of the eyelid. Precise three-dimensional alignment of the lid margin is crucial to the health of the eye. Silk sutures (5–0) are placed in the gray line and lash line and then draped away from the ocular surface (**Fig. 62.7**). A third silk suture may be placed in the mucocutaneous junction if needed. The lid margin tissue is everted with a vertical mattress suture in the gray line, so that as healing takes place the eyelid margin will become smooth and flat rather than contracting into a notched contour. The eyelid margin sutures should be left in place for 10 to 14 days because earlier removal may lead to dehiscence, eyelid notching, and trichiasis.[13] Absorbable sutures (polyglactin, 6–0) are placed in the tarsus and orbicularis. The skin is approximated with absorbable or nonabsorbable sutures.

Larger defects may require canthotomy, cantholysis, and a semicircular flap as described by Tenzel and Stewart.[14] The canthotomy is a straight, horizontal incision that splits the lateral canthal tendon down to the level of the periosteal insertion at Whitnall's tubercle. The cantholysis is performed across the lower crus of the tendon behind the skin. If a semicircular flap is anticipated, the skin incision is located entirely above the level of the lateral canthal angle, and includes skin and orbicularis. This flap is rotated medially to form the new eyelid margin. The lateral edge of the conjunctiva may be sutured to the edge of the semicircular flap with 6–0 plain running suture. The remaining healthy eyelid margin, now mobilized,

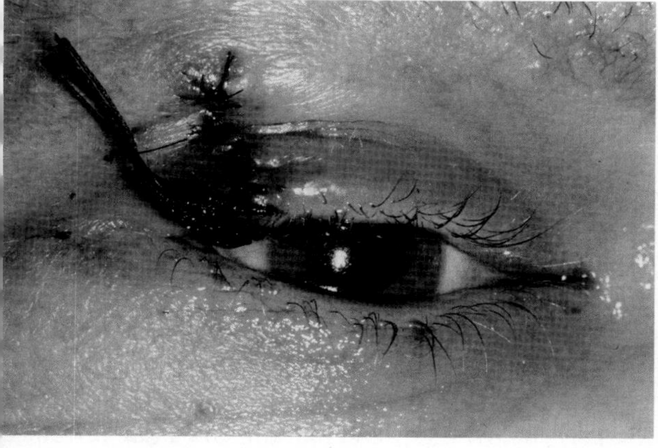

Fig. 62.7 This figure shows a lid margin closure with silk sutures in the lid margin. Eversion of the eyelid margin is enhanced by a vertical mattress suture in the gray line.

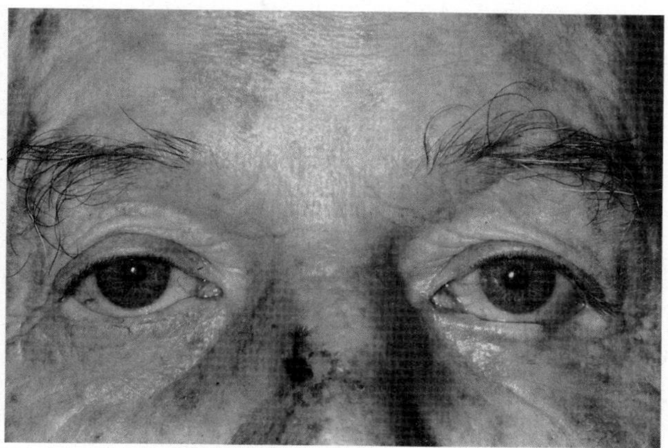

Fig. 62.8 This patient has had resection of multiple skin carcinomas of the left face, left ear, and left medial lower eyelid. He also has a history of radiation to the left temple and ear. Therefore, a vascularized rotational flap was used for reconstruction of the medial defect (Tenzel semicircular flap). One can see the abnormal contour and the retraction of the lateral left lower lid. Despite these residual eyelid abnormalities, the patient's eyelids are functional and he has no lagophthalmos.

may be sutured to the medial eyelid as described previously if the medial edge is lateral to the punctum and residual tarsus is present medially. If the medial edge of the remaining eyelid tissue is medial to the punctum, the closure is accomplished with subcutaneous 5–0 absorbable (polyglactin) skin sutures. In the latter case, the canaliculus may be preserved if it is in close proximity to the tear film. Silicone intubation is also a consideration. A common complication of the Tenzel semicircular flap is retraction of the reconstructed lateral eyelid margin, as seen in the patient in **Fig. 62.8**.

Composite grafts may also be used to fill moderate-sized defects that are too large to be reconstructed by direct closure or the Tenzel procedure.[15,16] A full-thickness block of tissue is taken from the opposite eyelid; the orbicularis and skin are removed up to the subciliary area and sutured to the defect (**Fig. 62.9**). Minimal cautery is used, so that damage to the lash follicles is avoided and a healthy vascular supply to the grafted eyelid is maintained. Lash survival is often disappointing, but an excellent lid contour may be achieved in a one-stage procedure. Double composite grafts, and a combined composite graft and temporal semicircular flap are other possibilities for the treatment of large defects.[17,18]

A variety of techniques may be used for reconstruction of large or total full-thickness defects. Procedures are lid sharing or non–lid sharing, one-stage or two-stage. Visual function should be taken into account when selecting the technique. For example, a one-stage procedure (which does not require closure of the eyelids for an extended period) should be used for reconstruction of an eyelid in a monocular or amblyopic patient (if the reconstruction is ipsilateral to the good eye).

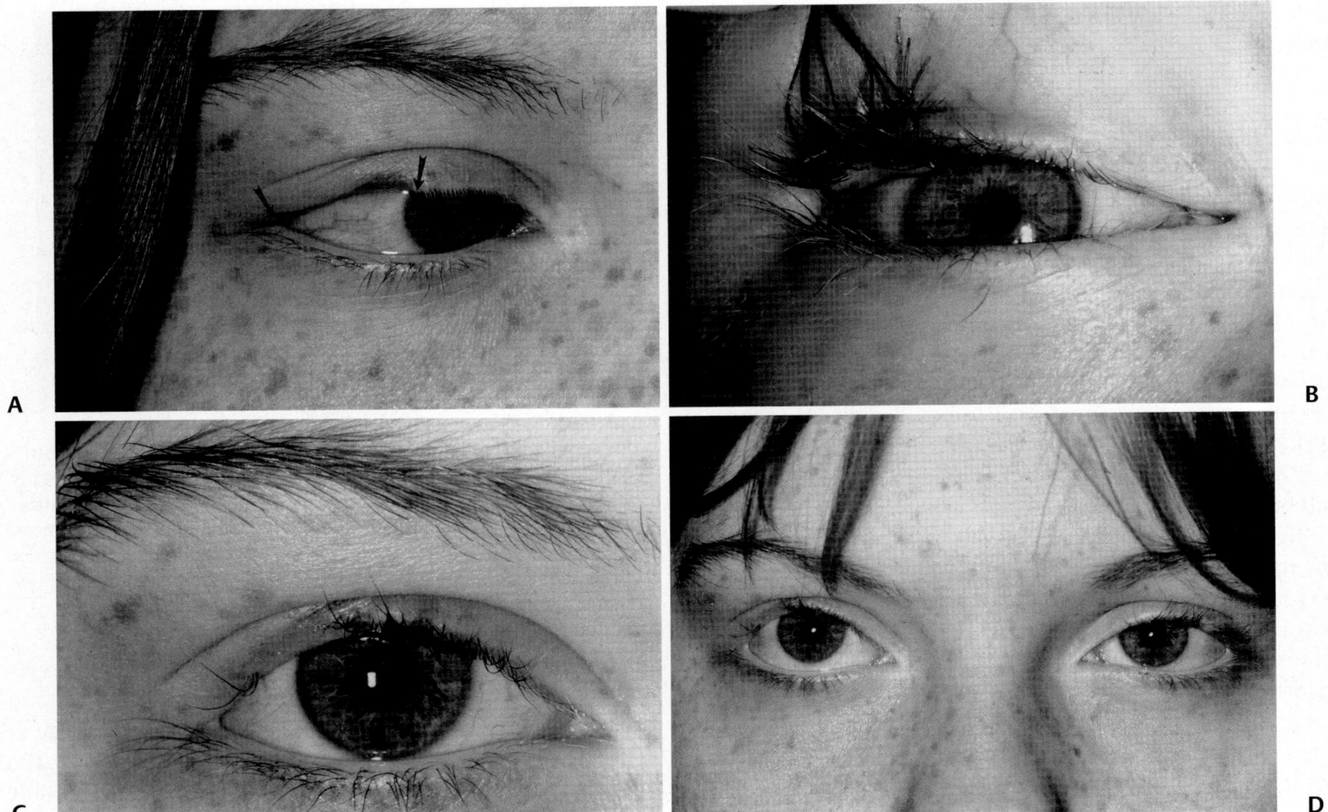

Fig. 62.9 This young patient lost the lateral half of the right upper eyelid margin in an automobile accident (**A**, *arrows* show extent of eyelid margin defect). A full-thickness composite graft was retrieved from the left upper eyelid and placed in the defect in the right upper eyelid (**B**). No cautery was used intraoperatively, and a flap of vascularized orbicularis was placed over the composite graft near the level of the lash follicles. The contour of the eyelid margin is restored, but only a few of the lashes within the composite graft survived (**C,D**).

The Hughes procedure is a superb two-stage reconstructive technique for treatment of total full-thickness lower eyelid defects and consists of a tarsoconjunctival flap with an overlying full-thickness skin graft or myocutaneous flap (**Fig. 62.10**).[19] The second stage takes place 3 to 6 weeks later to allow contraction to run its course, thereby minimizing the retraction of the newly constructed eyelid. Intraoperatively, the lower eyelid level is adjusted ~1 mm higher than the desired height to allow for additional contraction. This technique, carefully performed, is less likely than some other techniques to produce lagophthalmos or retraction, and it may be used for reconstruction of the upper or the lower eyelid. Complications include ptosis, retraction of the donor eyelid, lagophthalmos and retraction of the reconstructed eyelid, eyelid margin instability, necrosis of the donor eyelid, eyelid notching, and medial or lateral canthal deformity.[20]

A one-stage technique described by Leone and Van Gemert allows replacement of lower eyelid anterior and posterior lamellae with a pedicle tarsoconjunctival flap covered by a myocutaneous flap.[21] Both transposition flaps are based laterally.

A technique for total upper eyelid reconstruction analogous to the Hughes procedure for the lower eyelid is the Leone procedure.[22] This is a two-stage, lid sharing technique in which a tarsoconjunctival flap is mobilized from the lower eyelid into the upper eyelid defect. The lower edge of the tarsus will be the new upper eyelid margin once the flap is severed. A full-thickness skin graft is placed over the tarsoconjunctival flap, and the flap is separated after 4 weeks.

The Cutler–Beard technique is an eyelid sharing procedure in which a full-thickness flap from the lower eyelid is inserted into the upper eyelid defect.[23] A transverse horizontal blepharotomy incision is made several millimeters below the eyelid margin, and a full-thickness flap is brought upward behind the bridge of lower eyelid margin and sutured to the defect in the upper lid. The flap is severed 3 or more weeks later. Complications

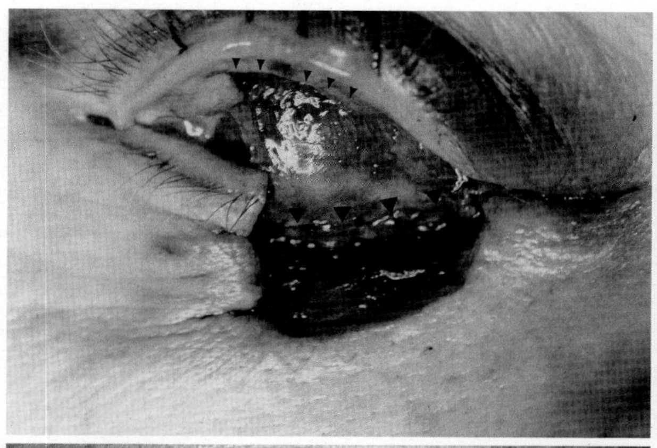

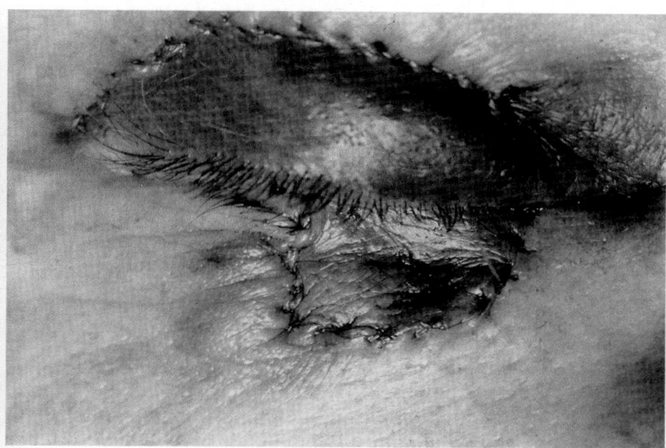

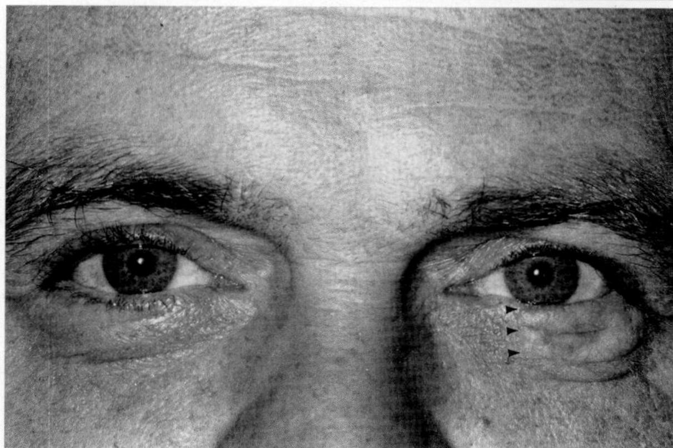

Fig. 62.10 Total or near-total eyelid defects may require a two-stage procedure, such as a Hughes procedure. A tarsoconjunctival flap is sutured to the remaining conjunctiva in the inferior fornix (*large arrowheads*) and the residual tarsus, tendon, or periosteum medially and laterally (**A**). The *small arrowheads* define the initial incision in the tarsus, 2 to 3 mm above the eyelid margin on the posterior surface of the eyelid. A myocutaneous flap or full-thickness skin graft from the retroauricular area or upper eyelid is sutured over the tarsoconjunctival flap (**B**). Three to 6 weeks later, the flap is detached from the posterior aspect of the upper eyelid. The upper and lower eyelids are adjusted intraoperatively to achieve good lid levels, contour, and symmetry, as seen in the patient in (**C**) who underwent left lower eyelid reconstruction. The reconstructed eyelid extends from the *arrowheads* medially to the lateral canthus.

include necrosis of the lower eyelid margin, retraction of the lower eyelid, retraction or ptosis of the upper eyelid, and decreased mobility of the upper eyelid.

Medial Canthal Defects

Specific anatomical considerations in the medial canthus are the lacrimal excretory apparatus, the complexity of the medial canthal tendon, soft tissue webbing, and deep defects requiring vascularized flaps. Certain techniques applicable to reconstruction involve the lacrimal excretory apparatus and the medial canthal tendon.

Careful examination of the defect will reveal whether or not the canalicular system is involved. If sufficient canalicular tissue remains, then microsurgical repair with silicone intubation is indicated (**Fig. 62.11**).[24,25] The silicone stent should remain in place for ~6 weeks. However, if only a tiny remnant of canaliculus remains, then the remaining tissue cannot be restored to a functional passageway from the tear film to the sac.

If both canalicular systems are absent, then a conjunctival dacryocystorhinostomy (DCR) with placement of a Jones tube is indicated, as seen in the patient in **Fig. 62.12**.[26] This glass tube serves as a permanent prosthetic device to drain tears from the medial canthal angle into the nasal cavity.

If the anterior crus of the medial canthal tendon is disrupted, it should be reattached to its normal location along the anterior lacrimal crest. If both anterior and posterior projections of the medial canthal tendon are disrupted, as in nasoethmoidal fractures, then unilateral or transnasal wiring is indicated.[27,28] The patient shown in **Fig. 62.13** has traumatic telecanthus and epiphora following a gunshot injury directly over the nasal bridge. Bilateral DCR and transnasal wiring were performed. The transnasal wiring was done through the DCR incisions using an awl to pass the 28 gauge wire between the canthi. Unilateral wiring may be performed using a microdrill to create an attachment site just behind the anterior lacrimal crest.

Telecanthus and epiblepharon are effectively treated with Z-plasties, Y- to V-plasties, or Mustarde flaps.[29] The Mustarde flap consists of two Z-plasties and a Y- to V-plasty. The patient in **Fig. 62.14** is a Caucasian female with congenital epiblepharon repaired with Mustarde flaps. Alternatives for deep and extensive soft tissue defects in the medial canthal area include the glabellar flap and the midline forehead flap (**Fig. 62.15**).[30] These defects require thicker tissue with a vascular supply that is provided by the supratrochlear and supraorbital vascular supply.

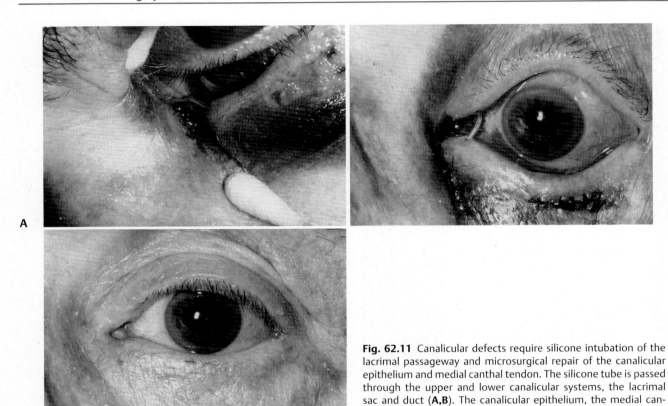

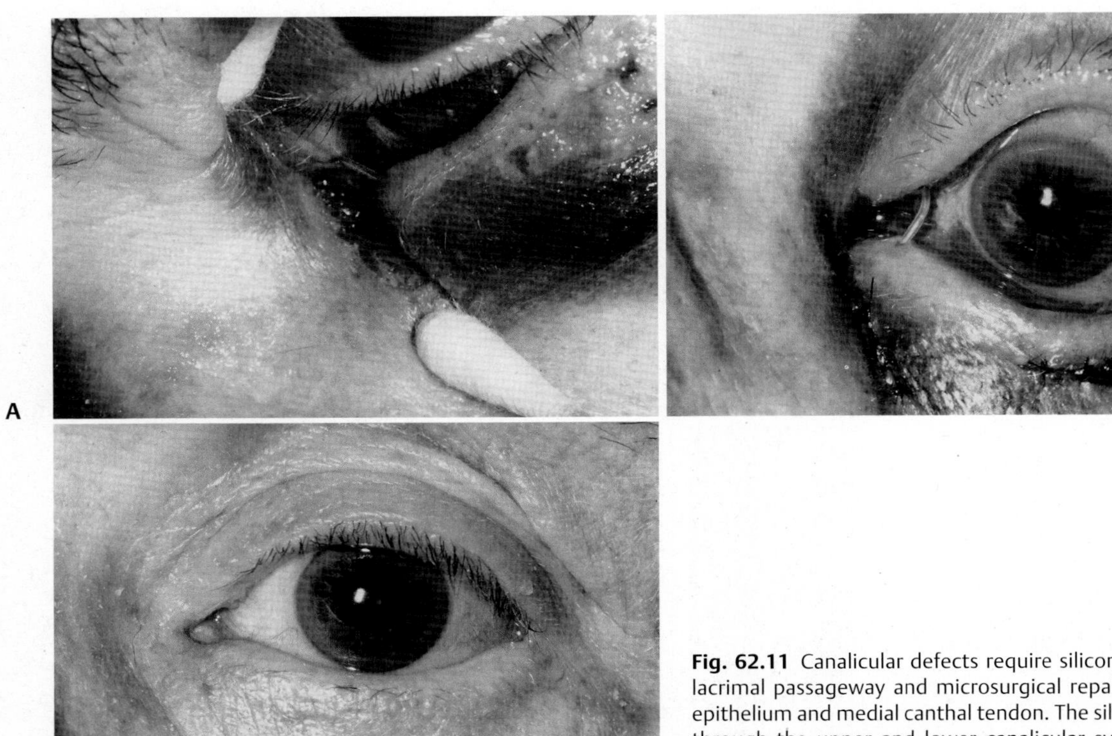

Fig. 62.11 Canalicular defects require silicone intubation of the lacrimal passageway and microsurgical repair of the canalicular epithelium and medial canthal tendon. The silicone tube is passed through the upper and lower canalicular systems, the lacrimal sac and duct (**A,B**). The canalicular epithelium, the medial canthal tendon, orbicularis, and skin are sutured. The silicone tube is removed after 6 weeks (**C**). The patient has no epiphora.

Complications include thickened flap, rounded medial canthal angle, and necrosis of the tip of the flap.

Lateral Canthal Defects

Anterior lamellar defects in the lateral canthal area are reconstructed with sliding, O to Z, rotation, transposition, or rhomboid flaps. Generally, redundancy of skin in this area and the lack of fixation of the tissues to the orbital rim allow mobilization of skin to cover small and moderate defects. The lateral canthal tendon attaches to Whitnall's tubercle, and this structure should be restored to its normal location if it has become disrupted. A periosteal strip or a tarsal strip may be used for reconstruction if the tendon is absent.[31,32]

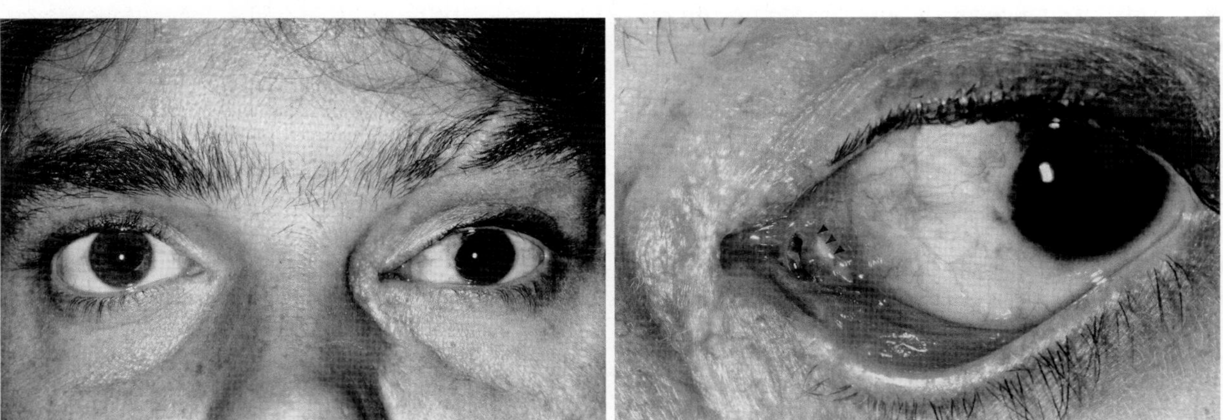

Fig. 62.12 The Jones tube, a Pyrex tube connecting the medial canthal angle to the nasal cavity, can be seen in this patient who sustained severe bicanalicular lacerations and ocular trauma (**A,B**). The *arrowheads* in (**B**) show the posterior edge of the flange of the tube.

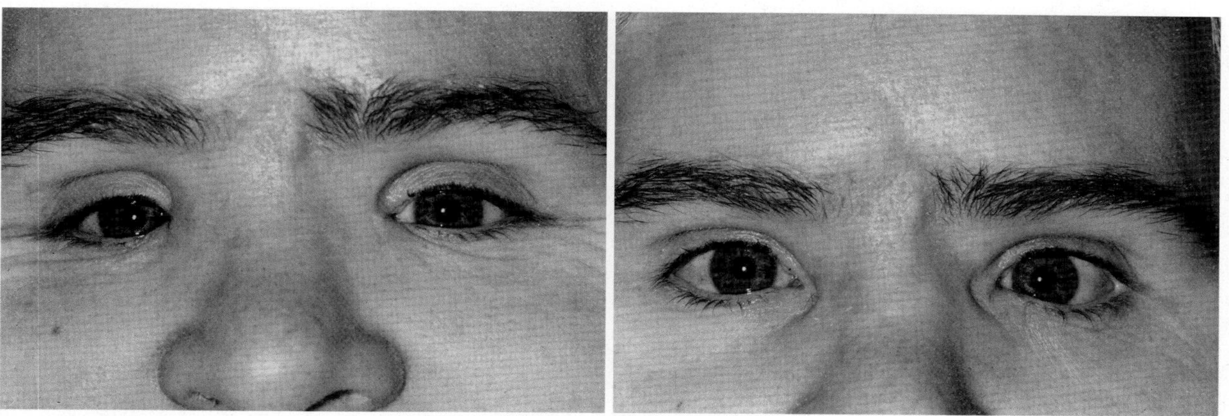

Fig. 62.13 Preoperative (A) and postoperative (B) photographs of a patient who underwent bilateral dacryocystorhinostomy and transnasal wiring following a gunshot wound. The intercanthal distance is diminished, and the patient's epiphora was resolved.

Eyelid shortening often prevents the complication of ectropion following reconstruction of the anterior lamella of the lower eyelid. A wedge of the eyelid margin and tarsus may be removed following canthotomy and cantholysis. The remaining tarsus may be sutured to the periosteum at Whitnall's tubercle using 5–0 polyglactin in the upper and lower tarsus to provide stability of the eyelid position. Alternatively, a periosteal

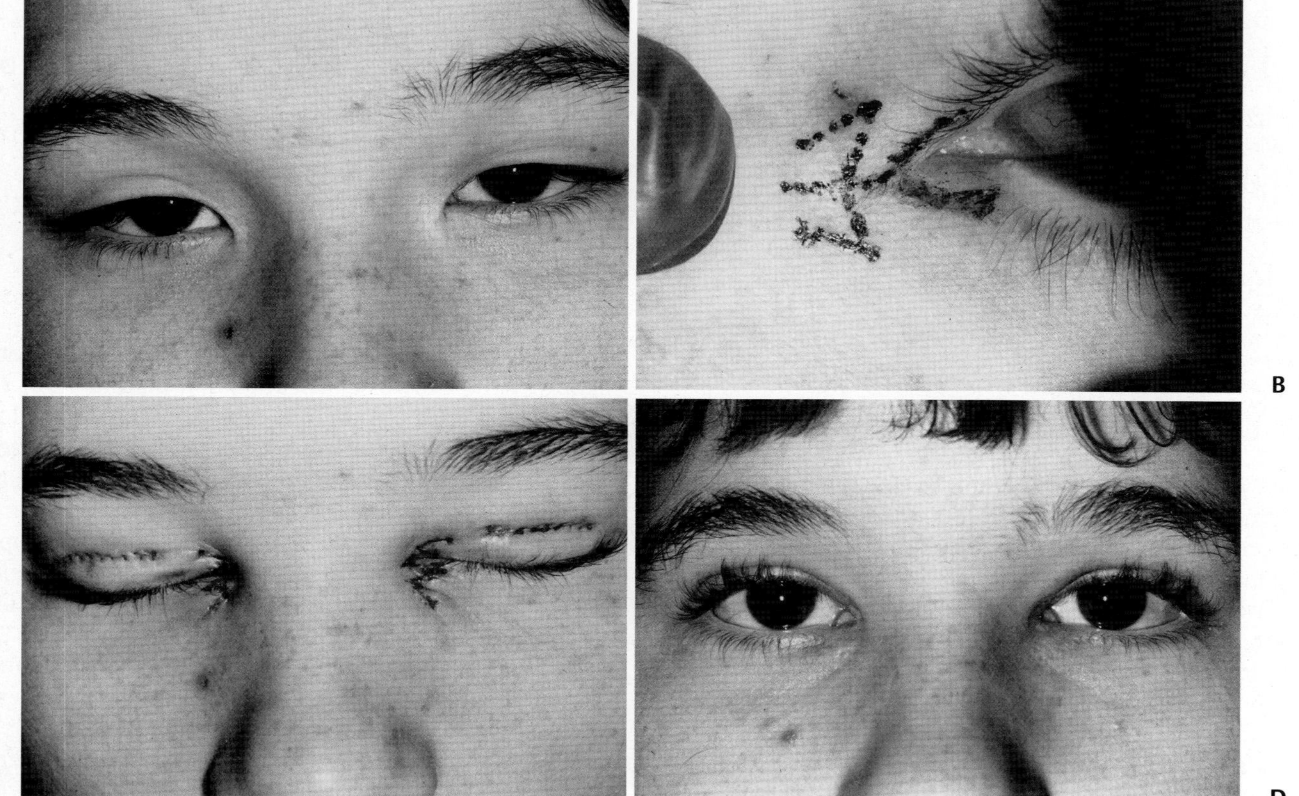

Fig. 62.14 This patient with congenital epiblepharon (A) underwent a Mustarde medial canthoplasty. Note the components of the canthoplasty include a Z-plasty in the upper and the lower eyelids, and a Y- to V-plasty to mobilize the medial canthal angle toward the nose (B). Fixation of an eyelid crease was performed by suturing the skin and orbicularis to the levator aponeurosis (intraoperative photograph, C). Postoperative appearance is seen in (D).

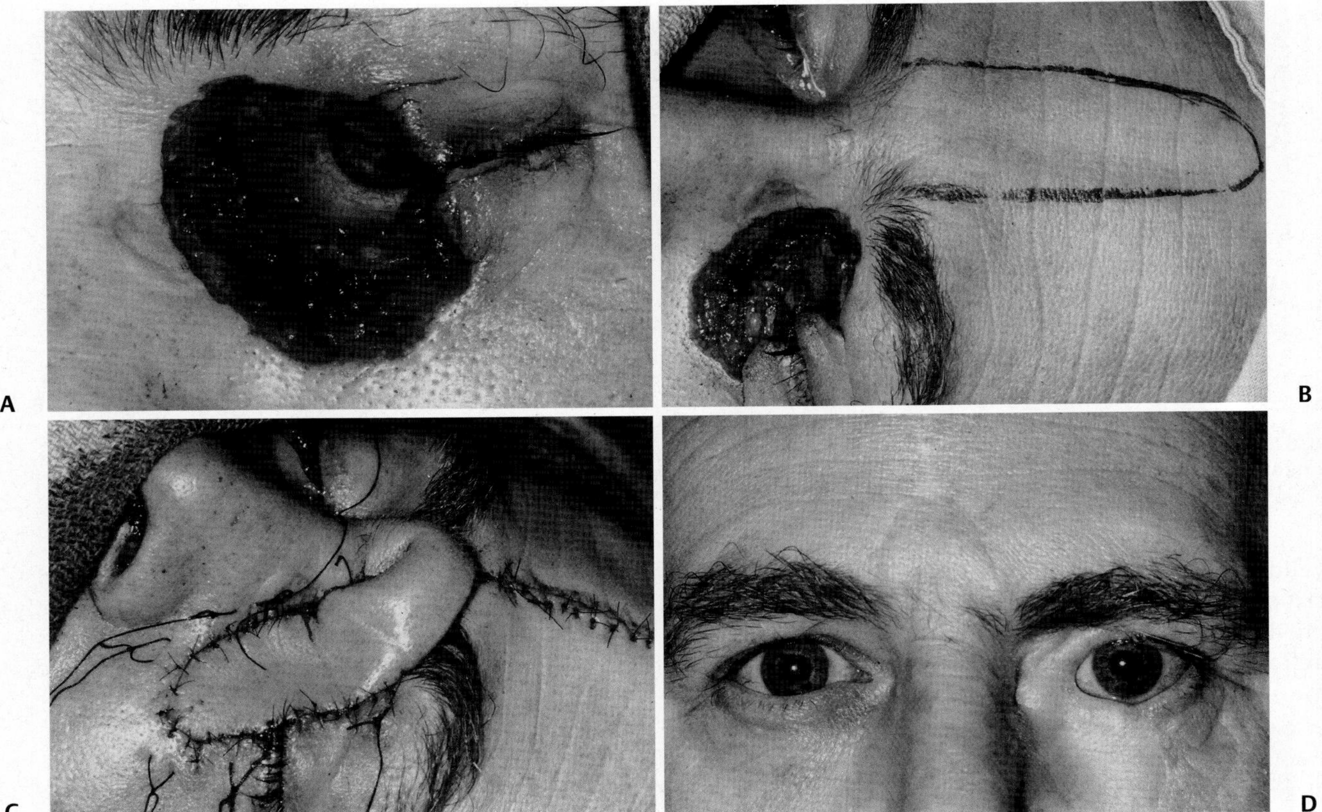

Fig. 62.15 This patient had an extensive and very deep defect following excision of a recurrent basal cell carcinoma (**A**). The defect involved the medial canthus, lacrimal excretory apparatus, medial half of the upper eyelid, and medial half of the lower eyelid. A sliding tarsoconjunctival flap and an overlying midline forehead flap were used to reconstruct the missing tissue (**B,C**). A Jones tube was placed beneath the medial canthal angle to drain the tears into the nose. Six months after the procedure, the patient has good eyelid function and no tearing (**D**).

or tarsal strip may be used following shortening of the eyelid.

Eyelid Retractors

The eyelid retractors, the levator in the upper eyelid and the capsulopalpebral fascia in the lower eyelid, must be restored to normal position at the time of reconstruction. The levator muscle inserts on the lower two thirds of the anterior surface of the tarsus. Absorbable or nonabsorbable sutures may be used for reattachment. Careful attention to eyelid contour, level, and symmetry will prevent complications postoperatively. Likewise, the capsulopalpebral fascia in the lower eyelid attaches to the inferior border of the tarsus, and this anatomy should be maintained for stability of the eyelid margin position. Inadvertent plication of the septum in the upper or the lower eyelid will cause retraction, tethering of the eyelid, and lagophthalmos. Therefore, one should avoid closure or tethering of this structure during reconstruction of the eyelids.

Anophthalmic Defects

The initial stage of reconstruction in anophthalmic patients begins at the time of enucleation and placement of the intraconal implant. Enophthalmos and superior sulcus deformity are the hallmarks of poor volume replacement and poor volume distribution in the socket. Adequate replacement of volume by the intraconal implant placed in the posterior compartment of the socket avoids enophthalmos and superior sulcus deformity in most cases.[3] Orbital bony asymmetry and socket contraction are factors that might limit optimal volume replacement. The balance of the volume deficit after enucleation and intraconal implant placement is provided by the prosthesis. The prosthesis is custom-fitted after the socket heals in ~4 to 6 weeks. Meticulous surgical technique at the time of enucleation provides a foundation for successful prosthetic fitting by the ocularist.

Enophthalmos and superior sulcus deformity are common findings in anophthalmic patients, and may be addressed by removing the intraconal implant and replacing

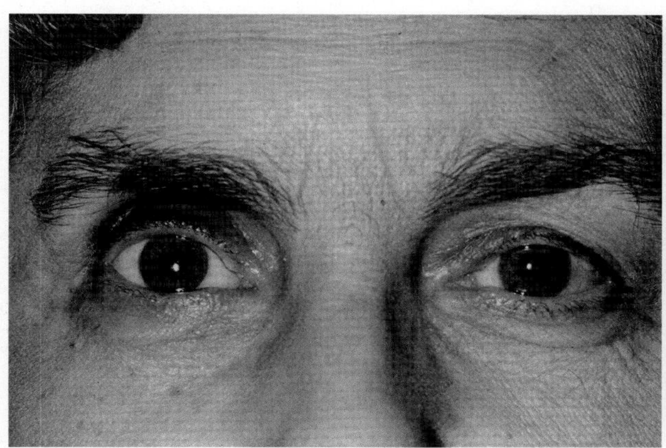
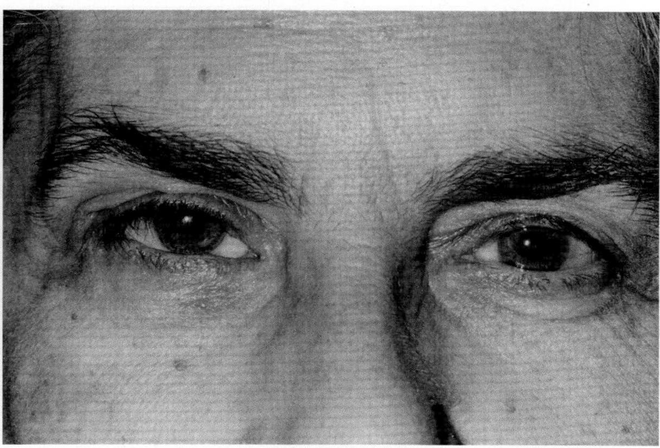

Fig. 62.16 This patient has severe enophthalmos and superior sulcus deformity (**A**). The superior sulcus deformity resolved following placement of a subperiosteal orbital floor implant through a transconjunctival approach (**B**).

it with a larger intraconal implant, or inserting a subperiosteal orbital floor implant. The former approach is extremely difficult if the primary implant is porous with fibrovascular ingrowth. Removal of porous implants risks damage to the extraocular muscles and their innervation. Subperiosteal implants for augmentation of volume should be placed far enough posteriorly that they effectively replace volume and at the same time do not cause shortening of the inferior fornix.[34–37] The anterior edge of the implant should rest behind the orbital rim. The patient in **Fig. 62.16** underwent subperiosteal implant placement by a transconjunctival approach.

Procedures that attempt to place material in the upper eyelid to fill the superior sulcus should be avoided because of risk of tethering the levator muscle and impairing upper eyelid function. A more conservative approach to achieve improved symmetry of the superior sulcus area is a blepharoplasty on the contralateral side.

Adequate surface area and good eyelid tone must be present for normal retention of the prosthesis and complete closure of the eyelids over the prosthesis. Lack of adequate surface area is generally manifested by cicatricial entropion, an early sign of socket contraction. Severe contraction precludes retention of the prosthesis in the anterior socket. Additional surface area is provided by mucous membrane grafting from the lip, buccal mucosa, or hard palate mucosa (**Fig. 62.17**).[38] One or both fornices may require reconstruction.

Dermal fat grafts provide both volume and surface area in selected cases, although control of volume replacement and motility is not as precise as other methods of volume replacement.[39] Keratinized epithelium should not be used as grafting material in the socket because of the presence of skin appendages that produce a malodorous discharge.

Optimal motility may be provided by porous implants, which may be integrated with the prosthesis if desired. Porous polyethylene and hydroxyapatite implants are available for patients whose priority is motility.[40,41] Implant exposure is a challenging problem associated with the porous implants, and results from anterior malposition of the implant, infection, or insufficiency of vascularized tissue over the anterior surface of the implant.[42] The advantages of these implants are a decreased risk of extrusion and migration, and the ability to integrate the implant and the prosthesis by way of a peg (**Fig. 62.18**).

Anophthalmic patients may develop entropion, ectropion, ptosis, and lid retraction. These problems are generally addressed in the same fashion as in ophthalmic patients, except for ptosis repair. Ptosis repair by a conjunctival approach should be avoided because of the risk of losing surface area and instigating socket contraction. An anterior approach to the levator should be used; a frontalis sling will suffice when no levator function exists.

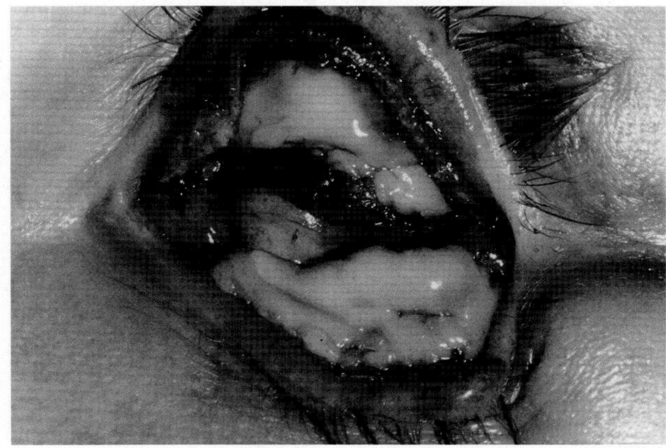

Fig. 62.17 Socket contraction is treated with mucous membrane grafting (buccal mucous membrane or hard palate mucosa) in one or both fornices. Entropion and lagophthalmos generally resolve after augmenting the surface area of the socket.

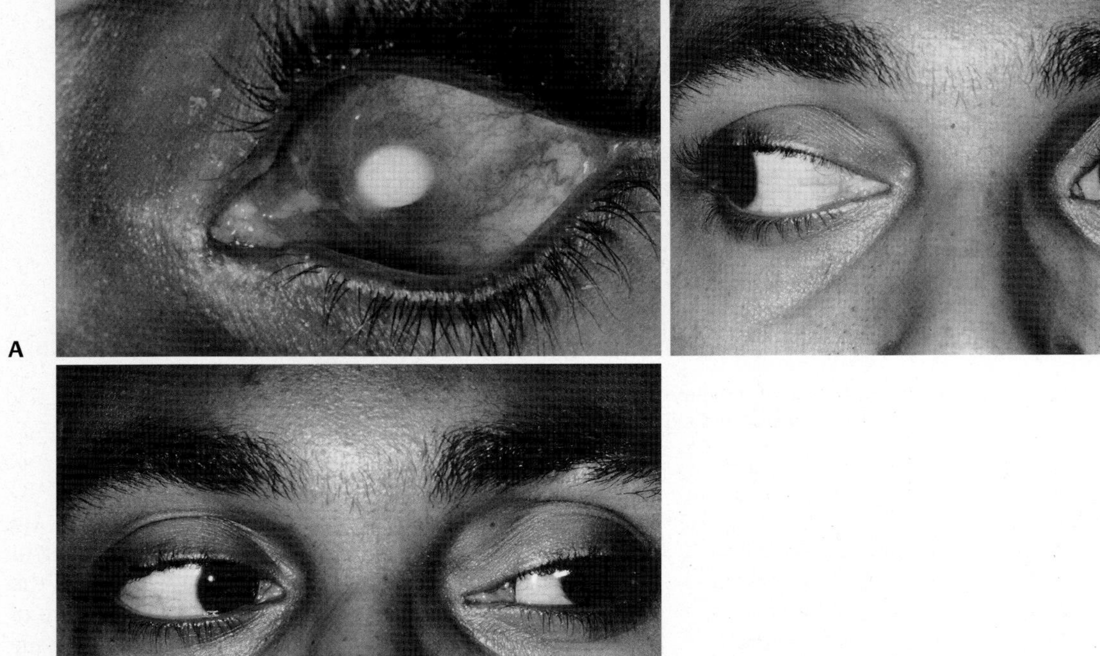

Fig. 62.18 A motility peg is seen in the left socket of this patient who underwent enucleation and placement of a hydroxyapatite implant (**A**). The peg transmits motility from the implant to the prosthesis (**B,C**).

Cosmetic optics provide noninvasive means of disguising the stigmata of anophthalmos.[43] Plus lenses augment and minus lenses minimize the image of the prosthesis. Plus cylinder lenses augment the image in the direction 90 degrees from the axis of the lens. Tint in the upper lens hides the superior sulcus deformity. Most importantly, all anophthalmic patients should wear protective glasses at all times while awake to protect the functioning eye. Anophthalmic patients should be examined thoroughly by an ophthalmologist at least once a year.

The optimal prosthesis is made by the modified-impression technique.[44] An alginate cast of the patient's socket is made with an impression tray. The prosthesis is made of polymethylmethacrylate in a reverse mold of the alginate cast. An iris disk custom-painted by the ocularist to match the appearance of the normal eye is embedded in the plastic. The prosthesis is modified as necessary to alter the position of the eyelids and to augment volume. Maintenance by cleaning and buffing at 6- to 12-month intervals is important for the health of the eye socket. The patient may leave the prosthesis in place for months unless mucous buildup occurs, whereupon more frequent removal and periodic cleaning may be necessary. Many patients experience giant papillary conjunctivitis related to prosthetic wear. Treatment with a mast cell inhibator ophthalmic solution and an ophthalmic steroid ointment usually eliminates the symptoms of chronic discharge and irritation.[45] Patients often require ophthalmic lubricant drops and ointment on a long-term basis for comfort.

References

1. Lemke BN, Della Rocca RC. Surgery of the Eyelids and Orbit: An Anatomical Approach. Norwalk, CT: Appleton & Lange; 1990
2. Kikkawa DO, Lemke BN. Orbital and eyelid anatomy. In: Dortzbach RK, ed. Ophthalmic Plastic Surgery: Prevention and Management of Complications. New York: Raven Press; 1994:1–29
3. Zide BM, Jelks GW. Surgical Anatomy of the Orbit. New York: Raven Press; 1985
4. Lowry JC, Bartley GB, Garrity JA, et al. The role of second-intention healing in periocular reconstruction. Ophthal Plast Reconstr Surg 1997;13:174
5. Patrinely JR, Marines HM, Anderson RL. Skin flaps in periorbital reconstruction. Surv Ophthalmol 1987;31(4):249
6. Shotton FT. Optimal closure of medial canthal surgical defects with rhomboid flaps: "rules of thumb" for flap and rhomboid defect orientations. Ophthalmic Surg 1983;14(1):46
7. Callahan MA, Callahan A. Ophthalmic Plastic and Orbital Surgery. Burmingham, AL: Aesculapius; 1979:3–32
8. Smith B, Lisman R. Preparation of split thickness auricular cartilage for use in ophthalmic plastic surgery. Ophthalmic Surg 1982;13:1018
9. Bartley GB, Kay PP. Posterior lamellar eyelid reconstruction with a hard palate mucosal graft. Am J Ophthalmol 1989;107:609
10. Stephenson CM, Brown BZ. The use of tarsus as a free autogenous graft in eyelid surgery. Ophthal Plast Reconstr Surg 1985;1:43

11. Wies FA. Spastic entropion. Trans Am Acad Ophthalmol Otolaryngol 1955;59:503
12. Shorr N, Christenbury JD, Goldberg RA. Tarsoconjunctival grafts for upper eyelid cicatricial entropion. Ophthalmic Surg 1988;19:317
13. Kaltreider SA, Sherman DD, McGetrick JJ. Eyelid trauma. In: Dortzbach RK, ed. Ophthalmic Plastic Surgery: Prevention and Management of Complications. New York: Raven Press; 1994:157–173
14. Tenzel RR, Stewart WB. Eyelid reconstruction by the semicircular flap technique. Ophthalmology 1978;85:1164
15. Callahan A. Free composite eyelid graft. Arch Ophthalmol 1951;45:539
16. Werner MS, Olson JJ, Putterman AM. Composite grafting for eyelid reconstruction. Am J Ophthalmol 1993;116:11
17. Beyer-Machule CK, Shapiro A, Smith B. Double-composite lid reconstruction. Ophthal Plast Reconstr Surg 1985;1:97
18. Putterman AM. Combined viable composite graft and temporal semicircular skin flap procedure. Am J Ophthalmol 1984;98:349
19. Hughes WL. Reconstructive Surgery of the Eyelids. 2nd ed. St. Louis: CV Mosby; 1954
20. Stasior GO, Stasior OG. Eyelid and canthal reconstruction. In: Dortzbach RK, ed. Ophthalmic Plastic Surgery: Prevention and Management of Complications. New York: Raven Press; 1994:125–140
21. Leone CR, Van Gemert JV. Lower eyelid reconstruction with upper eyelid transpositional grafts. Ophthalmic Surg 1980;11(5):315
22. Leone CR. Tarsal-conjunctival advancement flaps for upper eyelid reconstruction. Arch Ophthalmol 1983;101:945
23. Cutler NL, Beard C. A method for partial and total eyelid reconstruction. Am J Ophthalmol 1955;39:1
24. Dortzbach RK, Angrist RA. Silicone intubation for lacerated lacrimal canaliculi. Ophthalmic Surg 1985;16:639
25. Hawes MJ, Segrest DR. Effectiveness of bicanalicular silicone intubation in the repair of canalicular lacerations. Ophthal Plast Reconstr Surg 1985;1:185
26. Jones LT. Lacrimal surgery. In: Tessier P, Callahan A, Mustarde JC, Salyer KE, eds. Symposium on Plastic Surgery in the Orbital Region. St Louis: CV Mosby; 1976:129–135
27. Beyer CK. Unilateral medial canthal wiring technique. In: Wesley RE, ed. Techniques in Ophthalmic Plastic Surgery. New York: John Wiley and Sons; 1986:436–437
28. Smith B, Beyer CK. Medial canthoplasty. Arch Ophthalmol 1969; 82:3448
29. Mustarde JC. Epicanthus, telecanthus, blepharophimosis, and related conditions. In: Mustarde JC, ed. Repair and Reconstruction in the Orbital Region. New York: Churchill Livingstone; 1991:467–496
30. Dortzbach RK, Hawes MJ. Midline forehead flap in reconstructive procedures of the eyelids and exenterated socket. Ophthalmic Surg 1981;12:257
31. Weinstein GS, Anderson RL, Tse DT, Kersten RC. The use of a periosteal strip for eyelid reconstruction. Arch Ophthalmol 1985;103:357
32. Anderson RL, Gordy DD. The tarsal strip procedure. Arch Ophthalmol 1979;97:2192
33. Kaltreider SA, Jacobs JL, Hughes MO. Predicting the ideal implant size prior to enucleation. Ophthal Plast Reconstr Surg 1999;15(1):37
34. Spivey BE, Allen L, Stewart WB. Surgical correction of superior sulcus deformity occurring after enucleation. Am J Ophthalmol 1972;82:365
35. Dresner SC, Codere F, Corriveau C. Orbital volume augmentation with adjustable prefabricated methylmethacrylate subperiosteal implants. Ophthalmic Surg 1991;22:53
36. Nasr AM, Jabak MH, Batainah Y. Orbital volume augmentation with subperiosteal room-temperature-vulcanized silicone implants: a clinical and histopathologic study. Ophthal Plast Reconstr Surg 1994;10:11
37. Bilyuk JR, Rubin PA, Shore JW. Correction of enophthalmos with porous polyethylene implants. J Int Ophthalmol Clin 1992;32:151
38. Dortzbach RK, Kaltreider SA. Socket reconstruction. In: Dortzbach RK, ed. Ophthalmic Plastic Surgery: Prevention and Management of Complications. New York: Raven Press; 1994:269–290
39. Smith B, Petrelli R. Dermis-fat graft as a movable implant within the muscle cone. Am J Ophthalmol 1978;85:62
40. Perry AC. Integrated orbital implants. Adv Ophthalmic Plast Reconstr Surg 1990;8:75–81
41. Karesh JW, Dresner SC. High-density porous polyethylene (MEDPOR) as a successful anophthalmic socket implant. Ophthalmology 1994; 101:1688
42. Kaltreider SA, Newman SA. Prevention and management of complications associated with the hydroxyapatite implant. Ophthal Plast Reconstr Surg 1996;12(1):18
43. Strauss JV. Cosmetic optics. J Am Soc Ocularists 1993;24:8
44. Allen L, Webster HE. Modified impression method of artificial eye fitting. Am J Ophthalmol 1969;67:189–218
45. Meisler DM, Berzins UJ, Krachmer JH, Stock EL. Cromolyn treatment of giant papillary conjunctivitis. Arch Ophthalmol 1982;100:1608

63 Management of the Paralyzed Face

J. Madison Clark and William W. Shockley

Facial paralysis is a potentially catastrophic condition. Unfortunately, the facial nerve is the most commonly paralyzed nerve in the human body.[1] This impairment imposes a devastating effect on the cosmetic, functional, social, psychological, and economic aspects of a person's life. The facial nerve is responsible for emotional and voluntary facial expression, protection of the eye, lacrimation, oral competence, salivation, taste, and sensation. Even in cases where the actual disability is not severe, the accompanying disfigurement may result in a sense of isolation and alienation from one's community. Not surprisingly, depression is a common sequela of facial paralysis.

In addition to the role of facial movement in physical appearance and beauty, an intact facial motor system is essential for effective human communication, both spoken and unspoken. Facial movements provide a supplement to speech and help control the flow of dynamics in conversation. The constancy of facial expression during conversation is cross-cultural. The expressions of happiness, sadness, interest, disinterest, surprise, anger, and fear are universally understood. As originally proposed by Darwin in 1872, human facial expressions of emotion have evolved, are innate, and therefore are universal.[2]

Any distortion or disfigurement of an individual's facial features may have major social and psychological consequences. The sequelae of facial disfigurement, specifically facial paralysis, are complex and unpredictable. Clinical observation demonstrates that some patients with mild facial paresis display severe maladjustment, whereas others with complete facial paralysis demonstrate only mild negative reactions. The facial plastic surgeon must understand and anticipate a continuum of psychosocial adjustment in patients with facial paralysis. As with facial aesthetic surgery, reanimation surgery requires extensive preoperative counseling with regard to realistic expectations.

Facial paralysis not only impacts on appearance, self-image, and nonverbal communication, but also results in predictable functional sequelae. These include ophthalmologic disturbances, difficulty with speaking, nasal obstruction from valve collapse, as well as oral incompetence and the inability to maintain effacement of the gingivobuccal sulcus, leading to problems with mastication.

Of greatest concern to the facial plastic surgeon are the potentially devastating ophthalmologic consequences, such as exposure keratitis and corneal ulceration, leading to decreasing visual acuity and potentially to blindness. The fundamental deficits are loss of the blink response and incomplete eye closure. The primary goal in ocular rehabilitation is to protect the cornea from these sight-threatening complications. A staged approach to the management of the eye in facial surgery has been developed and will be discussed later.[3]

Paralysis of the orbicularis oris muscle leads to oral incompetence, which manifests as ipsilateral spillage of food and liquids and difficulty with pronunciation of words that require pursing of the lips. Loss of tone in the buccinator muscle leads to masticatory problems due to difficulty with clearance of food from the ipsilateral gingival buccal sulcus.

Nasal obstruction occurs due to loss of tone in the dilator nasi and nasalis muscles with subsequent valve collapse. This may be compounded by midface skin laxity. The resulting nasal symptoms may be an independent problem or may exacerbate a previously subclinical septal deformity or inferior turbinate hypertrophy.

The overall effect of facial paralysis on static and dynamic facial appearance, verbal and nonverbal communication, functional issues such as ocular dryness and epiphora, oral incompetence, nasal obstruction, and the resultant impairment in the patient's self-image results in significant global disability. Many patients withdraw from their normal lives. They may cease to interact socially, change to jobs that require minimal person-to-person contact, and avoid sexual relationships.[4,5] Not surprisingly, depression is a common emotional response to facial paralysis. It is incumbent on the facial plastic surgeon to recognize these psychosocial manifestations and be prepared to discuss them with the patient. If clinically significant maladjustment to the facial deformity is recognized, then professional referral may be necessary, preferably to a psychologist or psychiatrist with experience in treating patients with facial paralysis.

Etiology

The most complete differential diagnosis of facial palsy in literature was compiled by May and Klein[6] (**Table 63.1**). These authors classified the etiologic factors as follows: birth, trauma, neurologic, infection, metabolic, neoplastic, toxic, iatrogenic, and idiopathic. The four most common causes—trauma, Bell's palsy, iatrogenic, and idiopathic—merit further discussion. These are more commonly associated with permanent deficits and therefore frequently require facial reanimation.

Table 63.1 Causes of Facial Palsy Identified in a Review of Medical Literature (1900–1990)

Birth
Molding
Forceps delivery
Dystrophia myotonica
Möbius syndrome (facial diplegia associated with other cranial nerve deficits)
Trauma
Basal skull fractures
Facial injuries
Penetrating injury to middle ear
Altitude paralysis (barotrauma)
Scuba diving (barotrauma)
Lightning
Neurologic
Opercular syndrome (cortical lesion in facial motor area)
Millard-Gubler syndrome (abducens palsy with contralateral hemiplegia caused by lesion in base of pons involving corticospinal tract)
Infection
External otitis
Otitis media
Mastoiditis
Chickenpox
Herpes zoster oticus (Ramsay Hunt syndrome)
Encephalitis
Poliomyelitis (type 1)
Mumps
Mononucleosis
Leprosy
Influenza
Coxsackievirus
Malaria
Syphilis
Scleroma
Tuberculosis
Botulism
Acute hemorrhagic conjunctivitis (enterovirus 70)
Gnathostomiasis
Mucormycosis
Lyme disease
Cat scratch
AIDS
Metabolic
Diabetes mellitus
Hyperthyroidism
Pregnancy
Hypertension
Acute porphyria
Vitamin A deficiency
Neoplastic
Benign lesions of parotid
Cholesteatoma
Seventh nerve tumor
Glomus jugulare tumor
Leukemia
Meningioma
Hemangioblastoma
Sarcoma
Carcinoma (invading or metastatic)
Anomalous sigmoid sinus
Carotid artery aneurysm
Hemangioma of tympanum
Hydradenoma (external canal)
Facial nerve tumor (cylindroma)
Schwannoma
Teratoma
Hand-Schüller-Christian disease
Fibrous dysplasia
Neurofibromatosis type 2
Toxic
Thalidomide (Miehlke's syndrome, cranial nerves VI and VII with congenital malformed external ears and deafness)
Ethylene glycol
Alcoholism
Arsenic intoxication
Tetanus
Diphtheria
Carbon monoxide
Iatrogenic
Mandibular block anesthesia
Antitetanus serum
Vaccine treatment for rabies
Postimmunization
Parotid surgery
Mastoid surgery
Posttonsillectomy and adenoidectomy
Iontophoresis (local anesthesia)
Embolization
Dental
Idiopathic
Bell's, familial
Melkersson-Rosenthal syndrome (recurrent alternating facial palsy, furrowed tongue, fasciolabial edema)
Hereditary hypertrophic neuropathy (Charcot-Marie-Tooth disease, Déjérine-Sottas disease)
Autoimmune syndrome
Amyloidosis
Temporal arteritis
Thrombotic thrombocytopenic purpura
Periarteritis nodosa
Guillain-Barré syndrome (ascending paralysis)
Multiple sclerosis
Myasthenia gravis
Sarcoidosis (Heerfordt syndrome–uveoparotid fever)
Osteopetrosis

Source: Adapted from May M, Klein S. Differential diagnosis of facial nerve palsy. Otolaryngol Clin North Am 1991;24: 613–644.

In adults, blunt head injury is the most common cause of traumatic facial nerve injury. Approximately 7 to 10% of temporal bone fractures are associated with facial nerve dysfunction.[7]

Overall in children, trauma is second to Bell's palsy as a cause of facial palsy.[8] The more lateral position of the stylomastoid foramen and facial nerve renders it a higher risk factor in neonates and children. In neonates, the most common cause is birth trauma. A complete return of facial nerve function without sequelae was found in more than 90% of neonatal cases.[9] Facial paralysis in neonates with congenital malformations, such as Möbius syndrome, has a poor prognosis for recovery.

Iatrogenic facial paralysis following middle ear and mastoid surgery ranges in incidence from 0.2 to 1.4%.[10,11] The most common segment of the nerve to be iatrogenically injured is the tympanic segment.

Controversy remains regarding the difference between Bell's palsy and idiopathic facial palsy. However, formerly regarded as synonymous terms, most experts currently believe that Bell's palsy is caused by a herpes simplex virus (HSV) infection.[12–14] Statistically significant improvement in facial nerve function with acyclovir in a double-blind, prospective, randomized trial[15] is also suggestive of HSV causality. Despite the improved outcomes reported with treatment with antiviral agents and steroids, only a small percentage of patients with Bell's palsy have a poor outcome, with incomplete return of facial movement.[12]

Patient Evaluation and Workup

As with any disease or injury, a detailed history and physical examination precedes therapeutic intervention. The history and physical examination are directed to identification of the cause and topographic location of the injury, the degree of injury, and the optimal choice of neural repair or reanimation techniques.

After a complete history, physical examination, electrodiagnostic studies, and imaging studies have been obtained, the facial plastic surgeon is faced with the decision of when and how to proceed with facial reanimation. The complex decision-making involved in facial reanimation is not unlike that faced by the head and neck surgical oncologist. The decision must include consideration of both disease-specific factors and patient-specific factors. Disease-specific factors include prognosis for recovery (such as from resection of tumors involving the brain stem or cerebellopontine angle, or from parotid gland malignancies) and likelihood of recurrence or progression of disease (such as in neurofibromatosis). Patient-specific factors include age, medical status, skin type, motivation for rehabilitation, and likelihood of appropriate follow-up.

State-of-the-art rehabilitation of persons with facial paralysis involves a comprehensive program that includes medical management, physiotherapy, and psychosocial support, in addition to the myriad of surgical procedures available for reanimation. However, there is no universally accepted management tool for evaluation of these facial reanimation procedures.[16]

Radiologic Testing

Radiologic studies are occasionally necessary in patients with facial paralysis. Generally, the extratemporal facial nerve is usually made visible with fine-cut computed tomography (CT) scanning, whereas the intratemporal and intracranial portions are best seen with magnetic resonance imaging (MRI).

MRI has contributed significantly to improved imaging of the facial nerve. Gadolinium-enhanced MRI allows detection of inflammation and edema of the facial nerve, as well as differentiation of facial nerve tumors or hemangiomas from Bell's palsy.[17] Gadolinium enhancement centered at the geniculate ganglion on the side of the paralysis is often seen in patients with Bell's palsy. In addition, MRI findings may also carry prognostic significance in these patients. Murphy reported that patients with Bell's palsy who had enhancement extending to the mastoid segment of the facial nerve had more severe inflammation and, consequently, a poorer chance for recovery.[17] Some authors have recommended gadolinium-enhanced MRI prior to any reanimation procedure for facial nerve paralysis.

Radiologic testing should also be considered in the following clinical scenarios: (1) a patient with facial paralysis with a palpable mass in the parotid gland; (2) a patient with a suspected lesion in the internal auditory canal (IAC) or cerebellopontine angle; and (3) a patient with atypical idiopathic facial paralysis or Bell's palsy.

Electrodiagnostic Testing

Electrodiagnostic testing is a method of evaluating the degree of injury to the facial nerve and the integrity of the facial musculature. This battery of tests adds valuable information to the history and physical examination with regard to choice of method of facial reanimation. Electrical testing of the facial nerve is unique in the following ways: (1) as most causes of facial nerve injury occur proximal to the stylomastoid foramen, the electrical stimulation point is distal to the site of injury; (2) as the nerve distal to the lesion responds normally to stimulation as long as the axon is intact, the nerve will continue to respond to stimulation even in the presence of paralysis; and (3) with axonal disruption or complete transection, the ability to transmit any impulse is gradually lost over a period of 3 days, corresponding to the timing of Wallerian degeneration.

Electrodiagnostic testing is particularly helpful in differentiating a Sunderland first- or second-degree neural injury from more severe injury.[18] Compression of nerve trunks tends to block the larger fibers first because the smaller ones are more resistant to compression.[19] Initially, compression slows conduction through the area of injury, but conduction proximal and distal to the area of injury remains normal. Further compression will cause a complete block of transmission, first in the less resistant larger fibers and then in the smaller ones. As long as axonal flow remains intact, the nerve responds to stimulation distal to the area of compression. When axonal flow is completely blocked (axonotmesis, or Sunderland second degree), response to stimulation distal to the lesion decreases.

A variety of electrical tests are available, but the most commonly used tests are the maximum stimulation test (MST), the nerve excitability test (NET), electroneuronography (ENOG), and electromyography (EMG).

Maximum Stimulation Test

The MST is an appropriate test for facial nerve degeneration soon after onset of injury. The test is not useful during the first 3 days after injury because the nerve with complete proximal transection will continue to conduct impulses distally for up to 3 days. The test is performed using the Hilger nerve stimulator and involves subjective observation of the facial musculature in response to electrical stimulation. The technique for performing the MST is described in detail by Blumenthal and May.[19] The parameter of significance for the interpretation of the results of the MST is the amount of muscle twitch in response to supramaximal stimulation with the nerve stimulator. The response on the paretic side is compared with that on the normal side.

Because the test is uncomfortable for the patient, and because patients with incomplete paralysis have a favorable prognosis, the test should not be performed unless there is complete (House-Brackmann grade 6) paralysis. May found that when the MST was absent within 10 days of injury, the test was 100% reliable in predicting an incomplete return of facial function. When the response was markedly decreased, 73% of patients had an incomplete return of facial function.[20]

Nerve Excitability Test

The NET is based on the same principle as the MST, except that the NET measures the current (in amperage) required to obtain a minimal visible response at a standard square-wave pulse duration. Like the MST, the test is not useful during the first 3 days after injury because the distal segment of the nerve, even with complete proximal transection, will continue to conduct impulses distally for up to 3 days. The test is also performed using the Hilger nerve stimulator, which measures the difference in the amperage required to produce a barely visible twitch on the paretic side compared with that required on the normal side. A side-to-side difference of greater than 3.5 mA indicates a poor prognosis.[19]

Electromyography

EMG is the study of depolarization potentials of muscle fibers and groups of fibers that make up motor units. EMG measures the response to needle insertion and electrical activity of the muscle/motor unit at rest. As the needle is inserted in the muscle, a short burst of electrical activity normally occurs. Insertion activity is decreased when muscle has atrophied. With denervation, activity is usually increased and positive sharp waves are often present.

After insertion of the stimulating electrode, the muscle is measured at rest. Normal resting muscle exhibits no spontaneous electrical activity. With denervation, spontaneous fibrillation potentials and positive sharp waves are present. The presence of fibrillation potentials is the strongest electromyographic evidence that denervation has occurred.[19] Fibrillation potentials are not present immediately after injury, however. It may take up to 2 or 3 weeks for fibrillation potentials to be detected by EMG. The farther the recording electrode is placed from the site of the lesion, the longer it takes for the fibrillations to appear.[21]

Polyphasic action potentials (PAPs) refer to simultaneous discharge of a group of nerve fibers in the motor unit in the field of the stimulating electrode. PAPs are the best indication that regeneration is occurring.

EMG is most useful when significant nerve degeneration has occurred and the responses to the MST and ENOG have been lost. EMG can demonstrate the presence or absence of viable facial muscle tissue, as well as the gross functional integrity between nerve and muscle.

Electroneuronography

ENOG evaluates the integrity of the nerve and muscle together. ENOG is similar to the MST and the NET, except that instead of relying on observation of the response, the response to a supramaximal stimulation is recorded by the distal recording electrodes in ENOG. Fisch used ENOG to determine which facial nerve disorders would be best treated by facial nerve decompression.[22]

Using surface electrodes, a stimulating electrode is placed over the main trunk of the facial nerve on the skin at the stylomastoid foramen and a recording electrode is placed over the distal facial musculature. If intact axons are present over the branch of the nerve being tested then an action potential will be generated and recorded. If axonal degeneration or transection has occurred, then the ability to transmit an impulse will be lost after ~3 days. As in the MST and the NET, ENOG compares the response on the paretic side of the face with that on the normal side; however, ENOG is more sensitive.[23] The results are expressed as a percentage of the amplitude of the action potentials on the abnormal side as opposed to the normal side. This is believed to correlate with the percentage of nerve degeneration.[24]

ENOG results are most commonly used to stratify patients into surgical decompression versus observation following nerve injury. A 90% degeneration of the nerve is considered to be the threshold for consideration of surgical decompression.

Medical Treatment

Protection of the Eye

The primary goal of medical management in patients with facial paralysis is to protect the cornea from sight-threatening complications. As such, it should begin immediately following facial nerve injury. Correction of eyelid malpositions, reduction of epiphora, and improvement of cosmesis are therefore secondary goals, although they are of great importance to the patient.[4,25] It is vitally important for the facial plastic surgeon to emphasize the serious nature of eye protection when discussing the reconstructive possibilities because the patient may be more concerned with aesthetic aspects.

Corneal protection begins with patient education about the eyelids and their function. Eyelids provide a physical barrier to trauma and desiccation, and they inhibit adherence of organisms to the ocular surface. The tear film contains antimicrobial substances, such as immunoglobulin A, and provides mechanical lubrication to wash away organisms. If eyelid closure is defective, as with facial palsy, then the tear film may not provide adequate coverage and the epithelium may become susceptible to desiccation. This reduction in mechanical protection and tear production is especially dangerous in patients with concurrent ipsilateral corneal hypesthesia.

After adequate evaluation of the eye, treatment of the paralytic eye begins with a regimen of regular ocular lubrication. At a minimum, the regimen should include the use of artificial tears or the equivalent 5 to 10 times per day, with ophthalmic ointment at night. About one third of patients require lubrication only, and such patients do not require ophthalmic referral.[3]

Other adjunctive measures include the use of a moisture chamber and taping. A moisture chamber is used in addition to drops and ointment and has been found to be most useful whenever the patient is outdoors (to prevent mechanical trauma). Taping must be atraumatic, as corneal injury may result from poor taping technique. The nonallergenic tape should be applied from superomedial to inferolateral and should not contact the cornea or invert the eyelids. Again, taping is used in addition to drops and ointment.

Our recommendations regarding ophthalmologic referral are to refer (1) any patient with symptoms or signs of ocular irritation; (2) any patient with concurrent ipsilateral corneal hypesthesia; and (3) any patient being considered for surgical intervention.

Physical Therapy

Physical therapy is an underutilized modality in the comprehensive treatment of patients with facial nerve paralysis. Many patients with Bell's palsy are told, "Relax, it will get better on its own." Indeed, the natural history of Bell's palsy is that most patients recover fully, without any intervention. As previously alluded to, the goal in the management of patients with Bell's palsy is identifying those patients early who will not achieve full recovery. Those patients predicted to have adverse sequelae should have intervention designed to maximize their functional outcome. Several investigators have shown that outcomes may be improved with the use of physical therapy.[26–28] Additional research suggests that physical therapy also improves outcomes in patients who have undergone neural procedures or reanimation surgery for facial paralysis.[26,29–35]

Methods of rehabilitation for facial paralysis have included massage, electrical stimulation, and repetition of common facial expressions. This "generic" form of therapy has been found to be of little benefit.[36,37] In fact, some authors have suggested that certain nonspecific interventions may affect recovery adversely, perhaps by disrupting reinnervation patterns and leading to greater synkinesis and mass movement of the facial muscles.[29,37–39]

The most promising physical therapy treatment technique for patients with facial paralysis appears to be facial neuromuscular reeducation using surface electromyography (sEMG) or mirror biofeedback. Randomized clinical trials have demonstrated that qualitative and quantitative improvements in facial movement occurred after this method of treatment. Facial neuromuscular reeducation is a process of relearning facial movement using specific and accurate feedback to (1) enhance facial muscle activity in functional patterns of facial movement and meaningful expression and (2) suppress abnormal muscle activity and synkinesis interfering with normal facial function.[37] The program is highly individualized and has been validated, based on classification of patients according to one of four treatment-based categories.[37]

Comprehensive management of patients with facial paralysis should include the vital involvement of a physical therapist on the multidisciplinary team. The therapist should be involved early in the evaluation, as physical therapy techniques, like most surgical procedures, are most effective when implemented early in the course of the disease.

Botulinum Toxin

Botulinum toxin (botox) is an adjunctive treatment in the medical armamentarium for the management of facial paralysis. In patients with facial neuromuscular disorders, botox was initially introduced to treat patients with hemifacial spasm and hyperkinetic blepharospasm following Bell's palsy.[26] The use of botox in facial paralysis patients now includes selective medical neurolysis, treatment of hyperlacrimation after Bell's palsy, and treatment of synkinesia[40–42]

Aberrant regeneration of fibers after facial nerve injury leads to several untoward effects, as previously mentioned, such as involuntary synkinesia between the orbicularis oculi and orbicularis oris muscles, or increased lacrimation of the affected eye. Botulinum toxin blocks the presynaptic release of acetylcholine and causes a functional denervation of neuromuscular end plates. Collateral sprouting reestablishes the pathological state after 3 to 5 months.[40]

Local injection of botox into the orbicularis oculi muscle has been found by many researchers to be an effective means of controlling facial synkinesis.[41,43,44]

The toxin affects the neuromuscular junction as well as the autonomic cholinergic transmission, as in the lacrimation pathway. Secremotor fibers of the facial nerve innervate the lacrimal gland through greater superficial petrosal nerve via the nervus intermedius. After a facial nerve injury or Bell's palsy, aberrant fibers originally destined for the submandibular and sublingual glands may develop and travel to the lacrimal gland, causing a hyperlacrimation syndrome whenever the patient salivates (crocodile tears, or Bogorad syndrome). Because the fibers to the lacrimal gland utilize acetylcholine as a neurotransmitter, local injections of botox into the gland can remedy hyperlacrimation.

In fact, Boroojerdi et al have reported nearly total resolution of hyperlacrimation in a cohort of patients using this technique.[40] The authors found successful response in most patients with subcutaneous injection in the superolateral part of the orbicularis oculi muscle, and when this was suboptimal, injection into the lacrimal gland was more effective.

Surgical Reanimation

Eye Procedures

From a surgical perspective, the primary goal is to continue medical protection of the eye against sight-threatening complications. When considering the surgical options for improvement in cosmesis of the eye, this primary goal must not be compromised.

A multitude of surgical procedures have been described to correct paralytic lagophthalmos and ectropion, the main surgically correctable ocular features in patients with facial paralysis. Techniques include tarsorrhaphy as well as use of Silastic (Dow Corning, Midland, MI) or wire-spring implants, gold weights, magnets, ear cartilage grafts, and various muscle–tendon slings or grafts.[45–49] Reanimation may require surgery on the upper eyelid alone or on the lower lid as well. The method of "dual reanimation," or addressing the eye and the mouth with independent surgical procedures, provides the best functional and cosmetic results.[50]

Before any reanimation procedures are attempted, it is necessary to ascertain the baseline function of the eye and its supporting structures. A complete eye examination should include assessment of visual acuity, assessment of presence or absence of a Bell's phenomenon, assessment of tear production with a Shirmer's test, evaluation of the lacrimal excretory system with a Jones test, and measurement of the margin gap (the distance between the borders of the upper and lower eyelids on closure).[48]

Lower Eyelid Procedures

Although much attention has been directed to rehabilitation of upper lid lagophthalmos, assessment and treatment of the paralyzed lower eyelid has largely been neglected. The amount of lower lid laxity is best assessed by the snap test. The decision whether or not to address the lower medial canthus as part of the ectropion correction depends on the position and function of the inferior punctum. Medial lower lid laxity, or medial ectropion, causes the punctum to evert. With the inferior punctum no longer against the globe, drainage of the lacrimal system is interrupted, resulting in pooling of tears at the inferior lid margin.[48]

Correction of medial lower lid laxity requires that the inferior punctum be moved back into its native position against the globe to avoid collection of tears in the inferior cul-de-sac. This may be accomplished by the use of a Gore-Tex (W. L. Gore & Associates Inc., Flagstaff, AZ) sling procedure[48] or a medial canthoplasty.[51]

There are numerous procedures that exist for medial lid tightening. In the traditional technique, the procedure is performed under local anesthesia with intravenous sedation. The cornea is topically anesthetized with tetracaine, lubricated, and a corneal protector applied. The cutaneous incision is marked prior to injection of local anethesia. After the flaps have been raised, the tarsal components of the superior and inferior canthal tendons are dissected. The lateral portion of the inferior canthal tendon is plicated to the medial portion of the superior canthal tendon. Excess skin is excised prior to skin

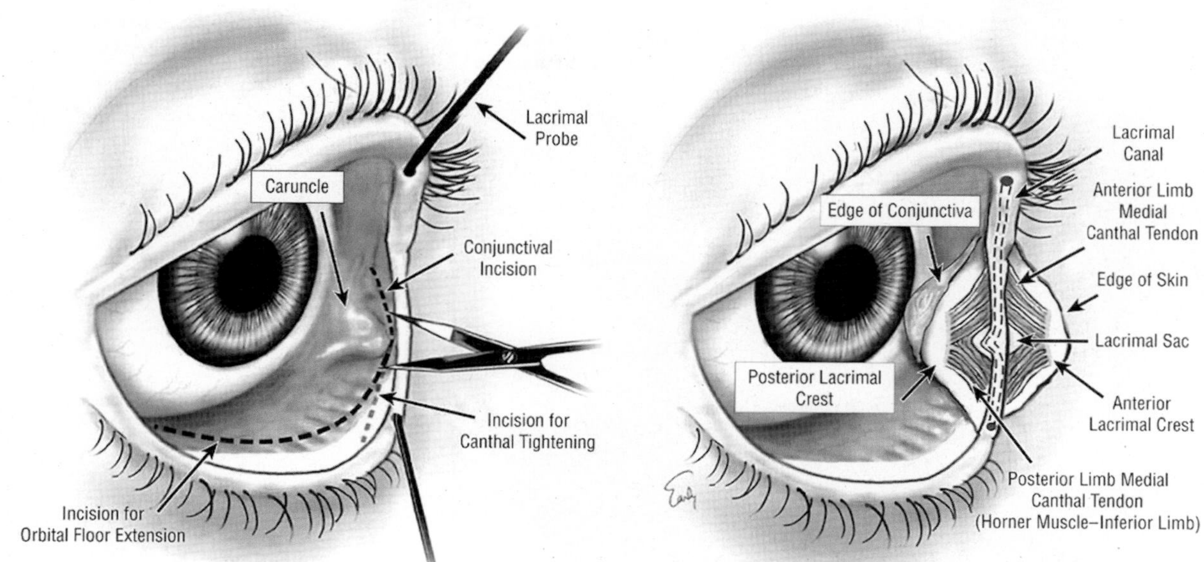

Fig. 63.1 (**A**) Conjunctival incision for the precaruncular approach. Lacrimal probes are placed in the superior and inferior lacrimal puncta. The scissors demonstrate the initial conjunctival incision. The incision may be continued laterally for additional access to the orbital floor (*dark dashed line*) or anteriorly for full access to the medial canthal tendon and tarsal plate (*light dashed line*). (**B**) The anterior and posterior limbs of the medial canthal tendon are illustrated, with the caruncle and adjacent conjunctiva reflected laterally. The lacrimal canaliculi are shown entering the lacrimal sac (medial to the canthal tendon). (From the Archives of Facial Plastic Surgery. Copyright 2003, American Medical Association. Reprinted by permission.)

closure.[51] Recently Moe has described the precaruncular approach as seen in **Fig. 63.1**.[52,53] This procedure affords the advantage of adding a posterior and superior vector to the traditional medial vector, as well as avoiding a skin incision (**Fig. 63.1**). The patient in **Fig. 63.2** has a medial canthoplasty through the precaruncular approach.

Laterally, the extent of laxity ranges from scleral show, defined as greater than 1-mm distance between the margin of the lower lid and the inferior limbus, to ectropion. When lateral lower eyelid laxity is excessive, a horizontal lid-shortening procedure is indicated. This procedure usually uses some variation on the classic tarsal strip technique.[48] A lateral canthotomy and inferior cantholysis are performed, preserving the insertions supplied from the upper lid. The anterior lamella of skin and muscle is separated from the posterior lamella, and

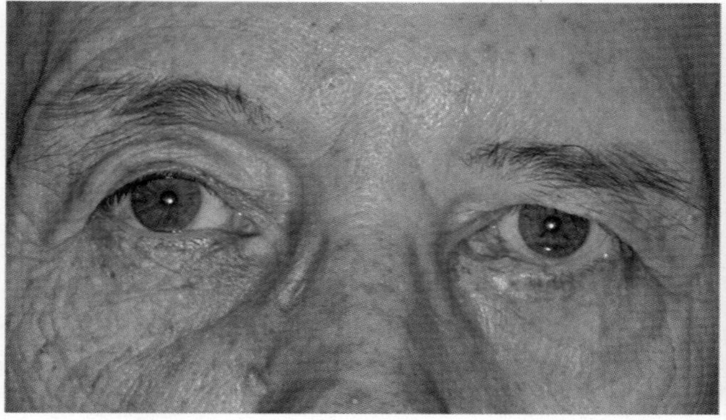

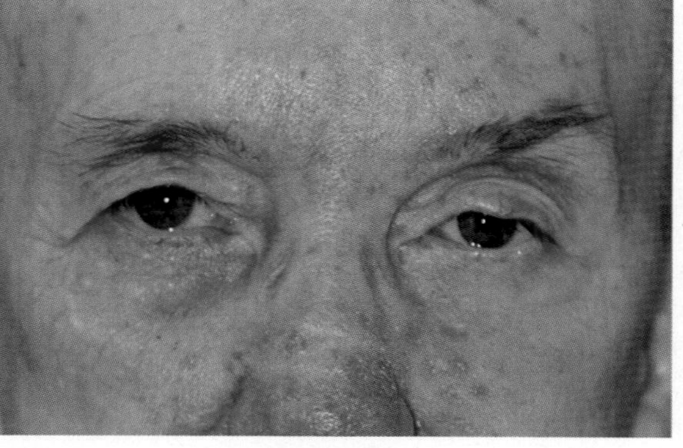

Fig. 63.2 Transcaruncular medial canthoplasty in a patient with left facial paralysis. The preoperative photograph (**A**) demonstrates that despite a positive canthal tilt, there is significant medial canthal laxity with resultant conjunctival irritation and inflammation. The postoperative photograph (**B**) demonstrates significant improvement of medial canthal position with complete resolution of conjunctival inflammation. Note also that the patient has undergone midforehead unilateral browlift and platinum upper eyelid weight.

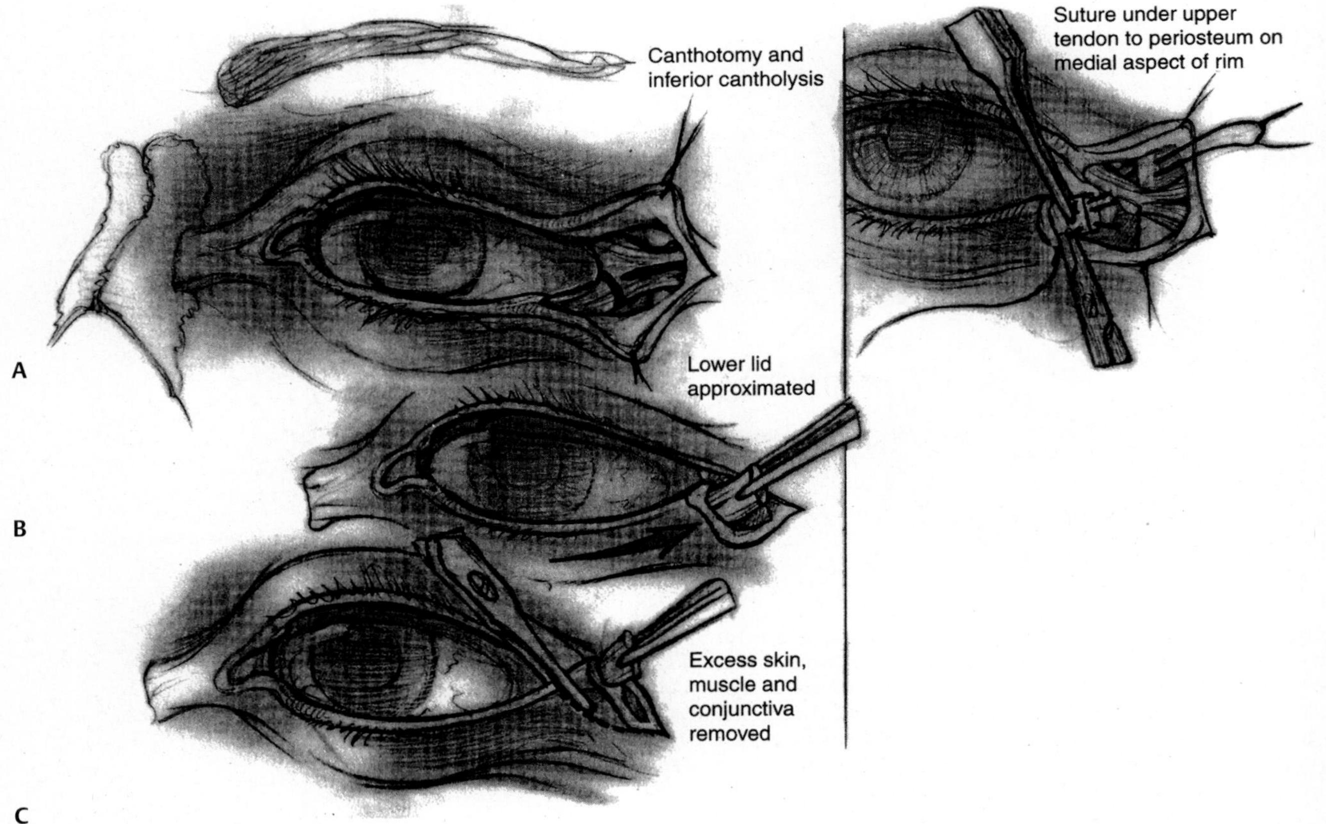

Fig. 63.3 Lateral tarsal strip. (**A**) Exposure and division of inferior lateral canthal tendon. (**B**) Lateral retraction of tendon to correct lid malpositioning. (**C**) Skin, muscle, and conjunctiva stripped from tendon as necessary. (**D**) Resuspension of tendon to medial aspect of lateral orbital rim.

the skin and conjunctiva are removed. The lateral canthal ligament is then trimmed appropriately and resuspended from periosteum from the medial surface of the lateral orbital rim superior to Whitnall's tubercle (**Fig. 63.3**). Moe and Linder have recently described a lateral transorbital canthopexy for the correction of lower lid laxity and ectropion that avoids any eyelid incisions.[54]

Upper Eyelid Procedures (Platinum or Gold Weight)

Originally conceived by Sheehan,[55] lid loading was later refined by Jobe,[56] who also introduced gold as the material of choice. The primary advantage of lid loading over other upper eyelid techniques is the superior success rates and low complication rates.[45,51,57] Gold weight lid loading has emerged as the standard surgical management of the paralytic upper eyelid and lagophthalmos. The advantages of gold are its low reactivity, high density, and good color match with skin. The gold weights are easily selected for proper placement and are reversible. This relatively simple procedure is usually performed under local anesthesia. The disadvantages are threefold: (1) Gold is a foreign body and could possibly extrude; however, extrusion rates are extremely low. (2) Lid loading is gravity-dependent, so when the patient is supine, it can be counterproductive. However, most of our patients do not require lubrication while sleeping after placement of gold weights. (3) The gold weight leaves a visible bump on the upper eyelid when it is closed. In response to the aesthetic disadvantage of the gold weight, lower profile solid platinum weights have been developed (MedDev Corp, Sunnyvale, CA). Like gold, platinum implants are inert but because they are more dense than gold, the implants are significantly thinner and smaller (**Fig. 63.4**).[45]

The technique begins with a small amount of local anesthetic injected in the supratarsal fold and over the tarsal plate. The incision is slightly longer than the implant and is centered over the junction between the medial and middle thirds of the upper eyelid. The skin is elevated to the superior edge of the tarsal plate. The orbicularis is sharply incised, and a pocket is formed over the tarsal plate to within 2 mm of the lash line. The weight is placed in the pocket so that the side with two fenestrations faces cephalad. The implant is sutured to the levator aponeurosis over the tarsal plate, using the fenestrations (**Fig. 63.5**). Platinum flexible chain implants resemble

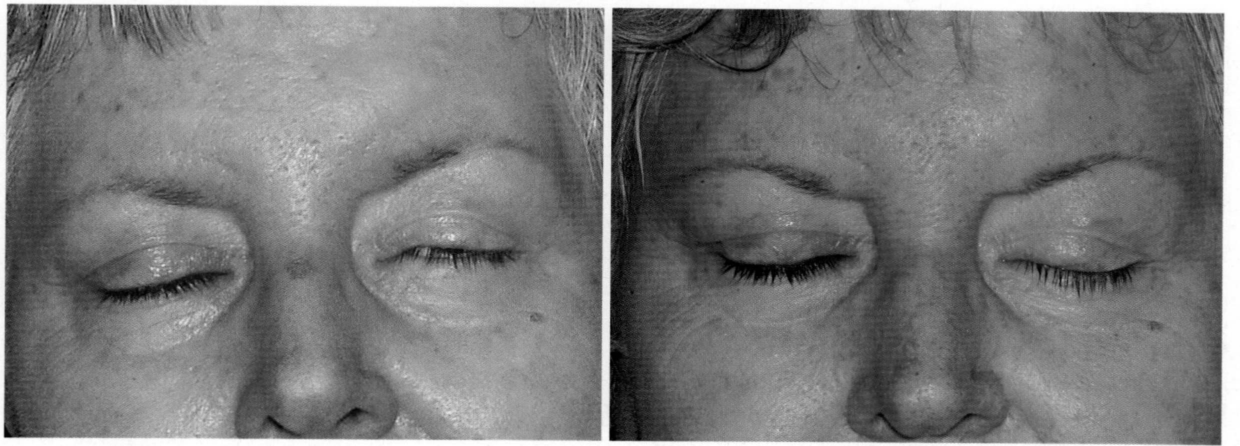

Fig. 63.4 Upper eyelid low profile platinum weight in a patient with left facial paralysis. The preoperative photograph (**A**) demonstrates 2 to 3 mm of lagophthalmos on the left with eyes closed position. The postoperative photograph (**B**) demonstrates complete resolution of lagophalmos and minimal distortion of pretarsal aesthetic with the lower profile platinum weight.

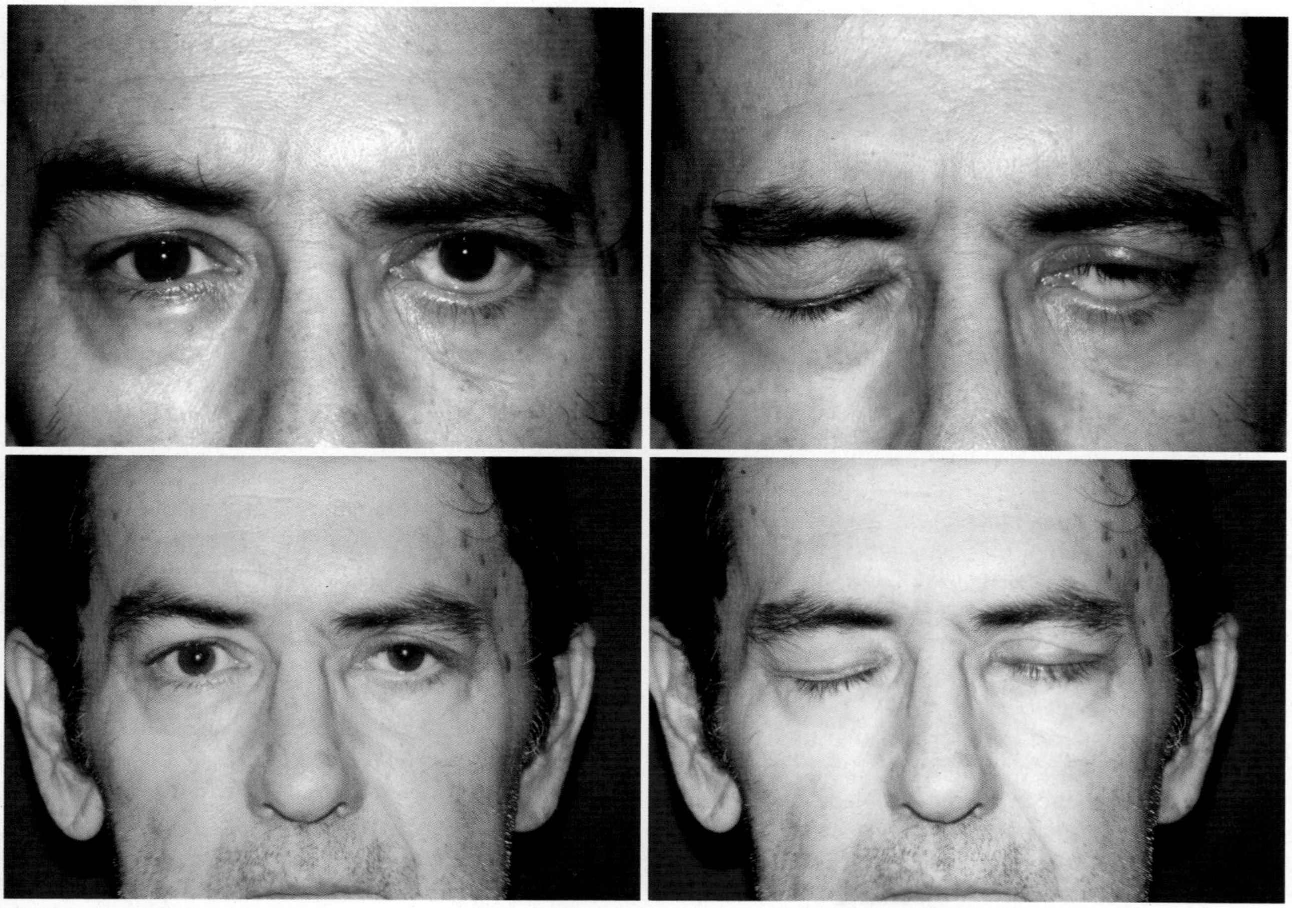

Fig. 63.5 A 52-year-old patient with injury to upper division of left facial nerve following penetrating trauma. (**A**) Scleral show and obvious lower lid laxity. (**B**) Lagophthmos despite previous placement of gold weight to left upper lid. (**C**) Improvement in left lower lid contour following lateral tarsal strip procedure. (**D**) Complete eye closure following placement of heavier gold weight to left upper eyelid.

watch band, allowing the implant to flex with the natural motion of the upper eyelid. Kao and Moe describe a retrograde technique for insertion of the platinum chain.[58] A supraciliary incision is used to place the implant in a precise pocket, centered at the medial limbus. The authors point out that the chain is especially useful in patients with increased tarsus curvature.

Neural Procedures

Regardless of the cause of facial paralysis, the most successful outcomes for reanimation were brought about by procedures intended to restore neural input to a functionally intact neuromuscular junction. Restoring impulses from the ipsilateral facial nerve is the first choice.[59–64] This could occur in the setting of facial nerve preservation/exploration for tumor removal, facial nerve decompression after trauma or Bell's palsy, neurorrhaphy with or without rerouting, and cable grafting. Nerve crossover procedures are a secondary consideration, with variations of XII to VII most commonly in use today. Cross-facial nerve grafting is another consideration, but this technique without free-muscle transplantation has largely been abandoned due to poor results.

Extratemporal Neurorrhaphy

It is currently accepted that the optimal timing of primary neurorrhaphy is immediately following injury to permit coaptation of the nerve ends before scarring and retraction require more extensive mobilization and grafting. Some authors have advocated waiting until 21 days after injury based on the belief that the greatest degree of axonal regeneration occurs at 21 days. Barrs reviewed the literature pertaining to this question, concluding that the best functional results are found with early repair. He also investigated optimal timing of repair in micropigs and found that there is a linear decrease in axonal counts and lower regeneration rate with delay of repair.[60]

The repair may be performed with either a perineural (fascicular) or epineural repair (**Fig. 63.6**). Most surgeons have abandoned the perineural repair because of its increased technical difficulty without proof of its superiority over epineural repair.

The technique for extratemporal primary neurorrhaphy is performed under the operating microscope. The nerve edges are freshened with a microblade on a tongue depressor. Because both proximal and distal (wallerian) axon degeneration occurs, the resection back to normal nerve is probably the most important surgical consideration in delayed nerve grafting.[60] Two sutures are placed 180 degrees apart and used as traction sutures. Based on the study by Szal and Miller, a total of six interrupted sutures is optimal for epineural repair.[65]

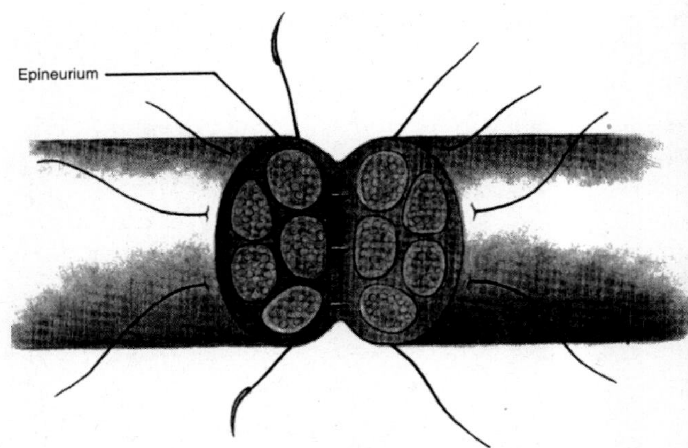

Fig. 63.6 Epineural nerve repair is performed under the operating microscope using microneural techniques with 9–0 monofilament. A tapered needle is preferred over a cutting needle. The nerve edges are freshened with sharp microscissors. A small square is used beneath the nerve ends to improve visibility during suturing. Most repairs are sutured free hand without the frame used in vessel anastomosis. Normally, six sutures are used and spaced 60 degrees apart. Three sutures are placed from top to bottom on the underside of the nerve; then three sutures are placed from top to bottom on the surface closest to the surgeon. Fewer sutures could be used for smaller peripheral nerve branches. Based on the study of Szal and Miller, the use of six sutures is probably closer to the optimal number for epineural repair.[65]

Intracranial and Intratemporal Neurorrhaphy

A complete discussion of advantages, disadvantages, and techniques of intracranial and intratemporal facial nerve neurorrhaphy is beyond the scope of this chapter, but a few salient points can be made. The interested reader is referred to an excellent review by Fisch and Lanser.[66]

A recent article by Malik et al compared the outcomes of three facial neurorrhaphy techniques: end-to-end anastomosis, cable nerve interposition, and XII-to-VII transposition.[67] It is accepted that end-to-end anastomosis, with tension-free coaptation yields the best results, and this concept was supported in Malik's study. The authors examined the rate of improvement with each technique and found that end-to-end anastomosis not only achieves the best results (85% of patients reached a House-Brackmann grade III or better), but also was associated with the fastest rate of improvement. Cable graft interposition was next fastest, but by 36 months, XII-to-VII anastomosis achieved the same level of success (66%).

Cross-Face Grafting

Since its introduction in the early 1970s,[68] cross-face grafting has fallen out of favor except as part of staged free-muscle transplantation. In this procedure, 30 to 50% of the buccal and zygomatic branches on the nonparalyzed side are severed and anastomosed to the corresponding branches on the paralyzed side. Theoretically, this produces minimal deformity on the normal side while restoring symmetry and some mimetic function on the paralyzed side. However, disappointing results with respect to incidence and amount of movement were reported by several respected authors.[69–71]

The technique can be performed in one or two stages. The second stage was originally added by Anderl, who postulated that fewer axons would grow through the second suture line if the scar had already formed before the axons arrived.[72]

In the first stage, the zygomatic and buccal branches of the nonparalyzed facial nerve are exposed through a preauricular, melolabial, or direct incision. The branches are stimulated electrically and blocked with local anesthesia to determine the dominant branches on the nonparalyzed side. These branches are preserved, and others (~50%) are cut cleanly. The branches are anastomosed to the sural nerve grafts and crossed to the other side. The sural grafts are tunneled through the upper lip and forehead with the help of midline incisions in the philtrum and glabella, respectively. Several sural cross-face grafts can be used. However, buccal grafts are the most important and most likely to be successful. The distal ends of the sural grafts are brought out beyond the edge of the parotid gland and marked with colored sutures that are brought out through the skin and cut near the surface.

The second stage is performed 4 to 6 months later. Through a preauricular incision on the paralyzed side of the face, the distal ends of the sural grafts are identified and the neuromas resected cleanly. The grafts are then anastomosed to the paralyzed branches of facial nerve as they exit the parotid gland. Alternatively, the nerve ends can be directly implanted into the atrophying muscle on the paralyzed side after the neuromas have been excised.

Cable Grafting

Interposition facial nerve grafting is used when the proximal and distal ends of the nerve cannot be coapted without tension. Techniques have been developed for grafting anywhere along the length of the facial nerve, from the cerebellopontine angle to the parotid gland.[66]

The most complicated segment to graft is the intracranial segment, due to the lack of an epineural sheath, as well as the deep and limited exposure and the background of constant cerebrospinal fluid flow. Most commonly indicated after removal of a large acoustic neuroma, results obtained with splinting in the cerebellopontine angle have been reported to compare favorably with those at more distal segments.[66]

A more common clinical situation in which cable grafting is employed is extratemporal grafting, such as following the removal of parotid malignancy with involvement of the facial nerve. For cases in which less than 10 cm in length of nerve graft is used, a contralateral greater auricular nerve graft is harvested. Ipsilateral nerve grafts can be used as well, provided tumor-free integrity can be established. For more than 10 cm and up to 35 cm, a sural nerve graft is used.

According to the method of Fisch and Lanser, two branches are used—one to the upper and one to the lower branch. They recommend clipping the branches of the digastric muscle, the retroauricular muscle, the platysma, and most of the buccal branches. This is based on laboratory work done on rats by Mattox et al,[73] which demonstrated that ligation of peripheral facial nerve branches concentrates regenerating axons in still "open" ramifications. By this method, regeneration is directed to the more important upper and lower regions of the face while minimizing mass movement in the midface.[74]

Nerve Crossover: Cranial Nerves XII-to-VII and Others

Nerve crossover procedures have been useful in facial reanimation for more than a century.[75] Several cranial nerves have been utilized for nerve crossover, including trigeminal, glossopharyngeal, and phrenic, all of which have been essentially abandoned.[76] The crossover techniques that remain in clinical use include XII-to-VII, XII-to-VII jump graft, and, rarely, XI-to-VII. These techniques, of which XII-to-VII crossover (**Fig. 63.7**) and XII-to-VII jump graft

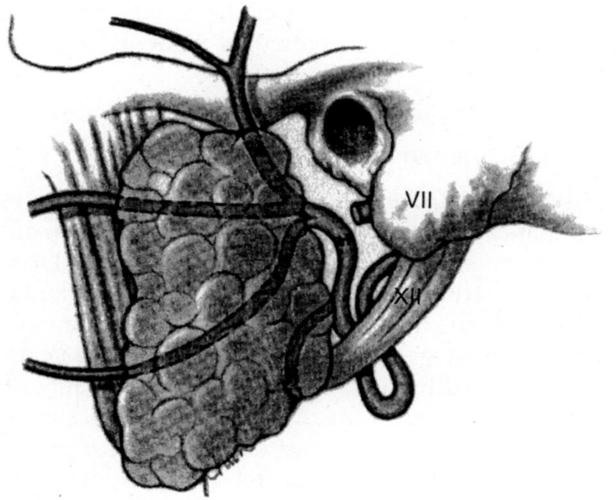

Fig. 63.7 Cranial nerve XII-to-VII crossover. Through a parotidectomy approach, cranial nerve XII is sectioned, rotated deep to the digastric muscle, and sutured to the pes. The nerve can also be split after sectioning and sutured to the main upper and lower branches of the facial nerve. (From Burgess LPA, Goode RL. Reanimation of the Paralyzed Face. New York: Thieme Medical Publishers; 1994:20. Reprinted by permission.)

(**Fig. 63.8**) have been the most popular,[76] remain a dependable and effective treatment for situations in which the proximal facial nerve is unavailable but the distal nerve remains anatomically intact. Advantages include relatively low degree of technical difficulty, relative short time to movement (usually 4 to 6 months), one anastomotic suture line (as opposed to cable grafting with two), and motion that can resemble mimetic function with practice (**Fig. 63.9**). Disadvantages of all crossover techniques include donor site morbidity and some degree of mass movement.

The major problem specific to XII-to-VII crossover is the paralysis of the ipsilateral tongue musculature, which can result in significant speech, mastication, and swallowing difficulties. In one study, more than 15% of patients complained of these difficulties.[77] Although most patients can tolerate such deficits without significant morbidity, they can be incapacitating for patients who may develop other cranial nerve deficits—particularly those who may be at risk for tenth or contralateral twelfth cranial nerve loss. In these patients, another cranial nerve, such as the spinal accessory, or the XII-to-VII jump graft, or the XI-to-VII (eliminates risk to cranial nerve XII), offers an alternative that can spare the morbidity of sacrificing the twelfth nerve.[64,75,78]

It is important that the crossover be accomplished before significant atrophy of the facial musculature and distal facial nerve has occurred. Most clinical studies have shown that crossover procedures performed within a year of facial paralysis are successful.[59] In general, the earlier the procedure is done, the better the results; however, good results have been reported as many as 10 years following injury.[79]

Dynamic Reanimation

Transposition of the temporalis or masseter muscles for dynamic reanimation of the face has been the mainstay technique in the otolaryngology and facial plastic surgery literature, whereas free-muscle transplantation has been the more commonly described technique in the plastic surgery literature. In the past 20 years, temporalis transfer has been used more frequently than masseter transfer. As previously discussed, dual-system reanimation produces the most successful outcomes.[50] Temporalis transfer is now reserved almost exclusively for the lower region, specifically for the mouth, whereas the eye is rehabilitated with a gold weight.

The major objectives of lower facial reanimation are to achieve symmetry at rest, oral sphincteric competence, and facial movement. Temporalis muscle transposition is ideally suited for this purpose if nerve grafting is not possible or to augment facial nerve or hypoglossal–facial nerve grafting.[80]

Surgical Technique for Temporalis Transposition to Oral Commissure

The technique described is fashioned after that of May and Drucker.[80]

The patient's hair on the operative (paralyzed) side of the face is parted over the temporalis muscle along the proposed incision line extending from the helical crus superiorly, and slightly posteriorly, and a narrow swath of hair is trimmed as close to the skin as possible. The incision is made down to the superficial temporalis fascia (**Fig. 63.10**). This layer is divided with scissors to expose the deep temporalis fascia immediately adjacent to the muscle. The middle one third of the muscle is outlined with a needle-tip cutting cautery and is elevated deep to the periosteum from the zygomatic arch superiorly to the temporal line.

A pocket is then created superficial to the superficial musculoaponeurotic system (SMAS) to receive the flap, down to the oral commissure. The pocket may be "hydrodissected" by saline injection prior to scissors dissection.

Next, the incision at the vermilion border or the lip–cheek crease is made. The incision extends to the orbicularis oris muscle, if present, or to the submucosa. This incision is then communicated with the preauricular incision in the supra-SMAS plane (to avoid damage to any residual functional facial nerve). The tunnel should accommodate two fingers or be wide enough to allow the transposed muscle to lie flat within it.

The distal end of the temporalis muscle is then bisected for a distance of 2 cm and figure-of-eight sutures are placed at each end. The sutures are then passed through the tunnel, thereby passing the temporalis muscle, which is sutured to the orbicularis oris muscle or the submucosa at the oral commissure. If additional length is needed to reach the oral commissure, then either periosteum or Gore-Tex strips may be used. There should be sufficient overcorrection, which resolves by 3 to 6 weeks, to achieve the desired long-term resting symmetry.

The defect left by the harvest of the middle third of the temporalis muscle may be filled with a prefabricated Silastic implant, if necessary. Alternatively, the defect may be filled with a temporoparietal fascial flap, raised prior to the temporalis transfer. The wounds are closed over a small suction drain.

May and Drucker have reported one of the largest series of temporalis transfers in the recent literature. They described several modifications over the originally described techniques that improved the outcome and

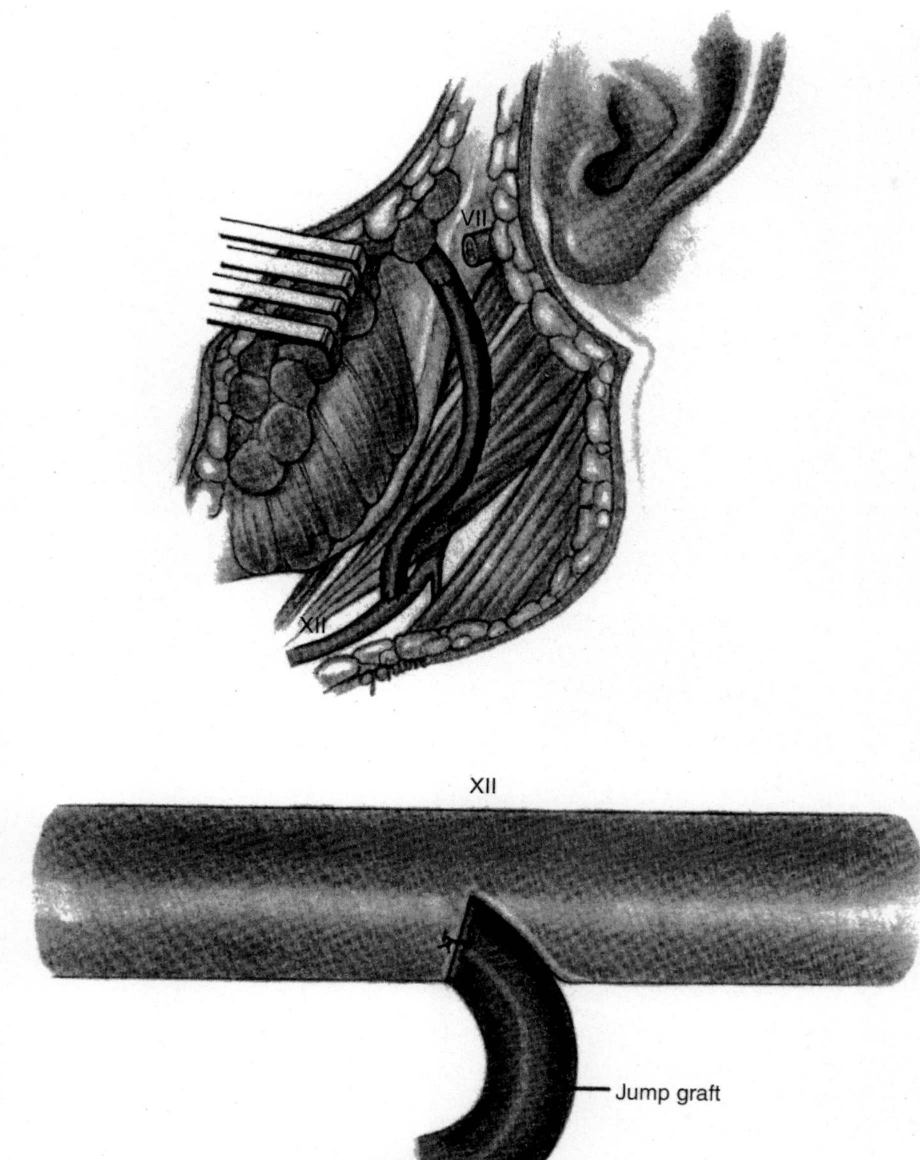

Fig. 63.8 Cranial nerve XII-to-VII crossover with jump graft. (**A**) Cranial nerve XII is isolated and exposed. (**B**) The adventitia and nerve sheath are incised. One third of the diameter of the nerve is sectioned with a slight inward bias toward the center of the cut. A deeper incision may allow for a better match in caliber between the incised hypoglossal and the facial nerve. In this situation, the proximal trunk of XII is stimulated electrically to assess whether the major motor fibers of XII remain intact. If they do remain intact, up to one half of XII can be incised to provide more donor axons. The incision in the nerve is widened 3 to 4 mm by gently pushing the distal portion of the incised nerve trunk away from the incision. The proximal portion of the sectioned nerve is not disturbed or back-elevated. A greater auricular nerve graft is sutured between the cut segment of XII and VII. Two sutures are placed between the graft and XII, one on each side of the incision. The graft is gently looped upward and anastomosed to VII. The greater auricular jump graft should be as long as possible to allow for two tensionless suture lines. (From Burgess LPA, Goode RL. Reanimation of the Paralyzed Face. New York: Thieme Medical Publishers; 1994:22. Reprinted by permission.)

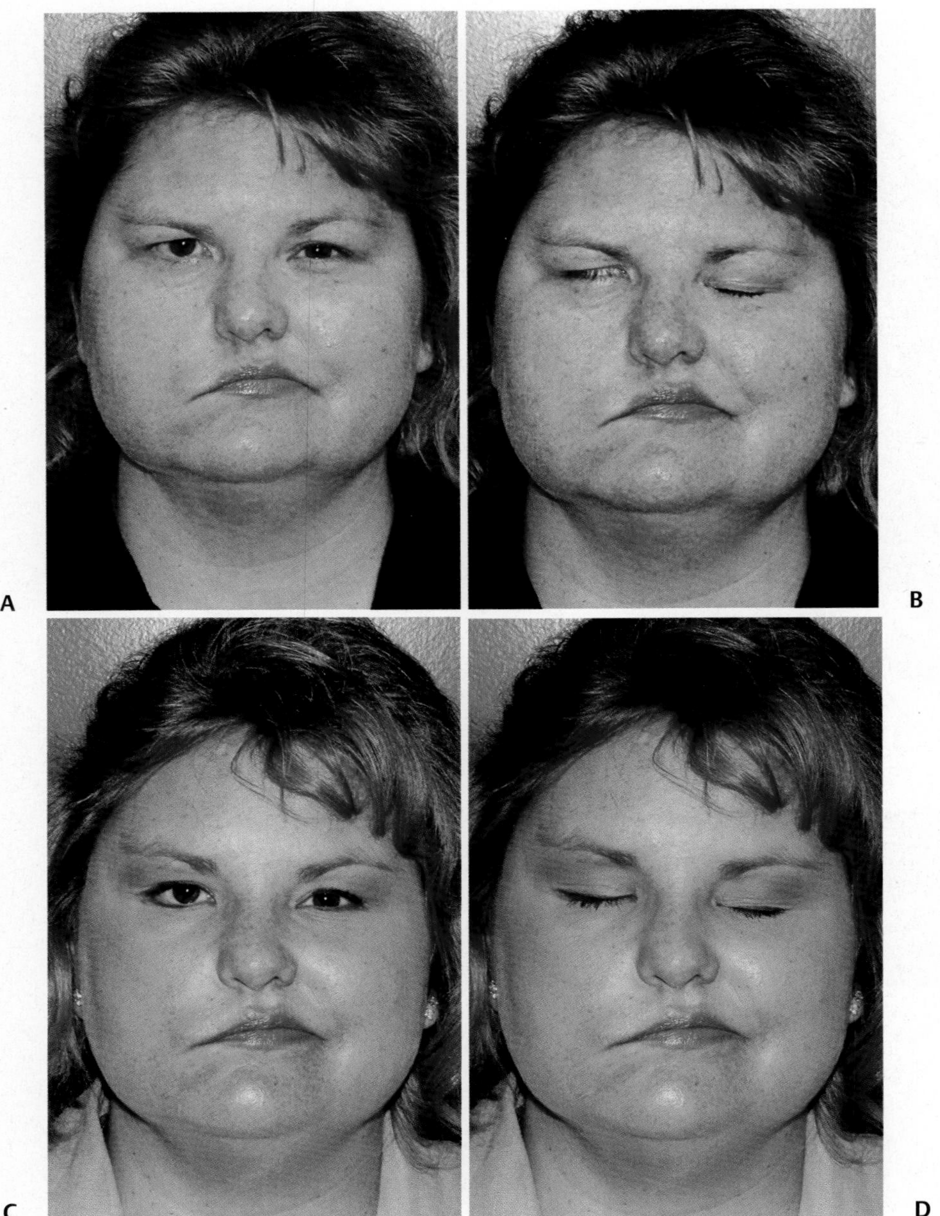

Fig. 63.9 Cranial nerve XII-to-VII "jump graft." Photographs **A** and **B** show patient before XII-to-VII jump graft, short flap facelift platinum upper eyelid weight, and endoscopic browlift. Photographs **C** and **D** are 4 years postoperative.

decreased the morbidity of the procedure.[80] They also concluded that better reanimation of the eye was achieved by techniques other than temporalis transfer and that they now use temporalis transfer exclusively for lower facial dynamic reanimation. Used as part of a comprehensive program to improve facial function, temporalis transfer provided good or excellent results in 80% and improved function in 96% of more than 200 patients.[80] Sherris has published a technical refinement of the temporalis muscle transfer that provides additional anchor points for the fascia at the midportion of the upper and lower lip.[81] This appears to further enhance lip contour of the paralyzed side.

Traditionally, one of the major criticisms of temporalis transfer has been about the bulge of muscle over the zygomatic arch, as well as the temporal defect. These problems were worse when the entire temporalis muscle was used; now most authors report transfer of only the middle third of the muscle. May and Drucker point out that making the tunnel wider so that the muscle lies

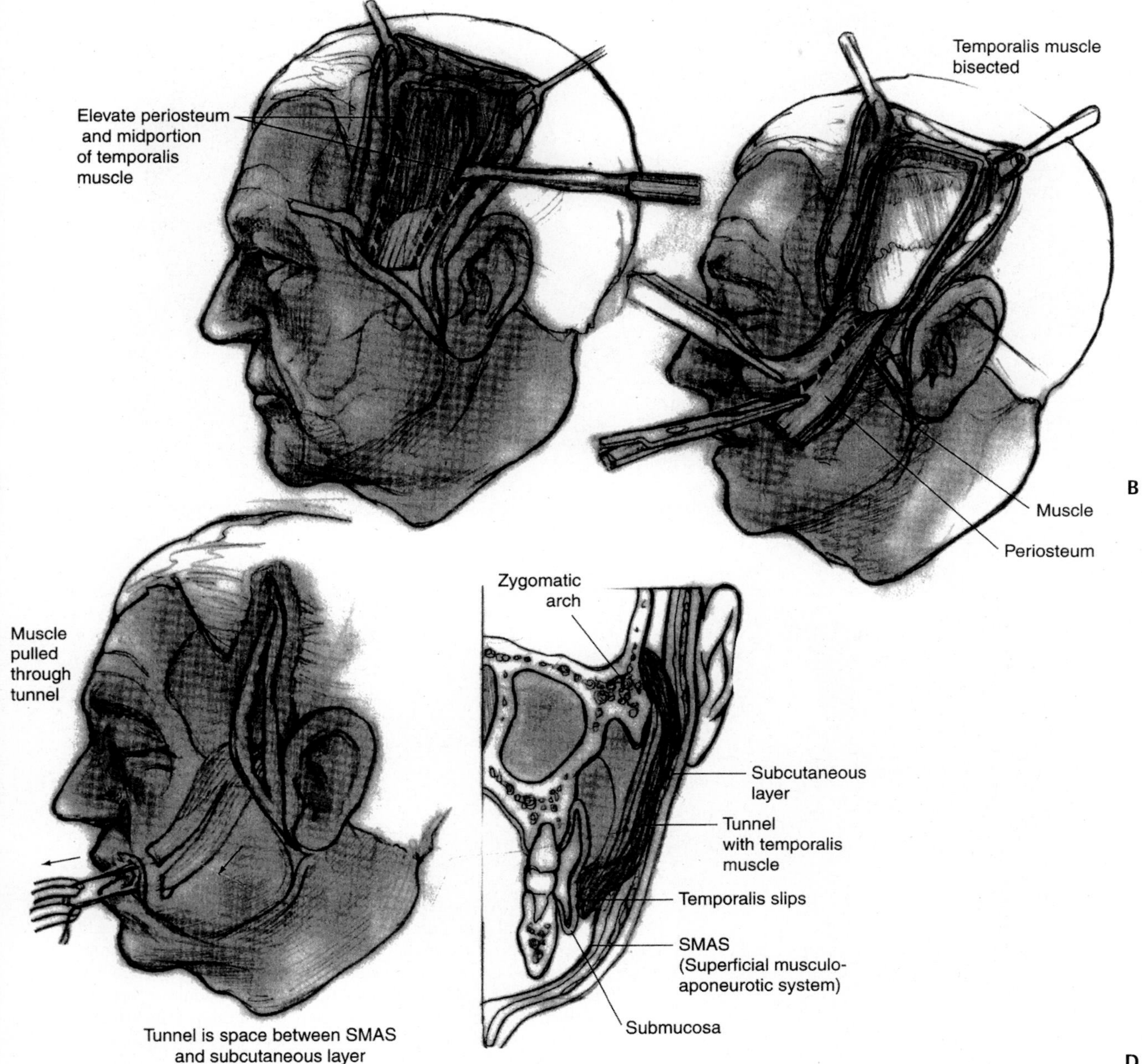

Fig. 63.10 Temporalis muscle transfer. (**A**) Elevate periosteum and middle one third of the temporalis muscle. (**B**) Periosteum and distal aspect of the bisected muscle are rotated inferiorly. (**C**) Tunnel to the ipsilateral oral commissure. Suture of the periosteum and muscle to the orbicularis oris muscle. (**D**) Coronal view of the tunnel.

flat in the tunnel significantly decreases the residual asymmetry.[80] Another problem is the gradual stretching of the muscle and loss of symmetry at the mouth. This may require a revision procedure to tighten the muscle.

The major drawback that remains with temporalis transfer is the persistent zygomatic bulge. Recently several authors have proposed alternative procedures using the temporalis muscle for facial reanimation. One of the most innovative solutions has been proposed by Labbé and Huault.[82] The "lengthening temporalis myoplasty" is based on a technique described by McLaughlin[83] and modified by Briedahl et al.[84] In this procedure, the entire temporalis muscle is mobilized and resuspended. After an osteotomy, the coronoid process and attached tendon

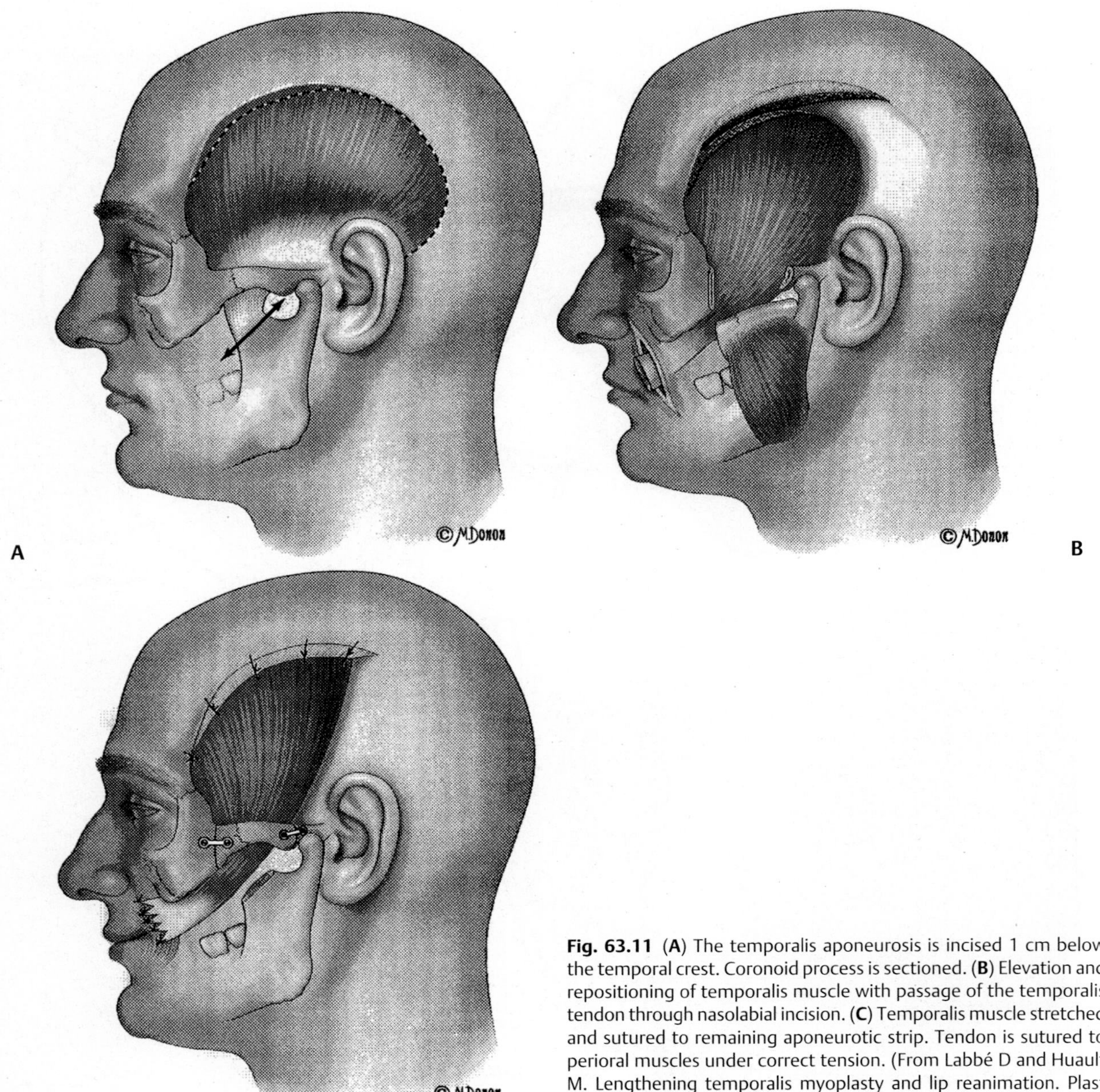

Fig. 63.11 (**A**) The temporalis aponeurosis is incised 1 cm below the temporal crest. Coronoid process is sectioned. (**B**) Elevation and repositioning of temporalis muscle with passage of the temporalis tendon through nasolabial incision. (**C**) Temporalis muscle stretched and sutured to remaining aponeurotic strip. Tendon is sutured to perioral muscles under correct tension. (From Labbé D and Huault M. Lengthening temporalis myoplasty and lip reanimation. Plast Reconstr Surg 2000;105(4):1289-1297. Reprinted by permission.)

are transferred through a cheek tunnel to the oral commissure. The coronoid is excised after pulling the tendon through a nasolabial incision, and the tendon is anchored to the perioral muscles, based on the patient's smile type (**Fig. 63.11**). The authors report favorable results in 10 patients.[82] Contreras-García et al have further modified Labbé's procedure by performing the temporalis lengthening through an endoscopic approach.[85]

An interesting phenomenon of trigeminal neoneurotization may be responsible for several cases reported in the literature in which patients achieved mimetic and more organized facial movement than would be expected following spontaneous facial nerve regeneration or segmental temporalis muscle transfer alone.[86,87] Rubin et al[86] recently reported 27 patients who after temporalis or masseter transfer could smile spontaneously without clenching their teeth. Cheney et al[87] recently reported a case in which a patient obtained lower facial muscle movement innervated by neurites from the ipsilateral masseter muscle. The literature pertaining to trigeminal neoneurotization is reviewed in this report.[87] In patients who have undergone facial nerve transection without attempt at nerve grafting but who later regain some mimetic movement, several authors have demonstrated reinnervation of the lower muscles of facial expression by the ipsilateral trigeminal nerve.[87] This reinnervation is enhanced by manipulation of the muscles of mastication, such as with temporalis muscle transfer. If this phenomenon were more predictable and reproducible, it would be very useful in the management of patients with facial paralysis.[88]

Static Rehabilitation

Although the static sling is used for lower facial rehabilitation to restore resting symmetry of the cheek and mouth and may improve oral sphincteric competence, it provides no dynamic change during smiling. This technique is generally thought to provide inferior functional outcomes in comparison with free-muscle transplantation or temporalis transposition, but it may be employed when the other techniques are not feasible.

Autologous tissue, such as fascia lata, has been used as a sling material but requires overcorrection during placement and may cause poor results due to unpredictable stretching, in addition to donor site morbidity and increased surgical time.[89] Other authors have reported favorable results, with less need for overcorrection using Gore-Tex[45,90,91] (see **Fig. 63.13**). However, patients receiving radiation therapy may be at increased risk for infection and extrusion of alloplastic implant material, such as Gore-Tex.[89]

Fisher and Frodel reported the use of acellular human dermal allograft (AHD allograft; AlloDerm, LifeCell Corp., Branchburg, NJ) for static facial slings in 11 patients.[89] They found that in addition to the fact that AHD allograft allows ingrowth of host tissue and the eventual replacement of the facial sling by host tissue, there was no need for overcorrection, which allowed for much more predictable results and no initially poor cosmetic results. Ninety percent of the patients in their series eventually had good or excellent results, and 100% reported functional improvements in mastication and oral competence. No patient had an infection or implant extrusion, despite exposure to radiation therapy in more than half.

Surgical Technique for Static Facial Sling

The technique outlined below is described by Fisher and Frodel.[89]

The preauricular incision is made in the temporal region just anterior to the base of the helical crus. A subcutaneous tunnel to a second incision located in the proposed new nasolabial fold is created. This incision is indicated in patients with a well-developed contralateral nasolabial fold; no nasolabial incision is created in patients without a well-developed nasolabial fold. The sling material of choice is then sutured to the orbicularis oris muscle, if present, or to the subcutaneous tissue, and to the lateral aspects of the upper and lower lips. Tension is then applied in a superoposterolateral direction to assess for symmetry with the contralateral side. Overcorrection is necessary for implant materials other than AHD allograft. Then the sling is secured to the periosteum of the zygoma with permanent sutures (**Fig. 63.12**).

The authors have utilized an alternative approach in some patients, making a small incision over the malar eminence and initiating the tunnel at this location. A screw can then be placed in the bone if Gore-Tex is used. The small zygomatic incision and larger melolabial incisions are closed, and drains are generally unnecessary.

Microvascular Free Tissue Transfer

The plastic surgery literature advocates free-muscle transplantation as the treatment of choice for longstanding facial paralysis.[92–98] Free-muscle transplantation offers the advantage of restoration of some emotional animation in addition to good tone in repose and some voluntary facial movement. Despite the theoretical advantages over transposition flaps, and despite immense efforts in both basic science and clinical research, prediction of the functional capability of the transferred muscle unit is as yet unattainable.[92] There have been no studies comparing the functional outcomes of free-muscle transplantation and muscle transposition techniques. Comparison of studies that use muscle transposition with free-muscle transplantation is difficult due to the lack of uniformity of grading systems to assess the functional and cosmetic results. In fact, there are nearly as many grading systems as there are techniques for reanimation.[98]

The evolution toward free-muscle transplantation for facial paralysis began nearly 30 years ago with the introduction of the cross-facial nerve graft, popularized by Anderl.[68] In 1976, Harii et al were the first to describe the use of free-muscle transplantation for reanimation of the paralyzed face, connecting a branch of the ipsilateral deep temporal nerve to the nerve of the transferred gracilis muscle.[99] Although the ipsilateral facial nerve would be the most desirable motor source for innervation of the transferred muscle, the clinical situations in which this would be applicable are quite limited. In subsequent reports, many different donor muscles have been utilized in two-stage procedures employing a cross-facial nerve graft in the first procedure and a free-muscle transplant in the second stage.[92,97,98]

The technique for cross-facial nerve grafting was originally described as an independent reanimation technique. However, as previously mentioned, the results in cases of longstanding paralysis were poor due to denervation

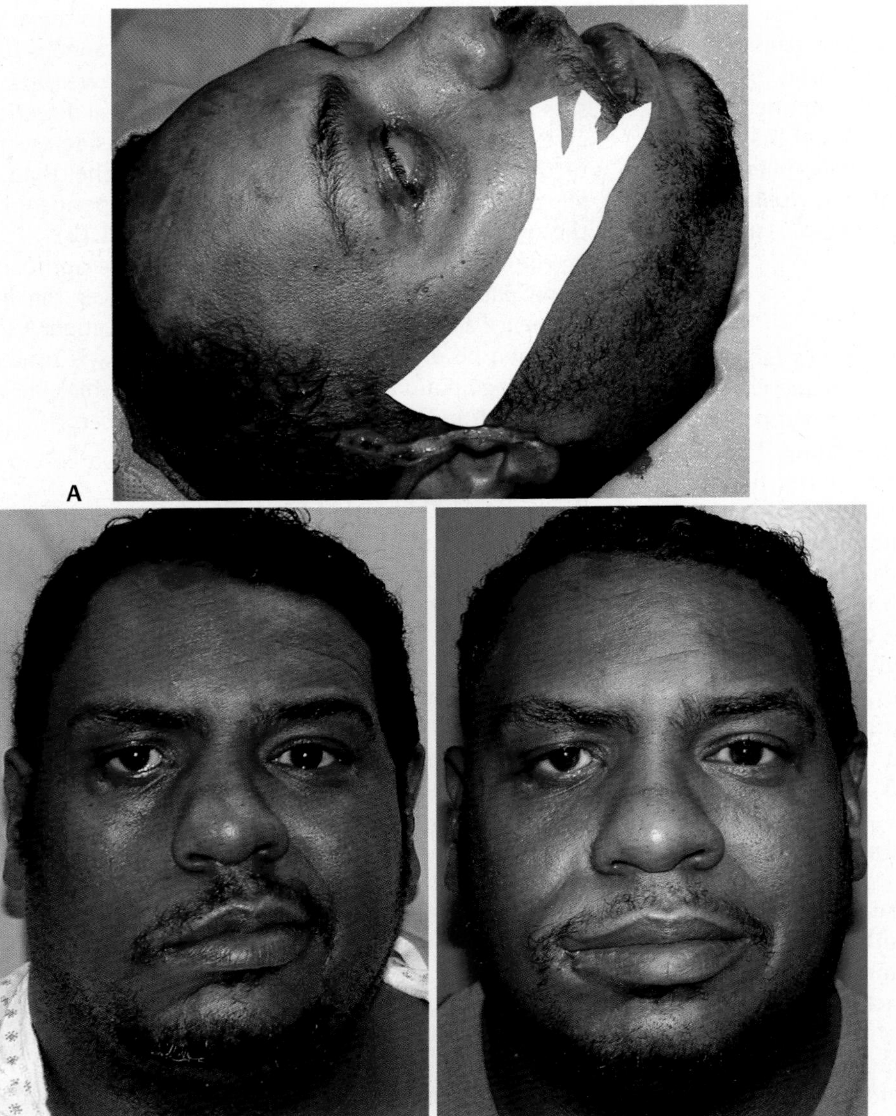

Fig. 63.12 Gortex static sling. (**A**) demonstrates proper vector and placement of Gortex intraoperatively through a male facelift incision. (**B**) and (**C**) demonstrate overall improvement in facial symmetry before and after static sling procedure.

atrophy and because of the time required for regenerating axons to traverse the nerve graft and reach the paralyzed side of the face.[100] Also, the number of axons is halved through each anastomosis; therefore, two anastomoses are felt by some to provide an inadequate neurite cell population to create detectable movement.

For successful reanimation with cross-facial grafting, an additional procedure may be necessary to maintain the paralyzed muscles until the regenerating axons can reach the motor end plates. Facial muscle tone can be maintained with nerve transposition techniques (as described previously). For example, a split XII-to-VII transposition can maintain the tone of the facial muscles and therefore "baby-sit" the paralyzed side of the face while the regenerating nerve fibers traverse the cross-face nerve graft.[101] Once the cross-facial nerve graft is in place, the XII–VII transposition can be divided.

Currently, the state of the art in free-muscle transplantation is in flux. Some favor a two-stage procedure, using a cross-face nerve graft in the first stage and anastomosis to a free-muscle transfer in the second stage. A more recently described single-stage procedure uses a long nerve pedicle that is grafted to contralateral buccal branches at the time of the free-muscle transfer.

General Plan for Two-Stage Technique

The two-stage technique employs a sural nerve graft from the contralateral buccal branches of the intact facial nerve, tunneled subcutaneously to the cheek on the paralyzed side.

After 4 to 6 months, Tinel's sign is used to clinically assess the growth of the axons along the nerve graft. This sign is elicited by percussing the nerve graft from distal to proximal until percussion produces distal tingling.[102] The zone of distal tingling does not exceed 2 to 3 cm, and the location of this zone corresponds to the location of the regenerating axons. It is generally recommended that an additional 3-month delay be allowed before beginning the second stage so that the maximum number of axons are available at the time of free-muscle transplantion.[98] Therefore, the total time between the two stages is usually 9 to 12 months.

The second stage involves a two-team approach whereby one team prepares the paralyzed side of the face for receiving the graft and the other team harvests the donor muscle and its neurovascular pedicle.

The disadvantages to the two-stage approach are unpredictability of the function of the transplanted muscle, sural nerve donor site scar, lower leg and foot hypesthesia, long delay awaiting the second stage, vascular anastomotic complications, and scar formation on the nonparalyzed side of the face.

Surgical Technique for Two-Stage Technique

Stage One

The sural nerve is located posterior to the lateral malleolus and anterior to the Achilles' tendon deep to the lesser saphenous vein system. The nerve is identified in this location and can be traced proximally and distally through either stair-step or longitudinal incisions. It may also be harvested endoscopically. The nerve may be raised with scissors and a nerve hook or by the use of a small tendon stripper.[59]

While the harvest site is closed, peripheral buccal branches of the facial nerve on the normal side are exposed through a preauricular approach. Others have used incisions immediately over the peripheral branches or through the melolabial folds.[59] Several fascicles (~50% of fibers) are transected and anastomosed to the sural nerve graft (which is in reverse orientation). The distal end of the sural nerve graft is tunneled subcutaneously to the other side (paralyzed side) of the face, usually through the upper lip, although forehead and lower lip tunnels have also been used. The distal end of the sural nerve graft is then tagged with a hemaclip for ease of identification at the second stage.

Stage Two

The technique described below is that of O'Brien et al.[97]

The most commonly used muscle in the two-stage technique is the gracilis muscle. It is exposed through an incision made posterior to the line joining the adductor tubercle to the medial condyle. This corresponds to the posterior margin of the adductor longus muscle, which is tensed on abduction of the thigh. The vascular pedicle is identified on the anterior border of the gracilis at the junction of the upper quarter and lower three quarters of the muscle. The vascular pedicle is then traced to the lateral side of the adductor longus, where it meets the profunda vessels. It is then mobilized, with division of all branches from it to the adductor longus muscle. The nerve to the gracilis from the anterior branch of the obturator nerve is traced to the obturator foramen. Reduction of the muscle is performed prior to transfer in situ, securing hemostasis before the vascular pedicle is divided and thereby reducing the risk of facial hematoma following transfer.

The length of the muscle required is measured and marked on the donor muscle. The neurovascular pedicle divides into two or three branches before entering the muscle. One of these vascular branches is ligated, and a nerve branch is divided. The segment of muscle supplied by them is separated by splitting of the muscle along its fibers. About one half to two thirds of the muscle with the main vascular pedicle is used as the graft.

If the graft is used to reanimate the whole hemiface, it is necessary to separate the muscle as two motor units; one third of the muscle is used for the upper face, and the other two thirds is used for the lower face. However, as previously discussed, better functional results are obtained when different methods are used to address the eye and the mouth.

The paralyzed side of the face is exposed by a modified facelift incision. The skin flap is elevated anteriorly to expose the upper lip and angle of the mouth, carefully preserving the cross-face nerve graft. The superficial temporal vessels are then exposed and prepared for anastomosis. The gracilis muscle is transferred to the face with the neurovascular pedicle on the deep surface, facilitating further debulking, if necessary. The distal end of the gracilis is divided into two segments and sutured with 4–0 Prolene (Ethicon, Inc., Somerville, NJ) to the muscles of the lateral aspect and angle of the mouth. Intraoperative traction on the orbicularis muscle determines the most appropriate area for attachment of the gracilis muscle. In the lip, this lateral attachment avoids adherence of the central lip. Insertion into the dermis of the nasolabial line is not recommended because this concentrates the muscle action into this line, creating asymmetry. The proximal muscle is then attached to the zygomatic arch, extending medially below the orbital margin to give a more vertical lift to the upper lip. The muscle is sutured under slight tension to slightly overcorrect the deformity.

The vessels are sutured to the facial or superficial temporal vessels and the nerve graft is joined with epineural sutures to the appropriate segment of the nerve to the gracilis. The wounds are closed with two suction drains placed above and below the muscle graft, lightly sutured in place to avoid proximity to the vessels.

General Plan for Single-Stage Procedure

To overcome the drawbacks of the two-stage method of free-muscle transfer, several authors have more recently reported the one-stage free-muscle transfer, in which the motor nerve is directly crossed through the face and sutured to the contralateral facial nerve branches. This technique has been described using several different donor muscles: the latissimus dorsi, the gracilis, the rectus femoris, and the abductor hallucis longus muscles.[93] The relative advantages and disadvantages of use of the most popular muscles for free-muscle transfer are summarized in **Table 63.2**. Because there is anatomical support for the latissimus dorsi,[93,96] and because the largest series of patients reported to date employing the single-stage method used the latissimus dorsi muscle,[93] this is the technique that will be discussed.

The advantages of the single-stage technique over the two-stage are one neural anastomosis, no sural nerve donor site morbidity, and most importantly, earlier time to facial movement with diminished duration of the psychological, social, and economic sequelae.

Surgical Technique for Single-Stage Procedure

The technique described here is drawn from the work of Harii et al.[93]

Through a preauricular incision on the paralyzed side of the face, the subcutaneous tissues of the cheek are elevated superficial to the parotid fascia and SMAS. This creates a subcutaneous pocket to accept the subsequent muscle transfer. The undermining subcutaneously extends ~1 to 2 cm beyond the nasolabial fold to the upper and lower lips. The lateral portion of the atrophied orbicularis oris muscle and the modiolus are also exposed. Several stay sutures are then placed at the lateral border of the atrophying orbicularis oris muscle, in the upper and lower lips, and in the modiolus. A newly created nasolabial fold, which should correspond to the contralateral nasolabial fold, is made visible by pulling these stay sutures toward the zygomatic region. Thus the fixation position of the end of the transferred muscle segment is determined. To secure the muscle fixation to the appropriate position in the nasolabial and lateral lip regions, a pull-out suspension suture is placed between the deep subcutaneous tissue at the corner of the mouth and the skin either behind the ear lobe or in the temporal region. A small portion of the subcutaneous tissue over the zygoma is excised to accommodate the bulkiness when the other end of the transferred muscle segment is anchored to the zygoma.

Another small incision, ~2 to 3 cm long, is placed at the submandibular region to expose the facial artery

Table 63.2 Muscles Used for Facial Reanimation with Microvascular Techniques

Donor Site	Blood Supply/Pedicle Length and Anatomical Reliability	Nerve Supply and Length	Advantages	Disadvantages
Extensordigitorum brevis	Dorsalis pedis artery and vein, 3–4 cm, reliable	Lateral branch, deep peroneal nerve, 3–4 cm	...	Insufficient bulk, inadequate contraction strength, short pedicle
Gracilis	Branches of profunda femoris, 5–8 cm, reliable	Anterior branch, obturator nerve, 10 cm	Can trim muscle in situ independent neuromuscular units	Bulky
Latissimus dorsi	Thoracodorsal artery and vein, 8–10 cm, reliable	Thoracodorsal nerve, 13–14 cm	Segmental innervation, can trim in situ	Bulky
Pectoralis major	Thoracoacromial artery and vein, 4–6 cm, reliable	Lateral pectoral nerve, 4–5 cm	...	Bulky, short pedicle
Pectoralis minor	Axillary artery and vein (direct branches) or lateral thoracic artery or vein or thoracoacromial artery and vein, 4–5 cm, variable	Medial and lateral pectoral nerve, 4–5 cm	Dual nerve supply, ideal form, weight, and shape	Debulking not possible in situ; short, complex neurovascular pedicle
Rectus abdominis	Deep inferior epigastric artery and vein, 6–10 cm, reliable	Segmental thoracic intercostal nerve, 3–15 cm	Tendinous inscriptions, segmental innervation	Bulky
Serratus anterior	Branches of thoracodorsal artery and vein, 4–5 cm, reliable	Long thoracic nerve, 9 cm	Segmental innervation	Bulky

Source: Adapted from Aviv JE, Urken ML. Management of the paralyzed face with microneurovascular free muscle transfer. Arch Otolaryngol Head Neck Surg 1992;118:909–912.

and vein as the recipient vessels. The final incision, ~2 cm in length, is then made on the nonparalyzed side of the face at the anterior margin of the parotid gland to expose several zygomatic and buccal branches of the intact nerve. With a nerve stimulator, a few branches innervating mainly the zygomatic and levator labii muscles are made ready for the recipient motor nerve from the free graft.

During preparation of the recipient cheek, the other team harvests the latissimus dorsi muscle segment. Through an incision along the posterior axillary line, the neurovascular pedicle of the latissimus dorsi muscle is first exposed. To obtain sufficient length of the thoracodorsal nerve (usually ~15 cm), the nerve is traced proximally to its origin from the posterior cord of the brachial plexus and distally to the muscle. If necessary, more proximal smaller twigs of the nerve may be sacrificed to obtain adequate length. After complete dissection of the neurovascular pedicle, a muscle segment of the appropriate size (usually 3 to 4 cm wide and 8 to 10 cm long in moderate stretch of the muscle) is harvested, dividing the proximal and distal muscle with a disposable stapler. Any sculpting of the muscle should be performed prior to dividing the vascular pedicle in situ to secure hemostasis and minimize risk for postoperative hematoma in the recipient cheek.

The harvested muscle is transferred to the recipient cheek pocket. The proximal end is fixed to the nasolabial region with the previously placed stay sutures, with the neurovascular pedicle positioned proximally and in reversed orientation. The thoracodorsal nerve is passed through the upper lip using a nerve passer and anastomosed to the contralateral intact nerve branches. Microvascular anastomoses are then performed between the thoracodorsal vessels and the recipient facial vessels in an end-to-end fashion. Finally, the distal end of the muscle is fixed to the zygoma, giving proper tension to the muscle.[92] The wounds are closed with suction drainage in both the donor and recipient wounds.

Adjunctive Procedures

The procedures described previously constitute the fundamental, or "workhorse," procedures in reanimation. Those procedures provide basic symmetry to the two major segments of the paralyzed face (eye and mouth). The following are "touch-up" procedures, valuable in attempting to return the patient with facial paralysis to as close to a normal appearance and function as possible. In general, these procedures can be performed separately or concurrently with the previously described procedures, and with experience, the facial plastic surgeon can visualize the optimal combination of workhorse and touch-up procedures for a specific patient's situation.

Upper Face Procedures

Brow ptosis can contribute significantly to the overall asymmetry of the paralyzed face and may be even more noticeable after the mid- and lower face have been addressed. Correction of the ptosis is accomplished with a unilateral or bilateral browlift. The browlift can be approached using an endoscopic, direct, midforehead, or pretrichial approach. In addition to the static lift, Rubin has added a slip of contralateral frontalis muscle to provide some motion and correction to the medial brow (**Fig. 63.13**).[103]

One important consideration regarding the browlift is that the lift must be conservative, due to the tendency of the browlift to potentially impede eye closure. As long as a gold weight is used and the browlift is conservative, eye closure is usually not a problem.[59] Simultaneous browlift and insertion of an upper lid weight require preoperative manual elevation of the brow to the desired location while the gold weight is being sized.

Blepharoplasty may also be performed, but, as with browlift, it must be conservative.

The techniques for browlift and blepharoplasty are otherwise the same as for the nonparalyzed face and are described in Chapters 16 and 17.

Midface Procedures

Facelift has become a standard adjunctive procedure for facial reanimation. Due to the inherent skin laxity in the paralyzed face, even young patients often benefit significantly from a conservative facelift. The technique is similar to that used for the nonparalyzed face and is described in Chapter 15.

An endoscopic (or subciliary) subperiosteal midface lift is valuable in management of the paralytic lower eyelid/midfacial ptosis. Restoration of the lower eyelid position provides improved symmetry as well as alleviation of symptoms of exposure.[104]

Longstanding moderate or severe facial paralysis can result in ipsilateral nasal collapse, leading to nasal obstruction. Several techniques have been described to correct paralytic nasal obstruction. In the technique by Goode,[105] a carved piece of irradiated rib cartilage is placed in a pocket just cephalad to the ala from the piriform aperture to the nasal tip region to provide nasal valve support. In the technique by May,[47] the alar base is widened by using a strip of fascia lata or Gore-Tex to suspend the alar base from a hole in the lateral zygomatic prominence.

The technique that has been most successfully used by the primary author (JMC) is the "butterfly" graft. Conchal cartilage is used to support the caudal margin of the upper lateral cartilage as well as the cephalic margin of the lower lateral cartilage, usually inserted through an intercartilaginous incision.[106] The senior author (WWS) typically treats nasal valve collapse as a part of the static

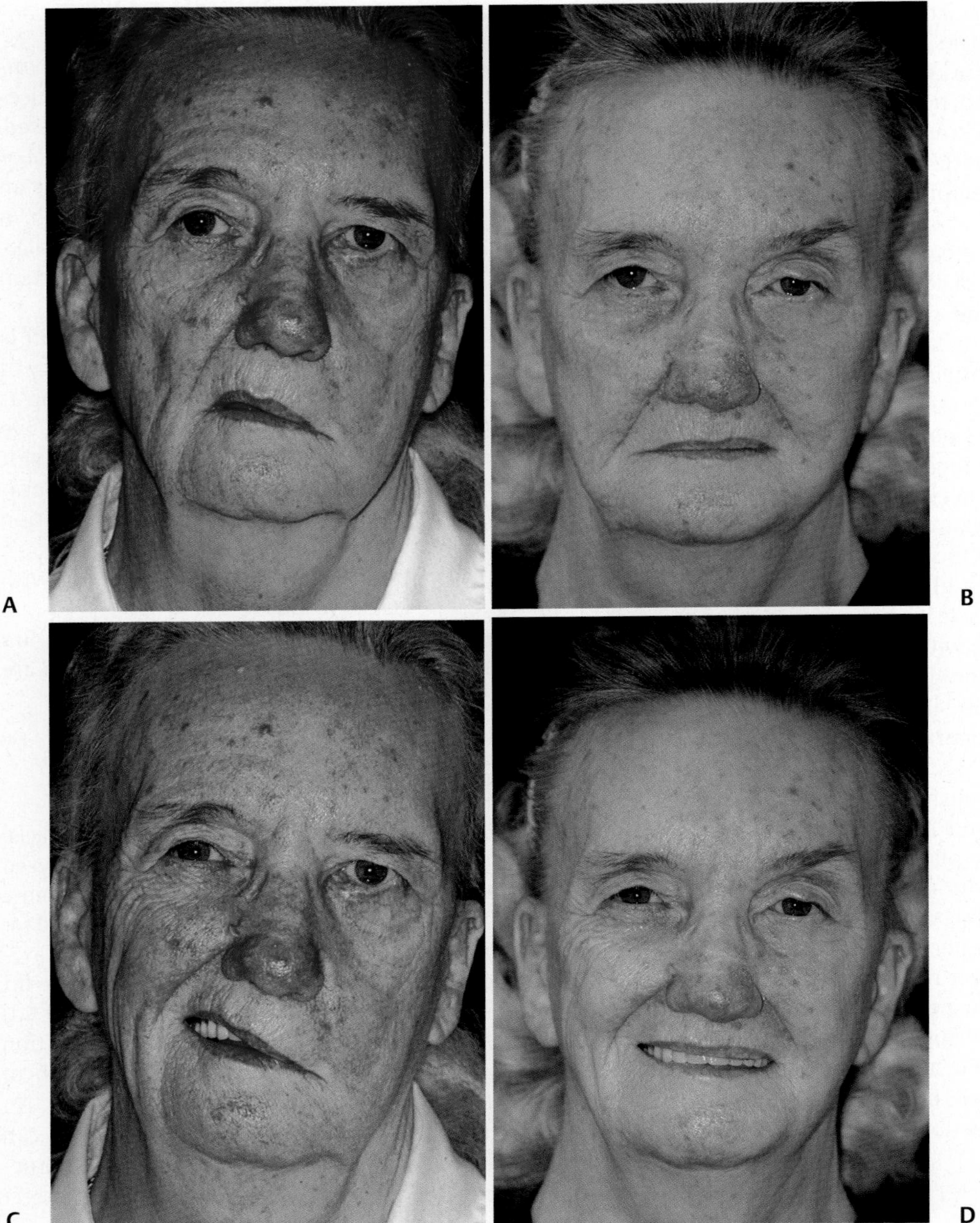

Fig. 63.13 Midforehead browlift and facelift for left facial paralysis. These photographs demonstrate the overall improvement of the face in repose and with smiling before and after left midforehead browlift, facelift, precaruncular canthoplasty, and upper eyelid weight. (**A**) and (**C**), and (**B**) and (**D**).

facial sling, with one of the Gore-Tex limbs anchored to the ipsilateral alar base, through a small perialar incision.

Lower Face Procedures

Loss of the action of the depressor anguli oris and the depressor labii inferioris results in an elevation of the lower lip, resulting in asymmetry, especially during smiling. This can be corrected by digastric transposition, as described by Conley et al.[107] In this procedure, the digastric tendon is identified and divided from the hyoid through a submandibular approach. The tendon is then split, transposed, and rotated upward to the lower lip and sutured to the orbicularis oris ~2 cm from the commissure through a separate vermilion border incision. This procedure, while innovative, is seldom used (**Fig. 63.14**).

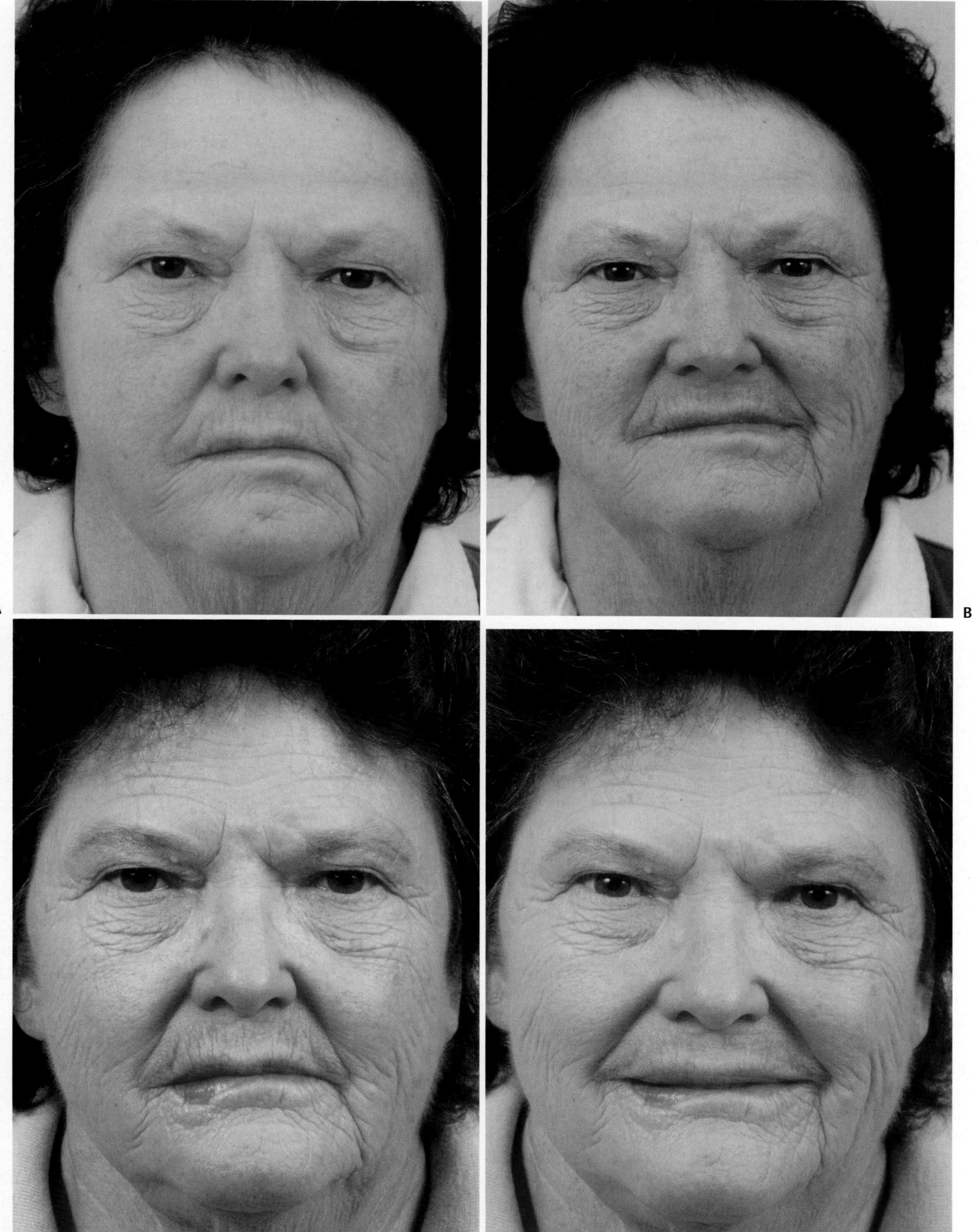

Fig. 63.14 A 62-year-old woman with an isolated right marginal mandibular nerve paralysis following resection of a parotid malignancy. (**A**) Weakness of the depressors of the right lower lip at rest. (**B**) Attempted smile. (**C**) Improved symmetry of the mouth and lips following digastric tendon transfer at rest. (**D**) Improved symmetry on attempted smile.

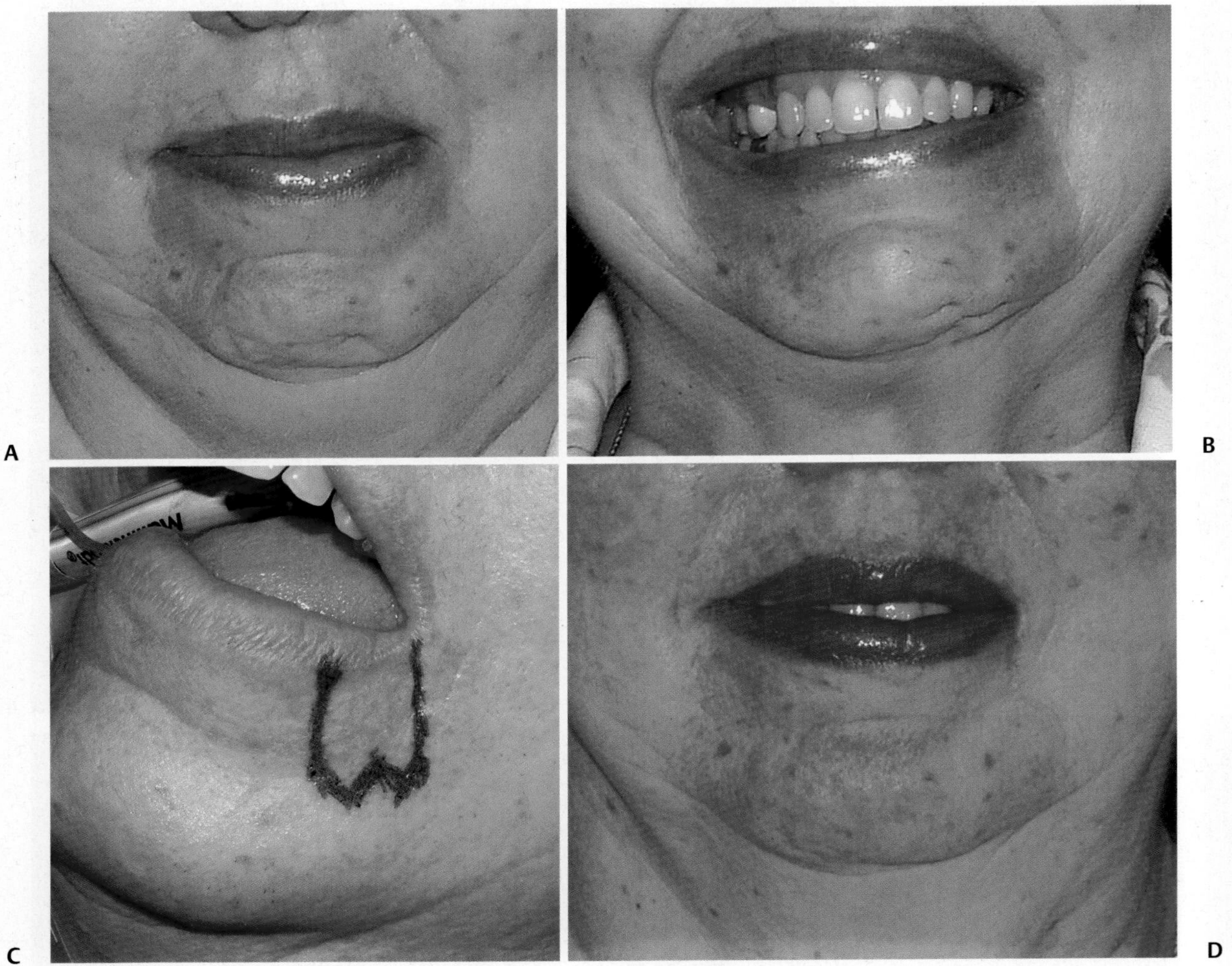

Fig. 63.15 Lower lip wedge excision. This 62-year-old patient with long-standing left facial paresis and difficulty with oral competence is shown in repose (**A**) and smiling (**B**). In (**C**), the proposed incisions are placed to avoid crossing the mentolabial crease. In (**D**), the scar from the wedge excision is well healed and placed in the marionette line.

Symmetry and oral competence can also be improved using the cheiloplasty technique, as described by Glenn and Goode.[108] In this procedure, a 2- to 2.5-cm full-thickness wedge is resected, with the lateral limb of the wedge 7 to 10 mm from the commissure (**Fig. 63.15**). For additional lower lip eversion, the vermilion border is advanced by excision of a horizontal ellipse of skin from the commissure to near-midline (**Fig. 63.16**).

Two final adjunctive procedures that can be used to achieve symmetry or to limit synkinesis are contralateral selective neurectomy[109] and selective myectomy.[110] The risk in performing either procedure is the potential loss of function, especially in oral competence, when the nonparalytic marginal mandibular nerve or its muscles are ablated. Recent evidence provided by Breslow et al suggests that selective marginal mandibular neurectomy of the nonparalyzed side in patients with unilateral facial paralysis improves symmetry with smiling without compromising oral competence.[111]

Summary

In conclusion, the patient with facial paralysis presents a challenging problem for the facial plastic surgeon. It is incumbent on those of us treating this complex disorder to be familiar with the psychosocial sequelae, the classification systems, the etiologic factors, the workup, the medical management, and the myriad of surgical procedures available to improve function and cosmesis in this patient population.

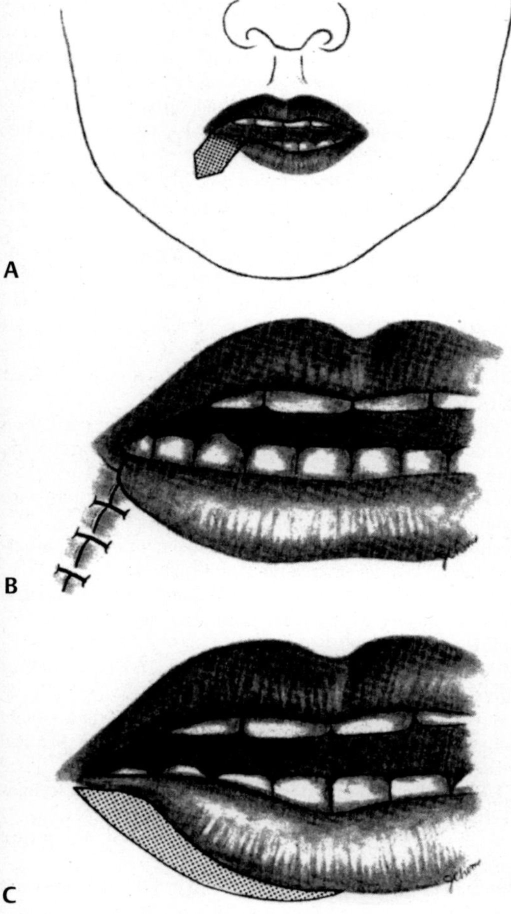

Fig. 63.16 Marginal mandibular nerve paralysis—cheiloplasty. (**A**) A wedge excision is outlined, with the lateral limb of the wedge placed 7 to 10 mm medial to the commissure. The wedge extends inferiorly ~2 cm and is 2.0 to 2.5 cm wide depending on the overall lip dimensions. These incisions do not cross the mentolabial crease. (**B**) The lateral incision is made first, and the exact amount of skin excision is determined by pulling the lip laterally. After excising the wedge, closure is accomplished in layers with interrupted 3–0 chromic or Vicryl (Ethicon, Inc.), similar 4–0 sutures in the subcutaneous layer, and 6–0 everting fast-absorbing gut sutures for skin closure. The vermilion is intentionally mismatched to produce the desired eversion of the lower lip medial to the incision line. Because this mismatch is placed laterally near the commissure, it is noted only on close inspection. (**C**) As an alternative to mismatching the vermilion or to add additional eversion, a horizontal cheiloplasty technique can be used to evert the lower lip. The amount of skin to be resected is carefully marked with the mouth half open. A horizontal ellipse of skin is excised from the lateral commissure to the midline or near the midline. This should not be overcorrected. (From Burgess LPA, Goode RL. Reanimation of the Paralyzed Face. New York: Thieme Medical Publishers; 1994:50. Reprinted by permission.)

Through an integrated approach, each patient may be offered a series of individualized surgical techniques to provide the optimal functional and cosmetic outcome.

References

1. Jackson CG, von Doersten PG. The facial nerve: current trends in diagnosis, treatment, and rehabilitation. Med Clin North Am 1999;83(1):179–195
2. Darwin C. Expression of emotions in man and animals. New York: Philosophical Library; 1955
3. Sadiq SA, Downes RN. A clinical algorithm for the management of facial nerve palsy from an oculoplastic perspective. Eye 1998;12(pt 2): 219–223
4. Kane N, Kazanas S, Maw A, et al. Functional outcome in patients after excision of extracanalicular acoustic neuromas using the suboccipital approach. Ann R Coll Surg Engl 1995;77:210–216
5. Jorgensen B, Pedersen C. Acoustic neuroma: follow-up of 78 patients. Clin Otolaryngol 1994;19:478–484
6. May M, Klein S. Differential diagnosis of facial nerve palsy. Otolaryngol Clin North Am 1991;24:613–644
7. Chang CY, Cass SP. Management of facial nerve injury due to temporal bone trauma. Am J Otol 1999;20(1):96–114
8. May M, Fria RJ, Blumenthal F, et al. Facial paralysis in children: differential diagnosis. Otolaryngol Head Neck Surg 1981;89:84–88
9. Smith JD, Crumley RL, Harker LA. Facial paralysis in the newborn. Otolaryngol Head Neck Surg 1981;89:336–342
10. House HP. The fenestration operation, a survey of 500 cases. Ann Otol Rhinol Laryngol 1948;57:41–54
11. Lee KJ, Schuknecht HF. Results of tympanoplasty and mastoidectomy at the Massachussetts Eye and Ear Infirmary. Laryngoscope 1971; 81:529–543
12. Gantz BJ, Rubinstein JT, Gidley P, Woodworth GG. Surgical management of Bell's palsy. Laryngoscope 1999;109:1177–1188
13. Murakami S, Mizobuchi M, Nakashiro Y, et al. Bell's palsy and herpes simplex virus: identification of viral DNA in endoneural fluid and muscle. Ann Intern Med 1996;124:27–30
14. Burgess RC, Michaels L, Bale JF Jr, et al. Polymerase chain reaction amplification of herpes simplex viral DNA from the geniculate ganglion of a patient with Bell's palsy. Ann Otol Rhinol Laryngol 1994;103:775–779
15. Adour K, Ruboyianes J, Von Doersten P, et al. Bell's palsy treatment with acyclovir and prednisone compared with prednisone alone: a double-blind, randomized, controlled trial. Ann Otol Rhinol Laryngol 1996;105:371–378
16. Tomat LR, Manktelow RT. Evaluation of a new measurement tool for facial paralysis reconstruction. Plast Reconstr Surg 2005;115:696–704
17. Murphy TP. MRI of the facial nerve during paralysis. Otolaryngol Head Neck Surg 1991;104:47–51
18. Sunderland S. Nerve and nerve injuries. 2nd ed. London: Churchill Livingstone; 1978:88–89, 96–97
19. Blumenthal F, May M. Electrodiagnosis. In: May M, ed. The facial Nerve. New York: Thieme Medical Publishers; 1986:241–263
20. May M, Blumenthal FS, Klein SR. Acute Bell's palsy: prognostic value of evoked electromyography, maximal stimulation, and other electrical tests. Am J Otol 1983;5(1):1–7

21. Luco JV, Eyzaquirre C. Fibrillation and hypersensitivity to Ach in denervated muscle: effect of length of degenerating nerve fibers. J Neurophysiol 1955;18:65
22. Fisch U. Total facial nerve decompression and electroneurography. In: Silverstein H, Norrell H, eds. Neurological surgery of the ear. Birmingham, AL: Aesculapius; 1977:21–33
23. Fisch U. Maximal nerve excitability testing vs electroneuronography. Arch Otolaryngol 1980;106:352–357
24. Coker NJ. Facial electroneuronography: analysis of techniques and correlation with degenerating motoneurons. Laryngoscope 1992;102: 747–759
25. Kartush J, Lundy L. Facial nerve outcome in acoustic neuroma surgery. [review] Otolaryngol Clin North Am 1992;25:623–647
26. May M, Croxson GR, Klein SR. Bell's palsy: management of sequelae using EMG rehabilitation, botulinum toxin, and surgery. Am J Otol 1989;10(3):220–229
27. Brady J. Biofeedback in facial paralysis: electromyographic rehabilitation. In: (ed). Reanimation techniques for the paralyzed face.
28. Brach JS, VanSwearingen JM. Physical therapy for facial paralysis: a tailored treatment approach. Phys Ther 1999;79(4):397–404
29. Miehlke A, Stennert E, Chilla R. Postoperative management of facial paresis. Clin Plast Surg 1979;6:465–470
30. Balliet R, Shinn JB, Bach-y-Rita P. Facial paralysis rehabilitation: retraining selective muscle control. Int Rehabil Med 1982;4:67–74
31. Brown DM, Nahai F, Wolf S, et al. Electromyographic biofeedback in the reeducation of facial palsy. Am J Phys 1978;57(5):183–190
32. Brudny J, Hammerschlag PE, Cohen NL, et al. Electromyographic rehabilitation of facial function and introduction of a facial paralysis grading scale for hypoglossal–facial nerve anastomosis. Laryngoscope 1988;98:405–410
33. Hammerschlag PE, Brudny J, Cusumano R, et al. Hypoglossal–facial nerve anastomosis and electromyographic feedback rehabilitation. Laryngoscope 1987;97:705–709
34. Walravens S. Using EMG biofeedback in the treatment of facial paralysis. Acta Otorhinolaryngol Belg 1986;40(1):1974–1977
35. Balliet R. Facial paralysis and other neuromuscular dysfunctions of the peripheral nervous system. In: Payton OD, ed. Manual of Physical Therapy Techniques. New York: Churchill Livingstone; 1987:41–76
36. Ross B, Nedzelski JM, McLean JA. Efficacy of feedback training in long-standing facial nerve paralysis. Laryngoscope 1991;101:744–750
37. Van Swearingen JM, Brach JS. Validation of a treatment-based classification system for individuals with facial neuromotor disorders. Phys Ther 1998;78(7):678–689
38. Mosforth J, Taverner D. Physiotherapy for Bell's palsy. BMJ 1958;2: 675–677
39. Jansen JK, Lomo T, Nicolaysen K, et al. Hyperinnervation of skeletal muscle fibers: dependence on muscle activity. Science 1973;181:559–561
40. Boroojerdi B, Ferbert A, Schwartz M, et al. Botulinum toxin treatment of synkinesia and hyperlacrimation after facial palsy. J Neurol Neurosurg Psychiatry 1998;65:111–114
41. Borodic GE, Pearce LB, Cheney M, et al. Botulinum A toxin for treatment of aberrant facial nerve regeneration. Plast Reconstr Surg 1993;91:1042–1045
42. Buncke HJ. Facial paralysis. In: Buncke HJ, ed. Microsurgery: transplantation—replantation. Philadelphia: Lea & Febiger, 1991: 488–506
43. Putterman AM. Botulinum toxin injections in the treatment of seventh nerve misdirection. Am J Ophthalmol 1990;110:205–206
44. Dressler D, Schonle PW. Botulinum toxin to suppress hyperkinesias after hypoglossal-facial nerve anastomosis. Eur Arch Otorhinolaryngol 1990;247:391–392
45. Moser G, Oberasher G. Reanimation of the paralyzed face with new gold weight implants and Gore-Tex soft-tissue patches. Eur Arch Otorhinolaryngol 1997;254(suppl 1):S76–S78
46. Inigo F, Chapa P, Jimenez Y, et al. Surgical treatment of lagophthalmos in facial palsy: ear cartilage graft for elongating the levator palpebrae muscle. Br J Plast Surg 1996;49:452–456
47. May M. Surgical rehabilitation of facial palsy: total approach. In: May M, ed. The facial nerve. New York: Thieme Medical Publishers; 1986:695–777
48. Ellis DA, Kleiman LA. Assessment and treatment of the paralyzed lower eyelid. Arch Otolaryngol Head Neck Surg 1993;119:1338–1344
49. Gilliland GD, Wobig JL, Dailey RA. A modified surgical technique in the treatment of facial nerve palsies. Ophthal Plast Reconstr Surg 1998;14(2):94–98
50. Casler JD, Conley J. Simultaneous "dual system" rehabilitation in the treatment of facial paralysis. Arch Otolaryngol Head Neck Surg 1990;116:199–203
51. Freeman MS, Thomas JR, Spector GJ, et al. Surgical therapy of the eyelids in patients with facial paralysis. Laryngoscope 1990; 100:1086–1096
52. Moe KS. The precaruncular approach to the medial orbit. Arch Facial Plast Surg 2003;5(6):483–487
53. Moe KS, Kao CH. Precaruncular medial canthopexy. Arch Facial Plast Surg 2005;7(4):244–250
54. Moe KS, Linder T. The lateral transorbital canthopexy for correction and prevention of ectropion: report of a procedure, grading system, and outcome study. Arch Facial Plast Surg 2000;2(1):9–15
55. Sheehan JD. Progress in correction of facial palsy with tantalum wire and mesh. Surgery 1950;27:122–129
56. Jobe R. A technique for lid-loading in the management of lagophthalmos in facial palsy. Plast Reconstr Surg 1974;53:29–31
57. Sobol SM, Alward PD. Early gold weight lid implant for rehabilitation of faulty eyelid closure with facial paralysis: an alternative to tarsorrhaphy. Head Neck 1990;12:149–153
58. Kao CH, Moe KS. Retrograde weight implantation for correction of lagophthalmos. Laryngoscope 2004;114:1570–1575
59. Burgess LPA, Goode RL. Total facial paralysis. In: Burgess LPA, Goode RL, eds. Reanimation of the paralyzed face. New York: Thieme Medical Publishers; 1994:11–26
60. Barrs DM. Facial nerve trauma: optimal timing for repair. Laryngoscope 1991;101:835–848
61. May M. Facial reanimation after skull base trauma. Am J Otol 1985;(suppl):62–67
62. May M. Management of cranial nerves I through VII following skull base surgery. Otolaryngol Head Neck Surg 1980;88:560–575
63. Anonsen CK, Duckert LG, Cumming CW. Preliminary observations after facial rehabilitation with the ansa hypoglossi pedicle transfer. Otolaryngol Head Neck Surg 1986;94:302–305
64. Griebie MS, Huff JS. Selective role of partial XI–VII anastomosis in facial reanimation. Laryngoscope 1998;108:1664–1668
65. Szal GJ, Miller T. Surgical repair of facial nerve branches. Arch Otolaryngol 1975;101:160–165
66. Fisch U, Lanser MJ. Facial nerve grafting. Otolaryngol Clin North Am 1991;24(3):691–708
67. Malik TH, Kelly G, Ahmed A, Saeed SR, Ramsden RT. A comparison of surgical techniques used in dynamic reanimation of the paralyzed face. Otol Neurotol 2005;26:284–291
68. Anderl H. Cross-face nerve grafting: up to 12 months of seventh nerve disruption. In: Rubin LR, ed. Reanimation of the Paralyzed Face. St. Louis: CV Mosby; 1977:241–277
69. Conley J, Baker DC. Hypoglossal–facial nerve anastomosis for reinnervation of the paralyzed face. Plast Reconstr Surg 1979;63:63–72
70. Gary-Bobo A, Fuentes JM. Long-term follow-up report on cross-facial nerve grafting in the treatment of facial paralysis. Br J Plast Surg 1983;36:48–50
71. Fisch U. Cross-face grafting in facial paralysis. Arch Otolaryngol 1976;102:453–457
72. Anderl H. Rehabilitation of the face by VIIth nerve substitution. In: Fisch U, ed. Facial Nerve Surgery. Amstelveen, the Netherlands: Kugler Medical Publications BV; 1977: 245–249
73. Mattox DE, Felix H, Fisch U, et al. Effect of ligating peripheral branches on facial nerve regeneration. Otolaryngol Head Neck Surg 1988;6: 558–563

74. Fisch U, Esslen E. The surgical treatment of facial hyperkinesia. Arch Otolaryngol 1972;95:400–405
75. Stennert E. Hypoglossal facial anastomosis: its significance for modern facial surgery. Clin Plast Surg 1979;6:471–486
76. Poe DS, Scher N, Panje WR. Facial reanimation by XII–VII anastomosis without shoulder paralysis. Laryngoscope 1989;99:1040–1047
77. Baker DC. Hypoglossal–facial nerve anastomosis indications and limitations. In: Portmann M, ed. Proceedings of the Fifth International Symposium on the Facial Nerve. New York: Masson; 1985: 526–529
78. May M, Sobol SM, Mester SJ. Hypoglossal–facial nerve interpositional-jump graft for facial reanimation without tongue atrophy. Otolaryngol Head Neck Surg 1991;104(6):818–825
79. Conley J. The treatment of long-standing facial paralysis—a new concept. Trans Am Acad Ophth Otol 1974;78:386–392
80. May M, Drucker C. Temporalis muscle for facial reanimation. Arch Otolaryngol Head Neck Surg 1993;119:378–382
81. Sherris DA. Refinement in reanimation of the lower face. Arch Facial Plast Surg 2004;6:49–53
82. Labbé D, Huault M. Lengthening temporalis myoplasty and lip reanimation. Plast Reconstr Surg 2000;105(4):1289–1297
83. McLaughlin CR. Surgical support in permanent facial paralysis. Plast Reconstr Surg 1953;11:302
84. Breidahl AF, Morrison WA, Donato RR, Riccio M, Theile DR. A modified surgical technique for temporalis transfer. Br J Plast Surg 1996; 49:46–51
85. Contreras-García R, Martins PD, Braga-Silva J. Endoscopic approach for lengthening the temporalis muscle. Plast Reconstr Surg 2003;112:192–198
86. Rubin LR, Rubin JP, Simpson RL, et al. The search for the neurocranial pathways to the fifth nerve nucleus in the reanimation of the paralyzed face. Plast Reconstr Surg 1999;103(6):1725–1728
87. Cheney ML, McKenna MJ, Megerian CA, et al. Trigeminal neoneurotization of the paralyzed face. Ann Otol Rhinol Laryngol 1997;106: 733–738
88. Dellon L, Mackinnon SE. Reanimation following facial paralysis by adjacent muscle neurotization: an experimental model in the primate. Microsurgery 1989;10:251–255
89. Fisher E, Frodel JL. Facial suspension with acellular human dermal allograft. Arch Facial Plast Surg 1999;1:195–199
90. Petroff MA, Goode RL, Levet Y. Gore-Tex implants: applications in facial paralysis rehabilitation and soft-tissue augmentation. Laryngoscope 1992;102:1185–1189
91. Biel M. Gore-Tex graft midfacial suspension and upper eyelid gold-weight implantation in rehabilitation of the paralyzed face. Laryngoscope 1995;105:876–879
92. Terzis JK, Noah ME. Analysis of 100 cases of free-muscle transplantation for facial paralysis. Plast Reconstr Surg 1997;99(7):1905–1921
93. Harii K, Asato H, Yoshima K, et al. One-stage transfer of the latissimus dorsi muscle for reanimation of a paralyzed face. Plast Reconstr Surg 1998;102(4):941–951
94. Koshima I, Tsuda K, Hamanaka T, et al. One-stage reconstruction of established facial paralysis using a rectus abdominus muscle transfer. Plast Reconstr Surg 1997;99(1):234–238
95. Kumar PAV. Cross-face reanimation of the paralysed face, with a single stage microneurovascular gracilis transfer without nerve graft: a preliminary report. Br J Plast Surg 1995;48:83–88
96. Bove A, Chiarini S, D'Andrea V, et al. Facial nerve palsy: which flap? Microsurgical, anatomical, and functional considerations. Microsurgery 1998;18:286–289
97. O'Brien BM, Pederson WC, Khazanchi RK, et al. Results of management of facial palsy with microvascular free-muscle transfer. Plast Reconstr Surg 1990;86(1):12–22
98. Aviv JE, Urken ML. Management of the paralyzed face with microneurovascular free muscle transfer. Arch Otolaryngol Head Neck Surg 1992;118:909–912
99. Harii K, Ohmori K, Torii S. Free gracilis muscle transplantation with microvascular anastomoses for the treatment of facial paralysis. Plast Reconstr Surg 1976;57:133–143
100. Freilinger G. A new technique to correct facial paralysis. Plast Reconstr Surg 1975;56:44–48
101. Mackinnon SE, Dellon AL. A surgical algorithm for the management of facial palsy. Microsurgery 1988;9:30–35
102. Mackinnon SE, Dellon AL. Facial nerve injury. In: Mackinnon SE, Dellon AL, eds. Surgery of the Peripheral Nerve. New York: Thieme-Stratton; 1988:393–422
103. Rubin LR. Reanimation of the paralyzed eyelid. In: Rubin, LR, ed. The Paralyzed Face. St. Louis: Mosby Year Book; 1991:234–242
104. Sullivan SA, Dailey RA. Endoscopic subperiosteal midface lift: surgical technique with indications and outcomes. Ophthal Plast Reconstr Surg 2002;18(5):319–330
105. Goode RL. Surgery of the incompetent nasal valve. Laryngoscope 1985;95:546–555
106. Clark JM, Cook TA. The "butterfly" graft in secondary funcational rhinoplasty. Laryngoscope 2002;112(11):1917–1925
107. Conley J, Baker DC, Selfe RW. Paralysis of the mandibular branch of the facial nerve. Plast Reconstr Surg 1982;70:569–577
108. Glenn MG, Goode RL. Surgical treatment of the "marginal mandibular lip" deformity. Otolaryngol Head Neck Surg 1987;97:462–468
109. Clodius L. Selective neurectomies to achieve symmetry in partial and complete facial paralysis. Br J Plast Surg 1976;29:43–52
110. Guerrissi JO. Selective myectomy for postparetic facial synkinesis. Plast Reconstr Surg 1991;87(3):459–466
111. Breslow GD, Cabiling D, Kanchwala S, Bartlett SP. Selective marginal neurectomy for treatment of the marginal mandibular lip deformity in patients with chronic unilateral facial palsies. Plast Reconstr Surg 2005;116(5):1223–1232

64 Craniofacial Approaches to the Anterior Skull Base

Scott A. McLean and Lawrence J. Marentette

Craniofacial surgical approaches developed by Obwegeser, Tessier, and many other pioneers, are designed to address the anatomically complex junction between intracranial and extracranial compartments. The anterior cranial fossa lies in close proximity to both the orbit and the paranasal sinuses. Likewise, the middle cranial fossa is intimately related to the pterygomaxillary space, the infratemporal fossa, and the temporomandibular joint. Surgical access to these regions is required for removal of a variety of benign and malignant neoplasms as well as for correction of traumatic or congenital anomalies. Traditional approaches to the anterior skull base have required transfacial incisions and removal of vital neurovascular and support structures, which have been associated with significant postoperative morbidity. Over the past four decades craniofacial approaches have been refined with three goals in mind: (1) maximize exposure allowing direct access to the skull base; (2) preservation or anatomical reconstruction of vital structures; and (3) aesthetically acceptable incisions with avoidance of unnecessary facial scars.

Collaboration among surgical specialists in otolaryngology–head and neck surgery, facial plastic and reconstructive surgery, neurosurgery, plastic surgery, and craniomaxillofacial surgery has lead to the development of skull base surgical teams. Many of the approaches and fixation methods used today developed out of experience gained in treating patients with frontobasal trauma or congenital craniofacial anomalies.[1,2] Significant reductions in morbidity and mortality have been achieved with advances in reconstruction of skull base defects, which help prevent postoperative cerebrospinal fluid leak. Many reports have now documented the decreasing incidence of complications associated with skull base surgery.[3–5]

As in any surgical specialty, a thorough understanding of anatomy and physiology is crucial to the success of craniofacial surgery. This chapter will discuss some of the pertinent anatomy for craniofacial approaches. However, a detailed discussion of the complex anatomy of the skull base is beyond the scope of this chapter.[6] The purpose of this chapter is to outline surgical approaches to the anterior skull base, infratemporal fossa, pterygomaxillary space, and orbit. These approaches are used in the treatment of patients with tumors, trauma, or congenital anomalies.

Subcranial Approach to the Anterior Skull Base

Traditional craniofacial resection of anterior skull base lesions requires frontal craniotomy to provide access to the skull base from superiorly coupled with transfacial incisions to approach the skull base from inferiorly. This combined superior and inferior approach allows for improved control of tumor margins. The limits of this approach, however, include a significant need for frontal lobe retraction, complete anosmia, and the potential for obvious facial scar formation. The subcranial approach, also referred to as the transglabellar or subfrontal approach, was initially described by Raveh et al for treatment of skull base trauma.[7] By disarticulating the frontonasoorbital complex, access is gained to the nasal cavity, paranasal sinuses, medial and superior orbit, and floor of the anterior cranial fossa without the need for transfacial incisions or frontal lobe retraction. The utility of this approach in management of skull base tumors lies in the broad anterior and inferior exposure of the skull base. This broad exposure allows precise control of tumor margins and reconstruction of the skull base defect.

Incisions and Soft Tissue Anatomy

The subcranial approach is begun by completing a bicoronal incision that extends from the preauricular crease anterior to the tragus, up to the root of the helix, then superiorly over the vertex to the root of the helix and preauricular crease on the contralateral side.[8] The incision should be 3 to 4 cm posterior to the hairline with care taken to avoid the receding temporal hair line in men. The incision is carried down through skin, subcutaneous tissue, and the occipitofrontalis/galeal layer to the level of the subgaleal loose areolar tissue (**Fig. 64.1**). The coronal flap is then sharply elevated in a subgaleal fashion being careful to leave the pericranium as thick as possible with loose areolar tissue. Elevation proceeds in this manner to within 2 cm of the superior orbital rims.

As dissection proceeds laterally over the temporal region the surgeon must be careful to protect the frontal branch of the facial nerve as well as the superficial temporal artery and vein. The fascial layers overlying the temporalis muscle have been given many names making

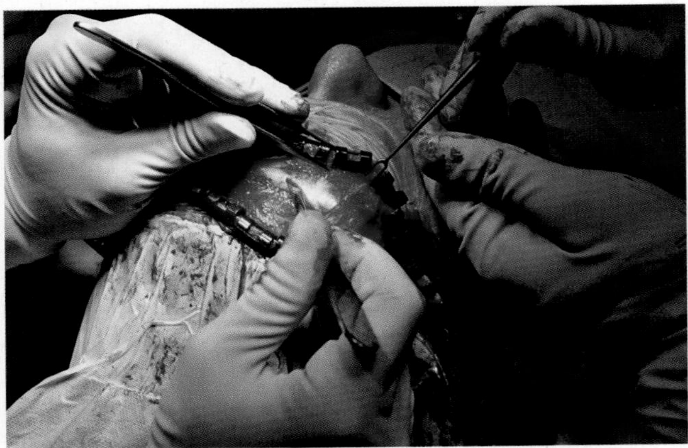

Fig. 64.1 Elevation of the coronal flap in the subgaleal layer.

communication concerning these layers difficult. The temporoparietal fascia is the superior extension of the superficial musculoaponeurotic system (SMAS) of the midface. The temporoparietal fascia is continuous with the occipitofrontalis/galeal layer superiorly. The superficial temporal artery and vein lie within the temporoparietal fascia. The frontal branch of the facial nerve is adherent to the undersurface of the temporoparietal fascia as it crosses over the zygomatic arch.

The deep temporal fascia is continuous with the pericranium superiorly above the temporal line. Below the temporal line, overlying the temporalis muscle, the deep temporal fascia is thick. Further inferiorly, at about the level of the superior orbital rim the deep temporal fascia splits to form the superficial layer of the deep temporal fascia and the deep layer of the deep temporal fascia. The superficial layer of the deep temporal fascia continues inferiorly to fuse with the anterior periosteum over the zygomatic arch. The deep layer of the deep temporal fascia continues inferiorly to fuse with the medial surface of the zygomatic arch. Between the two layers of the deep temporal fascia is a small fat pad called the superficial temporal fat pad.

As the coronal flap is elevated inferiorly toward the zygomatic arch the dissection should be deep to the temporoparietal fascia and superficial to the deep temporal fascia. This is continuous with the subgaleal dissection medially and attention is made to proceeding on a wide surgical front to maximize exposure. Once the flap is elevated to within 2 cm of the zygoma, a horizontal incision from the lateral orbital rim to the root of the helix should be made through the superficial layer of the deep temporal fascia (**Fig. 64.2**). Dissecting below this layer to the zygoma will help protect the frontal branch of the facial nerve. The zygoma can then be dissected in a subperiosteal plane from lateral to medial where the dissection can be connected to the subperiosteal plane along the lateral orbital rim.

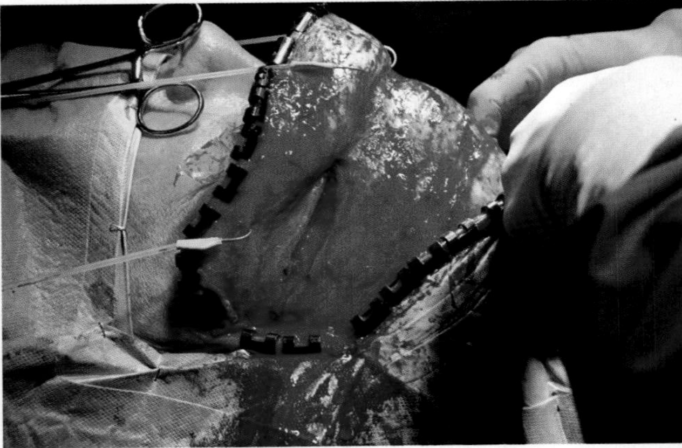

Fig. 64.2 The superficial layer of the deep temporal fascia is incised ~2 cm above the zygomatic arch. Dissection remains deep to this layer toward the zygoma to protect the frontal branch of the facial nerve.

Attention is then turned to elevation of the pericranial flap. Typically, the pericranial flap is bipedicled based on the supraorbital arteries and extends 15 cm cephalic to the supraorbital rims. The flap can be designed to extend posterior from the temporal line on each side to the vertex of the skull (**Fig. 64.3**). After incising the periosteum with either the knife or electrocautery the pericranial flap is carefully elevated using a wide periosteal elevator. As the pericranium is elevated up to the superior orbital rims the supraorbital neurovascular bundles must be identified and protected. In the majority of patients these will lie

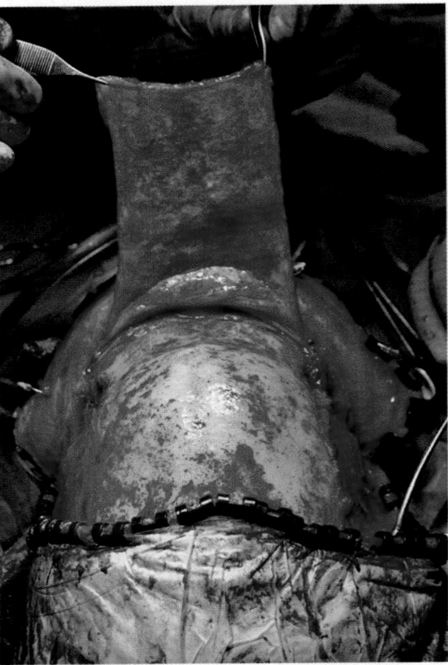

Fig. 64.3 The pericranial flap elevated to the level of the superior orbital rims.

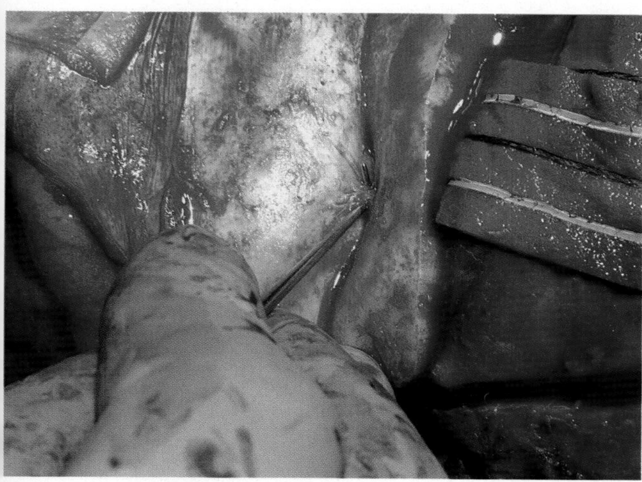

Fig. 64.4 Supraorbital neurovascular bundle identified within a true supraorbital foramen.

within the supraorbital notch found along the medial aspect of the supraorbital rim. In a minority of patients, the supraorbital neurovascular bundle will lie within a true foramen (**Fig. 64.4**). If this is the case, a small osteotome can be used to notch out the foramen allowing anterior displacement of the neurovascular bundle (**Fig. 64.5**).

To facilitate maximum exposure, the periorbita is dissected free from the orbital roof posteriorly 3 to 4 cm. This is done safely knowing that the orbital depth from the rim to the optic strut is 45 to 55 mm. Care is taken not to disrupt the periorbita as this will expose orbital fat and make visualization more difficult. Also, the superior branch of the oculomotor nerve (CN III) can be injured with disruption of the periorbita and cause postoperative levator dysfunction. Medially, the subperiosteal dissection continues down the medial orbital wall. The frontoethmoid suture marks the level of the cribriform plate and transmits the anterior and posterior ethmoid arteries through their respective foramen. The anterior ethmoid artery is found roughly 24 mm from the anterior lacrimal crest. The posterior ethmoid artery is 12 mm behind the anterior ethmoid artery. The optic nerve is then another 6 mm behind the posterior ethmoid artery. The anterior ethmoid artery is ligated using either bipolar electrocautery or small clips. Centrally, the periosteum and soft tissue over the glabella and nasal dorsum are elevated all the way down to the bony cartilaginous junction. With the soft tissue elevation now complete attention is turned to the bony anatomy.

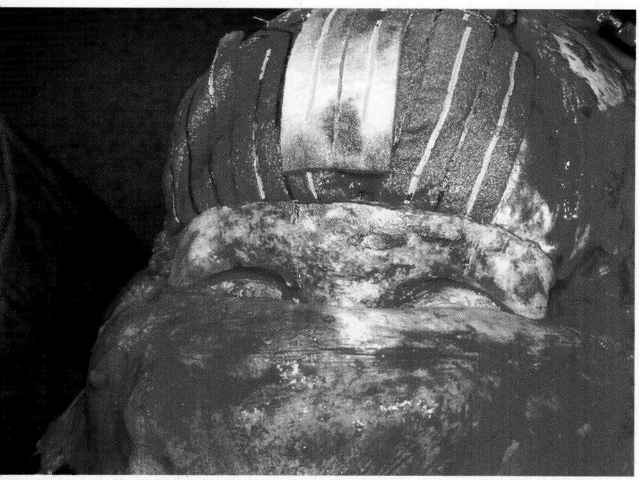

Fig. 64.5 The supraorbital foramens have been notched out allowing anterior displacement of the neurovascular bundles. The periorbita has been freed off of the medial and superior orbital walls.

Osteotomies and Bony Anatomy

Intracranial exposure begins with a wide bifrontal craniotomy performed by the neurosurgical service. Typically, the craniotomy is designed to extend from temporal line to temporal line just superior to the aerated frontal sinus. The bone cuts then gently curve posteromedially to meet in the midline ~10 cm cephalic to the glabella. The frontal bone flap is then turned with careful attention to preservation of dura and the superior sagital sinus.

The dura of the anterior cranial fossa is then carefully elevated beginning anteriosuperiorly with elevation off the frontal bone making up the posterior wall of the frontal sinus. Anteriolaterally the dura is elevated off the frontal bone making up the superior orbital rim and orbital roof bilaterally. Centrally, dissection is carried posterior to the level of the foramen cecum, just anterior to the crista gali and the cribriform plate.

Depending on the location of the lesion, osteotomies are then planned for removal of the frontonasoorbital complex. The frontal lobes and orbital contents are protected with malleable retractors. Using an oscillating saw sagital cuts are made through the superior orbital rim and orbital roof to a depth of ~2 cm bilaterally (**Fig. 64.6**). Using a side-cutting bur, cuts are then extended medially along the orbital roof and extended to meet in the midline at the foramen cecum (**Fig. 64.7**).

The roof of the orbit meets the medial orbital wall at the frontoethmoid suture. Inferior to the frontoethmoid suture, the lamina paprycia of the ethmoid bone constitutes the medial orbital wall. Anteriorly, the lacrimal bone constitutes a small portion of the media orbital wall and is seen as the posterior lacrimal crest lying posterior to the lacrimal fossa. Anterior to the lacrimal fossa is the frontal process of the maxilla and it is seen as the anterior lacrimal crest. This bony prominence marks the insertion of the medial canthal tendon. Using the side-cutting bur, an osteotomy is brought forward from the medial extent

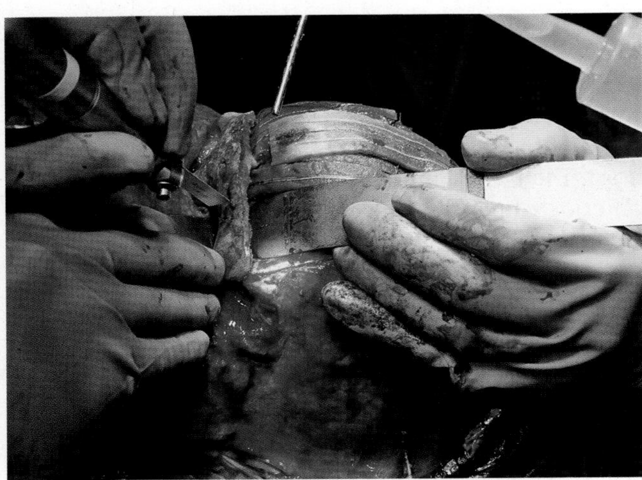

Fig. 64.6 An oscillating saw is used to make an osteotomy through the superior orbital rim. Malleable retractors are used to protect both the orbital contents as well as the frontal lobes.

of the orbital roof osteotomy along the medial orbital wall to extend anterior to the anterior lacrimal crest and thus avoid disrupting the insertion of the medial canthal tendon (**Fig. 64.8**).

Anterior to the frontal process of the maxilla lie the paired nasal bones with the upper lateral cartilages of the nose attached to their caudal ends. Continuing with the side-cutting bur, the osteotomy is continued caudally along the lateral aspect of the nasal bones to within 2 to 3 mm of the bony cartilaginous junction. Here, a transverse osteotomy is performed using a thin oscillating saw (**Fig. 64.8**).

Finally, the frontonasoorbital complex is disarticulated from the bony nasal septum using a sharply curved osteotome placed directly through the previously cut bone at the level of the foramen cecum. With removal of the frontonasoorbital complex the nasal vault, ethmoid sinus, and medial and superior orbit are easily visualized (**Fig. 64.9**). The floor of the anterior fossa is composed of the ethmoid bone making up the cribriform plate. Depending on the site of the lesion, the olfactory apparatus can be sectioned off of the cribriform plate either unilaterally or bilaterally. If done unilaterally, olfaction can be preserved on the contralateral side.

Posterior to the cribriform plate lays the planum sphenoidale of the sphenoid bone, which extends further posteriorly terminating at the anterior clinoid processes.

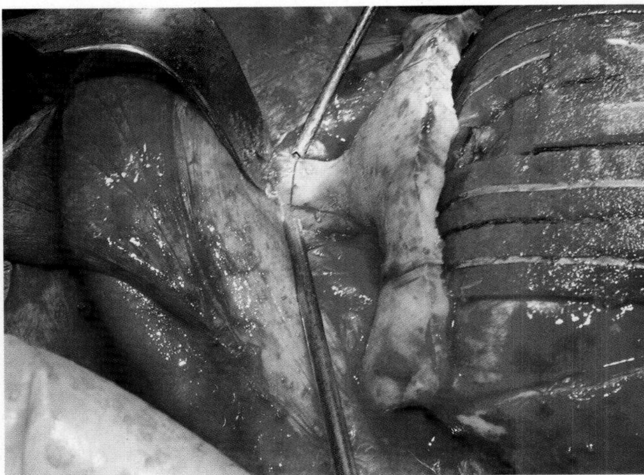

Fig. 64.8 Within the orbit, the orbital roof osteotomy is brought medially along the medial orbital wall just anterior to the anterior lacrimal crest. The cuts are then brought inferiorly along the nasal bones to within 2 to 3 mm of the nasal bony–cartilaginous junction where a transverse osteotomy is completed.

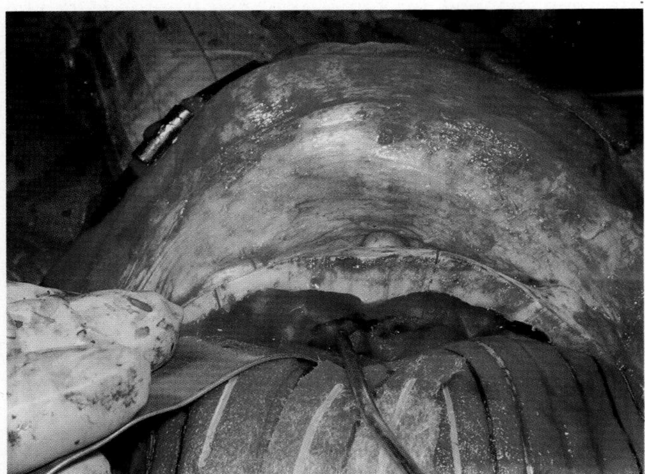

Fig. 64.7 A side-cutting bur was used to bring the orbital roof cuts medially to meet at the foramen cecum, just anterior to the crista gali and cribriform plate.

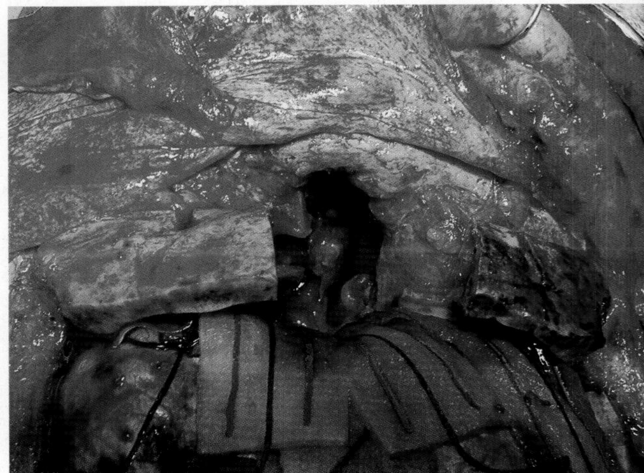

Fig. 64.9 With the frontonasoorbital complex removed there is excellent exposure of the sinonasal cavity, orbits, and anterior skull base.

From here the optic nerves can be appreciated as well as the optic chiasm. If needed the sphenoid sinus can be opened allowing direct visualization of the internal carotid arteries in the lateral wall of the sphenoid.

Reconstruction

The subcranial approach allows for wide exposure of the superior orbit, medial orbit, nasal cavity, paranasal sinuses, and anterior cranial fossa. After removal of pathological lesions in these areas it is critical to reconstruct the anterior skull base separating the intracranial contents from the paranasal sinuses. All dural defects are repaired using grafting material of choice by the neurosurgical service. If there are bony defects of the superior or medial orbit, these can be repaired with bone harvested from the inner table of the frontal craniotomy. Bone grafts are typically plated into place using microplates and screws.

Next, the frontonasoorbital complex is plated back into position using microplates and screws along the supraorbital rims bilaterally. If the frontal sinus was not involved, this structure is left intact. If there has been involvement of the posterior wall of the frontal sinus the posterior wall is completely taken down and all mucosa is removed from the sinus. A diamond bur is used to ensure that all mucosal remnants are removed. The nasofrontal ducts are then obliterated with fascia or muscle grafts.

Finally, the pericranial flap is rotated down over the frontal bone into the anterior skull base defect. If needed, the flap can be placed all the way back to the anterior clinoid processes. This provides robust tissue that will seal off the sinonasal cavity from the anterior cranial fossa. The bony cribriform defect does not require bony reconstruction. Nasal trumpets are placed to divert airflow away from the skull base for the first 3 postoperative days.

LeFort I Osteotomy

LeFort I osteotomy was initially described as a method of exposure for tumors of the nasopharynx. The osteotomy then was adapted by maxillofacial surgeons to reposition the maxilla for orthognathic correction of dental facial deformities. Initially this was done as a two-stage procedure; however, Obwegeser[9] described a one-stage mobilization and repositioning of the maxilla. It is currently useful not only in orthognathic procedures but also in gaining access to the nasopharynx and the mid- and lower clivus as well as the retromaxillary space. It is used in combination with the transzygomatic approach to remove tumors involving the nasal cavity and nasopharynx, with infratemporal and postzygomatic space extension.

Incisions and Soft Tissue Anatomy

Exposure involves skeletonizing the lower part of the maxilla up to the level of the infraorbital nerves. An incision is made in the gingivobuccal sulcus leaving a 1 cm cuff of mucosa away from the gingival–mucosal junction to allow for two-layer everted closure. The incision is carried down through mucosa, submucosa, and through the periosteum. This extends from the first molar to first molar bilaterally. After the incision is made, the periosteal elevator is then used to elevate the periosteum in the subperiosteal plane of the pyriform aperture, canine fossae, and the lateral or zygomaticomaxillary buttress (**Fig. 64.10**). This dissection is carried laterally around the posterior aspect of the lateral buttress until the pterygomaxillary fissure is palpated with the elevator. Next, a Freer elevator is used to elevate the mucosa from the pyriform aperture to the posterior nasal spine at the level of the nasopharynx, thus exposing the floor of the nose and the lateral nasal wall below the inferior turbinate.

Osteotomies

The location of the LeFort I osteotomy through the medial and lateral buttresses is outlined taking care to stay below the infraorbital foramen and above the tooth root apices. Prior to creating this bone cut, plates are placed on the medial and lateral buttresses and holes are predrilled so as to reposition the maxilla at the end of the procedure and maintain the presurgical occlusion. However, if orthognathic repositioning is required, the amount of maxillary repositioning is marked and later used to facilitate repositioning of the maxilla following tumor removal. A nasal tracheal tube would be employed instead of an oral tracheal tube.

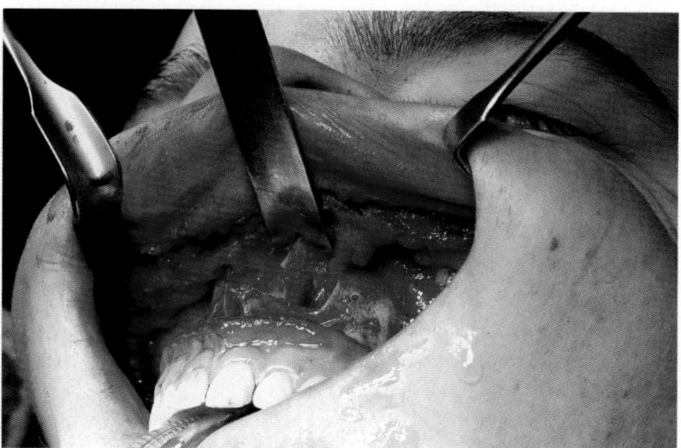

Fig. 64.10 The maxilla is exposed from pyriform aperture to lateral buttress bilaterally up to the level of the infraorbital foramen.

An osteotomy is then created through the medial buttress extending through the canine fossae and through the entirety of the lateral buttress. This may be accomplished with a reciprocating saw, sagittal saw, or a fissure side-cutting bur, the choice of which is totally at the preference of the surgeon. The osteotomy must be placed more than 5 mm above the apices of the teeth or else tooth devitalization will occur. The osteotomies through the medial buttress must extend posteriorly through the entirety of the lateral wall of the nose. Likewise, the lateral buttress osteotomies must also extend to the posterior wall of the maxillary sinus. Next, the nasal septum and vomer is separated from the maxillary crest. The nasal septal osteotome is placed between the caudal portion of the nasal septum and the anterior nasal spine and used to separate the nasal septum from the floor of the nose. During this portion of the osteotomy, a finger must be placed in the nasopharynx at the posterior nasal spine so as to prevent the osteotome from lacerating the endotracheal tube or injuring the cervical spine.

The pterygomaxillary suture line is then separated from the pterygoid plates to allow ease of downfracture of the maxilla. This can be accomplished with a curved pterygomaxillary osteotome or an oscillating saw. These must be placed carefully on the lateral aspect of the pterygomaxillary suture and low on the suture so as to avoid entering the pterygopalatine fossae and lacerating terminal branches of the internal maxillary artery. A finger is placed medial to the maxillary tuberosity of the hard palate and once the osteotome or saw blade is palpated the osteotomy is complete. Any further cuts medially of the osteotome or the saw blade could result in laceration of the palatal mucosa and the greater palatine artery.

Using the thumbs and forefinger or a bone hook, the maxilla is gently downfractured (**Fig. 64.11**). If any significant degree of force is required, all osteotomies must be rechecked for their completeness. Caution must be used when utilizing the Rowe forceps to downfracture the maxilla as this may injure the vascular pedicle and potentially lead to a slough of the lower maxilla. Once the maxilla is downfractured the mucosa of the floor of the nose is incised and the tumor is exposed. Approximately every 15 to 20 minutes, the maxilla should be released and placed back into its original position to ensure that its blood supply is maintained. If during the resection the gingiva of the maxilla becomes cyanotic or white, the maxilla must be replaced immediately, secured in position, and irrigated with warm saline. White mucosa can signify an impending slough of the maxilla.

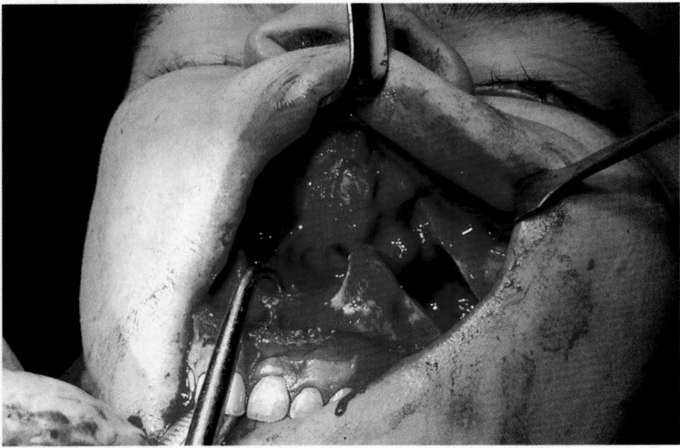

Fig. 64.11 LeFort I osteotomy completed bilaterally with downfracture of the maxilla.

Reconstruction

Once the resection is completed the maxilla is repositioned to achieve the planned occlusion. Plate fixation of the medial and lateral buttresses is then completed. Next, two-layered soft tissue closure is performed using a horizontal continuous mattress suture of a resorbable material through the mucosa, submucosa, and periosteum so as to allow for eversion of the edges of the maxillary incision. This is followed by a second continuous running suture of the mucosa. Finally, the nasal septum should be inspected to ensure that it is brought back to the midline. The septum and the nasal mucosa can be held in place with light nasal packing.

Transzygomatic Approach to the Infratemporal Fossa, Lateral Orbit, and Pterygomaxillary Space

Traditional approaches to the infratemporal fossa, lateral orbit, and pterygomaxillary space required transfacial incisions and removal of important functional and support structures. Although exposure was adequate, postoperative morbidity was not acceptable. After gaining experience with exposure of the temporomandibular joint (TMJ), Obwegeser described the temporal, or transzygomatic, approach to the TMJ, lateral orbit, infratemporal fossa, and pterygomaxillary space.[9] In his description of this approach he stressed the importance of avoiding facial incisions, preserving the TMJ, and preventing injury to the facial nerve. When combined with middle fossa craniotomy exposure can be brought medially all the way to the cavernous sinus.

Incision and Soft Tissue Anatomy

The transzygomatic approach is begun with a standard bicoronal incision that begins in the preauricular crease on the ipsilateral side. The incision is essentially the same as that used for the subcranial approach except that it may stop short of the root of the helix on the contralateral side. The arc of rotation needed for adequate elevation of the coronal flap will dictate how far inferiorly the incision should extend on the contralateral side. The coronal flap is elevated in the subgaleal plane as previously described (**Fig. 64.1**). As the dissection is carried laterally over the temporal fossa careful attention is paid to stay in the proper surgical plane. As noted previously, 2 cm above the level of the zygoma the plane of dissection should transition to below the superficial layer of the deep temporal fascia (**Fig. 64.2**). The pericranial flap can then be raised and brought forward to the superior orbital rim (**Fig. 64.3**). The supraorbital neurovascular bundle is identified and preserved and the periorbita is raised off the orbital roof (**Fig. 64.4**). The zygoma can then be exposed in a subperiosteal fashion from lateral to medial exposing the malar eminence and lateral orbital rim. If the frontal process of the zygoma is to be included in the osteotomy, then the periorbita is freed from the lateral orbital wall. The lateral canthal tendon is incised and tagged for later reattachment. Exposure of the lateral orbital wall is carried inferior and posterior until the inferior orbital fissure is identified.

Osteotomies and Bony Anatomy

Depending on the site and size of the target lesion a decision is made regarding the need for middle fossa craniotomy. For lesions not involving the skull base, the zygomatic arch can be removed by making osteotomies just anterior to the glenoid fossa and just posterior to the malar eminence. The arch is left pedicled to the masseter muscle and swung inferiorly thus exposing the insertion of the temporalis muscle on the coronoid process of the mandible.

If wider exposure is desired, the anterior osteotomy is made further forward on the malar eminence at the level of the zygomaticofacial branch of the maxillary division of the trigeminal nerve (V2). This anterior osteotomy is brought to just inside the lateral orbital rim. An osteotomy is then made superiorly at the zygomaticofrontal suture and connected inferiorly to allow displacement of the lateral orbital rim (**Fig. 64.12**). Again, the preparation can be left pedicled to the masseter muscle and reflected inferiorly. This approach allows excellent access to the infratemporal fossa, lateral orbit, and pterygomaxillary space (**Fig. 64.13**). For even greater exposure, the coronoid process can be separated from the ramus of the mandible and reflected superiorly pedicled to the temporalis muscle. Alternatively, maximum exposure is achieved by performing a horizontal

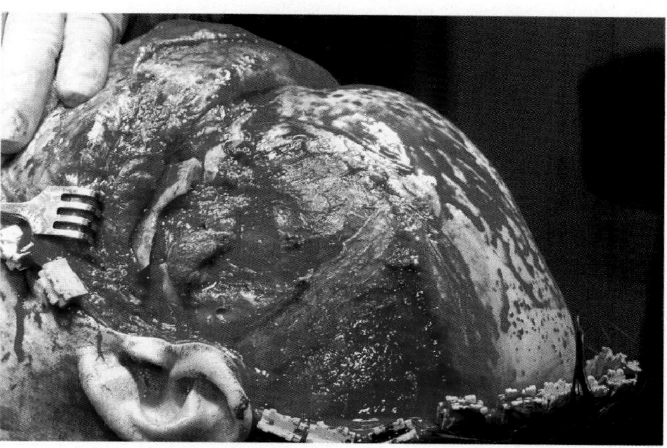

Fig. 64.12 Transzygomatic approach utilizing osteotomies at the lateral zygomatic arch, malar eminence, and zygomaticofrontal suture.

osteotomy of the ramus superior to the antilingular prominence. By performing a subcondylar osteotomy or disarticulating the temporomandibular joint, the entire upper ramus is reflected superiorly, pedicled on the temporalis tendon. This allows direct visualization of the pterygomaxillary space.

Palpation of the bony landmarks of the skull base will help protect the internal carotid artery. The spine of the sphenoid is a reliable marker. Proceeding anteromedially at a 45-degree angle from this point the surgeon will encounter the foramen spinosum, foramen ovale, and lateral pterygoid plate. Posterior and medial to the spine lays the internal carotid artery.

When using this approach for lesions with known or suspected intracranial involvement a temporal or frontotemporal craniotomy must also be performed. This can be performed separately or as a one-piece frontotemporal orbitozygomatic approach.

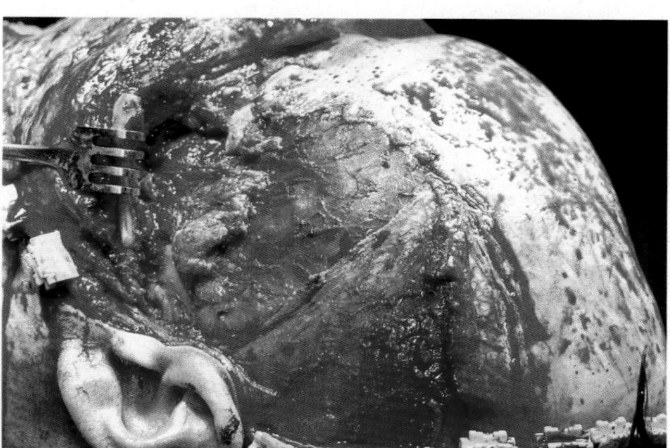

Fig. 64.13 Inferior displacement of the zygoma and lateral orbital rim allows excellent exposure of the infratemporal fossa and lateral orbit.

Reconstruction

Once the pathology has been removed, reconstruction can be performed as needed. Dura is repaired as needed by the neurosurgical team. If there is a bony dehiscence of the skull base this can be reinforced using the pericranial flap, a temporoparietal fascia flap, or temporalis muscle. In some cases a fat graft is used to provide bulk to the infratemporal fossa. The zygoma is plated back into anatomical position using microplates and screw fixation.

Summary

Modern craniofacial surgical techniques allow for extensive exposure of the upper and midfacial skeleton while preserving function and maintaining or improving cosmesis. These techniques have benefited children and adults afflicted with tumors, trauma, and congenital anomalies. These approaches are definitely within the realm of facial plastic and reconstructive surgery and the facial plastic surgeon is an integral part of any successful skull base surgical team.

References

1. Raveh J, Imola M, Ladrach K, Zingg M, Vuillemin T. Update on the correction of craniofacial anomalies. Facial Plast Surg Clin North Am 1995;3(1):17–38
2. Ladrach K, Annino DJ, Raveh J, Zingg M, Vuillemin T, Leibinger K. Advanced approaches to cranio-orbital injuries. Facial Plast Surg Clin North Am 1995;3(1):107–130
3. Kelly MBH, Waterhouse N, Slade DE, Carr R, Peterson D. A 5-year review of 71 consecutive anterior skull base tumors. Br J Plast Surg 2000;53:184–190
4. Kellman R, Marentette L. The transglabellar/subcranial approach to the anterior skull base. Arch Otolaryngol Head Neck Surg 2001;127:687–690
5. Vrionis FD, Kienstra MA, Rivera MR, Padhya TA. Malignant tumors of the anterior skull base. Cancer Control 2004;11(3):144–151
6. Lyons BM. Surgical anatomy of the skull base. In: Donald PJ, ed. Surgery of the Skull Base. Philadelphia, PA: Lippincott-Raven Publishers; 1998:15–30
7. Raveh J, Laedrach K, Iizuka T, Leibinger F. Subcranial extended anterior approach for skull base tumors: surgical procedure and reconstruction. In: Donald PJ, ed. Surgery of the Skull Base. Philadelphia, PA: Lippincott-Raven Publishers; 1998:239–261
8. Frodel JL, Marentette L. The coronal approach: anatomic and technical considerations and morbidity. Arch Otolaryngol Head Neck Surg 1993;119:201–207
9. Obwegeser H. Temporal approach to the TMJ, the orbit, and the retromaxillary–infracranial region. Head Neck Surg 1985;7:185–199

V

Trauma

65 Acute Soft Tissue Injuries of the Face

Christian L. Stallworth and G. Richard Holt

Acute soft tissue injuries of the face assume great importance to the patient and to the surgeon, owing to the potential functional and cosmetic outcome abnormalities. Resultant scarring from facial trauma may pose significant detriment to otherwise healthy individuals as evidenced by a significantly more negative perception of body image, a higher incidence of alcoholism and depression, unemployment, and an overall dissatisfaction with life, when compared with control groups, all of which have social and functional implications.[1] Because the face has such prominence in human social engagement, surgeons who manage facial trauma have both the opportunity and the responsibility to make a difference. This responsibility requires that the surgeon understand the biomechanics of tissue wounding, the biochemistry and molecular biology of wound healing, and the art of tissue repair, as well as a fundamental understanding and appreciation of basic mental health.

Soft tissue wounding can have a wide spectrum of etiologies, from knife wounds to gunshot wounds, from cat scratch to dog mauling, from fisticuffs to motor vehicle accident. Although most cases of facial soft tissue trauma are minor to moderate in nature and result, those involving massive injuries require thorough analysis and careful surgical planning. Many patients can undergo repair in the emergency room or outpatient surgery facility under local anesthesia with or without anesthetic monitoring. More difficult or complicated cases usually require operative intervention under general anesthesia, particularly in young children or in those patients with polytrauma or life-threatening injuries.

In cases of massive soft tissue trauma, the initial challenge may be to sort out what tissues are missing and which are still present, albeit in a different form or location. With lesser degrees of injury, the history of the injury and indirect evidence become very important in reconstructing the angle and depth of penetration or the application of force. In addition, a complete head and neck examination is vitally important, with special attention paid to neurological findings. The ultimate goal is to have the best understanding of the mechanics of the forces involved as well as knowledge of the involved facial tissues prior to formulating a surgical plan. A complete understanding of head and neck anatomy and physiology is essential to diagnosing and managing soft tissue wounds of the face.

Facial Soft Tissue Wound Management

Timing of Repair

It is not always necessary to repair a facial wound at the immediate time of injury. However, if it is possible to do so, this "primary" closure should be accomplished within ~4 to 6 hours after wounding. If the wound appears to be contaminated and a concern exists that infection might occur with primary closure (even after extensive debridement and copious irrigation), then a "delayed primary" closure can be performed. Here the wound is debrided, irrigated, packed, or cleansed over 24 to 72 hours, followed by a detailed closure, usually in the operating room. Parenteral antibiotics are commonly employed in this type of delayed closure.

Finally, healing by secondary intent is permissible, wherein good wound care is undertaken by both patient (or surrogate such as a family member or a visiting nurse) and surgeon, allowing for slow but steady closure of the defect. This latter approach may be required in uncontrolled diabetes, chronic hypoxia due to cardiopulmonary disease, or any other significant wound healing deficit. Additionally, adjunctive therapies such as the implementation of wound healing factors or the use of hyperbaric oxygen may also be required. After the wound is healed, then the scar can be dealt with in an appropriate fashion.

It is important for the surgeon to understand that, although the commonly observed factors (extent of wound, presence of bleeding or foreign bodies) tend to dictate timing of wound closure, other, perhaps more subtle factors should also be considered. A surgeon who is caring for a patient with an extensive soft tissue facial wound in the middle of the night after a long day of surgery should determine if he or she is really capable of doing a top-notch job. Additionally, such a wound closure might require special skills (microsurgery), special equipment, special technical support, or other factors that are not optimal at that time of the night. Under those conditions, it might be wise to dress the wound, begin parenteral antibiotics, and wait up to 12 hours until the correct situation is present and the surgeon is rested.

Anesthesia

Minor lacerations can be closed using injectable local anesthesia. Ideally, regional nerve blocks (i.e., infraorbital, mental, supratrochlear, and supraorbital) should be performed, thereby achieving excellent wide-field anesthesia and minimizing tissue distortion that results from subcutaneous permeation of significant fluid volume. Once the blocks have taken effect, local infiltration with a limited volume should be administered for targeted local anesthesia and hemostasis. If the procedure is likely to take longer than 1 to 1.5 hours, then 0.25% bupivacaine can be added to the local anesthetic to prolong its effect. It is also helpful, particularly with children, to buffer the anesthetic solution with sodium bicarbonate (10% of the total volume of anesthetic) to reduce the discomfort of local wound infiltration.

In extensive wounds, and in many children, a general anesthetic may be warranted (and humane). However, age alone does not preclude small children from tissue repair using local anesthetics. Parents must be counseled regarding the steps required and given factual information in an honest but empathetic manner. If appropriate, one parent may be allowed to stay with the child for support, but only if the surgeon feels the parent would be of positive benefit and be able to cope with observing the procedure. Again, nerve blocks or field blocks around the laceration aid in decreasing the discomfort of eventual infiltration into the wound itself. EMLA (Eutectic Mixture of Local Anesthetics) Cream (lidocaine 2.5% and prilocaine 2.5%; AstraZeneca, Wilmington, DE) can also be applied to the area of planned local nerve block if time allows. Usually after the child has cried enough in restraint and there is no longer any discomfort, she or he will fall asleep for most if not all of the procedure.

For extensive injuries involving tissue avulsion, or when underlying osseous or neurovascular structures are injured or at risk, more definitive sedation may be required in a child. Academic medical centers usually have the benefit of pediatric intensivists who are available to provide conscious sedation in the emergency department. However, if these services are not available, or the wound mandates an operating theater, general anesthesia will be indicated. Concern about aspiration seems to be more cogent in children owing to the shorter esophagus and the less protective capability of the gastroesophageal sphincter. The surgeon should discuss with the anesthesiologist whether evacuating the patient's stomach before administering the anesthetic or waiting several hours would be preferred—remembering that an upset child may also develop a relative ileus. For these reasons, the authors prefer to evacuate the stomach directly with a nasal or oral gastric tube before intubation, and not wait 6 to 8 hours for gastric emptying.

Most adults will not require sedation for primary closure of a wound prior to its anesthetization. However, if anxiety is an issue, certain patients may benefit from parenteral sedation (diazepam) or an antianxiety/antiemetic medication (promethazine). Again, any patient whose wounds are extensive should be considered for intraoperative management under general anesthesia.

General Considerations

Although the general principles of wound care—assessment, debridement, cleansing, and meticulous closure—comprise the foundation of facial soft tissue injury management, because of the specialized structures in this area specific techniques are applicable. Both functional and cosmetic considerations must be taken into account, with the former taking immediate precedence. However, the ultimate appearance of the repair (i.e., scarring) must be recognized for its importance to the patient.

Foremost is the need to assess a patient's airway, breathing, and circulation according to standard cardiopulmonary life support protocol. Neurological injuries can be present involving the nerves of the orbit and sympathetic chain, but may also involve the spinal cord, nerve roots, and intracranial contents via the infratemporal fossa.[2] A cervical spine injury should be deemed present with all significant facial traumas until ruled out by radiographic studies, and confirmed by a radiologist. Should there be a spinal cord injury; expanding hematoma in the lateral pharyngeal space; penetration of the brain or brain stem; or damage to the tongue, palate, or floor of the mouth, the airway becomes an issue. The latter would especially include fractures of the mandible and maxilla from gunshot wounds. The airway should be secured with an endotracheal tube or tracheotomy as necessary.

Once the patient has been stabilized and evaluated, tetanus prophylaxis and intravenous antibiotics should be given. For patients less than 7 years of age, or if greater than 5 years have lapsed since their last tetanus vaccination, tetanus toxoid (Td) or the DTP vaccine should be administered. For those with an unknown vaccination history, or who have received fewer than three vaccinations in the tetanus series, tetanus immune globulin (TIG) should be administered (250 to 500 units IM). These patients, together with those having not been vaccinated in more than 10 years, should be given Td as well.[3,4] This immunization should be given early in the emergency visit so it will not be forgotten. For very minor wounds where tetanus infection is an extremely low risk, the TIG need not be given.

The mainstays of successful soft tissue wound management include irrigation and debridement. Particularly in the case of human or animal penetrating wounds copious irrigation is essential. Depending on availability, sterile saline or tap water from a clean outlet can be utilized to decrease the bacterial load in tissues.[5] Although several liters of saline irrigation are adequate, the authors prefe a 2:1 solution of saline and povidone, usually in the volume of 1.5 L. For larger wounds, a bulb syringe or intravenous tubing irrigation will suffice, but for smaller penetrations or puncture wounds, a plastic intravenous catheter on a 20 cm^3 syringe works well. Additionally, commercial products such as the Pulsavac (Zimmer, Inc., Warsaw, IN) are available for simultaneous, aggressive lavage and microdebridement of wounds. Macrodebridement of wounds is an equally critical step in management of soft tissue injuries and may be performed with Adson pickups or hemostats for large particulate matter (e.g., glass or gravel) or a Betadine scrub brush (Cardinal Health, Dublin, OH) for abrasions. Unfortunately, these steps can generate significant discomfort for the patient. For this reason, the authors advocate pretreatment local anesthesia whenever possible.

Prior to definitive closure, all obviously devitalized soft tissue should be debrided, as well as any suspicious, marginally viable tissue. This may include skin, subcutaneous tissue, and even muscle. The wound edges of the skin should also be sharply debrided and the wound closed in layers. If a large dead space exists, or if an avulsed flap is replaced, it may be necessary to place a small drain, with or without suction. Finally, prior to definitive closure, wounds should again be copiously irrigated to reduce the risk of local infection and inflammation in response to the presence of foreign materials or dead cells.

Following the repair of traumatic soft tissue injuries, infections of the face are uncommon, owing primarily to the excellent blood supply available. In summary, the main deterrents to infection include copious irrigation in the emergency room and operating room, judicious debridement of devitalized tissue, wound drainage if indicated, and perioperative administration of antibiotics for 7 to 10 days, depending on the extent of the tissue damage. Hypertrophic scarring is more likely to occur with traumatic injuries than with surgical incisions and can be lessened by using silicone gel applied twice daily for up to 2 months after initial wound healing.

Specific Wound Management

Animal and Human Bites

Dog, cat, and human bites account for 99% of bite wounds, with facial bites in general accounting for less than 1% of all visits to the emergency department. Of these, dog bites are most common, particularly in children.[6] Lacerations from bites occur three times more frequently than puncture wounds. In the past, animal bites were treated in a manner similar to that for human bites; that is, very few were closed primarily. Copious irrigation was performed, the wound was minimally debrided, and delayed primary closure was performed (as opposed to healing by secondary intent). This often resulted in scars that were less than ideal or even unacceptable. Scar revision was an almost certainty, and functional disturbances from cicatrix formation were common.

Current standard of care has progressed significantly, particularly with respect to animal bites, based primarily on emergency wound care and antibiotic utilization.[7] Human bites remain problematic, and primary closure is selected only in the most favorable of wounds. A polymicrobial population, including anaerobic and aerobic organisms, contaminates most bites. Thus it is common to utilize broad-spectrum antibiotics with excellent anaerobic and microaerophilic efficacy. When bites become infected, though, specific culprits can be predicted based on the aggressor. Infected dog and cat bites, for example, are likely to be populated by *Pasteurella multocida*, *Staphylococcus aureus*, and *Streptococcus viridans*. Of these, cat bites are exceedingly more likely than dog bites to become infected (80% vs $< 5\%$). Human bites, on the other hand, are more likely to become complicated by *Eikenella corrodens* or *Bacteroides* sp.[3,8] We recommend that an intravenous bolus of a second-generation cephalosporin be administered for all penetrating soft tissue bite wounds. If penicillin sensitivity cross-reaction is a major concern with a cephalosporin, then parenteral ciprofloxacin is a good choice. Alternatively, clindamycin can be considered. This parenteral dose should be given in advance of any surgical care, so that rising blood levels can be available. If the wounds are severe, then consideration should be given to continued parenteral antibiotic therapy, either as inpatient treatment or home intravenous therapy. Usually, after the wounds have been cared for on an emergency basis, the patient may be discharged with an oral antibiotic that is effective against a wide range of organisms, including anaerobes. Good choices would include amoxicillin-clavulanate, cephalexin, clindamycin, and ciprofloxacin.

Viral transmission is also concerning for all bites. An overriding concern in animal bites is the risk of the rabies virus. If rabies is a possibility, the patient should receive a first dose of immune globulin on the day of the injury, followed by the vaccine at days 0, 3, 7, 14, and 28. Because povidone is a known virocidal and can eliminate 90% of the rabies risk, wound irrigation and cleansing with this agent should be done as well.[9] Human bites, on the other hand, are concerning for hepatitis B and C, herpes virus, and human immunodeficiency virus (HIV) transmission. It is good practice to treat a human bite as a possible HIV exposure, and an HIV test should be performed on both patient and attacker, if possible. Eliciting a history of other communicable diseases in both patient and attacker is also prudent.

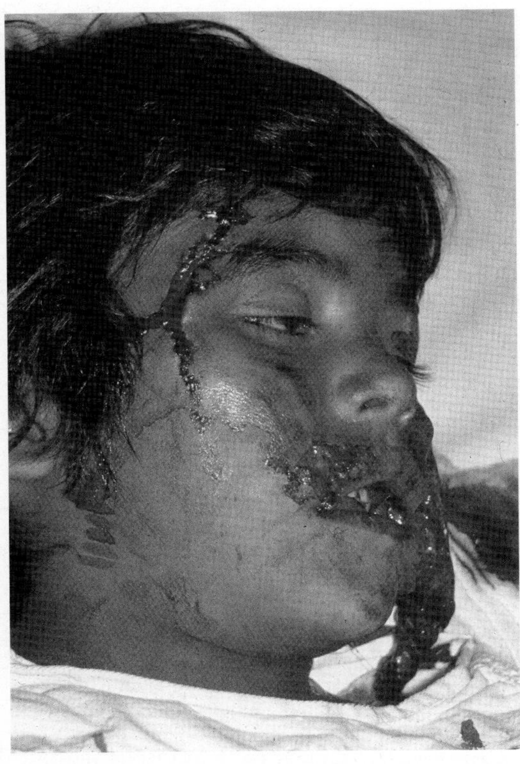

Fig. 65.1 Multiple tissue avulsions of child's face due to dog mauling.

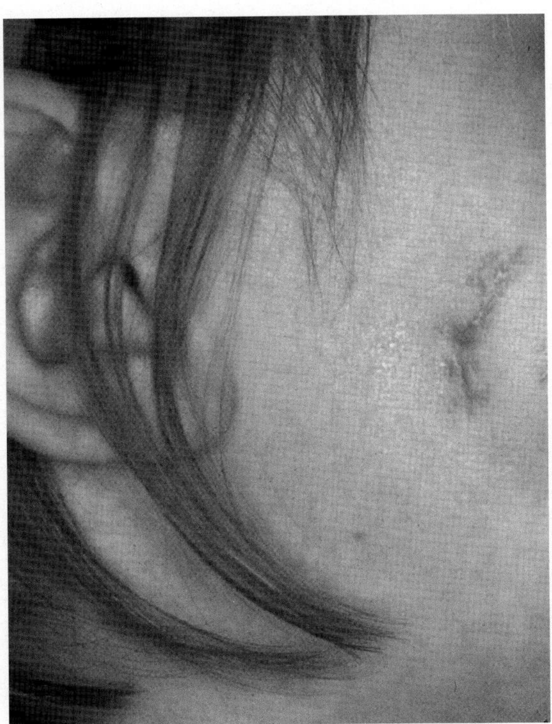

Fig. 65.2 Presence of hematoma and/or salivary secretions 1 week after animal bite repair.

Bite wounds are usually a combination of penetration and avulsion, due to the tearing action of the teeth on tissue (**Fig. 65.1**). Tissue loss is minimal unless a piece is missing from a protruding structure, such as the ear or nose. Depth of penetration varies depending on the resistance of the skin as well as the force of jaw contracture and shearing from the animal or human bite. In general, human bites are less likely to penetrate deeply into facial tissue than animal bites, owing to the length and shape of the anterior human teeth. In addition, humans are loath to draw much blood during a bite due both to an aversion to having someone else's blood in their mouth and the fear of contracting a bloodborne disease. All in all, human bites are significantly less common than animal bites because of the availability of more sophisticated instruments of injury (knife, gun, baseball bat). When they do occur, human bites are often associated with lovers' quarrels and typically involve a single region of injury (ear, nose, lip), whereas animal bites may reflect a recurring-attack pattern in multiple sites.

The most urgent priorities are to assess the airway (especially in bites involving the neck and floor of the mouth), assess the risk for a life-threatening incident, and determine the neurological and vision status. Particularly in children, there is a relatively short distance from the face to the neck, so coexisting neck injury should be considered, and a thorough assessment should be performed.[10] Fortunately, most penetrating wounds due to bites involve soft tissue only. However, an initial deep-penetrating animal bite may be masked by an avulsive injury of more superficial tissues, or a bite by an older dog might result in implantation of a loose tooth deep in the wound. Thus exploration of the wound after anesthetization is always warranted.

The level of penetration should be assessed and estimated, with particular attention paid to damage to underlying structures, such as muscles, ducts, and neurovascular bundles (**Fig. 65.2**). Certain vascular regions are at risk due to their superficial locations over bony prominences (e.g., the superficial temporal, facial, and angular arteries). Included in the neurological concerns would be facial nerve function, vision and ocular movement, and tongue motion. Because a tremendous amount of force can be delivered to the tissue through a bite, it is also possible for bony injury to occur. When a large-mouthed dog attacks a small child, fractures of the skull or face must be ruled out through computed tomography (CT) if indicated. Microscopic injury to adjacent tissues is expected, and one must assess tissue viability, based not only on the initial evaluation but also on an evolving evaluation throughout the emergency care process. Radiographic imaging is mandatory if physical findings raise a concern for neurological or osseous damage

Appropriate consultations should also be obtained early, especially a pediatric consultation if the victim is a child.

For small punctate penetration wounds from animal or human bites, the authors prefer to excise the puncture tract with a 2-, 3-, or 4-mm dermatologic punch for the purpose of removing damaged and contaminated tissue. This converts the tract to a clean, cylindrical wound that can be irrigated and loosely closed with one or two dermal sutures after instillation of antibiotic ointment, preferably mupirocin, within its depth.

Flaps of tissue should be minimally debrided and cleansed with irrigant. Then the surrounding tissue to which the flap will be sutured should be irrigated and slightly elevated to facilitate dermal closure with rather loosely placed 4–0 or 5–0 chromic catgut suture (or polyglactin suture if some tension exists). Loosely placed epidermal sutures of 6–0 polypropylene or 5–0 fast-absorbing catgut (in children) then complete the repair. Mupirocin ointment can be applied topically to the wound and utilized for approximately 1 week postoperatively. It may not be wise to apply sterile adhesive strips to a bite wound because it is important to observe the wound for infection and to allow a slight laxity of the wound margins for seepage of serous fluid.

Human bites deemed not safe for primary closure may be packed open with frequent dressing changes and application of topical antimicrobials, then closed in a delayed fashion 2 to 4 days after wounding (if clean) or left to heal by secondary intent. The latter will likely require subsequent scar revision. Replacement of completely avulsed tissue is generally not productive unless the facial part is an entire ear, nose, eyelid, or lip, wherein microvascular reanastomosis should be attempted, if feasible.

When the above wound care precautions are utilized appropriately, most penetrating wounds due to human bites heal reasonably well. However, the patient and family should be prepared for a less than ideal result from the beginning and understand that subsequent scar revision will likely be required. This might include one or more of the following: excision of the scar and reapproximation; steroid injection(s); dermabrasion; laser resurfacing; and reorientation of the scar. There is some clinical evidence that the use of silicone gel or sheeting may affect the subsequent scar in a positive manner. For movable areas, such as the lips, the gel is more practical than the sheeting. Scar revision is a process that may extend over several years, with multiple procedures, and such a possibility should be explained very early in the counseling process, usually in the emergency room.

In addition to caring for the physical sequelae of an animal bite, particular attention must be paid to the psychological impact of injury to the child by a family pet, if that is the case. The child may blame himself or herself, especially if the animal is euthanized, and the surgeon should be supportive and seek counseling for the child and family if the child becomes withdrawn or generally fearful.

Soft Tissue Injuries of the Lateral Face

The cheek is a common site for facial injuries because of its large surface area. Knife wounds, gunshot wounds, and automobile accidents account for the majority of the soft tissue injuries in this region, with animal bites further down the list. Both penetrating and avulsive injuries may be seen, although the relative resistance of cheek tissue, and the fact that it is "tethered" between fixed points of the zygoma, ear, and mandible, may favor a reduced risk for major avulsion. When penetrating wounds occur, though, there is considerable concern for the risk to the parotid gland; facial nerve; the glossopharyngeal, vagus, hypoglossal, and spinal accessory cranial nerves as they exit the skull base; the facial vasculature; and underlying bony structures.

Penetrating injuries to the lateral face require inspection prior to irrigation to reveal possible salivary leaks from the body of the parotid gland or from its duct anterior to the masseter muscle. Should a duct or gland injury be identified, definitive wound exploration, debridement, and surgical repair are often necessary through a parotidectomy and facial nerve dissection approach. The deep lobe of the parotid can usually be left intact because it will not be a likely source of salivary leakage. If, however, the parotid duct has been severed, the surgeon has the choice of repairing the duct or removing the gland. In most cases, it is possible to perform a ductal anastomosis using 6–0 or 7–0 nylon and loupe magnification. It may be necessary to cannulate the duct through the Stenson orifice because one can then perform the anastomosis circumferentially, taking care not to suture the duct closed. A suction drain may be preferred, though not required, if the duct or parotid gland has been injured or removed. Postoperatively, the wound should be compressed to reduce the stasis of saliva and a bland diet utilized for 7 to 10 days. If reanastomosis is not successful, the duct may be ligated to effectively stenose, following which the gland will become engorged and inflamed. Treatment with antibiotics, massage, heat, and sialogogues may help with the acute obstruction, but the gland either will atrophy or will require secondary parotidectomy. Because of the protracted course of parotid inflammation after traumatic stenosis of the duct, the surgeon may elect to perform a preemptive primary parotidectomy at the time of surgical exploration and repair of the wound to avoid that complication.[11]

Facial nerve injury should be presumed and ruled out in lateral facial lacerations or penetrations, particularly when the examiner can demonstrate parotid gland or duct injury. Since the parotid duct and the buccal branch of the facial nerve are closely aligned in their courses, both structures may be simultaneously injured. Fortunately, the thickness of the parotid gland and the overlying superficial musculoaponeurotic system provide relative protection for the facial nerve, leading to injury with only the deepest penetration. As is the case of typical knife or gunshot wounds, though, it is rare not to have sufficient penetration to involve at least one branch of the facial nerve. Elicitation of voluntary motion in the conscious patient is the best means of determining which, if any, branches are involved. It is worth mentioning that, even in the face of an intact nerve, severance of a specific facial mimetic muscle (i.e., zygomaticus or depressor labii inferioris) may mimic facial nerve injury on physical exam. Peripheral electrical stimulation of the facial nerve in the emergency room may be necessary in this case, or in that of the unconscious or uncooperative patient. Facial nerve testing is usually limited to the peripheral trunk and branches after exit from the stylomastoid foramen, when it is indicated.

In the case of facial nerve disruption, wounds should be explored as soon as feasible and the extent of injury identified (**Fig. 65.3**). It is usually necessary to perform a superficial parotidectomy to expose the proximal branches and trunk of the facial nerve. If exploration is performed within 72 hours of injury, it will be possible to utilize the nerve stimulator intraoperatively to assist in the identification of the distal branches of the severed nerve(s). The use of loupe magnification (4 to 4.5 power) or the operating microscope is essential for identifying the nerve endings in the traumatized tissues and in facilitating repair of the nerve(s). It is unusual to be able to perform a primary anastomosis of a nerve severed by a traumatic penetration because it is necessary to sharply trim the ends of the cut nerve to obtain undamaged neural bundles for repair. Thus a cable or interposition graft will likely be required. This graft can be obtained from a sensory nerve, such as the greater auricular nerve or, if that is not available due to the trauma, the sural nerve in the calf. Unfortunately, these nerves are not similar to the facial nerve and its branches in cross-sectional diameter, therefore necessitating that one or more fascicles be "stripped" from the donor nerve and sutured into interposition. No tension should be placed on the interposed graft, but if the nerve is too long, then reaxonization will be delayed; therefore only a slight laxity should be planned. An epineural closure should be performed using 8–0 or 9–0 nylon, or a single fascicle can be used with only a few fine nylon sutures at the periphery.

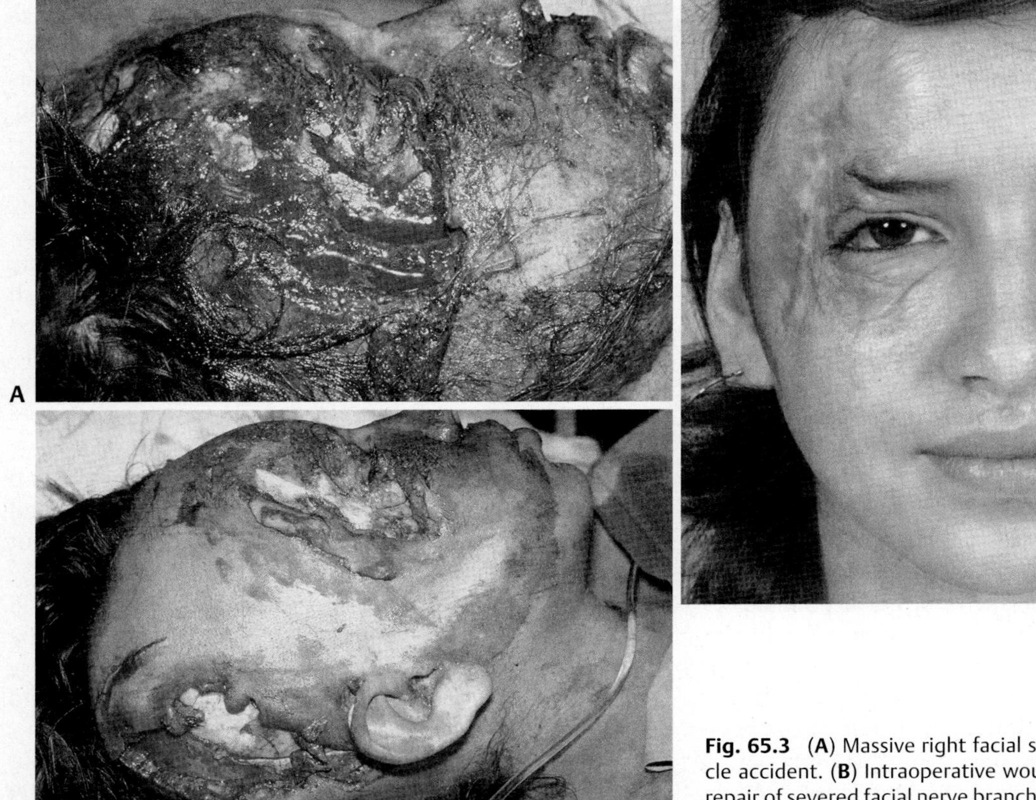

Fig. 65.3 (**A**) Massive right facial soft tissue injury due to motorcycle accident. (**B**) Intraoperative wound cleansing, debridement, and repair of severed facial nerve branches to eye. (**C**) One year postrepair and scar revision with normal eye closure.

Primary anastomosis should lead to early recovery within 12 months. If an interposition graft is used, then the length of time to potential recovery varies directly with the length of the graft and how far distally the injury was located. The longer the graft, the more likely the length of recovery is to approach 24 months; a distal injury is more likely to recover in just over half that time. The entire nerve, including the grafted segment, must undergo Wallerian degeneration and macrophagocytosis before reaxonitization occurs; thus the length of time expected for recovery must take this process into account. If a long recovery time is anticipated, one should consider a static rehabilitation of the face in the interim, including a gold weight to the upper eyelid, canthoplasty (in an older individual), and re-creation of the nasolabial fold with suspension of the nasal ala and oral commissure. This will provide a pleasant appearance in repose yet not interfere with the chance of later motion. If recovery does not occur or is incomplete, then one has a viable static support in place. The use of transcutaneous electrical stimulation of the facial musculature to maintain bulk and prevent atrophy has been advocated. There is no apparent contraindication to this, and the patient may feel comfortable performing some self-assistance.

In the lateral face, just anterior to the jaw and auricle, vascular injury to the superficial temporal artery and internal maxillary artery can arise. Active bleeding may be encountered and can typically be controlled by compression in the emergency room setting. However, severe epistaxis or an expanding hematoma in the pterygomaxillary space may arise from an internal maxillary artery injury. Injury to larger vessels, such as the internal maxillary artery, internal carotid artery, or jugular vein, requires arteriography for precise diagnosis and embolization or emergency exploration to repair or ligate the vessel. It is not wise to randomly clamp these vessels in a facial wound unless absolutely necessary because of the risk to the facial nerve and its branches.

Many facial injuries, particularly of the lateral face, will typically involve any number of significant structures, making evaluation, repair, and recovery that more complex. A gunshot wound to the lateral face, for example, can directly injure the mandible, maxilla, and internal carotid artery. If this is suspected by virtue of the location of the entry wound and likely course of the projectile, as well as other signs on the physical examination, then the patient should undergo angiography (if stable) to evaluate vascular integrity and CT scanning to assess for possible osseous damage. Some trauma surgeons are also using magnetic resonance arteriography and venography (MRA/MRV) to screen for vascular injury. Radiographic evaluation is also helpful in identifying foreign bodies present deep in the wound that remain "invisible" to the examining surgeon.

If osseous trauma is present, then the bone should be debrided, occlusion obtained, and internal stabilization plates applied. Even if the wound appears to be contaminated, small plates and mandibular/maxillary fixation can still be utilized, in conjunction with wound drainage, high-dose parenteral antibiotics, and copious irrigation.

Once healed, if persistent cosmetic problems ensue relating to scars of the cheek caused by avulsions or puncture injuries, management will typically involve scar reorientation into the lines of relaxed skin tension, geometric broken line closure, and dermabrasion. Makeup or cosmetic camouflage is also helpful from the beginning.

Soft Tissue Injuries of the Midface

Soft tissue injuries of the midface may present with bleeding, edema, difficulty with speech, and airway or muscle injury. In this area, the lips, nose, and periorbital structures are the main structures of concern. Because the lips are mobile; they are subject to stretch and avulsion. Penetrations may affect the teeth and attached gingiva and oral cavity. Nasal injuries occur because of the projecting position of the nose on the face, making it the first contact structure in most full-face wounding episodes.

It cannot be emphasized enough that the airway must first be controlled if at risk, especially in the event of edema, hematoma, or laceration involving the floor of the mouth or soft palate. This may require something simple, such as an oral airway or placement of a suture retraction for the tongue. If severe obstruction exists, though, nasal intubation, cricothyrotomy, or formal tracheotomy should be performed in the emergency department to secure the airway before any other diagnostic or therapeutic procedures are performed. Of all penetrating facial trauma, suspicion of airway compromise is greatest in cases of gunshot wounds to the face (**Fig. 65.4**).

Nasal evaluation should begin with identification of potential bleeding and hematoma. Septal hematoma is an emergency and must be identified and treated immediately. An attempt may be made to aspirate the hematoma using an 18-gauge needle, and if positive, the mucosa overlying the hematoma can be formally incised. In either case, once the fluid collection has been evacuated, a quilting mattress suture should be placed through the septum to tack down the mucoperichondrium and prevent reaccumulation. When anterior epistaxis is encountered, it is typically the result of trauma to the soft tissues of the nasal tip, alae, and columella (**Fig. 65.5**). Posterior bleeding is more dangerous, however, and may herald an injury to the greater palatine or sphenopalatine arteries in association with fractures. Inspection after suctioning, using either a fiberoptic headlight and nasal speculum or a nasal endoscope, will usually identify the source of the injury. If a bleeding source remains elusive and the

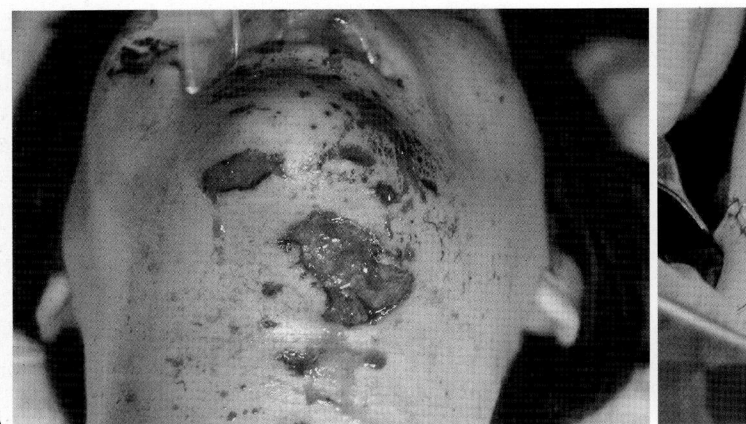

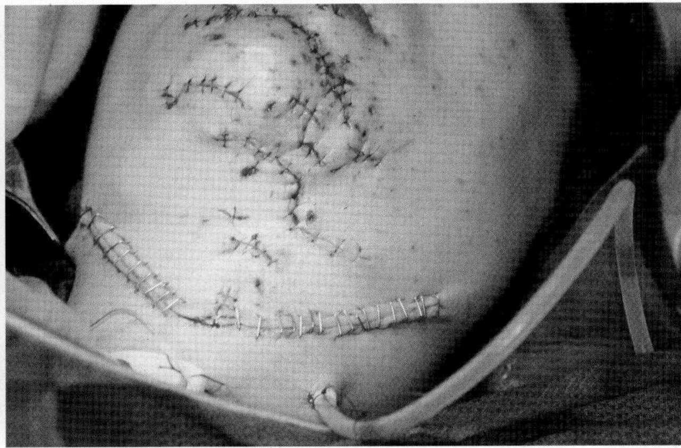

Fig. 65.4 (A) Gunshot wound to chin and lips, causing hematoma of sublingual tissue (**B**) Post–soft tissue repair, exploration of upper neck, and control of bleeding.

patient is stable, the source of significant bleeding may best be identified through carotid angiography. Nasal bleeding will often require urgent packing (either nonadhesive pads or microfiber surgical sponges soaked with Otrivin [Novartis International AG, Basel, Switzerland] and topical thrombin) or the insertion of nasal tamponading balloons.

For operative control of significant intranasal bleeding, the location of the bleeding, as identified by nasal cavity endoscopy, will guide the surgical approach. If the bleeding is in the inferior nasal cavity, then the internal maxillary artery can be ligated using fine metallic ligature clips via a transantral approach. The greater palatine artery can also be injected via its foramen in the oral cavity for temporary cessation until the internal maxillary artery can be ligated. If bleeding is found to be high in the nasal cavity, then an external ethmoidectomy approach can be utilized to identify both the anterior and posterior ethmoid arteries. These vessels may be clipped or cauterized with insulated bipolar bayonet forceps. The anterior artery must be divided after ligation or cautery to approach the posterior ethmoid artery, but the latter need not be divided after control is obtained. It provides a valuable guide for the distance to the optic foramen.

Also at risk for damage from penetrating wounds to the nose and nasal cavity are the palate, nasopharynx, paranasal sinuses, cribriform plate, and intracranial contents.

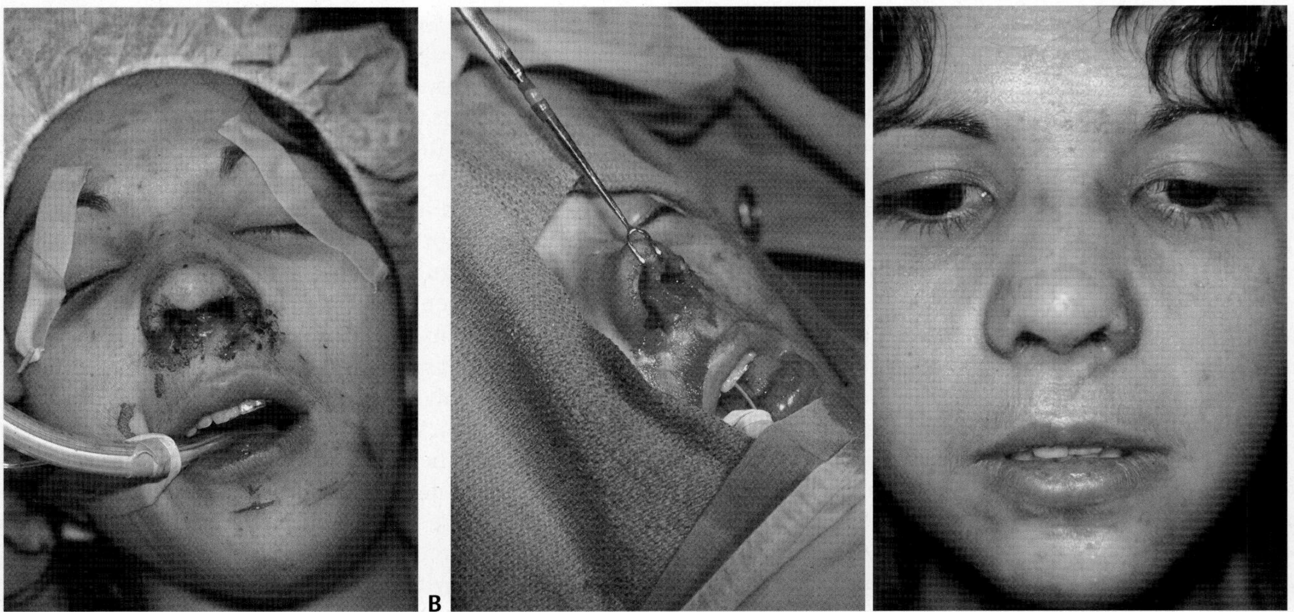

Fig. 65.5 (**A**) Avulsion of distal nasal tip from motor vehicle accident. (**B**) Exposure of extent of injury at time of surgery. (**C**) One-month satisfactory result without stenosis.

If a cerebrospinal fluid leak is suspected, then nasal packing should be used only as a temporary measure to control bleeding until the patient can undergo surgical vessel ligation or embolization. A cerebrospinal fluid leak can be identified through the crude "halo test" or via chemical analysis of clear nasal drainage for β-2-transferrin.

If the alar cartilages have been split or avulsed, then the cartilage should be minimally debrided and surgically reapproximated. The cartilages can be replaced in their anatomical position using 4–0 chromic catgut. Puncture wounds of the nose generally heal well with minimal debridement and loose closure. For through-and-through nasal punctures, only one surface—usually the skin surface—need be closed. Special care must be taken to carefully reapproximate the alar margin (rim) if it is severed because any misalignment will be noticed. The skin wounds may be closed with 6–0 polypropylene.

Nostril stenosis is perhaps the most common complication of soft tissue injuries to the nasal tip and may require Z-plasty or composite grafting from the auricle to widen the vestibule. Dilations, steroid injections, and soft nostril stents fabricated by a maxillofacial prosthetist can be helpful as well. If the nasal valve region has been damaged and is incompetent, then internal splinting using onlay (Batten) or underlay (alar stiffening) cartilage grafting usually works well.

Evaluation of the lips must identify through-and-through injuries, that is, involving the labial mucosa. If the penetration is close to the vermilion border, the labial artery may have been severed. The status of the orbicularis oris muscle must be ascertained; if separated in continuity, a deficit of closure will result. Deeper injuries may avulse teeth or implant them in the surrounding soft tissues, mandating that all teeth must be accounted for. Soft tissue wounds may be associated with alveolar or segmental fractures of the dental arches as well. Thus lip injury should raise one's suspicion of injury to underlying structures within the oral cavity.

The management of lip lacerations depends on the depth of penetration. If the lip is only partially involved, then dermal and skin closure will suffice. If the muscle is violated, then it should be reapproximated with either 4–0 chromic catgut or 4–0 polyglactin suture, taking care to close its entire dehiscence so that a continuity defect does not occur. If the penetration is full thickness, then the inner mucosal layer should be loosely closed with buried 4–0 chromic catgut sutures to prevent saliva from becoming entrapped and inciting infection. Special care should be taken to reapproximate the vermilion-skin border. Loupe magnification can be quite helpful in discerning this line. The vermilion can be sutured with 6–0 silk because the suture "tails" lie down flat on the vermilion surface and are not irritating to the patient. The nonvermilion epidermis is sutured with 5–0 or 5–0 polypropylene sutures.

If sutured properly, lip penetrations heal well and the sphincter effect of the oral stoma is maintained. If the oral commissure has been blunted, a commissuroplasty using intraoral mucosa can be performed. Notching of the lip ("whistle deformity") from incomplete closure of the orbicularis oris muscle can be reconstructed by excising the notch deformity and reapproximating the muscle and dermis well. The vermilion border, if misaligned, must be revised and realigned as closely as possible.

Additionally, neural injury to the infraorbital, mental, or supraorbital nerves should be elucidated through pinprick tests in the area of their distribution (**Fig. 65.6**).

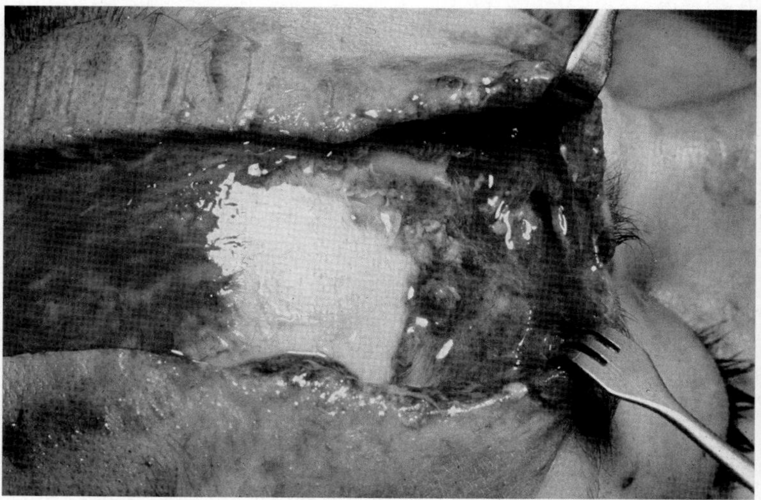
A

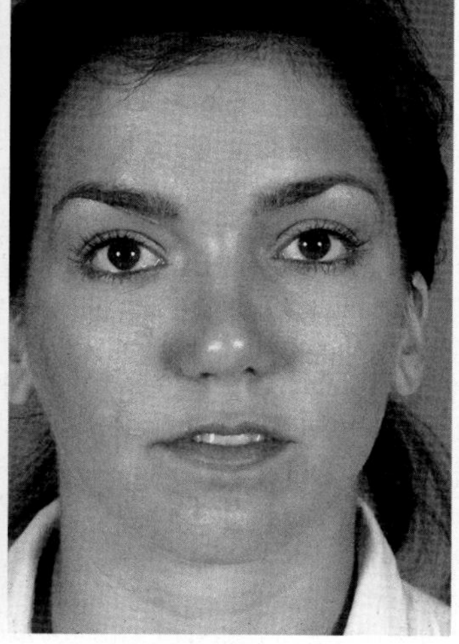
B

Fig. 65.6 (**A**) Motor vehicle accident injury to forehead with tissue separation, and damage to supraorbital and supratrochlear neurovascular bundles. (**B**) One year post–nerve repair and scar revision with improving sensation of forehead.

These nerves may be directly injured through severance by penetration, may be rendered neuropraxic from edema or shock, or may be involved in a fracture site.

CT scans may again help elucidate which, if any, of the aforementioned injuries are present. The surgeon should not be distracted by extensive overlying soft tissue injuries and neglect potential underlying bony injury. Holmgen et al proposed the acronym LIPS-N (*l*ip laceration, *i*ntraoral laceration, *p*eriorbital contusion, *s*ubconjunctival hemorrhage, and *n*asal laceration) to delineate midface zone injuries that have a greater likelihood of underlying fracture.[12] We advocate facial imaging when these injuries exist and/or clinical suspicion for underlying injury exists based on mechanism of injury and physical exam.

Periorbital Lacerations

Perhaps the most difficult of all, eyelid and periorbital lacerations require expert surgical care by a facial surgeon knowledgeable in the anatomy and physiology of these specialized structures. Additionally, in the authors' opinion, every periorbital soft tissue injury mandates an ophthalmology consultation to identify ocular or deeper orbital injuries. When these exist, an operative plan and repair as a team are often prudent.

With respect to lacerations of the eyelids, it is important to determine whether the laceration is horizontal or vertical. Horizontal lacerations are more likely than vertical lacerations to involve the elevators of the upper eyelid (levator and Müller muscles) or the retractors of the lower eyelid and violate the orbital septum. Conversely, vertical lacerations will likely involve the tarsus and possibly the lacrimal drainage system. Medial and lateral lacerations might also result in injuries to the canthal tendon attachments, with rounding of the palpebral fissures.

When a horizontal laceration is present, the most critical evaluation is to determine the patient's ability to raise the upper eyelid on upward gaze, and to slightly retract the lower eyelid on downward gaze. Should there be an inability to do so, then a presumptive injury to the eyelid elevators or retractors must be entertained. Also, fat identified in the wound raises the suspicion for orbital septum violation, thus foreshadowing further injury to underlying structures. This will require an open exploration of the laceration, identifying the layers of the eyelid, and locating the lacerated ends of the structures. Of primary concern is the reapproximation of the levator muscle and/or levator aponeurosis of the upper eyelid. Because the Müller muscle (sympathetically innervated) is attached fairly superiorly to the posterior aspect of the levator muscle and the upper portion of the aponeurosis, good repair of these structures will also likely include this special muscle. Often, it is necessary to perform the exploration and repair under local anesthesia and sedation in the operating room, so that the patient will be capable of looking upward during the exploration to facilitate identification of the superior or proximal end of the levator muscle for closure. Repair can be performed using interrupted 4–0 Vicryl (Ethicon, Inc., Somerville, NJ) sutures across the width of the muscle/aponeurotic complex. If necessary, the orbicularis muscle can be loosely reapproximated with a few Vicryl sutures as well. The skin can be closed with 6–0 polypropylene interrupted sutures.

Lower eyelid horizontal lacerations should be explored to identify any penetration that might have injured the inferior orbital muscles (inferior oblique, inferior rectus), particularly if there is evidence of decreased range of motion of the globe on ocular examination. Because of the potential for diplopia with inadequate reapproximation of the inferior orbital muscles, it is again wise to have this repair performed by an ophthalmologist.

Vertical lacerations of the eyelids are usually more straightforward, although they can appear to be very complex. These wounds tend to gape and spread apart, unlike horizontal lacerations, which can be nearly sealed and not raise concerns about deep tissue involvement. For any vertical laceration of the eyelid, the most important part of the closure is meticulous reapproximation of the eyelid margin. This is accomplished by realigning the anterior and posterior margins of the opposing sides of the laceration with 6–0 silk sutures. Additionally, silk sutures are placed through the Meibomian glands of the midmargin and tied, leaving the "tails" long. The suture tails are then tied beneath polypropylene sutures of the eyelid skin, below the lash line. These sutures should be left in place for at least 2 weeks to prevent a V-shaped deformity of the eyelid, which could cause epiphora. Following closure of the margin, the tarsus can be reapproximated with 4–0 or 5–0 Vicryl interrupted sutures. If the aponeurosis of the upper eyelid is separated, closure is performed in a similar fashion.

Lacerations involving one or both of the canthi should be explored to repair the attachment of the canthal tendon to the periosteum of the orbital wall using 4–0 Vicryl sutures. Lateral canthus repair should reestablish a nice lateral palpebral angle. For medial canthal lacerations, not only is the medial canthal tendon at risk but also the lacrimal drainage system. The latter structure is very important to the proper physiology of the globe mandating its repair. The lacrimal canaliculi and/or duct are typically repaired over a silicone tube-shaped stent which is tied within the nasal cavity. The stent can be removed in 6 weeks using a nasal endoscope.

Severe lacerations of the eyelids and periorbital structures require close attention to identify those structures remaining in the wound site, and an understanding of the intricate native anatomy, which will dictate where each

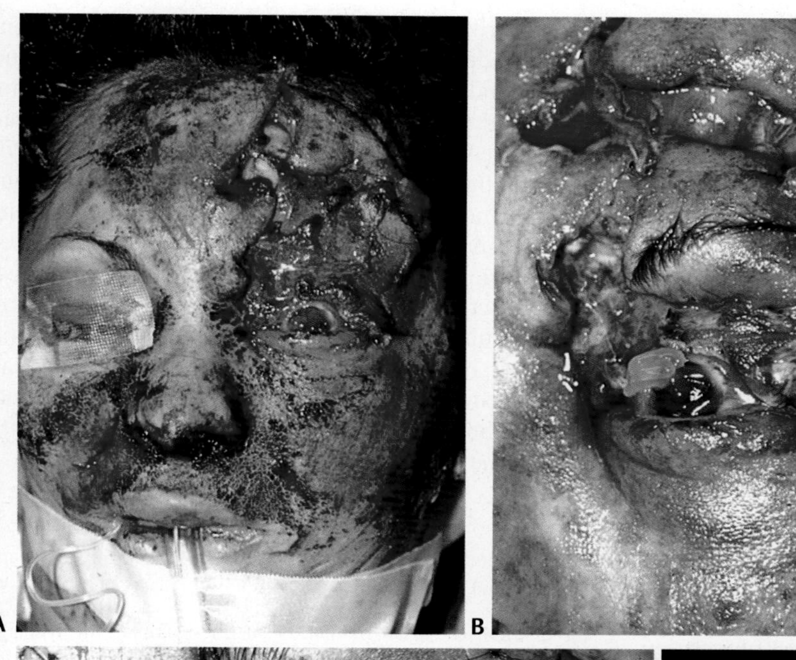

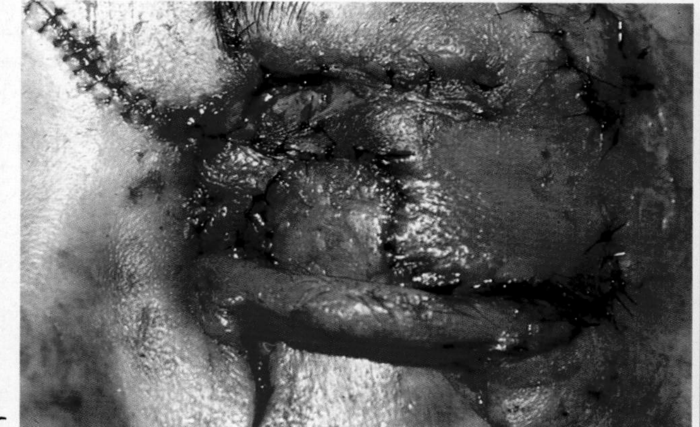

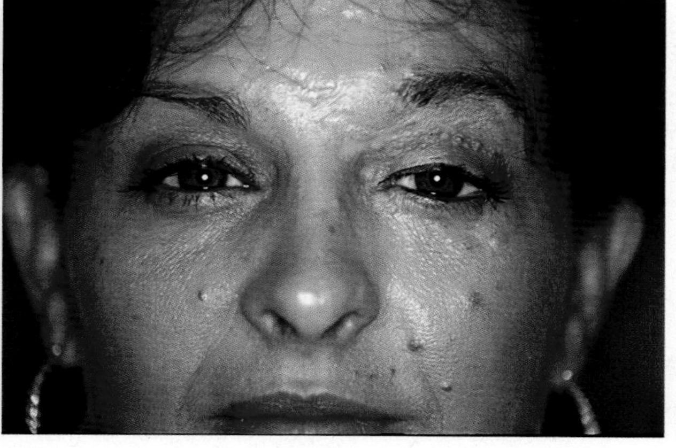

Fig. 65.7 (**A**) Multiple periorbital lacerations/avulsions from motor vehicle accident. (**B**) Closer view of periorbital lacerations. (**C**) Closure of eyelid lacerations with lower eyelid composite pedicle flap to upper eyelid defect. (**D**) Final result after release of lower eyelid flap and scar revision.

structure needs to be replaced. The distorted anatomy often found in these complex lacerations can be confusing, but, except for total avulsion of the eyelid(s), it is usually possible to locate and reposition all of the necessary structures. Should an avulsion occur, an inner/outer lamellae pedicle flap can be advanced to repair a full-thickness defect in the involved eyelid (**Figs. 65.7A–D**). Later revisions of the periorbital structures may be required to achieve optimal function and physiology of these special structures. The patient will also need to be followed closely by an ophthalmologist.

Before any repair of a complex or potentially complicated periorbital soft tissue injury is performed, a CT scan of the orbit may be required to identify a potential foreign body in the orbit that might have been introduced during the penetration. One must also consider that the globe itself may have been penetrated, hence further need for ophthalmological evaluation and assistance.

Soft Tissue Injuries to the ear

The ear, like the eyelids and lips, requires special attention to closure of lacerations. Most ear injuries are lacerations or avulsions, although blunt trauma can cause hematoma formation that requires incision and drainage. The two main concerns during repair are providing perichondrial coverage to the cartilaginous superstructure and maintaining a patent external auditory meatus and canal.

Most partial thickness lacerations can be easily managed by suture closure of the perichondrium with 4–0 or 5–0 Vicryl and the skin with 5–0 or 6–0 polypropylene. It is usually advisable to gently compress the ear postrepair with cotton, antibiotic ointment, and a loose mastoid dressing.

With full-thickness or avulsive injuries the repair is a bit more complex. Usually the skin and perichondrium will retract a few millimeters from the severed edge of the cartilage. To be able to close the perichondrium well, the free edge of the cartilage needs to be trimmed "inside" the free edge of the perichondrium. Prior to closing the perichondrium, "key sutures" should be placed in the skin to align the important anatomical landmarks of the ear—helix, antihelix, meatus, and so forth. This is similar to the key suture concept of closing the eyelid margin and white line of the lip. The cartilage need not be included in the sutures, as long as the anterior and posterior perichondrial layers are closed well. Following skin closure, a mastoid compressive dressing is helpful in reducing edema of the auricle. Because of the poor blood supply to the ear, a parenteral antibiotic such as ciprofloxacin or clindamycin should be initiated, before closure, and given orally for at least 10 days postclosure. Copious wound irrigation is also very important. The ear must then be closely observed for any signs or symptoms of perichondritis.

A laceration that involves the external auditory meatus should be carefully reapproximated and stented with a cotton or a Merocel sponge (Medtronic ENT, Jacksonville, FL) covered with mupirocin antibiotic ointment to reduce the risk of both infection and stenosis. Careful closure of the epidermis will reduce the risk of the formation of granulation tissue, which is associated with narrowing of the canal. Stenosis secondary to scar contracture is a vital concern in this area. Continued observation with appropriate splinting or steroid injections may be indicated.

Summary

Soft tissue injuries of the face can be complex, requiring careful identification of the involved structures and extent of damage, a careful analysis of options, and the development of a surgical plan, keeping in mind options for future reconstruction. Obtaining adequate comfort for the patient through specific anesthesia techniques allows the surgeon to focus on the wound care and closure. Copious irrigations, careful debridement of devitalized tissue, reapproximation of anatomical structures, and meticulous skin closures are key features of optimal wound care. Injuries to important and vital underlying structures should be suspected and identified, and then treated appropriately. Topical and oral or parenteral antibiotics, good wound care, use of silicone gel to reduce scar formation, and selected techniques for scar camouflage and revision complete the postsurgical management. Finally, an extensive knowledge of the functional and three-dimensional anatomy of the face and underlying structures is critical to achieving the best possible functional and cosmetic result. Psychosocial and emotional support must also be given to the patient and family. Scar revision and functional rehabilitation may require long-term care, multiple procedures, and commitment, and the patient should understand this possibility as early in the course of care as possible.

References

1. Levine E, Defutis L, Pruzinskky T, Shin J, Persing JA. Quality of life and facial trauma: psychological and body image effects. Ann Plast Surg 2005;534:502–510
2. Kornblut RM, Spetka LM, Heffner D. Penetrating injuries involving the anterior cranial fossa. Arch Otorhinolaryngol 1989;246:411–416
3. Dire DJ. 2005. "Tetanus" *http://www.emedicine.com/emerg/topic574.htm*
4. Atkinson W, Hamborsky J, McIntyre L, Wolfe S, eds. Epidemiology and Prevention of Vaccine-Preventable Diseases. 10th ed. Washington, DC: Public Health Foundation; 2008
5. Angeras MH, Brandberg A, Falk A, Seeman T. Comparison between sterile saline and tap water for the cleaning of acute traumatic soft tissue wounds. Eur J Surg 1992;158:347–350
6. Stefanopoulos PK, Tarantzopoulou AD. Facial bite wounds: management update. Int J Oral Maxillofac Surg 2005;34:464–472
7. Schultz RC. Animal bites. In: Facial Injuries. 3rd ed. Chicago: Year Book Medical Publishers; 1988:207–227
8. Stierman KL, Lloyd KM, De Luca-Pytell DM, Phillips LG, Calhoun KH. Treatment and outcome of human bites in the head and neck. Otolaryngol Head Neck Surg 2003;128:795–801
9. Manning SE, Human rabies prevention—United States, 2008. Recommendations of the Advisory Committee on Imuzination Practices (ACIP). MMWR 2008;57:1–26, 28
10. Mutabagani KH, Beaver BL, Cooney DR, Besner GE. Penetrating neck trauma in children: a reappraisal. J Pediatr 1995;30:341–344
11. Lewis G, Knottenbelt JD. Parotid duct injury; is immediate surgical repair necessary? Injury 1991;22:407–409
12. Holmgren EP, Dierks EJ, Assael LA, Bell RB, Potter BE. Facial soft tissue injuries as an aid to ordering a combination head and facial computed tomography in trauma patients. J Oral Maxillofac Surg 2005;63:651–654

66 Basic Principles of Craniofacial Bone Healing and Repair

Craig D. Friedman

This chapter will review basic concepts and principles of bone formation and repair important for facial plastic surgeons. Surgery of the craniofacial skeleton is an integral part of facial plastic surgery and thus a critical knowledge of fundamental bone biology and applied biotechnology including cellular, genetic, and molecular biology of bone formation and repair has become a requirement for successful clinical care. From this expanding knowledge increasingly sophisticated surgical techniques of bone repair and fixation have permitted the development of more effective treatments and resultant unprecedented successful patient outcomes.

Bone Formation and Structure

Bone tissue is a specialized composite of extracellular matrix proteins that is mineralized under the surveillance of associated cells, which maintain the structural integrity of the bone while responding to the metabolic requirements of the organism.

Formation

During embryological development there are two primary processes of bone formation. *Intramembranous* bone formation occurs independently of a preexistent model or structure; *endochondral* bone formation occurs via replacement of a cartilaginous structure or model/template.

In membranous bone formation, the ossification process takes place by direct mineral deposition into the organic matrix of mesenchymal tissues. The mesenchymal cells receive signals to induce differentiation to an osteoblastic lineage. Within the craniofacial skeleton, this is the major process observed. The frontal and parietal bones, nasal bone, maxilla, zygoma, and mandible are all of membranous origin.

In endochondral bone formation, mesenchymal cells differentiate to form a cartilage template. The cartilaginous structure proceeds through a hypertrophic state to become mineralized and ultimately replaced by differentiated bone cells. The removal and replacement of the mineralized cartilage is accomplished by the invasion of the template structure by osteoclast (large multinucleated) cells and blood vessels. Following removal of the mineral matrix, osteogenic precursor cells repopulate the template structure and form bone. This mechanism of bone formation is the basis of the axial skeleton; in the craniofacial region, endochondral origin is observed in the nasal septum and portions of the nasal bone complex, the occipital bone, skull base, and mandibular condyle.

Appositional growth in all bones (of either embryological origin) proceeds via membranous bone formation. Due to ongoing metabolic modeling and remodeling processes, no remnants of calcified cartilage are detected. The role that bone origin might play in healing and repair versus the impact of local regulatory factors has not been fully established. Many new insights regarding the molecular biology of bone formation are now being revealed, such as the interplay between developmental gene control for limb development (e.g., hox/HOM gene network) and local regulation (e.g., parathyroid hormone–related protein). Platelet-derived growth factor (PDGF) plays a role in inducing proliferation of undifferentiated mesenchymal cells. PDGF-AA and PDGF-BB have been shown to enhance proliferation of multiple types of bone cells, including both osteoblast and osteoclast lineages. The stimulatory effect of PDGF on bone proliferation appears dependent on the donor age and stage of cellular differentiation in that responsiveness to PDGF is decreased in more differentiated cells. Insulin-like growth factors (IGFs) are partly responsible for the general growth and maintenance of the body skeleton, with high levels of IGF-1 rapidly activating bone turnover with an increase in serum osteocalcin and carboxyterminal propeptide of collagen I as a marker of bone formation as well as an increased urinary ratio of calcium/creatinine and desoxypyridinoline excretion (a marker of increased bone resorption). Transforming growth factor β (TGF-β) has a biphasic effect, with enhancement of bone formation at low concentrations and suppression of proliferation and osteoblastic differentiation at high concentrations. Bone morphogenic proteins (BMPs), especially BMP2, BMP4, and BMP7, appear to be the most important and potent growth factors in terms of osteogenesis. Although beyond the scope of this chapter, further elucidation of the biology of bone formation will have an impact on clinical bone repair in the future.

Gross Structure

Grossly bone can be descriptively classified as either *cortical* or *cancellous*. These terms refer only to the structural architecture, not cellular origin or composition. Cortical (or compact) bone is immediately beneath the periosteum, adjacent to the endosteum, and these surfaces are lined with envelopes providing vascularity and osteoprogenitor cells for repair. The envelopes form a system of lacunae and canaliculi around the mineralized matrix for the transport of metabolites; this limits the outer diameter of the osteon (or basic bone unit) to ~100 μm of maximum diffusion and 200 μm of trabecular plate width. Within the cancellous bone, trabecular architecture is often described. The size, volume density, and dimension are variable and depend on the age, site, and loading of the bone. The transitions between the compact and cancellous bone are an area of flux; thus osteoclast cells may erode cavities inside of compact bone, allowing for cancellous bone to form. Conversely, osteoblasts may fill spaces within the trabeculae of cancellous bone to form new compact bone.

On the next level of microscopic exam, bone is usually classified as *woven* or *lamellar*, although some authors take the classification still further. Woven bone is characterized by its random collagen fibril orientation. Woven bone forms rapidly on the order of 3 to 5 μm/day in humans and can cover a relatively large physical territory, with resultant diminished biomechanical properties. Lamellar bone is characterized by elaborate orientation, and therefore its formation is more demanding and time consuming. Lamellar bone requires a preformed solid scaffold for its deposition; there is strict parallelism of the lamellae to the underlying surface. Any irregularities of the surface are usually addressed by woven bone prior to lamellar bone deposition. The linear appositional bone formation of lamellar bone is ~1 to 2 μm/day.

Remodeling of bone is a concerted and coupled action of bone resorption and formation that takes place on the surface and interior of compact bone. During remodeling, osteoclasts drill or create tunnels. Local signals (growth factors and their regulators) induce osteoblasts to follow and deposit lamellar bone, thereby contracting the tunnel walls around the nutrient capillary, forming secondary osteons, or Haversian systems. Bone remodeling allows for continued renovation and metabolic restoration while preserving functional capacity of the bone structure.

The blood supply to bone in the craniofacial region is abundant. Within the bony structure, the vascular supplies follow the Haversian system and are cross-connected by the Volkmann canals. Peripheral to the capillaries are the canalicular envelopes. These are related spatially to the osteocyte-perfusion exchange as noted earlier, limited to 100 μm. The blood supply to compact bone, especially as its thickness increases, is dependent on long low-pressure connections, thus making it more susceptible to disruption and longer recovery. In contrast, in cancellous bone the vascular supply reaches its anatomical destinations more directly without significant branching. Therefore, all processes of healing and remodeling that would require reestablishment of vascularization occur more rapidly and efficiently. Within the craniofacial bones, the vascular supply is more consistent with the cancellous bone model, with a relatively large surface area to bone volume; as such, these bones are less prone to vascular compromise. The mandible is a mixture of vascular supply types and therefore somewhat more susceptible to compromise. Overall, the plentiful blood supply of the craniofacial skeleton decreases the risk of infective complications in comparison with the extremities and appendicular skeleton.

Biochemical Structure

The noncellular composition of bone matrix is usually divided into organic and nonorganic components. The inorganic bone matrix makes up ~70% of the dry weight of the bone. The major constituent of the inorganic or mineral phase is calcium and phosphate in a unique biological crystal structure termed hydroxyapatite. Although hydroxyapatite conveys a specific chemical stoichiometry [$Ca_{10}(PO_4)_6(OH)_2$], various apatitic species of calcium phosphate exist (such as amorphous), with hydroxyapatite the most prevalent. The remainder consists of additional ionic species of sodium and magnesium as well as very small concentrations of other inorganic ion species.

The *organic* matrix of bone is usually divided into *collagenous* and *noncollagenous proteins*. Collagen composes 90% of the organic matrix in the form of a bone-specific type I unique in its specific glycosylation and cross-linking. The direct fibril–apatite interaction gives rise to the special biomechanical properties of bone. The remainder of collagen species present in bone are associated with blood vessels or are known to influence fibril diameter (types III, V, XII, and XIII).

The noncollagenous proteins make up the remaining 10% of the organic matrix. They are generally divided into proteoglycans, glycoproteins, Gla-containing proteins, and growth factors. The proteoglycans are composed of glycosaminoglycans (GAGs) covalently linked to core proteins. Examples of proteoglycans are decorin and fibromodulin with associated GAGs such as chondroitin and heparin sulfate. These proteoglycans are thought to play a role as binding reservoirs for various growth factors, such as basic fibroblast growth factor and transforming growth factor β (TGF-β).

Glycoproteins are represented by fibronectin, osteonectin, osteopontin, and bone sialoprotein. Glycoproteins share an arginine–glycine–aspartic acid (RGD) cell attachments sequence. A major role of these proteins is in modulating cell attachment and adhesion and mediating mineralization of the organic matrix.

Gla-containing proteins, represented by ostecalcin, take part in vitamin K–dependent enzymatic reactions. The final grouping of proteins is that of growth factors such as TGF-β, BMPs, insulin-like growth factors, and an ever-growing list of growth factors and their associated binding proteins. These factors, though present in small amounts, are thought to play important roles in bone formation and repair. Specifically, these factors can induce cellular differentiation of mesenchymal cells to osteoblastic lineage. In addition, they have complex interactions locally on the genetic control of repair and development of tissue. In summary, the extracellular matrix of bone is an extremely complex solid-state matrix that interacts with cellular components for the regulation of bone physiology.

Biomechanical Properties

The composite nature of bone affords it unique mechanical properties to support its physiological role. Bone also has anisotropic properties, meaning different properties along different axes. Measurements of bone strength are subject to various modeling and experimental considerations; however, comparison to steel places it at 10% relative strength. Compression of bone can be achieved because of the structural makeup, which permits force transduction. The result of compressibility is shortening or deformation of the bone; clinically, the response to such compression is resorption, or "creep." When bone is deformed by elongation, deformation is limited to ~2% before fracturing. The structure of bone, whether compact or cancellous, affects its strength, with cancellous bone having less than 10% the strength of compact bone. Measurements of bone strength have reported cortical bone with a compressive strength of up to 140 MPa and torsional or elastic modulus of 14 GPa. Various pathological conditions, such as osteoporosis, affect the microstructure of bone and thus the mechanical strength, which in turn affects the potential for fracture.

The craniofacial skeleton has evolved to provide protection to neurosensory structures (brain and eyes) and allow mastication. The structure of the calvarium, midface, and mandible allows for efficient function and protection. The skull and midface perform protective functions; therefore, repairs of these are usually less dependent on mechanical factors during healing.

Force transduction within the mandible occurs at the attachment of the muscles of mastication and at the dental occlusal plane. Model analysis of the mandible reveals that the muscles' forces are translated maximally at the angle and vertical ramus. The reactive forces generated in the occlusal plane bend the mandible forward, creating zones of tension in the alveolar region. When repairing mandibular disruption, attention to these zones of tension is imperative. Bite forces (up to 700 newtons) are generated along the occlusal planes. Calculation of the force and force-moment should be considered in the selection of fixation repair with certain minimum load resistance. These considerations are important in the design and placement of fixation devices, particularly in the mandible to maintain active function.

Fractures

Fractures are the result of mechanical overload, that is, failure to resist deformation under loading, resulting in the loss of structural integrity. Detailed analysis of fracture configuration has been done in terms of the force or load, energy release, and specific tissue characteristics. Torque, avulsion, bending, and compression result in specific patterns such as transverse, oblique, impacted, or comminuted. The structural disruption is accompanied by disruption of the osseous blood supply and is dependent on the dynamic nature of the injury disruption of soft tissues and associated neurovascular injuries. The vascular compromise is more significant in the mandible due to the relative thickness of the compact bone component affecting intracortical blood supply. However, the overall abundant blood supply aids in the healing and resistance to infection.

Fracture Healing

Restoration of function and original structure can be understood and evaluated on a biological and mechanical basis. Most fractures reach mechanical functional healing prior to histological or biological restoration of premorbid structure. The basic tenets of wound healing in bone are the requirement for functional cells, adequate nutrition (i.e., vascular supply), and mechanical environment to support the fragment ends in apposition. The initial events result in a process of internal and surface remodeling; increased DNA synthesis and cell proliferation in the subperiosteal region begin almost immediately. Nonperfused bone is replaced by vital bone via remodeling, and proliferating cells secrete osteoid (extracellular matrix), which is then mineralized and forms bone spicules. With progressive healing and osteoclast remodeling, the bone spicules are replaced by mature lamellar bone, and trabecular marrow spaces develop.

Within the extremes of interfragmentary motion, two general patterns of healing are described. This is in fact a continuum; however, it is best to consider the two classically described processes. With limited interfragmentary motion, the conditions for bone formation exist as already described; the contact zones of the fragments are not deformed and permit the osteoclasts in the "cutting cone" to cross the contact zone and connect newly formed osteons, which link the fragments. This is described as *primary bone healing* or *union*. Gaps across the contact zone allow for primary lamellar bone formation if immobilization is maintained; larger gaps induce a pattern of woven bone, which is then secondarily remodeled to lamellar bone. Larger but still immobilized gaps reach a critical defect size, which cannot support bone formation conditions and are therefore filled with fibrovascular tissue.

Under conditions of greater interfragmentary motion, the distractive forces in the fracture gap exceed the level of requisite stability necessary for primary healing across the gap. A process or "cascade" of tissue differentiation ensues, with the formation of granulation tissue to connective tissue, fibrocartilage, mineralized cartilage, woven bone, and finally compact bone. This process involving formation of a cartilaginous callus is considered *secondary bone healing*, or the extraperiosteal reaction to fracture with chondrogenesis and eventual endochondral ossification (**Fig. 66.1**). The cellular events are well documented based on experimental studies. Attached muscle and other soft tissues immediately outside of the periosteum show increased activity. Extravasated blood

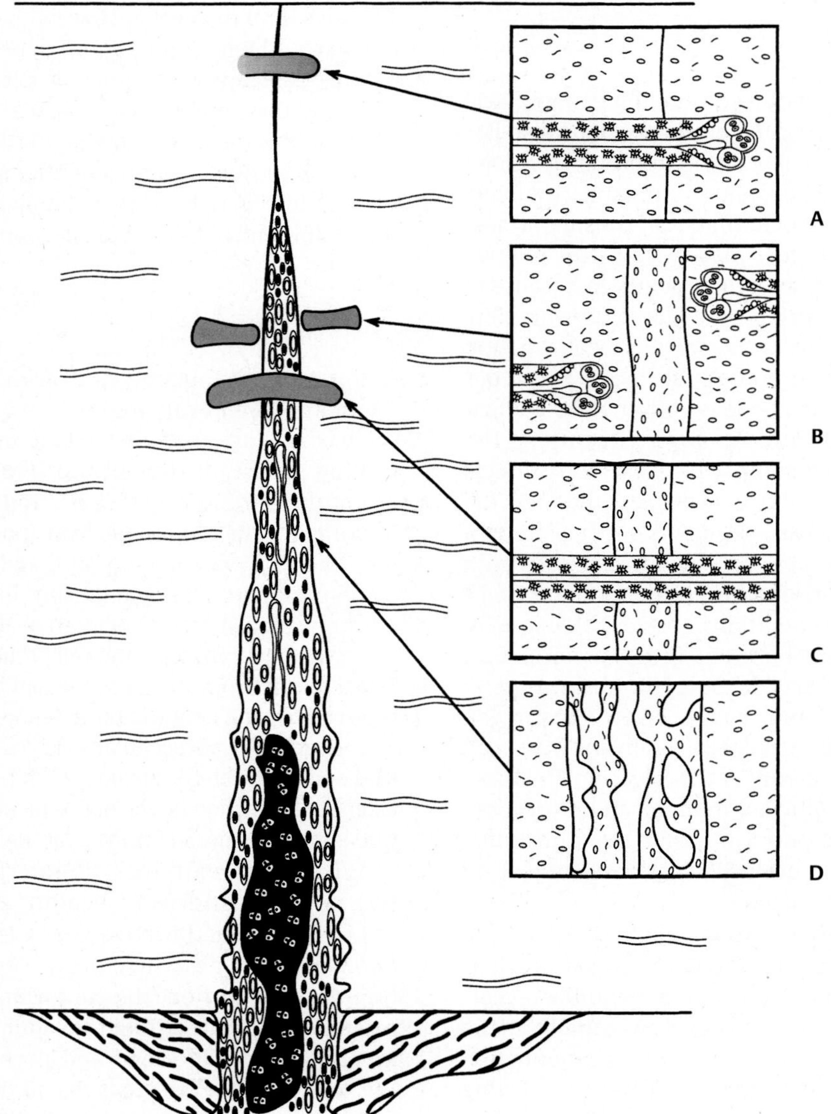

Fig. 66.1 Patterns of fracture healing. The appearance of a healing fracture is determined by the geometry of the fracture zone, the degree of immobilization at various sites, and their changes occurring over time. An absolutely perfect alignment of the entire fracture is not possible; direct contact between the fragment ends is restricted to only small portions. The remainder consists of a gap of varying width. Complete absence of interfragmentary motion is possible only in contact areas and in gap zones in their close vicinity. (**A**) If this zone is completely immobilized, whether from the beginning or as a sequel to bony bridging at other sites, direct intracortical remodeling across the fracture plane may take place at contact sites. (**B**) In a first step small immobilized gaps are filled directly with lamellar bone. (**C**) Then secondary remodeling in the axis of the bone gradually leads to reconstruction of the original integrity. This phenomenon of fracture healing without intermediate steps of tissue differentiation is called direct, or primary, bone healing. Pure direct healing, an extreme healing pattern on the one side of the scale, seems to be relatively rare. The farther away from the contact areas, the higher is the chance of interfragmentary motion of various degrees, and usually the higher is the gap. The healing pattern in these zones is characterized by resorption of the fragment ends, callus formation, and interfragmentary ossification via a cascade of tissue differentiation. This leads to a gradual immobilization during the healing process. This pattern, found on the other extreme of the scale, is common. (**D**) Intermediate stages, for instance, the subdivision of a wide gap by the formation of woven bone, may be observed between the two extremes. At a specific phase during the healing process it may happen that some sites of the same fracture are under relative motion while others become immobilized. Thus in a single fracture it is possible to observe a broad spectrum of different healing patterns. As a routine, however, only a narrow band from the full range of healing patterns reflects the situation of that specific fracture.

(or hematoma) is noted between the muscle fibers and periosteum. Inflammatory cells are noted in the hematoma (polymorphs and then macrophages). This follows the changes in the adjacent muscle with proliferation of fibroblasts and other cells within the degenerating muscle fibers. The basement membrane of the muscle fibers loses its structural integrity, allowing the fibroblasts to intermix with the hematoma cells and periosteal cells, forming a greater callus mass. The callus mass is then quickly vascularized with formation of small arterioles and venules.

The next stage in the tissue cascade is formation of cartilage within the callus and adjacent to areas of membranous bone formation near the junction between the cortex and subperiosteal bone. The cell proliferation decreases and a basophilic matrix is secreted devoid of blood vessels. The area becomes more avascular and lacunae form around the cells with hypertrophy of nuclei consistent with chondrocytes. Chondrogenesis continues in the same fashion as growth-plate formation during bone formation or maturation. The mature matrix and hypertrophic cells are calcified and invaded by blood vessels from the immediately adjacent membranous bone, then remodeled to woven and ultimately lamellar bone indistinguishable from subperiosteal bone formed via membranous ossification.

Cartilage formation is the primary mechanism of fracture healing in long bones and within the craniofacial region. It is usually seen in the mandible, but is also seen at other sites where conditions do not favor primary bone healing. Clinical conditions, including interfragmentary motion, can affect the local healing response. Diabetes and metabolic insult (chemotherapy), which impair cartilage formation, also play a role. It has been noted that within a given fracture, both types of healing may be noted.

Local regulation of fracture repair has received considerable attention. Growth factors important in local control can be produced by the associated inflammatory cells and found within the bone matrix itself. Osteoblasts, macrophages, or chondrocytes within the callus can also synthesize the factors. Growth factors prevalent in the fracture site are presented in **Table 66.1**. What has been initially discerned by various investigations is that TGF-β released from platelets initiates callus formation. Acidic fibroblast growth factor appears to regulate the proliferation of chondrocytes, and as the callus matures, synthesis of TGF-β is increased in the matrix and, along with other factors, induces chondrocyte maturation and initiation of endochondral ossification.

There is significant interplay among these local regulators of bone repair with the bone morphogenic proteins. BMPs are a subdivision of the TGF-β superfamily and play a crucial role in the process of cell growth and differentiation during bone regeneration. There are eight BMPs[2–9] (BMP1 is a proteinase and is not part of the TGF-β superfamily). When a bone is fractured, pluropotent progenitor cells are activated by the local immune response. The BMPs then bind to membrane receptors on these cells, resulting in activation of the osteocalcin gene, which transcribes a signal protein that

Table 66.1 Growth Factors Found in the Fracture Callus

Growth Factors*	Source	Matrix Location	Responding Cells	Unique Characteristics
TGF-β	Platelets, inflammatory cells (monocytes, macrophages), osteoblasts, chondrocytes	Bone is the most abundant source of TGF-β in the body	Most cells have TGF-β	Inactive precursor peptide, most potent chemoattractant identified for macrophages, promotes angiogenesis, activates a serine–threonine receptor
BMPs (BMP-2, BMP-4, BMP-5, and BMP-7)	Chondrocytes, urinary bladder, epithelium, brain	BMPs were originally identified in bone, but now are known to be widely distributed throughout the body	Unknown	TGF-β-like structure; may be involved in cartilage formation, important regulator during embryogenesis
Fibroblast growth factors (aFGF, bFGF)	Inflammatory cells, osteoblasts, chondrocytes	Binds HSPG in bone and cartilage matrix	Most cells of mesoderm or neuroectoderm origin	Stimulates neovascularization, evidence for an autocrine, intracellular function; stimulates type IV collagenase
Platelet-derived growth factors (PDGF-AA, AB, or BB)	Platelets, monocytes, activated macrophages, endothelial cells	Interactions unknown	Most cells of mesoderm origin	Activates a tyrosine kinase receptor

Abbreviations: TGF, transforming growth factor; BMP, bone morphogenetic protein; aFGF, acidic FGF; bFGF, basic FGF; HSPG, heparin sulfate proteoglycan.
Source: From Bolander, ME. Regulation of fracture repair and synthesis of matrix macromolecules. In: Brighton CT, Friedlander G, Lane JM, eds. Bone Formation and Repair. Rosemont, IL: American Academy of Orthopedic Surgeons; 1994. Reprinted by permission.

eventually leads to differentiation of the cell into an osteoblast. BMP3 (osteogenin) has been localized in perichondrium, cartilage, periosteum, and bone, as well as the membranous bones of the craniofacial skeleton, and has been shown to have the highest bone-inductive activity of all the BMPs. Further elucidation of osseous wound healing will undoubtedly aid in the development of new strategies for fracture repair.

Clinical Considerations in Fracture Healing

The clinical monitoring of fracture healing has been by the utilization of conventional radiological imaging. After reduction, the fracture line is minimally visible. Subsequent to the internal remodeling process, there is a decrease in the radiological density, and the fracture site becomes increasingly diffuse in appearance. Over time, there is characteristic loss of the visible fracture line. Determination of when healing is sufficient to enable progressive functioning has evolved from clinical experience and experimental models. Remodeling to full load bearing in the craniofacial skeleton can take up to 6 months in the mandible. Other areas of the facial skeleton may require significantly less time for healing. Reduced and fixated fractures can be returned to progressive function and loading beginning at 4 weeks. With the advent of rigid internal fixation plates, the time to function recovery has been decreased to essentially immediate limited functioning.

Potential complications of fracture healing include infection, refracture, delayed healing, nonunion, implant failure, and implant loosening. Due to the proximity and likely involvement of the oral cavity, infections that do occur usually involve oral flora and begin in the soft tissue adjacent to bone. Neurosensory injury is most likely secondary to the initial injury and most commonly involves trigeminal nerve branches and facial nerve.

Delayed healing is defined by clinical experience and can be said to occur in the midface after 6 weeks and in the mandible after 12 weeks if little or no healing has occurred. The management of delayed healing can be a spectrum from the replacement of the fixation apparatus to the curettage of the fibrous union with or without bone grafting. Implant failures usually stem from technical deviations during placement. Some common etiologic factors are use of monocortical screws lacking stability, insufficient number of screws, stripping of screws (when using self-tapping screws), and bone damage when inserting into an incompletely or poorly placed pilot hole.

Indications for Fracture Treatment

The goal in operative treatment of facial fractures is to promote rapid recovery of form and function. Stability of the reduction and fixation needs to be optimal for the specific anatomy. When this can be achieved, normal healing can be maximally stimulated. The decision to treat a fracture with closed or open techniques will always be individualized for the patient and the specific condition. Conservative closed splinting with maxillary mandibular fixation using interdental arch bars can successfully correct fractures that are closed and simple in nature. Internal fixation of fractures is best used for complex injuries in which return to function can be expedited. Functionally stable internal fixation is indicated for the following:

- Multiple or comminuted fractures
- Panfacial fractures
- Fractures with bone loss
- Open-wound fractures
- Severe midface dislocation
- Geriatric atrophic mandible fracture
- Infection or nonunion due to conservative treatment

Social factors, such as mental or cognitive variations that make conservative treatment more difficult, must be considered. In summary, open internal fixation of fractures should be carefully considered when warranted by the clinical status.

Fixation Technology for Fracture Treatment

Materials used for fixation implants must be strong and ductile, adaptable to fit the bone surface, and biocompatible. Metals have been used extensively in skeletal surgery; stainless steel, chromium–molybdenum alloys, and commercially pure titanium are the most commonly used. Titanium is now almost exclusively utilized for craniofacial repair, though resorbable miniplate systems are becoming a viable alternative. The advantages of titanium are (1) its resistance to corrosion by the formation of a surface oxide layer and (2) excellent tissue tolerance, providing a practically inert physiological status. Over time small amounts of particulate metallic debris from either natural degradation processes or from imperfections in metal implant can be noted within the reticuloendothelial system. This can produce instances of lymphadenopathy and measurable metal ion deposition in the liver.

Biodegradable polymeric materials have been introduced in recent years. Their use in fixation is preferred to titanium due to the anticipated resorption of the implant over time, precluding any need for implant removal. Internal titanium fixations have several disadvantages, including stress shielding and subsequent bone weakening near the implant site, palpable plates or screws and poor cosmesis, as well as extrusion and/or infection. Most biodegradable polymeric materials are based on various copolymers of ortho esters of lactic acid, although newer formulations with novel polymer constituents are also in development. One of the widely available resorbable miniplate systems is the amorphous 70:30 poly-L/DL-lactide copolymer plate, which has the advantage of continuous hydrolysis through the first 6 months. This breaks the copolymer chains into smaller particles that later become degraded by phagocytotic cells. Preliminary studies have found that these systems provide reliable stability for mandibular osteosynthesis after fracture. However, drawbacks include the increased costs, larger diameter, screw breakage, and the need to place screws into the plates. Due to the limited functional biomechanical capacity of biodegradable polymeric plates, these implants are best utilized in the areas of the craniofacial skeleton with the least amount of stress loading, such as the skull and orbitomaxillary region, or in the pediatric population, where concerns regarding growth inhibition with metal implants exist. Long-term follow-up of newer absorbable implants continues, and concern over local healing effects remains unresolved to date.

Splinting is the connecting of a stiffer device to the fractured bone. In craniofacial surgery, this most often consists of interdental arch bars that serve as an external splint. The goal of such splinting is to reduce fracture fragments without surgical intervention. There will always be mobility at the fracture site with this technique. Internal splinting in the form of wire suture or plate is more effective in reducing the interfragmentary motion and aiding the healing process.

Compression is a method of further reducing interfragmentary motion. Compression fixation consists in pressing the two surfaces together, bone to bone, or implant to bone. Compression produces a preload in the fracture plane and increases interfragmentary friction. Maintaining an axial preload greater than the tensile load produced by function and interfragmentary friction prevents displacement by shear forces, thereby keeping the fracture immobilized. Bone compression can theoretically be maintained for weeks to months, aiding bone healing between the fragments. The biological and mechanical advantage of compression for fracture healing is that it allows stability for the primary bone healing process to happen, and it allows for the load sharing between the implant and bone permitting function. Compression may be achieved with a screw or a combination of a screw and plate. In the craniofacial area the mandible is the primary bone to benefit from fracture compression. In the midface and orbitocranial region, compression is not necessary and is technically difficult to achieve. Onlay and inlay bone grafts are best fixated with compression when possible.

Compression with a screw (**Fig. 66.2**) can be achieved using the "lag screw" technique developed by woodworkers. Ideally, the screw should cross the fracture plane at a perpendicular angle. The outer cortex or surface is drilled to create a "gliding hole" by overdrilling, thereby allowing the screw to only engage at the cortical surface–screw head interface; the second surface or cortex is drilled and threaded to create a hole that accepts the screw threads intimately. Placement of the screw then produces interfragmentary compression. The use of screws to produce compression is efficient; however, clinical situations usually require application of more than one lag screw or their use in conjunction with a plate to overcome shear forces causing fragments to distract in very obliquely angled fractures.

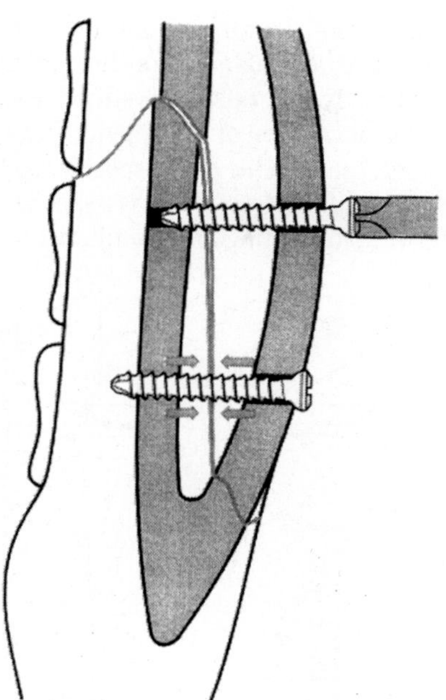

Fig. 66.2 Compression of oblique mandible with "lag screw."

Compression with a plate and screw (**Fig. 66.3**) is achieved by the combination of the design of the screw hole in the plate and the eccentric placement of the screw, which then allows interfragmentary compression in an axial direction when the screw is driven into the screw hole. Compression-plate screw holes are inclined horizontal cylinder shapes that permit the downward and horizontal movement of the screw head. The screw head engages the outer rim of the plate hole. The screw then glides horizontally toward the opposite (inner aspect) of the plate hole. The screw also engages the underlying bone, which is in turn moved toward the inner aspect and the fracture line. Only one eccentrically placed screw is used on either side of the fracture line. The remainder of the screws are placed centrally so as not to produce additional forces that would counteract the compression or distract the fracture fragments. Complete reduction of the fracture occurs only beneath the plate and at the opposite side of the bone; a gap may result, necessitating the use of a tension band in the form of a small plate or dental splint.

Screws function as a basic element in conjunction with plates to hold bone fragments together. The correct selection and placement of screws are essential for the successful stabilization of fragments. Screws are designated according to the outside diameter of their threads. **Fig. 66.4** shows the basic elements of a screw. Tapping, or creation of a recipient thread for the screw in the solid bone, can be achieved by specific tapping instruments or by a self-tapping screw that has a specialized distal tip design, allowing for cutting and simultaneous

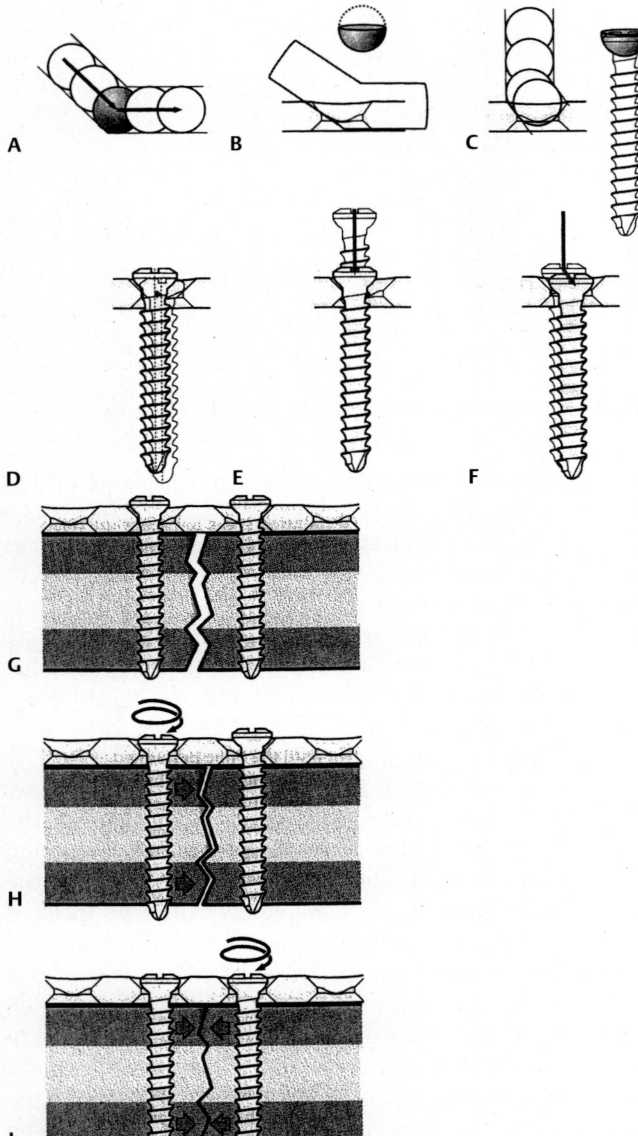

Fig. 66.3 Compression with plate and screw. (**A**) The screw head moves in the oval-shaped plate hole like a ball in an angled cylinder. (**B**) The screw hole is a section from of an inclined and a horizontal cylinder. (**C**) Movement of the screw head with its spherical undersurface in the DC hole of the plate. (**D**) The eccentrically placed screw arrives at the rim of the platehole. (**E**) As the screw is driven in, it glides within the platehole to (**F**) its final position. (**G**) The two innermost screws should be placed eccentrically within the DC holes. (**H**) As these screws are driven in, they approximate the fragments. (**I**) With final tightening of the screws compression is achieved.

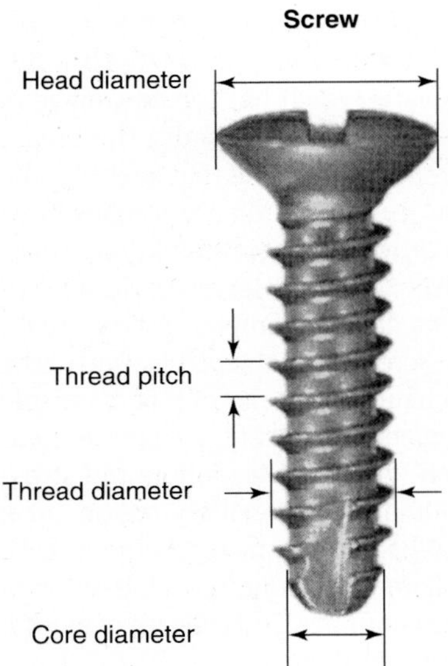

Fig. 66.4 Basic elements of a screw.

placement of the screw. Screws impart vector forces to engage the plate downward toward the bone; an additional screw configuration used in mandibular plates is that of the locking screw head, which is an expanding screw head that locks the plate and screw together as a single unit. The advantage is less loosening of mandible screws over the long term.

Plates have been designed in various configurations for craniofacial surgery. The adaptation of plates for specific sites, such as orbit, midface, and mandible, does not preclude maintaining the basic design to ensure stable fixation and screw placement. Specialized plates for compression and mandibular replacement share the same basic components.

Summary

Principles of craniofacial bone healing are important to the knowledge base of every facial plastic surgeon. An understanding of bone biology allows for successful treatment of various clinical states. Fracture repair as well as reconstruction for oncologic or developmental pathologies requires application of these principles. The basics of bone formation and repair aid the surgeon in selecting appropriate and effective therapies. Further elucidation of the interrelationship between bone formation development and wound repair will lead to more effective techniques and treatment strategies.

Suggested Reading

Blierzilkian JP, Raisz LG, Rodan GA, eds. Principles of Bone Biology. San Diego: Academic; 1996

Brighton CT, Friedlander G, Lane JM, eds. Bone Formation and Repair. Rosemont, IL: American Academy of Orthopedic Surgeons; 1994

Lynch SE, Genco RJ, Marx RE, eds. Tissue Engineering: Applications in Maxillofacial Surgery and Periodontics. Carol Stream, IL: Quintessence Books; 1999

Prein J, ed. Manual of Internal Fixation in the Craniofacial Skeleton. Berlin: Springer-Verlag; 1998

Additional Reading

Anderson R. Femoral bone lengthening. Am J Surg 1936;31:479

Ashhurst DE. The influence of mechanical conditions on the healing of experimental fractures in the rabbit: a microscopical study. Philos Trans R Soc Lond B Biol Sci 1986;313:271–302

Assael LA. Considerations in rigid internal fixation of midface trauma. Atlas Oral Maxillofac Surg Clin North Am 1990;1:103–119

Brunner U, Kessler S, Cordey J, Rahn B, Schweiberer L, Perren SM. Defektbehandlung langer Rohrenknochen durch Distraktionsosteogenese (Ilizarov) und Marknagelung. Unfallchir 1990;93:224–250

Champy M, Lodde JP. Synthesis mandibulare: location de synthese aux function de contraints mandibulaires. *Stomat* (Paris) 1971.

Claes L, Palme U, Palme E, Kirschbaum U. Biomechanical and mathematical investigations concerning stress protection University of Ulm; 1982

Coleman J. Osseous reconstruction of the mid-face and orbits. Clin Plast Surg 1994;21:113

Cordey J, Perren SM, Steinemann S. Parametric analysis of the stress protection in bone after plating. In: Bergmann G, Cordey J, Schwyzer HK, Brun S, Matter P. Bone loss following plate fixation of fractures? Helv Chir Acta 1985;52:181–184

Danckwardt-Lillieström G, Grevsten S, Olerud S. Investigation of effect of various agents on periosteal bone formation. Ups J Med Sci 1972; 77:125–128

Dannis R. Theorie et pratique de l'osteosynthese. Paris: Masson; 1979

Day TA, Vuillemin T, Laedrach K, Raven J, Stucker FJ. Theuse of Calvarial bone grafting in craniofacial reconstruction. Facial Plast Surg Clin North Am 1995;3:241–257

Frodel J, Marentette L. Lag screw fixation of the upper craniomaxillofacial skeleton. Arch Otolaryngol Head Neck Surg 1993;119:297

Fuji N, Yamashiro M. Classification of malar complex fractures using computed tomography. J Oral Maxillofac Surg 1983;41:562–567

Gautier E, Cordey J, Liithi U, Mathys R, Rahn BA, Perren SM. Knochenumbau nach Verplattung: biologische oder mechanische Ursache? Helv Chir Acta 1983;50:53–58

Gautier E, Cordey J, Mathys R, Rahn BA, Perren SM. Porosity and Remodelling of Plated Bone after Internal Fixation: Result of Stress Shielding or Vascular Damage? Amsterdam: Elsevier Science; 1984

Goodship AE, Kenwright J. The influence of induced micromovement upon the healing of experimental fractures. J Bone Joint Surg Br 1985;67:650–655

Gotzen L, Haas N, Strohfeld G. Zur Biomechanik der Plattenosteosynthese. Unfallheilk 1981;84:439–443

Greenberg AM, Prein J, eds. Craniomaxillofacial Reconstruction and Corrective Bone Surgery. Berlin: Springer-Verlag; 1970

Gruss JS, Mackinnon SE. Complex maxillary fractures: role of buttress reconstruction and immediate bone grafts. Plast Reconstr Surg 1986;78:9–22

Gunst MA, Suter C, Rahn BA. Die Knochendurchblutung nach Plattenosteosynthese. Helv Chir Acta 1979;46:171–175

Haas N, Gotzen L, Riefenstahl L. Biomechanische Untersuchungen zur Plattenfixation an die Hauptfragmente. Orthopedics 1985;123:591

Haug RH. Basics of stable internal fixation of maxillary fractures. In: Greenberg AM, ed. Craniomaxillofacial Fractures: Principles of Internal Fixation Using the AO/ASIF Technique. Berlin: Springer-Verlag; 1993:135–157

Hayes WC. Basic biomechanics of compression plate fixation. In: Uhthoff HK, Stahl E, eds. Current Concepts of Internal Fixation of Fractures. Berlin: Springer-Verlag; 1980:49–62

Hutzschenreuter P, Perren SM, Steinemann S, Geret U, Klebl M. Some effects of rigidity of internal fixation on the healing pattern of osteotomies. Injury 1969;1:77–81

Ilizarov GA. The tension–stress effect on the genesis and growth of tissues. Clin Orthop Relat Res 1989;238:249–281

Jackson IT. Classification and treatment of orbitozygomatic and orbitoethmoidal fractures: the place of bone grafting and plate fixation. Clin Plast Surg 1989;16:77–119

Kellman R. Recent advancements in facial plating techniques. Facial Plast Surg Clin North Am 1995;3:227–239

Klotch DW, Gilliland R. Internal fixation vs. conventional therapy in midface fractures. J Trauma 1987;27:1136–1145

Kolbel R, Rohlmann A, eds. Biomechanics: Basic and Applied Research. Dordrecht: Nijhoff; 1987:387–392.

Krompecher S, Kerner E. Callus Formation: Symposium on the Biology of Fracture Healing. Budapest: Academiai Kiado; 1979

Kroon FMH, Mathisson M, Cordey JR, Rahn BA. The use of miniplates in mandibular fractures: an in vitro study. J Craniomaxillofac Surg 1991;19:199–204

Kuhn A, McIff T, Cordey J, Baumgart FW, Rahn BA. Bone deformation by thread-cutting and thread-forming cortex screws. Injury 1996;26(Suppl l):12–20

Kuntscher G. Das Kallus-Problem. Stuttgart: Enke; 1970

Lane WA. The Operative Treatment of Fractures. London: Medical Publishing, 1913.

Lanyon LE, Rubin CT. Functional Adaptation in Skeletal Structures. Cambridge: Harvard University Press; 1985:1–25

Manson PN. Some thoughts on the classification and treatment of the Le Fort fractures. Ann Plast Surg 1986;17:356–363

Manson PN, Hoopes JE, Su CT. Structural pillars of the facial skeleton: an approach to the management of Le Fort fractures. Plast Reconstr Surg 1980;66:54

Marx RE. Clinical application of bone biology to mandibular and maxillary reconstruction. Clin Plast Surg 1994;21:377

Matter P, Brennwald J, Perren SM. Biologische Reaktion des Knochens auf Osteosyntheseplatten. Helv Chir Acta 1974;12(Suppl):1

Mueller ME, Nazarian S, Koch P. Classification AO des fractures: 1 Les os longs. New York: Springer; 1987

Muller ME, Allgower M, Schneider R, Willenegger H. Manual of Internal Fixation. Berlin: Springer-Verlag; 1991

Muller ME, Nazarian S, Koch P, Schatzker J. The Comprehensive Classification of Fractures of Long Bones. Berlin: Springer-Verlag; 1990

Pauwels F. Biomechanics of the Locomotor Apparatus. Berlin: Springer-Verlag; 1980

Perren SM, Cordey J. The concept of interfragmentary strain. In: Uhthoff HK, Stahl E, eds. Current Concepts of Internal Fixation of Fractures. Berlin: Springer-Verlag; 1980:63–70

Perren SM, Rahn BA, Liithi U, Gunst MA, Pfister U. Aseptische Knochennekrose: sequestrierender Umbau? Orthopade 1981;10:3–5

Phillips JH, Rahn BA. Comparison of compression and torque measurements of self-tapping and pretapped screws. Plast Reconstr Surg 1989;83:447

Rahn BA. Direct and indirect bone healing after operative fracture treatment. Otolaryngol Clin North Am 1987;20:425–440

Rhinelander FW. Physiology of Bone from the Vascular Viewpoint. Vol 2. San Antonio: Society for Biomaterials; 1978:24–26

Rudderman RH, Mullen RL. Biomechanics of the facial skeleton. Clin Plast Surg 1992;19:11–29

Ruedi TP. Titan and Stahl in der Knochenchirurgie. Berlin: Springer-Verlag; 1975;3

Schatzker J, Tile M. The Rationale of Operative Fracture Care. Berlin: Springer-Verlag; 1987

Schenk R. Cytodynamics and histodynamics of primary bone repair. In: Lane JM, ed. Fracture Healing. New York: Churchill Livingstone; 1987

Schenk RK. Biology of fracture repair. In: Browner BD, Jupiter JB, Levine AM, Trafton PG, eds. Skeletal Trauma. Philadelphia: WB Saunders; 1992:31–75

Schenk RK, Willenegger H. Zum histologischen Bild der sogenannten Primarheilung der Knochenkompakta nach experimentellen Osteotomien am Hund. Experientia 1963;19:593

Schliephake H. Bone growth factors in maxillofacial skeletal reconstruction. Int J Oral Maxillofac Surg 2002;31:469–484

Schmoker RR. Management of infected fractures in nonunions of the mandible. In: Yaremchuk M, Gruss J, Manson P, eds. Rigid Fixation of the Craniomaxillofacial Skeleton. Stoneham, MA: Butterworth-Heinemann; 1992:233–244

Schwenzer N, Steinhilber W. Traumatologie des Gesichtsschadels. Richtlinien für die kieferbruchbehandlung. Munchen; 1974

Spiessl B. Osteosynthese des Unterkiefers. Berlin: Springer-Verlag; 1988

Spiessl B. Internal Fixation of the Mandible: Manual of AO/ASIF Principles. Berlin: Springer-Verlag; 1989

Spiessl B, Schroll K. Spezielle Frakturen und Luxationslehre. Vol 1, Gesichtsschadel. Stuttgart: Thieme; 1972

Steinemann S. In: Greenberg AM, Prem J, eds. Craniomaxillofacial Reconstructive and Connective Bone Surgery: Metal for Craniomaxillofacial Internal Fixation Implants and Its Physiological Implication. Berlin: Springer-Verlag; 1998

Steinemann S, Mausly PA. Titanium alloys for surgical implants: biocompatibility from physicochemical principles. Sixth World Conference on Titanium, Cannes, 1988

Tonino AJ, Davidson CL, Klopper PJ, Linclau LA. Protection from stress in bone and its effects: experiments with stainless steel and plastic plates in dogs. J Bone Joint Surg Br 1976;58:107–113

Uhthoff HK, Dubuc FL. Bone structure changes in the dog under rigid internal fixation. Clin Orthop Relat Res 1971;81:165–170

Weber BG, Brunner C. The treatment of nonunions without electrical stimulation. Clin Orthop Relat Res 1981;161:24–32

Weber BG, Cech O. Pseudarthrosen: Pathophysiologie Biomechanik–Therapie–Ergebnisse. Bern: Huber; 1973

Wolf J. Das Gesetz der Transformation der Knochen. Berlin: Hirschwald; 1892

Wolff J. The law of bone remodelling. Berlin: Springer-Verlag; 1986

Woo SLY, Akeson WH, Coutts RD, Rutherford L, Jemmott GF, Amiel D. A comparison of cortical bone atrophy secondary to fixation with plates with large differences in bending stiffness. J Bone Joint Surg Am 1976;58: 190–195

Yamada H, Evans FG. Strength of Biological Materials. Baltimore: Williams and Wilkins; 1970

Yaremchuk MF, Gruss JS, Manson PN. Rigid Fixation of the Craniomaxillofacial Skeleton. London: Butterworth–Heinemann; 1992

67 Principles of Facial Plating Systems

Peter D. Costantino, Monica Tadros, and Matthew Wolpoe

In 1968, Hans Luhr was the first to introduce the idea of plate fixation in the craniomaxillofacial skeleton when he used compression plating adapted from orthopedic surgery to repair a mandibular fracture.[1] In the time since Luhr's innovation, plating of this region has become a highly reliable tool employing a complex combination of technique and technology. This is due in large part to the understanding of the mechanical forces affecting various areas of the craniomaxillofacial skeleton coupled with the fabrication of specialized hardware. The metals now used for rigid internal fixation have physical and mechanical properties that maximize both stability and flexibility while minimizing corrosiveness and tissue reactivity. Current plating systems are adaptable to a wide variety of skeletal defects as well as having reduced size and visibility. However, regardless of the type of plates employed, it is essential that the craniomaxillofacial surgeon have an understanding of the principles of rigid internal fixation. This chapter describes the various plating systems now available, the principles guiding their application, and the basic indications for their use.

History and Development of Rigid Internal Fixation for the Craniomaxillofacial Skeleton

Hansmann is credited by most as the first person to apply the concept of rigid internal fixation (RIF) when he used a metal implant in 1886 to repair a defect in the extremities. However, numerous technical difficulties prevented this method of skeletal stabilization from being practical until the latter half of the twentieth century.[2] In 1949, a Belgian surgeon, Danis, advanced the previously unrecognized concept that bones immobilized by rigid internal fixation devices could heal primarily.[3] In 1958, a group of 15 Swiss surgeons under the direction of Maurice Miller formed the Association of Osteosynthesis and the Association for the Study of Internal Fixation (AO and ASIF). These groups went on to perform many ground-breaking experiments using RIF in the extremities. On the basis of this research, the AO and ASIF derived four basic concepts that they deemed essential to rapid recovery of form and function with RIF. These principles were (1) anatomical reduction of bone fragments; (2) functionally stable fixation of the bone fragments; (3) preservation of the blood supply to bone fragments by utilization of atraumatic surgical techniques; and (4) early, active, and pain-free mobilization.[4–6]

Incorporating these principles, RIF soon became a widely employed method for treating traumatic injuries in the extremities. Although this is true, adapting these techniques to the craniomaxillofacial skeleton proved more difficult. Finally, after years of experimentation, Hans Luhr successfully adapted the AO and ASIF rigid fixation principles to treat mandibular fractures in 1968. Luhr, concurrently with Shenck and Willenegger, solidified the earlier theories of Danis and showed that it was possible to achieve primary healing in rigidly fixed bone ends. In 1973, Michelet presented the alternative hypothesis based on the physiological properties of osteosynthesis.[7] Unlike the AO and ASIF, which is based on the idea that bone ends should remain tension-free during the healing process, Michelet proposed that some forces could be beneficial. Based on the understanding that the physiological process of bone formation occurs along lines of stress, Michelet suggested that suboptimal healing might result from the historic concept of "stress shielding," where the transfer of forces to bone across a fracture site is prevented. Michelet designed a miniplate system that allowed micromotion at the fracture site and pioneered a new philosophy that opened the doors to present-day semirigid fixation. Studies conducted by Champy in 1976 verified the soundness of Michelet's theory. Initial experimentation in cadaveric mandibles confirmed that plating devices could withstand the masticatory forces and functional loading present at mandibular fracture sites.[8] Subsequent experiments by Champy et al successfully expanded on these principles in the clinical setting.[9–11] Later, with the use of smaller plating systems with lower visibility, Champy demonstrated the applicability of these principles in the midface.[12]

Despite these advances, rigid internal fixation of the craniomaxillofacial skeleton did not gain wide popularity until the 1980s. Contributing to this surge in popularity was the development of smaller plates and screws, including the newer microplating systems for infants and children.[13] In the early 1990s, Eppley pioneered the use of resorbable plating systems for use in the adult midface, as well as in infants and children.[14] Eppley's work in children followed from studies by Yaremchuk and others, which found that metallic plating systems could limit growth and potentially be extruded from the growing craniomaxillofacial skeleton.[15] As a result, the first commercially available resorbable plating system, composed of poly-L-lactic and polyglycolic acid became available in 1996 (Lactosorb, Walter Lorenz Surgical Corp.,

Jacksonville, FL). The culmination of these efforts and the refinement of available materials have made plating of the craniomaxillofacial skeleton a widely employed and effective method for achieving reduction and primary union of fractured bone ends as well as bone grafts in the postablative setting.

Anatomical Considerations

The craniomaxillofacial skeleton is not a homogeneous entity, but rather is composed of bones of different sizes and thickness exposed to a disparate array of forces. Therefore, it is helpful to have an understanding of these differences to facilitate proper application of RIF equipment in the most efficacious anatomical location.

Mandible

The region of the craniomaxillofacial skeleton exposed to the greatest amount and variety of stresses is the mandible. This is the result of its primary role in both mastication and articulation of speech, which expose the mandible to many torsional, compressive, and tensile forces. The masticatory forces of the mandible are generated by its shape, the position of the teeth, as well as the insertions of the major muscles of mastication. These factors are distributed in such a way that tensile forces are felt at the upper border of the mandible and compressive forces at the lower border. This concept is critical to an understanding of the requirements of plates applied for mandibular reconstruction. A line separating the anatomical regions subjected to these various forces, known also as the ideal line, is the plane where compressive forces equal tensile forces, and is located at the base of the alveolar processes just under the root apices (**Fig. 67.1**). In addition to these tensile and compressive forces, in the region anterior to the canines, the mandible is also subjected to a variety of torsional forces.

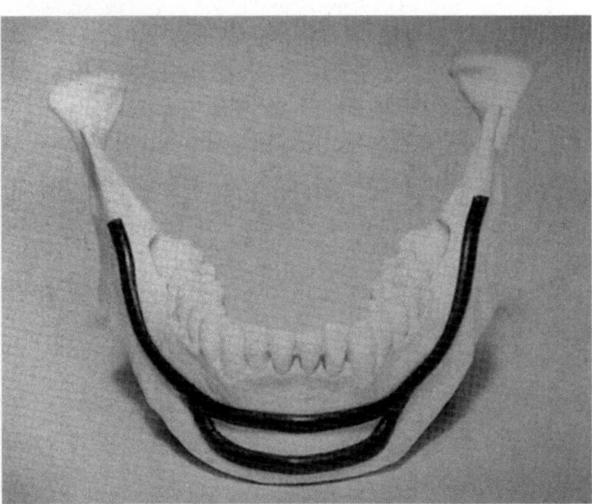

Fig. 67.1 Model of mandible with depiction of the ideal line.

The cortex of the mandible is of varying depths throughout its length. Specifically, thick cortical bone is found anteriorly in the region of the chin and laterally along the superior margin anterior to the third molar and along the inferior margin posterior to the third molar. Knowledge of these various anatomical differences will allow screw placement and plate application in a configuration that maximizes their fixation strength. Plates used in the mandible are typically thicker than those used in the midface, ranging from 2.0 to 2.7 mm, and generally require larger cortical screws. Imprecise plate selection in a stress-bearing location may loosen and act as a foreign body, leading to inflammation and an increased risk of infection and nonunion. Besides the forces of mastication, screw-and-plate application must also take into account the location of the apical processes of the teeth and the position of the inferior alveolar nerve that runs within the mandibular canal.

Many of these fundamental principles were incorporated by a group of French surgeons who founded the Groupe d'Etudes en Biomecanique osseuse et articulaire de Strasbourg (GEBOAS). GEBOAS proposed that because of the presence of the mandibular canal, specifically in the dentulous mandible, it is necessary to place plates beneath the alveolar processes near the inferior mandibular border. When this traditional plating technique is employed, the upper border of the mandible remains subject to distractive tensile forces. Because of this force distribution, they introduced the concept of using an upper plate as a "tension band" in addition to a lower plate to stabilize the fixation. Furthermore, in the area of the mandible anterior to the mental foramen, where torsional forces are greatest, it may be prudent to use both a subapical plate and a plate at the lower border to achieve stable mandibular fixation.[2]

Despite the fact that the plating principles put forth by GEBOAS are still employed, it was later found that use of a tension band can be avoided in situations where eccentric compression plating is used. This system utilizes oblique compression holes, set at an angle of ~75 degrees from the main axis of the plate. By orienting the screw holes in this manner, compression is applied at a vector such that it counters the tensile forces present at the upper border (**Fig. 67.2**). As a result, it is possible to position eccentric plates below the ideal line and achieve both a good reduction and stable fixation, without the use of a tension band.

Midface and Upper Cranium

Although this region of the craniomaxillofacial skeleton is subject to lesser forces than the mandible, various considerations must be kept in mind when plating in this

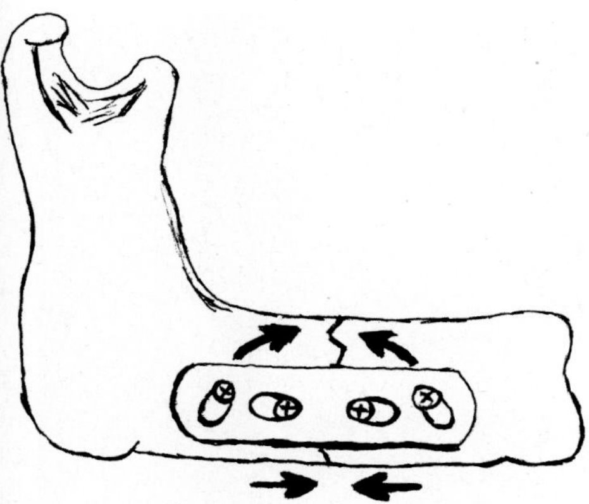

Fig. 67.2 Depiction of eccentric compression plating showing how orientation of oblique holes produces compression at upper border mandible when plate is placed below ideal line.

region. The area of the midface most exposed to the tensile forces of mastication is the zygomatic complex, particularly due to attachment of the masseter muscle. Rigid fixation in this region must be sufficient to overcome these forces and stabilize the zygomatic buttress. In addition, anatomical variability should be kept in mind when contemplating reconstruction of the midface and cranial vault.

Only a few regions in the midface have cortex of sufficient thickness to accommodate secure placement of most screws. These include the cranium, nasal bones, orbital rim, zygomatic bone, zygomatic buttress, and piriform aperture. Newer, smaller microplating systems, offer some flexibility to stabilize thinner areas of bone.

Materials and Equipment for Rigid Internal Fixation

Metals Used for Screws and Plates

Many factors must be considered when evaluating metals for use in craniomaxillofacial fixation. Sufficient strength and flexural resistance are important to ensure stabilization of the fractured bone ends and maintenance of a three-dimensional anatomical position. Biocompatible and immunologically nonreactive metals resist corrosion and help avoid adverse local tissue reactions and systemic toxicity over time. Materials that are somewhat malleable provide ease for intraoperative contouring to the skeletal surface. Lastly, the metals used for plating should produce a minimal amount of scatter on computed tomography (CT) and magnetic resonance imaging (MRI). This allows accurate monitoring of fracture-healing, plate placement, and in the case of reconstruction following tumor ablation, evaluation for recurrence.

Although several materials have been evaluated for use in craniomaxillofacial fixation, currently only three metal alloys are widely used commercially: titanium, vitallium, and stainless steel. Stainless steel, which is primarily composed of iron with lesser amounts of chromium, nickel, molybdenum, and manganese, was first used in orthopedic surgery in 1926.[6,16] Steel is available in several forms on the basis of the ratio of the aforementioned materials; however, the austenitic form, which minimizes corrosion and scatter on radiograph, is the primary form used currently for rigid fixation. Although stainless steel is still used on a limited basis, it has fallen out of favor and been replaced by titanium and vitallium, which have more favorable mechanical and physical properties such as the ability to osseointegrate with adjacent bone (**Fig. 67.3**).[17]

Scientists have appreciated the favorable qualities of titanium for a variety of purposes for several hundred years. However, it was not until the 1950s that an effective extraction and purification system for this metal was developed. Titanium, which is available primarily as an alloy mixed with small amounts of aluminum and vanadium, has found widespread use in craniomaxillofacial fixation. It is the metal alloy used most commonly in plating systems in the United States, such as the Stryker-Leibinger Universal Fixation System (Kalamazoo, MI) and the Synthes Maxillofacial Fixation System (Paoli, PA).

The success of titanium as an implant material is due to its remarkable biocompatibility and resistance to corrosion and infection. Studies reveal resistance of titanium to in vitro biofilm formation when incubated with *Staphylococcus aureus*, supporting the safety of titanium even in contaminated areas of the head and neck, such as the paranasal sinuses.[18] In addition, it is a remarkably light

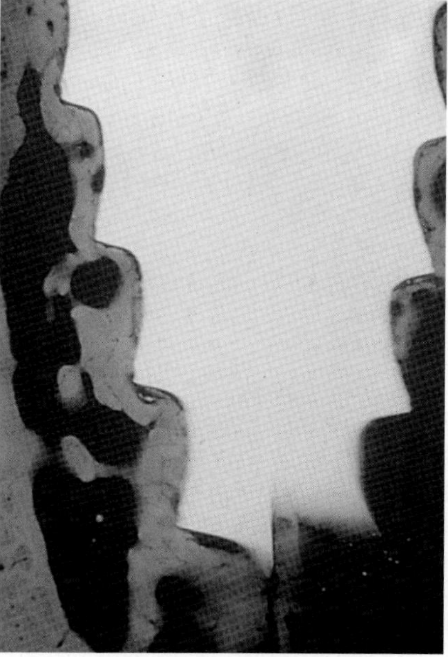

Fig. 67.3 Histological preparation showing osseointegration of bone into a titanium metal plate.

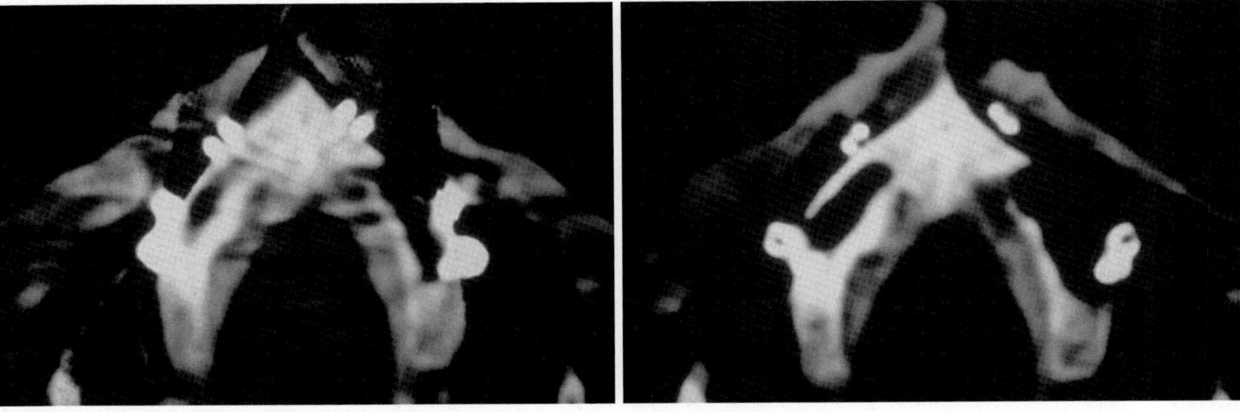

Fig. 67.4 Computed tomographic scans comparing degree of radiographic scatter produced by (**A**) vitallium versus (**B**) titanium implants.

material that possesses high tensile strength and produces minimal scatter on MRI and CT scans. Of the three currently used metals, however, titanium has the lowest elastic modulus. This necessitates the use of a slightly thicker implant to yield the same degree of stability as other alloys, such as chromium-molybdenum and stainless steel.

Vitallium used in the Luhr Maxillofacial Plating System (Stryker-Leibinger Corp., Kalamazoo, MI) was the metal alloy originally developed by Luhr for mandibular compression. It is composed of cobalt and chromium with small amounts of molybdenum, nickel, tungsten, and occasionally other elements. Vitallium has a biocompatibility and susceptibility to corrosion similar to that of titanium. In contrast, vitallium possesses a higher elastic modulus and is 1.5 times stronger than titanium, making it similar in strength to stainless steel. This allows vitallium plates to be thinner, with less visibility, than most other metals. Despite this fact, it is important to recognize that these vitallium plates produce significantly more radiographic scatter on CT scans than the larger titanium plates (**Fig. 67.4**).[19,20]

Screws

Characteristics

The properties of the screw used for rigid fixation determine much of the holding power and stability of the plating unit. There are several components of the screw that may impact its ability to provide this stability. These include the size and shape of the screw head, the length and diameter of the screw, the pitch and width of the threads, as well as the presence or absence of flutes. The height of the screw head and, in part, the shape of the screw hole determine the visibility of the screw. Specifically, thinner, flatter screw heads result in less vertical dimension than thicker, more conical screw heads. Therefore, screw heads of this type are less likely to be palpable in regions with limited soft tissue coverage. In addition, there are numerous types of slots available for screw heads that accommodate different styles of screwdrivers. These include hexagonal, cruciate, single, or Phillips slots. The shape of the slot determines both the axial pressure necessary for screw insertion as well as its tendency to strip. Phillips slots have the highest axial pressures and therefore require the most force to secure the screw head during insertion. In contrast, hexagonal slots have low axial pressure and are applied more easily than Phillips slots but conversely have a greater tendency to strip. Cruciate slots have low axial pressure and low risk of stripping, making this an effective screw design.[21,22]

External screw diameter and thread width in large part determine holding power. However, studies have shown that outer screw diameters greater than 2.0 mm do not improve the stability of screws in thin cortical bone.[2] The pitch of the threads determines the amount of bone purchase per turn. However, in thin cortical bones, especially those of the midface, a large pitch means in essence that only one or two threads may engage the cortex after insertion, making the screw potentially unstable. Therefore when screws are designed for rigid fixation equipment one must try to maximize screw purchase and holding power (i.e., screws for microplates have threads with a smaller pitch than those for standard plates).

Another factor that varies depending on the type of screw is whether or not it requires tapping or placement of a pilot hole prior to screw insertion. In contrast to screws requiring holes, self-tapping screws have three cutting flutes at their tips. These screw flutes shave bone of the internal surface of the screw hole as the screw is turned into the hole. This avoids binding and accumulation of bony debris in the screw hole, thus decreasing purchasing power. The disadvantage of self-tapping screws is that the cutting flutes reduce the tension at the head of the screw ınd therefore must extrude through the bone edge to ıchieve the same degree of stability as a pretapped screw. n addition, these screws require more torque for placenent and therefore risk stripping during insertion.

ag Screws

ag screw osteosynthesis is a method of screw placement vherein the screw purchases only the distal bone segnent as it crosses a fracture line (**Fig. 67.5**). This allows ompression of the two bone ends toward one another, hereby holding these fragments in stable union. The ompression results from the force that is generated as he distal bone segment (which is caught by the screw hreads) is pulled against the screw head, thereby trapping the proximal segment of bone between those two oints. The main indication for the use of lag screws, vhich can be used with or without an intervening plate, is or sagittal fractures caused by shearing forces. Lag screws vork best in an environment with thicker cortical bone nd therefore are useful in almost any region of the manible. Although the midface has thinner cortical surfaces, ıg screws still may be used in selected situations, such as he periorbital and subnasal regions.[23,24]

There are several technical considerations when mploying lag screw osteosynthesis. First, when implantng a lag screw across an oblique fracture, the two bone ragments are first held in motionless continuity using nodified towel clips (bone reduction forceps). These crews are not self-tapping, so the proximal segment is rst drilled utilizing a bit as wide as the outer diameter f the screw to be implanted. The ideal angle of this hole said to be found by drawing two imaginary lines, one erpendicular to the bony surface and the other to the blique fracture, and drilling the hole halfway between nem. Most surgeons contend that good compression can e achieved by simply drilling at a 90-degree angle from ne fracture line. After a hole has been drilled through ne proximal segment, a guide is inserted to protect the anal. Next, the distal segment is drilled using a bit the ze of the core diameter of the screw to be inserted. If the drill hole in the proximal segment is too small, then the screw threads will engage the proximal bone segment, and nonunion of the two fragments will occur. This is analogous to screwing in a bolt utilizing a washer and a nut. In this setting, screwing in the bolt will advance the nut and washer toward one another, thereby achieving compression. However, if two nuts are used on the same bolt, then these nuts will move in parallel and no compression will occur.[23] Overall, it is generally accepted that for wide sagittal fractures a lag screw alone will suffice, whereas for short sagittal fractures an intervening plate may be necessary to achieve an adequate reduction.

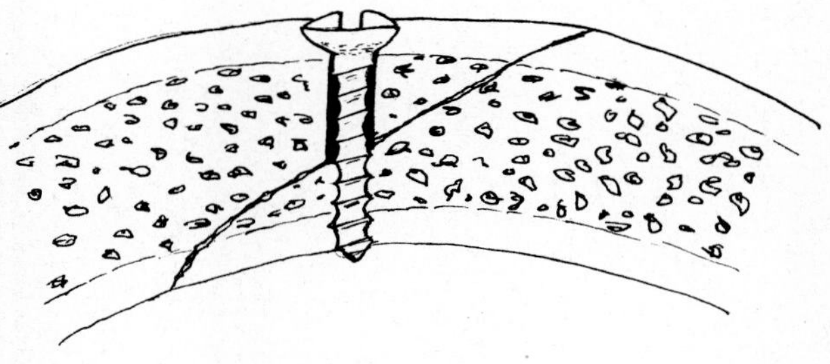

g. 67.5 Lag screw osteosynthesis. Notice that the hole in the oximal fracture segment does not engage the screw threads, hereas the distal segment does.

Emergency Screws

Included in all commercially available plating systems are emergency screws that can be used in the event that the initial screw stripped the bony cortex during insertion. An emergency screw is simply one that has an inner or core diameter that is equal to the outer diameter of a regular screw that was initially inserted. This allows rescue of a screw hole that has been stripped, which can be critical in certain situations.

Plates

Prior to the use of plates, it was customary to wire fractured bony fragments together (**Fig. 67.6**). Although this practice still has its indications, it has been shown that rigid internal fixation with plates promotes superior healing, and in contrast to wire interfragmentation, allows primary union of fractured bone fragments. Primary healing is defined as direct healing across a site of osteosynthesis without deposition of osteoid (immature bone). When this type of union occurs, there is no chance that an interpositional callus from fibrous healing will occur. In contrast, secondary osteosynthesis is defined

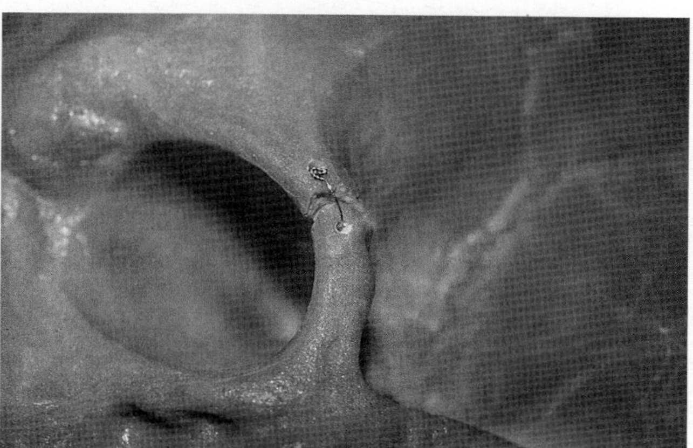

Fig. 67.6 Interfragmentary wire fixation.

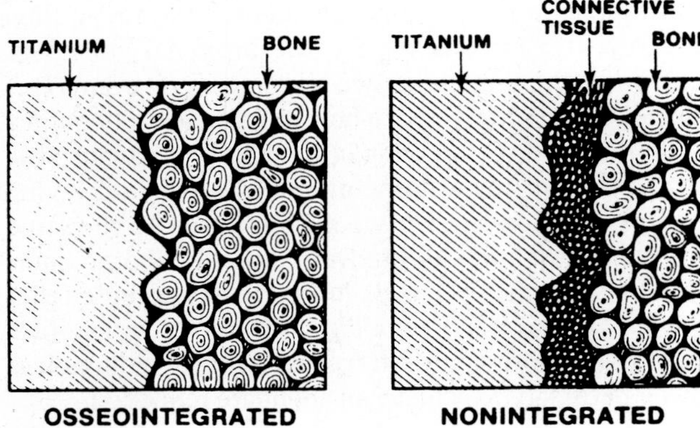

Fig. 67.7 The local environment as well as reactions to metallic implants in large part determine the success of a reconstructive procedure. On the left is depicted successful integration and primary healing of a titanium implant. In contrast, on the right the titanium implant has failed to integrate and therefore a stable reduction cannot occur.

as healing by deposition of osteoid across a gap in the fracture site and its subsequent remodeling into mature bone. In this situation, there is the potential for fibrous healing and instability as a pseudarthrosis. Thus, depending on the local environment during the healing process, metallic implants may be incorporated or osseointegrated into surrounding bone, or may remain nonintegrated and become a nidus for pseudarthrosis (**Fig. 67.7**).

Primary union is not possible with wires because with these fixation devices it is only possible to reduce motion in two dimensions; therefore, rotational and torsional forces still occur. By using plates and screws, with the caveat that at least two screws must be used on either side of a fractured segment, macromotion in three dimensions can be prevented. This allows the bone fragments to be held in close continuity in a relatively motionless environment, thereby encouraging healing by primary union.

Selection of the appropriate plating system and materials is fundamental to the success of facial fracture fixation. There are several types, shapes, and sizes of plates available commercially. These plates vary in size and configuration based on different indications and location of implantation. From a practical standpoint, it is very important to be familiar with the various categories of plating systems along with their primary indications. This will ensure the best possible reduction and will maximize healing and minimize morbidity.

Compression Plates

Danis was the first to advocate the use of compression plating to reduce the incidence of fractured bone fragments.[3] It was shown later by Luhr that with compression it was possible to achieve primary union following mandibular fractures.[1,25,26] As the name implies, compression plates are designed to apply a reducing force to close the gap between two fractured bone ends. This compression produces a preload, which counters the functional loading forces that promote distraction of fractured bone ends. In addition, if adequate compression is achieved, a frictional force is also generated between the two bone ends that reduces torsional and translational motion.

Compression is achieved by using the "spherical gliding principle." The compression plate has oval holes and is configured in such a way that the smaller end of the hole is too small for the upper portion of a conical screw. Therefore, if the screw is inserted at the smaller end of the compression hole, as it is advanced it will become progressively larger and thereby move toward the larger end of the hole. By advancing in this manner the screw forces the two bony segments to slide toward one another and achieves compression (**Fig. 67.8**). On a standard compression plate there is usually a compression hole on either side of a fracture segment as well as a round or neutral hole. However, some plates may have two compression holes on either side, allowing for greater

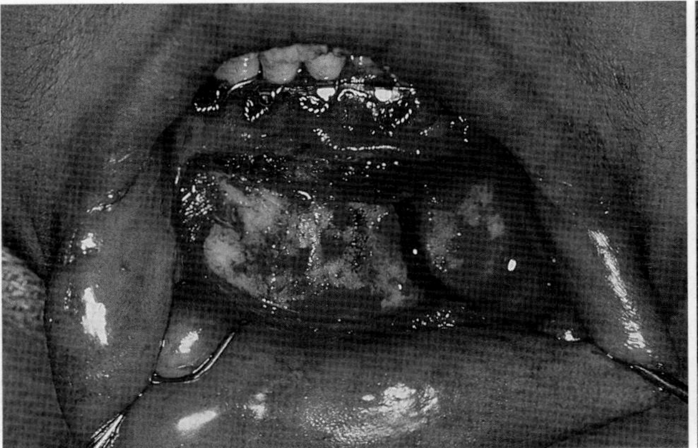

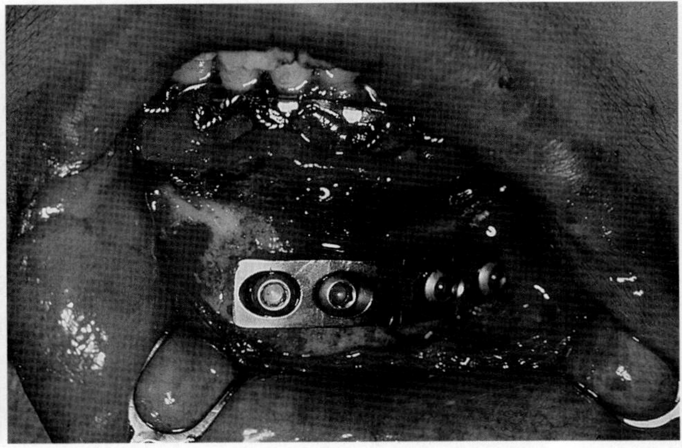

Fig. 67.8 Reduction of displaced fracture of mandibular body. (**A**) Application of compression plate reduces larger gap in body of mandible to produce a good occlusion with aid of (**B**) a tension band.

tension. In addition, it is possible to use compression plates in a neutral fashion if the screw is applied at the larger end of the hole in the compression plate.

There are two types of compression plates: dynamic compression plates (DCPs) and eccentric dynamic compression plates (EDCPs), both designed to achieve compression in a plane perpendicular to the plate itself. In mandibular plating, to protect the inferior alveolar nerve and tooth roots, plates are placed along the inferior border of the mandible. When using DCPs this often necessitates the use of a tension band across the upper alveolar border to avoid superior distraction of the fractured bone segment during mastication. A tension band can consist of either a miniplate along the alveolar border of an edentulous mandible or an arch bar segment attached to the teeth adjacent to the fracture site.

In contrast, EDCPs were designed to counter these distracting tensile forces when placed at the inferior mandibular border. This is achieved by utilizing two types of compression holes. The inner compression hole is the same as that in dynamic compression plates and achieves tension in a plane perpendicular to the plate, along the lower mandibular border. The outer holes of these plates have compression holes placed at oblique angles. These oblique holes are oriented in a manner that promotes compression along the superior mandibular border, thus obviating the need for a tension band. Although this is true, it should be noted that EDCPs are much more technically demanding to use and therefore are not favored by most surgeons.

Compression plates are indicated in edentulous mandibles for virtually all types of fractures, with the exception of highly comminuted fractures, fractures of the condylar neck, for fixation of bone grafts, or in highly atrophic mandibles. In these cases, a mandibular compression plate or titanium hollow-screw reconstruction plate system may be necessary (see the following). In dentulous mandibles, compression plates are indicated in displaced fractures of the mandible, fractures of the mandibular body and temporomandibular joint, moderately comminuted fractures, when maxillomandibular fixation is not desirable, and in cases of polytrauma.[27,28] In the midface, where there are fewer masticatory forces and thinner cortices, the indications for compression plates are much narrower. However, these plates can still be used in complex fractures of the zygoma and periorbital region, as well as following craniomaxillofacial trauma.[28]

Mandibular Reconstruction Plates

The mandibular reconstruction system (MRS) was described by Reuther in 1975 to provide static fixation rigid enough to bridge bony defects after tumor ablation, with or without a bone graft (**Fig. 67.9**).[29] The plates

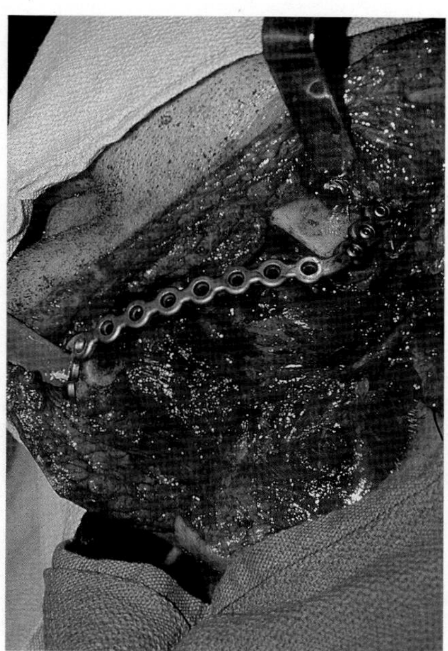

Fig. 67.9 Mandibular reconstruction plate bridging a postablational mandibular defect.

are constructed with a low modulus of elasticity to maximize strength, stability, and compression. They are either straight or curved and have two neutral and two compression holes on each side, a configuration designed to provide the greatest overall holding power. It should be remembered that when applying plates of this type, the lateral compression holes and screws are always placed first, followed by the more medial neutral holes. If this is not done, compression will not result.

There are three main indications for the MRS: alloplastic bridging of mandibular defects following tumor ablation, reduction of highly comminuted mandibular fractures as in shotgun wounds, and rigid fixation of bone grafts. The MRS is particularly suited for situations where long-term mandibular fixation is required and in injuries involving the mandibular symphysis.[28–30] When applied for these indications, the MRS provides support for the tongue as well as structures of the oropharynx and larynx. Often when using MRS, maxillomandibular fixation may also be indicated, at least for the short term. Furthermore, it is imperative when using the MRS plates that bicortical fixation be used, that the plates be contoured exactly to the defect to be bridged, and that four screws be used on each side of the injury. This avoids the high tendency for these types of injuries to result in distraction and nonunion. Though monocortical fixation has been described as effective, we believe that bicortical stabilization is intuitively superior and should be used in most circumstances.

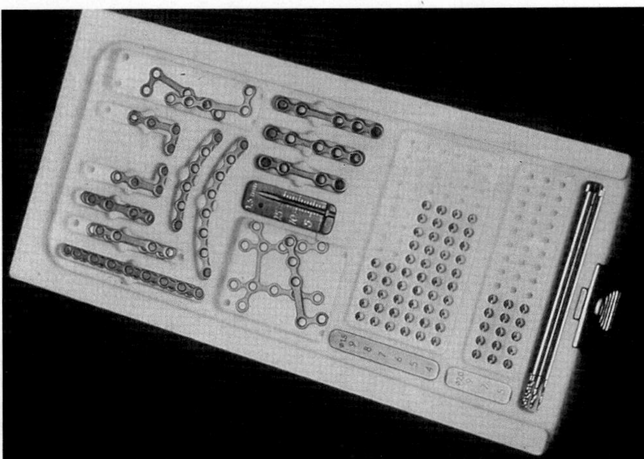

Fig. 67.10 Miniplates for Luhr vitallium maxillofacial system.

Miniplates and Microplates

Although traditional plating systems were found to work well in the mandible and for limited indications in the rest of the craniomaxillofacial skeleton, they proved too bulky for use in the majority of midfacial injuries, the cranial vault, or in infants and children. Miniplates, first introduced in 1973 by Michelet, followed soon after by Luhr, Champy, and Wurzberg, thereby widened the indications for rigid internal fixation of the craniomaxillofacial skeleton.[7,30] Miniplates are now widely accepted and employed for a variety of applications.

When compared with traditional-sized plates and screws, miniplates are thinner and have lower-profile screw heads (**Fig. 67.10**), allowing for use in areas with minimal soft tissue covering. Miniplates are available in compressive and noncompressive forms. Although they may be used in most mandibular fractures, their use is contraindicated in highly comminuted fractures or those in which delayed healing is expected. In terms of the midface and cranial vault, miniplates are available in a variety of shapes for the fixation of fractures in a wide variety of locations. Nevertheless, most contend that these plates should be used primarily in areas subject to masticatory forces, such as the frontonasal region, and zygomatic and sphenoid buttresses. Miniplates also provide a good reduction of complicated midfacial fractures and fractures in children, especially those in teeth-bearing regions, and have demonstrated wide utility in general orthognathic surgery.[30]

Microplates, which, as their name implies, are smaller with even less visibility than miniplates, represent the newest technology employed for craniomaxillofacial fixation (**Fig. 67.11**). Though very useful, miniplates can still be seen beneath the thin skin of the midface (periorbital region) and forehead.[31] Anything thicker than 0.5 mm and placed below the dermis can be seen in these areas. As a result, microplates were developed. Though not usually visible, microplates can still frequently be palpated beneath the skin's surface.

Whereas larger plates and screws are needed in areas subject to forces of mastication, several areas of the craniomaxillofacial skeleton are not subject to such stresses and may be repaired with microplates. These include midfacial fractures at sites other than the zygomatic buttress, nasoethmoidal region, supraorbital area, infraorbital area, and frontal sinus, and in skull reconstruction. Microplates are particularly useful in the repair of fractures in areas with minimal soft tissue covering, such as the glabellar region, as well as in infants and small children.[30] As with traditional mandibular plates, meticulous contouring and two-point fixation are important for stable reduction. In addition, the smaller microplates and miniplates may be used to join multiple small fracture fragments into larger segments for rigid fixation to framework buttresses.[32]

Three-Dimensional Plates

Although these plates are some of the newer adjuncts in rigid internal fixation, they have gained wide popularity and have been used for a variety of indications (**Fig. 67.12**). By

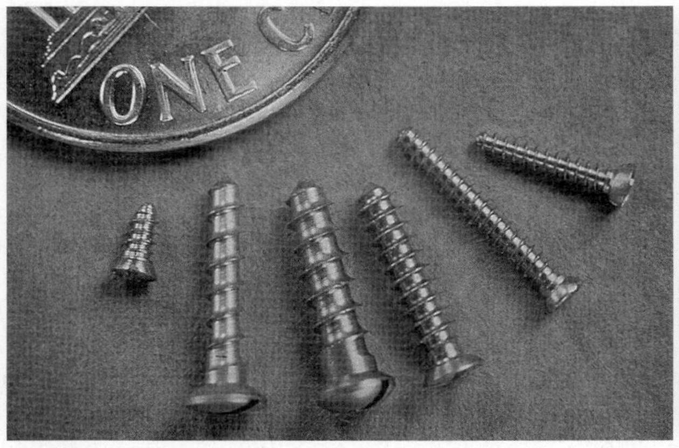

A

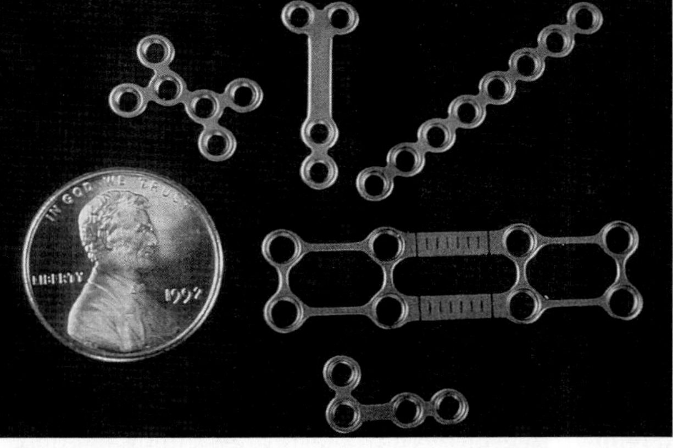

Fig. 67.11 (**A**) Microscrews and (**B**) microplates with penny for size comparison.

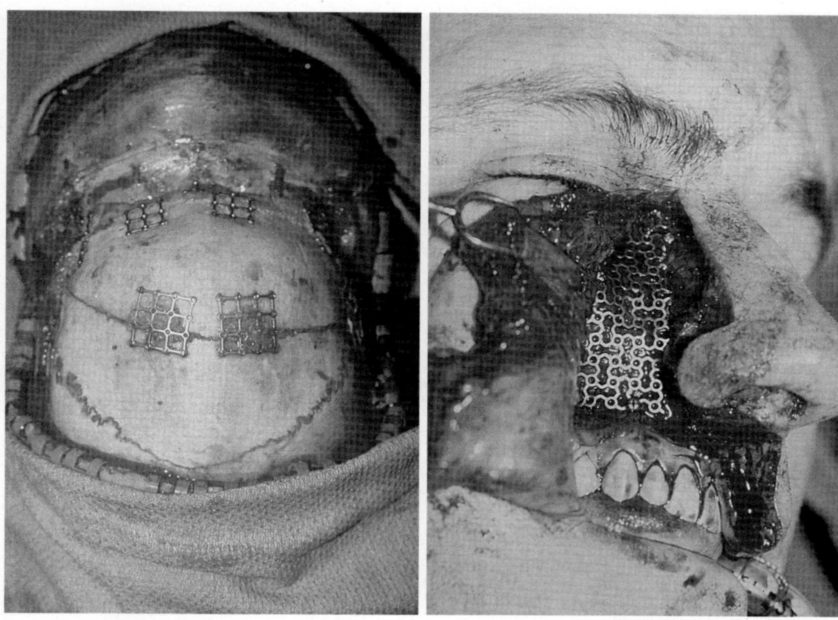

Fig. 67.12 Uses of three-dimensional plates. (A) These plates have many uses, including repair of large or comminuted calvarial and (B) orbital defects.

design these plates offer a great stability in both horizontal and vertical dimensions. This feature offers distinct advantages when a variety of defects are being repaired. This is especially true in the mandible, which is exposed to a disparate array of forces requiring support in multiple directions to achieve proper occlusion. When used in the mandible, the three-dimensional plates are capable of countering both distractive and torsional forces to produce a stable reduction. This type of fixation is particularly useful in the region of the mandibular body, which is exposed to more of these forces than any other region of the mandible.

In addition to mandibular reconstruction, three-dimensional plates have demonstrated utility in the midface and upper cranial vault. This is especially true in the orbital floor, where a stable reduction is essential to avoid herniation of orbital contents. Specifically, three-dimensional plates can be used after orbital blow-out fractures, as well as in the postablation setting to rigidly fix bone grafts. In addition to the orbital floor, three-dimensional plates are used for rigid fixation of heavily comminuted fractures of almost every part of the craniomaxillofacial skeleton. This is because in these situations there are multiple distracting forces that can cause instability if sufficient support is not generated by the plating unit. As the three-dimensional plates offer stability in multiple directions, they are ideally suited for these types of defects.

Ancillary Equipment

A variety of equipment can be employed to achieve a proper reduction of fractured bone ends (**Fig. 67.13**). This includes a plethora of tools besides the plates and screws themselves. Among these are screwdrivers that accommodate specific head types, including Phillips, hexagonal, cruciate, and simple slots. In addition, some screwdrivers have a sleeve designed to pick up the screw in the box and hold it until insertion is complete, allowing the surgeon to maintain a free hand (**Fig. 67.14A**). Depth gauges are designed to measure the depth of a hole after drilling to facilitate selection of the proper screw length. Taps are threaded instruments with the same dimensions as the screw in a particular kit that are designed to cut grooves into the bone hole into which the screw threads will fit for screws without self-tapping flutes. Drill bits are available in several sizes depending on the particular kit,

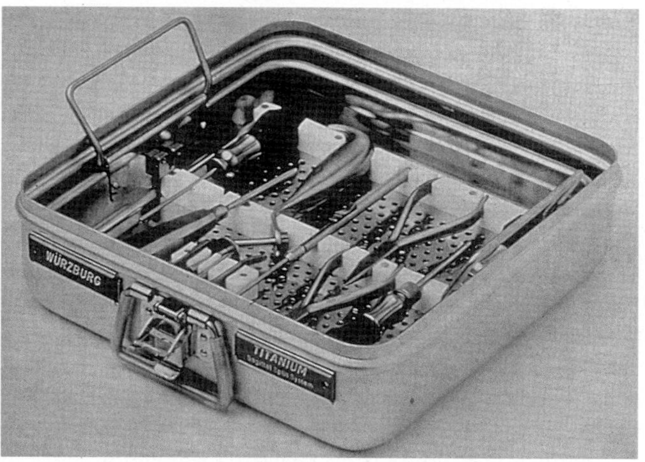

Fig. 67.13 General ancillary equipment for use in Wurzberg titanium system.

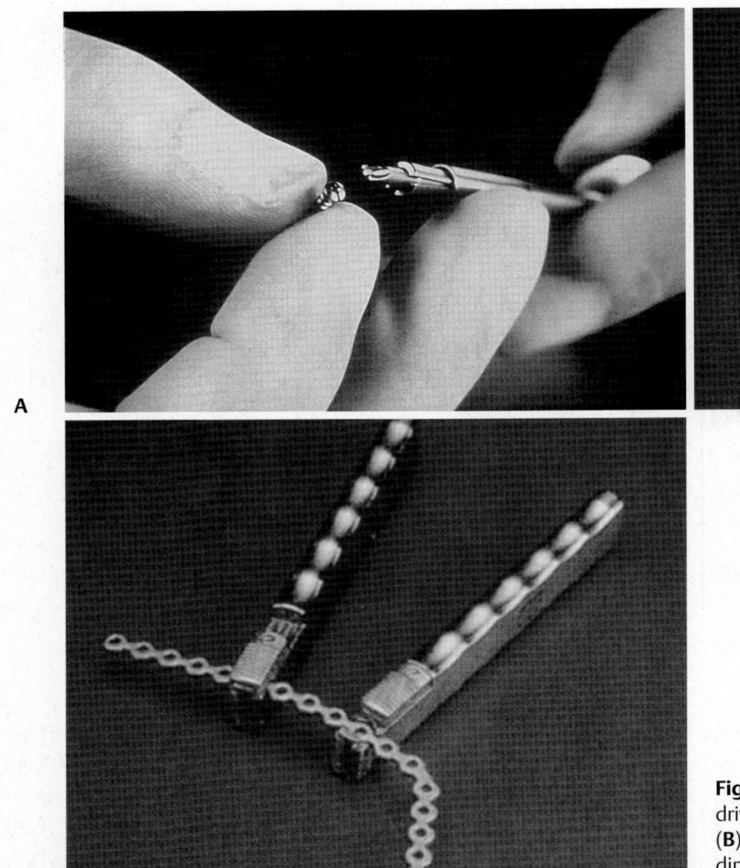

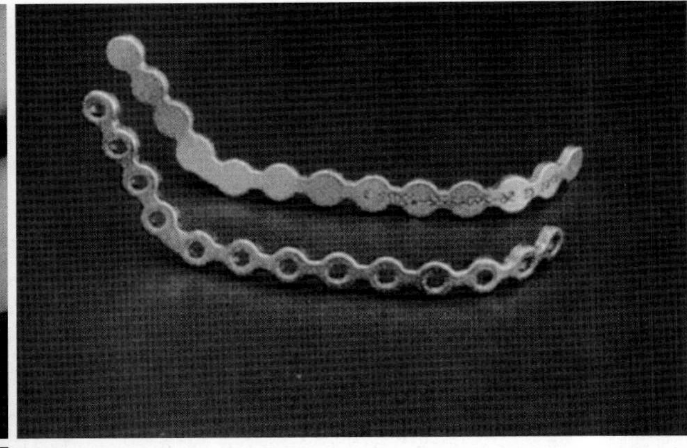

Fig. 67.14 Various pieces of ancillary instrumentation. (**A**) Screwdriver equipped with sleeve to allow screw placement with one hand. (**B**) Tin template for a mandibular reconstruction plate. (**C**) Three-dimensional plate benders demonstrating protection of screw hole shape during manipulation.

with diameters that correspond to the inner diameters of the screws to be inserted. These bits are often used in conjunction with a guide so the drill head does not wobble during insertion. When wobbling is allowed to occur during drilling, an irregularly shaped screw hole is created that will ineffectively engage the screw head.

There are several devices designed to bend and shape plates to correspond to the three-dimensional configuration of the fracture site. However, before this occurs a template may be used as a guide to mold the plate into the dimensions of the fracture site. These devices are usually composed of tin, which is malleable but also maintains its shape after bending. To mold the plate into the necessary configuration, first the template is applied to the fracture site and molded into the necessary shape. Then, using plate benders and the template as a guide, the plate itself is conformed to the dimensions of the fracture site (**Fig. 67.14B**). There are several different types of plate benders available, and which one is used depends on the plate to be bent and the preference of the surgeon. These include bending irons that are designed to work in pairs; flat, pronged, and side-bending pliers; as well as 90-degree bending pliers. In addition, there are bending pliers with a post, and three-pronged pliers designed to protect the shape of a hole during the three-dimensional bending process (**Fig. 67.14C**). Most kits also include a plate cutter in case a fracture requires fixation with a plate size that is not included in the kit. Finally, most rigid fixation kits include instruments designed to hold bone in a motionless and reduced state during plate-and-screw application. These include towel clip–like bone-holding forceps, bone-holding clamps, reduction/compression pliers, and reduction/compression pliers with side rollers (for applying tension on the alveolar border of the mandible when a tension band cannot be placed).

Plating Systems

Complications associated with rigid internal fixation include hardware prominence or exposure, plate migration, infection, inadequate reduction, or fracture instability. Proper plate selection and application may help minimize these occurrences. Several different plating systems have been developed and each system is usually marketed by more than one commercial dealer. The following section gives a general description of the equipment that is included in various commonly used systems.

Luhr Vitallium Maxillofacial Systems

Luhr developed an extensive plating system for broad indications including a mandibular compression system, a mandibular reconstruction system, as well as miniplates and microplates. Taken as a whole, the equipment of the Luhr system is sufficient to address almost all fractures within any region of the craniomaxillofacial skeleton. As stated previously, the Luhr maxillofacial system is composed of vitallium, which is one and a half times stronger, but produces three times as much scatter as titanium plates used in other systems. Therefore, although the Luhr plates are smaller than those of other systems, they produce more radiographic distortion (**Fig. 67.15A,B**). All Luhr systems are currently sold by Stryker-Leibinger Corporation (Kalamazoo, MI).

The mandibular compression system (MCS) has plates composed of vitallium that are either straight or curved, and each has two eccentric compression and two neutral holes. The straight plates are mainly applied to fractures of the mandibular body, whereas the curved plates are generally indicated for fractures involving the mandibular angle. Also included in the MCS kit are three-dimensional plates that are designed to reduce the occurrence of multiple mandibular fractures.[28,29] Like DCPs the three-dimensional plates provide compression perpendicular to the angle of the fracture site and therefore require placement of a tension band to achieve a good reduction. The screws in the MCS are self-tapping and designed for bicortical insertion.

The minisystem was developed mainly for implantation in the midface and cranial vault. The plates are smaller and have a lower profile than the mandibular plates and screws, and can be used with or without compression. These plates are available in a variety of shapes, including straight, curved, L, T, and double-T. The screws are self-tapping and have a flat head that fits into the countersink of the plate to reduce the vertical profile.

The MCS microsystem is mainly indicated in areas not subject to masticatory forces, and for use in infants and small children. As in the other Luhr kits, the screws are self-tapping but have a much narrower diameter. By the same token, like the screws in the minisystem, the screws in the microsystem have flat heads and are designed to fit into the countersink of the plate hole to minimize vertical profile. The plates for the Luhr microsystem are straight or T-, L-, or H-shaped. Also in the microsystem kit is micromesh, which is mainly used in periorbital reconstruction.[31]

The Wurzberg Titanium System

Similar to the Luhr system but composed of titanium, the Wurzberg system (Synthes Corp., Paoli, PA) is based on the adaptation of principles of rigid internal fixation of the long bones to the mandible, and later to the midface. Included in the Wurzberg system is a compression plate system, a mandibular reconstruction system, a miniplate system, and a dental implant system. The compression plate system has several indications but it is used primarily for badly comminuted mandibular fractures, fixation of bone grafts, and anticipated delayed healing.[30,33] The screws for this system are designed to be bicortical and can be pretapped (recommended for highly comminuted fractures) or self-tapping. The system includes both DCPs and EDCPs and is available in either curved or straight configurations.

The MRS is used primarily for stable bridging of bone segments in the postablation setting. The screws for the MRS are pretapping, with conical heads, and are available

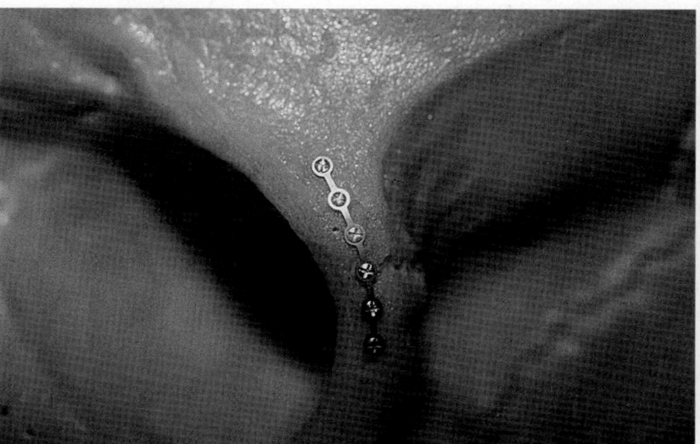

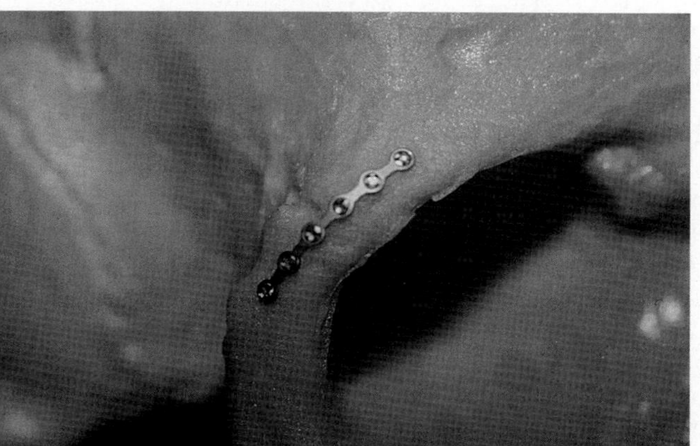

A B

Fig. 67.15 Difference in profile between plates made with various metals. (**A**) Notice that vitallium plates have a significantly smaller profile than (**B**) the larger titanium plates.

as straight as well as right- or left-angled plates. The plates have two compression and two neutral holes on each side but also can be used for neutral plating when fixing an implant in place.

The miniplate system, which was designed based on the work of Champy, is intended for use in the upper margins of the mandibular region of the alveolar crest as well as in the midface. The screws are self-tapping and have a flat head with a single slot that fits within the screw hole in a manner that minimizes screwhead visibility. The miniplates are designed for three-dimensional deformation and are available as straight; T; right and left L; Y; X; and complexly shaped plates.[30,33]

The Champy System

There are two original schools of thought that developed in parallel with regard to rigid fixation of the craniomaxillofacial skeleton. The first plating philosophy extrapolates the AO and ASIF principles originally intended for fixation of long bones for use in the craniomaxillofacial region. The main principle of this system is that any extrinsic forces that are present at a fracture site are potentially disruptive. As a result of this, the rigid fixation system must assume all of these stresses and strains, thereby keeping the fracture site absolutely motionless.[4–6] In contrast to this school of thought, Michelet in 1973 developed a craniomaxillofacial plating system based on the notion that in the course of normal osteosynthesis, bone is laid down along lines of stress.[7] Therefore, he maintained, it is unnatural to maintain absolute rigidity at the fracture site. He proposed that if properly channeled, micromotion in this region would encourage primary union in planes that maximize bone stability. Among the proponents of Michelet's principles was Champy, who developed a rigid internal fixation system composed of titanium for fixation of mandibular fractures. In the Champy system, as in other systems, the miniplates have minimum profile and are available as straight in a variety of sizes, as well as in Y, T, and L shapes. More recently, the Champy system has come to include separate plates specifically designed for fixation of orbital fractures, sagittal split osteotomies, and mandibular reconstructions. The screws for the Champy system are monocortical, self-tapping with conical heads. The head of the screw is designed to accommodate insertion at a maximal angle of 30 degrees from the bony surface, thus maximizing hold while allowing nondistractive micromotion to occur.[34]

Association of Osteosynthesis and Association for the Study of Internal Fixation System

As mentioned previously, the AO and ASIF system is based on extrapolation of principles of rigid internal fixation of the long bones for use in the craniomaxillofacial skeleton. Therefore, the system relies on the principle of "absolute stability," meaning it is designed to assume all forces transmitted across the fracture site. Included in this system are plates and screws designed for mandibular compression, mandibular reconstruction, and application to the midface and the rest of the cranium. All components are composed of stainless steel or titanium.[4–6]

Two types of plates are used in the mandible: linear and reconstruction. Linear plates are designed either as EDCPs or as DCPs. To achieve eccentric plating, the EDCP plates are equipped with oblique holes set at a 75-degree angle from the bony surface. The reconstruction plates are available in straight or curved shape and are designed for three-dimensional bending. Screws for the mandibular system are bicortical, with hemispherically shaped head with a hexagonal recess, allowing angling of the screws with respect to the bone surface. The screws have no flutes and therefore must be pretapped.

All equipment in the AO and ASIF craniofacial system is composed of titanium. This system is indicated for use in the craniofacial skeleton and for orthodontic applications. The plates for this system are designed for three-dimensional bending to accommodate the disparate regions of the cranium and upper face.[5] Also included are plates designed for use in the orbital floor, which can be cut and molded in a variety of configurations to achieve good stability in this region. The screws for the AO and ASIF craniofacial plating system are self-tapping with a conical tip. They have a low-profile hemispheric head and a cruciform slot to allow angulation of the screw head with the bone surface.

Titanium Hollow-Screw-Reconstruction Plate System (THORP)

It has long been noted that as a consequence of natural bony remodeling screws lose stability over time. Therefore, in situations where a long-term reduction is necessary, normal screws may prove inadequate. As a result of this, in 1987 a new system of screws was developed to optimize mechanical and physical forces necessary to achieve a long-term reduction. Indications for this system include complex fractures of the mandible where long-term reduction is needed, and for reducing postablation mandibular defects.[35,36] However because the THORP system is significantly more expensive than traditional rigid internal fixation systems, the added expense is not justified for the plating of simple fractures in which rapid healing is likely.

Overall, it is the screws of the THORP system that make it unique. These screws are designed to disperse local stresses and strains over a maximal area, to inhibit completely any micromotion at the screw–plate interface and to encourage maximal osseointegration of the fixation

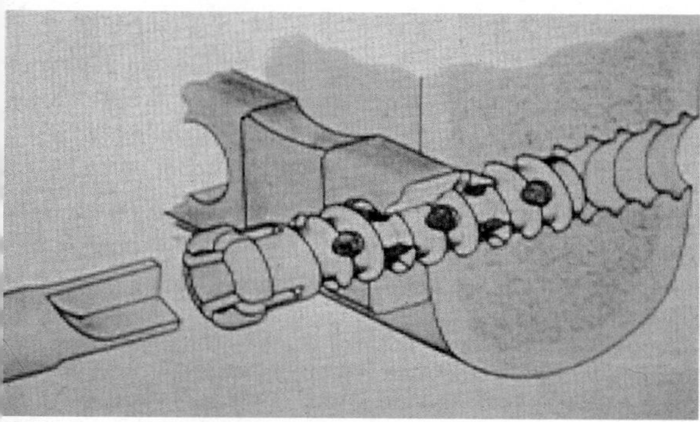

Fig. 67.16 Insertion of titanium hollow-screw reconstruction plate system (THORP) screw into bone. Notice that the shaft of the screw is hollow to allow osteointegration and that the screw head accommodates an expansion bolt to reduce micromotion at the screw–bone interface.

device. Inclusively, these properties give the THORP system many of the same advantages as an external fixation device. The THORP screws are available in two basic types: a normal full-bodied titanium screw and a perforated, hollow, argon-coated screw (**Fig. 67.16**). The screws are designed with a small thread pitch to allow maximal holding power, even when used in thin cortical bone. Although this is effective, a high bone to metal ratio is preserved by decreasing the overall thread depth. The screw is also equipped with lateral perforations and is coated with argon. This facilitates bony ingrowth into the screw, which produces great long-term stability (**Fig. 67.17**).[37] Furthermore, the hollow screw head is expandable and accommodates an expansion bolt that is inserted after the screw has been tightened in place. This produces complete rigid fixation of the screw head and minimizes motion at the screw–bone interface. In contrast to the THORP screws, the normal titanium full-body screw is indicated when the surgeon intends to initiate early screw removal.

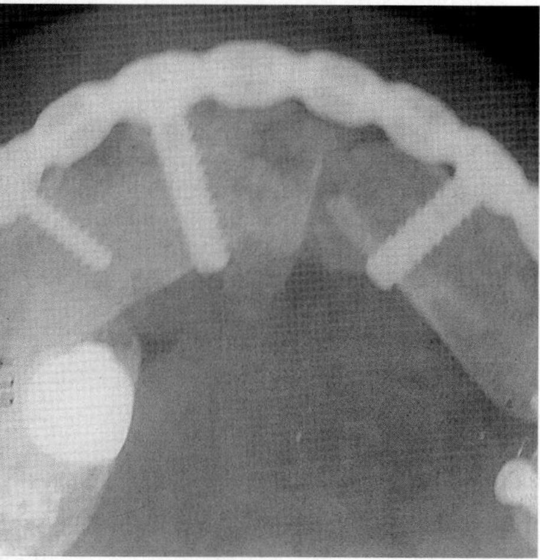

Fig. 67.17 Radiograph showing differences in shape between titanium hollow-screw reconstruction plate (THORP) and traditional screws.

Although it is the THORP screws that account for most of the long-term stability of this system, the plates also have physical properties that contribute to this longevity. One such property is that the THORP plates were designed to evenly disperse the force of functional loading throughout their length. This in theory should increase the plate strength and its ability to achieve a long-term reduction.[37] These plates are available in a variety of sizes, several shapes, including straight and curved, and can be used with a temporomandibular junction endoprosthesis.

Titanium Mesh

Titanium mesh, first used in the Vietnam War in 1968, has proven successful in the semirigid fixation of craniofacial fractures.[38] Due to its semirigid nature, it is easily contoured and affords great utility in several settings. This adaptability has considerable advantage over wire and plate osteosynthesis. Titanium mesh is time efficient and invaluable in reconstituting areas of bony curvature, especially under circumstances of absent or comminuted fragments of bone. Even three-dimensional reconstruction of large non–load-bearing craniofacial defects can be successfully performed without the need for bone or cartilage grafting.[39] Numerous studies assert that this material is extremely well tolerated, with minimal incidence of infection or extrusion,[38–40] and maintains excellent long-term contour stability.[39] Cases of reexploration confirm no substantial scarring or soft tissue adhesions, even when used adjacent to the periorbita in orbital floor reconstruction.[40] Rather than stress shielding and bony resorption seen with rigid fixation, the semirigid nature of the mesh fixation allows micromovements at the fracture site, which may promote callus formation and theoretically accelerate bone healing.[38,39]

Studies report complication rates from craniofacial reconstruction ranging from 7 to 17% with the use of older metal plates,[38,41] such as steel, which do not osseointegrate.[18,42] In comparison, appropriate selection of titanium mesh in cases of craniofacial reconstruction with or without titanium plates has proven advantageous at decreasing the rate of complication to less than 2%.[38,40] Titanium has a low rate of infection in part because of its biocompatibility and osseointegration. Titanium is chemically similar to calcium (elements 22 and 20, respectively) and histological analysis confirms the osseointegration of bone to titanium screws occurs by bonding on a molecular level.[43,44] Furthermore, a soft tissue fibrous reaction occurs around the screw heads, which facilitates hardware integration and diminishes extrusion.[40] The fear that mesh plating presents a larger foreign body than miniplates with a subsequent risk of increased rates of infection remains unsubstantiated.[38]

The inaccurate contouring and placement of plates at fracture sites is also a leading cause of complications such as infection, loosening of hardware, and foreign body reactions.[40] Alternatively, titanium mesh may afford easier application and has multiple holes to allow screw placement at the most optimal points and alternative holes to drill and screw securely in the event of stripping. The lattice-work of newer titanium mesh designs facilitate the passing of suture needles through spacers in the event that reconstruction in tight areas or areas of thin bone preclude drilling and require stabilization to adjacent soft tissue.

Titanium mesh is available in standard-thickness (0.6-mm profile) and low-profile malleable (0.3-mm profile) for use with 1.2-mm or 1.7-mm screws. The preangled connecting bars of the dynamic mesh act as spacers and allow for expansion and contraction of the mesh and facilitate stable three-dimensional contouring by keeping the holes from wrinkling or overlapping. Additionally, micromesh is available with 0.1-mm and 0.2-mm ultrathin profiles for use with a screw range of 1.0 mm to 1.9 mm.

Titanium mesh varieties are relatively thinner than most plates and are easily contoured with bending pliers or by hand allowing versatility in resculpturing bony curvatures. Thicker profiles should be selected for cranioplasty, and reconstruction of orbital wall, frontal sinus, and skull defects. Thinner profiles may be selected for reconstruction of the orbital floor, skull base, or areas underlying thin skin to avoid postoperative palpability, such as lateral orbital wall and sinus wall defects.

Good exposure, precise mesh positioning, and careful trimming of sharp edges are key principles to the success of fixation with titanium mesh. A sheet of mesh may be cut to the desired shape and size and contoured to resculpt even large defects spanning up to 25 cm^2 with excellent cosmetic results.[39] Convexity in contouring may be facilitated by trimming alternate holes along the perimeter of a curved piece of mesh prior to bending the edges forward. Screw holes should be placed as near to the periphery as possible. As the screws are tightened, the adaptable nature and lack of elastic memory of titanium mesh allow it to be reduced to the underlying bone. This optimally minimizes the risk of fracture site distortion that may otherwise occur from minor imprecisions in standard plate shaping.

Resorbable Plates and Screws

Although metal plating systems are the standard of care and have proven effective over the last several decades for a variety of clinical applications, they do have some disadvantages. First, the permanence of metal plates may affect long-term safety in infants and children. Specifically, there has been concern that these systems may limit growth when implanted into the immature craniofacial skeleton or erode through the calvaria into the intercranial space. Although the results of animal studies done by Yaremchuk and others suggest that metallic plates provide modest growth retardation if placed at suture sites, they remain associated with other problems, such as translocation into the inner table of the calvaria, and extrusion.[16] In addition, there are areas of the craniomaxillofacial skeleton where soft tissue covering is limited (e.g., the glabellar region), and therefore metallic screws may be palpable below the skin surface.

Based on these concerns, a great deal of time and effort have been invested in the development of resorbable plating systems. Resorbable plates and screws are intended to provide the same stability and support for fractured bone segments as do permanent implants, while undergoing resorption over time. Plate resorption avoids plate migration, bone growth restriction, and imaging artifact. Resorbable plates are indicated in comminuted fractures of the nasoethmoidal and infraorbital areas as well as of the frontal sinus wall, in trauma and reconstructive procedures of the midface or craniofacial skeleton, in mandibular osteotomies and graft fixation, in browlift procedures as well as in infant and pediatric craniofacial surgery.

In 1971, Cutright and Hunsuck were the first to report experimental use of resorbable fixation devices composed of polylactic acid (PLA) to repair blowout fractures in rhesus monkeys.[45] In 1994, Salyer et al were among the first to examine the effects of resorbable plates in a pediatric animal model.[46] They compared the outcome of facial plating using either titanium or a commercially available resorbable plating system in growing beagle dogs. At the conclusion of their study, Salyer and colleagues found the bioresorbable plates and screws provided the same degree of support as the titanium plating system, and were entirely resorbed, leaving no residual scar tissue. Eppley has since performed a plethora of animal and clinical studies that have demonstrated the utility of resorbable systems, primarily in the growing craniomaxillofacial skeleton.[14,15] More recent adult clinical studies report equal efficacy when compared with metal plating systems with respect to rigidity of fixation, functional results, and frequency of complications and suggest greater ease of contour and higher cosmetic satisfaction after plate resorption in head and neck reconstruction.[47,48]

Overall, although complications have been reported with resorbable systems, these systems seem to offer several of the advantages of metal rigid fixation while forgoing many of their shortcomings. The resorbable plates and screws facilitate primary bone healing, and allow three-dimensional control while not interfering with radiological imaging. They also may be conveniently used in conjunction with metal fixation at the discretion of the operating surgeon, especially in areas underlying thin skin to avoid postoperative contour irregularity.[49] Furthermore, because resorbable plating systems are eventually broken down by the body, they do not restrict long-term growth and drastically reduce the risk of migration or extrusion. With continual refinement of bioresorbable materials these devices are quickly becoming the treatment of choice for internal fixation of facial fractures in the pediatric population.

Several companies now offer resorbable fixation systems composed predominantly of PLA: Macropore (San Diego, CA), Lactosorb (Walter Lorenz Surgical Corp., Jacksonville, FL), Resorbable Fixation System (Synthes Corp., Paoli, PA), and Delta System (Stryker/Leibinger Corp., Kalamazoo, MI).[48] Studies show resorbable plates and screws maintain ~70% strength at 6 weeks and are completely resorbed at 12 to 36 months.[48] These materials are normally degraded by hydrolysis into glycolic acid and lactate, which are incorporated directly into the citric acid cycle. Extreme cases of severe inflammatory reaction with a localized foreign body reaction, and cyst formation has been reported for resorbable plates composed of polyglycolide, but has not been described in association with PLA and polyglycolic acid (PGA) used in current resorbable systems.[14]

The first commercially available resorbable system, Lactosorb (Walter Lorenz Surgical Corp., Jacksonville, FL), was introduced in 1996. The Lactosorb system is composed of 82% PLA and 18% PGA. The system has a wide variety of plates available and also three-dimensional panels for repair of intraorbital and some orbital floor defects (**Fig. 67.18**). The plates are available as straight, curved, T, X, or L shapes. The Lactosorb plates are somewhat malleable but must be heated to the transition temperature of the material (~60°C). This can be done using a commercially available heat pack (Biomet Inc., Warsaw, IA) into which distilled water is injected to initiate a chemical reaction. The plates are then immersed into the pack for 10 to 15 seconds, after which they can be easily molded into the necessary shape with a plate bender. The resorbable screws used as part of this system are of two types: standard and suspension. The standard resorbable screws have almost identical dimensions as metal screws used for similar indications. The suspension screws are specifically indicated for endobrow applications and have an eyelet that can accommodate a suture for brow suspension. Overall, when used for the proper indications and with sufficient surgical experience, resorbable plates and screws have shown a great deal of efficacy.

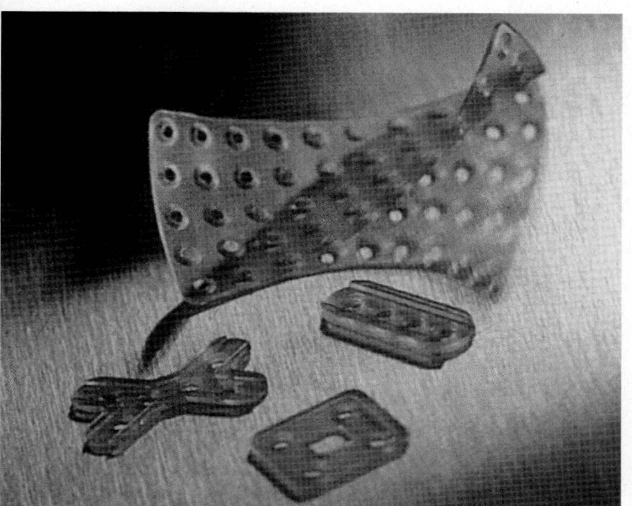

Fig. 67.18 Resorbable mesh and plates for use with Lactosorb system (Walter Lorenz Surgical Corp., Jacksonville, FL).

Summary and Conclusions

Since its inception in the late 1960s craniomaxillofacial plating has undergone an impressive revolution in technique and technology. Currently available plating systems can be used to repair almost any type of defect in any area of the craniomaxillofacial skeleton. These systems have been shown to provide a superior functional and aesthetic outcome over the older interfragmentary wire fixation devices. This is the direct result of the ability of plating systems to provide three-dimensional control of fractures and other defects. Although metallic systems now dominate the market, resorbable plating systems are gaining wide popularity, especially for use in the pediatric population. Familiarity with the technique and the equipment used for rigid internal fixation in the craniomaxillofacial region is essential for proper application and maximal efficacy, and is best obtained with long-term exposure to the diverse clinical situations in which these devices are employed.

References

1. Luhr HG. Zur stabilen Osteosynthese bei Unterkieferfrakturen. Dtsch Zahnarztl Z 1968;23:754
2. Phillips JH. Principles in compression osteosynthesis. In: Yaremchuk MJ, Gruss JS, Manson PN, eds. Rigid Fixation of the Craniomaxillofacial Skeleton. Boston: Butterworth-Heinemann; 1992:7
3. Danis R. Theorie et Prata que de L'Osteosyntheses. Paris: Libraries de L'Academie de Medicine; 1949
4. Prien J, Kellman R. Rigid internal fixation of mandibular fracture: basics of AO technique. Otolaryngol Clin North Am 1987;20:3
5. Yaremchuk MJ, Prein J. The AO/ASIF maxillofacial implant system. In: Yaremchuk MJ, Gruss JS, Manson PN, eds. Rigid Fixation of the Craniomaxillofacial Skeleton. Boston: Butterworth-Heinemann; 1992:124
6. Spiessl B. Internal Fixation of the Mandible: A Manual of AO/ASIF Principles. Berlin: Springer-Verlag; 1976
7. Michelet FX, Deymes J, Dessus B. Osteosynthesis with miniaturized screwed plates in maxillofacial surgery. J Maxillofac Surg 1973;1:79

8. Champy M, Lodde JP, Jaeger JH, Wilk A. Osteosynthes manbidulaires selon la technique de Michelet, I: Bases biomechaniques. Rev Stomatol Chir Maxillofac (Paris) 1976;77:569
9. Champy M, Lodde JP. Etude des contraintes dans la mandibule fracturee chez l'homme: mesures theoriques et verification par jauges extensometriques in situ. Rev Stomat (Paris) 1978;78:545
10. Champy M, Lodde JP, Wilk A, et al. Dehnungsmebstreifen am prepartieren Unterkiefer und bei Patient mit Untkierfrakturen. Dtsch Z Mund Kiefer Gesichtschir 1978;2:41
11. Champy M, Wilk A, Schnebelen JM. Die Behandlung der Mandibularfrakturen mittels Osteosynthese ohne intermaxillare Ruhigstellung nach der von F.X. Michelet. Dtsch Zahn Mund Keferheilk 1975;63:339
12. Champy M. Surgical treatment of midface deformities. Head Neck Surg 1980;2:451
13. Costantino PD, Wolpoe ME. Short- and long-term outcome of plating in the pediatric population. Clin Fac Plast Surg 1999;7:231
14. Eppley BL. Effects of resorbable fixation on craniofacial growth. J Craniofac Surg 1994;5:110
15. Yaremchuk MJ. Experimental studies addressing rigid fixation in craniofacial surgery. Clin Plast Surg 1994;21:517
16. Altobelli DE. Implant materials in rigid fixation: physical, mechanical, corrosion, and biocompatibility considerations. In: Yaremchuk MJ, Gruss JS, Manson PN, eds. Rigid Fixation of the Craniomaxillofacial Skeleton. Boston: Butterworth-Heinemann; 1992:28
17. Bothe RT, Beaton KE, Davenport HA. Reaction of bone to multiple metallic implants. Surg Gynecol Obstet 1980;71:598
18. Emery B, Dixit R, Formby C, et al. The resistance of maxillofacial reconstruction plates to biofilm formation in vitro. Laryngoscope 2003;113:1977
19. Fiala TG, Paige KT, Cambell TA, et al. Comparison of artifact from craniomaxillofacial internal fixation devices: magnetic resonance imaging. Plast Reconstr Surg 1994;93:725
20. Shellock FG. MR imaging of metallic implants and materials: a compilation of the literature. AJR Am J Roentgenol 1988;151:389
21. Rahn BA. Theoretical considerations in rigid fixation of facial bones. Clin Plast Surg 1989;16:21
22. Schilli W, Ewers R, Niederdellman H. Bone fixation with screws and plates in the maxillofacial region. Int J Oral Surg 1981;10:329
23. Niederdellmann H, Shetty V. Principles and technique of lag screw osteosynthesis. In: Yaremchuk MJ, Gruss JS, Manson PN, eds. Rigid Fixation of the Craniomaxillofacial Skeleton. Boston: Butterworth-Heinemann; 1992:22
24. Niederdellman H, Schilli W, Duker J, et al. Osteosynthesis of mandibular fractures using lag screws. Int J Oral Surg 1976;5:117
25. Luhr HG. Vitallium Luhr systems for reconstructive surgery of the facial skeleton. Otolaryngol Clin North Am 1987;20:573
26. Luhr HG. The compression osteosynthesis of mandibular fractures in dogs: a histologic contribution to "primary bone healing." Eur Surg Res 1969;1:3
27. Algower M, Perron S, Matter P. A new plate for internal fixation: the dynamic compression plate (DCP). Injury 1970;2:40
28. Luhr HG. Specifications, indications, and clinical applications of the Luhr vitallium maxillofacial systems. In: Yaremchuk MJ, Gruss JS, Manson PN, eds. Rigid Fixation of the Craniomaxillofacial Skeleton. Boston: Butterworth-Heinemann; 1992:79
29. Munro IR. The Luhr fixation system for the craniofacial skeleton. Clin Plast Surg 1989;16:105
30. Reuther JF. The Wurzburg titanium system for rigid fixation of the craniomaxillofacial skeleton. In: Yaremchuk MJ, Gruss JS, Manson PN, eds. Rigid Fixation of the Craniomaxillofacial Skeleton. Boston: Butterworth-Heinemann; 1992:134
31. Luhr HG. Indications for use of a microsystem for internal fixation in craniofacial surgery. J Craniofac Surg 1990;1:35
32. Evans G, Clark N, Manson P, et al. Role of mini-and microplate fixation in fractures of the midface and mandible. Ann Plast Surg 1995;34:453
33. Marsh JL. The use of the Wurzberg system to facilitate fixation in facial osteotomies. Clin Plast Surg 1989;16:49
34. Kahn JL, Khouri M. Champy's system. In: Yaremchuk MJ, Gruss JS, Manson PN, eds. Rigid Fixation of the Craniomaxillofacial Skeleton. Boston: Butterworth-Heinemann; 1992:116
35. Hellem S, Oloffson J. Titanium coated hollow screw and reconstruction plate system (THORP) in mandibular reconstruction. J Craniomaxillofac Surg 1988;16:173
36. Vuillemin T, Raveh J, Sutter F. Mandibular reconstruction with the titanium hollow screw reconstruction plate (THORP) system: evaluation of 62 Cases. Plast Reconstr Surg 1988;82:804
37. Raveh J, Sutter F, Vuillemin T. The titanium hollow screw reconstruction plate system (THORP). In: Yaremchuk MJ, Gruss JS, Manson PN, eds. Rigid Fixation of the Craniomaxillofacial Skeleton. Boston: Butterworth-Heinemann; 1992:620
38. Patel M, Langdon J. Titanium mesh (TiMesh) osteosynthesis: a fast and adaptable method of semirigid fixation. Br J Oral Maxillofac Surg 1991;29:316
39. Kuttenberger JJ, Hardt N. Long-term results following reconstruction of craniofacial defects with titanium micromesh systems. J Craniomaxillofac Surg 2001;29:75
40. Gear A, Lokeh A, Aldridge J, et al. Safety of titanium mesh for orbital reconstruction. Ann Plast Surg 2002;48:1
41. Brown J, Trotter M, Cliffe J, et al. The fate of miniplates in facial trauma and orthognathic surgery: a retrospective study. Br J Oral Maxillofac Surg 1989;27:306
42. Costantino P, Friedman C, Lane A. Synthetic biomaterials in facial and reconstructive surgery. Facial Plast Surg 1993;9:1
43. Albrektsson T, Branemark P, Hansson H, et al. The interface zone of organic implants in vivo: titanium implants in bone. Ann Biomed Eng 1983;11:1
44. Albrektsson T, Branemark P, Hansson H, et al. Osseointegrated titanium implants. Acta Orthop Scand 1981;52:155
45. Cutright DE, Hunsuck EE. The repair of fractures of the orbital floor using biodegradable polylactic acid. Oral Surg Oral Med Oral Pathol 1972;33:28
46. Salyer KE, Bardach J, Squier CA, et al. A comparative study of biodegradable and titanium plating systems on cranial growth structure: experimental study in beagles. Plast Reconstr Surg 1994;93:705
47. Bhanot S, Alex J, Lowlicht R, et al. The efficacy of resorbable plates in head and neck reconstruction. Laryngoscope 2002;112:890
48. Moe K, Weisman R. Resorbable fixation in facial plastic and head and neck reconstructive surgery: an initial report on polylactic acid implants. Laryngoscope 2001;111:1697
49. Tomasz Majewski W, Yu J, Ewart C, et al. Posttraumatic craniofacial reconstruction using combined resorbable and nonresorbable fixation systems. Ann Plast Surg 2002;48:471

68 Applications of Bone Plating Systems to Facial Fractures

Robert M. Kellman

Whether repairing fractures, fixing osteotomies, or reconstructing skeletal defects, the goal of the surgeon is to effect a bony union as rapidly and dependably as possible with limited morbidity and complication rates. Recent experience indicates that rigid skeletal fixation, when properly applied, is most likely to achieve these goals. There are numerous plating systems in use today, each with its own unique designs, instruments, plates, screws, and metals. Yet all systems have in common the following central principle: a screw screwed into a bone can remain tight and withstand functional stress over time. With this demonstrated, the following three principles support the various methods of rigid fixation in use throughout the craniofacial skeleton: (1) overlapping bone fragments can be screwed together stably with lag screws; (2) stability of fixation can be increased when fragments are compressed together with compression plates; and (3) plates screwed to bone fragments maintain and replace the structural integrity of damaged bone, even across a significant gap (bony defect). These principles form the foundation for the successful use of any bone plating system.

Initial attempts at plate fixation failed because of a lack of understanding of the biomechanical principles involved in bone repair. The earliest attempts at rigid fixation in facial bones were in mandible fractures, where improper plate positioning resulting from a lack of understanding of the tension and compressive forces acting on the mandible in function resulted in instability and, frequently, infection and failure. These failures were misunderstood and were thought to be due to excessive stability failing to provide the motion needed to effect bone healing. This misconception was corrected by research in orthopedic surgery. It was found that failures were due to inadequate (rather than excessive) stabilization. With a better understanding of the dynamic forces acting on bones, more stable fixations and high success rates were achieved. It was then some years before the biomechanical principles upon which proper stabilization of mandible fractures depends were elucidated. In the last 2 decades, facial plating techniques have gained wide acceptance as the advantages of rapid and effective healing with early function have become commonplace.

Bone Healing

Although osseous healing has been addressed in chapter 54, a few comments are appropriate here. Bone healing depends on the stabilization of fractured or osteotomized fragments. Whether guided by medical intervention (e.g., cast, splint, fixation device) or allowed to occur spontaneously, bone healing generally ensues. Healing depends on the growth of osteons across the fracture or defect so that the injury is bridged by new bone. This new bone remodels in response to physiological stresses, and healing is complete. However, motion disrupts the growing osteons. The body therefore produces a callus that stabilizes the fragments, allowing osteon growth and healing to proceed. The callus is nature's rigid fixation device. Casting and splinting [e.g., mandibulomaxillary fixation (MMF)] and even interosseous wiring and external fixation partially immobilize the fracture and guide the position that the fragments will be in when the callus stabilizes them. If the degree of motion is too great or if infection intervenes, stabilization may not occur at all, and the gap may widen and fill with fibrous tissue. If this occurs, a nonunion (fibrous union, pseudarthrosis) frequently results. A pseudarthrosis, as its name implies, is essentially a fibrous union, and motion occurs where the bone fragments are held together by fibrous tissue, thus creating a "false joint" or pseudarthrosis.

When bone injury occurs, bleeding results in a fracture hematoma. Early ingrowth of blood vessels and fibroblasts begins the differentiation cascade of bone healing. The development of chondroblasts, the conversion of fibrous tissue to fibrocartilage, and ultimately the ingrowth of osteoblasts that lay down osteoid result in callus formation.[1] This process begins subperiosteally on either side of the fracture, and the callus grows across from both sides, bridging and stabilizing the fracture. The same process is repeated across the fracture site. Finally, osteons grow across this area, and remodeling completes the healing process. This natural process, like surgically assisted healing, is dependent on the ability of the callus to stabilize the fragments, which in turn allows for the ultimate bridging of the fracture by bone. If the forces acting on the fragments are so great that stabilization cannot occur, ultimate bony union will be unlikely. Furthermore, in the absence of surgical guidance, even if healing does take place, it will often be in a poor anatomical alignment (malunion). [Note that although remodeling in response to stress can result in normal bone strength, it will not correct a malocclusion, a problem unique to malunions (malpositions) of mandibular and maxillary fractures.]

Rigid fixation techniques are designed to stabilize the fractured fragments, thereby increasing the likelihood that bony union will take place (in the correct position) and minimizing the chance for nonunion. As mobility leads to callus formation, the greater the stability of the surgical fixation, the less callus that develops. Though microscopically there is always some callus formation, when a very rigid fixation is accomplished there will not be enough callus to show on x-ray. Therefore, the finding of a callus at the fracture site on radiographic evaluation of a patient after surgical repair has been used as an indication of inadequate stabilization of the fragments.

Rigid Fixation of Mandibular Fractures

General Principles

Occlusion

In any discussion of facial bone repair, a discussion of occlusion must take a central role. Regardless of the stabilization techniques used, the surgeon must reestablish occlusal relationships between mandibular and maxillary dentition before repairing fractures of the related bones. MMF is generally applied before fracture repair, and the occlusion is periodically assessed to make certain that a malocclusion has not been created by osseous repositioning and repair. When a malocclusion is detected, the bones should be repositioned because a rigidly fixed malocclusion will not be improved by healing and bony remodeling. Proper occlusion is necessary for function; therefore, establishing a proper and functional occlusal relationship should be the priority in all but the severest of traumas. This generally means that if the appropriate position cannot be defined, use of a less rigid fixation (e.g., MMF alone) should be considered. When severe disruption of bone makes healing unlikely without rigid fixation, then the need to achieve healing and prevent infection may sometimes take priority over establishing the exact occlusion. This difficult and controversial clinical decision must be made by the facial plastic surgeon at the time of repair. Note that screws can be used for establishing occlusion. Two screws can be placed in the maxilla and two in the mandible, and wires can be tightened around these, thereby establishing MMF. Specially designed screws with large, protruding heads and holes through which the wires can be passed have been produced specifically for this purpose. Note that although this method is fast and simple, it is not an ideal technique because tightening of the wires tends to create lingual version of unstable fragments due to the buccal positioning of the fixation points.

Biomechanics

Proper use of rigid fixation requires placement of fixation devices so that immobilization of the fracture fragments is accomplished during motion as well as when the bones are at rest. The forces acting on the mandible are complex and variable, shifting depending on the site of the food bolus being chewed and the status of the dentition. To effectively stabilize the fragments, the surgeon must have some understanding of the forces of distraction that will be generated by muscle activity so that these can be overcome. Failure to accomplish this adequately can lead to motion around the implant during function. Not only does this increase the likelihood of implant failure and nonunion; it also increases the probability of wound infection and, ultimately, osteomyelitis. (The surgeon, believing that the plate has created stability, may be unaware that adequate fixation was never accomplished, and rigid fixation will be blamed for the failure.) Proper understanding of the biomechanics of the mandible in function will lead the surgeon to apply the appropriate number of plates of the correct size and strength in the proper position. When the forces of distraction are overcome by the fixation appliance, healing occurs most dependably and frequently, and the failure rate is kept to a minimum. Therefore, it is necessary to be familiar with the functional forces operating on the mandible in each anatomical area, and plate fixation techniques must be applied in each area to overcome the distracting forces and to take advantage of the naturally occurring compressive forces.

Most bones do not bear weight symmetrically, so that in function there are generally areas that are under pressure and areas that are under tension. **Fig. 68.1** is an oversimplified depiction of the forces affecting the mandible during chewing. In **Fig. 68.1A**, the plus signs indicate the compressive forces acting on the mandible during mastication and the minus signs show areas under tension. When a fracture occurs, these forces tend to distract the tension side of the fracture, whereas the fragments will be compressed together at the pressure side (**Fig. 68.1B**). Although this represents a markedly oversimplified description of the forces acting on the functioning mandible, the concept of tension and compression areas is fundamental to the proper placement of miniplates and compression plates for the repair of mandible fractures. This important biomechanical concept was first appreciated in the study of long-bone fracture repair.[2] Initially, it was thought that a rigid plate fixed to two pieces of bone with two fixation points in each fragment would create a stable fixation and prevent movement of the fragments relative to the plate and to each other. Early clinical failure in both the long bones and the mandible can be attributed to this misconception. Thoughtful analysis reveals that a rigid plate with two fixation points in each of two fragments can provide stability only if the forces transmitted to the plate and screws in functional loading are less than the strength of the plate and the forces holding the screws in place. When plates and screws of proper design and tensile strength are correctly positioned and applied according to biomechanical

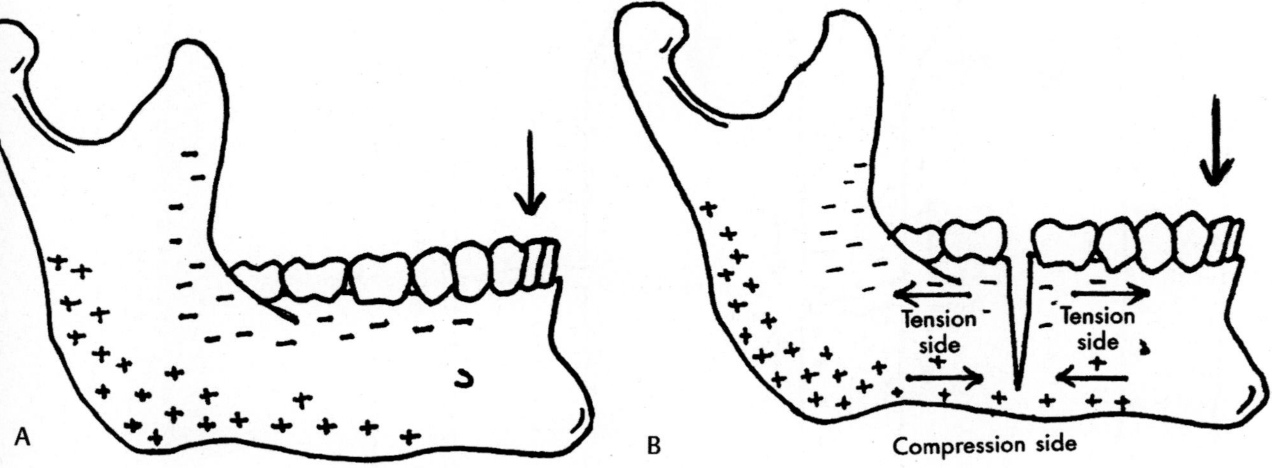

Fig. 68.1 (**A**) Commonly accepted diagram of the forces of tension and compression occurring in the mandible in function. Minus signs indicate areas of traction or tension; plus signs indicate areas of compression (when a force is directed as indicated by the *arrow*). (**B**) The effects of tension and compression forces on a fracture occurring in the mandibular body (when a force is directed as indicated by the *arrow*). (This is a marked oversimplification that nonetheless serves as an aid to proper fixation.)

principles, stability is achieved and healing usually results. In fact, adequate plate and screw design was achieved early; proper plate positioning was understood later, when tension and compression forces were appreciated.

Using the femur as an example (**Fig. 68.2**), it should be intuitively apparent that weight bearing on the femoral head produces distracting forces on the lateral cortex and compresses the medial cortex. A plate placed on either cortex (across a fracture) holds the fragments together at rest, and a compression plate adds a positive (compressive) force across the fracture. In function, however, the distracting forces on the lateral cortex generally exceed the compressive forces of a medially placed plate; therefore, the dynamic forces vary from positive (rest) to negative (weight bearing). Screw loosening frequently results, and motion leads to nonunion and even osteomyelitis. On the other hand, when the plate holds the tension side together, distraction cannot occur unless a screw fails, and the compressive forces of weight bearing are added to any static compressive forces applied by the plate and distributed across the fracture. Although the forces across the fracture vary, they never become negative (distracting), and healing generally ensues.

It should also be apparent that the more biomechanically advantaged the repair, the less dependent it will be on the size and strength of the hardware. When repairing a fracture in an area of tension, so long as there is extensive bony contact in the compressive area and minimal torque on the fixation point, small fixation appliances (so long as they can overcome the distracting forces at the site of placement) will generally prove adequate. On the other hand, when large distracting and rotational forces are found in areas with weak bone or minimal contact areas between the fragments (as in the atrophic mandible), larger fixation devices will generally be necessary. The most extreme example is an area of bone loss, in which case the implant used (if no bone replacement is performed at the time of repair) must be large and fixed with large screws using multiple fixation points.

Armed with an understanding of the above principles, the reader should see why certain techniques of mandibular repair succeed and why others fail.

Techniques

Arch Bar Fixation with Mandibulomaxillary Fixation

It has long been thought that MMF splints the mandible in a fixed position and puts it at rest. This is not entirely true, and even swallowing generates large forces across the mandible. However, because a well-placed mandibular arch bar puts tension across the teeth, it holds the area of distraction together. If there is large bony contact, and the torsional forces are minimal, the mandibular arch bar creates enough stability to allow a callus to form, and healing results. Of course, the significant failure rate seen when MMF alone is utilized has led to a need for more dependable fixation techniques (along with a desire to avoid prolonged periods of MMF).

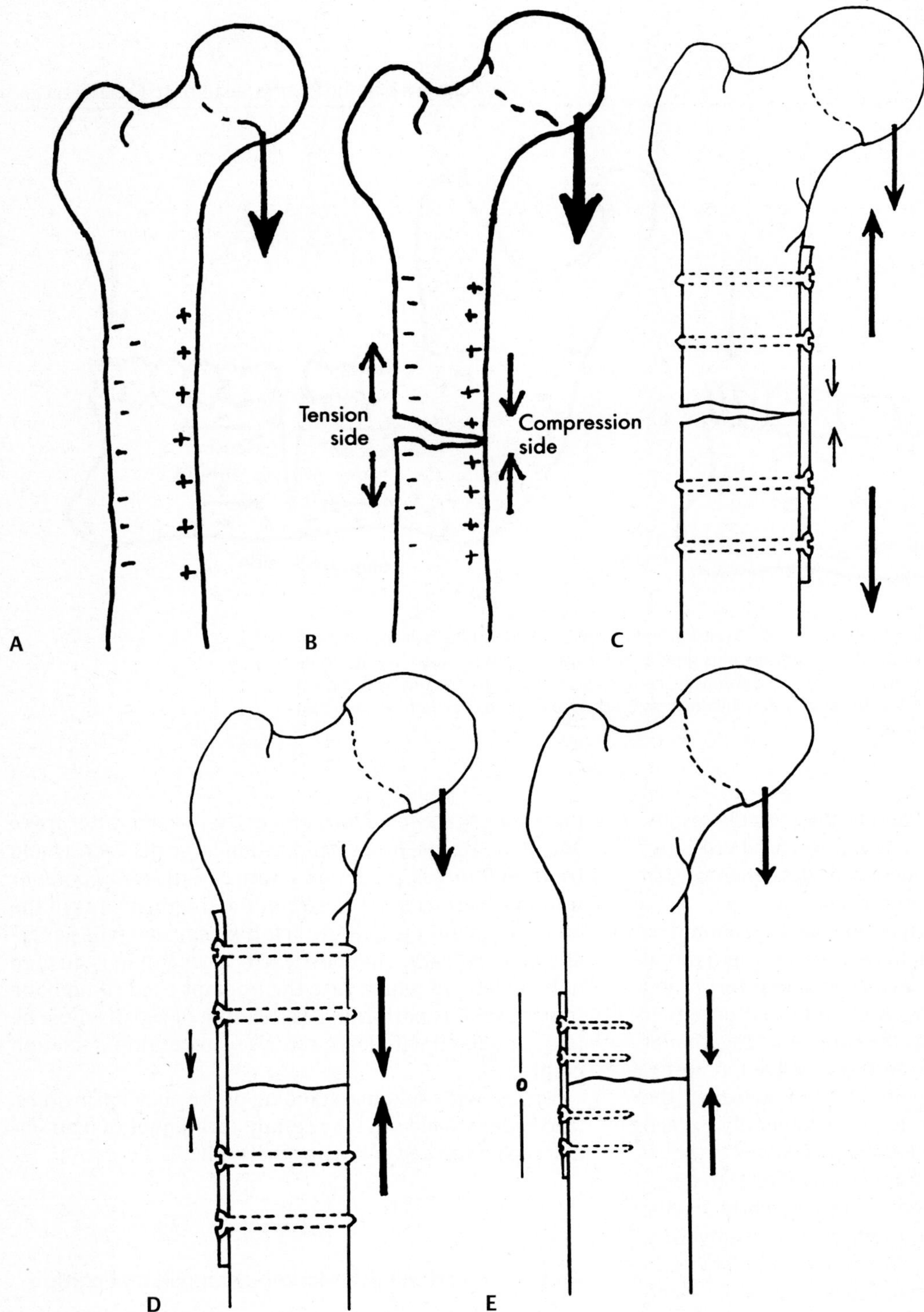

Fig. 68.2 The femur illustrates the effect of tension and compression forces on an intact and fractured bone. (**A**) It should be apparent that the weight-bearing force acting on the femoral head is positioned medially so that a compression force (plus signs) is directed along the medial side of the bone, and a distracting force (minus signs) is distributed along the lateral portion of the bone. In the absence of a fracture the full bone supports weight. (**B**) In the presence of fracture the force of weight bearing results in compression of the medial side and distraction of the lateral side. (**C**) Placement of a compression plate along the compression side will not overcome the stronger distracting forces of weight bearing. The small arrows represent the compression force applied by the plate, and this compression force is exerted across the fracture at rest. The large arrows represent the sum total force experienced across the fracture with weight bearing. Thus a compression plate placed across the compression side of the fracture does not prevent distraction at the tension side. (**D**) In this case, the compression plate has been placed along the tension side of the fracture. Again, the small arrows represent the static compression force applied by the plate. The heavy arrows represent the compressive force across the entire fracture that results from weight bearing. The stenting of the tension side of the compression plate prevents any distracting force from acting across the fracture, and the sum total is a stronger compressive force. (**E**) Schematic representation using a miniplate. The screws are monocortical. The force across the fracture at rest is 0. However, this plate (if strong enough) will hold the traction side of the fracture together, allowing the force of weight bearing to act across the entire fracture as a compression force. (This is an illustrative diagram and does not represent a technique used for the femur in clinical practice.)

Mandibulomaxillary Fixation with Interosseous Wire Fixation

Interosseous wire fixation was added to MMF in an effort to overcome the high failure rates seen when MMF was used for unstable fractures. When the wire repair was placed in the biomechanically advantaged tension areas of the mandible, success rates improved. However, when failures occurred, the presence of the wire frequently resulted in a foreign-body infection and osteomyelitis was common. Prolonged periods of MMF were also required and when delayed union occurred, MMF could be needed for as long as 6 to 12 months. Furthermore, although many surgeons believed that complex, basket-weave types of wire placement provided marked stability, the early work of Luhr[3] demonstrated the weakness of wire fixation—and even external fixation—compared with fixation with plates and screws (**Fig. 68.3**).

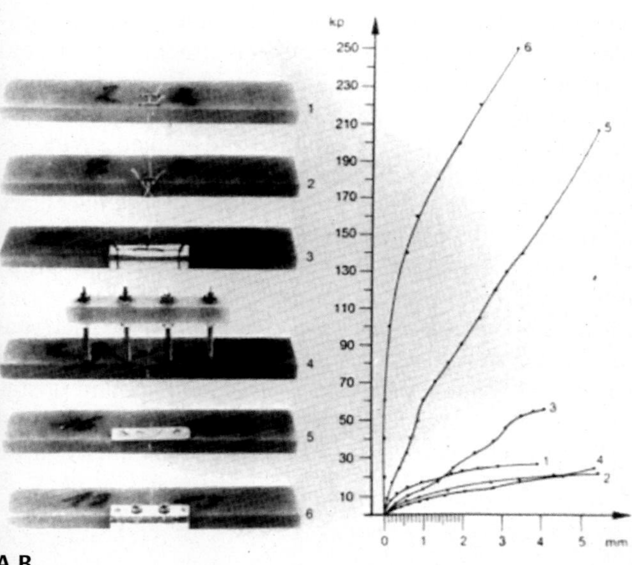

A,B

Fig. 68.3 (**A**) Models of osteosynthesis tested. (1) Two parallel wire ligatures (wire thickness of 0.5 mm). (2) Horizontal wire ligature combined with figure-of-eight ligature. (3) Groove-shaped, 0.5-mm, stainless steel splint 38 mm in length attached with three 0.5-mm wire ligatures (similar to the method advocated by Haward, 1962). (4) Pin fixation as modified by Becker (1958). Four percutaneous osteosynthesis screws are connected by a 10 × 10-mm bar of cold-curing acrylic (Paladur, Heraeus Kulzer, Hanau, Germany). (5) Normal four-hole bone plate (Venable bone plate, 38 mm vitallium). (6) Compression screw plate, 38 mm. (**B**) Stability of different types of osteosyntheses under bending stress. Shown is the gap width between pairs of test pieces as a function of load. Even relatively small loads of 20 kP lead to loosening of osteosyntheses (1–4; gap widths, several millimeters). The usual screw plate system (5) is considerably more stable, but it is far exceeded by a compression screw plate. (From Luhr HG. Compression plate osteosynthesis through the Luhr system. In: Kruger E, Schilli W, eds. Oral and Maxillofacial Traumatology. Vol 1. Chicago: Quintessence Publishing; 1982. Reprinted by permission.)

Miniplate Osteosynthesis

In an effort to improve techniques of mandibular fracture repair, Champy studied the biomechanics of mandibular fractures and found that a properly positioned miniplate can often take advantage of the dynamic compressive forces occurring in function.[4] A miniplate placed along the tension side of a fracture holds it together at rest without compression; under functional loading, when the fixation is strong enough to hold (i.e., to merely withstand the distracting forces), compression of the fracture fragments results (**Fig. 68.2E**).

The success of this approach for the repair of mandibular fractures depends on several factors. First, it is critical to determine where the miniplates must be applied to effect the stabilization necessary for healing. This was painstakingly accomplished by studying the lines of force generated by various miniplate fixation points, using araldite models to simulate mandible fractures. Using this approach, Champy was able to define the areas for miniplate fixation along the so-called ideal osteosynthesis line[5] (**Fig. 68.4**). This line corresponds to the line of tension along the mandibular body. From parasymphysis to parasymphysis, two miniplates are required to overcome the torsional forces affecting this area. Posteriorly, a single miniplate along the oblique line or below it was thought to be effective; however, Kroon[6] has shown that the forces in this area vary from positive to negative during function, necessitating the use of a second plate inferior to the first if dependable stabilization and healing are to be achieved. Whether to use one or two miniplates when repairing a fracture at the mandibular angle remains controversial. Levy et al[7] have shown that the complication rate when repairing mandibular angle fractures with miniplates drops from 26% when a single plate is utilized to 3% when a second plate is added. This is consistent with the findings of Kroon.[6] Ellis and Walker,[8] on the other hand, found a single plate not only to be adequate but to yield better results. However, they encountered a 16% complication rate in this group (compared with 28% when they used two miniplates), which is not as good as the 3% rate of Levy et al when two miniplates were used. Until this controversy is resolved, the author recommends the use of two plates if a miniplate technique is utilized to repair a fracture of the mandibular angle region.

With the ideal plate position identified, the osteosynthesis line overlying the inferior alveolar nerve and tooth roots remains a problem. The solution is the monocortical screw. A monocortical screw penetrates only the lateral cortex of the mandible, and great care is exercised to avoid deeper penetration into the alveolar nerve and tooth roots. When performing these procedures, the surgeon must be aware of the location of the tooth roots and of the inferior alveolar nerves. It should also be clear that the use

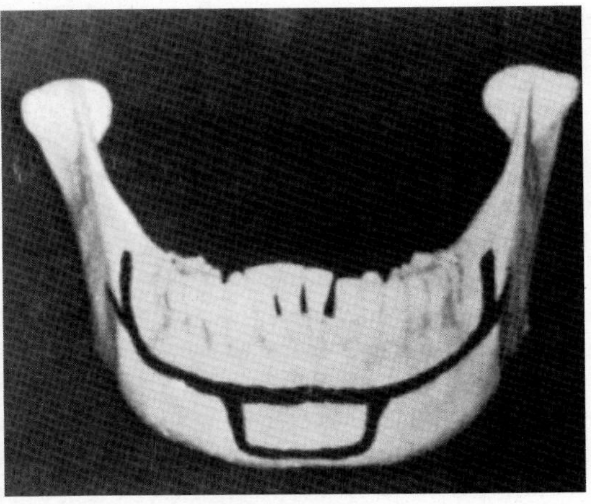

A

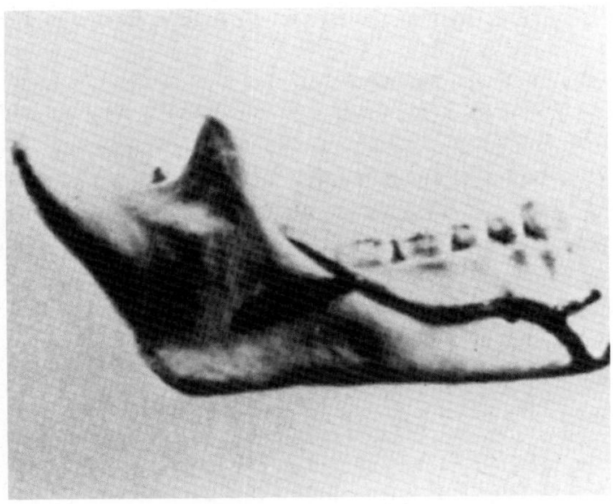

B

Fig. 68.4 Ideal osteosynthesis line for mandibular body. (From Champy M, et al. The Strasbourg miniplate osteosynthesis. In: Kruger E, Schilli W, Worthington P, eds. Oral and Maxillofacial Traumatology. Vol 2. Chicago: Quintessence Publishing; 1985.)

of monocortical screws precludes the application of compression because compression plating puts pressure on the screw shaft at its entry point into the bone; the thin monocortical fixation of the screw to the bone will likely be inadequate to prevent shifting of the screw, which would lead to loosening and failure. Nonetheless, the plates and screws used must be strong enough to resist the distracting forces that occur in function. Two-millimeter mandibular miniplates are designed to overcome these forces, and, when properly applied, fixation failure is uncommon. However, many failures have resulted from the use of inadequate fixation, as may be seen when weaker plates designed for midfacial applications are applied to the mandible. The facial plastic surgeon must be familiar with the systems and must be sure to select implants designed for the particular indications for which they are being used. Similarly, the screws must be of appropriate size, strength, and number, and they must hold tightly in the bone. If a screw hole strips during screw tightening, it must be abandoned because it will not provide fixation. A larger ("emergency") screw may be utilized or the plate must be moved and new holes used. A variation of the miniplate technique is the use of the "three-dimensional plate" applied along the line of tension as described by Farmand.[9] The three-dimensional plate is actually a miniplate that has been strengthened by being produced in geometric assemblies of squares and rectangles (**Fig. 68.5**). Although the plates are slightly more difficult to bend, the results using them have been excellent.

Compression Osteosynthesis

As the name implies, compression osteosynthesis involves the application of a force across the fracture such that the fractured fragments are compressed together by the fixation. Thus at the time of fixation there is a compressive force between the fragments at rest. This is in contrast to miniplate fixation, in which case the bone fragments are held together without compression, so that compressive forces are only seen across the fracture during function (if the plate has been properly positioned and applied). Whereas it was originally believed by the proponents of compression plating that the compressive forces were necessary for direct bone healing, it is now clear that healing takes place quite dependably when neutral fixation is properly applied. However, compression certainly increases the area of bone-to-bone contact as well as the frictional forces between the fragments, so that the likelihood of successful healing, particularly in a complex and unstable fracture, is probably increased. Compression fixation may also be accomplished with lag screws, as will be

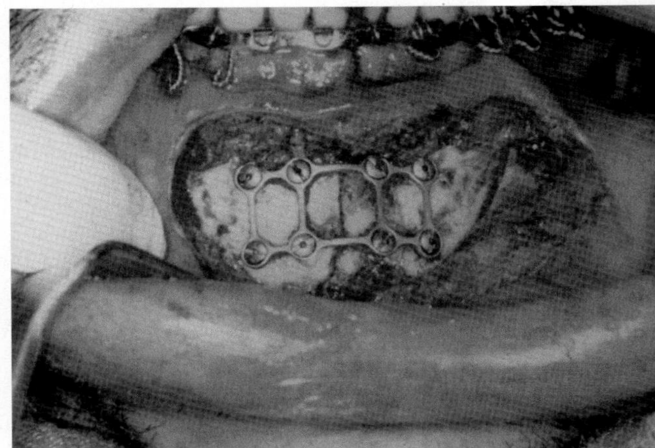

Fig. 68.5 A mandibular symphyseal fracture repaired using a 2.0-mm geometrical plate. Note the similarity to two miniplates that are connected together, thereby creating greater fixation strength.

described below. Note that when compression is applied across a fracture, the bone remodels under the stress to eliminate the force until the plate and/or screws are ultimately exerting no force on the bone. However, this remodeling is occurring during healing, so that a complete bony union has resulted by the time the force exerted by the fixation appliance has dissipated.

Compression Using a Plate

The technique for compression using a plate is described at the end of this chapter. As noted earlier, compression plate stability requires the use of bicortical screws (to prevent motion of the screws in the bone and failure of the fixation). Because the presence of the tooth roots and the inferior alveolar nerve prevents the placement of bicortical screws in the biomechanically correct position along the line of tension, compression plates are placed along the basal border of the mandible (below the inferior alveolar nerve). Despite the use of strong plates and large screws, this biomechanically incorrect positioning is frequently inadequate to overcome the distracting forces that develop across the fracture during function (**Fig. 68.6**), and, in fact, early experiences using this technique resulted in unacceptably high failure rates and frequent condemnation of the technique.

However, this problem was overcome by Spiessl with the use of tension banding.[2,10] A tension band is applied to hold the traction side of a fracture together. This is analogous to the miniplate applied along the ideal osteosynthesis line. Compression can then be applied to the pressure side without distracting the traction side. Furthermore, the compressive force applied will be distributed along the full length of the fracture. This compressive force increases the friction and contact between the fragments, thereby increasing the rigidity of fixation and the likelihood that bone healing will occur.

A tension band can be applied in several ways. When a fracture occurs in a dentulous area of the mandible, an arch bar attached to the teeth across the fracture line can serve as a tension band. This must be tightly applied so that distraction does not occur along the alveolar segment when compression is applied at the basal border. Behind the dentition, a plate can be placed above the level of the inferior alveolar nerve to serve as a tension band, and a compression plate can then be placed at the basal border. This is similar to the miniplate approach, and, in fact, a miniplate can also serve as a tension band for use in conjunction with a basally positioned compression plate for any mandibular fracture.

Compression Using a Lag Screw

The technique for using a lag screw is described at the end of the chapter. When fragments overlap (e.g., in an oblique fracture or sagittal split osteotomy), a compression plate tends to cause the fragments to glide past each other and override each other (**Fig. 68.7**). A lag screw, on the other hand, is placed through both overlapping fragments, thereby bringing the damaged surfaces together. Properly applied, a lag screw compresses these surfaces together, resulting in rigid fixation.

The key to the lag screw is that its threads bypass the first fragment and engage the second fragment. As the

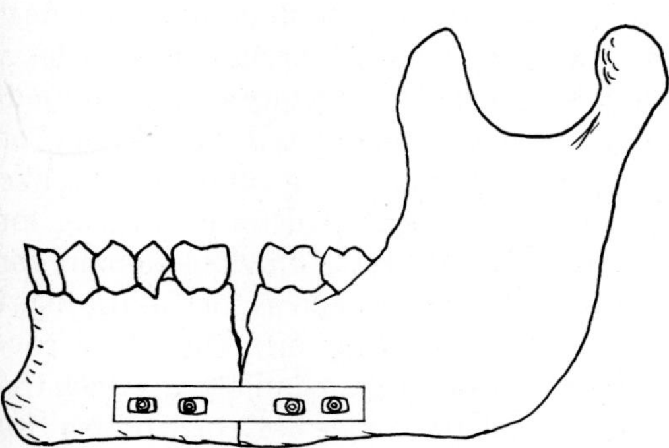

Fig. 68.6 Diagrammatic representation of the effect of placing a compression plate across the basal border (compression side) of the mandible in the presence of a fracture. In the absence of a tension band across the traction side of the fracture, functional forces overcome the weak compressive forces applied by the plate, resulting in an unstable fixation and gapping of the alveolar portion of the fracture.

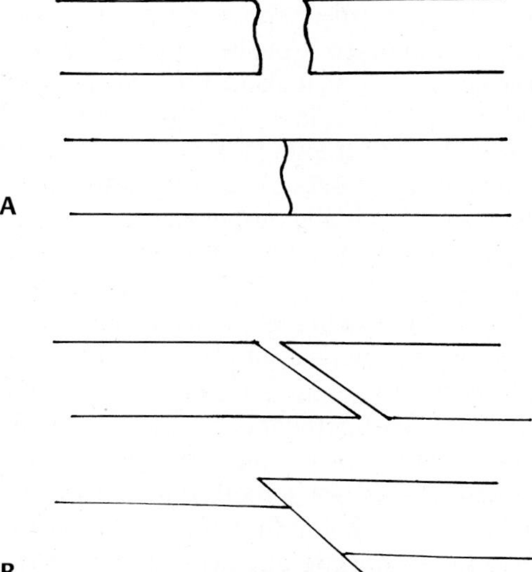

Fig. 68.7 This shows why a compression plate is ineffective and harmful in the presence of an oblique or overlapping fracture. (**A**) The ends of the fractured bones abut each other and compression will be accomplished by a compression plate. (**B**) The oblique fragments overlap, and if an attempt is made to compress them, they will glide over each other, resulting in a malposition.

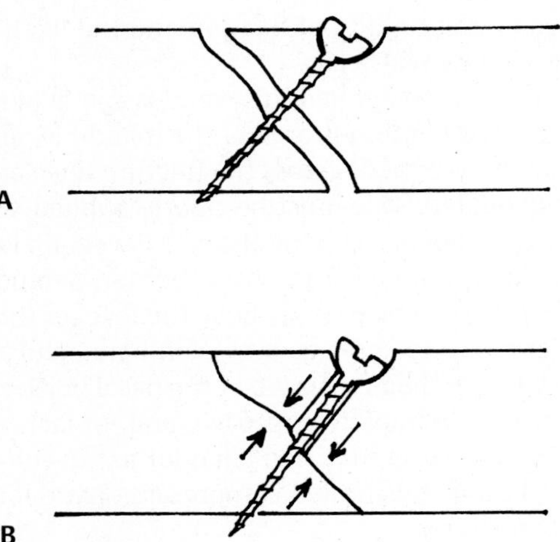

Fig. 68.8 **(A)** The screw catches in both fragments of bone. The screw first passes through the first fragment and encounters the second fragment. Initially, it pushes the second fragment away and then the thread catches. The screw can then be tightened until the head is firmly positioned in the first fragment and can no longer progress. Because the screw threads are holding tightly in both fragments of bone, the gap between the two fragments will never be closed. **(B)** In this case, the threads will not catch in the first piece of bone because the hole has been overdrilled. When the screw passes through the first piece of bone, it will similarly hit the second piece of bone and push it away, and then the thread will catch. However, the screw continues to tighten until its head is compressed firmly against the first piece of bone. Because the first piece of bone will not catch the threads of the screw, tightening results in compression of the first fragment between the head of the screw and the second fragment. Compression is thus achieved.

screw is tightened, the head of the screw cannot pass through the first fragment, so it pushes against the first fragment, thereby compressing it against the second fragment (**Fig. 68.8**). Compression fixation is thus achieved. If the screw engages the first fragment, fixation will occur without compression (**Fig. 68.8A**). When the screw exits the first fragment, the tip initially pushes the second fragment away slightly and then engages it. As the screw is tightened further, the threads hold in both pieces of bone, maintaining the gap between them unchanged. Tightening is complete when the head of the screw becomes firmly fixed in the first fragment, and thus compression is precluded. As the two fragments are held in a fixed relationship to each other, this is termed a "positioning screw." Positioning screws are sometimes used in sagittal split osteotomies to maintain a fixed relationship between the fragments and thereby avoid a shift in the position of the condylar head in the joint.

A single lag screw will not prevent rotation of the fragments around its axis. Therefore, when the lag screw is the only fixation device, two or three lag screws should be placed when feasible.[11] Note also that a lag screw can be used through a plate, but when this is done, any

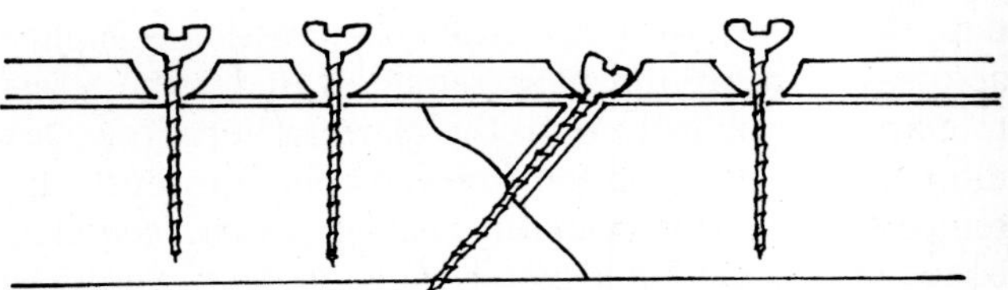

Fig. 68.9 A lag screw can be placed through a plate hole. The lag screw principle is followed and the first hole is overdrilled so that the screw thread will not catch in the first fragment of bone. All the remaining screws are placed neutrally in their holes so that there is no interaction between the screwheads and the plate.

screws through overlapping fragments must be lagged, and all other screws must be neutrally applied (i.e., without compression) (**Fig. 68.9**).

Use of a Mandibular Reconstruction Plate

Mandibular reconstruction plates (MRPs) are designed for reconstruction of mandibular defects. Unlike miniplates and compression plates, they do not rely on the intrinsic integrity of the mandible to stabilize the defective area. On the contrary, these plates are designed to replace the structural integrity of a defective area of the mandible. They must be compact enough and strong enough for use in mandibular reconstruction, and they must contain many holes so that numerous fixation points can be applied. The strength of the repair is increased by the placement of additional screws for fixation. Generally speaking, when a gap is being bridged with an MRP, at least three and preferably four or five screws on either side of the defect are preferred.

Because MRPs are strong enough to bridge defect areas, they are obviously strong enough to be used to repair fractures or relative defect areas. Whenever a fracture cannot be properly stabilized with a miniplate or compression plate (e.g., because of comminution or technical difficulty), the MRP can be used. Therefore, it provides a fall-back technique whenever difficulty is encountered. It provides rigid fixation without tension banding or compression. Areas of comminution often behave like areas of bone loss, lacking the structural integrity for compression plating. The MRP also provides stability for thin and biomechanically complex areas such as the mandibular angle and in atrophic mandibles. The MRP is particularly useful in the pencil-thin mandible, in which the weakened, poorly vascularized bone has a high propensity for nonunion after fracture. A reconstruction plate can be applied with minimal devascularization (periosteum is not stripped), and the functional stress is removed from the fractured areas, resulting in a high rate of healing.

The MRP is excellent for reconstructing areas of osteomyelitis. The area can be aggressively debrided, and the plate can be applied during the same procedure, or application can be delayed until the infection has cleared. It is important to place all screws in healthy bone at a distance from the osteitic area. Sometimes cancellous bone is placed in the defect during the same procedure.

For extensive traumatic defects with both soft tissue and bone loss (e.g., shotgun injuries), the MRP allows for the immediate reconstitution of the skeletal framework. The MRP seems to be stable enough to tolerate prolonged exposure without screw loosening and plate failure. It is therefore possible to provide a framework for later reconstruction, whether soft tissue reconstitution (e.g., pedicle or free flaps) is performed initially or not. The ease and simplicity of reconstruction plate placement make this possible even when the patient is too unstable to tolerate a lengthy reconstructive procedure.

For the reconstruction of oncologic mandibular defects, the MRP allows for the maintenance of the precise preresection relationship of the mandibular stumps. In most instances, the plate can be preapplied before the mandibular resection. The plate is then removed, carefully noting the screw and hole positions. After the resection and soft tissue reconstruction has been completed, the MRP can be reapplied using the previously drilled holes. The preresection relationship of the stumps is thus maintained. Bony reconstruction can be accomplished primarily or secondarily, depending on individual circumstances.

Recent advances in design have made the mandibular reconstruction plate more dependable and easier to use. With the traditional design, precise bending of the plate to match the bone was critical because the plate was stabilized only by its fixation to the bone by tightening of the screws. In more recent designs, the screw heads are fixed directly to the plate, so that as long as the screw threads are firmly held by the bone, the screw and plate are tightly fixed in place. This not only serves to make the plate more stable when the bend is less precise but keeps the screw stable if there is any bone resorption around the thread, thereby decreasing the likelihood of foreign-body reaction and infection (and thus fixation failure), so long as some of the screws remain fixed. Various designs include screws with expandable heads that are fixed to the plate by the insertion of expansion bolts and plates with threaded holes in which the threaded screw head tightens directly into the plate itself.

Repair of Specific Mandibular Fractures

Nonoverlapping Fractures

Occlusion should first be established. If an arch bar serves as a tension band, a single compression plate with at least two screws on either side of the fracture can be used anywhere along the symphysis and body of the mandible, so long as the alveolar portion of the fracture is held together by the tension band. At the mandibular angle, two plates should be used: a tension band plate above the nerve and a compression plate below. When inadequate dentition prevents the use of an arch bar as a tension band, a tension band plate can be used. Otherwise, an alternative technique should be utilized. When a tension band plate cannot be applied, a mandibular reconstruction plate is a good alternative. [Note that the eccentric dynamic compression plate (EDCP) is rarely used today and so it is not discussed.] These plates can be placed from an intraoral or an extraoral approach.

If miniplate osteosynthesis is preferred, two plates are necessary in the symphysis and parasymphysis, whereas a single plate is adequate along the mandibular body. At the mandibular angle, a single plate should be placed intraorally along the oblique line, with care taken to ensure that at least two well-held screws are fixed to the bone on each side of the fracture. A second miniplate is recommended on the buccal surface of the mandible, generally positioned above the inferior alveolar nerve. Three-dimensional plates are placed similarly to miniplates. Note that most miniplates can be easily applied via the transoral approach, whereas larger plates may require an external incision, particularly in the region of the mandibular angle.

Lag screws may be applied to the solid bone in the symphyseal and parasymphyseal regions of the mandible. At least two screws should be placed, and to minimize the risk of microfracture between the screws, it may be helpful to bring them in from opposite directions (**Fig. 68.10**). A lag screw may also be used to fix selected mandibular angle fractures as described

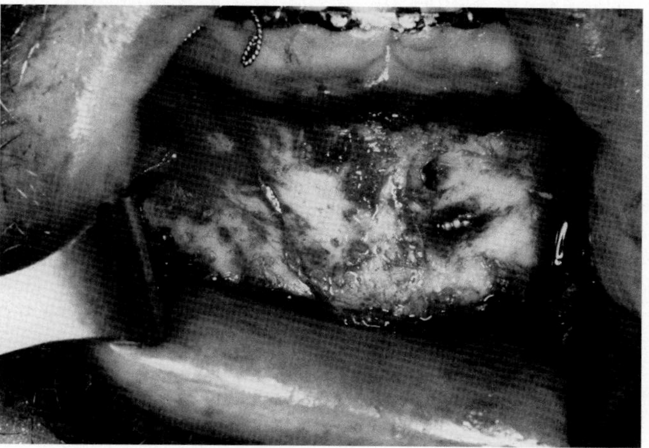

Fig. 68.10 Repair of a parasymphyseal fracture of the mandible using two lag screws. Note that the screws are placed in opposite directions to minimize the risk of microfracture of the bone between the two screws. Note also the countersinking of the hole to allow for insetting of the screwhead in the bone.

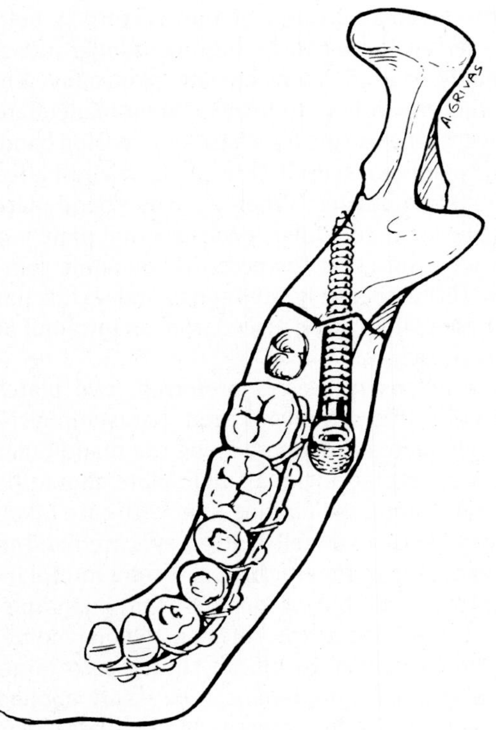

Fig. 68.11 View of a mandible from above with the bone transparent for visualization of a lag screw repairing a fracture of the mandibular angle. Note the positioning of the screw from buccal to lingual as it traverses the bone from the anterior to posterior direction. The screw was also directed somewhat superiorly, which cannot be seen from this view. When properly positioned, this screw provides compressive forces that bring the two fractured fragments directly together. (From Kellman RM, Marentette LJ. Atlas of Craniomaxillofacial Fixation. New York: Raven; 1995.)

by Niederdellmann et al[12] (**Fig. 68.11**). The screw must be placed transbuccally through the lower cheek, and it must pass in a superior, medial, and posterior direction while carefully avoiding the inferior alveolar nerve. This is a technically challenging technique.

Overlapping Fractures

As noted earlier, when bone fragments overlap, a lag screw can be placed through the fragments. Because the lag screw is only threaded in the second fragment, tightening the screw compresses the fragments together by compressing the first fragment between the second fragment and the head of the screw. Generally speaking, at least two and preferably three lag screws best stabilize the bones together. Alternatively, a lag screw technique may be combined with plate fixation (see **Fig. 68.9**).

Fractures in the Region of the Mandibular Angle

The mandibular angle is singled out because of the high complication rates seen when repairing fractures in this region.[7,8] The ideal repair remains quite controversial. Champy et al[4] and Ellis and Walker[8] recommend using a single miniplate along the oblique line. Kroon,[6] Levy et al,[7] and Fox and Kellman[13] recommend the use of two miniplates. Ultimately, the strongest repair of any mandible fracture is probably a well applied mandible reconstruction plate because it is strong enough to repair bone defects. Ellis[14] found the mandibular reconstruction plate provided the most dependable repair of mandibular angle fractures, though he preferred not to use this technique unless absolutely necessary given that it generally requires an external approach and is more technically demanding and time consuming. However, due to the thinning of the bone posteriorly, when in doubt, it is probably wise to use an angled reconstruction plate in this region, with at least three bicortical screws on each side of the fracture.

Subcondylar Fractures

The treatment of subcondylar fractures of the mandible remains controversial. Thus far, most surgeons continue to advocate a conservative (i.e., closed) approach to most fractures. However, with the advent of endoscopically assisted, minimally invasive techniques, the reluctance to open subcondylar fractures may diminish. Various new instruments have been designed to facilitate the endoscopic approach, which can be performed transorally or via a small incision below the angle of the mandible or by combination of these two approaches. Sleeves on the endoscope enlarge the optical cavity, and specially designed retractors allow for easier stabilization of the fragments prior to fixation. Devices that stabilize and advance the plate into position allow for easier placement of the screws through the transbuccal trochar (**Fig. 68.12**). One or two small (2.0-mm) plates are applied; the position of the bones should be checked radiographically to assure proper repositioning.[15,16]

Fractures with Severe Comminution, Bone Loss, and Atrophic Mandibles

Miniplates, compression plates, and lag screws all rely on the structural integrity of the underlying bone; by taking proper advantage of biomechanics, the fixation devices force the bones together so they can heal. When the bone is severely comminuted or missing, it cannot be adequately supported by these methods. The strength of the bone must be replaced with bone (e.g., via microvascular free-tissue transfer) or with an implant strong enough to support the defective area. Mandibular reconstruction plates are designed to replace the structural

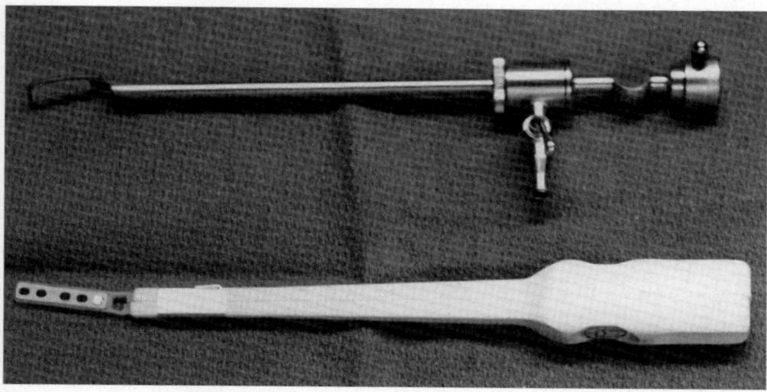

Fig. 68.12 Photo of an endoscopic retractor designed for forehead lifts that has served effectively for creating the optical cavity during the endoscopic repair of subcondylar fractures of the mandible. (Note that retractors designed specifically for this purpose are currently being developed.) The device below the retractor is a plate advancer designed to deliver the plate into position during the endoscopic procedure. The plate position can be rotated left to right by moving the sliding plastic handpiece sides against each other. Also note that a rotating rivet holds the plate in the holder. A half turn of the screw releases the plate so that it stays in the wound and the introducer can be removed.

integrity of the defective bone. When used to repair an area of comminution, the area should be treated as a defect and at least four screws should be placed into the solid bone on either side of the involved area. Small fragments can be pieced together with wires or small plates, or they may be discarded, depending on the circumstances (**Fig. 68.13**). An MRP works well for the repair

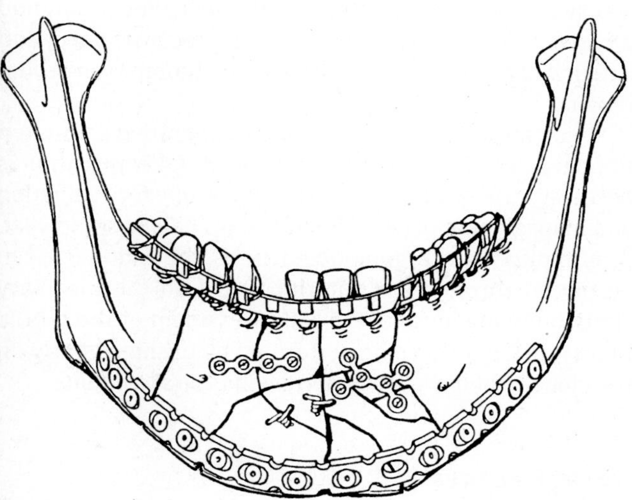

Fig. 68.13 Artist's depiction of a comminuted mandible fracture. Note that a single large reconstruction plate bridges the comminuted area fixing the solid, stable fragments to each other. Screws from the plate in essence lag the smaller fragments to the plate. Smaller monocortical miniplates and/or wires can be used to fix small fragments in place. (From Kellman RM, Marentette LJ. Atlas of Craniomaxillofacial Fixation. New York: Raven; 1995.)

of fractures of the severely atrophic mandible, which is not only difficult to stabilize but, due to the paucity of bone-to-bone contact and the poor blood supply, is very prone to nonunion. Use of the MRP for these injuries has minimized the occurrence of nonunions in these difficult situations.

Rigid Fixation for Fractures of the Midface and Upper Face

General Principles

Occlusion

As noted earlier, re-creating the proper (premorbid) occlusal relationship is a primary functional concern. This is as true for maxillary fractures as it is for mandibular fractures. Of course, it is not an issue for fractures that do not in any way involve the maxilla or mandible.

Biomechanics

Like mandibular fractures, midfacial fractures and osteotomies can be repaired reliably using plate fixation. However, many of the bones are thinner, the shapes are more variable, and the areas for application are smaller, with thinner overlying skin in most areas as well. Therefore, much smaller and more variously shaped plates have been developed for middle and upper facial repairs. Compression plates and neutral plates are available.

Generally speaking, even the thinnest bones can be held in place with screw fixation. It has been demonstrated that stable fixation can be accomplished in bone as thin as 2 mm,[17] which is available in most facial areas. However, plate fixation should not be used until the correct bone positions have been reestablished because rigid fixation will be maintained despite malpositioning.[18] Once exact repositioning has been accomplished, rigid fixation allows for the removal of MMF. Furthermore, craniofacial suspension and the associated risks of facial foreshortening and rotation can be avoided.[19]

Unlike the mandible, areas of tension and compression do not seem to be a major factor, and biomechanical concerns relate to proper fixation and stabilization. Skeletal position must be carefully reconstructed in three dimensions, and enough fixation must be applied to assure stability and immobility in function. The vertical buttresses are reestablished to define facial height.[20] The anteroposterior dimension is defined along the zygomatic arches, and the lateral dimension is determined from zygoma to zygoma across the infraorbital rims and nose and across the palate.

Repair for Specific Midface and Upper Face Fractures

Zygomatic Arch Fractures

Although rigid fixation of the isolated arch fracture is currently rare, the introduction of endoscopic techniques has led some people to attempt fixation of this injury. Although the technology is not yet state of the art, as the equipment improves we may expect to see this area treated more frequently.

Zygomaticomaxillary–Orbital Fractures

The so-called tripod fracture centers around the solid malar eminence; the name *tripod* comes from the junctional supports between the zygoma and the temporal bone, frontal bone, and maxilla. It has also been referred to as a quadrapod fracture, separating the maxillary fracture into its orbital rim and maxillary buttress components. In fact, it is far more complex than that, frequently with significant orbital floor and lateral orbital wall components. Manson has classified these fractures by severity into low-energy, middle-energy, and high-energy injuries.[21] Obviously, the more displaced and comminuted the fracture, the more extensive the repair will be. For low-energy injuries, displacement may be so minimal that no repair is indicated. Still, the key to repair of even the simple zygomatic fracture is proper anatomical repositioning before rigid fixation. Minimally displaced fractures sometimes require minimal exposure; in fact, a bone hook under the eminence may occasionally be adequate and fixation may be unnecessary. However, before any plate fixation is contemplated, care should be taken to ascertain that the positioning is optimal. Sublabial exposure of the zygomaticomaxillary area often reveals malpositions that are frequently ignored when only lateral orbital rim exposures have been used. Once exposed, this area can be plated along with the frontozygomatic area, providing solid two-point fixation. Some have advocated single-point fixation at the frontozygomatic area,[19,22] whereas others have advocated single-plate fixation at the zygomaticomaxillary buttress. However, these approaches remain controversial because the strong masseter pull on the zygomatic arch makes single-point fixation less dependable. It is not clear whether failures of single-point fixation are due to inadequate fixation or improper positioning. The recent work of Davidson et al[23] suggests that single-point miniplate fixation at the frontozygomatic suture should provide acceptable stability. It is therefore recommended that whether one- or two-point fixation is planned, the zygomaticomaxillary area should be visualized to ensure that the alignment is correct. With the wide variety of plate and screw sizes now available, it is still unclear what constitutes adequate fixation. Because three-point fixation with wires seems to stabilize a zygomatic fracture,[23] certainly the smallest plates could be adequate if three points are fixated (assuming no bone loss). What is unclear is the size of the implant(s) required if one- or two-point fixation is to be used, particularly for a middle-energy injury. If after what appears to be adequate reduction the malar eminence still appears flattened, it may be posteriorly displaced. Proper reduction may then require exposure of the zygomatic arch via a coronal incision, so that its proper shape and alignment can be reconstituted.

For high-energy injuries, severe displacement and comminution mandate wide exposures and multiple fixation points. A comminuted arch must be exposed via a coronal approach. It may be repaired with microplates, though even the smallest plates may alter the facial contour. Sometimes the shape of the arch can be reconstituted with multiple interosseous wires, and, after rigid stabilization of the remainder of the zygoma via reconstruction of the frontozygomatic continuity, the infraorbital rim, and the zygomaticomaxillary buttress, the wired arch will maintain its shape. The infraorbital rim should be repaired with the smallest implants possible, though great attention should be paid to assuring solid bony fixation along the lateral orbital rim (and frontal bone) and the zygomaticomaxillary buttress. If this buttress is deficient, a bone graft should be utilized to reconstruct it.

The orbital walls should be directly approached and repaired. The lateral orbital wall can sometimes prove very helpful when the alignment of the zygoma is difficult to determine. Although some have placed small bone plates across the intraorbital lateral wall, this is not a common technique. The orbital floor should be reconstructed, and a deficient medial wall should not be ignored (see orbital repair).

It is not always clear from the preoperative computed tomographic (CT) scan when direct orbital exploration is necessary. The availability of the endoscope for evaluation and management of facial fractures has helped somewhat. After reduction of zygomatic fractures, the endoscope can be placed through the anterior wall into the maxillary sinus, allowing for direct visual assessment of the orbital floor. A pulse test can be performed by pushing gently on the globe to help visualize herniated orbital contents.

Le Fort Fractures

Le Fort I

The Le Fort I or horizontal maxillary fracture separates the lower maxillae and palate from the upper face. It traverses the pyriform apertures and nasal septum and is completed posteriorly across the lower portion of the pterygoid plates, thereby separating the upper teeth and the bones

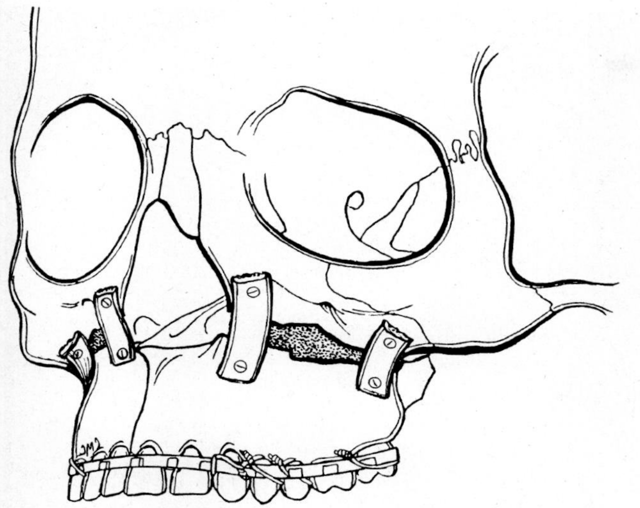

Fig. 68.14 Artist's depiction of a Le Fort I fracture with bone loss repaired using bone grafts as plates. When the buttresses are deficient, bone grafts should be used. Otherwise the same areas can be fixed directly with plates. (From Kellman RM, Marentette LJ. Atlas of Craniomaxillofacial Fixation. New York: Raven; 1995.)

holding them from the remainder of the craniofacial skeleton. Repair requires reattachment of the lower face to the upper face, with care taken to assure proper reestablishment of the occlusion. Rigid fixation must be accomplished along the four vertical buttresses that support the face with exposure via the sublabial approach. These are the bones on either side of the pyriform apertures and the solid zygomaticomaxillary buttress regions. Significant bone loss along these buttresses should be replaced with grafts (**Fig. 68.14**). The 1.5-mm or 2.0-mm plates are commonly used to prevent shifting of the bones, though 1.3-mm and 1.0-mm plates, particularly those with the three-dimensional geometrical designs, have been used as well. Careful attention must be paid to avoiding the tooth roots when placing screws. After adequate fixation, MMF may be released.

Split Palate

A split palate must be repaired to maintain the horizontal width of the lower midface and to prevent rotation of the maxillary dentition either lingually or buccally. Proper MMF is critical when these are adequately available, and a maxillary dental splint can also function well to maintain the relationship of the dental arches (alveoli). A plate across the anterior maxilla may stabilize these fragments. Rarely, it is possible to microplate or wire the palate itself.

Le Fort II

This fracture starts at the zygomaticomaxillary buttress and continues on a diagonal through the orbital floor and medial orbit, then crosses the nasal root before continuing down the contralateral orbit and maxilla. As in all Le Fort fractures, the proper occlusion must first be established. Stabilization requires repositioning of the nasal root if it is displaced and fixation to the frontal bone if it is unstable. This is generally accomplished via small plates placed on either side of the nasal root, though "x" plates and even single nasofrontal plates have been used. The zygomaticomaxillary buttresses are then plated via the sublabial approach, along with horizontal repair of the fractured maxillae. The orbital floors and medial walls are explored as needed, generally utilizing a transconjunctival approach. Bone defects are repaired with bone grafts. Once fixation is satisfactory, MMF may be released.

Le Fort III

The true Le Fort III fracture or craniofacial separation crosses the zygomatic arch; traverses the orbit through the lateral wall, floor, and medial wall; separates the nose from the frontal bone; crosses the upper septum; includes similar fractures on the contralateral side; and is completed posteriorly by crossing the top of the pterygoid plates, essentially separating the face anteriorly from the frontal bone and posteriorly from the sphenoid, leading to a complete craniofacial separation. In practice, most Le Fort III fractures are complex and include components of Le Fort I and II fractures. These are best approached by working from stable to unstable[24] or, as Champy et al state it, from the periphery toward the center.[25] When possible, mandibular stabilization should be completed first because the mandible can provide an excellent template for midfacial repair. Occlusion must be established at the outset using MMF. When necessary, subcondylar fractures are opened and repaired to help reestablish the vertical dimension.[20,26]

An important aspect of skeletal repair is adequate exposure. The bicoronal approach provides access to the frontal area, the nasofrontal junction, the lateral orbital rims, the malar eminences, and the zygomatic arches. Exact repositioning of multiply fractured bones is difficult, and the fragments are often first loosely approximated with wires. When anatomical alignment is satisfactory, plates are used to fix the bones rigidly in position. The thick lateral orbital rims can be fixed with minicompression plates or neutral plates as desired, with care taken to place at least two screws in each fragment. The nasofrontal area can be fixed with wires or plates; a single midline plate or two plates on either side of the nasal root will prevent facial rotation and loss of the nasal dorsum. The zygomatic arch is repaired with lag screws, plates, or wires as needed, thereby reestablishing the anteroposterior facial shape. At this point, the Le Fort III fracture has been converted to a Le Fort II fracture and can be fixated as already outlined. In fact, with adequate exposure, the key to facial skeletal repair is

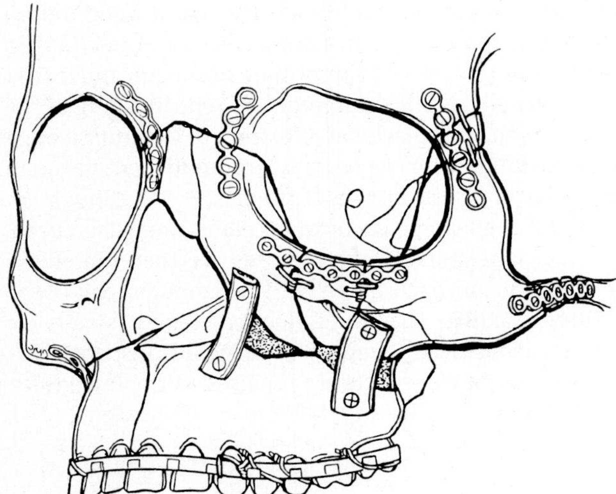

Fig. 68.15 Artist's rendering of a Le Fort III fracture repaired using a combination of wires, plates, and bone grafts. Note that fixation is necessary at the buttresses using plates or, when the bone is deficient, bone grafts that function as plates when lagged to the more solid bone above and below. (From Kellman RM, Marentette LJ. Atlas of Craniomaxillofacial Fixation. New York: Raven; 1995.)

the careful and painstaking reapproximation of all of the skeletal structures using the smallest plates and screws that can adequately stabilize each fracture area. All defect areas are reconstituted with bone grafts, and once complete stabilization has been accomplished, MMF should no longer be necessary (assuming adequate stabilization of the fragments has been achieved) (**Fig. 68.15**).

Note that with complex skeletal injuries, visualization of the repair may sometimes prove inadequate. The addition of intraoperative CT has been shown to enhance the ability of the facial plastic surgeon to assess the correctness of the repair at the time of surgery and to correct any malpositions during the initial procedure.[27]

Orbital Fractures

Rigid fixation has enhanced our ability to reconstruct the orbit as well. Fractures of the orbital floor and medial walls are generally explored via the transconjunctival approach, although subciliary incisions are still used as well. Defects are generally bone grafted, though many surgeons use a variety of alloplastic materials. The orbital floor plate (**Fig. 68.16**) or various forms of titanium mesh have been used to support bone grafts during reconstruction of extensive defects. Another alternative is to fix a microplate to a bone graft so that the plate will extend over the infraorbital rim. Fixing the plate to the rim with screws then stabilizes the graft. Microplates can also be used to fix pieces of calvarial bone together and thereby create a curved graft using the quite unmalleable calvarial bone.

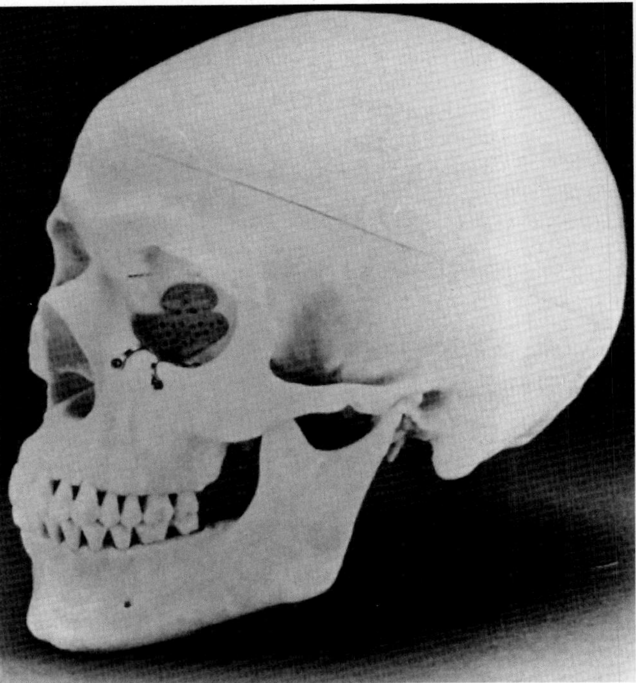

Fig. 68.16 Orbital floor plate.

Frontal Fractures

Rigid fixation has proved helpful for managing comminuted frontal sinus fractures. Severely comminuted areas can be reconstructed on the back table and then reimplanted into the defect. The smallest plates possible should be utilized to minimize the potential for later prominence of the implants through the skin. Management of the sinus is discussed in chapter 59, but it is worth mentioning that the recent development of calcium phosphate bone cements has simultaneously provided what appears to be an excellent material for frontal sinus obliteration while also providing contour for anterior frontal sinus wall defects (**Fig. 68.17 and 68.18**).

Naso-Orbital-Ethmoid Fractures

Naso-orbital-ethmoid fractures involve the nasal bones, lacrimal bones, and ethmoid lamina, with displacement of the medial canthal attachments and posterior telescoping of the nasal dorsum. There are numerous classifications of these fractures, but most significantly, if there is a single large central fragment with the medial canthal ligament still attached, then fixation of this fragment superiorly to the frontal bone and inferiorly to the maxilla will restabilize the medial canthus. When there is marked comminution, or when the medial canthus is detached, direct repair of the canthus is required. Transcanthal wiring is possible, though so-called centripetal suspension, as described

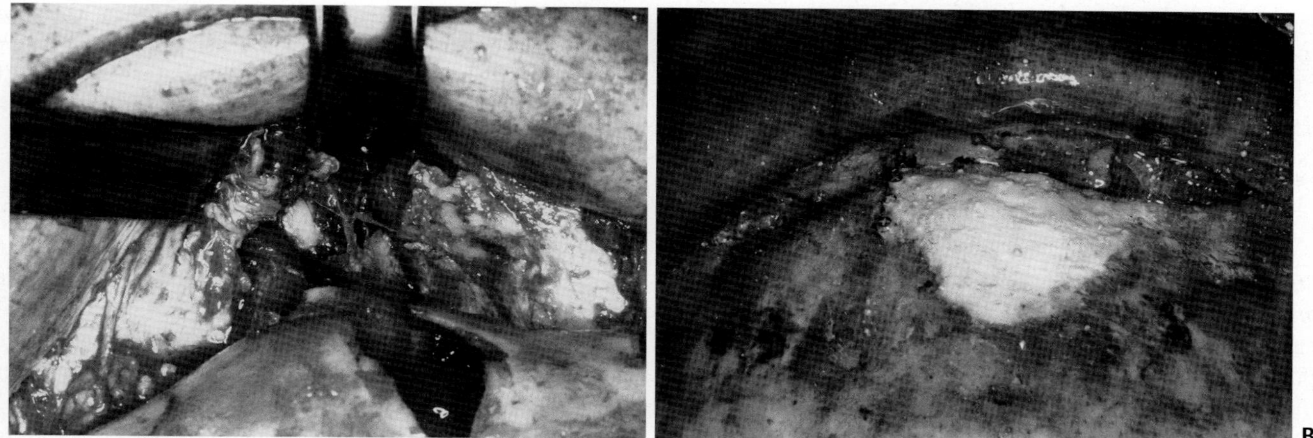

Fig. 68.17 Naso-orbital-ethmoid (nasoethmoid complex) and frontal sinus fractures. (**A**) The losses of the structural integrity of the nasal bone as well as a portion of the frontal sinus are demonstrated. (**B**) After repair of the medial orbits and medial canthal ligaments and reconstruction of the nasal bone with a bone graft, the frontal sinus was obliterated and the frontal contour re-created using bone cement.

by Raveh et al,[28] allows controlled positioning of the misplaced ligaments. In this approach, the medial canthus is sutured to the contralateral frontal bone, with the suture passing posteriorly behind the nasal bone and through the nasal septum. It is important to replace missing bone in the anterior medial orbit so that there is bone to which the repositioned ligament can adhere. When present and reducible, the nasal root is fixed to the frontal bone.

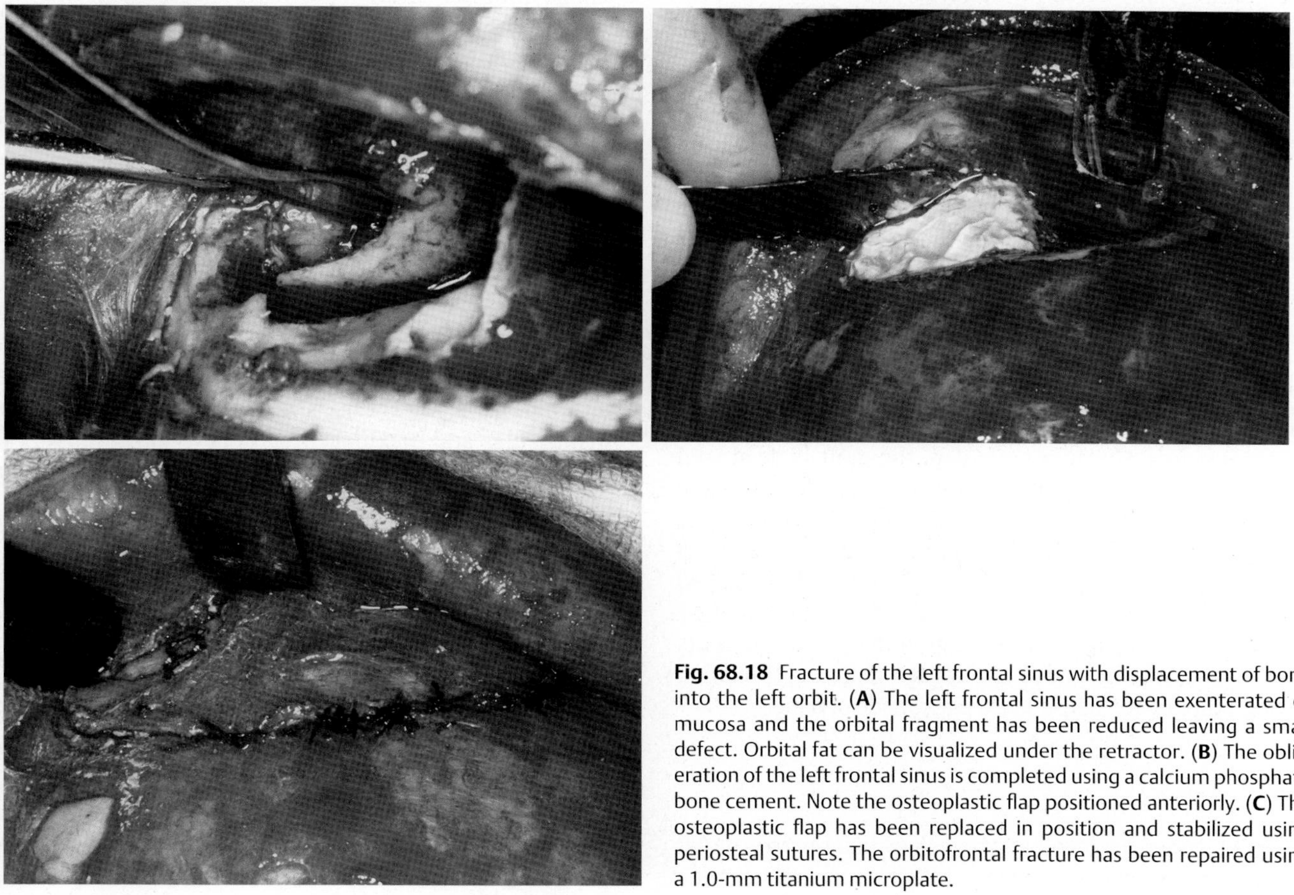

Fig. 68.18 Fracture of the left frontal sinus with displacement of bone into the left orbit. (**A**) The left frontal sinus has been exenterated of mucosa and the orbital fragment has been reduced leaving a small defect. Orbital fat can be visualized under the retractor. (**B**) The obliteration of the left frontal sinus is completed using a calcium phosphate bone cement. Note the osteoplastic flap positioned anteriorly. (**C**) The osteoplastic flap has been replaced in position and stabilized using periosteal sutures. The orbitofrontal fracture has been repaired using a 1.0-mm titanium microplate.

Typically, in severe injuries, bone grafts are lag-screwed to the depressed nasal bone or plated to the frontal bone to provide adequate nasal projection.

Grafts and Implants

Bone Grafts

Small areas of bone loss in the midface can be bridged with plates. However, when defects occur in the buttress areas, these should be reconstructed with bone grafts. Bone grafts are also necessary when deficient bone results in cosmetic and/or functional deformities. This is seen in the orbit, where significant structural loss results in cosmetically deforming enophthalmos and, often, a limitation in extraocular motion as well. The deformity from a naso-orbital-ethmoid fracture can be severely exaggerated by a loss of nasal dorsal height. Bone grafting of the nasal dorsum corrects this deformity and also minimizes the tendency toward epicanthus formation. Bone grafts are also frequently necessary to bridge the defects created by secondary repair of facial fractures via osteotomies.

Split calvarium is readily accessible when a coronal approach is used for facial repair. Studies have shown that the membranous calvarial bone persists for years with minimal resorption when it is rigidly fixed, as compared with much higher resorption rates when rigid fixation is not utilized.[29] Onlay grafts are best fixed with lag screws to the underlying bone. At least two lag screws should be used whenever possible. This not only provides rigid fixation but also compresses the graft against the underlying bone. Note that this is not the same as using a plate and screws in the bone graft because the lag screw through the graft is not dependent on the thread of the screw holding in the graft. An onlay implant, such as a malar implant, can be handled in the same manner, with lag screws preventing motion or displacement of the implant.

When a graft is spanning a defect, it can be carved to fit snugly into the defect and then held in place with a plate across the area. Unlike a bone flap, the graft is dead, and therefore screws in the graft are likely to loosen. It is therefore unwise to fix a graft with a plate that depends on the screws in the graft for stability. This is in contrast to a living bone flap (see next section). When possible, the graft can be designed to overlap the native bone on each side of the defect, and lag screws can then be used to fix the graft in place at each end. In this situation, the graft doubles as a graft and a fixation device, bridging the defect like a plate made of bone.

Bone Flaps

When live bone is placed in a defect, as in a microvascular free flap, the repair sites behave like fractures rather than graft sites because the bone is alive. These can therefore be repaired with small plates at each osteotomy site or with larger, bridging reconstruction plates according to the surgeon's preference. Contrast this with fixation of a bone graft (see earlier discussion).

Distraction Devices

Although beyond the scope of this chapter because distractors are considered variants of rigid-fixation appliances, they will be mentioned here. A distractor is generally applied across an area of bone to be lengthened with either pins or screws, after a corticotomy has been made at the site to be distracted. The corticotomy is then extended into an osteotomy. Distraction of the bone is then performed by advancing the space between the osteotomy at a rate of 1 mm/day (usually 0.5 mm b.i.d., though new programmed distractors can work continuously). After distraction is complete, the distractor serves as a rigid-fixation appliance to allow the completion of bony healing. Defects can be repaired by moving one or more transport disks of bone from one or both ends of the osseous defect. Multivector distractors allow for both vertical and horizontal lengthening of the mandible. Midfacial distractors can be utilized instead of extensive mobilization and repositioning of the midfacial skeleton. As the devices become smaller and more completely implantable, they will be used more commonly because the major drawback currently is distraction of the scar when distractors are placed using transcutaneous pin fixation.

Exposure for Fracture Fixation

Generally speaking, to avoid making visible scars, most facial fractures are repaired using incisions that are often not directly overlying the fracture to be repaired. Intraoral incisions are used whenever possible to expose mandibular and maxillary fractures. When exposing the mandibular body, care should be taken to avoid injury to the inferior alveolar nerve. The sublabial incision provides wide access to the maxilla. When elevating the mucoperiosteum, care should be used to avoid lifting bone fragments with the flap as well as to protect the infraorbital nerves. Nasal penetration should be avoided when possible. The orbit is now commonly approached transconjunctivally. Therefore, it is important for the facial plastic surgeon to understand the anatomy of the skin and lid retractors so as to avoid injury to these structures, which could lead to lower lid malpositions. Upper facial structures as well as the nasal root, nasoethmoid complex, and zygomas are often approached via coronal scalp incisions. The surgeon should understand the anatomy of the deep temporal fascia and its relationship to the frontal branch of the facial nerve. Dissection between the superficial and deep layers of the deep temporal fascia will minimize injury to the temporalis muscle (and, it is hoped, minimize temporal wasting) while simultaneously protecting the frontal branch of the facial nerve. Great care should also be used to protect the supraorbital and supratrochlear nerves, which may have to be dissected from their bony foramina in the supraorbital rim. The coronal flap not only provides wide access to the upper midface and upper face but also allows the surgeon to utilize a pericranial or galeal/pericranial flap to repair defects in the floor of the anterior fossa. Finally, it is important to pay attention to the repositioning of the soft tissues once the repair has been completed. Otherwise, a bony malposition may be replaced by a soft tissue anomaly. The facial soft tissues must be resuspended, particularly with reattachment of the severed portion of the temporalis fascia.

If the lateral canthal ligament has been detached, it should be reattached in its natural position inside the lateral orbital rims (Whitnall tubercle). A Frost stitch left for 24 to 72 hours from the lower lid taped to the forehead will stretch the lower lid upward and potentially decrease the likelihood of later malpositions.

Complications of Rigid Fixation

A brief list of complications specifically related to rigid fixation is included. First is a rigid fixation without proper reduction. Rigid fixation is considered an “unforgiving” technique, so that improper reduction that is rigidly fixed will result in a permanent malunion. If fragments of bone carrying teeth are involved, this will result in a malocclusion. Implant failure is usually a result of selecting too small a device for the indication, though occasional plate fractures, particularly when defects have been bridged by mandibular reconstruction plates, have been encountered. Screw loosening can occur, and this is most likely if a stripped screw is left in place or if the fixation is unstable. Some patients complain of persistent pain at the site of plate fixation, particularly in cold climates. Removal of the plates generally resolves this problem.

Infection and nonunion are the most serious complications. A localized abscess can sometimes be drained, at which time the fixation can be evaluated; if it is solid, it may tolerate drainage and antibiotic treatment. However, if infection persists, the implant may be serving as a colonized foreign body and should be removed. Unstable appliances must be removed. Infection may lead to osteomyelitis, which requires prolonged antibiotic treatment along with aggressive surgical debridement. Finally, there are iatrogenic injuries, such as injury to sensory and motor nerves, as well as soft tissue injuries.

Future Developments

As already noted, minimally invasive techniques are currently being utilized with endoscopic assistance. With ongoing advances in endoscopic technology, intraoperative imaging and computer-driven image-guided systems, it is likely that less invasive approaches will be applied to more anatomical regions and more complex fractures. The development of better implant technologies will allow placement of rigid fixation through smaller incisions as well.

Absorbable technology is progressing as well, and many facial fractures and osteotomies are now being repaired with biodegradable plates and screws. Development will continue in the area of bone replacement materials, along with growth-stimulating proteins that will affect the rate and quality of bone healing and possibly eliminate the need for bone grafts and flaps.

Appendix 68.1

Function and Application of Plates and Lag Screws

Plates

When screws are placed though a plate into bone across a fracture or osteotomy, a certain degree of stability is imparted. A two-hole plate prevents axial distraction at the plate site but does not prevent rotation. A four-hole plate prevents distraction and rotation when placed along the traction side. No compressive force is imparted, only neutral fixation.

A compression plate creates axial compression across a fracture or osteotomy. It is designed so that proper positioning of screws in the plate holes produces compressive forces simply and maintains them during the healing process.

The key to this device is a planned interaction between the screw head and the plate that results in a predictable relative movement between the screw and the plate. The plate hole and screw head are therefore designed so that the screw head does not rest on the plate but rather slides into the plate hole. If a curved (spherical) or slanted (conical) plate hole is used, then as the screw is tightened, the screw head will slide into its seated position in the plate hole, resulting in a relative motion between the screw and the plate. This predictable relative motion results in axial compression.

Axial compression occurs because as it moves relative to the plate, the screw carries the bone with it. Before drilling any holes, the plate has been placed over the site to be compressed. Once the screw is screwed into the bone, any movement of the screw will bring the bone with it; thus a "screw–bone unit" has been formed. The screw is placed in the plate hole so that the shaft of the screw rests against the plate as far away from the fracture site as possible but is not tightened (**Fig. 68.19**). The opposite screw is similarly placed away from the fracture site on the other side of the fracture. At this point two screw–bone units have been formed, and each is in contact with the plate so that they cannot possibly move apart. When a screw is tightened, the interaction between the screw head and the plate forces the screw head toward the fracture site, thereby bringing the bone with it. Because the opposite fragment cannot move away, compression is accomplished. When the second screw is tightened, it is similarly forced by the plate to move toward the fracture site, bringing its bony counterpart with it, which results in further compression at the fracture site.

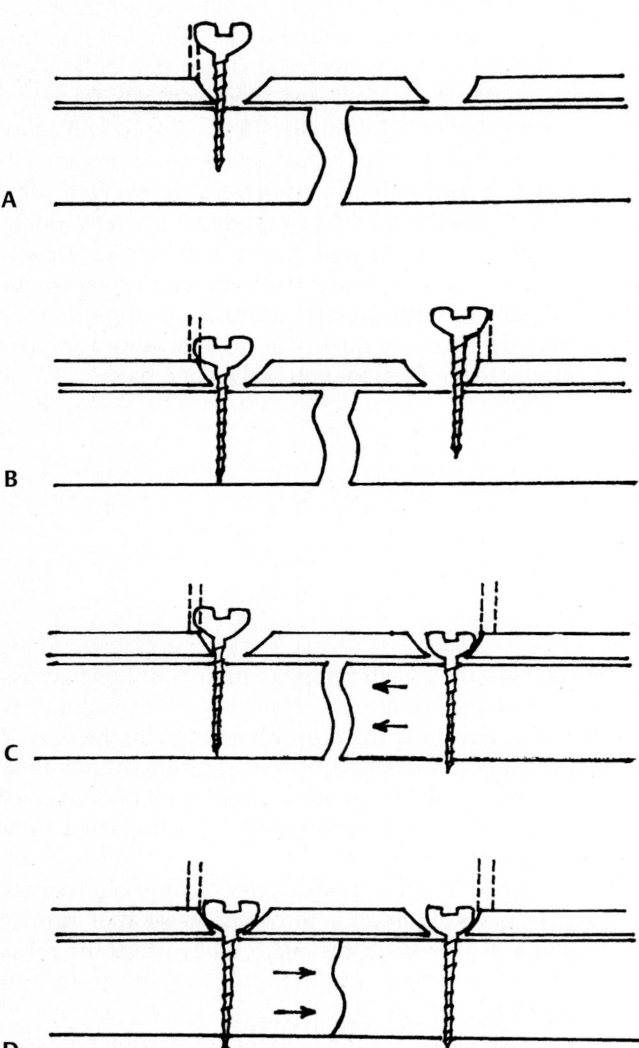

Fig. 68.19 Mechanism of action of a compression plate. (**A**) The screwhead overlaps the plate when the shaft of the screw is positioned in the hole so that it is as far away as possible from the fracture. (**B**) The first screw is screwed in until the head reaches the plate, but no compression is obtained. The second screw (right) is placed eccentrically in the plate hole similarly to the first screw (i.e., so that the shaft is positioned in the hole so that it is as far away from the fracture as possible). No compression has been accomplished. (**C**) The second screw is tightened, and the interaction between the head of the screw and the plate forces the screw (and the bone to which it is attached) to move to the left. When the bone fragments make contact, the piece of bone on the left cannot move away from the piece of bone on the right because the screw shaft in this fragment is up against the plate on the left side. (**D**) The first (left) screw is now tightened, and as the screwhead slides against the plate, it moves to the right bringing the bone with it. Again, the interaction between the screw and bone on the right with the plate prevents it from moving away. Thus compression is accomplished.

Lag Screws

Lag screw placement is fairly straightforward. The fragments are reduced and compressed together (frequently with a towel clip), and the site for screw placement is determined. An oversized gliding hold is drilled in the outer fragment (usually the size of the outside diameter of the screw thread), and a smaller-diameter hole is drilled through both fragments. This is the key to lag screw fixation. The larger hole in the first fragment prevents the screw from holding in it. The smaller hole in the second fragment catches the screw thread. As the screw is tightened, it only holds in the second fragment. Thus the first fragment is compressed between the head of the screw and the second bone fragment (see **Fig. 68.8**). Thus the two bones are forced tightly together. The first fragment can be an overlapping fracture segment, a bone graft or even an alloplastic implant. When available, drill guides are used for drilling the holes. The outer hole is then enlarged with a countersink. The screw is placed and tightened, and additional lag screws are similarly placed as needed.

References

1. Rahn BA. Direct and indirect bone healing after operative fracture treatment. Otolaryngol Clin North Am 1987;20:425
2. Pauwels F. Gesammelte Abhandlungen zur funktionellen Anatomie des Bewegungapparates. In: Spiessl B, ed. New Concepts in Maxillofacial Bone Surgery. New York: Springer-Verlag; 1976
3. Luhr HG. Compression plate osteosynthesis through the Luhr system. In: Kruger E, Schilli W, eds. Oral and Maxillofacial Traumatology. Vol 1. Chicago: Quintessence Publishing; 1982
4. Champy M, Lodde JP, Jaeger JM, et al. Osteosyntheses mandibulaires selon la technique de Mechelet, I: Bases biomecaniques. Rev Stomatol Chir Maxillofac 1976;77:569
5. Champy M, Pape HD, Gerlach KL, et al. The Strasbourg miniplate osteosynthesis. In: Kruger E, Schilli W, Worthington P, eds. Oral and Maxillofacial Traumatology. Vol 2. Chicago: Quintessence Publishing; 1986
6. Kroon F. Effects of three-dimensional loading on stability of internal fixation of mandible fractures. In: Spiessl B, ed. Internal Fixation of the Mandible. Berlin: Springer-Verlag; 1989
7. Levy FE, Smith RW, Odland RM, et al. Monocortical miniplate fixation of mandibular angle fractures. Arch Otolaryngol Head Neck Surg 1991; 117:149–154
8. Ellis E III, Walker LR. Treatment of mandibular angle fractures using one noncompression miniplate. J Oral Maxillofac Surg 1996;54:864–871

9. Farmand M. Three-dimensional plate fixation of fractures and osteotomies. Facial Plast Surg Clin North Am 1995;3:39–56
10. Spiessl B, ed. New Concepts in Maxillofacial Bone Surgery. New York: Springer-Verlag; 1976
11. Leonard MS. The use of lag screws in mandibular fractures. Otolaryngol Clin North Am 1987;20:479
12. Niederdellmann H, Akuamoa-Boateng E, Uhlig G. Lag-screw osteosynthesis: a new procedure for treating fractures of the mandibular angle. J Oral Surg 1981;39:938
13. Fox AJ, Kellman RM. Mandibular angle fractures: two-miniplate fixation and complications. Arch Facial Plast Surg 2003;5:464–469
14. Ellis E III. Treatment of mandibular angle fractures using the AO reconstruction plate. J Oral Maxillofac Surg 1993;51:250–254
15. Kellman RM. Endoscopic approach to subcondylar mandible fractures. Facial Plast Surg 2004;20:239–247
16. Kellman RM. Endoscopically assisted repair of subcondylar fractures of the mandible: an evolving technique. Arch Facial Plast Surg 2003;5:244–250
17. Harle S, Duker J. Druckplotten-osteosynthesen bei Jochbeinfrakturen. Dtsch Zahnarztl Z 1975;30:71
18. Schilli W, Ewers R, Niederdellmann H. Bone fixation with screws and plates in the maxillofacial region. Int J Oral Surg 1981;10(Suppl 1):329
19. Kellman RM, Schilli W. Plate fixation of fractures of the mid- and upper-face. Otolaryngol Clin North Am 1987;20:559
20. Manson PN, Hoopes JE, Su CT. Structural pillars of the facial skeleton: an approach to the management of Le Fort fractures. Plast Reconstr Surg 1980;66:54
21. Manson PN. Dimensional analysis of the facial skeleton: avoiding complications in the management of facial fractures by improved organization of treatment based on CT scans. In: Cranio-maxillofacial Trauma: Problems in Plastic and Reconstructive Surgery. Philadelphia: JB Lippincott; 1991
22. Eisele DW, Duckert LG. Single-point stabilization of zygomatic fractures with the minicompression plate. Arch Otolaryngol Head Neck Surg 1987;113:267
23. Davidson J, Nickerson D, Nickerson B. Fractures: comparison of methods of internal fixation. Plast Reconstr Surg 1990;86:25
24. Kellman RM, Woo P, Leopold DA. Rigid internal fixation of mid- and upper-facial fractures. Paper presented at the Middle Section of the Triological Society, Cleveland, January 1987
25. Champy M, Lodde JP, Muster D, et al. Osteosynthesis using miniaturized screw-on plates in facial and cranial surgery. Ann Chir Plast Esthet 1977;22:261
26. Kellman RM. Midfacial fractures. In: Gates GA, ed. Current Therapy in Otolaryngology–Head and Neck Surgery. Vol 4. Toronto: BC Decker; 1990
27. Stanley RB Jr. Use of intraoperative computed tomography during repair of orbitozygomatic fractures. Arch Facial Plast Surg 1999;1:19–24
28. Raveh J, Laedrach K, Vuillemin T, et al. Management of combined frontonaso-orbital/skull base fractures and telecanthus in 355 cases. Arch Otolaryngol Head Neck Surg 1992;118:605–614
29. Phillips JH, Rahn BA. Fixation effects on membranous and endochondral onlay bone-graft resorption. Plast Reconstr Surg 1988;82:872

69 Orbitozygomatic Fractures

Lisa E. Ishii, Patrick J. Byrne, and Robert B. Stanley Jr.

Traditionally, fractures of the facial skeleton resulting from trauma in the orbital and cheek areas were evaluated and treated in a segmentalized fashion. Fractures were classified simply as zygomatic arch, malar or tripod, or orbital blowout fractures. This simplistic approach produced acceptable results in most injuries that were due to suburban-based or low-velocity impact causes, such as sports injuries or fistfights. However, acceptable results were frequently not achieved in victims of urban-based or high-velocity impact injuries seen with high-speed motor vehicle deceleration crashes, interpersonal violence involving blunt instruments other than fists, and gunshot wounds.

Unfortunately, in modern society, the ratio of urban- to suburban-type injuries seen in both community hospitals and inner-city trauma centers has been increasing steadily. Nasal and zygomatic complex (ZMC) fractures are the most common facial fractures following motor vehicle accidents. Although the use of airbags and seat belts, especially together, significantly reduces facial fractures in severe motor vehicle accidents, the pattern of the fractures is not greatly altered.[1] In accidents severe enough to cause facial fractures air bags are least protective of the ZMC, in part due to the prominence of the zygoma, which predisposes it to injury.

Experienced maxillofacial trauma surgeons have shown that suboptimal results often cannot be attributed to the severity of the injury but rather to the segmentalized approach to the injury. Zygoma fractures can result in disruption of orbital contents, the maxillary sinus, and the coronoid process of the mandible, and result in significant functional and cosmetic deformities. Therefore, all fractures of the facial skeleton resulting from trauma in the orbital and cheek areas should be evaluated as potential orbitozygomatic or even cranioorbitozygomatic fractures, and repair of the injury must be directed to restoration of an anatomically correct skeletal unit. To achieve optimal results there must be an understanding of the anatomy, comprehensive diagnosis of fractures, and accurate reduction and stabilization with limited harm to unaffected surrounding tissues when possible.

Anatomy and Fracture Characteristics

Zygoma and Malar Prominence

The zygoma is a relatively sturdy bone that provides the aesthetically important malar eminence. It joins the surrounding craniofacial skeleton through four superficial and two deep projections. Superficially, the projections contribute to two critical external arcs of contour (**Fig. 69.1**). The vertical arc runs from the zygomatic process of the frontal bone over the zygoma to the ZM buttress area of the lateral wall of the maxillary antrum above the first molar. The longer horizontal arc runs from the maxilla in the area of the lacrimal fossa around the zygoma to the root of the zygomatic process of the temporal bone. It is parallel to, but slightly below, the Frankfort horizontal plane. Because the height of contour of the malar eminence is also just at or slightly inferior to the Frankfort plane, the point of intersection of these arcs of contour defines the position of the malar eminence, typically 2 cm inferior to the lateral canthus (**Fig. 69.1**). The two deep projections are the sphenoid projection that articulates along the lateral orbital wall with the orbital plate of the sphenoid bone and the orbital projection that articulates with the orbital surface of the maxilla in the extreme lateral aspect of the orbital floor. The sphenoid and orbital projections lie beneath and perpendicular to the external arcs of contour in the area of the inferolateral orbital rim, thus greatly strengthening this portion of the rim.

The zygoma is the main buttress between the maxilla and the cranium. It also serves as the principal component of the superficial lateral pillar of a buttress system of

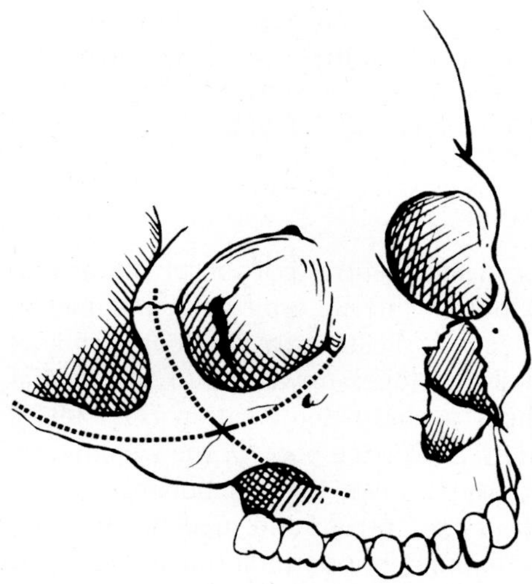

Fig. 69.1 Vertical and horizontal external arcs of contour of the zygomatic complex. Intersection at X marks the position of the malar prominence. (From Stanley RB. The zygomatic arch as a guide to reconstruction of comminuted malar fractures. Arch Otolaryngol Head Neck Surg 1989;115:1459. Reprinted by permission.)

platforms and pillars that surround and protect the orbit.[2] Because its convex outer surface creates the prominent contour of the cheek, it is highly susceptible to injury.

The term *tetrapod fracture* refers to the fracture of all four suture lines (zygomaticofrontal [ZF], zygomaticotemporal, zygomaticomaxillary, and zygomaticosphenoid) that occurs with blunt trauma to the zygoma. Typically the weaker bones with which the zygoma articulates absorb the strong impact forces directed to the zygoma and fragment. The weakest bone is the orbital floor, which can collapse into the maxillary sinus. In contrast, the ZF is the strongest buttress and it typically separates cleanly. The ZM buttress area and the medial aspect of the inferior orbital rim are frequently comminuted.

The Zingg classification system of ZMC injuries can be used to describe these fractures with clarity and simplicity.[3] Type A injuries, the least common, are isolated to one component of the tetrapod fracture. They are further divided into types A1, A2, and A3, depending on whether the area of involement is the zygomatic arch, lateral orbital wall, or inferior orbital rim, respectively. Type B fractures involve injury to all four of the supporting structures, and type C fractures are complex fractures with comminution of the zygomatic bone. Types B and C account for 62% of the ZMC injuries.[4]

The zygomatic arch typically either fractures near its midpoint in a single location or in two places resulting in a central fragment susceptible to displacement and rotation. Therefore, fracture dislocations of the zygoma may fragment both ends of the horizontal arc of contour and the lower end of the vertical arc. The degree of this disruption and the amount of displacement of the zygoma determine the severity of the injury and thus the complexity of the needed repair. Reconstruction of the horizontal arc restores anterior and lateral projection of the cheek, and reconstruction of the vertical arc restores the height of the malar eminence in relation to the Frankfort plane.

Orbit

The bone in the concave, central portion of the orbital floor lies 3 mm below the inferior orbital rim and may be as thin as 0.5 mm or less.[5] Posteriorly the floor is convex and posteromedially it slopes upward into the medial orbital wall without a sharp demarcation (**Fig. 69.2**). Impact forces centered over the body of the zygoma are transmitted inferiorly through the ZM buttress to the anterolateral wall of the antrum and medially through the orbital process to the inferior orbital rim and the floor of the orbit. The antral wall and the inferior rim frequently suffer a comminuted injury that results in multiple delicate fragments lying between the ZM suture line and the lacrimal fossa. The floor of the orbit almost always suffers a comminuted injury, the severity of which varies with the strength of the impact force. This injury usually involves the concave central portion. High-velocity periorbital impact forces may be transmitted to the convex posterior floor and even to the medial wall, causing serious displacement of the bone in these areas. Although the globe itself rests anterior to the convexity, evaluation and reconstruction of this area and the adjacent medial wall are as important as repair of the more accessible concave anterior portion of the floor.

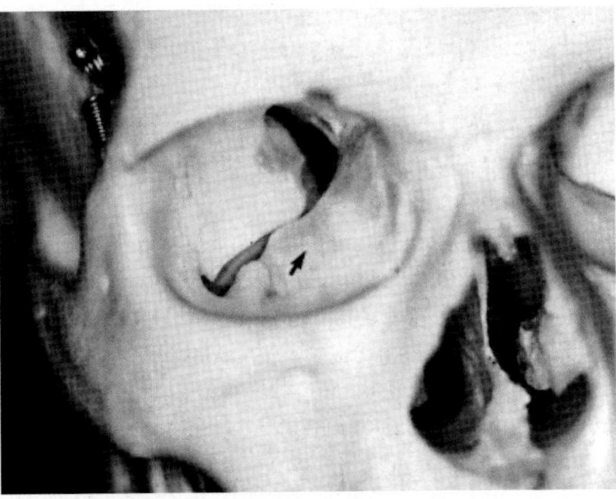

Fig. 69.2 Arrow in right orbit points to convex posterior orbital floor. Although the globe rests anterior to this convexity, reconstruction of this area and the adjacent medial wall is essential (see Fig. 68.4).

The sphenoidal and orbital processes of the zygoma transmit impact forces centered over the zygoma to the deeper structures within the orbit. The weak sphenotemporal buttress formed by the zygoma, orbital plate of the greater sphenoid wing, and the squamous portion of the temporal bone absorbs impact forces directed over the lateral orbital rim. When the impact force exceeds the capacity of this buttress to absorb it, fracture dislocations of the lateral orbital wall result and, at a minimum, comminution occurs at the zygomaticosphenoid suture line. When impact forces are directed in a medial superior direction the orbital plate of the sphenoid bone moves toward the orbital apex and decreases the orbital volume. This impaction may cause injuries to structures in the orbit, superior orbital fissure or optic canal. More commonly, laterally and inferiorly displaced ZMC fractures correspond with fractures of the inferior or medial orbital walls. This displacement increases the orbital volume and may allow orbital fat to herniate into the maxillary or ethmoid sinuses. Reduction of the bony injuries may be necessary to restore the volume of the orbit and the contour of the orbital rim and also to remove bony impingement on vital neurological structures.[6]

Globe Position

The position of the globe is determined by the integrity of the orbital walls and the extensive network of ligaments

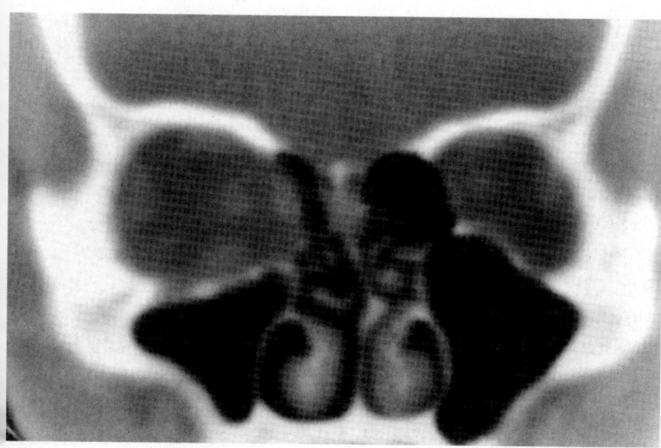

Fig. 69.3 Computed tomography scan shows altered orbital shape and volume resulting from displaced posterior convex floor and adjacent medial wall. Failure to correct both defects will lead to enophthalmos.

that suspend it.[7] Recession (enophthalmos) or depression (hypopthalmos) of the globe within the orbit results from injuries that push one or more orbital walls outward, increase the orbital volume, and also damage the network of suspensory ligaments. The orbital soft tissues are then displaced by both gravitational forces and the remodeling forces of fibrous scar contracture. This usually changes the shape of the orbital soft tissues from a modified cone to a sphere, and the globe sinks backward and downward.[8] Probably the most common cause of this posttraumatic enophthalmos is the incomplete repair of a defect in the normally convex posterior aspect of the floor or failure to recognize and correct a medial wall component of the injury (**Figs. 69.2 and 69.3**). Less commonly, the globe is displaced superiorly (hyperophthalmos) and anteriorly (exophthalmos) by medial and superior impaction of the ZMC that decreases orbital volume.

Diagnosis and Radiological Evaluation

The initial assessment of the patient with facial fractures must include an evaluation of the airway, the hemodynamic stability, and the cervical spine. Once these have been appropriately managed attention is focused on the head and neck examination, keeping in mind the mechanism of injury. Patients with ZMC fractures may have palpable step-offs at the zygoma or orbital rim, or malar flattening due to medial displacement of the ZMC. These findings become less apparent as the overlying soft tissue swells. Patients may experience trismus from compression of the coronoid process of the mandible and the temporalis by the depressed ZMC. Hypoesthesia or anesthesia may result from injury involving the infraorbital nerve (V_2). Associated facial fractures occur in 25% of patients sustaining ZMC fractures.[4]

A thorough ocular examination is required to assess the orbital soft tissues. Upward gaze restriction and diplopia may occur as a result of entrapment of the inferior rectus muscle. Forced duction testing can reveal entrapment of any of the extraocular muscles. Globe position should be evaluated for enopththalmos, hypophthalmos, hyperophthalmos or exophthalmos. The latter two globe malpositions indicate a decrease in orbital volume, which may be accompanied by optic nerve injury. An ophthalmologic consultation should be obtained for all patients with ZMC fractures.

Axial computed tomography (CT) scans should be considered the gold standard for radiological diagnosis of ZMC fractures.[9] Many trauma patients undergo CT scan of the brain to assess intracranial injury, and additional facial views to evaluate the facial bones can be included at this time. Axial images can be reformatted into coronal cuts with good resolution, thus obviating the need for neck flexion or extension. These CT scans provide valuable information about the fractures to guide surgical decisions.

The preoperative choice of the appropriate surgical approach for all but the most minimally displaced orbitozygomatic fractures can be made only if the horizontal and vertical arcs of contour and the lateral, inferior, and medial orbital walls are evaluated by CT. Although axial CT provides valuable information about the lateral and medial walls of the orbit, coronal CT or good coronal reconstructions are essential for evaluation of the orbital floor. This is especially true for the convex posterior floor and the area of sloping of the floor into the medial wall. Fracture dislocations in these areas can be studied in detail and decisions made regarding the need for orbital exploration and repair to prevent delayed enophthalmos. Approximately 1-cm^3 displacement of orbital soft tissue or increase in orbital volume produces 1 mm of enophthalmos.[10,11] A change of at least 3 cm^3 of orbital volume increase or orbital soft tissue loss is usually required before clinically perceptible enophthalmos occurs.[12]

It should be noted that acute enophthalmos may not be seen in association with severe orbitozygomatic fractures. An intact but medially impacted zygoma may compensate for the increased orbital volume caused by blowout fractures of other walls, and the globe may appear normal in anterior projection and vertical position, or even be proptotic. However, reduction of the zygomatic component of the injury to restore the malar eminence unmasks the traumatic increase in orbital volume and leads to delayed-onset enophthalmos if the other fractures are not treated. Careful review of the axial and coronal CT scans will prevent this error.

Before CT scans were routinely obtained for ZMC fractures, orbital exploration was performed for diagnosis as well as reconstruction of orbital floor defects. The acceptance of CT scans as the gold standard imaging modality for patients with suspected ZMC fractures has contributed to a significant change in the treatment algorithm. Shumrick and colleagues assessed pretreatment scans to determine which ZMC fractures required orbital exploration/reconstruction. They reported a 70% decrease in orbital explorations in this group.[13] Ellis and Reddy, in reviewing their treatment of isolated, unilateral ZMC fractures over a 10-year period, determined that the preoperative CT scan can be used to assess the amount of internal orbital disruption for purposes of developing a treatment plan in patients with ZMC fractures.[12] For fractures with minimal soft tissue herniation and minimal disruption of the internal orbit, ZMC reduction without orbital floor reconstruction was adequate treatment. A posttreatment increase in orbital volume was noted in eight of 65 cases where the floor was not reconstructed, but these increases were considered too small to result in clinically perceptible enophthalmos.

Surgical Technique

Restoration of the External Arcs of Contour

The precise relocation of the displaced zygoma is simplified by concentrating on reconstruction of the two main external arcs of contour. Restoration of the horizontal arc reestablishes anterior and lateral projection of the cheek, and restoration of the vertical arc reestablishes the height of the malar eminence in relation to the middle third of the face. The repositioned zygoma can then be used as a framework for repair of any associated orbital wall fractures. Treatment required to attain multidimensional restoration of the position of the zygoma becomes increasingly complex as the injury to each arc of contour increases in severity. Together, comminution of the bones with which the zygoma articulates (i.e., the lateral and medial ends of the horizontal arc and the inferior end of the vertical arc) and the amount of displacement of the zygoma itself determine the complexity of the injury and therefore the complexity of the needed repair.

Simple Fractures

Only rare cases without comminution of any of the projections of the arcs of contour should be managed with closed-reduction techniques, such as the Gilles method with or without transzygomatic Steinmann pin fixation. If the adequacy of reduction of this type of injury is in doubt because of difficulty in palpating the zygomatic arch and lateral antral wall, a small gingivobuccal sulcus incision may be used for direct visualization of the lateral wall. If this is employed, a single 2.0 miniplate can be placed across the reduced fracture line in lieu of the transzygomatic pin to stabilize the zygoma against the downward pull of the masseter.

Because any type of limited-access technique relies heavily on palpation and external visualization of the position of the zygoma and its projections, it is helpful to delay these procedures for at least 7 days to allow for maximal resolution of edema. In addition, preoperative steroids may reduce intraoperative edema and further facilitate evaluation of the reduction. The repair should not be delayed more than 10 days because the masseter begins to shorten after this time and elevation of the zygoma becomes more difficult.[13] For cases where there is a surgical delay and elevation of the ZMC is difficult due to the onset of healing, McGivern and Stein recommend a method of reduction using two points of elevation. An elevator is passed through an upper buccal sulcus incision to elevate the zygoma while also elevating from the outside with a temporary malar eminence screw placed through a handle/cannula complex.[14]

Frequently, the lateral wall of the maxillary antrum is comminuted even when the other projections of the arcs of contour suffer simple fractures or separation of a suture line. In such cases, a single craniofacial miniadaptation plate attached across the comminuted area is sufficient for lateral wall reconstruction (**Fig. 69.4**). Because

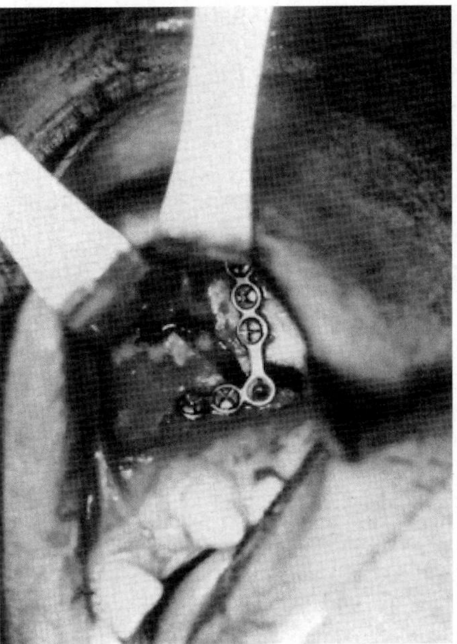

Fig. 69.4 L-shaped miniadaptation plate positioned across the comminuted lower end of the zygomaticomaxillary buttress. In this location it can serve as the sole means of fixation for the body of the zygoma.

the fixation device is not resisting heavy occlusal forces, as would be the case with a Le Fort fracture, insertion of only two screws into the body of the zygoma above and at the maxilla below is required for stability. In addition, a prebent L-shaped plate may be used to facilitate placement of screws below the fracture lines if there is concern for the root tips of the maxillary teeth.

If the adequacy of reduction is in doubt, another projection of the zygoma can be directly visualized by means of a tunnel dissection superior to the inferior rim, with identification and protection of the infraorbital nerve, or laterally over the malar eminence to expose the zygomatic arch. Adequate reduction can then be confirmed with palpation of the lateral orbital rim and direct visualization of the inferior rim or arch fracture. Thus the position of the zygoma after less severe injuries can be restored and fixation obtained without violating the lower eyelid, assuming that no serious floor component is present. This avoids the potential iatrogenic injuries most often associated with open reduction of zygomatic fractures, lower lid retraction, and eversion. Even the experienced operator notes occasional increased scleral show or even gross ectropion in a patient who underwent a transconjunctival incision for exposure of the inferior orbital rim, a step that can often be avoided with thorough preoperative CT evaluation.

Complex Fractures

The progression to more complex fractures usually involves comminution of one end or both ends of the horizontal arc of contour (i.e., the inferior orbital rim and zygomatic arch). Traditional three-point reduction restores the entire vertical arc of contour and the medial end of the horizontal arc. Approximation of the relatively intact bones at the ZF suture moves the point of intersection of the arcs superiorly along the vertical arc to restore the height of contour of the malar eminence to a more normal relationship to the Frankfort plane. However, comminution at the two other points of alignment prevents accurate restoration of the normal anterior and lateral projections of the prominence. Typically, the eminence is displaced posterior and lateral to its normal location (**Fig. 69.5A,B**), and failure to recognize the extent and direction of the displacement at the time of reduction will leave a flattened cheek and a widened face. In these situations, direct visualization of the entire fracture line from the frontozygomatic and orbitozygomatic points by exposing the medial side of the lateral orbital wall is helpful. This allows for the most accurate three-dimensional reduction of the zygoma.

Reduction begins with exposure of the ZF suture through an extended upper lid blepharoplasty-type incision or by way of a coronal or hemicoronal incision if the severity of the injury indicates that exposure of the entire length of the zygomatic arch is required. The ZM buttress is exposed through a gingivobuccal sulcus incision, and initial reduction is accomplished by placement of an elevator or bone hook deep to the anterior arch with lifting upward and outward. This initial reduction often facilitates placement of the transconjunctival incision for inferior rim exposure by bringing the rim fragments into better alignment.

In the case of the inferior rim, simple fractures usually cross it in the region of the infraorbital canal, and thus transcutaneous palpation can be used to confirm reduction. However, comminuted rim fractures usually have a

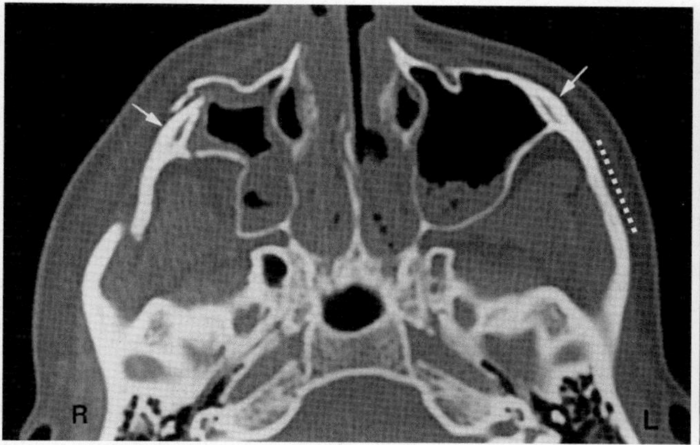

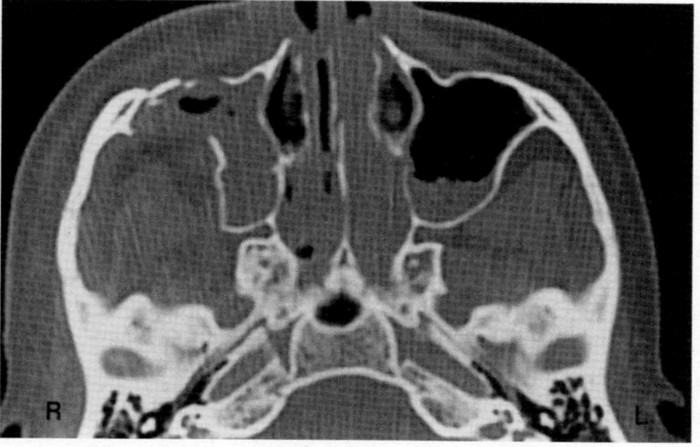

Fig. 69.5 (**A**) Correctly positioned axial CT scan showing fracture dislocation of right zygoma with comminution of the medial inferior orbital rim and double fracture of the zygomatic arch. Dotted white line on normal side indicates the straight central segment of the arch that must be reconstructed to accurately reposition the malar prominence (*arrow*). (**B**) Postreduction scar of the same patient, showing that the right arch has a contour that now corresponds to the normal left arch. This automatically restores anterior projection of the malar prominence. (From Stanley RB. Use of intraoperative computed tomography during repair of orbitozygomatic fractures. Arch Fac Plast Surg 1999;1:19. Reprinted by permission.)

component through the medial most aspect of the rim in the area of the lacrimal fossa. The free-floating central rim fragment is usually depressed and frequently associated with a serious medial orbital floor injury, thus mandating an approach through the lower lid for repair. The transconjunctival incision is the preferred incision for this.

Visualizing the medial surface of the lateral orbital wall as a guide, the initial realignment of the zygoma is performed at the ZF suture line. This realignment can be held in place temporarily with a single stainless steel wire through holes placed well away from the thick portion of the rim that will later be used for a rigid-fixation implant. Because this temporary wire allows for rotational movement of the zygoma, the point of intersection of the arcs can be appropriately adjusted in the lateral and anterior dimensions. This adjustment is accomplished by realignment of the orbital rim and lateral antral wall fragments. Resistance to the pull of the masseter muscle is again accomplished with a miniadaptation plate positioned over the lower end of the ZM buttress. Additional stability can be obtained with microadaptation plates placed on the inferior rim and across the ZF suture line.

Thicker plates at these sites may gradually become visible through the thin overlying skin. It is possible to avoid this complication and other plate-related complications altogether by using bioresorbable plating systems. In a quantitative biomechanical study comparing different combinations of titanium and resorbable plates for three-point ZMC fixation all combinations were sufficiently strong to overcome masseter displacement forces.[16] When resorbable systems were used clinically for ZMC fixation there were no differences in intraoperative or postoperative bone stability.[17,18] These systems are also advantageous for their radiolucency which allows postoperative imaging without artifact, low profile, and malleability for contouring. Regardless of the system used, care must be taken to reapproximate the periosteum over the inferior orbital rim to prevent scar contracture.

If the inferior rim and lateral wall fragments are too small to manipulate or are missing, the fourth point of alignment, the zygomatic arch, can be used to reposition the point of intersection of the arcs of contour. If the arch has a single displaced fracture or two greenstick fractures with bending of the arch, dissection may be performed over the malar eminence through the transconjunctival incision to expose the fractures. If there is a displaced central segment of the arch, then access to the full length of the horizontal arc will be required, and a coronal, hemicoronal, or extended pretragal incision will be necessary in addition to the transconjunctival incision (**Fig. 69.6**).[19,20] Dissection toward the lateral orbital rim and the zygomatic arch should be in a plane deep to the superficial layer of the deep temporal fascia so that the frontal and orbital branches of the facial nerve are automatically elevated with the flap. The periosteum is then incised along the orbital rim and along the arch fragments deep to the attachment of the superficial layer of this fascia. A subperiosteal dissection is carried over the body of the zygoma to connect with the anterior dissection, and all of the components of the zygomatic arch are exposed.

The zygomatic arch components are elevated and realigned, with emphasis placed on proper realignment of the straight middle portion of the arch. Surprisingly, although the bone of the arch is thin, an accurate end-to-end realignment can usually be obtained to reconstruct the true length of the arch and thus the anterior projection of the malar prominence. Fixation is accomplished with miniscrews and low-profile, multihole, miniadaptation plates (**Fig. 69.7**). Final bending and attachment of the plates is done after the lateral projection of the prominence has been established by realignment of the inferior rim fragments. If these fragments are missing or too small to manipulate, lateral projection can usually be established by realignment of the ZM buttress. If the bone fragments of the lateral antral wall are also too small or missing, restoration of the lateral projection of the prominence, like the anterior projection, must be based on the accurate restoration of the contour of the zygomatic arch, in particular its straight central portion. Fixation is then applied at the other three points of reduction. The soft tissues must be accurately draped over the repositioned malar prominence. This is best accomplished by simultaneous upward traction on the skin flap and the incised temporal fascia.

A tight closure of the fascial incision ensures that the periosteum is held in correct position over the zygoma and arch. Large defects in the inferior orbital rim or the anterolateral wall of the maxillary antrum should be reconstructed with bone grafts to prevent collapse of the soft tissues of the lower eyelid or upper buccal sulcus area into these defects. If the defect is not corrected, subsequent scar contracture may produce a noticeable depression of the lower lid or the midcheek area.

Occasionally, the zygoma itself will be fractured. Fortunately, the edges of any fracture traversing the body of the zygoma will be broad and strong and realignment is a simple function. After reduction and fixation of the zygoma are accomplished, the remaining fractures of the arcs of contour can be approached as previously described. If extreme difficulty is encountered in mobilizing the zygoma to its correct position even with the extended-access approaches, the masseter can be detached from the zygoma and the zygomatic arch. This is often necessary in patients not treated within the recommended 7 to 10 days. This maneuver should not have long-term effects on jaw mobility or masticatory

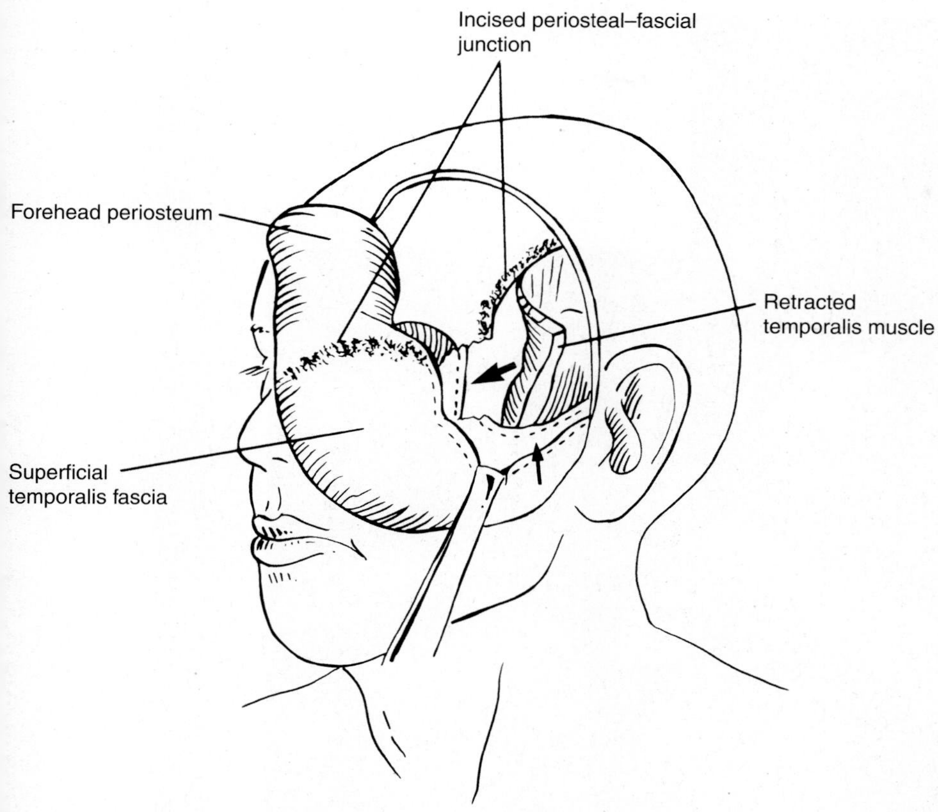

Fig. 69.6 Temporal approach to the lateral orbital wall (*large arrow*) and entire length of zygomatic arch (*small arrow*), using a hemicoronal incision and a frontotemporal flap. Elevation of the superficial layer of the two-layered fascia that overlies them. Temporalis protects all branches of the facial nerve. Use of a full bicoronal incision reduces the amount of flap retraction needed for full exposure and further reduces the chances of postoperative neuropraxia of the frontal branch of the nerve. Dashed line corresponds to incision of the fascial and periosteal attachments along the orbital rim and zygomatic arch. (From Stanley RB. The temporal approach to impacted lateral orbital wall fractures. Arch Otolaryngol Head Neck Surg 1988;114:551. Reprinted by permission.)

function, but the additional soft tissue trauma and subsequent scarring may cause accentuation of the prominence of the reconstructed arch, especially if a plate spans the length of the arch. Therefore, surgery for more severe injuries should be undertaken as expeditiously as possible.

Reconstruction of the Orbital Floor

The orbital floor projection of the zygoma usually remains intact and is restored to a normal position when the zygoma itself is repositioned. The medial floor (orbital plate of maxilla) can then be reconstructed using the intact lateral floor as a stable landmark. Reconstruction of a defect involving only the concave anterior aspect of the floor can usually be adequately accomplished with an alloplastic implant. Dissection of the floor must completely expose at least two of the opposing quadrants of the defect for stable support of the implant.

Of the various alloplasts available, porous polyethylene (MEDPOR, Porex Surgical, Inc., Newnan, GA) has many properties that make it an ideal choice.[21] It is readily available, easily trimmable, and tends not to migrate even without fixation of the implant to the orbital rim or residual floor. High-density polyethylene implants (MEDPOR Barrior implants) are impermeable to fibrovascular ingrowth and may be superior for use in the orbit where ingrowth may lead to tethering of orbital contents. The MEDPOR Titan implant is a newer, thinner product of titanium mesh covered with either porous or high-density polyethylene. As compared with the standard MEDPOR orbital implant, it is thinner and radiopaque so that its position can be confirmed on CT. As compared with standard titanium mesh, the polyethylene coating prevents the risk of sharp edges after cutting and contouring.

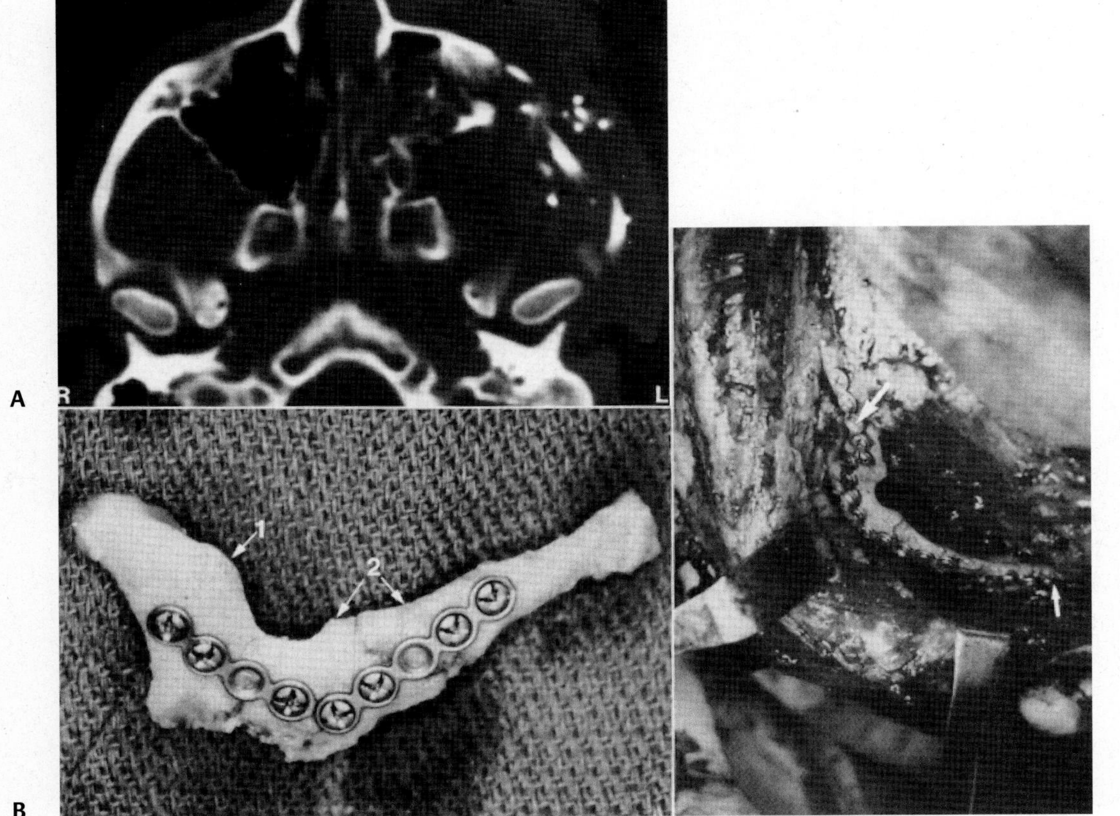

Fig. 69.7 (**A**) Preoperative CT scan showing severe comminution of the left zygomatic complex resulting from a gunshot wound. (**B**) Fragments of the lateral orbital rim (1) and zygomatic arch (2) were retrieved from the temporal fossa and parotid gland and realigned out of field. (**C**) Reconstructed segment has been reimplanted with fixation at the zygomaticofrontal suture line (*large arrow*) and the temporal root of the zygomatic arch (*small arrow*). The bony malar prominence has been restored, and the reimplanted bone will serve as a scaffolding as the surrounding soft tissue undergoes contracture invariably seen with this type of wound. This view closely approximates the schematic in Fig. 68.7.

For reconstruction of defects of both the concave anterior and convex posterior floor, an implant with rigidity greater than that offered by MEDPOR may be required. This is due to the frequent lack of a ledge of residual floor to stabilize the implant posteriorly and medially, even when the orbital floor dissection is carried well into the posterior third of the orbit. Use of MEDPOR in these cases requires exposure of the medial orbital wall through either a medial canthal or coronal incision so that the material can be draped along the medial wall for support of the floor repair. A graft material that is ideally suited for reconstruction of these larger defects is outer-table calvarial bone. This bone is easily harvested and contoured to match most large floor defects, and its rigidity eliminates the need for medial and posterior support. The graft may be stabilized by attachment to the orbital floor projection of the zygoma with one or two lag screws or to the reconstructed orbital rim with miniplates and screws in a cantilevered fashion (**Fig. 69.8**).

It should be noted that the calvarial bone graft will not restore accurate position of the globe if the surgeon is hesitant in floor dissection and does not venture the sometimes necessary 35 to 40 mm into the posterior third of the orbit to allow for maximal reconstruction of the convex posterior floor.[22] However, the orbital apex must not be compromised by the posterior end of a bone graft. A decrease in orbital apex volume can produce a compressive optic neuropathy with resultant blindness.

Reconstruction of defects that involve the concave anterior floor, convex posterior floor, and medial orbital wall (lamina papyracea) offer the greatest challenge. Although these severe orbital injuries are usually seen as the orbitozygomatic component of panfacial fracture, they may occur as isolated injuries. Complete exposure of the medial wall of the orbit is mandatory and is best accomplished through a coronal incision. Reconstruction is made difficult by the need to restore not only the

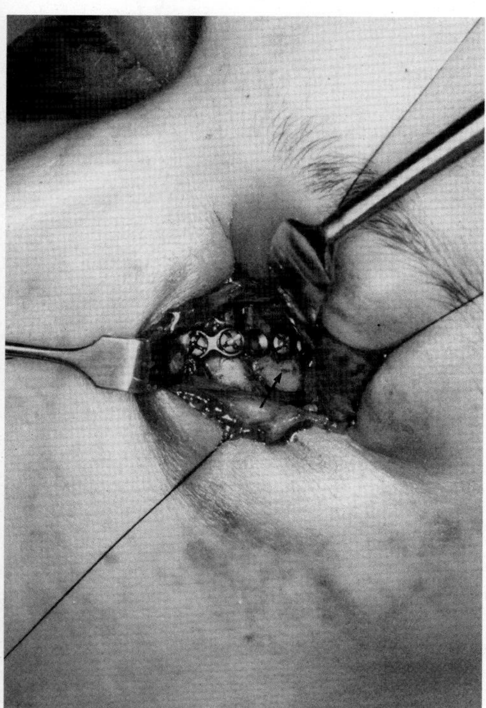

Fig. 69.8 Split cranial bone graft (*arrow*) that has been cantilevered from the inferior rim to repair a large blowout fracture of the orbital floor. Silk sutures have been placed to retract the conjunctiva inferiorly and superiorly over the cornea. (From Stanley RB. Maxillofacial trauma. In: Cummings CW, ed. Otolaryngology Head and Neck Surgery. Vol 1. 3rd ed. St. Louis: CV Mosby; 1996. Reprinted by permission.)

integrity of walls themselves but the exact relationship of one wall to the other. An accurate restoration of globe position requires restoration of bony orbital volume and shape so that the soft tissues will resume their normal shape and position.[19] The medial wall may also be reconstructed with a cranial bone graft that is cantilevered from the medial superior orbital rim. In some cases, a prefabricated titanium orbital floor plate that acts as a cradle for the multiple bone grafts may be used to facilitate placement stabilization.

As with orbital floor projection of the zygoma, the zygomatic contribution to the lateral orbital wall almost always remains attached to the body of the zygoma and is correctly rearticulated to the greater sphenoid wing with reconstruction of the arcs of contour. The orbital plate of the sphenoid bone is often comminuted and should not be relied on as a landmark for evaluation of realignment of the zygoma. However, in the event of a displaced sphenoid wing fracture, the intact lateral wall component of the zygoma can be used as a landmark for repositioning the orbital plate of the sphenoid bone. Only rarely will an alloplastic or autogenous graft be needed to reconstruct a lateral wall defect to correct herniation of orbital soft tissues into the temporal and infratemporal fossae. If a high-impact injury produces comminution and displacement of the lateral orbital wall, a split calvarial graft is the ideal graft material. Because a lateral approach must be used to safely expose these retrobulbar bone injuries, the calvarial donor site is already in the surgical field. In addition, a relatively flat area of skull can usually be found to produce a graft that closely matches the contour of the lateral orbital wall.

The use of a transconjunctival incision rather than a subciliary incision has eliminated the need for a Frost suture to suspend the lower eyelid from the forehead during early healing. However, when the soft tissues overlying the inferior orbital rim, malar prominence, and anterior maxillary wall have been completely elevated during reconstruction, slow-absorbing suspension sutures should be placed from the periosteum of the cheek tissues to the reconstructed rim. This pulls the elevated tissues superiorly to ensure that the infraorbital soft tissues redrape appropriately over the underlying skeleton. Periosteum that is incised during orbital floor exploration is not sutured so that the chance of tethering the orbital septum to the reconstructed rim is reduced.

Low profile (1.0- or 1.3-mm) titanium plates should not be visible under the skin of the lateral orbital rim and zygomatic arch. Therefore, these fixation devices can be left in place permanently. A plate positioned on the inferior rim may, however, produce an irregular contour visible through the thin skin of the lower eyelid. Therefore, it is preferable not to use rigid fixation devices on the inferior orbital rim unless absolutely necessary for stability of the reconstruction. If such a plate is placed and is visible after healing is complete, a second surgical violation of this lower lid to remove the plate exposes the patient to an even higher risk for lid complication. Bioresorbable plates may be ideally suited for fixation of the orbital rim to prevent this complication.

Evaluation of Ocular Injuries

Obtaining a complete preoperative ophthalmologic evaluation of every victim of an orbitozygomatic fracture is an unrealistic expectation and by no means mandatory. However, the reconstructive surgeon must be sensitive to the possibility of direct ocular trauma and obtain proper consultation when indicated. A minimal preoperative examination should include testing of visual acuity (subjective and objective in both eyes), pupillary function, and ocular motility; inspection of the anterior chamber for hyphema; and visualization of the fundus for gross abnormalities. A decrease in visual acuity or abnormality noted on the other phases of this screening examination warrants a more detailed examination by an ophthalmologist before reconstruction of the bony injuries is undertaken.

Occasionally, an ocular injury may prevent treatment of the bony injuries if any manipulation of the globe might worsen the ocular injury and precipitate total loss of vision in the eye. The potential hazards of orbital reconstruction around an only-seeing eye must be recognized by the surgeon and explained in detail to the patient. In general, reconstruction should be limited to returning the globe to a functional position in cases involving severe disruption of the orbit and marked displacement of the globe. Bone grafting should be directed to providing basic support for the globe rather than to total reconstruction of the orbital volume and shape. Intraoperative tonometry and funduscopic examination should be considered in these cases and in all other cases in which large implants are placed in the posterior orbit. Occasionally, forward positioning of the globe by an oversized implant causes an acute increase in intraocular pressure, and the implant must be removed and reduced in size.

Complications

Ophthalmologic

Diplopia occurs in ~7% of patients with orbitozygomatic injuries and is the most common ophthalmologic complication.[23] It is usually gaze-evoked with extreme upward or lateral gaze, and results from entrapment, neuropraxia, or muscle contusion. A release procedure should be performed for diplopia caused by entrapment. For neupraxia or muscle contusion an observation period of 6 months prior to any intervention is recommended.[24] Blindness is the most serious complication of orbitozygomatic injury. It may occur at the time of the injury or in rare instances be iatrogenic. An ophthalmologic evaluation is therefore indicated prior to surgical intervention.

Lower Eyelid Malposition

Lower lid ectropion results from scarring of the anterior lamella after a subciliary incision. It is often associated with preoperative lower lid laxity, which may be corrected with a tarsal strip procedure. Ectropion may manifest clinically in a spectrum ranging from scleral show to injected conjunctiva and corneal ulceration. Entropion results from scarring in the posterior lamella, typically associated with a transconjunctival approach. The resultant turn in of the lower lid may lead to corneal abrasion by the eyelashes and corneal exposure. Lower lid massage may help reduce the contracture, or placement of a spacer graft may be needed for correction.

Enophthalmos

Zygoma malposition and inadequate reconstruction of the orbital floor and medial wall, in combination or separately, may cause enophthalmos. Patients typically have globe position and malar eminence asymmetry. It is easily corrected in the early postoperative period by removing the hardware and repositioning the fragments. When patients present late after reconstruction when healing has occurred osteotomies must be performed to reposition the bones.

Plate-Related Complications

Titanium implants may result in soft-tissue irritation and cold intolerance, creation of a distortion artifact on CT and magnetic resonance imaging, and interference with facial growth. They may be palpable and ultimately become exposed. These problems may ultimately necessitate a second procedure for plate removal. The use of bioresorbable plate and screw systems can prevent these plate-related complications.

Summary

Fractures of the bones that provide support for the globe and the soft tissue contours of the cheek must be evaluated thoroughly and treated aggressively if posttraumatic deformities are to be avoided. The trauma surgeon should use detailed preoperative CT to formulate a complete treatment plan before beginning the reconstruction. Reduction and fixation of each fracture line or fracture dislocation should not be viewed in a segmentalized fashion but rather as a progressive step in reconstruction of the entire orbitozygomatic complex as a single unit. However, the surgeon should not attempt these procedures without a thorough understanding of the anatomy of the bony and soft tissue structures of the orbital and periorbital areas and also the ability to three-dimensionally conceptualize the reconstruction while it is in progress.

References

1. Simoni P, Ostendorf R, Cox AJ. Effect of air bags and restraining devices on the pattern of facial fractures in motor vehicle crashes. Arch Facial Plast Surg 2003;5:113
2. Sturla F, Absi P, Buquet J. Anatomical and mechanical considerations of craniofacial fractures: an experimental study. Plast Reconstr Surg 1980;66:815
3. Zingg M, Laedrach K, Chen J, et al. Classification and treatment of zygomatic fractures: a review of 1,025 cases. J Oral Maxillofac Surg 1992;50:778
4. Ellis E, El-Attar A, Moos FK. An analysis of 2,067 cases of zygomatico-orbital fracture. J Oral Maxillofac Surg 1985;43:417
5. Crumley RL, Leibsoh J, Krause CF, et al. Fractures of the orbital floor Laryngoscope 1977;87:934

6. Funk GF, Stanley RB, Becker TS. Reversible visual loss due to impacted lateral wall fractures. Head Neck Surg 1989;11:295
7. Koorneef L. Current concepts on the management of orbital blow-out fractures. Ann Plast Surg 1982;9:185
8. Manson PN, Grivas A, Rosenbaum A, et al. Studies on enophthalmos, II: the measurement of orbital injuries and their treatment by quantitative computed tomography. Plast Reconstr Surg 1986;72:203
9. Strong EB, Sykes JM. Zygoma complex fractures. Facial Plast Surg 1998;14:105
10. Whitehouse RW, Batterbury M, Jackson A, et al. Predication of enophthalmos by computed tomography after "blow out" orbital fracture. Br J Ophthalmol 1994;78:618
11. Ploder O, Klug C, Voracek M, et al. Evaluation of computer-based area and volume measurement from coronal computed tomography scans in isolated blowout fractures of the orbital floor. J Oral Maxillofac Surg 2002;60:1267
12. Ellis E, Reddy L. Status of the internal orbit after reduction of zygomaticomaxillary complex fractures. J Oral Maxillofac Surg 2004;62:275
13. Shumrick KA, Kersten RC, Kulwin DR, et al. Criteria for selective management of the orbital rim and floor in zygomatic complex and midface fractures. Arch Otolaryngol Head Neck Surg 1997;123:378
14. McGivern BE, Stein M. A method of reduction of zygomaticomaxillary complex fractures. J Oral Maxillofac Surg 2000;58:1188
15. Stanley RB. The zygomatic arch: a guide to reconstruction of comminuted malar fractures. Arch Otolaryngol Head Neck Surg 1989;115:1459
16. Hanneman M, Simmons O, Jain S, et al. A comparison of combinations of titanium and resorbable plating systems for repair of isolated zygomatic fractures in the adult. Ann Plast Surg 2005;54:402
17. Eppley BL. Zygomaticomaxillary fracture repair with resorbable plates and screws. J Craniofac Surg 2000;11:377
18. Moe KS, Weisman RA. Resorbable fixation in facial plastic and head and neck reconstructive surgery: an initial report on polylactic acid implants. Laryngoscope 2001;111:1697
19. Kawamoto HK. Late posttraumatic enophthalmos: a correctable deformity. Plast Reconstr Surg 1982;69:423
20. Mizuno A, Toril S, Akiyama Y, et al. Preauricular (tragus) skin incision in fracture of the malar arch. Int J Oral Maxillofac Surg 1987;16:391
21. Wellisz T. Clinical experience with the Medpor porous polyethylene implant. Aesthetic Plast Surg 1993;17:339
22. Markowitz BL, Manson PN. Panfacial fractures: organization of treatment. Clin Plast Surg 1989;16:105
23. Karlan MS, Cassisi NJ. Fractures of the zygoma, a geometric, biomechanical, and surgical analysis. Arch Otolaryngol 1979;105:320
24. Jelks GW, La Trenta G. Orbital fractures. In: Foster CA, Sherman JE, eds: Surgery of Facial Bone Fractures. New York: Churchill Livingston; 1987:67

70 Frontal Sinus and Naso-Orbital-Ethmoid Complex Fractures

E. Bradley Strong

The anterior wall of the frontal sinus is extremely resistent to injury. The majority of injuries involving the frontal sinus and naso-orbito-ethmoid region are the result of high-velocity impacts such as motor vehicle accidents, assaults, and sports injuries. The anatomy and surgical treatment of frontal sinus and naso-orbital-ethmoid fractures is distinct, however the anatomical proximity of these two areas warrants a combined discussion. Patients with frontal sinus and naso-orbital-ethmoid complex fractures often have associated injuries. The initial evaluation should be focused on airway maintenance and hemodynamic stability. Once the patient is stabilized, the brain, spine, orbits, and facial skeleton should be evaluated. This requires a team approach involving the facial plastic surgeon, neurosurgeon, and ophthalmologist. The goal of frontal sinus and naso-orbital-ethmoid complex fracture treatment is avoidance of short- and long-term complications as well as the return of normal sinus function and aesthetic facial contour. A treatment algorithm for frontal sinus and naso-orbito-ethmoid complex injuries will be presented.

Frontal Sinus

Embryology and Anatomy

The frontal sinus is absent at birth. At 2 years of age the anterior ethmoid air cells invade the frontal bone to form a rudimentary cavity. By 6 years of age, the frontal sinus can be detected radiologically. At 15 years of age the frontal sinus is adult size (**Fig. 70.1**). The floor of the sinus forms the medial portion of the orbital roof. The posterior table forms a portion of the anterior cranial fossa. The anterior table forms part of the forehead, brow, and glabella[1,2] (**Fig. 70.2**). The frontal sinus is most commonly bilateral, asymmetric in shape, and divided by one or more intersinus septations. However, the size and shape of the adult frontal sinus is highly variable. Ten percent of individuals have a unilateral sinus, 5% have a rudimentary cavity, and 4% have no sinus at all.[3] The average dimensions are: height 30 mm, width 25 mm, depth 19 mm, and volume 10 mL. The anterior table thickness may be as great as 12 mm (average 4 mm), whereas the posterior table ranges in thickness from 0.1 to 4.8 mm.[4]

The nasofrontal recess (NFR) is the sole outflow tract for the frontal sinus. The distance from the frontal sinus to the hiatus semilunaris is usually very short. It is therefore most accurately described as a recess rather than a true duct. Each ostium is ~3 × 4 mm in diameter and located on the posterior, inferior aspect of the sinus floor. The ostium lies anterior to the anterior ethmoid air cells, medial to the orbit, lateral to the intersinus septum, and posterior to the frontal bone. The true ostia represents the narrowest point of an hourglass configuration, with the frontal sinus infundibulum above and the nasofrontal recess below.[5]

The vascular supply to the frontal sinus is from the supraorbital and supratrochlear arteries via the internal carotid system. Venous drainage occurs through three pathways: the facial vein, the ophthalmic vein (to the cavernous sinus), and the foramina of Breschet (to the subarachnoid

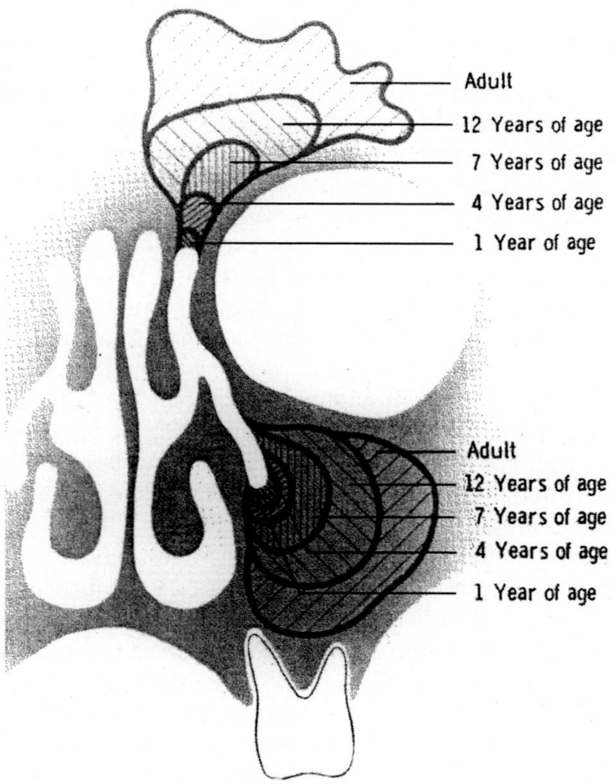

Fig. 70.1 Frontal sinus development. (From Nauman HH. Development of the frontal sinus. In: Nauman HH, ed. Head and Neck: Indications, Techniques, and Pitfalls. Vol 1. Philadelphia: WB Saunders; 1980. Reprinted by permission.)

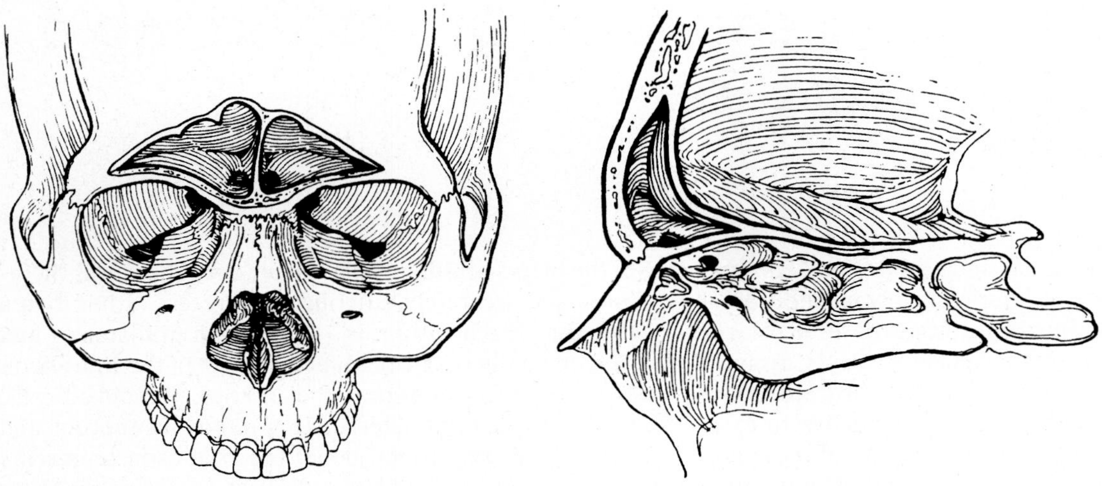

Fig. 70.2 Anterior (**A**) and lateral (**B**) views of the frontal sinus demonstrating the relative thickness of the anterior and posterior tables, as well as the relationship of the frontal sinus to the orbits, ethmoid sinuses, and anterior cranial fossa. (From Donald PJ. Maxillofacial Trauma: Management of the Difficult Case. Philadelphia: WB Saunders; 1984. Reprinted by permission.)

space).[6] The ophthalmic branch of the trigeminal nerve provides sensory innervation to the frontal sinus.

Frontal Sinus Fractures

The frontal sinus is protected by thick cortical bone and is more resistant to fracture than any other facial bone[7] (**Fig. 70.3**). Consequently, frontal sinus fractures account for only 5 to 15% of maxillofacial injuries and are most commonly associated with motor vehicles accidents, sporting events, and assaults.[8] The extreme force required to fracture the anterior table of the frontal sinus results in serious associated injuries in 75% of patients.[9] Sixty-six percent of patients will have associated facial fractures.[10] Mortality rates as high as 25% have been reported with severe through-and-through injuries.[10] Isolated anterior table fractures occur in approximately 50% of patients, while combined anterior/posterior table fractures occur in approximately 50% of patients.[11] Isolated posterior table fractures are uncommon (~1%).

Improper management can result in aesthetic deformity, chronic sinusitis, pneumocephalus, mucopyocele, meningitis, and brain abscess. Unfortunately, treatment of frontal sinus fractures remains one of the most controversial areas of maxillofacial trauma. When the frontal sinus mucosa is injured, it has a propensity to form mucoceles. Complications can occur years after the injury, and long-term follow-up is often difficult. Consequently, a surgeon may be confident in a particular surgical technique and have few known complications. However, the same surgeon may have a long list of cases done "elsewhere" that ultimately resulted in mucocele formation. When any type of an obliterative procedure is performed, cutting and diamond burs must be used to meticulously remove all mucosal remnants from the sinus and free bone fragments

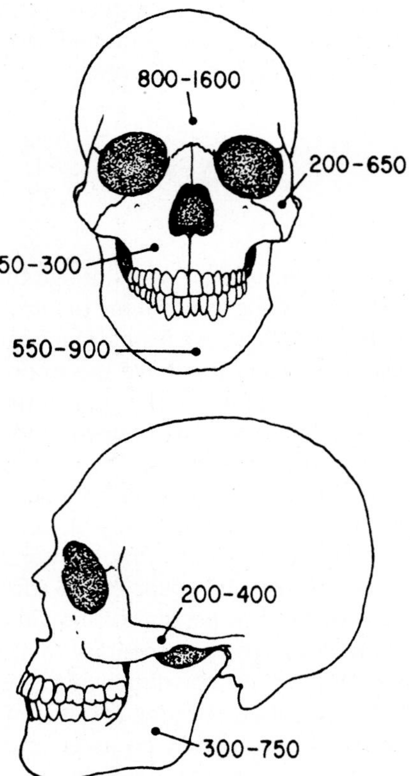

Fig. 70.3 Force (pounds) necessary to fracture different facial bones (From Nahum AM. The biomechanics of maxillofacial trauma. Clin Plast Surg 1975;2:63. Reprinted by permission.)

to avoid mucocele formation. Surgeons must continue to be diligent and emphasize long-term follow-up of frontal sinus injuries.

Diagnosis

The accurate diagnosis of frontal sinus fractures and NFR injuries is crucial to the appropriate treatment. After the patient has been stabilized and any associated injuries have been evaluated, a thorough head and neck examination should be performed. Patients with frontal sinus fractures often complain of forehead pain and swelling. Other findings that may suggest a frontal sinus injury include supratrochlear and supraorbital paraesthesias, epistaxis, diplopia, forehead abrasions, and forehead hematoma. Forehead lacerations should be examined under sterile conditions to assess the integrity of the anterior table, posterior table, and dura. Through-and-through injuries of the frontal sinus have high morbidity and prompt surgical treatment is indicated. If the patient is awake, he or she should be questioned regarding the presence of clear rhinorrhea or salty postnasal drainage. Drainage suspicious for cerebrospinal fluid (CSF) rhinorrhea can be grossly evaluated with a "halo test." The bloody fluid is allowed to drip onto filter paper. If CSF is present, it will diffuse faster than blood and result in a clear halo around the blood. The definitive test for CSF is β-2 transferrin. The presence of β-2 transferrin is very specific for CSF. The only other locations where β-2 transferrin is found are the vitreous humor of the eye and perilymph of the inner ear.

Radiological Evaluation

Historically, plain sinus x-rays have been used to evaluate facial fractures. Thin cut (1.5-mm) axial and coronal computed tomography (CT) scans are now the gold standard for diagnosis of frontal sinus fractures. The axial images provide excellent information about anterior and posterior table injury as well as pneumocephalus. The coronal images provide information about the frontal sinus floor and orbital roof. Unfortunately, the compact anatomy of the NFR makes an accurate fracture diagnosis in this area difficult. Three-dimensional (3-D) reconstructions with sagittal sections can be helpful to assess this area.

Treatment

The treatment goals for frontal sinus fractures include protection of intracranial contents, prevention of early and late complications, restoration of aesthetic forehead contour, and return of normal frontal sinus function. Accomplishing all of these goals is not always possible. However, reconstruction of a "safe" sinus is imperative. Once this has been accomplished, the aesthetic and functional repair can be addressed. Specific treatment options include observation, endoscopic fracture reduction or camouflage, open reduction and internal fixation, sinus obliteration, sinus exenteration (Riedel procedure), and sinus cranialization. The indications and techniques for each will be discussed below.

Appropriate treatment decisions can be made by assessing the status of four anatomic parameters: (1) anterior table fractures, (2) posterior table fractures, (3) nasofrontal recess injury, and (4) dural integrity (i.e., presence of a CSF leak).

Nasofrontal Recess Fractures (**Fig. 70.4**)

The compact structure of the NFR makes accurate diagnosis of isolated fractures difficult. A thorough physical examination and a thin cut CT scan with 3-D reconstructions should be performed. Sagittal and coronal sections of the 3-D reconstructions can be very helpful. Fractures involving the floor of the frontal sinus or the anterior ethmoid region should raise suspicion for NFR injury.[12] In the absence of fracture displacement or associated frontal sinus injuries, close observation and a repeat CT scan at 4 to 6 weeks is warranted.

If the NFR is found to be obstructed, or the frontal sinus is noted to be opacified after a period of observation, frontal sinus obliteration is indicated (see technique below).

Some authors have advocated reconstruction of the NFR with mucoperiosteal flaps (Sewell-Boyden). An intersinus septectomy has also been described for unilateral injuries. This theoretically allows the injured sinus cavity to drain into the uninjured NFR.[13,14] Although these techniques are successfully used by some surgeons, they have not gained significant popularity. More recent literature has suggested that open reduction and internal fixation of fractures involving the frontal recess (followed by close postoperative observation) may be efficacious.[15] If outflow obstruction becomes apparent weeks to months after the injury, an endoscopic sinusotomy can be performed. The author has had some success with this technique, but with limited long-term follow-up. This approach is still being investigated and should be reserved for surgeons with extensive experience with traditional approaches to the frontal sinus and the endoscopic approach to the frontal recess.

Surgical Technique for Frontal Sinusotomy and Endoscopy

After infiltration of local anesthesia, a 1.0- to 1.5-cm skin incision is placed midway between the medial canthus and the glabella, ~1 cm inferior to the brow (**Fig. 70.5**). The incision is best hidden by placing it inferior and deep to the curve of the brow. A guarded needle point

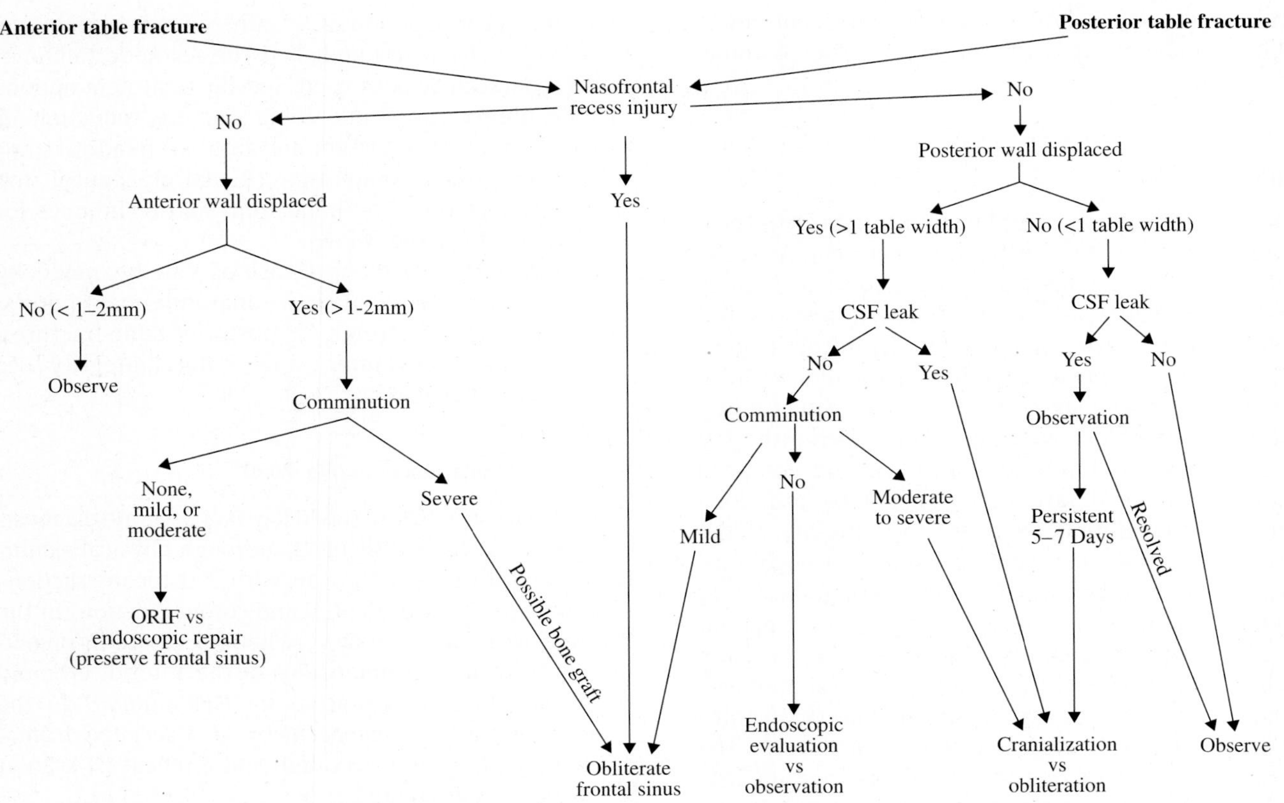

Fig. 70.4 Algorithm for treatment of frontal sinus fractures. CSF, cerebrospinal fluid.

monopolar electrocautery is used to expose the periosteum. Care is taken to avoid the supratrochlear neurovascular pedicle. The location of the frontal sinus is confirmed on the CT scan and a cutting bur is used to open a 4- to 5-mm frontal sinusotomy ~1 cm medial and inferior to the medial brow. The mucosa is incised sharply. Direct visualization of the posterior table and NFR is performed with a 30-degree nasal endoscope. Methylene blue or fluorescein can be instilled into the frontal sinus to assess patency. Intranasal endoscopy will reveal the presence of dye if the NFR is patent.[16] However, it does not rule out fracture, or assess the long-term risk of frontal recess stenosis, and there have been no studies to confirm efficacy of this technique. The procedure is completed with a meticulous, layered closure. Trephination can be performed bilaterally, if necessary.

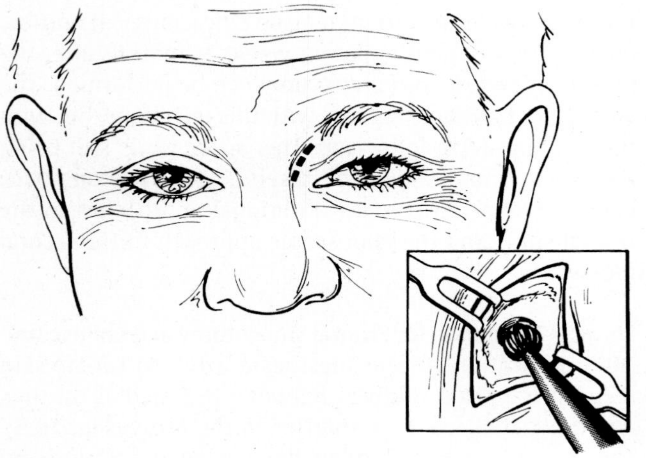

Fig. 70.5 Frontal sinus trephination.

*Nondisplaced Anterior Table Fractures (**Fig. 70.4**)*

Isolated, nondisplaced fractures of the anterior table pose little risk for mucocele formation, and rarely result in aesthetic or functional deficit. These injuries are best managed nonoperatively. The small risk of external deformity should be discussed with the patient.

Displaced Anterior Table Fractures

In the past, the long-term risk of mucocele formation was felt to be high enough to warrant open reduction and internal fixation in nearly all displaced frontal sinus fractures. This required a coronal incision and rigid internal fixation. Although the success rates are very high, the procedure results in postsurgical stigmata including a large scar, parasthesias, possible alopecia, and, uncommonly, facial nerve injury. Whereas the gold standard for isolated anterior table fractures remains open reduction and internal fixation, several authors have recently described an endoscopic approach for repair of moderately displaced fractures, eliminating the need for a coronal incision.[17-19] Strong et al evaluated the endoscopic technique in a cadaver model and found that fracture camouflage was easier and more efficacious than fracture reduction.[20] The camouflage technique has two advantages: (1) the repair does not require endoscopic manipulation or stabilization of the bone fragments, which can be extremely challenging; and (2) the repair need not be done in the acute setting. This is important because once the soft tissue edema resolves, there may be no aesthetic deformity and the patient may not require any surgical intervention (**Fig. 70.6**). However, this determination cannot be made until 3 to 4 months after the injury. Using this approach, only those patients with a true aesthetic deformity will require surgery. The author uses the endoscopic approach to treat isolated, moderate displacement fractures (2–6 mm) of the anterior table.

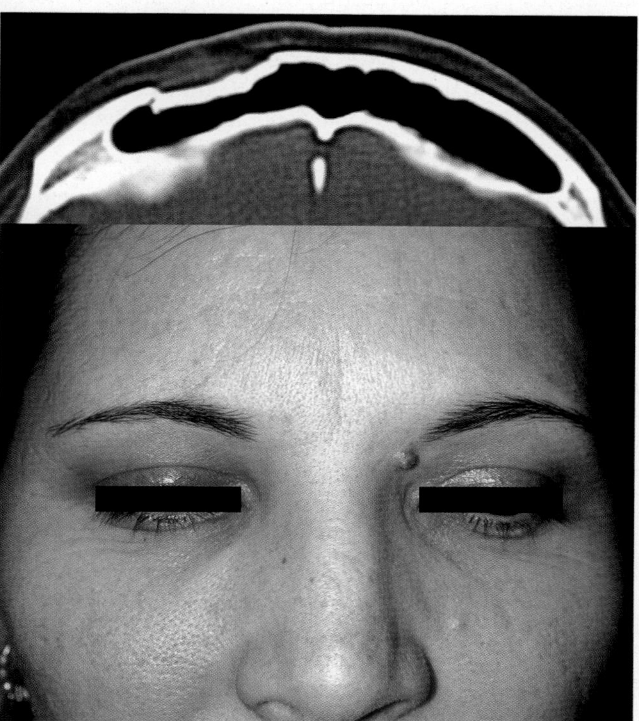

Fig. 70.6 (**A**) Coronal CT scan of a patient with an anterior table frontal sinus fracture with enough displacement to be considered for traditional open repair. (**B**) Four-month post-injury photograph of the same patient without any visible cosmetic deformity. The patient received no treatment for the injury.

Surgical Technique for Endoscopic Repair

Appropriate consent is obtained for the procedure including the risks of bleeding, infection, paraesthesia, alopecia, poor aesthetic result, and possible need for open approach if an endoscopic repair cannot be performed. A 3- to 5-cm parasagittal "working" incision should be placed above the fracture, 3 cm behind the hair line (**Fig. 70.7**). Care should be taken to avoid trauma to the hair follicles and cautery should be avoided if possible. The incision length should be kept to a minimum, but will vary depending on the size of the fracture and implant to be inserted. A second 1- to 2-cm endoscope incision is then placed at the same height, 6-cm medial to the working incision. In patients with a prominent forehead or receding hair line, the incisions may need to be closer to the hairline to allow visualization around the forehead curvature.

The technique is similar to an endoscopic browlift. A "blind" subperiosteal dissection is performed down to the level of the fracture. A 4.0-mm, 30-degree endoscope (with rigid endosheath and camera) is inserted to visualize the optical cavity. The periostum is carefully elevated over the defect. The elevation is generally not difficult because the procedure is performed 3 months after the injury and there is a fibrous layer preventing entry into the sinus. Once the entire fracture is exposed, a 0.85-mm thick porous polyethylene sheet (MEDPOR, Porex Surgical, Inc., Newnan, GA) is trimmed to approximate the defect. The superior edge of the implant is marked with a pen to maintain the orientation endoscopically. The implant is inserted through the working incision and manipulated over the defect. This process is repeated until the diameter of the implant is ~2.0 to 3.0 mm larger than the

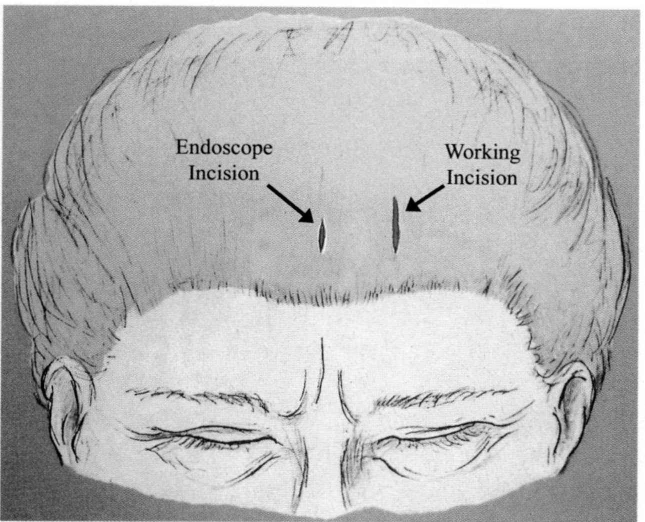

Fig. 70.7 Illustration of scalp incisions used for endoscopic repair of a left-sided frontal sinus fracture.

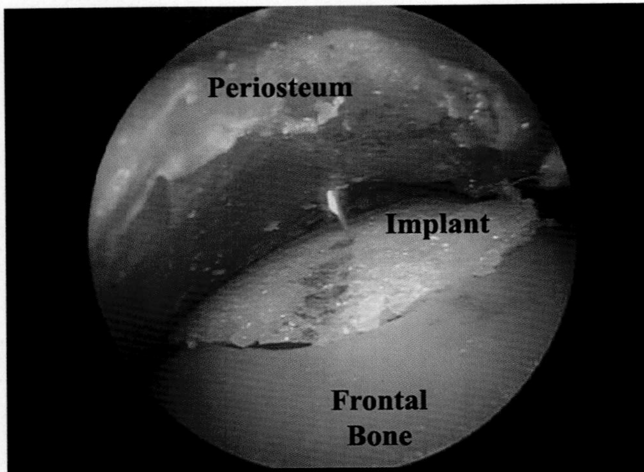

Fig. 70.8 Endoscopic view of a porous polyethylene implant inserted over a frontal sinus fracture. Note the pen mark placed on the implant to maintain the orientation and the needle being passed through the skin to determine the best location for the transcutaneous screw insertion.

defect (**Fig. 70.8**). At time, the author has sutured two to three layers of porous polyethylene together to more accurately fill the defect. A 25-gauge needle is then passed through the skin over the fracture site and endoscopically visualized to determine the best site for percutaneous screw placement. A no. 11 blade is used to make a 2-mm, through-and-through stab incision. A 1.7-mm self-drilling screw (length 4–7 mm) is passed through the stab incision, through the edge of the implant, and into the frontal bone (**Fig. 70.9**). If the implant is not completely stable, a second screw is placed on the contralateral side. The self-drilling screw must be placed at least 0.5 to 1.0 mm away from the implant edge, or the implant may tear. The scalp incisions are then closed in layers and a head dressing is applied.

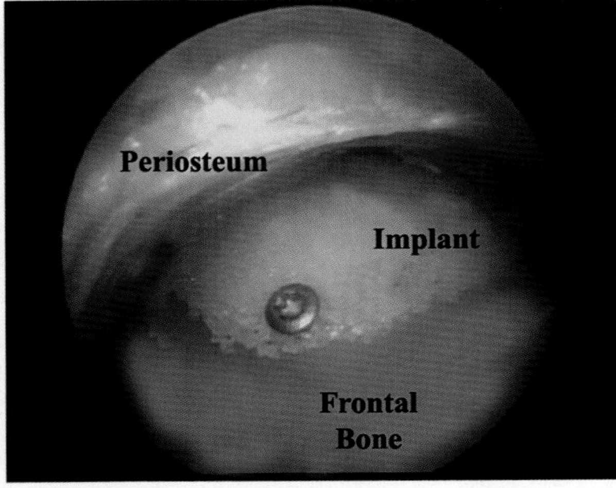

Fig. 70.9 Endoscopic view of a porous polyethylene implant stabilized over the bone defect with a self-drilling screw.

Not all isolated anterior table fractures are appropriate for this technique. Injuries with severe comminution and marked mucosal injury may require open reduction or even frontal sinus obliteration. Fractures that extend over the orbital rim may be difficult or impossible to visualize endoscopically, and may also require an open technique.

Surgical Technique for Open Reduction and Internal Fixation

Consent is obtained from the patient for the procedure including the risks of bleeding, infection, paraesthesia, CSF leak, meningitis, external deformity, and late mucocele formation. The coronal incision must be described in detail particularly in those patients with male pattern baldness. Once in the operating room, the bed is turned 180 degrees away from anesthesia and a coronal flap is drawn out at least 4 to 6 cm behind the anterior hairline. The author generally uses a zig-zag pattern in patients who wear their hair longer than 3 to 4 cm because the hair will fall down over the transverse arms of the incision (**Fig. 70.10**). If patients cut their hair extremely short a zig-zag incision has little advantage. The traditional coronal incision works equally well and is easier to perform. A 1- to 2-cm strip of hair can be shaved along the incision site, but this is not necessary. Brow incisions should be avoided due to the prominent scar and associated forehead anesthesia. If large lacerations are already present on the forehead, they should be explored and used for fracture repair if possible. However, forehead lacerations are often inadequate for exposure and repair of frontal sinus fractures. Significant extension of forehead lacerations should generally be avoided.

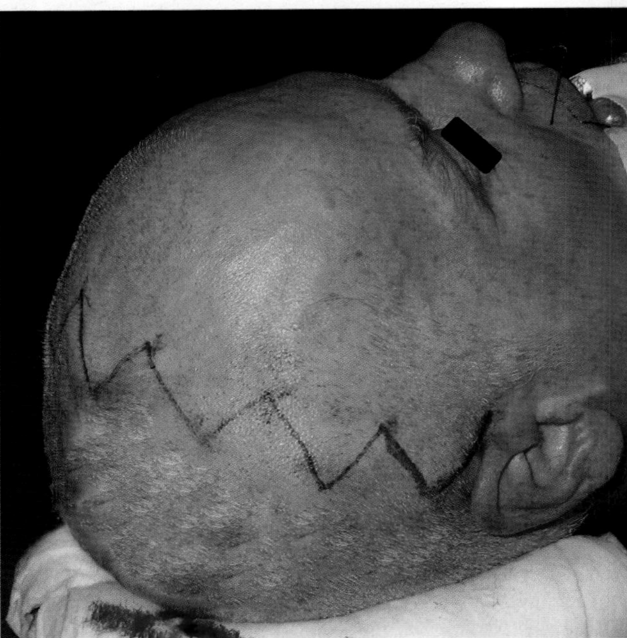

Fig. 70.10 Zig-zag scalp incision place 4 to 6 cm behind the hair line.

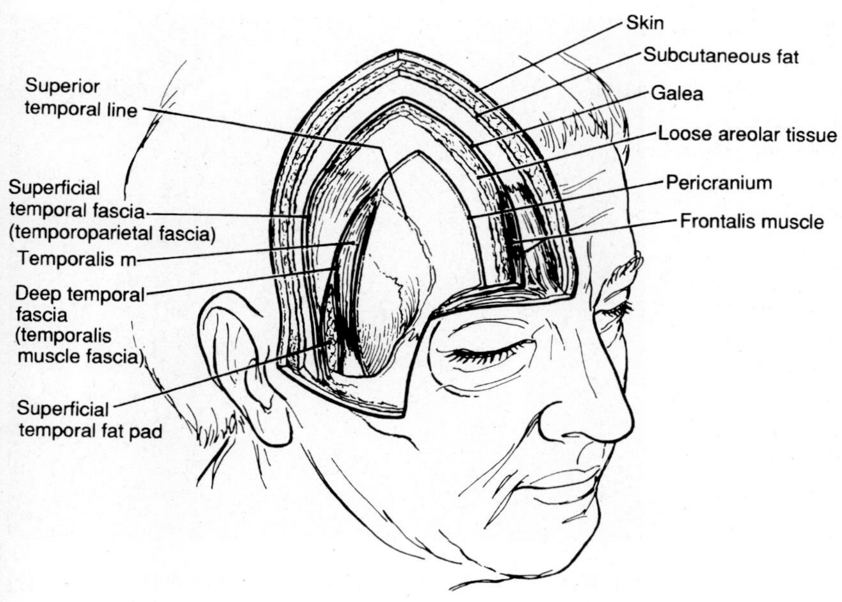

Fig. 70.11 Illustration depicting the fascial planes of the forehead and temple. The temporal branch of the facial nerve runs within the temporoparietal fascia (superficial temporal fascia).

After injection of local anesthetic, the scalp is incised and elevated in a subgaleal plane with scissors, scalpel, or finger dissection. Lateral dissection of the flap must be meticulously performed between the temporoparietal fascia (superficial temporal fascia) and the temporalis muscle fascia (deep temporal fascia) (**Fig. 70.11**). The temporoparietal fascia and frontal branch of the facial nerve are elevated with the flap. The supraperiosteal frontal dissection is discontinued just above the superior orbital rims, avoiding injury to the supraorbital and supratrochlear neurovascular pedicles. The pericranium is then incised 1 to 2 cm above the sinus and elevated below the fracture. The supraorbital and supratrochlear neurovascular pedicles are easily defined in the subperiosteal plane. If there is any concern about a posterior table injury or dural tear, the entire pericranial flap should be elevated from the level of the initial incision. The vascularized pericranial flap may then be used for a dural repair if necessary.

The frontal sinus contour has an intrinsic convex shape. As a perpendicular traumatic force is applied to the sinus, the convex shape is flattened. The bone is horizontally compressed until it fractures, and then it releases into a concave shape (**Fig. 70.12**). Reduction of noncomminuted, compressed fractures can be difficult. If the segments overlap at the fracture site, a bone hook can be insinuated between the fragments and elevated. If the bone fragments do not overlap, reduction can be accomplished by placing a 1.5- to 2.0-mm screw in the depressed segment, grasping the screw with a heavy hemostat, and pulling the segment anteriorly (**Fig. 70.13**). It may be necessary to carefully remove a bone fragment, release the tension, and make room for reduction of the remaining bone fragments. An attempt should be made to keep the majority of the fragments in place. This will allow a

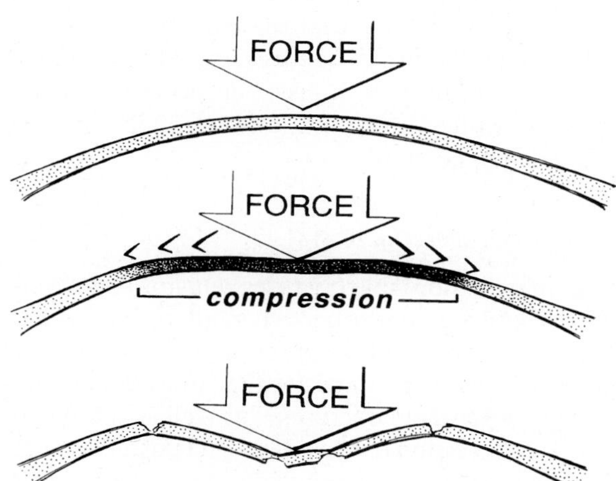

Fig. 70.12 Illustration of the compressive forces on frontal sinus as it is deformed from a convex to a concave shape.

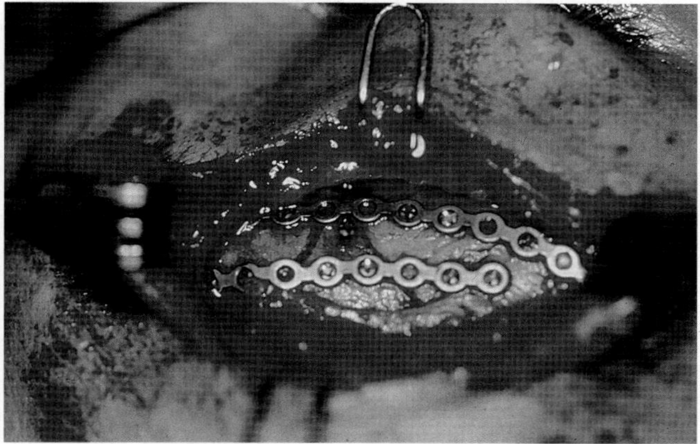

Fig. 70.13 Intraoperative photo of a single miniscrew placed in the anterior table bone and used to reduce/stabilize the fracture fragments while rigid fixation was applied.

more accurate repair. After the bone fragments are mobilized, an attempt should be made to assess the sinus mucosa. A 30-degree endoscope can be helpful to visualize the sinus and the nasofrontal recess through a small bone defect. Any torn mucosa should be removed from fracture lines to avoid entrapment. The reduced fragments are then plated with 1.0 to 1.3 microplates or micromesh.

Missing bone is uncommon. However, high-velocity injuries may result in small, comminuted fragments, which cannot be reapproximated. Small gaps (4–10 mm) can be reconstructed with titanium mesh. After the reconstruction is complete, the pericranium is reapproximted and sutured closed, followed by the galea aponeurosis and skin. A tight galeal closure is important to obtain hemostasis and avoid hematoma. Bilateral Penrose drains are placed beneath the scalp, exiting the coronal incision above each ear, and sutured to the skin. A pressure dressing is applied. Care should be taken to ensure that the ears are not rolled forward under the pressure dressing. The Penrose drains are removed at 24 hours, the pressure dressing are discontinued at 3 days, and the skin sutures/staples are removed at 10 days.

*Posterior Table Fractures (**Fig. 70.4**)*

Treatment of posterior table fractures remains controversial.[9,10,15,16] There are no prospective, randomized studies to validate the techniques proposed by various authors. A literature review reveals articles that support exploration of all posterior table fractures,[21] as well as those that recommend observation of even displaced posterior table fractures.[14] The author presents a conservative algorithm for treatment of these injuries.

Nondisplaced Posterior Table Fractures

Nondisplaced posterior table fractures (i.e., less than one table width) are felt to have a reduced risk of complications (i.e., dural tears, CSF leak, meningitis, and mucocele formation), when compared with displaced posterior table fractures.[22] Therefore, nondisplaced fractured can be managed more conservatively. The patient should be questioned for the presence of clear, watery drainage from the nose or salty tasting drainage into the nasopharynx. Patients with no evidence of CSF leak can be observed. If there is a question of a more severe injury, frontal sinus trephination and endoscopy can be used to evaluate paramedian fractures for mucosal injury, dural tear, CSF leak, or NFR injury. Nondisplaced fractures with a confirmed CSF leak may be observed for 5 to 7 days. Approximately half of these patients will have spontaneous resolution.[3,14] If the CSF leak is persistent, an obliteration procedure is indicated depending on the degree of injury noted at the time of surgery.

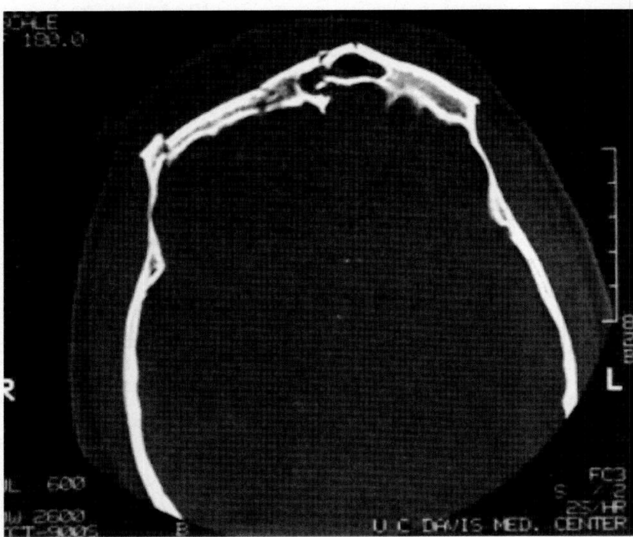

Fig. 70.14 Axial CT scan demonstrating a comminuted anterior and posterior table frontal sinus fracture.

Displaced Posterior Table Fractures

Fractures displaced greater than one table width (**Fig. 70.14**) require a more aggressive approach because the risk of long-term complications is increased. The presence of a CSF leak should be carefully evaluated. Patients without a CSF leak should be categorized by the severity of posterior table comminution. In the absence of significant comminution or NFR involvement, the surgeon may consider observation. Mild comminution noted on the CT scan is an indication for sinus obliteration. Moderate to severe comminution, involving more than 25% of the posterior table, is an indication for cranialization of the sinus.[13] The external contour is maintained with a bony reconstruction of the anterior table using titanium microplates and mesh to cover small defects. Larger defects may require bone grafts from the posterior table or calvaria. Neurosurgical consultation should be obtained for assistance with brain debridement and dural closure.

Surgical Technique for Frontal Sinus Obliteration

Informed consent is obtained from the patient including the risks of bleeding, infection, paraesthesia, CSF leak, meningitis, diplopia, external deformity, and late mucocele formation. Preoperatively, an anterior-posterior plain radiograph (Caldwell view) of the skull is obtained. The patient should be positioned 6 feet from the film to avoid magnification of the image. Alternatively, a surgical navigation system can be used intraoperatively to localize the sinus. The patient is prepared for a coronal flap (see "Surgical Technique for Open Reduction and Internal Fixation") and the abdomen is prepped for a fat graft. If a template is to be used, the orientation of the Caldwell x-ray is confirmed by comparison with the CT scan. An "R" is scratched into the template on the right side to confirm intraoperative positioning, and the template is cut out. A second template is usually cut in case one copy is contaminated during the procedure. Both templates are then sterilized.

A zig-zag coronal incision is performed (see "Surgical Technique for Open Reduction and Internal Fixation"). The pericranial flap should be maintained intact to repair any CSF leak that may be noted. If the anterior table of the frontal sinus is not comminuted, the frontal sinus template or navigation system is used to perform a frontal sinusotomy. If there is comminution of the anterior table, a bone fragment can be removed and one tine of a bipolar cautery can be placed on each side of the anterior table. The internal tine is then used to "walk" around the outline of the sinus while the outer tine is used to outline the sinus externally (**Fig. 70.15**). Traditionally, a drill is used to perforate the upper border of the flap. The drill should be angled toward the sinus cavity to avoid intracranial penetration and injury. The perforations are then joined with an oscillating saw. The author prefers a high-speed Midas Rex drill (Medtronic, Inc., Minneapolis, MN) and a B-1 bit. This bit can drill and cut laterally, obviating the need for an oscillating saw.

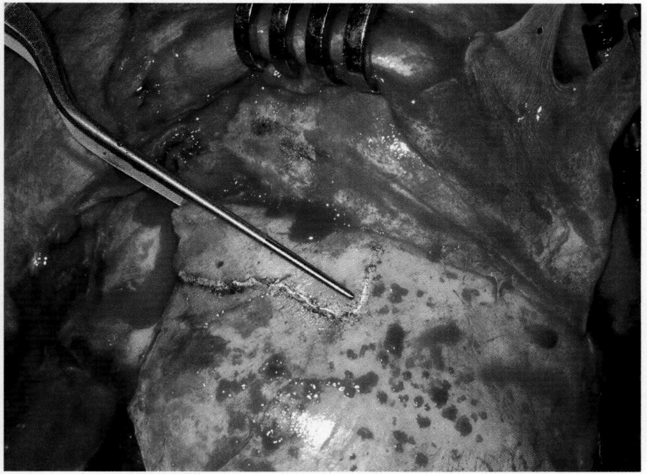

Fig. 70.15 Intraoperative photo of a frontal sinus fracture. A bipolar electrocautery is being used to determine the outline of the sinus by placing one tine on each side of the anterior table. The internal tine is then "walked" around the sinus while the outer tine is used to mark the sinus outline.

A 4-mm osteotome is then used to fracture the superior orbital rims and glabella at the periphery of the sinus. Care should be taken to avoid injuring the supraorbital/supratrochlear neurovascular pedicles. An osteotome is then placed through the saw kerf and the intersinus septum is fractured. This step is then repeated around the periphery of the sinus until the anterior table of the sinus is hinged open inferiorly at the level of the orbital rims.

After completion of the sinusotomy, posterior table comminution is assessed and a decision is made regarding sinus obliteration or cranialization. If the sinus is to be obliterated, meticulous debridement of all mucosa is accomplished with both cutting and diamond burs. The frontal sinus infundibulum mucosa is elevated inferiorly and a temporalis muscle plug is placed to occlude each ostia. The fat graft is obtained through a left lower quadrant (or periumbilical) incision using a sterile set of instruments. When the bone flap is replaced, the fat should meet but not extrude into the saw kerf. Other materials that have been used for frontal sinus obliteration include cancellous bone, muscle, and pericranium. Spontaneous osteoneogenesis with autoobliteration has also been described.[3] Hydroxyappatite bone cement should be avoided. Anterior table stabilization is achieved with ~1.3-mm microplates. Bone paté can be harvested from the frontal bone and used to fill the saw kerf or other small defects. The paté is then covered with Gelfoam (Pfizer, Inc., New York, NY) to maintain its position. This reduces the risk of postoperative frontal irregularities. The pericranium and scalp are then closed in layers.

Sugical Technique for Frontal Sinus Cranialization

The surgical approach for cranialization is identical to that described for frontal sinus obliteration. However, these injuries are often more severe and the pericranium is usually lacerated at the glabella. Special care should be taken to maintain the inferiorly based pedicle because the pericranial flap may be needed for closure of dural tears. Exposure of the sinus rarely requires osteotomies due to the severity of the anterior table injury. Any free bone fragments from the posterior table are removed and the dura is inspected. Simple lacerations of the dura can be repaired with interrupted 5–0 nylon sutures. More complex injuries may require neurosurgical debridement and dural closure. The remaining portion of the posterior table bone is then removed using elevators and rongeurs. Large pieces of posterior table bone should be preserved for possible use in reconstruction of the anterior table. All fragments of the anterior and posterior table are divested of mucosa with a cutting bur. Through-and-through injuries are often grossly contaminated with road dirt. In such cases, the bone fragments are soaked in Betadine (povidone-iodine) until needed for reconstruction. The

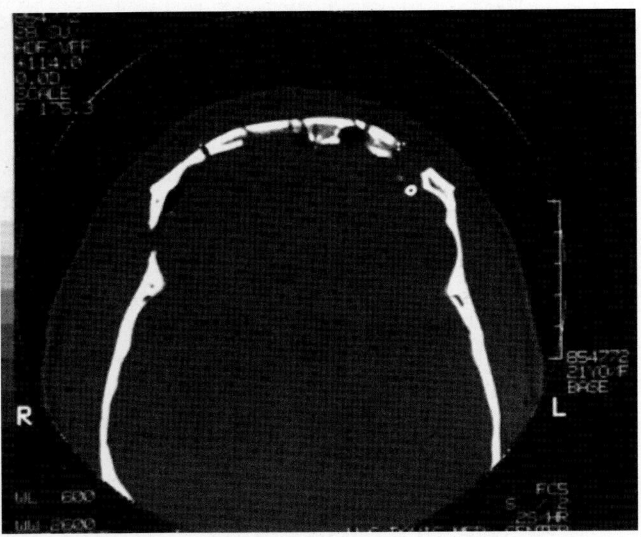

Fig. 70.16 Axial CT scan demonstrating previous frontal sinus cranialization and anterior displacement of the intracranial contents to fill the frontal sinus dead space.

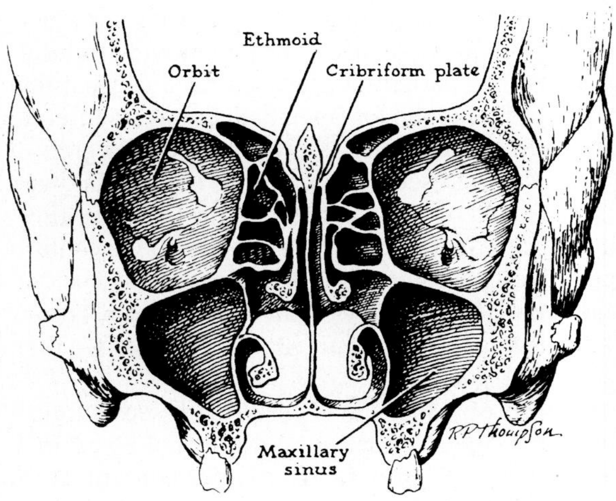

Fig. 70.17 Diagram of the naso-orbito-ethmoid complex. Note that the cribriform plate descends ~1 cm below the level of the ethmoid roof (fovea ethmoidalis). (From Kazanjian VH, Converse JM, eds. Surgical Treatment of Facial Injuries. 3rd ed. Baltimore: Williams & Wilkins; 1974. Reprinted by permission.)

posterior table bone is then drilled flush with the anterior sinus walls, floor, and anterior cranial fossa. Each frontal sinus infundibulum is drilled out, the mucosa is inverted, the ostia is occluded with a temporalis muscle plug, and a small bone fragment is placed on top to occlude each ostia. The pericranial flap can then be used to repair dural tears and cover the frontal recess. When replacing the anterior table bone, a small bony defect must be fashioned in the anterior table to allow the pericranial flap to pass intracranially without cutting off the blood supply. The preserved bone fragments are then cleansed with saline and the anterior table is reconstructed using ~1.3-mm microplates. Micromesh can also be very helpful. Outer-table calvarial bone grafts should be used as necessary to supplement native bone. The intracranial contents are then allowed to expand forward and fill the frontal sinus space (**Fig. 70.16**).

Naso-Orbital-Ethmoid Complex

Anatomy of the Naso-Orbital-Ethmoid Complex

The naso-orbital-ethmoid complex represents the confluence of the nasal, lacrimal, ethmoid, maxillary, and frontal bones. The paired nasal bones attach to the frontal bone superiorly and the frontal process of the maxilla laterally. The ethmoid bone is located posterior to the nasal bones. The ethmoid labyrinth separates the orbits laterally from the nasal cavity medially. The fovea ethmoidalis forms the roof of the ethmoid sinuses laterally. The cribriform plate, which is ~1 cm inferior to the fovea ethmoidalis, forms the roof of the nasal cavity (**Fig. 70.17**). The primary vertical buttress of the naso-orbital-ethmoid complex is the frontal process of the maxillary bone. The primary horizontal buttresses are the superior and inferior orbital rims. If these buttresses are violated, comminution of the entire complex may occur. Potential long-term sequelae include blindness, telecanthus, enophthalmos, midface retrusion, CSF fistula, anosmia, epiphora, sinusitis, and nasal deformity.

The medial canthal tendon (MCT) arises from the anterior and posterior lacrimal crests and the frontal process of the maxilla. It maintains the normal intercanthal distance, and is therefore the focal point of naso-orbital-ethmoid complex reconstruction. The MCT surrounds the lacrimal sac and diverges to become the pretarsal, preseptal, and orbital orbicularis oculi muscle (**Fig. 70.18**). Normal intercanthal distance is ~30 to 35 mm. Anatomically this equates to one half the interpupillary distance or equal to the width of the alar base (**Fig. 70.19**).

Fractures of the Naso-Orbital-Ethmoid Complex

Diagnosis

After any associated injuries have been evaluated, a complete head and neck examination should be performed. Ophthalmologic consultation is indicated in most cases. The naso-orbital-ethmoid fracture is primarily a clinical diagnosis. A high degree of suspicion must be maintained because failure to identify naso-orbital-ethmoid fractures often results in deformities that are extremely difficult to

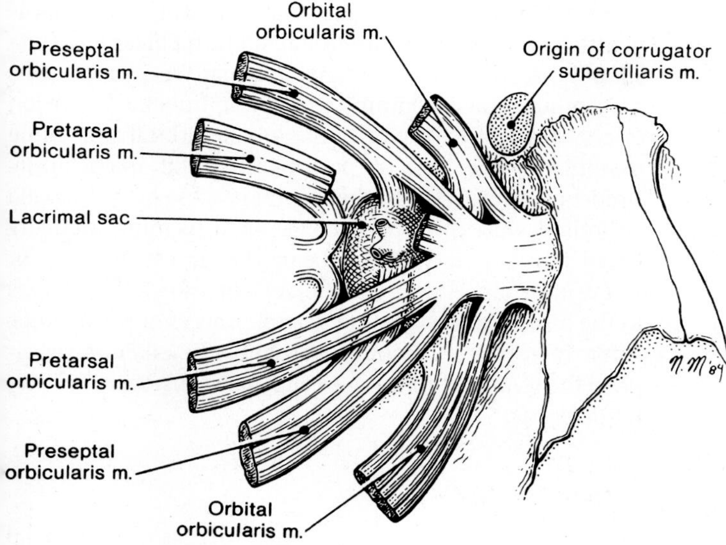

Fig. 70.18 Anatomy of the medial canthal tendon. The tendon splits around the lacrimal sac and attaches to the anterior and posterior lacrimal crests, as well as the frontal process of the maxilla. The canthal tendon diverges to become the pretarsal, preseptal, and orbital orbicularis oculi muscle. (From Bergin D, McCord CD. Anatomy relevant to blepharospasm. In: Bosniak S, ed. Advances in Opthalmic Plastic and Reconstructive Surgery: Blepharospasm. Philadelphia: Harper & Row; 1985.)

repair secondarily. The nasal cavity and any facial lacerations should be cleaned and examined for the possibility of a CSF fistula. The integrity of the medial canthal tendon should be evaluated by carefully applying lateral tension to each lower lid. Normally, there will be a defined end point to the maneuver, without palpable motion at the canthal insertion. A periosteal elevator can also be inserted through the nose to apply lateral pressure in the same area (however, this can result in epistaxis). A lax MCT, or medial orbital wall motion, is consistent with a naso-orbital-ethmoid complex fracture. Telecanthus, enophthalmos, pupillary response, and extraocular muscle mobility should be assessed and documented. The nasal bones should be palpated for crepitus and comminution. The degree of nasal or midface retrusion should be assessed. A complete cranial nerve examination will rule out trigeminal or facial nerve injury.

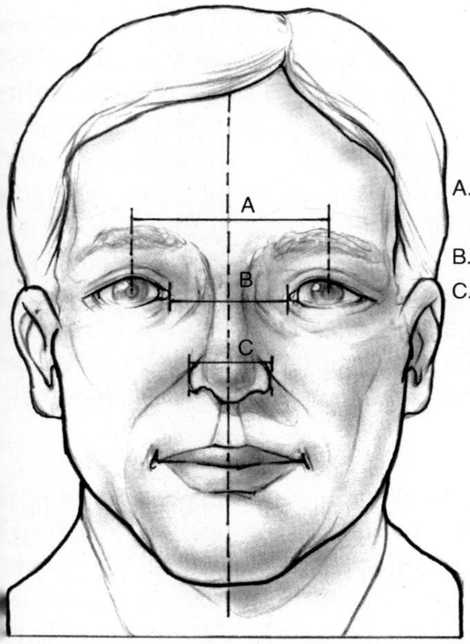

Thin-cut (1.5-mm) CT scans and 3-D reconstructions play an important role in defining the pattern and extent of injury. The surgeon must assess the cribriform plate, frontal recess/sinus involvement, orbital integrity, degree of naso-orbital-ethmoid complex comminution, and associated facial fractures. They are also very helpful in presurgical planning.

A. Normal interpupillary 60 mm
B. Telecanthus 45 mm
C. Normal intercanthal 30–35 mm

Fig. 70.19 Normal intercanthal distance is 30 to 35 mm. This is approximately one half the interpupillary distance and is equivalent to the width of the nasal base.

Classification

The anatomical focal point of naso-orbital-ethmoid reconstruction is the bony *central fragment* onto which the MCT inserts.[23] Markowitz et al devised a classification system describing the degree of bony injury[24] (**Fig. 70.20**). Type I fractures represent a single, noncomminuted central fragment without MCT disruption. Type II fractures involve comminution of the central fragment, but the MCT remains firmly attached to a definable segment of bone. Type III fractures are uncommon, and result in severe central fragment comminution with disruption of the MCT insertion. Each fracture type is subclassified as either unilateral or bilateral.

Treatment

Surgical Exposure

Naso-orbito-ethmoid complex injuries are the most challenging of all facial fractures, and surgical repair is often

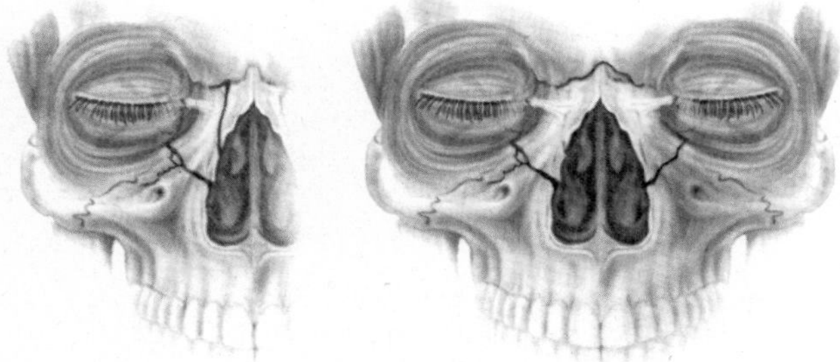

A

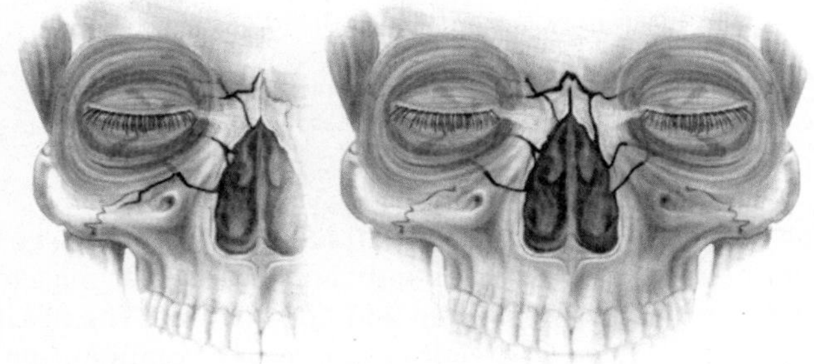

B

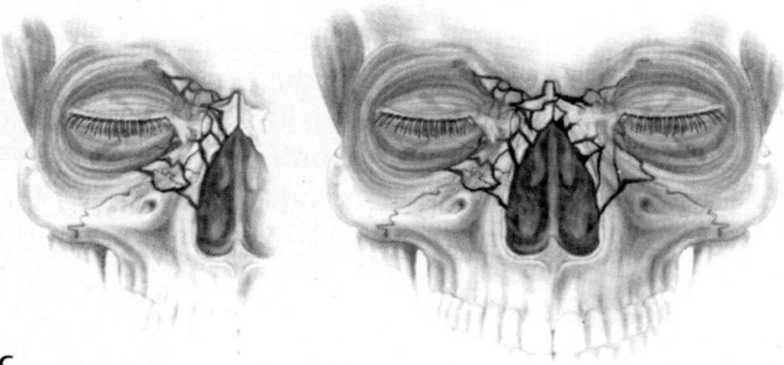

C

Fig. 70.20 Classification of naso-orbito-ethmoid complex fractures. (**A**) Type I injuries involve a single, noncomminuted central fragment without medial canthal tendon disruption (left-unilateral, right-bilateral), (**B**) Type II injuries involve comminution of the central fragment without medial canthal tendon disruption (left-unilateral, right-bilateral). (**C**) Severe central fragment comminution with medial canthal tendon disruption (left-unilateral, right-bilateral). (From Sargent LA, Rogers GF. Nasoethmoid orbital fractures: diagnosis and management. J Craniomaxillofac Trauma 1999;5(1):19–27. Reprinted by permission.)

complex and arduous. Inadequate exposure, imprecise fracture reduction, or poor MCT repair will almost certainly yield suboptimal results. Proper exposure can be obtained through coronal, transconjunctival, and sublabial incisions. Existing lacerations should be used to augment surgical access. Limiting the exposure to existing lacerations is usually inadequate. Glabellar and "open sky" incisions are generally avoided do to unfavorable external scars. The coronal incision should be elevated in a subperiosteal plane, taking care not to injure the supraorbital and supratrochlear nerves. The supraorbital/supratrochlear foramina should be released to obtain adequate exposure. This may require an osteotomy. A transconjunctival incision offers excellent exposure to the medial orbital rim, while minimizing the risk of postoperative lid malposition. Unfortunately, access to the frontal process of the maxilla is limited with this approach. A small (5-mm), medially based subciliary incision can be used to access this area for screw insertion. Finally, the sublabial incision allows access to the piriform aperture and frontal process of the maxilla. After the repair is complete, care must be taken to resuspend the temporal soft tissues and avoid postoperative soft tissue ptosis.

Fracture Reduction

Many authors recommend repair of associated facial fractures prior to naso-orbital-ethmoid complex repair. Reduction of maxillary and frontal sinus fractures often provides more accurate landmarks for subsequent naso-orbital-ethmoid fracture repair.

Type I Fractures

Nondisplaced single fragment injuries do not require surgical repair. Displaced type I fractures require superior (coronal) and inferior (transconjunctival and/or sublabial) exposure. Two separate microplates (1.0 to 1.3 mm) are applied from the frontal bone to the central fragment and from the maxilla to the central fragment (as previously mentioned, a 5-mm subciliary incision may be required to apply screw into the maxillary buttress plate). An accurate reduction must be maintained until both plates are placed or the lateral pull of the MCT may result in fracture displacement. Application of a single plate from the frontal bone, across the entire fragment and onto the maxilla, should be avoided. Such placement requires greater elevation of the periosteum on the central fragment, which may disrupt the MCT. Plates placed in this region may also widen the nasal root. Isolated superior or inferior displacement of the central fragment may require exposure and plating from only one direction. If there is significant suspicion of lacrimal injury, the lacrimal system should be cannulated, with the stent left in place for 1 to 3 months.

Type II Fractures

Comminuted fractures require more extensive surgical exposure, microplate reduction, and possible transnasal wiring. A subperiosteal dissection is used to locate, but not avulse, the MCT. If the central fragment is too small to be reduced and plated, transnasal wires must be used. Holes are drilled in the central fragment above and below the MCT. Both ends of a 28-gauge wire are passed from lateral to medial, leaving the free ends on the medial surface of

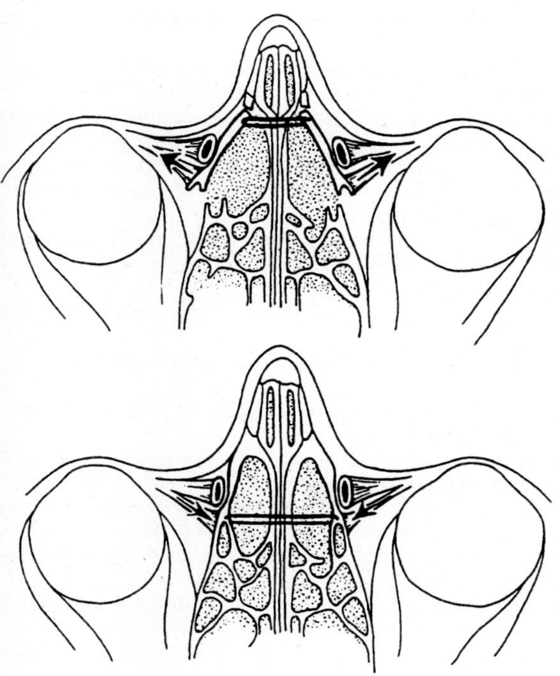

Fig. 70.21 (**A**) Placement of transnasal wires anterior to the lacrimal fossa results in rotation of the central fragment laterally, and postoperative telecanthus. (**B**) Placement of transnasal wires posterior and superior to the lacrimal fossa provides adequate support for the medial canthal tendon and avoids postoperative telecanthus. (From Markowitz BL, Manson PN, Sargent L, et al. Management of the medical canthal tendon in nasoethmoid orbital fractures: the importance of the central fragment in classification and treatment. Plast Reconstr Surg 1991;87(5):843–853. Reprinted by permission.)

the central fragment. The free ends are twisted tightly on the medial aspect of the central fragment. Once the central fragment is controlled with the wire, a contralateral hole is drilled posterior and superior to the contralateral lacrimal fossa and below the frontoethmoid suture line (to avoid intracranial injury) (**Fig. 70.17**). The contralateral holes ***must*** be drilled ***posterior and superior*** to the lacrimal fossa. Transnasal wires placed *anterior* to the lacrimal fossa will result in lateral rotation of the central fragment and iatrogenic telecanthus[25] (**Fig. 70.21A**). Wires placed appropriately will pull the canthus medially without rotation (**Fig. 70.21B**). A 14-guage spinal needle is then passed retrograde (from uninjured to injured side), through the ethmoid complex, toward the central fragment. The wires are passed through the lumen of the needle, and the needle is removed. The wires are then tightened while the central fragment is medialized with external pressure. The wire is then secured on a miniscrew previously placed on the superior orbital rim while maintaining the reduction. Some degree of bony overcorrection is desirable. It is difficult if not impossible to overcorrect the reduction. The transnasal wires can be joined in the midline for patients with bilateral injuries.

Type III Fractures

Type III fractures are associated with more severe trauma and may require primary bone grafting. There is greater risk of lacrimal duct injury. Wide surgical exposure is obtained and the MCT remnant is identified. A 3- to 5-mm horizontal skin incision just medial to the medial canthus can be used to identify and secure the MCT. A 28-gauge wire suture is then passed through the stump of the MCT twice. The wire is then passed through two drill holes in the central bone fragment, and twisted securely (see "Type II Fractures"). If the central bone fragment cannot be identified, an outer-table calvarial bone graft can be used instead. The wires are passed transnasally and fixated to the contralateral orbital rim. The transnasal wires can be joined in the midline for patients with bilateral injuries.

Type III injuries resulting in significant loss of nasal projection should be repaired with an onlay calvarial bone graft. After MCT reconstruction is complete, an outer-table calvarial bone graft should be fashioned to augment the nasal dorsum. The graft should be positioned to reconstruct a normal nasofrontal angle and extend as far as is necessary to provide a normal nasal contour. An open rhinoplasty approach can be very helpful for insertion and postioning of the graft. A horizontal groove should be drilled into the glabella to accept the superior aspect of the graft. A miniplate or two position screws are placed to cantilever the graft off the frontal bone[26] (**Fig. 70.22**). The inferior aspect of the graft should be inserted below the intermediate crura of the lower lateral cartilages.

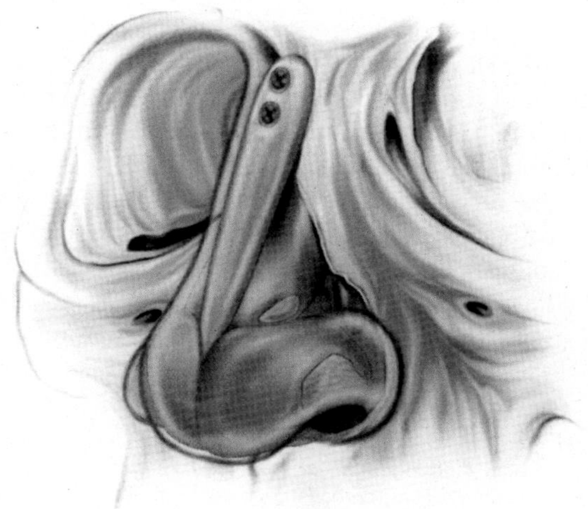

Fig. 70.22 Cantilevered calvarial bone graft fixated with two position screws. A horizontal groove should be drilled into the frontal bone at the superior aspect of the graft to accept the bone graft and reproduce an aesthetic nasofrontal angle. The bone graft should extend as far as is necessary to reconstruct the preinjury contour. (From Sargent LA, Rogers GF. Nasoethmoid orbital fractures: diagnosis and management. J Craniomaxillofac Trauma 1999;5(1):19–27.)

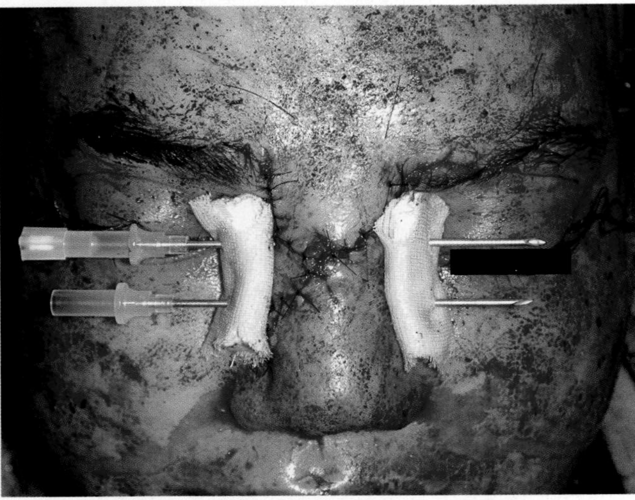

Fig. 70.23 Clinical photograph of nasal bolsters being applied to the lateral nasal side wall. Nasal bolsters help redrape the soft tissues and avoid postoperative hematoma and excessive soft tissue edema.

External bolsters are required for type II and III injuries to prevent hematoma formation and restore a normal nasal contour. Two-millimeter-thick lead plates (or thermaplast nasal splints) padded with several layers of Xeroform (Invacare, New York, NY) gauze are applied to the lateral nasal side wall. Fourteen-gauge angiocatheter needles (without the external plastic catheter) are passed transcutaneously across the nasal base at the level of the medial canthus, as well as at the inferior aspect of the nasal bones (**Fig. 70.23**).[24] One 26-guage wire is passed through each needle and bolster. The wires are twisted to apply mild pressure and reduce soft tissue edema. The underlying tissue should be closely observed to avoid tissue necrosis. The bolsters are removed at 7 to 10 days.

Disruption of the delicate ethmoid complex and comminution of the nasal bones can make the repair of naso-orbital-ethmoid fractures extremely difficult. These injuries often test the capabilities of even the most experienced surgeons. To obtain an aesthetic surgical result, the surgeon must meticulously identify, accurately reduce, and fixate the central fragment. Special attention must also be focused on the overlying soft tissue to avoid hematoma, induration, and telecanthus.

References

1. Donald PJ. Frontal sinus and nasofrontoethmoidal complex fractures, otorhinolaryngology self-instructional packages: Alexandria, VA: AAO/NH Surgery Foundation; 1980
2. Ritter TN. The Paranasal Sinues: Anatomy and Surgical Technique. 2nd ed. St. Louis: CV Mosby; 1978
3. Rohrich RJ, Hollier LH. Management of frontal sinus fractures, changing concepts. Clin Plast Surg 1992;19(1):219–231
4. Anon JB, Rontal M, Zinreich SJ. Anatomy of the Paranasal Sinuses. New York: Thieme; 1996
5. Stammberger HR, Kennedy DW. Paranasal sinuses: anatomic terminology and nomenclature. The anatomic terminology group. Ann Otol Rhinol Laryngol Suppl;1995;167:7–16
6. Mosher HP, Judd DK. An analysis of seven cases of osteomyelitis of frontal bone complicating frontal sinusitis. Laryngoscope 1933;43:153
7. Nahum AM. The biomechanics of maxillofacial trauma. Clin Plast Surg 1975;2(1):59–64
8. May M, Ogura JH, Schramm V. Nasofrontal duct in frontal sinus fractures. Arch Otolaryngol 1970;92:534–538
9. Donald PJ. Frontal sinus ablation by cranialization: a report of 21 cases. Arch Otolaryngol 1982;108:590
10. Wallis A, Donald PJ. Frontal sinus fractures: a review of 72 cases. Laryngoscope 1988;98(6):593–598
11. Grossman DG, Archer SM, Arosarena O. Management of frontal sinus fractures: a review of 96 cases. Lanjgoscope 2006;116:1357–1362
12. Heller EM, Jacobs JB, Holliday RA. Evaluation of the frontonasal duct in frontal sinus fractures. Head Neck 1989;11:46
13. Donald PJ, Gluckman JL, Rice DH, eds. The Sinuses. New York: Raven Press; 1995
14. Heckler FR. Discussion of frontal sinus fractures. Guidelines to Management of Plastic Reconstructive Surgery 1987;80:509
15. Smith TL, Han JK, Loehrl TA, Rhee JS. Endoscopic management of the frontal recess in frontal sinus fractures: a shift in the paradigm? Laryngoscope 2002;112(5):784–790
16. Luce EA. Frontal sinus fractures. Plast Reconstr Surg 1987;80(4):500–505
17. Forrest CR. Application of endoscopic-assisted minimal-access techniques in orbitozygomatic complex, orbital floor, and frontal sinus fractures. J Craniomaxillofac Trauma 1999;5(4):7–12
18. Graham HD III, Spring P. Endoscopic repair of frontal sinus fracture: case report. J Craniomaxillofac Trauma 1996;2(4):52–55
19. Lappert PW, Lee JW. Treatment of an isolated outer table frontal sinus fracture using endoscopic reduction and fixation. Plast Reconstr Surg 1998;102:1642–1645
20. Strong EB, Buchalter GM, Moulthrop T. Endoscopic repair of isolated anterior table frontal sinus fractures. Arch Facial Plast Surg 2003;5:514–521
21. Sykes JM, Donald PJ. Frontal sinus and nasofrontoethmoidal complex fractures. In: Papel ID, Nachlas N, eds. Facial Plastic and Reconstructive Surgery. Hanover, MD: Mosby-Yearbook, Inc.; 1980:485–495
22. McGraw-Wall B. Frontal sinus fractures. Facial Plast Surg 1998;14(1):59–66
23. Leipziper LS, Manson PN. Nasoethmoid orbital fractures: current concepts and management principles. Clin Plast Surg 1992;19:167–193
24. Markowitz BL, Manson PN, Sargent L, et al. Management of the medical canthal tendon in nasoethmoid orbital fractures. The importance of the central fragment in classification and treatment. Plast Reconstr Surg 1991;87(5):
25. Sargent LA, Rogers GF. Nasoethmoid orbital fractures: diagnosis and management. J Craniomaxillofac Trauma 1999;5(1):19–27
26. Hoffman JF. Naso-orbital-ethmoid complex fracture management. Facial Plast Surg 1998;14(1):67–76

71 Le Fort Fractures (Maxillary Fractures)

Timothy D. Doerr and Robert H. Mathog

Recent improvements in diagnostic imaging and craniofacial plating systems have led to significant advances in the management of midface fractures. With high-resolution computerized tomography (CT) allowing precise diagnosis, and low profile titanium hardware permitting stable fixation, midface fractures can now be managed in a single operation. These contemporary reconstructive techniques allow for rapid restoration of form and function with minimal treatment morbidity.

Etiology and Epidemiology

Maxillary fractures compose 10 to 20% of all facial fractures. These injuries usually result from motor vehicle accidents, interpersonal violence, or falls. The contribution from each category varies with the population sampled. In general, males predominate with fractures common in the second through fourth decades.[1] An expanding and increasingly active senior population is expected to add to facial fractures in the older age groups.[2] By comparison, children seldom sustain midface fractures. A proportionately larger mandible and frontal bone combined with a flexible facial skeleton, underdeveloped sinuses, and unerupted dentition protect against these fractures.[3,4] Further reductions in complex maxillary injuries is likely to be brought about by mandated improvements in automobile safety equipment.

Maxillary fractures are often associated with other bodily injuries. Serious intracranial injury occurs in up to 38% and serious ophthalmologic injury in 28% of midface fractures.[5–7] Trauma involving the cardiovascular, abdominal and orthopedic systems is also common especially in high-energy injury mechanisms.

Classification and Pathophysiology

The maxilla is the principle bone of the midface. It contains a large air-filled sinus cavity and fractures with far less force than what is required in the adjacent facial skeleton. The bony architecture of the midface is arranged in a latticework of vertical buttresses and horizontal beams with the vertical buttresses transferring masticatory loads from the mandible to the skull base (**Fig. 71.1**). This structural framework is also theorized to absorb impact forces and thereby avoid injury of the cranial and orbital contents. Thus impact forces directed to the midface can result in significant facial fractures with far less intracranial injury than the impact kinetics would otherwise predict.[8]

Fracture patterns of the facial skeleton are well described in the trauma literature with the most lasting contribution from René Le Fort. In his classic 1901 work, Le Fort described a series of characteristic fracture patterns produced in cadaver skulls.[9] This "linea minoros resistentiae" remains the basis of most contemporary classification systems. Traditionally, the maxillary fractures are classified as Le Fort I, Le Fort II, Le Fort III, segmental, palatal, and medial maxillary fractures.

Although pure Le Fort fractures are rarely encountered in clinical practice, Le Fort's original work provides an excellent description of the fracture patterns, which is invaluable in understanding the degree and level of injury. The Le Fort I, or Guèrin fracture, is a low horizontal fracture between the maxilla and palate/alveolar arch complex. It is usually the result of direct anterior-posterior impacts low on the midface that produce fractures of the paired nasomaxillary (medial) and zygomaticomaxillary (lateral) vertical buttresses. The fractures can continue

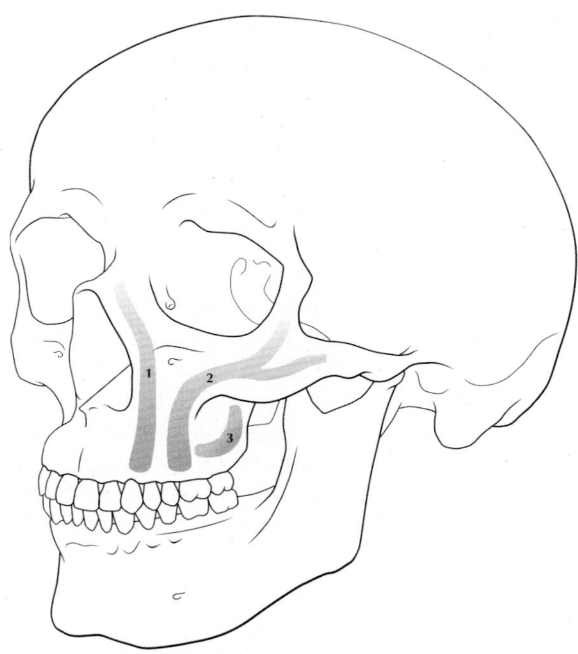

Fig. 71.1 Buttresses of the facial skeleton: (1) medial buttress, (2) lateral buttress, (3) posterior buttress.

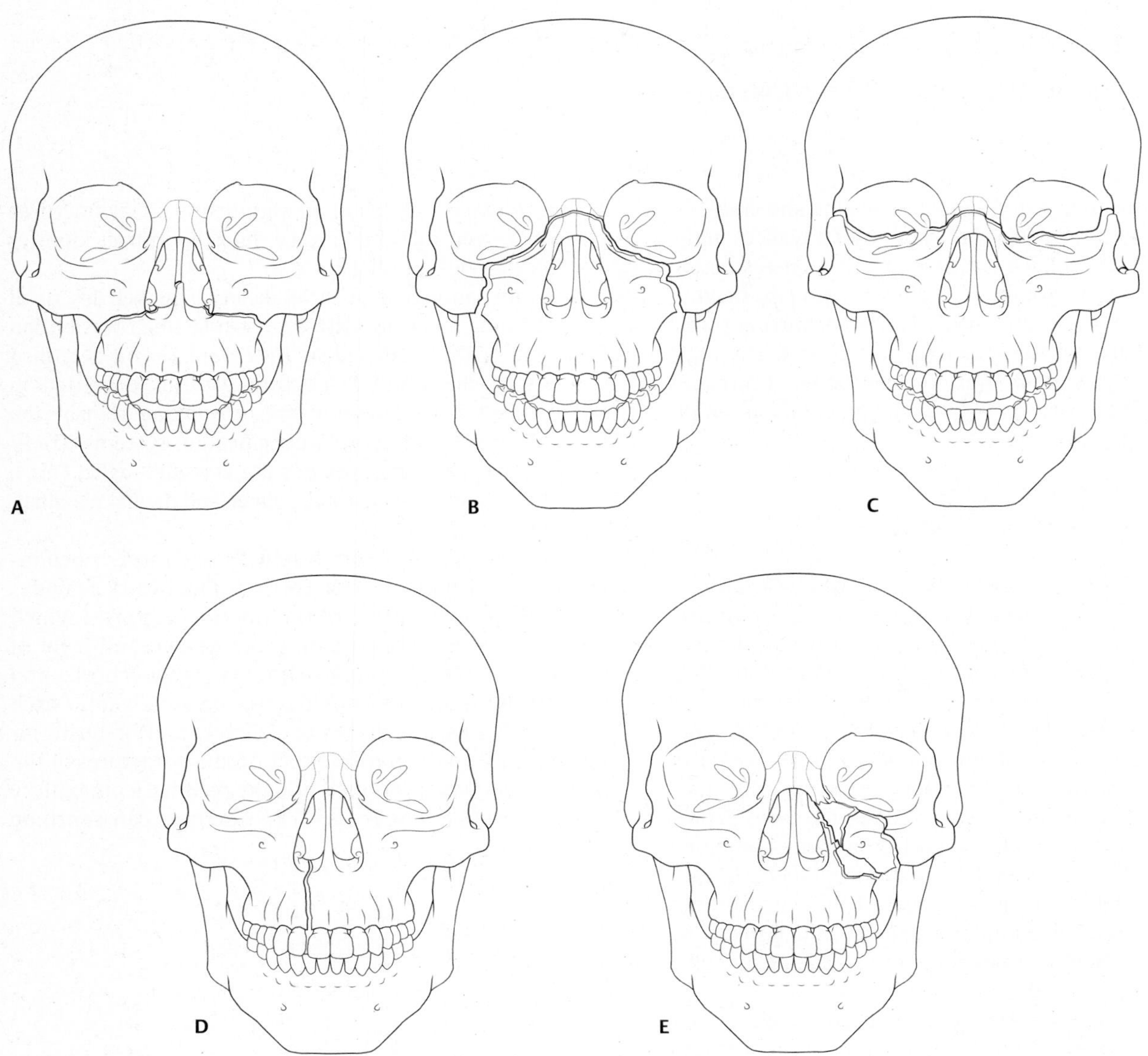

Fig. 71.2 Classification of maxillary fractures: (**A**) Le Fort I; (**B**) Le Fort II; (**C**) Le Fort III; (**D**) palatal split; (**E**) medial maxillary.

posteriorly through the pterygoid plates or between the palate and maxilla (**Fig. 71.2A**). A Le Fort I pattern is seen in ~30% of all Le Fort fractures.[1]

The Le Fort II, or pyramidal fracture, is the most common Le Fort fracture pattern seen in 60% of cases.[1] This injury can result from either direct horizontal forces to the midface, or from impacts to the chin point that are transmitted from the mandible to the midface. Classically, the fracture starts at the nasal bones and crosses the frontal process of the maxilla and lacrimal bones. Changing direction, the fracture descends through the floor of the orbit, infraorbital rim and lateral maxillary sinus wall. The Le Fort II often extends through the pterygoid plates (**Fig. 71.2B**).

The Le Fort III fracture, or craniofacial disjunction, is a relatively uncommon midface fracture. It is usually the result of forces directed obliquely to the vertical buttresses and is frequently seen in conjunction with other facial fractures. With a high-velocity impact mechanism there is significant comminution and, often, serious intracranial injury. The Le Fort III fracture typically passes through the nasal–frontal suture, frontal process of the maxilla, lacrimal bones, ethmoid sinus, and lamina papyracea before crossing the orbital floor to the inferior orbital fissure. From this point, the fracture extends in three directions: (1) across the lateral orbital wall through the zygomaticofrontal suture; (2) through the zygomatic arch; and (3) through the pterygoid plates thereby creating a separation of the midface from the skull base (**Fig. 71.2C**).

Palatal split fractures begin anteriorly at the incisor space and extend posteriorly. The fractures may be either a true sagittal split, which is more common in children, or a parasagittal fracture, which is more common in adults.[10] Although palatal fractures may be isolated, they usually accompany other midface fractures. A segmental or alveolar fracture is a fracture of the alveolar ridge. It can be anterior involving the incisors, or posterolateral involving the molars. Medial maxillary fractures result from impacts of small objects to the area between the nose and the cheek. The frontal process of the maxilla and usually the nasal bones are involved (**Fig. 71.2D,E**).

Despite the descriptive nature of the Le Fort classification system, most midface fractures are more complex, possessing components of several Le Fort injuries with differences in the degree of injury between sides. Furthermore, there is often comminution and displacement of the fracture that is not addressed in the Le Fort classification system. Because these complicated fractures are inadequately or inaccurately described using the Le Fort system other authors have suggested modifications. We now employ a schema that avoids the deficiencies of Le Fort's original classifications. This system uses a skeletal matrix of vertical buttresses and horizontal beams to simply and precisely describe all fracture patterns (**Fig. 71.3**). The system allows for easy communication between diagnosticians and surgeons so that injuries can be accurately assessed and repaired.[11]

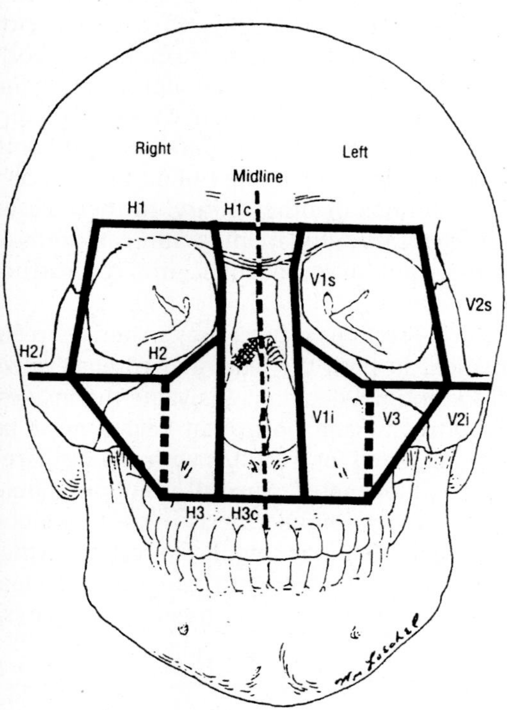

Fig. 71.3 Facial skeleton matrix: frontonasomaxillary (v1), frontozygomaticomaxillary (v2), pterygomaxillary (v3), supraorbital rims and glabella (h1), orbital rims and zygomatic arches (h2), alveolar process of maxilla (h3). (From Donat, Endress C, Mathog RH, et al. Facial fracture classification according to skeletal support mechanisms. Arch Otolaryngol Head Neck Surg. 1998;124:1308.)

To manage fractures of the midface a thorough analysis of the buttresses and beam framework is required. The vertical supports of the midface are three paired buttresses—the zygomaticomaxillary (lateral), nasomaxillary (medial) and pterygomaxillary (posterior)—along with a weaker, unpaired, midline, septovomerian buttress. These vertical supports are joined by less rigid, horizontal beams. These beams—the alveolus, orbital floor and rims, and supraorbital bar—collectively reinforce the vertical buttresses as well as maintain the vertical and lateral dimensions of the face.

Blows to the midface, especially high-energy impacts, result in a buckling and collapse of the midface structures. Therefore, repair of both the vertical buttresses and horizontal beams is critical to restore facial appearance and function.

Clinical Evaluation and Diagnosis

Facial trauma patients present a unique set of challenges for the clinician. Frequently, these patients sustain multiple-system traumas including intracranial injury with altered levels of consciousness. It is also common for more acute life-threatening conditions to delay a complete evaluation of facial injury for hours and even days. Because these potentially life-threatening injuries do occur, the facial trauma patient must be managed with a standardized approach. Use of an ABC (airway, breathing, and circulation) algorithm prioritizes the emergency intervention that is a prerequisite for facial skeleton evaluation.

Bleeding frequently complicates midfacial injuries. The bleeding may be minor, resulting from the disruption of septal, nasal, or sinus mucosa. Alternatively, it may be profuse from skull base vessels and require nasal packing or even temporary fracture reduction. In rare circumstances intravascular embolization of skull base vessels is required to control life-threatening hemorrhage.

Although difficult in the acute setting, the examiner needs to perform as complete a history and physical exam as conditions allow. The premorbid dental occlusion and any history of prior trauma are of particular importance. In addition, a brief ocular history will help avoid confusion if decreased vision is noted later.

Examination should include inspection and palpation of the entire facial skeleton. Despite the excellent imaging available, assessment of the mobility and stability of facial structures is only made through a physical examination. Reliance on radiological findings without an accurate clinical correlation will lead to treatment errors.

The examination begins with a visual inspection of the face for symmetry and proportion. Midface trauma usually produces significant soft tissue edema and ecchymoses that distort facial appearance. The forces of midface trauma usually drive the maxilla posteroinferiorly along the slope of the skull base creating a flat or "pan" face appearance. In other instances, separation at the frontozygomatic suture or an inferiorly displaced chin gives an elongated facial appearance. An extension of the injury to the orbits produces periobital edema and can result in abnormal globe position. Disruption of the medial canthi can produce telecanthus, whereas displacement of the zygomaticomaxillary complex can leave malar depression.

Palpation of the skeleton follows inspection. With a lower Le Fort injury there can be gingival buccal sulcus crepitance, or subcutaneous emphysema. Le Fort II fractures produce step-off deformities of the orbital rim and can have V_2 paresthesia. Le Fort III fractures often involve a diastasis and step deformity of the frontozygomatic suture and zygomatic arch. In medial maxillary fractures, the lateral nasal and medial maxillary bone are depressed, producing a palpable deformity.

Next, the examiner makes a careful assessment of the mandibular and maxillary dental relationship. A displaced maxilla will cause premature contact of the molars and an open-bite deformity. If there is lateral displacement a cross-bite can be seen. Additional occlusal disturbances are apparent in alveolar fractures and palatal split fractures. The occlusal evaluation is especially critical in nonmobile or minimally displaced fractures where few clinical signs are present, and a subtle malocclusion may be the only indicator of fracture.

The final step in evaluating maxillary trauma is an assessment of mobility. The mobility of the midface is best determined by using the thumb and forefinger to grasp the premaxilla while the other hand palpates the infraorbital rims. With a Le Fort I injury only the premaxilla is mobile, whereas a Le Fort II fractures separates at the infraorbital rims, which will move with the premaxilla. In a Le Fort III injury, the premaxilla, malar bones, and remainder of the facial bones are mobile at the nasofrontal and zygomaticofrontal sutures. Although clinical mobility is evidence of a maxillary fracture, nonmobile fractures are seen in 9% of Le Fort injuries.[12]

Ophthalmologic Evaluation

The prominent position of the orbits within the midfacial skeleton is responsible for the high incidence of ocular injuries with maxillofacial trauma. Eye injuries occur in as many as 90% of midface fracture patients, with vision threatening injuries (including hyphema, retrobulbar hemorrhage, and traumatic optic neuropathy) in 12% of cases.[8] When there is concern about decreased vision an ophthalmologic evaluation is needed. The early diagnosis of a serious eye injury allows for prompt treatment that may preserve sight. In addition it helps avoid fracture repairs that could threaten vision. Certainly the deterioration of vision following surgical repair demands an immediate ophthalmology assessment.

Neurological Evaluation

Neurological injuries are common in midface trauma, with most fracture patients having at least mild closed head injury. Serious intracranial injury occurs in up to 38% of midface fractures and is more common in injuries caused by motor vehicle accidents.[5,6] Those trauma patients presenting with loss of consciousness or altered sensorium need a CT scan of the head to properly evaluate for serious intracranial injury. Even with a normal head CT, clinical closed-head injury can produce long-term sequelae that may warrant evaluation and follow-up with a neurologist or neurotrauma specialist.

Radiological Evaluation

CT of the facial skeleton is the exam of choice in evaluating maxillofacial trauma. Ideally, all patients with suspected trauma should undergo scanning in both the axial and coronal planes with an appropriate bone window. This can be done with a head CT without adding significant imaging time. Many patients are unable to undergo coronal scanning because of intubation, cervical spine precautions or other injury. In these cases available contemporary software programs can produce excellent high-resolution coronal or sagittal reconstructive images.

Although thicker sections may serve as an initial screen, 2- to 3-mm slices in both the axial and coronal views are required for optimal detail. In analyzing the images, the vertical buttresses and horizontal beams must be systematically inspected for fractures with any displacement or comminution noted. Special attention should also be directed to the orbit and the skull base for globe or intracranial injury that may complicate repair. Further information can be obtained with three-dimensional reconstructed images and is beneficial in complicated cases.

Treatment

Objective

The reconstructive surgeon's primary objective is the restoration of form and function. In maxillary fractures it is critical to reestablish the projection and height of the face and to re-create the pretraumatic occlusion. In addition to treating the bony framework, the surgeon must also effectively manage the overlying soft tissue. The judicious use of incisions, careful handling of tissues and resuspension of the midface soft tissue are all important in minimizing postoperative complications. Optimal outcomes in maxillary fracture repair require a well-developed but adaptable surgical plan that encompasses anesthesia, exposure, reduction, and fixation.

Preoperative Assessment and Preparation

When initially seen, the maxillofacial trauma patient must be evaluated for any life-threatening process. The consistent use of the ABC algorithm will prevent the overlooking or compounding of existing injuries. Initially each patient needs a careful assessment of the airway. With the loss of consciousness, intracranial injury, or hemorrhage an artificial airway may be required to assure adequate oxygen delivery. If the maxilla is pushed back and blood and secretions obstruct the pharynx the airway can be improved with suctioning and temporary reduction of the maxilla. If this maneuver is not effective in relieving the airway problem then an oropharyngeal or nasal airway may be required. When any injury to the cervical spine is suspected, it is critical to protect the cervical spine and maintain appropriate precautions regardless of the method used to establish the airway.

Endotracheal intubation, when necessary, should be performed by a skilled anesthetist. Although there is some concern with nasal intubation in midfacial trauma, most authors report that it can be done safely. Nasal intubation is advantageous in that occlusion can be established without interference from the tube; however it can make reduction of nasal and maxillary fractures difficult. Oral intubation is simpler and less traumatic, but it can potentially interfere with occlusion. To avoid this, the tube can usually be placed behind the maxillary tuberosity and should not interfere with intermaxillary fixation. When conventional routes of intubation will not allow adequate fracture reduction and repair, the submental intubation technique does allow for intermaxillary fixation and avoids a tracheostomy.[13] The tracheostomy or cricothyroidotomy however, remains a safe alternative and should be considered if there is any question about establishing or maintaining an airway.

Timing of Surgery

The timing of midfacial fractures repair has moved toward earlier intervention. The classic dictum was to wait for the resolution of swelling, which would allow more accurate restoration of landmarks and presumably better surgical results. However, early intervention with open reduction and direct rigid fixation enables precise repair of fractures without the bone edge resorption or fibrous ingrowth seen with delayed repair. Additionally, authors report earlier function, less infection, decreased scarring, and fewer overall complications with prompt repair. There are also significant savings in hospitalization costs if surgery is not delayed.

Several other factors may influence the timing of surgery. Midfacial fracture patients often have concomitant intracranial and systemic trauma that can delay or interfere with plans for reconstruction. There has been debate whether early repair of fractures is safe in a patient with intracranial injury. The focus concerns the general anesthesia, supine positioning, and intraoperative fluid shifts that may exacerbate cerebral edema. Derdyn and colleagues addressed this question in reviewing clinical outcomes in 49 patients with facial fractures and significant intracranial injury. They found that patients with low Glasgow coma scale scores (<6), intracranial hemorrhage, or shift of midline cerebral structures did poorly. However, early surgical intervention did not negatively impact outcomes provided the preoperative intracranial pressure was less than 15 mm Hg.[14] The experiences of other investigators[5,15] also support safe early fracture repair in head-injury patients provided that they are carefully managed with close general surgical and neurosurgical support. In some instances where neurosurgical procedures are required, it may be safer to perform the facial fracture repairs under the same anesthesia rather than incur the risks of a second trip to the operating room.

In some circumstances early surgical intervention should be avoided. Any cervical spine injury must be thoroughly evaluated and stabilized before facial fracture repair. Likewise, any ocular injury where vision is threatened or could be threatened by surgical manipulation must be delayed. When it is necessary to postpone surgery, a primary repair can be successfully completed up to 3 weeks after injury.

Surgical Technique

Exposure

The bones of the facial skeleton can be exposed through concealed surgical incisions that produce little visible facial scars. Extended bicoronal, midfacial degloving, and transconjunctival incisions will allow accurate reduction of all the vertical buttresses and horizontal beams of the midface. The choice of incisions is dictated by the degree of maxillary injury, and by any extension of fractures into the zygomatic and naso-orbital-ethmoid complexes. In general, a Le Fort I fracture or isolated alveolar fractures can be managed through a wide sublabial incision.

A Le Fort II fractures may require the addition of a periorbital incision (subciliary, subtarsal, or transconjunctival). A bicoronal incision is usually necessary to expose the frontozygomatic and frontal nasal projections in Le Fort III fractures. Although these extended access approaches provide ample exposure to the facial skeleton, the surgeon should not ignore the traditional limited external incisions that offer direct exposure to the fracture sites. These incisions can be very well suited for fractures where minimal plating is required.

Reduction

Maxillary fractures may be loose, or impacted into the adjoining craniofacial skeleton. In many cases the fractured maxilla is pushed posteriorly along the incline of the skull base resulting in a face that appears retruded and lengthened. This creates an open-bite occlusion from premature molar contact. If there is a lateral displacement of the maxilla, an asymmetric deformity and cross-bite are seen.

When the fracture is loose, it can be reduced with digital or hook traction. In these instances an index finger or hook-like instrument (Army-Navy retractor or large bone hook) is placed behind the soft palate and used to pull the palate forward. The maxilla can then be manipulated into anatomical position.

When the maxilla is impacted into the adjacent bone greater force is needed to disimpact the segment. The Rowe forceps are designed for this task. These forceps have a right and left handle with both a straight and curved blade. The straight blades are placed along the nasal floor and the curved blade fits against the roof of the hard palate. With a handle in each hand, the surgeon rotates the maxilla into position vertically, then horizontally (**Fig. 71.4**). Brisk bleeding can accompany this maneuver but usually subsides in a few minutes. If the maxilla cannot be properly reduced with these techniques, a completion maxillary osteotomy may be necessary. After appropriate reduction the fractures can be fixated.

Fixation

Fixation of midface fractures has evolved with advances in plating systems. Previously the treatment included delayed repair through small incision with minimal exposure of fracture elements. Stabilization was with wires and/or external suspension with prolonged periods of intermaxillary fixation. Disappointment with suboptimal results led to our current practices. Superior outcomes are achieved by exposing, then precisely reducing and rigidly fixing the supporting bony buttresses of the midface. The use of rigid fixation provides stability with bone-to-bone contact that allows the midfacial bones to heal more rapidly with new bone formation and a true osseous union.[16]

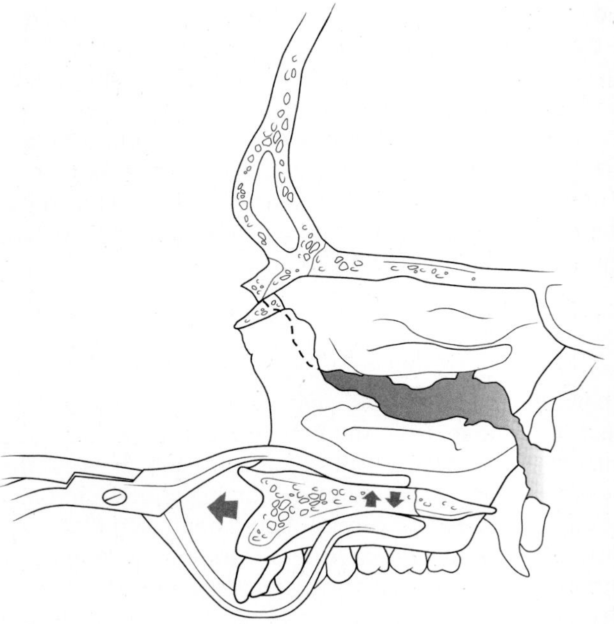

Fig. 71.4 Reduction of a maxillary fracture using Rowe forceps.

Most injuries are now managed using titanium plating systems. These thin, low-profile plates range in thickness from 0.8 to 2.0 mm and provide rigid (or more accurately semi-rigid) fixation with minimal tissue reactivity. The plates are secured with self-tapping screws. These plate and screw systems offer distinct biomechanical advantages with a superior ability to resist translation and rotation. Properly positioned plates with the appropriate number of screws on each side of the fracture line allow load-sharing between the plate and the bone. This results in less hardware failure and limits the need for postoperative intermaxillary fixation.[17]

More recently, plates made of bioresorbable polymers have been developed for midfacial fracture repair. These systems function as well as their metal counterparts provided there is not significant bony comminution. These plates appear to be well suited for pediatric fractures where the presence of permanent plating may interfere with facial growth.

Repair of Specific Maxillary Fractures

Le Fort I Fractures

Minimally displaced Le Fort I fractures can be reduced and stabilized with intermaxillary fixation. Elastic bands provide traction that maintains proper occlusion while the fracture lines heal. When there is displacement or mobility of the maxilla an open approach is necessary. Initially the occlusion is set using one of several techniques of intermaxillary fixation (ivy loops, arch bars, or cortical fixation screw)

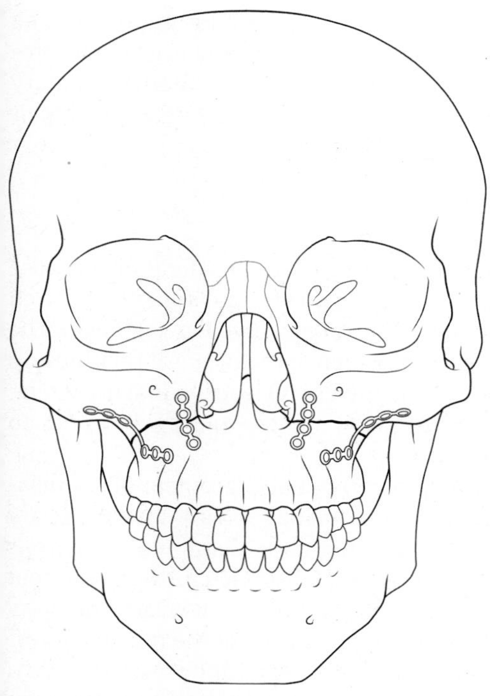

Fig. 71.5 Repair of a Le Fort I fracture by plating the medial and/or lateral buttresses.

The fractures are first exposed and then the lateral and medial buttresses plated using 1.5- to 2.0-mm miniplate. The plates should be oriented along the load-bearing pathways with ideally three screws on each side of fracture (**Fig. 71.5**).

The duration of postoperative intermaxillary fixation is dictated both by the degree of fracture and the stability achieved with repair. In cases where there is precise anatomical reduction with careful attention to the intraoperative occlusion postoperative intermaxillary fixation may be avoided. When there is comminution or questions about the established intraoperative occlusion the intermaxillary fixation hardware is maintained and the patient is followed closely for several weeks postoperatively. With careful follow-up occlusal problems can be identified and potentially corrected early. Frequently, reapplying elastic bands will be sufficient to direct the patient back into proper occlusion. Failing to correct even a subtle malocclusion can lead to problems with temporomandibular joint dysfunction. However, it is critical to recognize that intermaxillary fixation will not compensate for malocclusion resulting from inaccurate reduction or fixation.

An edentulous Le Fort I fracture that is minimally displaced and reasonably stable may be reduced without fixation. If there is displacement or appreciable mobility, the fracture should be plated. The techniques are generally the same as those for patients with teeth, although thinner atrophic bone and reduced masticatory forces permit the use of lower-profile plates.

Le Fort II Fractures

Nearly all Le Fort II fractures require an open reduction and fixation of the lateral buttress and possibly the infraorbital rims. After the proper occlusion is established the midface is exposed including the fractured zygomaticomaxillary buttresses. Additional exposure of the nasomaxillary buttresses may be needed and can be obtained through a periorbital incision that also allows exploration of the orbital floor. The lateral buttresses are repaired using miniplates directed along the pattern of flow (**Fig. 71.6**). In most instances the bony fracture segments are available for fixation; however, with severe comminution or bone loss, bone grafting may be required to reestablish the vertical buttress. If the superior portion of the fracture remains unstable, small plate fixation of the orbital rim is necessary. It is usually not necessary to plate the high nasomaxillary buttress. The guidelines for postoperative intermaxillary fixation are similar to those of Le Fort I injury.

In edentulous Le Fort II injury, the preferred repair is an open reduction with miniplate fixation. In rare instances when the fracture involves the alveolus and accurate reduction is uncertain, dentures or occlusal splints with arch bars can be used to establish intermaxillary fixation.

Le Fort III Fractures

Forces producing Le Fort III fractures are significant and the resultant injury is usually a complex maxillary fracture

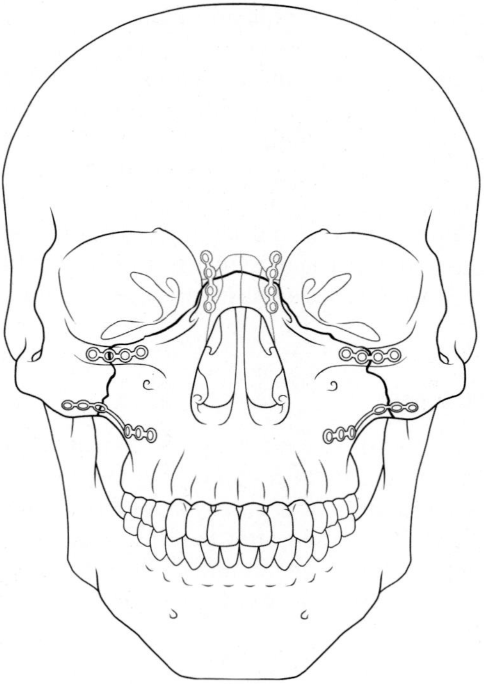

Fig. 71.6 Repair of a Le Fort II fracture by plating the lateral buttresses and orbital rim.

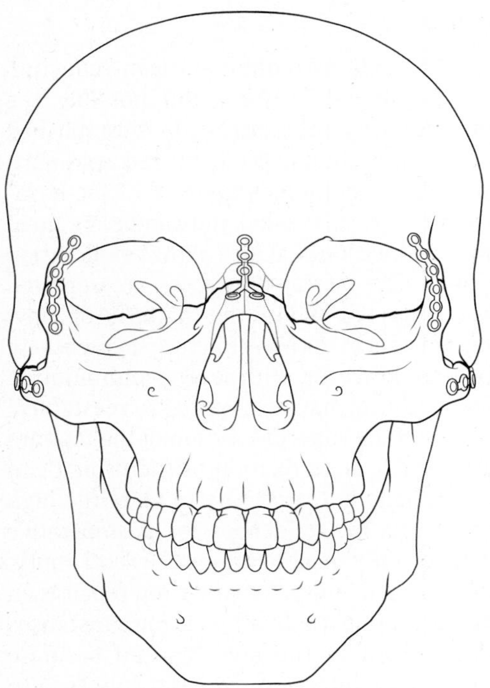

Fig. 71.7 Repair of a Le Fort III fracture by plating the nasofrontal suture, frontozygomatic process, and zygomatic arch.

requiring open reduction and direct fixation. Rarely there is a clean Le Fort III fracture with minimal displacement where occlusal fixation followed by plating of the buttresses through limited incisions is sufficient. Most Le Fort III injuries require wide surgical exposure with a bicoronal incision being used to access the zygomaticofrontal suture, zygomatic arch, and nasofrontal projections. After establishing occlusion, 1.0- to 1.5-mm plates are used to stabilize the superior components of the medial and lateral buttresses (**Fig. 71.7**). It is important to assess the zygomatic arch and restore its alignment when displaced to properly set the horizontal position and projection of the midface. The management of Le Fort III fractures in an edentulous patient is identical to a dentate counterpart.

Segmental Fractures

In segmental fractures where teeth are present an arch bar may be sufficient to stabilize the fracture. Alternatively this injury can be treated using a horizontally placed miniplate. If stability remains in question after plating, then intermaxillary fixation should be maintained. For edentulous segmental fractures miniplate fixation is the best.

Medial Maxillary Fractures

Fractures of the medial maxilla are best approached through a midfacial degloving. The nasomaxillary buttress should be stabilized with a low profile miniplate. The nasal fracture will require reduction, and if severely comminuted may require microplating or interfragmentary wiring. A periorbital incision may also be needed to repair the orbital rim or medial orbital wall.

Palatal Fractures

Palatal fractures deserve special consideration because this injury produces an irregular maxillary alveolar arch that allows rotation of the dental alveolar segments. The inability to properly reestablish the occlusal relationship between the upper and lower jaw leads to malalignment. It is therefore essential to restore the palatal arch to obtain proper occlusion.

If there is a fracture without displacement of the palatal arch, the injury can be managed with intermaxillary fixation. When the palatal arch is disrupted or there is injury to the adjacent vertical buttresses, further treatment is required. A horizontal plate placed beneath the nasal spine is used to join the two halves of the maxilla. Intermaxillary fixation is then established and when necessary, the medial and lateral buttresses are plated to support the posterior portion of the hard palate. Alternatively, sagittal and parasagittal palatal fractures can be managed by direct intraoral plating (**Fig. 71.8**). The direct plating of these fractures reestablishes palatal width but is not sufficient to prevent rotation of the alveolus. It is therefore necessary that intermaxillary fixation be maintained for 4 weeks after repair. Because of the large forces encountered, a larger 1.7- or 2.0-mm plate is required for fixation. The plates can become exposed intraorally and need to be removed after healing. In complicated cases where there is bone loss or severe comminution a dental splint can help maintain the palatal arch. In the edentulous fracture, the patient's denture secured with transpalatal screws will restore the palatal arch.

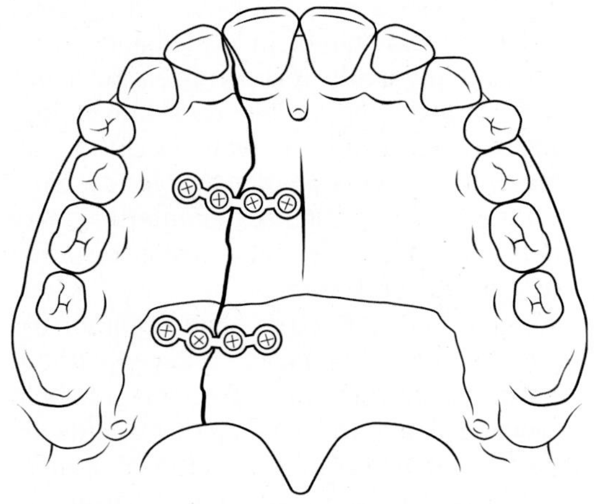

Fig. 71.8 Fixation of a split palate with direct intraoral plating.

Panfacial Fractures

Fractures that involve the upper, middle, and lower third of the facial skeleton are termed *panfacial fractures*. The fracture patterns are complex and affect both the vertical buttresses and horizontal beams. These complicated injuries call for a careful assessment and a logical approach to reduction and repair. To achieve optimal results the surgeon should work from a solid base using established landmarks.

Most panfacial fractures can be viewed as two areas of injury, one area above and one below the Le Fort I fracture line. The lower injury zone consists of the mandible and the lower half of the midface and is reconstructed by using the mandible as the stable base. The position of the lower half of the midface is then determined through the mandibular-maxillary occlusion. The upper injury zone is composed of the frontal bone and the upper half of the midface. The frontal bar acts as a solid base to establish the position of the upper half of the midface. These two upper and lower halves are then properly related to one another by accurate restoration of the vertical bony buttresses.[18] This sequence represents a logical approach for the repair of panfacial fractures. However, this is not absolute and the reconstructive surgeon must be able to adapt the repair to each injury.

Soft Tissue Repair

Many approaches for midface fractures use extensive degloving of soft tissues to gain wide exposure to the facial skeleton. Following bone fixation the soft tissues also must be repaired. Failure to do so can result in temporal hollowing, midface ptosis, and eyelid malpositioning. To prevent these aesthetic complications the periosteum and fascia of the midface must be resuspended to the bony skeleton with permanent or semipermanent sutures designed to inhibit downward migration of the overlying soft tissues.[19] In addition, incisions must be closed in multiple layers to prevent a soft tissue diastasis. Even with precise bone fixation, failure to adequately address the soft tissue can produce poor cosmetic outcomes.

Postoperative Care

Patients with maxillary fractures should be given preoperative broad-spectrum antibiotics directed against oral and sinus pathogens. The antibiotics are continued for 5 days postoperatively while oral hygiene is maintained with chlorohexadine oral rinses and pulsed irrigation. A close postoperative follow-up is important to monitor occlusion and make necessary adjustments. Postreduction imaging with CT scans is also helpful in confirming successful reduction and healing while serving as a valuable teaching aid.

Treatment of Pediatric Midface Fractures

Pediatric facial fractures are best managed using a conservative treatment approach. An aggressive approach with extensive periosteal stripping and plating should be avoided because these techniques can disrupt facial and dental growth centers. Plates are generally used only when there is considerable comminution. Because significant potential for remodeling exists, even displaced bones can remodel and assume normal position. When plates are used, they should be removed after healing to prevent any interference with bone growth. Because children exhibit rapid healing the window for fracture repair is only 7 to 10 days before complications from malunion are seen.

Most pediatric midface fractures can be managed by intermaxillary fixation with arch bars. Alternatively, dental mounts or circummaxillary splints can be used to lessen the damaging forces circumdental wires impart on short, deciduous tooth roots. When an open technique is required, plates and wires should be used sparingly, and when possible, a resorbable plating system is preferable.

Complications

The complications of midface fracture repair can be divided into bone and soft tissue sequelae producing either functional or cosmetic problems. Bony complications include delayed union, malunion, and nonunion. These almost invariably produce malocclusion. With a delayed union, the patient must be reduced to the preinjury occlusion and maintained in intermaxillary fixation for an additional 3 to 6 weeks. When a true nonunion or fibrous union occurs, the interposing fibrous tissue and any nonviable bone need to be removed. Bone grafts may be required to fill in gaps so the vertical buttresses can be restored.

Malunion resulting in a facial skeletal deformity needs a careful evaluation of occlusion and facial appearance. Reconstructive CT scans and cephalometric analysis are helpful in evaluating the degree of maxillary retrodisplacement and vertical midface collapse, whereas dental models can aid in surgical planning. When midfacial retrusion develops as a result of poor fixation or improper restoration of the craniofacial buttresses, correction is necessary. Usually this requires maxillary osteotomies and midfacial advancement using fixation plates and bone grafts to achieve proper occlusion and facial dimensions.

Subtle problems of malocclusion can initially be managed with intermaxillary fixation. If the malocclusion persists after healing, dental adjustments, orthodontics, and possibly osteotomies may be necessary to avoid chronic problems in the temporomandibular joints.

Malar flattening without any deformity or dysfunction of the adjacent orbit is best treated using onlay bone grafts or alloplasts. If the malar complex is rotated producing a disturbance in orbital volume, osteotomies and possibly bone grafts may be necessary to reestablish proper volume.

Soft tissue complications also occur following midfacial injury and fracture repair. Fortunately, because of an excellent blood supply, soft tissue infections are rare despite contamination from sinus and oral contents. When localized wound infections do occur they can usually be managed with systemic antibiotics. When an infection persists despite appropriate therapy osteomyelitis must be considered. In these cases removal of hardware and debridement of the underlying bone are necessary. If an oroantral fistula develops, it should be closed with excision of the fistula tract and any nidus of the infection.

Paresthesia or hypoesthesia of the infraorbital nerve is common with midface injury and after fracture repair. This is generally managed expectantly, but in rare cases nerve ablation has been required. A few patients will experience a hypersensitivity to cold at the site of a plate that may necessitate hardware removal.

There are also several cosmetic complications that can occur after the repair of maxillary fractures. Generally the cosmetic complications of midfacial fractures can be avoided by careful soft tissue handling and diligent resuspension of the midface to avoid temporal hallowing, cheek ptosis, and eyelid malposition. When there are significant concerns, cosmetic correction is an option. Problems with eyelid position including lower lid ectropion can occur after surgical repair. Initially the ectropion should be treated with massage and steroid injection. If conservative measures fail, a lid elevation or shortening procedure may be necessary. Entropion of the lower lid is less common but may follow a transconjunctival approach.

Summary

Le Fort fractures are a complex group of fractures that demand an understanding of buttresses of the facial skeleton. These injuries require open exposure and precise anatomical reestablishment of the bony skeletal matrix to restore form. Repairs can be made through camouflaged incisions with low profile plates that lessen the need for postoperative intermaxillary fixation. Restoration of the occlusion, bony buttresses, and the midfacial soft tissues optimizes outcomes and minimizes complications.

References

1. Haug RH, Adams JM, Jordan RB. Comparison of the morbidity associated with maxillary fractures treated by maxillomandibular and rigid internal fixation. Oral Surg Oral Med Oral Pathol Oral Radiol Endod 1995;80:629–637
2. Goldschmidt MJ, Castiglione CL, Assael LA, Litt MD. Craniomaxillofacial trauma in the elderly. J Oral Maxillofac Surg 1995;53:1145–1149
3. Ferreira P, Marques M, Pinho C, Rodrigues J, Reis J, Amarante J. Midfacial fractures in children and adolescents: a review of 492 case. Br J Oral Maxillofac Surg 2004;42:501–505
4. Haug RH, Foss J. Maxillofacial injuries in the pediatric patient. Oral Surg Oral Med Oral Pathol Oral Radiol Endod 2000;90:126–134
5. Brandt KE, Burruss GL, Hickerson WL, White CE, DeLozier JB. The management of midface fractures with intracranial injury. J Trauma 1991;31:15–19
6. Hohlreider M, Hinterhoelzl J, Ulmer H, Hackl W, Schmutzhard E, Gassner R. Maxillofacial fractures masking traumatic intracranial hemorrhage. Int J Oral Maxillofac Surg 2004;33:389–395
7. Al-Qurainy IA, Stassen LF, Dutton GN, Moos KF, el-Attar A. The characteristics of midfacial fractures and the association with ocular injury: a prospective study. Br J Oral Maxillofac Surg. 1991;29:291–301
8. Lee KF, Wagner LK, Lee YE, Suh JH, Lee SR. The impact-absorbing effects of facial fractures in closed-head injuries. J Neurosurg 1987;66: 542–547
9. Le Fort R. Etude experimental sur les fractures de la machoire superieure. Rev Chir Paris. 1901;23:208–227. Tessier P, trans. [Experimental study of fractures of the upper jaw.] Plast Reconstr Surg 1972;50:497–506
10. Hendrickson M, Clark N, Manson PN, et al. Palatal fractures: classification, patterns, and treatment with rigid internal fixation. Plast Reconstr Surg 1998;101:319–332
11. Donat TL, Endress C, Mathog RH. Facial fracture classification according to skeletal support mechanisms. Arch Otolaryngol Head Neck Surg 1998;124:1306–1314
12. Romano JJ, Manson PN, Mirvis SE, Dunham M, Crawley W. Le Fort fractures without mobility. Plast Reconstr Surg 1990;85:355–362
13. Meyer C, Valfrey J, Kjartansdottir T, Wilk A, Barriere P. Indications for and technical refinements of submental intubation in oral and maxillofacial surgery. J Craniomaxillofac Surg 2003;31:383–388
14. Derdyn C, Persing JA, Broaddus WC, et al. Craniofacial trauma: an assessment of risk related to the timing of surgery. Plast Reconstr Surg 1990;86:238–245
15. Piotrowski WP. The primary treatment of frontobasal and midfacial fractures in patients with head injuries. J Oral Maxillofac Surg 1992;50:1264–1268
16. Thaller SR, Kawamoto HK. A histologic evaluation of fracture repair in the midface. Plast Reconstr Surg 1990;85:196–201
17. Rudderman RH, Mullen RL. Biomechanics of the facial skeleton. Clin Plast Surg 1992;19:11–29
18. Manson PN, Clark N, Robertson B, et al. Subunit principles in midface fractures: the importance of sagittal buttresses, soft-tissue reductions and sequencing treatment of segmental fractures. Plast Reconstr Surg 1999;103:1287–1306
19. Frodel JL, Rudderman R. Facial soft tissue resuspension following upper facial skeletal reconstruction. J Craniomaxillofac Trauma 1996;2:24–30

72 Mandibular Fractures

Jaime R. Garza

Treatment of mandibular fractures can be a challenging endeavor and, at times, a frustrating one. The presence of teeth in an arched-shaped tubular structure and the need to restore accurate interdigitation with the opposing upper teeth makes management of these types of fractures very different from that of long-bone fractures. However, the principles of fracture reduction, fixation, and bone healing are the same.

Etiology

Mandibular fractures most often occur as a result of blunt trauma. Motor vehicle accidents, assaults, and falls constitute an array of possibilities for fracturing the mandible. A recent study from Austria reported that athletic competition was the most common cause of mandibular fractures, accounting for 31.5% of the series of 712 patients.[1] The prominence of the chin in the mature human makes this structure susceptible to injury. In the pediatric population, the cranium is the most projecting region of the head and neck. Therefore, in children, cranial injuries are more common than mandibular injuries.[2]

Anatomy

The mandible is an arched-shaped structure comprising vertical and horizontal components (**Fig. 72.1**). The majority of bone consists of a dense outer and inner cortex surrounding an inner layer of cancellous bone. Through the cancellous bone run the inferior alveolar neurovascular bundles and lymphatics that nourish the bone and the associated teeth. The inferior alveolar artery is a branch of the internal maxillary artery and enters the lingual aspect of the mandible high on the ascending ramus through the mandibular foramen. The inferior alveolar nerve is a branch of the mandibular nerve, which in turn is a branch of the trigeminal nerve. Its course in the mandible parallels that of the artery.

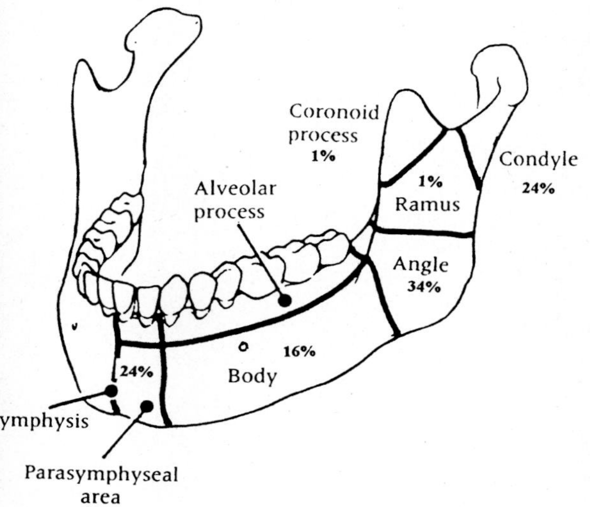

Fig. 72.1 Anatomy of the mandible.

There are 16 teeth in the fully developed mandible. There are two each of a central and lateral incisor; cuspids; first and second bicuspids; and first, second, and third molars. The horizontal portion of the mandible is divided into a superior or alveolar portion comprising spongy bone that surrounds and supports the roots of the teeth. The inferior or basal portion is where the inferior alveolar neurovascular bundle courses. The chin prominence at the midline of the mandible is called the symphysis. As the mandiblular arch continues proximally from midline, the area at the canine forms the parasymphysis. The horizontal region from the parasymphysis proximally is called the body. This horizontal body joins the vertical ascending ramus at the angle of the mandible. The ramus narrows superiorly to form the condylar neck and the coronoid process. The condylar neck flares superiorly to form the condyle, which articulates with the glenoid fossa of the temporal bone at the base of the skull. Interposed between the condylar head and the glenoid fossa is a fibrocartilaginous structure called the meniscus. This structure, the temporomandibular joint (TMJ), is an example of a diarthroidial or ginglymoarthroidial joint. This type of joint is capable of hinge, gliding, and rotational movements.

Although the mandible is a strong, dense bone, it has several areas of inherent weakness. The subcondylar region down to the angle is an area of naturally thin bone. The presence of a third molar at the angle further thins this area and makes it susceptible to fractures. The narrow portions of the condylar neck are frequently fractured when forces generated at the symphysis travel upward and overcome the compressive strength of the condylar neck, causing it to fracture. The presence of the canine tooth root and the mental foramen makes the parasymphyseal area susceptible to fractures. It is not surprising that the most common areas of fracture are the subcondylar, angle, and parasymphyseal regions.[3]

The muscles of mastication are mirror images bilaterally and attach to the mandible at various sites. The elevators of the jaw are the masseter, temporalis, and medial pterygoid muscles. The depressors are the suprahyoid muscles and the lateral pterygoid muscles. When a fracture occurs through the mandible, the unopposed pull of a particular muscle or muscle group can displace the fractured segments and keep them out of alignment.

Classification

Similar to long-bone fractures, fractures of the mandible can be described as closed, open, simple, complex, or comminuted. Fractures of the mandible that extend through the periodontal membrane surrounding the root of the tooth and communicate with the oral cavity are considered open fractures. Fractures can also be classified as favorable or unfavorable (**Fig. 72.2**). The direction in which the fracture line travels, the bevel of the fracture line, and the muscular forces acting on the fractured segments can either displace the segments to a position that is unfavorable for healing or reduce the fracture line to a position that is favorable for healing. In general, mandibular fractures that are directed inferiorly and anteriorly are classified as horizontally favorable. Fractures directed inferiorly and posteriorly are classified as horizontally unfavorable. Medial displacement can occur when a fracture runs from posterior to anterior because of the medial pull of the elevator muscles of mastication, thus making this a vertically unfavorable fracture. A fracture that passes from the outer surface of the mandible, posteriorly and medially, as in a sagittal split osteotomy, is a favorable fracture because the muscle pull prevents displacement. This is considered a vertically favorable fracture.

A fracture through the body of the mandible that contains a tooth in the posterior fracture segment, even if it is coursing in an unfavorable direction, can reduce itself when the tooth in the posterior fracture segment opposes a maxillary tooth and comes into contact with the opposing fragment. In this situation the tooth should be retained and used as an occlusal stop to prevent displacement of the fracture. Mandibular fractures that involve only the alveolar bone and the associated teeth are termed *dentoalveolar fractures*. These fractures are considered open fractures and should be managed as such. Treatment of all of these fractures must include fixation forces that are substantially greater than the displacing forces to optimize healing.

Diagnosis

Diagnosis of mandibular fractures can generally be made by a thorough clinical examination. Signs and symptoms of a mandibular fracture include intraoral bleeding, pain, swelling, trismus, malocclusion, and deviation of the jaw on opening. Palpation of the mandible may reveal step-offs at the fracture site as well as pain. An intraoral examination may reveal ecchymosis of the floor of the mouth in the region of a fracture, a step-off between the

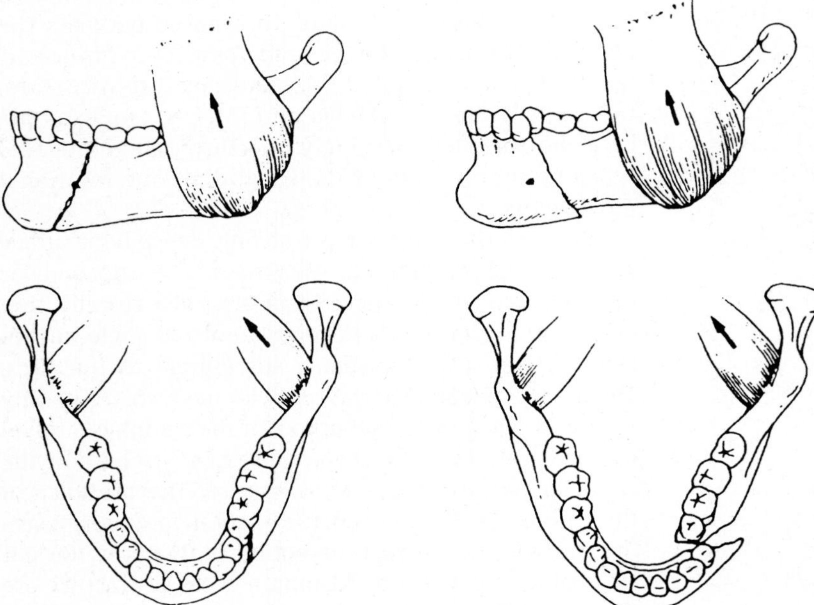

Fig. 72.2 Favorable and unfavorable fractures.

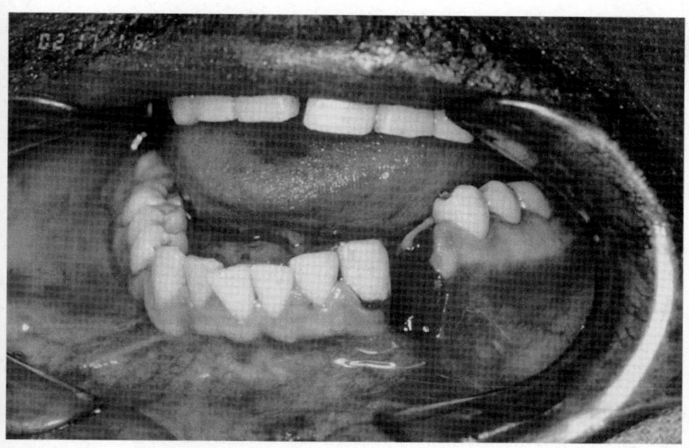

Fig. 72.3 Obvious step-off between the canine and first bicuspid in a parasymphyseal fracture.

teeth or bleeding (**Fig. 72.3**). The mandibular stress test can reveal subtle fractures. The stress test is performed by placing the volar pads of the examiner's thumbs on the lingual aspects of the body of the mandible and then pushing the thumbs outward. Pain elicited during this "stress" is usually indicative of a fracture at that site. This maneuver should obviously be performed only on cooperative patients.

Radiological examinations can delineate the locations and patterns of fractures. The most information for the least expense can be obtained from a panoramic radiograph of the jaws or panorex. A panorex is essentially a single tomogram that reveals the entire mandible in a two-dimensional panoramic view (**Fig. 72.4**). Due to the overlap of the x-ray at the mandibular midline, the symphyseal region is usually blurred. However, a Panorex cannot be obtained from an uncooperative or obtunded patient, and in that situation a mandibular series is indicated. This series of radiographs includes lateral obliques, a posterior-anterior view, and a Towne's view. Towne's view gives an excellent view of the condylar regions. Studies have shown that 92% of fractures in a given patient population can be detected on a Panorex, whereas only 66% were detected in a mandibular series.[4]

Computed tomography (CT) scans can give more detailed information of fractures in the condylar regions and the lingual aspect of the mandible (**Fig. 72.5**). However, their use as a screening tool is costly and unnecessary.

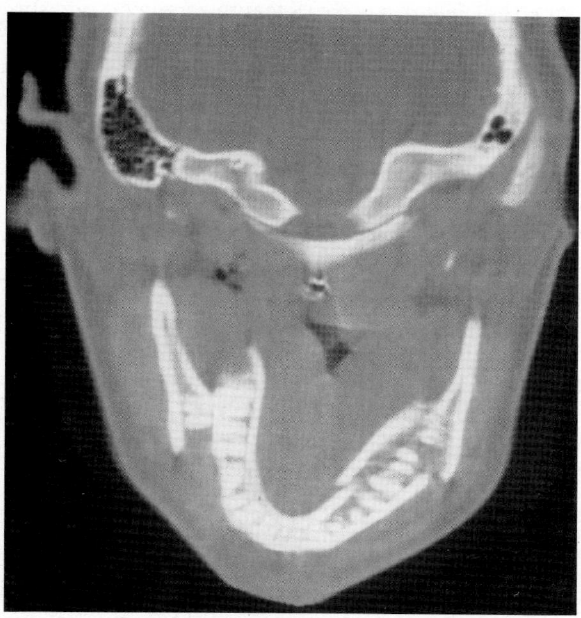

Fig. 72.5 CT scan demonstrating lingual fractures and their displacement.

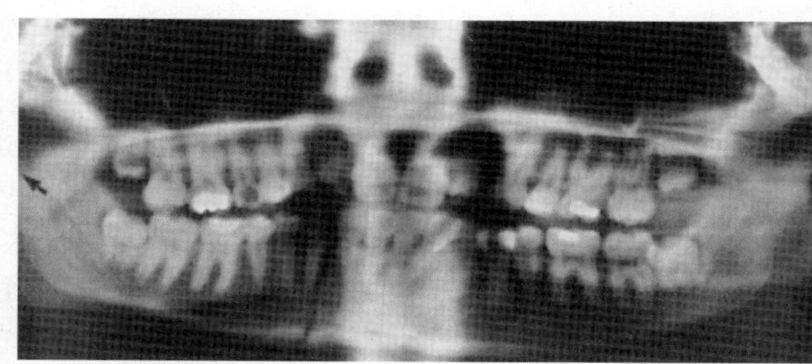

A

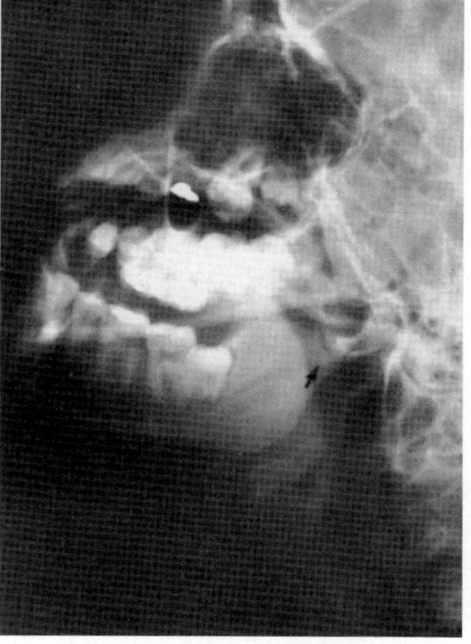

B

Fig. 72.4 Panorex demonstrating a right parasymphyseal fracture and subcondylar fractures.

Treatment Principles

General Principles

No matter what method of fixation is being considered for the repair, the principles of bone fracture management remain the same. After the appropriate diagnosis has been made, trauma to the remainder of the patient has either been ruled out or managed, and the patient is stable, there are several principles to which one should adhere. Open fractures should be treated with systemic antibiotics. This decreases the incidence of infection. Generally, the earlier a fracture can be reduced and fixated, the better is the outcome. If fixation of the fracture will be delayed, preliminary stabilization of the segments should be performed to decrease patient discomfort. Something as simple as an elastic band suspension device from the inferior border of the mandible to the top of the head could be used to bring the muscles of mastication to resting length and help decrease the amount of muscle spasm and movement of the fracture line.

The principles of mandible fracture management include establishment of the preinjury dental occlusion, anatomical reduction of the fractures, and stabilization of the fracture until bony healing has occurred. The question of how to manage teeth that are involved in the line of a mandibular fracture continues to be a point of controversy. Teeth that are fractured through the root or pulp chamber, teeth with significant amounts of carious decay and root abscesses, and loose teeth with severe periodontitis should probably be extracted prior to reduction and fixation of the fracture. The extraction sockets in the alveolar bone should be thoroughly curetted and irrigated with sterile saline solution. Another controversial issue regarding teeth in the fracture line is what to do with the third molar, which is in the line of a mandibular angle fracture. Some investigators recommend leaving teeth in the line of the fracture to provide a broader area of hard tissue contact and therefore provide stability.[5] In a study by Ellis and Sinn, of nine patients in whom teeth associated with a fracture were left in place, six developed infections, for an infection rate of 67%. On the other hand, in 46 fractures when the tooth was removed, 13 infections occurred, resulting in an infection rate of 28%.[6]

Techniques

Fixation

Fixation techniques can be described as either semirigid or rigid.

Semirigid Fixation

Semirigid fixation implies that because of the elasticity of these fixation devices, some movement occurs at the fracture line. Semirigid mechanisms of fracture fixation include maxillomandibular fixation (MMF) techniques, such as placement of arch bars with interdental wiring, four-screw intermaxillary fixation, ivy loops, and external fixation devices such as the Joe Hall Morris appliance. In general, minimally displaced, favorable fractures with easily reproducible occlusion can be managed with semirigid fixation (**Fig. 72.6**). MMF devices are placed, and heavy elastic or wire is then used to hold the teeth in their preinjury occlusion. Interdental fixation is then maintained for periods ranging from 2 to 6 weeks. The younger and healthier the patient, the less time required for bony healing to occur.

Although there are some advantages to the use of MMF, there are also distinct disadvantages. The advantages include simplicity of fixation and no need for soft tissue dissection. Disadvantages of interdental fixation include weight loss, tooth decay, gingivitis, and immobility of the TMJ, which can lead to stiffness and limitation of range of motion. A contraindication for the use of MMF is the patient's inability or unwillingness to cooperate with interdental fixation.[7] This can be the case with the elderly, obtunded patients, mentally retarded patients, alcoholics, drug addicts, or any patient predisposed to vomiting. Such patients are at risk for aspiration and should be treated with rigid-fixation techniques.

Rigid Fixation

Rigid fixation of the mandible involves the use of plates and screws for fracture fixation. Principles of rigid fixation include early anatomical reduction of the fracture segments, maintaining them in their anatomical reduction, and immobilizing the fracture segments with appropriate plates and screws or screws alone. The rigid-fixation devices should be of sufficient strength to neutralize loads that occur under normal functional requirements, such as

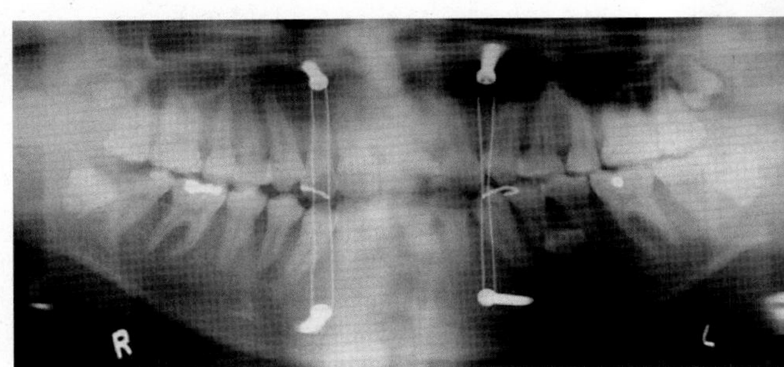

Fig. 72.6 Four-screw maxillomandibular fixation for minimally displaced subcondylar fracture.

mastication and speech. It is important not to underestimate the masticatory loading conditions because of the anger of plate fracture and nonunion or, worse, infection of the bone.

The majority of fixation plates used for the mandible are made of commercially pure titanium, which consists of titanium and oxygen. It is insoluble and therefore inert and biocompatible. Titanium has a high corrosion resistance due to the presence of a thin oxide layer that forms on the surface, which allows the material to behave passively.[7]

Techniques and principles that help to minimize complications of rigid fixation of the mandible are the same as for rigid fixation of any of the bones in the human skeleton. An extremely sharp drill bit is used at low speeds of less than 1000 rpm with constant irrigation of the drill bit with saline so that the temperature of the bone remains below 40°C. This prevents osteocyte necrosis, which can cause loosening of the screws. Loose screws are an absolute source of fixation failure and should never be left in place. The plate should be passively adapted to the underlying bone with a slight overbend of the plate just over the fracture site[8] (**Fig. 72.7**). This slight overbend helps to prevent lingual displacement of the fracture when the screws are placed. Accurate passive adaptation of the plate to the bone surface allows the fracture segments to remain in their reduced position. A poorly adapted plate forces the fracture segments out of position when the screws are placed and can lead to nonunion, malunion, and malocclusion. The screws should be placed through the bone so that at least one or two threads engage and exit the outer cortex of the bone to ensure engagement of the screws with as much cortical bone as possible. The plate must be of sufficient strength to overcome the tensile forces of the mandible.

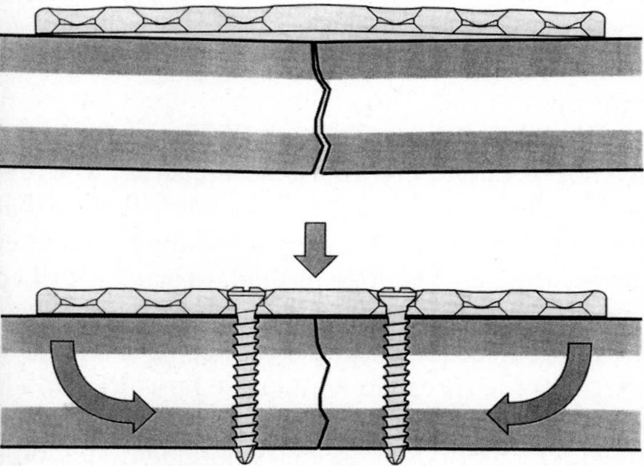

ig. 72.7 Correct passive adaptation of a plate to the mandible with a light overbend at the fracture site allows for accurate reduction of the racture during screw placement, as well as reduction of the lingual ıspect of the fracture.

Tension Band Principles in Fixation

As described in the anatomy section, there are multiple muscles acting and exerting forces on different areas of the mandible during function. During occlusal loading a zone of tension develops at the alveolar surface of the mandible and a zone of compression develops at the inferior border.[9] The depressor muscles acting at the symphysis pulling downward and the elevator muscles pulling upward at the angle and the coronoid process help to develop these tensile and compressive forces (**Fig. 72.8**). When a fracture occurs in the horizontal segments of the mandible, the tensile forces act to displace the fracture at the alveolar border and compress the fracture at the inferior border. Compressive forces can also cause the fracture segments to override at the zone of compression. Multiple forces acting at the symphysis allow for the development of torsion forces in this area.

Fixation systems should ideally be located at the superior border of the mandible across the fracture site. The fixation would function as a tension band that overcomes the distracting forces at the alveolar border. This tension band should therefore be strong enough to overcome the tensile forces at the superior border of the fracture line and resist separation of the fracture. The inferior border would remain closed due to the natural compressive forces.

Several methods are used to establish a tension band. The presence of the teeth and their roots in the alveolar portion of the mandible makes the use of bicortical fixation of plates and screws impossible. The two most used methods are bridging of the teeth across the fracture line with either an arch bar or direct wires (such as ivy loops) or placement of a monocortical miniplate across the fracture

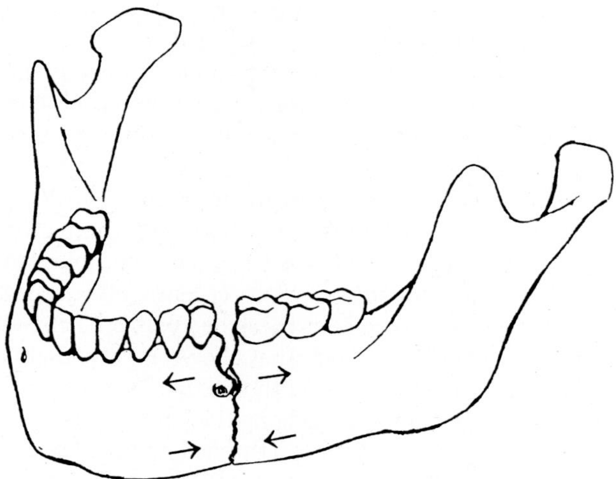

Fig. 72.8 During occlusal loading, tension forces cause the alveolar surface to separate and compressive forces cause the inferior border of the mandible to close at the fracture site.

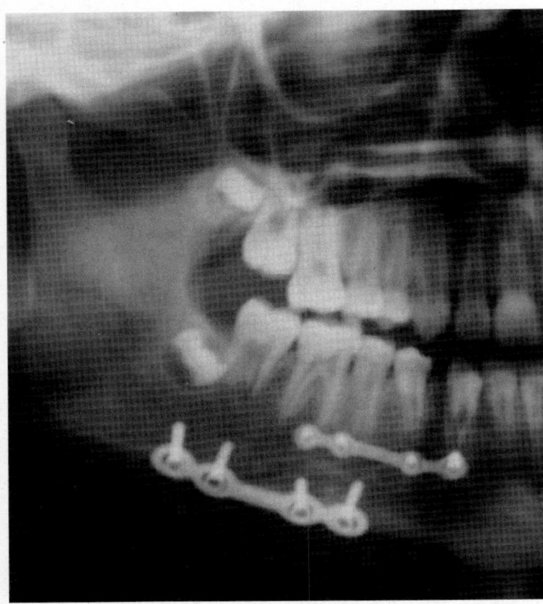

Fig. 72.9 Monocortical placement of a miniplate near the superior border of the mandible functions as a tension band.

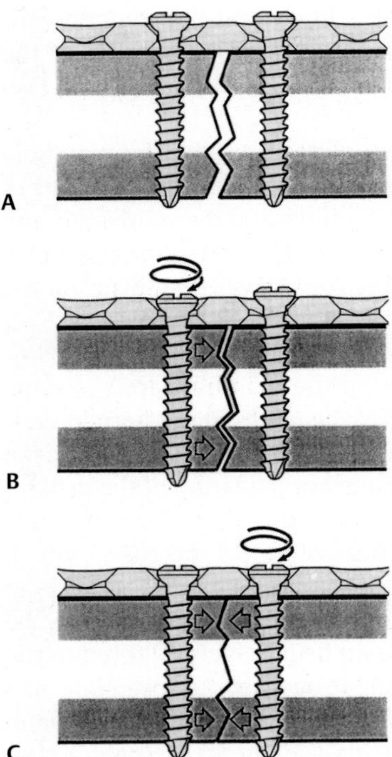

Fig. 72.10 Compression with a plate. (**A**) The two innermost screws should be placed eccentrically within the DC holes. (**B**) As these screws are tightened they approximate the fragment. (**C**) With final tightening of the screws, compression is achieved.

line (**Fig. 72.9**). Monocortical placement of the screws prevents damage to the tooth roots.

Compression and Compression Plates

A description of compression plating is important to the understanding of mandibular fracture fixation. Basically, compression is a method for preventing interfragmentary motion of the mandible fracture. Compression plating consists of the forcing together of two surfaces to produce an axial preload force in the fracture line and also acts by increasing interfragmentary friction. Therefore, the fracture remains immobile as long as the actual axial preload that has been placed with the plate is higher than the tensile forces produced by masticatory function.

Preloading with plates and screws mechanically allows load sharing to occur between the bone and the plate.[7] Compression plates are designed so that two holes on either side of the fracture line are eccentrically placed (**Fig. 72.10**). These two holes are designed with an inclined and horizontal beveled surface that allows a screw that is being threaded to glide toward the medial aspect of the plate. Because the screw is engaging the bone, the bone is moved medially as the screw is tightened and the bone is compressed against the opposite fracture segment. Only two screws, one on each side of the fracture, should be placed eccentrically. The remaining screws are placed in a centric or neutral fashion. This method of fixation is useful only when you have a noncomminuted, simple transverse fracture of the mandible. Bones that are fractured obliquely or are comminuted when compressed will override their fracture fragments, displace the comminuted segments, and lead to fracture instability and possibly malocclusion.

Compression can also be obtained with the use of a lag screw. Lag screw fixation is useful for uniting fracture segments and for fixating bone grafts.[10] The technique of lag screw fixation involves the establishment of a gliding hole in the outer cortex. This gliding hole allows the screw to pass through without engaging the bone. A second threaded hole is placed in the far or outer cortex. The first hole or the gliding hole is purposely overdrilled so that the hole is at a minimum the size of the outer diameter of the screw threads. The hole in the far cortex is drilled to the exact diameter of the size of the core of the screw. A screw is then placed through the gliding hole, and as the screw engages the threaded hole in the far cortex and is tightened, the two bone fragments are forced together and interfragmental compression is obtained. This type of compression is referred to as static interfragmental compression.[7] It is static because it does not change significantly with load. Lag screws can be used for fractures at the symphysis or oblique fractures of the body, angle and subcondylar regions that have significant overlapping

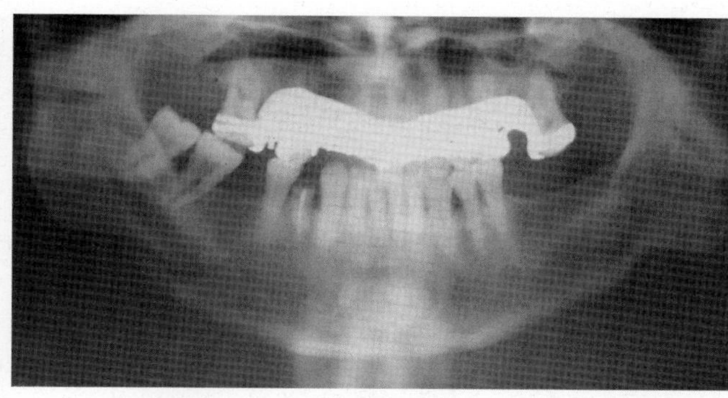

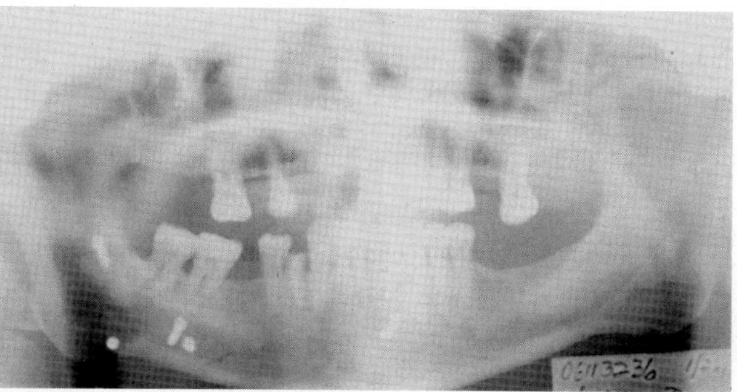

Fig. 72.11 (**A**) Oblique fracture of the mandible with overlapping segments. (**B**) Three lag screws placed to rigidly fixate the oblique fracture.

segments (**Fig. 72.11**). At least three lag screws are placed in fractures of the mandible. At the symphysis, two screws may be used. Rarely should only a single lag screw be applied. A single lag screw does not provide a great deal of strength, though it does provide stability.

Neutralization and Neutralization Plates

When a fracture of the mandible is more than a simple transverse fracture and compression plates are contraindicated, then a neutralization plate should be used. A neutralization plate is a plate of sufficient length and strength to overcome the functional forces acting on the mandible. The use of noncompression holes in the plate and an adequate number of screws with a minimum of two on either side of the fracture provides sufficient rigidity to allow bony healing to occur (**Fig. 72.12**).

Soft Tissue Approaches to the Mandible

A wide unobstructed view of the mandible at its fracture site is a key component of anatomical fracture reduction and fixation. With the advent of new craniofacial surgical techniques and the utilization of incisions adapted from facial aesthetic surgery, soft tissue approaches to the mandible can be chosen to minimize nerve injury and scarring of the patient.

In general, intraoral incisions should be utilized whenever feasible. Intraoral incisions made in the vestibule leaving a 5- to 10-mm cuff of mobile mucosa and wide periosteal dissection of the mandible allow for excellent exposure of the mandible from the symphyseal region back to the angle and ascending ramus. Care should be taken at the level of the bicuspids. The mental nerve exits the mental foramen and travels just under the mucosa toward the skin. Blunt dissection over this

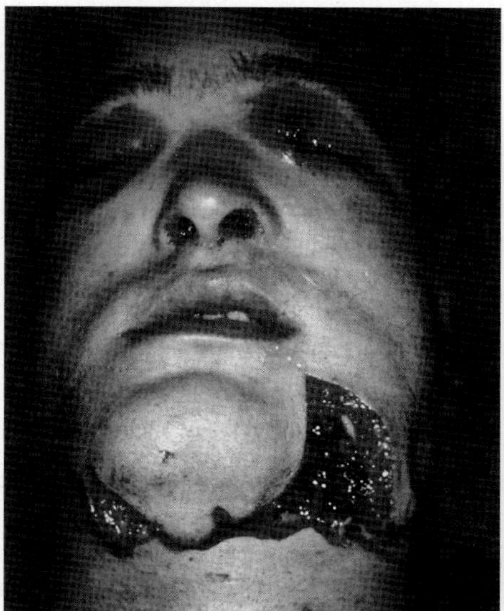

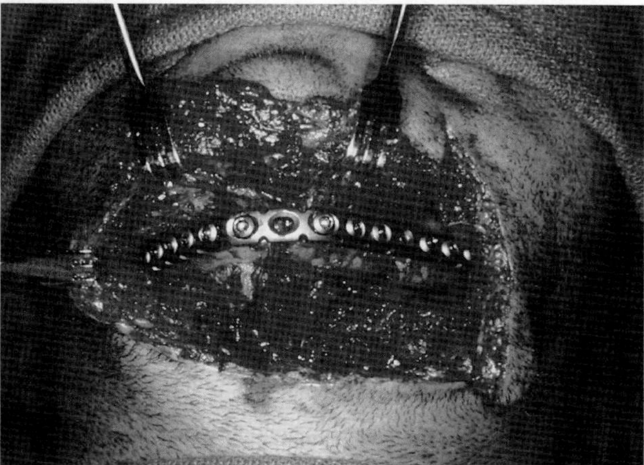

Fig. 72.12 (**A**) Gunshot wound to the mandible after debridement of damaged soft tissues. (**B**) Neutralization plate used to reduce the severely comminuted mandible.

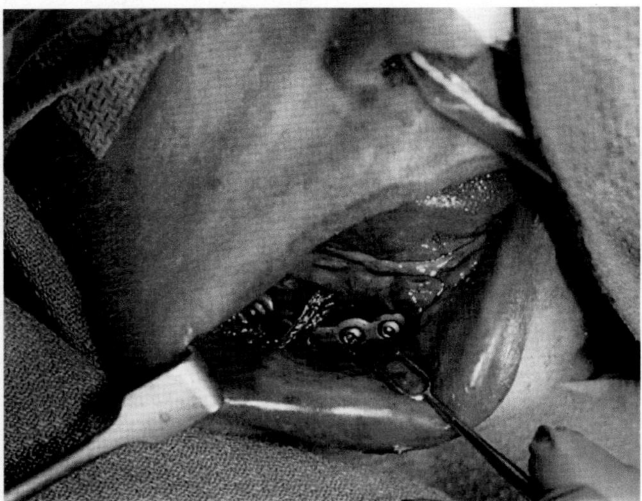

Fig. 72.13 Knowledge of anatomy and careful dissection allow for preservation of the mental nerve and adequate exposure of the mandible fracture for plate and screw placement.

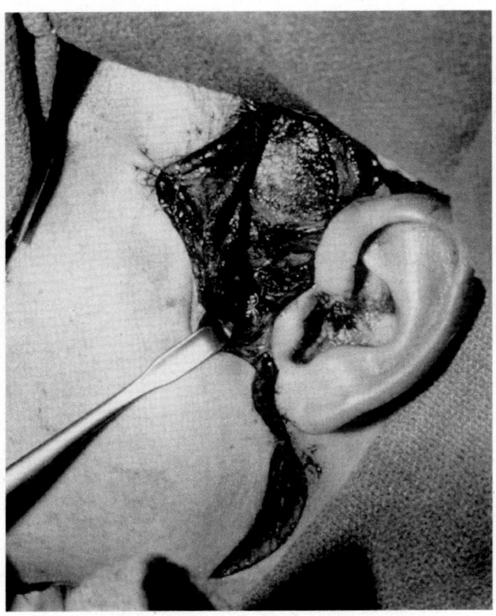

Fig. 72.14 Extended facelift incision combined with a modified Risdon incision exposes the glenoid fossa, condylar head, and subcondylar regions of the mandible.

area with a hemostat will expose the nerve (**Fig. 72.13**). With enough experience and the use of percutaneous drill and screw placement methods, low subcondylar fractures can also be approached from this direction. The intraoral approach avoids damage to the facial nerves and leaves no external scarring. Disadvantages include limited visibility of the inferior border of the mandible, particularly as the fracture lines approach the angle. In addition, there is no visualization of lingual cortical fractures. In an arched structure such as the mandible, it is important to maintain three-dimensional reduction of the fracture at the buccal cortex, the inferior border, as well as the lingual cortex. Not accurately reducing the lingual cortex can lead to widening of the mandibular arch and therefore widening of the facial plane in a transverse dimension.

Extraoral approaches to the mandible are variations of standard facelift and parotidectomy incisions. The incisions in the temple region extending to the preauricular regions are useful for exposure of the condyle of the mandible as well as the glenoid fossa (**Fig. 72.14**). The inferior extent of the facelift incision around the lobule of the ear and extended to the neck in a horizontal crease line is called the Risdon incision. The neck incision should be placed at least one finger breadth below the angle of the mandible to avoid injuring the marginal mandibular nerve. This incision exposes the angle of the mandible, the ascending ramus, and the subcondylar regions. The temporal extension of the preauricular incision is made deep to the superficial layer of the deep temporal fascia to avoid damage to the frontal branch of the facial nerve. Retraction of these flaps can also injure these facial nerves and should be done with care.

In the edentulous patient with a thin, atrophic mandible, an intraoral approach will strip the periosteum from the mandible. This increases the risk of complications due to devascularization of this thin, atrophic bone. Therefore, an extraoral approach is usually indicated in fractures of the edentulous mandible. The plane of dissection is above the level of the periosteum. The plate is screwed directly on top of the periosteum, allowing as much blood supply as possible to remain intact. In severely comminuted fractures and some bilateral fractures with displacement, a "cervical smile" incision has been used (**Fig. 72.15**). This is a transcervical incision that is made in a horizontal crease of the neck between the hyoid and the thyroid cartilage. Such dissection allows visualization of the mandibular branch of the facial nerve bilaterally with safe reflection of the nerve upward. Direct visualization of the inferior, buccal, and lingual borders of the mandibular fractures bilaterally is easily obtained.

The soft tissue approaches to the fractured mandible should be individualized to each patient and carefully chosen to optimize visualization, reduction, and fixation of the fractures and minimize facial scarring and damage to neurovascular structures.

Repair of Mandibular Fractures

Symphysis Fractures

Fractures of the symphysis can be difficult to detect, particularly if they are nondisplaced. Because of blurring at the midline, a Panorex usually cannot delineate a nondisplaced symphysis fracture. A sublingual hematoma or ecchymosis of the anterior floor of the mouth may

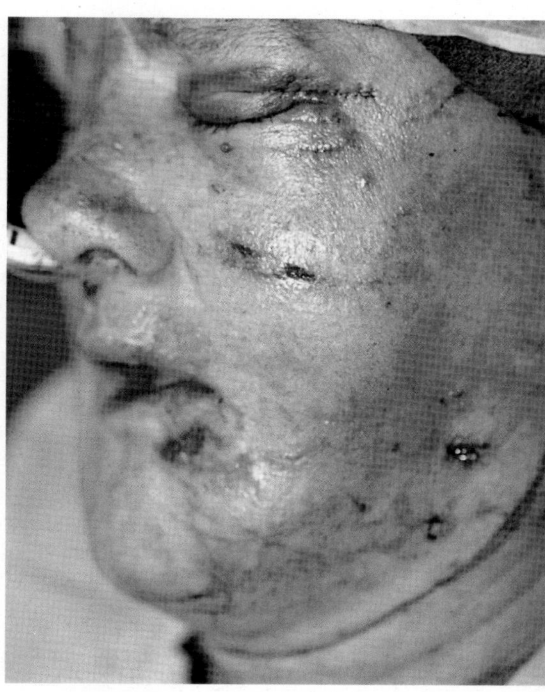

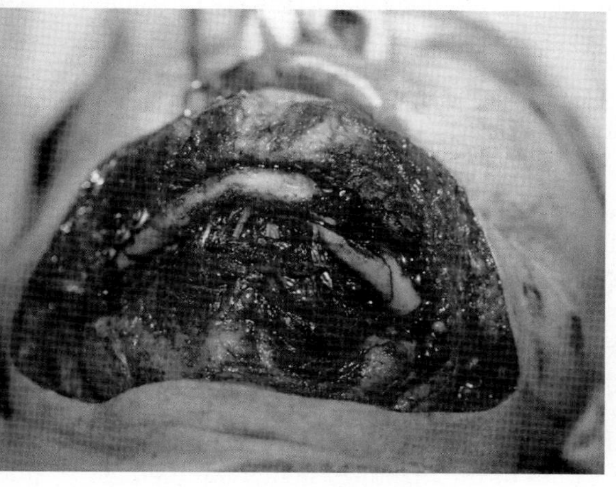

A B

Fig. 72.15 (**A**) A cervical incision allows for wide exposure of the mandible when extensive comminution or severe bilateral mandible fractures exist. (**B**) The "cervical smile" incision approach to severe bilateral mandible fractures. Note the excellent exposure of the lingual aspects of the mandible.

be the only sign of a fracture (**Fig. 72.16**). An intraoral approach is used for exposure of the symphysis. A large laceration at the chin, if present, may be used for the approach instead of the intraoral incision. When a symphysis fracture is identified, subcondylar fractures should be highly suspected until ruled out. In children presenting with a chin laceration because of a fall or other blunt trauma, a symphysis fracture should be sought and condylar head or subcondylar fractures ruled out (**Fig. 72.17**).

Arch bars or their equivalent should serve as tension bands and be used to set the teeth into their preinjury occlusion. Either the arch bar may be used as a tension band, or a four-hole miniplate can be placed in a monocortical fashion at the alveolar border. A mandibular fracture plate is then placed at the midportion of the symphysis. There is no inferior alveolar neurovascular bundle coursing through this portion of the mandible, and as long as the plate is placed below the roots of the teeth this will suffice.

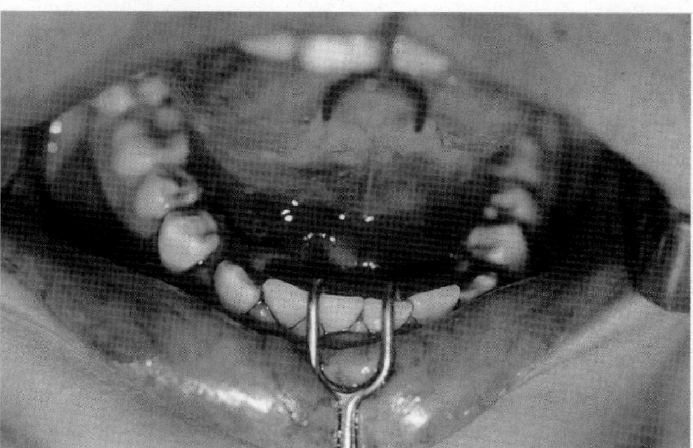

Fig. 72.16 Ecchymosis of the anterior floor of the mouth can be indicative of a symphyseal fracture.

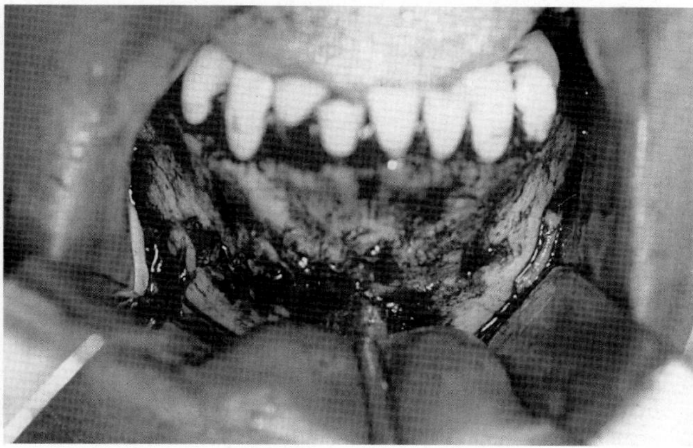

Fig. 72.17 Wide exposure of the symphysis is possible through an intraoral incision.

When a symphysis fracture is combined with subcondylar fractures a longer and stronger reconstruction plate should be considered. This stronger plate will help to overcome the torsion forces that develop at the symphysis and will also prevent widening of the mandibular arch. Lag screws may also be used for the symphysis. A minimum of two screws should be used. As previously stated, these screws should be placed perpendicular to the fracture line and parallel to each other.

Parasymphysis Fractures

Fractures of the parasymphyseal region are managed in a similar fashion to symphyseal fractures. An intraoral approach should be used. The mental nerve courses very close to the mucosal surface in the area of the canine and first bicuspid. Careful blunt dissection of the mental nerve will preserve its function. The mental nerve should be dissected free from the surrounding tissues and gently retracted from the dissection field. A tension band should be placed and a mandibular fracture plate positioned at the inferior border of the mandible below the mental nerve (**Fig. 72.18**).

Mandibular Body Fractures

An intraoral approach is usually employed for these fractures. It is important to remember that the inferior border and the lingual cortex cannot be visualized intraorally. Careful evaluation and diagnosis of the fractures will determine if an intraoral approach is adequate or if an external approach should be used. After preinjury occlusion has been reestablished a monocortical tension band can be placed. The mandibular fracture plate is then adapted to the inferior border and screwed into position. The inferior alveolar neurovascular bundle travels near the inferior border in this region and should be avoided. A Panorex is helpful in identifying the path of this structure.

When a sagittal or oblique fracture occurs through the parasymphysis or the body of the mandible, lingual tipping of the occlusal surfaces of the mandibular teeth can occur when the patient is placed in occlusion with arch bars and wires. As the MMF wires are tightened, the obliquely fractured segment can tilt lingually leading to a malocclusion. A custom acrylic splint fabricated from study casts is placed along the lingual borders of the mandibular teeth and wired into position, thus preventing lingual displacement of the fracture segment when the patient is placed in MMF.

Sagittal or oblique fractures of the body of the mandible and parasymphysis can be fixated using the lag screw technique. At least three screws should be placed to obtain sufficient fixation to allow for bony consolidation and healing.

Fractures of the Mandibular Angle

Fractures of the angle of the mandible tend to be difficult to reduce and fixate accurately. The combination of the location of the fracture, the thinness of the proximal segment, and usually the lack of a tooth in that segment makes anatomical reduction difficult. The approach can be an intraoral incision with wide stripping of the periosteum. The difficult area to visualize is usually the inferior border. The use of a dental mirror from the intraoral approach or an endoscope can help make visible the inferior border and often the lingual border to ensure adequate reduction of the fracture. When this has been done, preinjury dental

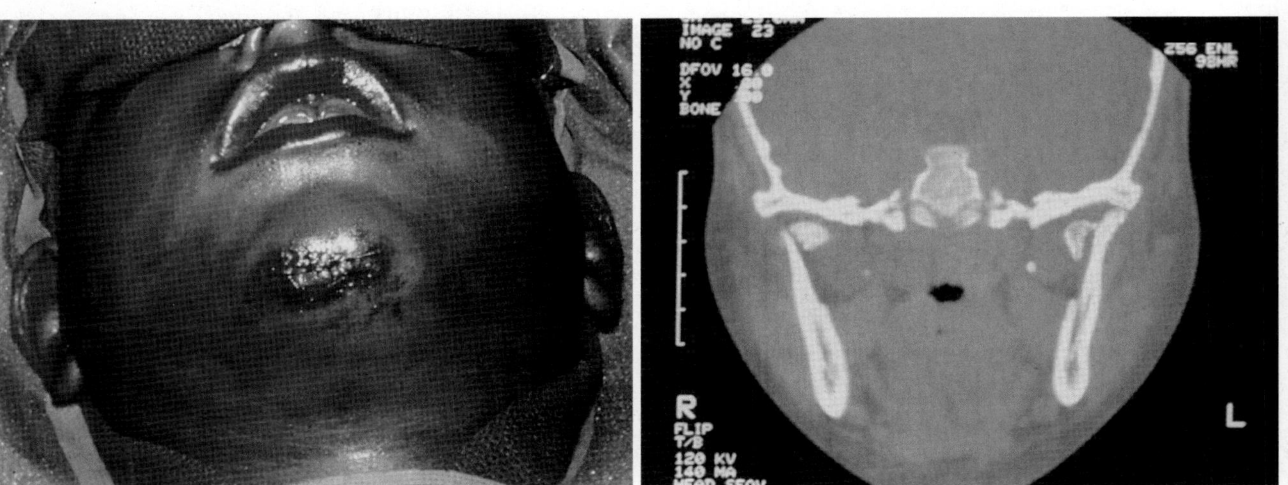

Fig. 72.18 (**A**) A repaired chin laceration in a 5-year-old child who suffered a fall from a bicycle. (**B**) CT scan of the same patient demonstrating medially displaced bilateral condylar head fractures.

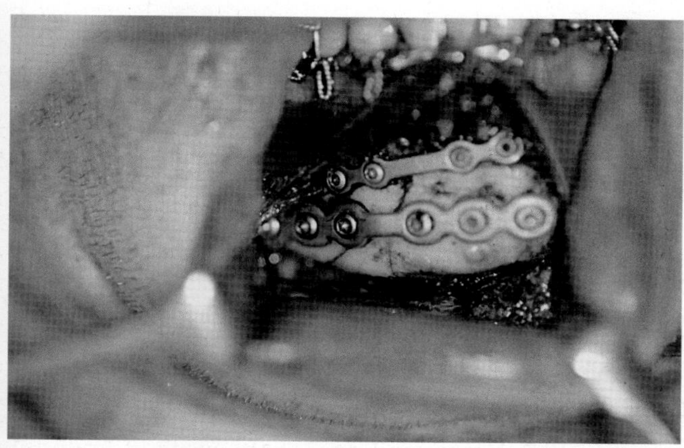

Fig. 72.19 Monocortical tension band and mandibular fracture plate placed for a parasymphyseal fracture.

occlusion is obtained and held in place with MMF. A curved or L-shaped mandibular plate is then placed across the fracture segment at the inferior border, with care taken to avoid the inferior alveolar nerve as well as the roots of the teeth (**Fig. 72.19**). Fixation is performed percutaneously. It is important that at least two screws be present on either side of the fracture. In a large, muscular patient, three screws should be placed on either side of the fracture segment. A monocortical 2–0 miniplate is placed at the superior border to function as a tension band (**Fig. 72.20**). Ellis and colleagues have described their experience using one noncompression miniplate at the external oblique ridge for fractures of the angle of the mandible. The theory behind this is that a plate positioned across the external oblique ridge functions as a tension band to prevent displacement of the superior border during function and that the inferior border will be compressed and remain reduced. In their patient population, treatment of angle fractures with traditional methods produced a high rate of complications (~17%).[11] Their study recommends an intraoral approach with an incision at the external oblique ridge. Dissection of the soft tissues over the fractures is performed, reduction is obtained, and the patient is placed in MMF. After adequate reduction of the fracture is obtained, a single noncompression miniplate is passively adapted to the external oblique ridge and a minimum of two screws are placed in a monocortical fashion on either side of the fracture line. As stated in their study, all biomechanical tests performed to date indicated that two plates are more stable than one. However, this author's clinical experience is the complete opposite. It is his belief that improved maintenance of the blood supply to the bone due to limited dissection may be a factor leading to successful use of this technique.

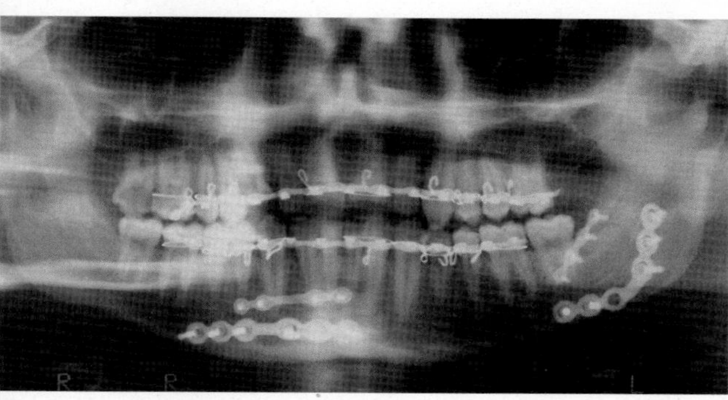

Fig. 72.20 Panorex of a rigidly fixated left mandibular angle fracture and a right parasymphyseal fracture with monocortical miniplates used as tension bands.

Condylar and Subcondylar Fractures

Perhaps no other fractures of the mandible generate as much controversy as condylar and subcondylar fractures.[12] Approaches to the fractured condyle inevitably involve areas of the face where the facial nerve is susceptible to injury. Multiple approaches are described in the literature, including preauricular, intraoral, Risdon, and a combination of a transexternal auditory canal approach and one of the above.[12] Again, the principles remain the same in treatment of condylar fractures (i.e., anatomical reduction of the fracture segments and stabilization of the reduced segments).

Fractures of the condylar and subcondylar region usually occur because of the inherent weakness of the condylar neck. Forces that are generated at impact, particularly at the symphyseal and parasymphyseal regions of the mandible, travel along the body and ramus of the mandible up to the condylar neck where they usually are sufficient to overcome the compressive strength of the bone in this region, and a fracture occurs. Condylar fractures can be classified as intracapsular, referring to fracture of the condylar head itself within its surrounding ligamentous capsule, or high subcondylar or low subcondylar, referring to fractures that occur at the level of the sigmoid notch. By definition, each of these fractures affects the TMJ and, as with any joint injury, early mobilization is recommended to prevent long-term problems. If a patient has easily reproducible occlusion and a nondisplaced or minimally displaced fracture, conservative management with a soft diet alone is indicated. A patient who has difficulty achieving occlusion but who has simple, minimally displaced fractures of the condylar or subcondylar region is usually treated with short-term MMF with heavy elastics for ~2 weeks. After release of the MMF, the patient is placed in lighter elastics to help guide the teeth into occlusion, and a postinjury physical therapy regimen is begun. Several treatment protocols are available. However, all essentially include opening and closing of the jaw and movement into lateral excursions, thus enabling the patient to open the jaws to their preexisting maximal interincisal opening.

Indications for open reduction of condylar and subcondylar fractures include (1) displacement of the proximal segment fragment of 30 degrees or more from the axis of the ascending ramus; (2) shortening of the ascending ramus with telescoping of the fragments and a resulting open bite; (3) dislocation of the condylar head from the temporomandibular fossa; and (4) inability to obtain adequate dental occlusion with closed reduction.[13] In addition, bilateral subcondylar fractures with loss of vertical height are usually an indication for open reduction and internal fixation of the condylar neck on at least one side to reestablish the posterior height of the mandible. Zide and Kent published their absolute indications for open reduction or the condylar neck fractures. These include (1) displacement of the condyle into the middle cranial fossa; (2) difficulty in obtaining adequate occlusion by closed reduction; (3) lateral capsular displacement of the condyle; or (4) invasion of the condylar neck by a foreign body, such as in a gunshot wound.[14] As previously stated, many techniques for stabilization of the condylar fracture have been described. These include traditional plate and screw fixation, direct wiring, extracorporeal removal of the proximal condylar fragment and placement of a plate and fixation to the distal fragment, lag screw placement, and replacement of the condyle with a rib graft. If the fracture occurs below the midlevel of the neck, it is often possible to perform an intraoral alignment and reduction of the fracture, stabilization with bone-holding clamps, followed by percutaneous placement of a passively adapted plate and screws. This author prefers the 2.4-mm titanium plate-and-screw system. A standard intraoral incision is made along the external oblique ridge wide dissection of the periosteum performed. Then the proximal segment is identified and reduced with bone-holding forceps. At this point, the patient is placed into preoperative dental occlusion and fixation with wires is performed. Then a 2.4-mm plate that has been appropriately adapted is placed along the lateral surface of the fracture supported by a single K wire that was driven percutaneously into the segment, and a standard transbuccal trocar system is used to screw the plate into position. When this has been performed, the bone-holding forceps is removed, the maxillomandibular fixation released, and the occlusion checked. It is important that during fixation the proximal segment be located in the glenoid fossa. If the condyle is out of the fossa and the fracture is fixated, the patient will be left with a posterior open bite.

Recent reports have described endoscopic techniques for approaching condylar and subcondylar fractures.[15] The endoscope allows visualization of the proximal segment and therefore manipulation of the segment into position. The use of endoscopic techniques combined with percutaneous screw placement is relatively recent but shows significant promise. The use of the endoscope therefore would avoid the need for large incisions, allow visualization of the fracture segments, and would prevent injury to the branches of the facial nerve. If a surgeon is skilled in the use of endoscopic techniques, the visualization is excellent and the remainder of the plating techniques remains the same.

Comminuted Fractures

Comminuted fractures of the mandible are usually the result of high-energy injuries. These types of fractures involve multiple fracture lines and small segments of free-floating bone. Gunshot wounds and motor vehicle accidents are responsible for the majority of comminuted fractures. It may be necessary and often wise to obtain preoperative study models and the fabrication of an acrylic splint to help guide establishment of the preinjury occlusion. An extraoral approach usually allows direct visualization of the fracture fragments. A stepwise anatomical reduction of the mandible fragments is then performed. Small fragments of bone are placed in their anatomical position and held there with monocortical miniplates. Wires may be used in a similar fashion. When the fracture segments have been reduced and held in position and the preinjury occlusion reestablished, a large reconstruction plate should be used to span all of the fracture fragments. Special attention should be paid to the extent of the lingual fractures. These fractures may extend further than the buccal cortex fractures. The reconstruction plate should be of sufficient length to span the length of all of the fractures. Any piece of bone that appears to be devascularized and nonviable should be removed prior to fixation. It is advised that fixation be obtained with at least three or preferably four screws on each side of these high-impact, high-energy fractures. There is often concomitant soft tissue loss over these fractures. Even in the area of soft tissue loss, bone reduction and reestablishment of mandibular contour should be obtained. Obtaining soft tissue closure in such a situation and not reestablishing the mandibular contour will lead to scarring of the soft tissue into the defect and render future mandibular reconstruction extremely difficult. Local, regional, and distant vascularized tissues for coverage of the fractured mandible and plate should be used to ensure healing.

Dentoalveolar Injuries

Injuries to the oral cavity are common in trauma patients. Of these injuries, 80% occur in the area of the four anterior maxillary teeth.[16] Any trauma to the lower face can result in injury to this dentoalveolar complex. Laceration of the lips and intraoral mucosa is often associated with injury to the teeth and their supporting structures. As in other mandibular fractures, signs and symptoms associated with dentoalveolar fractures include intraoral bleeding, tooth malposition, malocclusion, mobility of the affected structures, pain, and change of sensation in the teeth. It is extremely important that the physician always count the patient's teeth after an injury. Missing teeth should be noted and retrieved if at all possible. Damaged teeth may lodge in the surrounding soft tissue, such as lips and tongue, or may be caught in the airway or aspirated into the lungs. If there is any suspicion of aspiration, appropriate airway precautions should be taken along with x-ray films of the chest and neck.

Dentoalveolar fractures involve a fracture of the alveolar bone and the associated teeth. The teeth in turn may or may not have fractures at the crown of the root and may be luxated or avulsed. These injuries are open fractures and should be managed as such. Attention should be paid to tetanus prophylaxis, systemic antibiotics, and reduction and fixation of the fractures.

Tooth Fracture

Tooth fractures can involve the crown or the root or both. Ellis described a classification for tooth fractures.[17] Class I involves a fracture of the surrounding of the tooth enamel. Class I fractures are usually painless. The enamel has no sensory system. This is not an urgent problem. Appropriate referral to a dentist is encouraged. Class II fractures involve the dentin of the tooth that lies below the enamel and contains dentinal tubules. These are extremely sensitive, and the area should be treated with a medicated dental paste such as calcium hydroxide or an acid-etched composite resin to cover the exposed dentin and decrease the pain. A class III fracture involves the pulp or neurovascular center of the tooth and is extremely painful. Dental consultation should be sought urgently.

Tooth Luxation

Luxation of the tooth is described as malpositioning of a tooth in its alveolar bone socket. This type of injury is indicative of damage to the periodontal ligaments that surround the tooth roots as well as the neurovascular bundle that enters the apex of the tooth root. Treatment involves gentle manipulation of the tooth into position and digital manipulation of the surrounding alveolar bone into position. The prognosis for long-term damage of the tooth is dependent on the amount of displacement from its normal position.[18] Again, dental referral is strongly recommended. Treatment usually involves splinting of the affected tooth to the surrounding teeth with bonded acrylic, a monofilament nylon or wire, or placement of an arch bar segment.

Tooth Avulsion

An avulsion injury is described as subtotal or total separation of the tooth from the alveolar bone. This is a dental emergency. The prognosis for the long-term viability of the tooth in a successful replantation is inversely proportional to the length of time that it is out of its bony socket.[17] The tooth should usually be replanted into its bony socket within 20 minutes to 2 hours. The absolute key to success is the continued nourishment and maintenance of the periodontal ligament surrounding the roots of the tooth. If these periodontal ligament fibers become desiccated, necrotic, or avulsed due to rough handling, the tooth, if replaced in its bony socket, can ankylose to the surrounding bone and ultimately be lost. Therefore, gentle handling of the root of the tooth where the ligaments are attached is of utmost importance. The tooth root should not be scrubbed or brushed. The tooth should be handled by its crown and irrigated with normal saline. If the tooth cannot be immediately reimplanted in its bony socket, then it should be gently cleaned as previously described and placed in the buccal vestibule in the patient's mouth. Then the patient should be transported immediately to a dentist. If this is not possible, then the tooth should be placed in fresh cold milk, sterile saline, or cool tap water depending on the environment surrounding the injury. Milk is considered an ideal storage medium.[18] The periodontal cells have been shown to maintain mitotic activities for up to 6 hours when stored in milk. There are also commercial transport systems available for avulsed teeth. Treatment should be instituted by a dentist and involves replanting the tooth in its socket, splinting the tooth as previously described, placing the patient on a soft diet and antibiotics, and doing a close follow-up. Very often the tooth will require endodontic therapy for ultimate salvage.

Dentoalveolar Fractures

Fractures of the alveolar bone and the associated teeth may or may not be associated with fractures of the crown or roots of the teeth. The teeth may also be luxated or avulsed. A very careful examination will reveal the diagnosis. These types of fractures are to be treated as open fractures. Attention is paid to tetanus prophylaxis, antibiotic coverage, and reduction and fixation of the fractures.

Complications

Complications of the treatment of mandibular fractures are usually the result of improper surgical technique and operator error. The severity of the injury and poor patient compliance also contribute to development of complications.

Infection at the fracture site can result from a nonvital, damaged, or infected tooth in the fracture line, foreign body in the wound, poor oral hygiene, or inadequate reduction and fixation of the fracture. The issues of the tooth in line of a fracture have been addressed earlier. Most of the approaches to the fracture sites are now intraoral, thus avoiding an external skin incision. Intraoral contamination may theoretically increase the incidence of infection, though this has not been proven. Poor plate size selection, improper placement of the plate, or inadequate number of screws, which cannot withstand the forces of mastication, can lead to excessive movement at the fracture site. Plate failure, infection, and nonunion may result. When an infection is diagnosed, the source should be removed, the abscess drained, and an appropriate antibiotic administered. Rigid-plate fixation, an external pin device, or MMF should be used to maintain immobilization while preserving proper occlusion. If bony infection proceeds to sequestrum formation, sequestrectomy and bone graft to bridge the gap may be necessary.

Nonunion results when there is persistent motion at the fracture site, and bone necrosis occurs at the fracture site due to infection. Fibrous tissue fills the gap rather than new bridging bone. Treatment requires curetting of the intervening fibrous tissue and rigid fixation of the fresh bony ends together. If there is a persistent gap after the teeth have been placed in proper occlusion, the gap should be filled with a cancellous bone graft (or a corticocancellous bone graft for large defects).

Malunion occurs when the bone heals under poor anatomical reduction. Even the slightest step-off in the tooth-bearing region, or posteriorly in the angle or ramus, can result in malocclusion. Unfortunately, most of the titanium plates that are in use today are not forgiving enough to allow for realignment of teeth by the use of elastics. Therefore, it is important to achieve proper anatomical bony reduction, dental interdigitation, and passive plate adaptation prior to plate fixation. After fixation, the MMF is released; the jaw is manually opened and closed with the condyle seated in the fossa to double-check the occlusion. Any malalignment or open bite must be corrected at this time.

Damage to the tooth roots can occur if screws or pins are placed improperly. Although it is less likely to occur with the inferior border plates, indiscriminate placement of monocortical screws in the tension band plates at the superior border can damage the tooth roots. The inferior alveolar nerve is often contused, stretched, or even severed during injury. However, with proper fracture reduction and alignment of the mandibular canal, nerve regeneration may occur. Hence, further iatrogenic damage to the nerve should be avoided during screw placement. Finally, as an external approach to the mandible is occasionally required, placement of the preauricular incision to expose the condyle, and the submandibular incision for the angle, may risk injury to the temporal branch or the marginal mandibular branch of the seventh nerve. Resolution of traction injury may take 6 months to 1 year.

Summary

The treatment of the mandibular fracture has evolved from semirigid- to rigid-plate fixation, permitting immediate jaw opening. Percutaneous screw placement allows performance of most of the reduction and fixation through an intraoral approach, obviating the external incisional scar. There is also increasing awareness of the absolute importance of dental occlusion, bone healing principles, as well as a better understanding of rigid fixation using plates or lag screws. On the horizon appears to be the endoscopic approach to such difficult areas as the TMJ, distraction osteogenesis for bony transport to bridge a gap, and the use of resorbable plates.

References

1. Emshoff R, Schoning H, Rothler G. Trends in the incidence and cause of sport-related mandibular fractures: a retrospective analysis. J Oral Maxillofac Surg 1997;55:585–592
2. Hunter JG. Pediatric maxillofacial trauma. Pediatr Clin North Am 1992;39(5):1127–1143
3. Olson RA, Fonseca RJ, Zeitler DL, et al. Fractures of the mandible: a review of 580 cases. J Oral Maxillofac Surg 1982;40:23
4. Chayra GA, Meador LR, Laskin DM. Comparison of panoramic and standard radiographs for the diagnosis of mandibular fractures. J Oral Maxillofac Surg 1986;44(9):677–679
5. Niederdellmann H, Shetty V. Solitary lag screw osteosynthesis in the treatment of fractures of the angle of the mandible. Plast Reconstr Surg 1987;80:68
6. Ellis E, Sinn DP. Treatment of mandibular angle fractures using two 2.4-mm dynamic compression plates. J Oral Maxillofac Surg 1993;51:969–973
7. Prein J, Rahn BA. Scientific and technical background. In: Prein J, ed. Manual of Internal Fixation in the Craniofacial Skeleton. Berlin: Springer-Verlag; 1998:12,13,15,19
8. Schilli W, Ewers R, Niederdellmann H. Bone fixation with screws and plates in the maxillofacial region. Int J Oral Surg 1981; 10(suppl 1):329
9. Hackney F, Rohrich RJ, Sinn DP. Facial fractures II: lower third. In: Hackney F, Rohrich RJ, Sinn DP, eds. Selected Readings in Plastic Surgery. Dallas: 1998:14
10. Manson P. Facial injuries. In: McCarthy J, ed. Plastic Surgery. Vol 2. The Face. Part 1. Philadelphia: WB Saunders; 1990:961–965

11. Ellis E. Treatment methods for fractures of the mandibular angle. J Craniomaxillofac Trauma 1996;2(1):28–36
12. Ellis E, Dean J. Rigid fixation of mandibular condyle fractures. Oral Surg Oral Med Oral Pathol 1993;76:6–15
13. Klotch DW, Lundy LB. Condylar neck fractures of the mandible. Otolaryngol Clin North Am 1991;24(1):181
14. Zide MF, Kent JN. Indications of open reduction of mandibular condyle fractures. J Oral Maxillofac Surg 1983;41:89
15. Jacobovicz J, Lee C, Trabulsy PP. Endoscopic repair of mandibular subcondylar fractures. Plast Reconstr Surg 1998;101(2):437–441
16. Padilla RR, Felsenfeld AL. Treatment and prevention of alveolar fractures and related injuries. J Craniomaxillofac Trauma 1997;3:2–27
17. Elis RG. The Classification and Treatment of Injuries to the Teeth of Children. 4th ed. Chicago: Year Book Publishers; 1960
18. Camp JH. Diagnosis and management of sports-related injuries to the teeth. Dent Clin North Am 1991;35:733–756

VI

Congenital and Pediatric Facial Plastic Surgery

73 Embryology of the Head, Face, and Neck

George S. Goding and David W. Eisele

Prenatal life has been divided into an embryonic period, consisting of the first 8 weeks of gestation, and a fetal period, which encompasses the ninth gestational week to birth. The embryonic period is particularly important because it is the time during which most organ systems are established[1] and most congenital anomalies appear.[2] By the end of the embryonic period, the major features of the body form are recognizable. The fetal period is characterized by rapid growth and maturation of the tissues and organs.

In the Carnegie system of staging, the embryonic period is divided into 23 stages based on external and internal morphology.[3] This system is thought to provide greater accuracy in the sequencing of developmental events compared with other staging systems that are based on prenatal age or length. **Table 73.1** provides an overview of the 23 stages with reference to development of structures related to facial development. Where possible, developmental events are referenced to the embryonic stage in the first 8 weeks of development and to the gestational age in weeks during the fetal period.

This chapter concentrates on the aspects of normal prenatal development relating to facial plastic surgery. Emphasis is placed on development of external structures of the face, head, and neck. Such topics as the development of the orbital contents, the middle and internal ear, and the central nervous system are either abbreviated or omitted. The reader is referred to general texts on embryology for more detailed discussion of these topics.[1,4]

Early Development

Stages 1 to 5 fall within the first week of development. During these stages, the human organism changes from a single cell to a multicelled, hollow blastocyst embedded in endometrial stroma.[1,5] During the second week (stages 5 and 6), the bilaminar germ disc is formed with ectodermal and endodermal germ layers. The disc has bilateral symmetry, anterior and posterior ends, and dorsal and ventral surfaces.[5] The ectoderm gives rise to the cutaneous and

Table 73.1 Stages in the Embryonic Period

Embryonic Stage	Characteristic Structures and Size, Gestational Age, Developmental Events[a]
Stages 1 to 8	0 to 15 mm; 0 to 18 days. Based on the morphological appearance of the embryo or its covering.
Stage 9	1.5 to 2.5 mm; 1 to 3 pairs of somites; 20 days. Somites first appear, buccopharyngeal membrane, first pharyngeal pouch, otic disc present.
Stage 10	1.5 to 2.5 mm; 4 to 12 pairs of somites; 20 days. Neural folds begin to fuse, maxillary process, second pharyngeal cleft visible.
Stage 11	2.5 to 4.5 mm; 12 to 20 pairs of somites; 22 days. Rostral neuropore closes, third arch appears, buccopharyngeal membrane ruptures.
Stage 12	3.5 mm; 21 to 29 pairs of somites; 26 days. Caudal neuropore closes and upper limb buds appear. Cervical sinus visible.
Stage 13	4 to 6 mm; 30 or more pairs of somites; 28 days. Four limb buds are developing. 4th and 6th arches develop, nasal placode seen.
Stage 14	5 to 7 mm; 32 days. Optic cup forms.
Stage 15	7 to 9 mm; 33 days. Hard palate appears, olfactory pit is formed.
Stage 16	8 to 11 mm; 37 days. Footplate appears, auricular hillocks appearing, nasolacrimal groove forming.
Stage 17	11 to 14 mm; 41 days. Finger rays appear, inferior turbinate swelling present.
Stage 18	13 to 17 mm; 44 days. Toe rays appear. Choanae identifiable.
Stage 19	16 to 18 mm; 48 days. Changes in remaining stages more subtle.
Stage 20	18 to 22 mm; 51 days. Medial canthus established, merging of auricular hillocks complete.
Stage 21	22 to 24 mm; 52 days. Palatal processes separated by tongue.
Stage 22	23 to 28 mm; 54 days. Few specific changes.
Stage 23	27 to 31 mm; 57 days. The embryo is approximately 30 mm in crown-rump length and approximately 8 postovulatory weeks in age; palatal shelves reorient to horizontal position.
Fetus	Ninth to fortieth week. Bone marrow formation is present in the humerus.

[a]Especially as regards development of head, neck, and face.

Table 73.2 Derivatives of the Pharyngeal Arches

Arch	Cartilage	Muscle	Nerve
1	Maxillary process (premaxilla, maxilla, zygoma), Meckel cartilage (mandible), incus, malleus	Muscles of mastication, anterior of belly of digastric, mylohyoid, tensor tympani, tensor palatine	Mandibular branch trigeminal nerve
2	Hyoid or Reichert cartilage (stapes, styloid process, stylohyoid ligament, lesser horn and upper body of hyoid bone)	Stapedius, stylohyoid posterior belly of digastric, auricular, muscles of facial expression	Facial nerve
3	Greater horn and lower body of hyoid bone	Stylopharyngeus	Glossopharyngeal nerve
4 and 6	Thyroid, cricoid, arytenoid, corniculate, and cuneiform cartilage of larynx	4—cricothyroid, levator palatine constrictors of pharynx 6—Intrinsic laryngeal muscles	4—Superior laryngeal nerve 6—Recurrent laryngeal nerve

neural systems, and the endoderm develops into the lining epithelium of the digestive and respiratory systems and the secretory cells of the liver and pancreas.

During the third week of development (stages 7 to 9), folding of the embryonic disc occurs in the anteroposterior plane and the lateral plane. Ectodermal cells invaginate between the ectodermal and endodermal layers toward a primitive streak to form the mesodermal layer. The mesoderm becomes mesenchyme from which the cardiovascular system, connective tissues, and locomotor system of bones and muscles develop. Anterior to the primitive streak, the notochord is formewd from invaginating cells. Above the notochord, neural folds develop and begin to fuse in stage 10 to form the neural tube that detaches from the surface ectoderm.[1]

Ectodermally derived neural crest cells form an intermediate layer between the neural tube and the surface ectoderm. In the head the neural crest cells infiltrate the developing pharyngeal arch structures and proliferate extensively. The neural crest differentiates into mesenchyme, forming the majority of the facial structures but excluding the retina, lens, epithelial tissues, vascular endothelia, and most skeletal muscle.[6–9]

Development of the Pharyngeal Arches

The formation of the head and neck is intimately associated with the development of the pharyngeal arches. Development of the pharyngeal arches begins during stage 9 (20 days). By stage 13 (28 days), four well-developed pairs of arches are visible. Each arch contains an artery, a nerve, a cartilaginous bar, and a muscle component. Below each arch is an external groove (pharyngeal cleft) and a corresponding outpouching of the primitive pharynx (pharyngeal pouch).

In stage 14 (32 days), the second arch begins to grow rapidly over the third and fourth arches and clefts to form the cervical sinus. The second arch eventually fuses with the ectoderm in an area below the fourth arch. By day 48 (stage 18), the second, third, and fourth arches are obliterated along with the cervical sinus, giving rise to a smooth contour of the neck. Only the dorsal end of the first pharyngeal cleft remains to form the external auditory meatus.[9]

The derivatives of the pharyngeal arches are well described in general embryology texts[1,4] and are listed in **Table 73.2**.

Development of the Face

The development of the face can be first recognized in stage 9 with the appearance of stomodeum.[10] The majority of facial structures are near their final position by the end of the embryonic period, but gradual development of the face continues into adulthood.[11] The embryonic face is made up of grooves and bulges created by the uneven distribution of subepidermal mesenchyme. Developmental changes seem to be the result of a disappearance of the grooves, which gradually enlarge with proliferating mesenchyme, rather than the migration and fusion of distinct processes.[12,13] Development of the middle third of the face is closely associated with changes in the developing forebrain. The lateral and lower facial regions are formed by the maxillary and mandibular processes of the first pharyngeal arch.[13]

In the stage 11 embryo (**Fig. 73.1A**), the future region of the face is defined by an invagination of the surface ectoderm called the *stomodeum*. At the depth of the stomodeum is a bilaminar buccopharyngeal membrane consisting of surface ectoderm and endoderm from the anterior portion of the foregut. The buccopharyngeal membrane, which is first seen in stage 9, breaks down during this stage, giving rise to the primitive oral cavity.[10] The stomodeum is bounded by four masses of epithelially covered mesoderm. The cranial portion is the anterior end of the embryo, which contains the developing forebrain. The caudal portion is the mandibular process of the first pharyngeal arch, which meets its counterpart from the opposite side in the midline to separate the stomodeum from the developing heart. The maxillary process of the first pharyngeal arch is present on each lateral border.

In stages 12 and 13 (**Fig. 73.1B**), the third and fourth pharyngeal arches are well defined.[10,14,15] The forebrain

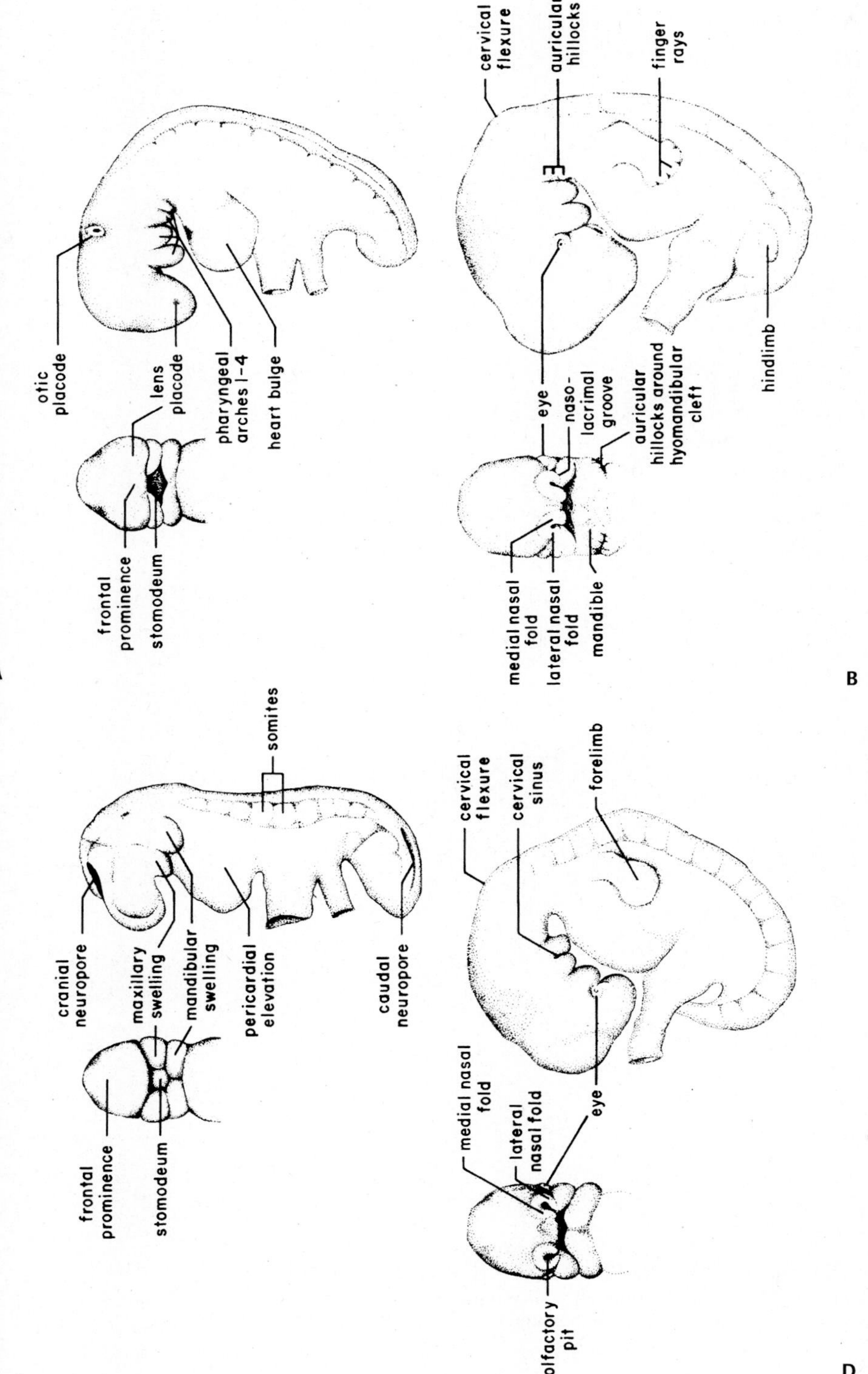

Fig. 73.1 Development of the face. (**A**) Stage 11. (**B**) Stage 13. (**C**) Stage 15. (**D**) Stage 16.

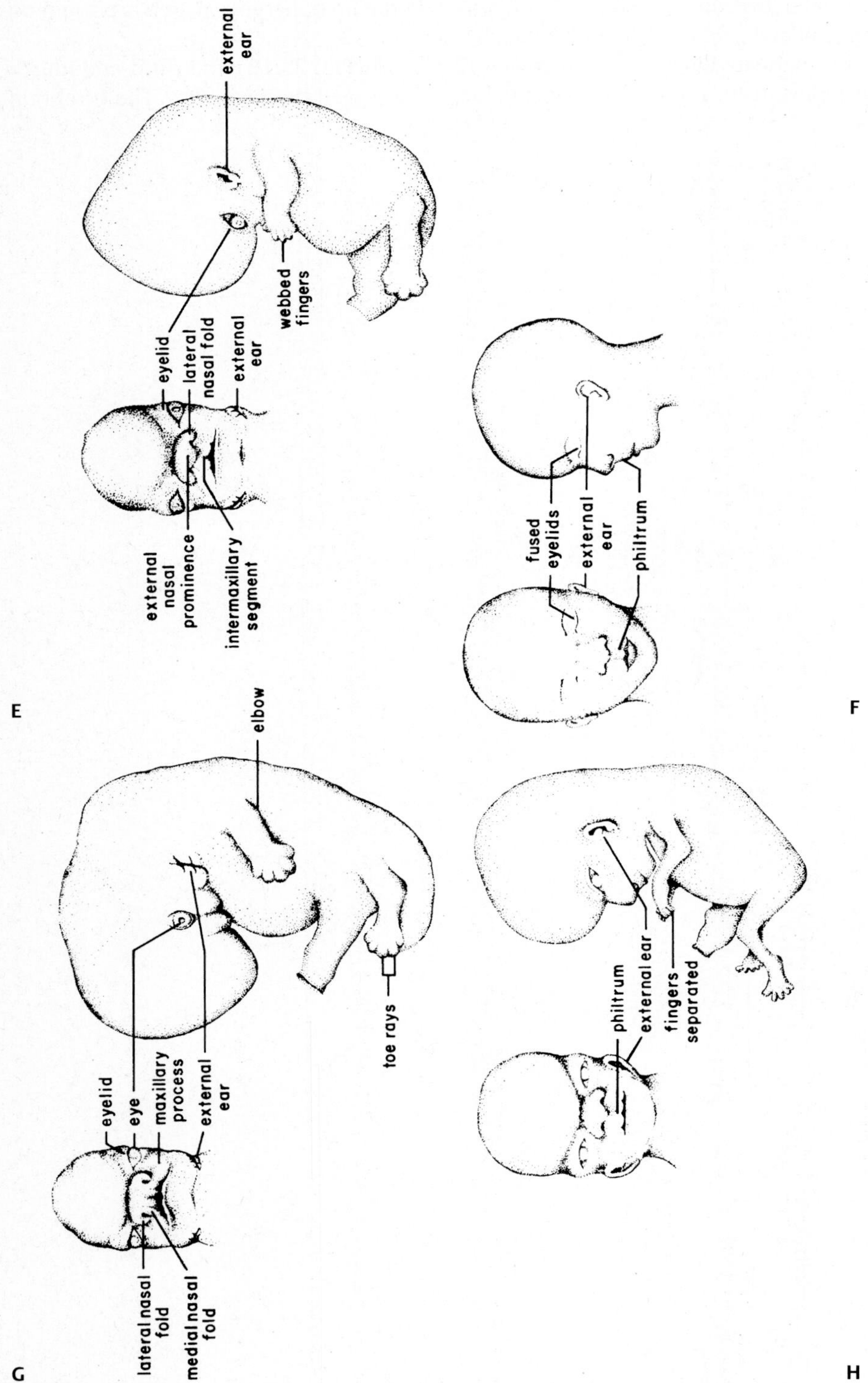

Fig. 73.1 (*Continued*) Development of the face. (**E**) Stage 18. (**F**) Stage 20. (**G**) Stage 23. (**H**) 19 weeks. (Modified from Patten W. The face and jaws and the teeth. In: Patten BM, ed. Human embryology. 3rd ed. New York: McGraw-Hill; 1968. Key. The embryonic period. In: Moore KL. The Developing Human. 2nd ed. Philadelphia: WB Saunders; 1977.)

begins to enlarge, and the upper end of the embryo begins to change from a conical shape and broadens to form the frontal prominence. The nasal placode has begun to develop and is seen as an ectodermal thickening on the frontal prominence.

In stages 14 and 15 (**Fig. 73.1C**), there is a proliferation of the mesoderm surrounding the nasal placodes, which leads to the formation of the lateral nasal fold and later, the medial nasal fold.[16] This process results in a depression of the nasal placodes, which are now referred to as *olfactory pits*. With the formation of the olfactory pits, the frontal prominence can be subdivided into upper and lower parts. The upper part is the primitive forehead, and the lower portion consists of the future external nose and prolabium.[13] While this process is occurring, the hemispheric vesicles expand, resulting in a broadening of the frontal prominence. This growth moves the nasal pits to the anterolateral border of the frontal prominence.

The maxillary prominences have become more distinct at the lateral border of the stomodeum in stage 15.[14] In stage 16 (**Fig. 73.1D**), the maxillary processes continue to develop medially and contact both the medial and the lateral nasal folds. Between the lateral nasal fold and the maxillary prominence is the nasolacrimal groove, which marks the site of the future nasolacrimal duct. The slit-shaped olfactory pits by this time have widened and deepened. The olfactory pits and their associated nasal folds move further toward the midline. The caudal portion of the two medial nasal folds forms the intermaxillary segment. Structures that are thought to arise from the intermaxillary segment include the philtrum of the upper lip and the anterior portion of the maxilla.[17] Beginning in stage 16, the region of the forehead enlarges because of the extensive growth of the developing brain. In stage 18, the eyes change their position from a lateral to a frontal oblique position. At the same time, the nostrils move medially from a frontolateral position.[14]

In stages 17 and 18 (**Fig. 73.1E**) the groove between the medial nasal folds begins to fill with mesoderm, and formation of the outer relief of the nose begins. The olfactory pits deepen further and open into the roof of the mouth during stage 18. The furrow between each medial and lateral nasal fold extends into the primitive oral cavity and begins to define the site of the palatal shelves.[14] Mesodermal proliferation begins to fill the grooves between the medial nasal folds and the maxillary processes to form the upper lip by stage 18. In addition, the maxillary processes merge with the lateral nasal folds, and the nasolacrimal groove is filled.

The origin of the nasolacrimal duct is controversial. Some believe the nasolacrimal groove is completely eliminated, with the nasolacrimal duct arising as a separate process.[11] Others believe the nasolacrimal duct to be a remnant of the nasolacrimal groove.[1]

The external changes that occur in stages 19 to 23 are gradual (**Fig. 73.1F, G**). Merging of the lateral portion of the maxillary processes with the mandibular processes occurs, thus reducing the opening of the oral cavity. Mesoderm from the second pharyngeal arch infiltrates the facial region and develops into the muscles of facial expression innervated by the facial nerve. Mandibular ossification is present lateral to Meckel's cartilage and extends posteriorly to form the coronoid and condylar processes of the mandible by stage.[11,12] At the end of the embryonic period, the temporomandibular joint can be identified.[11] In addition, muscles of mastication develop from the first pharyngeal arch and are innervated by the mandibular branch of the trigeminal nerve.

The nasal pits shift toward the middle of the face. There is no fusion of the median nasal folds; rather, a mesodermal filling between the nostrils occurs, which results in the external nasal prominence.[14] The external nose appears to develop from two distinct but contiguous mesodermal fields. One chondrifies at the end of the embryonic period and forms the cartilaginous skeleton for the nasal cavity. The other chondrifies at 10 weeks gestation to form the future alar cartilages.[18] At stage 22, an epithelial plug is present in the anterior nares, which regresses by week 24 of gestation, allowing patency of the nerves.[14] Near the end of the embryonic period, the epineural ectoderm in the roof of the nasal cavity differentiates into olfactory epithelium.[19]

The lateral wall of the nasal cavity first develops the inferior turbinate (stage 17) and, subsequently, the middle and superior turbinates.[11,16] By 12 to 14 weeks, the nasal region is fairly well developed. The paranasal sinuses develop much later as tiny diverticula from the lateral walls of the nasal cavity. The earliest sinuses to form are the maxillary, followed by the sphenoid. The ethmoid and frontal sinuses develop after birth.

Development of the Tongue

The floor of the primitive oral cavity in stage 12 to 14 embryos consists of a series of ridges formed by the first four pharyngeal arches (**Fig. 73.2A**). The first arch gives rise to two lateral lingual swellings and a midline tuberculum impar. The second ridge is the second pharyngeal arch, behind which the hypobranchial eminence forms a second midline structure made up of mesoderm from the second, third, and fourth arches.[1] The third and fourth arch derivatives do not meet in the midline, which is occupied by the epiglottic swelling.[20]

Over the next six embryonic stages, the lateral lingual swellings overgrow the tuberculum impar and form the anterior two thirds of the tongue[1] (**Fig. 73.2B**), the mucosa

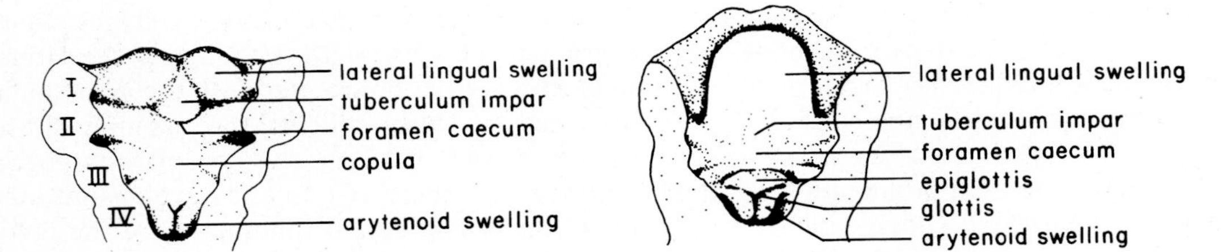

Fig. 73.2 Development of the tongue. (**A**) Horizontal section through pharynx at stage 14, showing ridges of pharyngeal arches. (**B**) Horizontal section at stage 20, showing formation of anterior tongue from fusion of lateral lingual swellings. (Modified from Patten BM. Human Embryology. 3rd ed. New York: McGraw-Hill; 1968.)

of which is innervated by the mandibular branch of the trigeminal nerve. The third pharyngeal arch contribution to the hypobranchial eminence develops into the posterior one third of the tongue, the mucosa of which is innervated by the glossopharyngeal nerve. The muscle of the tongue develops from occipital somites innervated by the hypoglossal nerve.[12]

The foramen cecum lies in the terminal sulcus, separating the anterior two thirds of the tongue from the posterior one third of the tongue. The presence of the foramen cecum marks the origin of the thyroid gland, which appears in stage 13 as an epithelial proliferation between the tuberculum impar and the hypobranchial eminence. The thyroid descends in stage 14 and detaches from the pharyngeal epithelium by stage 15.[10] The thyroglossal duct connects the thyroid to the tongue, becomes solid, and eventually disappears.[1]

From stage 20 to the tenth gestational week, the tongue descends from a position high in the oral cavity (**Fig. 73.3A**), allowing closure of the palatal shelves (**Fig. 73.3B**). During

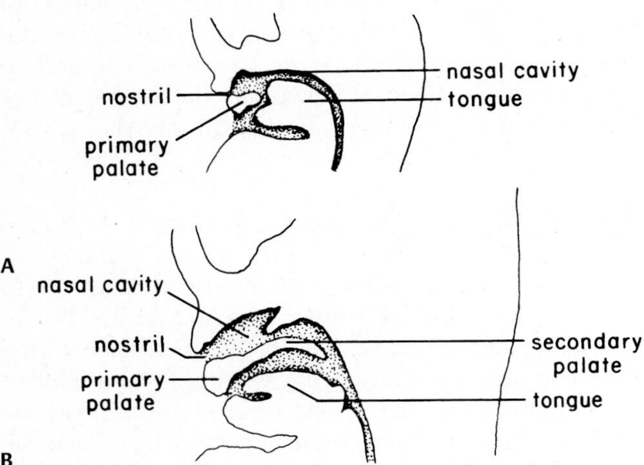

Fig. 73.3 Development of the tongue. (**A**) Sagittal section at stage 20. Note position of tongue high in oral cavity. (**B**) Sagittal section at stage 23 showing tongue descent. (From Diewert VM. A morphometric analysis of craniofacial growth and changes in spatial relations during secondary platal development in human embryos and fetuses. Am J Anat 1983;167:495. Reprinted with permission of Wiley-Liss, Inc., a subsidiary of John Wiley & Sons, Inc.)

this time, the length of the tongue does not increase but its position changes. The musculus genioglossus and musculus geniohyoideus are developed by stage 22 and are attached to the mandible, allowing anterior tongue protrusion.[21]

Development of the Palate

The palate develops over a relatively long period of time, with fusion of the palatal shelves delayed until after the embryonic period. The palate is divided into two components based on its formation. The primary palate is formed at least in part by the caudal portion of the medial nasal folds. The early development of the medial nasal fold has been described previously. The secondary palate develops from processes derived from the maxillary prominence.

In stage 17, the roof of the oral cavity is concave with the opening of Rathke's pouch placed posteriorly. The olfactory pits are prominent and in a frontolateral position. The groove between the medial and lateral nasal folds extends into the oral cavity and borders the middle portion of the roof. Lateral to the groove, swellings are developing that are the first indications of the future secondary palate.[14] There are no openings of the primary choanae at this stage.

As the medial nasal processes start to merge in stage 18, the future primary palate is present as a pair of small swellings, which develop in the anterior roof of the oral cavity (**Fig. 73.4A**).[14] The primary palate is further defined by the opening of the primitive posterior choanae of the nasal cavity into the roof of the oral cavity.[14,16]

In stages 19 to 22, the lateral palatine shelves of the maxillary processes lengthen bilaterally (**Fig. 73.4B**). Until stage 22, the shelves project inward and obliquely downward on either side of the developing tongue, which occupies the central portion of the oral cavity.[10,21] During this period, the paired primary palate becomes a single, triangular mass in the anterior roof of the oral cavity and is continuous with the primordium of the nasal septum above.[14]

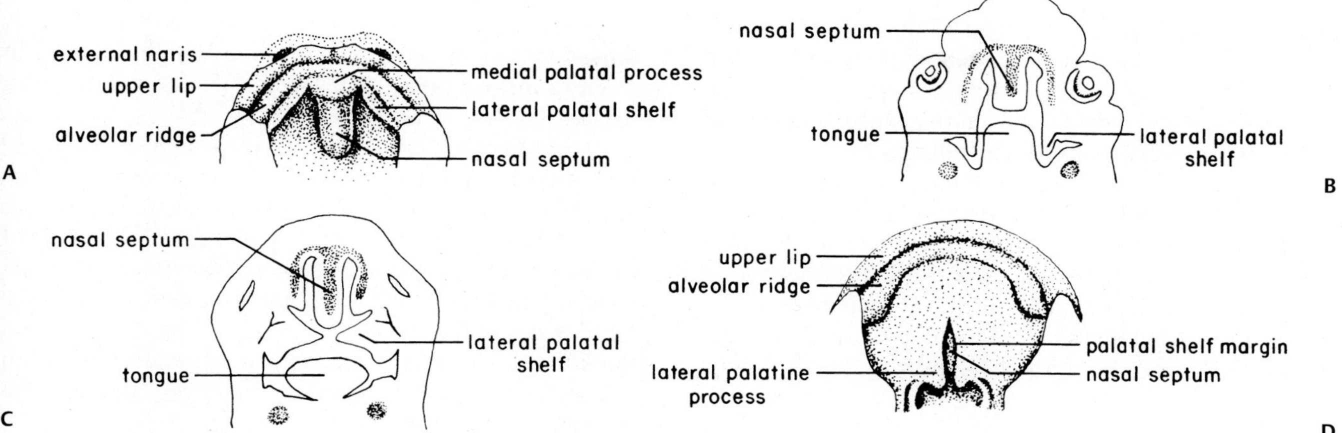

Fig. 73.4 Development of the palate. (**A**) Roof of oral cavity at stage 18. (**B**) Coronal section of palate at stage 22. Note separation of palatal shelves by tongue. (**C**) Coronal section of palate at stage 23. Note horizontal change of position of lateral palatine shelves. (**D**) Roof of oral cavity at 9 weeks with fusion of lateral palatal shelves. (From Dirske L. The face and jaws and the teeth. In: Patten BM, ed. Human Embryology. 3rd ed. New York: McGraw-Hill, 1968. Reprinted by permission.)

In stage 23, the palatal shelves swing upward to a more horizontal position (**Fig. 73.4C**). Debate continues over the mechanism whereby the reorientation of the palatal shelves occurs. Hydration and expansion of mesenchymal mucopolysaccharides within the palatal shelf may produce intrinsic tissue pressure that reorients the palate.[22] A direct role of palatal cell contractility to produce this effect has also been postulated.[23] Others believe that palatal shelf elevation involves a complex interaction between the shelves and the surrounding craniofacial complex.[21,24,25]

The mandibular process and tongue are relatively small in stage 19. In addition, the tongue is positioned high in the oral cavity. The head is rotated downward and forward with the nasomaxillary prominence near the developing heart. By stage 23, the facial profile has been reversed with increased growth of the mandible. With growth of Meckel's cartilage, the tongue is pulled forward and positioned under the primary palate where it no longer interferes with palatal shelf movement (**Fig. 73.3**). At the same time, extension of the head occurs relative to the body, which further separates the upper facial structures from the mandible–tongue complex.[21,24]

Fusion of the palatal shelves occurs during the fetal period. Growth of the horizontally positioned palatal shelves results in their midline approximation. Palatal fusion occurs in an anteroposterior direction beginning with fusion between the primary and secondary palates (**Fig. 73.4D**). During this process, the incisive foramina are formed. With continued fusion of the secondary palate, the oral and nasal cavities are separated. By the beginning of the tenth week, hard palate formation is complete.[21] Along the posterior border of the palatine processes, mesenchymal cells form the soft palate, which is closed in the midline by the end of the tenth week.[21]

Formation of the nasal septum during this period has traditionally been described to be a result of downward growth of a free process from the roof of the nasal cavity.[1] In contrast, others have proposed that the nasal septum develops in an anteroposterior direction in concert with palatal shelf fusion.[14]

Development of the Ear

The first indication of the developing ear can be seen in stage 9 with the presence of the otic disc.[26] The disc appears as a thickening of the surface ectoderm forming opposite the rhombencephalic fold. In stage 11, the otic disc has invaginated and is referred to as the *otic pit*. The pit's communication with the external surface narrows and by stage 13 is closed from the surface, forming the otic vesicle.[26] Under the influence of mesodermal and neural induction, the otic vesicle gives rise to the structures of the inner ear.[27]

The middle ear is derived from the first pharyngeal pouch and is endodermal in origin.[28] The distal end of the pouch grows toward the ectodermally derived external auditory meatus to form the tympanic cavity. The proximal end of the pouch forms the eustachian tube. The tympanic cavity expands and envelops the chorda tympani nerve and the middle ear ossicles, tendons, and ligaments, which develop from the first (incus and malleus) and second (stapes) pharyngeal arches.[1,9,28]

Like the middle ear, the external ear develops from the pharyngeal apparatus and begins development near the midline in the future region of the neck.[28] The dorsal parts of the first (mandibular) and the second (hyoid) arch show the beginnings of hillock formation by stage 16. Three hillocks develop from the caudal border of the first arch, and three develop from the cephalic border of the second arch (**Fig. 73.5A**). The hillocks increase in size secondary to mesenchymal proliferation, and by stage 17 the six hillocks reach their maximum size, move in a dorsolateral direction, and begin to merge (**Fig. 73.5B**).[9] The first auricular hillock gives rise to the tragus, and the second and third hillocks form the crus helicis. The fourth and fifth hillocks become the crura antihelicis and the helix, and the sixth develops into the antitragus (**Fig. 73.5C**).[9,26]

After obliteration of the cervical sinus by the second pharyngeal arch, only the first pharyngeal cleft (hyomandibular groove) remains. While the auricular hillocks are forming, the dorsal portion of the first pharyngeal cleft begins to widen (stage 17), and the ectodermal cells at its base begin to proliferate to form the meatal plug. The meatal plug extends medially and begins to approach the expanding tympanic cavity by the tenth week.[9] The central cells in the plug begin to dissolve in the eighteenth week to form a cavity that forms the external auditory meatus.[29]

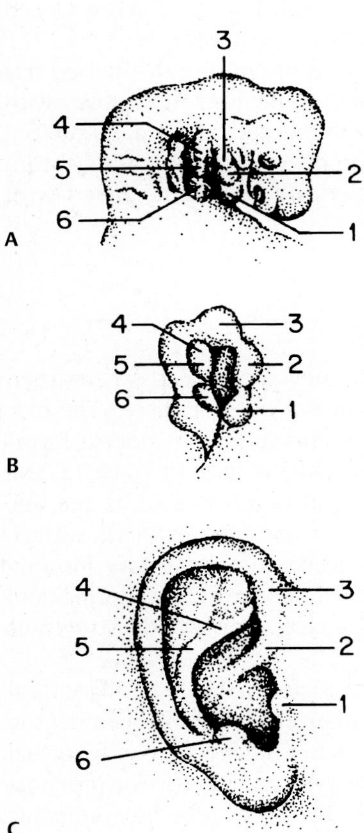

Fig. 73.5 Development of the auricle, lateral views. (**A**) Eleven-mm embryo; 1 to 3, first (mandibular) hillocks; 4 to 6, second (hyoid) hillocks. (**B**) Fifteen-mm embryo; hillock fusion begins. (**C**) Adult auricle; 1, tragus; 2 and 3, crus helicis; 4 and 5, antihelicis; 6, antitragus. (Modified from Anson BJ and McVay CB. Surgical Anatomy. 5th ed. Philadelphia: WB Saunders; 1971.)

A rudimentary pinna can be identified by stage 20 with differentiation of the fused auricular hillocks.[9] The auricle consists of a core of mesoderm covered by an epithelium of ectodermal origin. The mesodermal portion of the auricle develops from the bars of the first and second arches, which may begin to chondrify as early as stage 18.[26] At this point, the contributions of the first arch and the second arch to the auricle are roughly equal. With subsequent fetal development, however, the relative contribution of the second arch increases.[9]

The external ear is anatomically complete by the twentieth week of development. Mandibular growth during the late embryonic period and continued growth of the face during the fetal period allow the auricles to migrate to their final position.[28] The shape of the auricle is largely due to the plical folding of the cartilaginous plate, which is continuous with the cartilage of the external auditory canal. The pattern of plical folding of the auricular cartilage appears to be determined by the insertions of the intrinsic and extrinsic auricular muscles.[30]

Development of the Eye

The first indication of the developing eye occurs in stage 10 with the appearance of the optic sulcus at the level of the diencephalic portion of the brain.[26] In stage 11 the optic vesicles have formed as lateral evaginations. By stage 12, the optic vesicles have grown laterally to lie close to the surface ectoderm but remain attached to the brain by an optic stalk. The overlying surface epithelium thickens in response to the nearby optic vesicle to form the lens disc in stage 13. In stages 14 and 15 the optic vesicle flattens distally and invaginates to form the optic cup.[15] The invagination extends along the optic stalk to form a groove that will later encompass the hyaloid artery and vein (**Fig. 73.6A**). Thus the optic cup has two layers: a thin outer layer, which develops into the pigment layer of the retina, and a thick inner layer, which develops into the neural portion of the retina. Meanwhile, the lens disc invaginates and then separates from the surface epithelium to form the lens vesicle, which is situated in the opening of the optic cup (**Fig. 73.6B**).[28] The anterior one third of the optic cup near the lens vesicle develops into the iris and ciliary body, whereas the posterior two thirds of the optic cup develop into the pars optica retina containing rods, cones, bipolar cells, and ganglion cells.[1] The hyaloid vessels, which initially extend all the way to the lens, degenerate distally to become the central retinal artery

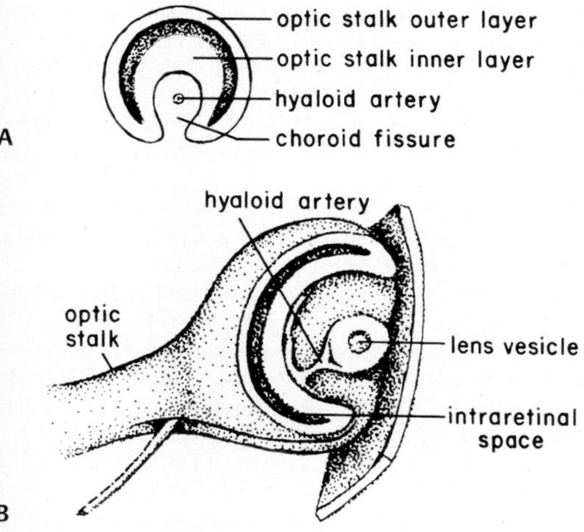

Fig. 73.6 Development of the eye. (**A**) Developing eye with optic cup, formed lens vesicle, and hyaloid artery. (**B**) Optic stalk transverse section with optic fissure. (From Reid G. The special sense organs. In: Moore KL. The Developing Human. 2nd ed. Philadelphia: WB Saunders; 1977. Reprinted by permission.)

and vein.[28] The choroid, sclera, and extraocular muscles develop from mesenchyme that envelops the optic cup.

Formation of the Cornea and Eyelids

After the lens detaches from the surface ectoderm in stage 15, the defect is restored by epithelium destined to participate in the formation of the eyelids, conjunctiva, and cornea. The presence of the eye does not appear to be necessary for formation of the lids.[31] In stage 16, the first indications of the eyelids are the formation of small depressions above and below the eye.[15] These grooves become more distinct in stage 17. The inferior groove is continuous with the nasolacrimal groove, which is forming between the maxillary process and the lateral nasal process.[15] During stages 17 to 19, mesodermal proliferation from the frontonasal process forms the upper lid and proliferation of mesodermal cells from the maxillary process forms the lower lid (**Fig. 73.1E**).[32] The mesoderm is contained by an epithelial layer with the outer epithelial layer and the inner epithelial layer destined to become eyelid skin and conjunctiva, respectively. By stage 19, the eyelid folds have developed into eyelids, and at the lateral canthus, the upper and lower lids meet. The medial canthus is established by stage 20 (**Fig. 73.1F**). During stages 21 to 23, the eyelids are rapidly encroaching over the globe, but fusion of the eyelids does not occur until approximately 1 week after the end of the embryonic period.[26]

During the last week of the embryonic period and the first 2 weeks of the fetal period, the developing eye is shifted medially from its original lateral position to the greatest extent.[28] This change in position appears to be closely related to the enormous development of the cerebral hemispheres and a general broadening of the head.[14]

Before fusion of the eyelids, the future lacrimal gland appears as a grouping of buds at the upper outer portion of the conjunctival ectoderm. At the same time, lacrimal ducts are forming medially in both upper and lower lids. The lacrimal sac is soon formed at the junction of the two lacrimal ducts.[28]

By the ninth week, fusion of the eyelids is complete. With fusion of the eyelids, the conjunctival sac is completely separated from the amniotic sac.[33] At this time, lacrimal gland secretion begins to fill the closed conjunctival sac. Soon after eyelid fusion, cilia hair bulbs are formed from epithelial ingrowths from the lid margins. During the tenth week of gestation, the first signs of the orbicularis oculi appear beneath the skin and the developing tarsus is indicated by an increased density of the connective tissue deep to the muscle.[33] The levator palpebrae superioris, rectus superior bulbi, and obliquus superior bulbi develop from the same mesodermal complex. The levator palpebrae superioris merges with the upper border of the tarsal plate at approximately 11 to 12 weeks and with the skin anteriorly at 13 to 14 weeks.[32] During the sixteenth to twentieth week, the glands of the lid margin develop. By the end of that period, the glands are producing lipid, and keratin is forming in the duct walls.[34] Separation of the eyelids begins at approximately 20 weeks gestation and takes 3 weeks to complete. Lid separation begins anteriorly and is completed with separation of the conjunctival ectoderm.

Both keratinization of the lid margin and lipid secretion, leading to breakdown of epithelial bridges, have been proposed as initiating mechanisms behind lid separation.[33] Epithelial growth factor may also play a role.[32] Eyelid separation may prevent keratinization of the epithelium of the conjunctiva and cornea, which is necessary for clarity of the cornea and a healthy mucous membrane.[33]

By the time lid separation is complete, all of the major elements of the developing eye and lid are present. Further development of the muscular, glandular, and connective tissue elements occurs during the remainder of the fetal period. The eyelashes appear to shed twice during fetal life, once at the beginning of the second month and again at the end of the seventh month.[33]

Acknowledgment

The authors gratefully acknowledge Gayle J. Eisele for the illustrations.

References

1. Langman J. Medical Embryology. Baltimore: Williams & Wilkins; 1981
2. O'Rahilly R, Muller F. Respiratory and alimentary relations in staged human embryos: new embryological data and congenital anomalies. Ann Otol Rhinol Laryngol 1984;93:421

3. O'Rahilly R. Early human development and the chief sources of information on staged human embryos. Eur J Obstet Gynecol Reprod Biol 1979;9:273
4. Moore KL. The Developing Human. Philadelphia: WB Saunders; 1977
5. Tucker JA, O'Rahilly R. Observations on the embryology of the human larynx. Ann Otol Rhinol Laryngol 1972;81:520
6. Johnston MC. The neural crest in abnormalities of the face and brain. In: Bergsma D, Langman J, Paul N, ed. Morphogenesis and Malformation of Face and Brain. New York: Liss; 1975. Birth Defects: Original Articles Series, vol 2, no. 7:1
7. Johnston MC, Millicovsky G. Normal and abnormal development of the lip and palate. Clin Plast Surg 1985;12:521
8. Ledouarin NM. The neural crest in the neck and other parts of the body. In: Bergsma D, Langman J, Paul N, eds. Morphogenesis and Malformation of Face and Brain. New York: Liss; 1975. Birth Defects: Original Articles Series, vol 2, no. 7:19
9. Melnick M, Myrianthopoulos NC. External ear malformations: epidemiology, genetics, and natural history. In: Bergsma D, Langman J, Paul N, eds. Morphogenesis and Malformation of Face and Brain. New York: Liss; 1979. Birth Defects: Original Articles Series, vol 15, no. 9:1
10. O'Rahilly R. The timing and sequence of events in the development of the human digestive system and associated structures during the embryonic period proper. Anat Embryol (Berl) 1978;153:123
11. Wilson DB. Embryonic development of the head and neck, III: the face. Head Neck Surg 1979;2:145
12. Ten Cate AR. Development of the dentofacial complexes. Dent Clin North Am 1982;26:445
13. Tondury G. The normal and abnormal development of the central facial areas. Rhinology 1979;17:133
14. Hinrichsen K. The early development of morphology and patterns of the face in the human embryo. Adv Anat Embryol Cell Biol 1985;98:1
15. Pearson AA. The development of the eyelids, I: external features. J Anat 1980;130:33
16. O'Rahilly R, Boyden EA. The timing and sequence of events in the development of the human respiratory system during the embryonic period proper. Z Anat Entwicklungsgesch 1973;141:237
17. Allard RH, van der Kwast WA, van der Waal I. Nasopalatine duct cyst: review of the literature and report of 22 cases. Int J Oral Surg 1981;10:447
18. Newman MH, Burdi AR. Congenital alar field defects: clinical and embryological observations. Cleft Palate J 1981;18:188
19. Bossy J. Development of olfactory and related structures in staged human embryos. Anat Embryol (Berl) 1980;161:225
20. O'Rahilly R, Tucker JA. The early development of the larynx in staged human embryos, I: embryos of the first five weeks (to stage 15). Ann Otol Rhinol Laryngol 1973;82(Suppl 7):3
21. Diewert VM. A morphometric analysis of craniofacial growth and changes in spatial relations during secondary palatal development in human embryos and fetuses. Am J Anat 1983;167:495–522
22. Ferguson MW. Palate development: mechanisms and malformations. Ir J Med Sci 1987;156:309
23. Zimmerman EF. Neuropharmacologic teratogenesis and neurotransmitter regulation of palate development. Am J Ment Defic 1984;88:548
24. Sandham A. Embryonic facial vertical dimension and its relationship to palatal shelf elevation. Early Hum Dev 1985;12:241
25. Sandham A. Embryonic head posture and palatal shelf elevation. Early Hum Dev 1985;11:69
26. O'Rahilly R. The timing and sequence of events in the development of the human eye and ear during the embryonic period proper. Anat Embryol (Berl) 1983;168:87
27. Melnyk AR, Weiss L. Mesodermal induction defect as a possible cause of ear malformations. Ann Otol Rhinol Laryngol 1983;92:160
28. Wilson DB. Embryonic development of the head and neck, IV: organs of special sense. Head Neck Surg 1980;2:237
29. Michaels L, Soucek S. Development of the stratified squamous epithelium of the human tympanic membrane and external canal: the origin of auditory epithelial migration. Am J Anat 1989;184:334
30. Zerin M, van Allen MI, Smith DW. Intrinsic auricular muscles and auricular form. Pediatrics 1982;69:91
31. Eayrs JT. The factors governing the opening of the eyes in the albino rat. J Anat 1951;85:330
32. Sevel D. A reappraisal of the development of the eyelids. Eye 1988 2:123
33. Hamming N. Anatomy and embryology of the eyelids: a review with special reference to the development of divided nevi. Pediatr Dermatol 1983;1:51
34. Andersen H, Ehlers N, Matthiessen ME. Histochemistry and development of the human eyelids. Acta Ophthalmol (Copenh) 1965;43:288

74 Craniomaxillofacial Deformities

Craig A. Vander Kolk, Benjamin S. Carson Sr., and Michael Guarnieri

Craniomaxillofacial deformities present a range of abnormalities based on congenital conditions, trauma, and tumors. This chapter concentrates on congenital deformities, which present as a continuum from nonsynostotic deformations (posterior plagiocephaly), to single-suture synostosis, to multiple-suture craniosynostosis (craniofacial dysostosis) **Table 74.1**. Treatment of the craniosynostoses extends from conservative to multiple complex reconstructions, which may require many years (**Fig. 74.1**).

We advocate a team approach to the management of pediatric patients. Brain development, vision, sinuses, and airways must be considered.[1,2] The craniomaxillofacial team evaluates midfacial growth in childhood and adolescence, as well as occlusion and mastication in the primary mixed and permanent dentition phase.[3,4] A typical evaluation includes pediatric neurology, radiology, neurosurgery, anesthesiology, ophthalmology, and orthodontics. The management of patients is diverse and requires a long-term plan for follow-up.[5] Information about the genes and mutations underlying syndromes affecting craniofacial bones is accumulating rapidly, and surgical outcomes have been associated with specific mutations.[6,7] Genetics undoubtedly will play a growing role in deciding surgical strategies and family counseling.[8,9] The demand for outcome-based studies and evidence-based medicine has also accelerated the team management approach.

Surgical procedures frequently involved extensive scalp dissection and bone osteotomies in children with low blood volumes. Advances in anesthesiology and hemostasis have significantly reduced morbidity.[10,11] Advances in distraction osteogenesis, endoscopic surgical techniques, and the technology of absorbable plates and screws continue to change surgical options.[12,13] Craniomaxillofacial surgery in pediatric patients focuses on syndromic and nonsyndromic craniosynostosis, craniofacial tumors, trauma, and aesthetics.[14-16] The present chapter discusses indications, methods, and outcomes for craniosynostosis surgery. Trauma, anesthesiology, aesthetics, and embryology are described in separate chapters.

Table 74.1 Craniomaxillofacial Deformities

Positional	Single Suture	Craniofacial Dysostosis–Multiple Suture
Positional	Uni- and bicoronal	Apert syndrome
	Metopic	Cruzon syndrome
	Sagittal	
	Lambdoidal	

Overview of Craniosynostosis

Craniosynostosis or premature fusion of the coronal, sagittal, metopic, or lambdoidal sutures (**Fig. 74.2**) may be primary or secondary to known teratogens, metabolic disorders, hematologic disorders, or malformations such as microcephaly.[17] Craniosynostosis can also be found when patients are overshunted and sutures subsequently override and fuse.[18,19] The condition may be "isolated," involving a single suture, or "complex," involving multiple sutures.[16,20] Approximately 100 different forms have been described. Pathophysiology may be heterogeneous because phenotypes do not always associate with specific mutations.[20,21] Phenotypes have been classified as nonsyndromic and syndromic; the latter have been linked to several chromosomes.[17,22] The common syndromic synostoses involve fibroblast growth factor receptor (FGFR) and transforming growth factor receptor (TGFR) activities.[23-26] Deletions in the *TWIST* gene have been detected in Saethre-Chotzen patients.[27] Because the same receptor can be involved in different "named" syndromes (e.g., Cruzon or Pfeiffer syndrome), it seems likely that syndrome eponyms will be replaced by designating the specific gene mutation.[28]

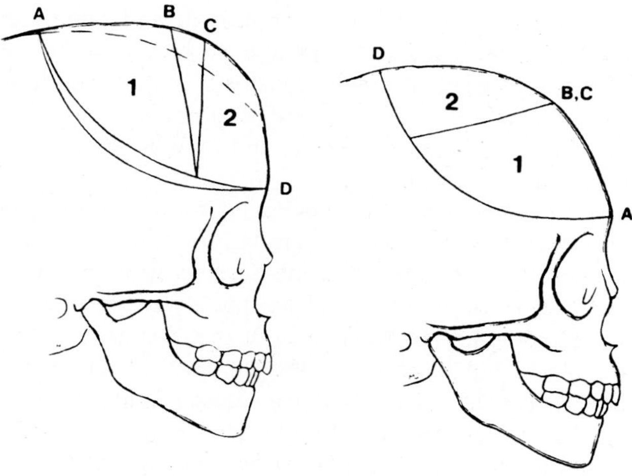

Fig. 74.1 Artistic demonstration of how bone pieces can be interchanged to dramatically alter cranial configuration. In this case, a towered forehead is given a more natural slope by interchanging pieces 1 and 2.

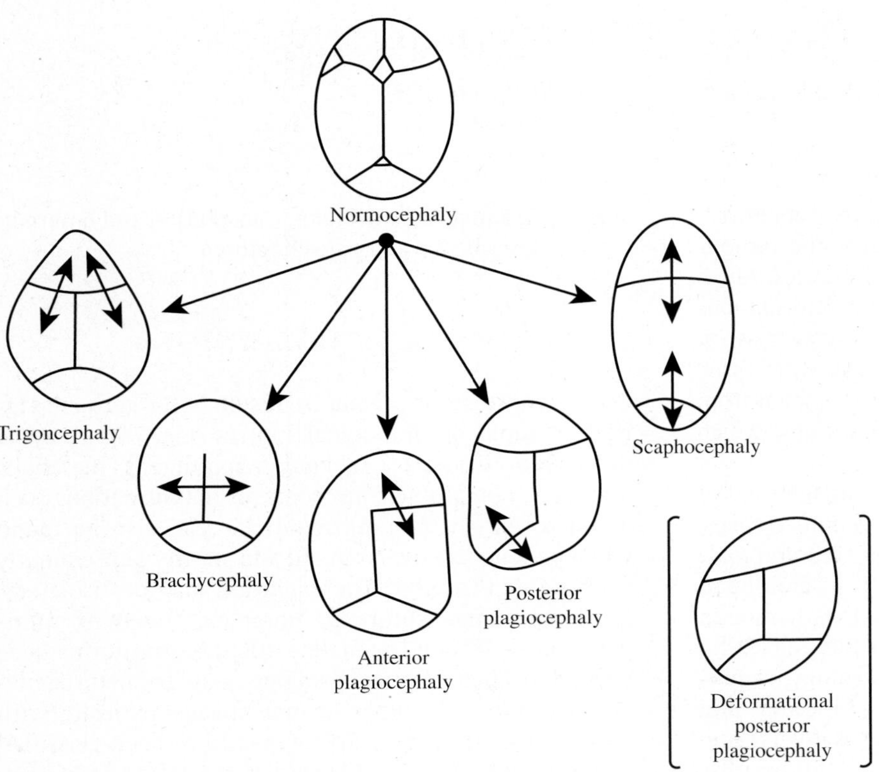

Fig. 74.2 Schematic illustration of suture changes in single-suture craniosynostosis.

Morphological studies are beginning to unravel the complex relations between intracranial pressure (ICP), skull shape, and skull volume. It has been postulated that a cranial base malformation was the primary anomaly. More recent studies lend support to the idea that the proximal cause is the premature closure of the cranial sutures, although the underlying dura may also play a role.[29,30] Computer-assisted morphological analyses have advanced the understanding of normal and abnormal growth. There are questions about intracranial volumes in patients with metopic craniosynostosis.[31,32] Many authors have concluded that intracranial volumes are normal in most forms of craniosynostosis and may be larger than normal in Apert syndrome.[33]

M. Michael Cohen has reviewed the epidemiology and pathophysiology of the craniosynostoses.[17] Briefly, incidence data are difficult to measure because the conditions are not often lethal and are not always recognized in newborns, or recorded in adults. Investigators have estimated 0.2 to 0.5 cases per 1000 births.[34,35] Such studies noted that rates appeared to be increasing, and suggested that the increase was due to enhanced awareness of the condition and improved diagnostic imaging technology. In the 1980s, a subset of the craniosynostoses, unilambdoidal synostosis, attracted particular interest because reports indicated a significant increase in the incidence, which generally had been considered to be about 1% of the craniosynostoses cases. Pediatric neurosurgeons observed that lambdoidal craniosynostosis and positional plagiocephaly (sometimes referred to as "occipital plagiocephaly" and "functional plagiocephaly") had similar morphological characteristics.[36] The suspected increase in lambdoidal synostosis was, in fact, an increase in positional plagiocephaly, an increase related to the American Academy of Pediatrics recommendation (in 1992) that healthy infants avoid the prone sleeping position. Asymmetric skull flattening tends to be perpetuated or accentuated by supine positioning of the infant; the head will turn to the flatter side by forces of gravity when any degree of torticollis exists.

Diagnosis

Pediatricians and family practitioners often request neurosurgical consultation for infants with abnormal head circumference in relation to standard growth curves yet who are otherwise normal in growth and development. Prenatal diagnosis has relied on the family's genetic information and fetal DNA analyses. Prenatal ultrasound measurements may play a role in confirming suspected cases.[37] Anomalies are frequently noted at birth; parents report a progressive worsening of the deformity and

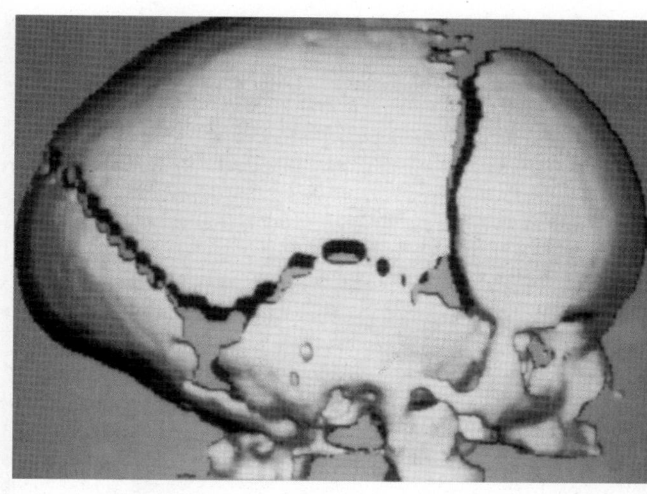
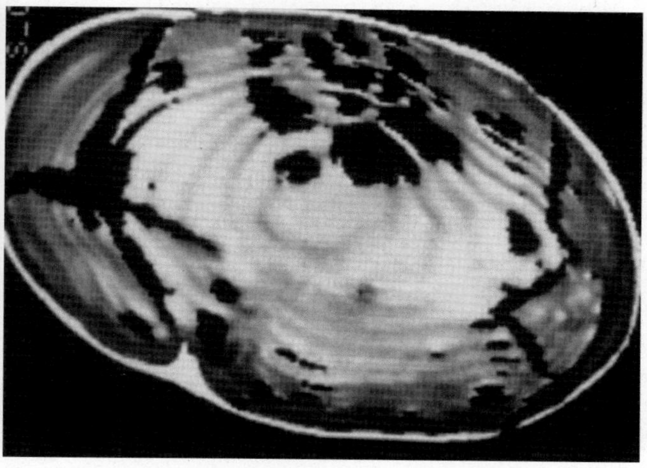

Fig. 74.3 (**A**) Sagittal three-dimensional computed tomographic reconstruction of a patient with sagittal craniosynostosis demonstrating the typical dolichocephalic configuration. (**B**) Three-dimensional CT reconstruction of the calvarial portion of the skull in a patient with sagittal craniosynostosis.

routinely express a concern about potential developmental problems.[38] The infants are usually seen by the age of 6 months. Preterm birth, which is associated with reduction in brain volume and poor cognitive outcomes, would signal a more frequent monitoring program.[39]

The evaluation of full-term infants with potentially misshapen heads is straightforward.[40] A long, narrow, "keel"-shaped head indicates sagittal synostosis (**Fig. 74.3**). Unilateral and bilateral coronal synostoses are recognized by their forehead deformities. **Fig. 74.4** illustrates metopic synostosis with the characteristic trigonocephaly-shaped forehead. At the time of examination, the child appeared to be developmentally normal. Examination revealed a prominent metopic suture with narrowing and elongation of the skull in the posterior direction. The child was hypoactive and not able to fix adequately on moving objects. A top view of the typical frontal distortion of unilateral coronal synostosis is shown in **Fig. 74.5**.

The large majority of misshapen heads seen in primary care relate to positional plagiocephaly. These anomalies are usually mild and noticed at birth or soon thereafter. Anatomically, the occipital region in positional plagiocephaly is flattened with anterior compensatory changes and asymmetry in the ear position. Contralateral anterior flattening and unilateral anterior bossing are generally mild. Unilateral cases have compensatory growth in the contralateral parieto-occipital region manifested by bossing and vertex elongation. This elongation is more prominent in bilateral deformities, which also have lateral parietal widening, and occipital flattening with anterior narrowing, and increased frontal projection. Infants may sleep on their back and have slight flattening of the occipital region. These problems generally correct themselves as the infant grows and begins to roll over. Sometimes assistive devices are useful.[41] Differential diagnoses include torticollis, positional molding, and craniosynostosis. Positional molding may have a clinical manifestation similar to an actual craniosynostosis, but the sutures appear open on plain x-rays and computed tomographic (CT) scans in the functional case. Torticollis involves a shortened sternocleidomastoid muscle, which can result in flattening of the temporal and occipital region. The anterior deformity is typically greater than the posterior deformity, and is on the side of the abnormality. The usually mild deformity improves with neck exercises and physical therapy. The muscle rarely needs to be divided or lengthened. Similar shaping can be seen in newborns with substantial developmental delays and in infants with torticollis, as well as with hypotonic infants who do not move their head. **Table 74.2** briefly outlines the differential diagnosis between lambdoidal synostosis and patients with posterior plagiocephaly.

Radiological Studies

Radiological studies are seldom needed to detect and characterize cranial deformities,[42,43] although imaging technology plays a key role in treatment decisions. CT imaging and three-dimensional reconstruction provide detailed information about the cranial anatomy and sutures that cannot be obtained with routine radiographs. The initial evaluation reveals the amount of asymmetry of the skull and the compensatory changes that have occurred.[44,45] The film frequently demonstrates an open anterior fontanelle and sutures. Reports have suggested that a deformed petrous bone may be a plain film diagnostic indicator of premature lambdoidal synostosis.

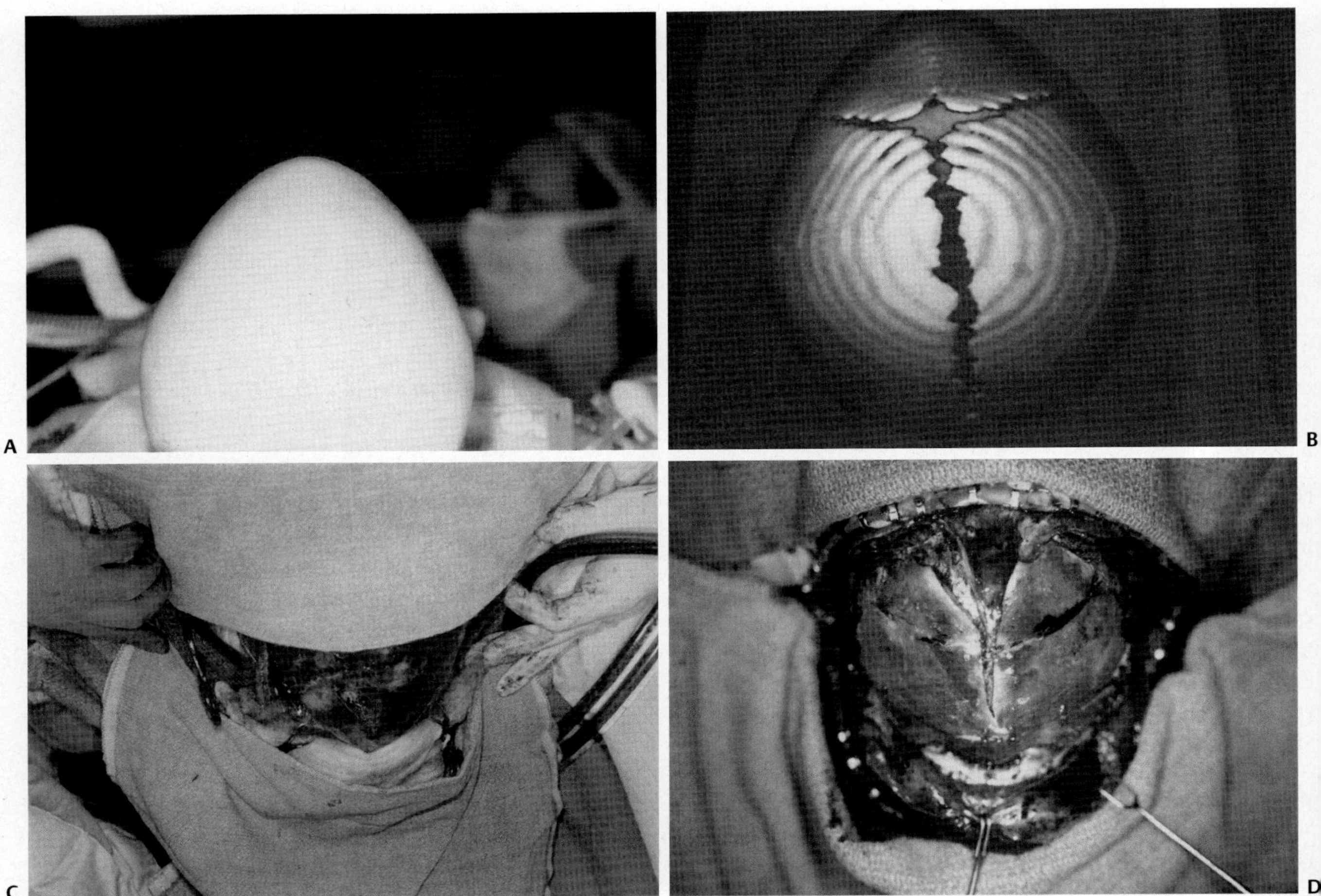

Fig. 74.4 (**A**) Preoperative photograph of the patient with metopic craniosynostosis. (**B**) Three-dimensional computed tomographic reconstruction of a patient with metopic craniosynostosis. (**C**) Intraoperative photograph of exposed, fused metopic suture. (**D**) Intraoperative photograph after correction of fused metopic craniosynostosis.

Usually there is sclerosis of the inferior inner aspect of the suture, which is evident on axial scans in this region. In our experience the shape of the suture is end-to-end rather than overlapping, as seen on the normal contralateral side. The CT scan in occipital deformities may also indicate abnormalities of the brain and the bone. We generally manage these cases conservatively. Infants with severe deformities typically show diminished posterior subarachnoid fluid similar to the changes seen with increased ICP, but on a more localized basis. This appears to extend into the ventricular system, resulting in ventricular effacement. Generalized subarachnoid space dilation per se anteriorly does not indicate neurological impairment, for it frequently is found in posterior plagiocephaly with normal neurological status. With severe compression, sometimes the ipsilateral perimesencephalic cistern is effaced also. The finding usually correlates with an irregular, patchy, diminished thickness of the occipital bone. The patchiness is greatest in bilateral cases and appears to be similar to the copper-beaten or thumbprinting appearance seen on plain radiographs. "Copper beating" may not be a good marker for raised ICP because it occurs late and is an inconsistent finding.[46]

Indications for Treatment

Several management protocols have been proposed. However, it is important to recognize that protocols cannot be viewed as absolute. For example, the decision not to operate can change rapidly with new information. Several protocols have focused on radiological descriptors of the skull. We believe that it is more important to focus on the brain and indications of its normal development, than on the bone that surrounds it. When plagiocephaly is severe enough to produce marked cerebral compression as demonstrated by clinical signs and the condition is progressive or nonrelenting, it is unwise to base all

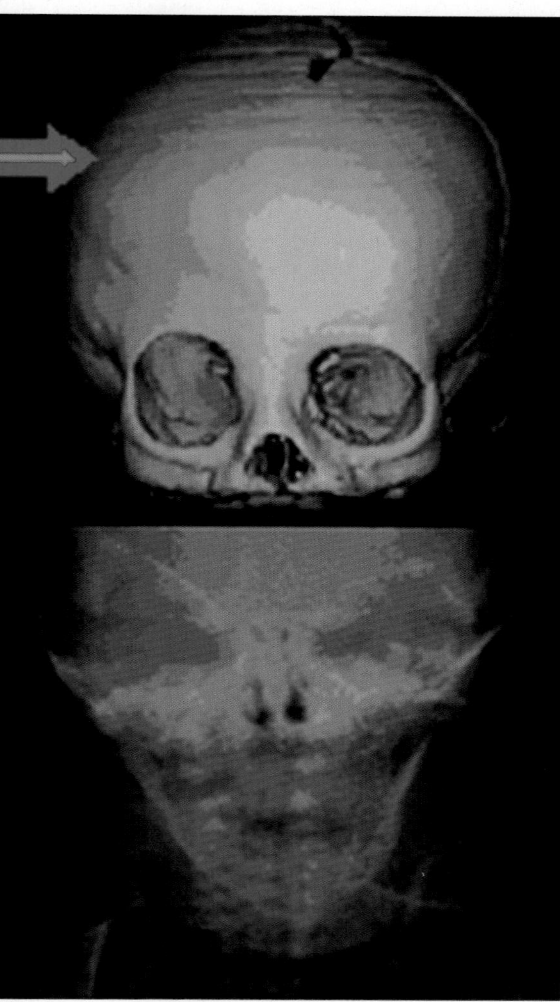

ig. 74.5 Three-dimensional computed tomographic reconstruction of a patient with unilateral coronal synostosis.

lecisions on whether sutures appear to be fused. Open utures on CT do not guarantee normal sutures or normal unction. Our experience suggests that children can have abnormal-appearing sutures with normal neurological status and normal-appearing sutures with neurological leficits or marked cerebral compression. In cases of plagiocephaly with only mild cerebral compression, we would not advocate surgical correction, whereas in other cases, where the suture abnormality is less clear but the brain is severely compressed, we would advocate surgical correction after failure of conservative management.

It should be emphasized that the majority of patients with posterior plagiocephaly can be managed conservatively. Parents are instructed to change the child's position slightly during naps and sleeping. Many therapists know how to carve out a pillow of foam rubber, which redistributes the weight of the head and is comfortable for the child. The costs are minor and the results appear to be excellent.[41]

Table 74.2 Clinical Differences between (Common) Positional Plagiocephaly and (Rare) Lambdoidal Craniosynostosis

Finding	Positional Plagiocephaly	Lambdoidal Craniosynostosis
Occipital bone	Flattening and ridging	Flattening with ridge along suture
		Frequently there is an ipsilateral inferior bulge.
Ipsilateral ear position	Displaced anteriorly	Displaced posteriorly
Forehead	Ipsilateral bossing	Little or no bossing, but if present, it is usually contralateral
Head circumference	Usually increased	Normal or decreased
Anterior subarachnoid spaces	Usually increased	Normal

Indications for procedures need to be considered by the craniomaxillofacial team for each case based on clinical signs, syndromic and genetic information, radiological indicators, and whether the child is stable or developing symptoms. Term newborns with mild localized bone deformities may develop normally despite their misshapen bones and appearance. Absent complications, one may take a wait-and-see attitude. Any benefits of routine imaging must be balanced against the considerable time and resources associated with CT investigations, especially in children.

Hydrocephalus is not usually found in single-suture, mild, nonsyndromic craniosynostosis.[47,48] The latter is thought by some to be an aesthetic problem with infrequent consequences for brain function and development. Mental development, measured by intelligence quotient tests, in infants with nonsyndromic, single-suture craniosynostosis appears to be normal in the absence of increased ICP and other pathologies.[49] However, clinical impressions have associated appearance with the adolescent's ability to socialize, school performance, and adult behavioral problems.[50,51] Postoperative developmental attainment scales improved in a group of 28 infants (mean age of 8 months) with sagittal synostosis who had significantly poorer gross locomotor function compared with normal controls.[52] Yet most available testing methodologies have detected little significant evidence associating surgical intervention in single-suture isolated craniosynostosis and ultimate intellectual outcome.[53,54] In this regard, it is of interest to note the anthropological studies of the many civilizations that practiced cranial deformation for appearance and political gains.[55,56] Such practices imply that an abnormal skull shape does not interfere with normal intelligence, although one cannot conclude that the physiological results of congenital and cosmetic deformations are the same.

Apparently well-tolerated craniosynostosis can abruptly worsen either spontaneously or following head injury. Craniosynostosis by definition may result in progressive deformities due to limitations of the growth of the skull perpendicular to the involved suture.[57] Multiple-suture synostosis and syndromic synostoses frequently associate with increased ICP, hydrocephalus, and visual impairment.[47,58,59] Multifactorial mechanisms underlie elevated ICP, including skull morphology and venous outflow obstruction.[60,61] The effects of craniosynostosis on the brain are not localized to structures immediately adjacent to the suture or to the endocranial surface of the skull. Visual loss can develop suddenly without other symptoms of ICP.[62] The actual size or changes in the size of the ventricles are not reliable predictors of ICP or changes in ICP.[63] Finally, severe cosmetic factors are in their own right a valid indication for surgery, especially as the intraoperative risks decrease with improved techniques and the increasing availability of biodegradable surgical tools.

Surgical Treatment

Use of Presurgery Models

Presurgery models should provide a better understanding of the anatomy, improved simulations for surgery, and more accurate fabrication of implants. Computer programs have been designed to analyze the cranial vault and to predict growth patterns of abnormal sutures.[64,65] Computer modeling of the surgical procedure offers the additional promise of reduced operating time and blood loss.[66] Stereolithography (STL) is a process for converting three-dimensional scans into solid models using liquid photopolymers and laser technology.[67] Initial assessments of STL models have suggested they can reduce operating time for complex surgeries, but there are several qualifications, including their use in designing bone replacement parts.[68,69] One may also consider whether improvements in surgical simulation software will make the use of plastic models redundant.[70,71]

Timing of Surgery

Much of the debate about the timing of surgery can be reevaluated because of the availability of biodegradable plates and screws. Because outcome data only recently became available, discussion must be considered as broad generalities.

The age to start craniofacial reconstruction is dependent on the philosophy of the craniofacial surgeons in each center. Many surgeons feel that early surgery releases the growth potential of the brain and skull. Therefore the goal is early surgery and reconstruction/repositioning of the abnormal cranial structures. Although this may be true in single-suture synostosis (metopic, sagittal, unicoronal synostosis), it is probably not true to the same extent in multiple-suture, syndromic craniosynostosis (Apert, Crouzon, Pheiffer syndromes). Therefore we recommend sagittal suturectomy before age 3 months for sagittal synostosis. Patients presenting after 3 months undergo partial calvarial reconstruction (**Fig. 74.6**), which uses a modified Pi technique with resorbable, rigid expansion of the reconstructed segments. In metopic (**Fig. 74.7**) and unicoronal synostosis, bilateral orbital reconstruction advancement is recommended between 6 and 9 months of age. Finally in multiple-suture synostosis involving frontal orbital advancement, we prefer to do this procedure as late as possible depending on functional issues. This usually ends up occurring between 9 and 12 months of age. Midfacial treatment is typically considered at age 4 years and older, depending on the deformation. Early correction is indicated for patients with tracheotomy. The final parts of the treatment protocol would include subsequent reconstruction of the minor anomalies during the school-age years if the cranium is involved. Le Fort I osteotomy for occlusal abnormalities, if they persist, can be considered in the teenage years. Most of the lower orbital problems occur early on because the majority of orbital growth occurs during the first 5 to 8 years. Occasionally, early correction can be considered for occlusal and aesthetic considerations. Frequently, subsequent growth anomalies can continue and require secondary revision at a later date, with definitive treatment at age 16 to 18 years.

Molding Helmets

Reports from several centers suggest that cranial molding devices can be used as an adjunct to surgical treatment, and that helmets can be used safely. They have been used for passive molding after endoscopic surgery,[72] and with extended strip craniectomy.[73] Helmet therapy appears to be useful in normalizing head shape in nonsyndromic scaphocephaly patients under the age of 12 months, but did not appear to be effective in children with positional brachycephaly.[74,75] It is our impression that molding devices provide the most benefit in infants with moderate-to-severe positional plagiocephaly when applied between the ages of 2 to 8 months.[41] Custom-fitted devices can be expensive, require frequent visits for adjustments, and can irritate the child's skin. We are unaware of randomized, prospective, controlled evidence for helmet efficacy.

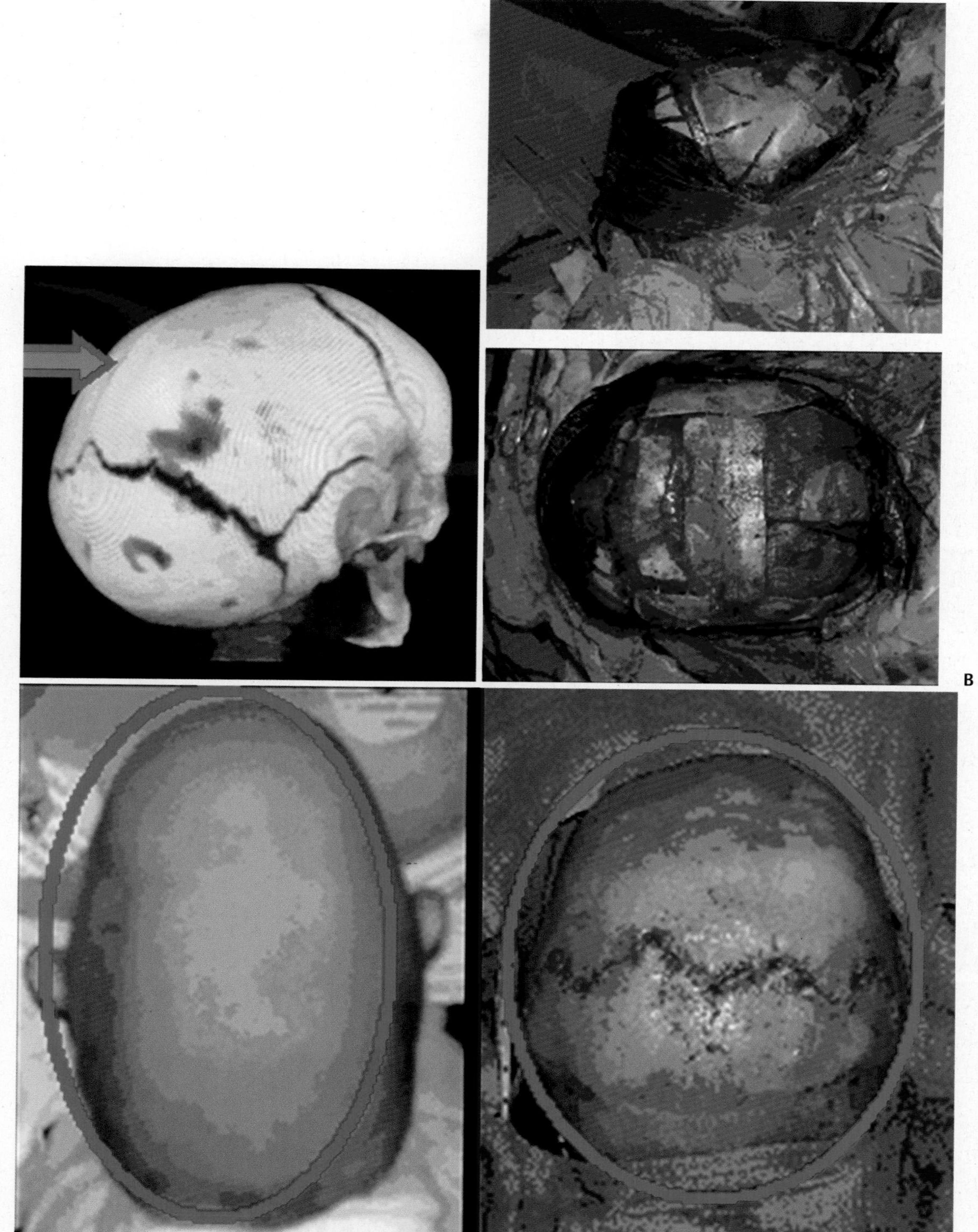

ig. 74.6 (A) Three-dimensional computed tomographic reconstruction of a patient with unilateral coronal ynostosis. (B) Intraoperative photograph of surgery. Pre- (C) and postoperative (D) photograph of same atient.

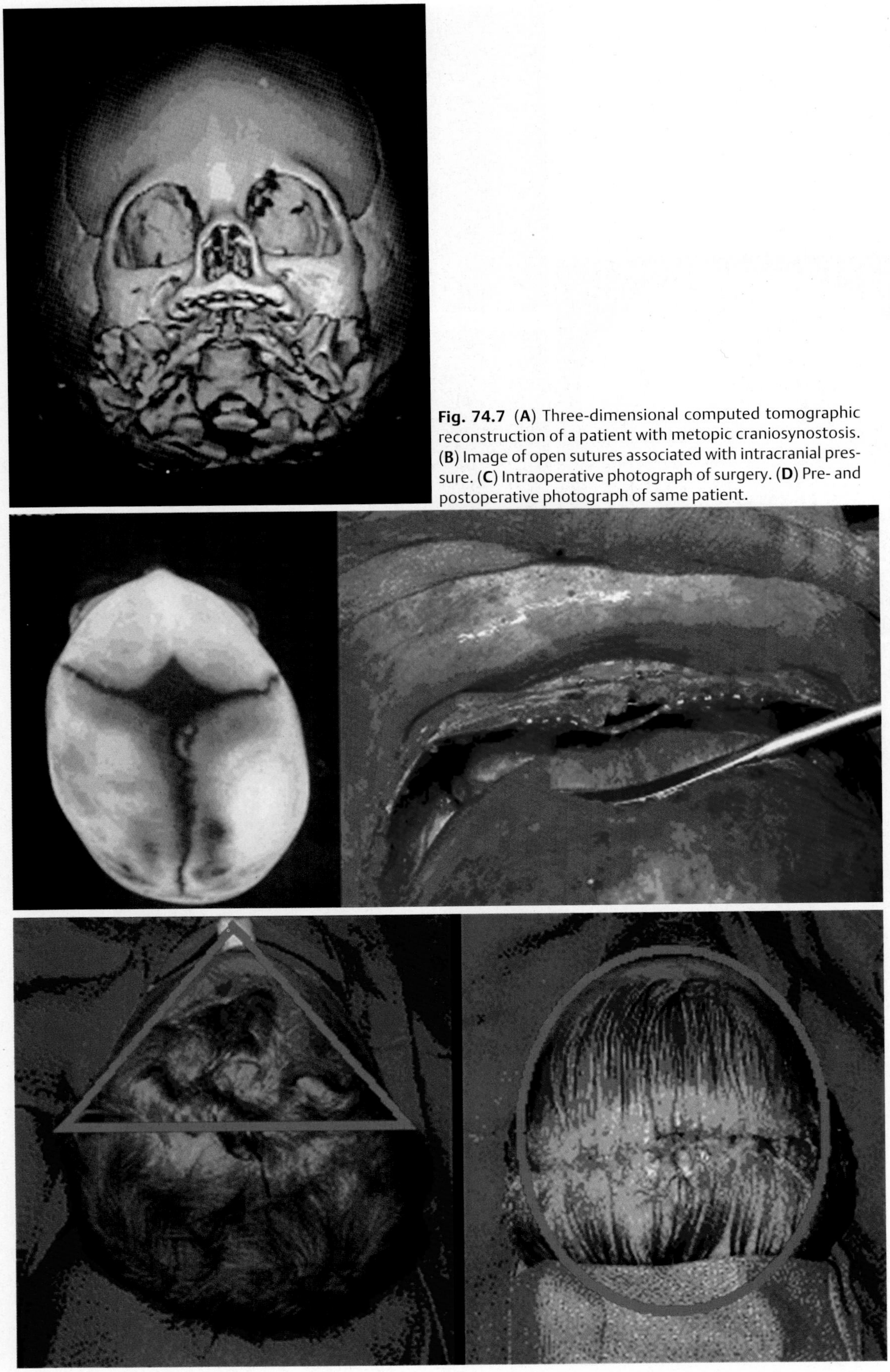

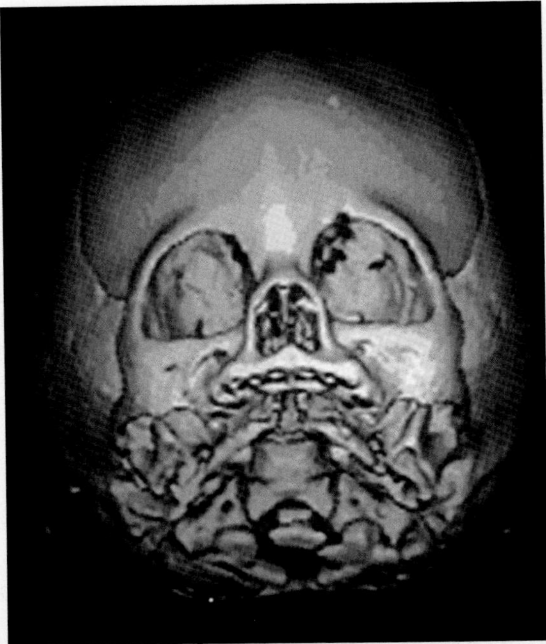

A

B

C

D

Fig. 74.7 (**A**) Three-dimensional computed tomographic reconstruction of a patient with metopic craniosynostosis. (**B**) Image of open sutures associated with intracranial pressure. (**C**) Intraoperative photograph of surgery. (**D**) Pre- and postoperative photograph of same patient.

Biodegradable Implants

Although there is no consensus on ideal management, resorbable polymers continue to extend approaches to craniomaxillofacial surgery first introduced by metallic biomaterials.[76,77] Metal implants improve aesthetic outcomes, speed rehabilitation, and facilitate substantially more complicated surgical reconstructions. Yet some devices require removal. Reoperations can be difficult and lead to postoperative problems. Biodegradable devices promise a significant technical advance because of the potential for their use beyond bone fixation to assist bone regeneration as well as to secure bone grafts in cranial defects.

Initial concerns about the use of biopolymers and bone substitutes can now be evaluated with accumulating experience. Short-term (0.5- to 3-year) studies had suggested that polymers could be used safely in a variety of procedures.[78–82] Midterm experience (5 to 10 years) supports this confidence in resorbable plates and screws.[83–86] Biodegradable screws are not self-tapping like metal screws and require an additional step for placement of screws. This limitation appears to have been solved by the development of biodegradable tacks.[87] Absorbable suture fixation has been described as another option for bone fixation in the treatment of craniosynostosis.[88] Despite the learning-curve requirements, informal reports suggest that complications requiring reoperation or significant intervention occur at similar rates with biopolymers and metallic implants. Published rates, which range from 0.5 to 8%, have been difficult to evaluate. Most reports represent small case series from a single institution, and various standards have been used to define complications and the bases for reoperation.

Calcium Phosphate Compounds

For more than 80 years, calcium phosphate compounds have been studied as a bone substitute. Hydroxyapatite (HA), a combination of several calcium phosphate compounds, was developed in the 1950s, and clinical use began in the 1970s.[89] Although HA and HA cements provide a good option for cranial contouring and filling of bone holes, current commercial preparations do not appear to be replaced by bone and are of little use below the calvarium.[89] Complication rates as high as 32% have been reported with HA preparations, although it has been suggested that newer commercial sources may improve outcomes.[90] Their use in pediatric craniofacial reconstruction is limited and contraindicated in sites that are contiguous with the sinus mucosa.[91,92]

Surgical Techniques

Until we have clinical guidelines based on well-defined input and output variables, the craniomaxillofacial team must consider indications for procedures for each case based on clinical signs, syndromic and genetic information, radiological indicators, and whether the child is stable or developing symptoms. Major issues to be considered are (1) frontal-orbital retrusion, usually manifest secondary to coronal or metopic synostosis affecting the frontal-orbital region; (2) posterior constraint occurring with growth anomalies in the parietal, lambdoidal, and squamosal sutures; (3) diffuse calvarial anomalies seen in sagittal or multiple-suture synostosis; and (4) midfacial anomalies. In addition, the evaluation frequently exposes Chiari malformations, hydrocephalus, hypertelorism, cleft palate, extraocular muscle movement, and ocular anomalies. Shunts further complicate reconstruction and increase opportunities for infection. Care must be taken to maintain the highest pressures possible to prevent large areas of dead space.

Unicoronal, metopic, bicoronal synostosis is treated with variations of a bilateral orbital advancement and frontal-temporal reconstruction. Surgical advances have addressed the question of technique through a union of multidisciplinary pediatric neurological and plastic surgical teams to achieve optimal cranio-orbital recontouring and appearance.[3]

Orbital advancement is usually bilateral, with attendant forehead and temporal remodeling for relatively symmetrical and bilateral craniofacial dysostosis. The floating forehead concept has not become a universal technique. Surgeons have gone to overcorrection and fixation to hold the reconstruction in place. Rigid fixation with titanium plates and screws has been replaced with biodegradable materials to provide three-dimensional constructs. No longer do temporal tenons need to be incorporated into the osteotomy segment, allowing segments to be individually osteotomized, subsequently contoured, and held in place. Specialized texts should be cited for details. Two strategies, which are being evaluated, are outlined here.

Endoscopy

In single-suture cases, the traditional aim has been to excise, or "strip," the fused suture in the hope that secondary changes would automatically correct themselves with normal development.[17] Jimenez and coworkers have examined endoscopy-assisted surgery to reduce blood loss and shorten postoperative stays. Two small incisions are made near the lambda and vertex to allow endoscopic visualization for wide-vertex craniectomies with bilateral temporal and parietal barrel-stave osteotomies. Postoperative treatment includes the use of a custom-fitted molding helmet for cranial reshaping and maintenance. In a series of

139 patients with sagittal synostosis, the mean craniectomy width was 5.4 cm and the length was 10 cm; the mean estimated blood loss was 29 mL, and 132 patients were discharged the day after surgery.[72] Similar results were reported for patients having coronal, metopic, and lambdoidal synostosis.[93] Initial evaluations have appreciated the advantage gained by decreased transfusion requirements and short hospital stays, but expressed the need for additional results before comparing the long-term safety and efficacy to other surgical approaches.[94] Helmet therapy itself has not been evaluated in prospective controlled trials.

Distraction Osteogenesis

Distraction osteogenesis of the midface alleviates many of the requirements of autogenous bone grafts and restriction of the soft-tissue envelope in remolding the midface. Potential advantages of distraction versus conventional LeFort III methods are less dead space with a reduced infection potential, decreased blood loss, shorter operating times, and the allowance for gradual expansion of facial soft tissue.[70,95–98] Modifications to the distraction procedure and hardware are the subject of several current studies.[99–102]

Cranial Vault Remodeling

Our preferred technique involves a combined neurosurgical and plastic surgery approach. Throughout, aesthetic considerations need to be considered (**Fig. 74.8**). The craniofacial procedure begins with a zigzag bicoronal incision followed by a subperiosteal dissection down to the brow region. A frontal craniotomy is performed followed by lateral temporal and anterior parietal craniotomies. The craniotomy is performed to allow advancement of these areas and more extensive remodeling of the forehead, temporal, and anterior parietal regions. The anterior cranial base is exposed. Most of the time, exposure can be assisted with lowering CO_2. However, occasionally this requires the use of mannitol. Spinal drainage is no longer utilized because pharmacological manipulation usually provides adequate exposure.

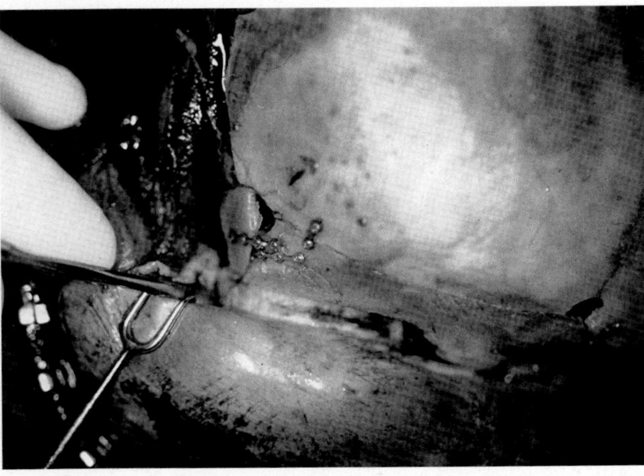

Fig. 74.8 Demonstration of use of small cranial pieces to obliterate cranial defects during the reconstruction process with the use of microplates and screws. This can be accomplished with absorbable plates and screws as well as with titanium products.

Subperiosteal dissection is further extended by the plastic surgery service down over the supraorbital ridge and brow, down to the nasofrontal region, and along the lateral orbital rim to the zygomatic arch. The temporalis muscle is included with the subperiosteal dissection, limiting the need to reposition this at the completion of the procedure. Because of the advancement of the orbital segments in the temporal region, the muscle routinely redrapes into the appropriate position and has less potential for atrophy with separate dissection. The osteotomy can extend into the temporal region because rigid fixation, originally with titanium plates, can bridge a defect in this region and provide stable fixation, which is augmented with bone grafting at the completion of the advancement.

The orbital osteotomy is performed by first cutting the anterior cranial base. This is accomplished by protecting the orbital contents because the subperiosteal dissection extended around the periorbita. One centimeter behind the orbital rim, the osteotomy is performed with a Lindeman bur. This side-cutting bur allows easy osteotomy of the anterior cranial base under direct vision. This is extended medially and laterally. Next, the osteotomy along the nasofrontal region is accomplished as low as possible without extending into the nose. Usually this is at the nasofrontal suture. This can be accomplished with a Lindeman bur or an oscillating saw. The lateral osteotomy begins as a Z osteotomy, allowing the maximum advancement and recruitment of bone. The Z allows the osteotomy to be performed low in the lateral orbital rim and permits stable fixation below the osteotomized segment. The connection between this Z osteotomy on the lateral orbital rim into the temporal area is accomplished with either the Lindeman bur or a reciprocating saw at ~7 to 10 mm, depending on the age of the patient. The segment is then fractured and brought out of the field. The brain and periorbita are checked for irregularities and cerebrospinal fluid (CSF) leakage. The orbital segment is then contoured. In the single-suture patient, this usually requires minimal contouring except perhaps for some bending and rounding. In severe cases of asymmetry or other abnormalities, biodegradable plates can be placed on the surface to get an improved three-dimensional shape.

The osteotomized segment is then advanced to a normal position. Often this requires up to 20 mm of advancement. Originally fixation was established with metal microplates and screws. Again, these have been replaced by biodegradables. Occasionally, to get a large advancement, metallic microplates and screws are used first to stabilize the advanced segment; then biodegradable plates are placed around the construct to stabilize it, and the microtitanium plates and screws are removed. Because systems such as the Synthes absorbable system (Synthes, Inc., West Chester, PA) allow contouring of the segments in situ, the plates can be placed on the segment on the near operating table and then brought up to the field where it can be contoured and held in place.

Because the procedure is performed on young patients, a portion of the temporoparietal bone can be used as a bone graft behind the advanced orbital segment and connected to the absorbable plate in the temporal advancement area. Following this, the frontal bone is contoured and attached to the orbital segment with wires or absorbable plates. The temporal bones are then brought to the forehead and orbital segments. If extensive advancement has been performed, this is further fixed to the native temporal bone to provide good stable fixation when the forces for closure may be excessive.

Closure proceeds in a routine fashion after it has been established that there is no bleeding or CSF leakage. Standard postoperative care includes monitoring of the patient in the intermediate care unit, and discharge usually is accomplished after 3 to 4 days. Erythropoietin injections reduce the need for transfusion. This can be supplemented by the use of the cell saver during the procedure. Frequently, not enough blood is lost to require this unless there is extensive bleeding from the sagittal sinus. Throughout the procedure, the patient is monitored for air embolism, with a central venous catheter in place for treatment.

Posterior reconstructions follow a similar pattern to that of the anterior cranial expansions. Occasionally, it is advantageous to use an occipital bar, similar to the orbital bar, for advancement. Asymmetries are corrected by rotation of the segments. Rigid absorbable fixation is particularly helpful in this region because, usually, extensive recontouring is necessary; stable fixation so that the patient can lie on his or her back is appropriate. The general goal of the procedure is to advance the posterior segment as much as possible along, with some expansion in width to decrease the towering. Occasionally the vertex cranial portions must be lowered to allow for posterior expansion. This can be accomplished by twisting wires down to the native bone and allowing the reconstructed segments to gradually decrease in volume.

Outcome Studies

The major challenges to outcome studies have been the absence of accurate methods to document the presenting deformity and to evaluate postoperative results. Guidelines for the evaluation of the results are few.[1,103] Some case review studies have been difficult to evaluate for several reasons, including uncertainties about the initial diagnosis. For example, earlier reports attempted to confirm craniosynostosis by histological studies. Yet histological samples can be misleading because craniosynostosis usually begins at a single point before spreading along the suture.[104] More recent radiological diagnosis appears to be remarkably accurate.[105] Suture abnormalities do not appear to exist as a continuum with normal development, and reports of uncertainties in the diagnosis may be attributed to inexperienced readers and ambiguous imaging rather than genuine similarities between abnormal and normal states.[106]

Approximately 1% of patients with single-suture synostosis eventually develop problems with multiple sutures.[107] Increased intracranial pressure may persist after reconstruction, despite a lack of clinical signs or symptoms of intracranial hypertension and normal imaging studies.[108] A review of 1297 cases with a 5-year follow-up showed abnormal CSF hydrodynamics in 8% of patients—less than half of whom had been shunted. Abnormalities included progressive hydrocephalus with ventricular dilation, nonprogressive ventriculomegaly, and dilation of the subarachnoid spaces. Hydrocephalus was found in 12% of complex syndromic patients and 0.3% of isolated suture patients.[109] Surgery itself may have to be repeated; ~6% of patients develop increased intracranial pressure after initial suture release and decompression.[104,110] Reoperation rates for syndromic and nonsyndromic patients were ~27% and 6%, respectively, in a series of 167 consecutive children with a mean length of follow-up of 2.8 years. Interestingly, age at initial surgery, length of operation, and estimated blood loss were not predictive of a higher reoperation rate.[111]

Clearly, mortality rates with experienced craniomaxillofacial teams are low. Morbidity increases with the presence of complex syndromes and tumors of the orbit and cranium. Morbidity includes loss of vision, infection, hydrocephalus, and CSF leakage. Hind-brain herniation has been reported in one series.[112] Complications may increase significantly with duration of surgery.[82] Surgical site infection rates can increase with the complexity of the diagnosis.[113] Surgical techniques that reduce operating time, blood loss, and inpatient days must be the focus of attention. It is difficult to see how techniques can be compared with randomized, prospective trials. However, genetic and morphological criteria can do much to standardize diagnoses and permit comparisons of single-institution case series by experienced investigators.

References

1. Longaker MT, Posnick JC, Rekate HL. Craniosynostosis and skull molding. J Craniofac Surg 1998;9:572–600
2. Vander Kolk CA, Carson BS Sr, Guarnieri M. Craniomaxillofacial deformities. In: Papel ID, ed. Facial Plastic and Reconstructive Surgery. 2nd ed. New York: Thieme; 2002:795–802
3. Vander Kolk CA, Toth BA. Syndromic craniosynostosis: craniofacial dysostosis. In: Vander Kolk CA, ed. Plastic Surgery: Indications, Operations, and Outcomes. Vol 2. St. Louis: Mosby; 2002:707–718
4. Goodrich JT. Skull base growth in craniosynostosis. Childs Nerv Syst 2005;21:871–879
5. Bristol RE, Lekovic GP, Rekate HL. The effects of craniosynostosis on the brain with respect to intracranial pressure. Semin Pediatr Neurol 2004;11:262–267
6. Arnaud E, Meneses P, Lajeunie E, et al. Postoperative mental and morphological outcome for nonsyndromic brachycephaly. Plast Reconstr Surg 2002;110:6–13
7. Thomas GP, Wilkie AO, Richards PG, et al. FGFR3 P250R mutation increases the risk of reoperation in apparent "nonsyndromic" coronal craniosynostosis. J Craniofac Surg 2005;16:347–352
8. Ibrahimi OA, Chiu ES, McCarthy JG, et al. Understanding the molecular basis of Apert syndrome. Plast Reconstr Surg 2005;115:264–270
9. Matsumoto K, Nakanishi H, Kubo Y, et al. Advances in distraction techniques for craniofacial surgery. J Med Invest 2003;50:117–125
10. Meara JG, Smith EM, Harshbarger RJ, et al. Blood-conservation techniques in craniofacial surgery. Ann Plast Surg 2005;54:525–529
11. diRocco C, Tamburrini G, Pietrini D. Blood sparing in craniosynostosis surgery. Semin Pediatr Neurol 2004;11:278–287
12. Habal MB. Technology that is driving the system for the coming decade. J Craniofac Surg 2003;14:1–2
13. Forrest CR. What's new in plastic and maxillofacial surgery. J Am Coll Surg 2005;200:399–408
14. Shermak MA, Carson BS, Dufresne CR. Issues in craniofacial surgery. In: Dufresne CR, Carson BS, Zinreich SJ, eds. Complex Craniofacial Problems. New York: Churchill Livingstone; 1992:137–150
15. Goodrich JT. Craniofacial surgery: complications and their prevention. Semin Pediatr Neurol 2004;11:288–300
16. Shin JH, Persing JA. Craniofacial syndromes. In: Winn HR, ed. Youmans Neurological Surgery. Vol 3. 5th ed. New York: Saunders; 2004: 3315–3330
17. Cohen MM Jr, MacLean RE. Craniosynostosis: Diagnosis, Evaluation, and Management. 2nd ed. New York: Oxford; 2000
18. Pudenz RH, Foltz EL. Hydrocephalus: overdrainage by ventricular shunts. A review and recommendation. Surg Neurol 1991;35:200–212
19. Chhabra DK, Agrawal GD, Mittal P. "Z" flow hydrocephalus shunt, a new approach to the problem of hydrocephalus, the rationale behind its design and the initial results of pressure monitoring after "Z" flow shunt implantation. Acta Neurochir (Wien) 1993;121:43–47
20. Keating RF. Craniosynostosis. In: Rengachary SS, Ellenbogen RG, eds. Principles of Neurosurgery. 2nd ed. Edinburgh: Elsevier; 2005: 157–180
21. Mathijssen IM, van Splunder J, Vermeij-Keers C, et al. Tracing craniosynostosis to its developmental stage through bone center displacement. J Craniofac Genet Dev Biol 1999;19:57–63
22. Vander Kolk CA, Beaty T. Etiopathogenesis of craniofacial anomalies. Clin Plast Surg 1994;21:481–488
23. Wilkie AO. Craniosynostosis: genes and mechanisms. Hum Mol Genet 1997;6:1647–1656
24. Gaudenz K, Roessler E, Vainikka S, et al. Analysis of patients with craniosynostosis syndromes for a pro246arg mutation of FGFR4. Mol Genet Metab 1998;64:76–79
25. Okakima K, Robinson LK, Hart MA, et al. Ocular anterior chamber dysgenesis in craniosynostosis syndromes with a fibroblast growth receptor 2 mutation. Am J Med Genet 1999;85:160–170
26. Hollway GE, Suthers GK, Haan EA, et al. Mutation detection in FGFR2 craniosynostosis syndromes. Hum Genet 1997;99:251–255
27. de Heer IM, de Klein A, van den Ouweland AM, et al. Clinical and genetic analysis of patients with Saethre-Chotzen syndrome. Plast Reconstr Surg 2005;115:1894–1902
28. Aleck K. Craniosynostosis syndromes in the genomic era. Semin Pediatr Neurol 2004;11:256–261
29. Bernardy M, Donauer E, Neuenfeldt D. Premature craniosynostosis: a retrospective analysis of a series of 52 cases. Acta Neurochir (Wien) 1994;128:88–100
30. Becker LE, Hinton DR. Pathogenesis of craniosynostosis. Pediatr Neurosurg 1995;22:104–107
31. Kolar JC, Salyer KE. Discussion re: intracranial volume measurement of metopic craniosynostosis. J Craniofac Surg 2004;15:1017–1018
32. Anderson PJ, Netherway DJ, Abbott A, et al. Intracranial volume measurement of metopic craniosynostosis. J Craniofac Surg 2004;15: 1014–1016
33. Sgouros S. Skull vault growth in craniosynostosis. Childs Nerv Syst 2005;21:861–870
34. David JD, Poswillo D, Simpson D. The Craniosynostoses: Causes, Natural History, and Management. Berlin: Springer-Verlag; 1982
35. Singer S, Bower C, Southall P, et al. Craniosynostosis in Western Australia, 1980–1994: a population-based study. Am J Med Genet 1999;83:382–387
36. Persing J, James H, Swanson J, et al. Prevention and management of positional skull deformities in infants. Pediatrics 2003;112: 199–202
37. Delahaye S, Bernard PP, Renier D, et al. Prenatal ultrasound diagnosis of fetal craniosynostosis. Ultrasound Obstet Gynecol 2003;21: 347–353
38. Panchal J, Uttchin V. Management of craniosynostosis. Plast Reconstr Surg 2003;111:2032–2048
39. Peterson BS, Vohr B, Staib LH, et al. Regional brain volume abnormalities and long-term cognitive outcome in preterm infants. JAMA 2000;284:1939–1947
40. Freeman JM, Carson BS. Management of infants with potentially misshapen heads. Pediatrics 2003;111:918
41. Carson BC Sr, Munoz D, Gross G, et al. An assistive device for the treatment of positional plagiocephaly. J Craniofac Surg 2000;11: 177–183
42. Agrawal D, Steinbok P, Cochrane DD. Diagnosis of isolated sagittal synostosis: are radiographic studies necessary? Childs Nerv Syst 2006;22:375–378
43. Cerovac S, Neil-Dwyer JG, Rich P, et al. Are routine preoperative CT scans necessary in the management of single-suture craniosynostosis? Br J Neurosurg 2002;16:348–354
44. Leboucq N, Montoya P, Martinez Y, et al. Lambdoid craniosynostosis: a 3D-computerized tomographic approach. J Neuroradiol 1993;20: 24–33
45. Fernbach SK. Craniosynostosis 1998: concepts and controversies. Pediatr Radiol 1998;28:722–728
46. Gault DT, Renier D, Marchac D, et al. Intracranial pressure and intracranial volume in children with craniosynostosis. Plast Reconstr Surg 1992;90:377–381
47. Collmann H, Sorensen N, Krauss J. Hydrocephalus in craniosynostosis: a review. Childs Nerv Syst 2005;21:902–912
48. Aldridge K, Kane AA, Marsh JL, et al. Brain morphology in nonsyndromic unicoronal craniosynostosis. Anat Rec A Discov Mol Cell Evol Biol 2005;285:690–698
49. Kapp-Simon KA. Mental development in infants with nonsyndromic craniosynostosis with and without cranial release and reconstruction. Plast Reconstr Surg 1994;94:408–410

50. Speltz ML, Kapp-Simon KA, Cunningham M, et al. Single-suture craniosynostosis: a review of neurobehavioral research and theory. J Pediatr Psychol 2004;29:651–668
51. Kapp-Simon KA, Leroux B, Cunningham M, et al. Multisite study of infants with single-suture craniosynostosis: preliminary report of presurgery development. Cleft Palate Craniofac J 2005;42:377–384
52. Bellew M, Chumas P, Mueller R, et al. Pre- and postoperative developmental attainment in sagittal synostosis. Arch Dis Child 2005;90: 346–350
53. Lekovic GP, Bristol RA, Rekate HL. Cognitive impact of craniosynostosis. Semin Pediatr Neurol 2004;11:305–310
54. Warschausky S, Angobaldo J, Kewman D, et al. Early development of infants with untreated metopic craniosynostosis. Plast Reconstr Surg 2005;115:1518–1523
55. Gerszten PC, Martinez AJ. The neuropathology of South American mummies. Neurosurgery 1995;36:756–761
56. Gerszten PC, Gerszten E. Intentional cranial deformation: a disappearing form of self-mutilation. Neurosurgery 1995;37:374–382
57. Martinez-Lage JF, Alamo L, Poza M. Raised intracranial pressure in minimal forms of craniosynostosis. Childs Nerv Syst 1999;15: 11–16
58. Persing J. Controversies regarding the management of skull abnormalities. J Craniofac Surg 1997;8:4–5
59. Tamburrini G, Caldarelli M, Massimi L, et al. Intracranial pressure monitoring in children with single-suture and complex craniosynostosis: a review. Childs Nerv Syst 2005;21:913–921
60. Hayward R. Venous hypertension and craniosynostosis. Childs Nerv Syst 2005;21:880–888
61. Hayward R, Gonsalez S. How low can you go? Intracranial pressure, cerebral perfusion pressure, and respiratory obstruction in children with complex craniosynostosis. J Neurosurg 2005;102:16–22
62. Bartels MC, Vaandrager JM, DeJong TH, et al. Visual loss of syndromic craniosynostosis with papilledema but without other symptoms of intracranial hypertension. J Craniofac Surg 2004;15:1019–1022
63. Eide PK. The relationship between intracranial pressure and size of cerebral ventricles assessed by computed tomography. Acta Neurochir (Wien) 2003;145:171–179
64. Richtsmeier JT, Valeri CJ, Krovitz G, et al. Preoperative morphology and development in sagittal synostosis. J Craniofac Genet Dev Biol 1998;18:64–78
65. Zumpano MP, Carson BS, Marsh JL, et al. A three-dimensional morphological analyses of isolated metopic synostosis. Anat Rec 1999;256: 1–12
66. Imai K, Tsujiguchi K, Toda C, et al. Reduction of operating time and blood transfusion for craniosynostosis by simulated surgery using three-dimensional solid models. Neurol Med Chir (Tokyo) 1999;39:423–426
67. Perez-Arjona E, Dujovny M, Park H, et al. Stereolithography: neurosurgical and medical implications. Neurol Res 2003;25:227–236
68. Chang PS, Parker TH, Patrick CW Jr, et al. The accuracy of stereolithography in planning craniofacial bone replacement. J Craniofac Surg 2003;14:164–170
69. Muller A, Krishnan KG, Uhl E, et al. The application of rapid prototyping techniques in cranial reconstruction and preoperative planning in neurosurgery. J Craniofac Surg 2003;14:899–914
70. Fearon JA. Halo distraction of the Le Fort III in syndromic craniosynostosis: a long-term assessment. Plast Reconstr Surg 2005;115: 1524–1536
71. Gateno J, Teichgraeber JF, Xia JJ. Three-dimensional surgical planning for maxillary and midface distraction osteogenesis. J Craniofac Surg 2003;14:833–839
72. Jimenez DF, Barone CM, McGee ME, et al. Endoscopy-assisted wide-vertex craniectomy, barrel stave osteotomies, and postoperative helmet molding therapy in the management of sagittal suture craniosynostosis. J Neurosurg 2004;100:407–417
73. Kaufman BA, Muszynski CA, Matthews A, et al. The circle of sagittal synostosis surgery. Semin Pediatr Neurol 2004;11:243–248
74. Baumgartner JE, Seymour-Dempsey K, Teichgraeber JF, et al. Nonsynostotic scaphocephaly: the so-called stick sagittal suture. J Neurosurg 2004;101:16–20
75. Teichgraeber JF, Seymour-Dempsey K, Baumgartner JE, et al. Moulding helmet therapy in the treatment of brachycephaly and plagiocephaly. J Craniofac Surg 2004;15:118–123
76. Haug RH, Cunningham LL, Brandt MT. Plates, screws, and children: their relationship in craniomaxillofacial trauma. J Long Term Eff Med Implants 2003;13:271–287
77. Ashammakhi N, Suuronen R, Tiainen J, et al. Spotlight on naturally absorbable osteofixation devices. J Craniofac Surg 2003;14:247–259
78. Goldstein JA, Quereshy FA, Cohen AR. Early experience with biodegradable fixation for congenital pediatric craniofacial surgery. J Craniofac Surg 1997;8:110–115
79. Tharanon W, Sinn DP, Hobar PC, et al. Surgical outcomes using bioabsorbable plating systems in pediatric craniofacial surgery. J Craniofac Surg 1998;9:441–444
80. Pensler JM. Role of resorbable plates and screws in craniofacial surgery. J Craniofac Surg 1997;8:129–134
81. Lin KY, Gampper TJ, Jane JA Sr. Correction of posterior sagittal craniosynostosis. J Craniofac Surg 1998;9:88–91
82. Edwards RC, Kiely KD. Resorbable fixation of Le Fort I osteotomies. J Craniofac Surg 1998;9:210–214
83. Ashammakhi N, Renier D, Arnaud E, et al. Successful use of biosorb osteofixation device in 165 cranial and maxillofacial cases: a multicenter report. J Craniofac Surg 2004;15:692–701
84. Losken A, Williams JK, Burstein FD, et al. Outcome analysis for correction of single suture craniosynostosis using resorbable fixation. J Craniofac Surg 2001;12:451–455
85. Eppley BL, Morales L, Wood R, et al. Resorbable PLLA-PGA plate and screw fixation in pediatric craniofacial surgery: clinical experience in 1883 patients. Plast Reconstr Surg 2004;114:850–856
86. Eppley BL. Use of resorbable plates and screws in pediatric facial fractures. J Oral Maxillofac Surg 2005;63:385–391
87. Cohen SR, Holmes RE, Amis P, et al. Tacks: a new technique for craniofacial fixation. J Craniofac Surg 2001;12:569–602
88. Fearon JA. Rigid fixation of the calvarial in craniosynostosis without using "rigid" fixation. Plast Reconstr Surg 2003;111:27–38
89. Eppley BL. Discussion. J Craniofac Surg 2004;15:594
90. Miller L, Guerra AB, Bidros RS, et al. A comparison of resistance to fracture among four commercially available forms of hydroxyapatite cement. Ann Plast Surg 2005;55:87–92
91. Matic D, Phillips JH. A contraindication for the use of hydroxyapatite cement in the pediatric population. Plast Reconstr Surg 2002;110:1–5
92. David L, Argenta L, Fisher D. Hydroxyapatite cement in pediatric craniofacial reconstruction. J Craniofac Surg 2005;16:129–133
93. Cartwright CC, Jimenez DF, Barone CM, et al. Endoscopic strip craniectomy: a minimally invasive treatment for early correction of craniosynostosis. J Neurosci Nurs 2003;35:130–138
94. Persing J. Endoscopy-assisted craniosynostosis. J Neurosurg 2004; 100:403–406
95. Meling TR, Due-Tonnessen BJ, Hogevold HE, et al. Monobloc distraction osteogenesis in pediatric patients with severe syndromal craniosynostosis. J Craniofac Surg 2004;15:990–1000
96. Bertele G, Mercanti M, Stella F, et al. Osteodistraction in the craniofacial region. Minerva Stomatol 2005;54:179–198
97. Robinson RC, Knapp TR. Distraction osteogenesis in the craniofacial skeleton. Otolaryngol Clin North Am 2005;38:333–359
98. Yonehara Y, Hirabayashi S, Sugawara Y, et al. Complications associated with gradual cranial vault distraction osteogenesis for the treatment of craniofacial synostosis. J Craniofac Surg 2003;14:526–528
99. Hirabayashi S, Sugawara Y, Sakurai A, et al. Frontal-orbital advancement by distraction: the latest modification. Ann Plast Surg 2002;49: 447–451
100. Shin JH, Duncan CC, Persing J. Monobloc distraction: technical modification and consideration. J Craniofac Surg 2003;14:763–766
101. Holmes AD, Wright GW, Meara JG, et al. LeFort III internal distraction in syndromic craniosynostosis. J Craniofac Surg 2003;13:262–272

102. Satoh K, Mitsukawa N, Hayashi R, et al. Hybrid of distraction osteogenesis unilateral frontal distraction and supraorbital reshaping in correction of unilateral coronal synostosis. J Craniofac Surg 2004; 15:953–959
103. Posnick JC, Lin KY, Jhawar BJ, et al. Crouzon syndrome: quantitative assessment of presenting deformity and surgical results based on CT scans. Plast Reconstr Surg 1993;92:1027–1036
104. Cohen SR, Dauser RC, Newman MH, et al. Surgical techniques of cranial vault expansion for increases in intracranial pressure in older children. J Craniofac Surg 1993;4:167–173
105. Fernbach SK, Feinstein KA. The deformed petrous bone: a new plain film sign of premature lambdoid synostosis. AJR Am J Roentgenol 1991;156:1215–1217
106. Pilgram TK, Vannier MW, Marsh JL, et al. Binary nature and radiographic identifiability of craniosynostosis. Invest Radiol 1994;29: 890–896
107. Reddy K, Hoffman H, Armstrong D. Delayed and progressive multiple suture craniosynostosis. Neurosurgery 1990;26:442–448
108. Campbell JW, Albright AL, Losken HW, et al. Intracranial hypertension after cranial vault decompression for craniosynostosis. Pediatr Neurosurg 1995;22:270–273
109. Cinalli G, Sainte-Rose C, Kollar EM, et al. Hydrocephalus and craniosynostosis. J Neurosurg 1998;88:209–214
110. Siddiqi SN, Posnick JC, Buncic R, et al. The detection and management of intracranial hypertension after initial suture release and decompression for craniofacial dysostosis syndromes. Neurosurgery 1995;36:703–708
111. Williams JK, Cohen SR, Burstein FD, et al. A longitudinal, statistical study of reoperation rates in craniosynostosis. Plast Reconstr Surg 1997;100:305–310
112. Thompson DN, Jones BM, Harkness W, et al. Consequences of cranial vault expansion surgery for craniosynostosis. Pediatr Neurosurg 1997;26:296–303
113. Yeung LC, Cunningham ML, Allpress AL, et al. Surgical site infection after pediatric intracranial surgery for craniofacial malformations: frequency and risk factors. Neurosurgery 2005;56:733–739

75 Congenital Auricular Deformities

Robert O. Ruder

Repair of the severely deformed auricle can be one of the most satisfying or frustrating experiences for both surgeon and patient. Microtia is a malformation of the auricle ranging from a small external ear with minimal structural abnormality to an ear with major external, middle, and inner ear aberrations. The literature is replete with descriptions of numerous malformations and techniques, which are often confusing to understand and frustrating to implement.[1,2] The terms *prominent, protruding, cupped, hooded, lidded, cryptotic, constructed*, and *peanut ear* have been used interchangeably for very different developmental problems. Auricular reconstruction requires a thorough understanding of the anatomy and the support elements of the normal ear. The surgeon needs to recognize and differentiate dysmorphic (deformational) development from dysplastic (arrested) development.

Embryology and Epidemiology

Adverse genetic, ototoxic, and environmental factors can interfere with the rapid sequence of developing auricle during the first trimester of pregnancy. However subtle these factors may be, they can cause catastrophic abnormalities. High fever, ototoxic substances such as alcohol, thalidomide, and retinoic acid are more common causes of congenitally malformed auricles when there is no family history of hereditary ear anomalies. Late gestational mechanical forces may also affect auricular shape and form. Abnormal intrauterine fetal positioning because of intrauterine masses (e.g., cystic hygromas), may displace the ear and cause excessive protrusion or constriction.

Six separate accumulations of mesoderm and epiderm, called hillocks, surround the first two branchial arches. The grooves and arches represent what were originally the primordial gill slits of a fish. Microtia is the consequence of arrested development of the hillocks on first and second branchial arches and the groove between them. The anlage of the external ear is first seen beneath the developing mandible by the fourth week of gestation. (**Fig. 75.1**). By the second month, the primordial ear tissue begins its migration from an inferior medial position beneath the mandible to a posterior-superior location on the mastoid (**Fig. 75.2**). The auricle reaches its adult configuration by the beginning of the second trimester.

The temporal association with other developing organ systems leaves more than 50% of these patients with additional congenital anomalies. Most often there is evidence of other maldevelopments of the first and second branchial arch and groove derivatives causing

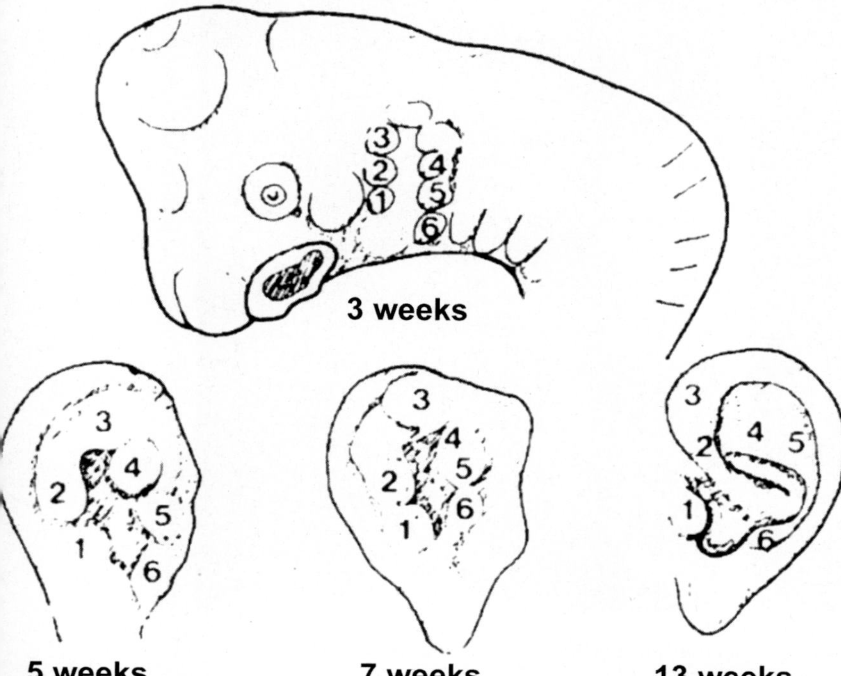

Fig. 75.1 The auricle develops from six hillocks of the first and second branchial arches. It is first seen in the third week of gestation and reaches adult configuration by the end of the first trimester.

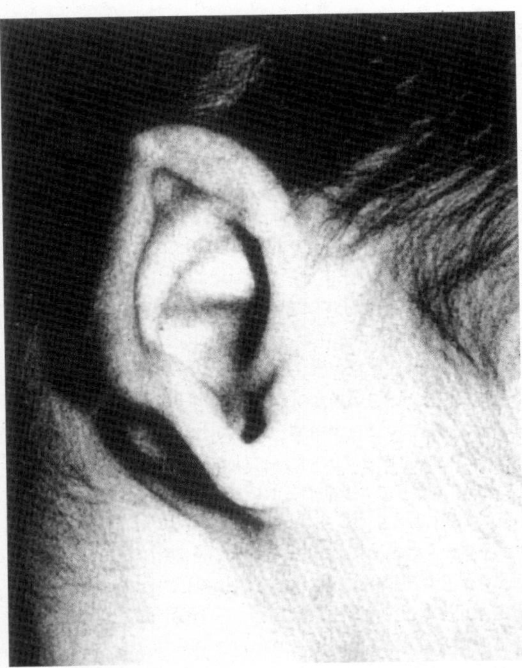

Fig. 75.2 The ear migrates from beneath the mandible in the midline to the mastoid area. In this patient the developing auricle failed to migrate posteriorly and lies in an inferior position on the mandible.

facial asymmetry, preauricular appendages, facial paresis, underdevelopment of the middle ear and external canal, and cervical vertebral anomalies. However, less than 15% of these patients have a family history of ear anomalies or have a recognized genetic syndrome. More distant concomitant anomalies can be seen in the kidneys and the conductive system of the heart. Because of the close association of ear anomalies with a variety of specific patterns of defects (syndromes), a comprehensive evaluation by an experienced dysmorphologist or clinical geneticist is mandatory.[3]

Classification

Auricular anomalies have been categorized and graded in numerous, often confusing ways. I use a grading system based on three levels of severity.[4]

Grade I

Grade I deformities (dysmorphic) include ears with all anatomical subunits present, but the ears are misshapen (**Fig. 75.3**). These seemingly severe deformities can often be corrected at birth with nonsurgical methods because of the excessive plasticity of the auricles within the first days after birth. During the first few days of life, the large amount of maternal estrogen still circulating in the neonate causes the hyaluronic acid content and the mucopolysaccharide matrix of the ear cartilage to remain soft and pliable.[5,6] If all anatomical subunits of the pinna

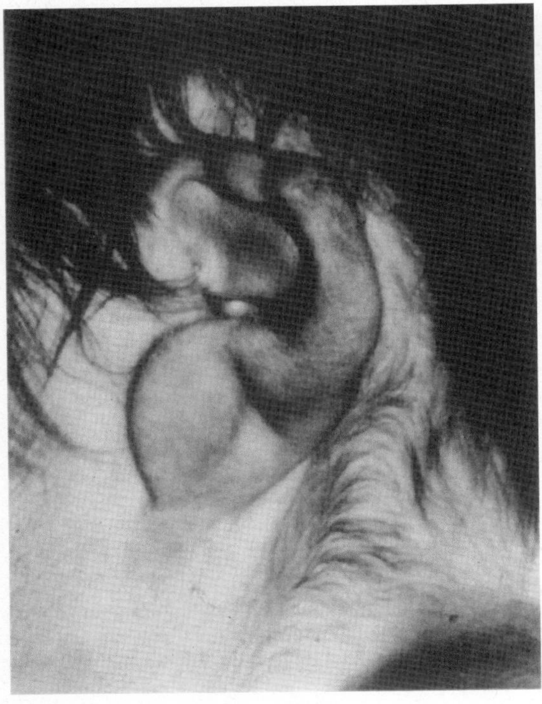

A

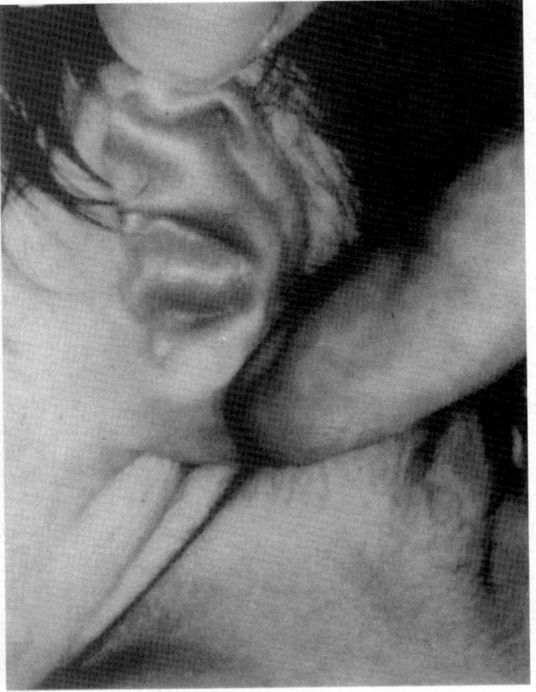

B

Fig. 75.3 Dysmorphic ear anomalies result from abnormal intrauterine positioning, which causes pressure on the developing auricle.

are present, even strikingly dysmorphic deformities can be resculptured with tape and cotton.

The protruding or prominent ear presents a special problem.[7] Although many minor anomalies spontaneously improve during the infant's first year, excessive ear protrusion can be an acquired deformity and may become more accentuated during the first year of life. Two different mechanisms may explain the excessive unfurling of the antehelical fold and the increased angulation of the concha present in the prominent ear: (1) weakness of the intrinsic auricular muscles, and/or (2) the forward displacement of one ear when the infant lies with the head turned to one side for an excessive length of time (e.g., plagiocephaly-torticollis deformation sequence). Whenever the rim of the helix protrudes more than 2 cm from the mastoid, one should consider placing a tubular elastic headband over the pinna when the child is lying supine. This "head banding" must be continued throughout the infant's first year. However, if ear molding is begun immediately after birth, prolonged head banding may not be necessary for some patients.

Remolding a dysmorphic ear after the first few months without surgery has not been successful. These children must wait until age 5 or 6 when the auricle attains 80% of its adult size. At this age, formal surgical otoplasty can readily improve both types of problems causing protrusion.

Case Example: The Dysmorphic Auricle

History and Diagnosis

A.J. was born at 39 weeks of gestation via cesarean section because of a breech presentation. The patient's bilaterally deformed ears appeared to have all of their anatomical components present, thus representing a dysmorphic ear caused by intrauterine malpositioning. The high concentration of circulating maternal estrogens in the first postpartum week kept the cartilage pliable, which allowed sculpting the auricles without surgery.[8]

Reconstruction

The ears were properly positioned (using fingers), and moistened cotton was secured into each deformed area for 1 week. The ears were then retaped for an additional 7 days (**Fig. 75.4**).

Grade II

The more severe types of congenital anomalies result when the primordial tissues that form the auricle fail to develop. The deformed (dysplastic) ears are small and constructed in configuration. Such defects do not respond to the molding approaches that are successful with the dysmorphic ear.[9]

Grade II anomalies result from dysplastic or aplastic development of the auricular hillocks of the first two branchial arches. One or more anatomical subunits of the three-layered auricle fails to develop (**Fig. 75.5**). Unlike overly prominent protruding ears, dysplastic or constricted ears do not worsen after birth. Most commonly, the scapha (the main supporting buttress of the ear) is weak and deficient. Without its support, the superior aspect of the pinna appears to fall over on itself, thus causing lidding and foreshortening. These defects must be surgically reconstructed with grafts of cartilage and skin, usually at the age of 6 (**Table 75.1**).

A–C

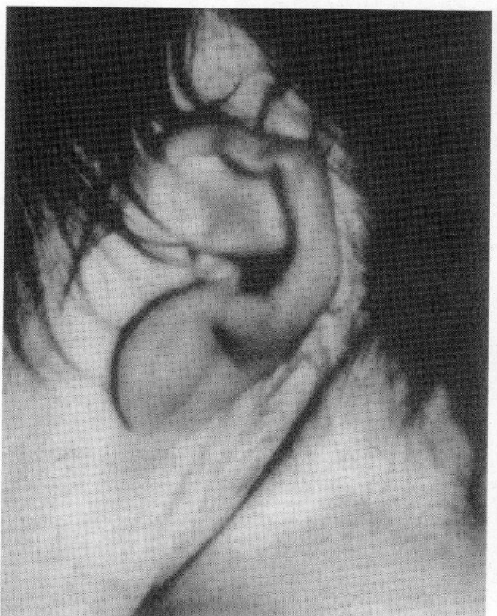

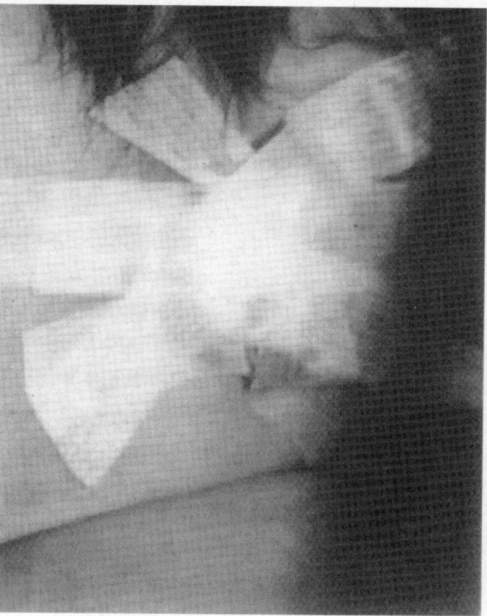

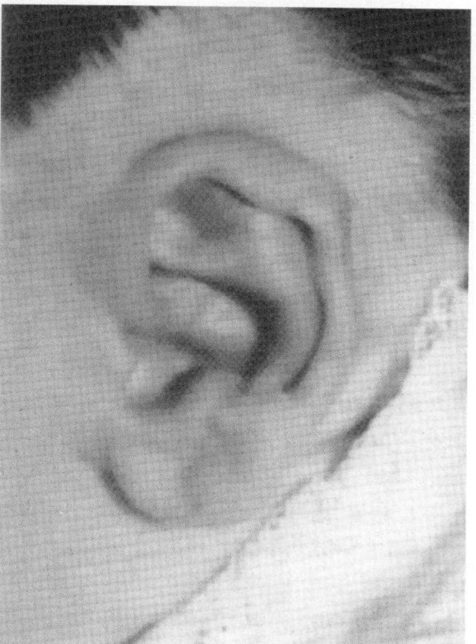

Fig. 75.4 (**A**) Moistened cotton is placed in the appropriate areas and (**B**) taped for 1 week. (**C**) Pre- and postmolding was done for 10 days after sculpturing by use of a nonsurgical technique.

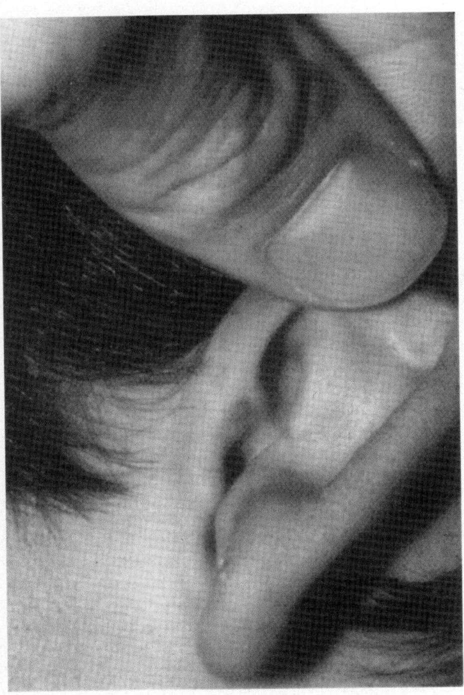

Fig. 75.5 Grade II deformities: Use fingers to evaluate absent anatomical subunits.

Table 75.1 Common Anatomical Auricular Deformities

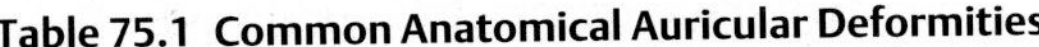

Unfurling of antehelical fold
Increased angulation of vertical portion of concha
Protrusion of ear
Flattening of helical fold
Low-lying crus helices
Absent fossa triangularis
Inadequate support of scapha, causing lidding of helical rim
Inadequate cartilage framework
Lack of adequate skin envelope

Case Example: Dysplastic Constricted Auricle

History and Diagnosis

R.M., an 8-year-old boy, presented with a constricted dysplastic right pinna. Several anatomical subunits were lacking. There was maldevelopment of the supporting scaphal layer with foreshortening of the fossa triangularis, folding over and flattening (lidding) of the superior aspect of the helix, unfurling of the antehelical fold, abnormal positioning of the crus helices, and an inadequate skin pocket.

Reconstruction

The crus helicis was detached and repositioned superiorly utilizing V to Y advancement, which opened the constricted portion of the superior scapha. Radial incisions were made in the scapha cartilage to allow it to open in a fanlike manner. The unfurled antehelical fold was corrected with a 4–0 clear nylon suture using a Mustarde technique. A postauricular skin graft was placed over the exposed scaphal cartilage and secured with Xeroform gauze (Patterson Medical Products, Inc., Bolingbrook, IL) and "tie-over" bolsters for 1 week (**Fig. 75.6**).

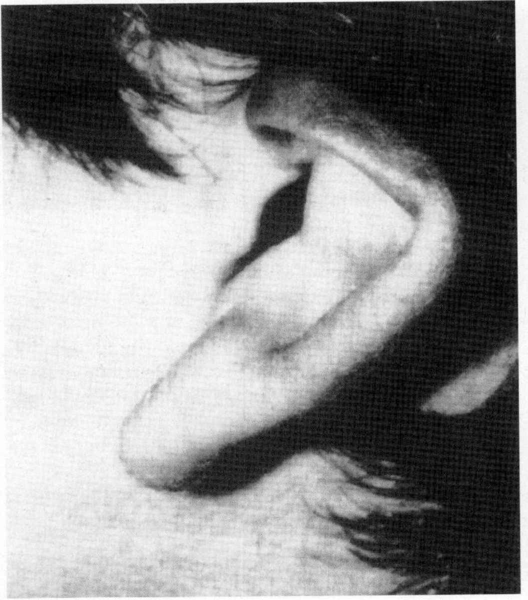

A

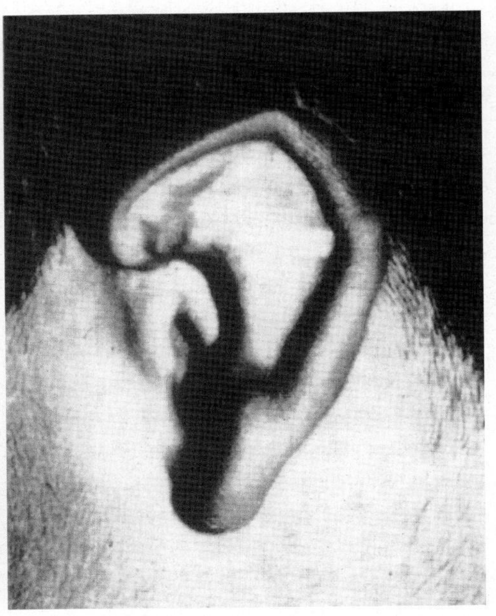

B

Fig. 75.6 Reconstructed grade II deformities need to be "augmented" with chondrocutaneous grafts from the opposite ear.

Grade III

The microtic auricle (grade III) results from arrested development of the first two branchial arches before the fifth gestational week. Classically, the microtic ear is a vestigial anlage of the six hillocks represented as a vertically oriented flap of tissue with cartilage remnants superiorly and a fibroadipose nubbin inferiorly (**Fig. 75.7**). The lobule of the hypoplastic ear usually lies at a different level than the normal lobule. Occasionally, the microtic auricle fails to complete its migration to its posterior-superior location on the mastoid. In most patients, the external canal also fails to develop. Such atretic ear canals are often associated with a moderate to profound unilateral conductive hearing loss. A definite correlation exists between the severity of the auricular deformity and the severity of the middle ear anomalies. These patients require early hearing evaluation with brain stem audiometry (ABR) before 3 months of age.

Philosophy and Timing of Reconstruction

Unlike the prominent, lop, or constricted ear, the microtic ear must have all its parts reconstructed and then be placed in a proper position for the sake of appearance. A delicately and carefully sculptured ear that is poorly positioned on the head is less attractive than a poorer configuration properly placed. In unilateral microtia the surgeon is fortunate to have the normal ear as a standard for size, position, and configuration. In the bilateral condition, sound knowledge of facial proportions, shape, and orientation of the auricle is necessary. Farkas has extensively assessed morphology of the ear and has established a detailed, uniform standard of measurements for planning and evaluation for surgery. However, for the reconstructed ear to look right, these measurements must be integrated with aesthetic guidelines. The ear must lie between the eyebrow and the base of the nasal columella, inclined somewhat parallel to the axis of the nasal dorsum, and then be placed equidistant in terms of the vertical height of the normal ear (5 to 6 cm) from the lateral orbital canthus (**Fig. 75.8**).

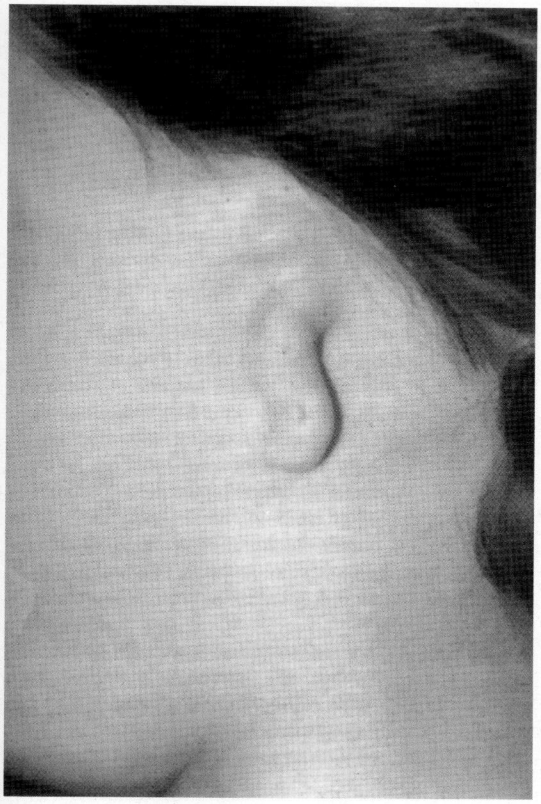

Fig. 75.7 Class III deformities: Classical microtic ear deformity with atresia of the canal has a nubbin of cartilage superiorly and an inferior lobule of fibroadipose tissue.

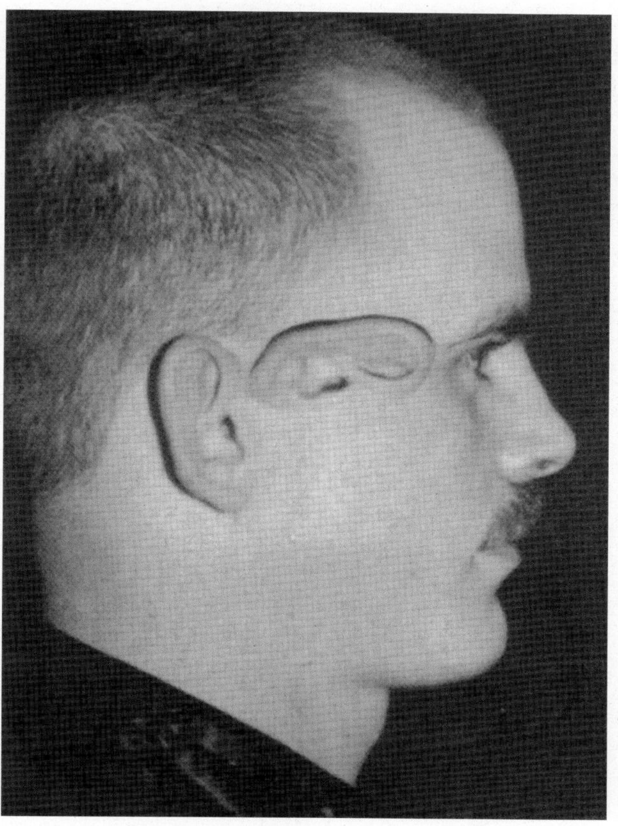

Fig. 75.8 The auricle must be properly positioned to lie a distance of one's ear length (6 cm) from the lateral canthus.

It is essential to have virgin, nonscarred, well vascularized skin in the mastoid area. In cases of unilateral microtia have compounded problems. In addition to the heightened incidence of other syndromic deformities, which also need investigation and treatment, hearing must be restored as early as possible. Most otologists and speech therapists agree that if the child's hearing cannot be brought to a communicable level with hearing aids, at least one ear should be explored to correct the bony atresia. If adequate hearing restoration cannot be achieved with amplification, the conductive component should be addressed surgically after the auricle is reconstructed. There must be considerable understanding of the full gamut of this problem and close communication between the facial plastic surgeon and the otologic reconstructive teams. One must consider this anomaly a problem of the first and second branchial arch development, and the pinna is regarded as part of this entire syndrome. If the teams are not well coordinated, the auricle and the canal may not be in the same place (**Fig. 75.9**).

Reconstruction usually begins when the child is 6 or 7 years old. Although age 8 or 9 may be more ideal, by age 6 the chest wall is of adequate size for harvesting ribs without leaving a significant cosmetic deformity. By this age, the normal auricle is almost 85% of adult size, and the patient is often asking for help. By age 5, children are extremely sensitive to their body image. Their deformity becomes an object of curiosity to school playmates. The emotional impact of this undue attention and ridicule often causes intense shame and devastating anguish.

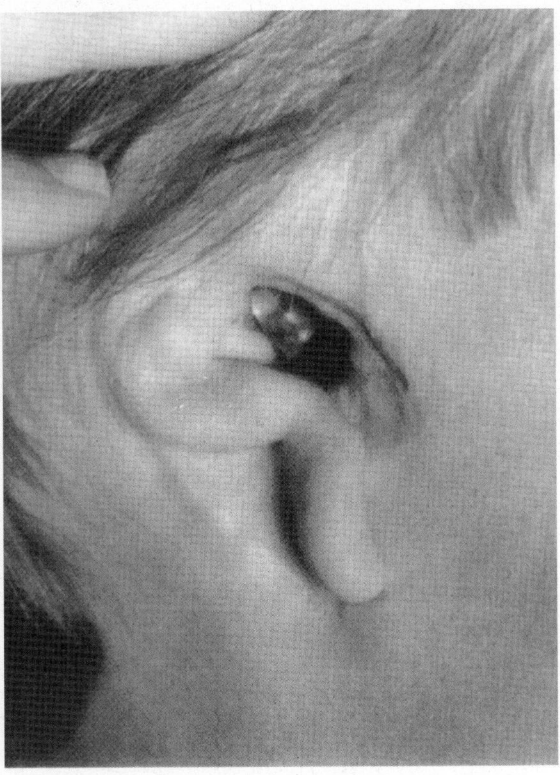

Fig. 75.9 The otologic and facial plastic surgeon must work closely to avoid abnormal placement of the canal.

Recommended Surgical Treatment

My method of microtia reconstruction usually involves four surgical stages separated by 3-month intervals. The first procedure entails harvesting and sculpturing of rib cartilage and placement in a thin skin pocket. During the second stage the inferior third of the pinna is constructed by rotating the fibroadipose remnant into a lobule. Stage three consists of constructing a tragus and neintroitus of the canal. In the final setting, the neoauricle is elevated and separated from the skull with a scalp advancement flap and skin graft. Treatment begins during the initial consultation with the family. Often the parents feel unjustified guilt that their genetic pool or behavior during pregnancy caused their child's deformity. Every child should be evaluated by geneticists, social workers, and craniofacial teams to help resolve these anxiety-provoking questions. The family must be comforted and introduced into a secure relationship with their surgeon for optimal patient compliance during the multistage postoperative periods.

Development of the reconstructed ear should parallel the growth of the normal side. Thus one should lengthen the lobular soft tissue. Brent's series suggested that 48% of constructed ears grew at an even pace with the opposite normal side. Only 10% of his patients had disparity of growth between the two sides in the youngest patients. I make the ear the same size or slightly larger than the normal ear. Proper placement of the neoauricle is critical. One should use landmarks from the normal side to ensure proper positioning, size, and configuration. Templates of exposed x-ray film are used to draw the proper distances from the lateral canthus, lip commissure, and nasal alae (**Fig. 75.10**). The template is reversed and tattooed into the skin of the microtic ear with methylene blue. A second template of x-ray film is then placed over the normal ear, and the ear's outline is drawn 2 mm smaller in all dimensions to allow for the thickness of the overlying skin. This template is cut for later use when one creates the shape and size of cartilage framework.

Patients with severe craniofacial asymmetry present additional problems in placement of the new auricle. A difference in facial height and other dimensions may require positioning at slightly different levels. The new ear may need to be larger or smaller than the unaffected side. The neoauricle must not be placed too close to

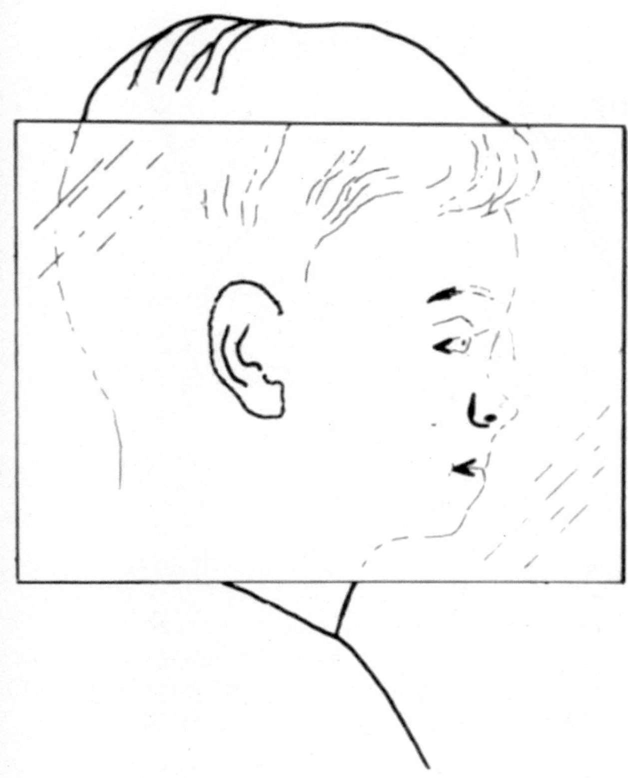

Fig. 75.10 Distances from the normal ear to the brow, nostril, and corner of the mouth are drawn on a template of clear exposed x-ray film from the normal side. These landmarks are tattooed to the microtic side to ensure proper placement of the reconstructed auricle.

the eye or too posteriorly on the mastoid. When both auricular reconstruction and craniofacial bony repairs are necessary, the surgical teams need to be integrated and well coordinated. Ideally, the auricular reconstruction should be done first to avoid scarred and unusable skin. If the craniofacial reconstruction is started first, incisions should be made peripherally to the mastoid skin.

Low-lying hairline is often troublesome. One should not avoid a low-lying hairline by placing the graft too low or anteriorly. A few options that do not compromise correct position are available. Depilation and electrolysis are helpful in light-skinned patients. Dark-skinned patients with thick hair may need to have the overlying hairline removed and replaced with temporoparietal fascia and a nonpilous skin graft. The reconstructed ear may have to be made smaller to avoid hair and the size of the normal ear later reduced for symmetry.

Surgical Technique

Rib cartilage is taken from the contralateral chest wall because its curvature allows better configuration of the sculptured framework (**Fig. 75.11**).[10–12] An incision is

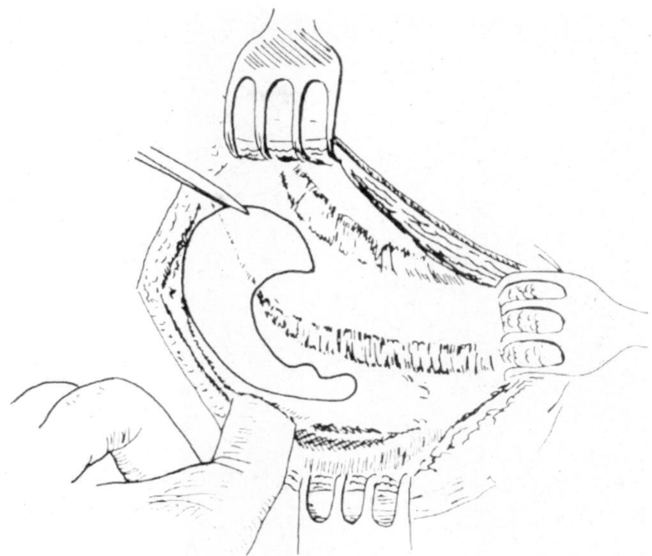

Fig. 75.11 Cartilage rib grafts are taken from the opposite side of the anterior chest wall.

made above and parallel to the inferior border of the rib cage. The rectus abdominis muscle and the rectus sheath are divided and dissected until the ribs are visualized. The previously made x-ray template is used to estimate the amount of costal cartilage necessary. All perichondrium should be carefully preserved in the extra perichondrial dissection. Iatrogenic tears in the pleura must be identified and can be repaired without chest tubes if intrathoracic air is suctioned with a red rubber catheter and syringe while the anesthesiologist inflates the lungs. The syndrotic region of ribs 7 and 8 are usually adequate for the framework. The ninth rib is separately dissected to create a helix.

Construction of the Auricle

While the cosurgeon is repairing the donor site, the cartilage grafts are taken to a separate "carving" table. A three-layered auricle (concha, scapha, and helix) is created by sculpturing and suturing the cartilages with 4–0 stainless steel wire (**Fig. 75.12**). The cartilage should be made 2 to 3 mm smaller than the opposite (normal) ear to allow for the thickness of the covering skin pocket. A common error is to make the framework too wide rather than too long. The shape and natural curvature of the ninth rib make it ideal for a helical rim. The helix is created by delicately removing perichondrium and cartilage from the convex side only, which allows the rib to bend away from the side of dissection. The rim must be gently thinned to create adequate curvature but maintain enough height to exaggerate the ridge. The new helix is connected to the base plate of cartilage with 4–0 and

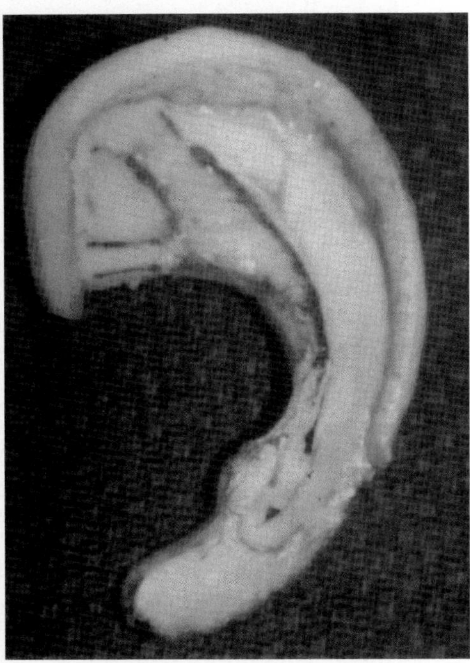

Fig. 75.12 The three-layered cartilage graft is sculptured to enhance definition. The concha, scapha, and helical rim are each a separate layer.

5–0 sutures. The rim should be placed a few millimeters beyond the base anteriorly to simulate the helical crus. The rim should reach the level of the antitragus inferiorly to resemble a cauda helix. The convolutions of the fossa triangularis and scapha are excavated into the framework with carving tools. This three-layered framework has been more reliable, sturdier, and more resistant to infection than have the "expansile" and monoblock frameworks, which tend to flatten with time.[13,14]

The outline of the previously contoured x-ray template is tattooed on the affected side with methylene blue and 18-gauge needles to ensure proper positioning and prevent erasure from the skin prep. An incision is placed anterior to the microtic nubbin and a thin, well-vascularized subdermal pocket is created. It is imperative not to infiltrate this area with adrenalin. Any blanching of the skin pocket suggests excessive tension and forebodes skin necrosis. However, skin blanching must not be confused with vasospastic effects of the infiltrate. The pocket is dissected 2 cm superior and 5 mm inferior to the skin markings to gain enough skin laxity to lie within the sculptured crevices. Vestigial microtic cartilage in the superior aspect is removed.[15] The graft is inserted into the pocket and rotated into position (**Fig. 75.13**). One or two Jackson-Pratt drains are inserted below the graft and are attached to continuous wall suction at 80 mm Hg for 2 days to remove inevitable accumulation of serum and prevent disastrous formation of a hematoma. The use of continuous suction avoids the use of bolsters and

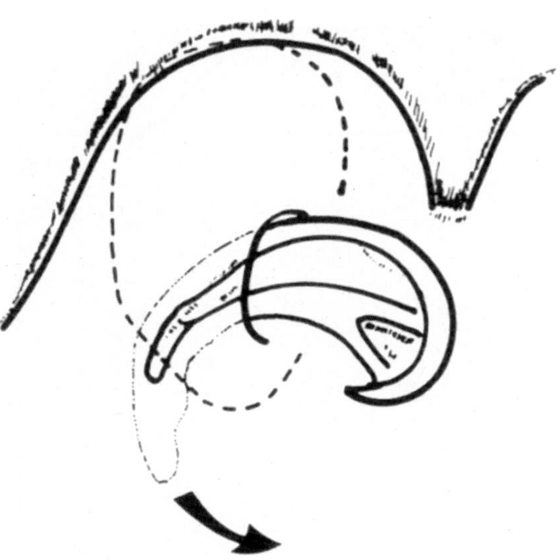

Fig. 75.13 The framework is inserted and rotated into proper position.

mattress sutures, maintaining adequate coaptation of the skin against the cartilage graft. The newly created sulci are packed with petrolatum gauze for 1 week. Antibiotics are also given until the packing is removed.

Reconstruction of the Lobule

After 3 months the inferior fibroadipose remnant is transposed into a lobule (**Fig. 75.14**). An inferiorly based flap is rotated posteriorly and repositioned onto the distal end of the cartilage graft. Skin is removed with care to preserve subcutaneous tissue coverage and to avoid exposure of the underlying bare cartilage. The lobular fibroadipose flap is further sculptured to lie along the inferior edge of the previously placed graft and sutured into place. This reconstructed lobule need not have internal support; however, any excessive tension in the closure will cause it to disappear by shrinkage. Redundant skin is redraped over the conchal area and extra amounts are removed. Steri-Strips are placed over the absorbable 5–0 catgut sutures.

Creation of the Tragus and Concha

The neoauricle now more closely resembles the opposite pinna. There is still no canal and there is considerable asymmetry because of the relative protrusion of the opposite ear compared with the microtic side. A composite skin–cartilage chondrocutaneous graft (1×3 cm) is taken from the anterior surface of the concha of the normal auricle. A defatted, circular, full-thickness 25-mm-diameter skin graft is also removed from the postauricular area. Closure of these defects lessens the relative excessive protrusion of this normal side and brings the auricle closer to the mastoid (**Fig. 75.15**).

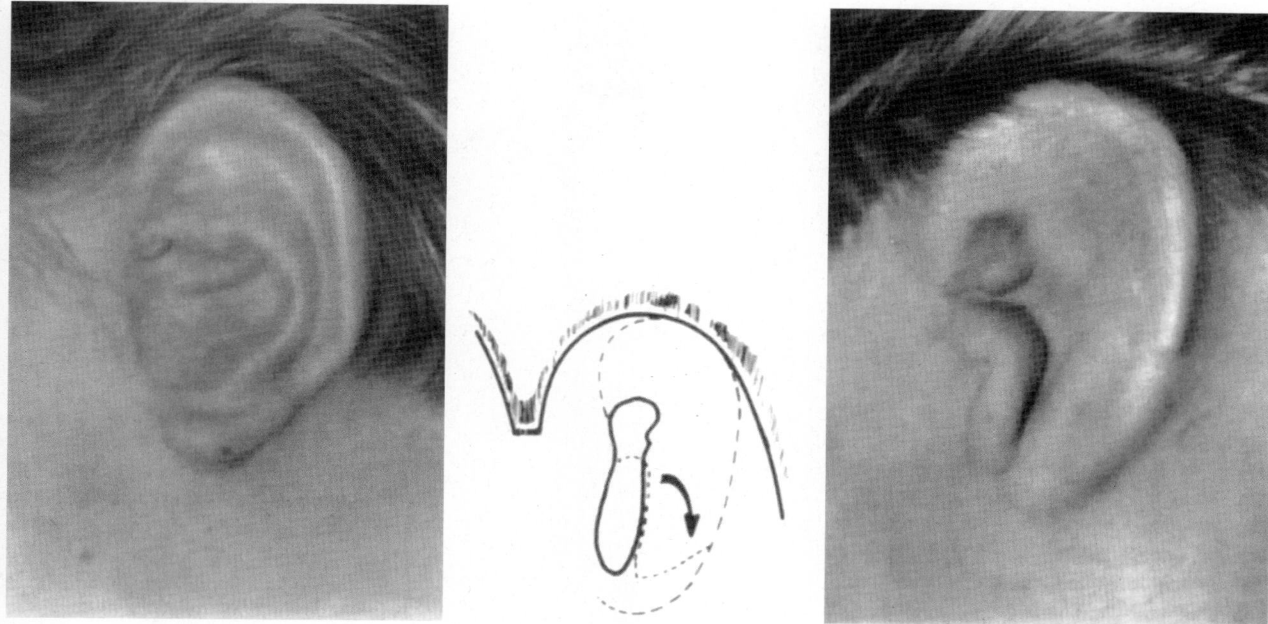

Fig. 75.14 The inferior fibroadipose remnant has been transposed to its proper location. No internal skeletal support is necessary to prevent contraction of the soft tissue.

A J-shaped incision is made in the conchal area of the new auricle where the tragus will be created. Only the anterior facial skin is elevated. The crescent-shaped composite auricular cartilage graft is sutured to the skin anteriorly and to the full-thickness skin graft posteriorly. The three tissues (anterior skin, composite graft, and skin graft) are folded on themselves in an accordion-like fashion with the supporting composite graft on the undersurface of the anterior facial skin.[16] The created bowl is packed with gauze for 1 week to prevent blunting. This tragus and concha resemble a meatus. I have not observed the shrinkage problems seen with other techniques that do not use a supporting cartilage graft. Patients with bilateral microtia have no available cartilage for grafting and may need to have their tragus constructed with less reliable soft-tissue flaps (**Fig. 75.16**).

Elevation of the Auricle

Adequate projection of the auricle has usually been accomplished in the prior reconstruction stages by exaggeration of the helical rim, placement of a crescent piece of cartilage beneath the sculptured cartilage, and relative flattening of the normal ear.[17] However, patients often need additional projection and a postauricular sulcus for glasses or hearing aids. Implantation of a hearing aid or creation of a true external canal by an otologist can be performed in conjunction with this stage of helical elevation. An incision is placed 5 mm outside the peripheral margin of the pinna. The posterior scalp is undermined 6 to 7 cm posteriorly in a subgaleal plane. The framework is then carefully dissected from the mastoid periosteum without exposure of the cartilage. If elevation is extended too far anteriorly beyond

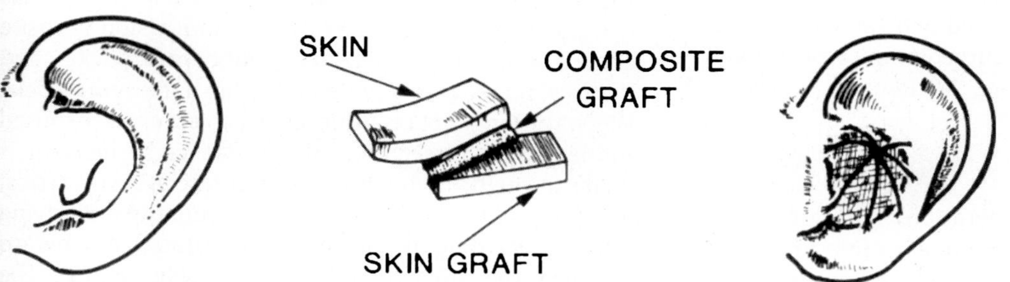

Fig. 75.15 The chondrocutaneous graft and postauricular skin grafts are folded in an "accordion-like" fashion to create a tragus.

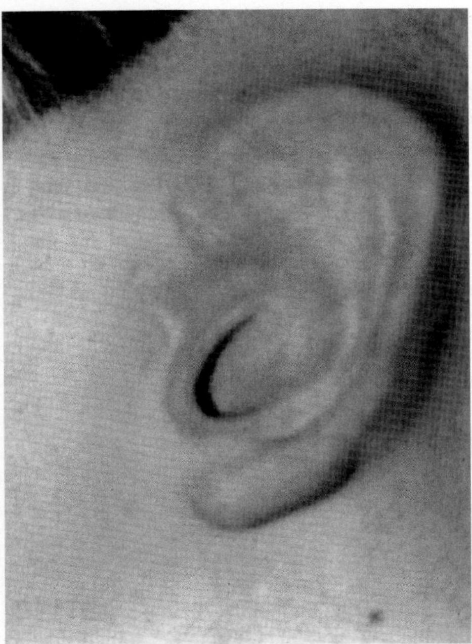

Fig. 75.16 Creation of a tragus and opening of a canal with "excavation" of the concha.

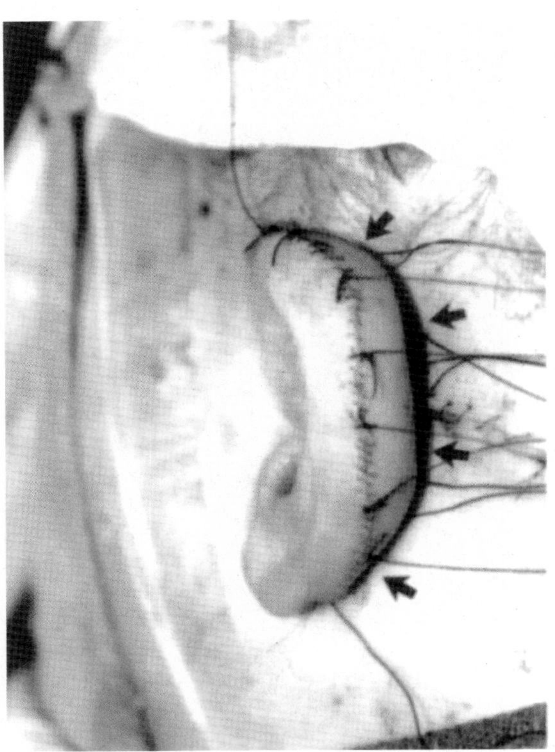

Fig. 75.17 A well-formed posterior auricular sulcus is created by advancement of the scalp and a skin graft.

the concha, the ear may become floppy and the upper pole may shift forward. Any minor exposure of cartilage must be covered with soft tissue for the skin graft to adhere. If a large amount of cartilage is inadvertently bared, the operation should be terminated and rescheduled in 3 to 4 months. The postauricular sulcus is created as the undermined skin is advanced forward and under the pinna. Under mild tension, the advanced scalp is secured to the mastoid periosteum with 2–0 Vicryl (Ethicon, Inc., Somerville, NJ). A 4 × 8 cm, 0.0016 in. skin graft is taken from the buttocks and is sutured to the mastoid and auricular skin margins. It covers the posterior aspect of the pinna and forms a sulcus. Compression is maintained for 10 days with Xeroform packing and tie-over sutures.[18] This maneuver avoids tenting of the skin graft and prevents a potential dead space with its potential complications of hematoma, loss of the graft, and ultimate exposure of the framework (**Fig. 75.17**).

If the hairline is low, this area is no longer replaced with skin grafts, nor is it elevated and the hair follicles excised. An experienced laser surgeon can conservatively remove the hair without injuring the tissue.

Atypical Microtia

Patients with previous operations present more difficult problems, and the results are often inferior to the results in patients who have not undergone prior surgery. Extensive scarring may make it impossible to create a thin subdermal skin pocket, which is essential for contour. Generally, the scarred remnants must be removed and a skin graft applied.[19–21] Well-vascularized tissue must be interposed between the avascular cartilage framework and the skin graft. A large flap of temporoparietal fascia, receiving its blood supply from the superficial temporal vessels, is created.

An attempt is made to create a subdermal pocket and remove all remnants of microtic cartilage.[22] The framework is placed in the pocket and unusable scarred skin is demarcated and excised (**Fig. 75.18**). The branches of the temporal vessels are marked on the shaven temporal scalp skin. No epinephrine solution is injected into the scalp or fascia to allow better evaluation of vascularity and to avoid necrosis of the most peripheral margins of the flap. A vertical 12-cm incision is made above the superior aspect of the subdermal pocket, and the parietal scalp is elevated from the underlying fascia. When the length of fascia necessary to cover the exposed framework is dissected, a 6-cm transverse incision is made through the temporoparietal fascia. Two vertical incisions are made to free the fascia from the underlying muscle. The flap is elevated and rotated downward to cover the embedded framework (**Fig. 75.19**). The facial flap is sutured to the undersurface of the superior

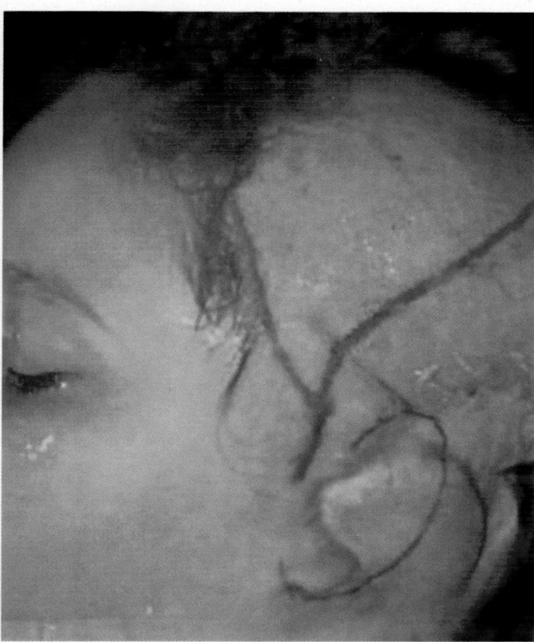

Fig. 75.18 Severely scarred skin must be removed. Vascularity for a facial flap is identified with a Doppler.

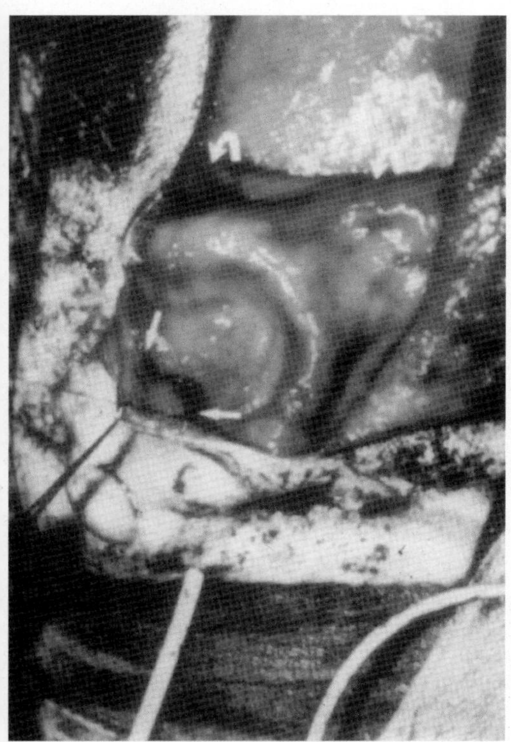

Fig. 75.19 The framework must be covered with a well-vascularized temporoparietal facial flap.

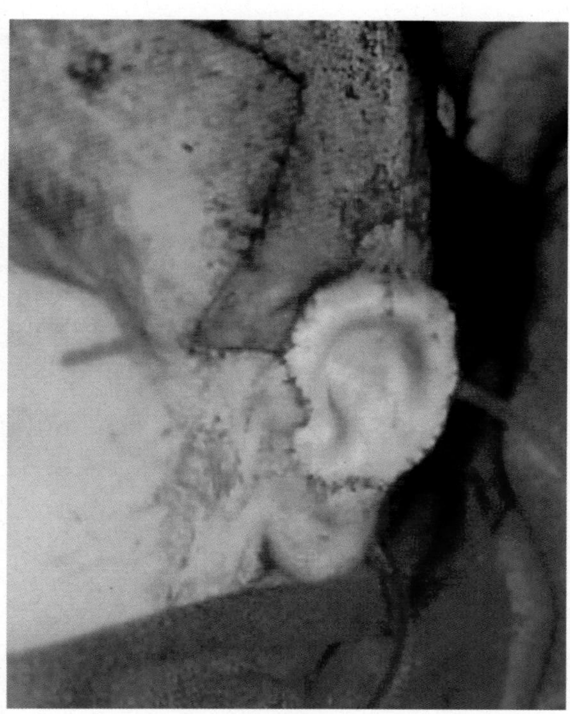

Fig. 75.20 The temporoparietal facial flap is covered by a full-thickness skin graft from the posterior aspect of the opposite ear.

margins of the skin pocket in two layers in a "vest-over-pants" fashion. One drain is inserted under the facial graft and continuous wall suction is started. A full-thickness skin graft is taken from the postauricular area of the opposite ear and is placed over the vascularized fascial flap (**Fig. 75.20**). A second suction drain is placed under the posterior aspect of the scalp and attached to continuous suction at 80 mm Hg for 3 days. After 3 months, any additional stages are started as with classical microtia reconstruction[24] (**Figs. 75.21, 75.22, and 75.23**).

Complications and Potential Pitfalls

Hematoma

I have not had problems with hematoma or seroma formation since I began using two continuous suction drains during the first stage when the framework is placed within the subdermal pocket. Continuous suction drainage at 80 mm Hg obviates the need for through-and-through compression sutures and tight external packing. No drains are necessary with any other stages if meticulous hemostasis is achieved intraoperatively. If a hematoma does occur, the area must be evacuated before the clot threatens the viability of the skin and cartilage.

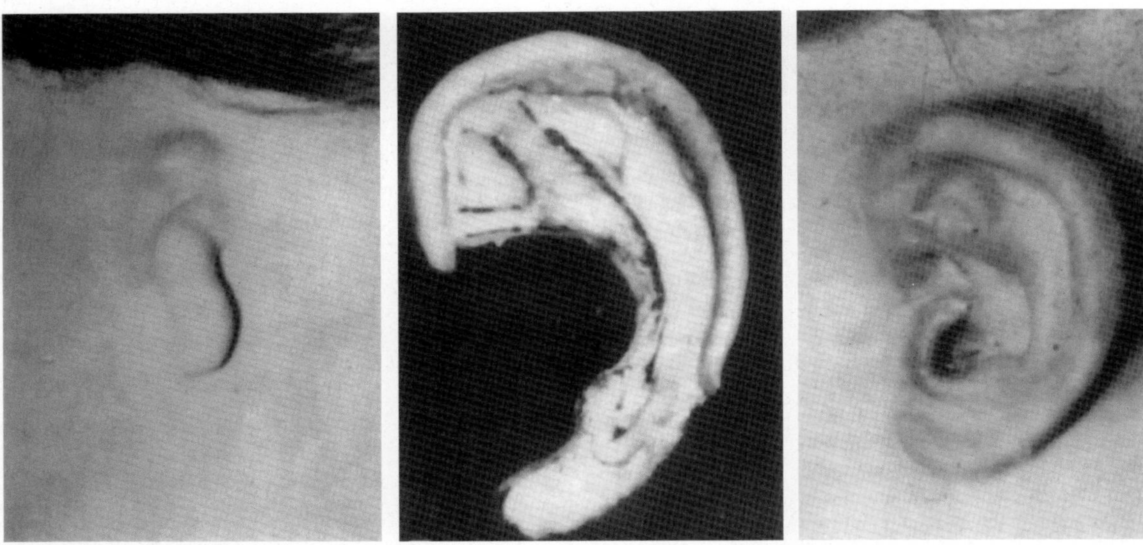

Fig. 75.21 Pre- and postoperative microtia reconstruction.

Infection and Tissue Necrosis

Infection can be the most devastating complication of all. The most common factors causing infection and skin necrosis are inadequate vascularity from too superficial dissection of the subdermal pocket and excessive tension on the overlying skin. Exposure of the cartilage is also a problem when the neoauricle is elevated and the postauricular skin graft fails to survive. Again, any exposure of the cartilage framework must be covered to have adequate nourishment for the skin graft. The most common cultured organisms have been *Pseudomonas*

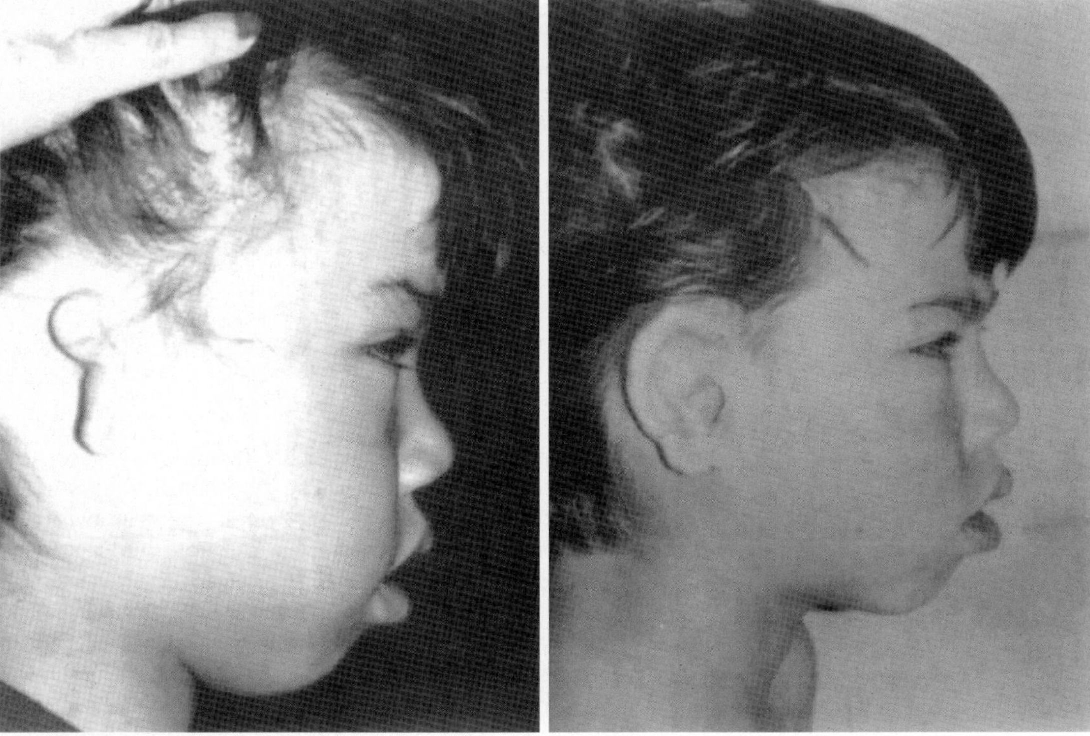

Fig. 75.22 Pre- and postoperative microtia reconstruction.

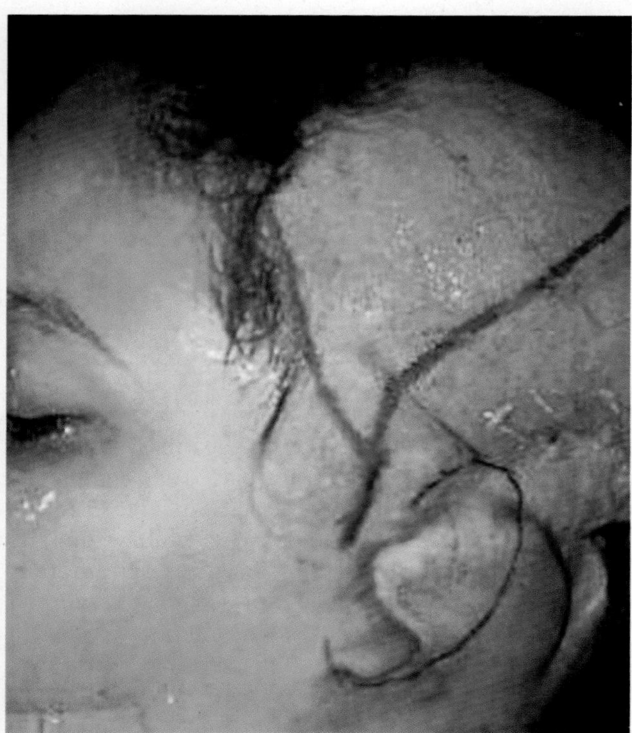

Fig. 75.23 Using a Doppler, the superficial temporal artery is identified and marked on the temporal scalp.

aeruginosa and *Staphylococcus aureus*. Antibiotic coverage with ciprofloxacin for infection and bacitracin ointment to prevent desiccation of the exposed cartilage helps avoid rapid resorption of the cartilage. If skin necrosis exposes more than 5 mm of the cartilage graft, the defect should be covered with a local advancement scalp flap. However, if no cartilage is exposed, a more conservative approach with antibiotics and local irrigations of 0.25% acetic acid has been successful.

Patients with prior canalplasty often have a moist, weeping canal cavity contaminated with *Pseudomonas*. It is imperative to create good vascular coverage with the temporoparietal fascia flap for the patients. Auricular reconstruction should not begin until all signs of infection and inflammation have been resolved for several months preoperatively.

Detachment of the Cartilage Framework

Early in my experience I encountered displacement of the helix (ninth rib) onto the scapha subunit of the framework. This problem was resolved by more aggressive thinning of the ninth rib helical rim on its convex side. Minimal tension in the helix lessens the "spring" of the tension, thus allowing it to conform to the curvature of the framework, and helps prevent its detachment.

Lateralization of the neotragus can be minimized by obtaining an adequately large chondrocutaneous graft, which can be folded onto the framework inferiorly and act as a stable skeletal support for the skin graft. If the chondrocutaneous graft is placed too anteriorly and not within the conchal bowl, it can migrate excessively.

Hypertrophic Scarring and Chest Wall Deformities

Healing of the chest wall determines whether mastoid scarring will be problematic. Excessive hypertrophic and keloid scarring of the chest will prohibit further surgeries to create a tragus and a postauricular sulcus. In these patients, further reconstruction has to be delayed until after the patient has reached puberty, when hypertrophic scarring appears to lessen.

Deformity of the chest wall donor site has not been a problem when reconstruction is delayed until the patient is age 6. I have not experienced severe retraction deformities in more than 600 patients.[25–27] Other authors have noted significant long-term chest wall retractions in 20% of patients who had rib grafts taken before age 5.

In 1996 John Reinish published his experience using MEDPOR (Porex Surgical, Inc., Newnan, GA), a nonautologous material, as a framework. He utilized prior experience of others that a well-vascularized tissue cover would be necessary to prevent problems of rejection, extrusion, and infection that so many prior investigators had encountered. A temporoparietal fascial flap proved to be a durable, reliable, and accessible well-vascularized "blanket" for the nonbiodegradable MEDPOR framework.

As with the other auricular reconstructive techniques, templates are made with clear x-ray film of the proper positioning and configuration of the normal opposite auricle. This is transferred and drawn onto the opposite microtic side. The graft must not be positioned vertically, but must be parallel to the dorsum of the nose and must lie between the eyebrow and the base of the patient's nose.

Using a Doppler, the vasculature superficial temporal artery is identified and marked on the temporal scalp (**Fig. 75.23**). The scalp is incised and meticulously dissected in a subdermal plane below the hair follicles, carefully avoiding the delicate vascularity of the temporoparietal flap. The temporoparietal fascial flap is measured to allow adequate length for complete coverage of the MEDPOR implant.

The prefabricated MEDPOR implant can be easily sculptured into a three-layered framework by "attaching" the helical rim to the scaphal supporting middle layer with nonabsorbable sutures. The constructed framework

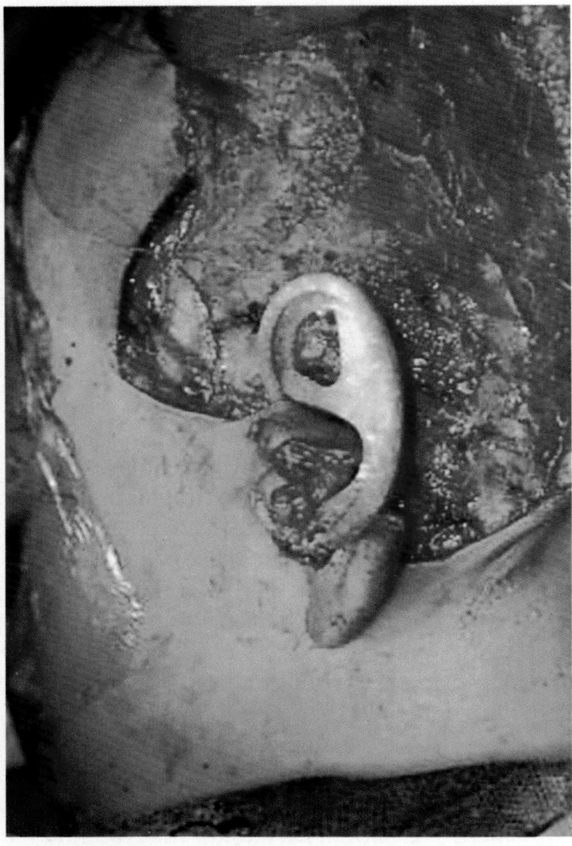

Fig. 75.24 The MEDPOR (Porex Surgical, Inc., Newnan, GA) implant is placed and the temporoparietal flap is measured and elevated to cover the entire implant.

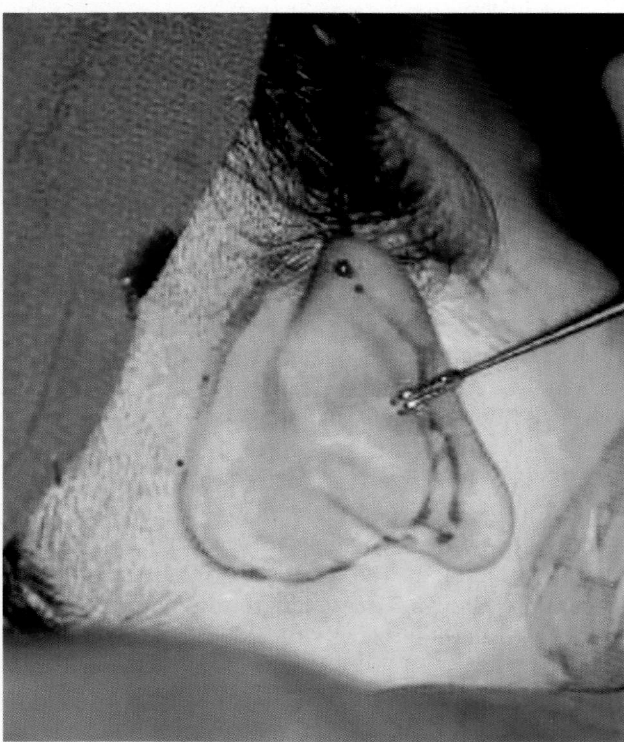

Fig. 75.25 A full-thickness skin graft is taken from the postauricular surface of the normal auricle.

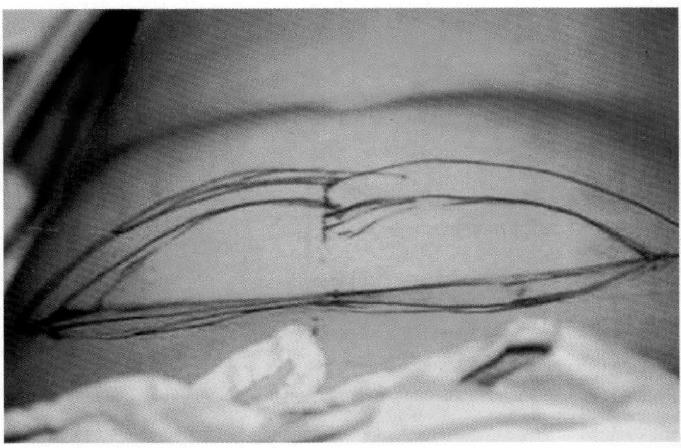

Fig. 75.26 A second skin graft is taken from the below the umbilicus.

is covered with Betadine (Cardinal Health, Dublin, OH) solution. The MEDPOR graft is then placed and completely covered by the temporoparietal fascial flap (**Fig. 75.24**).

The most natural skin coverage is grafts from the opposite normal auricle. A full-thickness skin graft is taken from the postauricular surface of the normal auricle (**Fig. 75.25**). A second skin graft is taken from the abdomen below the umbilicus (**Fig. 75.26**). The abdominal skin graft is used to recover both the denuded posterior surface of the normal donor auricle and the posterior aspect of the elevated reconstructed microtic ear (**Fig. 75.27**).

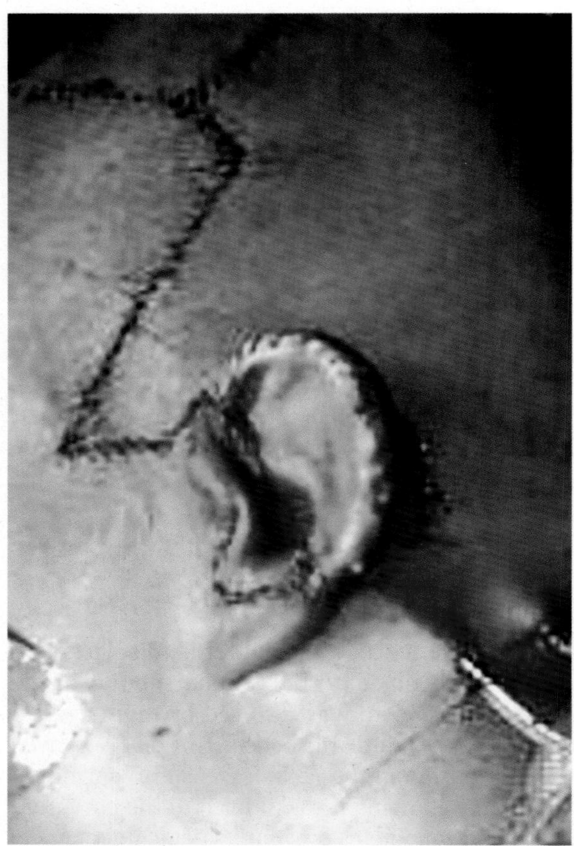

Fig. 75.27 Two suction drains are inserted and the incisions are closed.

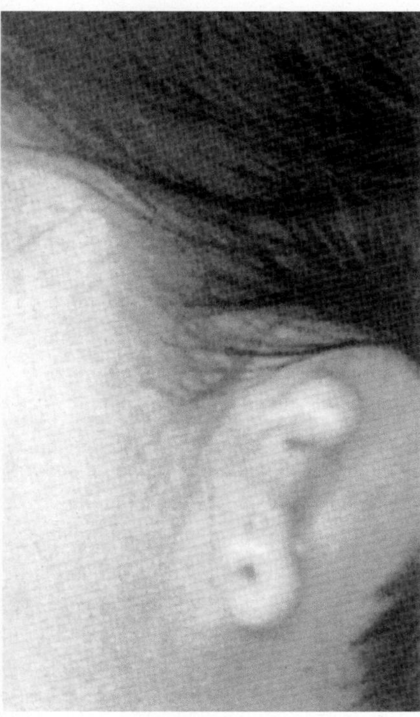
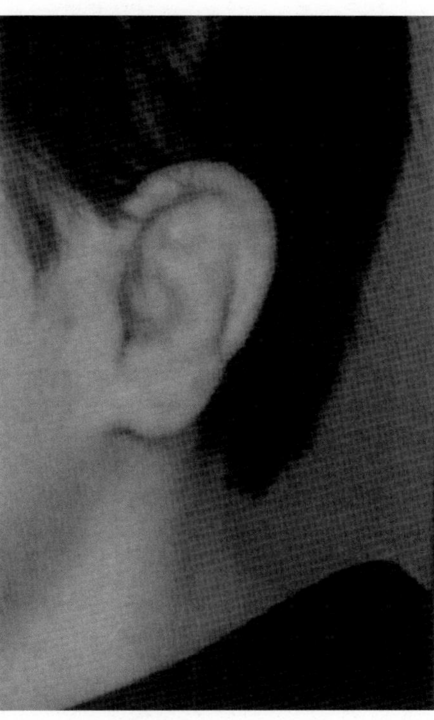

Fig. 75.28 Preoperative and postoperative reconstruction with a MEDPOR (Porex Surgical, Inc., Newnan, GA) implant.

Two suction drains are inserted and the incisions are closed (**Fig. 75.28**).

References

1. Anson B, Blast T. Developmental anatomy of the ear. In: Shambaugh G Jr and Glasscock M, eds. Surgery of the Ear. 3rd ed. Philadelphia: WB Saunders; 1980
2. Graham JM Jr. Smith's Recognizable Patterns of Human Deformation. 2nd ed. Philadelphia: WB Saunders; 1988
3. Berghaus A, Toplak F. Surgical concepts for reconstruction of the auricle: history and current state of the art. Arch Otolaryngol Head Neck Surg 1986;112:388
4. Farkas LG. Anthropometry of normal and anomalous ears. Clin Plast Surg 1978;5:401
5. Jahrsdoefer RA. Congenital ear atresia. In: Tanzer RC and Eadgerton MT, eds. Symposium on Reconstruction of the Auricle. St. Louis: CV Mosby; 1974
6. Derlacki EL. The role of the otologist in the management of microtia and related malformations of the hearing apparatus. Trans Am Acad Ophthalmol Otolaryngol;1968;72:980
7. Gorney M. Ear cartilage. In: Davis J, ed. Aesthetic and Reconstructive Otoplasty. New York: Springer-Verlag; 1978
8. Ruder RO. Congenital auricular deformities: dysmorphic and dysplastic ears. In: Lalwani A, Grunfast K, eds. Pediatric Otology and Neurotology. Philadelphia: Lippincott-Raven; 1998
9. Ruder RO, Maceri D. Management of congenital aural atresia and microtia. In: Johnson J, Mandel Brown M, Newman R, eds. Facial Plastic Surgery. St. Louis: CV Mosby; 1991
10. Cronin TD. Use of a Silastic frame for total and subtotal reconstruction of the external ear: preliminary report. Plast Reconstr Surg 1966; 37:399
11. Cronin TD, Ascough BM. Silastic ear construction. Clin Plast Surg 1978;5:367
12. Kirkham HLD. The use of preserved cartilage in ear reconstruction. Ann Surg 1940;111:896
13. Brent B. The correction of microtia with autogenous cartilage grafts, I: the classical deformity. Plast Reconstr Surg 1980;66:1
14. Brent B. Ear reconstruction with an expansile framework of autogenous rib cartilage. Plast Reconstr Surg 1974;53:619
15. Ohmori S, Sekiguchi H. Follow-up study of the reconstruction of microtia using Silastic frame. Aesthetic Plast Surg 1984;8:1
16. Cosman B. The constricted ear. Clin Plast Surg 1978;5:389–400
17. Ruder RO. Microtia reconstruction. In: Papel I, Nachlas N, eds. Facial Plastic Surgery. St Louis: CV Mosby; 1992
18. Giles H. Plastic Surgery of the Face. London: Frowde, Hodder, and Stoughton; 1920
19. David SK, Cheney M. An anatomical study of the temporoparietal flap. Arch Otolaryngol Head Neck Surg 1995;121:1153
20. Brent B, Byrd HS. Secondary ear reconstruction with cartilage grafts covered by axial random and free flaps of temporoparietal fascia. Plast Reconstr Surg 1983;72:141
21. Brent B. Auricular repair with autogenous rib cartilage grafts: two decades of experience with 600 cases. Plast Reconstr Surg 1992;90:355
22. Vernon J. Meeting of the Second International Symposium of Inner Ear, Denver, 1986
23. Ruder RO. Microtia reconstruction. In: Papel I, Frodel J, Holt GR, et al, eds. Facial Plastic Surgery. 2nd ed. New York: Thieme; 2003
24. Ruder RO, Graham JM Jr. Evaluation and treatment of the deformed and malformed auricle. Clin Pediatrr 1996;35:461–465
25. Brent B. Problems associated with total auricular reconstruction. In: Tanzer RC, Eadgerton MT, eds. Symposium on the Reconstruction of the Auricle. St Louis: CV Mosby; 1974
26. Tanzer RC. Reconstruction of microtia: a long-term follow-up. In: Goldwyn RM, Murray JE, eds. Long-Term Results in Plastic and Reconstructive Surgery. Boston: Little, Brown; 1980
27. Thomson HG, Kim TY, Ein SH. Residual problems in chest donor sites after microtia reconstruction: a long-term study. Plast Reconstr Surg 1995;95:961

76 Evaluation and Management of Cleft Lip and Palate Disorders

Randolph B. Capone and Jonathan M. Sykes

Of all facial plastic and reconstructive procedures, few are as rewarding as repair of cleft lip and palate deformities. Patients with these deformities experience difficulty with nursing, deglutition, and speech production, in addition to the social stigmata accompanying the obvious alterations in appearance and facial growth. The evaluation and treatment of patients with cleft lip, palate, and nasal deformities is a challenging task, requiring the care of a multidisciplinary team of providers to manage the myriad dental, psychosocial, speech, otologic, and aesthetic needs of these individuals. This chapter will review the embryology, anatomy, and classification of both the unilateral and bilateral cleft malformation. A treatment philosophy including the timing and technique of various cleft repairs is also described.

Embryology of the Lip and Palate

Normal development of the lip and palate occurs during the embryonic period (the first 12 weeks of intrauterine life). The midportion of the face develops anterior to the forebrain by the differentiation of the broad midline frontonasal prominence. The *primary palate* forms at ~4 to 6 weeks and forms the initial separation between the oral and nasal cavities. The primary palate, or median palatine process, is formed by the fusion of the paired *median nasal prominences* (MNPs), and is that portion of the hard palate anterior to the incisive foramen. In addition, fusion of the paired MNPs during the sixth week gives rise to the philtrum, the premaxilla, the columella, the nasal tip, and the central and lateral incisors (**Fig. 76.1**).[1,2] Development

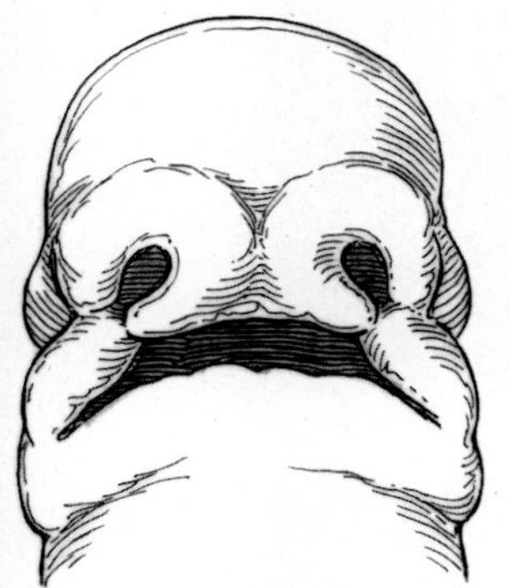

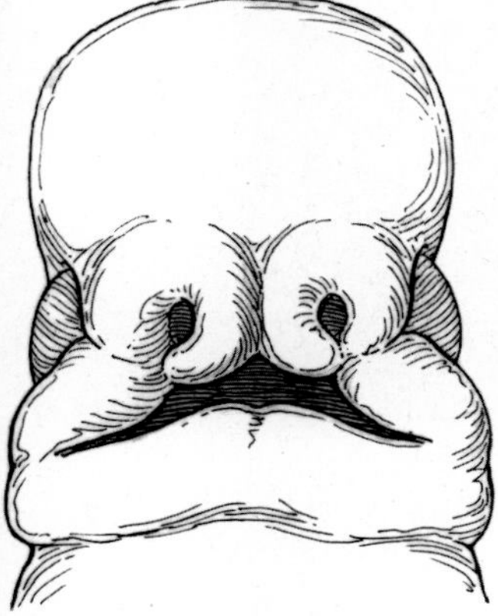

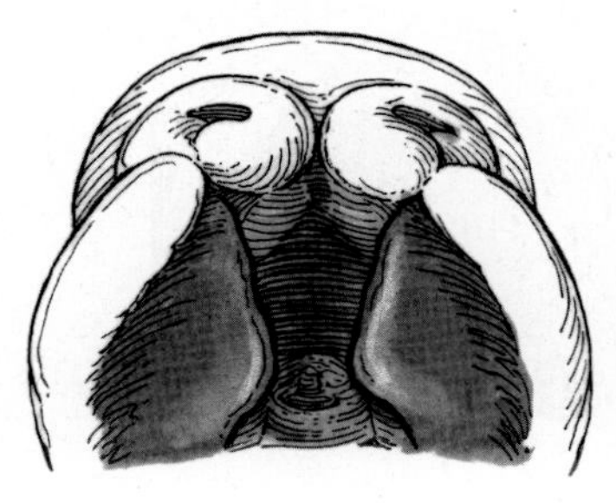

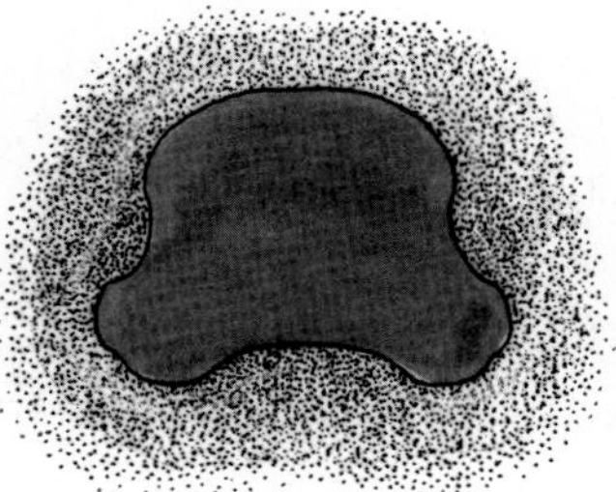

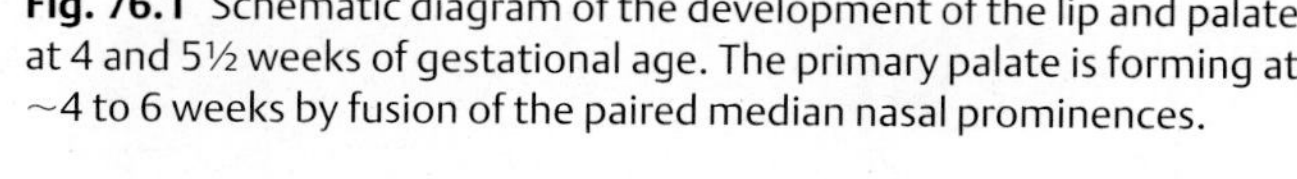
Fig. 76.1 Schematic diagram of the development of the lip and palate at 4 and 5½ weeks of gestational age. The primary palate is forming at ~4 to 6 weeks by fusion of the paired median nasal prominences.

of the primary palate is embryologically distinct from the formation of the palate posterior to the incisive foramen (the *secondary palate*). The lateral elements of the upper lip (lateral to the philtral columns) are derived from the paired *maxillary processes* (MXPs). The cheek, maxilla, zygoma, and secondary palate are also formed by the maxillary processes. The upper lip, therefore, is formed by both the median nasal and maxillary processes.[3]

The secondary palate begins developing at ~8 weeks of gestation, after development of the primary palate is complete (**Fig. 76.2**). Formation of the secondary palate occurs by inferomedial growth and migration of the palatal shelves (the medial projections of the maxillary processes). As the palatal shelves migrate inferiorly (similar to a drawbridge), the developing nasal cavities expand laterally and inferiorly.

The palatal shelves are initially separated by the developing tongue. Growth of the mandible with associated displacement of the tongue allows the palatal shelves to migrate inferiorly and assume a horizontal orientation. If fetal development and mandibular growth do not proceed normally, the palatal shelves cannot migrate inferiorly and medially. The resulting malformation can result in the Pierre Robin sequence (micrognathia, relative macroglossia, and U-shaped cleft palate) (**Fig. 76.3A,B**).[4]

Normal palatal formation begins when the palatal shelves and nasal septum contact each other and proceeds in an anterior-to-posterior direction. Palatal closure first occurs at the incisive foramen at ~8 weeks of gestation and is usually completed through the uvula by 12 weeks. The degree of clefting of the secondary palate is related to many factors, including when in fetal development the fusion process is interrupted. Therefore, a spectrum of palatal abnormality exists that can involve varying degrees of soft and hard palate clefting.[5]

Cleft Classification

The embryological development of the lip and palate serves as a natural mechanism to classify congenital clefts. The primary palate and lip develop between weeks 4 and 8.

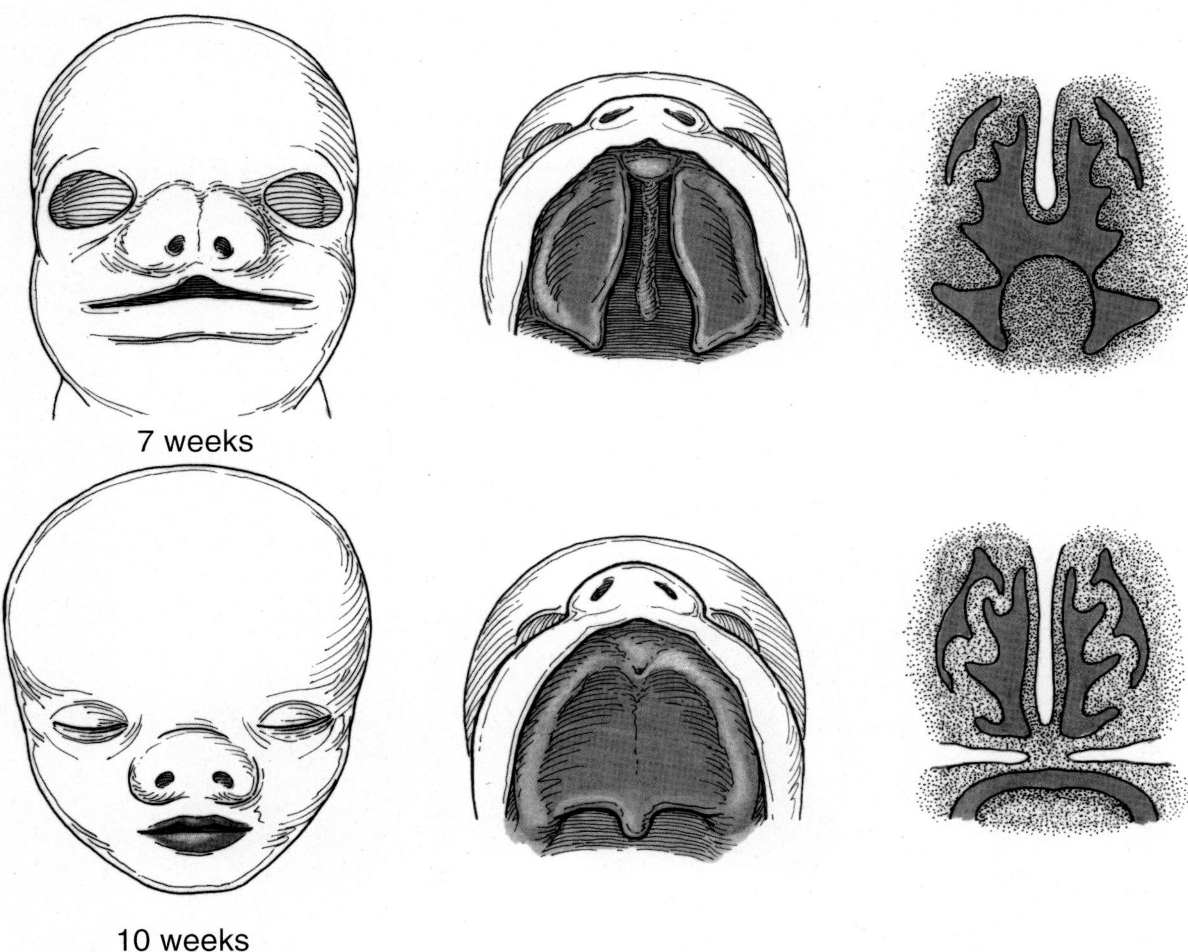

Fig. 76.2 Schematic diagram of the embryo at age 7 and 10 weeks during which time the secondary palate forms in an anterior-to-posterior fusion process beginning at the incisive foramen.

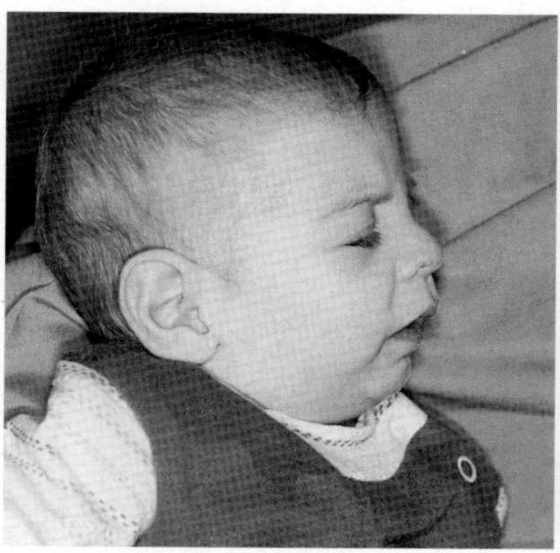

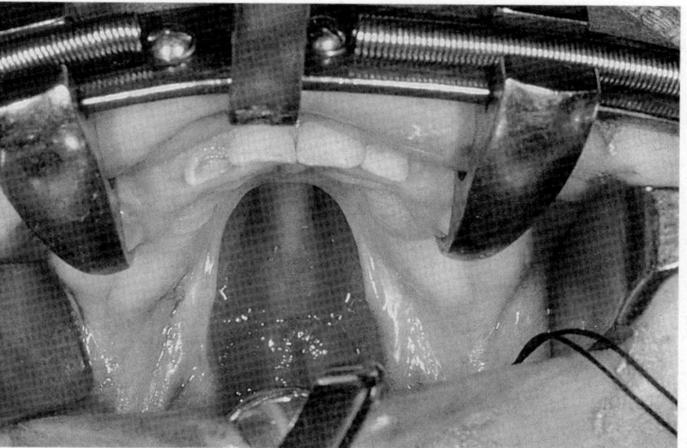

Fig. 76.3 (**A,B**) Child with Pierre Robin sequence including micrognathia, relative macroglossia, and a U-shaped cleft palate.

Interruption of this development can cause clefts of the lip and central alveolus (primary palate). Clefts of the lip may be unilateral or bilateral, complete or incomplete. They may be isolated, or associated with clefts of the palate or other malformations (syndromic clefts). Human cleft lip, with or without associated cleft palate, is caused by failure of the MNPs to make contact with the *lateral nasal processes* (LNPs) and MXPs during embryogenesis. Interruption of this embryonic process creates malformation of some or all of the upper lip, central alveolus, and primary palate. A minor malformation of normal development may cause diastasis of the central orbicularis oris muscle fibers, with no overt clefting of the epidermis of the upper lip. This condition is known as a *microform cleft lip* deformity (**Fig. 76.4**). An incomplete unilateral cleft lip involves a full-thickness deficit of skin, muscle, and mucosa, but does not extend superiorly through the entire lip height (**Fig. 76.5**). A *complete unilateral cleft lip* occurs when a full-thickness cleft extends through the entire height of the lip and floor of the nose (**Fig. 76.6**). A cleft of the alveolus is almost always associated with complete clefting of the lip.

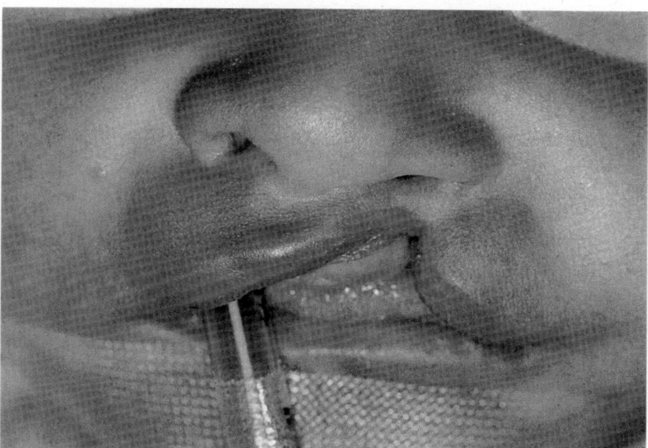

Fig. 76.5 A 3-month-old child with an incomplete left cleft lip.

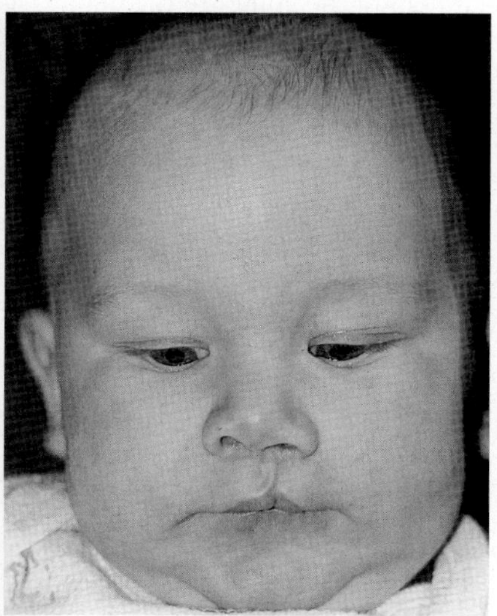

Fig. 76.4 A 3-month-old child with a microform left cleft lip.

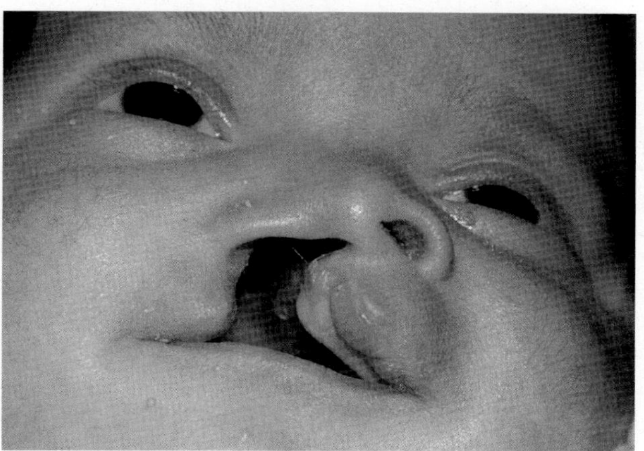

Fig. 76.6 A 2-month-old child with a complete cleft of the right lip and palate.

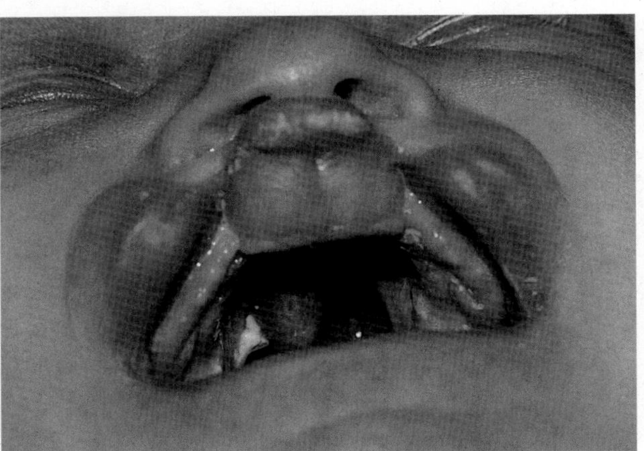

Fig. 76.7 Base view of a child with an incomplete bilateral cleft lip and palate.

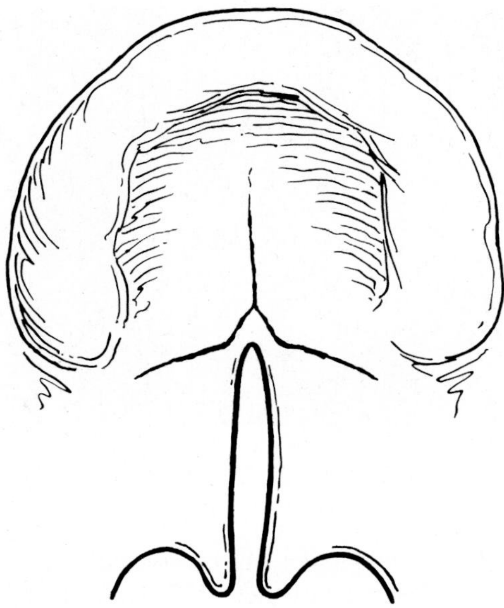

Fig. 76.9 Schematic diagram of a soft palate cleft.

The degree of clefting of the upper lip depends on the timing and degree of interruption of normal lip development. If disruption occurs on both sides of lip development, a bilateral cleft lip results. In the *incomplete bilateral cleft lip*, there is skeletal continuity and little or no protrusion of the premaxilla (**Fig. 76.7**). In the *complete bilateral cleft lip*, the premaxilla is totally detached from each maxilla (**Fig. 76.8A,B**).

Either the unilateral or bilateral cleft lip deformity may be isolated or associated with clefts of the alveolus or palate. Because a more substantial interruption of lip development is required to create a bilateral cleft lip, this deformity is more likely to be associated with clefting of the secondary palate than is the unilateral cleft lip.

As with cleft lip, clefts of the secondary palate display variable expression. A *bifid uvula* is the mildest expression of soft palate clefting. This common deformity occurs when there is a lack of normal uvular fusion. A *submucous cleft palate* occurs when there is diastasis of the soft palatal musculature. In this condition, the palatal mucosa is intact, but speech therapy and/or surgical repair are often required because of dysfunction caused by the associated muscle defect. Full-thickness clefting of the soft palate (incomplete secondary cleft palate) may also occur (**Fig. 76.9**). Finally, complete clefting of the secondary palate may result from total interruption of the normal formation of the palate posterior to the incisive foramen (**Fig. 76.10**).[6]

Clefts of the secondary palate may be associated with complete cleft lips and are termed *complete clefts of the lip and palate*. Complete cleft lip and palate may be unilateral or bilateral. The complete unilateral cleft lip and palate usually involves attachment of the vomer to the maxillary

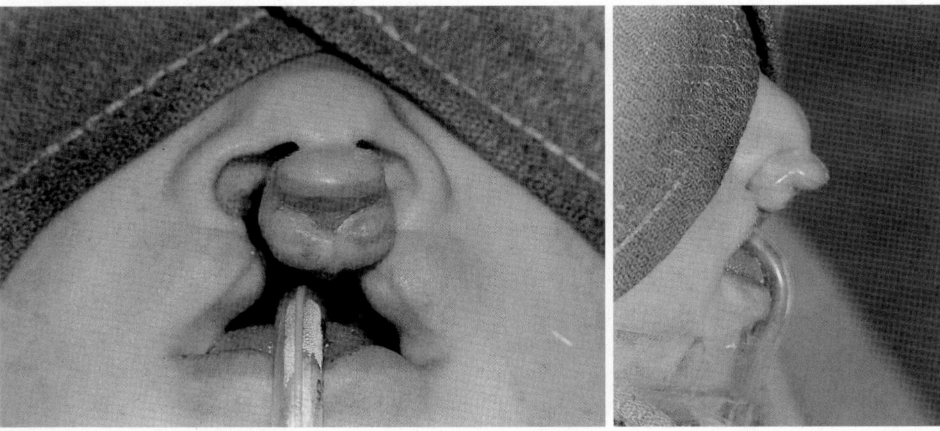

A B

Fig. 76.8 (**A,B**) A 3-month-old child with a symmetrical complete bilateral cleft lip and palate. Note the anterior protrusion of the premaxilla and prolabium and poorly projected nasal tip.

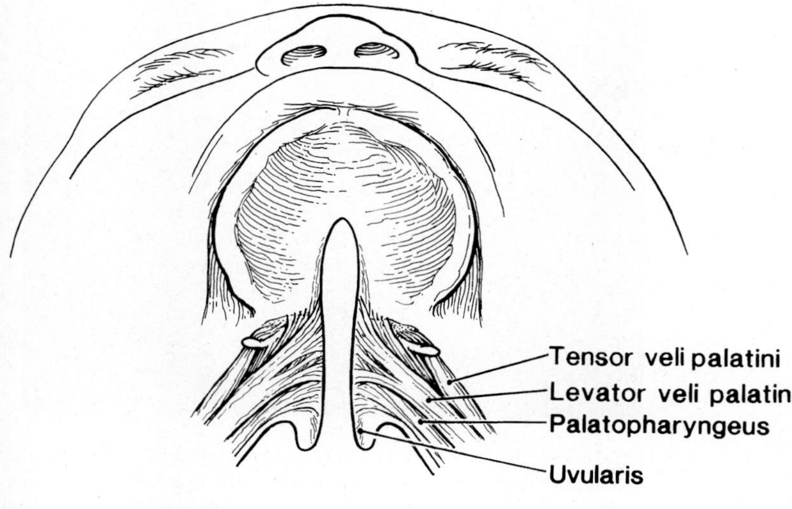

Fig. 76.10 Schematic diagram of a complete cleft of the secondary palate beginning at the incisive foramen.

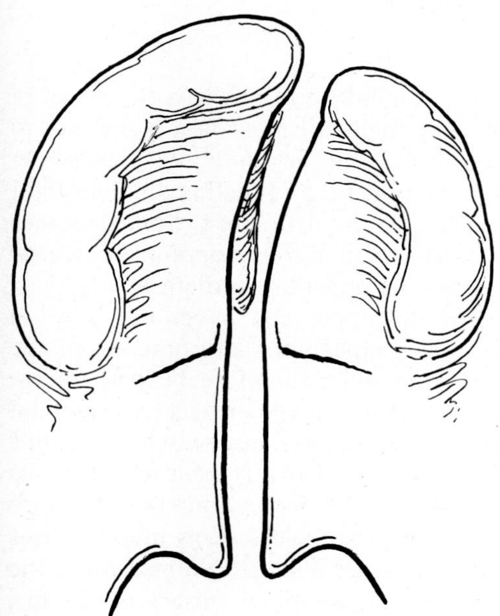

Fig. 76.11 Schematic diagram of a complete unilateral cleft palate.

palatal shelf of the noncleft side (**Fig. 76.11**), whereas complete bilateral cleft of the lip and palate usually exhibits vomerine and premaxillary detachment from the two lateral palatal shelves (**Fig. 76.12**). In all cases, clefting of the upper lip and palate is variable in expression and typically follows known embryological patterns.

Timing of Surgery and Philosophy of Cleft Repair

The decision when to repair a cleft lip or palate is based on a variety of factors, including patient growth and development, safety to undergo anesthesia, speech development, facial growth, and psychosocial impact. As always, the risks, alternatives, and benefits of repair need to be fully discussed with the parents or guardians prior to any procedure. The timing of cleft repairs is outlined in **Table 76.1**.[7]

In all patients with cleft palate, tympanostomy tube insertion is performed at age 3 to 6 months to overcome eustachian tube dysfunction, treat chronic otitis media with effusion, aerate the middle ear space, decrease conductive hearing loss, and minimize the likelihood of chronic ear disease. Because the literature increasingly supports early intervention in children with hearing loss and given that tympanostomy tube placement is associated with few complications, the benefits outweigh

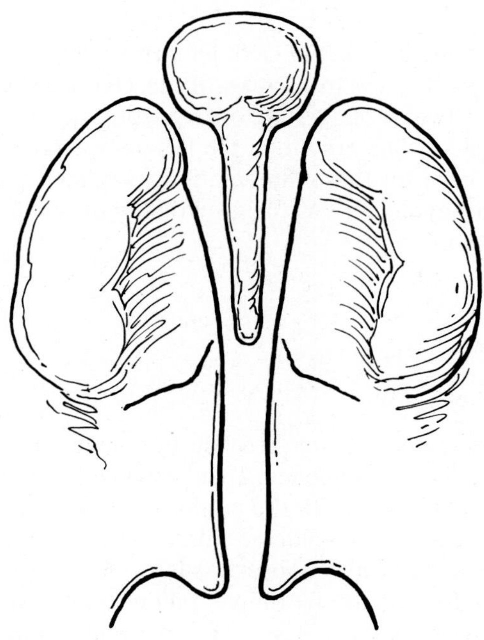

Fig. 76.12 Schematic diagram of a complete bilateral cleft palate.

Table 76.1 Timing of Cleft Repairs

Procedure	Age
Cleft lip repair	3 months
Tip rhinoplasty	
Tympanostomy tubes	
Palatoplasty	9–18 months
T-tube placement	
Speech evaluation	3–4 years
Velopharyngeal insufficiency workup and surgery (if necessary)	4–6 years
Alveolar bone grafting	9–11 years
Nasal reconstruction	12–18 years
Orthognathic surgery (if necessary)	At completion of mandibular growth (>16 years)

the risks of this additional procedure.[8–10] In patients with cleft lip and palate, the lip repair and tympanostomy tube placement are performed at ~3 months of age. Cleft palate repair is performed at 9 to 12 months, just prior to the initial development of speech to minimize the possibility of velopharyngeal dysfunction (VPD). Long duration tympanostomy tubes (e.g., Goode t-tubes) are placed at the time of palatoplasty.

After cleft palate repair, patients are monitored carefully for speech development, usually beginning at age 2 years. If VPD is identified, a VPD workup, including nasopharyngoscopy and videofluoroscopy, is performed. If the degree of VPD is significant and recalcitrant to speech therapy, surgical treatment is performed between 4 and 6 years of age.

Other surgical treatments for cleft deformities include alveolar bone grafting at 9 to 11 years of age, cleft rhinoplasty at 12 to 18 years of age, and orthognathic surgery after age 16 years, when growth of the facial skeleton is complete. The need for these interventions is related to the initial deformity as well as the growth and development of the patient.

Cleft Lip

Anatomy of the Lip

The upper lip can be divided into red (mucous membrane) and white (cutaneous) components. The *vermilion* (Latin *vermiculus*, "small worm") is the dry portion of the lip's red mucous membrane. It is a modified mucosal membrane lacking pilosebaceous units, salivary glands, or eccrine glands, bordered superiorly by the vermilion–cutaneous junction (i.e., the vermilion border). This mucocutaneous junction serves as an important aesthetic element

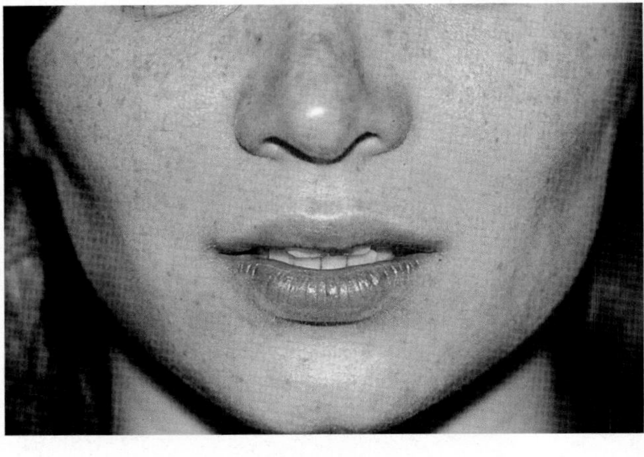

Fig. 76.13 Photograph of the perioral complex including the mucous membrane and cutaneous components of the upper and lower lips. Note the distinct white skin roll that reflects light just superior to the vermillion–cutaneous junction.

separating the convex red lip from the concave white lip. A round roll of epithelium is present just superior to the vermilion border, called the *white roll.*[11] The white roll spans the entire upper lip, reflecting ambient light (**Fig. 76.13**). Precise reconstruction of the mucocutaneous junction and white roll of the upper lip is essential in reestablishing normal upper lip aesthetics.

The muscles of the upper and lower lips play an important role in the appearance and function of the lips. Careful attention must therefore be paid to recreating muscle continuity in repair of any congenital or traumatic deformity. The principal muscle of the lips is the orbicularis oris (**Fig. 76.14**). This muscle encircles the oral orifice, forming a sphincter within the substance of the lips.[12] The superficial layer of this muscle arises from the dermis and passes obliquely to insert into the mucous membrane lining the inner surface of the lips. The fibers of the deep layer arise from the maxilla above and the mandible below.[13] The orbicularis oris is innervated by the buccal and marginal mandibular divisions of the facial nerve.

Unilateral Cleft Lip

The unilateral cleft lip deformity may involve any combination of skin, muscle, and underlying mucosa. As previously discussed, microform cleft lip involves clefting of the upper lip musculature. Incomplete cleft lip involves skin, muscle, and mucosa but often spares the nasal sill and underlying skeletal structures. Complete unilateral cleft lip deformities involve all tissue layers.

The orbicularis oris muscles associated with the unilateral cleft lip deformity are hypoplastic and incompletely

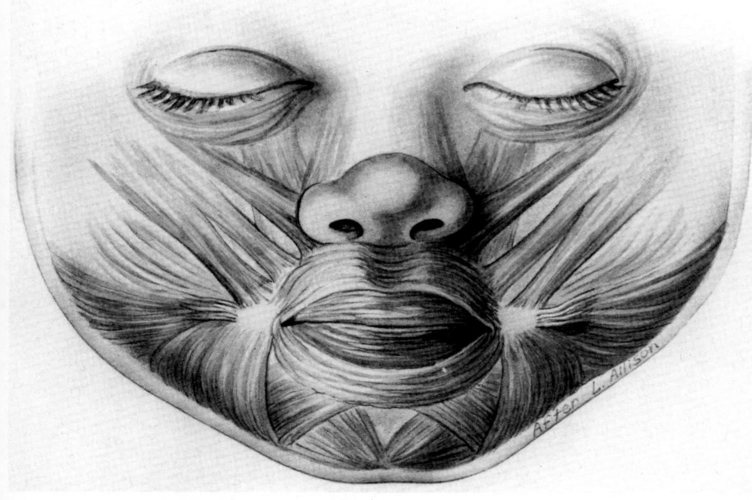

Fig. 76.14 Illustration of the orbicularis oris muscle as it relates to the other facial musculature.

developed when compared with their noncleft counterparts. In addition, the upper lip muscles are prevented from attaching to their normal insertions, finding unnatural insertions instead (**Fig. 76.15**). Although it is obvious that no muscle crosses the cleft in complete clefts, the skin bridge in incomplete clefts has also been found to contain no functional musculature. Muscle dissections by Fara et al on stillborn babies with incomplete clefts confirmed that the muscles in unilateral cleft lips are more hypoplastic on the medial side of the cleft than the lateral side.[14] Additionally, these dissections revealed that the upper lip muscles in incomplete clefts did not cross the cleft gap unless the skin bridge was at least one third the height of the lip. Even if the orbicularis oris muscle is present in the skin bridge of an incomplete cleft, however, the orientation of the fibers is abnormal.

The major vascular supply to the lips and nose arises from the facial artery, the fourth branch of the external carotid artery. The facial artery gives rise to the superior and inferior labial arteries at each oral commissure. The paired superior labial arteries anastomose in the midline of the upper lip, and the two inferior labial arteries behave similarly in the lower lip. In the unilateral cleft lip, the aberrant vascular supply parallels the findings of the unilateral cleft lip musculature (**Fig. 76.16**). As with the orbicularis oris, the blood supply on the lateral aspect of the cleft is better developed than the vasculature on the medial side. The superior labial artery courses along the margin of the cleft, anastomosing with either the angular artery or the lateral nasal artery at the base of the nose. In incomplete clefts, a thin, terminal branch of the superior labial artery crosses the skin bridge.

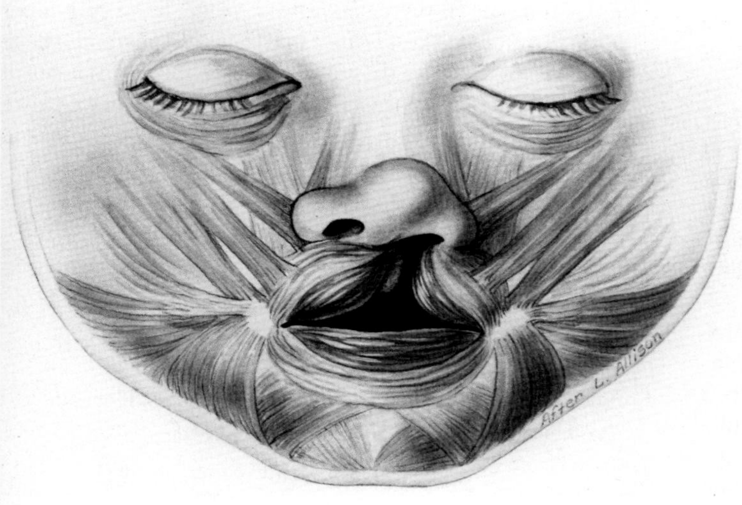

Fig. 76.15 Diagram of the orbicularis oris muscle associated with a unilateral cleft lip deformity. Note the abnormal insertions of the muscle along the cleft margin.

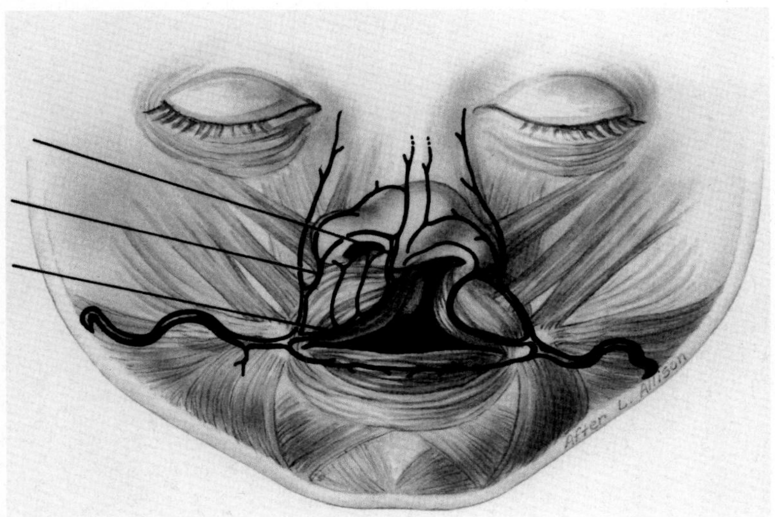

Fig. 76.16 Diagram of the aberrant vascular supply of the unilateral cleft lip.

Surgical Repair

Many techniques have been described over the years for repair of the unilateral cleft lip. Early descriptions of cleft lip repair utilized variations of straight-line closures. The main disadvantage of straight-line closure is the tendency for vertical scar contracture across the mucocutaneous junction, resulting in notching of the lip. Wide complete unilateral cleft lips are also difficult to repair by the straight-line method.

In the mid-twentieth century, various geometric closures were proposed for repairing the unilateral cleft lip. Geometrical techniques, such as modified Z-plasties, quadrangular flaps, and triangular flaps,[15–17] were designed to decrease the amount of lip shortening that occurred with cleft lip repair and to improve orbicularis oris realignment and function. LeMesurier[18] described the quadrangular flap and Tennison[15] described the triangular flap technique as a reliable method for decreasing vertical lip contracture in unilateral cleft lip repair.

The primary advantage of geometric repair techniques for cleft lip is that they provide a reproducible method of lip repair. Exact measurements can be taken with calipers to assure a tension-free closure of the lip. The basic disadvantage of these methods is that the incisions always violate the philtral column on the noncleft side, thereby creating a scar that does not respect boundaries of known anatomical subunits. In addition, geometric repairs require exacting presurgical measurement and often lack flexibility during surgical application.

In 1957, Millard incorporated aspects of multiple previously described repairs, and developed the *rotation-advancement flap* for repair of the unilateral cleft lip.[19] This method maximized surgical flexibility while facilitating elimination of a minimal amount of normal lip tissue. This method is now the most commonly utilized technique for repair of the unilateral cleft lip. The advantages and disadvantages of the Millard rotation-advancement flap technique are shown in **Table 76.2**.

Surgical Technique for Rotation-Advancement Repair

The important reference points of the rotation-advancement flap technique are summarized in **Table 76.3** and **Fig. 76.17**.[20] Some of these points are anatomical points (e.g., 1,2,4,5,6,10), whereas other points are "measured" (e.g., 3,5,8,9). Several measurements (**Table 76.4**) are used to idealize flap design and maximize lip aesthetics. The main objective of these measurements is to ensure that the length of the rotation flap (3 to 5 + x) equals the length of the advancement flap (8 to 9) (**Fig. 76.18**).

The reference points and premarked incisions create major flaps *A* (rotation) and *B* (advancement), and minor flaps *c* (skin), *m* (medial mucosa), and *l* (lateral mucosa) (**Table 76.5**). The uppercase letters indicate full-thickness flaps, and the lowercase letters refer to single-layer (skin or mucosa) flaps. After marking and incising these lip flaps, meticulous dissection and reapproximation of the orbicularis oris muscle are performed. This closure maximizes lip function while minimizing tension across the wound.

Table 76.2 Millard Rotation-Advancement Repair

Advantages	Disadvantages
Flexible	Requires experienced surgeon
Minimal tissue discarded	Possible excessive tension
Good nasal access	Extensive undermining required
Camouflaged suture line	Vertical scar contracture
	Tendency to small nostril

Table 76.3 Millard Rotation-Advancement Technique Reference Points

1. Center (low point) of Cupid's bow—NCS
2. Peak of Cupid's bow—lateral NCS
3. Peak of Cupid's bow—medial NCS
4. Alar base—NCS
5. Columellar base—NCS
X. Back-cut point—NCS
6. Commissure—NCS
7. Commissure—CS
8. Peak of Cupid's bow—CS
9. Medial tip of advancement flap—CS
10. Midpoint of alar base—CS
11. Lateral alar base—CS

Abbreviations: CS, cleft side; NCS, noncleft side.

Table 76.4 Measurements for Flap Design

1 to 2 = 1 to 3 = 2–4 mm
2 to 6 = 8 to 7 = 20 mm
2 to 4 = 8 to 10 = 9–11 mm
3 to 5 + X = 8 to 9

Table 76.5 Flap Labels and Designations

A: Rotation flap
B: Advancement flap
C: Columellar base soft tissue, NCS
D: Alar rim—CS
M: Medial mucosal flap
l: Lateral mucosal flap

Abbreviations: CS, cleft side; NCS, noncleft side.

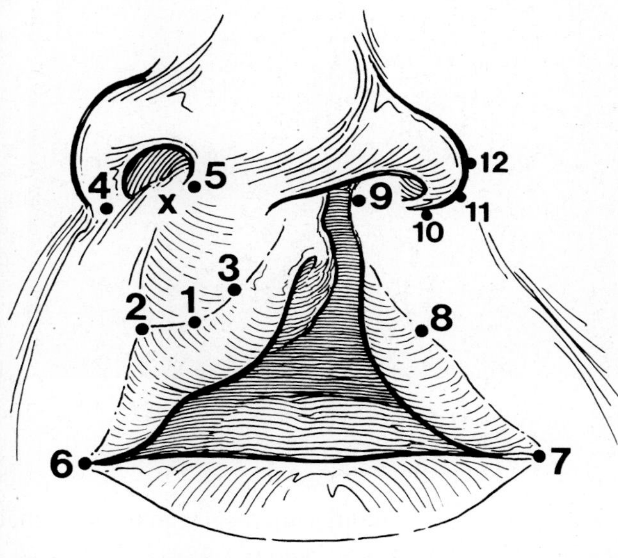

Fig. 76.17 The marked and measured points of the Millard rotation advancement unilateral cleft lip repair.

The Millard rotation-advancement lip repair also allows active closure of the nasal floor and concomitant tip rhinoplasty (**Fig. 76.19A,B**). These procedures create improved symmetry of the nasal tip and alar base. Complete access to the nasal tip can be obtained through the standard perialar and cleft margin incisions, without additional nasal incisions.

Bilateral Cleft Lip Deformity

There are several key anatomical differences between the unilateral and bilateral cleft lip deformities that must be considered before undertaking repair of the bilateral cleft lip (**Table 76.6**).

The shape and configuration of the two lateral segments of the bilateral cleft lip are similar to the lateral segment of the unilateral deformity; however, the central prolabium and premaxilla of the bilateral deformity are markedly different from those of the unilateral lip deformity. In a complete bilateral cleft, the premaxilla is totally detached from each maxilla. The central premaxilla and the attached prolabium (central segment of the bilateral cleft lip) may find their own position, unrelated to the position of the maxilla on either side. In an incomplete bilateral cleft lip, there is usually some skeletal continuity and very little protrusion of the premaxilla/ prolabium. The premaxilla in complete bilateral cleft lip usually protrudes more than in the incomplete deformity; therefore, the columella of the nose is usually shorter in the complete bilateral deformity.

The arterial network and musculature of the lateral elements of the complete bilateral cleft lip parallel that of the lateral segment in the unilateral anomaly. The abnormal insertion of the cleft lip musculature follows the margin of the cleft (**Fig. 76.20**).[21,22] The central prolabium in complete bilateral clefts contains no muscle. In incomplete bilateral cleft lip, some orbicularis oris muscle fibers cross the cleft from the lateral to the medial segment. The amount of muscle crossing the skin bridge is variable and related to the size of the skin bridge.[14]

The arterial supply in bilateral cleft lips is characterized by an aberrant course of the superior labial artery (**Fig. 76.21**). This artery runs superiorly along the edge of the cleft and forms an anastomosis with the angular and lateral nasal arteries. This abnormal course is similar to that in the lateral segment of the unilateral deformity. The prolabial segment receives its blood supply from the septal, columellar, and premaxillary vessels.

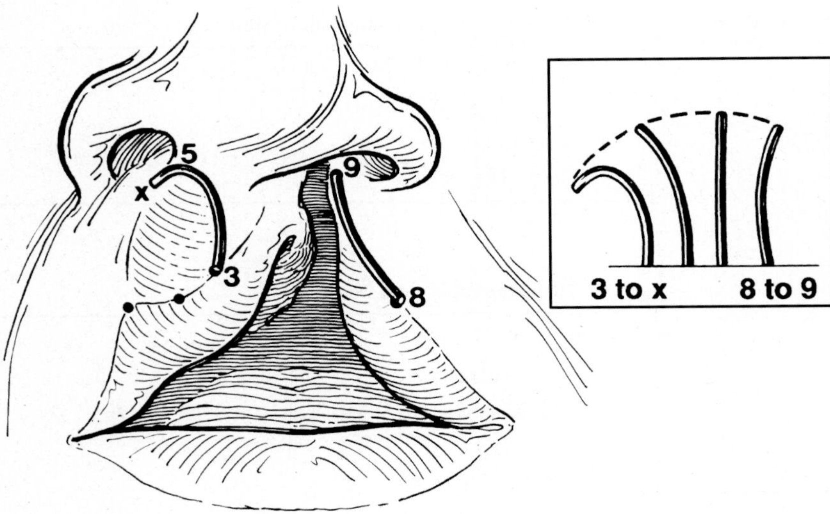

Fig. 76.18 Schematic representation of the rotation advancement incisions. Note the length of the rotation flap incision (3 to 5 + ×) should equal the length of the advancement flap incision (8 to 9).

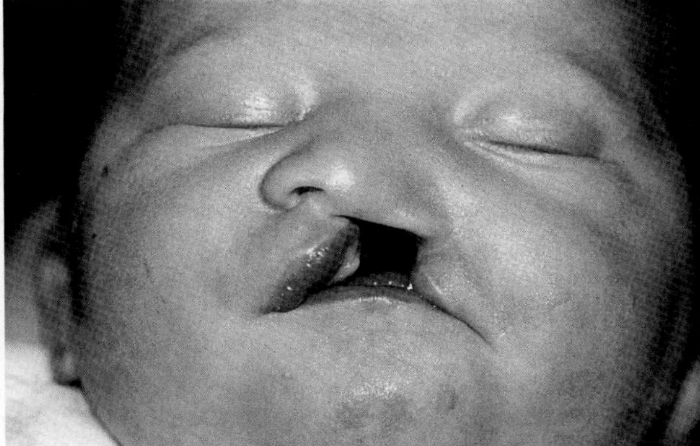

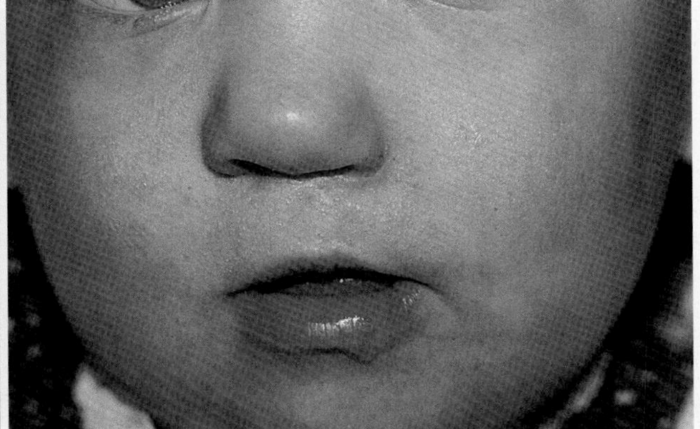

Fig. 76.19 (**A**) A 10-day-old patient with a complete left cleft lip/palate and (**B**) the same child at age 8 months (after Millard repair at age 3 months).

Surgical Repair

The timing and technique for repair of the bilateral cleft lip are related to the extent of the deformity and the philosophy of the operating surgeon. The repair can be performed after presurgical orthopedics or lip adhesion, both designed to narrow the cleft gap and to better align the cleft segments. Definitive lip repair can be performed in a single stage or in two separate surgical procedures.

Varying degrees of anterior premaxillary projection, rotation (creating asymmetry), and cleft width can be observed (**Fig. 76.22A–C**). In patients with a wide complete bilateral cleft lip, alveolus, and secondary palate, a two-stage closure may be indicated.[23] The first-stage lip

Table 76.6 Bilateral Cleft Lip Repair Characteristics

Characteristic	Surgical Approach
Wide, malpositioned nasal tip	Tip rhinoplasty (intermediate)
Short columella	V–Y advancement or delayed forked flap
Premaxilla may be "locked out"	Lip adhesion or lip repair
Prolabium contains no muscle	Lateral muscles sutured at midline (concentric orbicularis oris ring)
Orbicularis oris inserts superiorly	Reorient muscle under prolabium
More volume in lateral lip than prolabium	Lateral lip mucosal flaps rotate medially

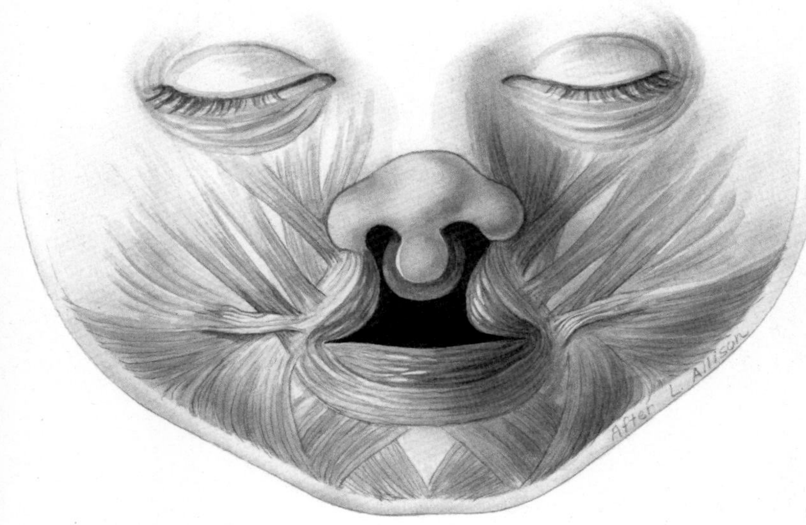

Fig. 76.20 Schematic diagram illustrating the abnormal orientation and insertions of the bilateral cleft lip musculature.

adhesion converts a complete cleft lip deformity to an incomplete deformity. The lip adhesion procedure also exerts an orthopedic force on the prolabium and premaxilla, inhibiting its forward growth. This orthopedic force retropositions the central premaxilla into an improved position in relation to the lateral lip segments.

The decision to perform a single-stage versus a two-stage lip repair is often related to the comfort and experience of the surgeon. The two-stage technique has the advantage of allowing better vascularity to the central prolabial segment and capability to apply the techniques of the Millard rotation–advancement technique to each side of the bilateral repair. However, the two-stage repair tends to create asymmetry of the lip and does not allow muscle to be advanced across the central prolabial segment. The single-stage bilateral cleft lip repair, as described by Millard in 1977, is designed to produce an intact lip with scars mimicking the philtral columns.[24] The single-stage repair maximizes the symmetry of the lip and is designed to reorient the orbicularis oris muscle from the lateral lip segment across the central prolabial segment. Intact lip musculature improves lip aesthetics and decreases tension across the vertical lip incisions.[25]

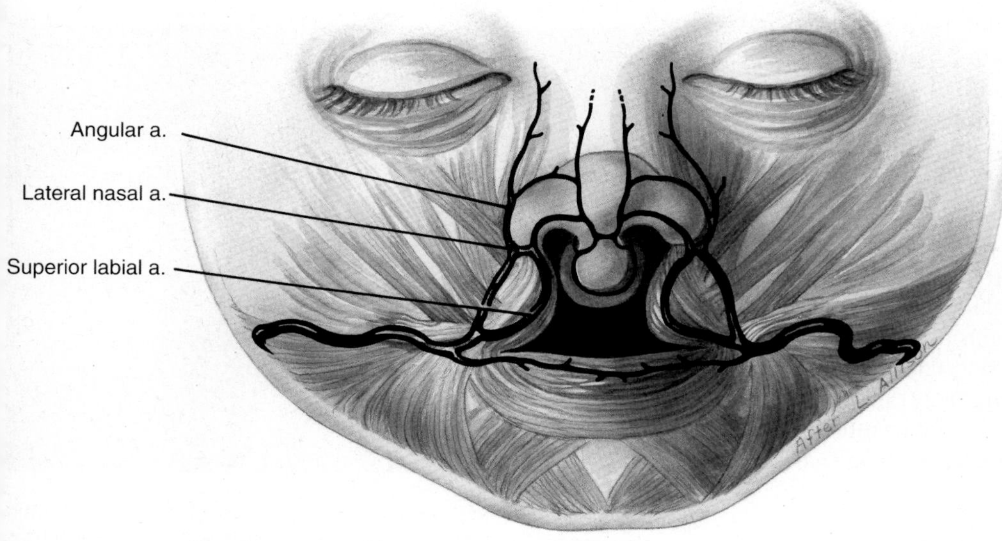

Fig. 76.21 Schematic diagram illustrating the aberrant arterial supply of the bilateral cleft lip deformity.

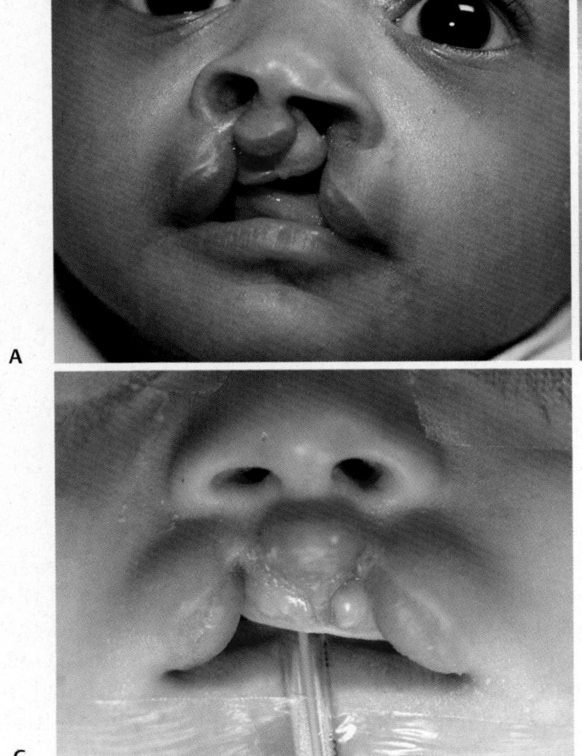

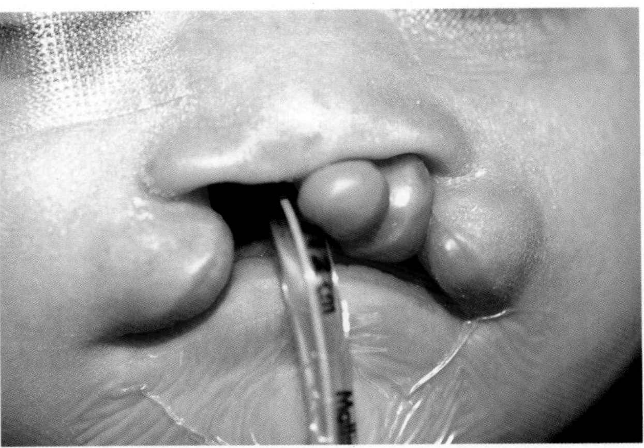

Fig. 76.22 (**A**) Photograph of a 4-month-old with bilateral complete cleft lip, left cleft alveolus, and cleft palate. Note the asymmetry of the alar base and rather large prolabial segment. (**B**) Intraoperative view of a bilateral cleft in 3-month-old illustrating the rotation of the premaxillary segment. (**C**) Intraoperative view of an incomplete bilateral cleft deformity illustrating the diminutive prolabium, but more normal alar base width.

Surgical Technique

Measurement and Design

A single-stage bilateral cleft lip repair and the unique characteristics of the bilateral cleft lip deformity will be described. First, the midline on the vermilion–cutaneous junction of the prolabial flap (p) is marked. The philtral width, which is expected to widen with growth, is measured using a caliper to mark 2.0 to 2.5 mm on each side of the midline (the total philtral width of 4 to 5 mm). Vertical markings are created to extend up to just superomedial to the columellar base. The lateral vermilion borders are then marked to create the prolabial forked flaps (f) which can be rotated laterally for closure of the nasal sill or banked as forked flaps for subsequent columellar lengthening.

Next, the lateral lip markings are designed to approximate the vertical height of the prolabial flap. This vermilion marking begins where the mucosa begins to thin superomedially. Marking and design of the mucosal flaps (m) is similar to those in unilateral cleft repairs (**Fig. 76.23**). Bilateral sublabial incisions were designed to extend from the mucosal flaps to allow release of the cheek–lip complex from the maxilla.

Incision and Flap Elevation

With the prolabial flap incised and elevated, the inferiorly based prolabial mucosa is sutured under the prolabial flap to create a labioalveolar sulcus. The forked flaps are incised and elevated in a subcutaneous plane to be rotated laterally into the floor of the nose as needed. Next, the mucosal flaps on the lateral lip segments are elevated with a conservative back-cut into the nasal–alar groove (**Fig. 76.24**). The lateral intraoral sublabial incisions are extended intraorally to release the

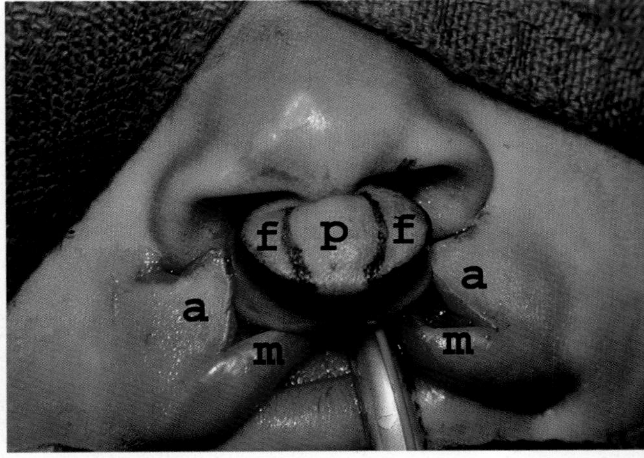

Fig. 76.23 Intraoperative view showing the marked prolabial flap (p) and forked flaps (f). The lateral lip advancement flaps (a) and mucosal flaps (m) have been elevated. The vertical heights of the prolabial and lateral lip advancement flaps are equal. (From Sykes JM, Tollefson TT. Management of the cleft lip deformity. Facial Plast Surg Clin N Am 2005;13:157–167.)

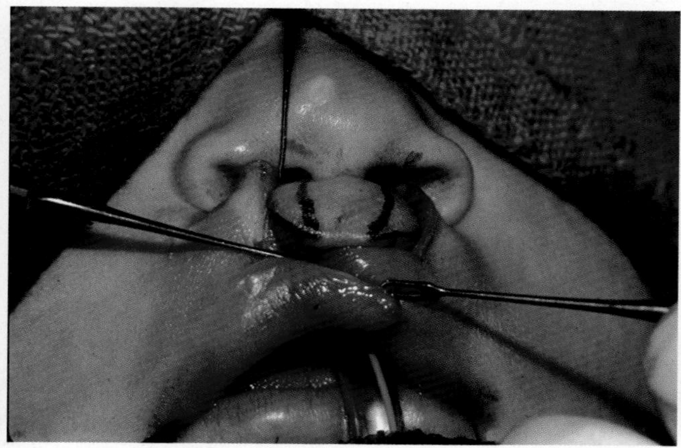

Fig. 76.24 Intraoperative view of the advanced mucosal flaps prior to elevation of the prolabial flap. The muscle layer closure will be performed anterior to the premaxilla, but deep to the prolabial flap. This minimizes tension on the skin closure and creates a concentric ring of orbicularis oris. (From Sykes JM, Tollefson TT. Management of the cleft lip deformity. Facial Plast Surg Clin N Am 2005;13:157–167.)

cheek–lip complex from the maxilla, with care to preserve the infraorbital neurovascular bundles. Care must be taken to fully release the aberrantly oriented orbicularis oris from the cleft margin of the pyriform aperture. Lastly, the lateral lip advancement skin flaps (a) are conservatively undermined from the reoriented orbicularis oris muscle fibers. The malpositioned lower lateral cartilages, including the shortened medial crus, are freed from the skin soft tissue envelope.

Nasal Floor Closure and Alar Base Width

The lateral lip segments' mucosal closure over the premaxilla but under the prolabial flap is performed with 5–0 chromic catgut sutures. The forked flaps can be rotated laterally to add to the nasal floor closure, or these flaps can be discarded. Release of the lateral nasal wall mucosa can help obtain nostril size symmetry. The alar base width is actively placed with a 4–0 monofilament absorbable suture.

Orbicularis Oris Closure

The orbicularis oris muscle should be reoriented over the premaxilla to create a concentric muscular ring, as well as to prevent dynamic inferior displacement of the alar base with muscle contraction. The "key suture" (4–0 long-acting monofilament absorbable) is placed at the vermilion–cutaneous junction to create vertical height symmetry and lip fullness. Two to three muscular closure sutures are placed using horizontal mattress to approximate the reconstructed orbicularis oris.

Skin Closure

After the mucosal and muscle approximation are completed, the Cupid's bow is created by aligning the prolabial flap vermilion with the lateral lip vermilion using a permanent 6–0 monofilament suture (**Fig. 76.25**). Often, a back-cut at the vermilion border of the lateral lip segment is helpful. Other than the vertical lip height and horizontal symmetry, the third dimension to be considered must be the lip fullness (**Fig. 76.26**). A mucosal Z-plasty can be used to distribute lip volume and prevent a "whistle" deformity that can be seen with central mucosal lip deficiencies.

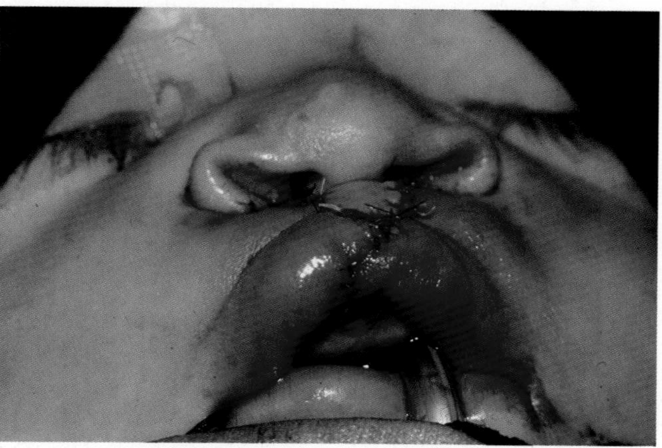

Fig. 76.25 Intraoperative view of the final closure prior to lower lateral cartilage bolster placement. (From Sykes JM, Tollefson TT. Management of the cleft lip deformity. Facial Plast Surg Clin N Am 2005;13:157–167.)

Tip Rhinoplasty

The nasal tip skin elevation is performed prior to lip closure to allow the lower lateral cartilages to be repositioned. After lip closure is completed, the lower lateral cartilages are sutured in a more cephalic and medial position using two to four bolsters secured with 4–0 permanent sutures and pledgets. The shortened columella will be addressed in subsequent surgeries with various techniques such as V-Y advancement (Bardach) or delayed inset of forked flaps to create columellar lengthening. Some surgeons prefer to perform this at the time of palatoplasty.

Palatoplasty

The goals of palatoplasty are restoration of normal speech development and cessation of nasal regurgitation through the oronasal fistula. Achievement of these goals requires (1) adequate flap mobilization to minimize wound tension, (2) atraumatic tissue handling to maximize flap viability and minimize vascular pedicle injury, (3) two-layer closure of oral and nasal mucosa to minimize fistula formation, and (4) re-creation of the velopharyngeal muscular sling to maximize palate function (**Table 76.7**).

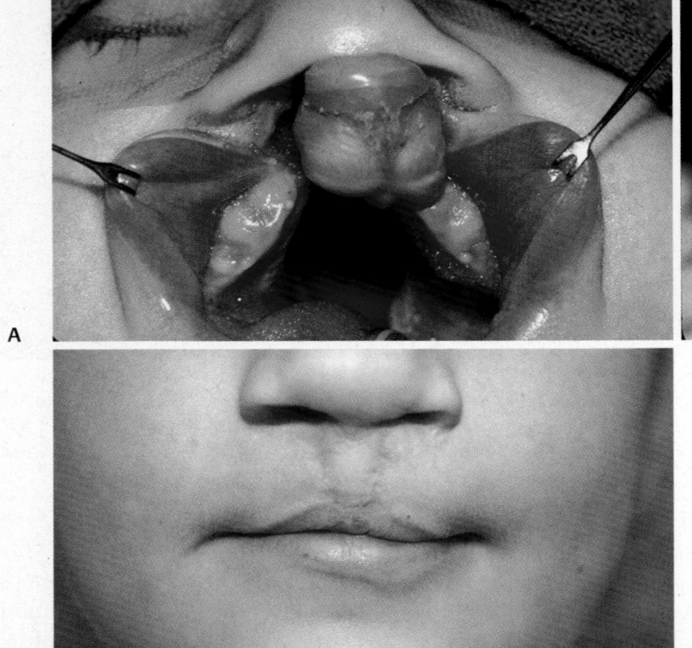

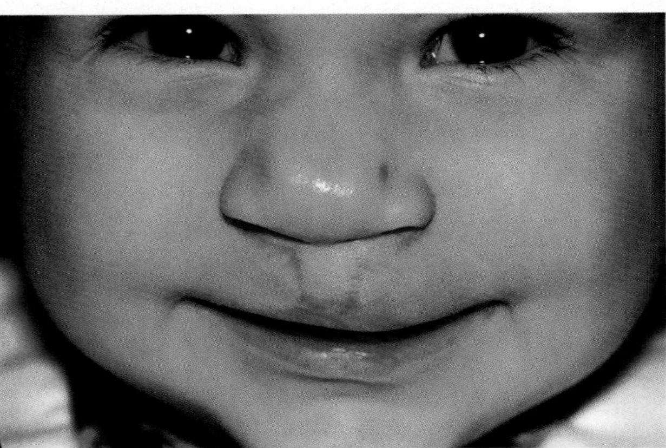

Fig. 76.26 (**A**) Intraoperative photograph of a 3-month-old patient with a bilateral cleft lip and palate deformity; (**B**) Eight-month postoperative photograph of this patient; (**C**) Ten-year postoperative photograph of this patient. (From Sykes JM, Tollefson TT. Management of the cleft lip deformity. Facial Plast Surg Clin N Am 2005;13:157–167.)

To maximize blood supply to the periphery of the palatal flaps, an atraumatic "no touch" technique should be used when elevating and advancing the flaps. The mucosal flaps are not grasped with tissue forceps, and monopolar electrocautery is avoided. Although different palatal clefts require different flap design, surgical techniques are maintained irrespective of the type of palatal repair utilized.

A summary of preferred palatoplasty techniques is listed in **Table 76.8**.

Table 76.8 Preferred Palatoplasty Techniques

Cleft Type	Technique
Complete unilateral	Two-flap
Complete bilateral	Two-flap (with vomerine flaps)
Complete secondary	Three-flap
Incomplete secondary	Double-reversing Z-plasty
Submucous cleft palate	Double-reversing Z-plasty

Von Langenbeck's Palatoplasty

In the early nineteenth century, elevation of bipedicled mucoperiosteal flaps to repair clefts of the hard palate was independently reported by Dieffenbach,[26] Warren,[27,28] and von Langenbeck.[29] Often referred to as the von Langenbeck repair (**Fig. 76.27**), bipedicle flap palatoplasty involves incisions along the cleft margin (medial) and adjacent to the alveolar ridge (lateral) (**Fig. 76.28A,B**). Undermining the flaps in a subperiosteal plane allows flap release, advancement, and approximation in a "drawbridge" fashion to achieve closure. This technique employs several important principles of palatoplasty, including two-layered closure and adequate flap mobilization to minimize wound tension. Closure of the oral and nasal layers independently decreases the incidence of postsurgical fistula when compared with single-layer closures. If there is breakdown of either the oral or the nasal layer, a fistula does not usually result because the other intact layer often prevents fistula formation.

Table 76.7 Principles of Palatoplasty

Minimization of wound tension
Atraumatic technique
Two-layer closure (oral and nasal mucosa)
Re-creation of soft plate muscular sling

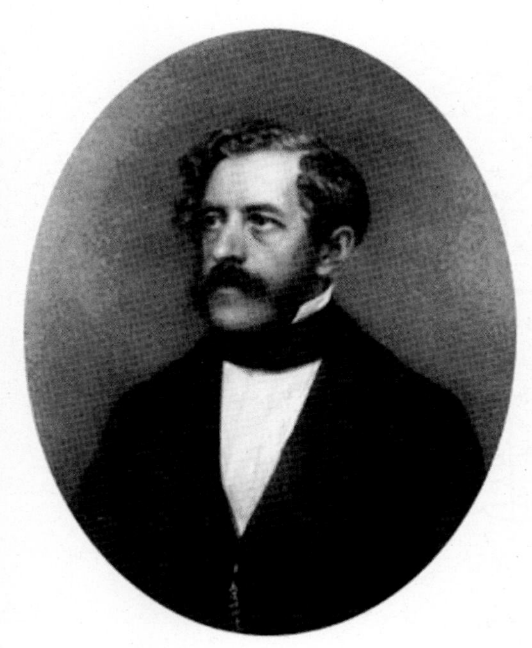

Fig. 76.27 Bernhard Rudolf Konrad von Langenbeck (1810–1887).

Although the von Langenbeck palatoplasty works well for many palatal clefts, it has a major disadvantage of not allowing visualization of the vascular pedicles of the palatal flaps. The greater palatine vascular pedicle is located ~1 cm medial to the upper second molar tooth. Identification of this pedicle allows far greater flap mobilization, and therefore less wound tension in wide palatal clefts. For this reason, most surgeons connect the medial and lateral cleft incisions, converting bipedicled flaps into posteriorly based unipedicled flaps. These three-flap (incomplete clefts) and two-flap (complete clefts) repairs allow visualization of the greater palatine pedicle and the resulting benefits.

Three-Flap Palatoplasty

The three-flap palatoplasty is used to repair clefts of the secondary palate (i.e., clefts posterior to the incisive foramen).[30,31] The medial cleft incisions are the same as those in the bipedicled flap technique, and the lateral incisions are made adjacent to the tooth crowns and carried around the maxillary tuberosity. The medial and lateral incisions are then connected anteriorly at the level of the canine teeth laterally. These anterior oblique incisions convert the flaps to posteriorly unipedicled flaps (**Fig. 76.29A**).

The flaps are elevated in a submucoperiosteal plane and contain the greater palatine vessels. Dissection and release of the malaligned soft palatal musculature is then performed from the posterior edge of the hard palate. This allows repositioning of the velopharyngeal muscular sling from an oblique to a more physiological transverse orientation.[32] The nasal mucosa is also elevated off the nasal cavity floor from medial to lateral, allowing medialization and complete closure of the nasal layer prior to oral mucosa closure.

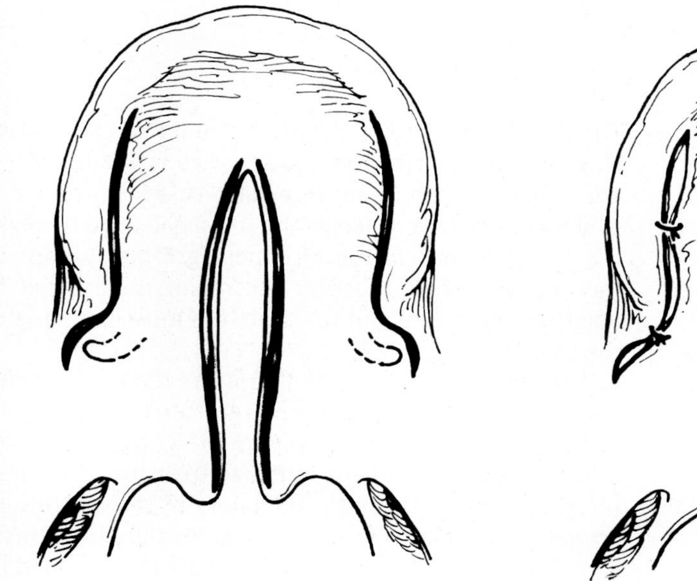

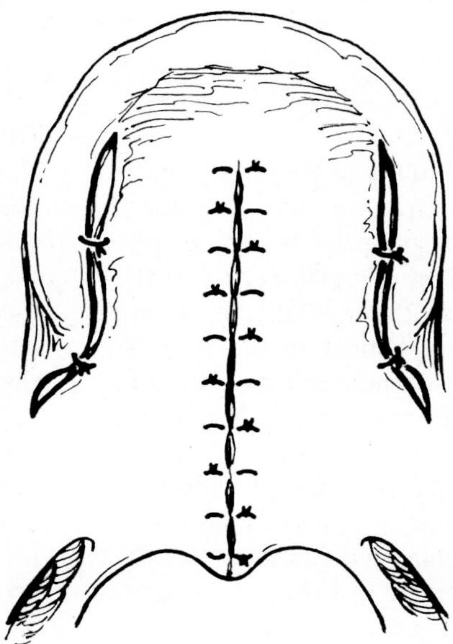

A B

Fig. 76.28 (**A**) Schematic diagram illustrating the incisions of the von Langenbeck cleft palate repair and (**B**) after closure.

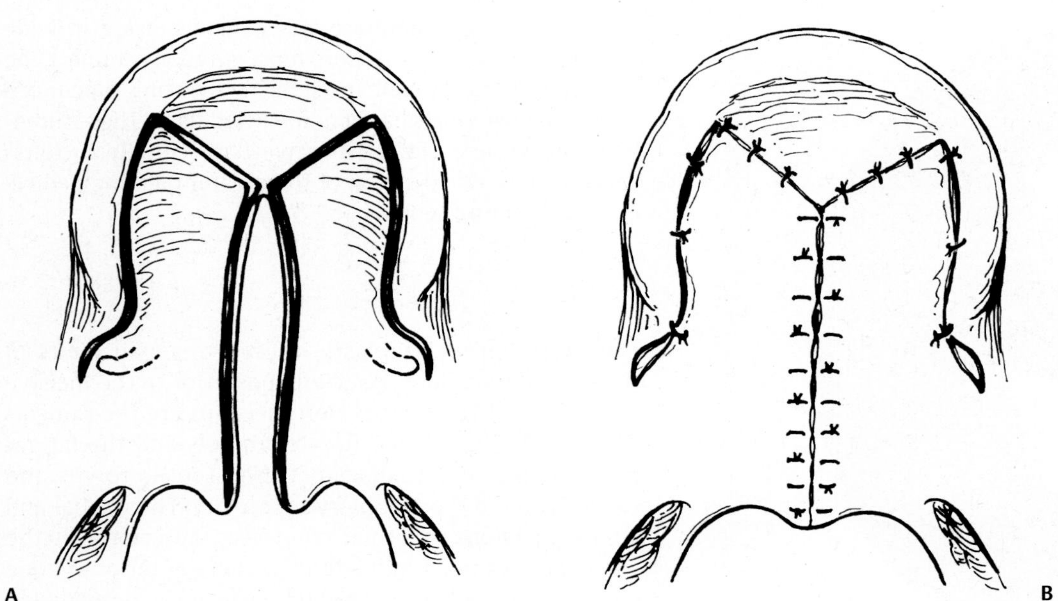

Fig. 76.29 (**A**) Schematic diagram of the incisions for the three-flap palatoplasty and (**B**) after closure.

Repair of the palate is thus performed in layers, beginning with reapproximation of the nasal layer, then closure of the muscle layer of the soft palate, and lastly closure of the oral mucosa overlying the hard palate. The strength of the repair is the closure of the muscle layer of the soft palate, which decreases overall tension on the midline repair. The oral layer is closed with alternating simple and vertical mattress sutures (**Fig. 76.29B**). At least one "tacking" suture is used to coapt the oral and nasal layers and prevent dead-space and hematoma formation.

Two-Flap Palatoplasty

The two-flap technique is used to repair complete palatal clefts (involving the entire primary and secondary palate). Modification of the two-flap technique may be used for both unilateral and bilateral palatal clefts. In the complete unilateral cleft palate, the medial cleft margin incisions are carried anteriorly almost to the alveolar cleft (**Fig. 76.30A**). These medial incisions are joined to the two curved lateral incisions, creating two posteriorly based palatal flaps.

Meticulous subperiosteal flap elevation with adherence to gentle tissue handling technique is performed to expose and isolate the neurovascular pedicles (**Fig. 76.30B**). Dissection posterior to the pedicle in the *space of Ernst* aids in further mobilization. The edges of the palatal flaps can be medialized with forceps to determine if adequate mobility has been achieved, helping to assure a tension-free closure.

After flap elevation, the palate is again repaired in layers, beginning with the nasal layer (**Fig. 76.30C**). The soft palate musculature is again closed with interrupted sutures, decreasing tension across the wound. Closure of the oral hard palatal mucosa is performed next, followed by a coapting suture (**Fig. 76.30D**). In complete cleft palate, the entire cleft with the exception of the alveolar cleft is thus accomplished.

Furlow's Palatoplasty

The double-reversing Z-plasty technique of cleft palate closure was described in 1978 by Leonard Furlow.[33,34] This elegant technique is usually used to repair a submucous cleft or a cleft of the soft palate, and involves the creation and closure of opposing Z-plasty flaps of the oral and nasal mucosa. The repair is designed to lengthen the palate and re-create the muscular sling of the soft palate.

The central limbs of the double-reversing Z-plasty technique are made at the margin of the soft palate cleft (**Fig. 76.31A**). If this technique is performed on a submucous cleft of the soft palate, a full-thickness incision is made through the palate in the midline to create a soft palate cleft. On one side, an oblique incision is made extending from the cleft margin toward the hamulus laterally. This leads to the creation of a

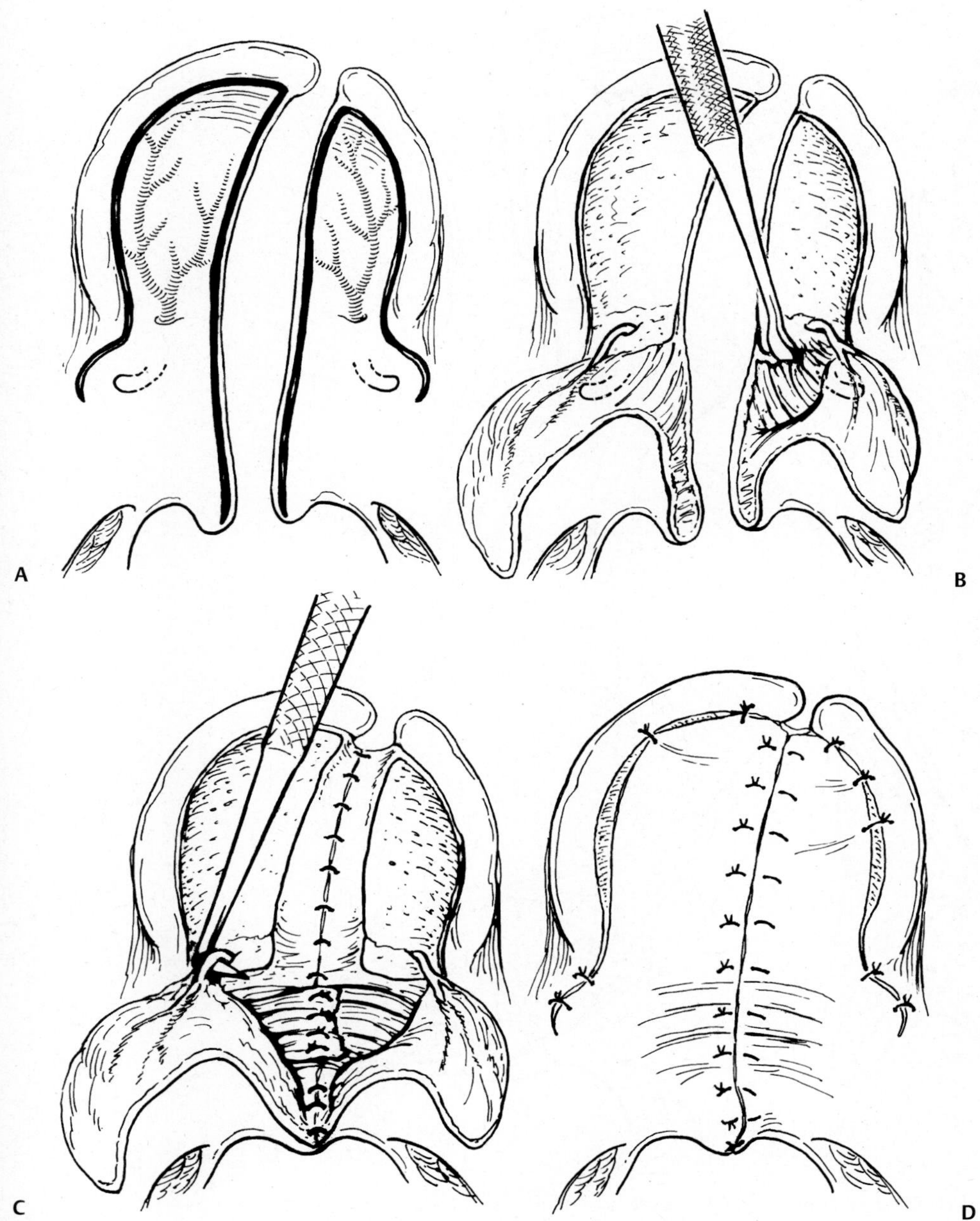

Fig. 76.30 (**A**) Schematic diagram of the incisions to create a two-flap palatoplasty for repair of the complete unilateral cleft palate. (**B**) Elevation of the flaps in a subperiosteal plane dissecting out the greater palatine vessels bilaterally. (**C**) Dissection posterior to the greater palatine vessels in the space of Ernst. (**D**) Repair of the oral mucosa and musculature after repair.

posteriorly based flap containing both oral mucosa and soft palate musculature (**Fig. 76.31B**). On the contralateral side, an oblique incision through oral mucosa only is made from the uvula toward the ipsilateral hamulus. The resultant flap contains no soft palate muscle.

On the nasal side, mirror-image incisions (relative to the oral mucosa incisions) are then made to create two triangular-shaped nasal flaps (**Fig. 76.31C,D**). The anatomy of the soft palate musculature is important in the dissection, elevation, and transposition of the oral and nasal flaps. Because the levator veli palatini muscles are

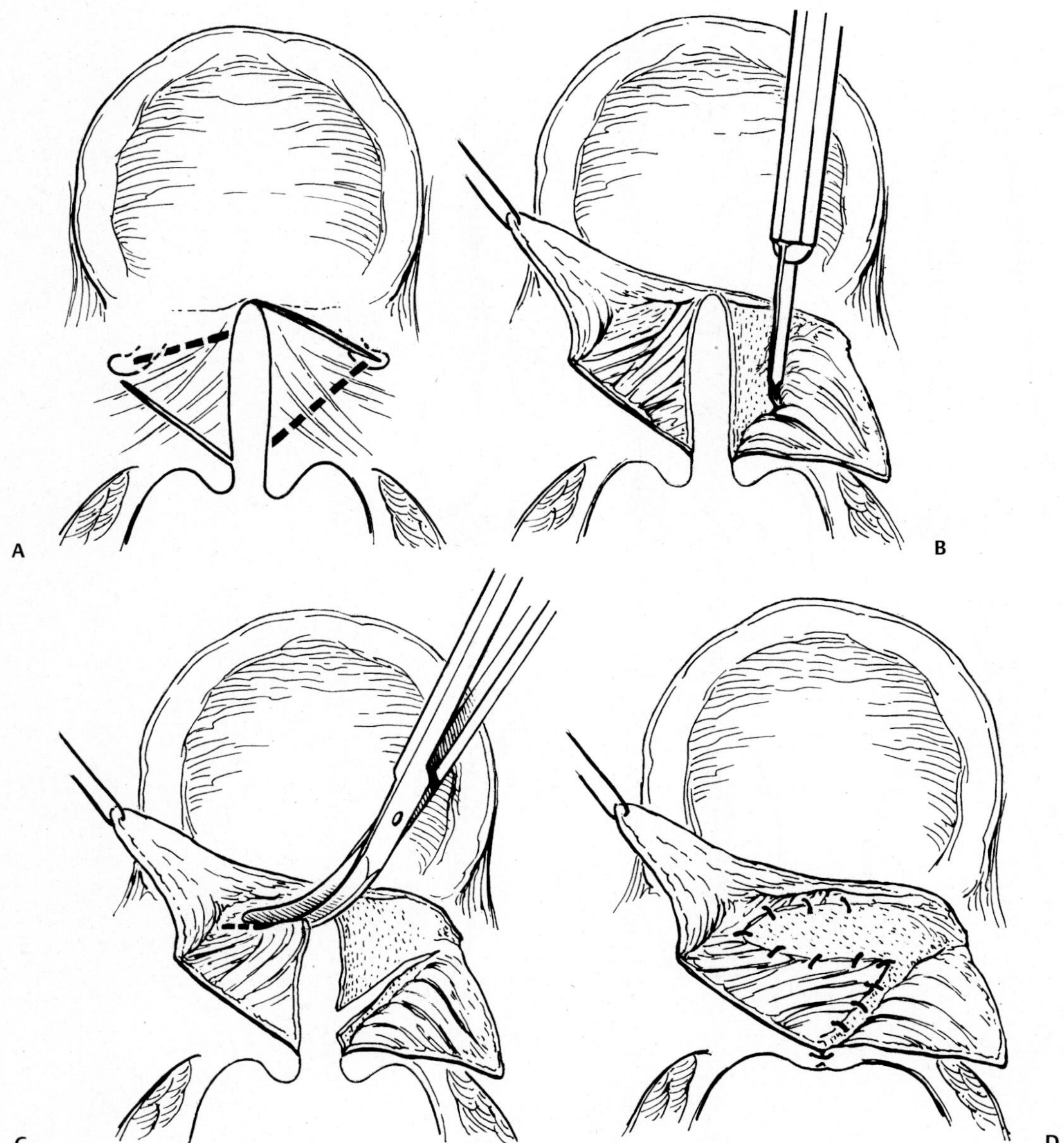

Fig. 76.31 (**A**) Schematic diagrams of the Furlow palatoplasty (double-reversing Z-plasty). Dotted lines indicate nasal mucosa incisions, and the solid lines indicate oral mucosa incisions. (**B**) Elevation of the oral flaps bilaterally. Note that the patient's left flap is elevated below the musculature (i.e., the oral flap contains both the oral mucosa and palatal musculature). The right flap contains only oral mucosa. (**C**) Incision of the flaps with curved scissors on the nasal side. (**D**) Closure of the nasal mucosa and palatal musculature.

located immediately adjacent to the nasal (not oral) mucosa, elevation of these muscles from the nasal mucosa is often difficult (**Fig. 76.32**). For this reason, right-handed surgeons may more easily perform the difficult dissection of the soft palate musculature from the nasal mucosa on the patient's left or contralateral side, whereas left-handed surgeons should design the incisions and flaps in the mirror image. After dissection of both oral and nasal flaps, transposition of all four flaps is accomplished. The nasal flaps are first transposed and reapproximated. The soft palate muscle sling is then reoriented and closed with 4–0 braided absorbable suture, prior to closure of the oral flaps (**Fig. 76.33**). An advantage of Furlow's technique is that the oral and nasal suture lines do not overlie one another, thereby reducing the incidence of postoperative fistulization.

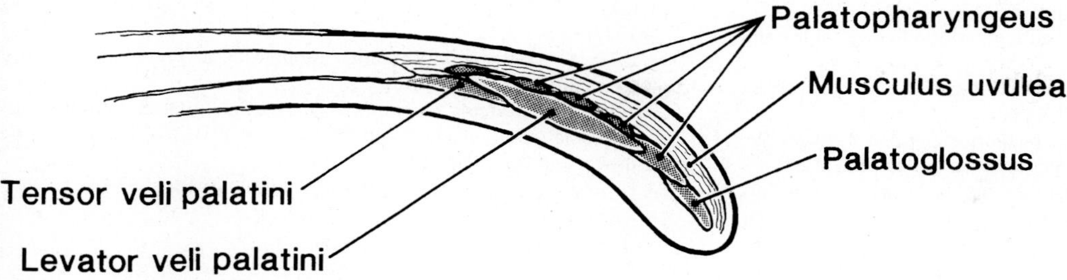

Fig. 76.32 Schematic sagittal view of the soft palate illustrating the position of the palatal musculature closer to the nasal mucosa than the oral mucosa.

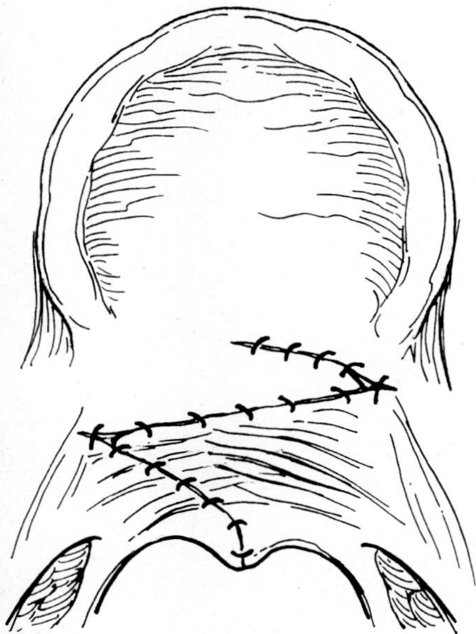

Fig. 76.33 Double-reversing Z-plasty (Furlow palatoplasty) after closure of the oral mucosa.

Summary

Congenital deformities of the lip and palate cause myriad difficulties for the affected individual, not limited to their inherent cosmetic and functional problems. Without doubt, proper repair of these anomalies also successfully treats their accompanying social and developmental sequelae. Thorough knowledge of the available techniques, attention to basic surgical principles, proper timing of surgical treatment, and experience with these operations will best assure most favorable outcomes and gratifying results.

References

1. Enlow DH. Facial Growth. 3rd ed. Philadelphia: WB Saunders; 1990:316–334
2. McCarthy JG. Plastic Surgery: Cleft Lip and Palate and Craniofacial Anomalies. Vol 4. Philadelphia: WB Saunders; 1990:2515–2552
3. Gaare JD, Langman J. Fusion of nasal swellings in the mouse embryo: surface coat and initial contact. Am J Anat 1977;150:461
4. Gorlin RJ, Pindborg J, Cohen MM. Syndromes of the Head and Neck. New York: McGraw-Hill; 1976
5. Sykes JM, Senders CW. Pathologic anatomy of cleft lip, palate, and nasal deformities. In: Meyers AD, ed. Biological Basis of Facial Plastic Surgery. New York: Thieme; 1993:57
6. Stark RB. Pathogenesis of harelip and cleft palate. Plast Reconstr Surg 1954;13:20
7. Sykes JM, Senders CW. Cleft palate. In: Practical Pediatric Otolaryngology. Philadelphia: Lippincott-Raven; 1999:809
8. Colletti V, Carner M, Miorelli V, Guida M, Colletti L, Fiorino FG. Cochlear implantation at under 12 months: report on 10 patients. Laryngoscope 2005;115:445
9. Waltzman SB, Roland JT Jr. Cochlear implantation in children younger than 12 months. Pediatrics 2005;116:4
10. Goldstein NA, Roland JT Jr, Sculerati N. Complications of tympanostomy tubes in an inner city clinic population. Int J Pediatr Otorhinolaryngol 1996;34:87–99
11. Millard DR Jr. Cleft Craft: The Evolution of Its Surgery, the Unilateral Deformity. Vol 1. Boston: Little, Brown; 1976:19–40
12. Barkitt AN, Lightoller GH. The facial musculature of the Australian aboriginal. J Anat 1927;62:33–57
13. Latham RA, Deaton TG. The structural basis of the philtrum and the contour of the vermilion border: a study of the musculature of the upper lip. J Anat 1976;121:151
14. Fara M, Chlumska A, Hrivnakova J. Musculus orbicularis oris in incomplete hare-lip. Acta Chir Plast 1965;7:125–132
15. Tennison CS. The repair of unilateral cleft lip by the stencil method. Plast Reconstr Surg 1952;9:115
16. Skoog T. A design for the repair of unilateral cleft lips. Am J Surg 1958;95:223–226
17. Randall P. A triangular flap operation for the primary repair of unilateral clefts of the lip. Plast Reconstr Surg 1959;31:95
18. LeMesurier AB. A method of cutting and suturing the lip in the treatment of complete unilateral clefts. Plast Reconstr Surg 1949;4:1
19. Millard DR Jr. A primary camouflage of the unilateral hare-look. Transactions of the First International Congress of Plastic Surgery, Stockholm, Sweden, 1957
20. Ness JA, Sykes JM. Basics of Millard rotation: advancement technique for repair of the unilateral cleft lip deformity. Facial Plast Surg 1993;9:167
21. Mullen TF. The developmental anatomy and surgical significance of the orbicularis oris. West J Med Surg 1932;20:134–141
22. Lee FC. Orbicularis oris muscle in double hare-lip. Arch Surg 1946;53:409
23. Seibert RW. Lip adhesion. Facial Plast Surg 1993;9:188
24. Millard DR. Adaptation of rotation-advancement principle in bilateral cleft lip. In: Wallace AB, ed. Transactions of the International Society of Plastic Surgeons, 2nd Congress, London, 1959. Edinburgh: Livingston; 1960:50–57
25. Schultz LW. Bilateral cleft lips. Plast Reconstr Surg 1946;1:338

26. Dieffenbach JF. Beitrage zur Gaumennath. Lit Ann Heilk 1928;10:322
27. Warren JC. On an operation for the cure of natural fissures of the soft palate. Am J Med Sci 1828;3:1
28. Warren JM. Operations for fissures of the soft and hard palate (palatoplastie). N Engl J Med 1843;1:538
29. von Langenbeck B. Operation der angebornen totalen Spaltung des harten Gaumens nach einer neuer Methode. Dtsch Klin 1861;3:321
30. Wardill WEM. Techniques of operation for cleft palate. Br J Surg 1937;25:117–130
31. Kilner TP. Cleft lip and palate repair technique. St. Thomas Hosp Rep 1937;2:127
32. Kriens O. Fundamental anatomic findings for an intravelar veloplasty. Cleft Palate J 1970;7:27–36
33. Furlow LT Jr. Double-reversing Z-Plasty for cleft palate. In: Millard DR Jr, ed. Cleft Craft, Alveolar, and Palatal Deformities. Vol 3. Boston: Little, Brown and Co., 1980:519.
34. Furlow LT Jr. Cleft palate repair by double-opposing Z-plasty. Plast Reconstr Surg 1986;78:724

77 Cleft Lip Rhinoplasty

John R. Coleman Jr. and Jonathan M. Sykes

Reconstruction of the cleft lip nasal deformity remains an ongoing challenge for the facial plastic surgeon. The deformity is a complex, three-dimensional alteration in nasal anatomy with defects in all tissue layers: skin, cartilage, vestibular lining, and bone. The extent of the deformity varies with the degree of lip abnormality; it may be unilateral or bilateral and subtle or complete.[1] The sheer number of publications and techniques reported in the twentieth century speaks to the difficulty of this reconstructive dilemma.[2]

This chapter provides the reader with an understanding of the pathophysiology of the cleft lip nasal deformity, discusses the timing of the various repairs needed, and highlights a selection of techniques currently used to repair the deformity.

Pathophysiology of the Cleft Lip Nasal Deformity

Etiology

The exact etiology of the cleft lip nasal deformity remains unknown. The two most common theories relate to intrinsic deficiencies and external pressures. Likely, the true answer is a combination of the two.

Veau proposed that the cleft lip nasal deformity is the result of agenesis of tissue within the lip and maxilla due to mesenchymal deficiency.[3] This leads to hypoplasia of the maxilla and lack of bone at the piriform margin and alar base and causes posterolateral displacement of the piriform margin and alar base. The abnormal position of the alar base is central to the overall formation of the defect. Other authors have contended that decreased growth or hypoplasia of the lower lateral cartilage contributes to the deformity.[4,5] These findings have been challenged by Park et al, who made direct measurements of the completely dissected lower lateral cartilages at the time of rhinoplasty in 35 patients (ages 6 to 40).[6] They found no difference between the cleft lower lateral cartilage and the noncleft cartilage when comparing thickness at the intercrural, middle and distal portion of the cartilage, width at the widest point, and overall length from the intercrural point to the distal end.

The extrinsic force theory holds that the abnormal insertions of ligaments and muscles lead to molding tension on the cartilage and soft tissue. Latham has postulated that the septopremaxillary ligament plays a critical role in the etiology of the unilateral cleft lip nasal defect.[7,8] This ligament binds the anterior septum to the premaxilla. Because the premaxilla is dissociated from the lateral maxilla by the cleft condition, these two growth centers are abnormally affected. The septopremaxillary ligament on the noncleft side provides unopposed tension on the caudal septum and columella causing deviation away from the cleft. Further, the disassociation of the growth centers leaves the lateral maxilla more posterior, which creates added tension on the lower lateral cartilage. Additional extrinsic force is applied by the discontinuity and abnormal insertion of the orbicularis oris muscle.[9,10] On the noncleft side in the unilateral cleft deformity, the muscle inserts into the columella and provides further distraction of the columella and anterior septum away from the cleft, and on the cleft side the orbicularis oris inserts into the alar base causing additional lateral pull on the alar base. Three-dimensional computed tomography scans of 12 3-month-old children with unilateral cleft lip confirmed four consistent and statistically significant findings related to the asymmetry of the nasal base.[11] All of the findings can be explained by the extrinsic force theory as already detailed: the columella is deviated to the noncleft side, the cleft alar base is more posterior than the noncleft, the noncleft alar base is further from the midline than the cleft, and the cleft piriform margin is more posterior than the noncleft. Finally, Fisher and Mann have been able to re-create the cleft lip nasal deformity in three dimensions with origami paper models.[12] Their models highlight the role that external tension places on the lower lateral cartilage and alar rim due to changes in the position of the piriform margin/alar base and columella in the development of the deformity.

These same theories can be applied to the bilateral cleft nasal deformity. The intrinsic deficiency theory allows for the absence of lip and maxilla to cause the posterolateral displacement of the alar base with the resulting widening of the nose but with little impact on columellar symmetry. On the other hand, the extrinsic force theory shows that the insertion of the septopremaxillary ligament is symmetric, thereby causing no alteration in the anterior septum/columella unit. The insertion of the orbicularis oris musculature into the alar base bilaterally contributes to the widening of the nose and flattening of the lower lateral cartilages.

Characteristics

Although the pathophysiology that causes the cleft lip nasal deformity has not been completely explained, the characteristics of the deformity have been well elucidated. The deformity begins with the deficiency of tissue in the nasal base related to the maxillary hypoplasia and continues with findings related to the external pressures applied after surgical repair and during development. The following discussion examines separately unilateral and bilateral defects and will subdivide the nose into thirds to illustrate the deformity and the repair of the deformity.

Unilateral

Lower One Third (Table 77.1)

The lower one third is the central portion of the cleft lip nasal deformity. Alterations from the noncleft nose are observed in the tip, the septum, and the external nasal valve. The nasal tip is the subunit composed of the alar bases, the columella, and the lower lateral cartilages. The position of both the columella and the alar base places distortional pressure on the lower lateral cartilage and influences the overall development of the deformity (**Fig. 77.1**). The columellar complex, which is created by the medial crura and feet of the lower lateral cartilage, the caudal septum, and the soft tissue, is typically deviated toward the noncleft side (**Fig. 77.2**). Although the total length of the lower lateral cartilage is the same on the cleft and noncleft sides, the medial crus on the cleft side is foreshortened, giving additional length to the lateral crus and creating a more obtuse angle to the dome. Further, the additional length leads to flattening of the dome and widening of the cleft nostril and nasal floor. The alar base is positioned posteriorly, inferiorly, and laterally when compared with the noncleft side. This changes the three-dimensional configuration of the entire tip.

Table 77.1 Characteristics of the Unilateral Cleft Lip Nose

Lower One Third
Nasal Tip
Deflects toward the noncleft side.
Columella deviates to the noncleft side.
Lateral steel of the lower lateral cartilage on the cleft side produces a long lateral crus and a short medial crus. This also causes blunting of the dome with a more obtuse angle.
Cleft side alar base is positioned posteriorly, laterally, and inferiorly.
Nasal floor and sill often absent on the cleft side.
Cleft nostril horizontally oriented and widened.
Septum
Caudal septum deflects toward the noncleft side.
Cartilaginous and bony septum deviates toward the cleft side.
External nasal value
Compromised by the introversion of the lower lateral cartilage and webbing of the nasal vestibule.
Middle One Third
Upper lateral cartilages
Weakened support leads to bowing or collapse with deep inspiration on the cleft side.
Abnormal relationship between the cleft upper and lower lateral cartilage.
Internal nasal valve
Frequently compromised by weakened support of the upper lateral cartilage and the deviation of the septum.
Upper One Third
Wide basal dorsum
Skeletal base
Bony deficiency on the cleft side

The nasal septum is deflected caudally into the noncleft nasal airway due to the unopposed pull of the orbicularis oris muscle and the septopremaxillary ligament (**Fig. 77.3**). Further posteriorly, the lack of these attachments to the middle and posterior cartilaginous septum leads to a bowing of the septum into the cleft side airway.[3] Moreover, Crockett and Bumsted found in a study of 140 cleft septums that the bony septum was deviated into the cleft airway in 80% of cases.[13] Therefore, in the unilateral cleft condition the nasal airway is compromised on both the cleft and the noncleft side.

The external nasal valve is created by the relationship of the columella, lower lateral cartilage, nasal ala, and nasal sill. In the unilateral cleft deformity the external nasal value is compromised by two related factors: introversion of the nasal ala and webbing of the nasal vestibule. Introversion of the cleft nasal ala is the result of posterior-inferior rotation of the lower lateral cartilage due to the distortional pressures on the cartilage from the position of the columella and alar base.[14] The introversion leads to hooding and thickening of the ala; it also contributes along with surgical scarring to webbing of the nasal vestibule. An oblique fold is formed by the posterolateral displacement of the piriform margin and the introversion of the lower lateral cartilage. This bulk influences airflow and alters the relationship of the upper and lower lateral cartilages.

Middle One Third

The middle one third of the nasal deformity can be characterized by interrelated changes to the upper lateral cartilages and to the internal nasal valve. On the cleft side there is limited attachment of the upper and lower cartilage and a side-to-side relationship rather than the more typical overlap seen on the noncleft side.[13] Both of these factors

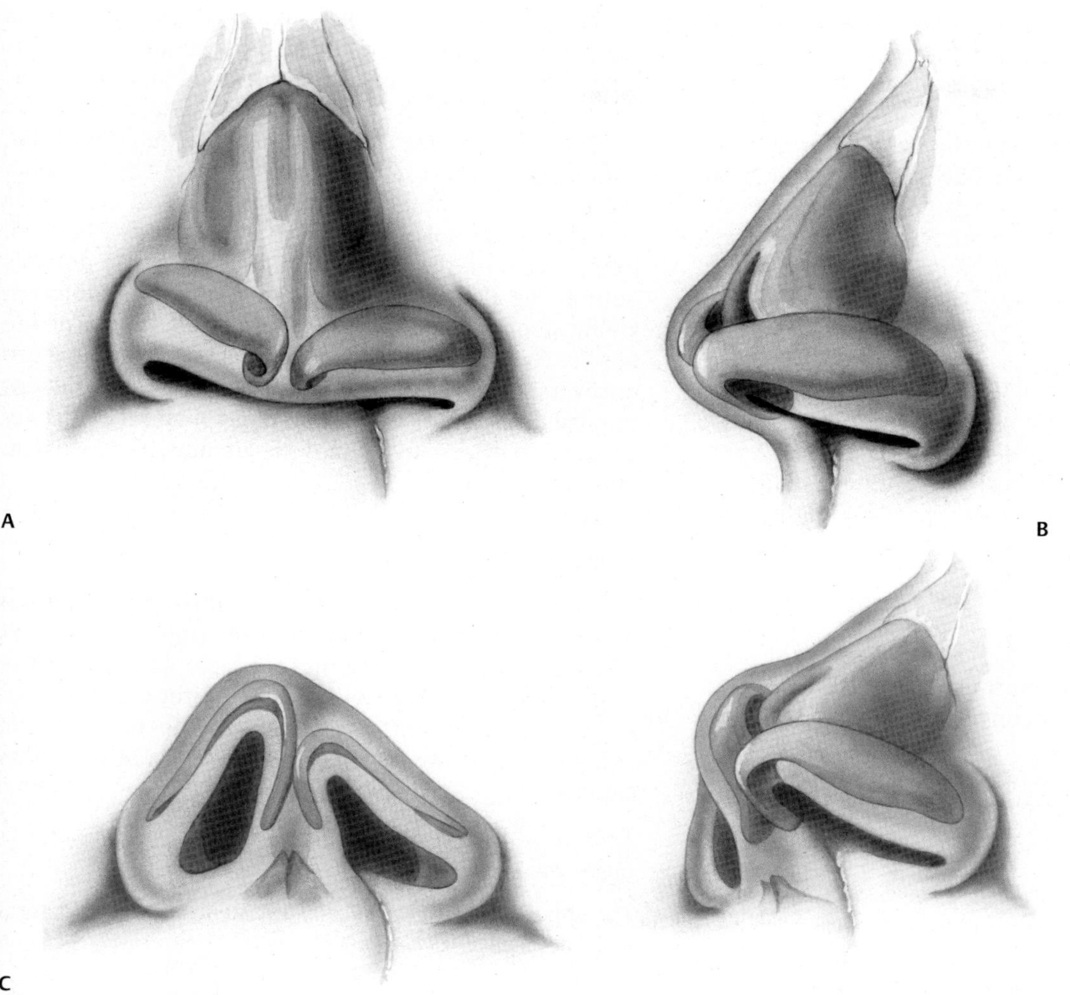

Fig. 77.1 Multiple views (anteroposterior, lateral, basal, and oblique) of the secondary unilateral cleft lip nasal deformity. Note the characteristic inferior, posterior, and lateral displacement of the alar base. (From Sykes JM, Senders CW, Wang TD, Cook TA. Use of the open approach for repair of secondary cleft lip nasal deformity. Facial Plast Surg North Am 1993;1:111–126. Reprinted by permission.)

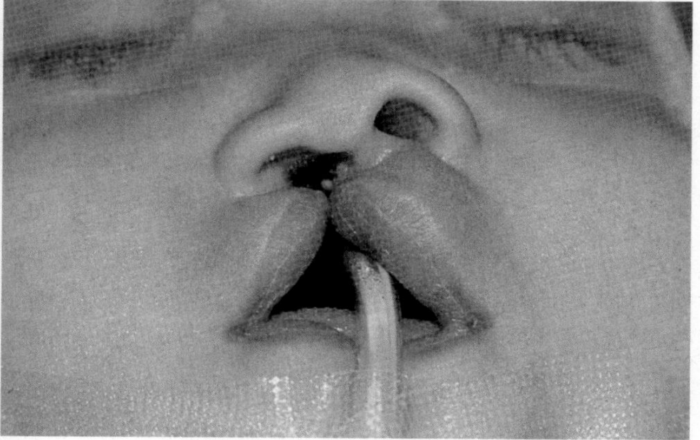

Fig. 77.2 Basal view of the primary unilateral cleft lip deformity demonstrating deviation of the columella toward the noncleft side, widening of the nasal floor, displacement of the alar base, and flattening of the lower lateral cartilage.

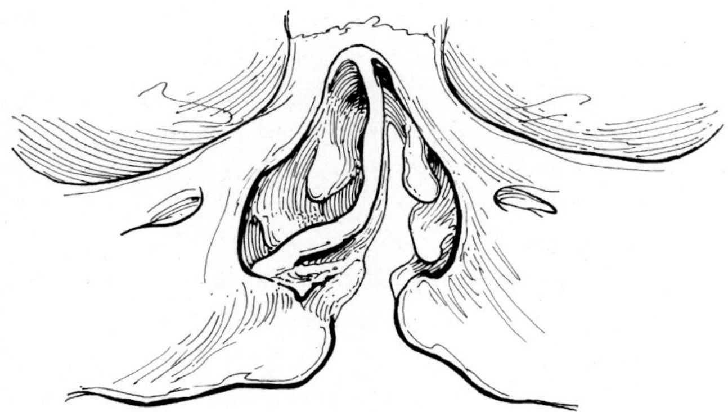

Fig. 77.3 Coronal section through the caudal septum showing deviation of the caudal septum to the noncleft side and more posterior bowing of the septum into the cleft side nasal airway. (From Jablon JH, Sykes JM. Nasal airway problems in the cleft lip population. Facial Plast Surg Clin North Am 1999;7:391–403. Reprinted by permission.)

lead to decreased support of the upper lateral cartilage and collapse of the upper lateral cartilage with deep inspiration. The internal nasal valve is formed by the relationship of the upper lateral cartilage, the nasal septum, and the inferior turbinate. In the cleft lip nasal deformity the septum is bowed into the cleft side at the internal nasal value, and the upper lateral cartilage support is weak, causing the cartilage to bow or collapse with respiration. Therefore, the internal nasal valve can significantly limit the nasal airway on the cleft side.

Upper One Third

Although there is no classic deformity to this portion of the nose in the cleft lip nasal deformity, the osseous pyramid is typically reduced in width at the time of definitive rhinoplasty to enhance the overall appearance of the nose.

Bilateral

Lower One Third (Table 77.2)

Similar to the unilateral deformity, the primary characteristics of the bilateral deformity revolve around the lower one third of the nose (**Fig. 77.4**). The nasal tip is typically in the midline in the bilateral complete deformity. If one side of the lip is more involved than the other, the short columella is typically deviated toward the less involved side, pulling the tip in that direction (**Fig. 77.5**). The lower lateral cartilages demonstrate short medial crura and long lateral crura. The domes of the lower lateral crura are splayed, contributing to a poorly defined, frequently bifid tip (**Fig. 77.6**). The angle at the dome is obtuse. The alar bases are posterior, lateral, and inferior, giving rise to flaring of the base and widening of the nostril. The tension on the lower lateral cartilage leads to introversion and webbing of the vestibular floor. The septum is in the midline in the complete bilateral deformity and deviated caudally toward the less involved side if an asymmetry exists.

Table 77.2 Characteristics of the Bilateral Cleft Nasal Deformity

Lower One Third
Nasal tip
Deviates toward less involved side if discrepancy exists.
Columella is short and deviates toward less involved side if discrepancy exists.
Lateral steel of lower lateral cartilage on the cleft side produces a long lateral crus and a short medial crus. This also causes blunting of the dome with a more obtuse angle.
Medial crura are splayed producing a poorly defined, bifid tip
Alar bases are displaced posteriorly, laterally, and inferiorly.
Nostrils are wide and horizontally oriented.
Septum
Deviated to less involved side if a discrepancy exists.
External nasal valve
Compromised by the introversion of the lower lateral cartilage and webbing of the nasal vestibule.
Middle One Third
Upper lateral cartilage
Weakened support leads to bowing or collapse with deep inspiration.
Abnormal relationship with the lower lateral cartilage.
Internal nasal valve
Compromised by weakened support of the upper lateral cartilage.
Upper One Third
Wide nasal dorsum.
Skeletal base
Bony deficiency on both sides.

Middle One Third

The middle one third is analogous to the unilateral deformity, with poor support to the upper lateral cartilage leading to bowing and possible collapse of the upper lateral cartilage with deep inspiration. However, because the septum is typically in the midline, the compromise of the internal nasal valve is often not as significant.

Upper One Third

The upper one third is typically not involved in the bilateral nasal deformity.

Timing of Repair of Cleft Lip Nasal Deformity (Table 77.3)

In Utero Repair

The potential advantages of in utero repair of the cleft lip nasal deformity are analogous to those described for lip and palate repair and include scarless healing, use of postrepair fetal growth to create symmetric results, elimination of social stigmata, and reduction in the number of surgeries required to obtain the desired results.[15–19] To date, experimentation has been limited to animal models, and recently, a paper has focused on the alteration of nasal anatomy with in utero surgery.[20] The authors placed a hypertonic sponge in the nostril of a fetal lamb, allowing it to function as a tissue expander. They measured increases in septal length, nostril area, and intranasal volume with no evidence of histological scarring at varying time intervals. They believe that they are able not only to induce scarless in utero change but actually to control that change. Their long-term proposal is to

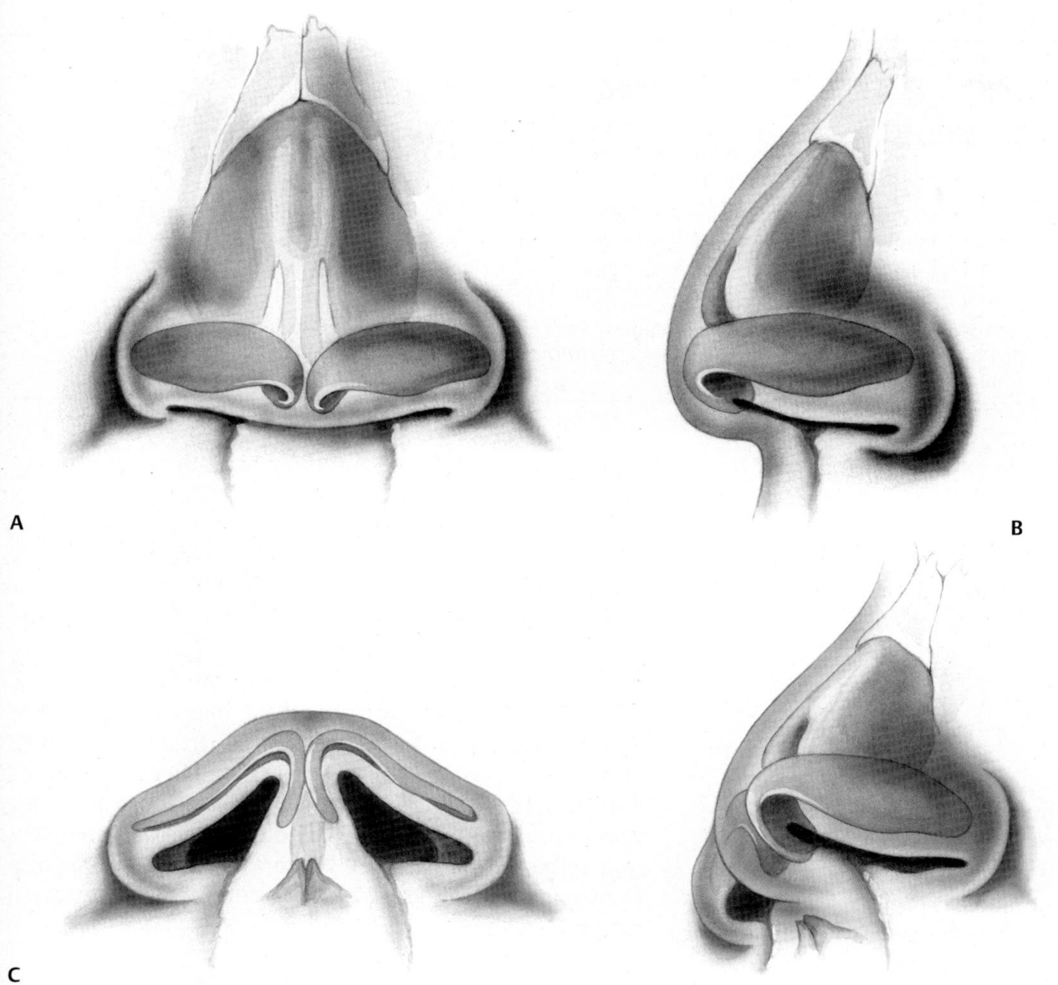

Fig. 77.4 Multiple views (anteroposterior, lateral, basal, and oblique) of the secondary bilateral cleft lip nasal deformity. Note the short columella and relative symmetric base. (From Sykes JM, Senders CW, Wang TD, Cook TA. Use of the open approach for repair of secondary cleft lip nasal deformity. Facial Plast Surg Clin North Am 1993;1:111–126. Reprinted by permission.)

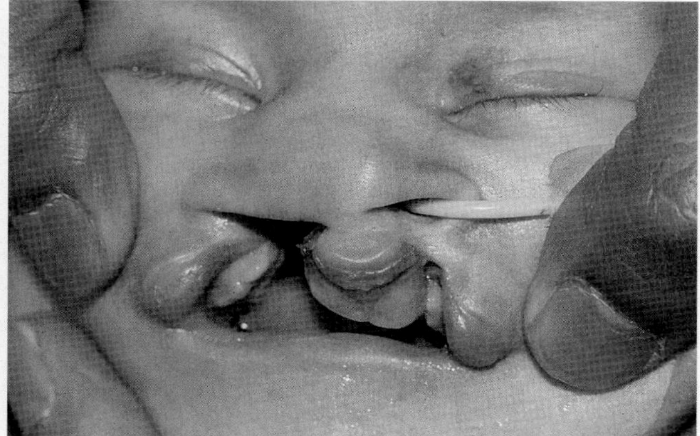

Fig. 77.5 Basal view of the asymmetric bilateral cleft deformity demonstrating deviation of the columella toward the less complete side of the cleft deformity.

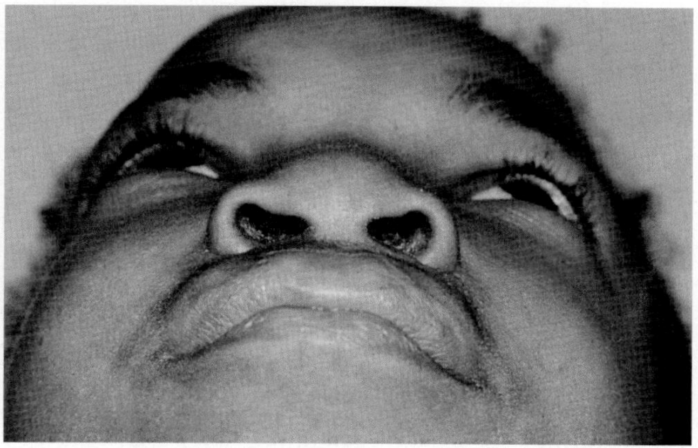

Fig. 77.6 Basal view of a secondary bilateral cleft lip nasal deformity demonstrating the wide, bifid tip and short columella.

Table 77.3 Timing and Goals of Cleft Lip Rhinoplasty

Type of Rhinoplasty	Timing of the Procedure	Goals of the Procedure
Primary	At the time of lip repair. Typically between 3 and 6 months of age.	Close the nasal floor, actively reposition the alar base, and reorient the lower lateral cartilage while minimizing scarring, which will affect future procedures. Some surgeons will also attempt to realign the septum and/or increase columella length.
Intermediate	From the time of lip repair until the definitive rhinoplasty is performed. Typically 1 year to 14 years of age.	Stabilize and support the nasal base, lengthen the columella, reposition the septum if obstruction is severe, and continue to improve the nasal tip symmetry. Procedures are typically smaller and designed to provide enhancements that can be used in definitive rhinoplasty.
Definitive	After the completion of nasal and midface growth. Typically age 14 in women and 16 in men.	Restore symmetry and definition to nasal tip and base; realign and open the nasal airway and prevent scarring and webbing from adversely affecting the results.

use specifically designed tissue expanders to impact the characteristic, anatomical abnormalities found in the cleft nasal deformity. As techniques improve with in utero surgery, repositioning of the alar base followed by controlled nasal expansion may become the principle treatment of this deformity.

Repair after Birth

Presurgical Orthopedics

There has been a growing trend toward the use of presurgical orthopedics to mold the palatal shelves into a more favorable position prior to lip repair. This has been accomplished with such simple methods as taping and parental finger pressure to more complex interactions such as lip adhesion, the Latham appliance, and nasoalveolar molding as proposed by Grayson et al.[21] The purpose of including the nose in the presurgical plan is to allow for molding of the deformed lower lateral cartilage and lengthening of the deficient columella.[22] This adjunct reduces the nasal deformity and allows for greater symmetry to be obtained with primary rhinoplasty.

Primary Rhinoplasty

One of the greatest movements in achieving consistent and improved results for cleft lip rhinoplasty was the acceptance and use of primary rhinoplasty in most cleft centers. Many authors now consider primary rhinoplasty to be the standard of care in cleft repair.[23,24] Early reluctance to accept primary rhinoplasty revolved around concerns related to future growth of the nose and midface. Experimental work by Sarnat and Wexler as well as Bernstein had demonstrated growth retardation of the nose and midface following aggressive resection of the nasal septum and mucoperichondrium.[25,26] McComb and Coghlan, however, have demonstrated with an 18-year longitudinal study that nasal and midface growth was not significantly different in children who underwent primary cleft rhinoplasty versus age-matched normal and age-matched cleft controls who did not have primary rhinoplasty.[27] Moreover, the symmetry obtained with primary rhinoplasty was maintained into adult life.

Primary rhinoplasty is then defined as alteration in the nose at the time of lip repair. The goal of the surgery is to close the anterior nasal floor; to relocate the posteriorly, inferiorly, and laterally displaced alar base; and to achieve early symmetry to the nasal base and tip. The advantage of a staged, nasal repair relates to smaller movements with each procedure and added opportunities to achieve a symmetric result.[28] The key is judicious use of maneuvers that reduce the deformity while avoiding incisions and excisions that might lead to scar contracture or growth retardation.[29]

Intermediate Rhinoplasty

Intermediate rhinoplasty refers to procedures that are performed from the time of the completion of the lip repair up to the time of the definitive rhinoplasty. These procedures are often grouped with the definitive repair and referred to as secondary rhinoplasty. Typically, the intermediate procedures are less involved and seek to correct inadequacies that will allow symmetric nasal growth and a more successful definitive procedure. More extensive procedures can be performed if the severity of the deformity warrants more aggressive intervention to prevent further mental or physical disability.

Definitive Rhinoplasty

Definitive rhinoplasty occurs after the completion of nasal growth around age 14 in women and 16 in men. At this point in time, complete and aggressive restructuring of the internal and external nasal anatomy can be performed. The goals of the surgery are the creation of symmetry and definition of the nasal base and tip, relief of nasal obstruction, and management of nasal scarring and webbing. The difficulty of the repair lies in the complex interaction of the original three-dimensional pathophysiology and the previous surgeries.

Surgical Techniques for Repair of Cleft Lip Nasal Deformity

Nasal Base

The first step in the repair of the nasal deformity, whether unilateral or bilateral, is the establishment of a solid nasal base upon which to build the remainder of the reconstruction. This begins with primary rhinoplasty and closure of the nasal floor. The next step is to correct the bone deficiency of the maxilla and premaxilla and restore the abnormal posterior-anterior position of the alar base.[3] Although the timing of alveolar bone grafting is controversial, it is most commonly performed between the ages of 7 and 11, when one fourth to three fourths of the adult canine root is formed, and should be considered an intermediate rhinoplasty procedure.[30] Further, augmentation of the nasal sill and base may be required at the time of the definitive rhinoplasty and can usually be accomplished with local tissue flaps.[31]

Unilateral Cleft Lip Nasal Deformity

Primary Rhinoplasty

The primary rhinoplasty is performed through the same incision used with the Millard advancement-rotation lip repair. The lateral dissection requires a complete alotomy with release of all of the attachments to the piriform aperature.[32] A lateral tunnel is then created with scissors dissection over the lateral crus up to the nasal dome (**Fig. 77.7**). A medial tunnel is also created from the original lip incisions with dissection superficial to the medial crus of the lower lateral cartilage. The subcutaneous tunnels free the lower lateral cartilage from the nasal skin–soft tissue envelope completely; the vestibular mucosal attachments are left undissected.[33] The floor of the nose is closed with the lip repair. If columella lengthening is needed on the cleft side, a back-cut onto the columella and rotation of the c-flap into this area can be used.[28] The closure of the floor begins the placement of the alar base; to place it exactly in a symmetric position with the contralateral ala, excision of skin inferiorly and laterally to the alar base is often required.[14] After the lip is closed and the alar base is positioned, the lower lateral cartilage is molded to its new configuration. This can be accomplished with interdomal sutures[28,34] or the application of nasal bolster(s) (**Fig. 77.8**).[14,35] The purpose of the interdomal suture or bolster is to re-create the dome of the lower lateral cartilage in a more lateral location. This is accomplished by stealing cartilage from lateral

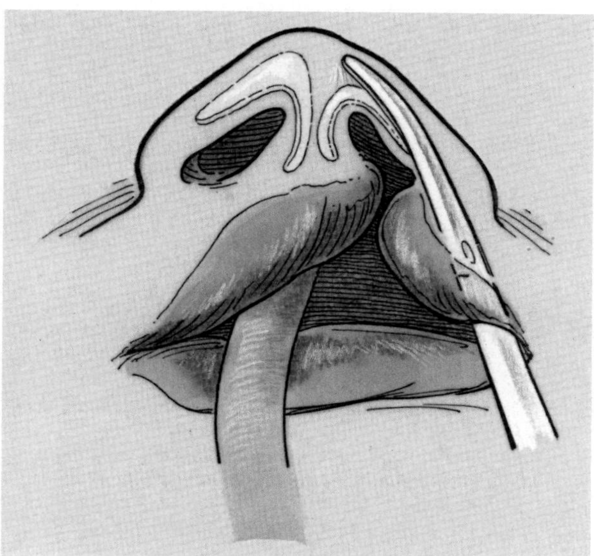

Fig. 77.7 Basal schematic demonstrating the lateral dissection to release the attachments of the lower lateral cartilage. (From Sykes JM, Senders CW. Surgery of the cleft lip nasal deformity. Oper Tech Otolaryngol Head Neck Surg 1990;1:219–224.)

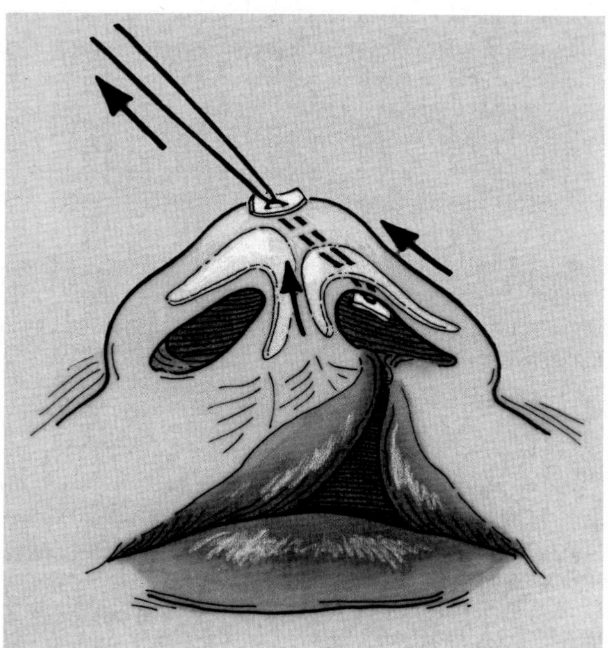

Fig. 77.8 Basal schematic demonstrating the application of bolsters to reposition the cleft lower lateral cartilage. The vectors of force of the repositioning are displayed. (From Sykes JM, Senders CW. Surgery of the cleft lip nasal deformity. Oper Tech Otolaryngol Head Neck Surg 1990;1:219–224.)

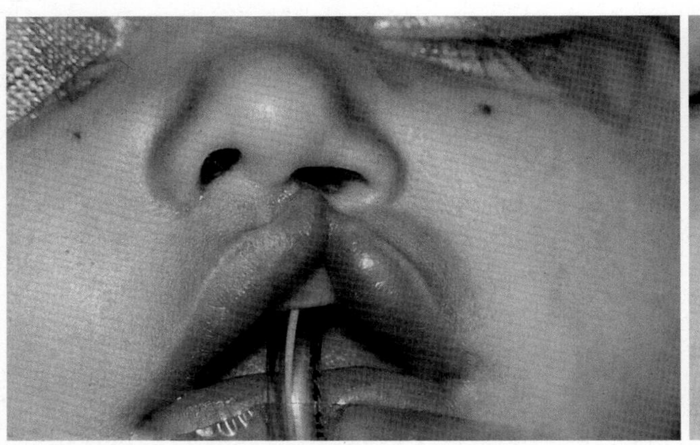

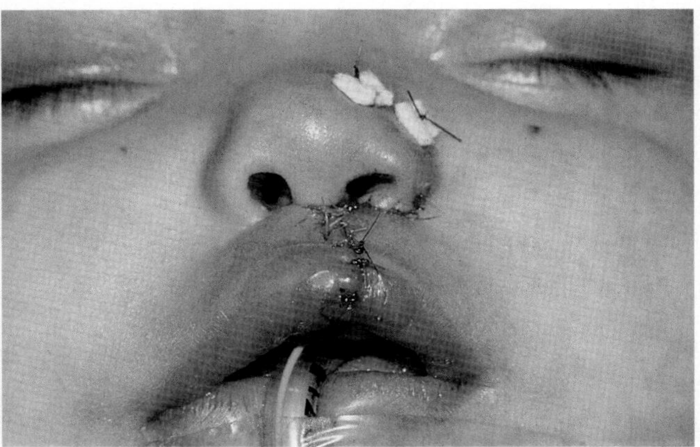

Fig. 77.9 Intraoperative photographs of primary cleft lip rhinoplasty at the time of lip repair. (**A**) Preoperative deformity. (**B**) Completed surgery. Note that the suture securing the bolsters is tightened until a slight blanch is seen.

to medial to increase tip projection and enhance tip symmetry. The complete release of the nasal skin from the lower lateral cartilage prevents tethering of the tissue and an incomplete reorientation. If the bolster technique is used, the suture is placed through the cartilage into the subcutaneous tunnel to come out of the nasal skin on the noncleft side of the midline and tied with the necessary tension to cause a slight blanching of the external nasal skin (**Fig. 77.9**). The bolster(s) can be removed at 1 week postoperatively. A novel, nonbolster technique has been proposed by Demirseren and colleagues using a 23-gauge needle as a suture passer.[36] Advantages to this technique are the length of hold before the suture dissolves and the lack of need to remove a bolster if follow-up is not consistent or ideal.

In those cases where significant caudal septal irregularity exists, the septum can be repositioned onto the nasal spine at the time of primary rhinoplasty.[34] This has the added positive effect of increasing the tip projection and enhancing the symmetry of the base. No significant removal of the septum and mucoperichondrium should be performed at this stage.

Intermediate Rhinoplasty

The use of intermediate rhinoplasty has decreased as surgeons have become more adept at primary rhinoplasty. Typically, in the unilateral cleft lip nasal deformity intermediate rhinoplasty serves to decrease the deformity and enhance the result of definitive rhinoplasty. Aggressive surgery is rarely performed at this time due to the potential negative aspects associated with scarring and growth retardation.

Three situations exist that warrant intermediate procedures in the unilateral deformity.[35] The first is severe nasal obstruction caused by caudal septal deviation. To correct this problem, the septum should be repositioned over the nasal spine with very limited resection of tissue. The second case is the child with a deformity not addressed at the time of primary rhinoplasty. Limited tip rhinoplasty and alar repositioning as described for the primary rhinoplasty can be performed to enhance nasal symmetry. The final indication is the child who is suffering severe emotional distress from ridicule related to the nasal deformity. In this patient a more complex and complete procedure may be warranted. If grafting material is needed for this stage of the repair, strong consideration should be given to banked, irradiated cartilage in an attempt to limit the long-term effect on nasal growth.

Definitive Rhinoplasty

Definitive cleft lip rhinoplasty is performed after the nose and midface have reached full growth. Both the original nasal deformity and the previous attempts at correction contribute to the secondary deformity and to the difficulties encountered with the procedure.

The rhinoplasty approach varies with the needs of the reconstruction. We use an open or external approach with or without an alotomy on the cleft side. The incision for the open approach has numerous configurations that reflect the specific needs of the reconstruction. The traditional inverted V incision can be modified to increase columella soft tissue with a V-Y closure,[37] or the incision can be made asymmetrically onto the nasal skin on the cleft side to recruit this skin inward to augment a superomedial alar web (**Fig. 77.10**).[38] Finally, techniques have been described related to the recruitment of tissue from the lip repair with a sliding chondrocutaneous flap.[2,39,40] This flap provides additional tissue to be used to augment the vestibular lining and reduce the alar–columellar web, and when it is combined with the open rhinoplasty,

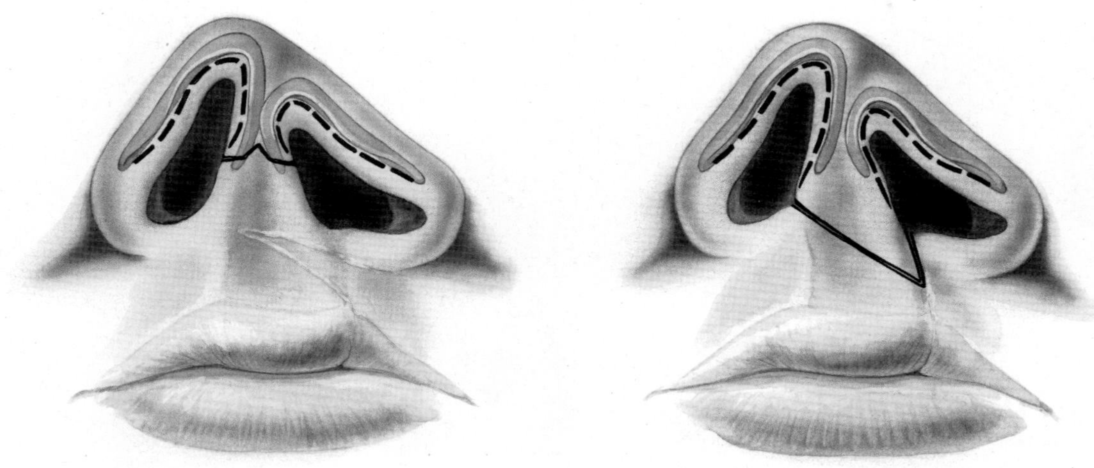

Fig. 77.10 (**A**) Basal view of the secondary cleft lip deformity demonstrating the modification of the standard external rhinoplasty incision. (**B**) Basal view demonstrating a modified Bardach incision. Closure of the incision in a V-Y fashion will recruit additional skin and soft tissue from the lip into the columella. (From Sykes JM, Senders CW, Wang TD, Cook TA. Use of the open approach for repair of secondary cleft lip nasal deformity. Facial Plast Surg Clin North Am 1993;1:111–126. Reprinted by permission.)

the chondrocutaneous flap can allow for tip stability and refinement.

The lower one third of the nose is addressed in open structure rhinoplasty by the complete evaluation of the lower lateral cartilage and the use of grafts to improve stability, enhance definition, and prevent wound contracture.[41] The first maneuver in the correction of the lower one third of the nose is septoplasty to relieve nasal obstruction and obtain grafting material. The septum can be accessed through a separate hemitransfixation incision or directly through the open approach. Adequate caudal and dorsal struts should be preserved while correcting the deviations in the cartilage and bone. To return the caudal septum to the midline, the surgeon must often remove a strip of cartilage inferiorly, allowing the septum to "swing" over the nasal spine (**Fig. 77.11**). This position can be maintained by suturing the cartilage to the spine.

The next step is to address the symmetry of the lower cartilages and to perform cephalic strip removal as necessary to correct asymmetries and reduce excessively large cartilages. A cartilaginous, columellar strut graft should then be placed between the medial crura of the lower

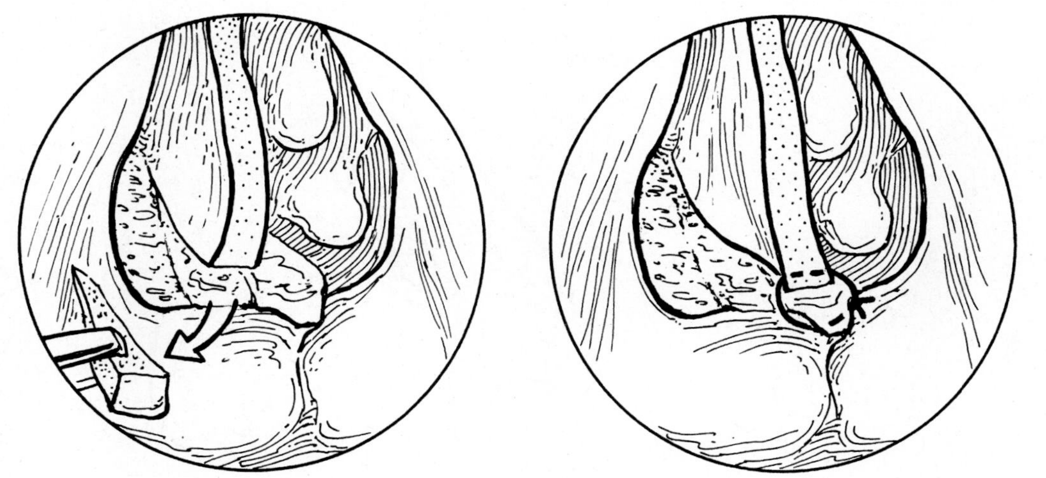

Fig. 77.11 Coronal drawings demonstrating (**A**) the release of the septum to allow it to "swing" over the maxillary crest and (**B**) suture fixation of the septum to the maxillary crest. (From Jablon JH, Sykes JM. Nasal airway problems in the cleft lip population. Facial Plast Surg Clin North Am 1999;7:391–403. Reprinted by permission.)

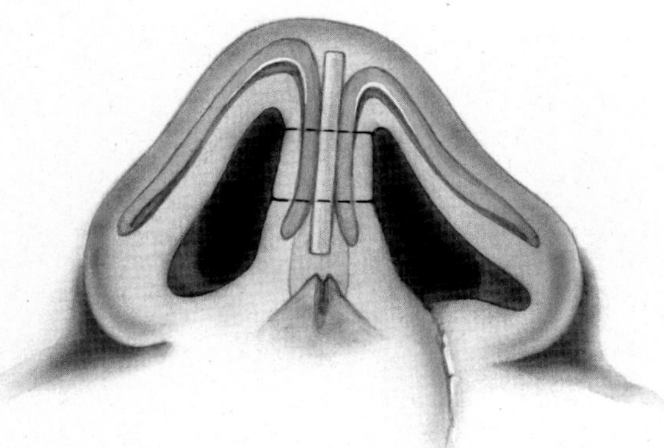

Fig. 77.12 Basal view depicting the placement of the cartilaginous columellar strut and asymmetric advancement of the lower lateral cartilages onto the strut. (From Sykes JM, Senders CW, Wang TD, Cook TA. Use of the open approach for repair of secondary cleft lip nasal deformity. Facial Plast Surg Clin North Am 1993;1:111–126. Reprinted by permission.)

cartilages. The lower laterals are sutured to the strut; advancement of the lower laterals onto the strut will enhance nasal projection (**Fig. 77.12**). Typically, the cleft side will need to be advanced more than the noncleft side to improve the flattening of the cleft lower lateral cartilage and enhance overall tip symmetry. The lower lateral cartilages are then divided and reconstituted. Division of the cartilages lateral to the dome increases the medial crural element and increases projection (**Fig. 77.13**). Once again, by vertically dividing the cartilages at different points and removing different amounts of cartilage, enhanced symmetry can be obtained. If there is still significant introversion of the cleft lower lateral cartilage after these maneuvers, the lower lateral can be sutured to the upper lateral cartilage to reposition the alar rim more superiorly (**Fig. 77.14**). Finally, a cartilaginous tip graft can be added to camouflage irregularities and improve tip definition.

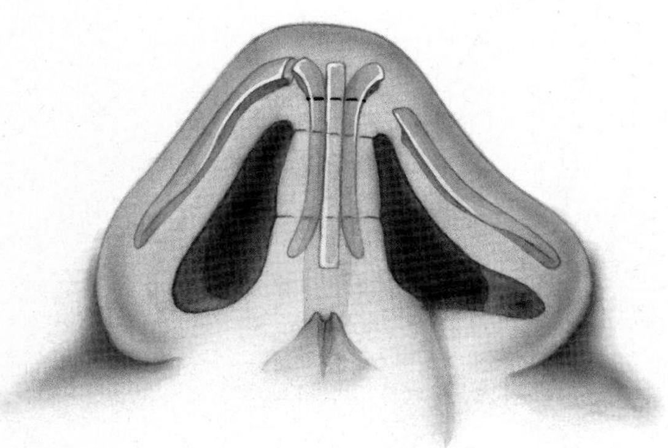

Fig. 77.13 Basal view demonstrating the asymmetric division of the lower lateral cartilages to increase projection and symmetry. (From Sykes JM, Senders CW, Wang TD, Cook TA. Use of the open approach for repair of secondary cleft lip nasal deformity. Facial Plast Surg Clin North Am 1993;1:111–126. Reprinted by permission.)

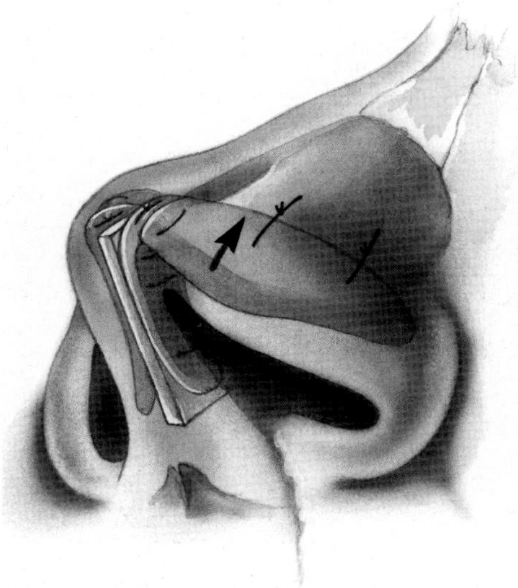

Fig. 77.14 Oblique view demonstrating suture fixation of the lower lateral cartilage to the upper lateral cartilage to alleviate vestibular hooding. The arrow demonstrates the vector of force applied by the suture fixation. (From Sykes JM, Senders CW, Wang TD, Cook TA. Use of the open approach for repair of secondary cleft lip nasal deformity. Facial Plast Surg Clin North Am 1993;1:111–126. Reprinted by permission.)

The obstruction at the external nasal valve caused by the introversion of the lower lateral cartilage and alar webbing is frequently improved by the approach chosen, the increased projection obtained with the strut and dome division, and the repositioning of the alar base.

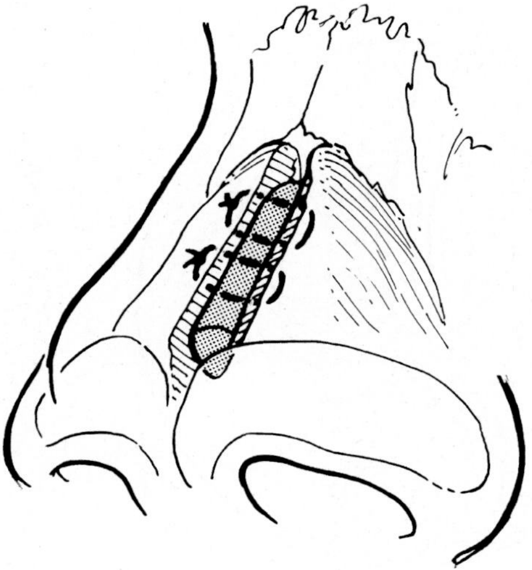

Fig. 77.15 Oblique view depicting the use of the unilateral spreader graft to improve the dynamics of the internal nasal valve. (From Jablon JH, Sykes JM. Nasal airway problems in the cleft lip population. Facial Plast Surg Clin North Am 1999;7:391–403. Reprinted by permission.)

Additional strategies that can be used include Z-plasty over the web, excision of redundant tissue with primary closure, and placement of bolsters to retract the tissue and promote lateral scarring of the tissue similar to the bolsters used in primary cleft lip rhinoplasty.

The middle one third of the nose is addressed with the stabilization of the upper lateral cartilage frequently by suturing the upper lateral to the lower lateral. Moreover, if compromise of the internal nasal valve exists, the use of a unilateral, cartilaginous, spreader graft between the septum and the upper lateral cartilage can improve the cross-sectional airway and stability of the upper lateral cartilage (**Fig. 77.15**).

The upper one third of the nose is treated in a standard fashion with hump reduction as needed and medial-lateral osteotomies to reduce width and straighten the osseous pyramid (**Fig. 77.16**).

Bilateral Cleft Lip Nasal Deformity

Primary Rhinoplasty

The role of primary rhinoplasty in the bilateral cleft nasal deformity is debated. The repair of the bilateral cleft nasal deformity has been frequently described. The evolution of the techniques described has ranged from staged repairs to simultaneous reconstruction with the labial repair. We favor alar repositioning only at the time of lip repair unless severe asymmetries of the nasal tip exist. Other authors prefer a more aggressive tip rhinoplasty at the time of lip repair.[42,43]

The Mulliken[42] and Trott[43] repairs of the bilateral cleft nasal deformity seek to repair the deformity at the time of the lip repair. Both authors feel that the length of the columella is within the nasal tissue and do not attempt to recruit additional columella length from the prolabium.[44] The columella length is determined by active positioning of the alar cartilages, interdomal approximation, and excision of excessive tissue in the superior-medial alar web. Their approaches vary, with Mulliken advocating a vertical, midline intradomal incision, and Trott preferring a more standard open incision approach. Long-term results have been good with both repairs, but definitive rhinoplasty is frequently required.

Intermediate Rhinoplasty

Intermediate rhinoplasty is more frequently used in the bilateral nasal deformity than in the unilateral deformity. The major goal of the intermediate rhinoplasty is columella

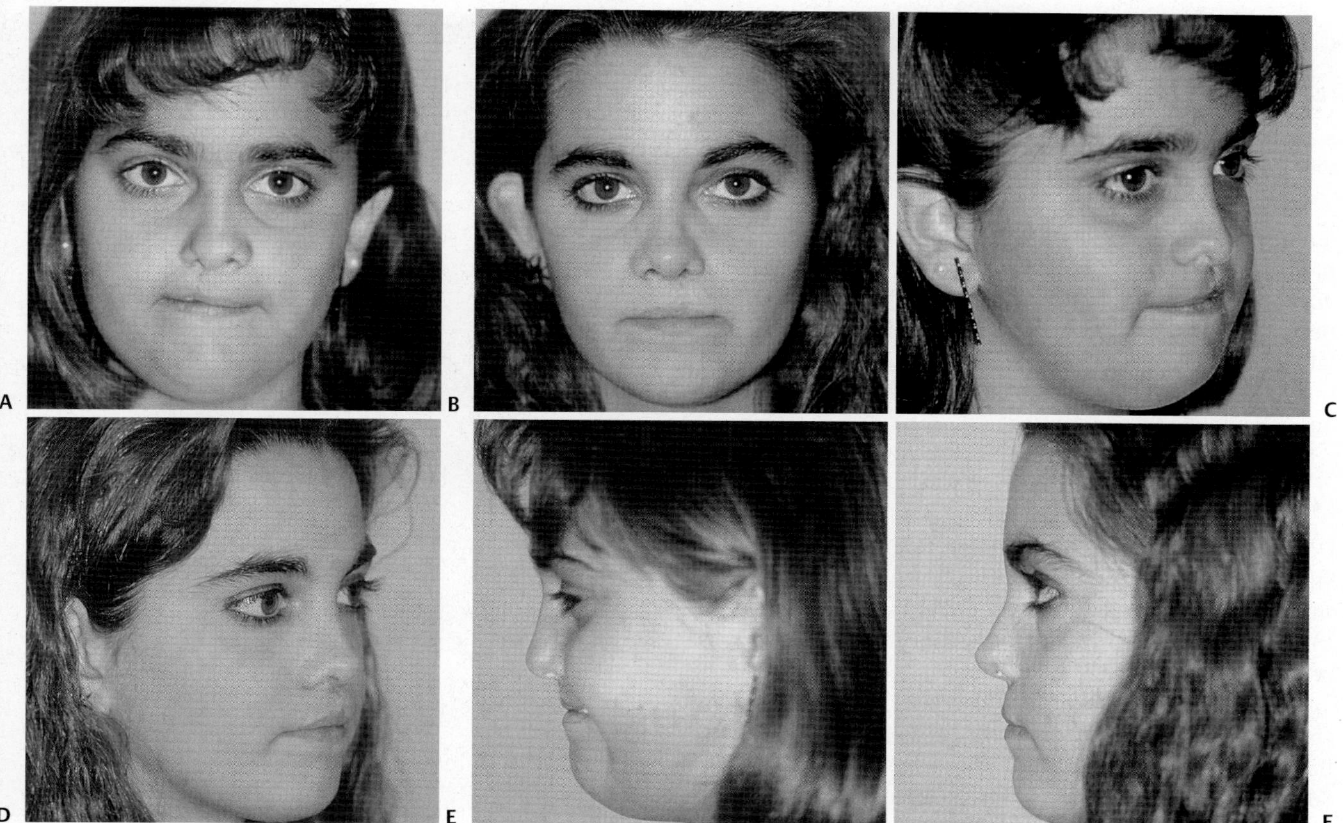

Fig. 77.16 **(A,C,E)** Preoperative anteroposterior, oblique, and lateral photographs of definitive cleft lip rhinoplasty. **(B,D,F)** Postoperative views.

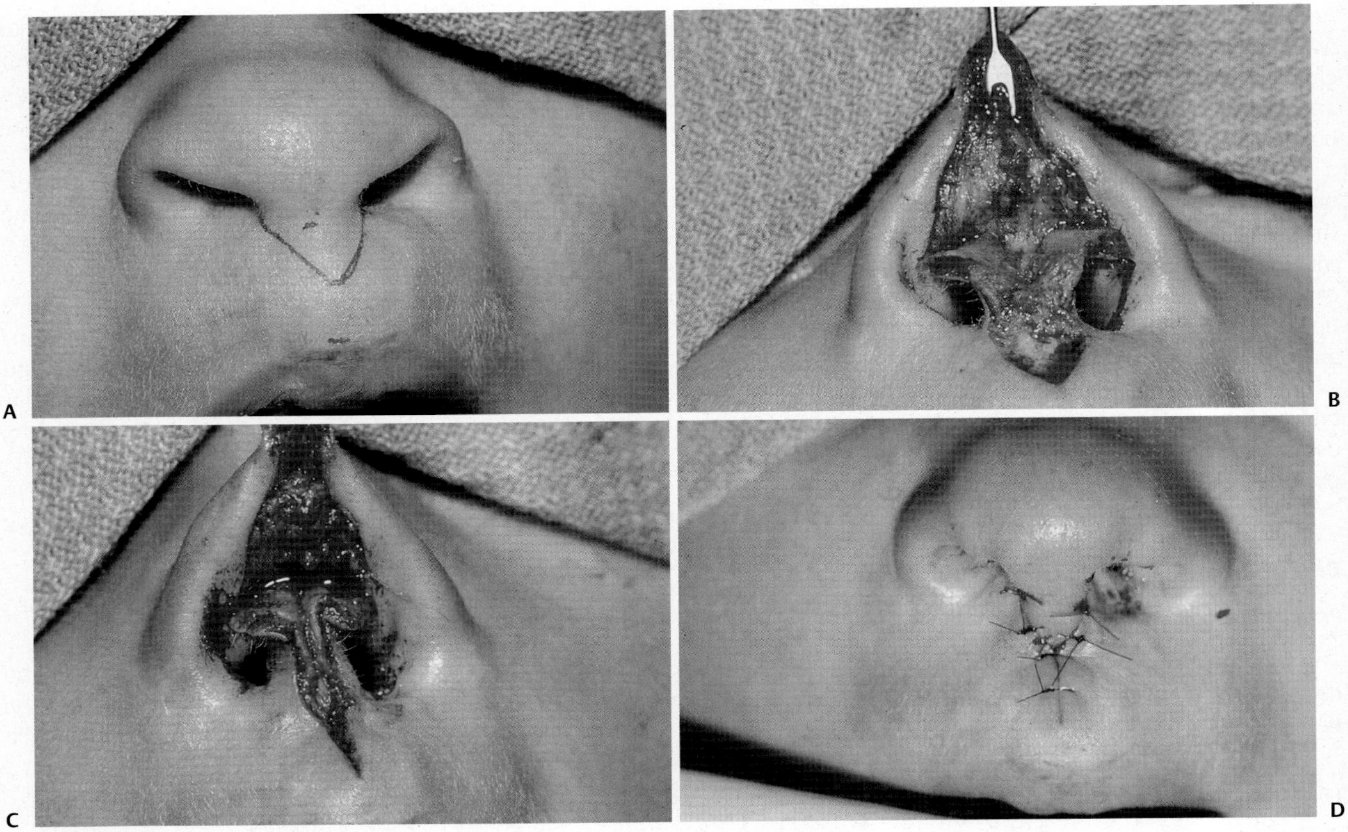

Fig. 77.17 Intraoperative photographs of intermediate bilateral cleft lip rhinoplasty approached with a V-incision (**A**), which recruits skin from the lip into the columella. (**B**) The splayed medial crura are approximated with an intradomal suture to (**C**) narrow the tip and improve symmetry. (**D**) The incision is then closed in Y-fashion.

lengthening by recruiting tissue from the lip into the columella. The intermediate rhinoplasty can be approached via a V-shaped incision, a central lip flap with a caudal V design, or bilateral forked flaps (**Fig. 77.17**).[35,45] The lower lateral cartilages are freed from the nasal skin, and an interdomal stitch is placed to aid with nasal tip projection and to enhance tip symmetry.

Definitive Rhinoplasty

Definitive rhinoplasty for the bilateral nasal deformity is similar to the unilateral deformity in that an open structure approach is used to correct remaining deficiencies and irregularities not addressed by primary and intermediate procedures.

The approach can be done through a standard open rhinoplasty inverted V incision or by using forked lip flaps if additional columellar tissue is needed (**Fig. 77.18**). Septoplasty is performed to correct any aspect of nasal obstruction and to obtain grafting material. The central concepts of the remainder of the lower one third of the repair include placing a cartilaginous tip strut, advancing

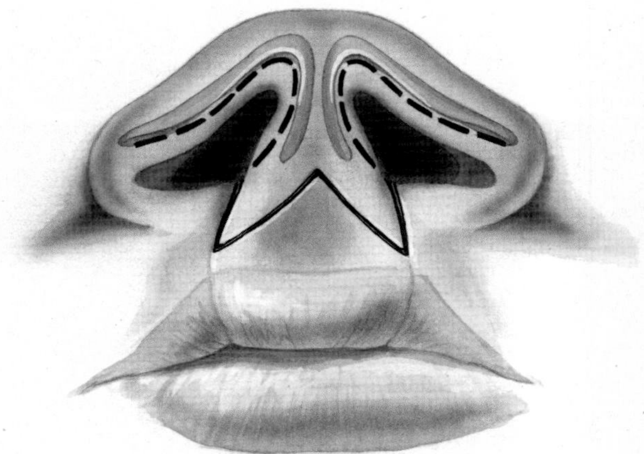

Fig. 77.18 Basal view demonstrating bilateral forked flap incisions to approach the definitive bilateral cleft lip rhinoplasty. (From Sykes JM, Senders CW, Wang TD, Cook TA. Use of the open approach for repair of secondary cleft lip nasal deformity. Facial Plast Surg Clin North Am 1993;1:111–126. Reprinted by permission.)

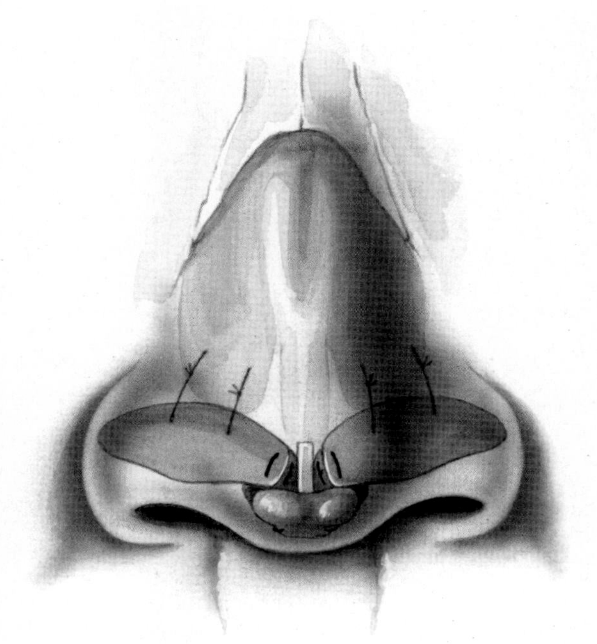

Fig. 77.19 Anteroposterior view depicting the cartilaginous tip strut, the reconstituted lower lateral cartilages, the suture fixation of the lower lateral cartilages to the upper lateral cartilages, and the use of a cartilaginous tip graft. (From Sykes JM, Senders CW, Wang TD, Cook TA. Use of the open approach for repair of secondary cleft lip nasal deformity. Facial Plast Surg Clin North Am 1993;1:111–126. Reprinted by permission.)

the lower lateral cartilages onto the strut, dividing the lower lateral cartilages lateral to the dome to increase projection, reapproximating these cartilages to obtain symmetry, and placing a cartilaginous shield tip graft to further improve projection and definition and to camouflage irregularities (**Fig. 77.19**).

The goals of the middle one third of the reconstruction are to improve the stability of the upper lateral cartilages and to ensure adequate cross-sectional airway at the internal nasal valve. Suturing the upper lateral to the lower lateral will improve stability and decrease the introversion of the lower lateral cartilage. The use of spreader grafts is unusual but should be kept in mind if internal nasal valve collapse is present.

The upper one third of the nose is addressed with hump reduction as needed, and medial-lateral osteotomies to improve the width and straightness of the nasal bones.

The final step is the active repositioning of the alar bases if needed. A complete alotomy is needed to free tissue and give the surgeon the ability to place the alar base in a symmetric position. The nasal floor must be reconstructed when the ala is moved. One, both, or neither side may be repositioned at the time of the definitive repair (**Fig. 77.20**).

Summary

The cleft lip nasal deformity will likely continue to frustrate and challenge reconstructive surgeons for years to come. The concepts seem clear: restore symmetry and definition to the nasal tip and base, realign and open the nasal airway, and prevent scarring and webbing from compromising the results. In practice, however, the three-dimensional nature of the deformity and the involvement of all nasal layers make a dependable result elusive.

The more extensive use of primary rhinoplasty without the fear of halting midface or nasal growth has dramatically changed the secondary deformity, reduced the need for intermediate rhinoplasty, and improved the results obtained with definitive rhinoplasty.[35] Whether the next major advance will occur with in utero surgery or a new technique or concept in definitive rhinoplasty is unknown, but if we continue to study our results, refine our techniques and develop new ones, uncover new truths in models, and

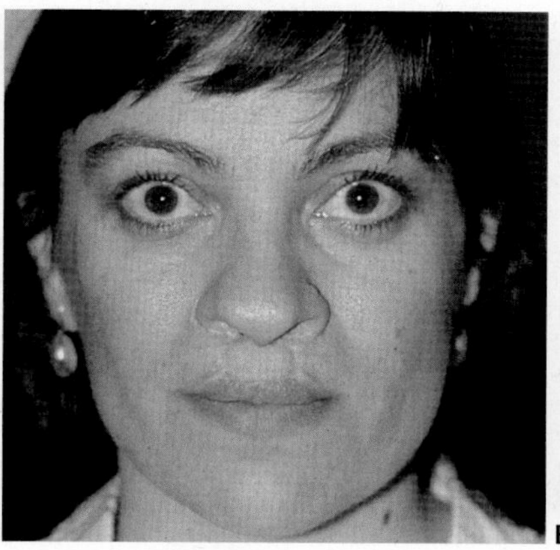
A

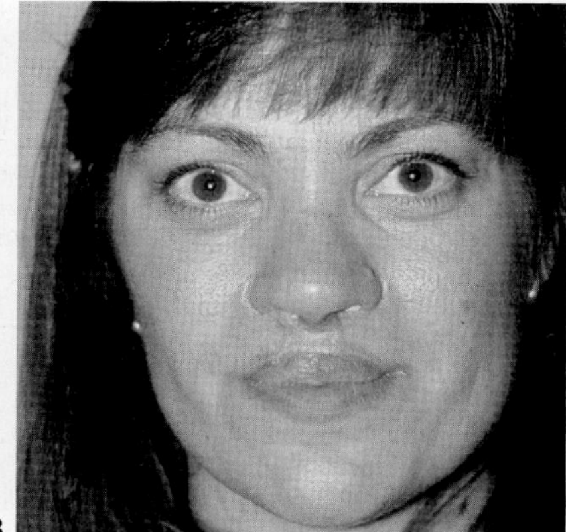
B

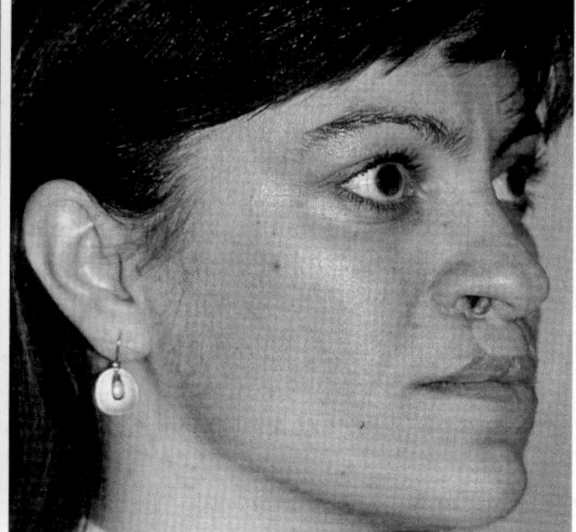
C

Fig. 77.20 (**A,C,E**) Preoperative anteroposterior, oblique, and lateral photographs of definitive bilateral cleft lip rhinoplasty. (**B,D,F**) Postoperative views.

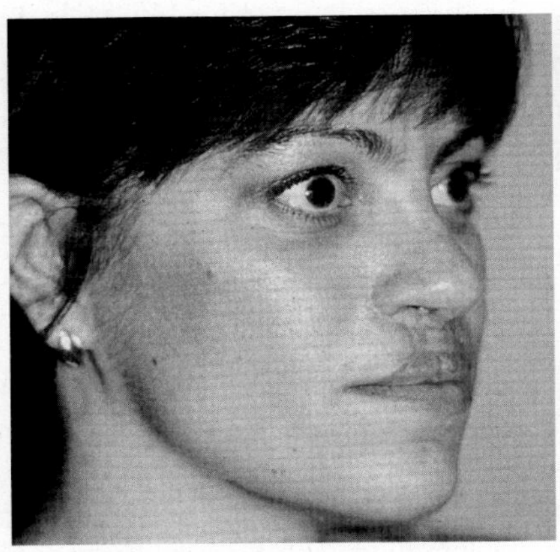
D

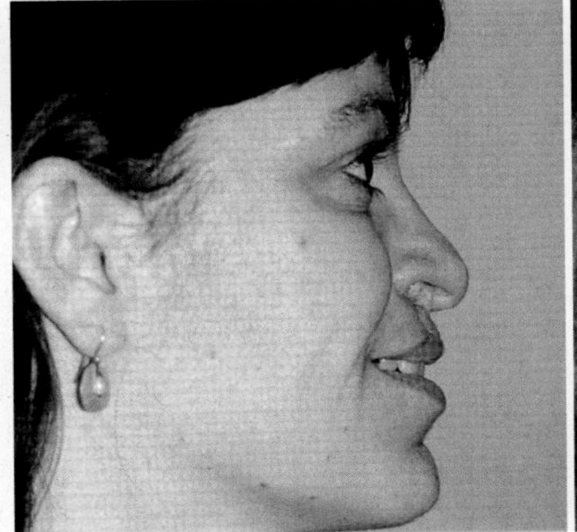
E

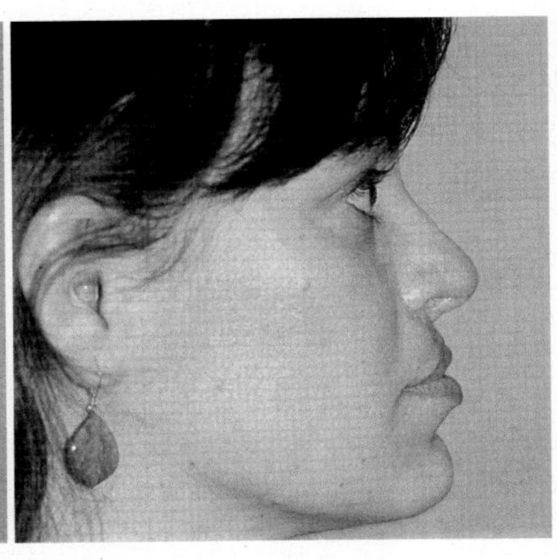
F

Fig. 77.20 *(Continued)*

challenge accepted principles, we will work toward more consistent and better results that improve both the functional and the aesthetic appearance of the cleft lip nasal deformity.

References

1. Sykes JM, Senders CW. Pathologic anatomy of cleft lip, palate, and nasal deformity. In: Meyers AD, ed. Biological Basis of Facial Plastic Surgery. New York: Thieme; 1993:57–71
2. Fisher DM, Mann RJ. A model for the cleft lip nasal deformity. Plast Reconstr Surg 1998;101:1448–1456
3. Madorsky SJ, Wang TD. Unilateral cleft rhinoplasty: a review. Otolaryngol Clin North Am 1999;32:669–682
4. Jablon JH, Sykes JM. Nasal airway problems in the cleft lip population. Facial Plast Surg Clin North Am 1999;7:391–403
5. Avery JK. The unilateral deformity. In: Millard RD, ed. Cleft Craft: The Evolution of Its Surgery. Boston: Little, Brown; 1976
6. Park BY, Lew DH, Lee YH. A comparative study of the lateral crus of alar cartilage in unilateral cleft lip nasal deformity. Plast Reconstr Surg 1998;101:915–919
7. Latham R. Anatomy of the facial skeleton in cleft lip and palate. In: McCarthy J, ed. Plastic Surgery. Vol 4. Philadelphia: WB Saunders; 1990
8. Latham R. The pathogenesis of the skeletal deformity associated with unilateral cleft lip and palate. Cleft Palate J 1969;6:404–414
9. Fara M. The musculature of cleft lip and palate. In: McCarthy J, ed. Plastic Surgery. Vol 4. Philadelphia: WB Saunders; 1990
10. Skoog T. Repair of unilateral cleft lip deformity: maxilla, nose, and lip. Scand J Plast Reconstr Surg 1969;3:109–133
11. Fisher DM, Lo LJ, Chen YR, et al. Three-dimensional computed tomographic analysis of the primary nasal deformity in 3-month-old infants with complete unilateral cleft lip and palate. Plast Reconstr Surg 1999;103:1826–1834
12. Fisher DM, Mann RJ. A model for the cleft lip nasal deformity. Plast Reconstr Surg 1998;101:1448–1456
13. Crockett D, Bumstead R. Nasal airway, otologic, and audiologic problems associated with cleft lip and palate. In: Bardach J, Morris HL, eds. Multidisciplinary Management of Cleft Lip and Palate. Philadelphia: WB Saunders; 1990
14. Sykes JM, Senders CW. Surgical treatment of the unilateral cleft nasal deformity at the time of lip repair. Facial Plast Surg Clin North Amer 1995;3:69–77
15. Hallock GG, Rice DC, McClure HM. In utero lip repair in the rhesus monkey: an update. Plast Reconstr Surg 1987;80:855–858
16. Longaker MT, Stern M, Lorenz HP, et al. A model for fetal cleft lip repair in lambs. Plast Reconstr Surg 1992;90:750–756
17. Estes JM, Whitby DJ, Lorenz HP, et al. Endoscopic creation and repair of fetal cleft lip. Plast Reconstr Surg 1992;90:743–746
18. Canady JW, Landas SK, Morris H, et al. In utero cleft palate repair in the ovine model. Cleft Palate Craniofac J 1994;31:37–44
19. Weinzweig J, Panter KE, Pantaloni M, et al. The fetal cleft palate, II: Scarless healing after in utero repair of a congenital model. Plast Reconstr Surg 1999;104:1356–1364
20. Levine JP, Bradley JP, Shahinian HK, et al. Nasal expansion in the fetal lamb: a first step toward management of cleft nasal deformity in utero. Plast Reconstr Surg 1999;103:761–767
21. Grayson BH, Santiago PE, Beecht LE, Cutting CB. Presurgical nasoalveolar molding in infants with cleft lip and palate. Cleft Palate Craniofac J 1999;36:486–498
22. Liou EJW, Subramanian M, Chen PKT, Huang CS. The progressive changes of nasal symmetry and growth after nasoalveolar molding: a 3-year follow-up study. Plast Reconstr Surg 2004;114:858–864
23. Salyer KE, Genecov ER, Genecov DG. Unilateral cleft lip–nose repair: a 33-year experience. J Craniofac Surg 2003;14:549–558
24. Wolfe SA. A pastiche for the cleft lip nose. Plast Reconstr Surg 2004;114:1–9
25. Sarnat BG, Wexler MR. Growth of the face and jaws after resection of the septal cartilage in the rabbit. Am J Anat 1966;118:755–767
26. Bernstein L. Early submucous resection of nasal septal cartilage: a pilot study in canine pups. Arch Otolaryngol 1973;97:272–285
27. McComb HK, Coghlan BA. Primary repair of the unilateral cleft lip nose: completion of a longitudinal study. Cleft Palate Craniofac J 1996;33:23–31
28. Mulliken JB, Martinez-Perez D. The principle of rotation advancement for the repair of unilateral complete cleft lip and nasal deformity: technical variations and analysis of results. Plast Reconstr Surg 1999;104: 1247–1249
29. Shih CW, Sykes JM. Correction of the cleft-lip nasal deformity. Facial Plast Surg 2002;18:253–262
30. TerKonda RP, Sykes JM. Controversies and advances in unilateral cleft lip repair. Curr Opin Otolaryngol Head Neck Surg 1997;5:223–227
31. Agarwal R, Bhatnagar SK, Pandey SD, et al. Nasal sill augmentation in adult incomplete cleft lip nose deformity using superiorly based turn over orbicularis oris muscle flap: an anatomic approach. Plast Reconstr Surg 1998;102:1350–1359
32. Ness JA, Sykes JM. Basics of Millard rotation–advancement technique for repair of the unilateral cleft lip deformity. Facial Plast Surg 1993;9: 167–176
33. Sykes JM, Senders CW. Surgery of the cleft lip nasal deformity. Oper Tech Otolaryngol Head Neck Surg 1990;1:219–224
34. Millard DR, Morovic CG. Primary unilateral cleft nose correction: a 10-year follow-up. Plast Reconstr Surg 1998;102:1331–1338
35. Sykes JM. Surgical management of the cleft lip nasal deformity. Curr Opin Otolaryngol Head and Neck Surg 2000;8:54–57

36. Demirseren ME, Ohkubo F, Kadomatsu K, Hosaka Y. A simple method for lower lateral cartilage repositioning in cleft lip nose deformity. Plast Reconstr Surg 2004;113:649–653
37. Bardach J, Sayler K. Surgical Techniques in Cleft Lip and Palate. Chicago: Year Book; 1986
38. Koh KS, Eom JS. Asymmetric incision for open rhinoplasty in cleft lip nasal deformity. Plast Reconstr Surg 1999;103:1835–1838
39. Wang TD, Madorsky SJ. Secondary rhinoplasty in the unilateral cleft lip nose. Arch Facial Plast Surg 1999;1:40–45
40. Clark JM, Skooner JD, Wang TD. Repair of the unilateral cleft lip/nose deformity. Facial Plast Surg 2003;19:29–39
41. Toriumi DM, Johnson CM. Open structure rhinoplasty. Facial Plast Surg Clin North Am 1993;1:1–22
42. Mulliken JB. Primary repair of bilateral cleft lip and nasal deformity. In: Goergiade GS, Riefkohl R, Levin LS, eds. Geogiade Plastic and Reconstructive Surgery. 3rd ed. Baltimore: Williams & Wilkins; 1997
43. Trott JA, Mohan N. A preliminary report on open tip rhinoplasty at the time of lip repair in bilateral cleft lip and palate: the Alor Setar experience. Br J Plast Surg 1993;46:215
44. Kohout MP, Aljaro LM, Farkas LG, Mulliken JB. Photogrammetric comparison of two methods for synchronous repair of bilateral cleft lip and nasal deformity. Plast Reconstr Surg 1998;102:1339–1349
45. Jackson IT, Yavuzer R, Kelly C, Bu-Ali H. The central lip flap and nasal mucosal rotation advancement: important aspects of composite correction of the bilateral lip nose deformity. J Craniofac Surg 2005;16:255–261

78 Orthognathic Surgery

Jonathan M. Sykes

The secret to facial beauty is balanced proportion of facial features. The overall attractiveness of the face is a composite of all of the anatomical elements, including skin, subcutaneous tissues, muscle, bone, and teeth. Facial plastic surgeons concern themselves daily with the achievement of this harmonious balance.

To achieve or approach an aesthetic ideal, the facial plastic surgeon must have a clear concept of proportion, a method to analyze deformities, and the ability to apply specific techniques to deformities. Although surgery of the nose involves correction of skeletal abnormalities, aesthetic surgery on the remainder of the face is mainly concerned with soft tissue deformities. In many instances, surgery of the soft tissues is sufficient; however, attention must often be paid to underlying skeletal deformities to correct many congenital and traumatic reconstructive problems.

Evaluation of facial deformities should include skeletal and soft tissue analysis. Soft tissue analysis can be done in an unstructured way through focused observation. It can also be achieved by careful study of consistent frontal and lateral photographs. Skeletal analysis involves evaluation of the facial bones and teeth. Generally, hard-tissue analysis is easier to quantify. It is achieved by determining the patient's dental occlusion and through the use of cephalometric radiography.

After careful skeletal and soft tissue analysis, a detailed, systematic treatment plan is established. This involves using dental and bony models and is often the product of input from multiple specialty fields. Surgical correction of the specific dentofacial deformities is then performed and, it is hoped, facial harmony is established.

Aesthetic Facial Analysis

Dental Analysis

The establishment of balanced facial proportions begins with good dental occlusion. Occlusion is the relationship of the maxillary to the mandibular teeth. This relationship largely depends on the relative position and angulation of the teeth to each other. Malocclusion refers to a dental relationship that is less than optimal. It can result from dental or skeletal deformities or a combination of both.

In 1899, Angle developed a classification system to describe normal and abnormal dental occlusion.[1] The reference point in the Angle classification is the relationship of the maxillary to the mandibular first molar teeth. Each molar tooth has four grinding surfaces, called cusps. The surfaces adjacent to each cusp are referred to as grooves. Cusps adjacent to the tongue are called lingual, and those adjacent to the cheek are called buccal. Cusps located anteriorly, or toward the midline, are referred to as mesial, and those situated posteriorly or away from the midline are called distal (**Fig. 78.1**).

There are three general categories of occlusion in the Angle classification system. In class I occlusion, the mesial buccal cusp of the first maxillary molar fits in the groove on the lateral or buccal surface of the first mandibular molar tooth (**Fig. 78.2**). However, this only represents the ideal relationship of the molar teeth. When the remainder of the teeth interdigitate perfectly, the occlusal relationship is said to be normal. Malocclusion can exist when the molar relationship is class I. This type of malocclusion is generally less severe and usually based on dental rather than skeletal deformities. Although the molar relationship is normal, crowding of the anterior teeth may occur. Another variation of class I malocclusion occurs when there is bimaxillary protrusion. In this situation the mandibular length is excessive, causing a protrusion of both upper and lower incisor regions.

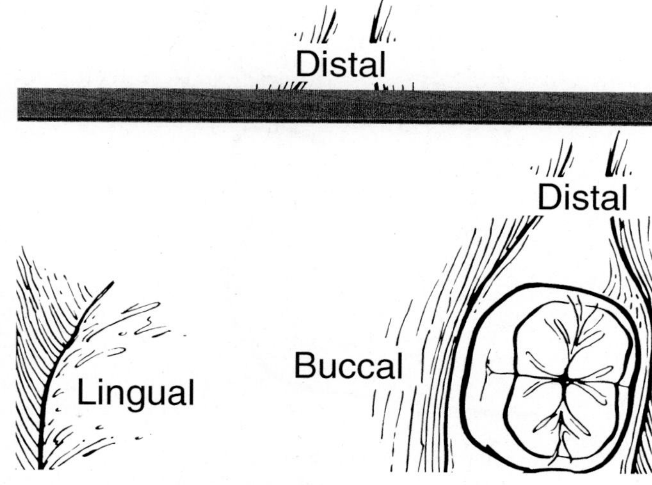

Fig. 78.1 Orientation of molar cusp. (From Donald PJ. The Surgical Management of Structural Dysharmony: A Self-Instructional Package. Washington, DC: American Academy of Otolaryngology–Head and Neck Surgery; 1985. Reprinted by permission.)

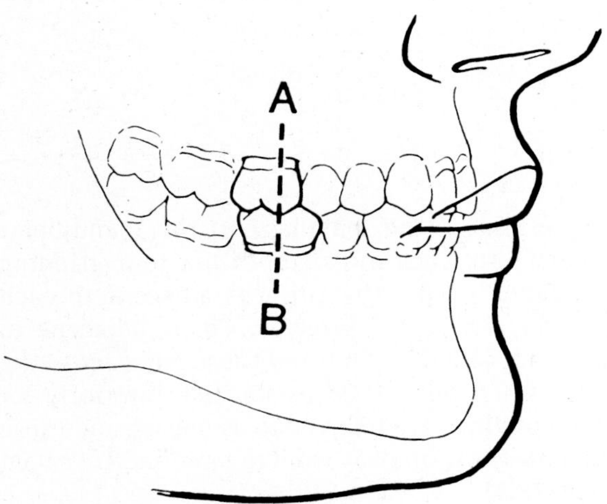

Fig. 78.2 Schematic diagram of class I molar occlusion. (A) The mesial buccal cusp of the first maxillary molar. (B) The buccal intercuspal groove of the mandibular first molar. (From Donald PJ. The Surgical Management of Structural Dysharmony: A Self-Instructional Package. Washington, DC: American Academy of Otolaryngology–Head and Neck Surgery; 1985. Reprinted by permission.)

Class II malocclusion is skeletally and dentally based. The mesial buccal cusp of the first maxillary molar is mesial, or in front of the first mandibular molar (**Fig. 78.3**).

There are two subtypes of class II occlusion. In the more common subtype, division 1, there is excessive overjet (anterior maxillary protrusion), and the maxillary incisors are quite protrusive. In division 2, there is a deep bite

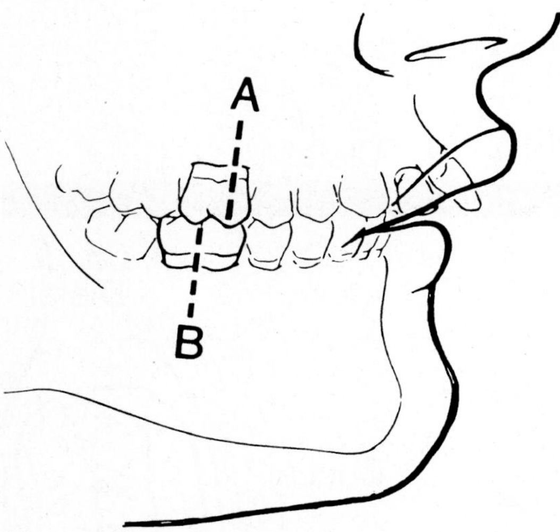

Fig. 78.3 Schematic diagram of a patient with class II malocclusion. The mesial buccal cusp of the first maxillary molar (A). The buccal intercuspal groove of the mandibular first molar (B). (From Donald PJ. The Surgical Management of Structural Dysharmony: A Self-Instructional Package. Washington, DC: American Academy of Otolaryngology–Head and Neck Surgery; 1985. Reprinted by permission.)

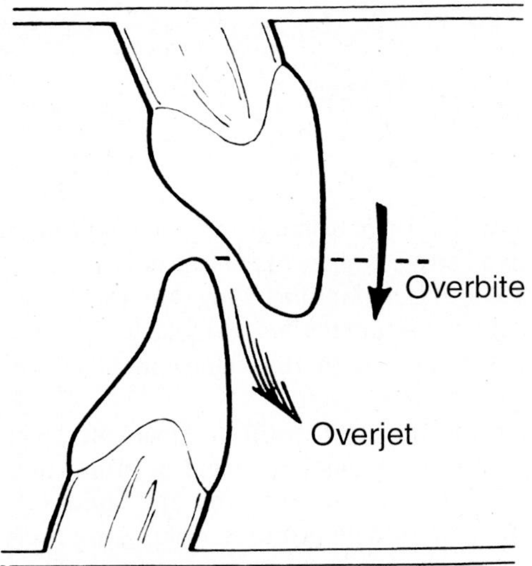

Fig. 78.4 Relationship of the central mandibular incisor. The difference between overbite and overjet is indicated by the schematic diagram.

(overbite) with the maxillary incisors overlapping and covering the mandibular front teeth by more than the usual amount. There is a posterior tilting of the central incisors and a flaring of the lateral incisors. A deep bite is present, but overjet is not as pronounced (**Fig. 78.4**).

Class II malocclusion may arise from a lack of mandibular development. The resulting posteriorly positioned mandible is termed retrognathia. This condition often prevents the upper lip from completely covering the upper incisor teeth. Lack of complete lip seal exposes the upper incisors, rendering them more vulnerable to injury. A class II molar relationship may also arise from an abnormally protuberant maxilla.

The class III malocclusion is primarily skeletally based. It is characterized by a large protrusive mandible or an underdeveloped, retrusive maxilla. The mesial buccal cusp of the first maxillary molar is positioned distal to its ideal position (**Fig. 78.5**). Protrusion of the mandible is called prognathism.

In addition to anteroposterior malocclusions, suboptimal relationships can exist in a medial to lateral direction (**Fig. 78.6**). The ideal relationship occurs when the buccal cusps of the maxillary molar teeth are just lateral to the opposing mandibular buccal cusps. If the maxillary and mandibular molar cusps contact end-to-end or the maxillary buccal cusps are medial to their mandibular counterparts, a lingual cross-bite is present. If the maxillary teeth are more lateral than is ideal, a buccal cross-bite exists.

Malocclusion can thus result from dental or skeletal abnormalities or a combination of both. The cause of malocclusion may be congenital, traumatic, or a consequence of extirpative surgery for neoplastic disease. The dentofacial deformities produced may cause both cosmetic and functional

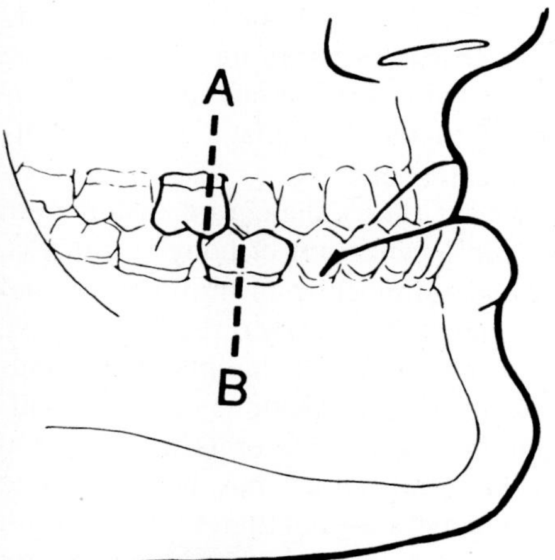

Fig. 78.5 Schematic diagram of a patient with class III molar occlusion. The mesial buccal cusp of the maxillary first molar (A). The buccal intercuspal groove of the mandibular first molar (B). (From Donald PJ. The Surgical Management of Structural Dysharmony: A Self-Instructional Package. Washington, DC: American Academy of Otolaryngology–Head and Neck Surgery; 1985. Reprinted by permission.)

problems. These include difficulties with speech, mastication, and swallowing. It is therefore imperative that the facial plastic surgeon carefully address the occlusal relationships when treating any facial deformity.[2]

Skeletal Analysis

The assessment of craniofacial dimensions is important in diagnosing structural facial dysharmony. Attempts have been made for years by artists, surgeons, and orthodontists to analyze and quantify the proportions of the face. Cephalometry, the scientific measurement of the dimensions of the head, was first used in orthodontics to assess craniofacial growth. Another method for craniofacial analysis based on cephalometry is cephalometric radiography. Although cephalometric radiography was originally introduced into

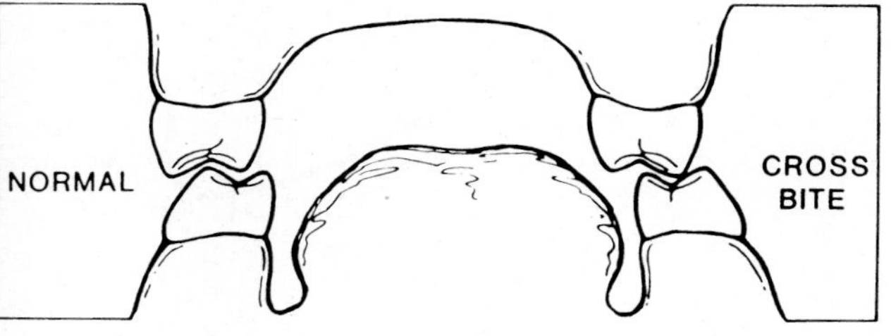

Fig. 78.6 Schematic diagram of the coronal view of the oral cavity at the level of the first molar. (Left) A normal molar relationship is shown with the maxillary buccal cusp related to the buccal surface of the underlying mandibular molar. (Right) A lingual cross-bite is indicated. (From Donald PJ. The Surgical Management of Structural Dysharmony: A Self-Instructional Package. Washington, DC: American Academy of Otolaryngology–Head and Neck Surgery; 1985. Reprinted by permission.)

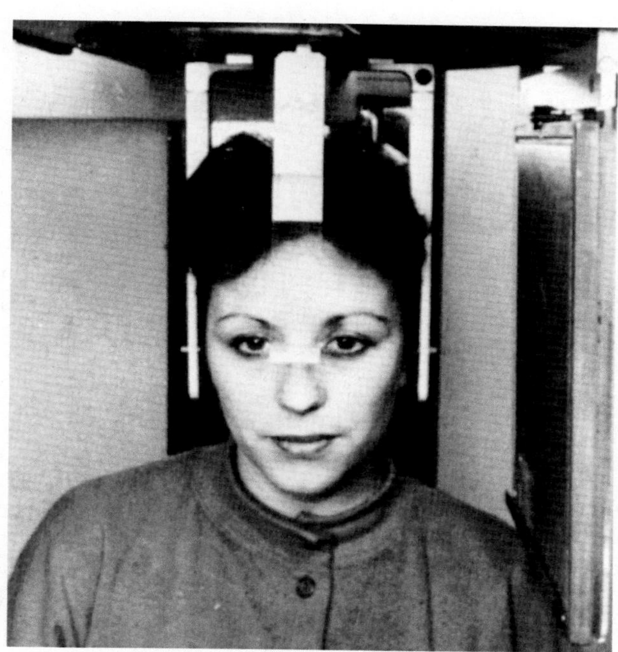

Fig. 78.7 The cephalostat holds the head in a fixed and reproducible position. Two rods are positioned in each external auditory meatus and a lucite bar rests passively at the nasofrontal angle. The x-ray cassette is positioned on the patient's left at a constant distance from the midline of the cephalostat and the head. (From Grayson BH. Cephalometric analysis for the surgeon. Clin Plast Surg 1989;16:10. Reprinted by permission.)

orthodontics during the 1930s, widespread acceptance of the method has only occurred during the past 20 years.[3] In 1931, Hofrath and Broadbent simultaneously and independently developed methods for the production of standardized cephalometric radiographs.[4] This standardization is achieved using a special head holder, known as a cephalostat, which holds the head in a fixed and reproducible position (**Fig. 78.7**).[5] The cephalostat stabilizes the head with three rods. One rod fits in each external auditory meatus, and a third rod rests passively on the inferior orbital rim or the nasofrontal suture. The radiograph taken is a true lateral view, with no head rotation in the sagittal plane. The cephalometric film should be taken with soft tissue technique to most clearly demonstrate the relationship between the soft tissues and the facial skeleton.[6] To further standardize the radiograph and to minimize distortion, a consistent subject-to-film distance and x-ray target-to-subject distance must be used.

The cephalometric radiograph obtained provides a two-dimensional outline of the lateral aspect of the craniofacial skeleton (**Fig. 78.8**). It can be traced onto a matte acetate sheet to provide a model on which various analyses may be performed. However, this radiograph is subject to image distortion. The acetate model is also subject to tracing error. The purpose of the cephalometric tracing is to provide objective data that assist in the diagnosis and treatment of facial skeletal deformities.

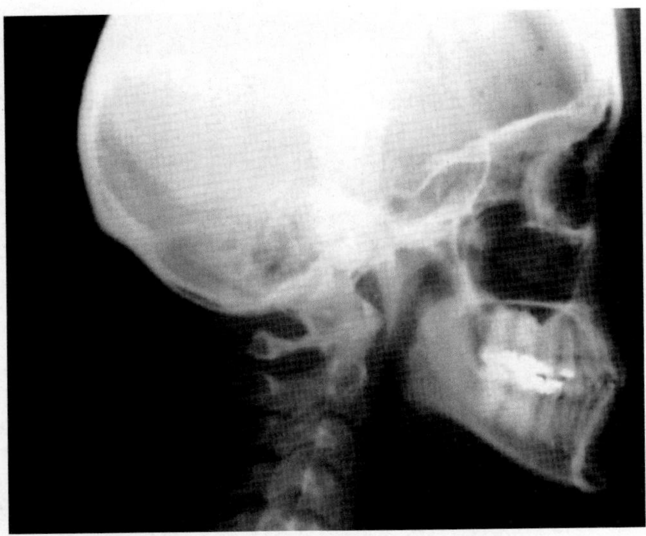

Fig. 78.8 The standard lateral cephalometric radiograph.

The cephalometric radiograph allows objective evaluation of bony and soft tissue morphology. To effectively use the lateral cephalometric tracing, standardized bony landmark points must be defined.[7] These skeletal landmarks may then be used to derive reference lines and angles (**Tables 78.1 to 78.3**).

Table 78.1 Cephalometric Reference Lines

Abbreviation	Term and Definition
S-N	sella–nasion—anteroposterior extent of anterior cranial base
N-A	nasion–height
P-O	Frankfort line (plane)—Plane should be parallel to ground; a reference for photographic analysis.
Me-Go	length of mandibular base
Cd-A	maxillary length
Cd-B	mandibular length
Pal	palatal plane (ANS-PNS)
Go-Me	extent of point A
N-B	nasion–point B
N-Id	nasion–infradentale
N-Go	nasion–gonion line, for analysis of the gonial angle
N-Pog	nasion–pogonion
N-Pr	nasion–prosthion
S-Go	posterior facial mandibular base (first measurement)
Go-Gn	extent of mandibular base (second measurement)
Cd-Go	length of mandibular ramus
S-Ar	lateral extent of the cranial base
FH	Frankfort horizontal—from porion (P) to orbitale (O)
S-Gn	y-axis

Source: From Rakowski T. An Atlas and Manual of Cephalometry Radiography. Philadelphia: Lea & Febiger; 1982. Reprinted by permission.

Linear measurements may be obtained between any two points, and angular measurements are made between three reference points. Various linear and angular analyses are then performed to aid in the diagnosis and treatment of dentoskeletal deformities.

Effective evaluation of the cephalogram depends on accurate definition and localization of bony landmarks. These points may be anatomical or anthropological and are located on or in the skeletal structures. In contrast, radiological or constructed reference points are secondary landmarks marking the intersections of x-ray shadows or lines. The points may be unilateral (in the sagittal plane) or bilateral. Bilateral points may be difficult to precisely determine and measure and therefore may result in slight loss of accuracy. The more commonly used skeletal reference points in cephalometric analysis are seen in **Table 78.2** and **Fig. 78.9**.

These reference points can be used to construct numerous reference lines, as described in **Table 78.1** (**Fig. 78.10**). Different lines are used for different linear analyses, with one particular line representing the reference plane on which

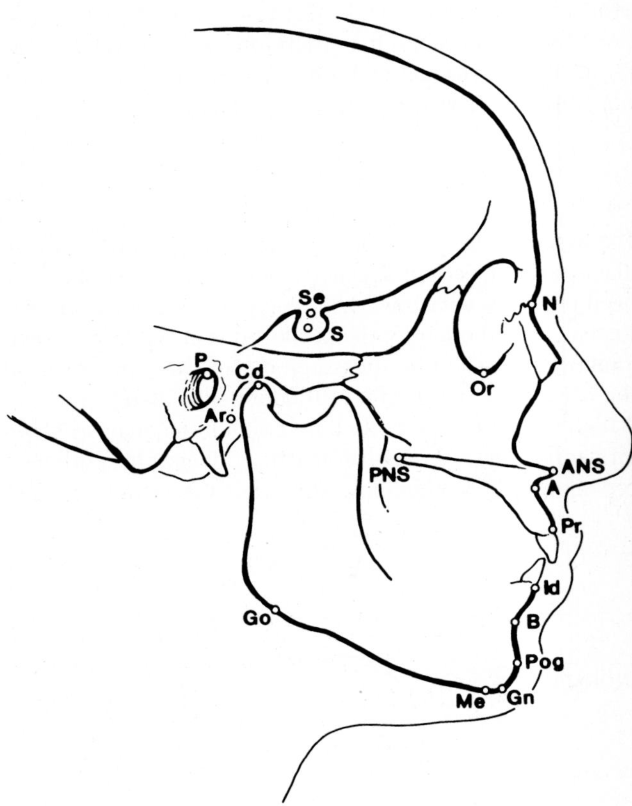

Fig. 78.9 Schematic diagram of the commonly used skeletal reference points in cephalometric analysis. N, nasion; S, sella; A, subspinale; Pr, prosthion; B, supramentale; Id, infradental; Pog, pogonion; Gn, gnathion; Me, menton; Go, gonion; Cd, condylion; Ar, articulare; ANS, anterior nasal spine; PNS, posterior nasal spine; Or, orbitale; P, porion. (From Rakowski T. An Atlas and Manual of Cephalometry Radiography. Philadelphia: Lea & Febiger; 1982. Reprinted by permission.)

Table 78.2 Cephalometric Bony Reference Points

Abbreviation	Term and Definition
N	nasion—The most anterior point of the nasofrontal suture in the median plane. The skin nasion (n) is located at the point of maximum concavity between nose and forehead.
S	sella—The midpoint of the hypophyseal fossa. The midpoint of the entrance of the sella (Se) represents the midpoint of the line connecting the posterior clinoid process and the anterior opening of the sella turcica.
Sn	subnasale—A skin point. The point at which the nasal septum merges with the skin of the upper lip.
A	point A, subspinale—The deepest point in the concavity of the maxilla. It is located between the anterior nasal spine (ANS) and the prosthion (Pr).
Pr	prosthion—The lowest, most anterior point on the alveolar portion of the premaxilla, between the upper central incisors.
B	point B, supramentale—The most posterior point in the outer contour of the mandibular alveolar process, in the median plane. It is located between the infradentale (Id) and the pogonion (Pog).
Id	infradentale—The highest, most anterior point on the alveolar portion of the mandible, in the median plane, between the central incisors.
Pog	pogonion—Most anterior point of the bony chin in the median plane.
Gn	gnathion—This point has been defined in many ways. It is best identified as a point between the most anterior (Pog) and inferior (Me) point of the chin.
Me	menton—The most caudal point in the outline of the symphysis (the lowest point of the mandible).
GO	gonion—A constructed point, defined as the intersection of the lines tangent to the posterior margin of the ascending ramus and the mandibular base.
Cd	condylion—Most superior point on the head of the mandibular condyle.
Ar	articulare—The point of intersection of the posterior margin of the ascending ramus and the outer margin of the cranial base.
ANS	anterior nasal spine—The tip of the bony anterior nasal spine in the median plane. It corresponds to the anthropolic acantion.
PNS	posterior nasal spine—This is a constructed point, represented by the intersection of the anterior wall of the pterygopalatine fossa and the floor of the nose. It marks the dorsal limit of the maxilla.
O	orbitale—The most inferior point on the infraorbital rim.
P	porion—The most superior point on the external auditory meatus.

Source: Modified from Rakowski T. An Atlas and Manual of Cephalometry Radiography. Philadelphia: Lea & Febiger, 1982, with permission.

the whole analysis is based. The Frankfort horizontal plane is based on a line joining the superior border of the bony external auditory canal with the inferior border of the infraorbital rim. The Frankfort plane is used as a reference when orienting medical photographs of patients. This plane should be oriented parallel to the floor with the patient in the upright position. However, the Frankfort plane is not usually used for cephalometric analysis because it is based on points that are not midline. As such, they are subject to error. The line connecting the nasion (N) and sella (S) is midline and is often used as the reference plane on which most cephalometric analysis is based.

Table 78.3 Soft Tissue Reference Points

Abbreviation	Term and Definition
tr	trichion (hairline)
n	skin nasion
no	nasal tip
sn	subnasal
ss	subspinale (concavity of upper lip)
Ls	labrale superius (border of upper lip)
Sto	stomion (central point of interlabial gap)
Li	labrale inferius (border of lower lip)
sm	submentale (labiomental fold)
pog	skin pogonion
gn	skin gnathion

Source: From Rakowski T. An Atlas and Manual of Cephalometry Radiography. Philadelphia: Lea & Febiger; 1982. Reprinted by permission.

Identification of standardized bony reference points and tines allows linear and angular measurements to be determined. These measurements can be compared with normative reference values. Deviation from these norms allows quantitation of the skeletal abnormality.

Angles SNA, SNB, and ANB are relatively simple to determine and provide valuable basic information in analyzing the relationship of the maxilla and mandible. These angles have a narrow range of normal values[3,8] (**Fig. 78.11**). If the angle ANB is greater than 4 degrees, a skeletal class II malocclusion is present. The maxillary versus mandibular contribution to this malocclusion may be determined by measuring the angles SNA and SNB. If ANB is greater than 4 degrees and SNA is greater than normal, the class II malocclusion is most likely secondary

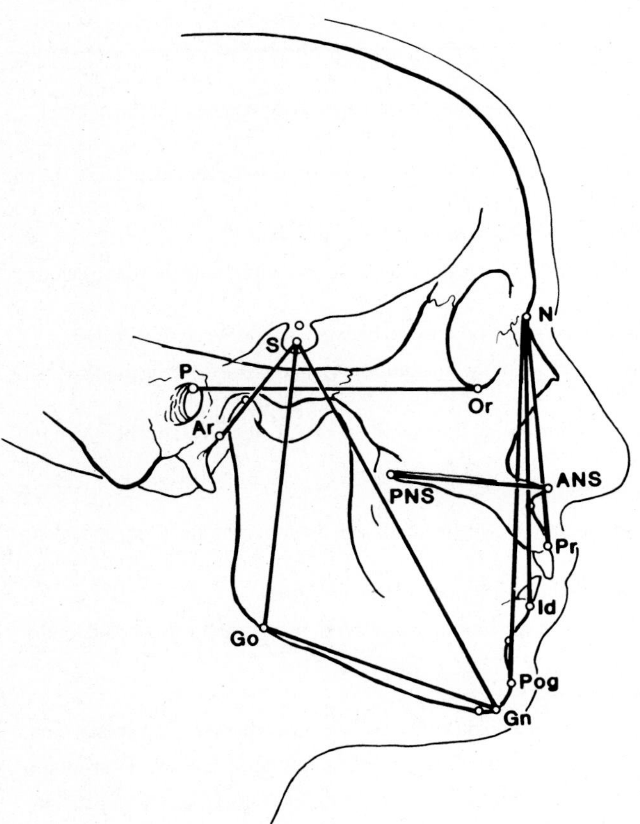

Fig. 78.10 Commonly used skeletal reference lines in cephalometric analysis. S, sella; P, porion; Ar, articular; Go, gonion; PNS, posterior nasal spine; Or, orbitale; N, nasion; ANS, anterior nasal spine; Pr, prosthion; Id, infradental; Pog, pogonion; Gn, gnathion.

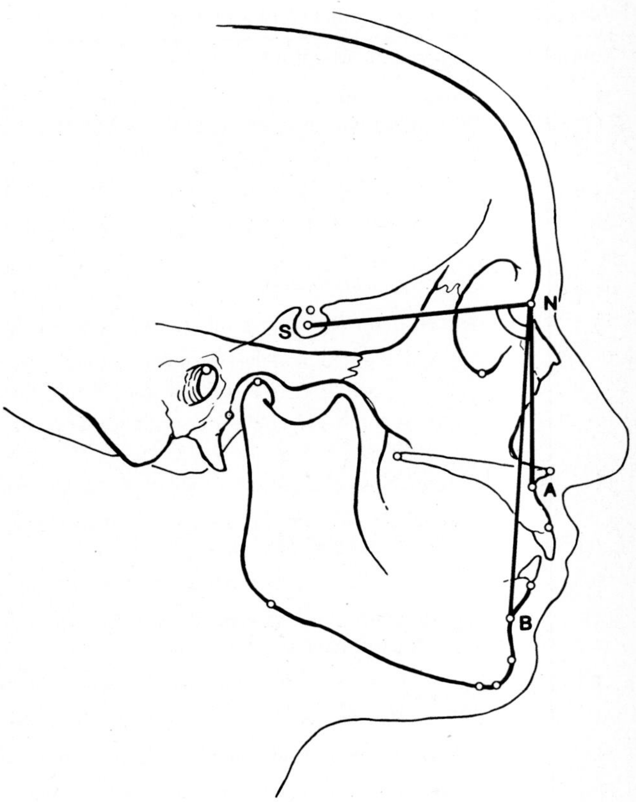

to maxillary protrusion. If ANB is greater than 4 degrees and SNA is less than normal, mandibular retrognathia probably exists.

Fig. 78.11 Cephalometric angular measurements. SNA, SNB, and ANB: these reference angles have a narrow range of normal values. S, sella; N, nasion; A, subspinale; B, supramentale.

Other important angles exist (**Table 78.4**). The Frankfort mandibular plane angle is created by the intersection of the Frankfort horizontal plane and the mandibular plane (from gonion to menton). It is defined by Tweed[9] as 20

Table 78.4 Cephalometric Angular Measurements

Points of the Angle	Definition	Mean Value (Degrees)
N-S-Ar	Saddle angle	123
S-Ar-Go	Articular angle	143
Ar-Go-Me	Gonial angle	128
Ar-Go-N	Upper gonial angle	52 to 55
N-Go-Me	Lower gonial angle	70 to 75
SNA	Anteroposterior position of maxilla	82
SNB	Anteroposterior position of mandible	80
ANB	Difference between SNA and SNB	22
SN-MP	Angle between SN and mandibular plane	35
Pal-MP	Angle between palatal and mandibular plane	25
O-P	Intersecting Frankfort mandibular plane angle	20 to 29

Source: From Rakowski T. An Atlas and Manual of Cephalometry Radiography. Philadelphia: Lea & Febiger; 1982.

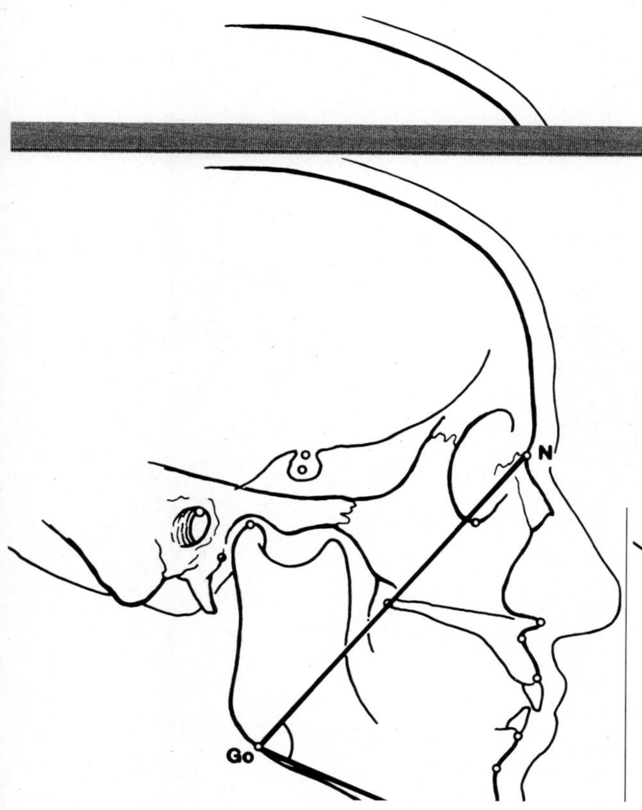

Fig. 78.12 Schematic diagram of the lower gonial angle. This angle can be an indicator of the direction of mandibular growth. N, nasion; Go, gonion; Me, menton.

to 29 degrees and by Burston[10] as 23 degrees. It reflects the inclination of the mandibular plane. The saddle angle is the angle between the anterior and posterior cranial bases. The articular angle (S–Ar–Go) can be affected by orthodontic treatment. It is reduced in all cases of mandibular prognathism. The gonial angle (Ar–Go–Me) plays a role in growth prognosis of the mandible and is affected by the relationship between the body and the ramus. It indicates the direction of mandibular growth, with a large gonial angle indicating posterior condylar growth. The gonial angle may be divided into upper and lower (**Fig. 78.12**) gonial angles.[11]

Various linear distances have also been described (**Table 78.5**). Again, these lines are measured by identifying the two connecting points on the cephalometric radiograph. The mandibular base is determined by measuring the distance between the gonion (Go) and pogonion (Pog) when projected onto the mandibular plane. The maxillary base is measured from the posterior nasal spine (PNS) to point A. The distance from the sella (S) to the nasion (N) is the anteroposterior extent of the anterior cranial base.

A variety of analyses using the previously mentioned skeletal points, lines, and angles have been described. These include the Zimmer aesthetic plane,[12] the Holdaway

Table 78.5 Cephalometric Linear Measurements

Distance	Definition	Mean Value (mm)
S-N	Anteroposterior extent of anterior cranial base	71
S-Ar	Extent of lateral cranial base	48
S-Go	Posterior facial height	87
N-Me	Anterior facial height	114
PNS-Point A	Maxillary base	48
Go-Po	Mandibular base	78

Source: From Rakowski T. An Atlas and Manual of Cephalometry Radiography. Philadelphia: Lea & Febiger; 1982.

ratio,[13] the Gonzales-Ulloa zero meridian line,[14,15] and others.[16] In all instances, these analyses represent an attempt to describe the normal relationship of the facial skeleton.

Soft Tissue Analysis

The overall form and structure of the human face are a product of many factors. Dental analysis and treatment directly address the relationship of the maxillary and mandibular teeth. Skeletal analysis demonstrates the relationship of the facial bones and illustrates any deformity in this relationship. However, dental and skeletal analyses alone are inadequate in evaluating and predicting facial form. Assessment of the soft tissues is crucial in preoperative facial analysis and in achieving harmonious facial balance after surgery.

Soft tissue analysis is the final determinant in evaluating the overall attractiveness of the face. It is the method used by the casual observer and therefore is generally more subjective and less easily quantified. However, the facial plastic surgeon must be able to set some standards of facial beauty; the casual observer also does this but in an unstructured manner. Successful correction of dentofacial deformities requires careful preoperative evaluation of soft tissues and accurate prediction of their response to skeletal surgery. Although the soft tissues are more difficult to standardize than dental or skeletal parameters, analysis may be performed by using fixed soft tissue reference points as described in the box at right (**Fig. 78.13**). These points are often direct correlates of associated bony reference points [e.g., n = soft tissue correlate to the nasion (N) or pog = soft tissue pogonion (Pog).] However, they also represent soft tissue points that are variable in their location and have no fixed skeletal correlate [e.g., the trichion (tr) or hairline]. It is the variable thickness of the soft tissues (e.g., skin of the lips or nose) and the relative position of nonfixed points (e.g., the trichion) that determine the overall facial structure and appearance.

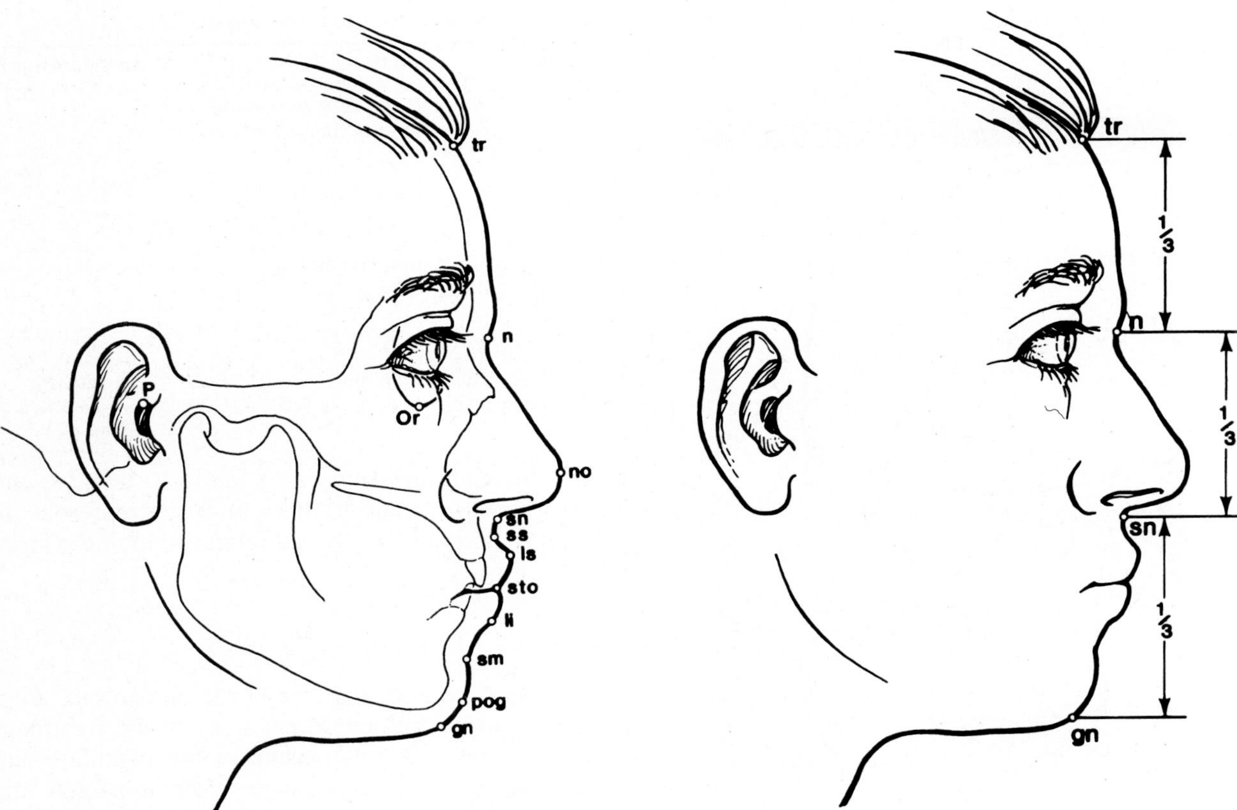

Fig. 78.13 Schematic diagram of soft tissue reference points. In some instances, these points are soft tissue correlates of fixed skeletal reference points. For example, the nasion (n) is the soft tissue correlate of the skeletal nasion (N). In other cases, these soft tissue points have a more variable position, such as the trichion (tr) or the nasal tip (no). N, nasion; Or, orbitale; P, porion; Gn, gnathion; Pog, Pogonion.

Fig. 78.14 Vertical facial height. Balanced facial proportion allows the face to be broken up into three relatively equal thirds. The upper facial third, from the trichion (tr) to the nasion (n), is the most variable because in individuals hairline is often quite variable. A ratio should exist between the middle and lower facial thirds.

The soft tissue reference points can be used to determine various lines and to calculate various angular measurements. This can be done in a similar manner to the cephalometric bony linear and angular measurements. The soft tissue points can also be used to analyze vertical facial height (**Fig. 78.14**).[6] In this analysis, the distance from the trichion to the gnathion may be subdivided into thirds by the nasion and subnasal soft tissue points. Because hairlines are variable, the upper third of the face is not usually a reliable measurement. However, the middle and lower thirds of the face are reliable and should approximately form a ratio. Ratios greater than 1 indicate vertical maxillary excess, foreshortening of the lower third of the face, or a combination of these elements. A vertical height ratio of less than 1 signifies a large lower facial third or vertical maxillary deficiency.

The lower third of the face may be further subdivided into two segments (**Fig. 78.15**). This allows further analysis of the soft tissues of the upper lips, lower lips, and chin.[17] The position and posture of the lips are determined by the dental and skeletal support and must be included in any complete evaluation of the lower third of the face. The upper lip length [from subnasale (sn) to stomion superius (stos)] should be approximately one half of the lower lip length [from stomion inferius (stoi) to gnathion (gn)]. When the ratio of the upper to lower lip is smaller than the vertical height of the lower lip and chin is excessive, a vertical reduction genioplasty may be indicated. Various other analyses have been developed for evaluating lip and chin position.[18–19] These analyses illustrate wide variation in the normal relationship between the teeth, lips, and chin. Lip and chin projection are perhaps best evaluated by drawing a vertical line from the subnasale (sn) to the pogonion (pog) (**Fig. 78.16**).

To accurately correct facial deformities, the facial plastic surgeon must understand the amount of soft tissue change gained by a given bony alteration. It is certainly clear that soft tissue responses to skeletal surgery vary in different regions of the face. It is the accurate

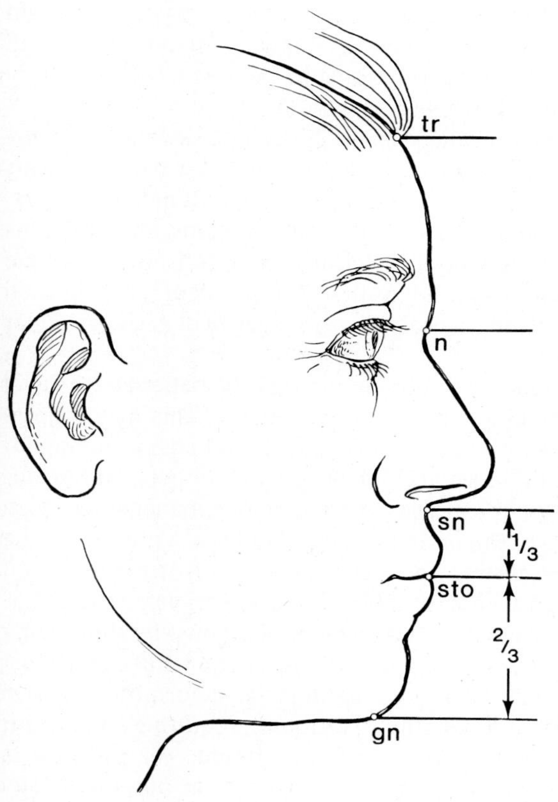

Fig. 78.15 Lower facial height. A ratio of 1:2 should exist between the height of the upper lip and height of the lower lip and chin.

prediction of these responses that determines the final aesthetic result.

In portions of the face where the overlying soft tissues are relatively thin, larger, and more predictable, soft tissue changes are usually obtained for a given bony alteration.[20] Additionally, different procedures on a given facial skeletal area may produce different soft tissue responses. For instance, mandibular advancement procedures increase the soft tissues in a ratio at the chin and approximately a ratio at the lower lip.[21,22] When augmentation genioplasty is used for less significant microgenia, the soft tissue response at the pogonion is ∼22. When augmentation genioplasty is used as an adjunct to mandibular advancement, the additional soft tissue advancement as a result of the genioplasty is only a response.[22] Similar response ratios of soft tissue to bony changes can be measured for mandibular setback surgery, and maxillary advancement and setback surgery (**Table 78.6**).[20] Although these ratios are not absolute, they can be used as a guide to predict the particular soft tissue response to surgery on a particular portion of the facial skeleton.

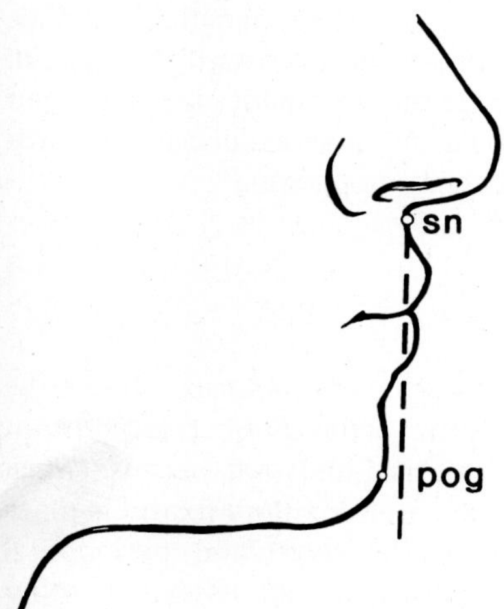

Fig. 78.16 Schematic diagram of anterior chin projection. Projection is best evaluated by dropping a vertical line from the lower lip perpendicular to the Frankfort horizontal. Pog, pogonion; sn, subnasale.

Table 78.6 Soft Tissue Changes after Maxillofacial Surgery

Procedure	Response Ratio of Soft Tissue to Bone
Mandible setback	
Pogonion (Pg)	1:1
Inferior labial sulcus (Si)	0.9:1
Labrale inferius (Li)	0.8:1
Labrale superius (Ls)	0.2:1
Mandible advancement	
Pogonion (Pg)	1:1
Labrale inferius (Li)	0.8:1
Labrale superius (Ls)	Variable
Chin advancement alone	
Pogonion (Pg)	0.8:1
Chin advancement with mandibular advancement	
Pogonion (Pg)	0.4:1
Chin setback alone	
Pogonion (Pg)	0.25:1
Menton (Me)	0.33:1
Maxilla setback	
Subnasale (Sn)	0.5:1
Labrale superius (Ls)	0.5:1
Maxilla advancement	
Subnasale (Sn)	0.5:1
Labrale superius (Ls)	0.5:1
Maxilla-superior repositioning	
Lip length–shortened	0.2:1
Maxilla-inferior repositioning	
Lip lengthened	Variable

Source: From Lehman JA. Soft tissue manifestations of aesthetic detects of the jaws: diagnosis and treatment. Clin Plast Surg 1987;14:4.

The overall appearance after correction of a facial deformity is therefore a result of both the skeletal correction and the redraping of the overlying skin soft tissue envelope. This fact has been well understood by surgeons who perform cosmetic rhinoplasty, where changes in the infrastructure of the nasoskeleton may be minimized or accentuated depending on the relative skin thickness.

Photographic Analysis

Consistent and reproducible photographs are essential when planning surgical correction of any facial deformity. They are an integral part of the preoperative soft tissue analysis. Photographs function as useful teaching aids for both patients and residents. They also provide accurate preoperative and postoperative medicolegal documentation. Photographs also give the surgeon a macroscopic view of the relationship between the individual's facial skeleton and the overlying soft tissues. Most importantly, however, photographs provide the surgeon with a visual record, which can be retrospectively analyzed. It is through such periodic critical assessment that surgical procedures are modified.

The most important aspect of useful medical photography is consistency. A 35-mm camera with a microscopic lens in the focal length range of 80 to 110 mm should be used. The Frankfort horizontal plane must be used religiously as a guideline when taking full-face portrait views. This plane can be constructed by connecting the porion (the superior aspect of the external auditory canal) with the orbitale (the most inferior point on the infraorbital rim). All photographs should be taken with this line parallel to the ground.

At least five full-face portrait views should be obtained. These include a posteroanterior, two lateral, and two oblique views. In addition, a submental-vertex (basal) view and close-up views of the occlusion from the posteroanterior and lateral orientation should be obtained.

Treatment of Dentofacial Deformities

Philosophy

Diagnosis and treatment of the patient with dentofacial deformities must occur in an orderly, systematic fashion. A careful medical and dental history and physical examination must be performed. This should include the patient's individual needs and expectations from orthognathic surgery. Specific concentration should be placed on the relative importance of functional versus cosmetic correction expected by the patient. After completion of the basic examination, photographic and radiographic analysis is obtained. Lastly, dental study models are constructed. These models may be mounted on an articulator, allowing analysis of static occlusion and the dynamic relationship between the maxillary and mandibular teeth.

After performing a thorough dental, skeletal, and soft-tissue analysis, a complete problem list is compiled. This complete problem list should include all medical or systemic problems, dental occlusal problems, and problems relating to the facial skeleton. In addition, any soft tissue abnormalities are identified. The problem list may then be prioritized according to the severity of each particular deformity.

A systematic treatment plan for the patient with facial dysharmony may then be formulated. This may require the cooperative efforts of many disciplines, including facial plastic surgeons, oral surgeons, dentists, and orthodontists. In most cases, more than one management plan is possible. The option chosen should be a product of the patient's desires and expectations from treatment and the surgical team's abilities and experience. The surgical options and final treatment plan must be thoroughly discussed with the patient. This is crucial because most management plans for dentofacial deformities involve complex and lengthy treatment, requiring significant patient cooperation and commitment. For instance, a patient with mandibular retrognathism may be ideally treated by combined orthodontic and orthognathic surgical treatment. However, after understanding the treatment and postoperative care, the patient may choose to have orthodontic treatment only. Alternatively, the patient may not complain of problems with occlusion and may only be concerned with cosmetic improvement of the retrusive mandible. In this instance, treatment with either a sliding genioplasty or an alloplastic chin augmentation may be appropriate.

It is imperative to discuss the risks, benefits, and limitations of potential treatment options with the patient. The patient, understanding the treatment plans and their limitations, may then make an informed decision regarding which management choice to pursue.[23]

Preoperative Dental Treatment

As a general rule, all routine dental care should be completed before initiating orthodontic treatment or orthognathic surgery. This is important because most orthodontic treatments or intermaxillary fixations place considerable demands on the teeth and periodontal tissues. Dental caries, periapical abscesses, or other intraoral inflammatory diseases must be treated. Fillings and extractions should also be completed. To facilitate orthodonture, temporary restorations may be necessary before placement of an orthodontic appliance. Placement of crowns or missing teeth is usually postponed until orthodontic and orthognathic treatment is completed.

Treatment of temporomandibular joint syndrome is usually begun before any orthodontic treatment. This may include analgesics or anti-inflammatory medication. It also may include dental splints to decrease pain and spasm. Pretreatment of these problems allows better evaluation of the patient's occlusion and facilitates more accurate treatment planning.

Preoperative Orthodontic Treatment

In most instances, preoperative orthodontic treatment is necessary to align the dental arches. This can minimize the occlusal deformity and often decreases the amount of movement necessary during orthognathic surgery. Preoperative orthodonture usually requires 12 to 18 months of treatment. It may require dental extractions to accommodate tooth movements and eliminate crowding.

The orthodontist should work closely with the maxillofacial surgeon to anticipate the postoperative position of the dental arches.[24–26] Careful dental analysis should occur, and the portion of malocclusion secondary to dental versus skeletal components should be identified. Plaster dental models are constructed (**Fig. 78.17**), and these models are placed on an articulator (**Fig. 78.18**). An articulator consists of two metal platforms that are hinged on one end to simulate the temporomandibular joint. This enables the two models to slide on each other. The amount of movement necessary to achieve class I occlusion can be determined. A facebow may also be used to improve the analysis of the occlusion (**Fig. 78.19**). This consists of a metal mount that is placed on the maxillary component of the articulator. This allows further examination of the relationship of the maxilla to the anterior cranial base. This improves analysis and treatment of the asymmetrical or obliquely oriented bite. Finally, a plan is made by the orthodontist to establish the maximal preoperative occlusal relationship.

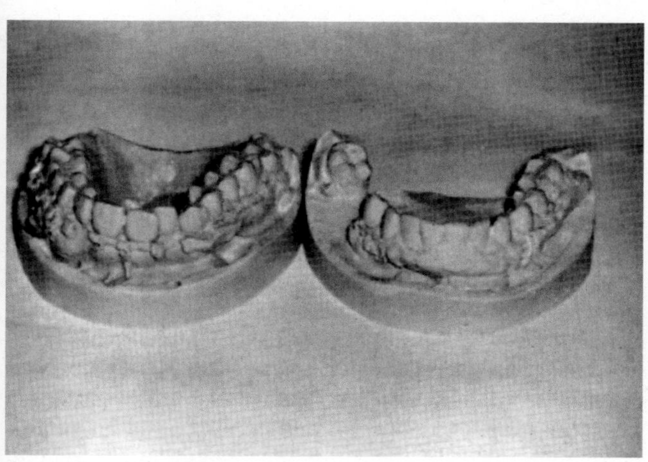

Fig. 78.17 Plaster dental study models.

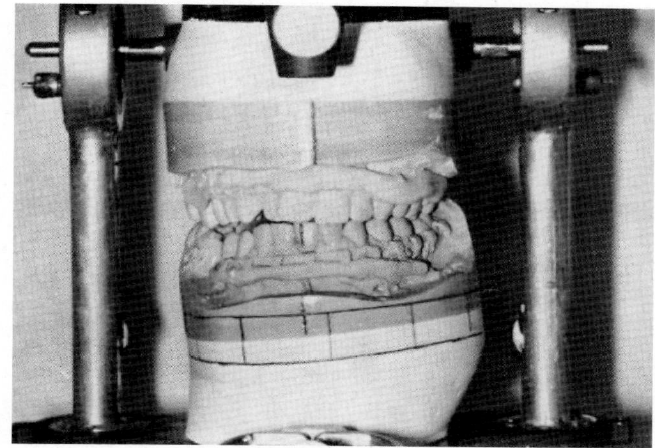

Fig. 78.18 Anteroposterior view of plaster dental models mounted on an articulator.

Preoperative Workup and Model Surgery

After maximal preoperative occlusal relationships are obtained, the plaster dental models are mounted and the amount of surgical correction is determined. An acrylic, interocclusal wafer splint is finished to be used during surgery. This splint provides an exact template on which the maxillary and mandibular dental arches may fit at the time of surgery.

If a single-jaw surgery is to be performed, a single interdental wafer splint is placed at the conclusion of the jaw movement. The patient is then placed in maxillomandibular fixation (MMF) with the wafer splint in position. If surgery

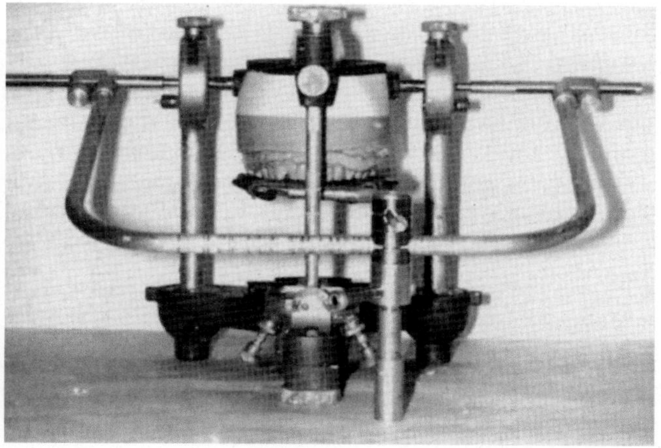

Fig. 78.19 Plaster dental model of the maxilla mounted on a facebow. Once mounted on the facebow, the model of the maxilla may be tilted in any direction to allow improved analysis and treatment.

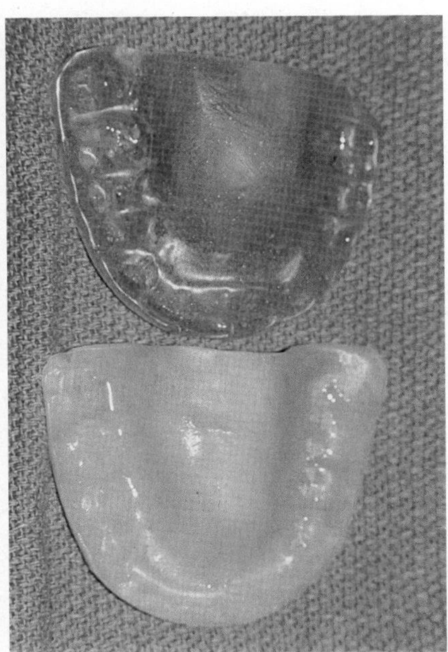

Fig. 78.20 Fabricated dental splints for patient undergoing two-jaw orthognathic surgery. The intermediate splint (above) is used after osteotomy, movement, and fixation of the maxilla and prior to mandibular osteotomy. The final splint (below) is used after both jaws are osteotomized, moved, and fixated.

involves both the maxilla and the mandible, two splints are fabricated prior to surgery (**Fig. 78.20**). The first splint (intermediate) is placed to indicate the position of the maxilla after movement but prior to mandibular osteotomy. The second splint (final) is used to identify the occlusion and jaw position after both the maxillary and mandibular osteotomies and movements. This final splint remains in place after repositioning of the entire maxillomandibular complex.

The interdental wafer splint is constructed to indicate the horizontal (anteroposterior) and transverse new position of both jaws after osteotomy and repositioning. However, the interdental splint does not dictate the new vertical (superior-inferior) position of the jaws. The vertical dimension is determined during presurgical planning and is accomplished by ostectomy (for shortening) and bone grafting (for lengthening) prior to final bony movement.

In cases of complex maxillary osteotomies, a splint with full palatal coverage (rather than a wafer splint) is constructed. The full palatal coverage splint enhances stability after bony osteotomy and movement. This type of splint would be used in a patient with maxillary transverse constriction. After a paramedian palatal split, a full palatal coverage splint would be placed.

The initial plan for correcting any dentofacial deformity should include the type of surgery, the amount of jaw movement planned, and whether the deformity is best treated with one- or two-jaw surgery. This treatment plan should specifically address the patient's problem list and will dictate surgical treatment.

Surgical Procedures

Mandibular Prognathism

Various surgical procedures exist for correction of mandibular prognathism, including the vertical-subcondylar osteotomy and the sagittal-split osteotomy. The vertical-subcondylar osteotomy may be performed through either an intraoral or an extraoral approach, whereas the sagittal-split osteotomy is usually done intraorally. Each approach and technique has specific advantages and disadvantages. The procedure chosen should be individualized for the specific needs of the patient.

The vertical-subcondylar osteotomy was first performed by Caldwell and Letterman in 1954.[28] Several modifications of the original procedure, which was performed through an external incision, have been made.[27–29] The major advantage of the vertical-subcondylar osteotomy is in avoiding injury to the inferior alveolar nerve. It may be performed through an intraoral or external incision. The intraoral approach has the advantage of avoiding the external cervical scar and the associated potential injury to the marginal mandibular branch of the facial nerve. However, the intraoral approach is technically more difficult. The more oblique the angulation of the mandibular rami in relation to the sagittal plane, the easier the exposure through the intraoral approach. It is performed through a mucosal incision in the gingivobuccal sulcus from the base of the coronoid to the second bicuspid. Care should be taken to avoid the buccal fat pad. Incision of the periosteum over the anterior aspect of the ramus is accomplished, and the periosteum is elevated posteriorly. The antilingular process is then carefully identified. This landmark is crucial because it is opposite the lingula, which is the entrance of the inferior alveolar neurovascular bundle on the medial aspect of the mandible.

The oblique osteotomy line is carefully marked from the sigmoid notch to the angle of the mandible. This line should be posterior to the antilingular process to avoid injury to the neurovascular bundle. The mandible is then scored with a cutting bur and the osteotomy completed with a reciprocating saw. After the osteotomy is performed bilaterally, the proximal segments are reflected laterally and the distal segment is allowed to recess medially (**Fig. 78.21**).

Occlusion is checked and the interocclusal wafer splint placed. Intermaxillary fixation is applied and maintained for 6 to 8 weeks. Sometimes rigid fixation of the mandibular segments is used, alleviating the need for intermaxillary fixation.

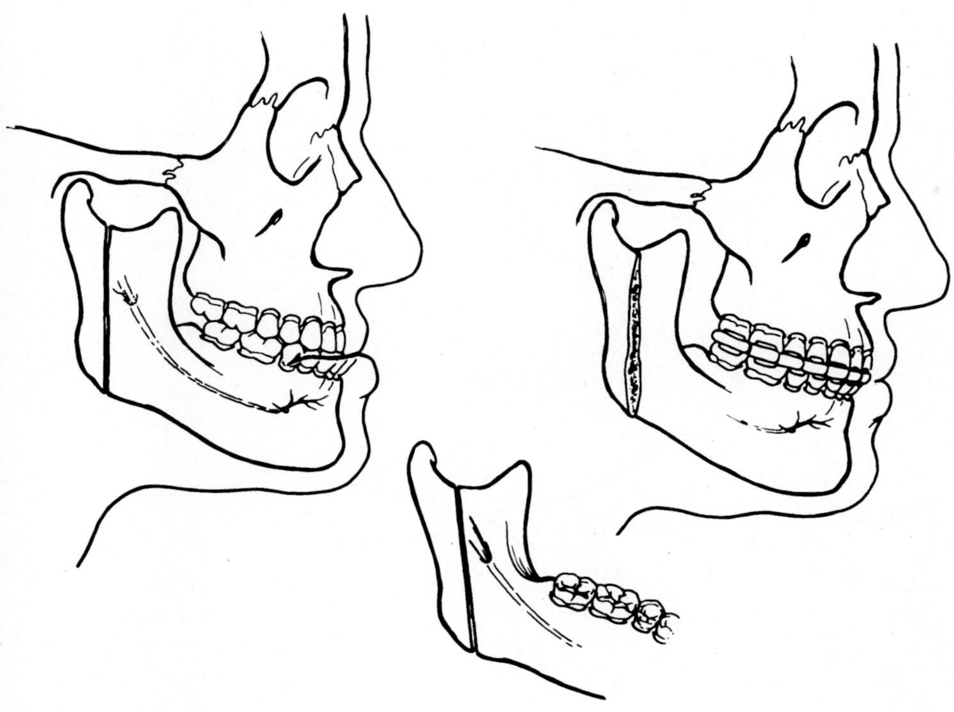

Fig. 78.21 Schematic diagrams of the vertical subcondylar osteotomy. The oblique osteotomy line is made from the sigmoid notch to the angle of the mandible. This osteotomy is posterior to the inferior alveolar neurovascular bundle. After bilateral osteotomies are performed, the proximal segments are reflected laterally and a mandibular setback is accomplished.

The external approach for vertical-subcondylar osteotomy has the disadvantage of a cervical scar and the potential for injury to the marginal mandibular branch of the facial nerve. It is the preferred approach for setbacks of greater than 10 mm and for asymmetrical setbacks. It is performed through a 3-cm cutaneous incision in the relaxed skin tension lines approximately one fingerbreadth below the angle of the mandible. Exposure and subperiosteal dissection are performed in a similar manner to the intraoral approach.

The sagittal-split osteotomy was first introduced by Obwegeser and Trauner in 1955.[30–32] Modified by Dal Pont in 1961,[33] it is a versatile procedure for correction of mandibular deformities because it can be used for both advancement and setback of the mandible. It is especially satisfactory when used in prognathic patients with an open-bite deformity. It is also well suited for rigid fixation.

A risk of the sagittal-split osteotomy is inferior alveolar nerve injury. The procedure is also associated with avascular necrosis of the proximal bony segment. The teeth adjacent to the sagittal fracture line may also be compromised and lost.

The sagittal-split osteotomy is done intraorally through a mucosal incision similar to that of the vertical-subcondylar osteotomy. Subperiosteal dissection is performed on both the medial and lateral surfaces of the mandible. The lingula and mandibular foramen are identified on the medial surfaces of the mandible. A horizontal osteotomy is made on the medial cortex 5 mm above the lingula. A vertical osteotomy is then made through the lateral cortex in the region of the second molar tooth. The osteotomies are connected along the oblique line, and separation of the medial and lateral segments is accomplished using a heavy osteotome as a lever. The inferior alveolar neurovascular bundle remains medially with the distal segment. A vertical segment of bone is then removed from the anterior aspect of the proximal lateral bony segment. The width of the segment to be removed should equal that of the setback to be achieved (**Fig. 78.22**).

The contralateral osteotomy is then accomplished in a similar manner, and occlusion is obtained with a wafer occlusal splint. The proximal segments are carefully positioned in each glenoid fossa. Intermaxillary fixation is again placed for 6 to 8 weeks.

The sagittal-split osteotomy is a versatile procedure for mandibular deformities. The distal (i.e., tooth-bearing) segment may be retruded, advanced, or rotated to close an anterior open bite (**Fig. 78.23A–L**). It is also the procedure of choice in patients requiring two-jaw surgeries. The wide surface contact between the proximal and distal segments ensures rapid bone healing; delayed union and nonunion are extremely rare. The main disadvantage of

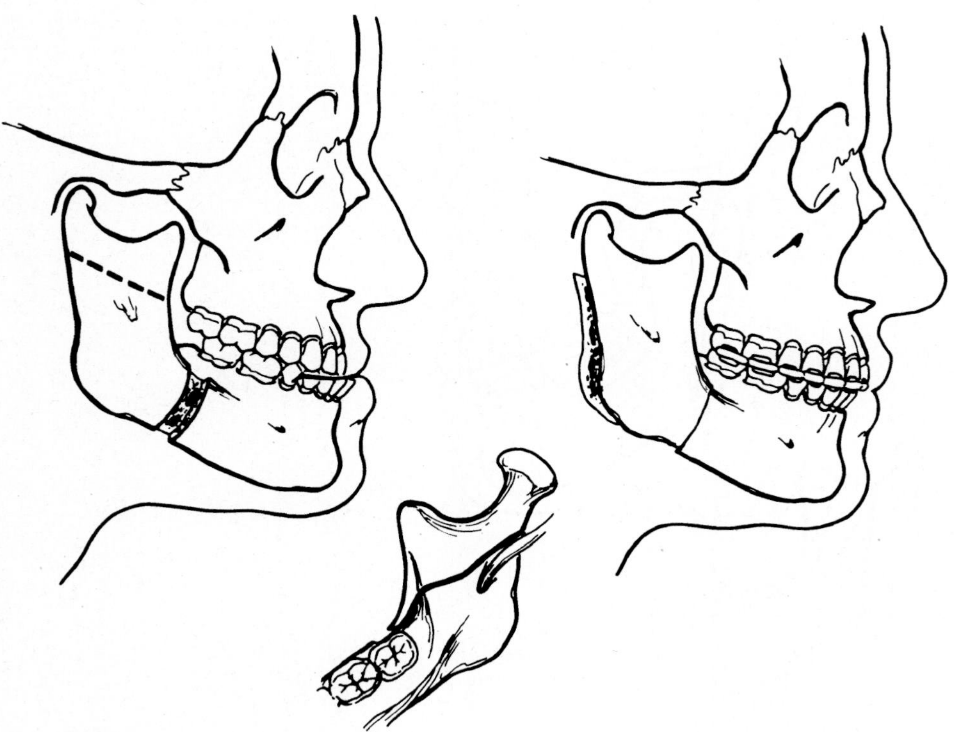

Fig. 78.22 Schematic diagrams of the sagittal-split osteotomy. This osteotomy consists of a horizontal osteotomy on the medial cortex 5 mm above the lingula. A second vertical osteotomy is made through the lateral cortex in the region of the second molar tooth. The sagittal split is completed by connecting the two osteotomies along the oblique line. The inferior alveolar neurovascular bundle remains medially with a distal segment.

this procedure is the incidence of permanent anesthesia of the lower lip, with reports as high as 45%.[34]

Mandibular Retrognathism

Retrognathism, or mandibular deficiency, defines a group of conditions in which the mandible is small, retruded, or both. The occlusion in retrognathism is class II and this malocclusion is generally skeletally based. There are many reasons for this condition, and it may be associated with many syndromes (e.g., Nager or Treacher Collins syndrome).

Many procedures have been developed for treatment of retrognathism. The sagittal-split osteotomy[33] is the most commonly used technique for correction of mandibular deficiency. This procedure allows for correction of significant bony retrognathism; in addition, correction of the soft tissue pogonion generally follows the bony alteration at a ratio.

The technique for sagittal-split osteotomy has been well described. A gingivobuccal-sulcus incision is made from the pterygomandibular raphe to the second molar tooth. Subperiosteal dissection is accomplished on both the lateral and the medial surfaces of the mandible. Care is again taken to avoid entering the buccal fat pad. The channel retractor is placed along the medial aspect of the ramus to expose the bone above the lingula.

A horizontal bony incision is made with the Lindemann side-cutting bur through the medial cortex of the ramus. This bony cut is made superior to the mandibular foramen, with care taken to protect the inferior alveolar neurovascular bundle. The vertical lateral osteotomy is performed at an oblique angle in the region of the second or third molar. The two osteotomies are joined on the anterosuperior margin with a reciprocating saw.

A thin osteotome is used to complete the sagittal split. The osteotome should angle toward the buccal cortex of the mandible, hugging the medial surface of the lateral bony table. This helps avoid injury to the inferior alveolar nerve. A similar procedure is performed on the contralateral side. The distal segment is then positioned with the condyles of the proximal segments held in the glenoid fossae. An acrylic wafer splint is again used to position the dental arches, and intermaxillary fixation is performed. If internal rigid skeletal fixation is used, intermaxillary fixation is not necessary (**Fig. 78.24A–G**).

Temporary or permanent injury to the inferior alveolar nerve is a recognized complication of sagittal-split osteotomy. Permanent lower-lip anesthesia has been reported in 2 to 45% of cases.[34] Relapse of some or all of the mandibular retrusion is also a known complication. Relapse is usually secondary to pull of the suprahyoid musculature. It may also result from improper positioning of the condylar head in the glenoid fossa at the time of mandibular advancement.

Some patients may have normal occlusion before surgery but a suboptimal aesthetic relationship between the chin and the remainder of the face. This can be determined by dropping a vertical line from the mucocutaneous (vermilion) border of the lower tip (**Fig. 78.16**). The soft tissue pogonion should almost reach this vertical line in men and is located just posterior to the vertical line in women. If the soft tissue pogonion falls significantly behind this line, microgenia may be diagnosed. In patients with mandibular retrusion and a normal occlusal relationship, osseous

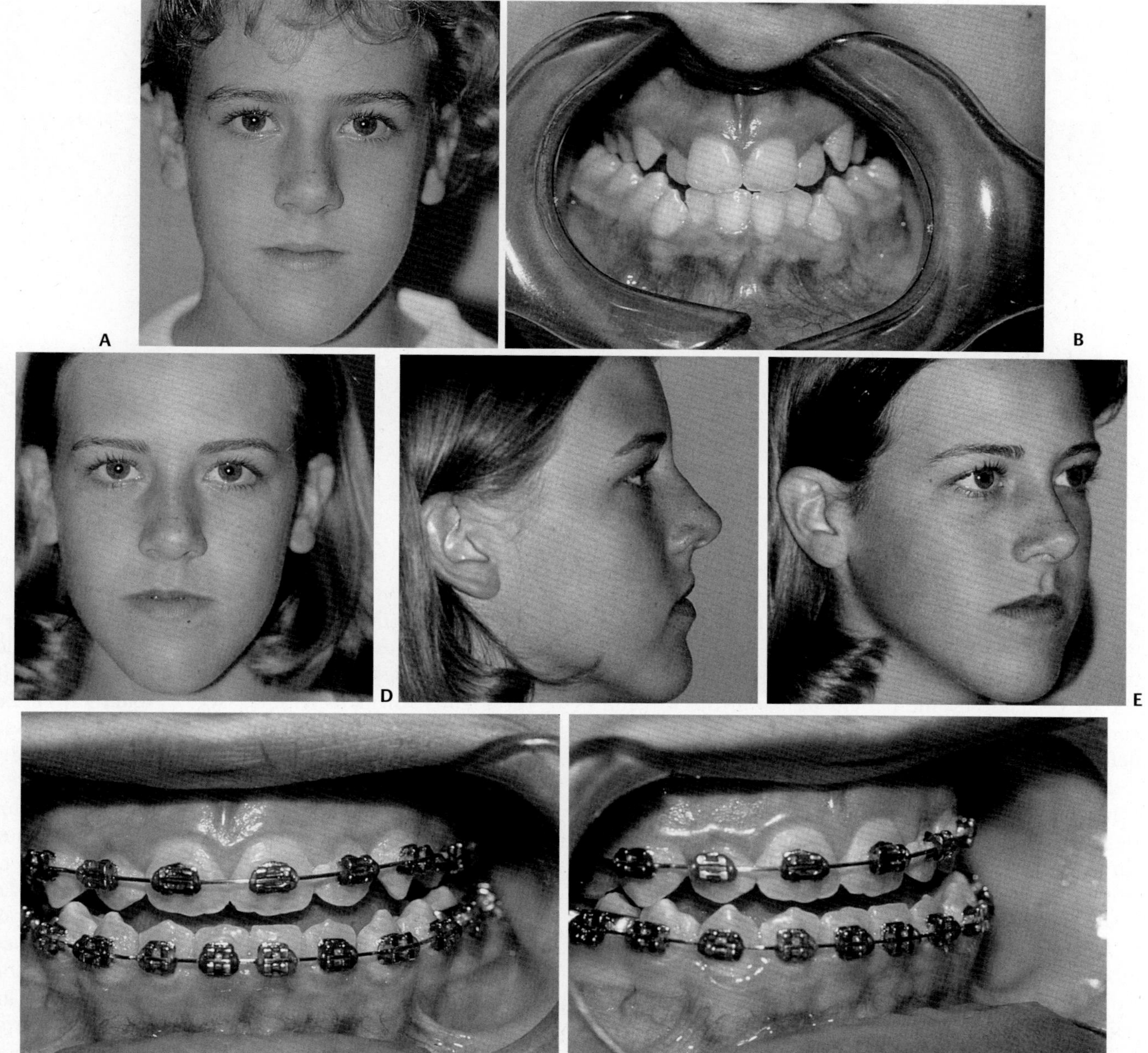

Fig. 78.23 (**A**) Full-face and (**B**) occlusion views of a 15-year-old patient with class III malocclusion, bilateral crossbite, maxillary hypoplasia, and mandibular prognathism. (**C–G**) The same patient after 15 months of orthodontic therapy and prior to two-jaw orthognathic surgery. Note that the orthodontic therapy has straightened the teeth and corrected malrotations but has accentuated the class III malocclusion.

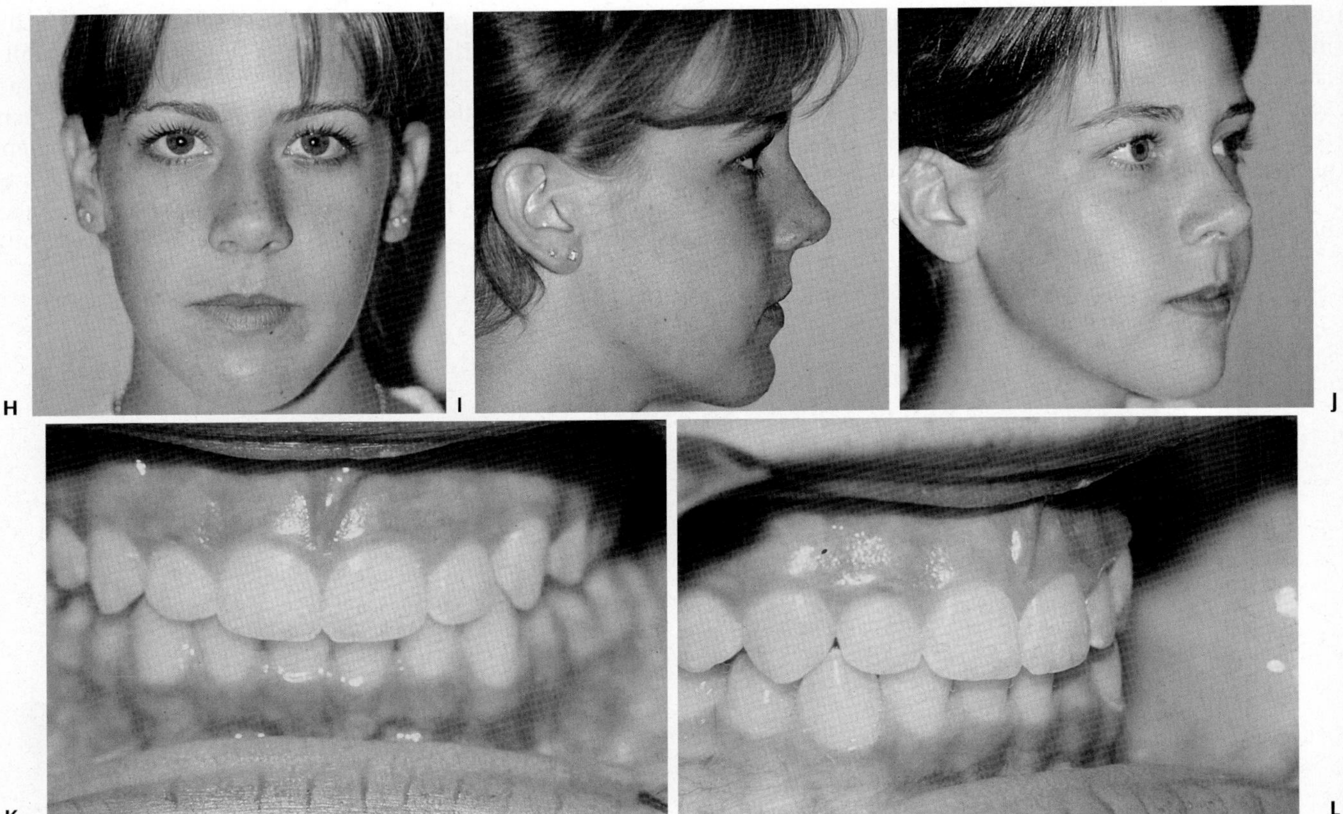

Fig. 78.23 (*Continued*) (**H–L**) Six months after two-jaw orthognathic surgery including Le Fort I maxillary osteotomy, bilateral sagittal split, ramus osteotomy of the mandible with setback, and rotation of the mandible.

genioplasty or chin augmentation may be performed to improve facial harmony. The decision to perform genioplasty versus placement of an alloplastic chin implant has been the subject of significant controversy. The choice should be made by the patient based on the surgeon's comfort with each procedure and the patient's specific deformity.

Horizontal sliding genioplasty has the advantage of achieving excellent aesthetic results without the potential risks of an alloplastic chin implant. It is performed through an intraoral gingivobuccal incision extending from one bicuspid to the other. A horizontal incision is made below the tooth roots, and subperiosteal elevation is accomplished. The mental nerves and inferior mandibular border are not usually exposed. A horizontal incision is outlined anterior to the emergence of the mental nerves. Horizontal incision is made with a series of bur holes, and these are connected with a sagittal saw or osteotome. The distal segment may then be repositioned anteriorly (**Fig. 78.25**).

The amount of anterior chin advancement is limited by the need to maintain good bony contact between the proximal mandible and the advanced distal segment. In extreme cases a bony onlay graft may be necessary to achieve adequate advancement. Stabilization of the bony segments may be accomplished with interosseous wiring or with lag-screw rigid fixation, Bell and Dann[21] demonstrated a 0.8:1 ratio of soft tissue response to skeletal change after sliding genioplasty (**Fig. 78.26**).

Chin augmentation has the advantage of being technically simple and reversible. It may be performed through an intraoral or external (submental) incision. A pocket is made centrally just above the periosteum to accommodate the implant. The implant may be tucked under the periosteum laterally to assist in fixation. Implants may be made of a variety of alloplastic materials, including expanded polytetrafluoroethylene, Silastic (Dow Corning, Midland, MI), Mersilene (Ethicon, Inc., Somerville, NJ), and porous materials such as porous polyethylene, Proplast (Vitek, Houston, TX) or MEDPOR (Porex Surgical, Inc., Newnan, GA). They may also be homografts (e.g., irradiated rib cartilage) or autografts (e.g., calvarial bone). Chin augmentation is often a useful adjunctive procedure to rhinoplasty

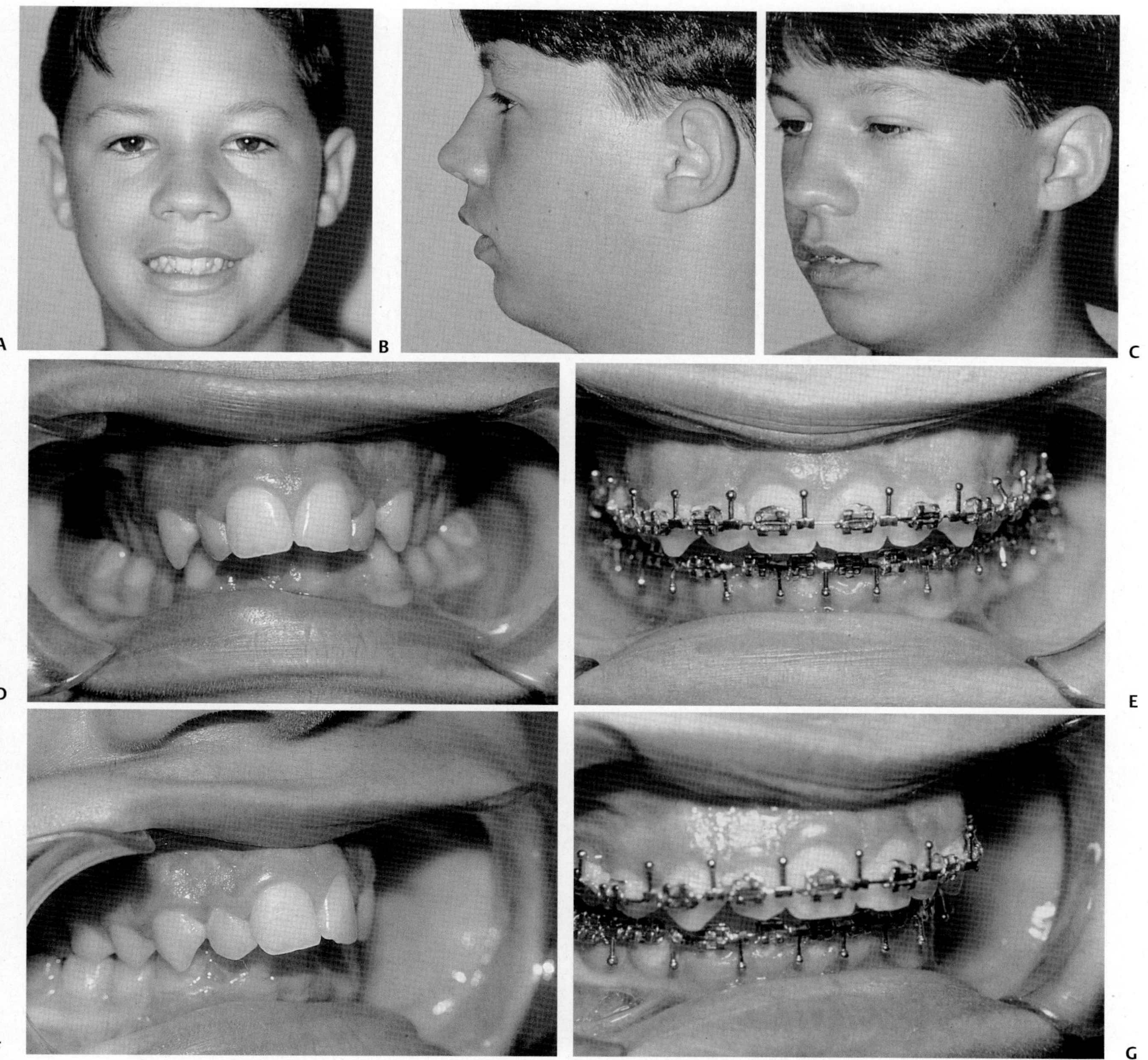

Fig. 78.24 (**A–C**) A 15-year-old boy with class II malocclusion maxillary constriction and retrognathia. (**D,F**) Pre-orthodontic occlusal views of the patient. (**E,G**) Postorthodontic two-jaw occlusal views after 12 months of orthodontic therapy. The patient ultimately underwent mandibular advancement and advancement genioplasty.

or surgical rejuvenation of the lower two thirds of the face (**Fig. 78.27**).

Maxillary Retrusion

Facial imbalance may also result when the middle third of the face is positioned suboptimally. The maxilla may be maldeveloped or malpositioned. It may be normal in architecture but malpositioned anteriorly or posteriorly (maxillary retrusion). Maxillary retrusion may also be associated with maxillar hypoplasia. Maxillary retrusion may be associated with either normal occlusion or class III malocclusion. It may also be present with a normal mandible or simultaneous mandibular malposition.

Diagnosis of midface retrusion may be difficult when the occlusion is normal or when there is simultaneous mandibular deformity. Cephalometric radiography is essential for diagnosis. An SNA angle of less than 79 degrees with

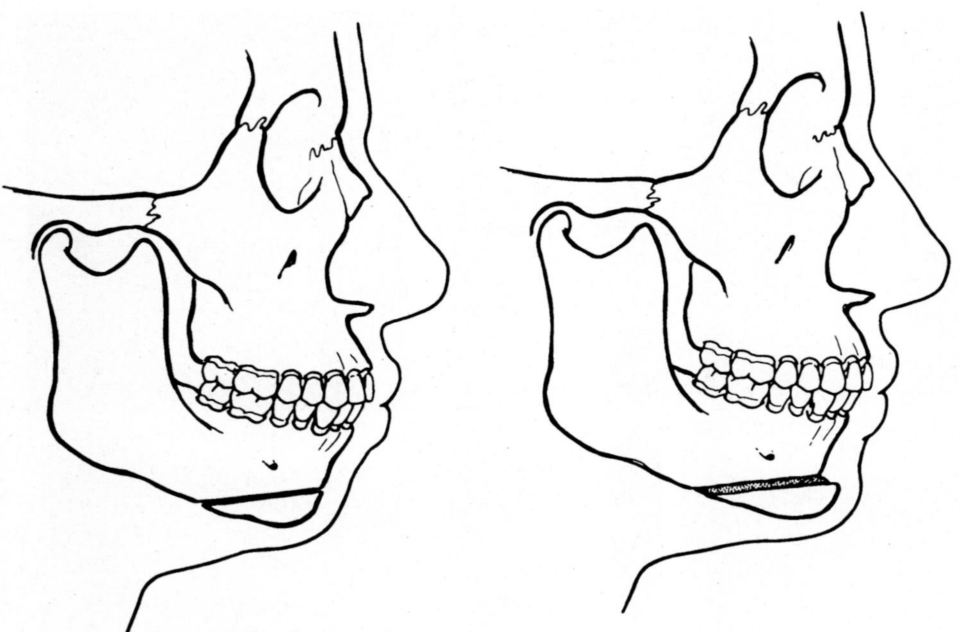

Fig. 78.25 Schematic diagram of a sliding genioplasty and anterior chin advancement.

a normal SNB angle establishes the diagnosis of maxillary retrusion. It is important to analyze not only the position of the skeleton but also its particular contour in patients with suspected maxillary retrusion. The maxillary deformity may be present inferiorly only, with abnormal angulation of the maxillary alveolar shelves. The entire maxilla may be hypoplastic or retruded, requiring attention to both the inferior and superior aspects of the maxilla.

When maxillary hypoplasia exists and occlusion is normal, onlay grafting is appropriate. Augmentation may be performed with autologous cranial or iliac bone or may be achieved with alloplastic materials. Maxillary and

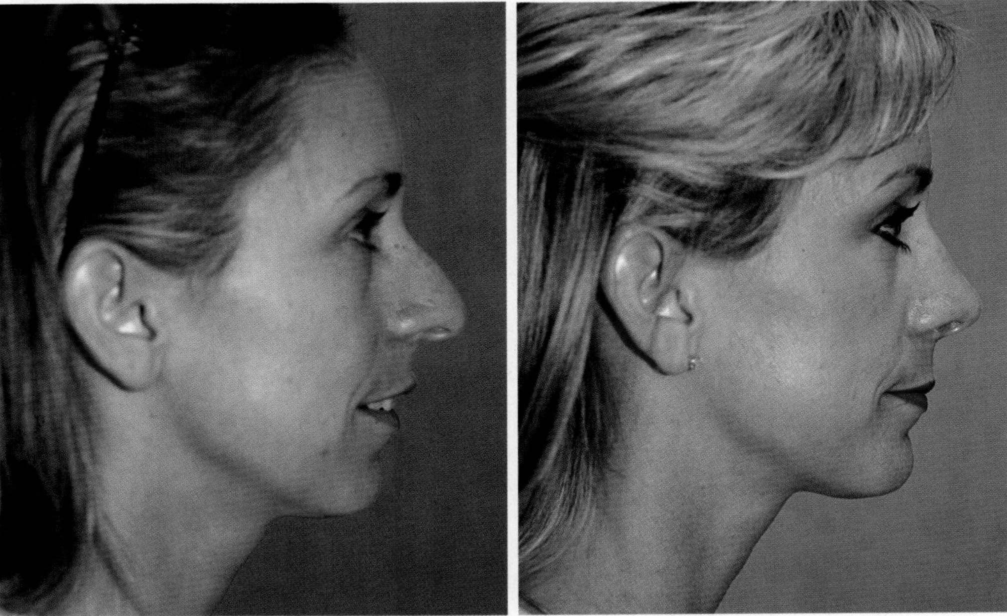

Fig. 78.26 (**A**) Preoperative lateral photograph of a patient with mild class II malocclusion, prominent nasal projection, and moderate microgenia. Note the incomplete lip closure. (**B**) Postoperative lateral photograph of the patient after rhinoplasty and sliding genioplasty with anterior chin advancement.

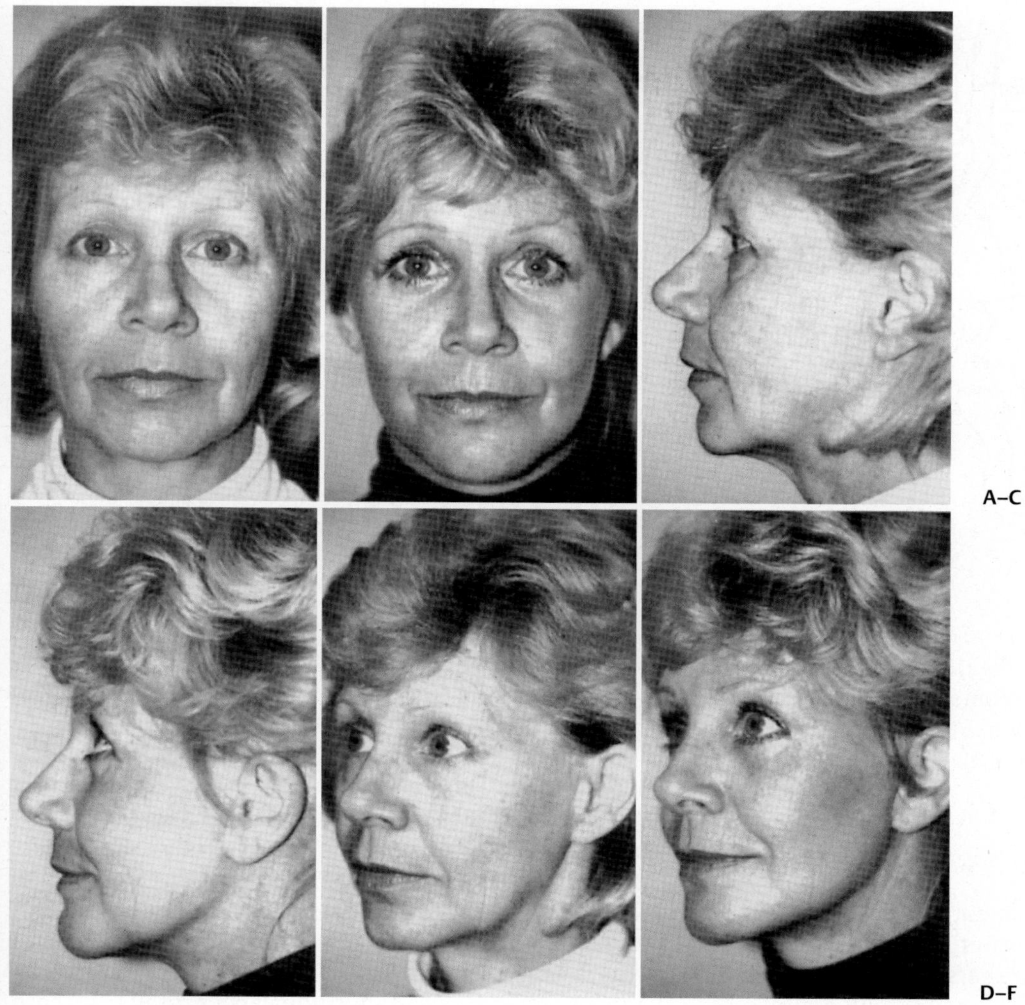

Fig. 78.27 (**A**) Preoperative anteroposterior view photograph. (**B**) Postoperative anteroposterior photograph of the patient 6 months after rhytidectomy, blepharoplasty, and alloplastic chin augmentation. (**C**) Preoperative left lateral photograph. (**D**) Postoperative result. Left lateral view 6 months after surgery. (**E**) Preoperative left oblique view. (**F**) Postoperative left oblique view.

premaxillary augmentation is a useful adjunct to facelift and rhinoplasty surgery.

In patients with retrusion of the inferior aspect of the maxilla, a standard Le Fort I osteotomy is indicated (**Fig. 78.28**).[33] This is a horizontal cut through the walls of the maxillary sinuses and the nasal septum, coupled with separation of the maxilla from the pterygoid plates. A gingivolabial-sulcus incision is made from the level of one second molar tooth to the opposite second molar. Periosteal elevation over the anterior nasal spine, pyriform aperture, and face of the maxilla is then accomplished. A decision must be made regarding the exact level at which to make the horizontal Le Fort I osteotomy. The osteotomy is started in the lateral wall of the pyriform aperture. The medial and lateral walls of the maxillary sinuses are cut, with the lateral cuts extending to the pterygomaxillary fissure. A curved osteotome is positioned in the pterygomaxillary fissure inferiorly and driven medially to separate the alveolar segment from the skull base. The maxilla is then downfractured and mobilized.

Advancement of the maxilla into the predetermined position is then accomplished. An acrylic, occlusal wafer splint is used, and the maxilla is wired to the mandible. The mandibular–maxillary complex may then be moved as a single unit. It is crucial to ensure that the mandibular condyles are well seated in the glenoid fossa before fixation of the maxilla. The maxillary segment may then be stabilized using miniplate rigid fixation.[7] Miniplates should be applied at the thickest portion of the maxilla at the pyriform aperture and zygomatic buttresses (**Fig. 78.29**). An alternative method of fixation is to use intermaxillary wires, with the acrylic occlusal splint as

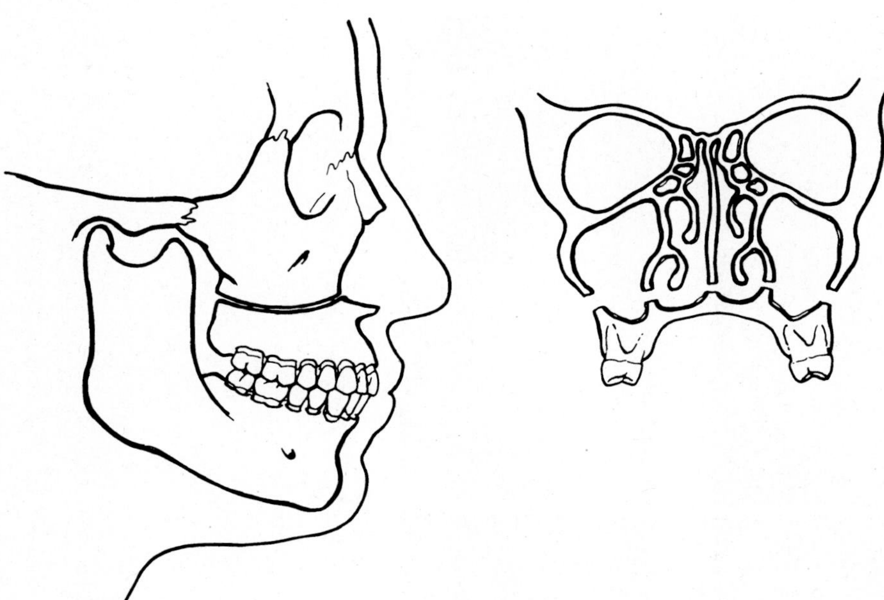

Fig. 78.28 Schematic diagram of a standard Le Fort I osteotomy of the maxilla. This osteotomy consists of cuts through the maxillary sinus, nasal septum, and pterygoid plates. This versatile osteotomy can be used for retrusion, advancement, or intrusion of the maxilla.

a guide. Controversy exists regarding posterior stabilization of the maxillary segments with bone grafts to prevent relapse of the retrusion. Some surgeons believe that bone grafts help maintain the alveolar segment in their advanced position.

Vertical Maxillary Dysplasia

The vertical maxillary component in the analysis and treatment of dentofacial deformities has become more important during the past 20 years.[35] Vertical maxillary excess is characterized by a short upper lip and excessive incisor show at rest. An anterior open bite may be present. Vertical maxillary deficiency is characterized by an apparent excess of upper-lip length, with a lack of incisor display at rest. The ideal lip position at rest shows ~2 to 3 mm of upper incisor. In both forms of vertical maxillary dysplasia, this relationship is disturbed.

Treatment of vertical maxillary dysplasias is usually accomplished using Le Fort I osteotomies. When the vertical dimension of the maxilla is excessive, superior positioning of the maxilla (maxillary intrusion) is accomplished. Bone may then be removed from the lateral aspect of the piriform rim to accommodate maxillary intrusion[20] (**Fig. 78.30**). Treatment of maxillary deficiency (short-face syndrome) is accomplished by downfracture of the maxilla and placement of interpositional bone grafts. In both instances, adequate bone contact must be maintained after osteotomy to ensure good bony healing.

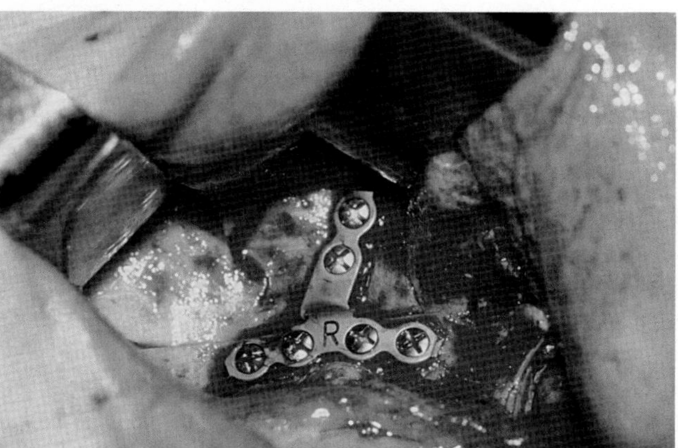

Fig. 78.29 Intraoperative view of a patient undergoing rigid fixation of the maxilla after Le Fort I maxillary osteotomy and advancement. The plate used is a T-shaped, stepped plate for fixation of the maxilla.

Transverse Maxillary Deficiency

Maxillary constriction was first described by Kole in 1959.[36] The maxillary corticotomy, in which the cortex alone is cut, aids in expansion of the palate. After corticotomy, the contour of the maxilla may be changed by using a palatal expander with a jackscrew appliance (**Fig. 78.31**). Surgically assisted rapid expansion is an alternative to segmental (multiple-piece) Le Fort osteotomies for correction of transverse maxillary deficiency.

Distraction Osteogenesis

The concept of lengthening the femur by distraction was introduced by Codivilla[37] in 1905 and expanded to use in the femur by Abbott[38] in 1927. Correction of dentofacial malocclusion was first reported in 1926 by the

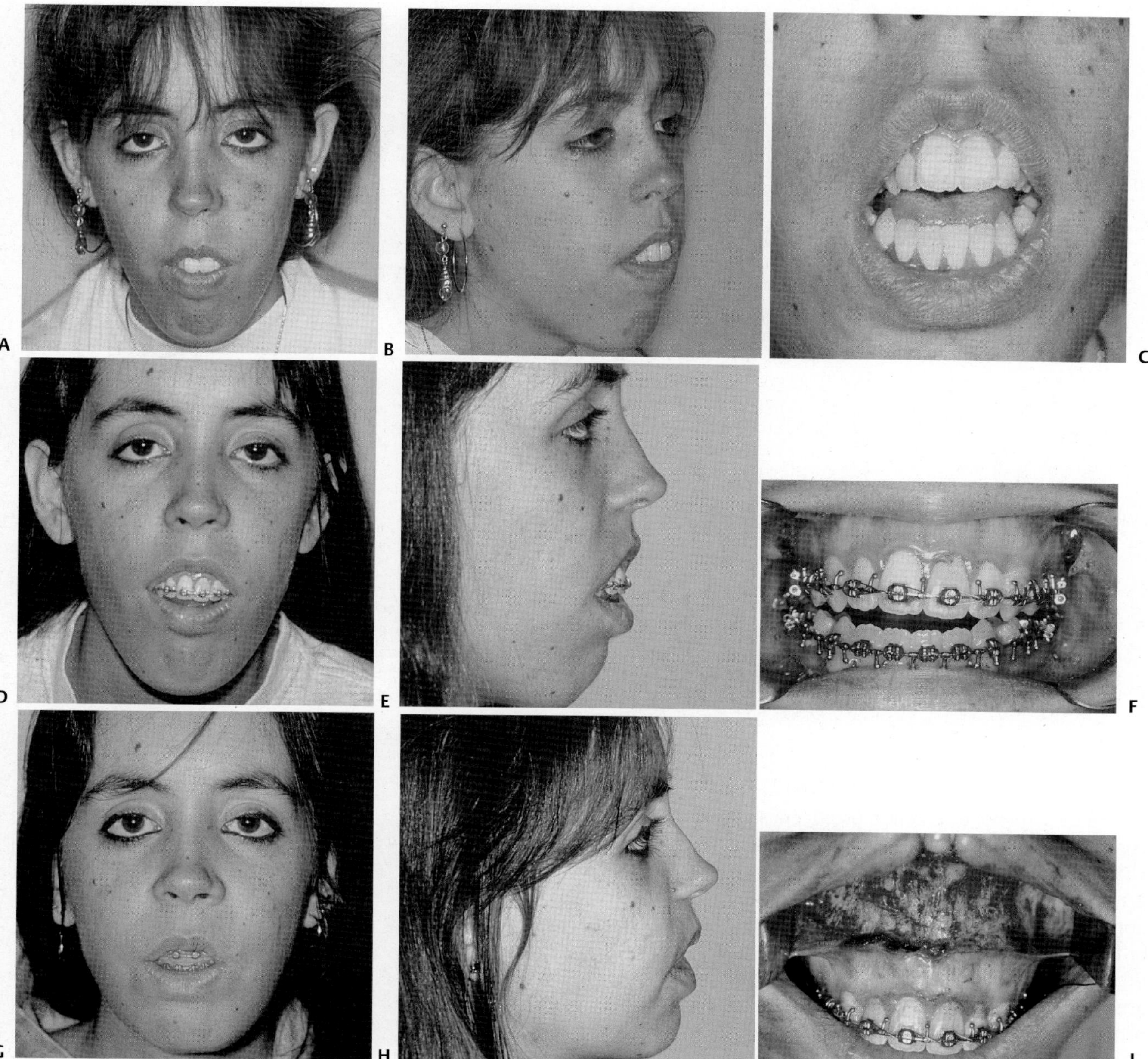

Fig. 78.30 (**A–C**) Preorthodontic photographs of an 18-year-old patient with myotonic dystrophy, severe vertical maxillary excess, and premature posterior contact of the occlusion. The patient has a severe open-bite deformity and labial incompetence. (**D–F**) An 18-year-old patient with myotonic dystrophy after preoperative orthodontic therapy in preparation for Le Fort I maxillary osteotomy with impaction. (**G,H**) Frontal and lateral photographs of the same patient after Le Fort I maxillary osteotomy with impaction and genioplasty with shortening of the chin. (**I**) Reveals intraoperative view of the maxilla showing a severely excessive maxilla in vertical dimension.

German craniofacial surgeon Wassmund for maxillary deficiency.[39,40] In 1927, Rosenthal introduced the term *distraction osteogenesis* when describing his technique of mandibular distraction in a patient with microgenia.[41] Craniofacial distraction osteogenesis was reinvigorated in the 1970s by Snyder, who described a canine mandible model.[42] The application of the technology has expanded to include the maxilla and cranial vault since 1992, when McCarthy reported a clinical series of distraction osteogenesis in human mandibles.[43] Multiple vectors of distraction can now be adjusted to more accurately treat the three-dimensional aspects of a deformity.

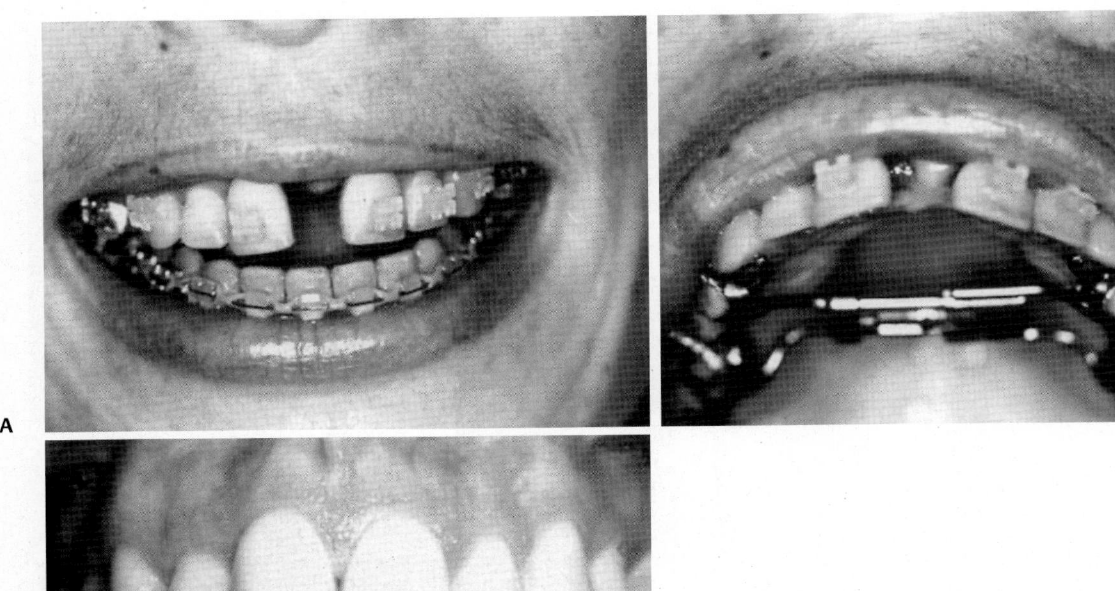

Fig. 78.31 (A) Preoperative occlusal views of a patient with transverse maxillary deficiency and maxillary construction. (B) Postoperative view after maxillary corticotomy with a palatal expander in place. (C) Postoperative occlusal view with palatal expander in place and improved occlusion after rapid palatal expansion. The patient will eventually have orthodontics to close the space between the incisor teeth.

The concepts of distraction osteogenesis have remained constant since being described by Ilizarov as the "the mechanical induction of new bone between bony surfaces that are gradually distracted."[44] The most common craniofacial application is on the mandible. The following description of the phases of distraction osteogenesis will concentrate on the mandible, but the process is similar for the other areas. External fixation devices are the most common and provide excellent control in multiple vectors (**Fig. 78.32**).[45] The resulting pin migration scars are the biggest drawback. On the other hand, internal devices lack the sophistication of external devices, but continue to develop.

In general, the process begins with a specific preoperative estimate of necessary distraction taking into account the soft tissue response that should be anticipated as the underlying bone is expanded. The procedure begins with exposure of targeted bone, which usually requires an external incision. After a periosteal incision, an osteotomy through the cortex protects the neurovascular bundles (e.g., inferior alveolar nerve). Care must be taken to assure bony separation before the distraction hardware is secured. The distraction phase has three important characteristics: latency, rate of distraction, and rhythm. The length of the latency period is the most debated. The callous formation in the original long

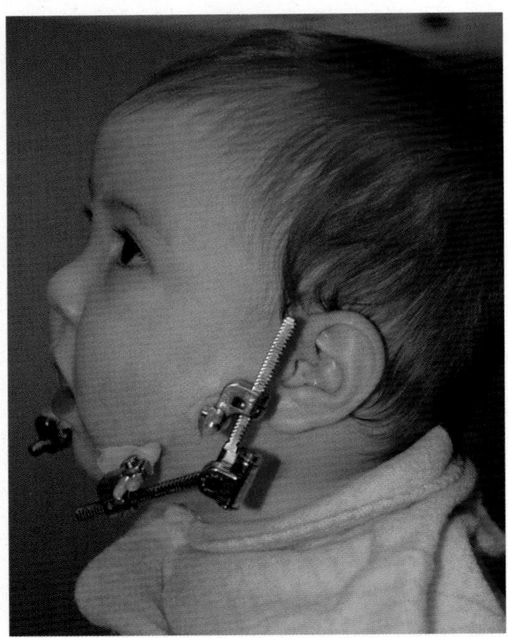

Fig. 78.32 Lateral postoperative photograph of 6-month-old infant with distraction device in place during the distraction phase of 0.5 mm twice a day. The pins will be removed after the consolidation phase.

bone studies is up to 4 to 7 days, whereas in craniofacial applications this time period can result in premature bone union, leading some to advocate only 24 hours latency. Most studies suggest an ideal rate of distraction of 1 to 3 mm a day because too little (<0.5 mm) will result in premature union and too much distraction will create a fibrous malunion. With the proper rate of distraction, immature bone is formed at the osteotomy edges. Ilizarov[44] suggests that a consistent separation provides the best rhythm; however, distraction is most often performed one or two times a day until the goal of distraction is reached. The consolidation phase involves bone remodeling and maturation, but also the soft tissue response to the gradual expansion. As a general rule, the distraction device is left in place for twice the time (4 to 8 months) that the distraction was performed.[46]

Summary

The goal in plastic and reconstructive surgery is to maximize form and function. The convergence of aesthetic and reconstructive concerns is most obvious in the patient with dentofacial deformities. With this in mind, the maxillofacial surgeon attempts to achieve balanced facial proportion. Consideration must be given to the teeth and how they relate to the bones that house them, and, most importantly, to the soft tissues that drape over this skeletal framework. Evaluation of dentofacial deformities should occur in a careful, systematic fashion, including dental, skeletal, and soft tissue analysis. Surgical correction is then performed and facial harmony reestablished.

References

1. Angle EH. Classification of malocclusion. Dent Cosmos 1899;41:248
2. Andrews LF. The six keys to normal occlusion. Am J Orthod 1972;62:296
3. Rakowski T. An Atlas and Manual of Cephalometry Radiography. Philadelphia: Lea & Febiger; 1982
4. Broadbent BH Sr, Broadbent BH Jr, Golden WH. Bolton standards of dentofacial development growth. St Louis: Mosby, 1975.
5. Grayson BH. Cephalometric analysis for the surgeon. Clin Plast Surg 1989;16(4):633
6. Donald PJ. The surgical management of structural facial dysharmony: a self-instructional package. Washington, DC: American Academy of Otolaryngology–Head and Neck Surgery, 1985.
7. Rosen HM. Miniplate fixation of the Le Fort I osteotomies. Plast Reconstr Surg 1986;78:748
8. Hinds EC, Kent JN. Surgical Treatment of Development Jaw Deformities. St Louis: Mosby; 1972
9. Tweed CH. The Frankfort mandibular plane angle in orthodontic diagnosis, classification, treatment planning, and prognosis. Am J Orthod Oral Surg 1946;32:175
10. Burstone CJ, et al. Cephalometrics for orthognathic surgery. J Oral Surg 1978;36:269
11. Jarabak JR, Fizzel JA. Light-Wire Edgewise Appliance. St Louis: Mosby; 1972
12. Hohl TH, Epker BN. Macrogenia: a study of treatment of results with surgical recommendations. Oral Surg Oral Med Oral Pathol 1976;41:454
13. Proffitt WR, Turvey TA, Moriarty JD. Augmentation genioplasty as an adjunct to conservative orthodontic treatment. Am J Orthod; 79:473
14. Gonzales-Ulloa M. Quantitative principles in cosmetic surgery of the face (profileplasty). Plast Reconstr Surg 1961;36:364
15. Gonzales-Ulloa M, Stevens E. The role of chin correction in profile plasty. Plast Reconstr Surg 1966;41:477
16. Bell WH, Proffit WB, White RP. Surgical Correction of Dentofacial Deformities. Philadelphia: WB Saunders; 1980
17. Burstone CJ. Lip posture and its significance in treatment planning. Am J Orthod 1967;53:262
18. Ricketts RM. Define proportion in facial esthetics. Clin Plast Surg 1982;9:401
19. Steiner CC. Cephalometrics as a clinical. In: Kraus BS, Reidel RA, eds. Vistas in Orthodontics. Philadelphia: Lea & Febiger; 1962
20. Lehman JA Jr.. Soft tissue manifestations of aesthetic defects of the jaws: diagnosis and treatment. Clin Plast Surg 1987;14: 763–783
21. Bell WH, Dann JJ. Correction of dentofacial deformities by surgery in the anterior part of the jaws. Am J Orthod 1973;64:162
22. Lines PA, Steinhauser EW. Diagnosis and treatment planning in surgical orthodontic therapy. Am J Orthod 1974;66:378
23. Vanarsdall RL, White RP. Editorial: diagnosis and patient expectations. Int J Adult Orthod 1988
24. Thomas P, Proffitt WR. Combined surgical and orthodontic treatment. In: Proffitt WR, ed. Contemporary Orthodontics. St Louis: Mosby;
25. White RP, Proffitt WR. Surgical orthodontics: a current perspective. In: Johnston LE, ed. New Vistas in Orthodontics. Philadelphia: Lea & Febiger; 1985
26. Worms FW, Isaacson RJ, Speidel TM. Surgical orthodontic treatment planning: profile analysis and mandibular surgery. Angle Orthod 1976;46:1
27. Hinds EC. Surgical correction of acquired mandibular deformities. Am J Orthod 1957;43:161
28. Robinson M. Prognathism correct by open vertical subcondylotomy. J South Calif Dent Assoc 1956;24:22
29. Winstanly RP. Subcondylar osteotomy of the mandible and the intraoral approach. Br J Oral Surg 1968;6:134
30. Obwegeser H, Trauner R. Zur Operationstechnik bei der Progenie und anderen Unterkieferanomalien. Deutsche Zahn-Mund-und-Kieferheillsunde 1955;23:1
31. Trauner R, Obwegeser HL. The surgical correction of mandibular prognathism and retrognathia with consideration of genioplasty I. Oral Surg Oral Med Oral Pathol 1957;10:677
32. Trauner R, Obwegeser HL. The surgical correction of mandibular prognathism and retrognathia with consideration of genioplasty II. Oral Surg Oral Med Oral Pathol 1957;10:787
33. Dal Pont G. Retromolar osteotomy for the correction of prognathism. J Oral Surg 1961;19:42
34. Zaytoun HS, Phillips C, Terry BC. Long-term neurosensory deficits following transoral vertical ramus and sagittal-split osteotomies for mandibular prognathism. J Oral Maxillofac Surg 1966; 44:193
35. West RA. Vertical maxillary dysplasia: diagnosis, treatment planning, and treatment response. Atlas Oral Maxillofac Surg Clin North Am 1990;2:11
36. Kole H. Surgical operations on the alveolar ridge to correct occlusal abnormalities. Oral Surg Oral Med Oral Pathol 1959;12:277
37. Codivilla A. On the means of lengthening in the lower limbs, muscle, and tissue which are shortened through deformity. Am J Orthop Surg 1905;2:353
38. Abbott LC. The operative lengthening of the tibia and fibula. J Bone Joint Surg. 1927;9:128
39. Wassmund M. Frakturen und Luxationen des Gesichtschadels. Berlin: Meuser; 1926:360
40. Honig JF, Grohmann UA, Merten HA. Facial bone distraction osteogenesis for correction of malocclusion: a more than 70- year-old concept in craniofacial surgery. Plast Reconstr Surg 2002;109:41

41. Rosenthal W. In: E Sonntag and W Rosenthal, eds. Lehrbuch der Mund und Kieferchirurgie. Leipzig: Georg Thieme; 1930:173–175
42. Synder CC, Levine GA, Swanson HM, Browne EZ. Mandibular lengthening by gradual distraction: preliminary report. Plast Reconstr Surg 1973;51:506
43. McCarthy JG, Schreiber J, McCarthy JG, et al. Lengthening the human mandible by gradual distraction. Plast Reconstr Surg 1992;89:1
44. Ilizarov GA. Basic principles of transosseous compression and distraction osteosynthesis. Ortop Travmatol Protez 1971;32:7–9
45. Mandell DL, Yellon RF, Bradley JP, Izadi K, Gordan CB. Mandibular distraction for micrognathia and severe upper airway obstruction. Arch Otolaryngol Head Neck Surg 2004;130:344–348
46. Imola MJ, Hamlar DD, Thatcher G, Chowdhury K. The versatility of distraction osteogenesis in craniofacial surgery. Arch Facial Plast Surg 2003;4:8–19

79 Classification and Management of Hemifacial Microsomia

Karin Vargervik

The mandible, the temporomandibular joint (TMJ), and the outer and middle ear structures are derived from the first and second branchial arches. Disruption of cell migration or proliferation such as could occur by a vascular insult have been implicated as etiologic factors in hemifacial microsomia (HFM), which is the most commonly occurring congenital anomaly affecting these structures.[1] Animal models mimicking clinical findings in humans have been developed by various experimental methods.[2–4]

HFM is primarily a unilateral congenital birth defect with involvement of several skeletal, neuromuscular, and other soft tissue components of the first and second branchial arches. The condition includes a wide spectrum of craniofacial anomalies and may also have ocular, renal, spinal, and cardiac components. Dysmorphologists and others have created a variety of terms to describe the broad spectrum of phenotypes, but HFM remains the most widely used name. Other terms include oculoauriculovertebral (OAV) spectrum, craniofacial microsomia, otomandibular dysostosis, and lateral facial dysplasia.[5–7] OAV dysplasia may be considered a separate category of HFM, also referred to as Goldenhar syndrome. The additional characteristics of this type are epibulbar dermoids and cervical spine abnormalities. There is also a higher incidence of oronasal clefting in this type, and most likely there are specific etiologic factors causing this constellation of birth defects. HFM is the second most common congenital craniofacial anomaly after cleft lip and palate. The most frequently quoted incidence estimate is 1 in 5600 live births.[6,8] There seems to be agreement that there is male predominance and a right side predominance as well.[9] For an extensive overview of the very heterogeneous phenotypes in this spectrum, the reader is referred to the work of Cohen et al[5] and Peterson-Falzone.[7] In the mildest form of HFM, the only clinical manifestation may be ear tags with or without malformed ears. The most severe cases may present with malformed ears, temporal bone involvement including missing glenoid fossa, malformed or absent joint structures, and mandibular ramus including both coronoid and condylar processes (**Fig. 79.1**).

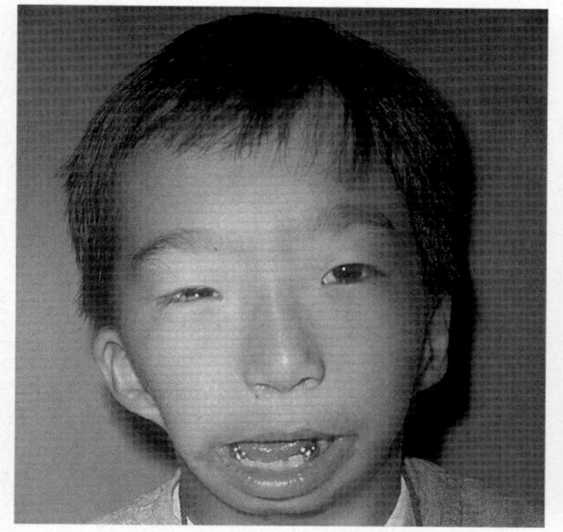

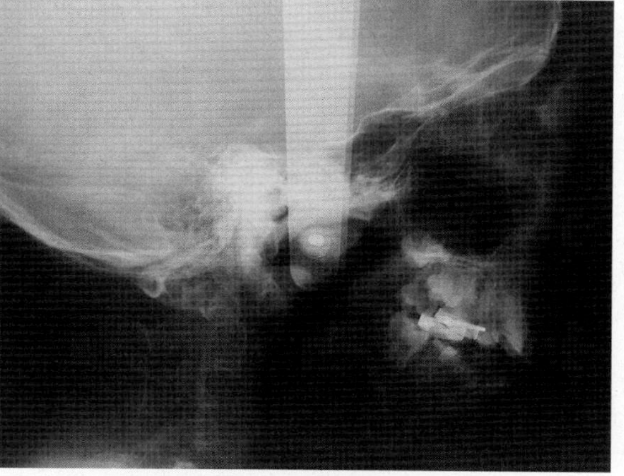

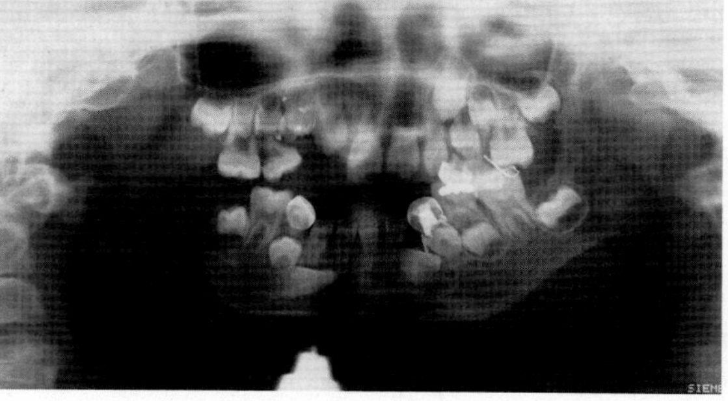

Fig. 79.1 (**A**) Goldenhar type of malformation with bilateral epibulbar dermoids, right macrostomia, chin deviation to right, deficient soft tissue development on right, mild ear deformity. (**B**) The lateral headfilm shows mandibular and cervical spine malformations. (**C**) The panoramic radiograph demonstrates bilateral mandibular involvement with type I malformation on the left side and type III on the right, with the entire mandibular ramus missing.

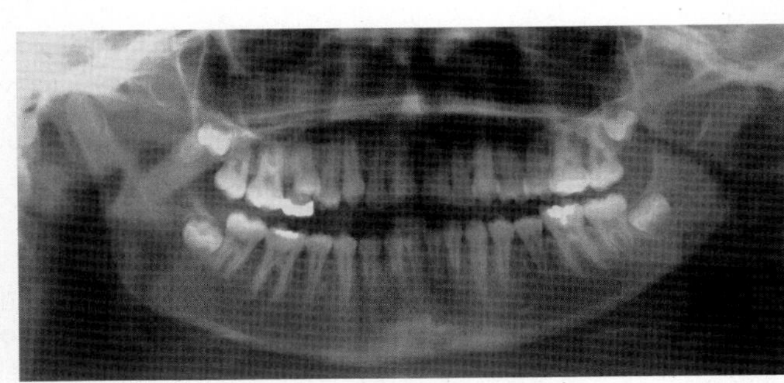

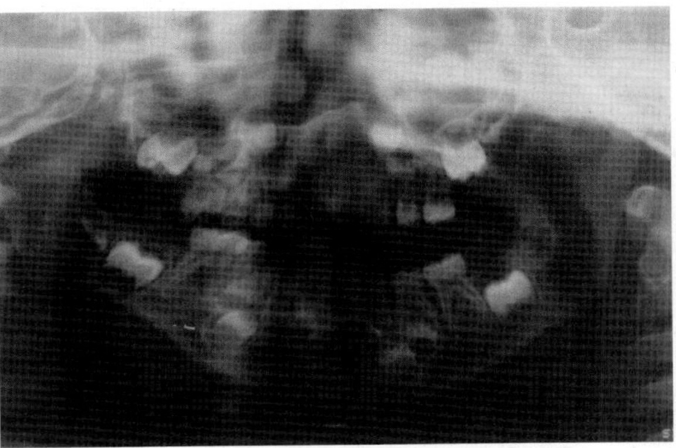

Fig. 79.2 (**A**) Left side type I, right side normal. (**B**) Right side type I with a very underdeveloped ramus, but all parts present.

Classification

By Phenotype

Tenconi and Hall[10] distinguished between the classic type, microphthalmic type, bilateral asymmetrical type, complex with limb deformity type, frontonasal type, and Goldenhar 3:2 type. The "infant of diabetic mother" type was recently added.[11–13] Of the 67 individuals included in the Tenconi and Hall study, 14.9% had some type of cardiac malformation, 5.9% had renal system malformations, 17.6% had microcephaly, and 13.3% had developmental delay. Cervical spine abnormalities were not assessed by them, but our finding and those of others indicate that close to 50% have some type of cervical spine abnormality.[14–17]

The OMENS classification represents an attempt to include all of the prominent features of HFM: *o*rbit, *m*andible, *e*ar, facial *n*erve, *s*keletal. Each entity is graded from 1 to 3 according to severity. Others have suggested that additions, such as the presence of noncraniofacial involvement, be annotated by an asterisk (OMENS*).[18–20]

The SAT classification system addresses only three main features: *s*keletal, *a*uricle, and soft *t*issue.[21] In this system, there are five levels of skeletal deformity (S1 to S5), four levels of auricular deformity (A0 to A3), and three levels of soft tissue deformity (T1 to T3). As an example, they indicate that an individual with minimal deformity might be classified as S1A0T1, whereas an individual with severe deformity would be S5A3T3. It does not appear that this classification system has clear advantages over the OMENS system, and it falls short of including all of the most essential elements.[20]

By Mandibular Involvement

This chapter emphasizes the mandibular and temporomandibular bone and joint malformations and malfunctions. The classification system we use is an amalgamation of the classifications described by Pruzansky,[22] Kaban and coworkers,[23] and Harvold, Vargervik, and coworkers.[24,25] Describing middle and lower face involvement, it is based on discrete findings of the presence or absence of critical elements of the mandible and temporomandibular joints and consists of types I, IIA, IIB, and III.

In type I, all parts of the affected side of the mandible and the attached muscles are present but are hypoplastic to varying degrees (**Fig. 79.2**). The glenoid fossa is usually missing, and translatory joint movement is minimal. Rotational movement of the condyle is usually not impaired, resulting in hinge movement on the affected side. During jaw opening, the mandible shifts to the affected side because translatory movement occurs on the contralateral side only. Frequently, the contralateral condyle moves excessively during maximum jaw opening.

Type IIA is characterized by a cone-shaped, anteriorly and medially displaced condyle, missing glenoid fossa, but presence of all masticatory muscles with varying degrees of hypoplasia (**Fig. 79.3**). The jaws and face are usually

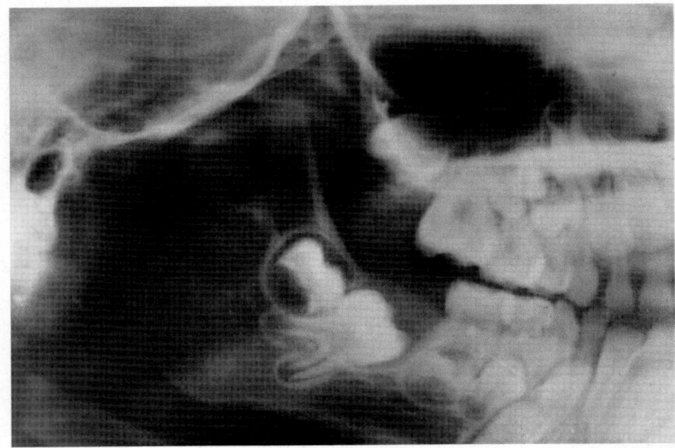

Fig. 79.3 Type IIA mandible with cone-shaped, anteriorly displaced condylar process.

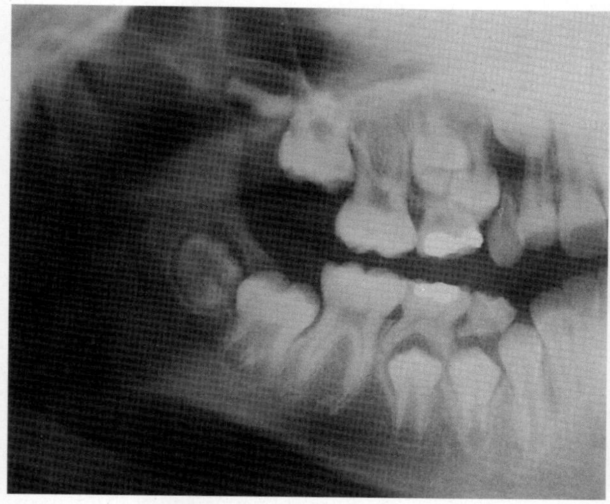
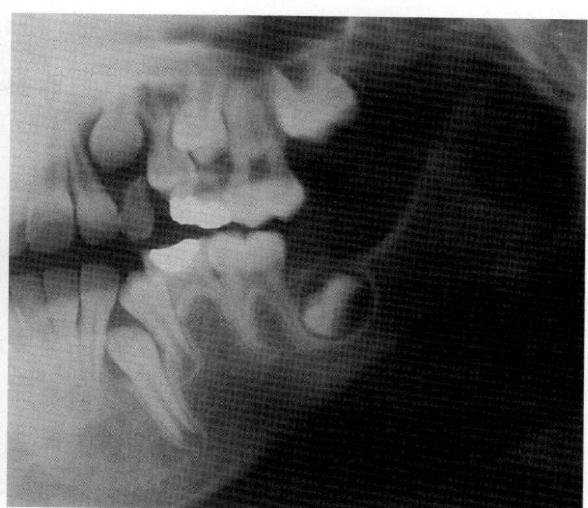

Fig. 79.4 Type IIB mandible with only one ramus extension.

highly asymmetrical. In type IIB, the condyle is missing along with the lateral pterygoid muscle (**Fig. 79.4**). The coronoid process is usually small and the temporal muscle hypoplastic. Jaw and facial asymmetry are usually quite marked.

Type III represents congenital absence of the entire ramus of the mandible and most of the masticatory muscles (**Fig. 79.1C**). The mandible can be guided freely into various positions because the movements of the affected side are not limited by either joint structures or muscles and ligaments. All joint structures are missing, and frequently the temporal region is flat or even concave, resulting in a poor platform for the ear, which is usually affected and requires reconstruction. **Tables 79.1** and **79.2**

Table 79.1 Morphological Characteristics of the Mandible and Associated Muscles in Hemifacial Microsomia

	Bony Characteristics				Muscle Characteristics		
Mandibular Type	**Glenoid Fossa**	**Condyle**	**Coronoid Process**	**Gonial Area**	**Masseter and Med. Pterygoid**	**Lateral Pterygoid**	**Temporalis**
I	Absent	Present but small	Present	Present to varying degree	Present but small	Present	Present but small
IIA	Absent	Cone-shaped and displaced	Present	Present	Present	Present	Present
IIB	Absent	Absent	Present	Absent	Rudimentary	Absent	Present
III	Absent	Absent	Absent	Absent	Rudimentary or absent	Absent	Rudimentary

Table 79.2 Functional Characteristics of Hemifacial Microsomia

		Jaw Movements				
Mandibular Type	**Rotation**	**Translation**	**Deviation on Opening**	**Palate Elevation**	**Other Facial Nerve Involvement**	**Hearing**
I	Unrestricted	Usually none	Toward affected side	Less on affected side	Varies	Loss on affected side
IIA	Unrestricted	None	Toward affected side	Less on affected side	Varies	Loss on affected side
IIB	Unrestricted	None	Toward affected side	Less on affected side	Varies	Loss on affected side
III	Unrestricted	None	Toward affected side	Less on affected side	Varies	Loss on affected side

summarize the morphological and functional characteristics of HFM.

Mandibular Growth

Normal

In the embryo, mandibular bone formation starts in association with the Meckel cartilage and around the developing tooth buds. The osseous areas expand, coalesce, and become the body of the mandible. The neuromuscular and vascular networks are well established before bone formation starts and are presumably prerequisites for osteogenesis. During these early stages of development, the mandibular structures are carried forward by the growing Meckel cartilage. The various muscle masses become attached to or included in the developing bone, probably by the same mechanisms by which muscle reattachment occurs.[26] The posterior muscles extending into the temporal region provide the environment for development of the ramus with the condylar and coronoid processes. The condylar process and the developing TMJ structures in association with the lateral pterygoid muscle presumably take over the propulsive action, which up to that point has been provided by the Meckel cartilage. This new propulsive mechanism continues postnatally throughout the growth period and presumably functions by sensorimotor feedback, primarily from the joint structures.[27] It appears that the periodic proliferation of condylar cartilage toward the glenoid fossa elicits activity in the lateral pterygoid muscle, which advances the condyle, thereby maintaining the optimal joint space. The various areas of the mandible remodel as the jaw is brought forward relative to its muscles and other structures. Bone apposition, which replaces cartilage in the interface between condylar cartilage and bone, appears to occur only when the cartilage is proliferating.[28] The condylar cartilage is therefore a controlling factor during growth.

Hemifacial Microsomia

In patients with HFM, the very structures that are essential to mandibular growth are affected; therefore, impairment of mandibular growth is always present, varying in degree according to the primary tissue deficiencies. Characteristically, in most individuals with HFM, the affected side of the mandible and the associated muscles grow less than the contralateral side. However, it is interesting to note that even in type III where the entire ramus is missing, the length of the mandibular body increases as bone forms around each successively developing tooth bud. This side of the mandible is gradually brought forward to a small degree, presumably by the presence and function of the tongue and tissues in the floor of the mouth. Because the main propulsive factors in advancing the mandible (condylar cartilage and lateral pterygoid muscle) are rudimentary or missing, it is understandable that jaw and facial asymmetry may increase rather than improve with growth.

Treatment of Craniofacial Abnormalities in Hemifacial Microsomia

The overall team management for a child with HFM involves attention to respiration, hearing, speech and language development, psychosocial issues, and management of associated problems, such as cervical spine fusions, scoliosis, epibulbar dermoids, and other eye problems. Every child with HFM should have a renal sonogram, cardiac evaluation, spinal radiographs, computed tomographic (CT) scans of ear structure, ophthalmology consultation, and management and intervention as needed.

Treatment of Mandibular Abnormalities

Early Intervention for Jaw Asymmetries

Our rationale for early treatment has been that some of the secondary unfavorable adaptations to deficient growth of the mandible could be prevented and that, where condylar and coronoid structures exist (types I and IIA), additional bone apposition could be achieved by providing a substitute for the normal advancing mechanisms.[29–32] A functional appliance of the activator type, with or without a buccal shield, has therefore been used routinely in our HFM patients as an initial treatment phase. Generally, this treatment is started at the time of the eruption of the 6-year molars. The expectations from this treatment phase include increased length of the mandible on the affected side and reduced vertical development of the maxilla on the contralateral side, resulting in an open bite (**Fig. 79.5**).

Mandibular Surgery

The second treatment phase is surgical lengthening or reconstruction of the affected mandibular ramus. If done during the mixed dentition stage, it is often possible to avoid a surgical procedure on the maxilla by minimizing the secondary growth inhibition on the affected side.[25,30,33] The exceptions are situations where the maxillary dental midline is severely deviated from the facial

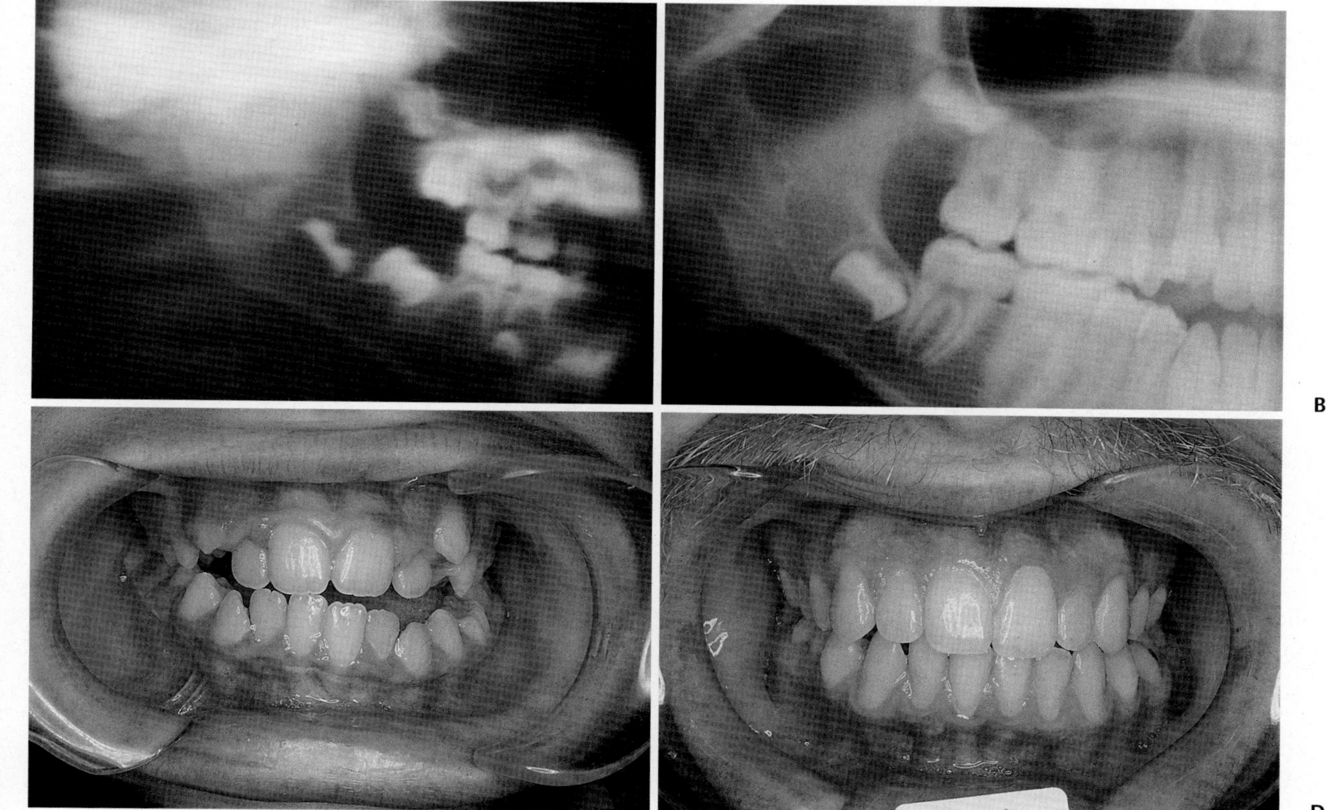

Fig. 79.5 (**A**) Age 6 years. Treatment with a functional appliance was started when the 6-year molars erupted. (**B**) Age 14 years. Note size increase and condylar development. (**C**) Open bite on contralateral side after functional appliance use. (**D**) Final occlusion after right mandibular lengthening and orthodontic treatment.

midline and orthodontic correction of the dental midline discrepancy is impossible, or where the vertical maxillary development on the contralateral side is excessive. It is generally not possible to correct a severely canted maxillary occlusal plane until an open bite has been created by surgical repositioning of the mandible. If maxillary surgery is anticipated due to severity of maxillary involvement, both jaw procedures can be postponed until most of the child's growth is complete. The more general growth there is remaining in the youngster, the higher the probability that the asymmetry will redevelop due to less growth on the reconstructed side than on the contralateral side of the mandible. A transplanted costochondral graft may also grow excessively, thereby creating an asymmetry to the opposite side. Following the mandibular surgery, the position of the mandible relative to the maxilla is secured by a bite registration splint and interarch fixation wires. Depending on the type of mandibular surgical procedure, the length of the fixation may vary from 2 weeks, if rigid or semirigid fixation was achieved, to 6 weeks if the entire mandibular ramus has been reconstructed. Following removal of the interarch fixation wires, the splint is attached to the maxilla with elastics to allow removal for cleaning. Lightweight guiding elastics are placed to the mandible to ensure precise and controlled mandibular movements into the splint.[25,30] This is a period for reattachment of muscles and ligaments, retraining of the neuromuscular system to a new position of the mandible, and formation of new bone as the bone graft is gradually replaced and remodeled. This very important adjustment period should last for several weeks. The progression of new bone formation and remodeling is monitored by panoramic radiographs. Continued growth of the reconstructed ramus/condyle unit is still unpredictable, and many factors are involved.[34,35]

Lengthening of the affected mandibular ramus by distraction has become popular lately.[36–38] Because this technique has both advantages and disadvantages, at this stage cases should be selected with care. When distraction osteogenesis can be applied in such a way that significant muscle lengthening is achieved, the approach will have

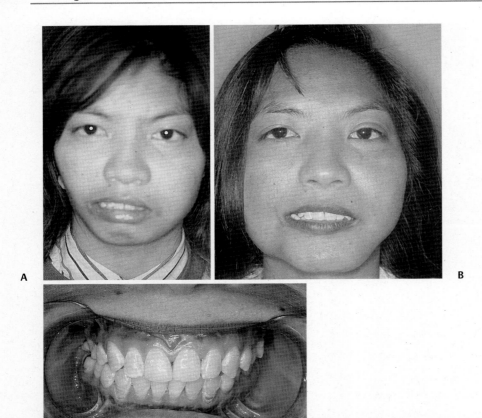

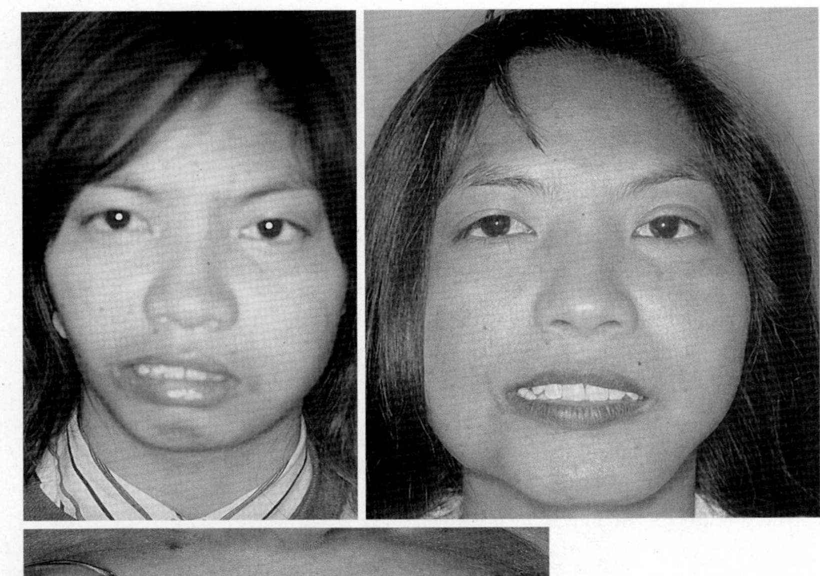

Fig. 79.6 (**A**) Before starting treatment, age 12 years. (**B**) After mandibular and maxillary reconstruction, orthodontic treatment, and soft tissue augmentation. (**C**) Final occlusion.

a major advantage over other lengthening procedures in selected cases.

Closure of Open Bite on the Affected Side

The postsurgical treatment phase blends into the next phase if it is expected that the unilateral maxillary underdevelopment can be corrected without a surgical procedure. The open bite created by lengthening of the affected mandibular ramus is protected by a maxillary bite plate. Auxiliary springs are placed on this plate for active extrusion of the maxillary teeth on the affected side.

Orthodontic Treatment

Full orthodontic treatment is started after eruption of the permanent teeth and after most of the jaw growth is completed. Standards for treatment outcome are the same for these patients as they would be for any other orthodontic patient. It is very important not to resort to interarch elastic mechanics that may contribute to redevelopment of the jaw asymmetry. It should be recognized that it may be very difficult, if not impossible, to correct unfavorable dentoalveolar adaptations completely. This is a particular challenge in the presence of an asymmetrical palate and tongue.

Table 79.3 Sequential Treatment Procedures in Hemifacial Microsomia

- Ear reconstruction (three procedures, starting at age 6–7)
- Presurgical jaw orthopedic treatment (phase I)
- Mandibular surgery (phase II)
- Lengthening/reconstruction of ramus with or without bone graft
- Interarch fixation with splint
- Controlled jaw movements with splint and guiding elastics
- Closure of open bite (phase III)
- Extrusion of maxillary teeth
- Alternatively, surgical correction of maxilla
- Orthodontic treatment (phase IV)
- Additional surgical procedures (optional phase V)
- Asymmetric genioplasty and nasal septal reconstruction
- Soft tissue augmentation

Table 79.4 Treatment Procedures for Hemifacial Microsomia by Age and Type

Type	0–6 years	6–12 years	12–14/15 years	>15 years
I	Team evaluations Hearing aid, if needed Ear tag removal Monitor eruption of teeth	Team evaluations Monitor eruption of teeth Treatment phases 1, 2, 3. May postpone phase 2 (mandibular surgery) if response to phase 1 (jaw orthopedic treatment) is favorable. Stages 1, 2, 3 ear reconstruction.	Team evaluations Phase 4 treatment (treatment phases 1, 2, 3 if not done previously)	If needed: Asymmetric genioplasty Rhinoplasty Soft tissue augmentation
IIA	Same as for I	Same as for I Mandibular surgery almost always necessary	Same as for I	Same as for I
IIB	Same as for I	Same as for I Mandibular surgery always necessary	Same as for I	Same as for I
III	Same as for I and macrostomia and ramus reconstruction if functional impairments dictate	Same as for I Ramus reconstruction always necessary	Same as for I	Same as for I

Surgical Treatment of Other Craniofacial Abnormalities

Reconstruction of a malformed or missing ear usually requires three surgical procedures, which are generally started at about age 6 years. Additional surgical procedures are often needed to correct bony chin asymmetry, nasal septal deviation, and soft tissue deficiency. The asymmetrical genioplasty and nasal septal reconstruction are done simultaneously. As the very last procedure, soft tissue augmentation may be indicated. If the soft tissue asymmetry is mild, the transferred tissue may be a double dermis graft obtained from the buttock.[24] However, if more tissue bulk is needed, a muscle flap transfer by microvascular procedures may be the choice[39] (**Fig. 79.6**). **Tables 79.3 and 79.4** summarize treatment interventions in HFM.

References

1. Poswillo D. The aetiology and pathogenesis of craniofacial deformity. Development 1988;103(Suppl):207
2. Johnston MC, Bronsky PT. Prenatal craniofacial development: new insights on normal and abnormal mechanisms. Crit Rev Oral Biol Med 1995;6:25–79
3. Cousley RRJ, Wilson DJ. Hemifacial microsomia: developmental consequence of perturbation of the auriculofacial cartilage model. Am J Med Genet 1992;42:461–466
4. Naora H, Kimura M, Otani H, et al. Transgenic mouse models of hemifacial microsomia: cloning and characterization of insertional mutation region on chromosome 10. Genomics 1994;23:515–519
5. Cohen MM Jr, Rollnick BR, Kaye CI. Oculoauriculovertebral spectrum: an updated critique. Cleft Palate J 1989;26:276–286
6. Gorlin RJ, Pindborg J, Cohen MM Jr. Syndromes of the Head and Neck. 2nd ed. New York: McGraw-Hill; 1976:546–552
7. Peterson-Falzone S. An introduction to complex craniofacial disorders. In: Berkowitz S, ed. Cleft Lip and Palate. Vol 2. San Diego: Singular Publishing Group; 1996:209
8. Grabb WC. The first and second branchial arch syndrome. Plast Reconstr Surg 1965;36:485–508
9. Rollnick BR, Kaye CI, Nagatoshi K, et al. Oculoauriculovertebral dysplasia and variants: phenotypic characteristics of 294 patients. Am J Med Genet 1987;26:361–375
10. Tenconi R, Hall BC. Hemifacial microsomia: phenotypic classification, clinical implications, and genetic aspects. In: Harvold EP, ed. Treatment of Hemifacial Microsomia. New York: Alan R Liss; 1983: 39–49
11. Grix A Jr. Malformations in infants of diabetic mothers. Am J Med Genet 1982;13:131–137
12. Johnson JP, Fineman RM. Branchial arch malformation in infants of diabetic mothers: two case reports and a review. Am J Med Genet 1982;13:125–130
13. Peterson-Falzone SJ, Seto S, Golabi M. Hemifacial microsomia in children of diabetic mothers. SENTAL annual meeting and personal communication, 1989
14. Avon SW, Shiveley JL. Orthopaedic manifestations of Goldenhar syndrome. J Pediatr Orthop 1988;8:683–686
15. Figueroa AA, Friede H. Craniovertebral malformations in hemifacial microsomia. J Craniofac Genet Dev Biol Suppl 1985;1:167–178
16. Gosain AK, McCarthy JG, Pinto RS. Cervicovertebral anomalies and basilar impressions in Goldenhar syndrome. Plast Reconstr Surg 1994; 93:498–506
17. Gibson JNA, Sillence DO, Taylor TKF. Abnormalities of the spine in Goldenhar syndrome. J Pediatr Orthop 1996;16:344–349
18. Vento AR, LaBrie RA, Mulliken JB. The OMENS classification of hemifacial microsomia. Cleft Palate Craniofac J 1991;28:68–76
19. Horgan JE, Padwa BL, La Brie RA, Mulliken JB. OMENS. Plus: analysis of craniofacial and extracraniofacial anomalies in hemifacial microsomia. Cleft Palate Craniofac J 1995;32:405–412
20. Cousley RR. A comparison of two classification systems for hemifacial microsomia. Br J Oral Maxillofac Surg 1993;31:78–82
21. David DJ, Mahatumarat C, Cooter RD. Hemifacial microsomia: a multisystem classification. Plast Reconstr Surg 1987;80:525–535
22. Pruzansky S. Not all dwarfed mandibles are alike. Birth Defects Orig Artic Ser 1969;1:120–129
23. Kaban LB, Mulliken JB, Murray JE. Three-dimensional approach to analysis and treatment of hemifacial microsomia. Cleft Palate J 1981;18:90
24. Harvold EP, Vargervik K, Chierici G, eds. Treatment of Hemifacial Microsomia. New York: Alan R Liss; 1983
25. Vargervik K, Kaban LB. Hemifacial microsomia: diagnosis and management. In: Bell WH, ed. Modern Practice in Orthognathic and Reconstructive Surgery. Philadelphia: WB Saunders; 1992:1533–1559
26. Chierici G, Miller AJ. Experimental study of muscle reattachment following surgical detachment. J Oral Maxillofac Surg 1984;42:485

27. Storey A. Temporomandibular joint receptors. In: Anderson OJ, Matthews B, eds. Mastication. Bristol, England: John Wright and Sons; 1976:50
28. Petrovic A, Stutzman J, Oudet C. Control processes in postnatal growth of condylar cartilage of the mandible. In: McNamara JAJ, ed. Determinants of Mandibular Form and Growth: Proceedings of a Sponsored Symposium Honoring Professor Robert E. Moyers. Ann Arbor: University of Michigan; 1975:100. Craniofacial Growth Series, no. 4
29. Melsen B, Bjerregaard J, Bundgaard M. The effect of treatment with functional appliances on a pathologic growth pattern of the condyle. Am J Orthod Dentofacial Orthop 1986;90:503–512
30. Vargervik K, Ousterhout DK. Factors affecting long-term results in hemifacial microsomia. Cleft Palate J 1986;23(Suppl):53–68
31. Silvestri A, Natali G, Iannetti G. Functional therapy in hemifacial microsomia: therapeutic protocol for growing children. J Oral Maxillofac Surg 1996;54:271–280
32. Kaplan RG. Induced condylar growth in a patient with hemifacial microsomia. Angle Orthod 1989;59:85–90
33. Kaban LB, Moses ML, Muliken JB. Correction of hemifacial microsomia in the growing child. Cleft Palate J 1986;23(Suppl 1):50–52
34. Peltomaki T. Growth of a costochondral graft in the rat temporomandibular joint. J Oral Maxillofac Surg 1992;50:851–857
35. Perrott DH, Vargervik K, Kaban LB. Costochondral reconstruction of mandibular condyles in nongrowing primates. J Craniofac Surg 1995; 6:227–237
36. McCarthy JG, Schreiber J, Karp N, et al. Lengthening of the human mandible by gradual distraction. Plast Reconstr Surg 1992;89:1–8
37. Molina F. Mandibular Distraction in Hemifacial Microsomia: Technique and Results in 56 Patients. Abstract of the Craniofacial Society of Great Britain, Cambridge, UK, 1994
38. Chin M, Toth BA. Distraction osteogenesis in maxillofacial surgery using internal devices: review of five cases. J Oral Maxillofac Surg 1996;54:45–53
39. Vargervik K, Hoffman WY, Kaban LB. Comprehensive surgical and orthodontic management of hemifacial microsomia. In: Turvey TA, Vig KWL, Fonseca RJ, eds. Facial Clefts and Craniosystosis: Principles and Management. Philadelphia: WB Saunders; 1996:537

80 Velopharyngeal Inadequacy

Marshall E. Smith, Steven D. Gray, and Judy Pinborough-Zimmerman

Velopharyngeal Anatomy and Function

The velopharynx comprises the structures that separate the nasopharynx from the oropharynx. *Velum* is a generic anatomical term for *covering* or *veil*, which usually refers to the velum palatinum or soft palate and uvula. These and adjacent pharyngeal structures work in concert to create a valve that opens for nasal breathing and closes for speech and swallowing. Normal velopharyngeal function varies depending on the type of activity or speech produced. Different patterns have been found in velopharyngeal closure for speech, blowing, whistling, swallowing, and gagging.[1] Greater velopharyngeal movement appears to accompany swallowing rather than blowing and phonation.[2] Physiologically, velopharyngeal movements in swallowing appear to be different from blowing and speech production. Physiological differences in movement between speech and nonspeech activities are consistent with the clinical observation that patients who are able to obtain complete velopharyngeal closure with swallowing (i.e., do not have nasal regurgitation of food) may have inadequate or variable closure during speech.

In speech production, the velopharynx can be viewed as an articulator in the same way that the jaw, tongue, oral cavity, lips, pharynx, and larynx all work in concert to produce the various sounds of speech. Normal velopharyngeal function varies according to the characteristics of the speech produced. Factors such as vowel height, consonant type, proximity of nasal sounds to oral sounds, utterance length, speaking rate, and tongue height can affect velopharyngeal patterns of opening and closing.

High vowels tend to be associated with greater velar height than low vowels. For example, velar height generally is higher for the high vowels < I > and < u > than for the low vowel < ah >.[3] No consistent differences have been found, however, for the front/back or tense/lax features of vowel sounds.[4] Magnitude of velar elevation has been found to be generally greater during production of the < s > sound than during production of low vowel sounds.[3,5]

During production of oral consonants and vowels, the velopharyngeal mechanism is generally closed, separating oral from nasal cavities. This directs acoustic energy and airflow out of the mouth. There may be incomplete closure during vowel production, particularly if the vowel production is in proximity to a nasal consonant. The English language has three nasal sounds: < n >, < m >, and < ng >. Low-level activity is seen during the production of these nasal consonants, usually somewhere between a relaxed and complete closure position. The velopharyngeal port therefore changes its relatively open and closed states depending on the balance of oral versus nasal consonants occurring in the speech stimuli (**Fig. 80.1**). Normal velar

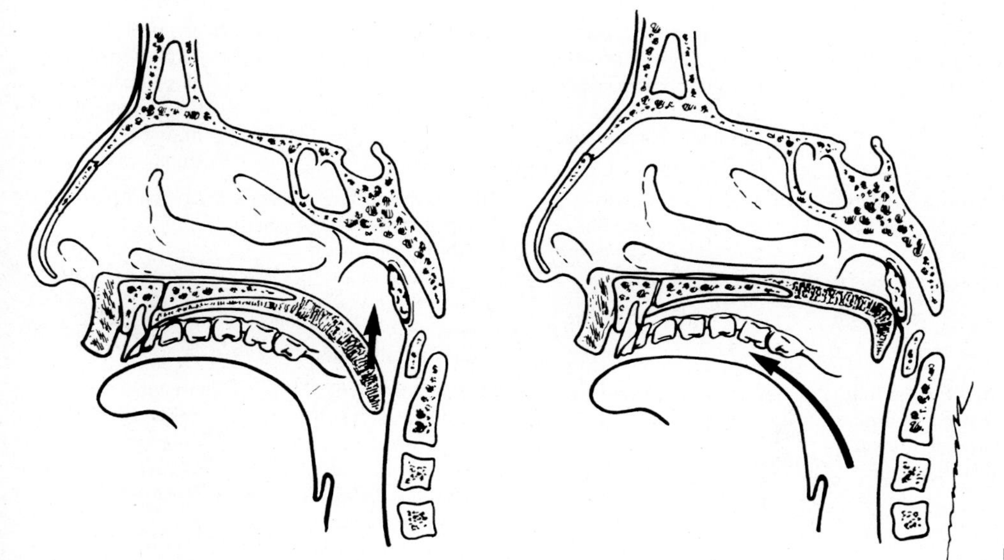

Fig. 80.1 For pressurized speech sounds the flow of air must be channeled to the oral structures. This is done by raising the palate and sealing off the nose from the oral cavity. (**A**) Velopharyngeal incompetence occurs when the velopharyngeal port is not sealed and leakage of air into the nasal cavity occurs. (**B**) Competency.

function may vary widely in velocity and displacement with the demand of the speaking situation. Velar displacement generally decreases with increased speaking rate.[6] The degree of velar elevation, however, is not significantly influenced by speech loudness.[7] Individuals achieve competent closure of the velopharyngeal port through a variety of sphincteric patterns utilizing muscles of the soft palate and pharynx. Muscles contributing to the function of the velopharyngeal sphincter include the five muscles composing the substance of the soft palate: the tensor veli palatine, levator veli palatini, musculus uvulae, palatoglossus, and palatopharyngeus. A sixth muscle, the superior constrictor of the pharynx, is also influential in velopharyngeal closure.[8]

During speech, the velopharyngeal port closes when the velum moves in a posterior-superior direction toward the posterior pharyngeal wall and the lateral pharyngeal walls move medially. In some individuals, the posterior pharyngeal wall may move anteriorly. Normal velopharyngeal closure involves variability in movement. **Table 80.1**

Table 80.1 Muscles of the Velopharyngeal Mechanism

Muscle	Origin	Attachment	Function	Innervation
Tensor veli palatine	Vertical portion arises from the scaphoid fossa at the base of the internal pterygoid plate, from the spine of the sphenoid, and from the outer side of the cartilaginous portion of the eustachian tube	Terminates in a tendon that winds around the hamular process	Tenses the soft palate; opens the auditory tube during swallowing	Mandibular branch of the trigeminal nerve
Levator veli palatini	Arises from the undersurface of the apex of the petrous portion of the temporal bone and from the inner surface of the cartilaginous portion of the eustachian tube; found to occupy the intermediate 40% of the length of the soft palate[106]	Fibers spread out in the soft palate where they blend with those of the opposite side	Acts as a sling when contracted to pull the velum in a postero-superior direction[107]; major elevator of the velum[108]; positions the velum[109]	Pharyngeal plexus derived from the glossopharyngeal and vagus nerves and the facial nerve[110]; course of the facial nerve is through the greater petrosal nerve[111]
Musculus uvulae	Palatal aponeurosis in a circumscribed area posterior to the hard palate[112]	Inserts into the uvula	Adds bulk to the dorsal surface of the soft palate	Pharyngeal plexus; pharyngeal plexus derived from the glossopharyngeal and vagus nerves and the facial nerve[110]
Palatoglossus	Has a fan-shaped attachment from the from the anterior surface of the soft palate[113]	Courses through loose connective tissue within the anterior faucial pillar and has a tapering termination in the side of the tongue[113]	Elevates the tongue upward and backward to constrict the pillars and probably lowers the velum[114]; positions the velum[109]	Pharyngeal plexus composed of from glossopharyngeus and vagus cranial nerves from the sympathetic trunk
Palatopharyngeal	Arises from the soft palate	Inserts with the stylopharyngeus into the posterior border of the thyroid cartilage	Adducts the posterior pillars, constricts the pharyngeal isthmus, narrows the velopharyngeal orifice, raises the larynx, and lowers the pharynx[115]; positions the velum[109]	Pharyngeal plexus
Superior constrictor	Arises from the lower third of the posterior margin of the internal pterygoid plate and its hamular process	Inserts into the median raphe	Medial movement of the lateral aspects of the pharyngeal walls[107]; high levels of activity are related to laughter[108]; may function to draw the velum posteriorly[108]; pulls the posterior wall and posterolateral angle anteriorly[109]	Pharyngeal plexus derived from the glossopharyngeal and vagus nerves and the facial nerve[110]

presents a summary of the muscles involved in velopharyngeal function—their origination, attachment, function, and innervation.

The back and upward movement of the velum has been attributed to the action of the levator veli palatini (LVP) muscle, the main muscle mass of the soft palate and the major elevator of the velum.[9] There is individual variability in the angle of velar insertion of the LVP relative to the cranial base.[10] Contraction of the palatoglossal and palatopharyngeal muscles probably serves to pull downward on the velum, thereby opposing the upward pull of the levator.[3] The palatopharyngeus also serves to stretch the velum laterally to increase available velar area and shape for contact.[10] Subtle adjustments in velar height have been attributed to the palatopharyngeus when the velum is in the elevated position.[4] Bulk to the dorsal side of the velum has been attributed to the musculus uvulae.[11]

Although the contribution of lateral pharyngeal wall movement to closure varies among individuals, it has generally been found to occur during speech and is related to the speech context. The greatest pharyngeal movement has been reported to be at the level of the full length of the velum and hard palate well below the levator eminence.[9] It has been suggested that lateral movement is a result of selective contraction of the uppermost fibers of the superior constrictor muscle. Laterally, the superior constrictor merges with fibers of the palatopharyngeus, so that an active role of this muscle in lateral wall movement is recognized.[12]

The Passavant ridge is a transverse elevation of the posterior pharyngeal wall seen during speech and swallowing in some individuals that has been associated with active lateral pharyngeal wall motion. It is felt to be due to contraction of the uppermost fibers of the superior constrictor, with merging fibers of the palatopharyngeus.[10] In some individuals it is the primary pharyngeal structure located on the posterior pharyngeal wall at the level of the velum. However, variations have been seen in the way the Passavant ridge is positioned relative to the velum. Findings suggest that in approximately one third of observed patients the Passavant ridge is one of the primary pharyngeal structures at the level of the velopharyngeal closure.[13] Velopharyngeal closure may or may not be assisted by the presence of the Passavant ridge in some individuals.

In summary, six muscles of the soft palate and pharynx are involved in velopharyngeal closure. Normal closure varies among individuals and is expressed by the varying contributions of the velum and the lateral and posterior pharyngeal walls. Types of velopharyngeal closure vary from individual to individual.[14,15] Open and closed states of the velopharyngeal port are relative to the demands of speech.

Causes of Velopharyngeal Dysfunction

There has been considerable discussion in medical and speech literature regarding the terminology used to describe dysfunction of the velopharyngeal mechanism. Definitions summarized by D'Antonio and Crockett are applied.[16] When referring to any type of abnormal velopharyngeal function, the term *velopharyngeal inadequacy* is employed. This can be separated into three etiologic categories: velopharyngeal insufficiency (VPI), velopharyngeal incompetence, and velopharyngeal mislearning. *Insufficiency* encompasses structural defects that result in insufficient tissue to accomplish closure. A common example of this is cleft palate. *Incompetence* describes impairment of motor control due to neurological dysfunction, such as paresis/paralysis. Causes of incompetence include skull base surgery or tumors around the jugular foramen and vagus nerve, or central nervous system impairment due to stroke, especially involving the brain stem. *Mislearning* includes etiologic factors that are independent of structural defects or neuromotor pathologies (i.e., functional).

Congenital

Congenital anatomical conditions affecting velopharyngeal function are most commonly attributable to clefting of the palate and associated anomalies. Cleft palates occur in ~1 of every 750 live births.[17] The incidence of VPI following repair of the cleft palate varies depending partly on how a particular research group is defining VPI. However, it appears that ~20 to 50% of children with cleft palates have perceptible hypernasality or nasal escape. Many of these patients can be successfully treated with speech therapy. Others require surgical intervention.

Palatal clefting can be considered on a continuum ranging from overt cleft palate to submucous cleft to occult submucous cleft. A submucous cleft is defined by a bifid uvula, muscular diastasis of the soft palate, and notching of the posterior border of the hard palate (loss of the posterior nasal spine). The bifid uvula and muscular diastasis are generally identifiable on visual inspection. The notch in the hard palate requires palpation for identification. The presence of a bifid uvula alone does not constitute a submucous cleft palate but rather serves as a harbinger; therefore, further inspection is warranted. Bifid uvulas have an incidence of one in 80 Caucasians.[17] Weatherley-White et al examined 10,836 school-age children and determined the incidence of submucous clefting to be 1 in 1200.[18] Only one in nine was symptomatic for VPI. An occult submucous cleft suggests that the usual triad of submucous cleft signs is not present.[19] In the occult submucous cleft palate, there is absence of the musculus uvulae and

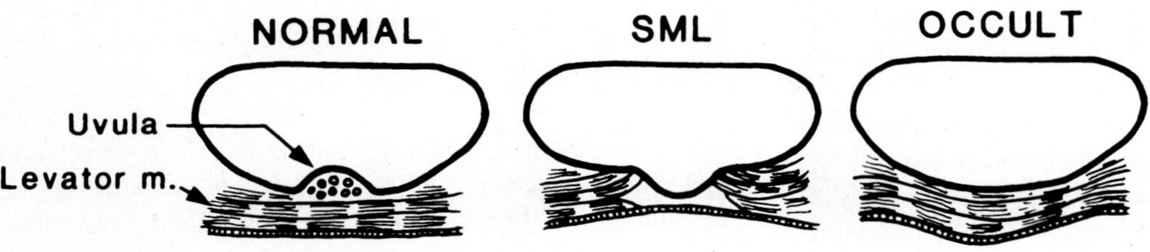

Fig. 80.2 Nasal endoscopic view of the soft palate.

diastasis of the levator palatini muscle. On the nasoendoscopic view, this finding is recognized as an absence of the bulge from the contraction of the musculus uvulae that is typically present on the nasal surface of the soft palate during speech (**Fig. 80.2**). Many children with VPI but no obvious cleft have been identified as having occult submucous cleft.

Occult submucous clefts or submucous clefts predispose children to VPI because of abnormal musculature of the velopharyngeal sphincter.[20] Consequently, these children may acquire VPI when changes to the anatomy of the velopharynx occur, such as an adenoidectomy or even involution of the adenoid pad.[21–23] For this reason, a preoperative evaluation for adenoidectomy should include a careful inspection of the palate, both visually and with palpation.[24]

Postadenoidectomy

VPI may occur following adenoidectomy even in children without a submucous cleft palate, but its occurrence in relatively healthy children can be hard to predict.[25] Huge adenoids may assist in easy velopharyngeal closure. When such adenoids are removed, considerable palatal motion may be required to obtain closure. Short palate, a relatively deep nasopharynx, and palatal hypotonia may all be factors in the development of VPI following adenoidectomy. Ren and colleagues showed that postadenoidectomy VPI is often associated with enlarged tonsils or remaining prominent adenoid tissue.[22] Incomplete removal of adenoid tissue can be a cause of VPI. If there is concern that the child's palate may not be capable of making the complete excursion back to the new position of the posterior pharyngeal wall, then a partial adenoidectomy can be performed. This has been described in various ways, but generally a superior half adenoidectomy is performed either with suction electrocautery or by using a Thompson-Sinclair adenoid forceps. If postadenoidectomy VPI exists, then our current recommendations are for a 3- to 6-month trial of speech therapy. Useful adjuncts to this therapy are biofeedback using nasometry and occasionally continuous positive airway pressure (CPAP) therapy for those with touch-closure VPI findings.[26–28] VPI due to hypertrophic tonsils has also been described. Observing tonsil interference with velopharyngeal closure on nasal endoscopy makes the diagnosis. The treatment is a tonsillectomy.[29–31]

Other Conditions or Syndromes

Many conditions or syndromes other than those associated with clefting can result in or predispose children to VPI. Furthermore, any condition that can affect the timing of the palate with speech, such as developmental delays, mental retardation, or traumatic brain injury, may result in velopharyngeal inadequacy. In the pediatric age group, velocardiofacial syndrome and Down syndrome warrant special comment.

Velocardiofacial Syndrome

Velocardiofacial syndrome (VCF) is diagnosed with increasing frequency. This is a result of increased awareness of the syndrome, as well as the availability of chromosome testing for diagnosis. This condition has characteristic facies: prominent nose, retruded mandible, cardiovascular anomalies, possibly cleft palate, and often learning disabilities.[32,33] Inheritance is autosomal dominant with variable expressivity. Failure to thrive in infancy is present in ~25%, and ~35% have short stature. Obstructive sleep apnea may also occur. Mental disability is experienced by nearly all. Childhood- or adult-onset schizophrenia has been reported.[34]

Facial appearance is fairly characteristic, consisting of a long face with vertical maxillary excess, malar flatness, and mandibular retrusion. Robin's sequence may be present. The nose is usually prominent with a square nasal root and narrow nasal passages.

Cardiac anomalies are present in more than 80% of patients. Ventricular septal defect is the most common, but other cardiac anomalies, such as right-sided aortic arch, tetralogy of Fallot, and aortic valve disease, are also found. Of significant consequence for the otolaryngologist is that the internal carotid arteries can be medially displaced along the posterior pharyngeal wall.[35] When considering velopharyngeal surgery in VCF patients, it is critical to consider internal carotid location. Often this is visible with nasoendoscopic examination. Radiographic techniques to precisely map the location related to the proposed surgery may be required.[36]

Diagnosis of VCF can be difficult. Finkelstein et al, reporting on 21 patients with VCF, found that only 11 (52%) had typical manifestations.[37] Fortunately, genetic testing for these patients is now possible. Microdeletions of the q11 region of chromosome 22 have been found in VCF patients. This is the same area in which microdeletions found in DiGeorge syndrome occur. The microdeletions in some patients with VCF syndrome have encompassed the DiGeorge chromosome locus.[38] The otolaryngologist providing care for such patients should recognize the possibility that features of both syndromes may coexist.

Down Syndrome

Down syndrome (trisomy 21) occurs in 1.5 in 1000 births and is associated with mental handicaps, hearing loss, and muscular hypotonia.[39,40] All of these can be risk factors for development of VPI. A review of 74 tonsillectomies and adenoidectomies in children with Down syndrome identified two children with postoperative VPI.[41] These authors point out the risk of possible VPI development in children with known hypotonia and known articulation problems. Considering their predisposing factors, it is somewhat surprising that postadenoidectomy VPI does not occur more often. The narrow oropharynx and velopharynx and the shallow skull base at the adenoid site (platybasia) seen in Down syndrome may offset these predisposing factors.

Evaluation of Velopharyngial Dysfunction

Evaluation of velopharyngeal dysfunction involves perceptual, instrumental, and physical examinations of the patient. The perceptual assessment of hypernasality and nasal emissions is aided by use of a commercially available instrument called the Nasometer (Kay Elemetries, Inc., Lincoln Park, NJ). This device measures the acoustic energy coming from the mouth and nose during production of standardized sentences or phonemes, and calculates the ratio of oral to nasal sound energy or nasalance. The subject's speech is then compared with normative data to assess the degree of hypernasality or hyponasality. Elevated nasalance scores on passages containing only oral sounds are significantly correlated to listener judgment ratings of hypernasality.[42] Reduced nasalance scores on passages containing primarily nasal sounds are correlated to listener judgment ratings of hyponasality.[43] In children with hypernasality, nasometric scores are also significantly correlated to aerodynamic estimates of velopharyngeal area and to nasoendoscopic findings.[42,44] Clinical judgment is important in interpretation because degrees of mixed resonance or imprecise articulation can affect results. When velopharyngeal inadequacy for whatever cause may be present, a direct examination of the velopharyngeal structures is indicated.

Two methods are advocated for velopharyngeal assessment: nasopharyngoscopy and multiview videofluoroscopy.[45] Each method has benefits and drawbacks. Nasopharyngoscopy allows a direct view of structures. This is very helpful in revision cases where prior pharyngoplasty has been done. But the procedure has some drawbacks as follows: (1) occasionally, patients may be uncooperative; (2) endoscopic images may be prone to distortion; and (3) vertical-level assessments may be relatively difficult.[46] Fluoroscopy is well tolerated and is felt to give a better view of lateral pharyngeal wall motion than endoscopy. However, ionizing radiation is required and the speech samples are necessarily brief. As with nasopharyngoscopy, experience and skill in performance of the study and interpretation of the images are needed. The availability of nasopharyngoscopy in cleft palate teams has increased from 8 to 90% during the last 2 decades.[47] We recommend its use in most cases.

Nasopharyngoscopy

Flexible nasopharyngoscopy is an effective way of viewing the velopharyngeal orifice. The contribution of the pharyngeal walls can be visualized, and a fairly accurate analysis of the closure patterns and deficiencies of velopharyngeal motion can be obtained. The motion of the velopharyngeal walls during closure has been classified into various patterns. Skolnick et al described three shapes of the persistent gap following closure: coronal, sagittal, and circular.[48] Croft et al studied closure patterns in both normal subjects and those with VPI.[49] They did not find a significant difference in the prevalence of particular closure patterns in normal subjects as opposed to those with VPI. Using both multivideofluoroscopic views and nasoendoscopy, Croft et al further refined these closure patterns. They include coronal (seen in ~55% of normal subjects), sagittal (in 10 to 15%), circular (10 to 20%), and circular with the Passavant ridge (15 to 20%) (**Fig. 80.3**).

Nasopharyngoscopy is usually performed so that both video and audio can be recorded. Most children, when properly prepared, can tolerate nasopharyngoscopy. Topical anesthesia is used for the nose, and systemic sedation is neither required nor advisable in nearly all cases. A speech pathologist is generally in attendance to assist in the speech examination. Both nasal chambers can be examined, followed by the nasopharyngeal area during speech. Despite the shortcomings of nasopharyngoscopy,

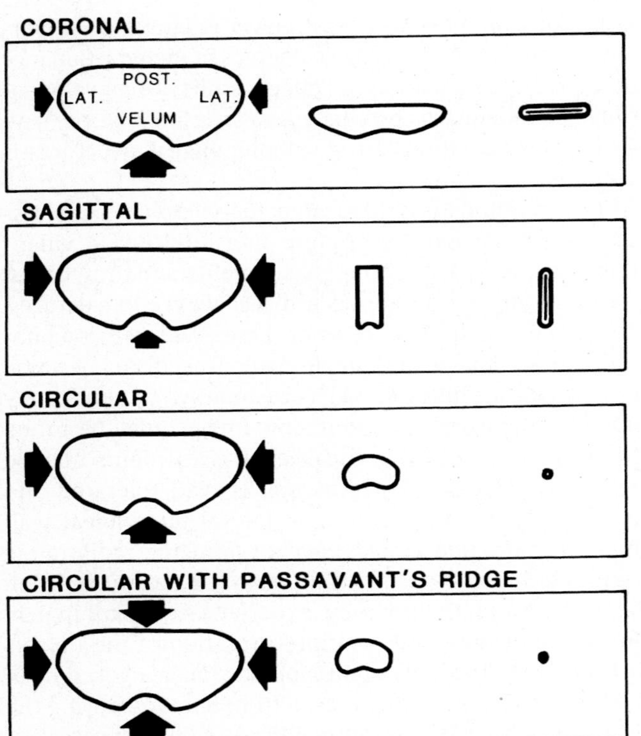

Fig. 80.3 Velopharyngeal closure patterns. Note that these descriptive patterns are based on the shape of the gap as it closes.

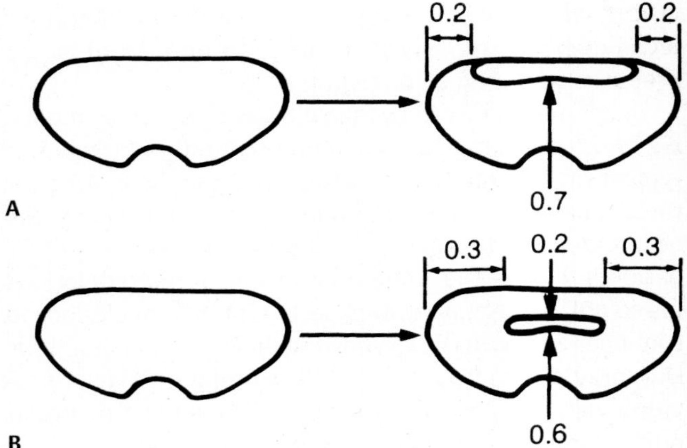

Fig. 80.4 Describing velopharyngeal closure patterns is performed by first naming the type of closure pattern involved and then showing with arrows the amount of motion present in each wall. A ratio of movement for the wall being described to the opposite wall is obtained. (**A**) A coronal closure pattern with the velum showing 0.7 motion and the two lateral pharyngeal walls showing motion rated at 0.2. (**B**) A circular closure with posterior wall motion. One could also argue that this is a coronal closure. It would be a very unusual closure pattern but is used here for descriptive purposes. In this case, the anterior wall shows 0.6 motion, both lateral pharyngeal walls show 0.3, and the posterior wall shows 0.2 with a resultant small corona-shaped gap.

it has been reliable in assessing VPI and is the standard method for viewing the nasopharyngeal area.

When the velopharyngeal mechanism is dysfunctional, nasopharyngoscopy includes an additional descriptive method. Besides describing the velopharyngeal closure pattern, the relative contributions of the pharyngeal walls are rated. Although absolute measurements of the velopharyngeal gap or pharyngeal wall motion have been performed, these are difficult in a clinical setting. In 1988, an international working group proposed rating pharyngeal wall contribution to closure as a ratio of motion from one wall to the other.[46] Therefore, pharyngeal wall motion is graded by the degree of movement of that wall to the opposite wall. If complete closure occurs to the opposite wall, then a ratio of 1 is given. If motion toward the opposite wall is only halfway, then a ratio of 0.5 is given. In this way pharyngeal wall dysfunction and resultant gaps in closure can be described (**Fig. 80.4**).

The vertical level of closure is an equally important anatomical location. In performing reconstructive velopharyngeal surgery, one would like to take advantage of already existing velopharyngeal motion. Videofluoroscopy or nasopharyngoscopy can be used to identify the point of maximal pharyngeal wall motion. This level of closure should be ascertained for each individual. This has generally been done using multivideofluoroscopy. Using this method, Finkelstein et al evaluated the Passavant ridge. They found that it exists in ~40% of individuals and is formed by fibers of the superior constrictor muscle.[32] Using the torus tubarius as a landmark, they found that the upper limit of lateral pharyngeal wall motion was ~1 cm below the torus. The vertical length of closure can be variable. It can be fairly short, making it necessary to be precise about the vertical level of any reconstructive sphincter, or it can be longer, in which case precise placement may be less critical.[8]

Nonsurgical Treatment

Successful treatment of velopharyngeal dysfunction depends on careful evaluation of both velopharyngeal function and speech. It is also influenced by the type and severity of defect; patient's age, cognitive ability, and motivation; availability of services; and expertise of service providers.[5,50] Integration of services provided by an interdisciplinary team of specialists is frequently required to develop and implement effective treatment plans. Treatment decisions must be based not only on subjective practitioner impressions but should also include data provided by objective procedures, such as nasopharyngoscopy, videofluoroscopy, aerodynamic or nasometric studies, and in-depth articulation analysis.[4]

For individuals who do not have the basic anatomy or function necessary to obtain adequate velopharyngeal closure for speech, surgical treatment is generally recommended.[51] Such patients often present with consistent lack of velopharyngeal closure with varied speech demands and have hypernasality measurements in the moderate to severe range.

Nonsurgical treatment options may be utilized prior to, in conjunction with, or in lieu of surgery. These options include, but are not limited to, prosthetic dental management, speech therapy, biofeedback treatment utilizing instrumentation, and resistance exercises performed while positive air pressure is introduced into the nasal cavities. To date, however, research data about the efficacy of these treatment options and factors affecting outcome are limited. For the past 30 years, prosthetic devices have been used successfully to assist with inadequate velopharyngeal closure.[52,53] These devices are particularly helpful when there are contraindications to surgery for significant velopharyngeal dysfunction, when dysfunction is secondary to neuromuscular involvement, or when velopharyngeal movements are poorly timed.[54,55] There are two basic types of prosthetic devices—obturators and palatal lifts.

An obturator is a device designed and constructed by a prosthetic dentist to substitute for missing or incomplete tissue; dental wires or bands attach it to the teeth.[56] Usually, the obturator used to improve velopharyngeal function is a thin acrylic plate that extends back to the pharyngeal area.

Customized fabrication and fitting of the obturator require the use of data provided by nasopharyngoscopy, aerodynamic measurements, videofluoroscopy, or nasometric studies.[27,57–60] A gradual reduction in obturator size has been advocated for some patients; usually, this involves adjusting the size of the original obturator. It is postulated that as the size of the obturator is gradually reduced, velopharyngeal function may improve and, in some cases, eliminate the need for the obturator or for surgical intervention.[52,54]

Unlike obturators, palatal lifts are designed to elevate the soft palate when the length of the palate is adequate. Lifts are particularly useful in patients with limited or no dynamic palatal movement. It is unclear at this time whether palatal lifts improve the neuromuscular ability of the velopharynx.[55] Use of obturators or palatal lifts can be difficult in young children, particularly if cooperation or cognitive ability is compromised.

Hypernasality, nasal emissions, and articulatory/phonologic deficits can be the result of mislearning rather than VPI. These problems respond well to speech treatment, particularly phoneme-specific nasal emissions occurring with a select group of sounds. *Surgical intervention is contraindicated in these cases.* For children, diagnostic speech therapy is often recommended prior to physical management, particularly in cases of borderline, mild, or inconsistent hypernasality.[59,60] Speech or language treatment is strongly recommended for children with severe articulatory/phonologic deficiencies or limited expressive language. Compensatory articulation error patterns, such as glottal stops, restrict airflow below the velopharyngeal valve.[61,62] Radiographic or nasopharyngoscopic observation of the velopharyngeal mechanism is appropriate for children who are able to demonstrate correct articulatory placement for some oral consonant sounds and who have enough language to provide a varied speech sample.

Diagnostic speech therapy frequently involves use of a Nasometer. This biofeedback device has proven effective in the reduction of nasality levels in some patients.[5,47] Treatment utilizing the Nasometer encourages such strategies as ear training, promoting a lower posterior tongue placement, increasing loudness, speaking at a lower pitch, using a more open mouth posture, controlling the type of consonants and vowels used in speech training, and lowering the rate of speech.[51,58] The duration of any speech therapy designed to reduce hypernasality should be carefully monitored. If continued improvement in hypernasality is not demonstrated within 3 to 6 months, speech therapy to reduce hypernasality should be discontinued and other treatment options explored.[60]

Videorecorded nasopharyngoscopy is used with success in biofeedback therapy for adults with VPI.[28,63] A case study involving an older child demonstrated correction of phoneme-specific nasal emissions using nasopharyngoscopy.[28] Nasopharyngoscopy biofeedback therapy may prove to be a useful tool in training some children to achieve better velopharyngeal function, but further research is necessary.

A new therapy for hypernasality uses CPAP, which is introduced into the nasal cavities during speech production.[26] It is theorized that in cases where hypernasality is related to physiological limitations, resistance training might strengthen muscles involved in velopharyngeal closure. It has been demonstrated that as positive air pressure is delivered to the nasal cavities, levator veli palatini muscle activity increases.[64] Therapy can take place in the patient's home—a major treatment advantage. Preliminary case reports suggest that CPAP therapy is useful for patients with mild to moderate hypernasality, regardless of the underlying etiologic factors.

Surgical Treatment

Palatoplasty

In a patient with overt cleft of the palate, repair of the cleft palate, usually done before 1 year, is expected to prevent VPI in most cases. These success rates average 80%.[64a] In treatment of VPI, an additional point to be made here is that palatoplasty may also be used in older children. Indications for this include (1) submucous cleft palate and (2) previously repaired cleft palate wherein an intravelar veloplasty was not performed. The technique of choice in these situations is the double opposing Z-plasty described by Furlow.[65] The success rate with this procedure both in primary cleft palate repair and in submucous cleft treatment has been excellent, as reported by a variety of centers.[66,67]

Pharyngoplasty

The principle behind surgical improvement of velopharyngeal competence is to narrow the velopharyngeal opening and essentially to create a partial nasopharyngeal stenosis. The key word is *partial* because an adequate airway must be maintained for nasal breathing and sleep to take place. Procedures have been developed to obturate the middle of the velopharyngeal area or the lateral portion of the velopharynx. Hynes first described an operation that obturated the lateral part of the velopharynx.[68] His goal in designing this was to construct a sphincter that would be dynamic. He felt that raising lateral flaps of superior origin would lead to a neuromuscular flap that would contract. Nearly 2 decades later, Orticochea reported using lateral-based flaps for the treatment of VPI.[69] According to his description of the Orticochea pharyngoplasty, he used the posterior tonsillar pillars as donor flaps and also created a recipient site by raising a small inferior pharyngeal flap. Again, nearly a decade later, Jackson modified the Orticochea technique.[70] It is essentially the latter version of the pharyngoplasty that has gained so much popularity. The posterior tonsillar pillars are still used as donor flaps to be sutured across the nasopharynx. However, an inferior pharyngeal flap is not created. Instead, the transverse incision is made higher in the nasopharynx, and a small superior pharyngeal flap can be created if needed. Further modifications of this technique have been made. Most have centered on obtaining an adequate superior placement and covering raw tissue areas. Several studies have assessed the success of a sphincter pharyngoplasty to improve VPI. In 1984, Riski et al reported correction of hypernasality in 78% of patients.[71] In 1992 a more complete evaluation of the sphincter pharyngoplasty had similar success rates, although during the study the surgical technique changed.[72] An objective study was performed by Witt et al who found that nasal resonance improved in 79% of patients.[73] In their study, sphincter pharyngoplasty was done to correct hypernasality in patients exhibiting all velopharyngeal closure patterns, rather than selecting certain patients for other techniques. This study also appropriately documented potential problems with all types of velopharyngeal obturating surgery. They found that 30% of their patients were judged to be hyponasal postoperatively. Sloan et al compared a modified Hynes pharyngoplasty with placement of inferiorly and superiorly based pharyngeal flaps and concluded that the sphincter pharyngoplasty was a better technique for management of VPI.[74]

Indications

A sphincter pharyngoplasty is considered when the nasal endoscopy study shows velopharyngeal insufficiency associated with good velar movement but poor to absent lateral wall motion.[71] A sphincter pharyngoplasty may also be indicated for those with poor motion of any of the pharyngeal walls, including the velum. Such persons have a relatively adynamic sphincter, and typically their velopharyngeal port is described as a black hole because there is no light reflection of the sphincter during nasoendoscopic examination.[75] Because the sphincter pharyngoplasty pulls the lateral pharyngeal walls medially and because the flaps are sewn across the back wall, both the lateral and posterior portions of the velopharyngeal port are obturated. The degree of obturation can be varied by adjusting the thickness of the flaps, the snugness or tightness with which the flaps are sutured together, and the extension of the flaps toward the uvula. The possibility of modifying the sphincter based on individual variations in VPI pattern is an appealing aspect of this procedure.[76] When needed, revisions of sphincter pharyngoplasty are generally successful.[77,78]

Surgical Technique

Proper patient preparation includes the surgeon's review of the nasoendoscopy tape and videofluoroscopic results, if applicable. If possible, a recording of the nasoendoscopic examination should be present in the surgical suite so that this may be reviewed at the time of operation. The potential necessity of a tonsillectomy or adenoidectomy should also have been previously determined from the nasal endoscopy study. If positioning and placement of the sphincter will be through the adenoid pad, an adenoidectomy should have been performed. Placement of a sphincter pharyngoplasty through the adenoid can increase the difficulty of the operation. We prefer to do an adenoidectomy ~8 weeks prior to placement of the sphincter pharyngoplasty. A tonsillectomy can be done prior to or at the time of pharyngoplasty. In doing this tonsillectomy, care is taken not to injure the posterior tonsillar pillars and to keep scarring of the palatopharyngeal muscle to a minimum. Use of extensive electrocautery should be avoided.

Following intubation with an oral RAE endotracheal tube, a Dingman or Davis mouth gag is used to obtain adequate exposure of the posterior tonsillar pillars. Exposure to the nasopharynx is obtained by use of a uvula retractor. With the soft palate retracted superiorly, the proper vertical level for the sphincter pharyngoplasty is determined by comparing anatomical landmarks found videofluoroscopically or nasoendoscopically with those directly visible or palpable during surgery. After the site has been determined it is injected with a vasoconstrictive agent such as 1% lidocaine with epinephrine. The posterior tonsillar pillars are likewise mildly injected to improve hemostasis. A no. 15 blade is used to make an incision along the anterior surface of the posterior tonsillar pillar. The posterior tonsillar pillar is detached inferiorly just above the inferior pole of the tonsil. A combination of a no. 15 blade and lower lateral crural right-angle scissors is used to elevate the palatopharyngeal muscle superiorly.

The posterior incision, which is close to the junction of the lateral and posterior pharyngeal wall, is carried superiorly to the level of the desired vertical placement across the nasopharynx. Then the palatopharyngeus flaps are elevated up to nearly this level. The anterior incision does not extend as superiorly as the posterior incision. In fact, the anterior incision of the palatopharyngeal muscle usually does not extend even as high as the superior pole of the tonsil because as a result of so doing the reconstructed velopharyngeal port can become quite narrow (**Fig. 80.5**). The blood supply to the flap may also be disrupted.[79]

As the anterior pillar incision extends superiorly and toward the uvula, the reconstructive port becomes narrower. If the intent is to keep the velopharyngeal port open and at the same time create significant obturation of the lateral and posterior portion of the nasopharynx, this anterior incision can be extended across the back of the tonsillar pillars and curved up along the posterior and

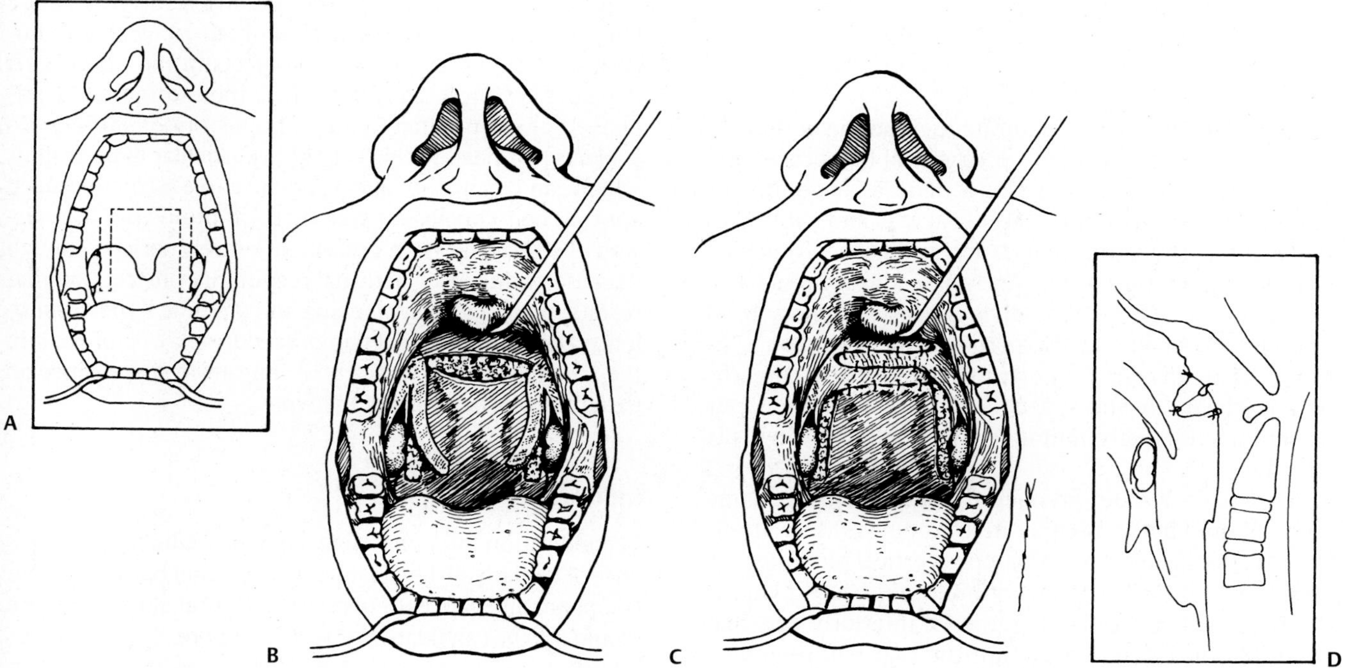

Fig. 80.5 Sphincter pharyngoplasty technique. (**A**) The height or vertical level of the sphincter must usually be placed in relation to the pharynx. The soft palate is retracted. *Broken lines* represent an approximation of the surgical incisions, although this is difficult to represent two-dimensionally. (**B**) The soft palate is retracted superiorly, and the posterior tonsillar pillars (palatopharyngeal muscle) have been elevated. Note that the anterior incision stops at the superior pole but may extend further vertically and medially along the nasal surface of the soft palate toward the uvula if the surgeon desires a narrow, tight port. Note also that the medial or posterior incision for the flaps extends up to the horizontal incision so that the flap can be easily rotated. (**C**) Flaps have been sutured into the sphincter position overlapped. The flaps may also be sutured end-to-end. This illustration better demonstrates that the sphincter could be closed by pulling the flaps in more tightly, by creating a larger posterior wall ridge (harvesting larger and thicker flaps), and by extending the anterior incision medially along the nasal side of the soft palate (this step is usually not needed and can lead to severe narrowing of the port). (**D**) Lateral view following pharyngoplasty. Note that the sphincter is in the nasopharynx, above the soft palate. (From Gray S, Pinborough-Zimmerman J. Diagnosis and treatment of velopharyngeal incompetence. Fac Plast Surg Clin North Am 1996;4:405–412. Reprinted by permission.)

superior (nasal) surface of the soft palate/pharynx. This extension allows for more superior elevation of the palatopharyngeus flap without necessarily constricting the velopharyngeal port.

With the two palatopharyngeal muscles elevated, an incision is made across the nasopharynx at the desired level of sphincter placement. This usually requires a palatal retraction with the uvula retractor. The palatopharyngeus flaps are sutured transversely across the nasopharynx. These flaps can either be sutured end-to-end or in an overlapping fashion, and to the nasopharyngeal mucosal flaps with 4–0 Vicryl (Ethicon, Inc., Somerville, NJ). (It is usually adequate to sew the posterior pillar edge to the inferior edge of the nasopharyngeal mucosa. Partial dehiscences that yield necklace bands usually function adequately.) If a very snug sphincter is created, then an obstructive breathing pattern may occur in the immediate postoperative state. In this case, a soft nasal trumpet is placed through the sphincter and kept there until the following morning.

Posterior Pharyngeal Flaps

An operation designed to obturate the midline of the velopharyngeal port is termed a pharyngeal flap procedure. In this procedure, a flap of tissue is pedicled superiorly or inferiorly to the posterior pharyngeal wall and sutured to the palate. Through the years, success has been reported using both inferiorly and superiorly based pharyngeal flaps. Placement in the midline divides the velopharyngeal port into two smaller lateral ports. Mobile lateral pharyngeal walls are needed for ports to be open during breathing and closed during speech. Posterior wall and velar motion are relatively unimportant when choosing this procedure.

In the last decade, preoperative nasopharyngoscopy has facilitated better preoperative planning. More attention has been focused on the proper vertical placement of flaps.[80] One of the criticisms of inferiorly based pharyngeal flaps is that the flap is tethered inferiorly and that with additional scar contracture the flap will be pulled from the optimal position.[81] For this reason, in the United States, the trend has been toward superiorly based pharyngeal flaps. Pharyngeal flaps have been effective in reducing hypernasality. Morris et al studied 65 subjects, over half of whom had had their surgery more than 10 years previously.[82] Eighty-three percent showed normal velopharyngeal function, and 66% showed normal or near-normal speech production. Eight of the 65 subjects had surgical revision of the flap. One required reduction in the size of lateral ports; the other seven had either flap takedowns or lateral port enlargements performed. Likewise, Hirschberg reported a series of 500 cases involving pharyngeal flaps wherein 90% of patients demonstrated improvement in hypernasality and 74% showed improvement in speech.[83] It was also emphasized that the best speech results were obtained when the width of the flap was appropriately matched with the relative motion of the lateral pharyngeal walls. Matching the width of the flap to obturate the remaining gap area, which is determined by maximal medial motion of the lateral pharyngeal walls, is termed "tailoring of the pharyngeal flap."[84] The theory of tailor-made flaps is a good one. In practice, achieving consistent, precise millimeter dimensions in the lateral ports due to the many forces of scar contracture is probably unrealistic. Variation of scar contracture between individuals leads to some of the complications that are reported regarding pharyngeal flaps.

Numerous long-term studies have thoroughly documented the drawbacks and benefits of this procedure.[85] Sleep apnea is a reported complication of pharyngeal flap placement.[86,87] Sleep apnea is more likely to occur in the early postoperative period, and within 3 months obstructed sleep problems should be substantially resolved.[88,89] In a long-term follow-up, Morris et al obtained electrocardiograms (ECGs) on 33 of the 65 subjects in the pharyngeal flap study.[82] Those chosen for ECG monitoring had complained of sleep difficulty or had a history of snoring. No subjects had clear findings of right ventricular hypertrophy, which can be a pathological response to obstructive sleep apnea. Their conclusion was that symptoms of nasal airway obstruction, when present, are rarely serious enough to cause pathology. Nocturnal respiratory obstruction that results in nocturnal awakening and daytime hypersomnolence after a pharyngeal flap procedure may be present in the absence of sleep apnea.[90] Its long-term significance on patients' well-being is not known.

Indications

The indication for a pharyngeal flap procedure is the presence of a relatively good lateral wall motion but with a central persisting gap. Patients with a sagittal closure pattern would also be candidates for this procedure.

Surgical Technique

The procedure is performed by placing a Dingman mouth gag and injecting the posterior pharyngeal wall and the palate with 1% lidocaine and 1:200,000 epinephrine. Two different techniques can be used for insetting the pharyngeal flap to the palate. One, termed a fish-mouth technique, essentially consists of by-valving the soft palate (separating nasal mucosa from oral tissue) to create a pocket into which the pharyngeal flap is pulled and sutured.[91] The pocket is usually placed just superior and anterior to the edge of the soft palate on the nasal side. This technique has not yielded consistent results.[92] The other technique involves splitting the palate and has been well described by Hogan[93] and Crockett et al.[94] Both of these articles describe adjustments to the lateral ports.

The width of the flap is determined from previous nasoendoscopic or videofluoroscopic procedure. The superiorly based flap is elevated a little higher than the level ascertained to be appropriate for maximum medial motion of the lateral pharyngeal walls. With scar contracture, the flap usually descends a couple of millimeters. The fish-mouth technique or the palatal splitting technique is used to sew the flap into position. Prior to suturing the flap, small endotracheal tubes are placed in both ports to assist in postoperative breathing and to provide guidance on lateral port size.

Postoperatively, after the small endotracheal tubes have been removed, the patient should be monitored for obstructive apnea. The tubes may be left in place the first night, and the patient should not be discharged from the hospital until indications are clear that serious obstructive apnea is not present. Parents should be cautioned that if obstruction seems to be worsening, the patient should be brought back to the hospital for monitoring and reevaluation.

Augmentation of the Posterior Pharyngeal Wall

The concept of augmenting the posterior pharyngeal wall in an effort to improve velopharyngeal competence has received and will continue to receive attention for several reasons: (1) the majority of persistent velopharyngeal gaps are continuous with the posterior pharyngeal wall, (2) in many VPI patients the velum or soft palate has relatively good motion, (3) the risk of inducing hyponasality and nasal obstruction is lower, and (4) the procedures are relatively easy to perform. The concept of simply bringing the posterior pharyngeal wall forward to correct the gap is appealing. However, in practice, many posterior pharyngeal wall augmentation techniques have failed to meet expectations. Currently, one of the best techniques to augment the posterior pharyngeal wall is a sphincter pharyngoplasty because a large shelf of tissue is placed across the posterior pharyngeal wall. However, this section focuses on techniques that augment the posterior wall.

Various materials have been used to augment the posterior wall by either injection or implantation.[95–97] Tissue implants, such as cartilage and fascia, have been used.[98–101] The most common injectable material used for treatment of marginal VPI over the last few decades has been Teflon.[102] Smith and McCabe injected Teflon into the posterior pharyngeal wall, thus creating a transverse ridge.[103] Disadvantages of Teflon include (1) the fact that it is not approved by the Food and Drug Administration for this indication and (2) the fact that migration may occur within the pharynx due to growth of the neck, or even elsewhere in the body. One inadvertent carotid artery injection with Teflon has occurred.

Obviously, it is important to palpate the posterior wall for great vessels prior to any sort of posterior pharyngeal wall procedure. An anecdotal advantage of Teflon injection is that as the Teflon migrates and the posterior wall bulges less, the velopharyngeal sphincter may gradually adapt to maintain competency, much like sphincter improvement with obturator reduction. However, if this does not occur, the Teflon will move to a position below the plane of velar closure, resulting in recurrence of hypernasal symptoms; this has also been noted anecdotally.

Because of the theoretical advantages of posterior wall augmentation, there is renewed interest in the use of posterior wall tissue to create a shelf or ledge along the posterior wall. In this procedure, a superiorly based pharyngeal flap is lifted and buckled to create a ridge across the posterior wall.[104,105] Results obtained with this procedure have been mixed. Witt et al reported experience with 14 patients and concluded that the procedure was ineffective.[104] On the other hand, Gray et al also reported 14 patients who had the same procedure.[105] Improvement in hypernasality by either perceptual assessment or nasometry was seen in 12 of 13 assessed. Only one patient had revision surgery. Though not statistically significant, the procedure was felt to be more effective in younger patients, postadenoidectomy VIP patients, and nonsyndromic patients in this series. In comparing this report with that of Witt et al, it appears that the patients in Gray's series had smaller (61-mm) gaps, whereas those in Witt's had somewhat larger gaps (up to 20%).

Indications

Posterior wall augmentation is indicated when there is a very small central midline gap and velopharyngeal closure could be made complete by simply bringing forward the posterior wall. Occasionally, a patient may achieve velopharyngeal closure that is not tight enough, whereupon pressure causes leakage of the air through the velopharyngeal port. This condition is referred to as a "touch closure" problem because the pharyngeal walls touch but do not achieve competent closure. Under these conditions, a small augmentation of the posterior pharyngeal wall is enough to provide a competent seal. If significant augmentation of the posterior pharyngeal wall is required, then a sphincter pharyngoplasty is usually a better alternative. Posterior wall augmentation works best for small central or off-center gaps in the area of 1 to 2 mm or for touch closure problems.

Surgical Technique

Posterior wall augmentation using a buckled or folded pharyngeal flap is relatively easy to perform. A superiorly based pharyngeal flap is raised and then folded on itself at the level of maximum pharyngeal wall motion in the area of the velopharyngeal port. A superiorly based pharyngeal flap is elevated to prevertebral fascia such that the constrictor muscle is present within the flap. Flap width is determined by ascertaining the width of the gap to be obturated and making the flap slightly larger. The flap shrinks once elevated; therefore, a wider flap than anticipated is usually required (**Fig. 80.6**).

The lateral incisions are made first and carried through the constrictor muscle until the white fascia is encountered posteriorly. At this point, a right-angle elevator can be used to elevate the remaining muscle off the fascia. The flap is detached inferiorly at about the level of the inferior pole of the tonsil. The flap is elevated superiorly to slightly above the level of the desired augmentation. When the flap is elevated above the level of augmentation, the buckle of the flap will be correctly positioned. The flap can then be sutured on itself or to the posterior wall so that the fold is in the desired location vertically. Usually three or four sutures are placed across the inferior edge of the flap to hold it in proper position, and then one or two sutures are placed on the lateral aspects of the folded flap for stability and to close any dead space between the two layers of the flap.

Drawbacks to this procedure include (1) variability in flap atrophy and (2) inadequate closure of large posterior gaps. Even when a large buckled flap is created, large folded flaps are functionally not very useful because a large buckle has a tendency to flap (move up and down) depending on air pressure in the vocal tract. For this reason, small gaps of 1 to 2 mm can be closed successfully, but large gaps are inconsistently closed because a large folded flap is not vertically stable.

Summary

In conclusion, treatment of VPI requires careful evaluation by a team of professionals consisting of a speech–language pathologist and a surgeon with expertise in speech disorders. Patient care should be individualized. Surgical care requires preoperative assessment of the velopharynx by nasoendoscopy, videofluoroscopy, or both. We generally support the approach that selection of the surgical procedure

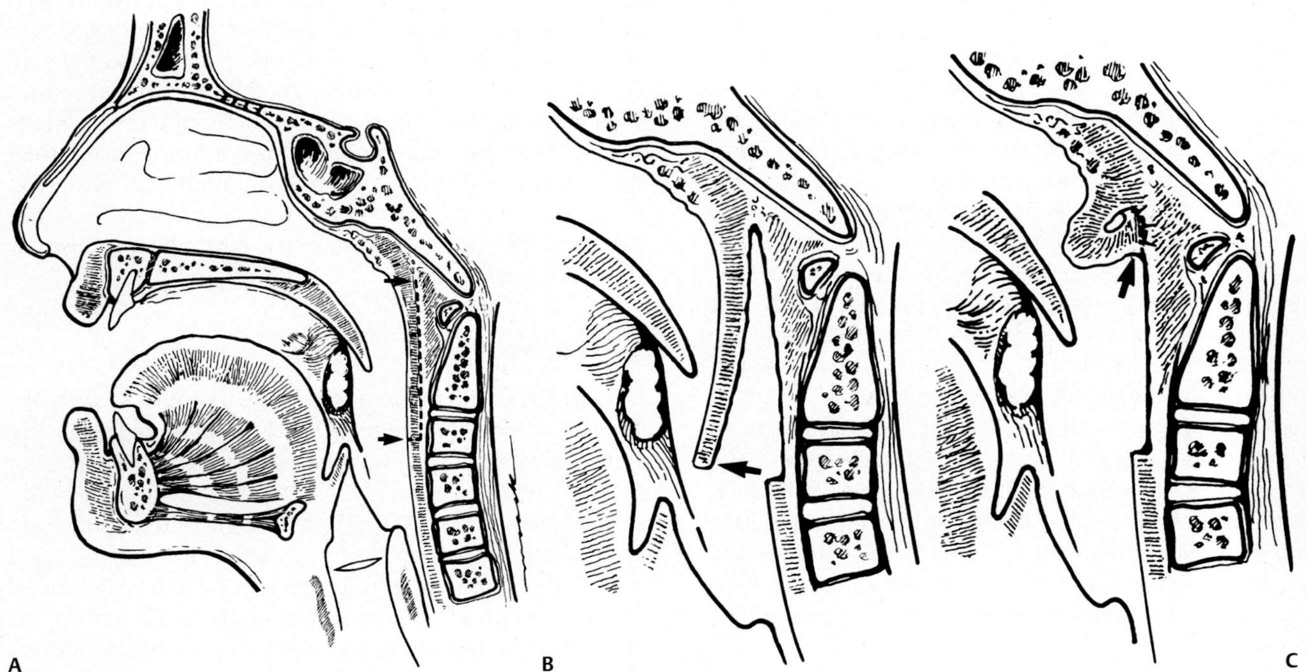

Fig. 80.6 Augmentation of the posterior pharyngeal wall. (**A**) The section of the posterior pharyngeal wall to be elevated; the inferior level is at about the inferior pole of the tonsil. (**B**) The constrictor muscle is raised with the flap and elevated quite superiorly. (**C**) The flap has been folded and sutured in place. Even though the flap was elevated higher, the fold and maximum area of augmentation occur a little lower. Although not shown in (**C**), sutures are often placed on the folded flap laterally to close some of the dead space; sometimes this seems to create a little more stability. (From Gray S, Pinborough-Zimmerman J. Diagnosis and treatment of velopharyngeal incompetence. Fac Plast Surg Clin North Am 1996;4:405–412. Reprinted by permission.)

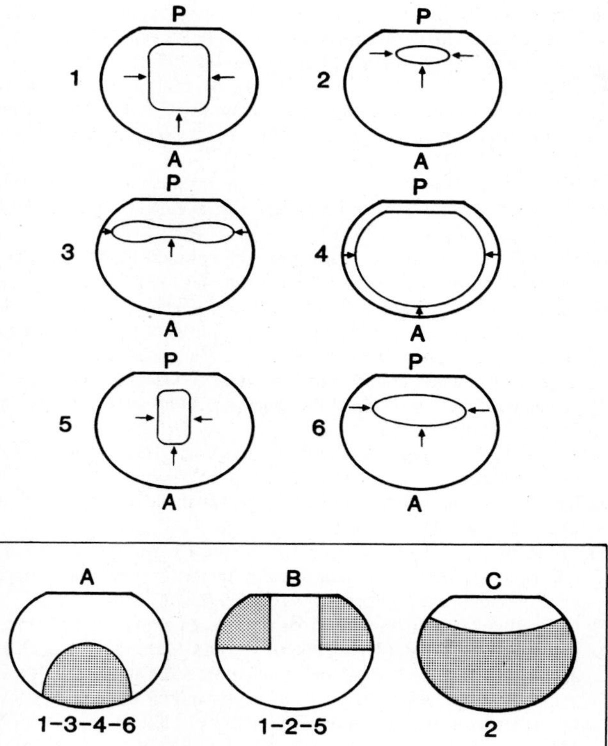

Fig. 80.7 The types of obturation that can be expected with these surgical methods described. *Shaded areas* represent parts of the velopharyngeal area left open following the surgery; *white areas* show what is obturated with tissue during the surgery. Remember that in all of these examples there are variations; with surgery more or less can be obturated than is demonstrated. (**A**) The type of obturation obtained with a sphincter pharyngoplasty. Significant augmentation and closure of the posterior and lateral pharyngeal walls occur. The area left open is midline and located just behind the uvula. This helps demonstrate why someone with good soft palatal motion will generally do well with a sphincter pharyngoplasty. A sphincter pharyngoplasty would work well in treating the patients in *1* (this sphincter would need to be a little bit snug), *3*, *4* (black-hole patterns are usually best treated with a very snug or tight sphincter or with a prosthetic obturator), and *6*. (**B**) Obturation following a pharyngeal flap attachment to the soft palate. Because the lateral areas (ports) are left open, it is apparent why this surgery works best in people with good lateral-wall motion. Matching the obturated pattern over *1* to *6*, it can be seen that a good match could be made in patients in *1* (wider pharyngeal flap would be needed), *2*, and *5*. (**C**) The folded or rolled pharyngeal flap mildly augments the posterior wall. The best match for this procedure is the patient in 2. Although this patient could be treated by any of the surgical methods, the described augmentation of the posterior wall is the least aggressive approach and leaves the most unobturated area. Therefore, it is less likely to cause airway obstruction. (From Gray S, Pinborough- Zimmerman J. Diagnosis and treatment of velopharyngeal incompetence. Fac Plast Surg Clin North Am 1996;4:405–412. Reprinted by permission.)

depends on the pattern of velopharyngeal closure, the degree of closure, and associated medical conditions.[92] A sample of common nasopharyngoscopic findings and selected surgical procedures is given for review (**Fig. 80.7**).

Acknowledgment

Portions of this material appeared in Gray SD, Pinborough-Zimmerman J. Velopharyngeal incompetence. In: Cummings CW et al, eds. Pediatric Otolaryngology: Head and Neck Surgery. 3rd ed. St. Louis: CV Mosby; 1998: 174–187.

References

1. Shprintzen RJ, Lencione RM, McColl GN, Skolnick ML. A three-dimensional cinefluoroscopic analysis of velopharyngeal closure during speech and nonspeech activities in normals. Cleft Palate J 1980;11: 412–428
2. Matsuya T, Miyazaki T, Yamaoka M. Fiberscopic examination of the velopharyngeal closure in normal individuals. Cleft Palate J 1974;11:286–291
3. Kuehn DP, Folkins JW, Cutting CB. Relationships between muscle activity and velar position. Cleft Palate J 1982;19:25–35
4. Seaver EJ, Kuehn DP. A cineradiographic and electromyographic investigation of velar positioning in nonnasal speech. Cleft Palate Craniofac J 1980;17:216–226
5. Fletcher SG. Diagnosing Speech Disorders from Cleft Palate. New York: Grune and Stratton; 1978
6. Hawkins CF, Swisher WE. Evaluation of a real-time ultrasound scanner in assessing lateral pharyngeal wall motion during speech. Cleft Palate Craniofac J 1978;15:161–166
7. Engelke W, Bruns T, Striebeck M, Hoch G. Midsagittal velar kinematics during production of VCV sequences. Cleft Palate Craniofac J 1996;33:236–244
8. McWilliams BJ, Morris HL, Shelton RL. Cleft Palate Speech. St. Louis: CV Mosby; 1990
9. Shprintzen RJ, McCall GN, Skolnick ML, Lencione RM. Selective movement of the lateral aspects of the pharyngeal walls during velopharyngeal closure for speech blowing and whistling in normals. Cleft Palate Craniofac J 1975;12:51–58
10. Huang MHS, Lee ST, Rajendran K. Anatomic basis of cleft palate and velopharyngeal surgery: implications from a fresh cadaveric study. Plast Reconstr Surg 1998;101:613–627
11. Huang MHS, Lee ST, Rajendran K. The structure of the musculus uvulae: functional and surgical implications of an anatomic study. Cleft Palate Craniofac J 1997;34:466–474
12. Iglesias A, Kuehn DP, Morris HL. Simultaneous assessment of pharyngeal walls and velar displacement for selected speech sounds. J Speech Hear Res 1980;23:429–446
13. Glaser ER, Skolnick ML, McWilliams BJ, Shprintzen RJ. The dynamics of Passavant's ridge in subjects with and without velopharyngeal insufficiency: a multiview videofluoroscopic study. Cleft Palate J 1979;16:24–33
14. Skolnick ML, McCall GN, Barnes M. The sphincteric mechanism of velopharyngeal closure. Cleft Palate Craniofac J 1973;10:286
15. Croft CE, Shprintzen RJ, Rakoff SJ. Patterns of velopharyngeal valving in normal and cleft palate subjects: a multiview videofluoroscopic and nasoendoscopic study. Laryngoscope 1981;91:265
16. D'Antonio LL, Crockett DM. Evaluation and management of velopharyngeal inadequacy. In: Smith JD, Bumsted RM, eds. Pediatric Plastic and Reconstructive Surgery. New York: Raven; 1993:173–196
17. Gorlin RJ, Cerrenk J, Pruzansky S. Facial clefting and its syndromes. Birth Defects 1971;1:3
18. Weatherley-White RCA, et al. Submucous cleft palate: incidence, natural history, and implications for treatment. Plast Reconstr Surg 1972;49:279
19. Kaplan EN. The occult submucous cleft palate. Cleft Palate J 1975; 12:356–368
20. Lewin ML, Croft CB, Shprintzen RJ. Velopharyngeal insufficiency due to hypoplasia of the musculus uvulae and occult submucous cleft palate. Plast Reconstr Surg 1980;65:585

21. Mason RM, Warren DW. Adenoid involution and developing hypernasality in cleft palate. J Speech Hear Disord 1980;45:469
22. Ren YF, Isberg A, Henningsson G. Velopharyngeal incompetence and persistent hypernasality after adenoidectomy in children without palatal defect. Cleft Palate Craniofac J 1995;32:476–482
23. Gibb AG. Hypernasality (rhinolalia aperta) following tonsil and adenoid removal. J Laryngol Otol 1958;72:433–451
24. Morris HL, Jrueger LJ, Bumsted RM. Indications of congenital palatal incompetence before diagnosis. Ann Otol Rhinol Laryngol 1982;91: 115–118
25. Witzel MA, Rick RM, Magar-Bacal F, Cox C. Velopharyngeal insufficiency after adenoidectomy: an 8-year review. Int J Pediatr Otorhinolaryngol 1986;11:15–20
26. Kuehn DP. New therapy for treating hypernasal speech using continuous positive airway pressure (CPAP). Plast Reconstr Surg 1991;88: 959–965
27. Pinborough-Zimmerman J. Nasometric and appliance treatment for hypernasality in one CVA patient. Paper presented at the American Speech-Language-Hearing Association Annual Meeting, Orlando, FL, December 1995
28. Witzel MA, Tobe J, Salyer K. The use of nasopharyngoscopy biofeedback therapy in the correction of inconsistent velopharyngeal closure. Int J Pediatr Otorhinolaryngol 1988;15:137–142
29. Sphrintzen RJ, Sher AE, Croft CB. Hypernasal speech caused by tonsillar hypertrophy. Int J Pediatr Otorhinolaryngol 1986;14:45–56
30. MacKenzie-Stepner K, Witzel MA, Stringer DA, Iaskin R. Velopharyngeal insufficiency due to hypertrophic tonsils: a report of two cases. Int J Pediatr Otorhinolaryngol 1987;14:57–63
31. Kummer AW, Billmire DA, Myer CM. Hypertrophic tonsils: the effect of resonance and velopharyngeal closure. Plast Reconstr Surg 1993; 91:608–611
32. Finkelstein Y, Zohar Y, Nachmani A, et al. The otolaryngologist and the patient with velocardiofacial syndrome. Arch Otolaryngol Head Neck Surg 1993;119:563–569
33. Ford LC, Sulprizio SL, Rasgon BM. Otolaryngological manifestations of velocardiofacial syndrome: a retrospective review of 35 patients. Laryngoscope 2000;10:362–367
34. Usiskin SI, Nicolson R, Krasnewich DM, et al. Velocardiofacial syndrome in childhood-onset schizophrenia. J Am Acad Child Adolesc Psychiatry 1999;38:1536–1543
35. D'Antonio LL, Marsh JL. Abnormal carotid arteries in velocardiofacial syndrome. Plast Reconstr Surg 1987;80:471–472
36. Witzel MA, Tobe J, Salyer K. The use of nasopharyngoscopy biofeedback therapy in the correction of inconsistent velopharyngeal closure. Int J Pediatr Otorhinolaryngol 1988;15:137–142
37. Finkelstein Y, Shapiro-Feinberg M, Talmi YP. Axial configuration of the velopharyngeal valve and its valving mechanism. Cleft Palate Craniofac J 1995;32:299
38. Scrambler PJ, Kelly D, Lindsay E. Velocardiofacial syndrome associated with chromosome 22 deletions encompassing the DiGeorge locus. Lancet 1992;339:1138–1139
39. Evans D. Language development in Mongols. Forward Trends 1974;1: 23–25
40. Strom M. Down syndrome: a modern otorhinolaryngological perspective. Laryngoscope 1981;91:1581–1594
41. Kavanagh KT, Kahane JC. Risks and benefits of adenotonsillectomy for children with Down syndrome. Am J Ment Retard 1986;91:22–29
42. Dalston RM, Warren DW, Dalston ET. Use of nasometry as a diagnostic tool identifying patients with velopharyngeal impairment. Cleft Palate Craniofac J 1991;28:184–189
43. Dalston RM, Warren DW, Dalston ET. A preliminary investigation concerning the use of nasometry in identifying patients with hyponasality and/or nasal airway impairment. J Speech Hear Res 1991;34:11–18
44. Pinborough-Zimmerman J. Relationship between nasalance and nasoendoscopy in children with hypernasality. Paper presented at the American Speech-Language-Hearing Association Annual Meeting, Orlando, FL, December 1995
45. Shprintzen RJ. Instrumental assessment of velopharyngeal valving. In: Shprintzen RJ, Bardach J, eds. Cleft Palate Speech Management: A Multidisciplinary Approach. St. Louis: Mosby; 1995:221–256
46. Golding-Kushner KJ, Argamaso RV, Cotton RT, et al. Standardization for the reporting of nasopharyngoscopy and multiview videofluoroscopy: a report from an international working group. Cleft Palate Craniofac J 1990;27:337–327
47. D'Antonio LL, Achauer BM, Vander Kam VM. Results of a survey of cleft palate teams concerning the use of nasoendoscopy. Cleft Palate Craniofac J 1993;30:35–39
48. Skolnick ML, McCall GN, Barnes M. The sphincteric mechanism of velopharyngeal closure. Cleft Palate Craniofac J 1973;10:286
49. Croft CB, Shprintzen RJ, Rakoff SJ. Patterns of velopharyngeal valving in normal and cleft palate subjects: a multiview videofluoroscopic and nasoendoscopic study. Laryngoscope 1981;91:265
50. Miyazaki T. Commentary on the use of videonasopharyngoscopy for biofeedback therapy in adults after pharyngeal flap surgery. Cleft Palate Craniofac J 1989;26:136
51. Boone DR, McFarlane SC. The Voice and Voice Therapy. Englewood Cliffs, NJ: Prentice Hall; 1994
52. Blakely RW. Temporary speech prosthesis as an aid in speech training. Cleft Palate Bull 1960;10:63
53. Wolfaardt JF, Wilson FB, Rochet A, McPhee L. An appliance-based approach to the management of palatopharyngeal incompetency: a clinical pilot project. J Prosthet Dent 1993;69:186–195
54. McGrath CO, Anderson MW. Prosthetic treatment of velopharyngeal incompetence. In: Bardach J, Morris HL, eds. Multidisciplinary Management of Cleft Lip and Palate. Philadelphia: WB Saunders; 1990
55. Witt PD, Rozelle AA, Marsh JL, et al. Do palatal lift prostheses stimulate velopharyngeal neuromuscular activity? Cleft Palate Craniofac J 1995;32:469–475
56. Adisman IK. Cleft palate prosthetics. In: Grabb WC, Rosenstein SW, Bzoch KR, eds. Cleft Lip and Palate. Boston: Little, Brown; 1971
57. Karnell MP, Rosenstein H, Fine L. Nasal videoendoscopy in prosthetic management of palatopharyngeal dysfunction. J Prosthet Dent 1987;58:479
58. Reisberg DJ, Smith BE. Aerodynamic assessment of prosthetic speech aids. J Prosthet Dent 1985;54:686–690
58a. Turner GE, William WN. Fluoroscopy and nasoendoscopy in designing palatal lift prostheses. J Prosthet Dent 1991;66:63
59. Gray S, Pinborough-Zimmerman J. Diagnosis and treatment of velopharyngeal incompetence. Facial Plast Surg Clin North Am 1996;4: 405–412
60. Gray SD, Smith ME, Schneider H. Voice disorders in children. Pediatr Clin North Am 1996;6:1357–1384
61. Broen PA, Doyle SS, Bacon CK. The velopharyngeally inadequate child: phonologic change with intervention. Cleft Palate Craniofac J 1993;30:500–507
62. Henningsson GE, Isberg AM. Velopharyngeal movement patterns in patients alternating between oral and glottal articulation: a clinical and cineradiographical study. Cleft Palate J 1986;23:1–9
63. Yamaoka M, Matsuya T, Miyazaki T, et al. Visual training for velopharyngeal closure in cleft palate patients: a fiberoscopic procedure. J Maxillofac Surg 1983;11:191–193
64. Kuehn DP, Moon JB, Folkins JW. Levator veli palatini muscle activity in relation to intranasal air pressure. Cleft Palate Craniofac J 1993;30: 361–368
64a. Bardach J. Palate repair: two-flap palatoplasty: research, philosophy, technique, and results. In: Bardach J, Morris HL, eds. Multidisciplinary Management of Cleft Lip and Palate. Philadelphia: WB Saunders; 1990:352–365
65. Furlow LT. Cleft palate repair by double-opposing Z-plasty. Plast Reconstr Surg 1986;78:724–736
66. Kirschner RE, Wang P, Jawad AF, et al. Cleft-palate repair by modified Furlow double-opposing Z-plasty: the Children's Hospital of Philadelphia experience. Plast Reconstr Surg 1999;104:1998–2010
67. Seagle MB, Patti CS, Williams WN, Wood VD. Submucous cleft palate: a 10-year series. Ann Plast Surg 1999;42:124–148

68. Hynes W. Pharyngoplasty by muscle transplantation. Br J Plast Surg 1950;3:128
69. Orticochea M. Construction of a dynamic muscle sphincter in cleft palates. Plast Reconstr Surg 1968;41:323
70. Jackson IT, Silverton JS. The sphincter pharyngoplasty as a secondary procedure in cleft palates. Plast Reconstr Surg 1977;59:518–524
71. Riski JE, Serafin D, Riefkohl R, et al. A rationale for modifying the site of insertion of the Orticochea pharyngoplasty. Plast Reconstr Surg 1984;73:882
72. Riski JE, Ruff GL, Georgiade GS, et al. Evaluation of the sphincter pharyngoplasty. Cleft Palate Craniofac J 1992;29:254–261
73. Witt PD, D'Antonio LL, Zimmerman GJ, Marsh JL. Sphincter pharyngoplasty: a preoperative and postoperative analysis of perceptual speech characteristics and endoscopic studies of velopharyngeal function. Plast Reconstr Surg 1994;93:1155–1168
74. Sloan GM, Reinisck JR, Nichter LS, Downey SE. Surgical treatment of velopharyngeal insufficiency: pharyngoplasty vs. pharyngeal flap. Plast Surg Forum 1990;13:128–130
75. Witt PD, Marsh JL, Marty-Grames L, et al. Management of the hypodynamic velopharynx. Cleft Palate Craniofac J 1995;32:179–187
76. Sie KCY, Tampakopoulou DA, de Serres LM, et al. Sphincter pharyngoplasty: speech outcome and complications. Laryngoscope 1998;108:1211–1217
77. Witt PD, Marsh JL, Marty-Grames L, Muntz HR. Revision of the failed sphincter pharyngoplasty: an outcome assessment. Plast Reconstr Surg 1995;96:129–138
78. Kasten SJ, Buchman SR, Stevenson C, Berger M. A retrospective analysis of revision sphincter pharyngoplasty. Ann Plast Surg 1997;39:583–589
79. Huang MHS, Lee ST, Rajendran K. Clinical implications of the velopharyngeal blood supply: a fresh cadaveric study. Plast Reconstr Surg 1998;102:655–667
80. Pigott RW. The results of pharyngoplasty by muscle transplantation by Wilfred Hynes. Br J Plast Surg 1993;46:440–442
81. Whitaker LA, Randall P, Graham WP III, et al. A prospective and randomized series comparing superiorly and inferiorly based posterior pharyngeal flaps. Cleft Palate J 1972;9:304
82. Morris HL, Bardach J, Jomes D, et al. Clinical results of pharyngeal flap surgery: the Iowa experience. Plast Reconstr Surg 1995;95:652–662
83. Hirschberg J. Pediatric otolaryngological relations of velopharyngeal insufficiency. Int J Pediatr Otorhinolaryngol 1983;5:199
84. Shprintzen RJ, Lewin ML, Croft CB, et al. A comprehensive study of pharyngeal flap surgery: tailor-made flaps. Cleft Palate J 1979;16:46
85. Valnicek SM, Zuker RM, Halpern LM, Roy WL. Perioperative complications of superior pharyngeal flap surgery in children. Plast Reconstr Surg 1994;93:954–958
86. Kravath RE, Pollak CP, Borowiecki B, Weitzman ED. Obstructive sleep apnea and death associated with surgical correction of velopharyngeal incompetence. J Pediatr 1980;96:645
87. Ysunza A, Garcia-Velasco M, Garcia-Garcia M, et al. Obstructive sleep apnea secondary to surgery for velopharyngeal insufficiency. Cleft Palate Craniofac J 1993;30:387–390
88. Orr WC, Levine NS, Buchanan RT. Effect of cleft palate repair and pharyngeal flap surgery on upper airway obstruction during sleep. Plast Reconstr Surg 1987;80:226
89. Sirois M, Caouette-Laberge L, Spier S, et al. Sleep apnea following a pharyngeal flap: a feared complication. Plast Reconstr Surg 1994;93:943–947
90. Wells MD, Vu TA, Luce EA. Incidence and sequelae of nocturnal respiratory obstruction following posterior pharyngeal flap operation. Ann Plast Surg 1999;43:252–257
91. Rosenthal W. Zur Frage der Gaumenplastik. Zentralbl Chir 1924;51:1621
92. Peat BG, Albery EH, Jones K, Pigott RW. Tailoring velopharyngeal surgery: the influence of etiology and type of operation. Plast Reconstr Surg 1994;93:948–953
93. Hogan VM. A clarification of the surgical goals in cleft palate speech and the introduction of the lateral port control (L.P.C.) pharyngeal flap. Cleft Palate J 1973;10:331
94. Crockett DM, Bumstead RM, Van Dmark DR. Experience with surgical management of velopharyngeal incompetence. Otolaryngol Head Neck Surg 1988;99:1–9
95. Blocksma R. Correction of velopharyngeal insufficiency by Silastic pharyngeal implant. Plast Reconstr Surg 1963;31:268
96. Eckstein H. Paraffin for facial and palatal defects. Dermatol Ztschr (Basel) 1904;11:772
97. Gersuny R. Euber eine subcutane Prostheses. Ztsch Heilk 1900;21:199
98. Halle M. Gaumennaht and Gaumenplastic. Arch Ohren Nasen Kehlkopfheilkd 1925;12:377
99. Hill MJ, Hagerty RF. Efficacy of pharyngoplasty for speech improvement in postoperative cleft palates. Cleft Palate Bull 1960;10:66
100. Perthes H. Reported by Hollweg E. Beitra a zur Behandlung von Gaumenspalten. Diss. Tubingen: 1912
101. Von Gaza W. Transplanting of free fatty tissue in the retropharyngeal area in cases of cleft palate. Lecture presented to the German Surgical Society, April 9, 1926
102. Ward PH. Uses of injectable Teflon in otolaryngology. Arch Otolaryngol Head Neck Surg 1968;97:637
103. Smith JK, McCabe BF. Teflon injection in the nasopharynx to improve velopharyngeal closure. Ann Otol Rhinol Laryngol 1977;86:559
104. Witt PD, Marsh JL, O'Daniel TG, et al. Surgical management of velopharyngeal dysfunction: outcome analysis of autogenous posterior pharyngeal wall augmentation. Plast Reconstr Surg 1997;99:1287–1296
105. Gray SD, Pinborough-Zimmerman J, Catten M. Posterior wall augmentation for treatment of velopharyngeal insufficiency. Otolaryngol Head Neck Surg 1999;121:107–112
106. Boorman JG, Sommerlad BC. Levator palatini and palatal dimples: their anatomy, relationship, and clinical significance. Br J Plast Surg 1985;38:326
107. Shprintzen RJ, McCall GN, Skolnick ML, Lencione RM. Selective movement of the lateral aspects of the pharyngeal walls during velopharyngeal closure for speech blowing and whistling in normals. Cleft Palate J 1975;12:51
108. Kuehn DP, Folkins JW, Cutting CB. Relationships between muscle activity and velar position. Cleft Palate J 1982;19:25
109. Finkelstein Y, Shapiro-Feinberg M, Talmi YP, et al. Axial configuration of the velopharyngeal valve and its valving mechanism. Cleft Palate Craniofac J 1995;32:299
110. Nishio J, Matsuya T, Machida J, Miyazaki T. The motor nerve supply of the velopharyngeal muscles. Cleft Palate J 1976;13:20
111. Ibuki K, Matsuya T, Nishio J, et al. The course of facial nerve innervation for the levator veli palatini muscle. Cleft Palate Craniofac J 1978;15:209
112. Azzam NA, Kuehn DP. The morphology of musculus uvulae. Cleft Palate J 1977;14:78
113. Kuehn DP, Azzam NA. Anatomical characteristics of palatoglossus and the anterior faucial pillar. Cleft Palate Craniofac J 1978;15:349
114. Matsuya T, Miyazaki T, Yamaoka M. Fiberscopic examination of the velopharyngeal closure in normal individuals. Cleft Palate J 1974;11:286
115. McWilliams BJ, Morris HL, Shelton RL. Cleft Palate Speech. Philadelphia: CV Mosby; 1990

Index

Note: Page numbers followed by *f* and *t* indicate figures and tables, respectively.

A

B

C

D

E

F

G

H

I

J

M

N

O

P

Q

R

S

T

U

V

W

Z